Principles of

Pathophysiology

THIRD EDITION

Pearson Australia
Building B, Level 1
459–471 Church Street
Richmond Victoria 3121

www.pearson.com

Pearson respects and honours Aboriginal and Torres Strait Islander Elders past, present and future. We acknowledge the stories, traditions and living cultures of the Traditional Custodians of the lands on which our company is located and where we conduct our business. Pearson is committed to honouring Australian Aboriginal and Torres Strait Islander peoples' unique cultural and spiritual relationships to the land, waters and seas and their rich contribution to society.

Aboriginal and Torres Strait Islander peoples are advised that this text may contain images, voices and names of deceased persons.

Senior Commercial Product Manager: Mandy Sheppard
Development Editor: Anna Carter
Senior Project Manager: Bernadette Chang
Content Producer: Nikhil Kumar
Digital Producer: Paul Ryan
Rights and Permissions Editor: Samantha Russell-Tulip
Lead Editor/Copy Editor: Kate Stone
Proofreader: Integra Software Services
Indexer: Integra Software Services
Cover and internal design by Natalie Bowra
Cover illustration by noicherrybeans/Shutterstock
Typeset by Integra Software Services

Printed in Malaysia by Vivar/01 (2023)

Print ISBN 9780655708377
eText ISBN 9780655708391
ePub ISBN 9780655708384

1 2 3 4 5 28 27 26 25 24

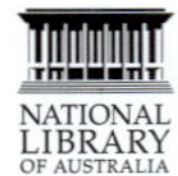

A catalogue record for this work is available from the National Library of Australia

Pearson Australia Group Pty Ltd ABN 40 004 245 943

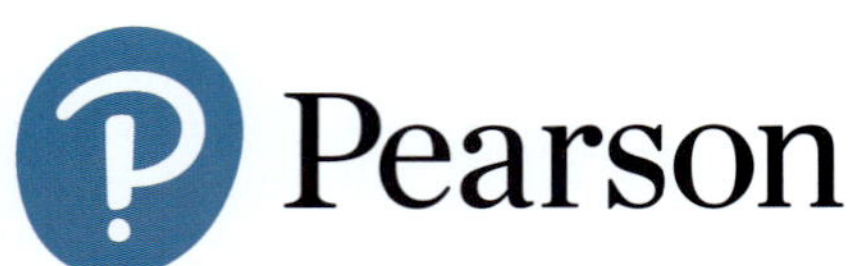

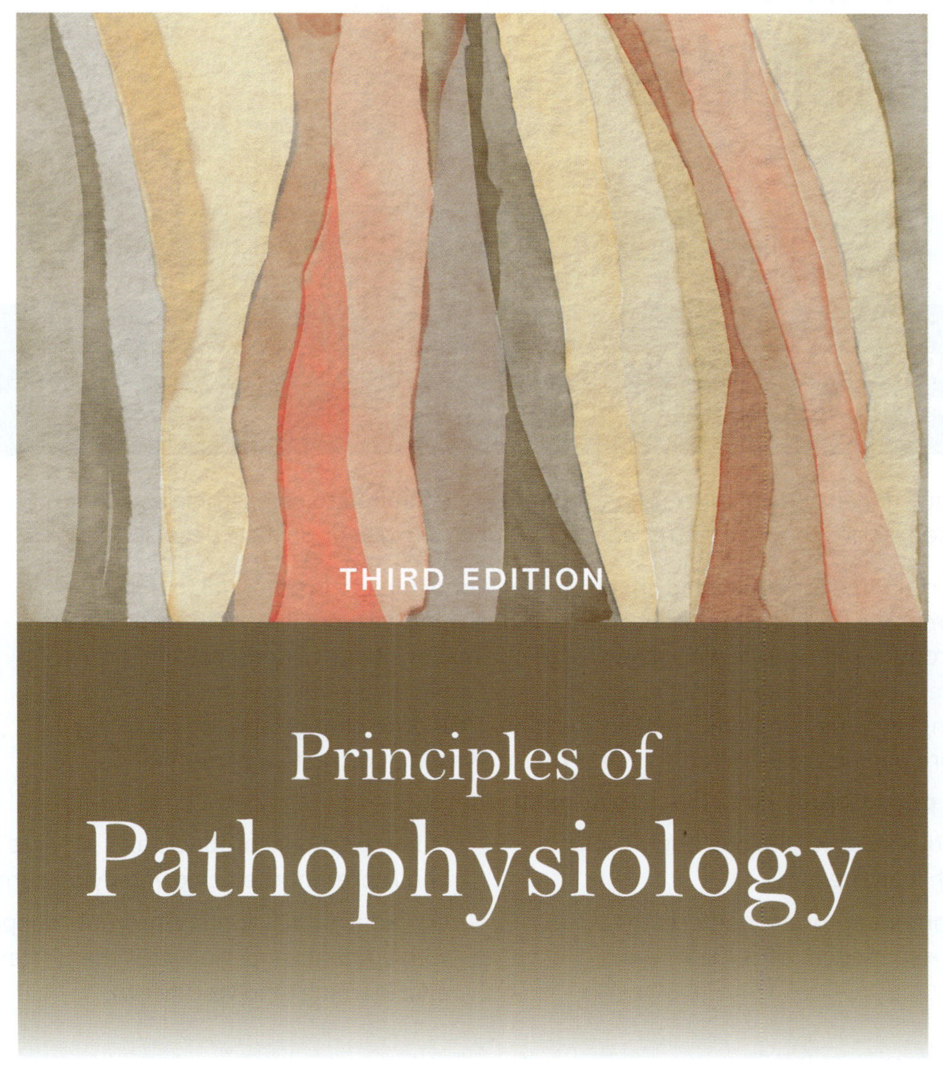

SHANE BULLOCK | MAJELLA HALES

Pearson's Commitment to Diversity, Equity, and Inclusion

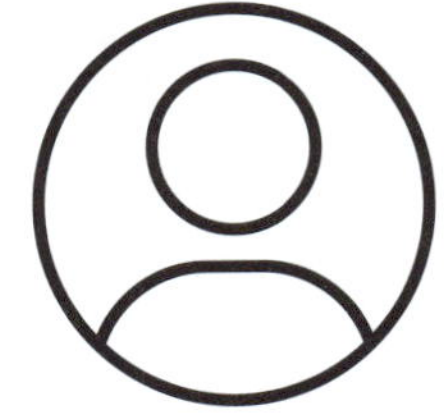

Pearson is dedicated to creating bias-free content that reflects the diversity, depth, and breadth of all learners' lived experiences.

We embrace the many dimensions of diversity, including but not limited to race, ethnicity, gender, sex, sexual orientation, socioeconomic status, ability, age, and religious or political beliefs.

Education is a powerful force for equity and change in our world. It has the potential to deliver opportunities that improve lives and enable economic mobility. As we work with authors to create content for every product and service, we acknowledge our responsibility to demonstrate inclusivity and incorporate diverse scholarship so that everyone can achieve their potential through learning. As the world's leading learning company, we have a duty to help drive change and live up to our purpose to help more people create a better life for themselves and to create a better world.

Our ambition is to purposefully contribute to a world where:

- Everyone has an equitable and lifelong opportunity to succeed through learning.
- Our educational content accurately reflects the histories and lived experiences of the learners we serve.
- Our educational products and services are inclusive and represent the rich diversity of learners.
- Our educational content prompts deeper discussions with students and motivates them to expand their own learning (and worldview).

Accessibility

We are also committed to providing products that are fully accessible to all learners. As per Pearson's guidelines for accessible educational Web media, we test and retest the capabilities of our products against the highest standards for every release, following the WCAG guidelines in developing new products for copyright year 2022 and beyond.

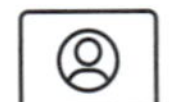

You can learn more about Pearson's commitment to accessibility at **https://www.pearson.com/us/accessibility.html**

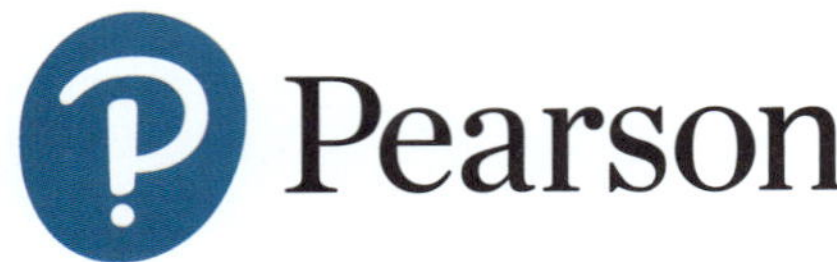

Contact Us

While we work hard to present unbiased, fully accessible content, we want to hear from you about any concerns or needs with this Pearson product so that we can investigate and address them.

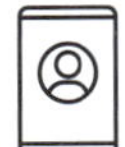

Please contact us with concerns about any potential bias at **https://www.pearson.com/report-bias.html**

For accessibility-related issues, such as using assistive technology with Pearson products, alternative text requests, or accessibility documentation, email the Pearson Disability Support team at **disability.support@pearson.com**

Brief table of contents

Detailed table of contents

PART 3
Nervous system pathophysiology 161

PART 4
Endocrine pathophysiology 333

PART 5
Cardiovascular pathophysiology 423

About the authors

Shane Bullock

Shane has been involved in the education of health professionals and science students for more than 30 years. He is currently the Head of the Monash University School of Rural Health, involved in rural health workforce preparation and development. Shane is the co-author of two Australian textbooks, *Fundamentals of Pharmacology*, now in its 9th edition, and *Psychopharmacology for Health Professionals*. He has also published a number of journal articles on health professional education and health service delivery.

Majella Hales

Majella has been nursing for over 30 years, much of this time in education roles both clinically and in academia. She is the co-founder of Sciencopia, a business producing and manufacturing educational resources for nurses and other undergraduate health care professionals. She maintains her clinical experience working with Queensland Health, offering rapid assessments to facilitate the provision of urgent community services to avoid hospitalisation. Majella authoured several chapters of Kozier & Erb's *Fundamentals of Nursing Vols 1–3* and LeMone and Burke's *Medical–Surgical Nursing.* Along with journal articles and conference presentations, she has also produced the original skills DVD for *Tollefson's Clinical Psychomotor Skills* text, and adapted the American case study resource *The Neighbourhood*. She is also co-author of the *Essential Aussie Drugs, Biology Translator* and *Common Antibiotics, Pathogens and Infections*.

Preface

Our goals

Principles of Pathophysiology is the first wholly local, comprehensive pathophysiology textbook written for students studying nursing and allied health in Australia and New Zealand. Where possible we have embedded throughout this text epidemiological data, lifespan issues, Indigenous issues, clinical practices, drug names, units of measurement and websites that are relevant to the Australian and New Zealand region.

Most of the existing pathophysiology books are unwieldy in both a physical and a readable sense. There is a common format—around half of the book comprises chapters on the normal anatomy and physiology of the body systems. In our view these chapters are redundant, as student health professionals purchase anatomy and physiology textbooks during their first year at university. Instead, the approach we have taken is to maintain the focus on pathophysiology, and to complement other textbooks that the students have at hand covering anatomy/physiology and pharmacology.

The book is designed to be very readable and accessible for students studying their chosen profession prior to registration. We have endeavoured to strongly link and integrate the science with clinical practice. To this end, each chapter is co-authored by a scientist and an expert clinician, given that few individuals possess both the scientific and the clinical expertise in any one field.

Organisation of the text

The book is organised into parts, the first of which contains chapters examining major pathophysiological concepts, such as cellular adaptations, inflammation and neoplasia, as well as the determinants of health and illness. The following parts cover the pathophysiology of the various body systems.

Chapters are structured with a consistent content framework for ease of accessing information about specific disorders associated with a particular body system. This is best reflected in the sequencing of chapter subheadings for each disorder, which are as follows: aetiology and pathophysiology, epidemiology, clinical manifestations, then clinical diagnosis and management.

New for this edition

The content of this textbook has been reviewed with respect to the recent literature, as well as current clinical practices and guidelines at the time of writing. This edition reflects the major effect on human health the COVID-19 pandemic has had. Where appropriate, we have given particular emphasis to the pathophysiological effects of COVID-19 infection, both generally and more specifically on major body systems.

INDIGENOUS HEALTH FAST FACTS AND CULTURAL CONSIDERATIONS

The Indigenous health fast facts and cultural considerations sections at the end of most chapters have been updated to reflect the most recent epidemiological data available.

NEW AND REVISED IMAGES

A significant number of new and revised images have been produced for this edition. These images provide clearer understanding or representation of either new or reconceptualised content. Several new and revised clinical snapshots have also been constructed to accommodate the latest in best practice, to clarify previously included material, or to expand on content not previously addressed.

Language and terminology

The use of correct scientific and clinical language is important in order to prepare student health professionals for the workplace. However, preparatory textbooks need to be accessible and readable for students developing their knowledge base. We believe that we have struck a good balance in a writing style that is easily understandable while not compromising the integrity of the scientific and clinical disciplines.

By their nature, pathophysiology textbooks contain jargon terms that pertain to the science and to the clinical practice. It is important for students to have ready access to definitions of this terminology. In this book, key terms are printed in bold type. All of these terms are defined in the glossary; many are described within the chapter text as well.

We have avoided using terminology usually associated with those accessing healthcare, such as 'patient', 'client' or 'customer', as they suggest power relationships. Instead, we have opted for terms such as 'person' or 'individual'.

Shane Bullock and Majella Hales

Acknowledgements

We sincerely thank all of those people who have contributed to the development of this textbook over the years, particularly our contributors to the first edition: Ralph Arwas, Judith Applegarth, Anna-Marie Babey, Melainie Cameron, Trisha Dunning, Elizabeth Manias, Anita Westwood and Alison Williams. We also thank the reviewers for their thoughtful and extremely valuable comments and suggestions on the text.

A major inclusion in this edition is the effects of SARS CoV-2 virus, the cause of COVID-19 infection. Our lives have changed in so many ways as a result of this pandemic. We have all been affected, and many of us have lost loved ones and friends directly or indirectly due to the pandemic. We acknowledge and pay tribute to the health care workers within our communities who have worked tirelessly to care for us during and since the pandemic.

Shane would like to acknowledge the support of his family during the writing of this edition. There have been tears and joy for us during these COVID-19 times. Nevertheless, it has been delightful watching some family members grow up into adulthood, while the rest of us just grow older with none of us necessarily growing any wiser. My grateful thanks to Majella, my co-author, with whom I buckled in for the rollercoaster ride in preparing this edition. I am in awe of Majella and her Sciencopia colleagues' skills in making the complex look so much simpler for students through creative diagrams, charts and concept maps.

Majella would like to extend her heartfelt thanks to her dear friends and business partners Robin Fisher and Eun Jeong Roh. Robin's valuable discussion and debate influenced clarity in expression and imagery. EJ's superpower is to turn largely indeterminate squiggles into beautiful illustrations for several new images in this text. Finally, Majella is ever so grateful for the humour, support and encouragement from Shane, who coped with the earnest but painstakingly slow progress (hopefully this did not require chemical psychomodulation). Thank you, Shane, for having the patience of a snail crawling through molasses on a cold day.

It has been a pleasure to work with the team at Pearson Australia. They have shown us tremendous support, flexibility, patience, encouragement, good humour and cajoling in equal measure. Our thanks to Anna Carter, Victoria Kerr, Lakshmi Balakrishnan, Nikhil Kumar, Samantha Russell-Tulip and Rebecca Pedley. We also thank Kate Stone for her excellent copyediting and proofreading, whose eagle eye for detail and a meme for every occasion are legendary.

Reviewers

Pearson would like to thank the reviewers for their contribution to this text:

Matthew Ireland, Charles Sturt University
Debra Carlson, Central Queensland University

We would also like to thank technical editor Natalie Colson of Griffith University for her insightful feedback.

Features of the text

WHAT YOU SHOULD KNOW BEFORE YOU START THIS CHAPTER

Can you name the main structures of the cell and their functions?

Can you describe how molecules are transported across the cell membrane?

Can you describe the cell cycle?

Can you define cellular metabolism?

Can you identify the major types of tissues and their functions?

CLINICAL BOX 11.3

Spinal shock versus neurogenic shock

It is imperative to understand the difference between spinal shock and neurogenic shock. *Spinal shock* is when reflexes are temporarily lost below the level of spinal cord injury.

Neurogenic shock is when bradycardia and vasodilation occur, resulting in a profound hypotension. This occurs because of the loss of sympathetic nervous system innervation below the level of spinal cord injury and the unopposed parasympathetic nervous system effects on heart rate. Neurogenic shock can only occur in those with injuries above the level of T6.

INDIGENOUS HEALTH FAST FACTS AND CULTURAL CONSIDERATIONS

ALTERED NUTRITIONAL STATE AS AN AGENT OF INJURY

- *Poor nutrition contributes to approximately 9.7% of the burden of disease for Aboriginal and Torres Strait Islander peoples.*
- *Estimations of food costs in rural and remote communities are considered to be approximately 30% higher than in major cities, which probably contributes to the very low fruit and vegetable intake described among Aboriginal and Torres Strait Islander groups.*
- *Poor nutrition results in the birth of low-birth-weight babies*

LIFESPAN ISSUES

CHILDREN AND ADOLESCENTS

- Cancer is the most common cause of death in children.
- Umbilical cord blood containing stem cells can be obtained from newborns and used for the treatment of cancer if no suitable bone marrow is available. Cord blood is beneficial for use in childhood cancers, and poses less risk of graft versus host disease (GvHD).
- Acute lymphocytic leukaemia is the most common childhood cancer.

OLDER ADULTS

- Almost 80% of all neoplasms occur in adults older than 50 years of age.
- The incidence of malignant tumours increases with age.
- Cellular senescence may contribute to the proliferation of malignant and premalignant cells; however, ageing increases the risk of some cancers and decreases the risk of others.

What you should know before you start this chapter

These questions ensure that students review the basic bioscience principles and concepts that provide the foundation for the pathophysiological knowledge they will gain in the chapter.

Clinical boxes

This feature highlights considerations specific to the successful clinical application of relevant knowledge to reduce the theory–practice gap.

Indigenous health fast facts and cultural considerations

Important health concerns for Aboriginal and Torres Strait Islander peoples, Māori and Pacific Islands people are highlighted in relation to the issues presented in each chapter. Selected information is expanded on in the following separate section, Cultural considerations, to reflect more on the qualitative influence of indigeneity on health and wellness.

Lifespan issues

Important health concerns or age-related principles specific to individuals across the age continuum—from neonates and children to older adults—are highlighted.

Clinical snapshots

These concept maps are designed to demonstrate the critical links between pathophysiology, clinical manifestations and management. They are a key feature for integrating the science and clinical practice components of the text. Ideal for visual learners, the boxes in the diagrams are colour-coded—pink (pathophysiology), blue (clinical manifestations) and yellow (management)—to enable quicker understanding and application.

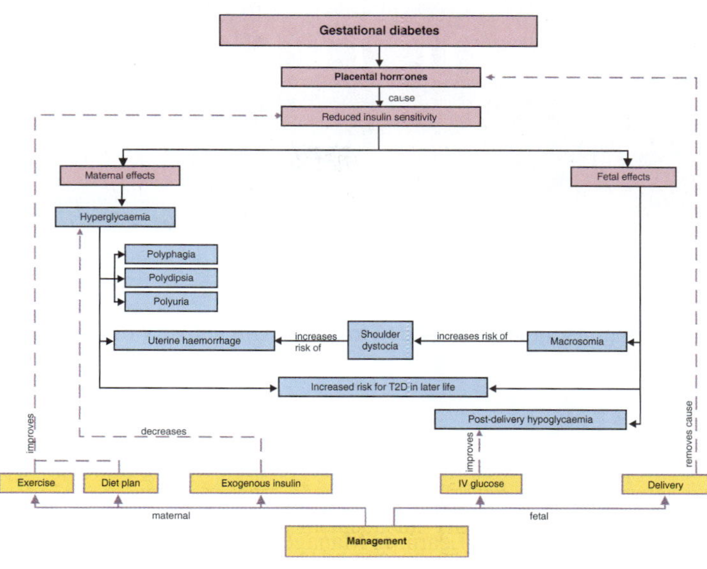

Figure 20.5
Common clinical manifestations and management of gestational diabetes
T2D = type 2 diabetes mellitus IV = intravenous.

Key clinical issues

This is a summary of the significant principles in each chapter that are central to providing safe, informed, clinical practice.

Chapter review and Review questions

A summary of the key content essential to understanding the pathophysiological knowledge in each chapter is provided. Questions enable the student to assess, review and consolidate what they have learnt in the chapter.

Health professional connections

This feature enables students to understand the roles and importance of the various health professionals with whom they will work in an inter-professional team. This information is presented in the context of the management of the specific disorders discussed in each chapter.

Case studies

Clinically accurate and realistic scenarios allow students to apply, synthesise and evaluate their knowledge, and in some instances predict clinical outcomes.

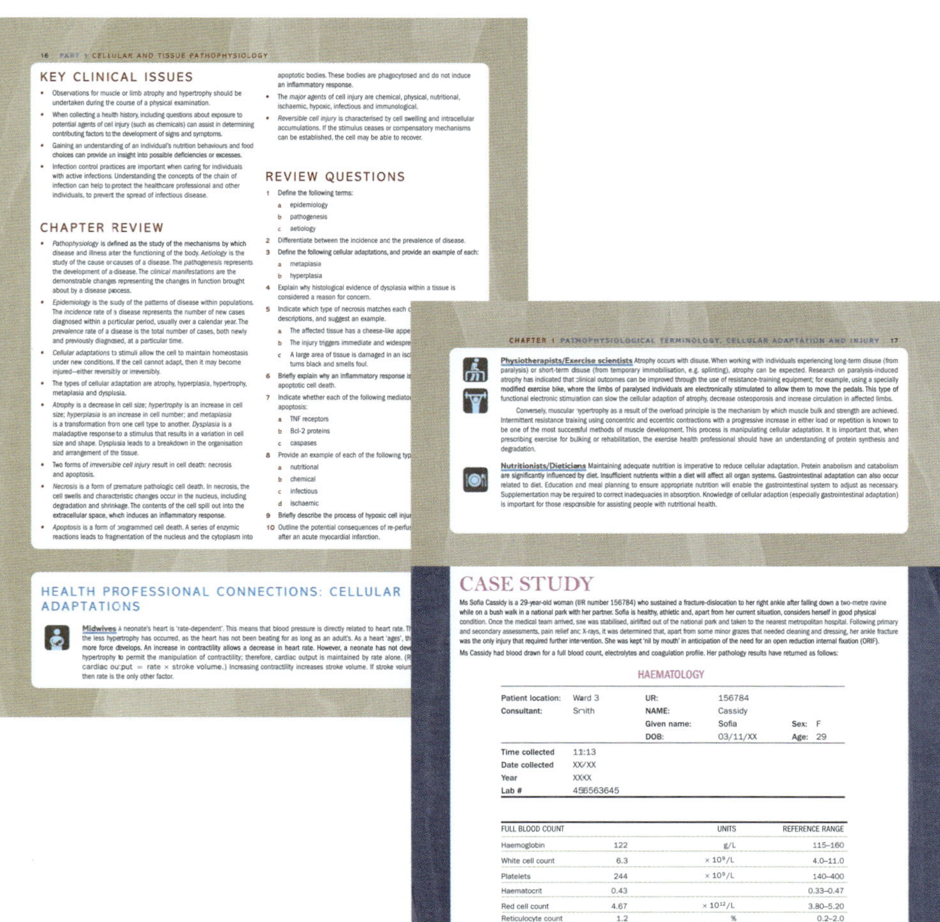

16 PART 1 CELLULAR AND TISSUE PATHOPHYSIOLOGY

KEY CLINICAL ISSUES

- Observations for muscle or limb atrophy and hypertrophy should be undertaken during the course of a physical examination.
- When collecting a health history, including questions about exposure to potential agents of cell injury (such as chemicals) can assist in determining contributing factors to the development of signs and symptoms.
- Gaining an understanding of an individual's nutrition behaviours and food choices can provide an insight into possible deficiencies or excesses.
- Infection control practices are important when caring for individuals with active infections. Understanding the concepts of the chain of infection can help to protect the healthcare professional and other individuals, to prevent the spread of infectious disease.

CHAPTER REVIEW

- *Pathophysiology* is defined as the study of the mechanisms by which disease and illness alter the functioning of the body. *Aetiology* is the study of the cause or causes of a disease. The *pathogenesis* represents the development of a disease. The *clinical manifestations* are the demonstrable changes representing the changes in function brought about by a disease process.
- *Epidemiology* is the study of the patterns of disease within populations. The *incidence* rate of a disease represents the number of new cases diagnosed within a particular period, usually over a calendar year. The *prevalence* rate of a disease is the total number of cases, both newly and previously diagnosed, at a particular time.
- *Cellular adaptations* to stimuli allow the cell to maintain homeostasis under new conditions. If the cell cannot adapt, then it may become injured—either reversibly or irreversibly.
- The types of cellular adaptation are atrophy, hyperplasia, hypertrophy, metaplasia and dysplasia.
- *Atrophy* is a decrease in cell size; *hypertrophy* is an increase in cell size; *hyperplasia* is an increase in cell number; and *metaplasia* is a transformation from one cell type to another. *Dysplasia* is a maladaptive response to a stimulus that results in a variation in cell size and shape. Dysplasia leads to a breakdown in the organisation and arrangement of the tissue.
- Two forms of *irreversible cell injury* result in cell death: necrosis and apoptosis.
- *Necrosis* is a form of premature pathologic cell death. In necrosis, the cell swells and characteristic changes occur in the nucleus, including degradation and shrinkage. The contents of the cell spill out into the extracellular space, which induces an inflammatory response.
- *Apoptosis* is a form of programmed cell death. A series of enzymic reactions leads to fragmentation of the nucleus and the cytoplasm into apoptotic bodies. These bodies are phagocytosed and do not induce an inflammatory response.
- The *major agents* of cell injury are chemical, physical, nutritional, ischaemic, hypoxic, infectious and immunological.
- *Reversible cell injury* is characterised by cell swelling and intracellular accumulations. If the stimulus ceases or compensatory mechanisms can be established, the cell may be able to recover.

REVIEW QUESTIONS

1 Define the following terms:
  a epidemiology
  b pathogenesis
  c aetiology
2 Differentiate between the incidence and the prevalence of disease.
3 Define the following cellular adaptations, and provide an example of each:
  a metaplasia
  b hyperplasia
4 Explain why histological evidence of dysplasia within a tissue is considered a reason for concern.
5 Indicate which type of necrosis matches each c… descriptions, and suggest an example.
  a The affected tissue has a cheese-like appe…
  b The injury triggers immediate and widespre…
  c A large area of tissue is damaged in an isc… turns black and smells foul.
6 Briefly explain why an inflammatory response is… apoptotic cell death.
7 Indicate whether each of the following mediato… apoptosis:
  a TNF receptors
  b Bcl-2 proteins
  c caspases
8 Provide an example of each of the following typ…
  a nutritional
  b chemical
  c infectious
  d ischaemic
9 Briefly describe the process of hypoxic cell inju…
10 Outline the potential consequences of re-perfu… after an acute myocardial infarction.

HEALTH PROFESSIONAL CONNECTIONS: CELLULAR ADAPTATIONS

Midwives A neonate's heart is 'rate-dependent'. This means that blood pressure is directly related to heart rate. Th… the less hypertrophy has occurred, as the heart has not been beating for as long as an adult's. As a heart 'ages', th… more force develops. An increase in contractility allows a decrease in heart rate. However, a neonate has not dev… hypertrophy to permit the manipulation of contractility; therefore, cardiac output is maintained by rate alone. (R… cardiac output = rate × stroke volume.) Increasing contractility increases stroke volume. If stroke volum… then rate is the only other factor.

CHAPTER 1 PATHOPHYSIOLOGICAL TERMINOLOGY, CELLULAR ADAPTATION AND INJURY 17

Physiotherapists/Exercise scientists Atrophy occurs with disuse. When working with individuals experiencing long-term disuse (from paralysis) or short-term disuse (from temporary immobilisation, e.g. splinting), atrophy can be expected. Research on paralysis-induced atrophy has indicated that clinical outcomes can be improved through the use of resistance-training equipment; for example, using a specially modified exercise bike, where the limbs of paralysed individuals are electronically stimulated to allow them to move the pedals. This type of functional electronic stimulation can slow the cellular adaption of atrophy, decrease osteoporosis and increase circulation in affected limbs.

Conversely, muscular hypertrophy as a result of the overload principle is the mechanism by which muscle bulk and strength are achieved. Intermittent resistance training using concentric and eccentric contractions with a progressive increase in either load or repetition is known to be one of the most successful methods of muscle development. This process is manipulating cellular adaptation. It is important that, when prescribing exercise for bulking or rehabilitation, the exercise health professional should have an understanding of protein synthesis and degradation.

Nutritionists/Dieticians Maintaining adequate nutrition is imperative to reduce cellular adaptation. Protein anabolism and catabolism are significantly influenced by diet. Insufficient nutrients within a diet will affect all organ systems. Gastrointestinal adaptation can also occur related to diet. Education and meal planning to ensure appropriate nutrition will enable the gastrointestinal system to adjust as necessary. Supplementation may be required to correct inadequacies in absorption. Knowledge of cellular adaption (especially gastrointestinal adaptation) is important for those responsible for assisting people with nutritional health.

CASE STUDY

Ms Sofia Cassidy is a 29-year-old woman (UR number 156784) who sustained a fracture-dislocation to her right ankle after falling down a two-metre ravine while on a bush walk in a national park with her partner. Sofia is healthy, athletic and, apart from her current situation, considers herself in good physical condition. Once the medical team arrived, she was stabilised, airlifted out of the national park and taken to the nearest metropolitan hospital. Following primary and secondary assessments, pain relief and X-rays, it was determined that, apart from some minor grazes that needed cleaning and dressing, her ankle fracture was the only injury that required further intervention. She was kept 'nil by mouth' in anticipation of the need for an open reduction internal fixation (ORIF).

Ms Cassidy had blood drawn for a full blood count, electrolytes and coagulation profile. Her pathology results have returned as follows:

HAEMATOLOGY

Patient location:	Ward 3	UR:	156784		
Consultant:	Smith	NAME:	Cassidy		
		Given name:	Sofia	Sex:	F
		DOB:	03/11/XX	Age:	29

Time collected	11:13
Date collected	XX/XX
Year	XXXX
Lab #	456563645

FULL BLOOD COUNT		UNITS	REFERENCE RANGE
Haemoglobin	122	g/L	115–160
White cell count	6.3	$\times 10^9$/L	4.0–11.0
Platelets	244	$\times 10^9$/L	140–400
Haematocrit	0.43		0.33–0.47
Red cell count	4.67	$\times 10^{12}$/L	3.80–5.20
Reticulocyte count	1.2	%	0.2–2.0
MCV	94	fL	80–100

Educator resources

A suite of learning resources is provided to assist with delivery of the content, as well as to support teaching and learning.

Test Bank

The Test Bank provides a wealth of accuracy-verified testing material. Updated for the new edition, each chapter offers a wide variety of question types, arranged by learning objective and tagged by NMBA standards. Questions can be integrated into Blackboard, Canvas or Moodle Learning Management Systems.

Digital image powerpoint slides

All the diagrams and tables from the course content are available for lecturer use.

Solutions manual

The Solutions Manual provides educators with detailed, accuracy-verified solutions to in-chapter and end-of-chapter problems in the book.

PART 1

Cellular and tissue pathophysiology

1 Pathophysiological terminology, cellular adaptation and injury

KEY TERMS

Aetiology
Apoptosis
Atrophy
Caseous necrosis
Clinical manifestations
Coagulative necrosis
Dysplasia
Epidemiology
Fat necrosis
Gangrene
Homeostasis
Hyperplasia
Hypertrophy
Hypoxia
Incidence
Ischaemia
Liquefactive necrosis
Metaplasia
Necrosis
Oxygen free radicals
Pathogenesis
Pathophysiology
Prevalence
Reactive oxygen species (ROS)

LEARNING OBJECTIVES

After completing this chapter, you should be able to:

1 Define the terms 'pathophysiology', 'aetiology', 'pathogenesis', 'clinical manifestations' and 'epidemiology'.

2 Distinguish between the incidence and the prevalence of a disease.

3 Describe the types of cellular adaptations, and suggest situations in which each may occur.

4 Define 'dysplasia', differentiate it from other cell adaptations, and outline its consequences.

5 Differentiate between the characteristics of reversible and irreversible cell injury.

6 Compare and contrast necrosis and apoptosis.

7 Differentiate between the types of necrotic cell death.

8 Identify the major agents of cell injury.

9 Describe the process of cell injury resulting from an ischaemic or hypoxic agent.

WHAT YOU SHOULD KNOW BEFORE YOU START THIS CHAPTER

Can you name the main structures of the cell and their functions?

Can you describe how molecules are transported across the cell membrane?

Can you describe the cell cycle?

Can you define cellular metabolism?

Can you identify the major types of tissues and their functions?

Introduction

LEARNING OBJECTIVE 1

Define the terms 'pathophysiology', 'aetiology', 'pathogenesis', 'clinical manifestations' and 'epidemiology'.

Pathophysiology is defined as an understanding of the mechanisms by which disease and illness alter body functioning. These changes represent a breakdown of **homeostasis**, the dynamic state of equilibrium characterised by constant adjustment to changing circumstances to maintain normal function. Health professionals require a sound knowledge of pathophysiology for competent clinical practice. This knowledge is important in that it provides the rationales for care, and informs the clinical assessment and management of those in your care.

In this chapter, you are introduced to the key principles and concepts of pathophysiology that underpin your understanding of the specific diseases encountered in later chapters. These concepts include cellular responses to stimuli, cellular adaptations, types of cell injury and agents of injury. First, important terms that provide the framework for describing the pathophysiology of specific diseases in subsequent chapters are defined.

Important terminology

It is important to familiarise yourself with the four key principles of pathophysiology that form the framework in this textbook for the descriptions of specific diseases. The four important terms are aetiology, pathogenesis, clinical manifestations and epidemiology.

AETIOLOGY

Aetiology is the study of the cause, or causes, of a disease. Identifiable reasons for the development of a disease can include a person's diet, environment, inheritance and other genetic factors, occupation, health and age. Disease can arise within the body as a result of cell injury caused by immunological, metabolic, nutritional, inheritable, psychological or cancerous agents. It can also arise external to the body, due to the action of infectious organisms or traumatic physical agents, such as extreme temperature or force (see the 'Agents of cell injury' section later in this chapter for more detail).

If the cause is unknown, then an illness will be classified as an *idiopathic disease*. Alternatively, if an illness is a direct consequence of medical treatment, it is called an *iatrogenic condition*.

PATHOGENESIS

The **pathogenesis** represents the development of a disease. It usually covers the mechanisms by which a disease becomes established and progresses. Pathogenesis can be described in both chronological and spatial terms. In this aspect, the way in which homeostatic mechanisms attempt to adapt and then collapse are detailed. In detailing the pathogenesis of a disease, acute and chronic phases can be identified and differentiated.

CLINICAL MANIFESTATIONS

The **clinical manifestations** are the demonstrable changes representing the changes in function brought about by a disease process. The clinical manifestations are the changes *observed* by the affected person, their families or other people, as well as the changes *felt* by the affected person. They are also known, respectively, as the *signs* and *symptoms* of a disease. In a book such as this, common signs and symptoms are stated, but in reality a person with a particular disease may not show all of the clinical manifestations at any time during the progress of the condition.

EPIDEMIOLOGY

LEARNING OBJECTIVE 2

Distinguish between the incidence and the prevalence of a disease.

Another important term associated with pathophysiology is **epidemiology**. This is the study of the patterns of disease within populations. The factors that are frequently used to describe patterns of disease at the population level include age, sex, ethnicity, location, socioeconomic status and lifestyle. Risk factors and the aetiology can emerge from epidemiological studies.

Such studies also reveal the **incidence** and the **prevalence** of diseases within our communities. The *incidence rate* represents the number of *new* cases of a disease diagnosed within a particular period, usually over a calendar year. The *prevalence rate* is the *total* number of cases of a disease, both newly and previously diagnosed, at a particular time. Prevalence can be affected by other factors, such as disease recovery, mortality, recurrence and emigration. Health measures, such as immunisation, can lead to reductions in incidence and prevalence. Figure 1.1 illustrates the relationships between incidence, prevalence and these other factors.

Where possible in this text, we have drawn on the population statistics available for our region—Australia and New Zealand—and we have highlighted Indigenous health issues. This information is drawn from government documents, the Australian Institute of Health and Welfare, the World Health Organization and recent published epidemiological research. Where these statistics are not readily available, we will draw on those from other Western industrialised nations.

Cellular responses to stimuli

LEARNING OBJECTIVE 3

Describe the types of cellular adaptations, and suggest situations in which each may occur.

In order to maintain homeostasis, the body must make adjustments to functioning in response to changes in its internal and external environments. These environmental changes are called *stimuli*. Examples of stimuli include changes in temperature, oxygen supply or demand, pH, energy demand and body water levels. Homeostatic imbalances can arise if the adjustments to the changed conditions prove to be inadequate.

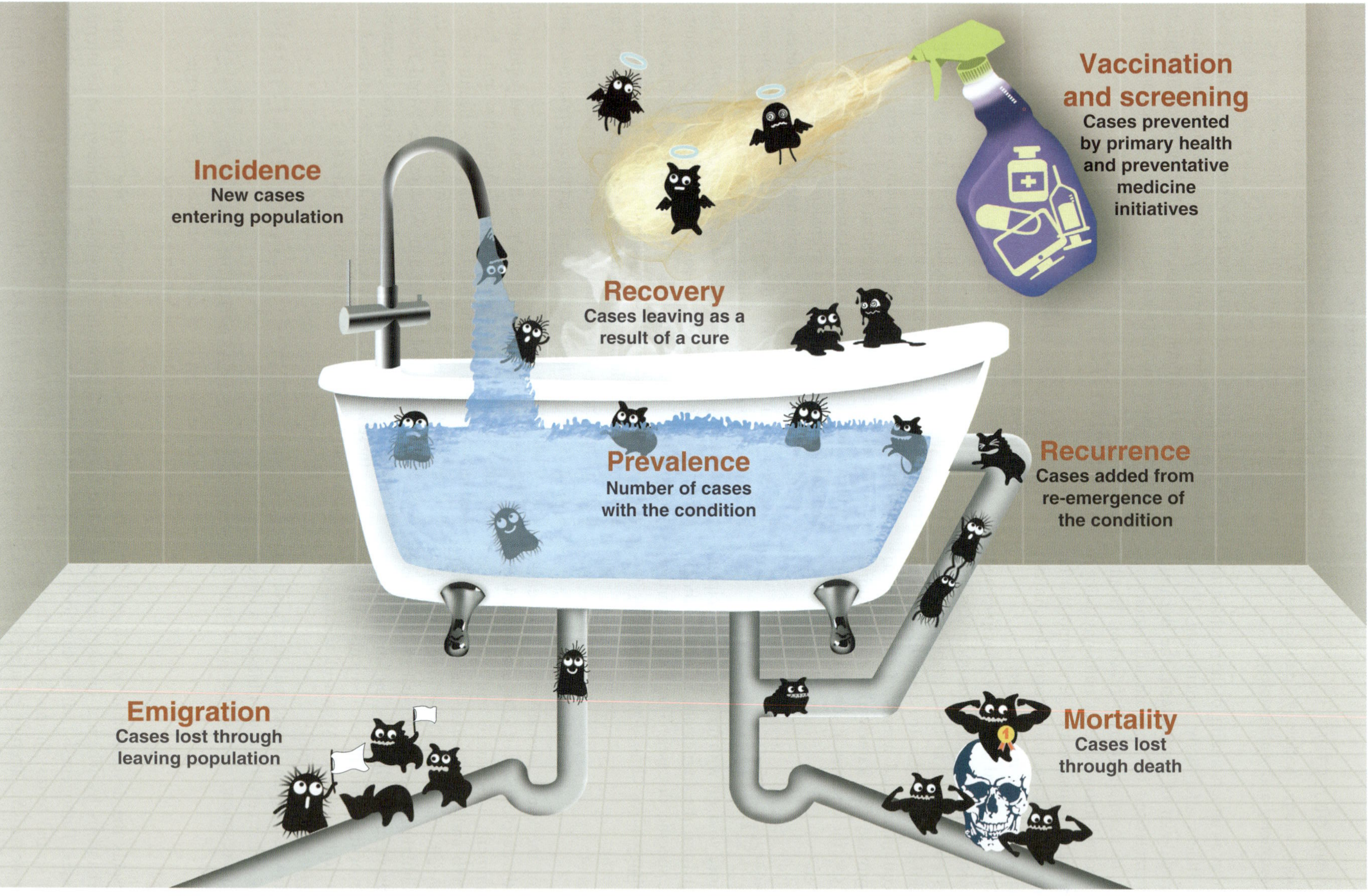

Figure 1.1

Epidemiological relationships

A conceptual representation of incidence and prevalence, and the effects of other factors and health measures on these rates.

Source: E.J. Roh & M. Hales © Sciencopia.

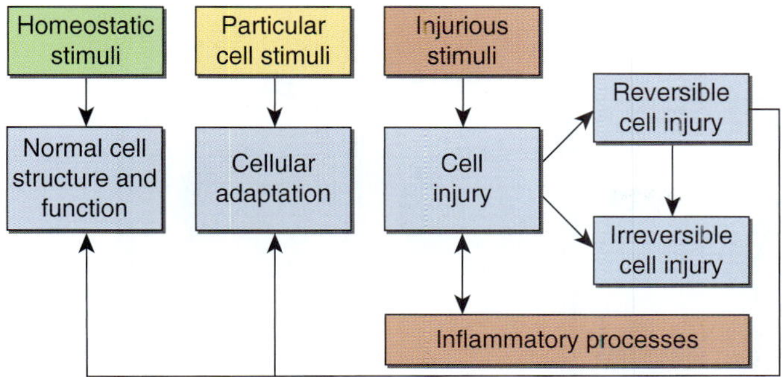

Figure 1.2

Continuum of cellular responses to stimuli

This is a representation of the interplay between normal cell structure and function, cellular adaptation and cell injury in response to stimuli. Inflammation plays an important role when cells are injured.

In response to persistent or intense stimuli, cells can adapt to the new conditions and maintain homeostasis. A number of *adaptations* are possible, and these are described.

Cellular adaptation and injury need to be considered across a continuum. If cells cannot adapt to current environmental conditions, then they may become injured. Cellular injuries can be *reversible*, where the affected cells recover after the stimulus is removed, or they can be *irreversible* and result in cell death. *Inflammation* is initiated in response to cell injury. Inflammatory processes can neutralise the agent of injury and promote healing. In some circumstances, the intensity or duration of inflammation can itself injure cells (see the chapter 'Determinants of health and illness'). The continuum of adaptation and injury is represented in Figure 1.2.

Cellular adaptations

Body cells are able to adapt to new conditions by increasing or decreasing their size, number, shape or arrangement within tissues. The terms associated with these adaptations are atrophy, hypertrophy, hyperplasia, metaplasia and dysplasia.

ATROPHY

Cell **atrophy** occurs when the demands on a population of cells decrease below normal or cannot be maintained at normal levels. The cells respond by *decreasing* in size (see Figure 1.3). An example of atrophy is during disuse when a person is bedridden for an extended period of time (i.e. disuse atrophy). The stretch and length of the skeletal muscle fibres involved decreases, which is known as *mechanical unloading*. Muscle fibres will decrease in size as an adaptation to the changed conditions. Functional changes accompany this structural adaptation so that muscle weakness can be a consequence. Muscle atrophy can also occur when a person has fractured a limb that is immobilised in plaster for months, or when astronauts are in space for a long period. Appropriate exercise/activity programs can assist in minimising the degree of atrophy experienced, or assist in the return of normal muscle function if and when the condition can be reversed.

Cell atrophy may also be induced when regulatory communication with another structure becomes compromised. Examples of this are in cases of spinal injury, when the neural stimulation of muscles is blocked, or when the hormones responsible for the maintenance of normal tissue function are not available. An example of the latter would be testicular atrophy as a result of the inhibition of luteinising hormone and follicle stimulating hormone secretion.

HYPERTROPHY

If the demands on cells are greater than normal, they may respond by *increasing* in size; this is called **hypertrophy** (see Figure 1.4). Again, skeletal muscle is a good example of a population of cells that readily undergo hypertrophy. When the mechanical loading on muscle fibres increases, they undergo hypertrophy. In skeletal muscle hypertrophy, an increase in nuclei and stem cells within the fibres is observed, and intracellular signalling and gene expression is altered, triggering the release of growth factors such as insulin-like growth factor-1 (IGF-1).

This effect can also occur in the heart. As the heart has more load placed on it, the cardiac myocytes will increase in size, which will cause cardiac hypertrophy. If the heart is diseased,

Figure 1.3

Cellular atrophy

The cells on the left are normal cells. Those on the right have undergone atrophy—a decrease in the size of the cells.

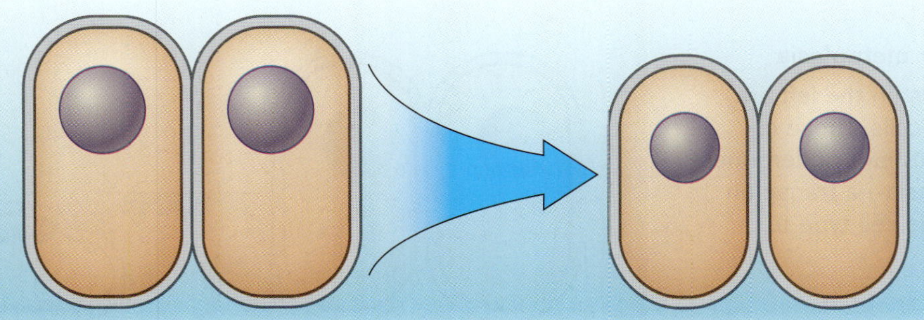

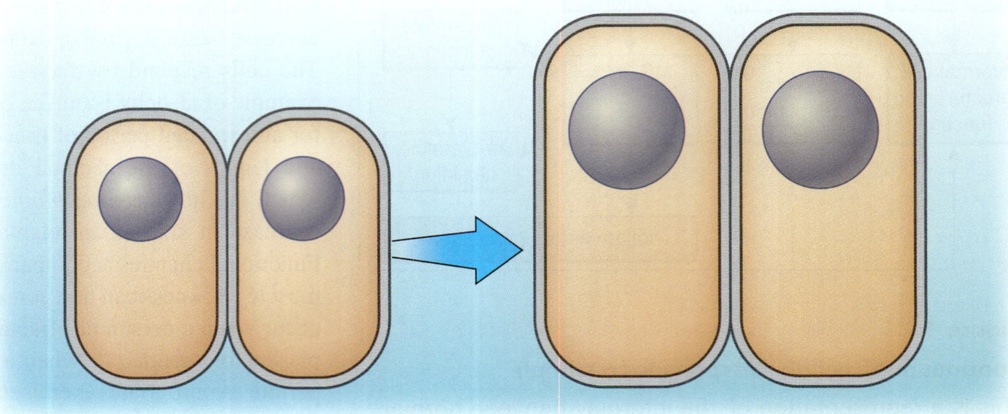

Figure 1.4

Cellular hypertrophy

The cells on the left are normal cells. Those on the right have undergone hypertrophy—an increase in the size of the cells.

such as in heart failure (see the chapter 'Cardiac muscle and valve disorders'), a normal workload is considered an increased load and results in hypertrophy. The increase in muscle mass creates an upsurge in demand on oxygen supply that cannot be met under these circumstances, worsening the cardiac impairment.

HYPERPLASIA

Hyperplasia is another form of cellular adaptation in response to increased demand. In **hyperplasia**, *cells increase in number* (see Figure 1.5); they do this by increasing their rate of mitosis. The capacity of cell populations for this is highly variable, with mature muscle cells and neurons lacking the capacity for this response. If hyperplasia occurs in these cell populations, it is usually due to a proportion of relatively undifferentiated stem cells within the tissue that proliferate in the right circumstances. Other cell populations, such as epithelial cells, can undertake hyperplasia more efficiently.

In reality, observed increases in the size of organs or other body structures are usually brought about through a combination of hyperplasia and hypertrophy. This can be demonstrated in examples where an increased exercise or mechanical loading can induce an enlargement of the heart, or the change in hormone levels during pregnancy leads to an enlargement of the uterus. In these cases, the change in organ size is largely due to hypertrophy.

METAPLASIA

In **metaplasia**, cells *change from one cell type to another* (see Figure 1.6). Importantly, these cells are fully differentiated,

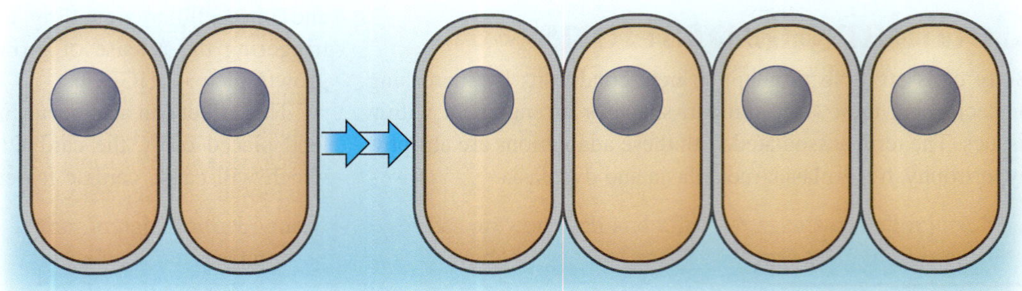

Figure 1.5

Cellular hyperplasia

The cells on the left are normal cells. Those on the right have undergone hyperplasia—an increase in the number of cells.

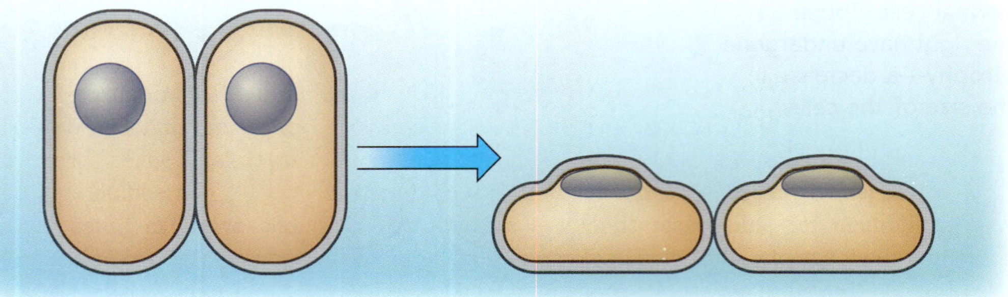

Figure 1.6

Cellular metaplasia

The cells on the left are normal cells. Those on the right have undergone metaplasia—a transition from one cell type to another.

and if the stimulus is removed the cells may revert back to their original type. However, metaplasia may also be a transitional form leading to pre-cancerous dysplasia (see 'Dysplasia'). Metaplastic transition is regulated by the altered expression of local transcription factors.

The most common example of this involves epithelial tissue. If the lining of the bronchial tree is exposed to persistent irritation (e.g. from cigarette smoke or exposure to air pollutants), the ciliated columnar epithelial cells can transform into stratified squamous epithelium. These cells endure the irritation better than the original cell type, but the downside may be some resultant localised deficit in the function of this region. This is brought about by the loss of the ciliated mucus-secreting cells, meaning debris is not cleared out of the airways as effectively. Metaplasia has also been observed in intestinal, glandular, cervical and skin tissue in response to noxious environmental stimuli.

DYSPLASIA

LEARNING OBJECTIVE 4

Define 'dysplasia', differentiate it from other cell adaptations, and outline its consequences.

In some instances, the adaptive response to a stimulus can be flawed, and the consequences can lead to a profound homeostatic imbalance and the onset of disease. An example of this maladaptive response is dysplasia. **Dysplasia** is characterised by a *variation in the size and shape of cells* within a tissue. This leads to a breakdown in the organisation and arrangement of the tissue (see Figure 1.7). Dysplasia is frequently identified by histological examination of tissue. In contrast to metaplasia, it can occur in undifferentiated and immature cell types.

In some circumstances, cell dysplasia may be considered a pre-cancerous stage. Dysplastic cells can show delays in maturation and differentiation that reflect the characteristics of cancer. Epithelial cell dysplasia in the cervix of the uterus is considered a potential sign of carcinoma in situ (where cancer cells proliferate in their native tissue without spreading to other sites) or invasive cancer, and when detected by a Pap smear is subjected to close monitoring. Dysplasias affecting liver cells, bronchiolar columnar cells and erythrocytes may also be linked to cancer development.

Cellular injury

LEARNING OBJECTIVE 5

Differentiate between the characteristics of reversible and irreversible cell injury.

A failure to adapt to a stimulus leads to cell injury. The injury can be reversible, eventually leading to a return to the pre-injured state, or irreversible, resulting in cell death.

REVERSIBLE CELL INJURY

Reversible injury is characterised by the cell swelling with water (*hydropic swelling*) or by the excessive inclusion of substances within the cell cytoplasm (*intracellular accumulations*). A common cause of these changes is the failure of the enzymes involved in normal cellular metabolism. The injury may be reversible if the stimuli can be extinguished or the cell develops compensatory processes to neutralise further damage. However, the tissue may not be able to return to full function if significant injury has occurred.

Hydropic swelling occurs when the membrane sodium pump (Na^+/K^+-ATPase) fails; more specifically, allowing sodium influx into the cell. As an energy-dependent pump, a poor supply of ATP (adenosine triphosphate), due to a deficient oxygen supply or the unavailability of glucose, often leads to this situation. As a consequence, sodium ions accumulate within the cell, creating an osmotic gradient that draws water into the cell. Cells undergoing hydropic swelling can enlarge as the cytoplasm and cellular organelles expand. If these conditions persist, the organelles may actually rupture and vacuoles appear in the cytoplasm (see Figure 1.8).

Substances that can accumulate within cells include the normal nutrients (lipids, carbohydrates and proteins), pigments and inorganic particles. These substances tend to accumulate due to excessive supply and/or metabolic dysfunction. Some of the compounds are naturally present inside cells (although not normally at these levels), whereas others are abnormal (see Figure 1.9).

When excessive levels of fats, carbohydrates or proteins occur in the body, some tissues will attempt to take them up and store them. An example of a condition where this occurs is diabetes mellitus (see the chapter 'Diabetes mellitus'). High blood lipid levels can lead to the uptake of fats into the walls of blood vessels, which may lead to the development of atherosclerosis (see the chapter 'Diabetes mellitus'), as well as into the liver (i.e. hepatosteatosis). Diabetes mellitus is also characterised by

Figure 1.7

Cellular dysplasia

The cells on the left are normal cells. Those on the right have undergone dysplasia—variability in size and shape of cells—which leads to an alteration in tissue arrangement.

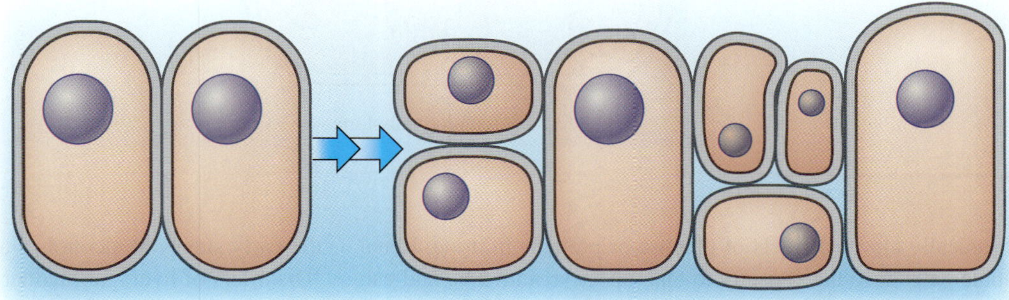

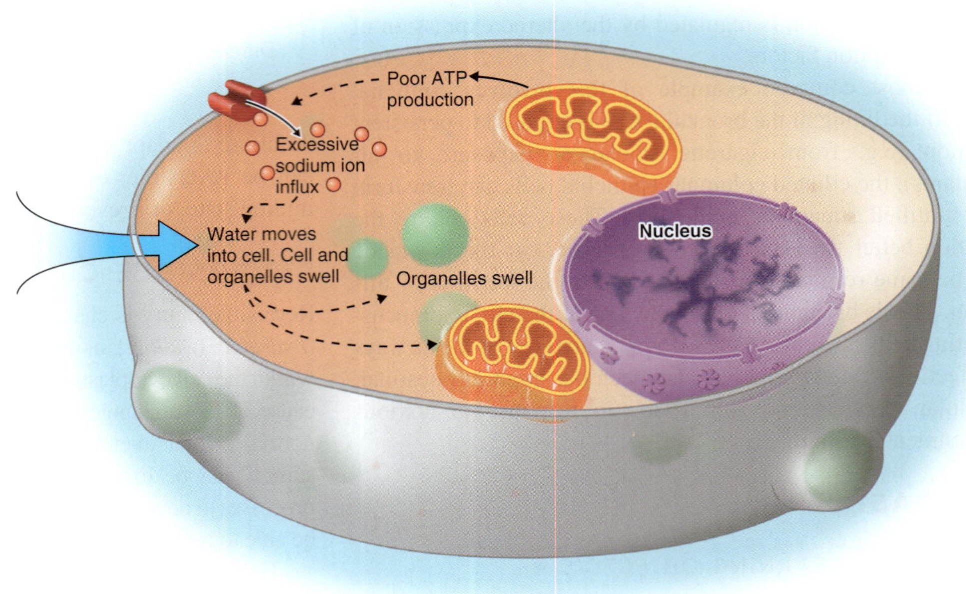

Figure 1.8

Hydropic swelling

Poor ATP production leads to dysfunction of the membrane pumps, resulting in reduced sodium ion influx. This exerts a strong osmotic pressure that draws water into the cell. The cell and its organelles swell. This swelling can lead to membrane rupture and irreversible cell injury.

ATP = adenosine triphosphate.

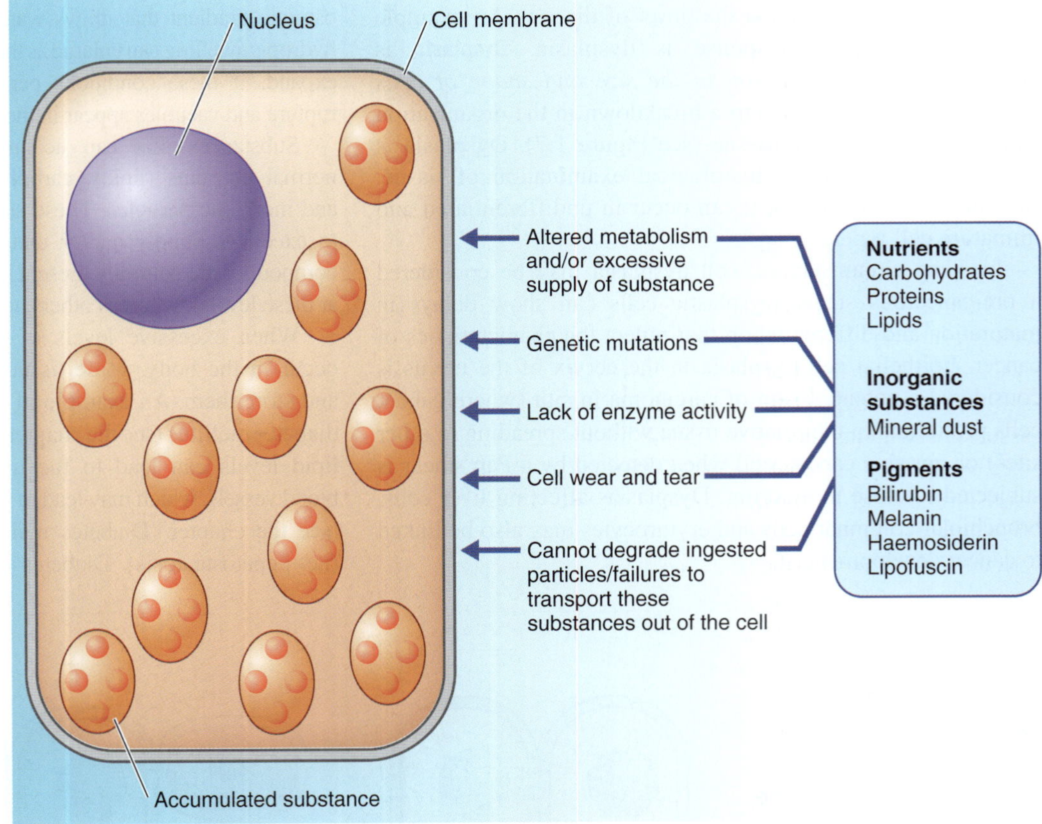

Figure 1.9

Examples of the types of substances that accumulate intracellularly, and some general causes

chronically elevated levels of glucose or proteins in urine. Renal tubule cells have the capacity to take up these nutrients, and can store them in excess; glucose is stored as glycogen.

Under some circumstances, the nutrient does not need to be present in surplus for excessive accumulation to occur. In the early stages of alcohol-related liver disease (see the chapter 'Disorders of liver, gallbladder and pancreas'), the liver appears to preferentially metabolise alcohol over lipids. This leads to the intracellular accumulation of fat particles within the liver, giving rise to a condition known as alcoholic fatty liver or alcoholic hepatosteatosis. It is a mild condition and may be asymptomatic. Unlike later stages in alcoholic liver disease, it is reversible if alcohol intake is reduced or stopped.

Proteins can accumulate inside cells in the presence of a persistent injurious agent. Under these circumstances, the proteins have become denatured, so they take up abnormal shapes, greatly altering their function. If they are not cleared from the cell, they will cause irreversible injury. This pathophysiological process is considered to be the basis of the development of some of the neurodegenerative diseases, such as Parkinson's disease and Alzheimer's disease (see the chapter 'Neurodegenerative disorders'). Intracellular entities, such as a group of chaperone proteins known as heat shock proteins, are present in the endoplasmic reticulum to assist in the reshaping of denatured proteins, but these can be overwhelmed by the rate of formation of the latter in the presence of the injurious agent.

Certain genetic disorders are characterised by cell accumulations, although these are not usually considered reversible. In these conditions, a key enzyme involved in intracellular nutrient metabolism is missing, giving rise to the term 'inborn errors of metabolism'. The substrate or some intermediate product (e.g. glycogen or lipid) accumulates in cells. Glycogen can accumulate in cells, particularly liver and/or muscle tissue, greatly diminishing the availability of glucose to these and other body cells. This group of conditions is called the *glycogen storage diseases (GSD)*. The form of GSD depends on which enzyme in the process is dysfunctional; currently, approximately 10 types of GSD have been identified.

Lipid storage diseases can also arise as inborn errors of metabolism. In these conditions, lipids accumulate in many body tissues, including the liver, kidneys, lung, spleen, brain and bone marrow, causing widespread deficits in function. Examples of inheritable lipid storage diseases include Gaucher disease, Niemann–Pick disease and Tay–Sachs disease (see the chapter 'Genetic disorders').

Natural body pigments can accumulate in cells when they are present in excess quantities. Melanin, a skin pigment responsible for tanned or darkened skin, can be present in the skin in excessive quantities during excessive pituitary activation associated with an endocrine disorder called Addison's disease (see the chapter 'Adrenal gland disorders').

Bilirubin and haemosiderin are pigments formed from the breakdown of haemoglobin in erythrocytes. Bilirubin can be present in excess within the body, and can be taken up by cells when there is a disproportionately large breakdown of erythrocytes, in obstructive biliary disorders or during liver disease. Body tissues take on a characteristic yellow hue, referred to as 'jaundice'.

Lipofuscin is an insoluble yellowish-brown pigment which accumulates in cells, especially muscle, skin and nerve cells. It is formed from the breakdown of the cellular organelles, called lysosomes, and is considered a normal marker of the ageing process and the 'wear and tear' of living, as more of it is observed in tissues as we get older. Pigmented blemishes, called liver spots, can be seen in the skin of the aged. Excessive lipofuscin accumulation has been implicated in diseases of the aged such as macular degeneration, where the lipofuscin accumulates in the retina, and in Alzheimer's disease, where it accumulates in the brain.

Mineral dust contains insoluble inorganic particles that can be very problematic once they enter the body. Once inhaled, these particles are taken up by lung cells and accumulate there, because they cannot be degraded by phagocytosis or cleared from the tissues. Their presence induces chronic inflammatory responses (see the chapter 'Inflammation and healing') that severely damage the lung tissue and lead to disease. Exposure to these agents is most commonly associated with the mining of coal, asbestos, iron and lead.

IRREVERSIBLE CELL INJURY

LEARNING OBJECTIVE 6

Compare and contrast necrosis and apoptosis.

Irreversible injury results in cell death. Two physiological processes are associated with cell death: necrosis and apoptosis.

Necrosis

LEARNING OBJECTIVE 7

Differentiate between the types of necrotic cell death.

Necrosis is the process whereby the injury directly leads to premature pathologic *cell death* and *autolysis* (self-digestion). Characteristic changes in structure accompany this process, affecting all parts of the cell: the plasma membrane, nucleus, cytoplasm and cellular organelles. Most of these changes can be observed histologically. Within the nucleus, the chromatin threads degrade and the organelle shrinks. This is called *pyknosis*. Mitochondrial membranes break down, causing the mitochondria to swell and rupture. Vacuoles form within the cytoplasm. The impairment of ATP production leads to the seizing up of the membrane pumps, allowing sodium ions to accumulate intracellularly. Water is drawn into the cell, expanding the cytoplasm. Ultimately, the cell ruptures (see Figure 1.10).

The contents of the cell, including intracellular enzymes, spill out into the extracellular fluid and eventually diffuse into the bloodstream. The level of these substances in the blood correlates to the degree of necrotic cell death. These intracellular substances, particularly enzymes, may be characteristic to particular cell types—representing a kind of cellular signature. As a result, their presence in the blood is indicative of necrotic cell death in specific organs, such as the heart or the liver (Table 1.1), and can be used in clinical diagnosis. The release of chemical mediators from dying cells during necrosis triggers an inflammatory reaction. The purpose of this reaction is to clear away the cellular debris and facilitate the healing process (see the chapter 'Inflammation and healing').

There are four identifiable types of necrosis: coagulative, liquefactive, caseous and fat. The type of necrosis induced can depend on the type of tissue affected and the nature of the injurious agent (Table 1.2). **Coagulative necrosis** is characterised by protein denaturation. A good everyday example of coagulative protein denaturation is when an egg is poached. The protein turns white and forms a firm, gelatinous mass that holds its shape well. Cells that undergo coagulative necrosis behave in a similar fashion, and because of this the affected tissue initially holds its shape before breaking down. Ischaemic injury affecting the heart or kidneys is a good example of coagulative necrosis.

Liquefactive necrosis occurs when lysosomal digestive enzymes are released rapidly in large amounts during cell death, which leads to immediate autolysis. Infections are often associated with

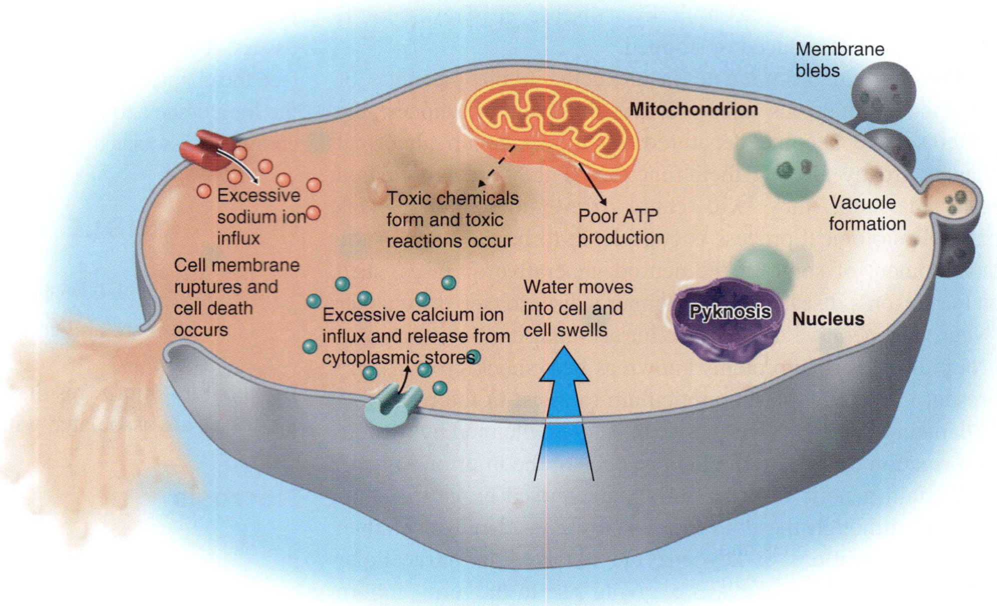

Figure 1.10

Necrotic processes

Poor ATP production leads to dysfunction of the membrane pumps, resulting in excessive sodium ion influx. This exerts a strong osmotic pressure that draws water into the cell. The cell and its organelles swell. Calcium ions are released from cytoplasmic stores, activating intracellular enzymes, which further impair mitochondrial function and damage membranes. The plasma membrane forms blebs (blisters), which weaken its integrity. Toxic chemicals accumulate inside the cell, which can also damage its structures. The nucleus shrinks and forms a dense structure (pyknosis), which breaks up. Numerous vacuoles form within the cell. Cell membranes rupture, and inflammation follows.

ATP = adenosine triphosphate.

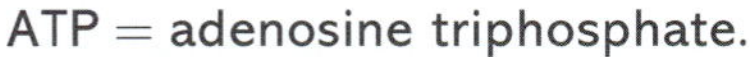

Table 1.1 Common intracellular enzymes released in cell injury

Enzymes	Tissue damage marker
Alanine aminotransferase (ALT)	Heart, liver and kidney
Alkaline phosphatase (ALP)	Liver and bone
Amylase	Pancreas
Aspartate aminotransferase (AST)	Liver, skeletal muscle, heart, pancreas and kidney
Creatine kinase (CK)	Brain, heart and skeletal muscle
Lactate dehydrogenase (LDH)	Liver, kidneys, skeletal muscle and erythrocytes
Cardiac troponin I (cTnI)	Heart
Troponin T (cTnT)	Heart and skeletal muscle

Table 1.2 Types of necrosis

Type	Features
Coagulative	Primarily characterised by protein denaturation. The cell holds its shape well during necrosis.
Liquefactive	Characterised by the rapid release of large amounts of lysosomal enzymes. The cell liquefies.
Caseous	Tissue framework not completely liquefied. The cell looks cheese-like.
Fat	Fat cell membranes are damaged, causing the release of triglycerides. The triglycerides are converted into free fatty acids that bind to calcium ions. The tissue becomes chalky and white.

this form of necrosis as the microorganism may release enzymes that contribute to the liquefaction. The affected tissue degrades rapidly, losing its framework and becoming a semi-solid mass. Irreversible ischaemic brain injury results in liquefactive necrosis.

Caseous necrosis is a combination of liquefactive and coagulative processes, where the tissue framework is not completely broken down by lysosomal enzyme action. The necrotic area is contained in an immune response, rather than being removed from the body. The affected tissue has the consistency of cottage cheese, giving rise to the term *caseous*, which means 'cheese-like'. An example is a chronic tuberculotic lesion in the lung, where the microbe escapes immune attack within infected macrophages (see the chapter 'Respiratory infections, cancers and vascular conditions').

Fat necrosis occurs in adipose tissue. Fat cell membranes are damaged, leading to a release of triglycerides into the tissue. Lipases act on the triglycerides to degrade them, leading to the formation of free fatty acids. Calcium ions bind to these tissue fatty acids, forming calcium soaps, a process called *saponification*. The affected tissue becomes chalky and white. Fat necrosis occurs in pancreatitis, when pancreatic lipasess attack surrounding adipose tissue as a result of injury caused by infection, trauma, toxin release or ischaemia. Another structure prone to fat necrosis is breast tissue as a result of traumatic injury.

Gangrene is a term associated with the necrosis of a relatively large amount of tissue as a result of ischaemia. The affected tissue usually turns black, and may feel cold and smell fetid; there is usually a clearly identifiable boundary between the affected and normal tissue. This distinctive boundary is due to necrotic cells releasing their concentrated contents, leading to injury to neighbouring cells. Gangrene can involve liquefactive or coagulative necrosis. Gangrene that develops in the skin, affecting a foot or toe, for example, usually undergoes coagulative necrosis. The affected area becomes wrinkled and black, and in this form is called *dry gangrene*. Internal organs when infected usually undergo liquefactive necrosis, and this is termed *wet gangrene*. In some cases of infection, the metabolic processes of the infective organism result in gas bubbles in the affected tissue area. This is called *gas gangrene*, and can occur in tissue infections caused by anaerobic *Clostridium* bacteria.

Apoptosis

Programmed cell death, **apoptosis**, is an integral part of the normal process of tissue maintenance and development during our lives. Within the nervous system, neurons that do not make the appropriate connections die. This also happens during developmental processes while we are in utero. We see it in the repair of a bone after a fracture as it is remodelled to its normal appearance. This physiological cell death is also a key part of immune system regulation, when a body cell is infected by a virus or an immune cell reacts against our own tissue. Apoptosis occurs rapidly in response to a specific stimulus that indicates that the cell is no longer required or has become redundant as a result of tissue maturation.

Upon receiving this stimulus, the cell initiates a cascade of enzymic reactions that leads to its death. Initially, the cell will decrease in size and the nucleus condenses. At this time, other cellular organelles remain normal in their appearance. As the reaction progresses, the cell membrane blebs, as the nucleus and its contents fragment. Eventually the whole cell fragments, forming apoptotic bodies that are engulfed by neighbouring phagocytes. In contrast to necrosis, the death of the cell does not induce an inflammatory response (see Figure 1.11).

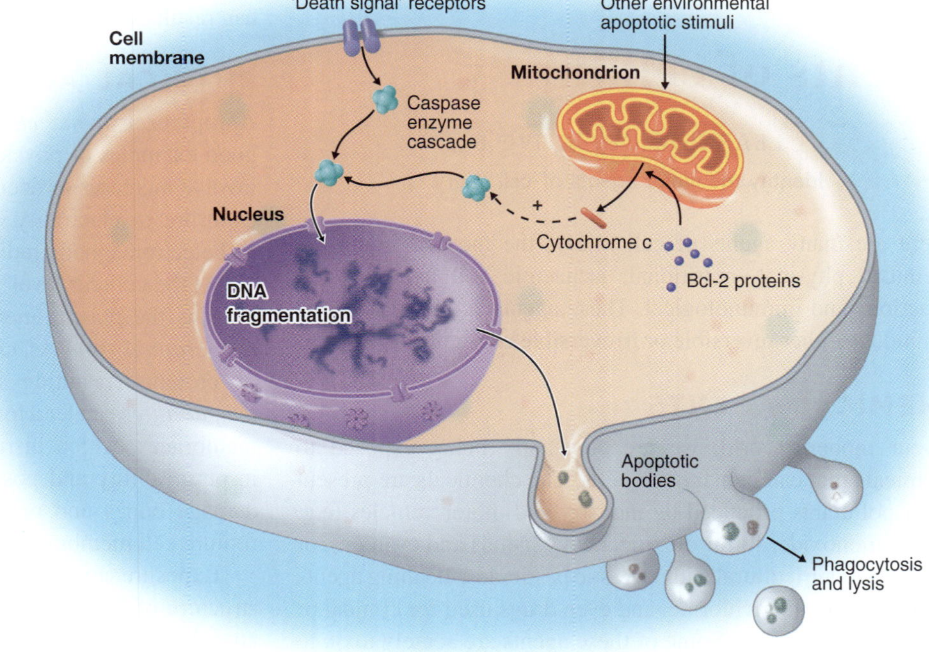

Figure 1.11

Apoptosis

Apoptosis can be triggered by the activation of so-called 'death signal' receptors (tumour necrosis factor [TNF] and Fas receptors) or a variety of other stimuli. These receptors activate a cascade of intracellular reactions, involving caspase enzymes. Other stimuli induce cytochrome c synthesis within the mitochondria. Cytochrome c can also activate the caspases. Within the nucleus, the cascade triggers the condensation of chromatin and nuclear fragmentation. The fragmented cell components are captured within membrane-bound structures called apoptotic bodies, which are phagocytosed. There is no subsequent inflammatory response. Bcl-2 proteins appear to have a key role in regulating apoptosis.

DNA = deoxyribonucleic acid.

Table 1.3 A typical comparison between necrosis and apoptosis

Necrosis	Apoptosis
Pathological cell death	Cell suicide or programmed cell death
Numerous cells in the tissue affected	One or a few cells in the tissue affected
Cells swell, organelles disrupted (including the nucleus), and loss of membrane integrity	Cells shrink, organelles remain normal, nucleus and organelles broken down into membrane-bound fragments
Induces inflammation	No inflammation

The differences between necrosis and apoptosis are summarised in Table 1.3.

Key mediators of the apoptotic process include the proteolytic enzymes called *caspases*, the tumour-suppressing gene *p53*, calcium ions and the so-called *'death signal' receptors* on cell surfaces—the *Fas receptor* and the *tumour necrosis factor (TNF) receptor*. On the other hand, a family of intracellular proteins grouped as *Bcl-2* have been shown to suppress apoptosis under a variety of conditions. It appears that the intracellular balance of Bcl-2 proteins may be important in the regulation of apoptosis.

Apoptosis has been linked to the development of certain diseases. If apoptosis does not occur when it should, is induced prematurely, or in the presence of the correct stimulus does not take place at all, disease may develop. Examples where evidence of this is apparent include certain cancers (see the chapter 'Neoplasia'), neurodegenerative diseases such as Parkinson's disease and Alzheimer's disease (see the chapter 'Neurodegenerative disorders') and some congenital abnormalities.

Agents of cell injury

LEARNING OBJECTIVE 8

Identify the major agents of cell injury.

There are many agents of cell injury; the most common are chemical, physical, nutritional, ischaemic and hypoxic, and infectious and immunological. These agents act as stimuli that can induce either reversible or irreversible cell injury.

CHEMICAL AGENTS

In our modern world, we are constantly being exposed to chemicals that can damage our cells. The chemicals are present as air pollutants produced by industry and motor vehicles (e.g. carbon monoxide, sulfur dioxide, heavy metals and cyanide), or available as agricultural and domestic pesticides, cleaning agents such as carbon tetrachloride, and even drugs used for clinical or recreational purposes. Some of these agents are acutely toxic to cells, while others accumulate in our bodies and become toxic after reaching a particular threshold level.

Some of these chemicals, such as the heavy metals, produce widespread toxicity affecting a number of body systems. Other chemicals target specific organs; for example, an overdose of paracetamol can irreversibly damage the liver. A chemical may even attack a specific population of cells within an organ, as the neurotoxin 1-methyl-4-phenyl-1,2,3,6-tetrahydropyridine (MPTP) does when it selectively destroys the dopaminergic neurons of the nigrostriatal motor pathway in the brain. MPTP has been implicated in some forms of Parkinson's disease pathophysiology (see the chapter 'Neurodegenerative disorders').

Some toxic environmental agents can react with oxygen molecules within the cell and lead to the formation of free radicals. *Free radicals* are highly **reactive oxygen species (ROS)** that can then disrupt cell membranes, intracellular lipid and deoxyribonucleic acid (DNA) structure. Fortunately, these free radicals can be neutralised by chemicals with antioxidant properties, such as some vitamins. Under certain conditions, cells can become saturated with free radicals, and, if the availability of antioxidants is exhausted, irreversible cell injury can result (see Figure 1.12).

PHYSICAL AGENTS

Abrupt or *extreme changes in temperature or pressure* are good examples of physical agents of injury. These changes can involve increases or decreases. Physical agents can also include exposure to electricity, significant mechanical force (trauma) and electromagnetic radiation.

At the cellular level, these agents can disrupt cell structures such as the plasma membrane, nucleus and organelles. *High temperatures and electricity* can lead to the denaturation of proteins, resulting in coagulation within the cell. *Low temperatures* can lead to the formation of ice crystals within cell membranes, which disrupt their integrity, leading to changes in permeability and possible cell death. *Mechanical force* can damage bones and organs. At the cellular level, trauma can rupture cell membranes, leading to cell death.

Exposure to *electromagnetic radiation* can change the structure of DNA such that it may induce gene mutations that alter the structure and/or function of the cell. Such an alteration can trigger the onset of cancer. Changes to DNA could also lead to impairments in cell growth or a breakdown in DNA

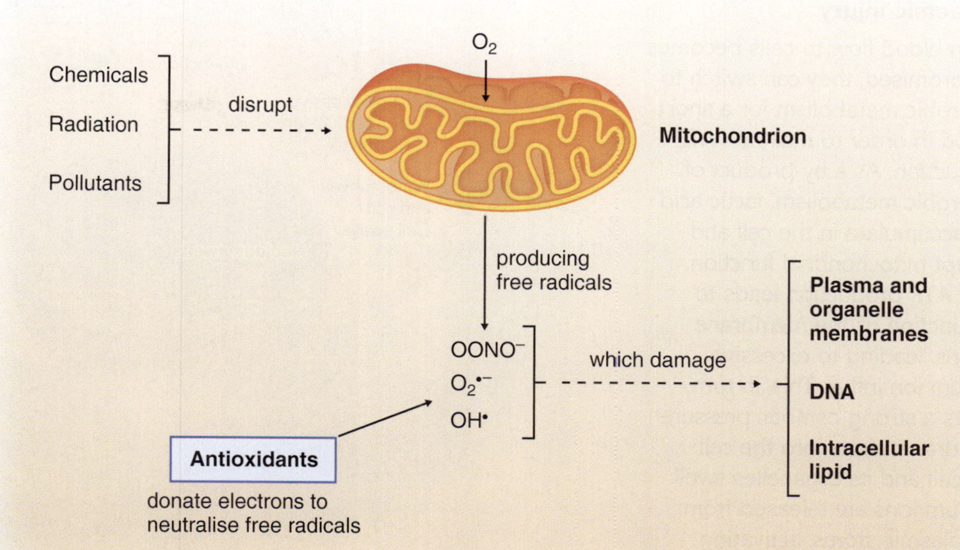

Figure 1.12

Free radical formation and antioxidant action

Oxygen free radicals are formed as part of aerobic metabolism. They are also formed when stimuli, such as those shown, disrupt mitochondrial function. These highly reactive chemicals interact with and damage cell structures to acquire electrons in order to form stable bonds. Antioxidant substances, such as vitamins and flavonoids, can neutralise free radicals by donating electrons without disrupting their chemical structures.

DNA = deoxyribonucleic acid; $OH^\bullet$ = hydroxyl radical; O_2 = oxygen; $O_2^{\bullet -}$ = superoxide radical; $OONO^-$ = peroxynitrite ion.

integrity that result in cell death. Like some of the chemical agents, radiation can also ionise oxygen molecules, leading to the formation of damaging free radicals.

NUTRITIONAL AGENTS

Nutrient balance is a key aspect of homeostasis. When nutritional *imbalances* develop, they can have a significant effect on the capacity of the body to maintain equilibrium, resulting in cell injury. Proteins, carbohydrates, lipids, vitamins and minerals are vital for normal cell function. Although the body can manufacture a number of these nutrients, most of these substances, or their precursors, must be obtained from our diet.

Nutrition-related cell injuries can arise as a result of nutrient deficiencies. Vitamin deficiencies can lead to a diverse range of conditions, including anaemia, bleeding disorders, dermatitis, skeletal and nervous system dysfunction, as well as altered immunity. Conditions associated with mineral deficiencies include anaemia (iron deficiency), hypothyroidism (iodine deficiency), tooth decay (fluoride deficiency) and impaired healing and immunity (zinc deficiency). Malnutrition develops when the macronutrients (proteins, lipids and carbohydrates) become unavailable to body cells. This can be the result of inadequate intake, absorption, distribution or cellular uptake (see the Part 'Gastrointestinal pathophysiology').

Cells can also be damaged in states of nutritional excess, resulting from higher intake or poor cellular uptake. Obesity as a result of the excessive intake of calories is a major concern today in most Western countries, and is considered a major risk factor for cardiovascular, joint and biliary diseases.

ISCHAEMIC AND HYPOXIC AGENTS

LEARNING OBJECTIVE 9

Describe the process of cell injury resulting from an ischaemic or hypoxic agent.

Body cells require a ready supply of oxygen for normal metabolism to occur, although oxygen requirements may vary greatly between cell types. Oxygen is required for normal energy production and storage in the form of *adenosine triphosphate (ATP)* molecules, and is delivered to cells via the bloodstream. The bloodstream is also the means by which cellular wastes are removed before they can accumulate.

When oxygen supply via the blood is compromised, a state of **hypoxia** will develop. The interruption of blood supply to a tissue is called **ischaemia**. Hypoxia will eventually develop as a result of ischaemia. This state can happen very quickly if the degree of interruption of blood flow is severe and the tissue's metabolic needs are high. Examples of ischaemic conditions are angina pectoris (see the chapter 'Coronary artery disease'), peripheral vascular disease (see the chapter 'Vascular disorders and circulatory shock') and the most common form of stroke (see the chapter 'Brain and spinal cord dysfunction').

Hypoxia can also develop in the absence of ischaemia. Examples where this can happen include *poor oxygen levels in the blood* (anaemia), *impaired oxygenation* (lung disease) or *heart disease*. A number of toxic agents can induce hypoxia through a *disruption of cellular respiration*. These agents include carbon monoxide, hydrogen sulfide and cyanide.

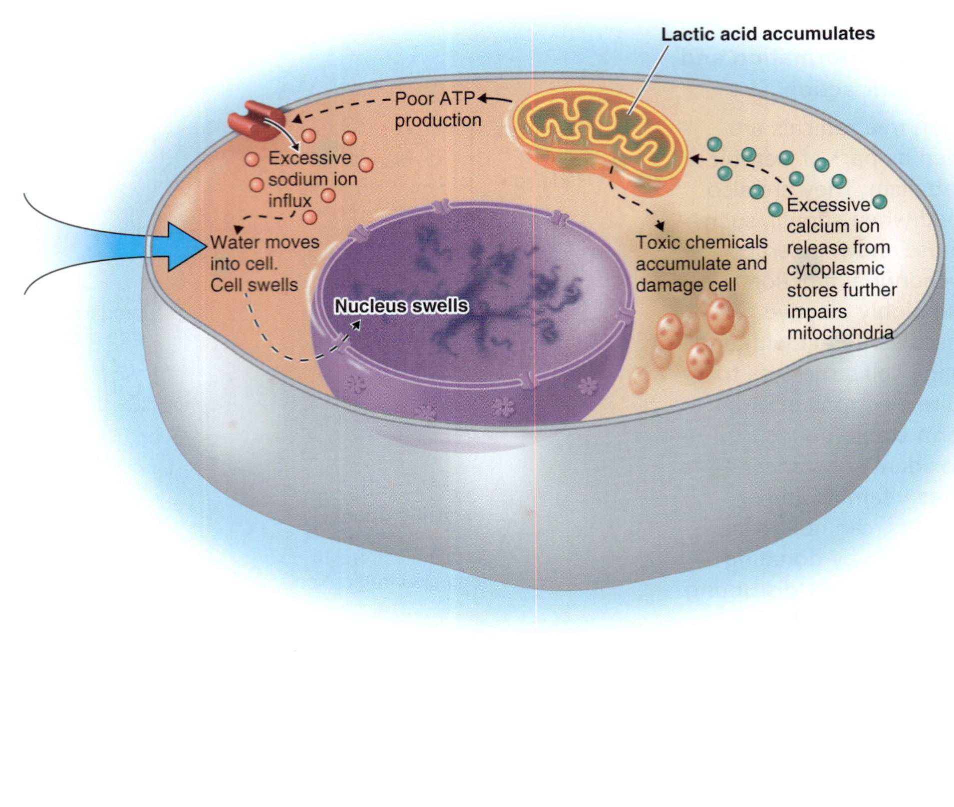

Figure 1.13

Ischaemic injury

When blood flow to cells becomes compromised, they can switch to anaerobic metabolism for a short period in order to maintain ATP production. As a by-product of anaerobic metabolism, lactic acid can accumulate in the cell and disrupt mitochondrial function. Poor ATP production leads to dysfunction of the membrane pumps, leading to excessive sodium ion influx. This, in turn, exerts a strong osmotic pressure that draws water into the cell. The cell and its organelles swell. Calcium ions are released from cytoplasmic stores, activating intracellular enzymes that further impair mitochondrial function and damage membranes. Toxic chemicals accumulate inside the cell, which can also damage its structures.

ATP = adenosine triphosphate.

Once the oxygen supply to cells is compromised, the production of ATP decreases markedly. Cells will attempt to compensate for this change by switching to anaerobic metabolism, which results in relatively lower levels of ATP production and the accumulation of lactic acid. This cannot be sustained, because high levels of lactic acid can be toxic to cells. Impaired ATP production leads to a failure of the membrane pumps controlling the movement of sodium, potassium and calcium into and out of the cell. Sodium ions accumulate intracellularly, drawing water into the cell, which causes the cell to swell, damaging membranes and disrupting organelle functions. Calcium ions are also released into the cytoplasm from intracellular stores, which further impairs mitochondrial function. In ischaemia, cellular waste products cannot be cleared away, and so accumulate in the cell's environment. These wastes can contribute to cell injury (see Figure 1.13).

Intuitively, one would think that simply restoring blood flow would allow the affected cells to recover and return to normal. Unfortunately, this is not the case. Re-perfusion of the tissue with blood can lead to further damage and cell death. This secondary injury is termed *re-perfusion injury*. As the cellular membrane pumps are still impaired, restoration of blood flow can lead to an uncontrolled influx of calcium ions. The calcium ions can trigger processes that result in the breakdown of membrane lipids and cell death. Large numbers of **oxygen free radicals** are produced, which can cause extensive and potentially irreversible cell injury by attacking cell membranes, denaturing proteins and damaging cell DNA (see Figure 1.14).

Re-perfusion injury plays a major role in the potentially catastrophic cell death associated with *stroke* and *acute myocardial infarction (AMI)*. Interestingly, research has shown that the degree of re-perfusion injury that occurs in AMI can be reduced by pre-exposure to a sublethal ischaemic state that primes the heart for a subsequent ischaemic episode. This process is called *ischaemic pre-conditioning*, and may have a role to play in the clinical management of someone at high risk of AMI.

INFECTIOUS AND IMMUNOLOGICAL AGENTS

Microbes are common and effective agents of cell injury. This group includes organisms such as bacteria, viruses and parasites. The earliest human records show that microbes have plagued us for aeons, most likely from the time that the first humans appeared on Earth.

Once microbes gain access to cells, they can cause extensive damage. They can do this by entering the cell and *disrupting normal function*, or they can remain in the extracellular space and *secrete powerful chemicals*, usually enzymes, that disable or kill cells. Viruses, comprised of the nucleic acids RNA or DNA, can enter a body cell and *change its programming* so that it becomes a factory for making new virus particles, or *alter its structure* in such a way that it is irreversibly damaged.

The immune system is responsible for neutralising and removing these microbial invaders. Infected body cells are recognised, and immune reactions then triggered. Immune cells

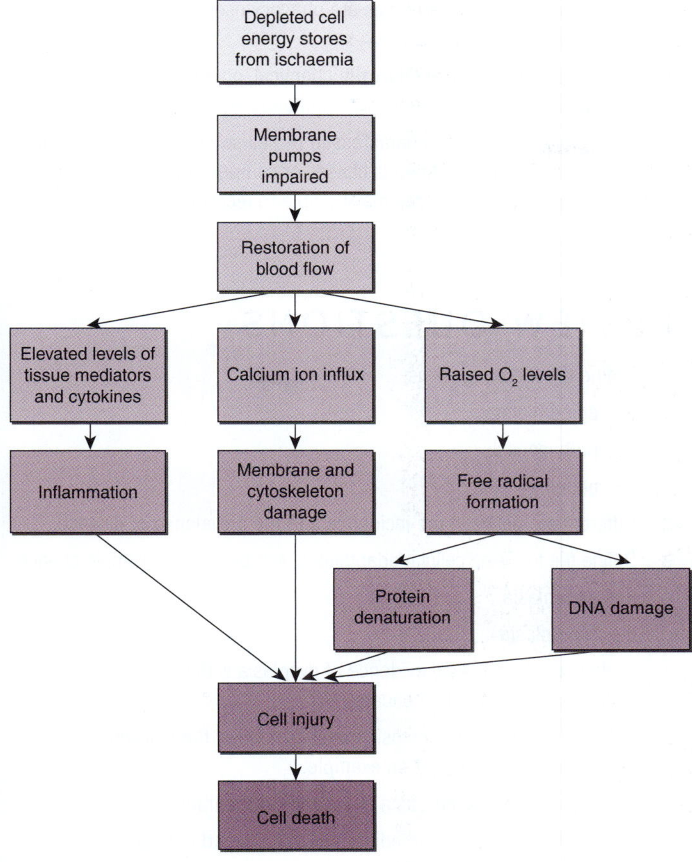

Figure 1.14

Reperfusion injury

DNA = deoxyribonucleic acid; O_2 = oxygen.

are recruited to the site, and release a range of chemicals (see the chapters 'Inflammation and healing' and 'Infectious diseases') that lead to the death of the infected cell. Unfortunately, the lack of specificity of this immune response and/or its magnitude may lead to injury to a significant number of normal cells that are in close proximity.

INDIGENOUS HEALTH FAST FACTS AND CULTURAL CONSIDERATIONS

ALTERED NUTRITIONAL STATE AS AN AGENT OF INJURY

- *Poor nutrition contributes to approximately 9.7% of the burden of disease for Aboriginal and Torres Strait Islander peoples.*
- *Estimations of food costs in rural and remote communities are considered to be approximately 30% higher than in major cities, which probably contributes to the very low fruit and vegetable intake described among Aboriginal and Torres Strait Islander groups.*
- *Poor nutrition results in the birth of low-birth-weight babies almost twice as frequently in Aboriginal and Torres Strait Islander women as in non-Indigenous women.*
- *Food security is a greater issue for Aboriginal and Torres Strait Islander peoples, with 22% of people reporting that at least one person went without food when the household ran out of food, compared to 3.7% in non-Indigenous Australian households.*
- *Māori or Pacific Islands babies are less likely than European New Zealand children to be breastfed.*
- *Based on a set of predetermined risk factors, Maori children make up 66% of children at risk of developing poor outcomes later in life, compared to 21% of European New Zealand children, 12% of Pacific Islands children and only 2.1% of Asian New Zealand children.*
- *European New Zealand babies are, on average, given their first solids at approximately 5½ months of age. Maori babies are more likely to be given solids before 4 months of age.*

Sources: Australian Bureau of Statistics (2019); Australian Health Ministers' Advisory Council (2017); Australian Indigenous HealthInfoNet (2022); Australian Institute of Health and Welfare (2020); National Health and Medical Research Council (2019); New Zealand Ministry of Health (2022).

CHILDREN AND ADOLESCENTS

- Assessment of a child's quadriceps femoris for atrophy or hypertrophy is a good clinical indicator of the need to continue investigations for the presence of neuromuscular disease.
- Hormonal changes from transition through growth stages can influence a child's tissue. Tonsils can hypertrophy during childhood and atrophy after puberty; many other tissues hypertrophy as a result of puberty (e.g. secondary sex characteristics).

OLDER ADULTS

- As an individual ages, significant atrophy occurs in most major organs. These changes result in the increased need to observe for drug toxicities, hydration status, malnutrition and changes to strength and balance.
- Exercise can moderate age-related muscular atrophy to some degree.
- Hyperplasia of the prostate gland occurs as a direct result of ageing, and can negatively affect an older man's urological and sexual function.

KEY CLINICAL ISSUES

- Observations for muscle or limb atrophy and hypertrophy should be undertaken during the course of a physical examination.
- When collecting a health history, including questions about exposure to potential agents of cell injury (such as chemicals) can assist in determining contributing factors to the development of signs and symptoms.
- Gaining an understanding of an individual's nutrition behaviours and food choices can provide an insight into possible deficiencies or excesses.
- Infection control practices are important when caring for individuals with active infections. Understanding the concepts of the chain of infection can help to protect the healthcare professional and other individuals, to prevent the spread of infectious disease.

CHAPTER REVIEW

- *Pathophysiology* is defined as the study of the mechanisms by which disease and illness alter the functioning of the body. *Aetiology* is the study of the cause or causes of a disease. The *pathogenesis* represents the development of a disease. The *clinical manifestations* are the demonstrable changes representing the changes in function brought about by a disease process.
- *Epidemiology* is the study of the patterns of disease within populations. The *incidence* rate of a disease represents the number of new cases diagnosed within a particular period, usually over a calendar year. The *prevalence* rate of a disease is the total number of cases, both newly and previously diagnosed, at a particular time.
- *Cellular adaptations* to stimuli allow the cell to maintain homeostasis under new conditions. If the cell cannot adapt, then it may become injured—either reversibly or irreversibly.
- The types of cellular adaptation are atrophy, hyperplasia, hypertrophy, metaplasia and dysplasia.
- *Atrophy* is a decrease in cell size; *hypertrophy* is an increase in cell size; *hyperplasia* is an increase in cell number; and *metaplasia* is a transformation from one cell type to another. *Dysplasia* is a maladaptive response to a stimulus that results in a variation in cell size and shape. Dysplasia leads to a breakdown in the organisation and arrangement of the tissue.
- Two forms of *irreversible cell injury* result in cell death: necrosis and apoptosis.
- *Necrosis* is a form of premature pathologic cell death. In necrosis, the cell swells and characteristic changes occur in the nucleus, including degradation and shrinkage. The contents of the cell spill out into the extracellular space, which induces an inflammatory response.
- *Apoptosis* is a form of programmed cell death. A series of enzymic reactions leads to fragmentation of the nucleus and the cytoplasm into apoptotic bodies. These bodies are phagocytosed and do not induce an inflammatory response.
- The *major agents* of cell injury are chemical, physical, nutritional, ischaemic, hypoxic, infectious and immunological.
- *Reversible cell injury* is characterised by cell swelling and intracellular accumulations. If the stimulus ceases or compensatory mechanisms can be established, the cell may be able to recover.

REVIEW QUESTIONS

1. Define the following terms:
   a. epidemiology
   b. pathogenesis
   c. aetiology
2. Differentiate between the incidence and the prevalence of disease.
3. Define the following cellular adaptations, and provide an example of each:
   a. metaplasia
   b. hyperplasia
4. Explain why histological evidence of dysplasia within a tissue is considered a reason for concern.
5. Indicate which type of necrosis matches each of the following descriptions, and suggest an example.
   a. The affected tissue has a cheese-like appearance.
   b. The injury triggers immediate and widespread autolysis of cells.
   c. A large area of tissue is damaged in an ischaemic injury. The tissue turns black and smells foul.
6. Briefly explain why an inflammatory response is not triggered by apoptotic cell death.
7. Indicate whether each of the following mediators triggers or suppresses apoptosis:
   a. TNF receptors
   b. Bcl-2 proteins
   c. caspases
8. Provide an example of each of the following types of injurious agents:
   a. nutritional
   b. chemical
   c. infectious
   d. ischaemic
9. Briefly describe the process of hypoxic cell injury.
10. Outline the potential consequences of re-perfusing the heart with blood after an acute myocardial infarction.

HEALTH PROFESSIONAL CONNECTIONS: CELLULAR ADAPTATIONS

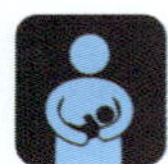

Midwives A neonate's heart is 'rate-dependent'. This means that blood pressure is directly related to heart rate. The younger an individual, the less hypertrophy has occurred, as the heart has not been beating for as long as an adult's. As a heart 'ages', the ability to contract with more force develops. An increase in contractility allows a decrease in heart rate. However, a neonate has not developed sufficient cardiac hypertrophy to permit the manipulation of contractility; therefore, cardiac output is maintained by rate alone. (Remember the equation: cardiac output = rate × stroke volume.) Increasing contractility increases stroke volume. If stroke volume cannot be increased, then rate is the only other factor.

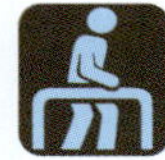
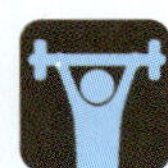

Physiotherapists/Exercise scientists Atrophy occurs with disuse. When working with individuals experiencing long-term disuse (from paralysis) or short-term disuse (from temporary immobilisation, e.g. splinting), atrophy can be expected. Research on paralysis-induced atrophy has indicated that clinical outcomes can be improved through the use of resistance-training equipment; for example, using a specially modified exercise bike, where the limbs of paralysed individuals are electronically stimulated to allow them to move the pedals. This type of functional electronic stimulation can slow the cellular adaption of atrophy, decrease osteoporosis and increase circulation in affected limbs.

Conversely, muscular hypertrophy as a result of the overload principle is the mechanism by which muscle bulk and strength are achieved. Intermittent resistance training using concentric and eccentric contractions with a progressive increase in either load or repetition is known to be one of the most successful methods of muscle development. This process is manipulating cellular adaptation. It is important that, when prescribing exercise for bulking or rehabilitation, the exercise health professional should have an understanding of protein synthesis and degradation.

Nutritionists/Dieticians Maintaining adequate nutrition is imperative to reduce cellular adaptation. Protein anabolism and catabolism are significantly influenced by diet. Insufficient nutrients within a diet will affect all organ systems. Gastrointestinal adaptation can also occur related to diet. Education and meal planning to ensure appropriate nutrition will enable the gastrointestinal system to adjust as necessary. Supplementation may be required to correct inadequacies in absorption. Knowledge of cellular adaption (especially gastrointestinal adaptation) is important for those responsible for assisting people with nutritional health.

CASE STUDY

Ms Sofia Cassidy is a 29-year-old woman (UR number 156784) who sustained a fracture-dislocation to her right ankle after falling down a two-metre ravine while on a bush walk in a national park with her partner. Sofia is healthy, athletic and, apart from her current situation, considers herself in good physical condition. Once the medical team arrived, she was stabilised, airlifted out of the national park and taken to the nearest metropolitan hospital. Following primary and secondary assessments, pain relief and X-rays, it was determined that, apart from some minor grazes that needed cleaning and dressing, her ankle fracture was the only injury that required further intervention. She was kept 'nil by mouth' in anticipation of the need for an open reduction internal fixation (ORIF).

Ms Cassidy had blood drawn for a full blood count, electrolytes and coagulation profile. Her pathology results have returned as follows:

HAEMATOLOGY

Patient location:	Ward 3	**UR:**	156784		
Consultant:	Smith	**NAME:**	Cassidy		
		Given name:	Sofia	**Sex:**	F
		DOB:	03/11/XX	**Age:**	29

Time collected	11:13
Date collected	XX/XX
Year	XXXX
Lab #	456563645

FULL BLOOD COUNT		UNITS	REFERENCE RANGE
Haemoglobin	122	g/L	115–160
White cell count	6.3	$\times 10^9$/L	4.0–11.0
Platelets	244	$\times 10^9$/L	140–400
Haematocrit	0.43		0.33–0.47
Red cell count	4.67	$\times 10^{12}$/L	3.80–5.20
Reticulocyte count	1.2	%	0.2–2.0
MCV	94	fL	80–100

Neutrophils	4.43	$\times 10^9$/L	2.00–8.00
Lymphocytes	1.1	$\times 10^9$/L	1.00–4.00
Monocytes	0.48	$\times 10^9$/L	0.10–1.00
Eosinophils	0.31	$\times 10^9$/L	< 0.60
Basophils	0.11	$\times 10^9$/L	< 0.20
ESR	2	mm/h	< 12
COAGULATION PROFILE			
aPTT	29	secs	24–40
PT	14	secs	11–17

BIOCHEMISTRY

Patient location:	Ward 3	**UR:**	156784		
Consultant:	Smith	**NAME:**	Cassidy		
		Given name:	Sofia	**Sex:**	F
		DOB:	03/11/XX	**Age:**	29

Time collected	11:13
Date collected	XX/XX
Year	XXXX
Lab #	456563646

ELECTROLYTES		UNITS	REFERENCE RANGE
Sodium	138	mmol/L	135–145
Potassium	4.1	mmol/L	3.5–5.2
Chloride	102	mmol/L	95–110
Bicarbonate	25	mmol/L	22–32
Glucose	5.9	mmol/L	3.5–5.4
Iron	15.6	μmol/L	11–30

Her neurovascular observations were acceptable, and once the orthopaedic team reviewed her X-rays she was given a 'procedural sedation' in the emergency department and underwent a closed reduction of her ankle fracture-dislocation. Her observations were as follows:

Temperature	Heart rate	Respiration rate	Blood pressure	SpO_2
36.9°C	92	18	142/84	96% (RA*)

*RA = room air.

A backslab splint was applied, and 12 hours post-procedure she was discharged into the care of her partner. A physiotherapist provided her with appropriate-sized crutches, and assessed Ms Cassidy's safety with mobilising and negotiating stairs. She was given analgesia, fracture care instructions and a fracture clinic appointment, and told to return to the emergency department or her local doctor if she had any concerns. Ms Cassidy is vegan, and she asked whether there were any dietary considerations that would influence the healing of her injury. The nurse discussed the importance of good nutrition and of selected macro- and micronutrients necessary for fracture repair.

Once the swelling in her ankle subsided, the plaster clinic applied a fibreglass cast, and her ankle remained immobilised for a further six weeks.

Finally, after X-rays, a consultation with the orthopaedic team, and waiting what seemed like an eternity, it was time for Ms Cassidy's cast to be removed. Once the technician removed her cast, she was able to see her lower leg again. She was surprised and a little embarrassed when she saw her very dry, scaly-skinned, hairy leg… but then she noticed the size of her gastrocnemius. She became a little teary, as she had prided herself on the size of her calf muscles. She always felt she had lovely, defined calves that any dedicated cyclist would envy. Now, her right calf seemed almost half the size of her left.

CRITICAL THINKING

1. Consider Ms Cassidy's physical condition prior to her accident and her dietary preferences. Discuss what and how these factors may influence her fracture healing.
2. Ms Cassidy was proud of the size of her gastrocnemius muscles prior to her accident. What do you think accounted for that physiological state?
3. Once Ms Cassidy's fracture has healed, the new bone tissue in the area surrounding the fracture will be larger than the normal continuity of the bone. By the end of the healing process the fracture zone will be continuous with the rest of the bone. What process has occurred to shape the bone?
4. When the cast was removed from Ms Cassidy's right leg, she noticed that her gastrocnemius was almost half the size of that of her left leg. Explain what has happened to her muscle at a cellular level. Why did this occur?
5. What interventions could have been implemented during Ms Cassidy's recovery to reduce the effects of immobilisation? What interventions are required now that this has occurred? Which healthcare professionals are best placed to assist Ms Cassidy with her current situation?

BIBLIOGRAPHY

Aguilar-Agon, K.W., Capel, A.J., Martin, N.R.W., Player, D.J. & Lewis, M.P. (2019). Mechanical loading stimulates hypertrophy in tissue-engineered skeletal muscle: molecular and phenotypic responses. *Journal of Cellular Physiology* 234:23547–58. https://doi.org/10.1002/jcp.28923.

Australian Bureau of Statistics (ABS) (2019). *Australian Aboriginal and Torres Strait Islander health survey, 2018–19*. Canberra: ABS. http://www.abs.gov.au.

Australian Health Ministers' Advisory Council's National and Aboriginal and Torres Strait Islander Health Standing Committee (2017). *Cultural respect framework 2016–2026: for Aboriginal and Torres Strait Islander health—a national approach to building a culturally respectful health system*. Canberra: Australian Government Department of Health. https://nacchocommunique.files.wordpress.com/2016/12/cultural_respect_framework_1december2016_1.pdf

Australian Indigenous Health*Info*Net (2022). *Overview of Aboriginal and Torres Strait Islander health status, 2021*. Perth, WA: Australian Indigenous Health*Info*Net. https://healthinfonet.ecu.edu.au/learn/health-facts/overview-aboriginal-torres-strait-islander-health-status.

Australian Institute of Health and Welfare (AIHW) (2020). *Aboriginal and Torres Strait Islander Health Performance Framework 2020 summary report*. Cat. No. IHPF 2. Canberra: AIHW. https://www.indigenoushpf.gov.au/publications/hpf-summary-2020.

Australian Institute of Health and Welfare (AIHW) (2021). *Australian Burden of Disease Study: impact and causes of illness and death in Australia 2018*. Cat. No. BOD 29. Canberra: AIHW. http://www.aihw.gov.au/reports/burden-of-disease/abds-impact-and-causes-of-illness-and-death-in-aus/summary.

Australian Institute of Health and Welfare (AIHW) (2022). *Australia's health 2022*. Australia's Health series No. 18. Cat. No. AUS 241. Canberra: AIHW. https://www.aihw.gov.au/reports-data/australias-health.

Best, O. & Fredericks, B. (2021). *Yatdjuligin: Aboriginal and Torres Strait Islander nursing and midwifery care* (3rd edn). Port Melbourne, VIC: Cambridge University Press.

Franchi, M.V., Reeves, N.D. & Narici, M.V. (2017). Skeletal muscle remodeling in response to eccentric vs. concentric loading: morphological, molecular, and metabolic adaptations. *Frontiers in Physiology* 8:447–62. http://doi.org/10.3389/fphys.2017.00447.

Jorgenson, K., Phillips, S. & Hornberger, T. (2020). Identifying the structural adaptations that drive the mechanical load-induced growth of skeletal muscle: a scoping review. *Cells* 9(7), 1658–89. https://doi.org/10.3390/cells9071658.

Marieb, E.N. & Hoehn, K. (2019). *Human anatomy and physiology* (11th edn). San Francisco, CA: Pearson Benjamin Cummings.

National Health and Medical Research Council (2019). *Eat for health—Australian dietary guidelines. Providing the scientific evidence for healthier Australian diets*. Canberra: National Health and Medical Research Council. https://www.eatforhealth.gov.au/guidelines.

New Zealand Ministry of Health (2021). *Annual update of key results 2020/2021: New Zealand health survey*. Wellington: Ministry of Health. https://www.health.govt.nz/publication/annual-update-key-results-2020-21-new-zealand-health-survey.

New Zealand Ministry of Health (2022). *Health and independence report 2020: the Director-General of Health's annual report on the state of public health*. Wellington: Ministry of Health. https://www.health.govt.nz/publication/health-and-independence-report-2020.

2 Determinants of health and illness

KEY TERMS

Alma Ata declaration
Burden of disease
Communicable diseases
Determinants of health
Healthcare gap
Infant mortality
Inverse care law
Life expectancy
Non-communicable diseases
Sociocultural factors
Socioeconomic factors

LEARNING OBJECTIVES

After completing this chapter, you should be able to:

1. Discuss the major factors contributing to health and illness.
2. Briefly explore disparities in worldwide disease burden and mortality.
3. Discuss the influence of the COVID-19 pandemic on global health.
4. Identify various biomedical and behavioural factors that influence a person's health.
5. Briefly describe how socioeconomic and sociocultural factors influence a person's health.
6. Discuss the environmental factors contributing to the health of a community and of an individual.
7. Briefly describe the challenges and gains associated with the healthcare gap experienced by Aboriginal and Torres Strait Islander peoples.

WHAT YOU SHOULD KNOW BEFORE YOU START THIS CHAPTER

Can you differentiate between mortality and morbidity?

Can you differentiate between incidence and prevalence?

Introduction

The World Health Organization (WHO) defines health as '*… a state of complete physical, mental and social well-being and not merely the absence of disease or infirmity*'. The WHO also believes that the attainment of maximal health is a fundamental human right. This chapter will focus on the multitude of aspects that can determine health status and the development of illness for an individual, community or population. This will be achieved in the process of exploring the **burden of disease**, which is the measure of how life is shortened by illness, injury, disability and premature death in a population. This chapter is not meant to be a deep exploration of the pathophysiological causes of all of the conditions mentioned, as this is done in the body of the text in the appropriate chapters; rather, its role is to highlight the complex and prolific influences of various factors that can affect health and illness, which may not otherwise be appreciated by a purely biomedical examination of the diseases and conditions explored in the text.

Determinants of health and illness

LEARNING OBJECTIVE 1

Discuss the major factors contributing to health and illness.

HEALTH AND ILLNESS

When planning illness prevention and disease management programs, organisations responsible for health promotion consider the **determinants of health**. These are factors that influence the likelihood of staying healthy or becoming ill. Although there are numerous factors that influence health, they may be distilled into three primary determinants:

1 *individual factors*—such as biomedical conditions or the behavioural choices made by the individual
2 *societal factors*—such as socioeconomic or sociocultural influences
3 *environmental factors*—which can contribute to the health and wellness of a person, community or population.

Figure 2.1 illustrates the complexity of various factors that can influence individual and population health. This diagram is by no means complete; however, it attempts to identify major contributors to health and illness. The diagram's construction also closely represents the structure and contents of the chapter.

In 1978, an international body co-sponsored by the WHO formulated a document called the **Alma Ata declaration**. Its fundamental goal was to achieve world health by the year 2000, and, although the goal was not achieved, the action marked the first steps towards identifying the need for world governments, local communities and healthcare workers to understand the importance of primary healthcare in the prevention of disease and the promotion of health and wellness.

While many diseases are preventable through the management of risk factors, the provision of basic nutrient and hygiene requirements or the use of vaccinations, other diseases are non-preventable, such as Parkinson's disease, type 1 diabetes or aortic aneurysm. *Preventable diseases* are often divided into communicable and non-communicable diseases. Although some **communicable diseases** will be discussed briefly in this chapter, see the chapter 'Infectious disease' for more in-depth discussion on various communicable or infectious diseases. **Non-communicable diseases** account for approximately 70% of all deaths, which equates to approximately 40 million people globally per year. Measurement of **life expectancy** and mortality rates can provide an insight into the health of a nation, and comparisons over time can measure the efficacy of programs or initiatives to improve the health of a population.

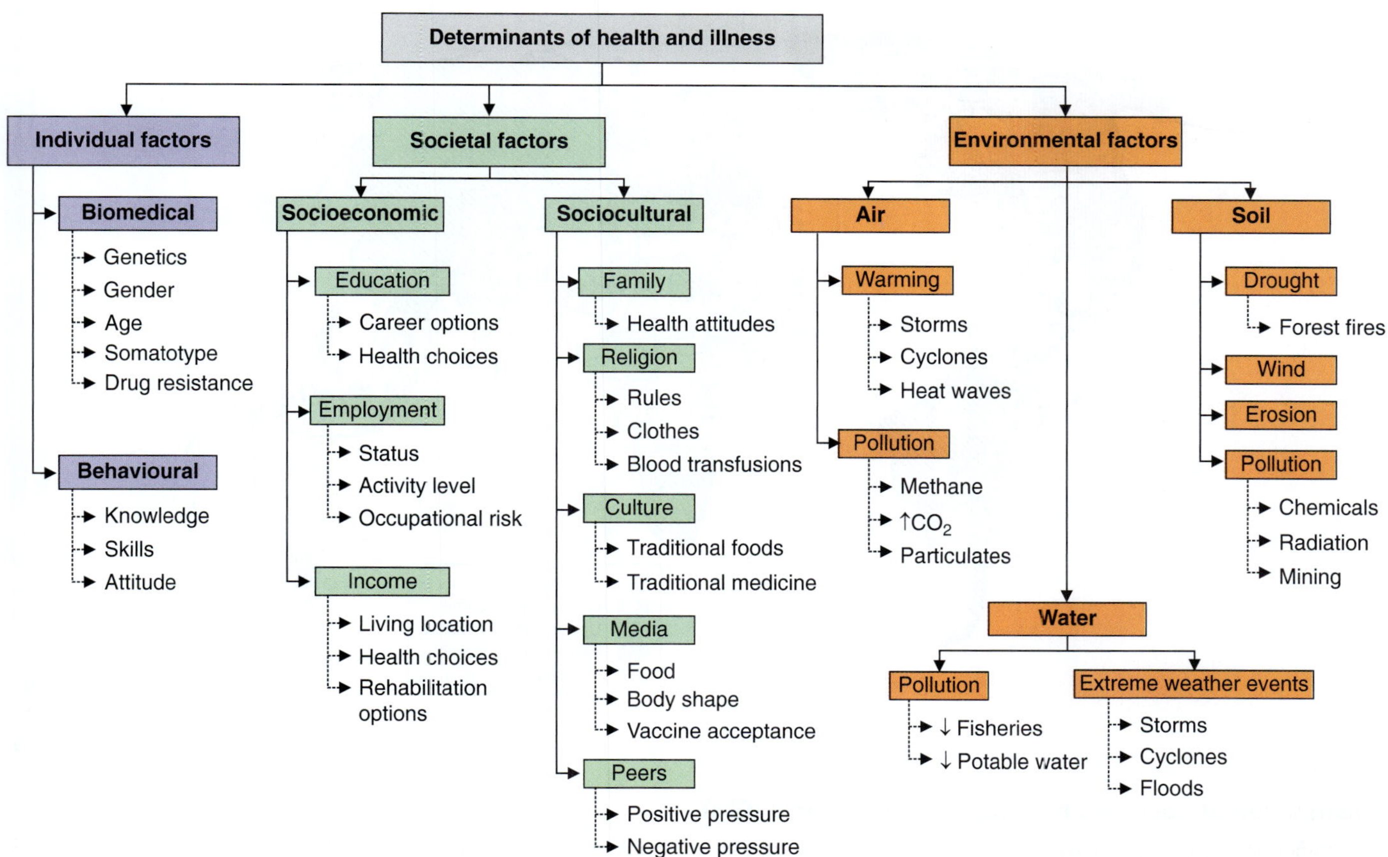

Figure 2.1

Determinants of health and illness

↓ = decrease; ↑ = increase; CO_2 = carbon dioxide.

Disease burden and mortality

LEARNING OBJECTIVE 2

Briefly explore disparities in worldwide disease burden and mortality.

A former Secretary-General of the United Nations, Kofi Annan, once said: 'The biggest enemy of health in the developing world is poverty.' It is estimated that more than 784 million people live on less than US$2 per day. The World Bank groups all countries by income, and has developed a classification based on gross national income (GNI) per capita, sorting each country into one of four GNI classifications: low, low-middle, upper-middle and high. Figure 2.2 illustrates countries' economies by GNI per capita for 2021. When reporting health statistics, many agencies now convey certain data by this metric. Although GNI per capita does not exactly encapsulate a country's level of development, it has been found to correlate well with important measures, such as quality of life, **infant mortality** and life expectancy.

The insight of Kofi Annan's words is readily demonstrated when contrasting the life expectancy and infant mortality rates to a country's income. The more impoverished countries with the lowest incomes experience significantly lower life expectancy and significantly higher infant mortality statistics compared to high-income countries (see Figures 2.3A and 2.3B). Unfortunately, these statistics support the existence of the **inverse care law**, which is the concept whereby those in the most need of medical care are the least likely to receive it.

Other distinguishing features between high-income and low-income economies are the *leading causes of death*. The WHO reports that low-income economies tend to experience more than 50% of their leading causes of death as communicable disease, nutritional deficiencies, and child and maternal health issues. However, high-income countries tend to experience non-communicable disease for almost all of their leading causes of death. Figure 2.4 represents a comparison of the top 10 leading causes of death between high-income economies and low-income economies.

LEARNING OBJECTIVE 3

Discuss the influence of the COVID-19 pandemic on global health.

In December 2019, a new coronavirus-related pneumonia emerged from Wuhan, the capital city of one of China's central provinces. By late January 2020, this new virus had been found in 18 countries, and by March the WHO identified the novel coronavirus (COVID-19) as a global pandemic. Figure 2.5 demonstrates the number of COVID-19 cases and deaths in a time series since the beginning of the outbreak. By mid-2022,

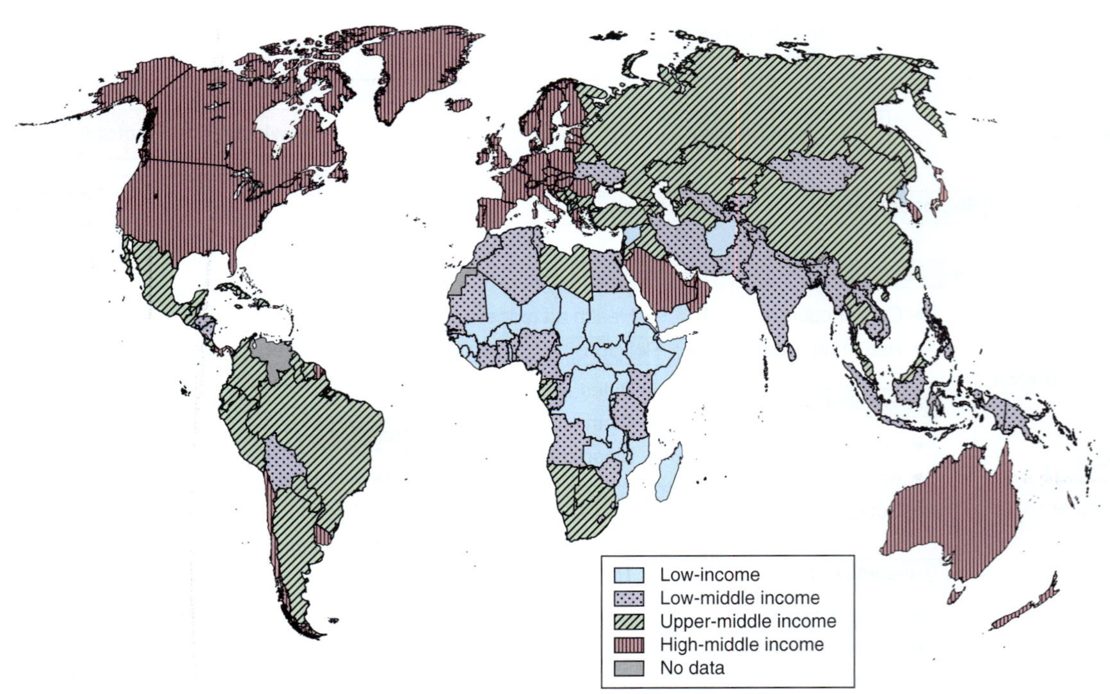

Figure 2.2

Distribution of countries by gross national income (GNI)

Classification according to World Bank estimates of gross national income per capita US$, 2021—Atlas method.

Source: Data adapted from The World Bank: World Bank Official Boundaries and World Development Indicators. Licenced under Creative Commons Attribution 4.0 International License https://creativecommons.org/licenses/by/4.0/.

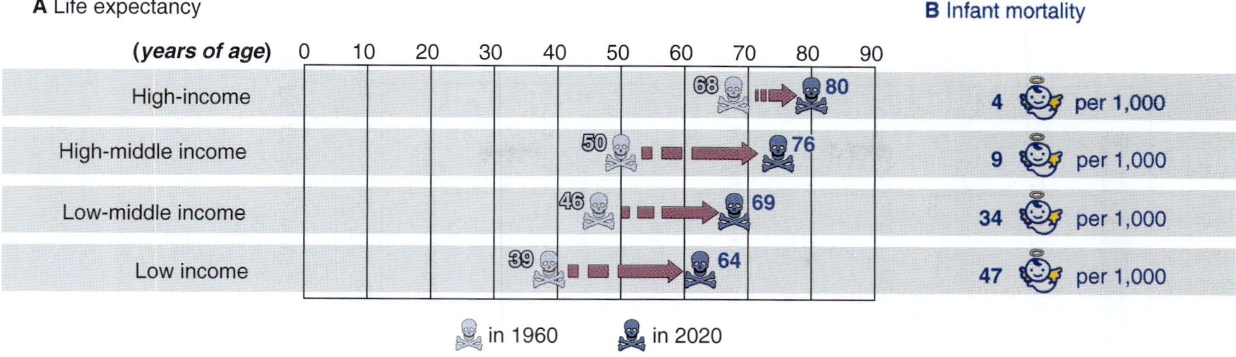

Figure 2.3

Life expectancy and infant mortality rate (per 1,000) by GNI economy

(A) Life expectancy data comparing countries' economies by gross national income per capita, 1960–2020.
(B) Infant mortality per 1,000 population comparing countries' economies by gross national income per capita, 2021.
GNI = gross national income.

Source: Data from The World Bank: UN Inter-agency Group for Child Mortality Estimation. Licenced under Creative Commons Attribution 4.0 International License https://creativecommons.org/licenses/by/4.0/.

there had been over 560 million cases and 6.4 million deaths. The new virus (later named SARS-CoV-2) causes an average case-fatality rate of 1.5% because the world population's immune systems are totally naïve to the pathogen. However, as expected, this value is influenced by age, health, somatotype (body shape), variant infection, and several other variables. Importantly, the fatality rate varied greatly across countries. For example, Peru's case-fatality ratio is 5.7% (with a mortality rate of 648 per 100,000); however, Australia and New Zealand's case-fatality rate is 0.1% with a mortality rate of 42 per 100,000 and 37 per 100,000, respectively.

It is important to note that data quality cannot be relied upon from all countries. Accuracy issues in the data are caused by factors such as: reporting lags; a country's capacity to count and maintain vital, accurate reporting systems; the potential impact of normal seasonal mortality changes; the motivation to purposefully misrepresent data; and the potential disparity of COVID-related mortality definitions between countries and regions. One primary difficulty faced by reporting authorities globally is the difficult distinction between a person dying *of* COVID-19 or dying *with* COVID-19 (i.e. did the person die as a direct result of the COVID-19 infection, or did another condition contribute primarily to the individual's death even though the person also happened to be COVID-positive). Notwithstanding all these factors, even the probably grossly under-reported 'official' worldwide statistics tell a story about the terrible impact and carnage that this infectious disease has had on global life, health and well-being.

Remarkably, unlike most of the common health challenges facing the world, loss of life from this pandemic across the various countries and regions was not distributed along the typical high-income versus low-income clusters. Many high-income countries (and regions within high-income countries) had phenomenally high mortality rates (see Figure 2.6). Collectively, sub-Saharan Africa reports a mortality rate of 7.2 per capita (although southern sub-Saharan Africa reports a rate of 71.6), yet the United States of America's rate is 121.5, Western Europe's rate is 94.7 and the United Kingdom reports a mortality rate of 130.1. Australia's reported rate is 4.0, and New Zealand's 0.5 per capita.

Notwithstanding data accuracy issues and potential underestimation, many low-income/lower-middle-income countries (LMICs) fared better in mortality rates than high-income countries despite poor infrastructure, technology and medical support. However, although there may have been potentially fewer lives lost during the pandemic when compared to high-income countries, declines in essential health services—including community nutrition support, antenatal care, vaccination, non-critical medical support, and disease surveillance—have been seriously affected. Disturbingly, this will ultimately translate to greater lives lost, as the declining population health related to pandemic disruptions undoes health gains from pre-pandemic years. Until LMICs can compensate for missed healthcare services and support opportunities, coupled with medical supply shortages, and financial resources redeployed to pandemic response, their populations are at risk of increased avoidable illness and death. The potential impacts are well represented in Figure 2.7, which identifies the various factors that will influence population health in the coming and post-pandemic years.

To reduce the mortality and morbidity from SARS-CoV-2 infections sweeping across their populations, public health officials began instituting control measures. Until effective, reliable vaccines and antiviral agents could be designed and manufactured in sufficient numbers to reduce the reproduction number (R_0) of the virus (the number of people that one infected

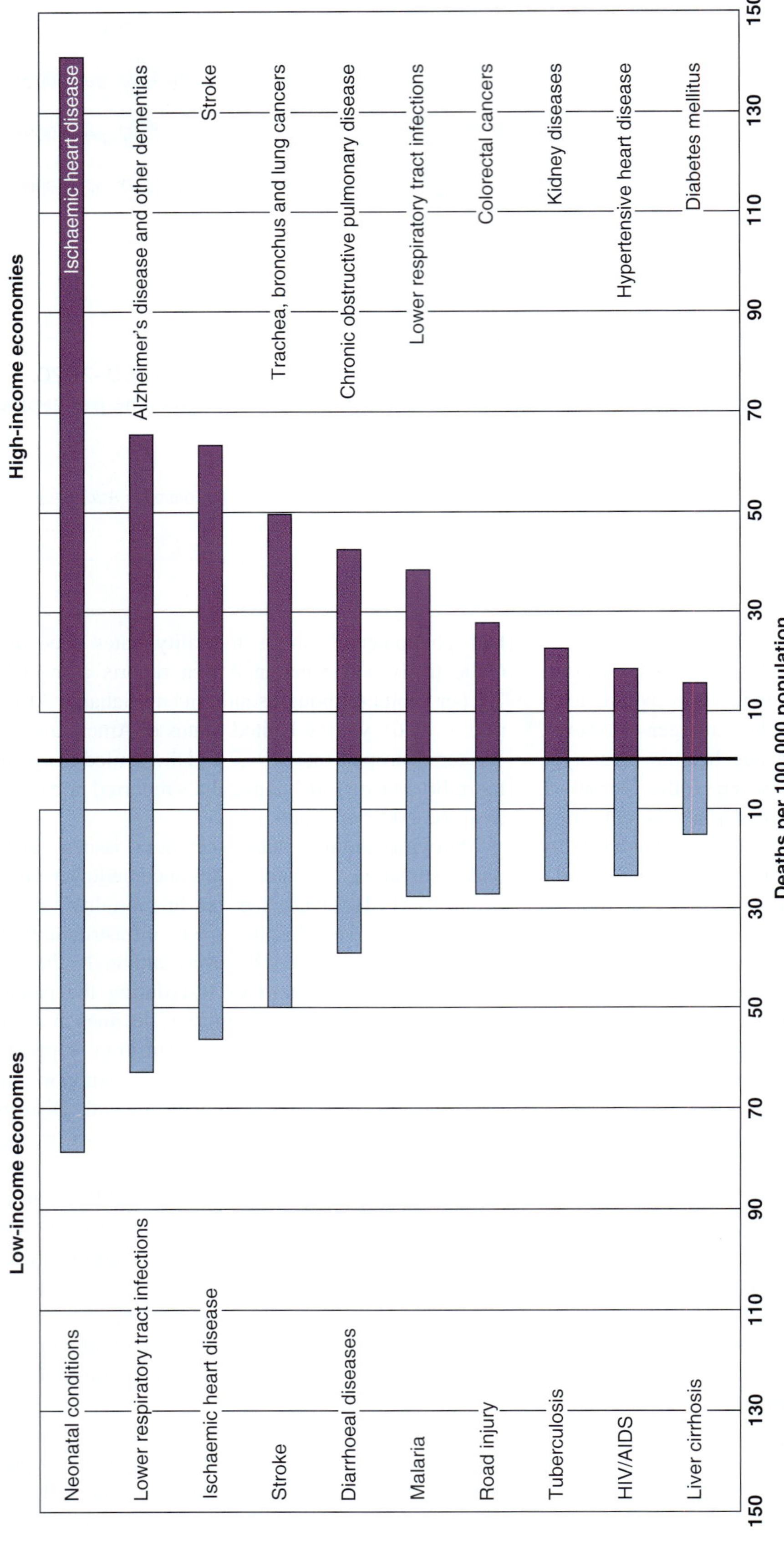

Figure 2.4

Leading causes of death in the lowest- and highest-income economies

The top 10 causes of death by economic income group for 2019.

AIDS = acquired immune deficiency syndrome; HIV = human immunodeficiency virus.

Source: Data from the World Health Organization (2020).

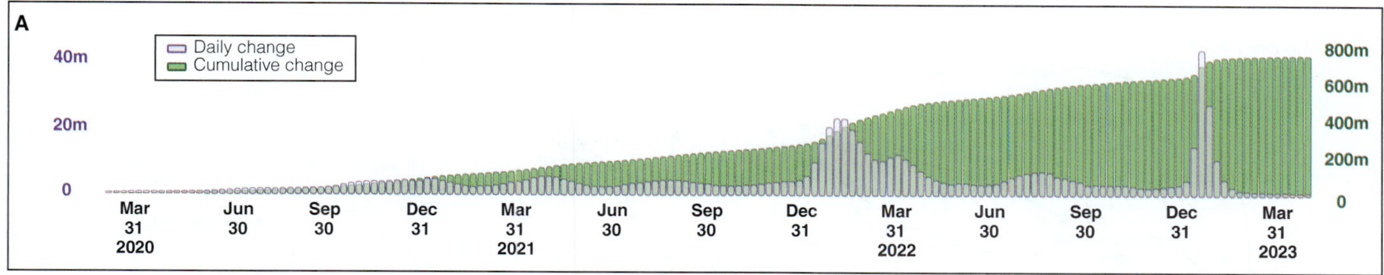

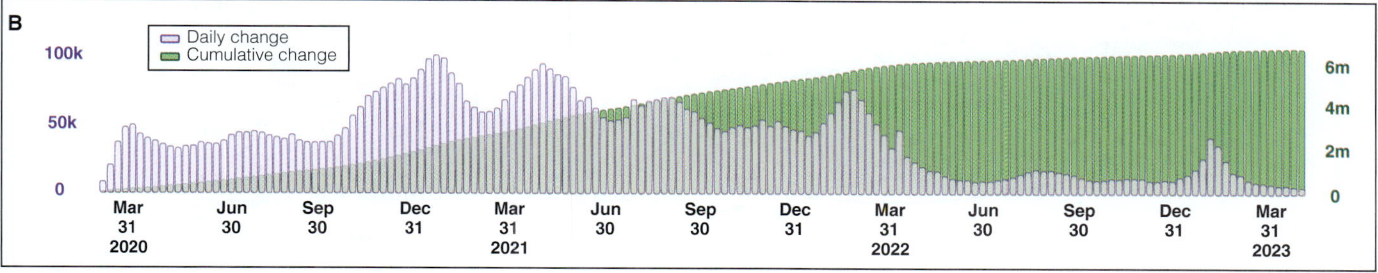

Figure 2.5

Time series of SARS-CoV-2 (COVID-19) representing global cases and deaths

(A) Global confirmed COVID-19 cases displayed as both a daily change (in pink) and also as a cumulative total (green) from March 2020 until April 2023.

(B) Global confirmed COVID-19 deaths displayed as both a daily change (in pink) and also as a cumulative total (green) from March 2020 until April 2023.

Source: Data from World Health Organization (2023). WHO Coronavirus (COVID-19) Dashboard. *https://covid19.who.int/.*

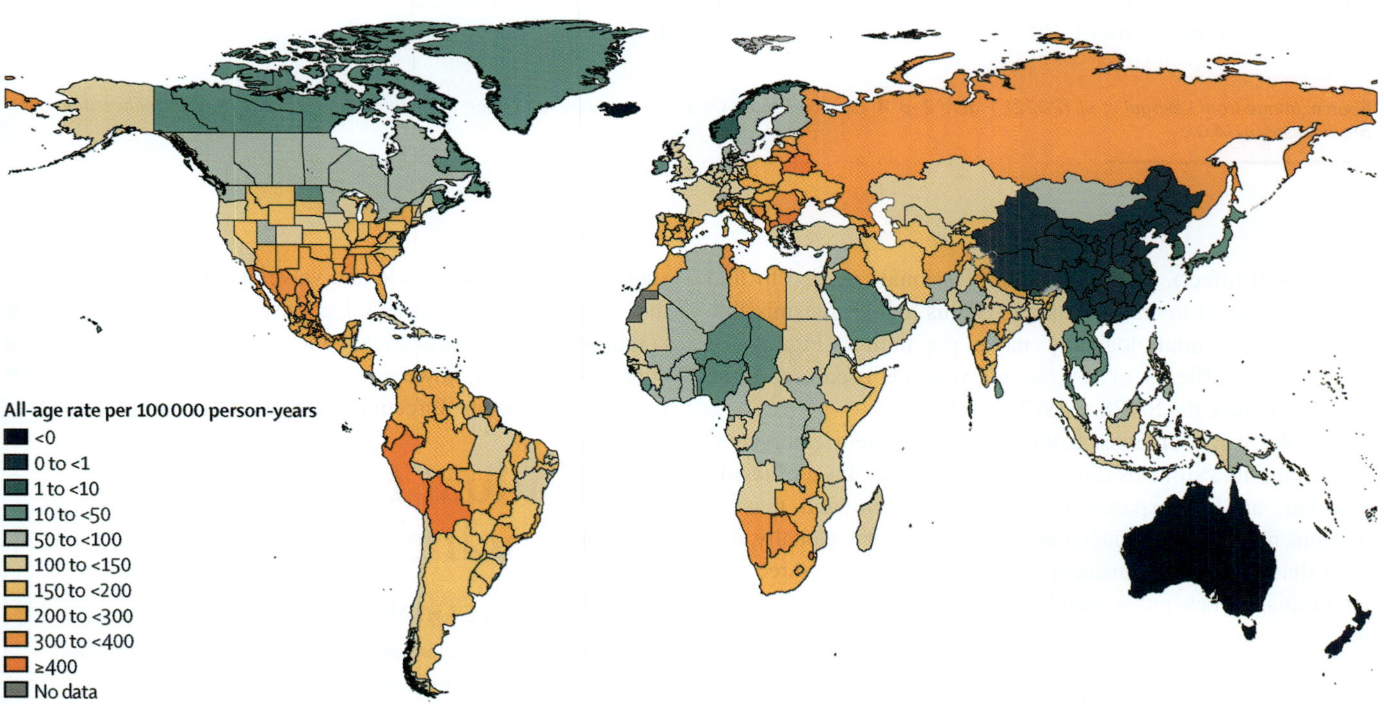

Figure 2.6

Global distribution of estimated excess mortality rate due to the COVID-19 pandemic for the cumulative period 2020–21

Source: Image from Wang et.al. (2022), Figure 2, p. 1517. Licenced under Creative Commons Attribution 4.0 International License https://creativecommons.org/licenses/by/4.0/.

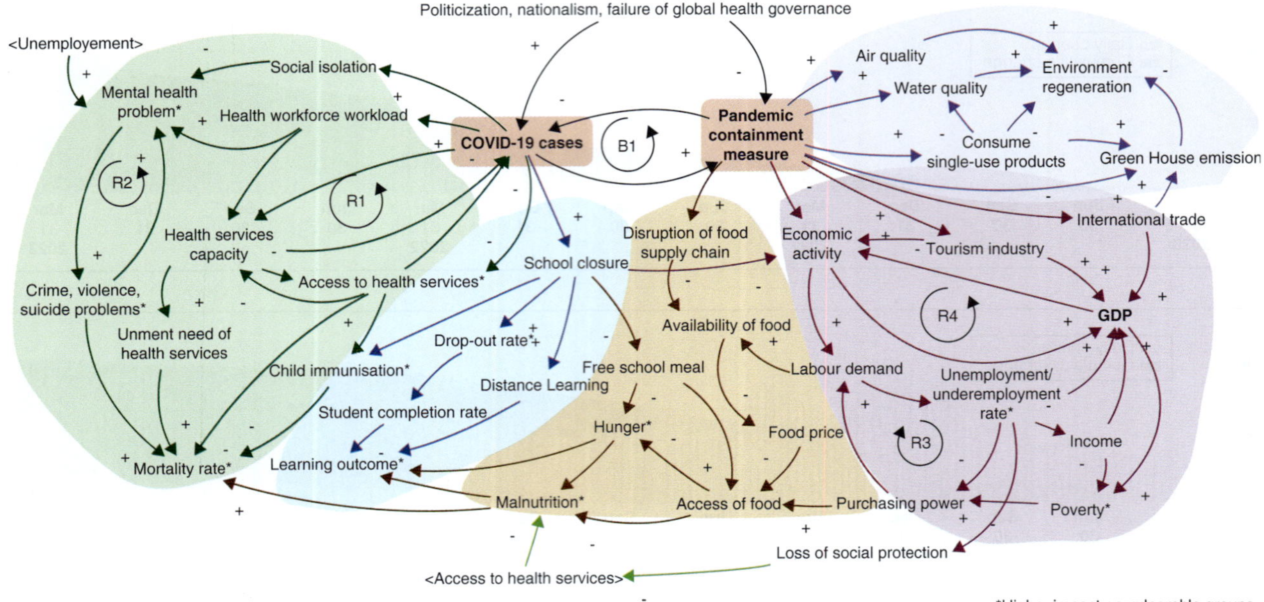

Figure 2.7

Multi-dimensional impacts of the COVID-19 pandemic on factors influencing population health

Although the actual 'health' section is in green, most factors displayed here, either independently or in concert with other factors, play a distinct role in influencing population health because of the disruption caused by the COVID-19 pandemic.

green = health; lilac = education; orange = food and nutrition; pink = economics and employment; royal blue = environment.

GDP = gross domestic product; R = feedback loops; R1 = diminished health care capacity due to surge; R2 = increased mental health issues; R3 = reduced labour demand resulting in increased unemployment; R4 = reduced economic activity diminishing labour demand.

Source: Image from Lekagul et al. (2022), Figure 2, p. 4. Licenced under Creative Commons Attribution 4.0 International License https://creativecommons.org/licenses/by/4.0/.

person will infect), public health professionals needed to find reliable methods to curb the spread of this highly transmissible virus in an immunologically naïve population. Figure 2.8 identifies the efficacy of several interventions used across the world to reduce the SARS-CoV-2 virus R_0.

As the world emerges from this public health emergency, with mortality estimates three times higher than those officially reported, an ever-expanding morbidity burden, and tens of millions more people plunged into extreme poverty globally, it is clear that it will take considerable time for the world to recover. Unfortunately, new public health burdens caused by SARS-CoV-2 infections continue to be unmasked. Chronic health issues affecting numerous organ systems continue to stretch the already fatigued healthcare workforce, and the devastated healthcare dollar. Large-scale mental health crises are developing, with an increase of more than 25% in anxiety and major depressive order statistics (see the chapter 'Mental health disorders'). More specific COVID-19 content can be found in various chapters where specific organs are affected (such as cardiovascular—the chapters 'Blood disorders', 'Vascular disorders and circulatory shock' and 'Cardiac muscle and valve disorders'; respiratory—the chapter 'Respiratory infections, cancers and vascular conditions'; and neurological—the chapter 'Brain and spinal cord dysfunction'); however, COVID-19 content can largely be found in the chapter 'Infectious disease'.

Individual factors influencing health

LEARNING OBJECTIVE 4

Identify various biomedical and behavioural factors that influence a person's health.

BIOMEDICAL

Factors such as genetics and sex may influence the health and wellness of an individual. It is sometimes difficult to separate these two concepts. It is also important to understand the distinction between gender and sex. Sex refers to the biological

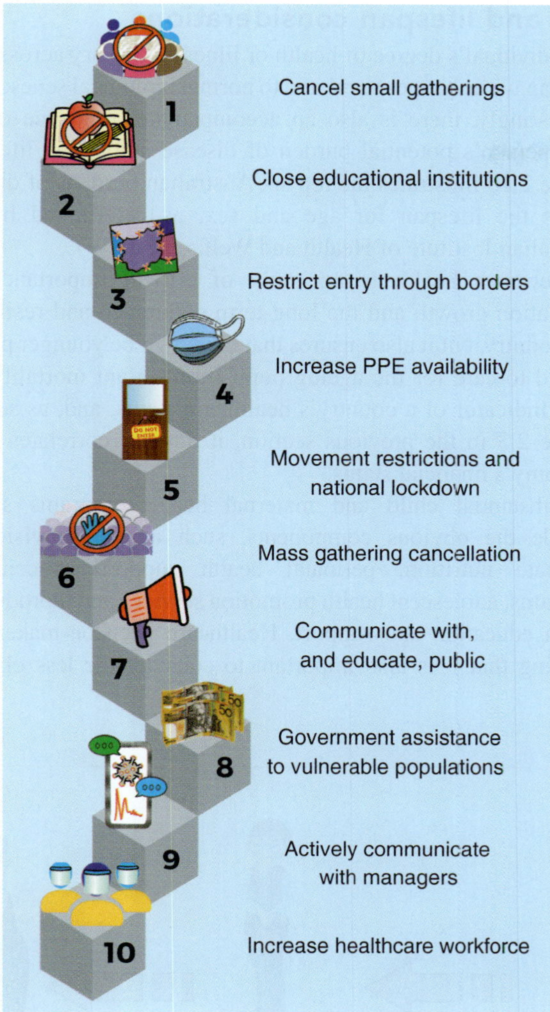

Figure 2.8

Top 10 interventions to reduce the SARS-CoV-2 R_0

These results were determined to be the most effective worldwide interventions as a result of a large research project by Haug and colleagues. It is important to note that this analysis took place in 2020, when there was no vaccination program available at that stage of the pandemic.
PPE = personal protective equipment.

Source: Data from Haug et al. (2020), Figure 1, p. 1304.

characteristics determined by chromosomes and genitalia, and is primarily associated with physical and physiological features; whereas gender refers to how the person identifies, often related to the socially constructed characteristics relating to concepts of femininity and masculinity, along a spectrum, or outside of that spectrum, or even self-identified.

Genetics

A person's sex is determined by their genetics and the presence or absence of a Y chromosome. The substitution of the Y chromosome instead of a second X chromosome in males may contribute to the likelihood of expressing an X-linked inheritable condition, such as haemophilia. However, elements of a person's sex may have nothing do with the sex chromosomes, and everything to do with the health opportunities provided, withheld or forced upon a person based on sex alone. This may be expressed through inequalities in nutrition, education or access to healthcare opportunities for girls, through to extreme sex bias procedures, including female genital mutilation, and selective abortion or female infanticide practised in some regions of the world.

As previously discussed, a person's chromosomal makeup may influence the expression of an inheritable condition (see the chapter 'Genetic disorders'). Genetic polymorphisms (chromosomal variations in a certain population that cannot be maintained by only recurrent mutation) have long been identified as explaining the varied metabolism of many drug-metabolising enzymes. This means that individuals may experience different values from the same therapeutic drug. Early research also suggests that these variances may contribute to certain individuals' increased propensity to develop liver disease. This genetic tendency is seen in myriad other health conditions, such as in atopy (an individual's tendency to be hyper-allergic). Atopy is commonly expressed as asthma, anaphylaxis and autoimmune disease. Figure 2.9 illustrates the sex chromosomes, showing a distinct difference in size and, therefore, potential genetic information related to sex.

Sex

Irrespective of genetics, sex still plays a considerable role in the determinants of health. Sex may influence access to healthcare, or even the conditions experienced. In the most simplistic terms, males develop conditions affecting sexual health structures and male genitalia, such as the testicles and the prostate, and females develop conditions affecting sexual health structures and female anatomy, such as breasts, the uterus and the ovaries. Nonetheless, sex may play an even more significant role in a person's health and wellness when considering access to healthcare, religious

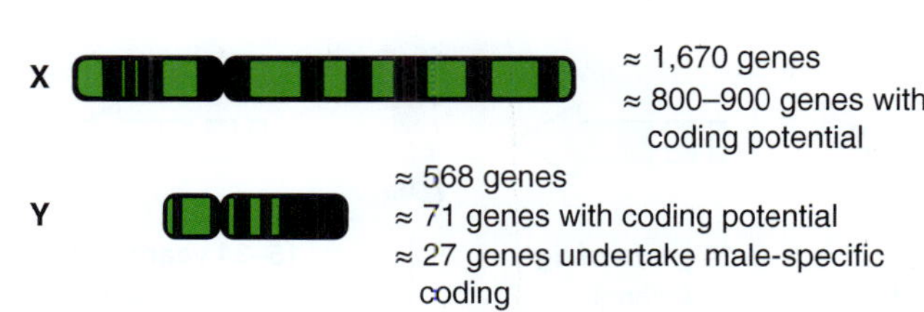

Figure 2.9

Sex chromosomes

The X chromosome is significantly longer and contains far more genes than the Y chromosome. Although modern medicine does not appreciate the entire implication of this, it is thought that this size differential may account for the significant variance in immunity, response to vaccinations and autoimmunity experienced by women compared to men.

or cultural practices performed on sex-specific anatomy, and governmental policy or regulation withholding, directing or dictating access or intervention.

Male and female circumcision have vastly different outcomes; however, some cultures and religions may hold strong beliefs about this practice. Attempts to legislate against access to reproductive health resources, such as fertility prevention measures or pregnancy termination interventions, may deprive a woman of the right to decide what happens with her own body. Poor maternal health programs and support also result in increased infant and maternal mortality. Therefore, the failure to provide and maintain resources to assist pregnant women will also result in poorer health outcomes for infants. Conversely, money well spent in supporting good maternal health will result in significant, long-term savings to an economy's finite health budget.

In some regions of the world, girls are excluded from the nutrients and resources necessary to facilitate conditions and opportunities to maximise their health potential. Also, for some individuals, gender identity and sexual orientation may influence the person's ability to access suitable healthcare for their needs.

Age and lifespan considerations

An individual's degree of health or illness may vary across their lifespan with changes unrelated to normal biological senescence. Interestingly, there is also an accompanying influence of sex on a person's potential burden of disease across the lifespan. Figure 2.10 illustrates the top six Australian burdens of disease across the lifespan for age and sex, as determined by the Australian Institute of Health and Welfare (AIHW).

Newborn health is not only of critical importance for population growth and the long-term endurance and resilience of a country, but it also ensures that there will be younger people around to care for the ageing population. Infant mortality is a good indicator of a country's healthcare status, and, as seen in Figure 2.3 in the previous section, it directly correlates to an economy's financial status.

Substantial child and maternal health programs should include the obvious components, such as the provision of adequate nutrition, perinatal health supports, vaccination programs, adolescent health promotion services and reproductive health education and support. Healthcare decision-makers are realising that it is also important to consider the less obvious

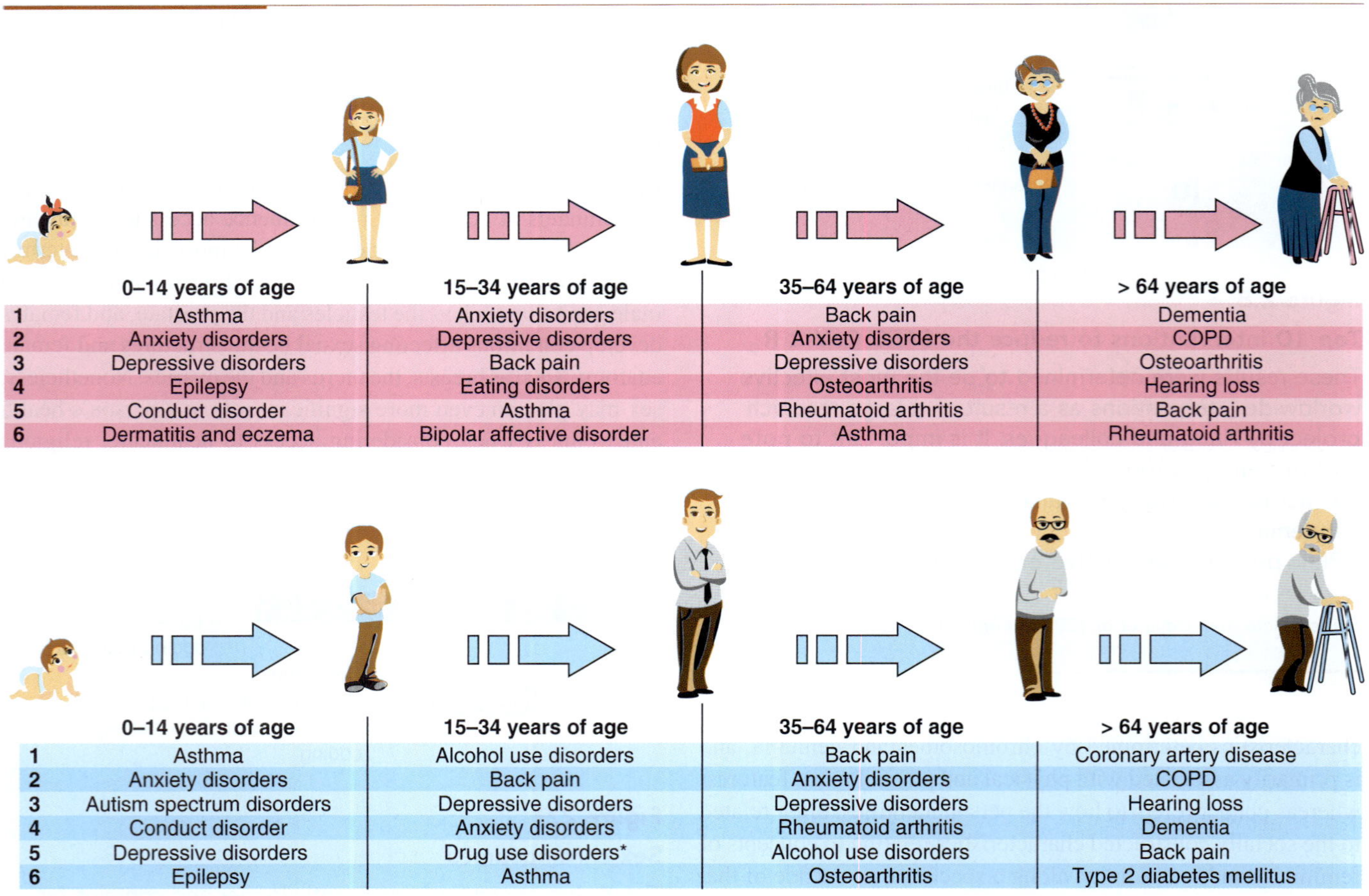

	0–14 years of age	15–34 years of age	35–64 years of age	> 64 years of age
1	Asthma	Anxiety disorders	Back pain	Dementia
2	Anxiety disorders	Depressive disorders	Anxiety disorders	COPD
3	Depressive disorders	Back pain	Depressive disorders	Osteoarthritis
4	Epilepsy	Eating disorders	Osteoarthritis	Hearing loss
5	Conduct disorder	Asthma	Rheumatoid arthritis	Back pain
6	Dermatitis and eczema	Bipolar affective disorder	Asthma	Rheumatoid arthritis

	0–14 years of age	15–34 years of age	35–64 years of age	> 64 years of age
1	Asthma	Alcohol use disorders	Back pain	Coronary artery disease
2	Anxiety disorders	Back pain	Anxiety disorders	COPD
3	Autism spectrum disorders	Depressive disorders	Depressive disorders	Hearing loss
4	Conduct disorder	Anxiety disorders	Rheumatoid arthritis	Dementia
5	Depressive disorders	Drug use disorders*	Alcohol use disorders	Back pain
6	Epilepsy	Asthma	Osteoarthritis	Type 2 diabetes mellitus

Figure 2.10

Top six burdens of disease in Australia across the lifespan, comparing sex

* = excluding EtOH; COPD = chronic obstructive pulmonary disease; EtOH = ethanol (ethyl alcohol)

Source: Data from AIHW (2021b).

requirements, such as intra-family violence prevention education and resources, and even healthcare worker education programs to ensure sufficient numbers of appropriately educated individuals.

As the world ages, and health improves and life expectancy extends, many upper-middle- and high-income economies face an ever-increasing obesity epidemic associated, with significantly diminishing population health resulting from myriad obesity-related disease processes. Therefore, with increased life expectancy not associated with sufficiently wise individual health choices, the health care budget is more burdened from chronically ill people living longer. Consequently, resource provision is taxed, and decisions about the best use of the healthcare dollar results in equity dilemmas when determining 'who' must miss out on 'what'.

As a person ages, changes associated with senescent body systems can affect every organ system, and may exacerbate disease or even influence the selection or effects of pharmacological interventions chosen for the individual (see Figure 2.11).

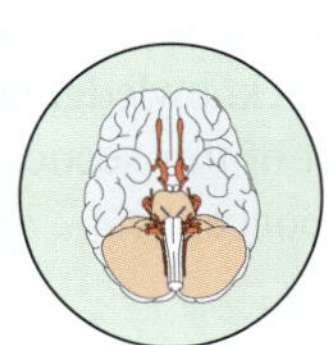

Nervous system

CNS - Brain mass ↓ ≈ 30% by 8th decade
↓ NT production & uptake (5-HT & DA)
PNS - ↓ in conduction velocity & transduction
Denervation & muscle atrophy
ANS - ↓ PSNS tone → ↑ SNS tone → ↑ SVR
↓ β-adrenergic response
↓ baroreceptor sensitivity

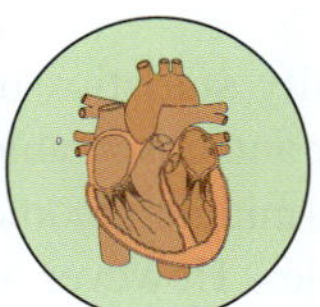

Cardiovascular system

↑ Vascular smooth muscle tone
↓ Vascular compliance yet ↓ elastin & collagen
↓ Response time to Δ in intravascular volume
↑ SVR & ↑ Afterload → ↑ SBP
↑ Left ventricular hypertrophy

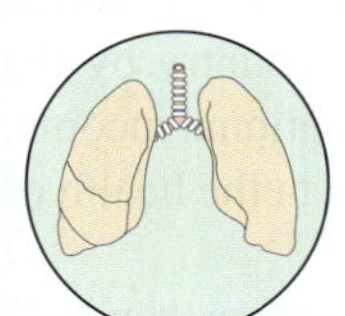

Respiratory system

↓ Thoracic compliance & ↑ kyphosis
Atrophy of respiratory muscles
↓ Tidal volume and vital capacity
↓ Cough strength & ↓ mucocilliary escalator
↓ β-adrenergic response → bronchoconstriction
↓ Alveolar surface area

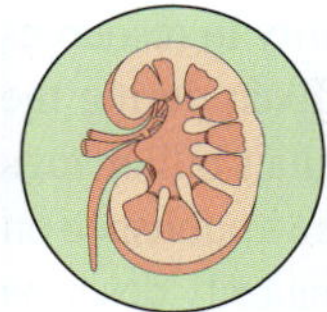

Renal system

Renal mass (cortical) ↓ ≈ 25% by 9th decade
Renal blood flow ↓ ≈ 10% per decade > 30 yo
↓ Filtration surface area → ↓ GFR
↓ Adaptation to ischaemia → ↑ risk for AKI

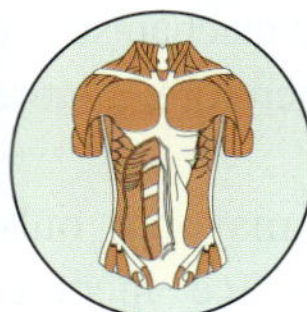

Musculoskeletal system

Muscle - Muscle mass ↓ ≈ 30% by 8th decade
Bone - Gender-specific loss by 8th decade
♀ - Cortical ↓ ≈ 35%; trabecular ↓ ≈ 50%
♂ - Cortical ↓ ≈ 21%; trabecular ↓ ≈ 30%
Joint - ↓ Flexibility & stability

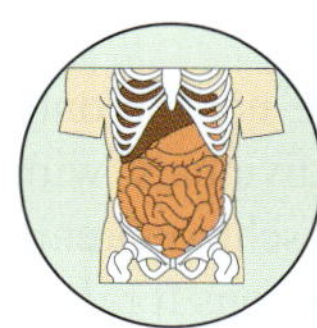

Gastrointestinal system

↓ Acinar cells & ? ↓ saliva → xerostomia
Oropharynx Δ → tooth loss & ill-fitting dentures
↓ Olfactory coordination → dysphagia
↓ Gastric wall elasticity → ↓ gastric volume
↓ Gastric mucosa & HCO_3^- → ↑ mucosal injury
↓ HCl acid secretion → slight ↑ gastric pH
↓ Absorptive surface area of small intestine
↓ Lactase → ↑ lactose intolerance
Microbiota Δ → ↓ Ca^{2+}, Fe^{2+} & Vit. B9 absorption
Liver mass & blood flow ↓ ≈ 40% by 8th decade
↓ Anorectal sphincter Fx → ↑ incontinence risk

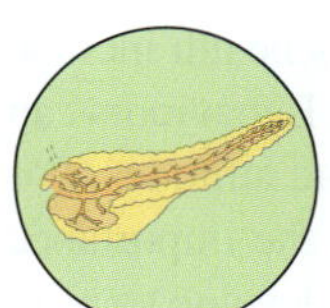

Endocrine system

↓ Target organ response from hormones
↓ Testosterone, oestrogen, GH & IGF-1
Cumulative results
↓ Protein synthesis
↓ Lean body mass & ↓ bone mass
Fatigue, depression & ↓ libido
↑ Fat mass
↑ Insulin resistance

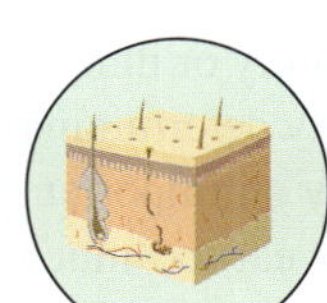

Other systems

Immune system
Innate - ↓ Macrophage Fx & antigen presenting
↓ Complement system Fx
↓ NT production & uptake (5-HT & DA)
↓ TNF, IL-1, & NO
Acquired - Thymic mass ↓ ≈90% by 6th decade
↓ Helper T-cell & B-cell Fx
↑ Antibodies → ↑ Autoimmunity risk
Skin - ↓ Epithelial turnover → ↓ barrier Fx
↓ Vascularity → Atrophy & ↓ repair
↓ Vit. D synthesis
↓ Dermal immune Fx → ↑ infection risk

Figure 2.11

Selected biological effects of ageing that may exacerbate disease conditions and reduce effectiveness of pharmacological interventions

≈ = approximately; ↑ = decreased; ↓ = increased; Δ = change; ♂ = female; ♀ = male; 5 - HT = serotonin; AKI = acute kidney injury; ANS = autonomic nervous system; β = beta; Ca^{2+} = calcium ion; CNS = central nervous system; DA = dopamine; Fe^{2+} = iron ion; Fx = function; GFR = glomerular filtration rate; GH = growth hormone; HCl = hydrochloric acid; HCO_3^- = bicarbonate ion; IGF-1 = insulin-like growth factor; IL-1 = interleukin-1; NO = nitric oxide; NT = neurotransmitter; pH = potential of hydrogen (acidity); PNS = peripheral nervous system; PSNS = parasympathetic nervous system; SBP = systolic blood pressure; SNS = sympathetic nervous system; SVR = systemic vascular resistance; TNF = tumour necrosis factor; vit. = vitamin; yo = years of age.

Drug resistance

A serious and developing global threat is the emergence of drug-resistant infections. Several infections that may have been managed easily a few decades ago are becoming increasingly difficult to treat, as the drug-resistant microorganisms responsible are developing and sharing mechanisms to defeat these drugs' effectiveness. Some individuals infected with multidrug-resistant organisms must rely entirely on their immune responses to fight the infection. However, the people who are most at risk of developing such infections are often those most immunocompromised, and possess minimal capacity to triumph over virulent, drug-resistant pathogens. Individuals with chronic disease and the youngest and oldest community members are most at risk. Healthcare professionals are also at greater risk, as they work in environments teeming with microbial exposure. Compounding this challenge are drug companies who display little interest in developing new antimicrobial substances.

It should also be understood that bacteria are not the only factor presenting drug-resistant challenges. Individuals with HIV, epilepsy or mental health conditions, such as schizophrenia and depression, can possess pharmacogenomic reasons for drug resistance, such as variations in drug transporters or the enzymes necessary for conjugation or other drug-metabolising processes (see the chapter 'Infectious diseases').

BEHAVIOURAL

Other individual factors contributing to a person's health include those that can be considered behavioural in nature. Behaviours can be particularly influenced by knowledge, skills and attitudes. For example, if people possess knowledge regarding the importance of good nutrition and adequate exercise, they may develop steps to incorporate these into their lifestyles. If a person possesses skills that enable them to manage stress, keeps themself and their family safe with accident prevention and first-aid knowledge, knows how to parent appropriately, and understands the basic measures to reduce their exposure to violence, they may be less likely to experience physical, emotional or psychological injury or illness.

However, knowledge and skills are not the only determining factors in relation to behaviour. Attitude can play an important part. For example, people may know that if they eat too much and don't exercise enough, they will become obese. Many individuals know that if they smoke cigarettes they are more likely to develop emphysema or any number of cancers; however, they still choose to undertake this risky behaviour. Although it is known that education level and financial status inversely correlate with levels of chronic disease and poor health choices, at least in Australia, many informed and affluent people still make poor health choices, evidenced by 67% of the population being overweight or obese in Australia in 2017–18.

Other attitudes that diminish the capacity to develop maximal well-being are decisions to reject important primary health initiatives, such as vaccination or screening measures for common, preventable diseases. In many preventable conditions, early diagnosis can result in reduced morbidity and mortality. Individuals may have a distrust of Western medicine and drugs, or unfounded beliefs in the putative dangers associated with vaccination. These people rely on herd immunity to keep them safe from vaccine-preventable diseases. However, as the numbers of unvaccinated people in a population increase, herd immunity will not keep them safe from diseases with high penetration.

Sociocultural and socioeconomic determinants of health

LEARNING OBJECTIVE 5

Briefly describe how socioeconomic and sociocultural factors influence a person's health.

Some **socioeconomic factors** contributing to a person's health status include their level of education, the type of employment they find and their level of income. **Sociocultural factors** may include family, religion, culture, the media or peers. As many of these factors interrelate, it is often hard to discuss one without acknowledging the influence of another. As a result, the construct of this section will be more fluid, with less delineation between concepts.

SOCIOECONOMIC

Employment

As can be seen by the morbidity and mortality statistics in Figure 2.3 earlier in the chapter, there is a clear and observable difference in the health of individuals in high-middle-income economies and those in lower-income economies. However, it would be interesting to explore whether there is a similar effect occurring within the same country. For example, even though Australia has been identified as a high-income country by the WHO and the World Bank with respect to gross national income, are there still marked and observable differences in the health of individuals within that same affluent country?

Given that in Australia the wealthiest 1% holds more than 14% of all wealth and have 50 times more wealth than the bottom 60%, it would be reasonable to conclude that such disparity in resources must also afford at least some health advantage. Even during the COVID-19 pandemic, the average wealth of Australia's billionaires increased 12% in a year. In numerous literature reviews published on various countries and regions, the overwhelming majority describe a positive correlation with health and wealth. Yet the mechanism by which this fact exists is not necessarily as clear. Therefore, a more focused analysis of possible influences is required.

The type of occupation a person chooses may not only determine their societal status, but also influence income, opportunity and risk. Although Australia's worker fatality rates have dropped by 50% since 2007, in 2020, 194 workers still died while doing their job. In 2020, 34.5% of all workplace fatalities involved machinery operators and drivers, and the two most common types of serious work injuries and fatalities come from the agriculture, forestry and fishing industry, and the transport, postal and warehousing industry. Conversely, the financial and insurance industry and the information, media and telecommunications industry are the safest. Labourers claimed the greatest number of serious injuries (24% of claims), with sales workers (4%), managers (5%) and clerical and administrative workers (4%) being least at risk. Musculoskeletal trauma, such as sprains and strains and muscle injuries, accounted for 56% of all occupational injuries. Lacerations and amputations accounted for 16%, and fractures for 11%. Fortunately, burns and nervous system/head injuries only represented 2% each. Other health effects that should be considered include the development of more long-term issues, such as osteoarthritis from repetitive strain for factory workers, or obesity risk and insulin resistance from individuals employed in sedentary occupations.

Education

Education level may influence health choices through access to health education campaigns or knowledge of primary health services and the resources available. In some countries, disparity in healthcare access can be directly associated with education. If insurance must be provided through employment or be paid for directly out of pocket, rather the being paid for by governmental funds raised through taxes, those who are the least educated are more likely to be uninsured, as they may be less likely to be employed, and even more unlikely to have sufficient funds to maintain adequate health insurance payments. In countries with universal healthcare, these disparities are less obvious.

Income

In countries without universal healthcare, income will most likely be a significant limiting factor for access to appropriate healthcare. Greater wealth may permit earlier intervention or greater choice of doctor and access to allied health services, such as physiotherapy, speech pathology or occupational therapy. Peripheral beneficial effects may also include easier access to transport (personal vehicle compared to public transportation) and more capacity to take time off work. With increasing wealth, the standard of living increases, and access to basic health needs, such as functioning sanitation and food security, is met. Although there are individual circumstances, overall, as income trends away from lower brackets, exposure to physical and environmental risks also reduces.

SOCIOCULTURAL

Family

The health attitudes of a family may have a significant influence on an individual, although it may be difficult to differentiate between this and the role genetics has played. For example, if the offspring of two obese parents are also obese, how much of the influence was genetics, and how much of the influence was food volume and selection or attitudes to healthy lifestyle choices? Nutrition is a pivotal factor in health and wellness, and a significant influence on a child's eating habits, which are formed in early life. When introducing a child to foods, providing a range of nutritious foods and limiting exposure to junk foods is only a small component of the task. Parents who understand the importance of promoting a healthy relationship with foods through not using it as a means of punishment, conveying simple messages about 'all-the-time foods' and 'sometimes foods', and involving children in the meal preparation, planning and the tasting process may begin to assist their child to embrace an open and interested relationship with classically unpopular foods.

However, few of these points are important when the capacity to provide any food is compromised by poverty, and access to even the most basic nutrients is limited. Although many people rightly reflect on the challenges of poverty and malnutrition faced by those in low-income countries, it is also important to acknowledge that there are individuals and families in every country who experience issues of food security, such as inadequate or inappropriate supply. In Australia, there are individuals and families who, because of circumstance, are unable to access nutritious food. The child living in a family that is unable to provide sufficient nutrition for growth or building immunological resilience due to unemployment, geographical isolation, mental health issues or knowledge deficits may experience life-long challenges because of their early experiences.

Nonetheless, nutrition is not the only family influence on a person's health. Family, domestic or sexual violence experiences may harm a person physically or emotionally in the acute phase, and also long-term. Enduring a family life of persistent disadvantage makes succeeding and rising from the potentially cyclical trap very difficult. As discussed in the chapter 'Stress and its role in disease', prolonged stress contributes to and exacerbates immune and neuroendocrine dysregulation and myriad health conditions.

The global COVID-19 pandemic has worsened the burden for people in poverty. In Australia in 2020, unemployment rates effectively rose from 5.1% to 17% during the lockdowns. However, because of the initial robust government support, income inequality actually declined and official poverty statistics reduced by half because of Coronavirus Supplements designed particularly to support low-income households. Unfortunately, in 2021, with the staged withdrawal of pandemic support payments, financial hardship increased, and is now in excess of pre-pandemic levels. Twenty-five per cent more people are living in poverty when compared to 2019 pre-pandemic levels. It is not clear how long medium- and low-income Australians will take to recover from the financial assaults experienced during this time, but it is already clear that this COVID-19 pandemic experience will have more than just far-reaching public health and financial implications on Australia and its people.

Religion

The effect of religion on health may manifest as regulation, preventing a person from consuming alcohol, or influencing when and what they eat. For example, certain religions may restrict food types or may require a follower to fast or feast for a period of time. Some religions may determine the clothing that the follower wears. If a religion requires a follower to cover themselves so they have limited exposure to sunlight, vitamin D metabolism will be affected. Some religions may prevent a follower from receiving all of the healthcare options available to them. For example, if a person with anaemia or suffering a severe haemorrhage following surgery belongs to a religious group that prohibits the administration of a blood transfusion, a positive outcome may be compromised. It is important for healthcare professionals to learn, understand and honour a person's religious wishes without judgment. However, religious beliefs should not prevent the healthcare professional from finding acceptable alternatives that may help the individual honour their religion while improving their morbidity or mortality risks.

Culture

Much like religion, culture may influence a person's health through food choice, reliance on traditional medicines, or embracing concepts such as holsim or tribal healing. For many cultures, food plays a central role in almost every aspect of society, from welcoming gestures and building relationships, to feasting and fasting. The composition of a culture's diet is also known to strongly influence or prevent disease. The effects of following a Western diet that is high in fat will have drastically different outcomes to following a Mediterranean or a Japanese diet. Reliance on traditional healing practices may be beneficial for proven interventions, or may be detrimental for people in the community if the belief contributes to ill health itself, or if it impedes a person's willingness to seek assistance from Western medicine.

Media and peers

Positive and negative health influences can be derived from the media and peer pressure. More recently, consumers of social media are less inclined to rely on critically reviewed and factually prepared reports, and instead rely more on random thoughts espoused by unknown individuals through anonymous social networks. As this trend increases, it becomes less likely that all of the health information a person is exposed to will be accurate, evidence-based, or even from an appropriately qualified person. Unfortunately, there is much erroneous or outright misinformation available to naïve and young individuals on social media networks, and following advice from some false 'experts' may ultimately cause negative effects to a person's health and well-being. To some extent we have observed this phenomenon during the COVID-19 pandemic.

Conversely, peer pressure and the use of social media can also have positive influences, such as inspiring and motivating perceptions away from risk-taking behaviours and towards constructive beliefs about exercise, lifestyle choices, sexual health, the dangers of illicit drugs, or even the need to heed natural disaster and storm warnings. Social media networks possess a remarkable capacity to permit movement away from or towards a belief. Some healthcare professionals and primary care organisations are already beginning to harness this power to drive positive health influences. For example, during the COVID-19 pandemic social media was harnessed to great effect to spread messages, regarding vaccination and infection minimisation measures, to communities that do not tend to engage with mainstream media and medical institutions.

Environmental determinants of health

LEARNING OBJECTIVE 6

Discuss the environmental factors contributing to the health of a community and of an individual.

The WHO reports that environmental conditions contribute to 13.7 million deaths per year (24.3% of all deaths). Major environmental influences on health can be categorised into three distinct factors: challenges originating from the air, water or soil. The primary focus here will be on common factors that have far-reaching, grand-scale influences over multiple populations and constitute a sustained risk. While it is acknowledged that large-scale, catastrophic, man-made events, such as wars and conflicts, radiation accidents, or terrorist activities involving large numbers of casualties, or natural disasters, such as earthquakes, tsunamis or volcanic eruptions, can have a major influence on the health and welfare of those involved, these are outside the purview of this resource.

AIR POLLUTION

As populations increase and more fossil fuel is burnt, air pollution rises from energy-generation processes, transportation and industrial emissions. Other sources of ambient pollution (outdoor air pollution) can be from forest fires, waste incineration and agriculture. Pollution may consist of high levels of carbon dioxide (CO_2), methane, ground-level ozone (O_3—a key ingredient of smog), volatile organic compounds (VOCs—e.g. fuels, cleaning products and industrial chemicals), nitrogen oxide gases (from motor vehicles and the residential, industrial and commercial burning of fuels) or even black carbon particles. In 2022, the WHO identified that 99% of the world's population is living in conditions that do not meet WHO air-quality guidelines. Figure 2.12 shows two examples of air pollution, one from industry and the other from forest fires.

It has been demonstrated that, even at very low concentrations, small particulate matter (PM) pollution can have an observable influence on a person's health. Unfortunately,

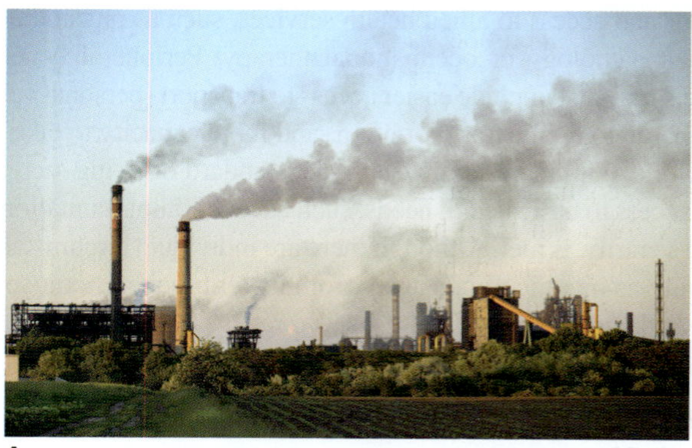

A

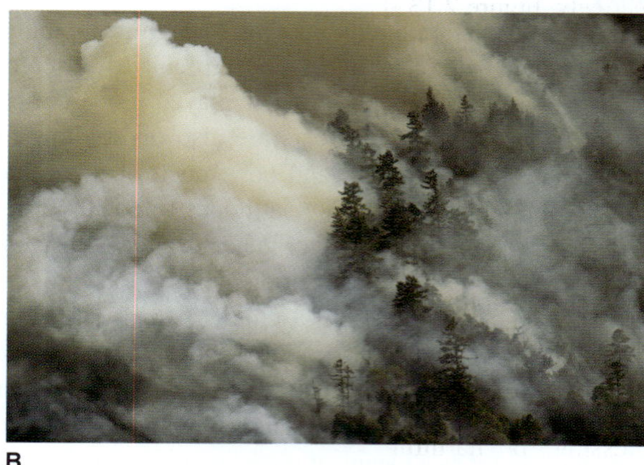

B

Figure 2.12

Air pollution from various sources

(A) A factory emitting pollution high in sulfur dioxide and particulate matter prior to the installation of emission-control equipment. (B) Particulates released into the air from forest fires can exacerbate symptoms for individuals with respiratory conditions for kilometres around the source.

Sources: (A) SvedOliver/Shutterstock. (B) N. F. Photography/Shutterstock.

Table 2.1 The World Health Organization's ambient air-quality targets

Particle size	Particle volume target 24-hour mean (max)	Particle volume target Annual mean
Small particles (≤ 2.5 microns in diameter—$PM_{2.5}$)	15 μg/m³	5 μg/m³
Large particles (≤ 10 microns in diameter—PM_{10})	45 μg/m³	15 μg/m³

m³ = cubic metres; PM = particulate matter; μg = micrograms.

Source: World Health Organization (2022c).

it is impossible to eliminate particulate pollution entirely. Therefore, targets for the lowest achievable concentrations have been established (see Table 2.1).

According to the WHO's Ambient Air Quality 2022 database, between the locations where air quality is being measured in particulate matter (PM), Australia's average annual PM_{10} is 16.8 μg/m³ (5.3–35.3 μg/m³), and average annual $PM_{2.5}$ is 7.5 μg/m³ (2.1–17.2 μg/m³). Compare these figures with the countries that have the highest average PM_{10} in the world: Basra (in Iraq) had a measure of 365 μg/m³, Jharia (in India) was second highest (322 μg/m³). However, during the lockdowns for the COVID-19 pandemic, air quality actually improved as people around the world were not permitted to move about, thus reducing particulate matter created by travel. The lowest average PM_{10} and $PM_{2.5}$ in the world is Todalen, a town in Norway, with measures of 2.9 μg/m³ and 1.9 μg/m³, respectively. Figure 2.13 shows how, even when the problem of pollution seems overwhelming, measures to reduce emissions can have dramatic effects over time.

WATER POLLUTION

Gastrointestinal tract (GIT) illness, the consumption of heavy metals, and chemicals are major factors in the health effects of water pollution. Major sources of water pollution include chemicals from industry, mining and farming, sewage, and other biological hazards such as toxic algae. When humans and animals consume water contaminated with heavy metals or chemicals, accumulation can result in poisoning, serious immune system suppression, or harmful reproductive effects. Exposure to inadequately treated water or water contaminated with sewage can cause water-borne infectious disease, such as gastroenteritis, cholera, skin infections and renal disease. Viral, bacterial and vector-borne parasitic infections are also common consequences of water pollution. Toxic algae blooms can contaminate water, affecting almost every body system, including the skin and the GIT, respiratory and nervous systems. Unfortunately, even the water treatment process used to manage these toxic algae blooms can harm health. Dangerous by-products produced when the water treatment chemicals react with the algae are linked to cancers and reproductive and developmental risks.

A

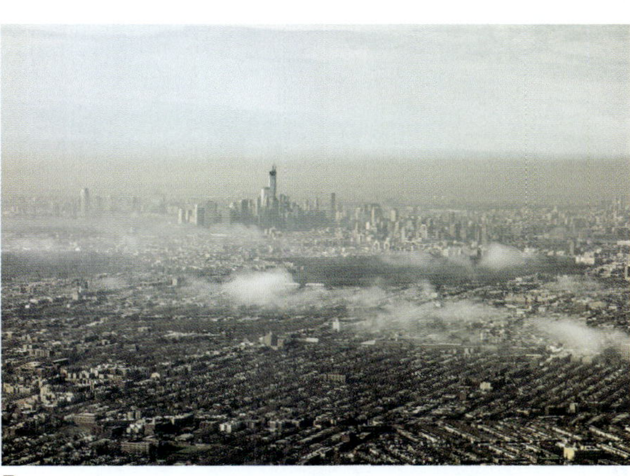

B

Figure 2.13

Active measures to reduce pollution can improve air quality

(A) New York City, 1973. (B) New York City, 2013.

Source: US Environmental Protection Agency.

A basic primary health requirement is the provision of adequately treated water suitable for human consumption. Figure 2.14 demonstrates the importance of dealing with various types of water pollution, as the effects on the environment may not only harm children now, but also in years to come.

SOIL POLLUTION

As with water pollution, soil may be contaminated with toxic heavy metals and chemicals. Such contamination can disrupt the soil–plant–human continuum normally important for flora, fauna and human health. Good-quality, unpolluted soil is essential for food security and the preservation of safe agriculture, and for inhabited and uninhabited land alike. The identification, remediation and management of soil pollution are critical to the health and wellness of individuals, communities and nations. Figure 2.15 demonstrates why soil pollution needs to be considered a population health priority.

Finally, an important component of the environment's influence on health comes directly from climate change. Figure 2.16 summarises the processes and interactions occurring as a result of increased population, the consumption of fossil fuel, and the industrial and mining contamination

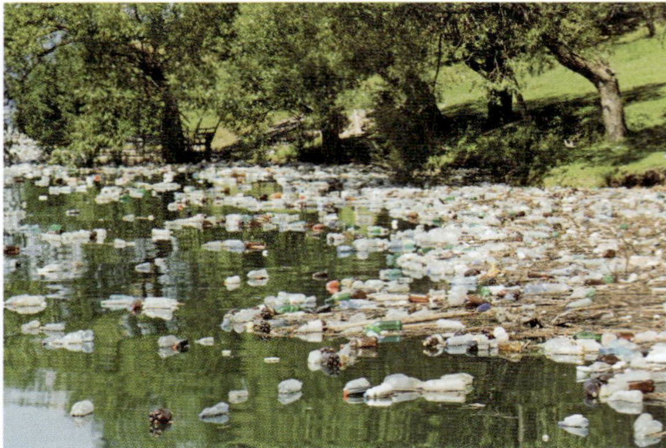

A

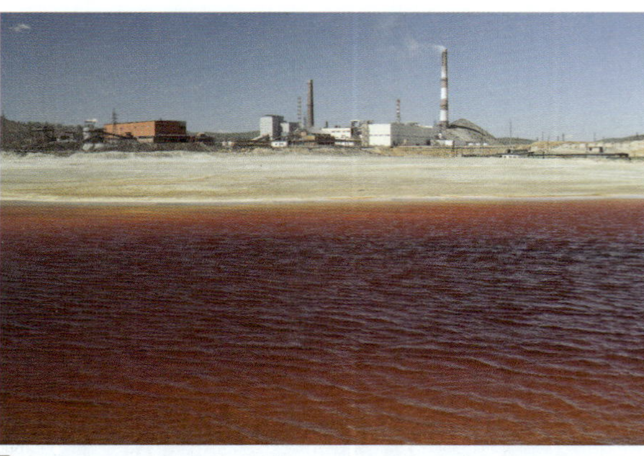

B

Figure 2.14

Water pollution

(A) River heavily contaminated with plastic pollution.
(B) The red water of a lake contaminated with copper-smelting waste.

Sources: (A) Stephane Bidouze/Shutterstock. (B) Salienko Evgenii/ Shutterstock.

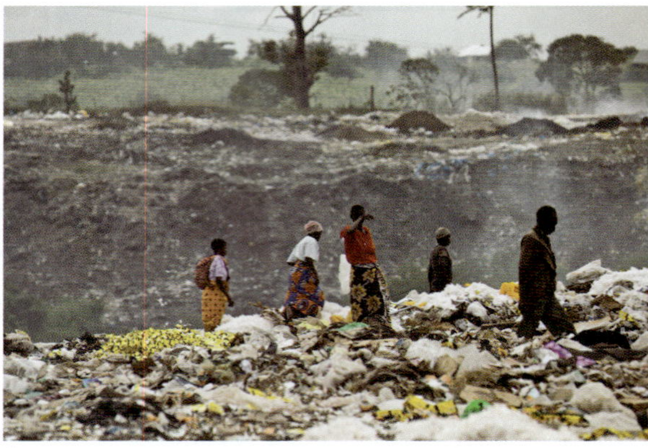

A

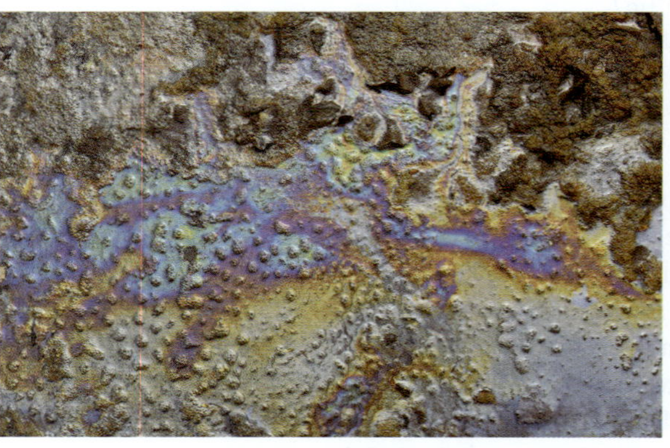

B

Figure 2.15

Soil pollution

(A) People scavenging on a mountainous rubbish tip.
(B) Soil pollution from an oil spill.

Sources: (A) Andrew Aitchison/Alamy Stock Photo. (B) Valery Orlov/ Shutterstock.

of the world's natural resources. These factors contribute to myriad negative health effects, such as infections, respiratory conditions and injury.

The Australian Indigenous context

LEARNING OBJECTIVE 7

Briefly describe the challenges and gains associated with the healthcare gap experienced by Aboriginal and Torres Strait Islander peoples.

Aboriginal and Torres Strait Islander peoples are the Indigenous peoples of Australia. They are made up of distinct cultural groups, each with their own languages, laws, customs and communities. An immense diversity results in more than 250 language groups encompassing the land. Aboriginal and Torres Strait Islander peoples may describe themselves as being from the regions from which they have come, by the language that they speak, or by the ecological characteristics of their People's land (e.g. 'Saltwater Peoples' or 'Desert Peoples'). Figure 2.17 identifies selected information regarding the distribution of Aboriginal and Torres Strait Islander peoples across Australia.

The AIHW suggests that 34% of the health disparity between Aboriginal and Torres Strait Islander peoples and non-Indigenous peoples—known as the **healthcare gap**—can be explained by social determinants.

In July 2020, the Coalition of Aboriginal and Torres Strait Islander Peak Organisations and all Australian governments agreed upon major reform to incorporate four priority reform targets: *P*artnership in decision making; *I*ncrease in government funding; *R*eduction in racism; and *P*rojects to assist Aboriginal and Torres Strait Islander communities to make decisions. Table 2.2 lists a further 17 socioeconomic outcomes on which the strategies will be developed or modified to achieve improvement that realise gains and close the gap.

After a slow start in relation to early attempts made to close the gap from approximately 2008, Australia has made some

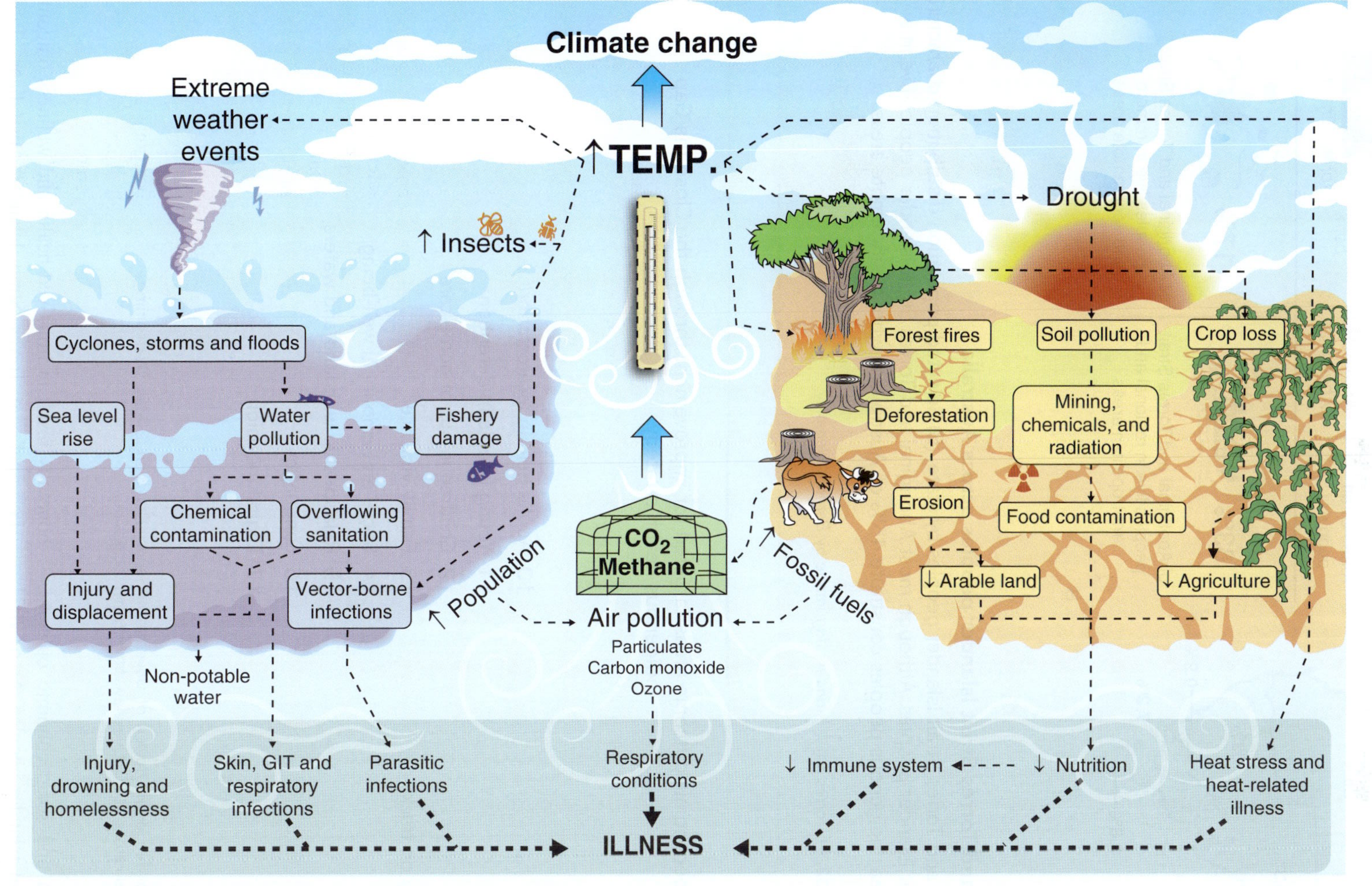

Figure 2.16

Environmental factors influencing health

Three major influences of the environment on health are those that affect water, air and soil, each with their own unique and critical contribution to the development of ill health.

↓ = decreased; ↑ = increased; CO_2 = carbon dioxide; GIT = gastrointestinal tract.

Source: Fisher & Hales © Sciencopia.

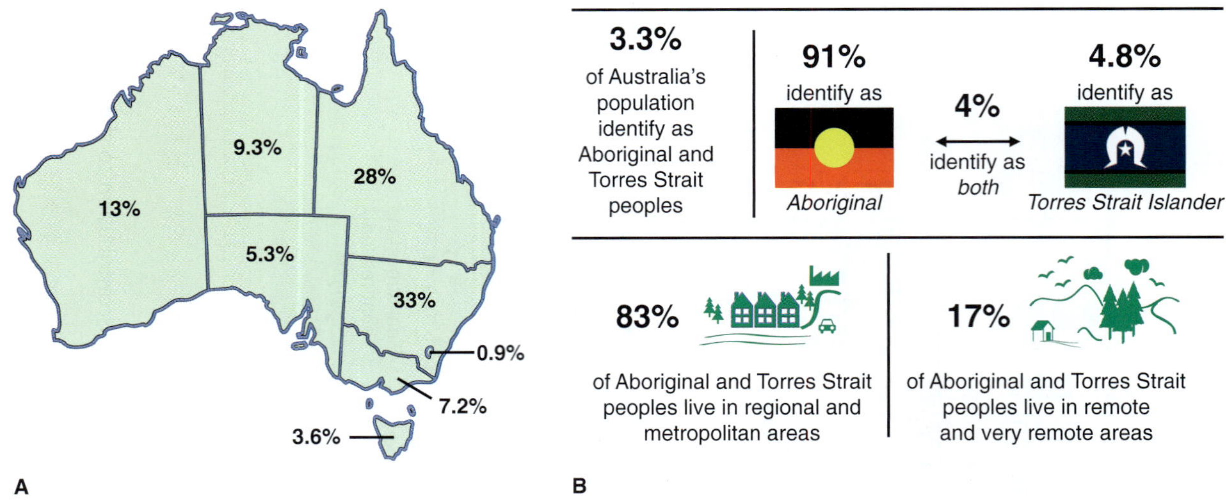

Figure 2.17

Distribution of Aboriginal and Torres Strait Islander peoples across Australia

(A) Distribution of Aboriginal and Torres Strait Islander peoples by state. (B) Selected population distribution characteristics of Aboriginal and Torres Strait Islander peoples. Although most Aboriginal and Torres Strait Islander peoples live in a metropolitan or a regional area, Indigenous peoples constitute 45% of Australians who live in remote areas.

Sources: Data from AIHW (2020, 2022e); Torres Strait Islanders flag image by Bernard Namok.

Table 2.2 Socioeconomic outcome areas targeted for improvement through the Close the Gap Indigenous health strategy

Target areas	
1 Life expectancy	10 Adults held in incarceration
2 Healthy birth weight	11 Young people in detention
3 Preschool program	12 Children in out-of-home care
4 Children developmentally on track	13 Family violence
5 Year 12 or equivalent	14 Social and emotional well-being
6 Tertiary qualification	15 Relationship with land and waters
7 Youth engagement	16 Languages
8 Employed	17 Digital inclusion
9 Appropriate housing	

Source: Data from Steering Committee for the Review of Government Service Provision (2020). Overcoming Indigenous Disadvantage. Key Indicators 2020: Overview. *https://www.pc.gov.au/.*

headway in improving health and socioeconomic outcomes for Aboriginal and Torres Strait Islander peoples. As of 2021, four targets are on track—improving birth weights, preschool enrolments, reduction of youth detention rates, and addressing interests in land mass rights and interests.

Although many targets across various activities have not yet been met, there have been some meaningful gains that will hopefully result in improved health and wellness outcomes for Aboriginal and Torres Strait Islander Australians. Table 2.3 identifies some gains achieved through education programs, improved finances, and changes in how targeted money is being spent.

In relation to the remaining Close the Gap targets, there has been no significant change in child and infant mortality rates

Table 2.3 Current outcomes of the Close the Gap initiative

Targeted activity	Current outcome
Mental health (suicide)	↑ 40% since 2008
Circulatory disease	↓ 18% since 2010
Kidney disease deaths	↓ 36% since 2010
Respiratory disease deaths	No significant change since 2010
Obesity	↑ 5% since 2012
Smoking rates	↓ 11% since 2001
Binge drinking	No significant change since 2012
Child mortality	No significant change since 2010

Percentage differences are represented from different time periods, depending on the targeted activity.

Sources: Data from National Indigenous Australian Agency (2020); Steering Committee for the Review of Government Service Provision (2020).

since 2010; however, non-Indigenous mortality rates have declined in the period, meaning the gap has actually widened by 58%. And while significant improvements in literacy and numeracy have occurred since 2008, one in four Aboriginal and Torres Strait Islander children remained below minimum standards for reading. Finally, there has been little change in the employment rates of Aboriginal and Torres Strait Islander peoples. Other comparisons related to specific diseases or conditions are discussed in greater length throughout various chapters of this book.

A model describing the complex inter-relationships between factors contributing to disparities in healthcare for Aboriginal and Torres Strait Islander peoples was initially conceptualised by Paradies and colleagues in 2013 from a comprehensive literature review. After minimal adaptation, it was included in the *2017 Aboriginal and Torres Strait Islander Health Performance Framework*, and appears to analyse and organise significant factors, such as the effects of racism, which need to be considered in the context of Aboriginal and Torres Strait Islander peoples' health and well-being (see Figure 2.18).

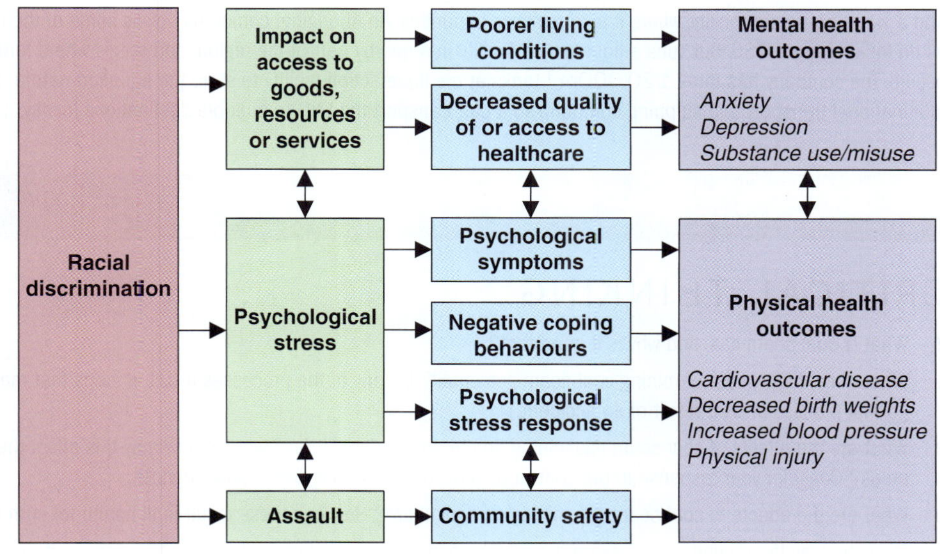

Figure 2.18

Pathways between racism and ill health

Various components of racism and physical and mental well-being are interconnected, complex and affect every aspect of healthcare design, provision and acceptance.

Source: Adapted from Australian Government (2017), Figure 40, p. 28. Licensed from the Commonwealth of Australia under a Creative Commons Attribution 3.0 Australia Licence. The Commonwealth of Australia does not necessarily endorse the content of this publication.

CHAPTER REVIEW

- Health is more than just the absence of disease. It encompasses *physical, mental and social well-being*.
- *Disease burden* and *mortality statistics* can be used as measures of a community's or a country's health status. This information may also influence the design and construction of primary healthcare programs.
- The three overarching determinants of health can be categorised as factors relating to individuals, social determinants and environmental factors.
- *Individual factors* that need to be considered in relation to health include biomedical issues related to genetics, sex, age and drug resistance. *Behavioural factors* include knowledge, skills and attitudes.
- The *societal factors* that may contribute to health include socioeconomic factors, such as employment, education and income, or sociocultural factors, such as family, religion, culture, media or peer pressure.
- *Environmental factors* contributing to health include those that affect air, water and soil quality.
- The *COVID-19 pandemic* has resulted in *significant loss of public health gains globally*, and has exacerbated the influences of poverty on health and well-being.
- The effects of *increasing populations and the use of fossil fuels* can play a significant role in the development of illness.
- The *healthcare gap* is an identifiable disparity between Aboriginal and Torres Strait Islander peoples and non-Indigenous Australians, which results in significantly poorer health outcomes for Indigenous Australians.

REVIEW QUESTIONS

1. In what ways could knowledge of the determinants of health influence your practice as a health professional?
2. Within your local area, find primary health services that directly address the socioeconomic and sociocultural factors associated with health.
   a. Create a table and list the services on the far-left column.
   b. Do any of these programs assess their influence or measure outcomes? If so, identify the measured outcomes in the next column of your table.
   c. Are any of these programs specifically designed for Aboriginal and Torres Strait Islander peoples? If so, identify these programs in the next column of your table.
   d. Review your results and form an opinion regarding the diversity, appropriateness and equity of the available services.
3. Find governmental resources that identify wealth within areas of Australia. Choose three areas—one that appears to represent high income, one that appears to represent middle income, and one that appears to represent low income. See whether you can determine other important demographics, such as average age, the healthcare services available, and any other factors that you deem to be appropriate for influencing the health of a community.
4. What environmental factors are relevant in your local area? (For example, is there a lot of bushland that might catch fire in summer and cause increased air pollution with the potential to affect individuals in the area?) Try to identify at least three potential environmental risks.
5. Imagine that you are single-handedly responsible for solving the health disparities experienced by a certain group of people in a community. You may choose to invent a simulated community—be as creative and specific as you like (it will make the next task easier). Design a plan that can address all of the appropriate aspects of the determinants of health associated with your imaginary community.

CASE STUDY

You live in a community where 'CSG-Bux', a coal-seam gas company, has its main plant nearby. CSG-Bux drills into the Tarus Basin in your region. It uses a series of mechanical rigs to drill the well and extract the gas and associated water. It owns a lot of land in the region, including a field compression station and a water treatment facility, where it also removes impurities. An Aboriginal community owns some of the land on which the plant has been established, as do local farmers. CSG-Bux runs a liquefaction facility in a nearby part of the region, and this is where further processing, impurity removal and storage occurs. The company has three $120{,}000 m^3$ tanks at the liquefaction facility to store the liquefied natural gas (LNG). CSG-Bux has a relationship with a multinational transport and shipping company, so it can transport the LNG to multiple destinations locally, nationally and internationally.

CRITICAL THINKING

1. What is coal-seam gas, and why is it important?
2. What does the process of mining coal-seam gas entail? Do any of the processes result in steps that may cause injury or illness? (This may occur in the normal process or as a result of an accident.)
3. What are the effects of coal-seam gas mining on the aquifer and surface water? How may this affect the health of people living in the surrounding areas? Consider your response in the context of short-term and long-term consequences.
4. What are the effects of coal-seam gas mining on agriculture? How can these result in ill health for current and future generations?
5. Describe how the mining of coal-seam gas might affect the health of its workers and the community with respect to the following aspects:
   a. individual factors
   b. societal factors
   c. environmental factors

BIBLIOGRAPHY

Australian Bureau of Statistics (ABS) (2021). *Causes of death, Australia, 2020*. Canberra: ABS. www.abs.gov.au.

Australian Health Ministers' Advisory Council (AHMAC) (2017). *Aboriginal and Torres Strait Islander Health Performance Framework 2017 Report*. Canberra: AHMAC. https://www.indigenoushpf.gov.au/publications/hpf-2017.

Productivity Commission (2022). *Closing the Gap annual data compilation report.* Canberra: Productivity Commission. https://www.pc.gov.au/closing-the-gap-data/annual-data-report/report.

Australian Institute of Health and Welfare (AIHW) (2020). *Aboriginal and Torres Strait Islander Health Performance Framework 2020 summary report.* Cat. No. IHPF 2. Canberra: AIHW. https://www.indigenoushpf.gov.au/publications/hpf-summary-2020.

Australian Institute of Health and Welfare (AIHW) (2021a). *Australian Burden of Disease Study: interactive data or risk factor burden.* Australian Burden of Disease Study series No. 23. Cat. No. BOD 35. Canberra: AIHW. Retrieved from Australian Burden of Disease Study 2018: Interactive data on risk factor burden, About - Australian Institute of Health and Welfare (aihw.gov.au).

Australian Institute of Health and Welfare (AIHW) (2021b). *Australia's welfare, 2021: data insights.* Australia's Welfare series No. 14. Cat. No. AUS 236. Canberra: AIHW. https://www.aihw.gov.au/reports/australias-welfare/australias-welfare-2021-data-insights/contents/summary.

Australian Institute of Health and Welfare (AIWH) (2021). *Profile of Indigenous Australians.* Canberra: AIHW. https://www.aihw.gov.au/reports/australias-welfare/profile-of-indigenous-australians.

Australian Institute of Health and Welfare (AIHW) (2022a). *Australia's health, 2022*. Australia's Health series No. 15. Cat. No. AUS 199. Canberra: AIHW. https://www.aihw.gov.au/reports-data/australias-health.

Australian Institute of Health and Welfare (AIHW) (2022b). *Australian Burden of Disease Study 2022: data tables. ABDS 2022 National estimates for Australia*. Canberra: AIHW. https://www.aihw.gov.au/reports/burden-of-disease/australian-burden-of-disease-study-2022/data.

Australian Institute of Health and Welfare (AIHW) (2022c). *Housing assistance in Australia.* Cat. No. HOU 326. Canberra: AIHW. https://www.aihw.gov.au/reports/housing-assistance/housing-assistance-in-australia/contents/about.

Australian Institute of Health and Welfare (AIWH) (2022d). *Overweight and obesity.* Canberra: AIHW. https://www.aihw.gov.au/reports/australias-health/overweight-and-obesity.

Bauldoff, G., Gubrud-Howe, P.M., Carno, M.-A., Levett-Jones, T., Hales, M., Berry, K., … Stanley, D. (2020). *LeMone and Burke's medical–surgical nursing: critical thinking for person-centred care* (4th [Australian] edition.). Sydney: Pearson Australia.

Bauserman, M., Thorsten, V.R., Nolen, T.L., Patterson, J., Lokangaka, A., Tshefu, A., … Bose, C. (2020). Maternal mortality in six low and lower-middle income countries from 2010 to 2018: risk factors and trends. *Reproductive Health* 17 (Suppl 3):173. https://doi.org/10.1186/s12978-020-00990-z.

Bullock, S. & Manias, E. (2022). *Fundamentals of pharmacology* (8th edn). Sydney: Pearson Australia.

Dassarma, B., Tripathy, S., Chabalala, M. & Matsabisa, M.G. (2022). Challenges in establishing vaccine induced herd immunity through age specific community vaccinations. *Aging and Disease* 13(1):29–36. https://doi.org/10.14336/AD.2021.0611.

Davidson, P. (2022). A *tale of two pandemics: COVID, inequality and poverty in 2020 and 2021.* Build Back Fairer Series Report No. 3. Sydney: ACOSS/UNSW Sydney Poverty and Inequality Partnership. https://povertyandinequality.acoss.org.au/wp-content/uploads/2022/03/Build-back-fairer-report-3_FINAL.pdf.

Davidson, P. & Bradbury, B. (2022). *The wealth inequality pandemic: COVID and wealth inequality.* Build Back Fairer Series Report No. 4. Sydney: ACOSS/UNSW Sydney Poverty and Inequality Partnership. https://povertyandinequality.acoss.org.au/wp-content/uploads/2022/07/The-wealth-inequality-pandemic_COVID-and-wealth-inequality_screen.pdf.

Department of Health and Aged Care (2020). *Clinical practice guidelines: pregnancy care*. Canberra: Australian Government. https://www.health.gov.au/resources/pregnancy-care-guidelines.

Flavel, J., McKee, M., Freeman, T., Musolino, C., van Eyk, H., Tesfay, F.H. & Baum, F. (2022). The need for improved Australian data on social determinants of health inequities. *Medical Journal of Australia 216*(8):388–91. https://doi.org/10.5694/mja2.51495.

Gao, Q., Prina, A.M., Ma, Y., Aceituno, D. & Mayston, R. (2022). Inequalities in older age and primary health care utilization in low- and middle-income countries: a systematic review. *International Journal of Social Determinants of Health and Health Services 52*(1):99–114. https://doi.org/10.1177/00207314211041234.

Haug, N., Geyrhofer, L., Londei, A., Dervic, E., Desvars-Larrive, A., Loreto, V., … Klimek, P. (2020). Ranking the effectiveness of worldwide COVID-19 government interventions. *Nature Human Behaviour* 4(12):1303–12. https://doi.org/10.1038/s41562-020-01009-0.

Heuveline, P. (2022). Global and national declines in life expectancy: an end-of-2021 assessment. *Population and Development Review* 48(1):31–50. https://doi.org/10.1111/padr.12477.

Johns Hopkins Coronavirus Resource Centre (2022). *Maps and trends: mortality analyses.* https://coronavirus.jhu.edu/data/mortality.

Kairuz, C.A., Casanelia, L.M., Bennett-Brook, K., Coombes, J. & Yadav, U.N. (2021). Impact of racism and discrimination on physical and mental health among Aboriginal and Torres Strait islander peoples living in Australia: a systematic scoping review. *BMC Public Health 21*:1302. https://doi.org/10.1186/s12889-021-11363-x.

Klein, S.L. & Flanagan, K.L. (2016). Sex differences in immune responses. *Nature Reviews Immunology 16*(10):626–38. https://doi.org/10.1038/nri.2016.90.

Laker, S.R., Blake, J.R. & Sullivan, W.J. (2022). Overuse injury. *Emedicine*. https://emedicine.medscape.com/article/313121-overview.

Lekagul, A., Chattong, A., Rueangsom, P., Waleewong, O. & Tangcharoensathien, V. (2022). Multi-dimensional impacts of Coronavirus disease 2019 pandemic on Sustainable Development Goal achievement. *Globalization and Health* 18(1):65. https://doi.org/10.1186/s12992-022-00861-1.

Levin, A.T., Owusu-Boaitey, N., Pugh, S., Fosdick, B.K., Zwi, A.B., Malani, A., … Meyerowitz-Katz, G. (2022). Assessing the burden of COVID-19 in developing countries: systematic review, meta-analysis and public policy implications. *BMJ Global Health, 7*(5):e008477. https://doi.org/10.1136/bmjgh-2022-008477.

Lu, R.J., Wang, E.K. & Benayoun, B.A. (2022). Functional genomics of inflamm-aging and immunosenescence. *Briefings in Functional Genomics* 21(1): 43–55. https://doi.org/10.1093/bfgp/elab009.

Murray, C.J.L., Ikuta, K.S., Sharara, F., Swetschinski, L., Robles Aguilar, G., Gray, A., … Ashley, E. (2022). Global burden of bacterial antimicrobial resistance in 2019: a systematic analysis. *The Lancet* 399(10325):629–55. https://doi.org/10.1016/S0140-6736(21)02724-0.

National Indigenous Australians Agency (NIAA) (2020). *Aboriginal and Torres Strait Islander Health Performance Framework: measures*. https://www.indigenoushpf.gov.au/measures /.

Priest, N., Doery, K., Truong, M., Guo, S., Perry, R., Trenerry, B., … Paradies, Y. (2021). Updated systematic review and meta-analysis of studies examining the relationship between reported racism and health and well-being for children and youth: a protocol. *BMJ Open* 11(6):e043722. http://dx.doi.org/10.1136/bmjopen-2020-043722.

Royal Australian College of General Practitioners (RACGP). (2022). The physiology of ageing. *RACGP aged care clinical guide (Silver Book)*. East Melbourne, VIC: RACGP. https://www.racgp.org.au/silverbook.

Safe Work Australia (2021). *Key work health and safety statistics, Australia, 2021*. Canberra: Safe Work Australia. https://www.safeworkaustralia.gov.au/doc/key-work-health-and-safety-statistics-australia-2021.

Steering Committee for the Review of Government Service Provision (SCRGSP) (2020). *Overcoming Indigenous disadvantage: key indicators, 2020: Overview.* Canberra: Productivity Commission. https://www.pc.gov.au/ongoing/overcoming-indigenous-disadvantage/2020.

Swihart, D.L., Yarrarapu, S.N.S. & Martin, R.L. (2022). *Cultural religious competence in clinical practice*. StatPearls. https://www.ncbi.nlm.nih.gov/books/NBK493216/.

Takahashi, T. & Iwasaki, A. (2021). Sex differences in immune responses. *Science* 371(6527):347–48. https://doi.org/10.1126/science.abe7199.

Tortora. G.J., Derrickson, B., Burkett, B., Peoples, G., Dye, D., Cooke, J., … Green, H. (2022). *Principles of anatomy and physiology* (3rd Asia-Pacific edn). Milton, QLD: John Wiley and Sons.

Wang, H., Paulson, K.R., Pease, S.A., Watson, S., Comfort, H., Zheng, P., … Castro, E. (2022). Estimating excess mortality due to the COVID-19 pandemic: a systematic analysis of COVID-19-related mortality, 2020–21. *The Lancet* 399(10334):1513–36. https://doi.org/10.1016/S0140-6736(21)02796-3.

Wilkinson, N.M., Chen, H.-C., Lechner, M.G. & Su, M.A. (2022). Sex differences in immunity. *Annual Review of Immunology* 40(1):75–94. https://doi.org/10.1146/annurev-immunol-101320-125133.

World Health Organization (WHO) (1978). *Declaration of Alma-Ata*. Geneva: WHO. https://www.who.int/teams/social-determinants-of-health/declaration-of-alma-ata#:~:text=The%20Alma%2DAta%20Declaration%20of,goal%20of%20Health%20for%20All.

World Health Organization (WHO) (2018). *Preventing disease through healthy environments: a global assessment of the burden of disease from environmental risks*. Geneva: WHO. https://www.who.int/publications/i/item/9789241565196.

World Health Organization (WHO) (2020). *The top 10 causes of death*. Geneva: WHO. https://www.who.int/news-room/fact-sheets/detail/the-top-10-causes-of-death.

World Health Organization (WHO) (2021a). *Antimicrobial resistance*. Geneva: WHO. https://www.who.int/health-topics/antimicrobial-resistance.

World Health Organization (WHO) (2021b). *WHO global air quality guideline values*. Geneva: WHO. https://apps.who.int/iris/handle/10665/345329.

World Health Organization (WHO) (2022a). *About WHO*. Geneva: WHO. http://www.who.int/about.

World Health Organization (WHO) (2022b). *Air quality database*. Geneva: WHO. https://www.who.int/data/gho/data/themes/air-pollution/who-air-quality-database/2022.

World Health Organization (WHO) (2022c). *Ambient air pollution data.* Geneva: WHO. https://www.who.int/data/gho/data/themes/topics/topic-details/GHO/ambient-air-pollution.

World Health Organization (WHO) (2022d). *Noncommunicable diseases*. Geneva: WHO. https://www.who.int/news-room/fact-sheets/detail/noncommunicable-diseases.

World Health Organization (WHO) (2022e) *Public health and environment*. Geneva: WHO. https://www.who.int/data/gho/data/themes/public-health-and-environment.

World Health Organization (WHO) (2022f). *World report on the health of refugees and migrants.* Geneva: WHO. https://www.who.int/publications/i/item/9789240054462.

Wozniak, T.M., Dyda, A., Merlo, G. & Hall, L. (2022). Disease burden, associated mortality and economic impact of antimicrobial resistant infections in Australia. *The Lancet* 27:100521. https://doi.org/10.1016/j.lanwpc.2022.100521

Inflammation and healing

3

LEARNING OBJECTIVES

After completing this chapter, you should be able to:

1. State the purpose of inflammation.
2. Name the key pro-inflammatory chemical mediators, and outline their roles.
3. Describe the vascular and cellular phases of acute inflammation.
4. Define an exudate, and differentiate between the types.
5. Compare and contrast acute and chronic inflammation.
6. Outline fibrosis and granuloma formation in chronic inflammation.
7. Outline the changes in inflammatory responses in SARS-CoV-2 coronavirus infection.
8. Describe the processes of healing and repair.
9. Compare and contrast first and second intention healing.
10. State the key factors that can impede the healing process.

WHAT YOU SHOULD KNOW BEFORE YOU START THIS CHAPTER

What are the main characteristics of the different types of tissues?

Can you describe the phases of the cell cycle?

Can you describe the mechanisms of reversible and irreversible cellular injury?

Can you name the major blood components and blood cell types?

Can you describe the coagulation process?

KEY TERMS

Acute inflammation
Adhesions
Chronic inflammation
Clotting
Coagulation
Complement system
Contracture
COVID-19 infection
Cytokines
Debridement
Epithelialisation
Exudate
Fibrosis
Granulation tissue
Granuloma
Healing
Hypertrophic scar
Keloid
Kinin–kallikrein system
Parenchyma
Pro-inflammatory chemical mediators
Repair
SARS-CoV-2 infection
Scar
Wound contraction

Introduction

Inflammation is an innate, non-specific, first-line body defence response to cell injury. It is non-specific in that the response is the same irrespective of the nature of the agent of cell injury: physical, chemical, ischaemic or infectious. As inflammation is in response to cell injury, the magnitude of the response depends on the degree of damage.

LEARNING OBJECTIVE **1**

State the purpose of inflammation.

The purpose of inflammation is to quickly *neutralise the injurious agent and stop further cell damage*, as well as to *clean up the tissue site to enable completion of the healing process*. If the agent of injury persists, the inflammatory response will become chronic. This is undesirable, as the healing processes cannot be completed, and the inflammatory reaction can lead to further tissue damage and deformity.

In this chapter, the acute and chronic inflammatory responses will be described and contrasted. Tissue healing processes will then be described. The factors affecting healing, and the clinical issues associated with the management of these, will also be discussed. Figure 3.1 describes inflammation and its association with common clinical manifestations and management.

Acute inflammation

Acute inflammation is a combination of vascular and cellular responses. It is characterised by an easily recognisable set of localised clinical manifestations, which are termed the *five cardinal signs of inflammation*: *redness, warmth, swelling, pain* and *loss of function*. Systemic manifestations such as fever also occur in inflammation (see the section on the cellular phase of inflammation). The nomenclature for inflammation is to attach the suffix *-itis* onto the medical term for the tissue or structure. For example, 'dermatitis' is an inflammation of the dermis or skin. Table 3.1 lists some well-known examples of inflammatory conditions.

LEARNING OBJECTIVE **2**

Name the key pro-inflammatory chemical mediators, and outline their roles.

The inflammatory process begins when injured cells release a range of intracellular substances into the tissue environment. These substances are called **pro-inflammatory chemical mediators**, because they *induce inflammation* and their levels determine the magnitude of the reaction. Histamine and prostaglandins are just two examples of inflammatory mediators. A list of key pro-inflammatory mediators and their specific roles is provided in Table 3.2.

LEARNING OBJECTIVE **3**

Describe the vascular and cellular phases of acute inflammation.

VASCULAR PHASE

The vascular phase of inflammation is the first stage. Pro-inflammatory mediators induce a *vasodilatory response* in the affected tissue. This involves relaxation of the pre-capillary arterioles and increases blood flow into the tissue, accounting for the cardinal sign of increased warmth. Capillaries increase permeability by increasing the gap between the endothelial cells that comprise their wall. This allows plasma to ooze into the interstitial fluid, carrying in it plasma proteins and other substances that participate in the inflammatory response. *Capillary permeability* accounts for the cardinal sign of swelling. Swelling can increase tissue pressure and cause pain by stimulating nociceptors. A number of the chemical mediators sensitise sensory nerves to increase the frequency of pain transmission to the brain, thus heightening pain. Pain transmission and the role of chemical mediators are explained further in the chapter 'Nociception and pain'.

Plasma protein levels are up-regulated during inflammation. These proteins enter the tissue site and bring about a series of linked cascading reactions that lead to complement formation, kinin production and localised **coagulation**. These reactions are cascades, because one plasma protein involved in a reaction is an inactive enzyme (a proenzyme) that is activated in inflammation, and sets off a series of subsequent reactions that lead to the formation of particular reaction products. Some of these products facilitate the continuation of the cascades, while others perform key inflammatory functions. The *main cascades* involved in inflammation are the complement system, clotting and the kinin–kallikrein system.

The **complement system** can be activated by a variety of triggers: plasma proteins, substances released from invading cells, and antigen–antibody complexes. Primarily, 10 proteins form the nine components of the complement system. These components can form *inflammatory activators called opsonins*, act as *chemotactic agents* (i.e. *attractants*) that induce white blood cell migration to the site of injury, cause the *release of histamine* from mast cells, *induce the vascular phase* of inflammation, and *create pores* in the membranes of cells (e.g. microorganisms, cancer cells), causing them to burst and die (see Figure 3.2).

There is an association between inflammation and coagulation. The **clotting** cascade is activated in inflammation primarily to form a *fibrin meshwork boundary* around the site of injury. This will trap the injurious agent in the site, concentrate the attack in this area, and prevent the spread of damage throughout the tissue. If there is damage to tissue blood vessels, the clot will *stop any bleeding*. It will also help restore the continuity of the tissue and build a *framework for its repair*. Activators of the clotting process during inflammation include the presence of proteolytic enzymes, collagen or bacterial toxins.

The activation of the **kinin–kallikrein system** leads to the production of a group of important chemical mediators called

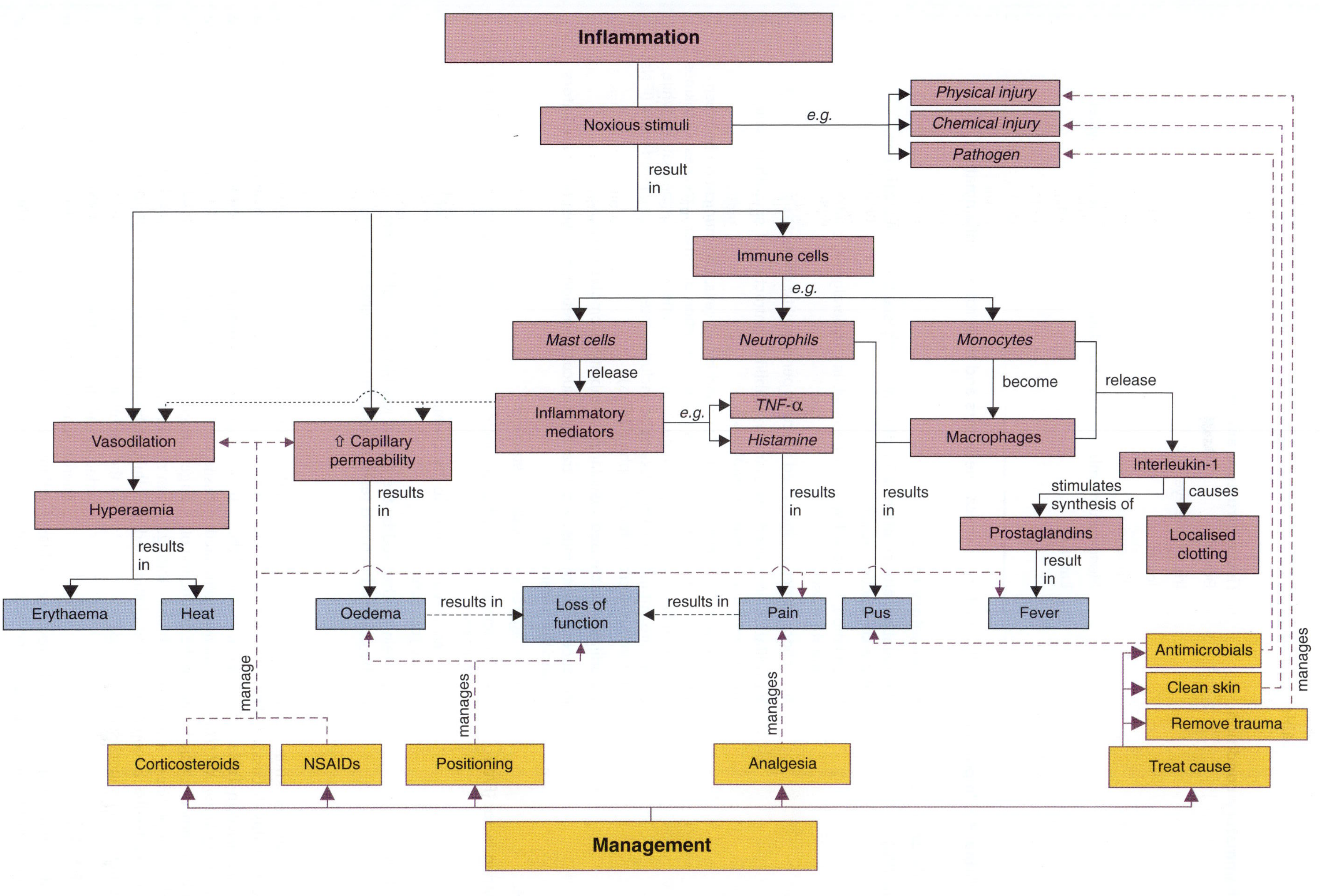

Figure 3.1

Clinical snapshot: Inflammation

↑ = increased; NSAIDs = non-steroidal anti-inflammatory drugs; TNF-α = tumour necrosis factor-alpha.

Table 3.1 Examples of common inflammatory conditions

Name of inflammatory condition	Tissue/structure affected
Colitis	Bowel
Iritis	Iris of the eye
Arthritis	Joints
Appendicitis	Appendix
Meningitis	Meningeal membranes surrounding the central nervous system
Laryngitis	Larynx

Table 3.2 Important pro-inflammatory chemical mediators and their roles in inflammation

Chemical mediator	Inflammatory roles
Prostaglandins (PG)	Vasodilation, altered platelet function, hyperalgesia, bronchoconstriction, uterine contraction, fever
Bradykinin	Vasodilation, increased vascular permeability, hyperalgesia, contraction of smooth muscle
Leukotrienes	Bronchoconstriction, increased vascular permeability, chemotaxis
Histamine	Vasodilation, increased vascular permeability, contraction of smooth muscle, stimulates PG synthesis, chemotaxis
Cytokines	Peptide secretions from inflammatory and blood cells, communication between inflammatory cells, some cytokines induce secretion of other cytokines. Cytokines regulate inflammatory and immune responses; some are pro-inflammatory, while others are antiinflammatory. Examples includes interleukins (ILs), interferons (IFNs) and tumour necrosis factor-alpha (TNF-α)
Nitric oxide	Vasodilation, increased vascular permeability, promotes PG action
Substance P	Produces smooth muscle contraction, mucus secretion, releases other mediators (especially histamine)
Thromboxanes	Platelet aggregation, vasoconstriction
Platelet-activating factor (PAF)	Platelet activation, vasodilation, increased vascular permeability, bronchoconstriction, chemotaxis
Complement	Increased vascular permeability, chemotaxis, bronchoconstriction, cellular lysis, allergic reactions
C-reactive protein	A protein synthesised by the liver. A key biomarker of inflammation or infection that can be detected in blood tests. Involved in complement activation

kinins. The most abundant kinin synthesised is *bradykinin*, which is the focus of this discussion. The roles of bradykinin in inflammation are listed in Table 3.2. A key activator of the kinin system is *clotting factor XII (Hageman factor)*, generated during the coagulation process, which leads to the production of kallikrein. *Kallikrein*, a protease, also activates blood clotting. This creates a positive feedback loop on the blood clotting and kinin systems during inflammation (see Figure 3.3).

CELLULAR PHASE

The next phase of inflammation is the cellular response. White blood cells are drawn to the site of tissue injury by chemical mediators. They can squeeze through the larger gaps in the capillary wall induced in the vascular response—this process is called *diapedesis*. *Phagocytic cells* play a key role in inflammation by directly *neutralising the injurious agent* and by *recruiting other immune cells*, such as lymphocytes, to participate in the response. *Neutrophils* are the first phagocytes to enter the tissue site, because they are smaller, followed soon after by the larger phagocytes, *monocytes/macrophages*. The macrophages can remain active for longer. The phagocytes ingest dead cells, cellular debris and foreign cells (if these are the injurious agent in the site of injury). Phagocytic cells release pyrogens (fever-inducing substances) that can inhibit the metabolism of some microorganisms, making them more susceptible to attack from inflammatory cells.

Other blood cells have roles in inflammation, and these roles are summarised in Table 3.3. Immune cell functions and interactions are explained in greater detail in the chapter 'Immune disorders'.

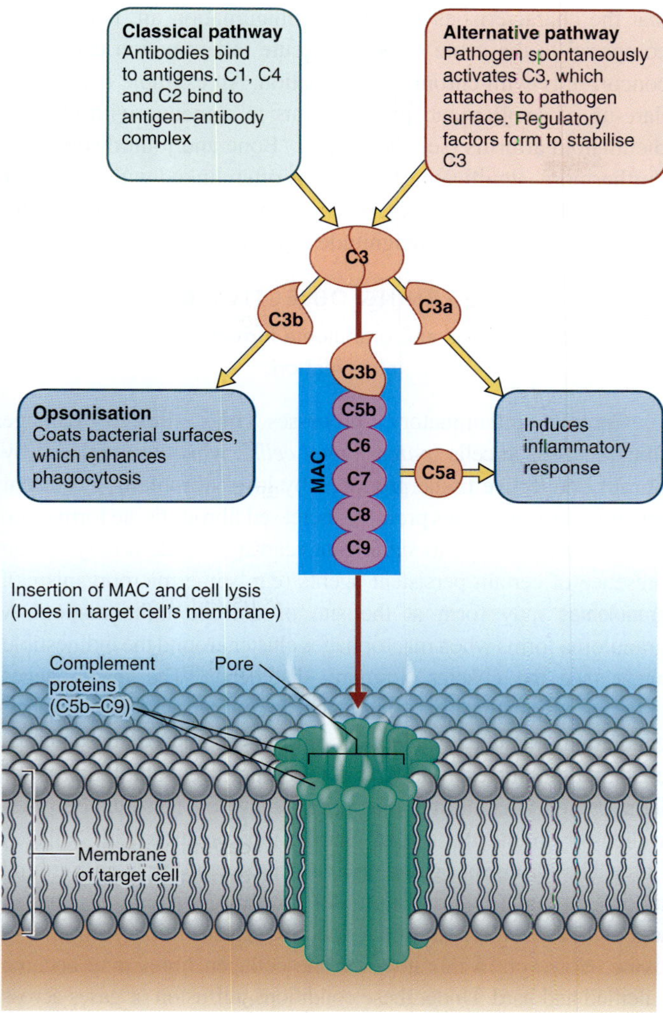

Figure 3.2

Complement activation

In the classical pathway of complement activation, antibodies coating the surface of a pathogen activate selected complement proteins, which in turn activate C3. In the alternative pathway, C3 spontaneously activates and attaches to pathogen membranes. The two pathways converge at C3, which splits into active pieces: one promotes inflammation, the other enhances phagocytosis. Other complement proteins can form a membrane attack complex (MAC) that inserts into the target cell membrane, creating a pore that can lyse the target cell.

Source: Adapted from Marieb & Hoehn (2019), Figure 21.6, p. 821.

Table 3.3 The roles of blood cells in inflammation

Blood cell type	Inflammatory role(s)
Neutrophils	Phagocytosis
Monocytes (blood)/ macrophages (tissues)	Sustained phagocytosis, antigen presentation to immune cells to activate them, produce cytokines, initiate healing
Eosinophils	Mediate allergic reactions, intestinal parasitic infection (especially helminths)
Basophils (blood)/ mast cells (tissues)	Concentrated source of histamine, mediate allergy
Lymphocytes	Immune responsiveness, cell–cell immune attack, antibody production, immune memory

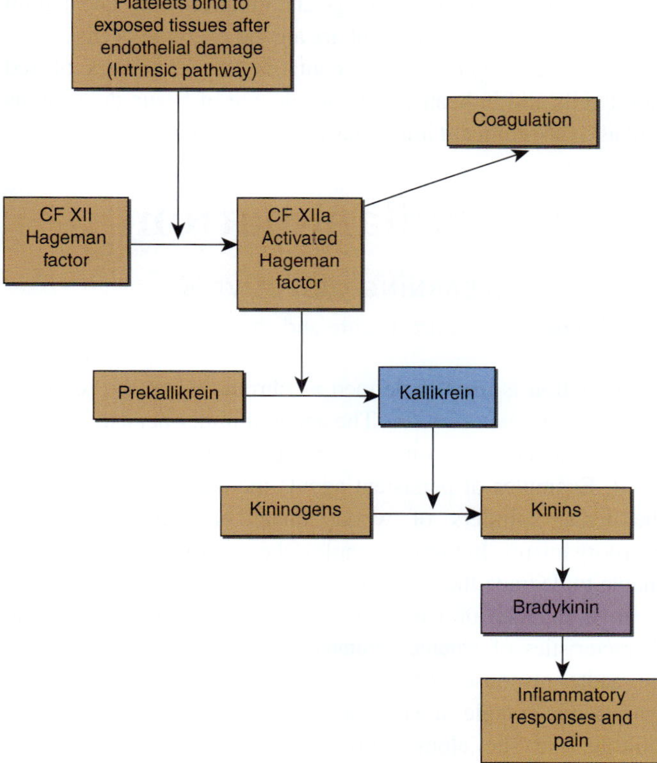

Figure 3.3

The role of kallikrein in coagulation and inflammation
CF = clotting factor.

EXUDATES

LEARNING OBJECTIVE 4

Define an exudate, and differentiate between the types.

During the vascular phase of inflammation, fluid moves out of the blood vessels and accumulates in the tissues. This fluid is called the **exudate**, and the process is termed *exudation*. The exudate transports cells and plasma components into the tissues that participate in inflammation and healing, and it *dilutes toxins*.

The composition of an exudate can vary greatly, and depends on the type of agent, the nature of the tissue damage and the intensity of the inflammatory response. There are four types of exudate: serous, fibrinous, purulent and haemorrhagic.

A *serous exudate* is watery and has a low protein concentration. This is because the inflammatory reaction is mild, with a dampened capillary permeability response. It is the kind of exudate that accumulates in a common skin blister.

A *fibrinous exudate* is characterised by a high rate of plasma protein exudation and the formation of fibrin at the site of injury. A fibrinous exudate can be problematic because of its very viscous and sticky consistency, which may greatly inhibit the healing process. It can also lead to adjacent tissue layers adhering to each other. These are called **adhesions**. Adhesions can sometimes require clinical intervention, such as when two adjacent sections of bowel wall or bowel and a pelvic structure adhere. Under these circumstances, there is risk of an obstructed passageway developing involving abdominopelvic structures, such as the gastrointestinal or reproductive tracts.

A *purulent exudate* contains pus. Pus consists of cellular debris, as well as living and dead cells. It is usually associated with injuries caused by invading bacteria. When a large amount of pus accumulates in a tissue, it is termed an *abscess*. Purulent exudates can be problematic, as some antimicrobial agents are unable to penetrate pus and so are rendered ineffective against the infectious agent at the injury site. Remember that the formation of a purulent exudate is part of the inflammatory response to the damage being done by an infectious agent, not to the presence of the microbe itself in the body. Microbes can be present in the body without causing cell damage and inflammation. The natural flora on our skin and in our gut are a good example of this.

A *haemorrhagic exudate* contains large numbers of red blood cells and indicates a greater degree of tissue damage, as well as that significant injury has occurred to local blood vessels.

Chronic inflammation

LEARNING OBJECTIVE 5

Compare and contrast acute and chronic inflammation.

Inflammation is usually defined as chronic when the response lasts for *two weeks or more*. The agent of injury persists because the inflammatory response has not been able to neutralise or kill it. Examples of persistent agents include inhaled particles, chemicals, splinters of wood, metal or glass, and some microorganisms. In these examples, the inflammatory process is unable to degrade the agent of injury.

In a number of cases, the physiological and histological characteristics of **chronic inflammation** are distinguishable from the acute response. The membranes of neutrophils rupture, cytoplasmic granules are released and the cells die. Lymphocytes infiltrate the site along with monocytes/macrophages—these become the dominant cell types in the chronic inflammatory site. By this stage, there is little evidence of the vascular phase of the acute inflammatory response. Fibroblasts are activated, leading to the production of fibrous connective tissue, part of the repair process. Fibroblasts also signal more infiltration by lymphocytes and macrophages. Macrophages and fibroblasts initiate the commencement of the healing process. However, healing and repair cannot be completed until the injurious agent is neutralised.

However, the delineation of acute and chronic inflammation based on time and histology are often rather simplistic and arbitrary, and can suggest a dichotomy. Students can be forgiven for developing the misconception that acute and chronic inflammation can be easily differentiated. The reality is that the two forms can overlap along a *continuum of inflammatory responses*, such that the characteristics of chronic inflammation are not distinct compared to the acute response. Acute inflammation can occur concurrently with chronic inflammation. An example is an acute flare-up of swollen and painful joints in someone with chronic rheumatoid arthritis (see the chapter 'Bone and joint disorders'). Furthermore, significant cell injury is often linked with persistent chronic inflammatory states, when it can also be observed in acute inflammation when the magnitude of the response is excessive.

LEARNING OBJECTIVE 6

Outline fibrosis and granuloma formation in chronic inflammation.

Chronic inflammatory processes may indeed damage functional tissue cells (*parenchymal cells*), which are replaced by fibrous connective tissue produced by local fibroblasts. Persistent inflammatory processes promote increased fibrous tissue formation. This **fibrosis** can lead to significant scarring and deformity. In the presence of certain persistent agents (e.g. some microorganisms), **granulomas** may form at the site of chronic inflammation. A granuloma forms when macrophages cluster around the indigestible agent (see the chapter 'Immune disorders'). The macrophages undergo a transformation into altered cell types. Some become epithelioid cells that have lost the capacity for phagocytosis but can endocytose particles. Others fuse into giant cells that phagocytose large particles that normal macrophages cannot. This area becomes walled-off around the site of chronic inflammation with collagen fibres. The purpose of a granuloma is not unlike the fibrin mesh around the site of acute inflammation—to keep the *infected site isolated* and *minimise the spread* of the infective organism into surrounding tissue. However, in this instance, the collagen fibres may become calcified and hard. Under these conditions, diffusion of gases across the granuloma wall becomes severely restricted. The cells inside the granuloma may eventually undergo *liquefactive necrosis*, leaving a hollowed-out structure. Granuloma formation is a characteristic feature of a number of conditions, including tuberculosis (see the chapter 'Respiratory infections, cancers and vascular conditions'), inflammatory bowel disease (see the chapter 'Intestinal disorders'), some neoplastic disorders (see the chapter 'Neoplasia') and a rare immunodeficiency disorder called chronic granulomatous disease (see the chapter 'Immune disorders').

INFLAMMATION AND SARS-CoV-2 INFECTION

LEARNING OBJECTIVE 7

Outline the changes in inflammatory responses in SARS-CoV-2 coronavirus infection.

The **SARS-CoV-2 coronavirus** is the causative agent in **COVID-19 infection**. The human body's response to this infection involves an aberrant inflammatory and immune reaction. In people with severe infection, massive inflammatory response is triggered through an excessive release of pro-inflammatory **cytokines** resulting in what is commonly referred to as a *hyperinflammatory cytokine storm*, which damages the lung and other body tissues and can disrupt normal coagulation. The pro-inflammatory cytokines released in excess include tumour necrosis factor-alpha (TNF-α), selected interleukins and γ-interferon. There

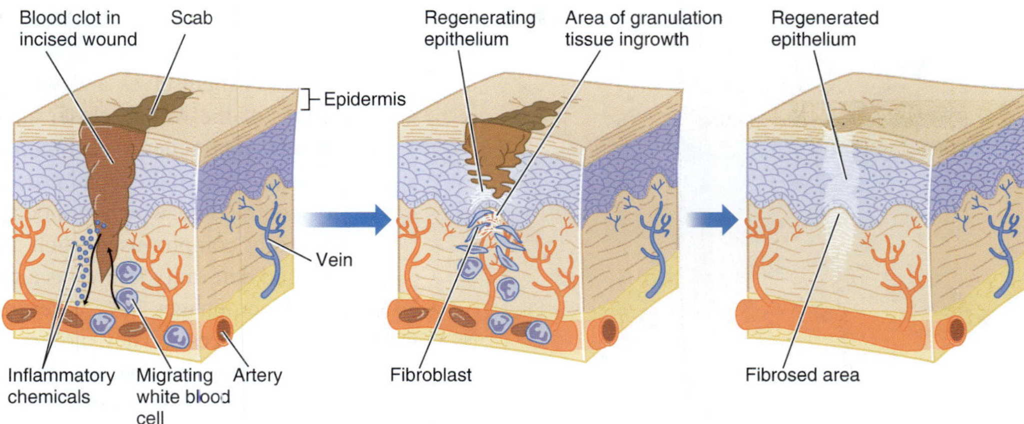

Figure 3.4

The process of tissue healing

Source: Adapted from Marieb & Hoehn (2019), Figure 4.15, p. 175.

is a loss of protective immunity due to disrupted immune cell numbers and functions with lymphocytes, phagocytes and eosinophil levels increased, while B cells, natural killer cells and certain T cell sub-populations are reduced.

For some people, post-viral fatigue symptoms and other complications can develop, a condition known as *long COVID* (for more detail, refer to 'Infection' chapter). These complications can affect the brain, thyroid, lungs, heart and muscles. While there is some uncertainty as to whether long COVID is due to the hyperinflammatory cytokine storm or a reduction in normal protective immunity, there is agreement that inflammation persists in people so affected.

Healing and repair

LEARNING OBJECTIVE 8

Describe the processes of healing and repair.

The purpose of these processes is the restoration, where possible, of the lost functional tissue cells (**parenchyma**) and the re-establishment of the continuity of the tissue framework through **scar** formation. These processes are called **healing** and **repair**, respectively. For these processes to reach their completion, the injurious agent must be neutralised and the site of injury cleaned up. This, of course, is the purpose of the inflammatory response, so there is significant overlap between inflammation and healing. Normally, healing commences within four days of an injury and, depending on the tissue affected, is largely resolved within weeks. However, scar maturation can continue for a couple of years.

Initially, the gap in the tissue created by the injury is filled by a fibrin clot, providing a temporary seal against haemorrhage and infection. It may also bring the edges of the wound closer together. In a skin wound, the clot will dry out (desiccate) as it is exposed to the air. The desiccated clot is called a *scab* (see Figure 3.4).

The injured area needs to be cleaned of debris and dead cells. This is the responsibility of the macrophages and any surviving neutrophils. This clean-up is referred to as **debridement**. As this is occurring, an epithelial layer begins to grow from the surrounding tissue under the clot, in order to form a more permanent bridge between the edges of the wound and to separate the clot from the wound surface underneath. This is known as **epithelialisation**. Once epithelialisation is established, the remaining clot dissolves. The restoration, or regeneration, of the parenchyma then occurs (see Figure 3.4). The degree of regeneration depends on the tissue type. Epithelial and connective tissues have a high capacity for regeneration, whereas mature muscle and nervous tissue have very limited capacity. Other factors that influence regeneration are the extent of damage to the tissue basement membrane and the number of undifferentiated 'reserve' cells, known as *stem cells*, present in the tissue.

Repair processes that result in scar formation begin during the regenerative phase. New connective tissue, called **granulation tissue**, grows into the wound; this consists of collagen fibres, new capillaries and lymphatic vessels, fibroblasts, myofibroblasts and macrophages. Initially, it is bright red in colour, but as it matures it turns pink (see Figure 3.4). The presence of granulation tissue is a key clinical indicator that healing is progressing.

Fibroblasts make *collagen*, a protein associated with tissue structure and strength. At first the collagen is deposited in a haphazard fashion, but then the fibres become cross-linked into an organised lattice within the affected body area (see Figure 3.4). However, if the degree of collagen synthesis in a skin wound is excessive, a raised or thickened scar that grows beyond the wound margin can develop; this is called a **keloid** (see Figure 3.5). Keloids can occur in anyone, but are more common in people

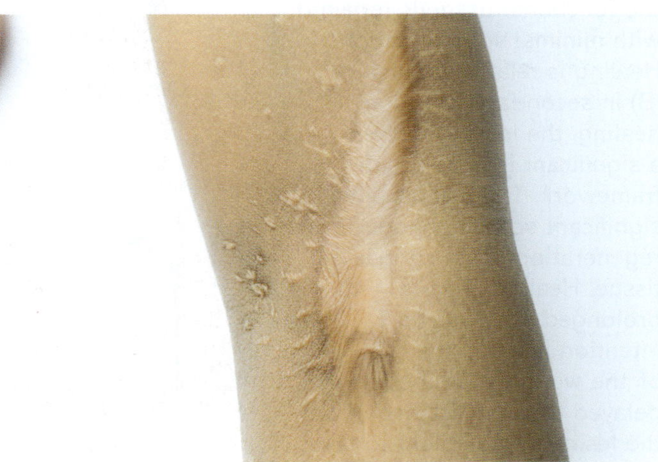

Figure 3.5

A keloid scar

Source: Big Mama/123R.

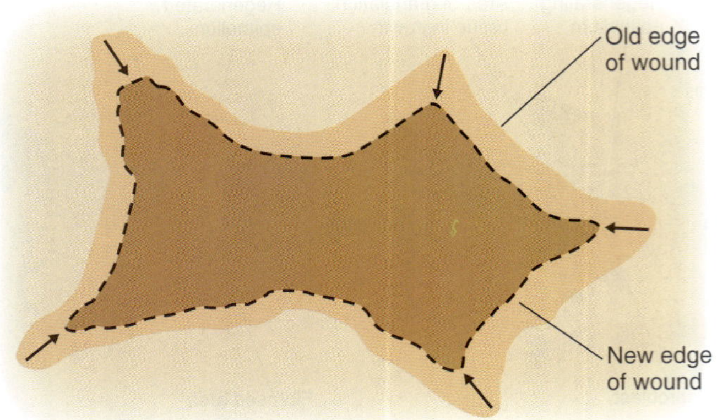

Figure 3.6

Wound contraction

In a wound where a significant amount of the tissue framework has been destroyed, the repair process will involve wound contraction. Myofibroblasts arrange connections between themselves and with neighbouring cells, to draw the edges of the wound closer and reduce its area (the dotted line).

of sub-Saharan African, Chinese or Polynesian origin. A similar condition is a **hypertrophic scar**, which is readily differentiated from a keloid because it remains within the wound margin.

Capillaries and lymphatic vessels bring the nutrients and cofactors necessary for normal healing, such as vitamin C, to the region, and promote appropriate drainage of fluid into the systemic circulation. *Myofibroblasts* are derivatives of fibroblasts that have contractile properties. They arrange connections between themselves and with neighbouring cells, to draw the edges of the wound closer and reduce its area. This is termed **wound contraction** (see Figure 3.6). Wound contraction is an essential part of the repair process. However, an excessive degree of contraction, which can occur when the tissue framework is severely compromised, such as in a large burn, can result in a wound deformity known as a **contracture**.

Macrophages have a key mediator role in the healing and repair process. They are responsible for debridement, and produce factors that facilitate fibroblast entry into the wound and activate collagen production in these cells.

As the scar matures, it will be remodelled to more closely approximate the normal form of the damaged tissue. This *remodelling phase* commences at about two weeks post-injury and can continue for years. The scar becomes avascular and turns white. As this happens, collagen fibre cross-links are dissolved and new cross-links are established to allow realignment of the tissue for greater tensile strength. However, the scarred area never regains the strength of the original tissue.

TYPES OF HEALING

LEARNING OBJECTIVE 9

Compare and contrast first and second intention healing.

Where healing involves minimal tissue loss, such as a cut with a scalpel blade, it is referred to as *primary intention healing* (see Figure 3.7A). This form of healing requires little scar

Figure 3.7

Primary, secondary and tertiary intention healing

(A) In primary intention healing, the lesion involves little loss of tissue. Most of the functional tissue is repaired with minimal scar formation. Healing is relatively quick. (B) In secondary intention healing, the lesion involves a significant loss of tissue framework. There is usually significant scarring and little regeneration of functional tissue. Healing is more prolonged. (C) In tertiary intention healing, the closure of the wound is deliberately delayed to allow drainage from the lesion or treatment to take effect.

Source: Averil Bellert © Sciencopia.

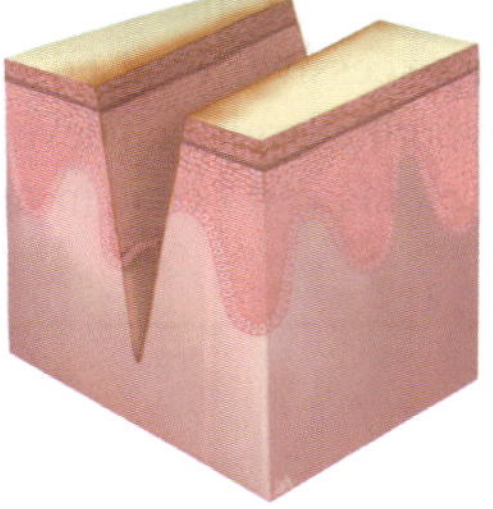

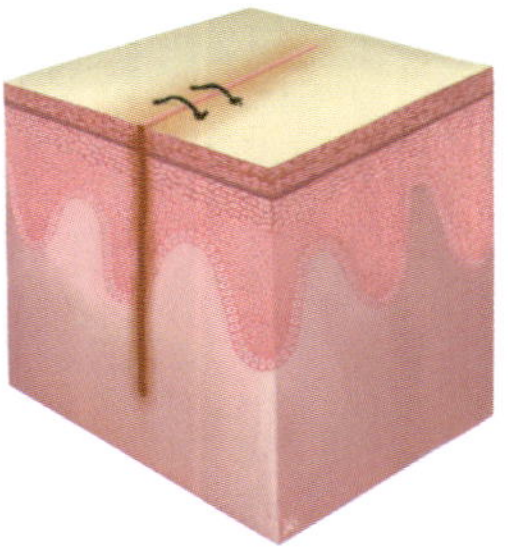

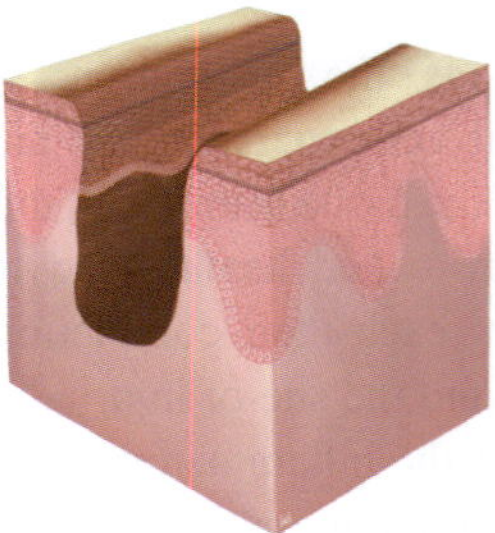

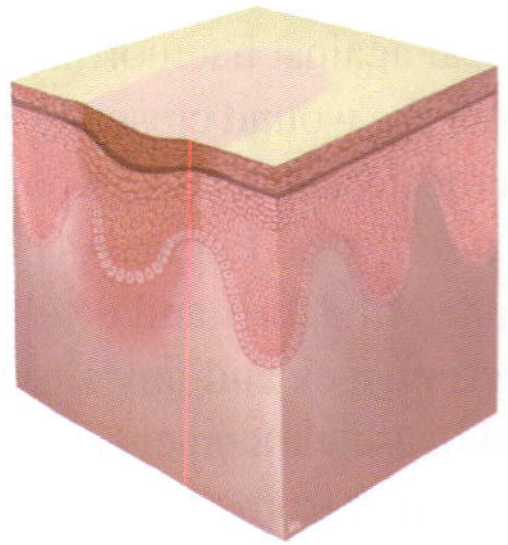

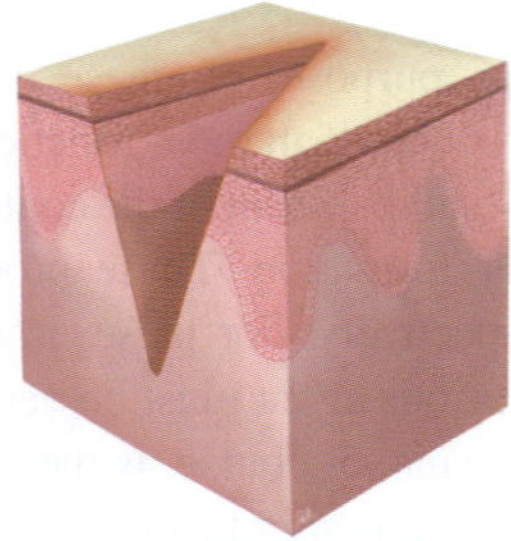

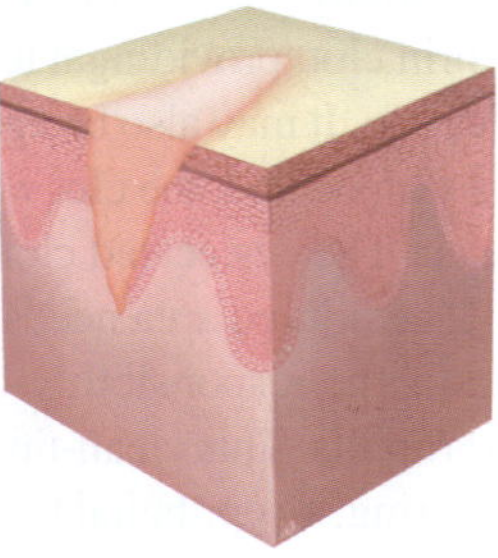

formation and involves minimal loss of functional cells. Healing is relatively quick and uncomplicated. Where a wound occurs that involves a significant loss of tissue framework, such as a skin ulcer or a severe burn, the healing is termed *secondary intention* (see Figure 3.7B). This form of healing is characterised by significant scarring and little parenchymal regeneration. Secondary intention healing is more prolonged, and is often associated with complications such as contractures. When the wound closure is delayed the healing is termed *tertiary intention* (see Figure 3.7C). When a wound becomes infected, terteriary intention healing allows drainage from the lesion or treatment to take effect.

FACTORS AFFECTING HEALING AND REPAIR

LEARNING OBJECTIVE 10

State the key factors that can impede the healing process.

A number of physiological factors can greatly influence the degree and rate of healing and repair. The factors that have been shown to have a significant effect clinically include blood supply to the affected area, the oxygen-carrying capacity of the blood, nutrition (especially glucose, vitamin C and protein availability), infection, drug therapy and movement. Examples of how these factors impede healing are provided in Table 3.4.

Table 3.4 Factors that impede healing processes

Factor	Consequences
Infection	Microorganisms damage cells, induce excessive accumulation of exudate in tissue, prevent the wound edges from adhering, triggering dehiscence (splitting open of the wound edges)
Movement	New tissues lack tensile strength, so movement can disrupt the integrity of the newly forming tissues
Poor nutrient supply	Newly forming tissue has increased metabolic demands—it requires higher levels of glucose, proteins, vitamins and other nutrients to sustain growth
Poor oxygen delivery	Newly forming tissue has increased metabolic demands—it requires higher levels of oxygen
Drug therapy	Anticancer drugs, immunosuppressants and glucocorticoid (cortisol-related) drugs impair healing processes
Poor blood flow	Inadequate blood flow cannot sustain the supply of oxygen and nutrients for growth and facilitate waste removal

INDIGENOUS HEALTH FAST FACTS AND CULTURAL CONSIDERATIONS

FAST FACTS

- *Aboriginal and/or Torres Strait Islander peoples are more likely than non-Indigenous Australians to experience conditions of infection or inflammation: otitis media (3.3:1), tuberculosis (5.5:1) and hepatitis C (3.6:1), and sexually transmitted infections, including syphilis (8:1), gonorrhoea (7:1, and 30:1 in remote areas).*
- *Māori and Pacific Islands New Zealanders are more likely than European New Zealanders to experience conditions of infection or inflammation: meningitis (Māori–2.6:1; Pacific Islands people–2.2:1), acute rheumatic fever hospitalisations (Māori–22 times more likely; Pacific Islands people–50 times more likely than European New Zealanders).*

CULTURAL CONSIDERATIONS

- *Sexual health education, prevention and management is complicated in Aboriginal and Torres Strait Islander communities, as it is often seen as shameful to seek help for such medical matters. Other difficulties can arise from the fact that the Aboriginal and Torres Strait Islander Health Worker is likely to be family or, in the case of remote locations, they may, because of cultural restrictions, not be permitted to talk to the affected person.*
- *As a result of four syphilis outbreaks among Aboriginal and Torres Strait Islander peoples in rural and remote Australia in recent years (Queensland in 2011, Northern Territory in 2013, Western Australia in 2014 and South Australia in 2016), the Communicable Disease Network of Australia has in place the Multijurisdictional Syphilis Outbreak Group (MJSO) to monitor and guide actions to further address barriers and issues resulting in outbreak response and control. Infection prevention and control remains an area of extreme disparity between Aboriginal and Torres Strait Islander Australians and non-Indigenous Australians, especially in the 15–34-year-old age bracket.*
- *Notwithstanding shame, other barriers that may contribute to inadequate sexual health services may be related to geographical limitations on healthcare, communication styles or abilities, or insufficient numbers of Aboriginal and Torres Strait Islander Health Workers to assist with culturally appropriate health promotion and education activities.*

Sources: Data from Australian Indigenous HealthInfoNet (2022); Australian Institute of Health and Welfare (2022); Bennett et al. (2021); Laird & Schultz (2021); New Zealand Ministry of Health (2022).

CHILDREN AND ADOLESCENTS

- Teenagers tend to experience acne, and, as a result of severe inflammation and delayed healing, acne scars can form. Using topical antiseptic and anti-inflammatory agents can reduce the risk of scarring associated with acne.
- Children scar more than adults because of the rapid collagen, fibroblast and elastin deposition, and epidermal immaturity results in quicker wound closure.

OLDER ADULTS

- As people age, the quality and volume of collagen available for rapid wound healing is reduced. Delayed healing and increased scar formation may occur as an adult ages.
- Older adults are at an increased risk of dehiscence as a result of poor-quality wound healing.

KEY CLINICAL ISSUES

- Following trauma or surgery, excessive inflammation can result in limb-threatening neurovascular compromise. Undertake frequent neurovascular assessment distal to the site of injury. During assessment, observe for changes in colour, warmth, movement and sensation.
- Appropriate positioning to promote venous return and lymphatic drainage will assist in reducing oedema.
- Oedema can result in challenges to skin integrity. Ensure that pressure area care is undertaken frequently in those with excessive inflammation.
- Use of non-steroidal anti-inflammatory drugs (NSAIDs) in the control of inflammation can be beneficial; however, NSAID therapy can also induce gastric ulcers, photosensitivity and kidney disease, depending on the dose and the duration of treatment. Use of NSAIDs in certain groups can be dangerous. Individuals with asthma have an increased risk of serious adverse reactions, and the use of aspirin in children is associated with Reye's syndrome.

CHAPTER REVIEW

- The *purpose of inflammation* is to neutralise an agent of injury and stop further damage. It also prepares the site of injury for healing.
- The *cardinal signs* of inflammation are swelling, redness, warmth, pain and loss of function. The suffix representing an inflammatory condition is *-itis*.
- A range of chemicals released into the site of tissue injury mediate the induction and magnitude of the process of inflammation. The key *pro-inflammatory chemical mediators* are prostaglandins, histamine, leukotrienes, kinins, cytokines, platelet-activating factor, thromboxanes, nitric oxide and neuropeptides.
- The *vascular phase* of acute inflammation comprises tissue vasodilation and increased capillary permeability. Three important *cascading reactions* contribute to the inflammatory response: the complement system, coagulation and the kinin–kallikrein system.
- The *cellular phase* involves the movement of *immune cells* to the site of the inflammation in order to neutralise the agent of injury and prepare the site for healing. The phagocytic cells, monocytes/macrophages and neutrophils play a key role in this phase.
- The fluid that accumulates in the site of inflammation is called an *exudate*. The four main types of exudate are: serous, fibrinous, purulent and haemorrhagic.
- *Chronic inflammation* is defined as the persistence of the response for more than two weeks. Chronic inflammation can be distinctly different from the acute response. When this occurs, neutrophils die out and lymphocytes can infiltrate the site along with monocyte/macrophages—these become the dominant cell types in the site. By this stage, there is little evidence of the vascular phase of the acute inflammatory response.
- The distinction between *acute and chronic inflammation* can be simplistic and arbitrary. In inflammation, a *complex interplay between states* occurs, which means that aspects of acute inflammation can be present during chronic states, and significant cell damage is not limited to only the chronic form.
- *Chronic inflammatory processes* may damage parenchymal cells, which are replaced by fibrous connective tissue produced by local fibroblasts. This fibrosis can lead to significant scarring and deformity. Walled-off areas within the site of chronic inflammation that are calcified and hard are called *granulomas*. Cells within a granuloma tend to undergo liquefactive necrosis, leaving a hollowed-out structure.
- *SARS-CoV-2 coronavirus* is the causative agent in COVID-19 infection. The virus can trigger a hyperinflammatory cytokine storm, which leads to tissue and organ damage. In 'long COVID' the inflammatory response persists.
- *Healing and repair processes* restore the lost parenchyma and re-establish the continuity of the tissue framework through scar formation. Healing and repair processes comprise debridement, epithelialisation, regeneration of parenchyma, formation of granulation tissue and wound contraction.
- *Primary intention* healing involves minimal loss of functional cells. Healing is relatively quick and uncomplicated. *Second intention* healing involves a significant loss of tissue framework and is characterised by significant scarring and little parenchymal regeneration. Secondary intention healing is more prolonged, and is often associated with complications such as contractures. *Tertiary intention* healing is when the wound closure is delayed to allow drainage or treatment effects to occur.
- A number of factors can greatly influence the *degree and rate of healing*. These include blood supply to the affected area, the oxygen-carrying capacity of the blood, nutrition (especially glucose, vitamin C and protein availability), infection, drug therapy and movement.

REVIEW QUESTIONS

1. Briefly outline the pathophysiological processes underlying each of the following cardinal signs of inflammation:
   - a swelling
   - b pain
   - c increased warmth
2. Determine the body tissue affected in the following inflammatory conditions (*Note:* You may have to do some research):
   - a laryngitis
   - b cellulitis
   - c blepharitis
   - d rhinitis
3. What are the roles for each of the following pro-inflammatory chemical mediators?
   - a histamine
   - b cytokines
   - c nitric oxide
   - d leukotrienes
4. In what ways does the complement system contribute to inflammation?
5. Which type of exudate is particularly associated with the following?
   - a abscesses
   - b blisters
   - c adhesions
6. In what ways is it possible to differentiate between acute and chronic inflammation?
7. Arrange the following in the correct sequence for the healing and repair processes:

   scar formation — debridement

   wound contraction — regeneration

   epithelialisation
8. Compare and contrast primary, secondary and tertiary intention healing.
9. How can movement and poor blood flow affect healing?

HEALTH PROFESSIONAL CONNECTIONS

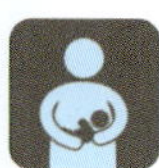

Midwives Intrauterine inflammation can occur as a result of microbial invasion of the amniotic cavity (MIAC). As a result, the risk of preterm labour is increased, and therefore issues relating to lung immaturity are also amplified. Premature rupture of membranes increases the risk of MIAC, and therefore preterm labour. These women are more likely to develop chorioamnionitis. The presence of microbes (or colonisation) alone will not necessarily result in poorer clinical outcomes; however, a fetal inflammatory response may occur, which will influence gestation time and premature delivery. Microbial contamination can occur by ascending through the cervix or, less commonly, as a haematogenous dissemination, or from instrumentation from invasive procedures such as amniocentesis. Midwives should be familiar with the signs of MIAC, and ensure that they seek assistance from other members of the healthcare team to ensure a positive outcome.

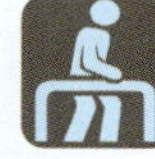

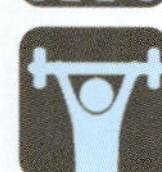

Physiotherapists/Exercise scientists Exercise can reduce C-reactive protein and inflammatory cytokines. It is well established that exercise can have anti-inflammatory effects; however, some important considerations—such as the type, duration and intensity of the exercise—can influence this effect. Strenuous exercise can induce pro-inflammatory mediators as well as anti-inflammatory cytokines. It is important to understand the influence of short-term strenuous exercise and also prolonged exercise on the immune system and the inflammatory response. Exercise professionals assisting people with inflammatory disorders must ensure that the individual effects of the disease process are considered when developing an exercise or rehabilitation program.

All allied professionals Inflammation can be a sign of infection. It is important that when working with a person, all observations of inflammation are reported to other members of the healthcare team so that further investigation and management can be instituted. Early treatment will often result in a less serious clinical outcome, reducing morbidity and mortality risks. Open communication with all members of the healthcare team will result in the provision of a better service.

CASE STUDY

Mrs Linda Carter is a 35-year-old woman (UR number 654238). She has been admitted for management of cellulitis on her right calf. She suspects the original insult was a spider bite, although she never saw the spider. However, she did see two small puncture marks when she first noticed the wound. Over the next few days, the site became red and inflamed, a red line began tracking up the inside of her right thigh, and she developed bilateral inguinal lymphadenopathy. Her observations were as follows:

Temperature	Heart rate	Respiration rate	Blood pressure	SpO_2
38°C	80	20	116/76	98% (RA*)

* RA = room air.

Mrs Carter was commenced on intravenous antimicrobials, paracetamol q6h PRN and daily dressings as necessary. Although no pus was observed, a swab was taken of the lesion. Her admission pathology results have returned as follows:

MICROBIOLOGY

Patient location:	Ward 3	**UR:**	654238	
Consultant:	Smith	**NAME:**	Carter	
		Given name:	Linda	**Sex:** F
		DOB:	02/02/XX	**Age:** 35

Time collected	09:27	**Organisms**	**1.** *S. epidermidis* colonisation (mild)
Date collected	XX/XX	**Isolated**	**2.**
Year	XXXX		
Lab #	434563455		

Specimen site	Swab from swelling on R) leg	**Antimicrobial sensitivities S = Sensitive R = Resistant**					
		Organism	1	2	**Organism**	1	2
Leukocytes	+ +	Ampicillin	R		Flucloxacillin		
Erythrocytes	+	Amoxicillin	R		Gentamycin	S	
Proteins	+	Cefotaxime	R		Rifampicin	S	
		Ceftriaxone	R		Sodium fusidate		
		Cephalothin			Ticarcillin	S	
		Chloramphenicol			Timentin	S	
		Cotrimoxazole			Trimethoprim	R	
		Erythromycin			Vancomycin	S	

Gram stain	**Gram negative**	–
	Gram positive	✔
	Bacilli	–
	Cocci	✔
	Other	–

HAEMATOLOGY

Patient location:	Ward 3	**UR:**	654238		
Consultant:	Smith	**NAME:**	Carter		
		Given name:	Linda	**Sex:**	F
		DOB:	02/02/XX	**Age:**	35

Time collected	09:35
Date collected	XX/XX
Year	XXXX
Lab #	42937428

FULL BLOOD COUNT		UNITS	REFERENCE RANGE
Haemoglobin	132	g/L	115–160
White cell count	13.6	$\times 10^9$/L	4.0–11.0
Platelets	320	$\times 10^9$/L	140–400
Haematocrit	0.41	L/L	0.33–0.47
Red cell count	4.23	$\times 10^{12}$/L	3.80–5.20
Reticulocyte count	0.8	%	0.2–2.0
MCV	92	fL	80–100
Neutrophils	8.43	$\times 10^9$/L	2.00–8.00
Lymphocytes	2.43	$\times 10^9$/L	1.00–4.00
Monocytes	0.42	$\times 10^9$/L	0.10–1.00
Eosinophils	0.32	$\times 10^9$/L	$<$ 0.60
Basophils	0.13	$\times 10^9$/L	$<$ 0.20
ESR	15	mm/h	$<$ 12

BIOCHEMISTRY

Patient location:	Ward 3	**UR:**	654238		
Consultant:	Smith	**NAME:**	Carter		
		Given name:	Linda	**Sex:**	F
		DOB:	02/02/XX	**Age:**	35

Time collected	09:35
Date collected	XX/XX
Year	XXXX
Lab #	456345356

ELECTROLYTES		UNITS	REFERENCE RANGE
Sodium	138	mmol/L	135–145
Potassium	4.3	mmol/L	3.5–5.2
Chloride	105	mmol/L	95–110
Bicarbonate	25	mmol/L	22–32
Glucose	4.7	mmol/L	3.5–5.4

CRITICAL THINKING

1. Mrs Carter thinks that a spider bite may have caused the cellulitis. What is the physiological mechanism leading to the inflammation of Mrs Carter's leg tissue? Describe what is occurring at a cellular level to cause Mrs Carter's discomfort.
2. Given your knowledge of the immune system's ability to cope with challenges, what immediate responses and what delayed responses would occur to 'fight' this attack? Is this different from an attack as a result of a pathogen?
3. Mrs Carter has developed bilateral swollen lymph glands in the groin (bilateral inguinal lymphadenopathy). Why is it occurring?
4. The pathology results have returned. What does the full blood count suggest is occurring? What values did you observe to come to this conclusion?
5. What interventions are required to assist Mrs Carter with her cellulitis? Identify all of the necessary interventions (including the ones stated in the case study), and explain the mechanism of each intervention listed.

BIBLIOGRAPHY

Anka, A.U., Tahir, M.I., Abubakar, S.D., Alsabbagh, M., Zian, Z., Hamedifar, H.,... Azizi, G. (2020). Coronavirus disease 2019 (COVID-19): an overview of the immunopathology, serological diagnosis and management. *Scandinavian Journal of Immunology* 93(4):e12998. https://doi.org/10.1111/sji.12998.

Australian Health Ministers' Advisory Council's National and Aboriginal and Torres Strait Islander Health Standing Committee (2017). *Cultural respect framework 2016–2026: for Aboriginal and Torres Strait Islander health—a national approach to building a culturally respectful health system.* Canberra: Australian Government Department of Health. https://nacchocommunique.files.wordpress.com/2016/12/cultural_respect_framework_1december2016_1.pdf.

Australian Indigenous Health*InfoNet* (2022). *Overview of Aboriginal and Torres Strait Islander health status, 2021.* Perth, WA: Australian Indigenous Health*Info*Net. https://healthinfonet.ecu.edu.au/learn/health-facts/overview-aboriginal-torres-strait-islander-health-status.

Australian Institute of Health and Welfare (2021). *Australian Burden of Disease Study: impact and causes of illness and death in Australia 2018.* Australian Burden of Disease Study series No. 23. Cat No. BOD 29. Canberra: AIHW. http://www.aihw.gov.au/reports/burden-of-disease/abds-impact-and-causes-of-illness-and-death-in-aus/summarywww.aihw.gov.au.

Australian Institute of Health and Welfare (2022). *Australia's health, 2022.* Australia's Health series No. 15. Cat. No. AUS 199. Canberra: AIHW. https://www.aihw.gov.au/reports-data/australias-health.

Bauldoff, G., Gubrud-Howe, P.M., Carno, M.-A., Levett-Jones, T., Hales, M., Berry, K.,... Stanley, D. (2020). *LeMone and Burke's medical–surgical nursing: critical thinking for person-centred care* (4th [Australian] edn). Sydney: Pearson Australia.

Bennett, J., Zhang, J., Leung, W., Jack, S., Oliver, J., Webb, R.,... Baker, M.G. (2021). Rising ethnic inequalities in acute rheumatic fever and rheumatic heart disease, New Zealand, 2000–2018. *Emerging Infectious Diseases* 27(1):36–46. https://doi.org/10.3201/eid2701.191791.

Best, O. & Fredericks, B. (2021). *Yatdjuligin: Aboriginal and Torres Strait Islander nursing and midwifery care* (3rd edn). Port Melbourne, VIC: Cambridge University Press.

Cerqueira, É., Marinho, D.A., Neiva, H.P. & Lourenço, O. (2020). Inflammatory effects of high and moderate intensity exercise—a systematic review. *Frontiers in Physiology* 10:1550. https://doi.org/10.3389/fphys.2019.01550.

Department of Health (2022). *National syphilis surveillance quarterly report: Quarter 1: 1 January – 31 March 2022.* Canberra: Department of Health. https://www.health.gov.au/sites/default/files/documents/2022/10/national-syphilis-surveillance-quarterly-report-jan-to-mar-2022.pdf.

Dykov, I., Hällqvist, J., Gilmour, K.C., Grandjean, L., Mills, K. & Heywood, W.E. (2021). 'The long tail of Covid-19'—the detection of a prolonged inflammatory response after a SARS-CoV-2 infection in asymptomatic and mildly affected patients. *F1000Research* 9:1349. https://doi.org/10.12688/f1000research.27287.2.

Fajgenbaum, D.C. & June, C.H. (2020). Cytokine storm. *New England Journal of Medicine* 383(23):2255–73. https://doi.org/10.1056/NEJMra2026131.

Lahra, M.M., Hogan, T.R., Shoushtari, M., Armstrong, B.H., for the National Neisseria Network, Australia (2021). Australian Gonococcal Surveillance Programme annual report, 2020. *Communicable Diseases Intelligence* 45. https://doi.org/10.33321/cdi.2021.45.58.

Laird, P. & Schultz, A. (2021). Tuberculosis in Australia's Top End First Nations highlights health and life expectancy gaps: a call to arms. *The Lancet Regional Health—Western Pacific* 15:100253. https://doi.org/10.1016/j.lanwpc.2021.100253.

Marieb, E.N. & Hoehn, K. (2019). *Human anatomy and physiology* (11th edn). San Francisco, CA: Pearson Benjamin Cummings.

New Zealand Ministry of Health (2021). *Annual update of key results 2020/2021: New Zealand Health Survey.* Wellington: Ministry of Health. https://www.health.govt.nz/publication/annual-update-key-results-2020-21-new-zealand-health-surveyhttp://www.health.govt.

New Zealand Ministry of Health (2022). *Health and independence report 2020: the Director-General of Health's annual report on the state of public health.* Wellington: Ministry of Health. https://www.health.govt.nz/publication/health-and-independence-report-2020.

Genetic disorders

4

LEARNING OBJECTIVES

After completing this chapter, you should be able to:

1. Differentiate between autosomal and X-linked inheritance.
2. Differentiate between recessive and dominant inheritance.
3. Explain the significance and the potential conditions resulting from monosomy and trisomy.
4. Differentiate between diploid and triploid.
5. Explain what occurs in a reciprocal translocation, and why this might contribute to cancer formation.
6. Distinguish between threshold traits and traits with variable penetrance.
7. Describe multifactorial inheritance, and outline its implications.
8. Briefly describe the frequency, development and consequence of selected common congenital malformations.

WHAT YOU SHOULD KNOW BEFORE YOU START THIS CHAPTER

Can you describe the basic structure of DNA?

Can you describe meiosis and mitosis, and contrast their processes?

What are the principles of transcription and translation required for protein synthesis?

KEY TERMS

Aneuploidy
Autosomal
Autosomes
Carrier
Complete lethal gene
Congenital malformations
Deletion
Diploid
Dominant inheritance
Duplication
Fragile chromosomal site
Genotype
Heterozygous
Monosomy
Mosaic
Multifactorial inheritance
Penetrance
Phenotype
Polygene traits
Polyploidy
Recessive inheritance
Reciprocal translocation
Sex chromosomes
Sublethal gene
Triploidy
Trisomy
X-linked

Introduction

Even before the availability of technology to rapidly sequence small amounts of *DNA (deoxyribonucleic acid)*, a variety of conditions were recognised as inherited and were often attributed to a gene, despite not knowing the location of that gene and its role. Once it was possible to visualise DNA in the form of chromosomes, it was possible to demonstrate that other conditions arose as the consequence of changes to, addition of or loss of chromosomes. Despite all of our technological advances, however, we still have difficulty understanding the roles of most genes within our genome in normal development and physiology, to say nothing of their contribution to the development of genetic disorders. Therefore, it is important to understand the inheritance of a condition so that the affected people and their families can be counselled about the risk of receiving the altered gene/s themselves, and the risks to any potential offspring.

Principles of genetic inheritance

With the exception of the gametes (i.e. sperm and egg cells), all of the cells of the body have 23 pairs of chromosomes, 22 of which are referred to as **autosomes**, and one pair representing the **sex chromosomes** (see Figure 4.1). The genetic instructions within this set of chromosomes represents the **genotype**, the genetic 'blueprint' required to create and maintain the human organism. By contrast, gametes have half the number of chromosomes, with one representative of each pair. When two gametes merge to form the cell that will become the embryo, the full set of 23 pairs of chromosomes is restored. Inherited conditions can arise from a change to the chromosomes in part or as a whole, or to individual genes on a specific chromosome. If a gene is located on an autosome, it is said to have **autosomal** inheritance. By contrast, if the gene is on the X chromosome, it is considered **X-linked**. Although small, the Y chromosome does carry genes, many with homology to the X chromosome; mutations to the Y-exclusive genes affect men only. **Aneuploidy** is when there is an abnormal number of chromosomes, generally either one too many or one too few, whereas **polyploidy** describes a situation in which there is a full additional set of chromosomes. Chromosomes can undergo structural changes, where parts are added, deleted, duplicated or swapped, with the resulting change leading to a disease state.

The majority of single-gene disorders are due to point mutations: the replacement of a single base pair with another that can change the identity of an amino acid, create a stop codon or create a new start codon. These changes can: inactivate a gene so that there is no protein product; stop transcription of the gene too soon, so that a truncated protein is produced; prolong transcription to create a protein that is too large and cannot function properly; increase the activity of, or add function to, a protein; or create a protein that interferes with the function of the normal protein if only one allele (second gene copy) is affected. Chromosomal abnormalities involve a portion of a chromosome, or even entire chromosomes, and therefore affect multiple genes, leading to more complex changes in the individual.

One aspect of the manifestations of genetic disorders that bears special mention is the effect of the condition on the ability of the affected individual to have offspring. A gene or chromosomal defect that is fatal to an individual before they reach reproductive age is referred to as a **complete lethal gene** or defect. By contrast, a gene or chromosomal defect that is fatal after the person achieves reproductive age, and allows that individual to reproduce, is referred to as a **sublethal gene** or defect.

We will examine these various changes to individual genes or to chromosomes, with specific examples of each. In addition, we will discuss the probability of offspring inheriting the condition from an affected parent.

Figure 4.1

Karyotype of the 23 pairs of human chromosomes

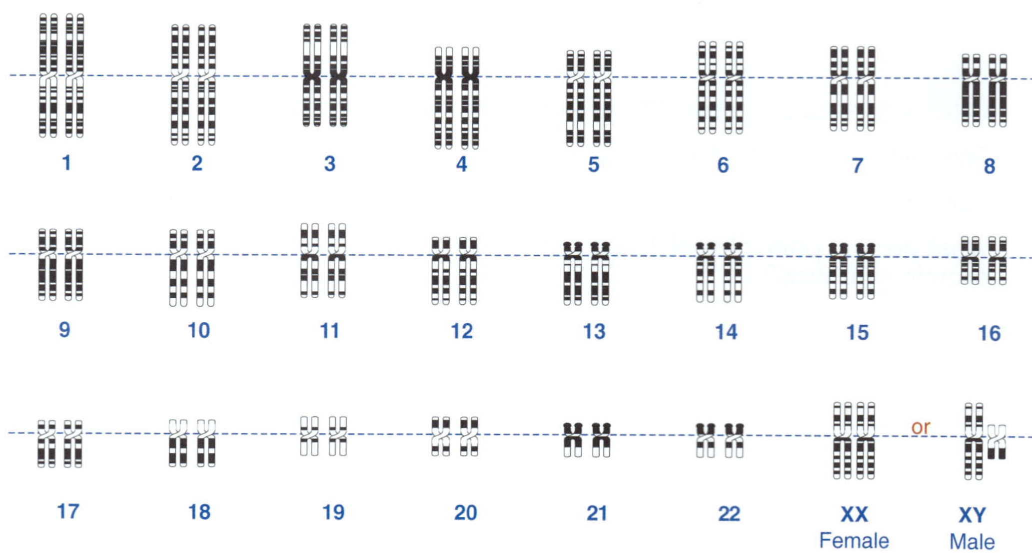

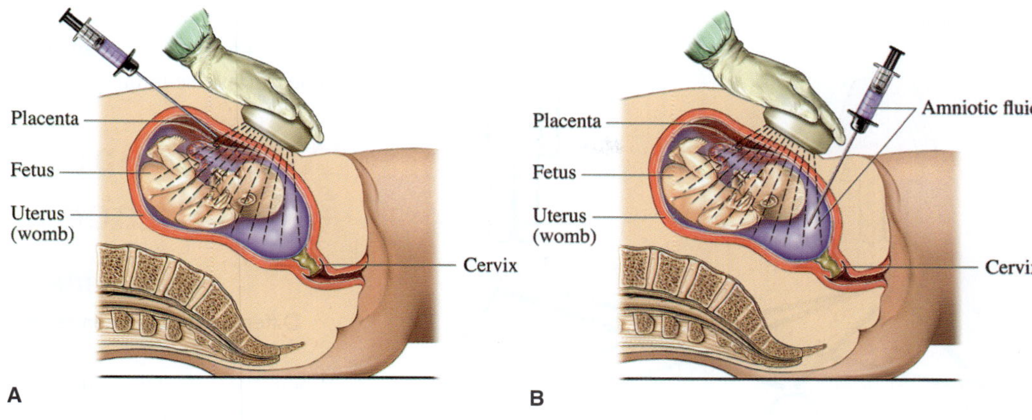

Figure 4.2

In-utero genetic testing

(A) Chorionic villus sampling.
(B) Amniocentesis.

Source: © Nucleus Medical Media/ Alamy Stock Photo.

Clinical diagnosis

The diagnosis of a genetic disorder in an affected person can be made on the basis of a presentation of a characteristic set of clinical manifestations, through the examination of the number and appearance of the set of chromosomes obtained from a sample body cell (called a *karyotype*), and, if possible, a molecular analysis of a recognisable gene mutation.

Gene mutations have been assessed using either non-invasive (sequencing fetal DNA that circulates in a pregnant woman's blood) or invasively through fetal DNA obtained by amniocentesis, chorionic villi sampling or cord blood. The oldest and most common protocol is Sanger sequencing technique. Although this formerly cutting-edge technology has guided many decisions in healthcare, it is slow and limited in scope. Now, as knowledge and technology are advancing, next-generation sequencing (NGS) techniques are helping to provide information on diagnosis, prognosis, molecular targets for treatment, and reproductive risks associated with genetic disorders.

The two types of NGS genetic testing becoming more prevalent are whole exome (WES) and whole genome sequencing (WGS). Whole WES sequences approximately 1% of a person's genome (as most disease-causing mutations occur in the exon—the sections which code for proteins). WGS determines the complete DNA sequence of the individual and detects any variation in a person's genome (because some gene activity outside of the exome can lead to genetic disorders).

Mapping the incidence of a particular genetic condition within a person's family over a number of generations (i.e. determining a disease pedigree) can be very useful in assessing risk and in making informed decisions about disease management, not only for living family members but also for potential offspring. This is the principal aim of genetic counselling. The risk is usually calculated as a probability of having the disorder or not, or, in case of single-gene mutations, remaining unaffected but being a **carrier**. The matrix for calculating the risks in single-gene disorders of classical Mendelian inheritance, such as autosomal dominant or recessive conditions, is known as a *Punnett square*.

In-utero genetic testing of offspring can be performed in situations where an increased risk of abnormality is predictable (e.g. familial history or ageing persons of child-bearing capacity). Testing the fetus can be undertaken through chorionic villus sampling or amniocentesis. *Chorionic villus sampling (CVS)* is when placental tissue is biopsied with a long needle that is inserted with the assistance of ultrasound equipment (see Figure 4.2A). The tissue can then be subjected to testing for genetic anomalies. *Amniocentesis* involves the removal of amniotic fluid contained within the amniotic sac that surrounds the fetus (see Figure 4.2B). This fluid can then be tested for genetic anomalies. It is also often undertaken with the assistance of ultrasound equipment to reduce the risk to the fetus.

Genetic testing can also be performed by sampling blood, urine, saliva, tissue or hair from the individual. This information may be used to diagnose a genetic anomaly, to inform individuals of their 'carrier' status, or to identify whether a future disease may develop.

Autosomal dominant inheritance

LEARNING OBJECTIVE 1

Differentiate between autosomal and X-linked inheritance.

When a change to a gene or genes on an autosome overwhelms the influence of the comparable gene or region on its autosomal pair (allele), it is referred to as a *dominant trait* and will be considered to have autosomal **dominant inheritance**. In this case, the affected parent is generally **heterozygous** for the trait, as only one chromosome is required to confer the condition. Therefore, their offspring have a 50% chance of inheriting the affected chromosome (see Figure 4.3). Depending on the gene involved, the individual might show the disorder or disease from infancy, or the condition might manifest later in life. Two excellent examples that show this contrast are achondroplasia and Huntington's chorea.

Achondroplasia, which is diagnosed in infancy through physical examination, is the most common form of skeletal dysplasia. It results from a 'gain-of-function' point mutation

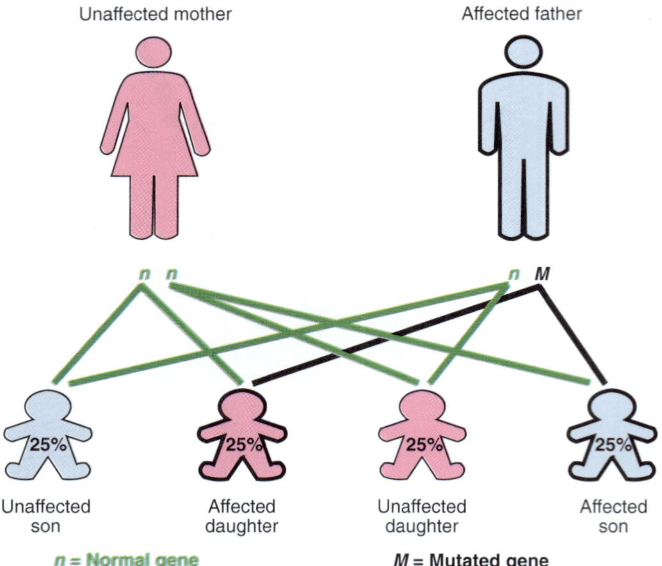

Figure 4.3

Autosomal dominant inheritance

(see the chapter 'Neoplasia') in the fibroblast growth factor receptor 3 gene, resulting in a new function, or a change in function, in the receptor when the gene is expressed. In this disorder, changes to cartilage and bone lead to limited growth of the bones of the arms and legs, but a slightly larger head, midface hypoplasia and inward curvature of the lumbar spine. However, cognitive development is completely normal, and these individuals have no problem with fertility. If two individuals with achondroplasia have children, their offspring have a 75% chance of inheriting the mutant gene, and therefore having achondroplasia themselves, and a 25% chance of inheriting two normal versions of the gene, assuming each parent is heterozygous for the fibroblast growth factor 3 receptor gene.

Huntington's chorea (see the chapter 'Neurodegenerative disorders' for a full discussion) is a neurodegenerative disorder marked by impulsive behaviour, impaired memory, mood changes, sudden involuntary jerky, writhing movements that will worsen over time, and eventually dementia and death. Symptoms do not manifest until the individual is between 40 and 60 years of age, generally well after they have had children, and therefore this condition is classed as sublethal. The gene defect involves increased numbers of tandem repeats of the CAG trinucleotide within the huntingtin protein gene, with the number of repeats directly proportional to the severity of the disease. The hallmark of the disease is the death of neurons within the brain, and it is assumed that a threshold level of neuronal destruction is required before symptoms manifest. Generally, affected individuals are heterozygous for the huntingtin gene mutation, so their children will have a 50% chance of inheriting the affected gene and developing the disorder. The affected offspring then have a 50% chance of passing their affected gene on to their own children. Interestingly, there is a degree of variability in the stability of the CAG repeat region, and therefore the disease can worsen over generations due to an accumulation of additional CAG repeats.

Autosomal recessive inheritance

LEARNING OBJECTIVE 2

Differentiate between recessive and dominant inheritance.

When the affected gene is found on an autosome and two copies of the affected gene are required to have the disease or disorder, the condition is said to have autosomal **recessive inheritance**. A child of an affected individual will automatically receive the mutated gene from this parent, but will not inherit the condition unless a second altered gene is inherited from the unaffected parent. If the unaffected parent has one affected gene and one normal gene, they are said to be a carrier for that trait (see Figure 4.4). Like autosomal dominant disorders, the manifestation of an autosomal recessive disorder can occur early in life or can be delayed until much later. Two examples of this disparity are Tay–Sachs disease and Friedreich's ataxia.

Tay–Sachs disease is common within the Ashkenazi Jewish population, and so individuals in this population are routinely tested in certain countries for carrier status before they have children. This condition is marked by a defect in metabolism that leads to the accumulation of lipids that are not broken down. Neurons and microglia become distorted and swollen, with a granular appearance. Cerebral white matter degenerates and the cerebral cortex atrophies. This deterioration of the brain is marked by seizures, muscle rigidity and blindness. Onset of

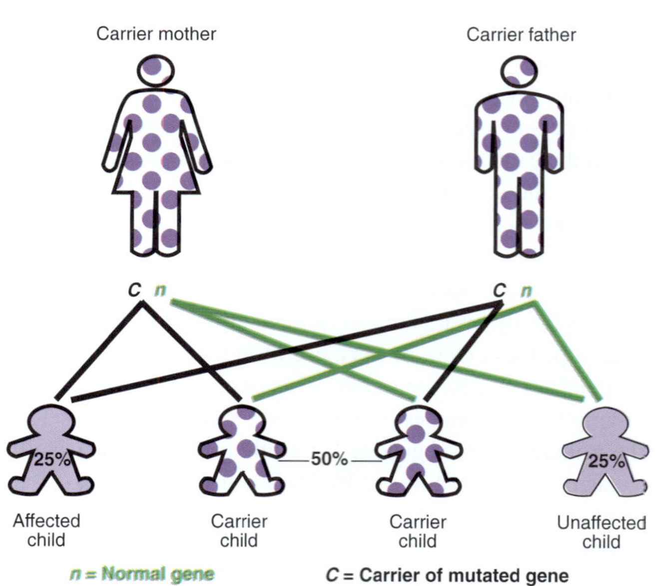

Figure 4.4

Autosomal recessive inheritance

symptoms begins at approximately 3–6 months of age, with death between 2 and 5 years of age; therefore, it represents an example of a complete lethal disorder.

Friedreich's ataxia is a rare neurodegenerative condition that causes adolescent- and adult-onset disability due to muscle weakness and a loss of coordination in the arms and legs. Those affected also develop visual and hearing deficits, dysarthria, scoliosis, diabetes mellitus and hypertrophic cardiomyopathy. These people generally die relatively young, at an average age of 37 years, due to the consequences of the cardiomyopathy and respiratory difficulties. The age of onset is late childhood or early adolescence, and is caused by an expanded trinucleotide repeat (GAA) mutation in the frataxin gene (FXN), which codes for a mitochondrial protein that regulates iron transport and respiration.

X-linked inheritance

X-linked inheritance occurs when the gene responsible for the disorder is carried on the X chromosome. It can be inherited as a dominant or a recessive trait, although this really only applies to female offspring; all X-linked disorders in male offspring are effectively dominant since they only have a single X chromosome (see Figure 4.5). The best-known X-linked disorder is *haemophilia A*, also known as 'classic' haemophilia, which results from the absence of clotting factor VIII. *Haemophilia B*, also known as *Christmas disease*, is inherited as an X-linked recessive disorder as well, but in this case the deficiency is in factor IX. By contrast, the other two bleeding disorders in this group—*haemophilia C* and *von Willebrand disease*—are autosomal recessive and autosomal dominant, respectively. Until the advent of blood donations and, more specifically, the transfusion of clotting factors, individuals with haemophilia generally did not live long enough to have children. Now, however, these individuals do live long enough to have children, meaning that all female children of a father with haemophilia A or B will be carriers of the condition, and their sons will then have a 50% chance of having haemophilia. A woman can develop haemophilia A or B if she has an affected father and a mother who is a carrier. This occurrence is relatively rare, but is more likely now that affected men are having children.

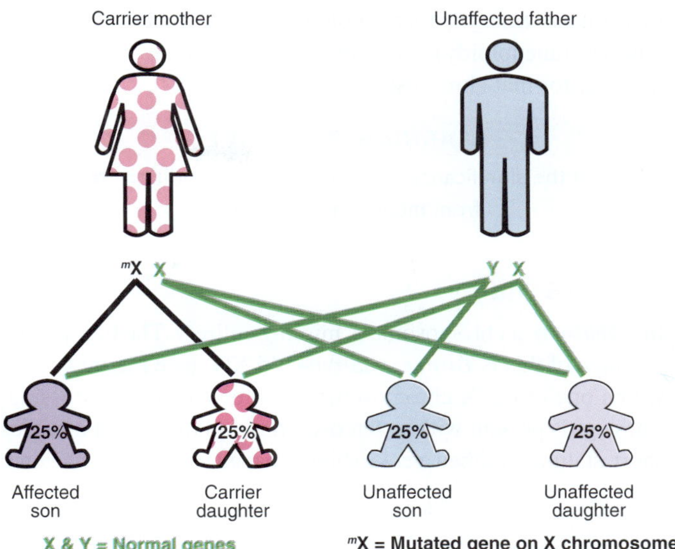

Figure 4.5
X-linked recessive inheritance

Chromosomal abnormalities

Chromosomal abnormalities can result from an additional chromosome, the loss of a chromosome or a change in a chromosome. In rare instances, they will arise due to a full set of additional chromosomes (known as **triploidy**). Generally, the addition or loss of a chromosome results from a non-disjunction event during the formation of gametes. In non-disjunction, the chromosomes do not separate evenly into the two forming gametes, which means that one gamete has two copies of a given chromosome whereas the other gamete has no copy of that chromosome (see Figure 4.6). When this gamete joins

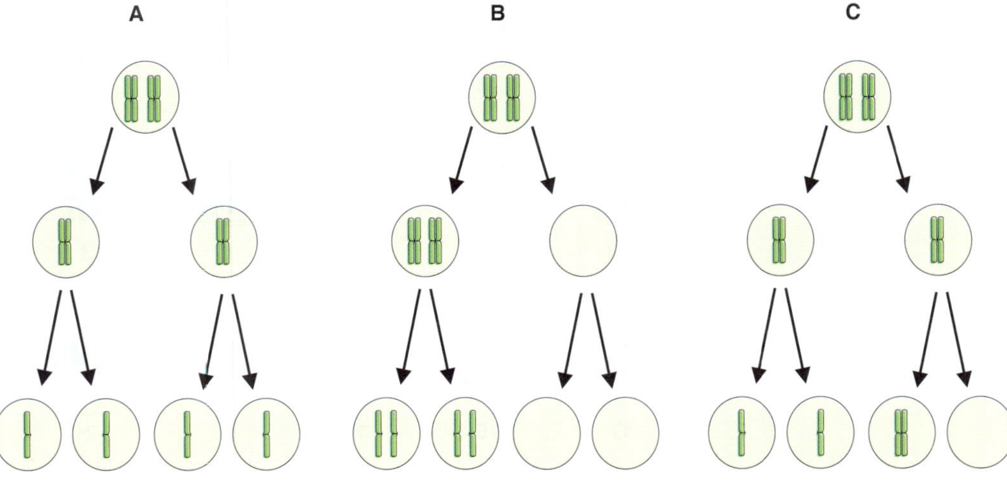

Figure 4.6
The process of non-disjunction during meiosis

(A) Normal meiosis.

(B) Non-disjunction in meiosis I.

(C) Non-disjunction in meiosis II.

to form an embryo, there will be an abnormal chromosome number (aneuploidy), and this will lead to a characteristic disorder for that chromosome.

LEARNING OBJECTIVE 3

Explain the significance and the potential conditions resulting from monosomy and trisomy.

MONOSOMY

In **monosomy**, a chromosome is missing entirely. The best known example of this is *Turner syndrome* (45,XO) (see Figure 4.7), in which one of the X chromosomes in a female child is missing. These girls present with a stereotyped morphology that includes short stature, webbed neck, shield-shaped chest, low hairline, lymphoedema and possibly congenital heart defects. Hormone treatment is generally required to ensure the proper development of secondary sex characteristics.

TRISOMY

Trisomy is when there are three copies of a particular chromosome. The best known example of this is *Down syndrome*, a condition in which there are three copies of chromosome 21 (see Figure 4.8). Virtually any chromosome can, in theory, create a trisomy, but not all of these conditions make it through gestation to produce a living baby. Common syndromes associated with a trisomy include *Patau syndrome* (trisomy 13) (see Figure 4.9), a condition of highly variable expression that can include cleft lip and/or cleft palate, congenital heart defects, polydactyly,

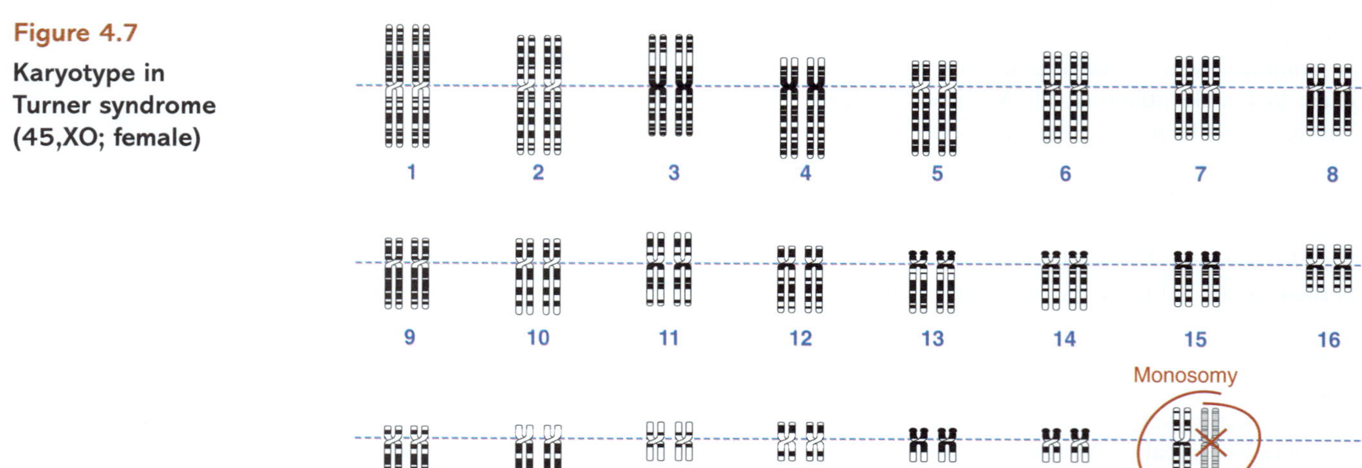

Figure 4.7
Karyotype in Turner syndrome (45,XO; female)

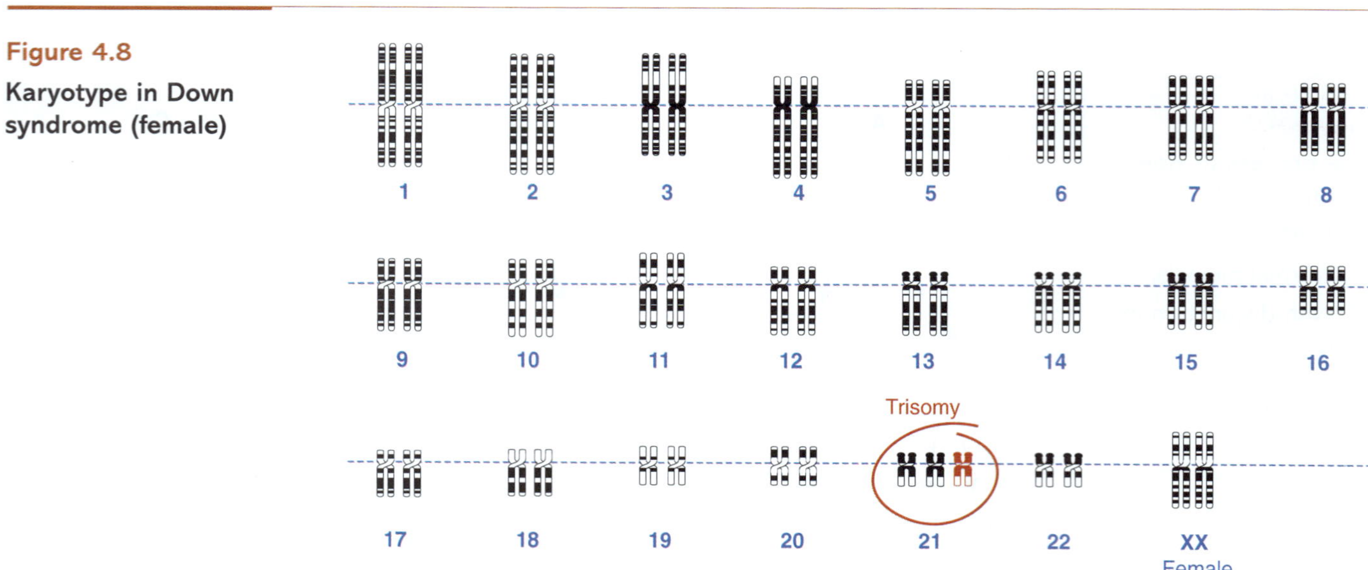

Figure 4.8
Karyotype in Down syndrome (female)

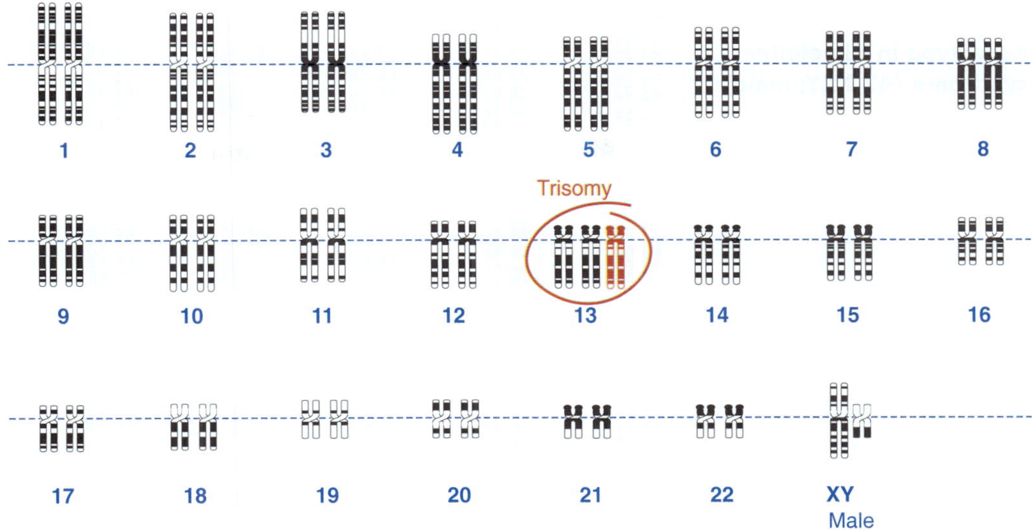

Figure 4.9
Karyotype in Patau syndrome (male)

intellectual disability and crypto-orchidism in affected males, but which can be quite severe and include holoprosencephaly (a failure of the forebrain to divide into left and right hemispheres) and microphthalmia (small eye or eyes); and *Edwards' syndrome* (trisomy 18) (see Figure 4.10), which is associated with rocker-bottom feet, leg position malformations and malformations of a number of organs, including the heart and kidneys.

Often forgotten in discussions of trisomy is the fact that a child can have three copies of the sex chromosomes. Two common syndromes included in this group are Klinefelter syndrome and Jacob's syndrome. *Klinefelter syndrome* (47,XXY) (see Figure 4.11) is often picked up during infertility testing, and manifests with hypogonadism, infertility, scoliosis, emphysema, diabetes mellitus, osteoporosis and possibly mild intellectual disability. *Jacob's syndrome* (47,XYY) (see Figure 4.12) has a highly variable presentation such that some individuals have normal **phenotypes**. Others are generally taller than average, but have an increased risk of learning disabilities, delayed acquisition of speech/language skills, behavioural and emotional problems, possibly delayed motor development, weak muscles, hand tremors and motor tics.

TRIPLOIDY

LEARNING OBJECTIVE 4

Differentiate between diploid and triploid.

In triploidy, the developing fetus has an additional full set of all chromosomes. Recall from earlier in this chapter that the normal number of chromosomes in human cells is 46; the **diploid** number. Triploidy is generally incompatible with life. The condition represents approximately 2% of all conceptions, and is associated with markedly low birth weight, disproportionately small trunk-to-head size, syndactyly (fusion of digits) and multiple congenital

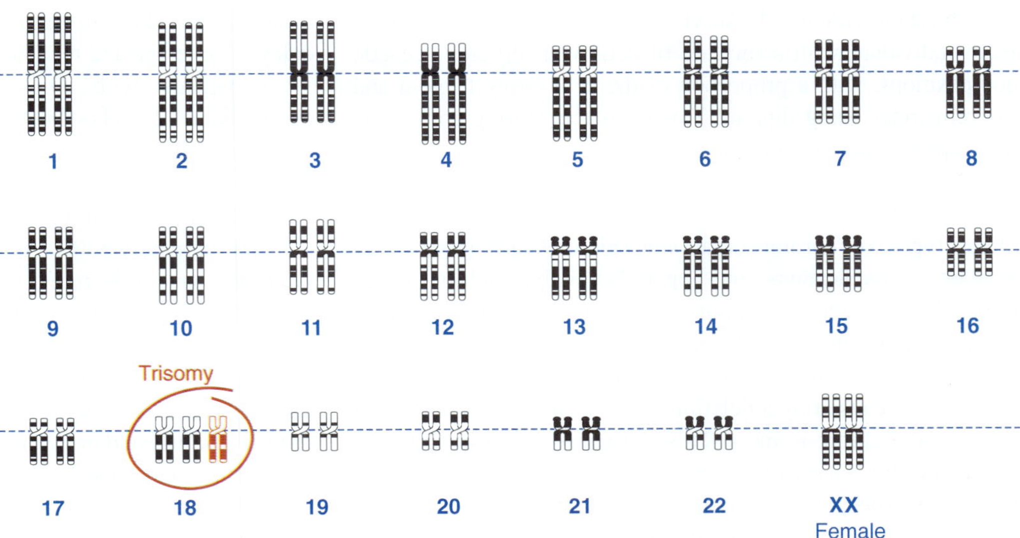

Figure 4.10
Karyotype in Edwards' syndrome (female)

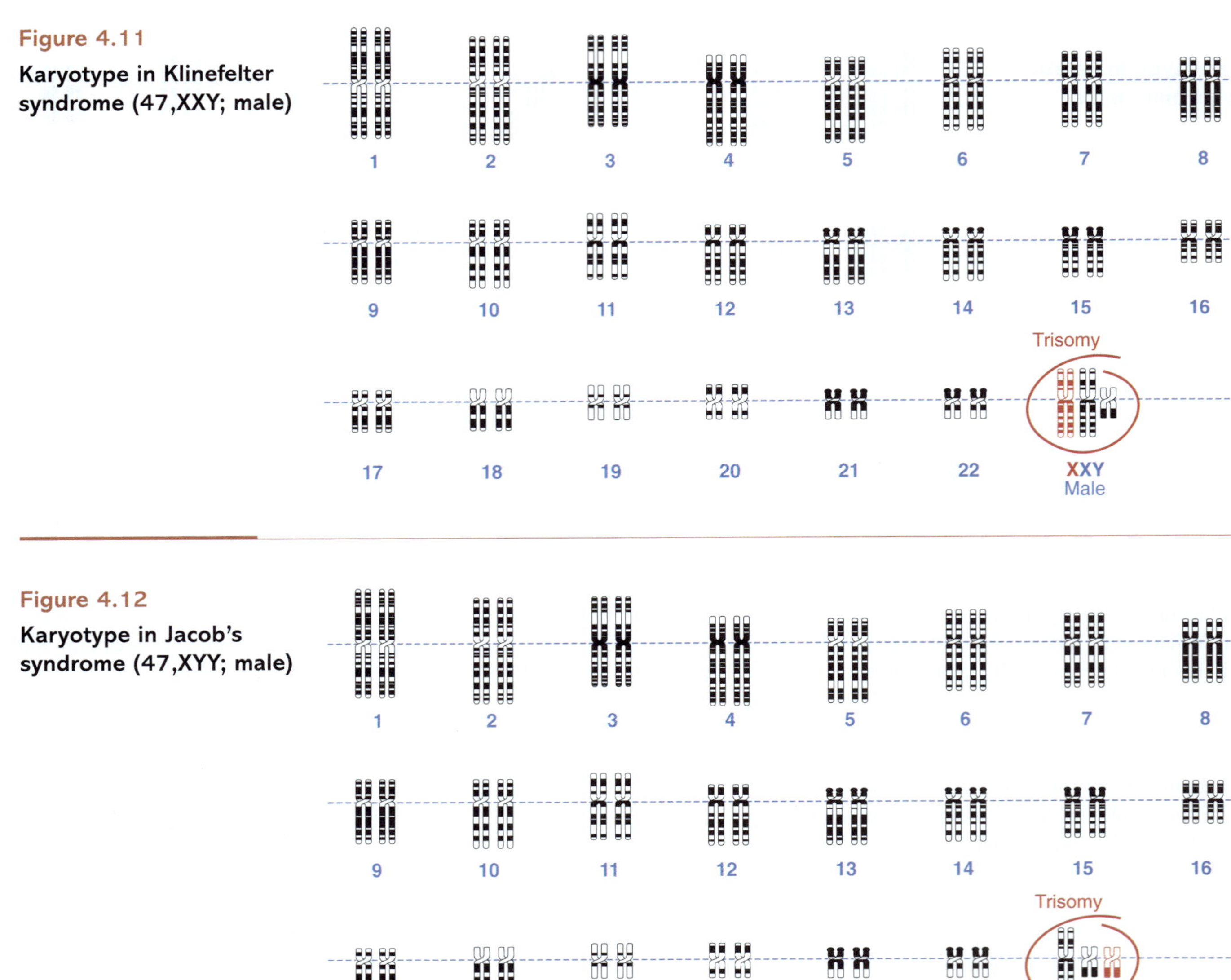

Figure 4.11
Karyotype in Klinefelter syndrome (47,XXY; male)

Figure 4.12
Karyotype in Jacob's syndrome (47,XYY; male)

defects. Survival past the first few days or weeks is extremely rare; those individuals who survive are usually mosaics. A **mosaic** is an individual with a mixture of cells with different genetic compositions, with a proportion of the cells being triploid and the remainder being diploid. This can occur during embryonic development due to a non-disjunction event in mitosis.

DELETIONS AND DUPLICATIONS

Other types of chromosomal abnormalities are grouped as **deletions** or **duplications**, and generally involve multiple genes rather than a single gene. Four well-known deletion syndromes are Wolf–Hirschhorn syndrome, DiGeorge syndrome, Prader–Willi syndrome and cri-du-chat syndrome. *Wolf–Hirschhorn syndrome* is caused by a deletion of the terminal portion of the short arm of chromosome 4. This loss causes a constellation of symptoms that varies significantly between individuals, but can include microcephaly, cleft lip and/or cleft palate, strabismus (crossed eyes), hypertelorism (increased distance between organs, particularly the eyes), a fish-like mouth and intellectual disability. In addition, heart defects, fused teeth, hearing loss, delayed bone age and renal abnormalities might also be seen.

Individuals with *DiGeorge syndrome* have a partial chromosome 22, also known as 22q11.2 (see Figure 4.13). Affected children experience numerous physical impairments, as well as intellectual disability, behavioural problems and immunological compromise (see the chapter 'Immune disorders').

Approximately 50% of individuals with *Prader–Willi syndrome* have a deletion on the long arm of chromosome 15 at 15q11-13, and have a highly variable presentation that is generally marked by hypotonia, poor muscle tone and balance, learning difficulties, a lack of sexual development, emotional instability and a lack of maturity. Characteristically, in this disorder the affected individuals generally manifest an obsession with eating and food, and can be capable of literally eating themselves to death. An individual with Prader–Willi syndrome is thought to have been the subject of a 17th-century painting

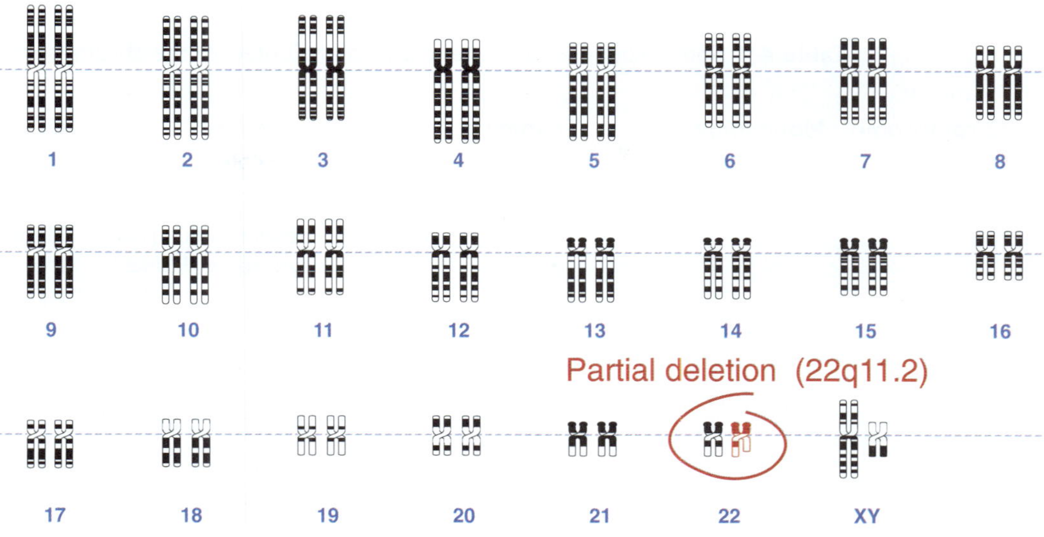

Figure 4.13
Karyotype in DiGeorge syndrome (male)

by Juan Carreño de Miranda, suggesting that the condition was relatively well known at this time, but possibly by a different name.

Cri-du-chat syndrome is named for the characteristic cat-like cry that these children make, which is due to abnormal larynx development. The condition is caused by a deletion of chromosome 5, the size of which varies between individuals, and individuals manifest with heart defects, muscular or skeletal defects, hearing or sight problems, behavioural problems (e.g. hyperactivity, aggression) and potentially significant developmental delay.

Syndromes and conditions that arise from duplications are less well known, but one interesting duplication is the reverse of the Prader–Willi deletion. Duplication of 15q11-13 has been associated with autistic spectrum disorders. Recently, three generations of a family with this duplication were described, in which the carriers of the duplication experienced intellectual disability, motor and visuo-motor skill impairments and adaptive functioning deficits that do not appear to be associated with autism.

FRAGILE SITES

Intriguingly, the region of chromosome 15 described in the previous section is a **fragile chromosomal site**, which is particularly prone to mutational events, including deletions, duplications, translocations and the creation of partial trisomies. Genes in this region may also be an inverted sequence as a consequence of mutations.

A very well-known condition associated with a fragile chromosomal site is the *fragile X syndrome*, which is associated with a constriction of the long arm of the X chromosome. This syndrome is second only to Down syndrome as a cause of intellectual disability, and male children affected by this chromosomal abnormality have unusually high foreheads, unbalanced faces, large jaws, long, protruding ears and large testicles, and are prone to violent outbursts. Interestingly, supplementation with folate modifies their behaviour. In female children, the impact of the abnormal X chromosome is modified by the presence of a normal X chromosome, and only about one-third of carriers have intellectual disability.

RECIPROCAL TRANSLOCATIONS

LEARNING OBJECTIVE 5

Explain what occurs in a reciprocal translocation, and why this might contribute to cancer formation.

The final group of chromosomal abnormalities to consider in this chapter are the **reciprocal translocations**. In these disorders, a piece of one chromosome changes position with a piece of another chromosome. Generally, it does not appear that any of the genetic material is missing, but the relocation of the genes, and even the merging of genes to form a compound gene, causes significant problems for the individual. The two best-known examples are both associated with the development of cancer: the Philadelphia chromosome and Burkitt's lymphoma.

The *Philadelphia chromosome* occurs when the end section of the long arm of chromosome 9 exchanges position with the majority of the long arm of chromosome 22. The point at which the piece of chromosome 9 joins chromosome 22 creates a gene construct comprised of a piece of the *bcr* gene, which encodes for a protein involved in phosphorylation activation, while the *c-abl* gene is a kinase that mediates phosphorylation associated with the control of cellular growth. Merging these two genes into the hybrid *bcr/abl* gene creates a fusion protein that contributes to the development of chronic myelogenous leukaemia.

In *Burkitt's lymphoma*, a piece of the terminal end of the long arm of chromosome 8 changes position with the terminal end of the long arm of either chromosome 2, 14 or 22. This reorganisation causes a gene called *c-myc*, which regulates the expression of other genes, to move into position near immunoglobulin genes, resulting in lymphoma.

Some examples of genetic issues are summarised in Table 4.1. This table identifies some syndromes related to monosomy,

Table 4.1 Some examples of genetic issues attributed to the chromosomes involved

Chromosome	Monosomy	Trisomy	Deletions	Other genetic issues
1			Neuroblastoma Thrombocytopenia-absent radius (TAR) syndrome (*RBM8A* gene)	Alzheimer's disease (*PSEN2* gene) Maple syrup urine disease (type II) Hereditary spherocytosis type 3 (*SPTA1* gene)
2		Acute myeloid leukaemia	2q37 deletion syndrome (*HDAC4* gene)	
3			3p deletion syndrome	Clear cell renal carcinoma Von Hippel–Lindau syndrome (*VHL* gene)
4		Trisomy 4	Wolf–Hirschhorn syndrome	Huntington's disease (*HHT* gene) Achondroplasia (*FGFR3* gene) Polycystic kidney disease (*PKD2* gene)
5		Trisomy 5p	Cri-du-chat syndrome 5q minus syndrome	Myelodysplastic syndromes
6				6q24-related transient neonatal diabetes mellitus Maple syrup urine disease (type Ib)
7	Familial monosomy 7 syndrome		Williams syndrome	Cystic fibrosis (*CFTR* gene)
8		Warkany syndrome	Mosaic trisomy 8	Burkitt lymphoma
9			Kleefstra syndrome	Galactosaemia Xeroderma pigmentosum (many types across several chromosomes) Tuberous sclerosis (*TSC1* gene)
10			10q26 deletion syndrome	Several leukaemias
11			Jacobsen syndrome	α- and β-thalassaemia (*HBA1* and *HBA2* genes) Sickle cell anaemia Ewing sarcoma
12		Chronic lymphocytic leukaemia		Pallister–Killian mosaic syndrome Phenylketonuria
13		Patau syndrome	Feingold syndrome (*MIR17HG* gene	Breast and ovarian cancer (*BRCA2* gene) Retinoblastoma
14			FOXG1 syndrome (*FOXG1* gene)	Alzheimer's disease (*PSEN1* gene) α-1 antitrypsin deficiency (*SERPINA1* gene) Hereditary spherocytosis type 2 (*SPTB* gene)

Table 4.1 Some examples of genetic issues attributed to the chromosomes involved (*continued*)

Chromosome	Monosomy	Trisomy	Deletions	Other genetic issues
15	Partial monosomy 15	Partial trisomy 15	Prader–Willi syndrome	Acute promyelocytic leukaemia Marfan syndrome (*FBN1* gene) Tay–Sachs disease Kartagener syndrome
16			Rubinstein–Taybi syndrome	Acute myeloid leukaemia Polycystic kidney disease (PKD1)
17	Partial monosomy 17	Partial trisomy 17	Koolen–de Vries syndrome	Breast and ovarian cancer (*BRCA1* gene) Neurofibromatosis
18		Edwards' syndrome	Distal 18q deletion syndrome Proximal 18q deletion syndrome	
19			19p13.13 deletion syndrome	Alzheimer's disease (*APOE* gene) Maple syrup urine disease (type la) Familial hypercholesterolaemia
20			Alagille syndrome (*JAG1* gene)	Polycythemia vera
21		Down syndrome		Alzheimer's disease (*APP* gene)
22		Cat eye syndrome	DiGeorge syndrome 22q11.2 deletion syndrome	Chronic myeloid leukemia (*BCR-ABL1* gene)
X	Turner syndrome (XO)	Klinefelter syndrome (XXY) Trisomy X	Microphthalmia with linear skin defects syndrome (*HCCS* gene)	Duchenne muscular dystrophy Rett syndrome (*MECP2* gene) Fanconi anaemia
Y		Jacob's syndrome (XYY)		Y chromosome infertility

trisomy and deletions. Table 4.1 also associates some diseases that are known to be directly caused by genetic mutations, and some predispositions that increase the risk to individuals who have these mutations in their genes.

Figure 4.14 summarises chromosomal abnormalities and how they may occur.

Threshold and penetrance

LEARNING OBJECTIVE 6

Distinguish between threshold traits and traits with variable penetrance.

For many conditions, the presence of a gene or chromosomal abnormality is insufficient to determine whether the individual will express the condition. For some disorders, there is a *threshold effect*, in which a certain minimum number of genes and possible environmental factors are required for the manifestation of a trait. These conditions are often referred to as *'either/or' conditions*: up to a certain gene/environment contribution you do not show the trait, but at threshold you do. This is not the case for other **polygene traits** for which there is a graded manifestation, such as with height or skin colour.

By contrast, the **penetrance** of a gene is a reflection of whether or not the trait is expressed if the person carries the gene, with no guarantee that inheriting the gene will cause the individual to express the condition. Thus far, most of the conditions we have discussed (e.g. autosomal dominant, autosomal recessive) have complete penetrance; that is, if you have the genotype, you have the phenotype. An example of a condition with incomplete penetrance is brachydactyly, a group of limb malformations marked by shortened index fingers and toes. There are a number of different types that tend to be

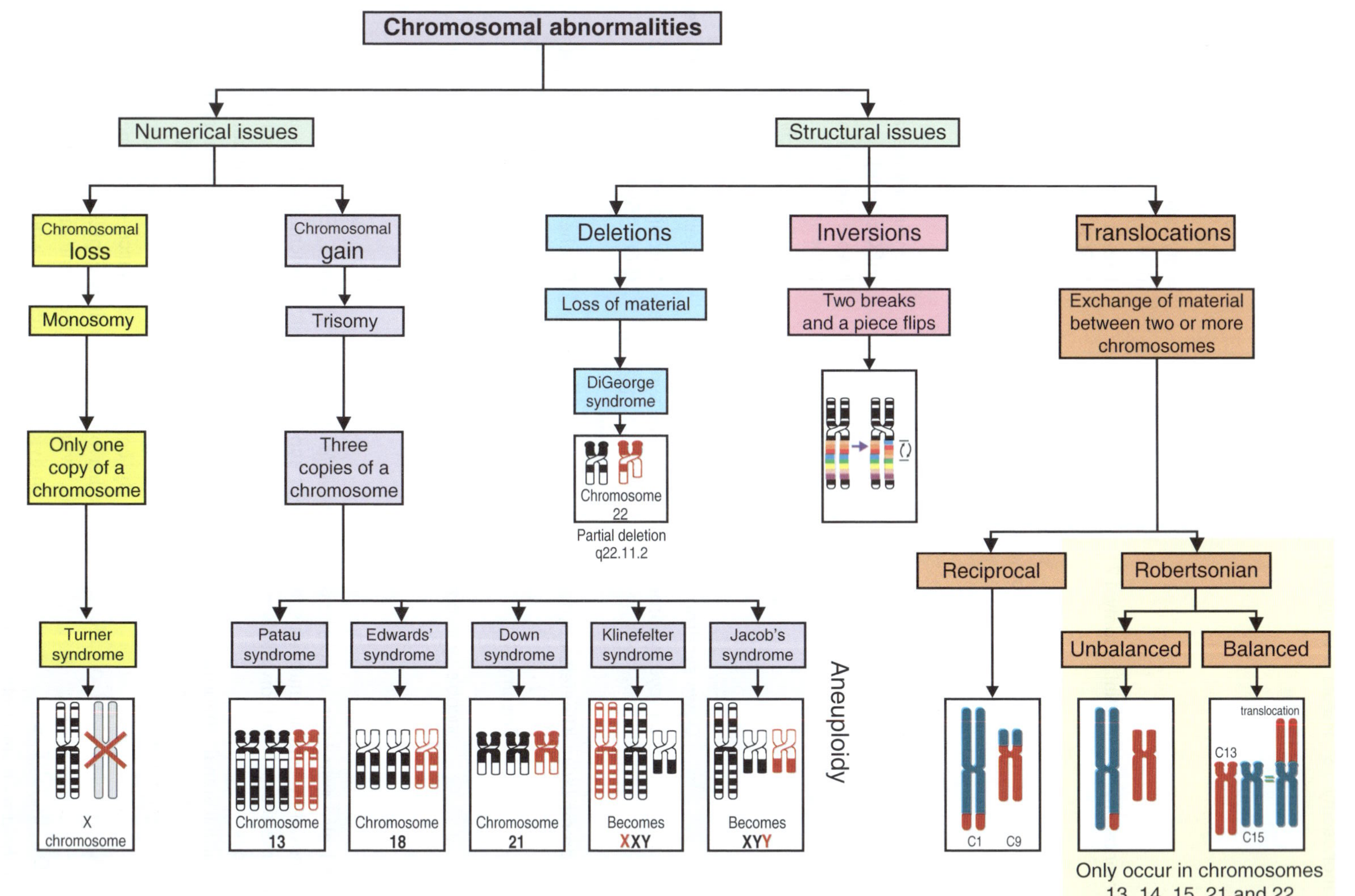

Figure 4.14

Chromosomal abnormalities

A Robertsonian translocation is typically defined as a translocation occurring between two acrocentric chromosomes (chromosomes with long and short arms) where the fusion point is near the centromere.

inherited in an autosomal dominant pattern. Several types have reduced penetrance, meaning that some people who carry the genetic defect (or mutation) will express the condition, while others do not.

Principles of multifactorial inheritance

LEARNING OBJECTIVE 7

Describe multifactorial inheritance, and outline its implications.

Although, as mentioned above, height and skin colour are polygene traits, they are also multifactorial traits: they require not only multiple genes but also environmental factors to determine their manifestation. **Multifactorial inheritance** creates a situation in which a trait has a continuous range of phenotypes rather than only two or three genes. If one considers height, for example, a substantial number of genes would be involved, including those for bone and muscle formation, growth factors, growth factor receptors and the signalling molecules involved in cell growth and duplication, as well as environmental conditions, such as the health of the mother during gestation, the child's diet, the standards of healthcare and the crowding index in the home environment. Many common disorders have, or are assumed to have, multifactorial inheritance. Some key examples include coronary artery disease, hypertension, breast and colorectal cancer, diabetes mellitus, obesity, Alzheimer's disease, alcoholism, schizophrenia and bipolar disorder.

Congenital malformations

LEARNING OBJECTIVE 8

Briefly describe the frequency, development and consequence of selected common congenital malformations.

Congenital malformations may or may not involve true chromosomal defects, as generally there is a contribution from in-utero restriction of development. In the case of congenital malformations, a malformation is defined as a *primary error of the normal development or morphogenesis of an organ or tissue*. This malformation can represent a single malformation or multiple malformations, and can be of minor or major concern. Examination of data across a number of studies argues that 14% of newborns will have a single minor malformation, 3% will have a single major malformation, and 0.7% will have multiple major malformations. The frequency of major malformations is higher at conception, and therefore spontaneous abortion of major malformations is estimated at approximately 7–10% of all conceptions. Some of the more common congenital defects include heart defects, hydrocephaly, neural tube defects, cleft lip and palate, club foot, isolated cleft palate and pyloric stenosis. A brief overview of congenital heart defects, hydrocephaly and neural tube defects is presented.

Although reports of the incidence of *congenital heart defects* varies considerably between studies, on average 8–10 out of every 1000 newborns have one or a combination of heart malformations, with ventricular septal defects representing up to 30% of all affected newborns. Twenty per cent of infants with severe malformations will not survive past one year of age. Interestingly, although the malformations are present from birth, septal defects can close by themselves over time, while compensatory mechanisms can manage other defects for a time, meaning individuals might not be aware until well into adulthood that they have a congenital heart defect.

Hydrocephaly is usually due to the blockade of normal cerebrospinal fluid (CSF) circulation (e.g. due to stenosis of the cerebral aqueduct), and this condition has a frequency of 1 in 1000 live births. This condition may be inherited as a multifactorial, X-linked recessive (< 1% of cases) or as an autosomal dominant disorder. If a shunt is provided to remove excess CSF fluid, 80% of affected children will have normal intelligence.

Neural tube defects are a group of disorders in which there is a failure of the neural tube to close at some point along its length. Neural tube defects fall into two categories: failure at the anterior (head) end, which generally results in *anencephaly* (no brain) and will lead to stillbirth or neonatal death; and failure at the posterior (rectal) end, which results in *spina bifida* (see the chapter 'Brain and spinal cord dysfunction'). In anencephaly, the top of the skull is missing, leaving nervous tissue exposed. This exposure leaves the developing brain vulnerable and leads to degeneration of nervous tissue. Further, the defective hypothalamus, deteriorating due to this generalised degeneration, triggers fetal adrenal atrophy and death. Spina bifida may be an open (no skin covering the lesion) or closed (the defect is hidden under skin) defect. Inadequate maternal folate intake plays a significant role in the pathogenesis (and is easily corrected). Between 15% and 20% of affected infants have closed lesions, and these individuals will experience only mild-to-moderate disability. Therapy will allow one-third of babies with open lesions five years of survival; 85% of these children will have severe disabilities, while 5% will have no impairment. However, it should be noted that neural tube defects represent multifactorial conditions that can be heavily influenced by environment or maternal state, and, besides the role of folate, other influencing factors that have been identified are the teratogenic influence of treatment drugs (e.g. anti-epilepsy medications), maternal diabetes mellitus, and chromosomal (e.g. trisomy 18) or single-gene disorders.

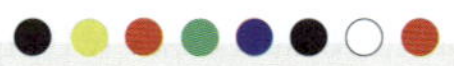

INDIGENOUS HEALTH FAST FACTS AND CULTURAL CONSIDERATIONS

FAST FACTS

- *Aboriginal and Torres Strait Islander peoples experience 1.9 times the number of infant deaths that non-Indigenous Australians experience. Data for chromosomal abnormalities comparing Australian Indigenous status is sparse. The Australian Bureau of Statistics reports perinatal mortality rates involving Edwards' syndrome and Patau syndrome accounted for 1.6% of deaths (8,600) between 2016 and 2020. The rate ratio between Aboriginal and Torres Strait Islander peoples and non-Indigenous people is 1.3:1.*
- *Prevalence rates for Down syndrome in Aboriginal and Torres Strait Islander peoples are equivalent to those in non-Indigenous people.*
- *In New Zealand, Down syndrome is the most frequent chromosomal abnormality, accounting for approximately 57% of chromosomal anomalies.*
- *Prevalence rates for Down syndrome are equivalent between Māori, Pacific Islands people and other New Zealanders.*

CULTURAL CONSIDERATIONS

- *In traditional language, there is no equivalent term for 'disability', so a community or an Aboriginal or Torres Strait Islander person may not identify with, or as, someone with a disability. The undesirable connotation or further negative label may also be a factor in reluctance to seek or embrace assistance or support services to promote an individual's optimum health and safety. The tyranny of distance, remote health service provision or the logistical implications of the infrastructure in a non-urban environment may also complicate optimum service provision.*
- *Culturally appropriate factors (including cultural, social and specific environmental considerations) should be reviewed in order to improve Aboriginal and Torres Strait Islander peoples' health and welfare.*

Sources: Data from Australian Institute of Health and Welfare (2022a, 2022c); Luke et al. (2022); Simpson et al. (2016); Steering Committee for the Review of Government Service Provision (2016).

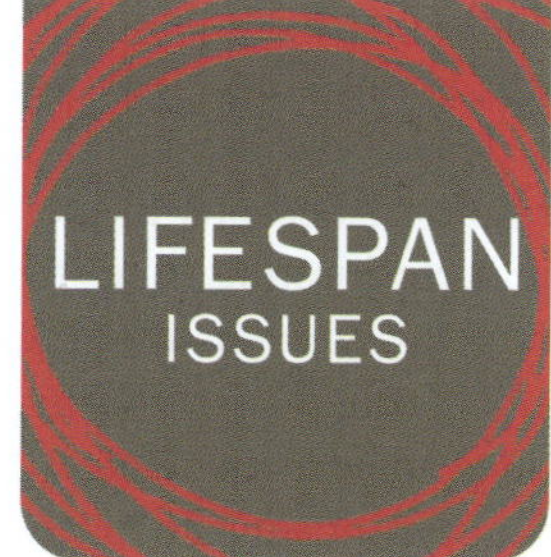

CHILDREN AND ADOLESCENTS

- Children with genetic disorders often experience difficulties with acceptance at school and in the community. Issues related to facial characteristics, behaviours or even cognitive function may directly influence a child's psychological development.
- Children and adolescents with chromosomal abnormalities may demonstrate deficits in cognitive, motor or language development. Developmental milestones will need to be adjusted in the assessment of their progress.
- Some chromosomal disorders may result in precocious puberty, while others may delay puberty. Irrespective of the influence, changes associated with sexual development can complicate the management of children with chromosomal abnormalities, especially in the context of cognitive deficit.
- In fertile adolescents with a chromosomal abnormality and cognitive deficit, appropriate protections to prevent pregnancy are often considered.

OLDER ADULTS

- Life expectancy for an individual with Down syndrome is approaching 55 years of age. Many other chromosomal anomalies also significantly reduce life expectancy.
- Older persons of child-bearing age have greater the risk of having a baby with chromosomal abnormalities.
- Maternal age plays a significant role in the increased risk of conceiving a baby with Down syndrome (see Table 4.2).

Table 4.2 Maternal age risk related to Down syndrome compared to any chromosomal abnormality

Maternal age	Down syndrome risk	Any chromosomal abnormality
20	1 in 1,667	1 in 526
25	1 in 1,250	1 in 476
30	1 in 952	1 in 384
35	1 in 385	1 in 192
40	1 in 106	1 in 66
45	1 in 30	1 in 21
49	1 in 11	1 in 8

Source: Data from Hill (2020).

KEY CLINICAL ISSUES

- A direct relationship between maternal age and chromosomal abnormalities exists. As women are choosing to start families later in life, an increased incidence in chromosomal abnormalities is expected.
- A carrier of a chromosomal abnormality does not have any symptoms.
- Individuals with chromosomal abnormalities may or may not be fertile, or have cognitive deficiencies or other symptoms. Each person must be assessed individually, and medical intervention and support measures determined as necessary.
- Congenital malformations may not involve chromosomal defects; rather, they may develop as a result of an insufficiency or restriction during the development of the fetus in utero.
- *Prenatal tests* can be undertaken to determine whether a fetus/embryo has a genetic condition. This information can be beneficial to parents who may consider the possibility of a therapeutic termination.

CHAPTER REVIEW

- Twenty-three chromosomes are required for human reproduction (a set from each parent), as normal human cells contain *46 chromosomes*.
- Twenty-two pairs of chromosomes are called *autosomes*, and one pair of chromosomes is called *sex chromosomes* (X and Y).
- *Chromosomal errors* can occur as a result of having too few, too many or altered chromosomes.
- The number, type and chromosome(s) affected will influence the outcome. A fetus with a *chromosomal abnormality* inconsistent with life will terminate. Some fetuses may be delivered at term and die soon after birth, yet other babies with chromosomal abnormalities may live long lives and not express any signs or symptoms of a condition.
- *Congenital malformations* may or may not occur as a result of chromosomal abnormalities.

REVIEW QUESTIONS

1. Define the following terms:
   a. chromosome
   b. autosome
   c. recessive inheritance
   d. dominant inheritance
   e. monosomy
   f. trisomy
   g. diploidy
   h. triploidy
   i. reciprocal translocation
2. What determines whether an individual will inherit a chromosomal abnormality?
3. Are all people with chromosomal anomalies infertile? Explain.
4. Are any chromosomal anomalies specific to a gender? Explain.
5. Down syndrome is the most common chromosomal abnormality. What are the characteristics of Down syndrome? What is the life expectancy of an individual with Down syndrome?
6. Can anything be done to cure an individual with a chromosomal abnormality? Explain.
7. Are congenital malformations a direct result of a chromosomal abnormality? Explain.

HEALTH PROFESSIONAL CONNECTIONS

Midwives Genetic testing brings with it an array of concerns for all involved. When caring for pregnant women of advancing years (especially nulliparous), consultation with genetic counsellors is important to ensure that all aspects of the testing and the results are understood before entering into the process. There are ethical, emotional and physical issues related to genetic testing, and healthcare professionals should seek the assistance of those with specific expertise in this area of specialisation. Neonates who are obviously 'different' in appearance may also be delivered. This will come as a surprise if it is unexpected. Again, parents will need much support and education to cope with the process of genetic testing. Issues surrounding fertility and the concept of being a 'carrier' for a disease may challenge couples.

All allied professionals Working with individuals who have genetic anomalies can be very challenging. Individuals with the same genetic anomaly can present with different issues. Common traits will generally be associated with each anomaly, but each individual will be confronted by different challenges. Often, those with genetic abnormalities show reduced intellectual development; however, individuals can also have higher intellectual functioning than expected. It is critical that each person is treated with respect, and that each management plan is developed based on the individual's goals and needs, rather than on generic ideas of what each 'genetic anomaly' may require. Multidisciplinary teams will manage the care of individuals with genetic issues. Interpersonal communication between all team members and the sharing of observations are important to enable the best care plan development and provision.

CASE STUDY

Mr Scott Jacoby is 25 years old (UR number 874916). He has many challenges in life because of his chromosomal abnormalities. He has an intelligence quotient (IQ) of 39. Characteristically, he has a small mouth and a protruding tongue. He has brachycephaly, his eyes are wide apart and his face appears flatter than usual. He has a flat nose and small ears. He is shorter than usual, and has a wide gap between his first and second toe. As a baby his muscle strength was hypotonic, and he required surgery for an endocardial cushion defect. As an adult he has hypogenitalism, with his penis, testes and scrotum all smaller than usual. His chromosome karyotype looks like this:

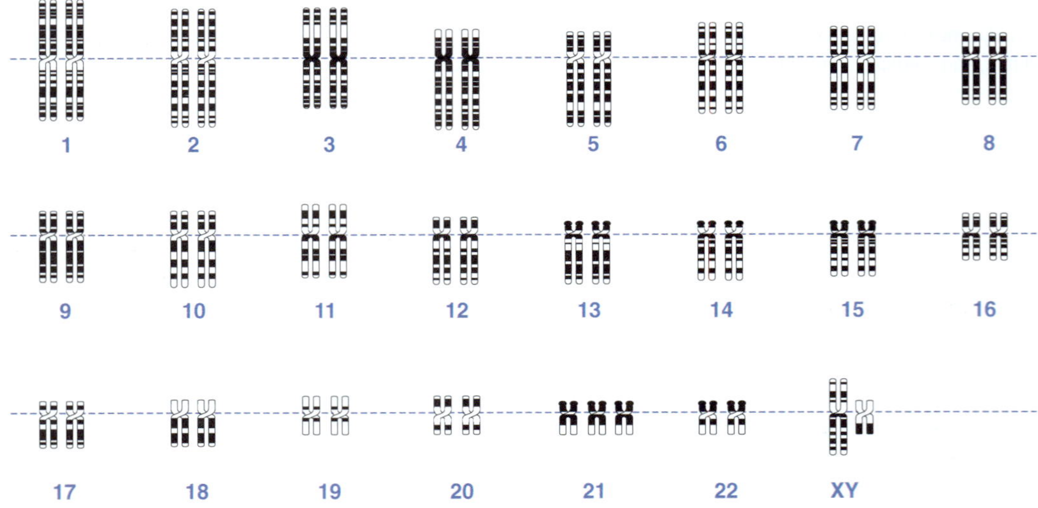

CRITICAL THINKING

1 Consider the history and the chromosomal study. What genetic anomaly does Mr Jacoby have?
2 How is this genetic anomaly diagnosed?
3 Is there an association between maternal age and this genetic anomaly? If so, what is it?
4 Are there any interventions that could assist Mr Jacoby? If so, what are they?
5 How does this anomaly occur? Use the following diagram to explain how this occurs.

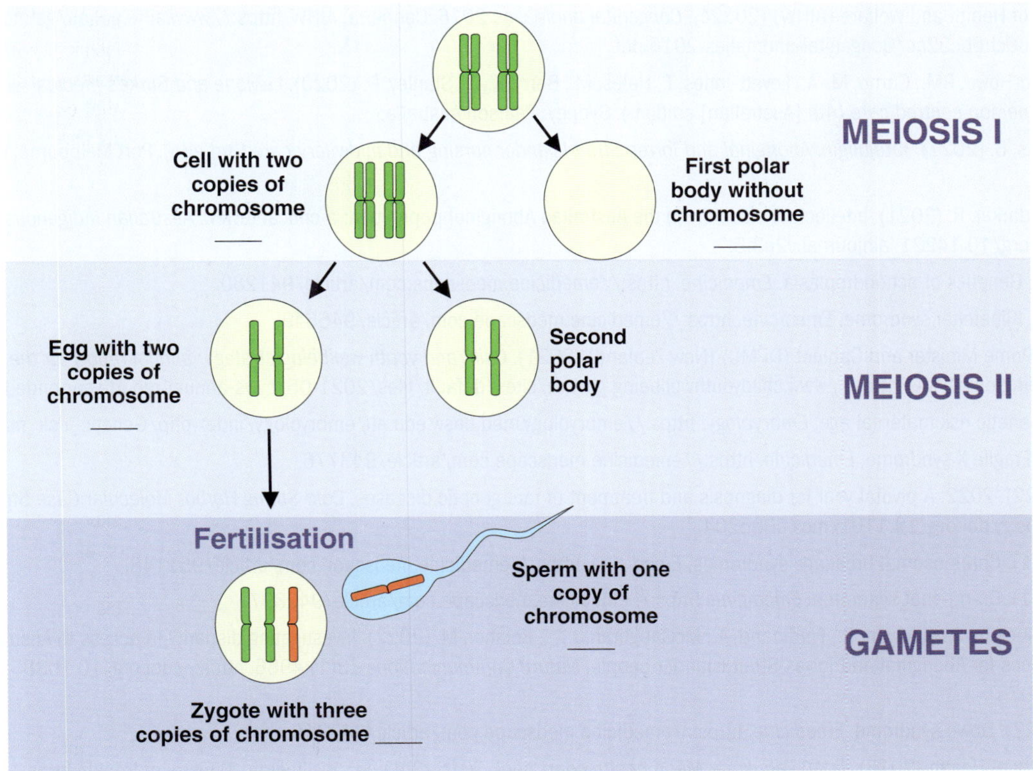

BIBLIOGRAPHY

Australian Bureau of Statistics (ABS) (2021). Table 15.19 Perinatal deaths by Aboriginal and Torres Strait Islander top causes of death, NSW, Qld, SA, WA, NT, by Aboriginal and Torres Strait Islander status, 2016–2020. *3303.0 Causes of death, Australia, 2020.* Canberra: ABS. https://www.abs.gov.au/statistics/health/causes-death/causes-death-australia/latest-release.

Australian Health Ministers' Advisory Council's National and Aboriginal and Torres Strait Islander Health Standing Committee (2017). *Cultural respect framework 2016–2026: for Aboriginal and Torres Strait Islander health—a national approach to building a culturally respectful health system*. Canberra: Australian Government Department of Health. https://nacchocommunique.files.wordpress.com/2016/12/cultural_respect_framework_1december2016_1.pdf.

Australian Indigenous Health*Info*Net (2017). *Overview of Aboriginal and Torres Strait Islander health status, 2016*. Perth, WA: Australian Indigenous Health*Info*Net. http://www.healthinfonet.ecu.edu.au.

Australian Indigenous Health*Info*Net (2021). *Overview of Aboriginal and Torres Strait Islander health status, 2020*. Perth, WA: Australian Indigenous Health*Info*Net. https://apo.org.au/sites/default/files/resource-files/2021-03/apo-nid311685.pdf.

Australian Indigenous Health*Info*Net (2022). *Overview of Aboriginal and Torres Strait Islander health status, 2021*. Perth, WA: Australian Indigenous Health*Info*Net. https://healthinfonet.ecu.edu.au/learn/health-facts/overview-aboriginal-torres-strait-islander-health-status/.

Australian Institute of Family Studies (AIFS) (2019). *The longitudinal study of Australian children annual statistical report, 2018*. Melbourne: AIFS. https://growingupinaustralia.gov.au/research-findings/annual-statistical-reports-2018.

Australian Institute of Health and Welfare (AIHW) (2012). *A picture of Australia's children, 2012*. Cat. No. PHE 167. Canberra: AIHW. https://www.aihw.gov.au/getmedia/31c0a364-dbac-4e88-8761-d9c87bc2dc29/14116.pdf.

Australian Institute of Health and Welfare (AIHW) (2016). *Australia's health, 2016*. Australia's Health series no. 15. Cat. No. AUS 199. Canberra: AIHW. https://www.aihw.gov.au/reports/australias-health/australias-health-2016/contents/summary.

Australian Institute of Health and Welfare (AIHW) (2020). *Australia's children*. Cat. No. CWS 69. Canberra: AIHW. https://www.aihw.gov.au/getmedia/6af928d6-692e-4449-b915-cf2ca946982f/aihw-cws-69-print-report.pdf.

Australian Institute of Health and Welfare (AIHW) (2022a). *Aboriginal and Torres Strait Islander Health Performance Framework. Health status and outcomes.* 1.20 Infant and child mortality. Canberra: AIHW. https://www.indigenoushpf.gov.au/measures/1-20-infant-child-mortality.

Australian Institute of Health and Welfare (AIHW) (2022b). *Australia's health, 2022*. Australia's Health series no. 15. Cat. No. AUS 199. Canberra: AIHW. https://www.aihw.gov.au/reports-data/australias-health.

Australian Institute of Health and Welfare (AIHW) (2022c). *Congenital anomalies 2016*. Canberra: AIHW. https://www.aihw.gov.au/getmedia/3743dd66-3aa9-4812-9bdf-db6cb6bc52ac/Congenital-anomalies-2016.pdf.

Bauldoff, G., Gubrud-Howe, P.M., Carno, M.-A., Levett-Jones, T., Hales, M., Berry, K., … Stanley, D. (2020). *LeMone and Burke's medical–surgical nursing: critical thinking for person-centred care* (4th [Australian] edition.). Sydney: Pearson Australia.

Best, O. & Fredericks, B. (2021). *Yatdjuligin: Aboriginal and Torres Strait Islander nursing and midwifery care* (3rd edn). Port Melbourne, VIC: Cambridge University Press.

Chong, R.Y. & Bhandarkar, R. (2021). Intellectual disability in the Australian Aboriginal population: a critical review. *Australian Indigenous Health Bulletin 2*(3). http://dx.doi.org/10.14221/aihjournal.v2n3.5.

Defendi, G. (2022). Genetics of achondroplasia. *Emedicine*. https://emedicine.medscape.com/article/941280.

Defendi, G. (2022). Klinefelter syndrome. *Emedicine*. https://emedicine.medscape.com/article/945649.

Department of the Prime Minister and Cabinet (DPMC) [New Zealand] (2021). *Child and youth wellbeing strategy: annual report for the year ending 30 June 2020.* Wellington: DPMC. https://www.childyouthwellbeing.govt.nz/sites/default/files/2021-05/cyws-annual-report-year-ended-june-2020.pdf.

Hill, M.A. (2020). Genetic risk maternal age. *Embryology.* https://embryology.med.unsw.edu.au/embryology/index.php/Genetic_risk_maternal_age.

Jewell, J.A. (2022). Fragile X syndrome. *Emedicine*. https://emedicine.medscape.com/article/943776.

Kingsmore S.F. (2022). 2022: A pivotal year for diagnosis and treatment of rare genetic diseases. *Cold Spring Harbor Molecular Case Studies 8*(2):a006204. https://doi.org/10.1101/mcs.a006204.

Kumar Lal, M. (2021). Chromosomal breakage syndromes. *Emedicine*. https://emedicine.medscape.com/article/951148.

Kumar Lal, M. (2021). Cri-du-chat syndrome. *Emedicine*. https://emedicine.medscape.com/article/942897.

Luke, J., Dalach, P., Tuer, L., Savarirayan, R., Ferdinand, A., McGaughran, J., … Kelaher, M. (2022). Investigating disparity in access to Australian clinical genetic health services for Aboriginal and Torres Strait Islander people. *Nature Communications 13*(1):4966. https://doi.org/10.1038/s41467-022-32707-0.

Mundakel, G.T. (2022). Down syndrome. *Emedicine*. https://emedicine.medscape.com/article/943216.

New Zealand Ministry of Health (2015). *Tatau kahukura: Māori health chart book 2015* (3rd edn). Wellington: Ministry of Health. https://www.health.govt.nz/publication/tatau-kahukura-maori-health-chart-book-2015-3rd-edition.

Parker, R. (2014). Dementia in Aboriginal and Torres Strait Islander people. *Medical Journal of Australia* 200(8):435–6. https://doi.org/10.5694/mja14.00259.

Revilla, F.J. (2019). Huntington disease. *Emedicine*. https://emedicine.medscape.com/article/1150165.

Rodriguez, K., Kobayashi, E.S., Coufal, N., Dimmock, D., & Kingsmore, S. (2022). 577: impact of rapid whole genome sequencing in the PICU. *Critical Care Medicine 50*(1):280. https://doi.org/10.1097/01.ccm.0000808632.68570.af.

Simpson, J., Duncanson, M., Oben, G., Adams, J., Wicken, A., Morris, S. & Gallagher, S. (2018). *The health of children and young people with chronic conditions and disabilities in New Zealand 2016 (National).* Dunedin: New Zealand Child and Youth Epidemiology Service. http://hdl.handle.net/10523/8478.

Simpson, J., Oben, G., Craig, E., Adams, J., Wicken, A., Duncanson, M. & Reddington, A. (2016). *The determinants of health for children and young people in New Zealand (2014).* Dunedin: New Zealand Child and Youth Epidemiology Service, University of Otago. http://hdl.handle.net/10523/6383.

Sperling, R. (ed.) (2020). *Obstetrics and gynecology*. West Sussex, UK: Wiley Blackwell.

Steering Committee for the Review of Government Service Provision (SCRGSP) (2020). *Overcoming Indigenous disadvantage: key indicators, 2020*. Canberra: Productivity Commission. https://www.pc.gov.au/ongoing/overcoming-indigenous-disadvantage/2020.

Sweeney, N.M., Nahas, S.A., Chowdhury, S., Batalov, S., Clark, M., Caylor, S., … Kingsmore, S.F. (2021). Rapid whole genome sequencing impacts care and resource utilization in infants with congenital heart disease. *NPJ Genomic Medicine 6*(1):29. https://doi.org/10.1038/s41525-021-00192-x.

Tortora. G.J., Derrickson, B., Burkett, B., Peoples, G., Dye, D., Cooke, J., … Green, H. (2022). *Principles of anatomy and physiology* (3rd Asia-Pacific edn). Milton, QLD: John Wiley and Sons.

Neoplasia

5

LEARNING OBJECTIVES

After completing this chapter, you should be able to:

1. Discuss the regional cancer statistics, including the influence of age and sex on cancer development.
2. Describe the ways in which cancer cells differ from normal cells.
3. Outline cancer aetiology, and describe the various factors predisposing someone to carcinogenesis.
4. Describe the types of genes that are known to contribute to cancer.
5. Describe the process of tumour invasion and metastasis.
6. Outline the common clinical manifestations of cancer.
7. Describe contemporary and emerging screening, diagnostic and management options for people with cancer.

WHAT YOU SHOULD KNOW BEFORE YOU START THIS CHAPTER

Can you identify the main structures of the cell, and describe their functions?

Can you describe the phases of the cell cycle?

Can you describe the processes of DNA synthesis and repair?

Can you describe how cells divide and differentiate?

KEY TERMS

Age-standardised
Anaplastic
Benign
Cancer
Carcinogen
Carcinogenesis
Constitutive activity
Malignant
Metastasis
Neoplasia
Oncogene
Oncology
Pleomorphic
Proto-oncogene
Senescence
Telomere
Teratoma
Transformation
Tumorigenesis
Tumour
Tumour markers
Tumour suppressor genes
Tumour suppressor proteins

Introduction

Few words generate the degree of fear that 'cancer' invokes, and rightly so, as it is the leading cause of death in Australia and New Zealand. Although often considered an alien entity divorced from the normal processes of the body, cancer is an all-too-common result of errors in normal cell growth, regulation and/or differentiation. These conditions cause uncontrolled cell division, resulting in the unrestrained growth of abnormal cells and sometimes their invasion into healthy tissue.

While it is true that external factors contribute to and even cause the development of cancer, such as the well-established link with smoking, the primary reason for cancer development is essentially changes to the cells. Changes to a cell's deoxyribonucleic acid (DNA) may lead to unchecked division and, ultimately, cancer may result.

In order to better understand cancer, it is necessary to appreciate that cells normally have stringent controls on their division, and are constantly monitored for errors in their DNA that will, if uncorrected, trigger cell 'suicide'. If any of these processes fail, then cells can become cancerous.

Before examining the nature and development of cancer, it is important to address some basic terminology. The term **neoplasia** literally means 'new growth'; it is a term that usually refers to the growth of a tissue, or the proliferation of cells, that serves no physiological purpose. Moles and warts are considered forms of neoplasia. **Tumour**, a term commonly linked to cancer, also refers to inappropriate cell growths, and is derived from the Latin word meaning 'a swelling'. The original medical usage of the term 'tumour' was in association with swelling due to inflammation. Interestingly, a tumour mass can be **benign** (no direct threat to life) or **malignant** (tending to produce death or deterioration). (For details on the characteristics and naming of benign and malignant tumours, see the section 'Classification of tumours' later in this chapter.) Importantly, the presence of a lump in the body does not necessarily mean that it is cancer.

The word **cancer** is derived from the ancient Greek word for crab (*karkinos*), referring to the projections outwards from a tissue, and is particularly used to refer to malignant growths (tumours), while **oncology** is the study of cancer and its treatment (from the Greek *onkos*, meaning 'mass'). Generally, tumours are derived from a single cell that has lost the ability to curtail its division; therefore, since all cells that form the tumour come from this single, original cell, the tumour is said to be *clonal*. However, that does not mean that all tumour cells will remain identical. The rapid rate of growth of many tumours can cause some cells to accumulate additional mutations that other cells do not, and therefore a tumour might end up with cells of different types, a condition referred to as **pleomorphic**. This is particularly true of tumours that form from totipotent stem cells of the reproductive tissues; literally, cells that can be anything. These tumours arise from so-called 'germ cells', the cells that form eggs or sperm, and these tumours, when opened, can contain such clearly defined structures as hair (very common), teeth, pieces of bone, pieces of neuronal tissue, or combinations of these. Historically, these tumours surprised and frightened their discoverers, who consequently named them **teratomas**, a word that means 'monstrous tumours'.

Epidemiology of cancer

LEARNING OBJECTIVE 1

Discuss the regional cancer statistics, including the influence of age and sex on cancer development.

According to a 2022 report from the Australian Institute of Health and Welfare (AIHW), cancer is responsible for 3 out of every 10 deaths annually, and accounts for 18% of Australia's disease burden. However, Australia's **age-standardised** mortality rate for cancer dropped from 209 per 100,000 in 1982 to 145 deaths per 100,000 in 2022. In relation to countries with Organisation for Economic Co-operation and Development (OECD) membership, in 2020 (when average mortality was 191 per 100,000), Australia ranked 15th highest in cancer mortality statistics, between the United States and Austria; and New Zealand ranked 30th between France and The Netherlands. The leading cause of cancer mortality is lung cancer, followed by colorectal, prostate, breast and pancreatic cancers.

The incidence of cancer in Australia rose from 383 per 100,000 people in 1982, peaked at 613 per 100,000 in 1994, and decreased to 507 per 100,000 in 2022. In comparison to world standards, Australia had the highest age-standardised cancer incidence, and New Zealand was ranked second highest, in 2020, when comparing incidence statistics to countries with OECD membership. This important distinction between high incidence and significantly lower mortality is primarily related to high skin cancer statistics; however, quality screening programs, medical care, and follow-up must also contribute to these statistics. Unfortunately, it is expected that future cancer incidence and mortality will be affected by the COVID-19 pandemic as routine cancer screening was delayed and elective surgeries were postponed in order to redistribute healthcare resources and funds towards management of the pandemic.

The five-year relative survival rate overall has improved to 70%, and the sex disparity in mortality statistics favouring females has now disappeared. However, age still plays an important factor in positive survival outcomes, as demonstrated by the high five-year survival rates for individuals between 20 and 25 years of age at 89%; yet for individuals over 85 years of age, the survival rates are as low as 39%. Such poor statistics for older adults are probably attributable to the type of cancer, disease comorbidity, and the failure of these older people to be included in clinical trials. Figure 5.1 demonstrates many improvements, and some regression, in the Australian five-year survival rates for selected cancers across three decades.

The most common newly diagnosed cancers in 2021 (excluding non-melanoma skin cancer) were breast (13.3%), prostate (12%), melanoma of the skin (11.2%), colorectal (10.3%) and lung (9.2%). Table 5.1 lists the 10 most common cancers in both men and women. Generally, cancer is a disease of older people, with 73% of new diagnoses occurring after the age of 60. It is important to note that the five most commonly diagnosed cancers account for almost 60% of all the cancers diagnosed.

Mortality statistics from the New Zealand's Te Aho o Te Kahu | Cancer Control Agency (2021) indicate an age-standardised mortality rate of 110 deaths per 100,000 people. This equates to approximately 9,770 deaths per year, and over 26,400 new cancer registrations. When observing all cancers, incidence rates overall are high in New Zealand, at 340 per 100,000. The most common newly diagnosed cancers (excluding non-melanoma skin cancer) are prostate (16%), breast (13.1%), colorectal (12.6%), melanoma of the skin (10.3%) and lung (8.9%).

Aboriginality appears to have an influence on incidence and mortality in both Australia and in New Zealand. Age-standardised

Figure 5.1

Five-year survival rate trends, comparing 1984–88 to 2013–17 for selected cancers, Australia, 2021

Source: Data from Australian Institute of Health and Welfare (2021), Figure 7.5, p. 84.

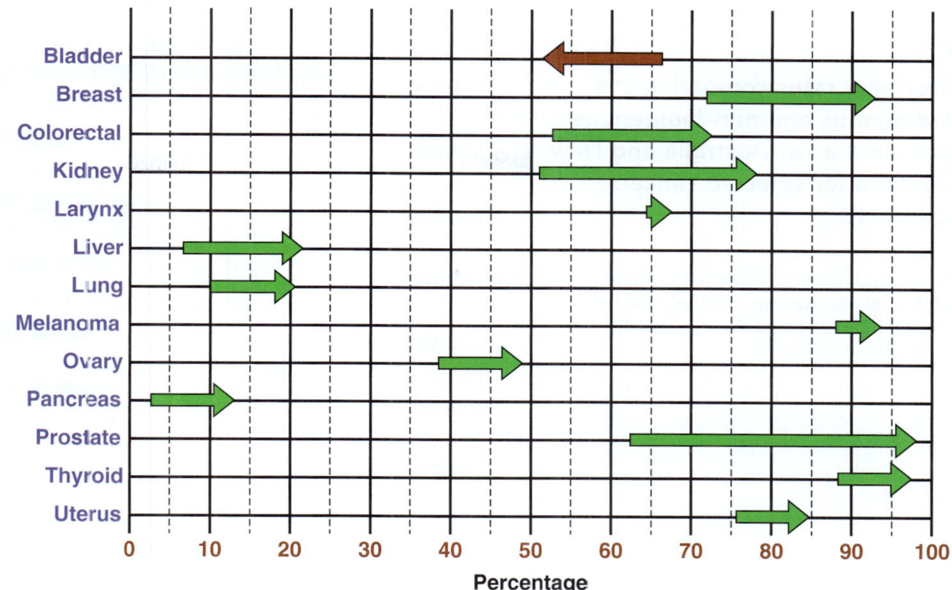

Table 5.1 The 10 most commonly diagnosed cancers by sex in Australia in 2021*

	Males			Females	
Site	Cases	5-year survival (%)	Site	Cases	5-year survival (%)
Prostate	18,110	95.5	Breast	19,866	91.5
Melanoma of skin	9,869	90.8	Colorectal	7,293	71
Colorectal	8,247	69.8	Melanoma of skin	7,009	94.3
Lung	7,460	17	Lung	6,350	24.7
Lymphoma	3,694	74.2	Uterine	3,267	83.5
Kidney	2,936	79.1	Thyroid	2,760	97.9
Bladder	2,369	57.6	Lymphoma	2,708	76.9
Pancreas	2,213	11.2	Pancreas	2,048	11.8
Liver	2,050	21.6	Ovary and fallopian tube	1,720	48.1
Stomach	1,558	32.5	Kidney	1,441	80.2
All cancers	**80,371**	68.5	**All cancers**	**70,411**	71.1

**The rates were standardised to the Australian population as at 2001, and are expressed per 100,000 population.*

Sources: Data from AIHW (2021a), Table 1, p. xi, and AIHW (2021b), Table 7.3, p. 86.

mortality rates of cancer are higher in Aboriginal and Torres Strait Islander Australians at 230 per 100,000, compared to 159 for non-Indigenous Australians. New Zealand statistics are marginally better, with a Māori cancer mortality of 176 per 100,000, compared to 103 per 100,000 for the non-Māori population. Figure 5.2 demonstrates mortality statistics comparing Aboriginal and Torres Strait Islander Australians', non-Indigenous Australians', Māori and non-Māori New Zealanders' cancers across selected cancers.

By the age of 85, half of all Australian men and women will have been diagnosed with cancer at some point in their life (excluding non-melanoma skin cancer), with prostate cancer the most common newly diagnosed cancer in men, and breast cancer the most likely cancer in women. Cancer risk changes through the lifespan. Figure 5.3 demonstrates the different types of cancer risks a person may face within broad lifespan categories, and Table 5.2 illustrates the most common cancers by age and sex.

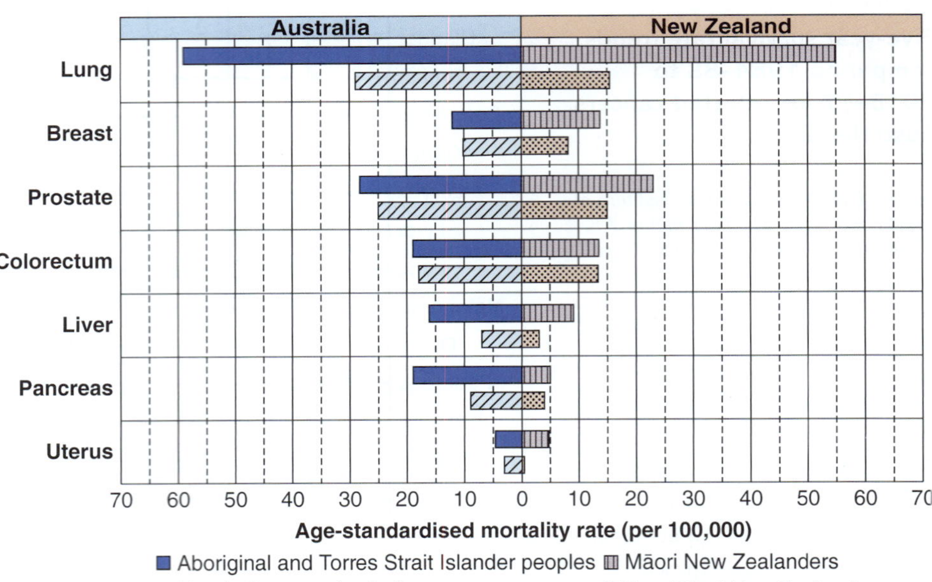

Figure 5.2

Mortality rates comparing the Indigenous and non-Indigenous populations of Australia and New Zealand for selected cancers, 2015–19

Sources: Data from Australian Institute of Health and Welfare (2022a); Cancer Australia (2022); Health New Zealand | Te Whatu Ora (2021).

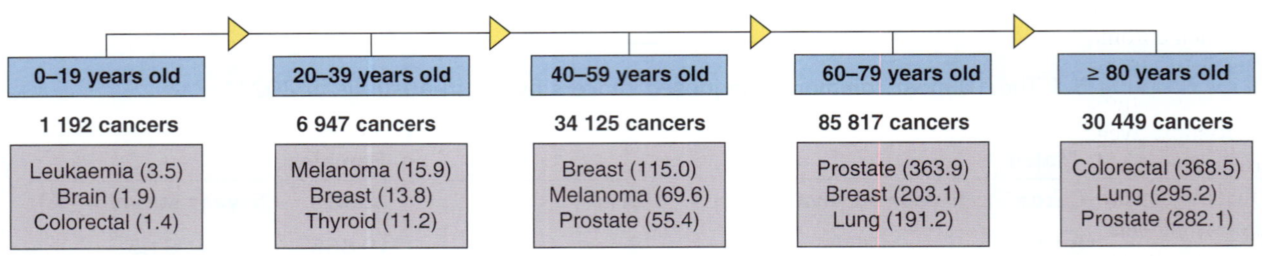

Figure 5.3

Common cancers across the lifespan

The numbers in parentheses represent age-standardised incidence (per 100,000) per cancer type.

Source: Data from AIHW (2021a).

Table 5.2 The 10 most commonly diagnosed cancers by sex in New Zealand in 2019

Males			Females		
Site	**Cases**	**Rate per 100,000***	**Site**	**Cases**	**Rate per 100,000***
Prostate	4,219	107.1	Breast	3,451	95.7
Colorectal	1,730	44.40	Colorectal	1,588	36.9
Melanoma of skin	1,481	39.2	Melanoma of skin	1,249	32.5
Lung	1,155	28.4	Lung	1,189	27.1
Lymphoma	595	16.1	Uterine	686	18.4
Leukaemia	465	12.9	Lymphoma	391	9.7
Kidney	376	10.4	Pancreas	345	**
Bladder	343	8.2	Leukaemia	314	8.7
Pancreas	378	9.6	Ovary	260	7.1
Stomach	266	7.0	Thyroid	258	8.7
All cancers	**14,021**	9.0	**All cancers**	**12,384**	4.7

*Rates were standardised to the WHO world standard population.
**Accuracy of data not confirmed.

Source: Data from New Zealand Ministry of Health (2021).

Carcinogenicity and cancer

NORMAL CELL DEVELOPMENT: CELL GROWTH, REGULATION AND DIFFERENTIATION

LEARNING OBJECTIVE 2

Describe the ways in which cancer cells differ from normal cells.

Normal cells grow, divide and differentiate into specialised cell types, such as myocytes, erythrocytes or neurons; have awareness of their neighbours and curb their growth to accommodate them; monitor their own growth, activity and DNA integrity; respond to their environment; and die when required. Each cell in the body has a limited ability to replicate, with a predicted number of doublings (generally 50–60 for the average cell, see Figure 5.4), after which the cell becomes growth-inhibited or senescent. Mature cells are fully capable of undertaking their roles and responsibilities in their tissue or organ, and are therefore referred to as *terminally differentiated*. In part, this **senescence** is controlled by the **telomeres**, or caps, on the ends of each chromosome, which are in place to prevent any loss of integrity of the chromosomes during cell division. As chromosomes undergo successive rounds of replication, the telomere is shortened. Eventually the telomere becomes too short to allow further division. In addition, senescence is controlled by proteins that are powerful inhibitors of cell growth, known as **tumour suppressor proteins**.

When normal cells experience errors in the duplication of their DNA, or when cells are exposed to chemicals or radiation that cause damage to parts of the cell, including DNA and cell membranes, a series of repair proteins are on hand to monitor and correct the damage where possible. However, if the damage cannot be repaired, the cell will undergo a form of suicide, known as *programmed cell death* or *apoptosis* (see Figure 5.5). For example, if chemicals punch holes in the mitochondrial membrane, a protein involved in the electron transport chain known as *cytochrome c* is released into the cytoplasm. The presence of cytochrome c, which should not be found outside the mitochondria, triggers a cascade of linked proteins to cause the death of the cell (see the chapter 'Pathophysiological terminology, cellular adaptation and injury').

CARCINOGENESIS: CELL GROWTH, REGULATION AND DIFFERENTIATION

A cell must violate three fundamental rules to become a cancer cell.

1 A cell must normally only divide in response to an appropriate signal. A hormone or growth factor is normally the method by which cell division is activated. A potentially cancerous cell needs to be successful in permanently activating cell division without appropriate signalling.

2 A cell must normally undergo apoptosis (programmed cell death) when faced with conditions that can cause aberrant or excessive cell division. Genes called tumour suppressors (such as *RB1*—retinoblastoma gene—and *PT53*, which makes p53 proteins that prevent cell division) are responsible for maintaining genomic integrity. Mutation in these genes may have permitted a potentially cancerous cell to avoid the activation of self-destruction programmes.

3 A cell must normally only divide a certain number of times. As previously discussed, this control is usually achieved through the shortening of the chromosomal end cap called a telomere. The telomere is a repeated DNA sequence which erodes and shortens with each cell division. Once all of the repeats in the telomere are gone, the cell is no longer capable of dividing. A potentially cancerous cell must have either activated an enzyme called telomerase or adopted a similar alternate strategy to permit the addition of new repeats to be added to the end of the chromosome, effectively bypassing the control of finite cell divisions.

If a cell does violate these three rules, it becomes capable of unrestrained growth independent of an initiating signal, and impervious to attempts to monitor and/or ameliorate the

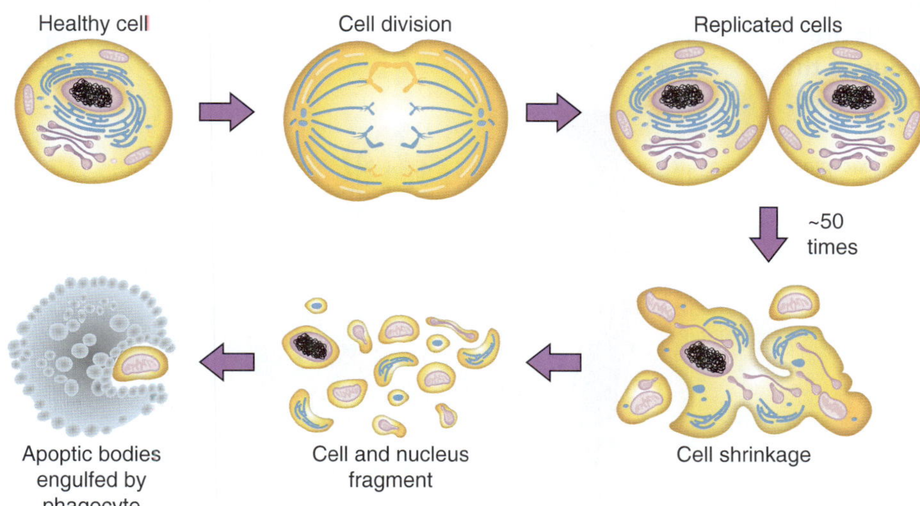

Figure 5.4

Cells become senescent and apoptic after 50–60 replications

Source: © Sciencopia.

Figure 5.5

Damaged cells undergo apoptosis

Source: © Sciencopia.

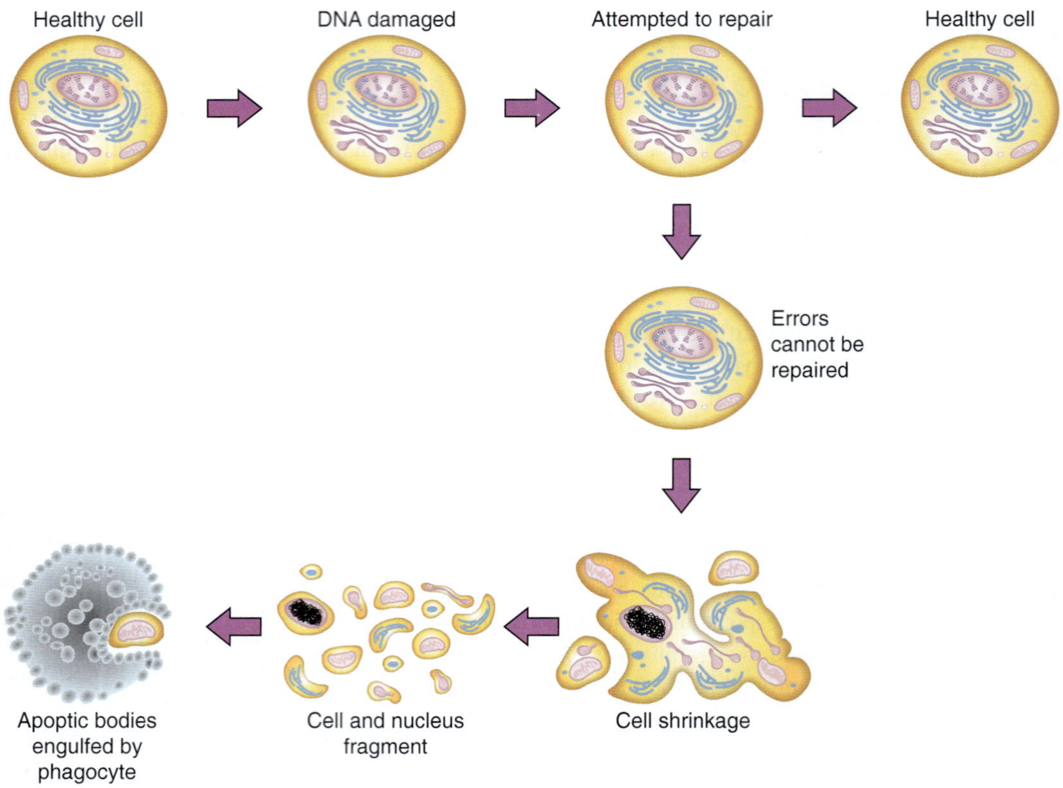

unrestrained growth. Because these cells are insensitive to attempts to activate apoptosis, they will encroach upon their neighbours. They will sequester nutrients for their own use at the expense of their neighbours, and, if circumstances permit, will migrate to other parts of the body (see Figure 5.6). There is evidence to suggest that many types of cancer cells can generate their own growth signals, creating a self-perpetuating loop, which allows practically limitless growth either by

Figure 5.6

When normal cells become damaged they undergo apoptosis, but cancer cells are impervious to the apoptosis signal

Source: © Sciencopia.

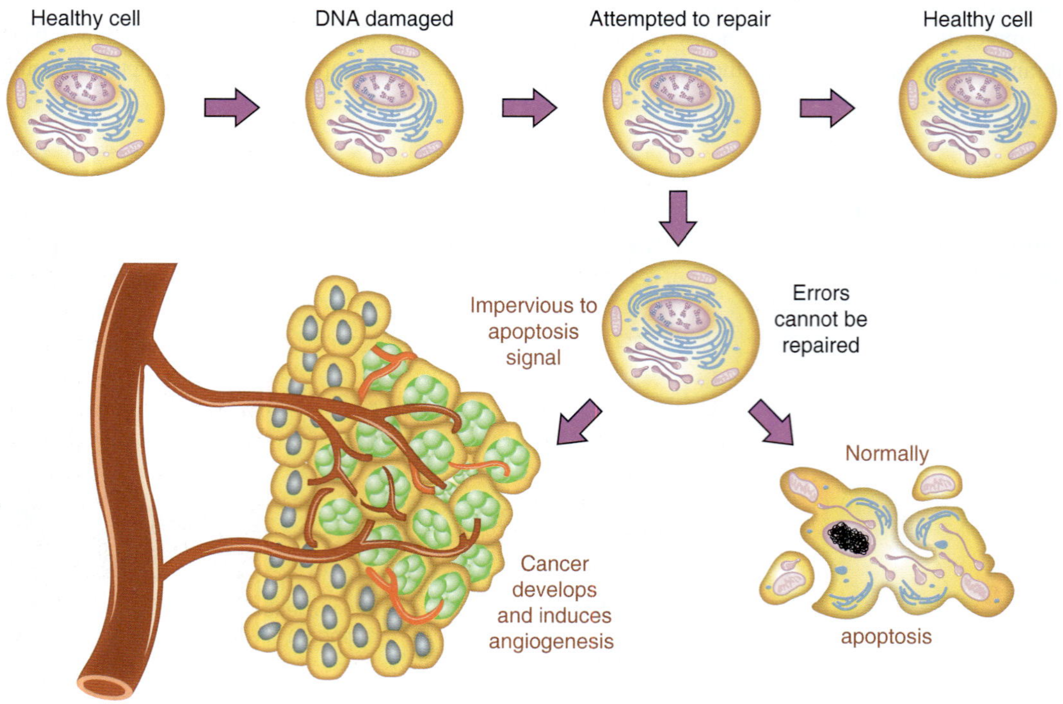

changing or over-expressing growth factor receptors (e.g. the epidermal growth factor receptor in stomach, brain and breast cancer) so that they are active in the absence of a signal (known as **constitutive activity**). Cells can also increase growth factor synthesis in certain cancers (e.g. platelet-derived growth factor and tumour growth factor-alpha in glioblastomas and sarcomas). Further, changes to the way in which a cell processes extracellular signals can also predispose a cell to cancer and/or promote tumour activity. In other words, the growth signals or receptors might be normal, but the internal protein cascade to which they are linked is irrevocably altered.

One of the first intracellular signalling molecules to be implicated in carcinogenesis were the RAS proteins, which are involved in everything from neurotransmitter release in neurons to cell growth. These proteins normally modulate the activity of G proteins, allowing an interaction between surface receptors and key intracellular cascades. Mutated RAS proteins have been found in more than 30% of all cancers, including pancreatic cancers (95%), carcinomas of the colon (45%) and adenocarcinoma of the lung (35%).

Although many epigenetic changes (those not arising from genetic influences) are a normal part of cellular function, when these events reduce or eliminate the activity of tumour suppressor proteins (for example), cell growth will be unchecked and/or apoptosis avoided. In this instance, cancer will result. A substance called pRB protein, from the retinoblastoma gene, normally arrests cell growth, and the activity of this protein is blocked by growth signals, such as the release of growth factors. If an epigenetic event, triggered by a carcinogen or internal signal, prevents the acetylation of certain histones, the stretch of DNA on which the retinoblastoma gene is found might not be made available, and so the signal to inhibit further cell growth is lost. In this case, the gene itself is normal, but the ability of the cell to access that gene is lost, and therefore the control of growth is reduced.

Caffeine has been demonstrated to increase levels of a protein called SC35, which controls the alternative splicing of genes (when DNA sequence is used to assemble different proteins). This protein controls the alternative splicing of genes such as *KLF6*, a tumour suppressor gene implicated in prostate cancer. Interestingly, caffeine has been proposed to be a protective substance in neurodegenerative diseases and certain cancers; it has been argued that its effect on alternative splicing might enhance the activity of normal *KLF6* or even reduce the impact of mutated *KLF6* genes. This data supports the proposal that lifestyle substances and not just environmental carcinogens could potentially contribute to and/or protect from carcinogenesis.

Inflammation (see the chapter 'Inflammation and healing') has been linked to mutational events in a variety of cells, with a key role played by reactive oxygen species, also known as oxygen free radicals (see the chapter 'Pathophysiological terminology, cellular adaptation and injury'). Chronic inflammatory conditions, such as chronic hepatitis and ulcerative colitis, are associated with increased levels of tumour necrosis factor-alpha (TNF-α), a potent endogenous mutagen, which is known to increase cancer risk. Although endogenous antioxidants, such as vitamin E (α-tocopherol), can significantly reduce the DNA damage caused by TNF-α–generated reactive oxygen species, in chronic inflammatory conditions it is not unusual for levels of antioxidants to be reduced. Further, up-regulation of enzymes such as inducible nitric oxide synthase, lipoxygenase and cyclo-oxygenase 2 will promote the availability of reactive oxygen species, as well as triggering the growth of tumours.

Characteristics of cancer cells

When a person encounters a lump or an unexpected growth, such as when a woman undertakes a routine breast self-examination, the lump might be benign or malignant. Benign tumours tend to grow more slowly than malignant tumours, are well-differentiated (i.e. they more closely resemble the surrounding tissue, upon examination of biopsy material) and are encapsulated. While it is true that malignant tumours, by contrast, generally grow more rapidly, this is not always the case. In fact, some benign tumours can grow very rapidly, while some malignant tumours grow slowly, inhibiting the effectiveness of many classic anticancer drugs, which often rely on rapid growth rates to be effective. Malignant tumours are also most often poorly differentiated, have many dividing cells within the mass, are not encapsulated and invade local tissues.

Generally, cancer cells are less differentiated than normal cells or become completely undifferentiated, which makes sense given that terminally differentiated normal cells such as neurons usually don't divide. Usually malignant cancer cells are less differentiated compared to benign cancer cells. When the cells are undifferentiated, they are referred to as **anaplastic**. Generally, the more malignant a tumour, the more anaplastic it is. Additionally, cancer cells might have defects in differentiation, allowing a cell that was of one type, such as a nerve, to acquire the characteristics of another type, such as muscle. This change in differentiation state means that the cells that comprise a tumour can be of different sizes, shapes and types, a status referred to as *pleomorphic*.

Changes to the characteristics of cells that make them cancerous often involve marked changes to the proteins and compounds that are produced within the cell and on the cell surface, and released from the cells. Depending on the identity of the chemicals and proteins released by these cancer cells, it is possible in some types of cancer to test a person's blood for the presence of these compounds, which are referred to as **tumour markers** or *biological markers*. An example of a common tumour marker that is tested routinely is prostate-specific antigen (PSA). Unfortunately, not all tumours of a given type will express the tumour marker; therefore, these screening methods, while valuable, must be used in conjunction with other testing. Also problematic is the fact that both malignant and benign tumours might release the same chemicals, and, therefore, while the presence of a tumour can be identified, its nature cannot.

Surprisingly, not all cells within a tumour are truly immortal; in other words, only certain cancer cells can divide indefinitely. This presents an interesting problem for cancer chemotherapy, as the cells within the tumour that are not immortal can be more sensitive to treatment than the immortal cells. Given that even a single cell, when active, can give rise to an entire tumour, a failure to kill all affected cells means that after treatment the cancer can re-emerge. As one of the key characteristics of malignancy is the ability of the tumour to invade neighbouring tissues and travel to other tissues, the presence of a single viable cancer cell is potentially life-threatening.

Cancer development is so complex that a framework to conceptualise the process is evolving. Through various cell function alterations, many of which we have already discussed, cancer cells develop properties unlike normal, healthy cells. These properties, known as the *hallmarks of cancer cells,* have been most recently updated by Hanahan to include two further hallmarks and two enabling characteristics (see Figure 5.7). (A) represents an evolution of normal cells to cancer cells through hyperplasia, dysplasia, cancer in situ and invasive malignancy. (B) represents the hallmarks and enabling characteristics that are present in most, if not all, cancer cells, and promote, enable or perpetuate cancer activity. The properties explained here include:

- *Genomic instability:* Cells that become cancer cells experience an increased rate of mutation that avoids the myriad safety mechanisms that normally prevent the use of damaged DNA.
- *Tumour promoting inflammation:* Increased inflammation in the tumour microenvironment from pro-inflammatory molecules released by the mutated cell promotes cell proliferation, contributes to genomic instability, and promotes the construction of new blood vessels (angiogenesis) that increase nutrient delivery, which increases the risk of metastasis.
- *Sustaining proliferative signalling:* When mutations cause the activation of the pathways or proteins responsible for the rapid and uncontrolled production of more cells, it creates an environment where there is less time for DNA repair, and also a greater volume of mutated cells to survive evolutionary selection.
- *Evading growth suppressors:* When cancer cells can resist the effects of proteins that halt the cell cycle at checkpoints that would normally prevent or repair mutation, they become capable of continued growth and proliferation.
- *Resisting apoptosis:* If the pathways that result in programmed cell death are inactivated by mutation, the cell can resist the need for cell suicide, which will further perpetuate the mutation.
- *Enabling replicative immortality:* When a cancer cell can override the process that results in a finite number of replications, usually provided by telomere length, the cell will not enter a state of senescence. This cell not only becomes capable of endless replication, but can also undertake the process faster, resulting from an increased transcription rate.
- *Angiogenesis induction:* With cell proliferation, increased tissue density results in a microenvironment that is rich in carbon dioxide and waste, and oxygen-poor. These conditions, along with molecules secreted by the cancer cells, can increase the production of new blood cells in the area.
- *Activation of invasion and metastasis:* When cancer cells can secrete molecules that are capable of degrading nearby tissue that may have contained them, they can invade surrounding tissue. This may give them access to nearly blood or lymphatic vessels.
- *Deregulating cellular energetics:* As cancerous tissue volume increases, a disparity in nutrient delivery and waste production can cause the cells in the overstressed microenvironment to change to less efficient energy systems, resulting in an increased need for glucose.

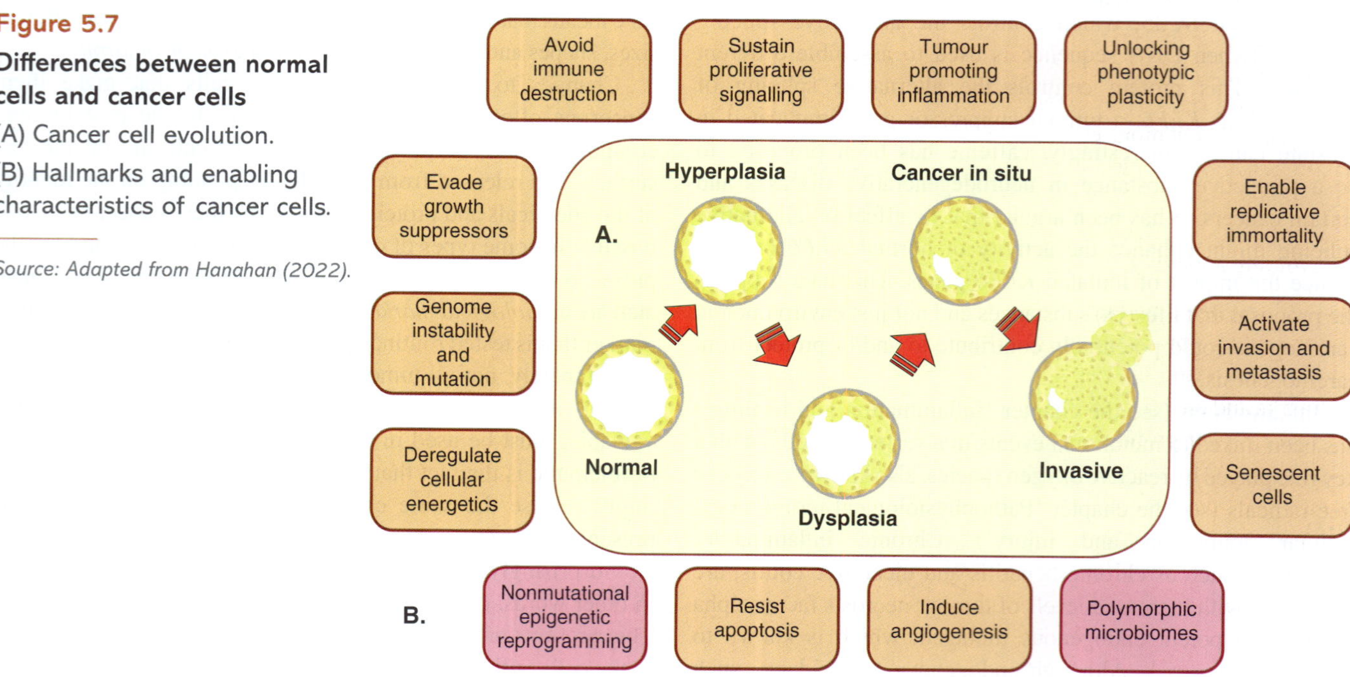

Figure 5.7

Differences between normal cells and cancer cells

(A) Cancer cell evolution.

(B) Hallmarks and enabling characteristics of cancer cells.

Source: Adapted from Hanahan (2022).

- *Avoiding immune destruction:* The persistence of cancer cells developing the capability of evading immune surveillance or resisting immune-mediated destruction means that the cells become evolutionarily superior and gain a selective advantage.

In recent years, several more mechanisms of tumour development have been attributed to the change from normal cells to cancer cells. The most recent four characteristics include:

- *Unlocking phenotypic plasticity:* During development, once cells have organised into mature tissue and are able to service the needs of the structure (organogenesis), progenitor cells may no longer need to differentiate (change). This process of *terminal differentiation* is known to be one of the factors preventing possible transformation from normal cells to cancer cells. Phenotypic plasticity suggests that some cells may short-circuit this process and evade the permanency of their correct shape and function to regain the ability to differentiate and therefore increase the likelihood of mutation resulting in neoplasm.
- *Nonmutational epigenetic reprogramming:* The concept of cells adjusting to environmental conditions can be likened to a mini-Darwinian 'survival of the fittest' experience, with cells that change to resist the challenges of the microenvironment prevailing over cells that are unable to adapt. To this end, there is a suggestion that this, initially physiological change, sets up the circumstance for proliferative expansion. With the addition of other pro-neoplastic factors, these cells are more likely capable of undergoing further mutation resulting in tumourgenesis.
- *Polymorphic microbiomes:* With advancement in our understanding of the genetic diversity of our microbiome (microbes which live in and on us), it has become clear that there are collections of bacterial species that are tumour-promoting which alter the environment and surrounding tissue, and subsequently influence tumourigenesis.
- *Senescent cells:* Having previously established that *resisting apoptosis* is a factor contributing to tumourigenesis, where senescent cells fail to commit cell suicide to prevent cancerous mutation, evidence is also now strengthening to suggest that, in some circumstances, cell senescence may also stimulate tumour development through signalling molecules, angiogenesis induction, suppressing tumour immunity, and avoiding apoptosis.

Quantifying these properties has become critical not only for understanding how cancer develops, but also in the search for finding therapeutic interventions to treat cancer. Each of these hallmarks and enabling characteristics represent a potential drug target for cancer prophylaxis or treatment. (See more on this in the section on the management of cancer, later in this chapter.) Excitingly, this knowledge enables the development of more targeted cancer treatment as opposed to historical imprecise approaches that can result in extensive damage and destruction to healthy tissue, which may ultimately result in unpleasant and potentially serious side-effects of treatment.

LEARNING OBJECTIVE 3

Outline cancer aetiology, and describe the various factors predisposing someone to carcinogenesis.

Cancers develop because of mutations, which may be inherited, induced by environmental factors or result from random DNA replication errors. A recent genomic and epidemiological investigation, culminating in some mathematical modelling, suggests that up to two-thirds of human cancers may be caused by random mutations in DNA replication. This major claim would suggest that most cancers are not preventable. There is still clearly much that we do not understand about carcinogenesis, and this new assertion highlights the need for more research. So, until more definitive, evidence-based answers with global acceptance develop, we should work on the concept that modifying or eliminating risk factors will significantly reduce the risk of developing cancer.

There are many risk factors that have been attributed to cancer development; however, one-third of cancer deaths can be directly associated with five modifiable factors. The primary modifiable factor causing over 8 million cancer-related deaths is the use of tobacco; the other factors include alcohol consumption, high body mass index, low fruit and vegetable intake, and lack of physical activity. The WHO focuses cancer prevention on systematic, evidence-based strategies for seven major risk factors. Figure 5.8 outlines these most common risk factors, details the mechanism by which the cancer develops, and suggests methods to prevent cancer by that cause.

LEARNING OBJECTIVE 4

Describe the types of genes that are known to contribute to cancer.

Ultimately, cancer development is proposed to occur as a result of a mutation to both alleles of a given gene. If someone has inherited one mutant allele, they only require one mutational event at the normal allele to trigger cancer, leading to the so-called *two-hit hypothesis* (see Figure 5.9). Subsequently, it was discovered that certain viruses could cause cancer in animals, such as leukaemia in cats, leading to the discovery of **oncogenes**; namely, genes that caused cancer. Human equivalents of these genes were found, coding for normal essential proteins. These normal genes were then referred to as **proto-oncogenes**, with the demonstration that mutations of these genes allowed them to contribute to cancer, and therefore to be referred to as oncogenes. Oncogenes tend to be dominant at the cellular level, where a mutation is needed in only one allele to trigger cancer.

However, these very straightforward examples of cancer development, or **carcinogenesis**, are not the most common processes through which cancer is established. Generally, a number of mutations, not just one or two, occur in a family of cells, referred to as a *cell lineage*, and many of these mutations occur in stem cells. In fact, it has been proposed that four to seven mutations, accumulated as a person ages, are usually necessary for most types of cancer to develop.

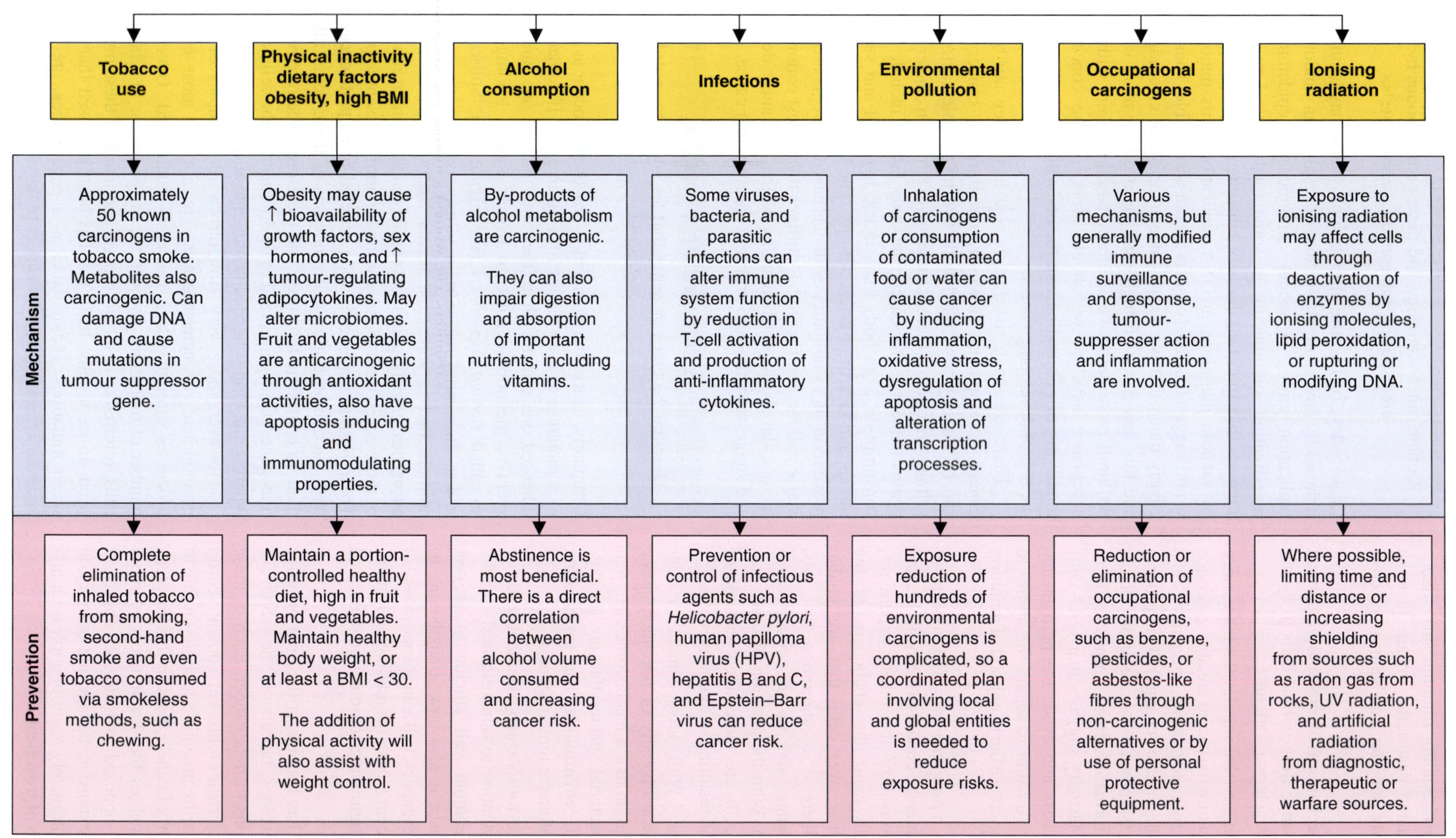

Figure 5.8

Major risk factors, mechanisms and prevention of preventable cancers

↑ = increased; BMI = body mass index; DNA = deoxyribonucleic acid; UV = ultraviolet.

Sources: Based on data from Belli & Tabocchini (2020); Cancer Council Australia (n.d.); Domenech (2017); Dyck & Mills (2017); Hosseini et al. (2021); Hussain et al. (2019); Papadimitriou et al. (2021); WHO (2022b); Yoo et al. (2022).

Figure 5.9

Knudson's two-hit hypothesis

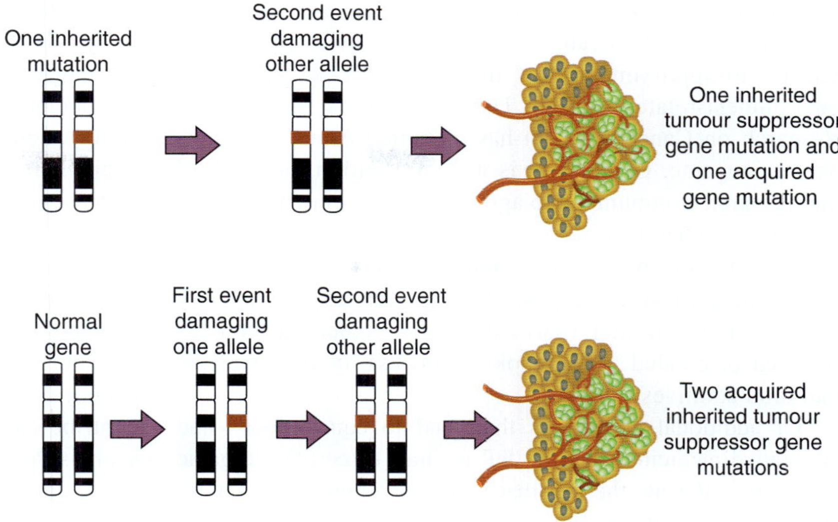

INHERITED CANCERS

The first human somatic gene mutation identified in association with cancer was a point mutation in the *HRAS* (human Ras) gene in a human bladder cancer cell line. Since that initial report in 1982, a small number of cancers have been shown to result from mutations in a single gene, referred to as *Mendelian cancers*, after the single gene inheritance model originally described by Gregor Mendel. As mentioned above, genes that involve a loss of function, such as **tumour suppressor genes**, are generally inherited as recessive conditions. This means that an individual must either inherit two copies of the mutated gene or, as shown with retinoblastoma, inherit a single copy and then experience a mutation in the other gene that leads to cancer formation. By contrast, if the gene is responsible for growth, such as a growth factor receptor, and the mutation allows a gain of function, such as activity of the receptor in the absence of a signal, these cancers are inherited as an dominant condition, meaning that only a single copy of the mutant gene is required. Mendelian cancers are much easier to screen than the majority of cancers, as only a single site within the genome needs to be evaluated. However, it is essential to note that different genes can contribute to the same type of cancer, and therefore more than one gene might need to be screened. The list of genes associated with cancer continues to expand, with examples of genes identified including breast cancer (*BRCA1, BRCA2, ERBB2, PTPRF*), retinoblastoma (*RB*), melanoma (*BRAF*) and colorectal cancer (*MSH6, PMS2, EPHA3, MLK4, PTPN3*). Interestingly, although the affected gene remains the same, the mutations identified often differ between families.

The majority of human cancer genes represent somatic mutations, with a small proportion due to mutations in germline cells or both. The nature of the mutations also differs between somatic and germline cells, with the majority of somatic mutations having dominant inheritance and representing translocations. By contrast, most germline mutations are inherited in a recessive manner. These data are interesting when considered in the context of the number and types of mutations that can occur and the causes of DNA mutation.

However, the situation is complicated by the fact that the overwhelming majority of single gene cancers have less than 100% penetrance; in other words, having the mutation does not necessarily mean that the person will have cancer. The demonstration of reduced penetrance for inherited cancers has sparked an enormous interest in genetic modifiers, which might provide new targets for chemotherapeutic or even preventative drugs.

In an excellent example of decreased penetrance, a family was identified with Lynch syndrome, or hereditary non-polyposis colorectal cancer, in which affected individuals have colorectal cancers that can also appear in other sites such as the face. A 26-year-old woman was diagnosed with colorectal cancer only days after her maternal grandfather, who had previously had four colorectal cancers removed and had just learnt that a tumour removed from his face carried the mutation associated with Lynch syndrome. The young woman was tested for the mutation, and it was found that she had the same mutation as her grandfather. The mutated gene in Lynch syndrome is inherited as an dominant disorder, meaning that only a single copy of the mutated gene is required. The woman's mother was completely healthy and had no history of cancer, and a colonoscopy performed after her father and daughter were diagnosed showed no signs of any abnormalities whatsoever. In order to have an dominant disorder, the young woman must have inherited the gene from her mother, but in this family the penetrance of the gene is highly variable.

Cancers that do not have a genetic basis (i.e. are not related to inherited gene changes) are called *sporadic* in origin. Sporadic cancers are caused by cellular errors, environmental exposures, diet and lifestyle choices, hormones, pathogens, or other influences. Most cancers are considered sporadic.

CARCINOGENS AND THE ROLE OF THE ENVIRONMENT

Carcinogens are factors that promote **transformation** of cells, leading to cancer formation. In some parts of the world, environmental exposure has been touted as a major contributor to carcinogenesis. The WHO estimates that 19% of total cancer deaths are due to the environment. This equates to approximately 1.7 million deaths per year from environment-related cancer. The International Agency for Research on Cancer (IACR) has classified over 100 agents as carcinogenic. Of concern is a failure within the medical and research communities to agree on whether environmental exposure to chemical, physical and/or biological agents is a major or minor contributor to **tumorigenesis** when compared to so-called lifestyle factors, such as tobacco use, alcohol consumption and diet (particularly fat content, chemicals released or created in the cooking process, or preservatives and food additives).

Of additional concern is the trend to equate foods and alternative medicines that are 'all natural' or certified organic with safety, despite the fact that many carcinogens are natural and organic. Aflatoxin B1 is a natural product of the fungus *Aspergillus flavus*, which is commonly found on a number of agricultural products, including cotton, peanuts, corn, grain and pistachios. It is a potent carcinogen implicated in liver cancer. When ingested, aflatoxin B1 is oxidised by cytochrome P450 enzymes in the liver and turned into aflatoxin-epoxide, which damages DNA through the introduction of errors in repair. While washing agricultural products is insufficient to remove the toxin, roasting, such as with peanuts, for example, will reduce the aflatoxin content of a sample of contaminated nuts, although it does not completely remove the toxin.

Another natural source of carcinogens is cooked food. Heterocyclic amines and polycyclic aromatic hydrocarbons are the product of heating protein-rich food, and are generated during such everyday activities as putting a steak on the barbecue or pan-frying a piece of meat. Heterocyclic amines cause DNA mutations similar to those caused by aflatoxin, and have been implicated in prostate cancer. A study of more than 57,000 people in the United States demonstrated a possible link between the ingestion of well-done or very-well-done meat and prostate cancer, with a 1.26-fold increase in the risk of prostate cancer and a 1.97-fold risk of advanced disease.

Another type of natural carcinogen is represented by ultraviolet (UV) rays and natural sources of ionising radiation. Most people are familiar with the concept that prolonged exposure to the sun or intense acute exposure, such as with a sunburn, can lead to melanoma. UV radiation causes the formation of covalent bonds in DNA, which, when corrected, introduces errors into the genome that accumulate over time and can lead to cancer formation. Ionising radiation can introduce strand breaks, covalent bonds and other damage to DNA, and natural sources of this carcinogen include long-distance flights and the geological properties of the places where people live or go on vacation. As an example, the background radiation in Townsville in North Queensland is twice that of neighbouring cities because of the presence of a small amount of uranium in Castle Hill, a prominent feature in the heart of the city. Additionally, medical sources of ionising radiation must be taken into account, including diagnostic X-rays and research experiments, or nuclear accidents such as that following the great east-Japan earthquake and tsunami.

Another natural source of carcinogens that is often ignored is viruses. Since the identification of the role of viruses in carcinogenesis was identified in animals, extensive research has demonstrated that viruses can cause cancer in humans as well. Among the best known of these viruses are: the human papilloma virus (HPV), which causes cervical cancer; Epstein–Barr virus (EBV), which is implicated in Burkitt's lymphoma, Hodgkin's lymphoma and nasopharyngeal carcinoma; hepatitis B and C viruses, which have been linked to hepatocellular carcinoma; and herpes virus type 8 (HHV-8), which contributes to Kaposi's sarcoma.

There is no question, however, that environmental chemicals provide a breadth of possible carcinogens that contribute to human disease. Polycyclic aromates are chemicals such as the 'tar' found in cigarettes. These compounds cause DNA damage similar to that caused by aflatoxin, and are primarily associated with lung cancer. However, it is important to remember that there are additional carcinogens in cigarette smoke, including aldehydes, nitrosamines, heavy metals and even the radioactive isotope polonium-210, the latter of which is known to be in cigarettes, but has generally been ignored since its initial discovery in 1964. Although excellent progress has been made in reducing tobacco use—with approximately 69 million fewer people currently smoking tobacco worldwide (compared to 2000), and more than 60 counties on track to reduce tobacco use by 30% by 2025—cigarette smoking still poses a large risk factor for cancer. The WHO estimates that tobacco accounts for an estimated 22% of all cancer deaths, equating to more than 8 million lives lost per year. The Global Burden of Disease Study 2019 equates it to 33.9% in males. Tobacco is also responsible for 90% of all lung cancer deaths. It is argued that the combination of tobacco smoke and the tar contained in cigarettes represents a 'complete carcinogen' because of the combination of chemicals involved. By contrast, asbestos, a well-recognised and feared carcinogen, is responsible for only approximately 10% of lung cancers, even though Australia has one of the highest rates of asbestos-related cancer in the world.

Tumour invasion and metastasis

LEARNING OBJECTIVE 5

Describe the process of tumour invasion and metastasis.

In order for cells to migrate from one location to another, they require certain characteristics, such as the ability to grow without being anchored in place or connected to other cells, the ability to create finger-like projections (e.g. filopodia, pseudopodia) to reach between other cells or into lymphatic or blood vessels (see Figure 5.10), and the capacity to produce proteins and enzymes to facilitate the breakdown of barriers to movement. Certain normal cells can do all of these things; namely, the cells of the immune system, such as macrophages. With the mutations that accumulate within the rapidly growing cells of a cancer, these

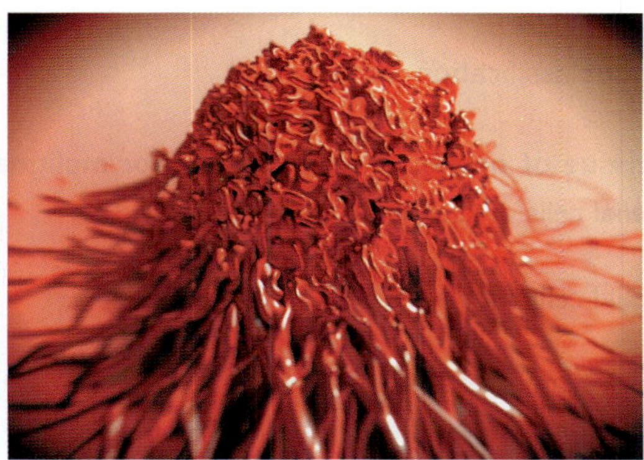

Figure 5.10

Coloured scanning electron micrograph of a prostate cancer cell showing the typical microvilli and filopodia

Source: royaltystockphoto.com/Shutterstock.

characteristics can be acquired, and the recruitment of blood vessels to facilitate the growing tumour provides a route through which its cells can spread to other parts of the body.

It has been proposed that the first step in the process of tissue invasion and subsequent **metastasis** is for the tumour cell to become detached from its neighbours. In part, this occurs due to a change in the expression of surface proteins, particularly fibronectin and cadherin, which reduce the connection between adjacent cells and render the cell unable to associate with its neighbours. The tumour cell must be able to express receptors, such as the laminin receptor, which allow it to recognise and bind to the basement membrane. Secretion of enzymes to degrade the proteins and collagen of the extracellular matrix that supports the tissue or organ, and gives it structure, allows penetration of pseudopodia through the interstitial connective tissue layer, which anchor to the walls of the blood and lymphatic vessels. The cell then literally pulls itself through the gap and into these vessels, to be carried to other tissues throughout the body, where the process acts partly in reverse, namely for the pseudopodia to penetrate back through the wall of the vessel and insert themselves into the new tissue, where growth begins anew.

Classification of tumours

The two primary issues associated with the classification of tumours are: the tissue and cell source, and therefore type of tumour; and the grading of the tumour. Although the source of many different types of cancer is often known, as we discussed in the 'Epidemiology of cancer' section earlier in this chapter, some tumours have unknown sources. Initial classification of the tumour requires identification of the tissue of origin. The suffix *-oma*, which is from the Greek, meaning a 'result' or 'outcome', is used to denote a tumour, and the primary part of each word denotes the source of the tumour. Therefore, a lymphoma is a tumour from lymphatic tissue, whereas a glioma is a glial cell tumour. It is common for the tumour name to be a compound word, such as lymphosarcoma, to denote a sarcoma that arises from lymph nodes, the spleen or the thymus. Table 5.3 provides an overview of common tumour types and names.

It should be noted that certain tumour types are benign while others are malignant, and the name given to the tumour denotes this. While both benign and malignant tumours are comprised of a rapidly growing parenchyma (functional core) and supportive stroma (framework), which is connective tissue and blood vessels, it is the nature of the parenchyma that determines whether a tumour is benign or malignant. A benign tumour is one that does not invade or destroy the tissue in which it originates, and does not spread, whereas one that is malignant does destroy tissue, will spread and can cause death. Therefore, lipomas or fibromas are common benign tumours that, while they might grow rapidly and cause pain and discomfort, have no lasting impact on the individual once they are removed, and do not cause disease.

Several grading systems are used to describe cancers, one of which was developed by the Union for International Cancer Control (UICC). This system, also known as the *TNM system*, classifies cancer according to the primary tumour (T), the regional lymph node involvement (N) and the presence or absence of metastases (M). The size is rated on a scale of 1 to 4 (T1–T4), where T0 denotes an in-situ (i.e. in place) tumour. If no lymph nodes are involved, the cancer is rated N0, but if lymph nodes are involved, an increasing number and range of nodes is denoted by an increasing number from 1 to 3 (N1–N3). If the tumour has not metastasised, then it is designated an M0 tumour, but if it has, then M1 or M2 will be used to identify whether there are some or many metastases. A more basic grading system comes from the American Joint Committee on Cancer Staging, which uses stages, designated 0–IV, wherein each stage is defined on the basis of the same characteristics used in the TNM system.

Clinical manifestations of cancer

LEARNING OBJECTIVE 6

Outline the common clinical manifestations of cancer.

PAIN

Pain in someone with cancer may occur for a number of reasons. The increased size of the neoplastic tissue may produce pressure on organs, nerves or bone. This pressure is then transmitted via afferent nerves to the brain, where it is interpreted as pain. Treatments administered to manage the cancer may also cause pain. Some chemotherapeutic agents can cause peripheral neuropathies, mucositis and abdominal pain. Surgery for investigation or for the resection of tumours can result in pain from the tissue trauma related to the surgery. External beam radiotherapy can also cause pain, as it causes local inflammation, which results in the release of prostaglandins, which irritate the nerve endings and are transmitted and interpreted as pain.

Table 5.3 Nomenclature for tumour classification

Tumour type	Word root	Cell/tissue of origin	Benign or malignant
Adenoma	New Latin *aden*, meaning 'gland'	Epithelial cells of glands or ducts	Benign
Adenocarcinoma	Conjunction of adenoma and carcinoma	Epithelial cells of glands or ducts	Malignant
Angioma	Greek *angieo*-, meaning 'vessel'	Blood or lymph vessels	Benign
Blastoma	Greek *blastos*, meaning 'bud' or 'shoot'; used to denote embryonic cells	Depends on the prefix: e.g. a neuroblastoma is a tumour derived from embryonic neural cells; a retinoblastoma is a tumour derived from the embryonic retina	Malignant
Carcinoma	Greek *karkinos*, meaning 'crab', and therefore 'cancer'	Epithelial cells	Malignant
Fibroma	Modification of French *fibreux*, meaning 'fibre'	Connective (fibrous) tissue or fibroblasts	Benign
Lipoma	Greek *lipos*, meaning 'fat'	Well-differentiated fat cells	Benign
Melanoma (*Note:* These tumours are more properly known as 'melanocarcinomas'.)	Greek *melas*, meaning 'black'	Melanocytes	Malignant
Neuroma	Latin *nervus*, meaning 'nerve'	Neurons	Benign
Osteoma	New Latin *oste*, meaning 'bone'	Bone	Benign
Papilloma	Latin *papas*, meaning 'nipple', or a 'nipple-like projection'	Epithelial cells on papillae of vascular connective tissue; also an epithelial tumour caused by a virus	Benign
Sarcoma	Greek *sarcoma*, meaning 'fleshy growth'	Tissue of mesodermal origin, such as connective tissue, bone, cartilage or striated muscle	Malignant

FATIGUE

A feeling of malaise or fatigue is commonly reported by people with cancer. Although the causes of cancer-related fatigue are not well understood, it is thought that many factors contribute to its development. Chronic exposure to stress and pain has been associated with fatigue. Alterations to diet resulting in poor nutrition can cause fatigue. Some healthcare professionals believe that there is an element of competition with the tumour for nutrients. Cancer treatment is also known to cause symptoms of fatigue. Some chemotherapeutic agents commonly cause fatigue for several weeks after treatment; other side-effects result from the impact of chemotherapy on the development of red blood cells, resulting in anaemia. Anaemia will also cause fatigue. Radiotherapy and other cancer-managing interventions can insult the body so much that they result in fatigue that often persists for weeks to months after treatments.

CACHEXIA

Cachexia—weakness or body-wasting—may develop in those with advanced or end-stage cancer. Although the mechanism for the development of cancer-related cachexia is not entirely established, several contributing factors are known. Some tumours can release proteolytic factors, such as proteolysis-inducing factor (PIF). PIF and several inflammatory mediators are thought to contribute to the development of cachexia.

ANAEMIA

Several factors are known to contribute to the development of cancer-related anaemia. Some tumours can secrete substances that cause a reduction in erythropoietin (EPO), which reduces red blood cell production. Iron storage may also be altered. An increase in the amount of blood lost through haemorrhage is possible, and an increase in haemolysis can also occur; therefore, more cells may be lost and fewer replaced. These factors independently or cumulatively can result in the development of anaemia. Unfortunately, some treatments, including chemotherapy and radiotherapy, can also induce anaemia. The mechanism of treatment-related anaemia is generally as a result of myelosuppression.

INFECTION

Although some infections can cause cancer, most cancer causes an increased risk of infection. Several factors are thought to contribute to the development of cancer-related infection, including the possibility that the immune system is so overwhelmed (distracted) by the presence of the cancer that the immunosurveillance for pathogens is compromised. A person with cancer will generally experience an increase in stress, a decrease in sleep and a poorer diet. All of these factors can increase the risk of infection. The stress response results in the release of cortisol. Cortisol causes immunosuppression. Finally, when cancer affects the bone marrow, or chemotherapy or radiotherapy are used, an increased risk of infection develops. Neutropenia is a common issue in people receiving chemotherapeutic agents. When the immune system is so compromised, even normal flora can become pathogenic.

Figure 5.11 explores the clinical manifestations and management of some common cancer-related signs and symptoms.

PARANEOPLASTIC SYNDROMES

Various symptoms can occur either as a direct result of immunological responses to the tumour presence or from substances secreted by the tumour. These are known as *paraneoplastic syndromes*. Biologically active substances can be released in large volumes due to ectopic production. As there are no nervous system connections to the tumour that can control the production and release of these substances, there is no negative feedback system to adjust secretion. Paraneoplastic syndromes are diverse and are often organised into systems. The diversity and effects of paraneoplastic syndromes are represented in Figure 5.12 and can be divided into endocrine, neurovascular, haematological, renal, gastrointestinal, rheumatological and cutaneous effects.

Screening, diagnosis and management

LEARNING OBJECTIVE 7

Describe contemporary and emerging screening, diagnostic and management options for people with cancer.

SCREENING

Population health initiatives such as the systematic cancer screening in asymptomatic populations are an important step in attempts to reduce the global burden of cancer. In Australia, three national screening programs are supported by various levels of government. These free programs aim to achieve early detection in three of Australia's highest-incidence cancers—breast, cervical and bowel cancer.

Other surveillance and detection opportunities outside of the national screening programs that are subsidised by Medicare, the Australian government's universal healthcare scheme, include the prostate-specific antigen (PSA) testing to detect prostate cancer in males, and breast imaging for women.

DIAGNOSIS

Primary prevention of cancer through the reduction of risk factors and carcinogen exposures constitutes an important step in reducing cancer morbidity and mortality; however, diagnostic interventions such as the early recognition of signs and symptoms, imaging and pathology are critical cancer control measures. Diagnostic modalities such as cytology, biopsy, histopathology, assessment of biomarkers, immunochemistry and various imaging technologies form the bulk of cancer investigations. Table 5.4 details the various methodologies used in the diagnosis of cancer.

In relation to diagnostic tests for the common signs and symptoms of cancer (pain, fatigue or cachexia), there are limited investigations. Observation and the collection of an in-depth history will assist in verifying that these signs and symptoms exist. Blood can be drawn for pathology to ascertain the presence of anaemia by observing red blood cell and haematocrit levels. Monitoring temperature, wounds and white blood cell counts can assist in the recognition of an emerging infection. Excessive pain at a surgical site can also be an early sign that an infection is developing. Pain can occur before erythema and swelling, and is commonly considered in retrospect after the infection has emerged.

MANAGEMENT

Conventional cancer management has included surgery, chemotherapy, radiotherapy, and bone marrow and stem cell transplants. Recently, there have been some major advances in the management of cancer, including new types of cancer drugs, hormone therapy and biological therapy. However, it needs to be noted that planning interventions for cancer are based on numerous factors. There are ultimately three possible courses a cancer management plan may take: the aims of the plan may be to cure, to control the cancer and prolong life, or to palliate the symptoms and facilitate comfort moving towards end-of-life care. Most people will receive a combination of treatments. The decisions leading up to treatment choices are complex, and are influenced by factors that can be grouped into three major variables. These include factors related to the:

- *individual*—including their mental and physical health, values and beliefs, sex, age, education, trust in medicine, previous medical experiences, and even the influence of family, friends and media
- *tumour*—including the size, type, staging, anatomical location, survival statistics, and ultimately potential for treatment success
- *treatment*—including local availability, effectiveness, affordability, and the existence of established guidelines.

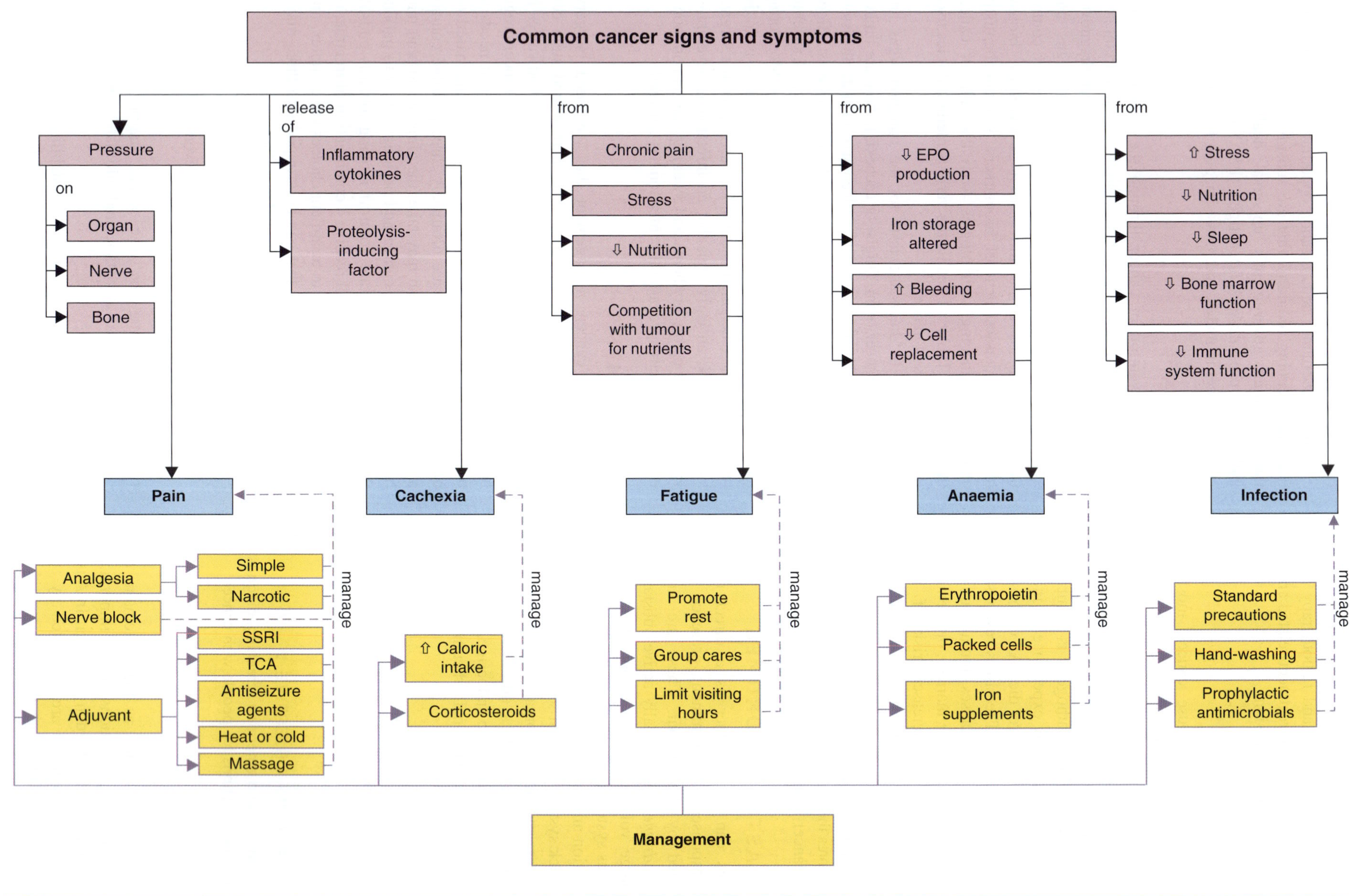

Figure 5.11

Clinical snapshot: Common cancer-related signs and symptoms.

↓ = decreased; ↑ = increased; EPO = erythropoietin; SSRI = selective serotonin reuptake inhibitor; TCA = tricyclic antidepressant.

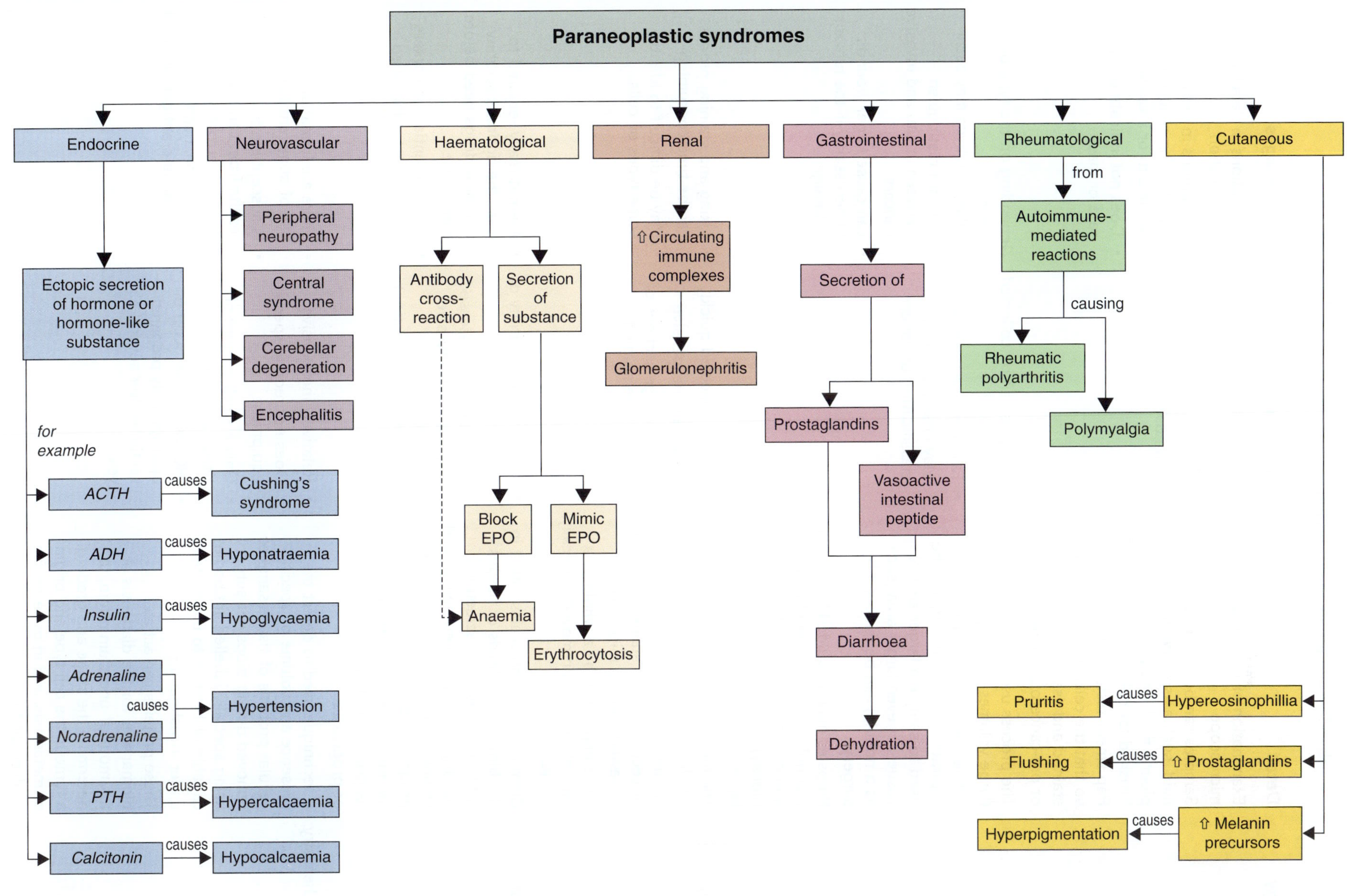

Figure 5.12

Summary of common paraneoplastic syndromes and effects

↑ = increased; ACTH = adrenocorticotropic hormone; ADH = antidiuretic hormone; EPO = erythropoietin; PTH = parathyroid hormone.

Table 5.4 Diagnostic methodologies utilised in cancer diagnosis

Methodology	Detail	Advantages	Disadvantages
Cytology	Examination of cells under a microscope Samples can be taken from body fluid, such as sputum, urine or pleural fluid, or can be scraped or brushed for collection, such as a Pap smear test, or oral scrapings, so that the cells collected can be stained and assessed for cancerous or pre-cancerous changes	• Less invasive • Less painful • Potential for more rapid diagnosis	• Limitations in detailed classification • Limitations in determining whether the cancerous cells are in situ or invasive • Does not indicate growth rate or mass
Biopsy	The process used to collect tissue (large volumes of cells) A fine needle can be used to aspirate, or a core needle can be used to sample a larger area of tissue. An even larger area (such as a nodule) can be removed by surgery Biopsies may be guided by imaging technology, such as an ultrasound, fluoroscopy, CT or MRI (stereotactic biopsy), or surgically via a laparoscope	• Samples can be collected quickly • Relatively inexpensive • May enable detailed classification of cancer	Depending on the type of biopsy: • false negatives may occur • may not distinguish between in-situ and invasive cancers • can cause larger wounds unnecessarily if the tumour is benign
Histopathology	The microscopic examination of whole tissue that has been sampled Tissue is generally prepared, sliced or sectioned, and stained and then reviewed under a microscope The sample may be a whole or a part of an organ removed surgically or via biopsy	• Can be collected quickly • Relatively inexpensive • Permits large sections of tissue to be studied	• Fixing and staining process can be time-consuming • May be difficult to identify some types of cells
Assessment of biomarkers	Biomarkers are molecules found in the blood, body fluids or tissues that can be used for screening, distinguishing between benign and malignant findings, determining prognosis, and potentially monitoring status for treatment response, or of cancer recurrence or progression	• There is a large variety of markers • Many are easily assessed and minimally invasive (i.e. detected in secretions or circulation)	• Are not really required to pass the rigorous scrutiny that new drugs need before clinical use • Many potential biomarkers have not yet established clinical utility
Immunohistochemistry (IHC)	A technique used to detect the presence and volume of specific cellular proteins of tissue samples removed during biopsy or surgery using specially labelled antibodies capable of binding to the proteins under investigation These proteins can act as biomarkers, for the diagnosis of a tumour of uncertain origin, to determine the stage and grade of a tumour, the cell type and origin or metastasis, and in gene profile analysis of tumours	• Relatively inexpensive • Does not require special equipment • Only a small amount of tissue is required • IHC testing can occur on appropriately prepared sections after several years	• There are limitations in the use of some antibodies • Is susceptible to unreliable results from various technical errors related to acquisition, handling, fixation and antigen retrieval

Table 5.4 Diagnostic methodologies utilised in cancer diagnosis (*continued*)

Methodology	Detail	Advantages	Disadvantages
X-ray	Uses a controlled beam of radiation which either passes through or is blocked by tissue to varying degrees The denser the structure, the whiter the image (e.g. bone); the less dense the structure, the blacker the image (e.g. air) Contrast may be added to increase the visibility of a structure	• Fast • Painless • Generally, no preparation needed • Inexpensive	• The tests expose a person to a dose of radiation (albeit a small dose) • Allergies to contrast materials, iodine or seafood render contrast imaging impossible • Unable to diagnose the tumour as a cancer, and will need further follow-up investigations to quantify the lesion
Ultrasound	Uses high-frequency sound waves that penetrate tissue and bounce (reflect) echoes that can be displayed in real time on a screen	• Fast • Painless • Good for imaging soft tissue that is less visible on X-ray • Good for solid tumours and cysts • No exposure to radiation	• Images not as detailed as CT or MRI • Image unable to determine whether the tumour is a cancer, and will need further follow-up investigations to quantify the lesion
Endoscopy	Uses a special camera in the shape of a long, flexible tube that can be introduced into the cavity requiring investigation Endoscopes can examine the respiratory, gastrointestinal, renal and reproductive systems via natural openings	• Quick recovery as minimally invasive • No scars • Minimal discomfort • Low-risk • Cost-effective	Small potential for: • excessive bleeding • infection • organ perforation
Computerised tomography (CT) scan	Uses a pencil-thin beam of radiation from multiple angles Creates a 3D image of the scanned area, and permits a tumour's shape, size and location to be easily quantified	• Painless • Images are clearer than X-ray • Can be used in conjunction with other diagnostic techniques, such as biopsy (to guide sampling) • Can create a 3D view that can be rotated for further investigation	• Expensive • Larger dose of radiation than with an X-ray • Children often require sedation • Limitations on size and weight, related to an individual's ability to fit into the scanner • Allergies to contrast materials, iodine or seafood render contrast imaging impossible
Magnetic resonance imaging (MRI)	Uses magnetic fields and radiowaves to create 3D images of the scanned area Permits a tumour's shape, size and location to be easily quantified	• Painless • Non-invasive • Images are clearer than X-ray • Does not require exposure to ionising radiation • Can be used in conjunction with other diagnostic techniques, such as biopsy (to guide sampling) • Can create a 3D view that can be rotated for further investigation	• Can be noisy and lengthy • Children often require sedation • Contraindicated for individuals with metal in situ (e.g. a pacemaker or orthopaedic fixations) • Expensive • Limitations on size and weight, related to an individual's ability to fit into the scanner • Allergies to contrast materials, iodine or seafood render contrast imaging impossible

(*continued*)

Table 5.4 Diagnostic methodologies utilised in cancer diagnosis (*continued*)

Methodology	Detail	Advantages	Disadvantages
Radionuclide imaging	Uses tracers (radionuclides or radiopharmaceuticals) which release a low level of radiation Types of radionuclide imaging include: • thyroid scans • bone scans • PET scans • gallium scans • MUGA scans	Shows internal organ and tissue function issues well, through 'hot spots' where metabolism is increased, or 'cold spots' where metabolism is decreased	• Exposure to a small amount of gamma radiation is necessary • May not locate small tumours well • Are not detailed images • Unable to distinguish whether the find is a tumour or something else (i.e. infection) • Often requires follow-up investigations to quantify the lesion

3D = three-dimensional; CT = computed tomography; IHC = Immunohistochemistry; MRI = magnetic resonance imaging; MUG = multigated acquisition; Pap = Papanicolaou; PET = positron emission tomography.

Sources: Data from information in AIHW (2017); Hacking et al. (2022); National Cancer Institute (2020); WHO (2017a).

Table 5.5 details various conventional, new, potential and future interventions in cancer treatment.

The past decade has seen many advancements in the understanding and success in cancer treatments. As knowledge and technology have progressed, the factors that make a cell exhibit neoplastic properties have become the focus of potential treatment targets. Figure 5.13 demonstrates clear links between the pathogenesis and the exciting and ever-expanding opportunities of future successful cancer treatments.

In relation to the management of common cancer symptoms, pain management is crucial, and the goal should always be to reduce an individual's pain to zero. Sometimes, total pain control may be difficult to achieve; however, various methods, including the appropriate use of analgesic agents (including opioids) and, occasionally, surgical interventions, may provide as much pain relief as is possibly achievable in the care of some individuals. Adjuvant therapies, including the use of heat packs or cold packs, massage, or even other medications—such as tricyclic antidepressants, some antiseizure medications and some selective serotonin reuptake inhibitors (SSRIs)—can assist with providing better pain control.

Fatigue management is generally achieved by promoting as much rest as necessary. A balance between sufficient rest and reducing inactivity can be important, as people with cancer have a significantly increased risk of developing stasis-related issues, such as deep vein thrombosis and emboli. Provision of rest periods is also important, especially in the control of visitors. Prolonged or successive visitation will increase fatigue and decrease defences. Another method of reducing fatigue is related to how healthcare professionals organise care. Frequent interruptions to sleep can exacerbate symptoms; however, grouping cares to enable longer periods of rest can be more beneficial.

Management of cachexia is complicated by the fact that many cancer treatments also cause changes in taste, loss of appetite, nausea, vomiting and abdominal pain. Some methods to assist a person with cachexia include the use of corticosteroids to increase appetite, increasing the caloric intake with supplements, and reducing the size of meals and increasing their frequency. Finally, making food aesthetically pleasing and reducing overwhelming aromas may assist in some way.

Cancer-related anaemia can be managed in many ways. Iron deficiency can be treated with oral iron supplementation. If haemoglobin levels get too low (< 80 mg/dL), blood transfusions of packed red blood cells may be administered. If a decrease in erythropoietin (EPO) is being influenced by the tumour, exogenous EPO can be administered subcutaneously every three weeks. There is still some debate about the use of EPO in people with cancer-related anaemia, as it is thought that there may be an increased risk of thromboemboli and renal failure. A cost–benefit analysis should be undertaken on a case-by-case basis to determine the most appropriate intervention.

Care of an individual with cancer-related infection requires basic infection control procedures. Frequent and careful hand-washing is paramount in the prevention of pathogenic transmission to already immunocompromised individuals. Standard infection control methods should be undertaken. Other methods to reduce the infection risks associated with cancer include the use of prophylactic antimicrobials. Bacterial, fungal and viral prophylaxis is generally directed towards the most common pathogens. Provision of care may be required in protected environments, especially in profoundly immunocompromised people.

Diagnosis of paraneoplastic disorders can be complex. Sampling of blood may assist in determining the presence of

Table 5.5 Conventional, new and future cancer treatments

Intervention	Detail	Use
Surgery	The use of scalpels, lasers, liquid nitrogen or argon gas (cryosurgery), heat (hyperthermia) or light (phototherapy) to remove or reduce the size (debulk) of the tumour. May also be done as a method to reduce pain or pressure from the presence of the tumour Achieved through an 'open' approach (via one large incision), or 'minimally invasive' (via a few small incisions and assisted by a laparoscopic camera)	• Primarily with contained, solid tumours
Radiotherapy	The use of high-dose radiation, either by an external beam precisely targeting the cancer location, or internally (brachytherapy), where radiation-emitting seeds, capsules or ribbons are inserted into or near the cancer tissue	• Used with many types of cancer • May be used before surgery to reduce tumour size, or after surgery on the remaining tissue with margins to the tumour
Chemotherapy	The use of anticancer drugs (cancer-killing) to stop or slow the growth of quickly dividing cancer cells Many chemotherapy drugs are taken orally or intravenously, but they may also be given into the peritoneal cavity (intraperitoneal), into the space between the brain and spinal cord (intrathecal), into an artery that leads to the cancer (intra-arterial) or topically onto the skin The route will depend on the type and location of the cancer	• Used with many types of cancer • May be used before surgery to reduce tumour size, or after surgery to destroy any possible remaining cancer cells • May be used prior to a stem cell transplant
Stem cell transplants	The administration of blood-forming stem cells intravenously (which migrate to the medullary cavity of the bone) after high doses of radiation and/or chemotherapy have been given to destroy the person's own cancerous stem cells The three different types of transplant involve cells that come from someone else (allogeneic), from an identical twin (syngeneic) or from the person's own body (autologous)	• Primarily with leukaemia and lymphoma • May also be used for multiple myeloma and neuroblastoma
Immunotherapy	The use of one of the six current classes of immune modifying agents such as: 1. *Monoclonal antibodies (mAb):* target tumour-specific antigens 2. *Cancer vaccines:* trigger the person's own immune response to the cancer 3. *Cytokine therapy:* Enhance non-specific immune reactions, such as interleukins and tumour necrosis factor 4. *Adoptive T-Cell Transfer (CAR-T):* where T cells are extracted, modified to respond to tumour-associated antigens (TAAs) expressed by the cancer cells, grown and reinfused into the person. These T cells then recognise that the cancer cells are foreign, and attack and kill them 5. *Checkpoint inhibitors:* prevent cancer cells from 'turning off' the immune activity of T cells 6. *Bacillus Calmette–Guérin (BCG):* Appears to induce a macrophage response that stimulates cytokine and direct cell-to-cell cytotoxicity	• The type of cancer drives the selection of immunotherapy
Hormone therapy	The use of agents to prevent the hormones from being produced by blocking the hormone from attaching to its receptor either by using another compound to antagonise the receptor, or by modifying the shape of the receptor Surgery to remove the hormone-producing glands—such as an oophorectomy (ovaries) or an orchidectomy (testis)—is also considered to be a type of hormone therapy	• Primarily with breast and prostate cancer
CRISPR-Cas9	The use of a new and evolving gene-editing technique called Clustered Regularly Interspaced Short Palindromic Repeat (CRISPR) and CRISPR-associated protein 9 (Cas9) enables precise, permanent targeting of oncogenic mutations to kill malignant cells	• Currently clinical trials are ongoing to treat various cancers such as leukaemia, lymphoma, advanced biliary tract cancer and gastrointestinal cancer

Sources: Data from information in Balon et al. (2022); Cancer Council Australia (2019); Liu et al. (2022); Mahadevan (2021); National Cancer Institute (2022); Rafii et al. (2022).

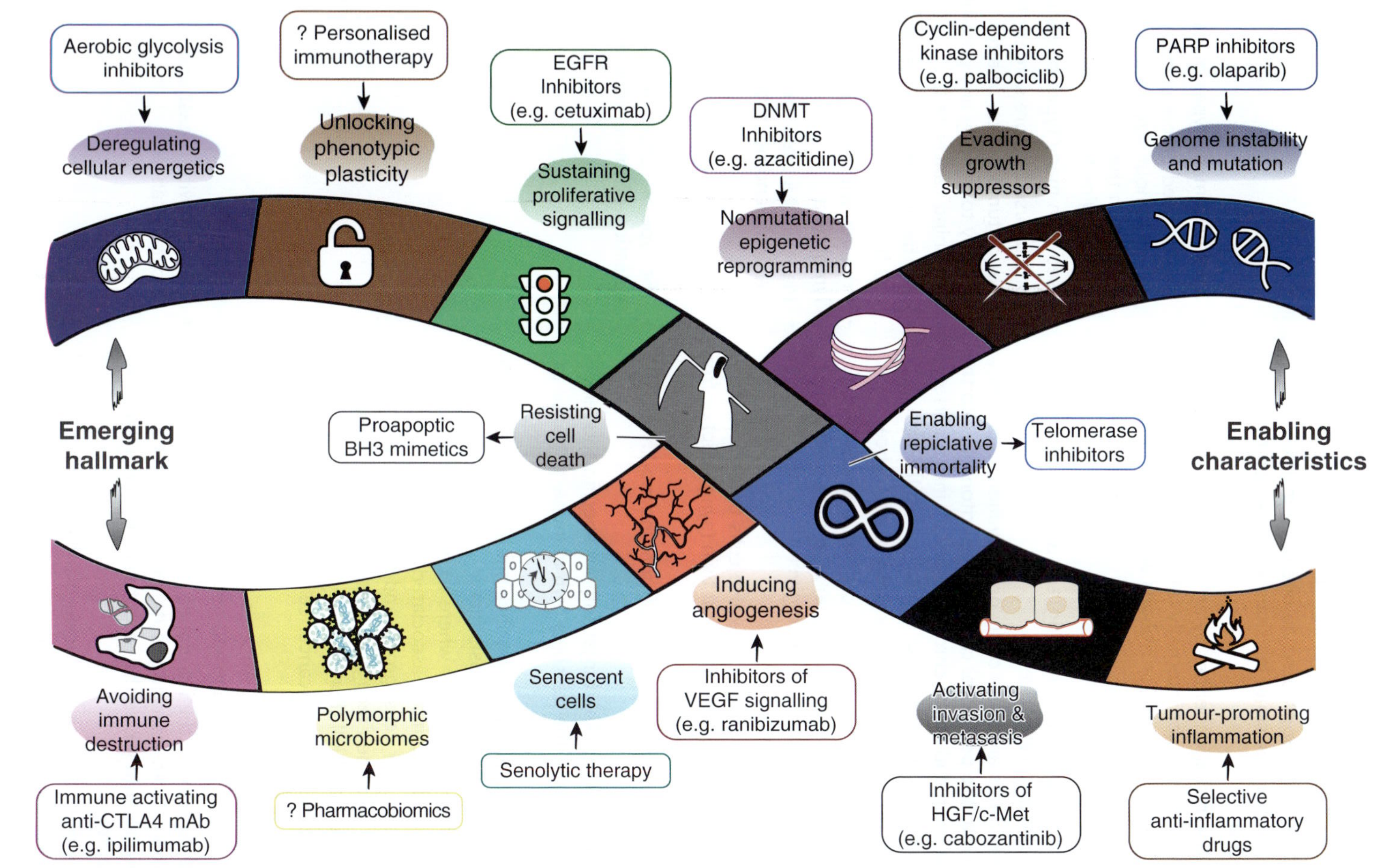

Figure 5.13

How current and emerging treatments are targeting the hallmarks of cancer cells

? = possible; ADP = adenosine diphosphate; anti-CTLA4 mAb = cytotoxic T lymphocyte antigen 4 monoclonal antibody; BCL-2 = B cell lymphoma-2; BH3 = BCL-2 homology; DNMT = DNA methyltransferase; EGFR = epidermal growth factor receptor; HDAC = histone deacetylase; HG*F*/c-Met = hepatocyte growth factor/mesenchymal-epithelial transition factor; PARP = poly-ADP ribose polymerase; VEGF = vascular endothelial growth factor.

Source: Adapted from Hanahan (2022), Figure 6, p. 668.

anaemia, erythrocytosis, electrolyte imbalances or any number of other various issues that can occur as a result of the ectopic release of substances. Specific investigation of tumour markers may be beneficial; however, as they are generally not specific, the location of the issue will still be unknown. Imaging studies determining changes to the structure or function of tissues or organs may assist in the detection of tumours.

Management of paraneoplastic syndromes varies depending on the cause. If the tumour is secreting hormone or hormone-like substances, tumour removal (if possible) will reduce the symptoms. This may be achieved by surgery, chemotherapy or radiation therapy. If the cause of the paraneoplastic disorder is immune-mediated, immunomodifying drugs, such as steroids or immunoglobulins, may be beneficial.

INDIGENOUS HEALTH FAST FACTS AND CULTURAL CONSIDERATIONS

FAST FACTS

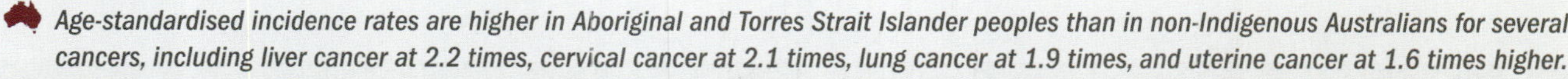

- *Age-standardised incidence rates are higher in Aboriginal and Torres Strait Islander peoples than in non-Indigenous Australians for several cancers, including liver cancer at 2.2 times, cervical cancer at 2.1 times, lung cancer at 1.9 times, and uterine cancer at 1.6 times higher.*

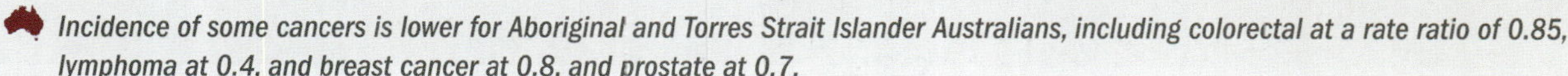

- *Incidence of some cancers is lower for Aboriginal and Torres Strait Islander Australians, including colorectal at a rate ratio of 0.85, lymphoma at 0.4, and breast cancer at 0.8, and prostate at 0.7.*
- *Māori have an overall cancer rate 1.7 times higher than that of European New Zealanders.*
- *Mortality rates for cancer in Māori are twice those of European New Zealanders.*
- *More Māori women experience melanoma (4.6:1), stomach cancer (4.5:1), lung cancer (3.8:1) and uterine cancer (16.2:1) than European New Zealand women. However, colorectal cancer was lower (1:1.5) when comparing female Māori and European New Zealanders.*
- *More Māori men experience lung cancer (3:1), pancreatic cancer (1.9:1) and lymphoma (1.2:1) than European New Zealand men. However, colorectal cancer (1:1.5) and prostate cancer (1:1.1) were lower when comparing male Māori and European New Zealanders.*

CULTURAL CONSIDERATIONS

- *The cancer mortality gap between Aboriginal and Torres Strait Islander peoples and non-Indigenous Australians is ever-increasing, although current efforts are reducing the disparity in some cancers. Cancer-related deaths of non-Indigenous Australians have decreased by 7%, whereas Indigenous Australian cancer-related deaths have increased by 4%.*
- *The cancer burden for Aboriginal and Torres Strait Islander Australians is 1.4 times higher than for non-Indigenous Australians. Cancer incidence is complicated by the presence of significantly higher cancer risk factors, most known for causing more than two-thirds of all cancers. These risk factors include 2.8 times the rate of smoking, 1.6 times the risky alcohol consumption, and a diet with low fruit and vegetable intake. Another serious risk factor in cancer development is obesity. Aboriginal and Torres Strait Islander Australians are 1.5 times more likely to be obese than non-Indigenous Australians. People in inner regional areas experience the highest rates of obesity, and lowest rates occur in outer regional and remote areas.*
- *Other important considerations include the fact that Aboriginal and Torres Strait Islander Australians are less likely than non-Indigenous Australians to be involved in cancer screening programs, and are less likely to be hospitalised, diagnosed early, or receive adequate treatment for cancer. These factors contribute to reduced five-year survival statistics and overall higher mortality statistics.*
- *It is critical that we, as a country, work harder to reduce the cancer morbidity and mortality of Aboriginal and Torres Strait Islander peoples, especially when so many preventable risk factors mean that great success is entirely achievable.*
- *Key emphasis needs to be on timely and equitable health delivery by skilled, caring staff with cultural competence, and an understanding of the social and cultural determinants of health. A strong community focus is required, with the involvement of Aboriginal and Torres Strait Islander leaders to help guide culturally appropriate education; person-, family- and community-centred plans; and an integrated, multidisciplinary, inclusive approach. Clearly, risk factors, screening participation levels and quality healthcare provision will be major influencers in closing this healthcare gap.*

Sources: Data from Australian Bureau of Statistics (2023); AIHW (2020, 2021a; 2022c); New Zealand Ministry of Health (2021, 2022); Te Aho o Te Kahu | *Cancer Control Agency (2021).*

CHILDREN AND ADOLESCENTS

- Cancer is the most common cause of death in children.
- Umbilical cord blood containing stem cells can be obtained from newborns and used for the treatment of cancer if no suitable bone marrow is available. Cord blood is beneficial for use in childhood cancers, and poses less risk of graft versus host disease (GvHD).
- Acute lymphocytic leukaemia is the most common childhood cancer.

OLDER ADULTS

- Almost 80% of all neoplasms occur in adults older than 50 years of age.
- The incidence of malignant tumours increases with age.
- Cellular senescence may contribute to the proliferation of malignant and premalignant cells; however, ageing increases the risk of some cancers and decreases the risk of others.

KEY CLINICAL ISSUES

- Early detection and diagnosis are critical to the clinical outcome related to a cancer diagnosis. Educating people and the community about screening programs, breast and testicular self-examination, and skin health can assist in reducing the high incidence of cancer.
- Relief of pain is a priority in the management of someone with cancer. Consultation with specialist pain services is imperative to provide as much pain relief as is achievable.
- Prevention and management of nausea will impact on many aspects of an individual's ability to cope with the treatment regimen. Nausea and vomiting can influence nutrition through the development of anorexia, and can even influence choices regarding compliance with the appropriate management plan.
- Not everyone can be cured. Those who cannot will require palliative care. Quality of life, assistance with decisions, and psychosocial and spiritual support are all key aspects of the provision of palliative care.
- Prevention of infection becomes a priority in the care of those with cancer, as various degrees of immunocompromise can occur. In neutropenic individuals, even a common, benign type of infection may have devastating consequences. Infection control measures must be undertaken at all times. Educating those around them about basic hand-washing skills and the importance of adhering to the required infection control regimens is important to increase the potential for compliance.

CHAPTER REVIEW

- A tumour (growth) may or may not be cancerous.
- The term *malignant* refers to cancerous tumours that can cause deterioration or death, whereas the term *benign* refers to a growth that does not generally cause death.
- The shortening of a telomere, the presence of tumour suppressor proteins and apoptosis assist in the prevention of cancer.
- When duplication errors occur and the replication of the faulty cell is not halted, cancer develops.
- As cancerous tumours enlarge, they may develop a blood supply and take nutrients away from nearby normally functioning cells.
- Cancer can have an *inherited* component to which an appropriate *environmental insult* must also occur for cancer to develop.
- Several *viruses* are linked to the development of cancer.
- Tumour cells may invade other areas of the body. Tumour growth in a secondary site is called *metastasis*.
- The *TNM classification* of cancer enables tumours to be staged. Staging directs the management plan, and also provides information about the statistical probability of recovering from the event.
- Pain, fatigue, severe weight loss and anaemia are significant issues related to the management of someone with cancer.
- *Paraneoplastic syndromes* occur when the tumour produces biologically active substances that can alter the function of other organs or homeostatic systems.

REVIEW QUESTIONS

1. Define the following terms:
   a. tumour
   b. malignant
   c. benign
   d. paraneoplastic
   e. proto-oncogenes
   f. tumour suppressor genes
2. How do cancer cells differ from normal cells?
3. What changes occur in cancer cells that contribute to the excessive growth of a tumour?
4. How do genes contribute to the development of cancer?
5. What viruses are associated with the development of cancer?
6. How do environmental and lifestyle factors contribute to the development of cancer?
7. How does a tumour metastasise?

HEALTH PROFESSIONAL CONNECTIONS

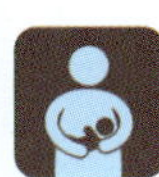

Midwives Fortunately, malignancy in neonates is rare; however, a woman may have cancer diagnosed at some stage within her pregnancy. The management of pregnant women with cancer is complex and requires very individualised management plans. The teratogenicity of chemotherapeutic agents is highly variable, and outcomes may range from as minor as low birth weight, to the more common craniofacial anomalies and limb deformity, to fetal death. Mechanisms contributing to the development of cancer may include pregnancy-related immunosuppression. To prevent rejection of the embryo, the placenta releases hormones to modulate the woman's immune system function. Although many changes occur within the uterus and feto-maternal interface, systemic maternal immunomodulation does occur. Pregnancy causes a unique state of simultaneous immunosuppression yet enhanced inflammatory response. T cells increase in number but become more tolerant, and natural killer cell activity is down-regulated. Leukocyte counts increase, and there is an increase in some pro-inflammatory cytokines, including tumour necrosis factor-α.

Whatever the cause of cancer, a woman's management is complicated by the presence of the fetus. The decision to terminate the pregnancy is complex for most people and impossible for others. Surgical resection of solid tumours is preferential, but leukemic and lymphoid cancers are more difficult to manage. Multidisciplinary support and significant counselling is required to assist a woman to make fully informed decisions about her cancer management.

Nutritionists/Dieticians People with cancer, especially in end-stage cancer, can develop changes that influence taste and appetite. This may be as a result of the cancer itself or be directly related to the treatment. Cachexia may develop. Healthcare professionals responsible for nutrition need to understand ways to influence caloric intake. Becoming familiar with the person's dietary preferences, and finding ways to encourage optimum nutrition, can have a positive influence on their outcome. Adequate nutrition will assist with the physical and emotional stress caused by cancer and its treatment.

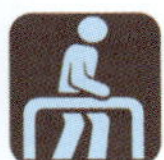

Physiotherapists A physiotherapist can play a major role in cancer management in relation to assisting with functional decline before, during and after cancer treatment. Each timeframe presents its own challenges. Before-treatment interactions may involve assisting with fitness prior to prolonged or consuming interventions. Interactions during treatment may focus on assisting with early recovery, management of functional decline, prevention of complications, and lymphoedema screening and education. Physiotherapeutic interactions in the post-treatment phase may simply include exercise and stretching prescriptions, provision of walking aides, and assistance with balance and mobility. More complex interactions post treatment may include cardiorespiratory care, external support for ongoing care, or even assistance with end-of-life support and palliation.

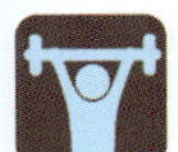

Exercise scientists It is clearly established that exercise can reduce the risk factors for many types of cancers. Just because someone has been given a diagnosis of cancer does not mean that exercise has to stop. Individually tailored, critically planned exercise can benefit those with cancer in numerous ways. Not only will the positive effects of the exercise-related release of endorphins assist with mood, exercise can also assist with fatigue and reduce muscle atrophy. Important considerations in the development and prescription of exercise in people with cancer include duration, intensity and frequency. These decisions should be made after consultation with other members of the healthcare team.

CASE STUDY

Mrs Evaline Galanovic (43 years of age; UR number 629840) had a modified left radical mastectomy for an invasive breast carcinoma. She has a Jackson-Pratt drain in situ on suction and her left arm is elevated on two pillows. Her observations are as follows:

Temperature	Heart rate	Respiration rate	Blood pressure	SpO_2
36.9°C	65	14	110/68	96% (4 L/min – HM*)

*HM = Hudson mask.

Mrs Galanovic has patient-controlled analgesia (PCA) of morphine 1 mg/mL with a background of 40 μg/h. The bolus is set for 1 mg with a lock-out time of five minutes. She has a naloxone standing order if required. Mrs Galanovic currently rates her pain as 3 out of 10, and she has subsequently been given further education on the use of her PCA. She has also been encouraged to give herself another dose of morphine. She has had q6h metoclopramide with effect. Mrs Galanovic has been tolerating her diet, and has sat out of bed for half an hour this morning. She has intravenous antibiotics and fluids. She will be reviewed by the oncology team this afternoon for planning regarding her chemotherapy and radiotherapy.

Her genogram (commonly known as a family pedigree) looks like this:

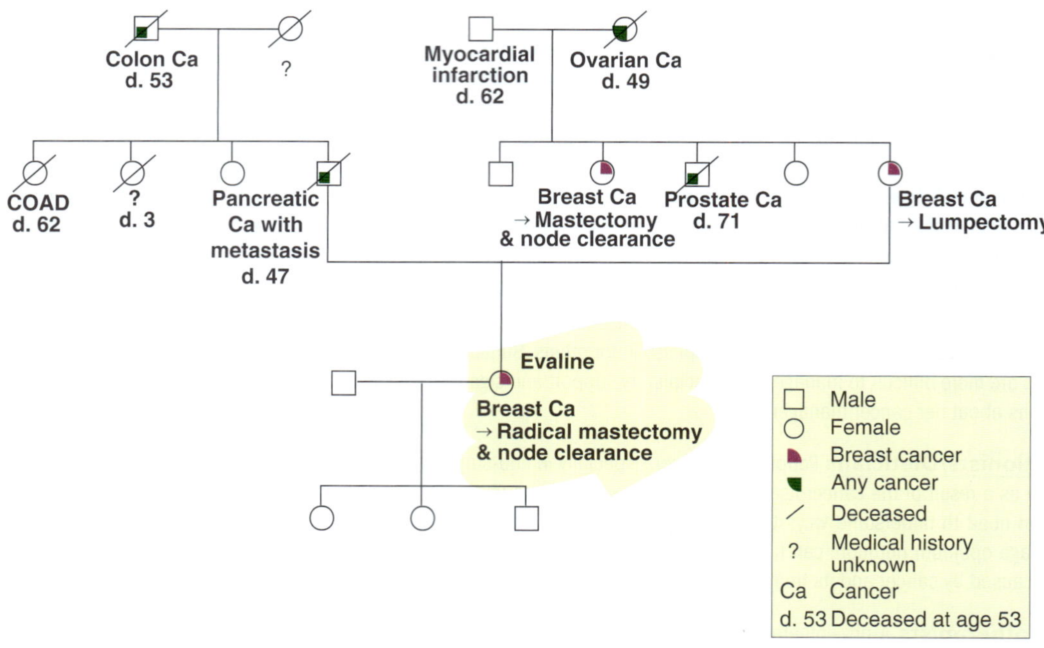

CRITICAL THINKING

1. Study Mrs Galanovic's genogram, paying specific attention to the maternal history. Is there a genetic component to the development of breast cancer? Explain. If so, what is the percentage of breast cancer development related to genetic risk? Considering Mrs Galanovic's genogram, do you think that genetic risk could be an issue in this family?
2. Is there an association with breast cancer and ovarian cancer? Explain. In your answer, discuss your observations of Mrs Galanovic's genogram. Is this a genetic or a sporadic concern? What does this mean?
3. Mrs Galanovic had a radical mastectomy. What does this mean in the context of anatomy? In relation to a mastectomy, compare and contrast the terms 'simple', 'total', 'radical' and 'radical modified'.
4. This type of surgery will mean that certain complications may develop, and certain cares may need to be modified. Discuss all of the possible complications of the surgery (*Hint:* Ensure that you mention something about interstitial fluid) and how the care may need to be modified (*Hint:* Ensure that you mention something about a sphygmomanometer cuff).
5. Analyse the case study above. Draw up a table that lists the interventions included in the case study in the far left-hand column (one intervention per row). In the next column, explain the reason that each intervention is required. In the third column, explain the mechanism of how each intervention achieves its objective.

BIBLIOGRAPHY

Abramson, R. (2019). Overview of targeted therapies for cancer. *My Cancer Genome*. https://www.mycancergenome.org/content/page/overview-of-targeted-therapies-for-cancer/.

Australian Bureau of Statistics (ABS) (2015). *Australian Aboriginal and Torres Strait Islander health survey: nutrition results—food and nutrients, 2012-13*. Canberra: ABS. https://www.abs.gov.au/ausstats/abs@.nsf/Lookup/4727.0.55.005main+features12012-13.

Australian Bureau of Statistics (ABS) (2023). *Closing the Gap and National Government Reporting*. Canberra: ABS. https://www.abs.gov.au/statistics/people/aboriginal-and-torres-strait-islander-peoples/closing-gap-and-national-government-reporting/2022-23.

Australian Health Ministers' Advisory Council's National and Aboriginal and Torres Strait Islander Health Standing Committee (2017). *Cultural respect framework 2016-2026: for Aboriginal and Torres Strait Islander health—a national approach to building a culturally respectful health system*. Canberra: Australian Government Department of Health. https://nacchocommunique.files.wordpress.com/2016/12/cultural_respect_framework_1december2016_1.pdf.

Australian Institute of Health and Welfare (AIHW) (2020). *Aboriginal and Torres Strait Islander health performance framework 2020 summary report*. Cat. No. IHPF 2. Canberra: AIHW. https://www.indigenoushpf.gov.au/publications/hpf-summary-2020.

Australian Institute of Health and Welfare (AIHW) (2021a). *Cancer in Australia, 2021*. Cancer series No. 133. Cat. No. CAN 144. Canberra: AIHW. https://www.aihw.gov.au/reports/cancer/cancer-in-australia-2021/summary.

Australian Institute of Health and Welfare (AIHW) (2021b). Chapter 7: Survival and survivorship after a cancer diagnosis. *Cancer in Australia, 2021*. Cancer series No. 133. Cat. No. CAN 144. Canberra: AIHW. https://www.aihw.gov.au/getmedia/0ea708eb-dd6e-4499-9080-1cc7b5990e64/aihw-can-144.pdf.aspx?inline=true.

Australian Institute of Health and Welfare (AIHW) (2022a). *Aboriginal and Torres Strait Islander Health Performance Framework—1.08 Cancer*. Canberra: AIHW. https://www.indigenoushpf.gov.au/measures/1-08-cancer.

Australian Institute of Health and Welfare (AIHW) (2022b). *Alcohol, tobacco and other drugs in Australia*. Cat. No. PHE 221. Canberra: AIHW. https://www.aihw.gov.au/reports/alcohol/alcohol-tobacco-other-drugs-australia/contents/about.

Balon, K., Sheriff, A., Jacków, J. & Łaczmański, Ł. (2022). Targeting cancer with CRISPR/Cas9-based therapy. *International Journal of Molecular Sciences* 23(1):573. https://doi.org/10.3390/ijms23010573.

Bauldoff, G., Gubrud-Howe, P.M., Carno, M.-A., Levett-Jones, T., Hales, M., Berry, K.,… Stanley, D. (2020). *LeMone and Burke's medical–surgical nursing: critical thinking for person-centred care* (4th [Australian] edn). Sydney: Pearson Australia. Belli, M. & Tabocchini, M.A. (2020). Ionizing radiation-induced epigenetic modifications and their relevance to radiation protection. *International Journal of Molecular Sciences* 21(17):5993. https://doi.org/10.3390/ijms21175993.

Best, O. & Fredericks, B. (2021). *Yatdjuligin: Aboriginal and Torres Strait Islander nursing and midwifery care* (3rd edn). Port Melbourne, VIC: Cambridge University Press.

Bullock, S. & Manias, E. (2022). *Fundamentals of pharmacology* (9th edn). Sydney: Pearson Australia.

Cancer Australia (2015). *National Aboriginal and Torres Strait Islander Cancer Framework*. Surry Hills, NSW: Cancer Australia. https://www.canceraustralia.gov.au/publications-and-resources/cancer-australia-publications/national-aboriginal-and-torres-strait-islander-cancer-framework.

Cancer Australia (2017). *Aboriginal and Torres Strait Islander cancer statistics.* Surry Hills, NSW: Cancer Australia. https://www.canceraustralia.gov.au/affected-cancer/indigenous/cancer-statistics.

Cancer Australia (2020). *Guide to implementing the Optimal Care Pathway for Aboriginal and Torres Strait Islander people with cancer.* Strawberry Hills, NSW: Cancer Australia. https://www.canceraustralia.gov.au/sites/default/files/publications/optimal-care-pathway-aboriginal-and-torres-strait-islander-people-cancer-guide/pdf/optimal_care_pathway_for_aboriginal_and_torres_strait_islander_people_with_cancer_the_guide.pdf.

Cancer Australia (2022). *Immunotherapy.* Strawberry Hills, NSW: Cancer Australia. https://www.canceraustralia.gov.au/impacted-by-cancer/treatment/immunotherapy.

Cancer Australia (2023). *EdCaN module: cancer treatment planning.* Surry Hills, NSW: Cancer Australia. https://www.edcan.org.au/edcan-learning-resources/supporting-resources/cancer-treatment-planning.

Cancer Council Australia (n.d.). *National Cancer Prevention Policy*. Sydney: Cancer Council Australia. https://www.cancer.org.au/about-us/policy-and-advocacy/prevention-policy/national-cancer-prevention-policy.

Cancer Council Australia (2019). *Alcohol and cancer: national position statement*. Sydney: Cancer Council Australia. https://www.cancer.org.au/about-us/policy-and-advocacy/position-statements/alcohol-and-cancer.

Chynoweth, J., McCambridge, M.M., Zorbas, H.M., Elston, J.K., Thomas, R.J.S., Glasson, W.J.H.,… Whitfield, K.M. (2020). Optimal cancer care for Aboriginal and Torres Strait Islander people: a shared approach to system level change. *JCO Global Oncology* 6:108–14. https://doi.org/10.1200/JGO.19.00076.

Debela, D.T., Muzazu, S.G.Y., Heraro, K.D., Ndalama, M.T., Mesele, B.W., Haile, D.C.,… Manyazewal, T. (2021). New approaches and procedures for cancer treatment: current perspectives. *SAGE Open Medicine* 9:205031212110343–20503121211034366. https://doi.org/10.1177/20503121211034366.

Domenech, H. (2017). *Radiation safety: management and programs*. Cham: Springer International. https://doi.org/10.1007/978-3-319-42671-6.

Dyck, L. & Mills, K.H.G. (2017). Immune checkpoints and their inhibition in cancer and infectious disease. *European Journal of Immunology* 47(5):765–79. https://doi.org/10.1002/eji.201646875.

García-Figueiras, R., Baleato-González, S., Padhani, A.R., Luna-Alcalá, A., Vallejo-Casas, J.A., Sala, E.,… Vargas, H.A. (2019). How clinical imaging can assess cancer biology. *Insights into Imaging* 10(1):28–35. https://doi.org/10.1186/s13244-019-0703-0.

GBD 2019 Cancer Risk Factors Collaborators (2022). The global burden of cancer attributable to risk factors, 2010–19: a systematic analysis for the Global Burden of Disease Study 2019. *The Lancet* 40(10352):563–91. https://doi.org/10.1016/S0140-6736(22)01438-6.

Hacking, S.M., Yakirevich, E. & Wang, Y. (2022). From immunohistochemistry to new digital ecosystems: a state-of-the-art biomarker review for precision breast cancer medicine. *Cancers* 14(14):3469. https://doi.org/10.3390/cancers14143469.

Hanahan, D. (2022). Hallmarks of cancer: New dimensions. *Cancer Discovery* 12(1):31–46. https://doi.org/10.1158/2159-8290.CD-21-1059.

Hanahan D. & Weinberg R.A. (2011). Hallmarks of cancer: the next generation. *Cell* 144(5):646–74. https://doi.org/10.1016/j.cell.2011.02.013. PMID: 21376230.

Health New Zealand | Te Whatu Ora (2021). *Mortality web tool: mortality by causes of death and demographics, 2015–2019*. Wellington: Health New Zealand | Te Whatu Ora. https://www.tewhatuora.govt.nz/our-health-system/data-and-statistics/mortality-web-tool/.

Hosseini, B., Hall, A.L., Zendehdel, K., Kromhout, H., Onyije, F.M., Moradzadeh, R.,… Olsson, A. (2021). Occupational exposure to carcinogens and occupational epidemiological cancer studies in Iran: a review. *Cancers* 13(14):3581. https://doi.org/10.3390/cancers13143581.

Hussain, A., Dulay, P., Rivera, M.N., Aramouni, C. & Saxena, V. (2019). Neoplastic pathogenesis associated with cigarette carcinogens. *Curēus* 11(1):e3955. https://doi.org/10.7759/cureus.3955.

Katti, A., Diaz, B.J., Caragine, C.M., Sanjana, N.E. & Dow, L.E. (2022). CRISPR in cancer biology and therapy. *Nature Reviews Cancer* 22:259–79. https://doi.org/10.1038/s41568-022-00441-w.

Klein, W.M., O'Connell, M.E., Bloch, M.H., Czajkowski, S.M., Green, P.A., Han, P.K.J.,… Vanderpool, R.C. (2022). Behavioral research in cancer prevention and control: emerging challenges and opportunities. *Journal of the National Cancer Institute* 114(2):179–86. https://doi.org/10.1093/jnci/djab139.

Little, M.P., Wakeford, R., Bouffler, S.D., Abalo, K., Hauptmann, M., Hamada, N. & Kendall, G.M. (2022). Review of the risk of cancer following low and moderate doses of sparsely ionising radiation received in early life in groups with individually estimated doses. *Environment International* 159:106983. https://doi.org/10.1016/j.envint.2021.106983.

Liu, J., Fu, M., Wang, M., Wan, D., Wei, Y. & Wei, X. (2022). Cancer vaccines as promising immuno-therapeutics: platforms and current progress. *Journal of Hematology and Oncology* 15:28. https://doi.org/10.1186/s13045-022-01247-x.

Lokeshwar, S.D., Lopez, M., Sarcan, S., Aguilar, K., Morera, D.S., Shaheen, D.M.,… Lokeshwar, V.B. (2022). Molecular oncology of bladder cancer from inception to modern perspective. *Cancers* 14(11):2578. https://doi.org/10.3390/cancers14112578.

Mahadevan, D. (2021). Targeted Cancer Therapy. *Emedicine*. https://emedicine.medscape.com/article/1372666-overview.

Marieb, E.N. & Hoehn, K. (2019). *Human anatomy and physiology* (11th edn). San Francisco, CA: Pearson Benjamin Cummings.

Markozannes, G., Kanellopoulou, A., Dimopoulou, O., Kosmidis, D., Zhang, X., Wang, L.,… Tsilidis, K.K. (2022). Systematic review of Mendelian randomization studies on risk of cancer. *BMC Medicine* 20:41. https://doi.org/10.1186/s12916-022-02246-y.

Memon, R., Prieto Granada, C.N., Harada, S., Winokur, T., Reddy, V., Kahn, A.G.,… Wei, S. (2022). Discordance between immunohistochemistry and in situ hybridization to detect HER2 overexpression/gene amplification in breast cancer in the modern age: a single institution experience and pooled literature review study. *Clinical Breast Cancer* 22(1):e123–e133. https://doi.org/10.1016/j.clbc.2021.05.004.

Monroy-Iglesias, M.J., Crescioli, S., Beckmann, K., Le, N., Karagiannis, S.N., Van Hemelrijck, M. & Santaolalla, A. (2022). Antibodies as biomarkers for cancer risk: a systematic review. *Clinical and Experimental Immunology* 29(1):46–63. https://doi.org/10.1093/cei/uxac030.

Muscaritoli, M., Arends, J., Bachmann, P., Baracos, V., Barthelemy, N., Bertz, H.,… Bischoff, S.C. (2021). ESPEN practical guideline: clinical nutrition in cancer. *Clinical Nutrition* 40(5):2898–913. https://doi.org/10.1016/j.clnu.2021.02.005.

National Cancer Institute (2020). *Cancer imaging basics*. Bethesda, MD: National Cancer Institute. https://imaging.cancer.gov/imaging_basics/cancer_imaging.htm.

National Cancer Institute (2022). *Targeted therapy to treat cancer*. Bethesda, MD: National Cancer Institute. https://www.cancer.gov/about-cancer/treatment/types/targeted-therapies.

New Zealand Ministry of Health (2021). *New cancer registrations 2019*. Wellington: Ministry of Health. https://www.health.govt.nz/publication/new-cancer-registrations-2019.

New Zealand Ministry of Health (2022). *Cancer: historical summary 1948–2018*. Wellington: Ministry of Health. https://www.tewhatuora.govt.nz/our-health-system/data-and-statistics/historical-cancer#publishing-information.

Organisation for Economic Co-operation and Development (OECD) (2021). Cancer incidence and mortality. In *Health at a Glance 2021: OECD Indicators*. Paris: OECD Publishing. https://doi.org/10.1787/6cfe5309-en.

Papadimitriou, N., Markozannes, G., Kanellopoulou, A., Critselis, E., Alhardan, S., Karafousia, V.,… Tsilidis, K.K. (2021). An umbrella review of the evidence associating diet and cancer risk at 11 anatomical sites. *Nature Communications* 12:4579. https://doi.org/10.1038/s41467-021-24861-8.

Rafii, S., Tashkandi, E., Bukhari, N. & Al-Shamsi, H.O. (2022). Current status of CRISPR/Cas9 application in clinical cancer research: opportunities and challenges. *Cancers* 14(4):947. https://doi.org/10.3390/cancers14040947.

Sleight, A., Gerber, L.H., Marshall, T.F., Livinski, A., Alfano, C.M., Harrington, S.,… Stout, N.L. (2022). Systematic review of functional outcomes in cancer rehabilitation. *Archives of Physical Medicine and Rehabilitation* 103(9):1807–26. https://doi.org/10.1016/j.apmr.2022.01.142.

Te Aho o Te Kahu | Cancer Control Agency (2021). *He pūrongo mate pukupuku o Aotearoa 2020 | The state of cancer in New Zealand 2020*. Wellington: Te Aho o Te Kahu | Cancer Control Agency. www.teaho.govt.nz/reports/cancer-state.

United Nations Scientific Committee on the Effects of Atomic Radiation (UNSCEAR) (2022). *Sources, effects and risks of ionizing radiation*. New York: UNSCEAR. http://www.unscear.org.

World Cancer Research Fund International (WCRF) (2022). *Global cancer data by country*. London: WCRF. https://www.wcrf.org/cancer-trends/global-cancer-data-by-country/.

World Health Organization (WHO) (2016). An estimated 12.6 million deaths each year are attributable to unhealthy environments. [News release.] Geneva: WHO. https://www.who.int/news/item/15-03-2016-an-estimated-12-6-million-deaths-each-year-are-attributable-to-unhealthy-environments.

World Health Organization (WHO) (2022a). *Cancer*. Geneva: WHO. https://www.who.int/health-topics/cancer#tab=tab_1.

World Health Organization (WHO) (2022b). Obesity causes cancer and is major determinant of disability and death, warns new WHO report. [News release.] Geneva: WHO. https://www.who.int/europe/news/item/03-05-2022-obesity-causes-cancer-and-is-major-determinant-of-disability-and-death-warns-new-who-report#:~:text=new%20WHO%20report-,Obesity%20causes%20cancer%20and%20is%20major%20determinant%20of,death%2C%20warns%20ne.

Yang, L., Ning, Q. & Tang, S. (2022). Recent advances and next breakthrough in immunotherapy for cancer treatment. *Journal of Immunology Research* 2022:8052212. https://doi.org/10.1155/2022/8052212.

Yoo, J.E., Han, K., Shin, D.W., Jung, W., Kim, D., Lee, C.M.,… Song, Y.-M. (2022). Effect of smoking reduction, cessation, and resumption on cancer risk: a nationwide cohort study. *Cancer* 128(11):2126–37. https://doi.org/10.1002/cncr.34172.

PART

2

Body defences and immune system pathophysiology

6 Stress and its role in disease

KEY TERMS

General adaptation syndrome
Stress
Stressor

LEARNING OBJECTIVES

After completing this chapter, you should be able to:

1. Define the stress response and the term 'stressor'.
2. Define the term 'general adaptation syndrome', and describe the three stages of the response.
3. Contrast the historical and current views of the stress response.
4. Outline how stress affects the brain.
5. Outline the roles of pituitary hormones, neuropeptides and sex hormones in the stress response.
6. State the implications of ageing on the stress response.
7. Contrast the stress response in males and females.

WHAT YOU SHOULD KNOW BEFORE YOU START THIS CHAPTER

Can you define the term 'homeostasis', and outline its purpose?
Can you describe the types of cellular adaptation?
Can you describe the mechanisms of cellular injury?

Introduction

LEARNING OBJECTIVE 1
Define the stress response and the term 'stressor'.

Stress is a response of the body to a change in demand. The change in demand disrupts the state of homeostasis, and the stress response is an attempt to return to equilibrium, to adapt to the challenge. Acute stress can be beneficial, as it can lead to enhanced physiological performance. However, an extreme or prolonged disruption in homeostasis can result in cell injury, which may progress to disease. In this chapter, we will explore the stress response and the process by which illness may arise. We will also discuss the stress response in terms of ageing and sex differences.

Stressors

Stimuli that trigger the stress response are called **stressors**. A stressor may be internal or external to the person; it may be real or imagined. Stressors can be classified as biological, chemical, physical, social or psychological. Examples of stressors are provided in Table 6.1. A number of these stressors are the same agents that cause cell injury (see the chapter 'Pathophysiological terminology, cellular adaptation and injury'). The degree of *homeostatic disruption* by a particular stressor (and the potential for damage to the body) varies greatly from person to person, and can depend on its magnitude, type, duration and personal meaning. Importantly, an individual's perception of the stressor influences the character of the stress response and its subsequent outcomes. This perception can be determined by the person's genetic makeup, their current health status, past experience of stress, cultural expectations, coping strategies and present life circumstances. Indeed, at different times in life a person can experience the same stressor and have totally dissimilar responses.

Historical perspectives on the stress response

LEARNING OBJECTIVE 2

Define the term 'general adaptation syndrome', and describe the three stages of the response.

Our current understanding of the stress response is derived from the classic experiments on rats conducted around 80 to 90 years ago by Dr Hans Selye, who coined the term the **general adaptation syndrome**. He determined that the stress response was non-specific and reproducible regardless of the physiological stimulus—stimuli as diverse as exposure to cold, hunger, physical trauma or noxious chemicals.

Dr Selye determined that the general adaptation syndrome consisted of three stages through which an organism passes if there is continuous exposure to the stressor: the alarm reaction, resistance (see Figure 6.1) and exhaustion.

ALARM REACTION

The *alarm reaction* is an acute heightened and alert state initiated at the level of the hypothalamus, and is primarily characterised by an activation of the sympathetic nervous system, incorporating the release of noradrenaline and adrenaline from the adrenal medulla (known as the *sympathoadrenal responses*). The fight-or-flight responses that result are directed towards increased energy production, enhanced cardiovascular and respiratory function, and heightened arousal. A summary of the key sympathetic responses is provided in Table 6.2.

The hypothalamus also stimulates the pituitary gland to release *adrenocorticotropic hormone (ACTH)* through its secretion of corticotropin-releasing hormone (CRH).

The alarm reaction is an important response in circumstances of physiological threat, such as hypoglycaemia, infection or injury, or psychologically testing situations, like exposure to a predator or in social dominance.

Importantly, the stress response should not be viewed as always noxious or injurious. Seyle originally proposed a term reflecting 'positive' stress called *eustress*; in his description this form of stressor produced less damage than a more noxious one. Short-term stress responses can have positive benefits on health, resulting in increased motivation, performance and well-being.

STAGE OF RESISTANCE

The purpose of the stage of resistance is to enable *adaptation* to the stressor and a *return to a state of homeostasis*. The alarm reaction is intensely energy-consuming and so cannot be maintained for a prolonged period. The consequences of a prolonged alarm reaction would be a severe disruption of homeostasis.

The resistance stage is initially characterised by elevated hormone levels from the adrenal cortex, under the influence of ACTH, and a waning of the fight-or-flight responses. The two main corticosteroids (hormones produced by the adrenal cortex) are the mineralocorticoid aldosterone and the glucocorticoid cortisol. *Aldosterone* is part of the renin–angiotensin system,

Table 6.1 Examples of stressors

Type of stressor	Examples
Biological	Microbial infection, injury, interrupted sleeping pattern
Chemical	Pesticides, fertilisers, industrial chemical waste
Physical	Loud noise, extremes of temperature
Social	Peer pressure, social isolation, the breakdown of a relationship
Psychological	Anxiety, anger

Table 6.2 Key sympathetic responses in the alarm stage

- Heightened arousal
- Increased heart rate
- Increased breathing rate
- Elevated blood glucose levels
- Vasoconstriction of major blood vessels
- Vasodilation of tissue blood vessels associated with heart, muscle and kidneys
- Increased blood pressure
- Decreased digestive processes

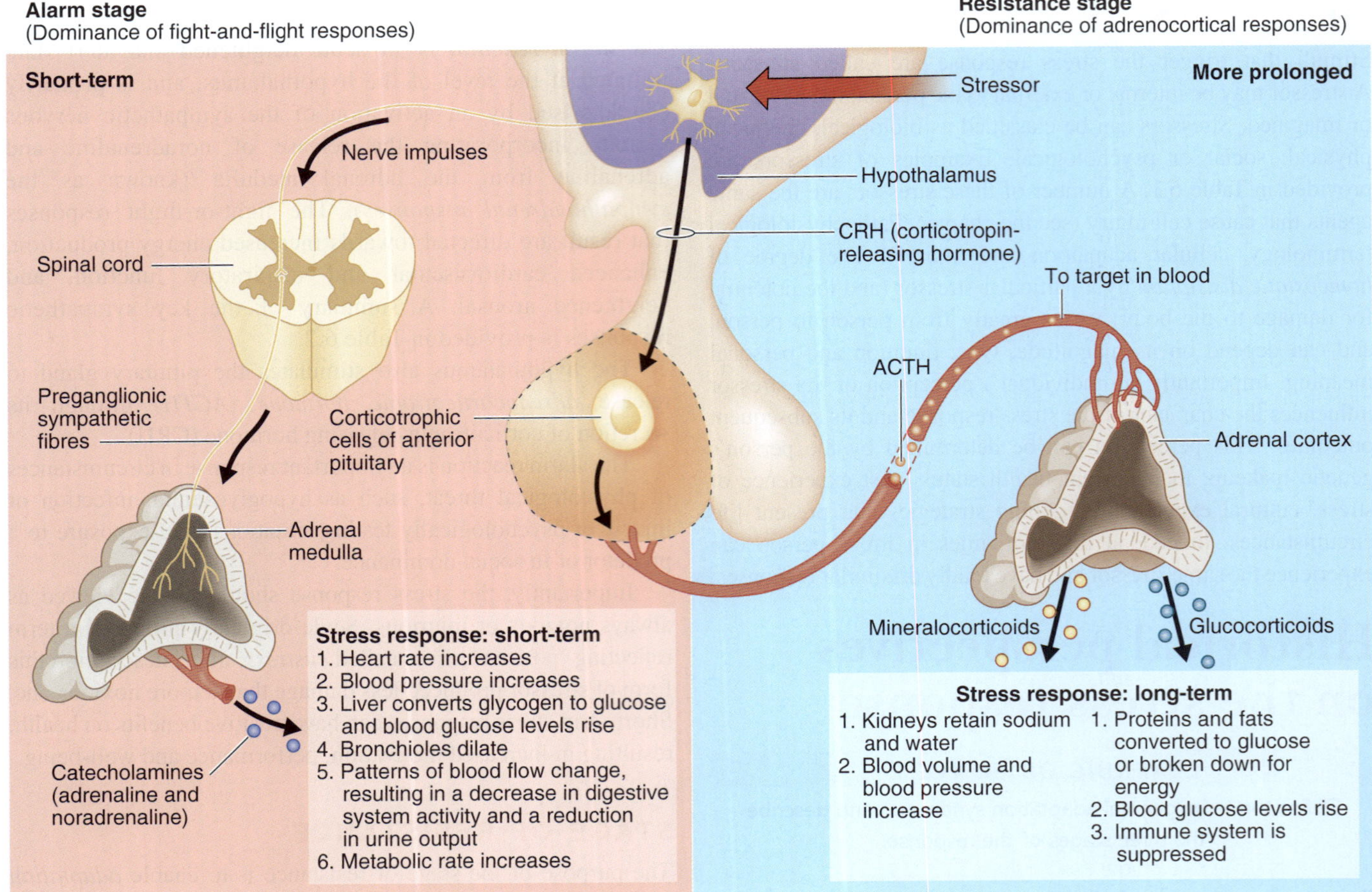

Figure 6.1

General adaptation syndrome: The alarm reaction and resistance stages

ACTH = adrenocorticotropic hormone.

Source: Adapted from Marieb & Hoehn (2016), Figure 16.16, p. 641.

and is responsible for sodium and water retention, which can enhance blood volume. The main functions of *cortisol* are to maintain elevated blood glucose levels for tissue metabolism (particularly the brain) and regulate the immune system. The effects of the corticosteroids are summarised in Table 6.3. Thus, the *hypothalamic–pituitary–adrenal (HPA) axis* is the key mechanism controlling the endocrine responses in stress.

Selye postulated that for adaptation to occur, the organism must maintain access to energy stores. If the stressor can be addressed and resolved while energy production can be maintained, then homeostasis will be re-established. The activity of the endocrine and nervous systems will then return to normal.

If neuroendocrine function does not return to a homeostatic level, immune dysregulation can ensue, which may be linked to an increased risk of infection and the development of autoimmune diseases such as rheumatoid arthritis, inflammatory bowel disease, Graves' disease or Hashimoto's thyroiditis.

Table 6.3 Summary of the effects of corticosteroids

Mineralocorticoids	Glucocorticoids
• Sodium and water retention: increased blood volume and blood pressure	• Modulation of immune system (immunosuppression) • Increased blood glucose levels • Mobilisation of fats • Protein catabolism • Enhanced tissue responsiveness to adrenaline and noradrenaline

EXHAUSTION

If adaptation to a persistent stressor cannot be achieved, the organism moves to the stage of exhaustion. In this stage, the stress response is maladaptive and leads to *dysfunction*. The characteristic pathology associated with this stage is hypertrophy of the adrenal glands due to excessive activation of the HPA axis. This leads to further increases in corticosteroid production. Coupled with this change is atrophy of lymphoid tissue, altered immune function and bleeding peptic ulcers.

Eventually, the adrenal glands fail, immune function becomes severely compromised, organ failure ensues and the organism dies. Figure 6.2 explores the general adaptation syndrome and its association with common clinical manifestations and management.

Current perspectives on the stress response

LEARNING OBJECTIVE 3

Contrast the historical and current views of the stress response.

Selye's concept of the stress response with the HPA axis and sympathoadrenal systems remains the cornerstone of our understanding of this response, even though it was found to be an incomplete description of the process. A number of other hormones and neuropeptides are now thought to contribute to the response. In particular, the release of a range of *chemokines* and *cytokines* occurs in selected regions of the brain, other tissues and in the blood, which have profound effects on neuroimmune processes.

Furthermore, investigators have since argued against the non-specificity of the response to all stressors. Different stressors can induce stress responses that are discernibly distinct from one another. For example, the sympathetic responses to thermal stimuli, as a part of the alarm reaction, are not the same. Part of the response to cold is peripheral vasoconstriction and shivering, whereas to heat it is peripheral vasodilation and sweating. We also now know that *psychological and experiential factors* are powerful stressors, equal to if not more powerful than some physiological stimuli. Indeed, physiological and psychological stressors can induce distinctive different stress responses; in some instances one category of stimuli produces no discernable response, whereas the other induces a significant response.

The characteristic pathology of the exhaustion stage has long been considered good evidence of the strong links between persistent stress, collapse of homeostasis and the development of disease. Prolonged stress has been considered an important risk factor for such diverse conditions as cardiovascular disease, peptic ulceration, anxiety disorders and depressive illness. The immune suppression induced by the excessive corticosteroid activity associated with prolonged stress has also been linked to an increased susceptibility to infection, autoimmune disease and cancer. Examples of the effects of prolonged or intense stress on body systems can be found in Figure 6.3.

LEARNING OBJECTIVE 4

Outline how stress affects the brain.

The role of the brain in the stress response has also been further elucidated in recent times. The brain has long been regarded as important in the interpretation of and the response to stressors. This is implicit in Selye's model, as it is the hypothalamus that initiates the physiological stress response. We now believe that *the brain has a central role in stress*, and is itself an important target for the stress hormones, particularly the glucocorticoids, and a number of immune mediators that can enhance or dampen immune processes. The interaction between these mediators and the HPA and sympathetic nervous system are yet to be fully teased out.

Acutely, the brain forms memories associated with the experience, as a part of the learning process in dealing with the situation should it arise again. This learning is dependent on brain plasticity, which is facilitated by glucocorticoid action in areas such as the hippocampus. The hippocampus is important in long-term memory formation and retrieval. This *adaptive brain plasticity* occurs throughout the lifespan, not just during childhood. In chronic stress, this plasticity becomes maladaptive, promoting hippocampal atrophy and impairments in memory and other cognitive functions. There is also evidence that chronic stress leads to alterations in the structure and function of other areas of the brain involved in cognitive, behavioural and emotional processing, including the amygdala, located within the temporal lobe, which plays an important role in the processing of fear and anger, and the prefrontal cortex, within the frontal lobe, which has a central role in decision-making and cognition.

LEARNING OBJECTIVE 5

Outline the roles of pituitary hormones, neuropeptides and sex hormones in the stress response.

A range of hormones and neuropeptides are released during stress to modulate the response. These include pituitary hormones (*antidiuretic hormone [ADH]*, growth hormone and prolactin), neuropeptides (endorphins, neuropeptide Y and angiotensin II), and the sex hormones oestrogen and testosterone.

PITUITARY HORMONES

When a stressor triggers activation of the hypothalamus, this initiates the release of ADH from the posterior pituitary. ADH induces water retention, which, along with aldosterone's action, will boost blood volume and increase blood pressure. It has also been shown that the action of CRH on ACTH secretion is potentiated by ADH during chronic stress. ADH has also been shown to stimulate the adrenal gland directly to increase cortisol secretion.

Intense stress has been found to trigger the release of growth hormone and prolactin from the anterior pituitary. *Growth hormone* induces increased blood glucose levels, promotes the

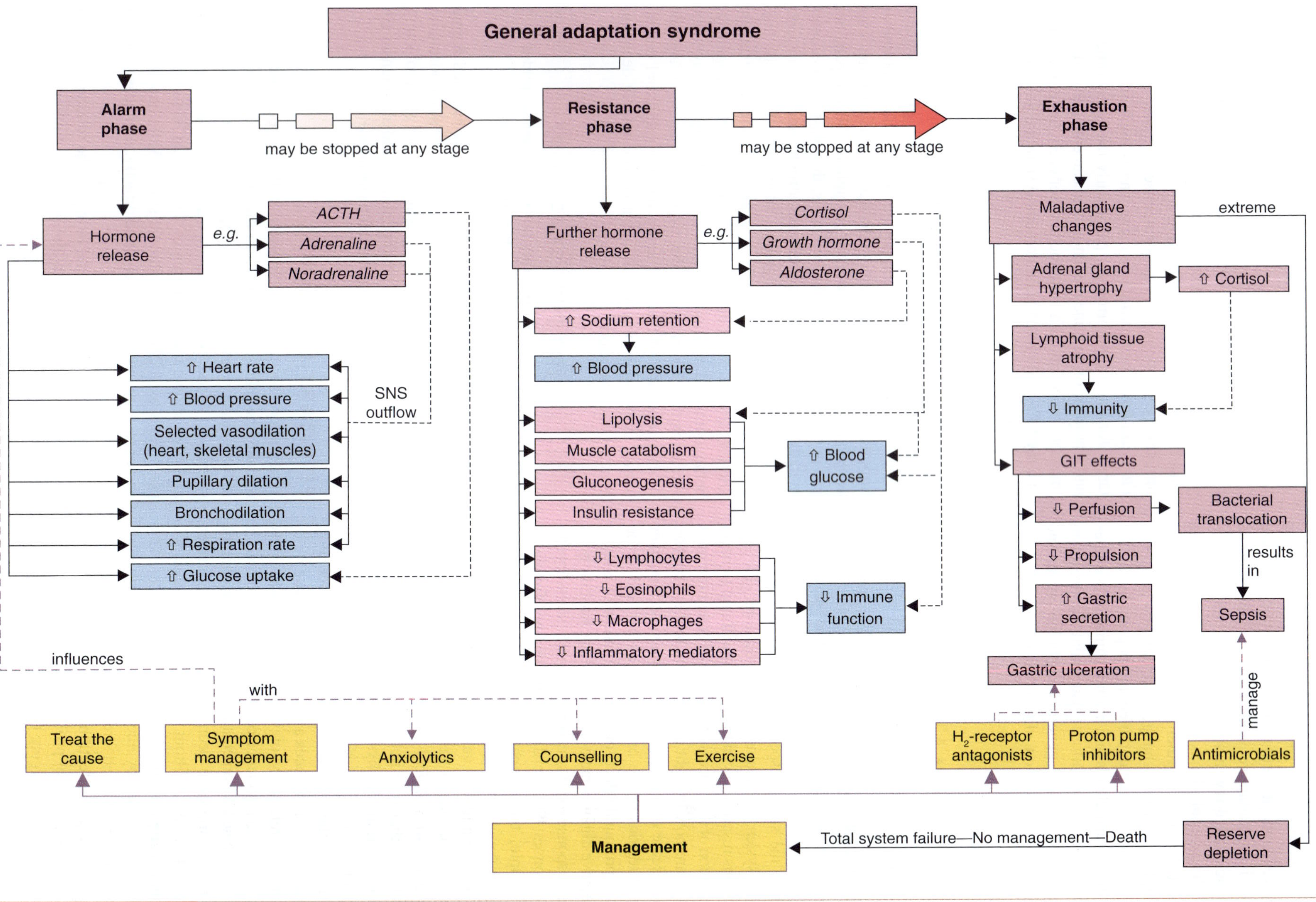

Figure 6.2

Clinical snapshot: General adaptation syndrome

↓ = decreased; ↑ = increased; ACTH = adrenocorticotropic hormone; GIT = gastrointestinal tract; SNS = sympathetic nervous system.

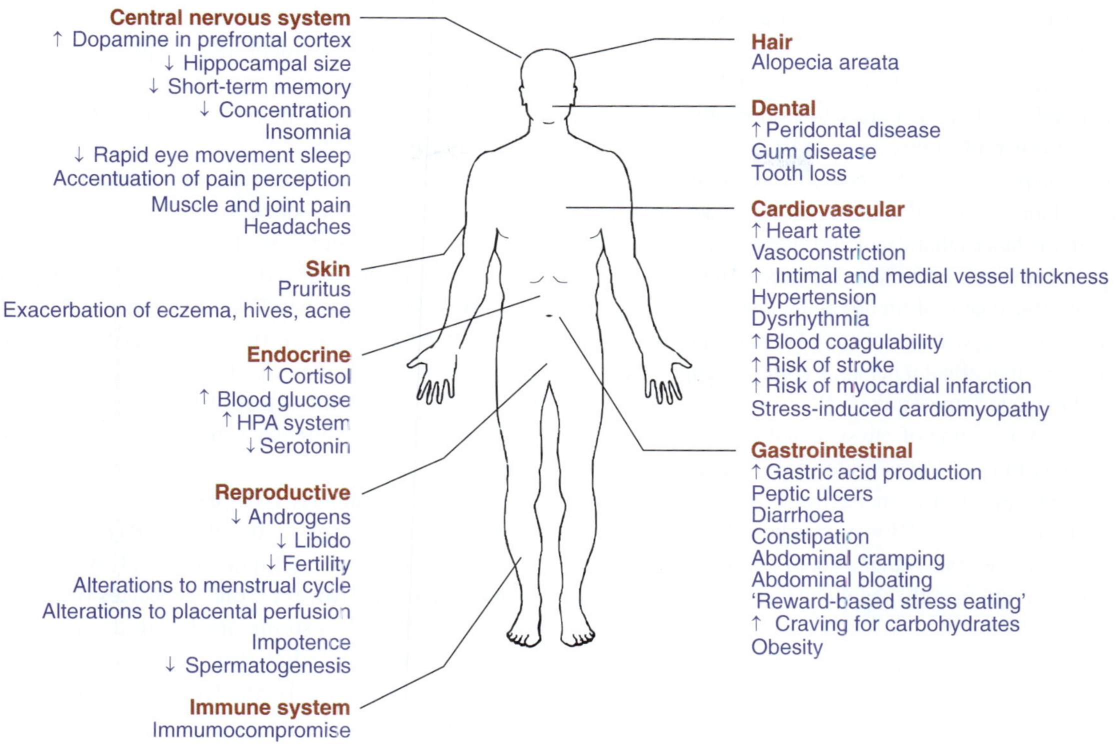

Figure 6.3

Examples of the effects of prolonged or intense stress on the body systems

↓ = decreased; ↑ = increased; HPA = hypothalamic–pituitary–adrenal axis.

breakdown of fats and facilitates protein synthesis. The role of *prolactin* in stress is unclear, as it is primarily associated with breast development and lactation.

NEUROPEPTIDES

Neuropeptide Y is known to act peripherally as a co-transmitter with noradrenaline at sympathetic terminals to trigger vasoconstriction as a part of the fight-or-flight responses. There is evidence to suggest that neuropeptide Y can also act on the amygdala and hippocampus to counteract an endogenous alarm system activated when an organism faces a stressful situation. It may also play a role in the adaptation of behavioural responses associated with chronic stress.

Endorphins are also released as a part of the stress response, and act as an endogenous morphine-like substance to induce analgesia and feelings of well-being. Increased levels of circulating *angiotensin II*, also a component of the renin–angiotensin system, appear to act centrally to enhance the activity of both the HPA axis and the sympathoadrenal systems during stress.

SEX HORMONES

Oestrogen and testosterone responsiveness appears to be quite different during stress. Studies have shown that *oestrogen* appears to decrease the activity of the HPA axis in stress, resulting in lower cortisol activity, while *testosterone* levels in men and women (secreted by the adrenal gland) decrease in response to stressful situations. Sex differences in stress responsiveness are further discussed later in this chapter.

Ageing and the stress response

LEARNING OBJECTIVE 6

State the implications of ageing on the stress response.

Stress can have a significant effect on ageing. The ageing process can also alter the stress response, and this has been demonstrated experimentally in rats and in humans. Older organisms show higher basal levels of glucocorticoid secretion than young organisms, and are slower to stop secretion after exposure to stress.

The functioning of body systems decreases with advancing age, even in healthy older people. Stress can exacerbate the wear and tear on body systems, and may accelerate the development of disease. A number of age-related diseases, such as Alzheimer's disease, diabetes mellitus and hypertension, have been shown to be associated with *elevated glucocorticoid levels*.

A particular focus for the effects of stress on ageing and its clinical implications is associated with the functioning of the immune system. *Immune function* decreases with age and can become further compromised in chronic stress. Under these circumstances, an elderly person may become more prone to conditions related to impaired immunity, such as infections. As an example, the development of a serious infection can lead to a downward spiral where the condition exacerbates the person's stress, especially if hospital admission for treatment is required, resulting in a greater deterioration in immune function and then further infections.

Once again, the perception of a potentially stressful situation discussed earlier in this chapter is worth revisiting. Older adults face changing life circumstances that can colour their perception of the situation and promote stress. Factors such as impending retirement, a change in income, the deaths of friends and relatives, deteriorating health, a loss of social support and increased dependence on others can become stressors that affect a person's ability to cope, when in the past they had managed stress quite well.

Adolescence, too, is a time of physical and emotional change, and the brain at this time of life is quite sensitised to stress. The common therapeutic approach in managing stress in adolescence has been on stress reduction. However, clinical research into adolescent well-being has shown that a focus on positive stress or eustress may produce significantly beneficial therapeutic outcomes.

Sex differences in the stress response

LEARNING OBJECTIVE 7

Contrast the stress response in males and females.

There is evidence in humans of sex differences in the responsiveness to stress. These differences in autonomic and HPA axis responses tend to be subtle in the unstressed state, but are more evident after exposure to a psychological stressor. The sex differences are more pronounced for females between puberty and menopause compared to males of the same age.

The character of the autonomic responses was found to be different between the sexes, with men showing increased blood pressure and greater catecholamine responses, and women showing more pronounced heart rates. With respect to the HPA axis, ACTH secretion was lower in women and was accompanied by smaller rises in salivary cortisol levels. The glucocorticoid response varied across the menstrual cycle, where it tended to increase during the luteal phase (i.e. post-ovulatory). There is also evidence of greater sensitivity of the pituitary to ADH in women.

During pregnancy, HPA axis activity is enhanced, with significant increases in baseline CRH, ACTH and cortisol levels. There is also enhanced basal sympathetic nervous system activity. However, the responses of the HPA axis and sympathoadrenal systems are blunted during pregnancy. It has been proposed that this is to protect the developing fetus from harm arising from an inappropriate stress response.

These sex differences have been largely accounted for in terms of the action of oestrogen on the HPA axis and sympathoadrenal systems. Supportive evidence has been obtained showing similar effects in women who take oral contraceptive agents and in postmenopausal women on oestrogen hormone replacement therapy.

INDIGENOUS HEALTH FAST FACTS AND CULTURAL CONSIDERATIONS

FAST FACTS

- *Aboriginal and Torres Strait Islander peoples are over three times more likely to experience high to very high levels of psychological stress compared to non-Indigenous Australians. Rates of suicide in Indigenous Australians are 2.4 times higher than in non-Indigenous Australians.*
- *Sixty-seven per cent of Aboriginal and Torres Strait Islander peoples had low to moderate levels of psychological distress, while 31% had high to very high levels.*
- *Aboriginal and Torres Strait Islander peoples are 1.6 times less likely to drink alcohol than non-Indigenous Australians; however, Indigenous Australians who do drink alcohol are 1.4 times more likely to drink at 'high-risk' levels.*
- *Māori are 1.6 times more likely to experience high to very high levels of psychological stress compared to European New Zealanders.*
- *Pacific Islands people are 1.5 times more likely to experience high to very high levels of psychological stress compared to European New Zealanders.*

CULTURAL CONSIDERATIONS

- *Multifactorial issues, including access to good nutrition, water quality, maternal health, genetics and biological factors, are not the only influencers in one's mental health. For Aboriginal and Torres Strait Islander peoples, the legacies of the events following colonisation contribute to the population's physical and mental health challenges. Historical experiences of exclusion, segregation and forced removal from family and community have contributed to enduring and transgenerational effects on Indigenous culture and society. Racism and social and economic disadvantage contribute to frequent and ongoing stress for Indigenous Australians. Yet, despite high levels of stress and suicide, targeted funding is limited for Aboriginal and Torres Strait Islander programs that support mental health.*

Sources: Data from: Australian Indigenous HealthInfoNet (2022); Australian Institute of Health and Welfare (2022); New Zealand Ministry of Health (2021, 2022).

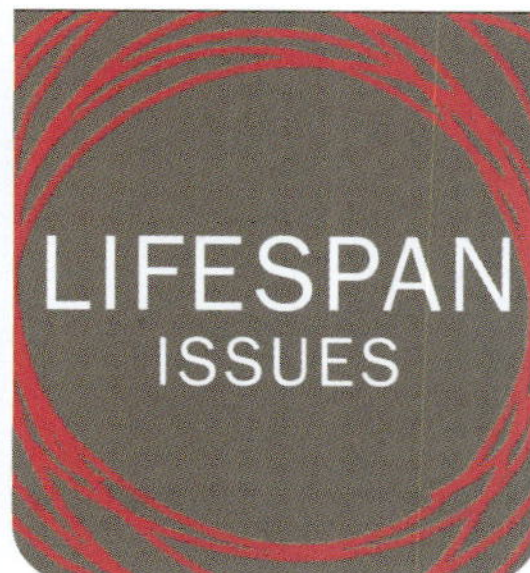

CHILDREN AND ADOLESCENTS

- Excessive and sustained stress in childhood can cause cortisol-induced damage to the hippocampus, resulting in cognitive deficits and low stress thresholds in adulthood.
- Stress and pain experienced in neonatal intensive care can cause anxiety disorders, heightened startle responses and abnormal pain thresholds as the child ages.
- The action of sucking a dummy or holding a comforter can assist in calming a young child, but is generally unnecessary after approximately 4 years of age.
- The use of a dummy (or finger-/thumb-sucking) after approximately 3 years of age can begin to hinder the normal development of a child's teeth and jaw.

OLDER ADULTS

- Age-induced changes to cell-mediated immunity can cause suppression of the cellular inflammatory response.
- Age-induced changes to the humoral response are blunted as antibody production reduces with advancing age.
- Stressors related to ageing (e.g. chronic illness) can exacerbate the immunological effects of ageing and cause further diminution of immunological function.

KEY CLINICAL ISSUES

- Educating someone on stress and coping skills will assist in their well-being.
- Reducing environmental, physical and financial stressors results in a decreased sympathetic nervous system response, which ultimately prevents the negative effect on an individual's immune system.
- Provision of pain relief and repositioning are two important methods of influencing physical stress related to pain.
- Excessive, unrelenting stress can result in exhaustion of nutrient stores, failure of the immune system, organ failure and, ultimately, death. Early identification of serious stressors will assist with instituting coping mechanisms and prevent more serious physical outcomes.

CHAPTER REVIEW

- *Stress* is a response of the body to a change in demand. Acute stress can be beneficial, as it can lead to enhanced physiological performance. However, an extreme or prolonged disruption in homeostasis can result in disease.
- Stimuli that trigger the stress response are called *stressors*.
- The *general adaptation syndrome* is considered a non-specific and reproducible response regardless of the physiological stimulus. It consists of three stages: the alarm reaction, resistance and exhaustion.
- The *alarm reaction* is an acute response initiated at the level of the hypothalamus, and is primarily characterised by an activation of the sympathetic nervous system, as well as the release of noradrenaline and adrenaline from the adrenal medulla.
- *Resistance* enables adaptation to the stressor and a return to the state of homeostasis. It is initially characterised by elevated hormone levels from the adrenal cortex, under the influence of ACTH, and a waning of the fight-or-flight responses.
- *Exhaustion* is maladaptive and leads to dysfunction. The characteristic pathology associated with this stage is hypertrophy of the adrenal glands, due to excessive activation of the HPA axis. This leads to further increases in corticosteroid production. Coupled with this change is deteriorating immune function.
- *Psychological and experiential factors* are powerful stressors, which are equal to, if not more powerful than, some physiological stimuli.
- The characteristic *pathology of the exhaustion stage* has long been considered good evidence of the strong links between persistent stress, collapse of homeostasis and the development of disease. Prolonged stress has been considered an important risk factor for such diverse conditions as cardiovascular disease, peptic ulceration, anxiety disorders and depressive illness. The immune suppression induced by the excessive corticosteroid activity associated with prolonged stress has also been linked to an increased susceptibility to infection, autoimmune disease and cancer.
- There is evidence in humans of *sex differences* in the responsiveness to stress. The sex differences are more pronounced for females between puberty and menopause compared to males of the same age. The character of the autonomic responses was found to be different between the sexes, with men showing increased blood pressure and greater catecholamine responses, and women showing more pronounced heart rates. With respect to the HPA axis, ACTH secretion was lower in women and was accompanied by smaller rises in salivary cortisol levels.

REVIEW QUESTIONS

1 Define the term 'stress'.

2 Define the term 'stressor', and give three examples of stressors.

3 For each of the following, indicate which stage (or stages) of the general adaptation syndrome it belongs to:
   a atrophy of lymphoid tissue
   b elevated aldosterone levels
   c heightened arousal and increased energy
   d compromised immune function
   e acute elevation in blood pressure

4 Briefly outline the role of each of the following mediators in the stress response:
   a ADH
   b endorphins
   c neuropeptide Y

5 How does basal glucocorticoid secretion differ between young and older people?

6 How do the autonomic effects associated with the stress response differ in men and women?

HEALTH PROFESSIONAL CONNECTIONS

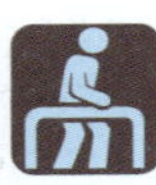

Physiotherapists Physiotherapists can be pivotal in assisting people to manage stress-related illness. Programs that promote health and well-being may include education in techniques such as progressive muscle relaxation, stretching and breathing techniques. Goals of treatment may include reducing muscle tension, reducing pain and discomfort, improving vigour, and potentially even reducing the doses of antihypertensives and psychoactive medications being taken.

Occupational therapists Occupational therapists can assist people to identify stressors, develop skills to manage stress, encourage desirable health behaviours and improve sleep. Techniques to achieve positive outcomes may include cognitive behavioural and solution-focused therapy. Other techniques that may prove beneficial include teaching fatigue management skills and relaxation or mindfulness-based meditation.

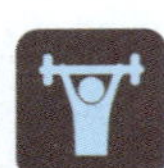

Exercise scientists Exercise prescription for those experiencing excessive stress must be approached with care. The cortisol released during the stress response diminishes the effectiveness of the immune system to some degree. Although physical exercise is good for the control of hypertension, excessive physical exercise can also modify immune system responses and metabolic needs. Considerations of gradual and measured programs would reduce the risk of tipping a person into the exhaustion phase before the benefits of exercise could contribute to their overall health improvement.

Nutritionists/Dieticians The stress response induces gluconeogenesis and glycogenolysis in an attempt to compensate for the increased metabolic requirements. Some people increase their carbohydrate consumption in times of stress. Education regarding blood glucose levels and low-glycaemic-index food is important.

Social workers People requiring hospital admission will experience an increase in psychological stress not only from their disease process, but also from the loss of control that they are faced with as a result of the admission. Financial factors, and logistical issues regarding child-minding, transport and meals, may all exacerbate the psychological stresses experienced by a person. Interventions to assist a person in their specific social needs will have a very positive impact on the stress response and decrease the amount of immunosuppression as a result of cortisol release.

All allied professionals Infection control principles are important to reduce the risk of hospital-acquired infections. The immunosuppressive effects of the stress response increase this risk. When caring for people with excessive physical and/or emotional stress, interventions that break the skin and bypass non-specific defences should be used judiciously. Education regarding personal hygiene and good respiratory hygiene practices will also assist in reducing the risk of exacerbating the physiological responses through exposure to pathogens from poor infection control measures.

CASE STUDY

Mrs Grace Schmidt is a 49-year-old woman (UR number 511672). She has been admitted for investigation of hypertension. Mrs Schmidt has a history of throbbing headaches and feelings that she might faint (pre-syncope). She is studying to be a teacher, and is completing her practical placement in a local high school. She finds the course and the work placement very stressful, especially after leaving a full-time job as a sales assistant at the local supermarket. She denies smoking, but has the occasional glass of wine. She is 111 kg in weight and 162 cm tall; her diet is high in fat and sodium. Mrs Schmidt is so busy with studying, undertaking practicum at the high school, and raising four teenage sons that she doesn't have time for any regular programmed exercise. The family has just had to move house as their previous rental property went into foreclosure. The landlord gave her only four weeks to find alternative accommodation. Her second-oldest son is being investigated for attention-deficit/hyperactivity disorder. Mrs Schmidt states that her whole family has had a 'string of chest infections and viruses over the past few months'. She denies any family history of hypertension and heart disease. Her observations were as follows:

Temperature	Heart rate	Respiration rate	Blood pressure	SpO_2
36°C	100	16	180/115	99% (RA*)

*RA = room air.

Mrs Schmidt's electrocardiogram demonstrated sinus tachycardia, and no dysrhythmia or ischaemic event was detected. She denies any pain. Her chest X-ray demonstrated clear lung fields, no focal consolidation, and normal hilar and pulmonary vasculature. Her costophrenic angles were clear, and the cardiac silhouette was within acceptable limits. Her admission pathology results have returned as shown below.

HAEMATOLOGY

Patient location:	Ward 3	**UR:**	511672		
Consultant:	Smith	**NAME:**	Schmidt		
		Given name:	Grace	**Sex:**	F
		DOB:	05/12/XX	**Age:**	49

Time collected	14:10
Date collected	XX/XX
Year	XXXX
Lab #	42937428

FULL BLOOD COUNT		UNITS	REFERENCE RANGE
Haemoglobin	128	g/L	115–160
White cell count	10.2	$\times 10^9$/L	4.0–11.0
Platelets	280	$\times 10^9$/L	140–400
Haematocrit	0.42		0.33–0.47
Red cell count	4.12	$\times 10^{12}$/L	3.80–5.20
Reticulocyte count	0.9	%	0.2–2.0
MCV	84	fL	80–100
Neutrophils	6.11	$\times 10^9$/L	2.00–8.00
Lymphocytes	3.81	$\times 10^9$/L	1.00–4.00
Monocytes	0.48	$\times 10^9$/L	0.10–1.00
Eosinophils	0.28	$\times 10^9$/L	< 0.60
Basophils	0.11	$\times 10^9$/L	< 0.20
ESR	2	mm/h	< 12
COAGULATION PROFILE			
aPTT	32	secs	24–40
PT	13	secs	11–17

BIOCHEMISTRY

Patient location:	Ward 3	**UR:**	511672		
Consultant:	Smith	**NAME:**	Schmidt		
		Given name:	Grace	**Sex:**	F
		DOB:	05/12/XX	**Age:**	49

Time collected	14:10
Date collected	XX/XX
Year	XXXX
Lab #	34579834

ELECTROLYTES		UNITS	REFERENCE RANGE
Sodium	147	mmol/L	135–145
Potassium	4.2	mmol/L	3.5–5.2
Chloride	101	mmol/L	95–110
Bicarbonate	24	mmol/L	22–32
Glucose	6.9	mmol/L	3.5–5.4
Iron	15.4	μmol/L	11–30
LIPID STUDIES			
Total lipids	7.9	g/L	4.0–8.0
Triglycerides	4.0	mmol/L	0.2–4.8
Total cholesterol	7.04	mmol/L	4.45–7.69
HDL cholesterol	1.8	mmol/L	0.98–2.38
LDL cholesterol	5.55	mmol/L	2.59–5.80

CRITICAL THINKING

1. Consider the admission history provided. Identify factors that could be considered stressors.
2. Given your knowledge of the immune system's response to long-term stress, discuss the statement regarding the family's experience with infections over the past few months.
3. Considering the history and observations provided, identify and discuss what stage of the general adaptation syndrome Mrs Schmidt is experiencing.
4. What other signs and symptoms will probably develop soon if the level of stress that Mrs Schmidt is experiencing continues?
5. What interventions could be implemented in order to reduce the risk of experiencing the exhaustion phase of the general adaptation syndrome? Draw up a table identifying the change, the intervention and the physiological rationale for its success.

BIBLIOGRAPHY

Australian Bureau of Statistics (ABS) (2019). *Australian Aboriginal and Torres Strait Islander health survey, 2018–19*. Canberra: ABS. https://www.abs.gov.au/statistics/people/aboriginal-and-torres-strait-islander-peoples/national-aboriginal-and-torres-strait-islander-health-survey.

Australian Health Ministers' Advisory Council's National and Aboriginal and Torres Strait Islander Health Standing Committee (2017). *Cultural respect framework, 2016–2026: for Aboriginal and Torres Strait Islander health—a national approach to building a culturally respectful health system*. Canberra: Australian Government Department of Health. https://nacchocommunique.files.wordpress.com/2016/12/cultural_respect_framework_1december2016_1.pdf.

Australian Indigenous Health*Info*Net (2022). *Overview of Aboriginal and Torres Strait Islander health status, 2021*. Perth, WA: Australian Indigenous Health*Info*Net. https://healthinfonet.ecu.edu.au/learn/health-facts/overview-aboriginal-torres-strait-islander-health-status/.

Australian Institute of Health and Welfare (AIHW) (2020). *Aboriginal and Torres Strait Islander Health Performance Framework 2020—summary report*. Cat. No. IHPF 2. Canberra: AIHW. https://www.indigenoushpf.gov.au/publications/hpf-summary-2020.

Best, O. & Fredericks, B. (2021). *Yatdjuligin: Aboriginal and Torres Strait Islander nursing and midwifery care* (3rd edn). Port Melbourne, VIC: Cambridge University Press.

Black, E., Kisely, S., Alichniewicza, K. & Toombs, M. (2017). Mood and anxiety disorders in Australia and New Zealand's indigenous populations: a systematic review and meta-analysis. *Psychiatry Research* 255:128–38. https://dx.doi.org/10.1016/j.psychres.2017.05.015.

Branson, V., Palmer, E., Dry, M.J. & Turnbull, D. (2019). A holistic understanding of the effect of stress on adolescent well-being: a conditional process analysis. *Stress and Health* 35(5):626–41. https://doi.org/10.1002/smi.2896.

Dhabhar, F.S. (2018). The short-term stress response—mother nature's mechanism for enhancing protection and performance under conditions of threat, challenge, and opportunity. *Frontiers in Neuroendocrinology* 49:175–92. https://doi.org/10.1016/j.yfrne.2018.03.004.

Marieb, E.N. & Hoehn, K. (2016). *Human anatomy and physiology* (10th edn). San Francisco, CA: Pearson Benjamin Cummings.

Marieb, E.N. & Hoehn, K. (2019). *Human anatomy and physiology* (11th edn). San Francisco, CA: Pearson Benjamin Cummings.

New Zealand Ministry of Health (2021). *Annual update of key results 2020/2021: New Zealand health survey*. Wellington: Ministry of Health. https://www.health.govt.nz/publication/annual-update-key-results-2020-21-new-zealand-health-survey.

New Zealand Ministry of Health (2022). *Health and independence report 2020: the Director-General of Health's annual report on the state of public health*. Wellington: Ministry of Health. https://www.health.govt.nz/publication/health-and-independence-report-2020.

7 Immune disorders

KEY TERMS

Acquired immune deficiency syndrome (AIDS)
Antibodies
Antigens
Autoimmune disease
B cells
Cellular immunity
Human immunodeficiency virus (HIV)
Human leukocyte antigen (HLA)
Humoral immunity
Hypersensitivity reaction
Immunity
Immunodeficiency
Immunosuppressants
Phagocytes
Self-antigens
T cells

LEARNING OBJECTIVES

After completing this chapter, you should be able to:

1 Outline the roles of the major antibody classes, immune cells and cytokines in immune processes.

2 Explain how immune dysfunction can be classified.

3 Outline the pathophysiology and risk factors of autoimmunity, and provide common examples.

4 Describe the characteristics of the main types of primary immunodeficiencies, and provide examples of specific conditions.

5 Identify the main environmental circumstances that can lead to secondary immunodeficiencies.

6 Describe the epidemiology, pathophysiology and complications associated with HIV/AIDS.

7 Identify the four types of hypersensitivity reactions, and give examples of specific conditions associated with these reactions.

8 Compare and contrast the characteristics of the hypersensitivity reactions.

WHAT YOU SHOULD KNOW BEFORE YOU START THIS CHAPTER

Can you describe the processes involved in inflammation and healing?

Can you describe the role of stress in disease?

Can you describe the main concepts associated with genetic disorders?

Can you describe the main concepts associated with infectious disease?

Introduction

Immune disorders are characterised by changes in the body's defence mechanisms that can leave humans either vulnerable to a range of opportunistic and serious infectious diseases or hyperreactive to benign stimuli, including our own tissue components. The consequences of altered immune function can be profound tissue damage leading to debilitating chronic disease or life-threatening illness.

The focus of this chapter is on conditions characterised by immune deficiency and excessive activity. An overview of autoimmunity is also provided. Common disorders of immune dysfunction will be covered, including humoral immunodeficiencies, cellular immunodeficiencies, combined immunodeficiency, HIV/AIDS and the immune hypersensitivity reactions.

The chapter commences with an overview of normal immune processes.

An overview of immune function

LEARNING OBJECTIVE 1

Outline the roles of the major antibody classes, immune cells and cytokines in immune processes.

The primary function of the immune system is *body defence*. It provides protection against foreign cells, organisms and non-living particles that enter our bodies and have the potential to injure cells and tissues. It also protects us against the development of cancerous cells that damage normal tissues through uncontrolled proliferation and then spread around the body. Fundamentally, the immune system acts through the recognition of **antigens**—markers on cells, organisms and particles that interact with immune components and trigger an immune response.

Immunity can be both cellular and humoral. **Humoral immunity** is enabled through the production of **antibodies**, which are immunoglobulins, and direct attack by immune cells. There are five classes of antibodies. Each class performs relatively specialised functions (see Table 7.1), and interacts with other protein-based systems, such as *complement*. **Cellular immunity** is provided by a range of immune cells. The key cell types involved in the immune response are the leukocytes, lymphocytes (T, B and natural killer cells), monocytes (which become macrophages after migrating into tissues), eosinophils and basophils (which become mast cells after migrating into tissues). The immune roles of each leukocyte subtype are summarised in Table 7.2.

The activity of the immune cells and the character of the response are influenced by chemical messengers, such as cytokines and other chemical mediators. A number of these mediators are also associated with nervous and endocrine functions. This highlights the interaction between neuroendocrine regulatory processes and immune function. Table 7.3 lists some key cytokines and their functions.

Table 7.1 Antibody classes and their functions

Class	Function
IgA	Major immunoglobulin in body secretions. Plays a role in local immunity in mucous membranes.
IgD	Low levels in serum. Binds to B cells to act as an antigen receptor.
IgE	Least common immunoglobulin in serum. Binds to basophils and mast cells. Involved in allergic reactions.
IgG	The major immunoglobulin in serum. Crosses the placenta. Activates complement. Binds to immune cells to enhance antigen recognition and activate cell functions.
IgM	Activates complement. Involved in the lysis and agglutination of microbes. Binds to B cells to act as an antigen receptor. First immunoglobulin in the primary immune response.

Table 7.2 Immune roles of leukocytes

Leukocyte cell type	Functions
GRANULOCYTES	
Neutrophils	Phagocytosis; important role in bacterial infection
Eosinophils	Modulate allergic reactions; important in parasitic infection
Basophils	Facilitate allergic reactions through the release of histamine, heparin and serotonin
AGRANULOCYTES	
Lymphocytes	Mediate cellular and humoral immunity. B cells differentiate into plasma cells, which secrete immunoglobulins (antibodies). T cells and natural killer cells attack microbes, foreign cells and cancerous cells
Monocytes	Phagocytosis

Table 7.3 Examples of cytokines and their functions

Cytokine	Functions	Secreting cell
Colony stimulating factors (CSF)		T cells, endothelium, fibroblasts
• Granulocyte CSF	Stimulates the proliferation and differentiation of granulocyte subpopulations	
• Macrophage CSF	Stimulates the proliferation and differentiation of macrophages and monocytes	
• Stem cell factor (SCF)	Synergises with other cytokines and erythropoietin to stimulate proliferation of blood cell lines	Bone marrow fibroblasts
Interferon-α and -β	Inhibit viral replication, stimulate T cell proliferation	Macrophages, viral-infected cells
Interferon-γ	Enhances cellular and humoral immunity	Th1 and Tc cells
Interleukin-1	Induces fever, stimulates B and T cells proliferation, mediates bone erosion in rheumatoid arthritis	Monocytes, macrophages
Interleukin-2	Stimulates lymphocyte proliferation, activates cellular immunity, stimulates cytokine production	Th cells
Interleukin-3	CSF that stimulates the production of many leukocyte populations	T cells
Interleukin-4	Stimulates B cells, plasma cell differentiation, increased IgE production in B cells, allergic reactions, T cell-mediated immunity, tissue repair and homeostasis	Th2 cells, mast cells, eosinophils, basophils
Interleukin-5	Stimulates B cells, increases IgA secretion	Th2 cells, mast cells
Migration-inhibiting factor	Inhibits macrophage migration away from a site of inflammation/infection	T cells
Tumour necrosis factor (TNF-α)	Chemotactic factor, pro-inflammatory, stimulates cytokine secretion, stimulates B cells, induces fever, mobilises calcium, activates neutrophils, antitumour activity	Macrophages, T cells

Tc = cytotoxic T cells; Th1 = type 1 helper T cells; Th2 = type 2 helper T cells.

Source: Adapted from Bullock & Manias (2022), Table 35.1, p. 415.

Types of immune dysfunction

LEARNING OBJECTIVE 2

Explain how immune dysfunction can be classified.

LEARNING OBJECTIVE 3

Outline the pathophysiology and risk factors of autoimmunity, and provide common examples.

Immune dysfunction can be classified broadly in two ways: deficient or hyperreactive. In *immunodeficient* states, a person loses the capacity for effective immune responsiveness and becomes susceptible to the development of serious infection and/or neoplasia. In hyperreactive immune responsive states, an affected person can experience localised or widespread tissue damage induced by immune processes.

Immune dysfunction should not be seen as dichotomous, resulting in only a deficient or hyperreactive state. Acute or chronic activation of immune cells shorten their lifespans, leading to immunodeficient states. Deficiencies in selected immune cells or mediators can induce an inappropriate immune attack on normal healthy tissues, and this is known as *autoimmunity*.

Autoimmunity is associated with the development of a loss of tolerance to 'self' antigens. These **self-antigens** are body cell markers that indicate to the immune system that they are not 'foreign' and should not be attacked. Self-tolerance arises at an early stage of human development. During the early differentiation of lymphocytes, B and T cells that bind to self-antigens undergo elimination through apoptosis or, alternatively, they remain viable but become profoundly inactive. Other ways in which tolerance of self can be maintained include the suppression of sensitised T cells by other immune cells, or through the establishment of a physical barrier between the blood and particular body compartments so that immune cells cannot gain access (see Figure 7.1).

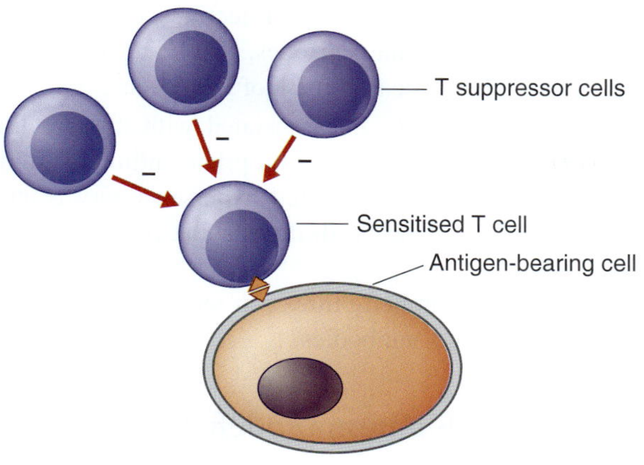

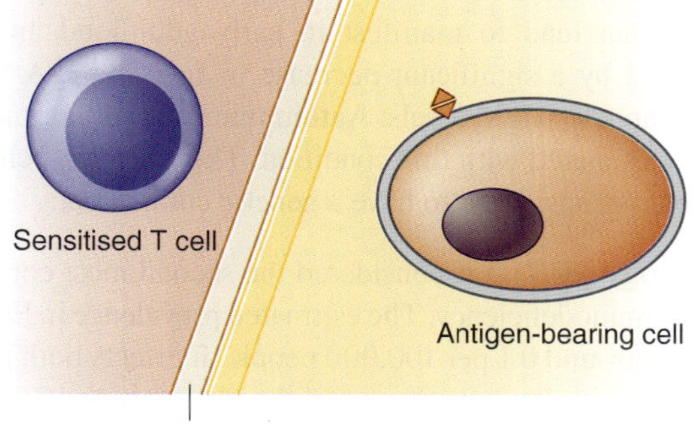

Figure 7.1

Immune tolerance of self

(A) The T cell comes into contact with a cell to which it is sensitised, but immune cell activation is suppressed by other immune cells.

(B) The T cell cannot access the body compartment (in this case, the brain) containing cells to which it is sensitised.

Examples of 'privileged' sites that normally exclude immune activity include the brain, the testicles and the pregnant uterus.

In **autoimmune disease**, the loss of self-tolerance may be associated with a number of mechanisms, such as disruption to the suppression of sensitised T cells, a breach in the barrier excluding immune processes from privileged sites, or antigens on infectious organisms and self-antigens on body cells being too similar, creating cross-reactivity between immune processes directed towards the infectious agent and body tissues. The immune attack leads to ongoing tissue damage through *chronic inflammatory reactions*. This leads to extensive damage and fibrosis over time, and a marked deterioration in the functions performed by the affected structure or structures.

Table 7.4 provides a list of some common autoimmune disorders. For some of these diseases, immune attack is primarily directed towards one structure, whereas for others the attack is widespread and affects a number of organs. Generally, the incidence of autoimmune disease tends to be greater in females than in males, although a condition called ankylosing spondylitis (see the chapter 'Bone and joints disorders') has its highest rates in young men.

Table 7.4 Common autoimmune disorders

Disorder	Primary target(s)
Type 1 diabetes mellitus (see the chapter 'Diabetes mellitus')	Pancreas
Rheumatoid arthritis (see the chapter 'Bone and joints disorders')	Joints
Graves' disease (see the chapter 'Thyroid and parathyroind disorders')	Thyroid
Hashimoto's thyroiditis (see the chapter 'Thyroid and parathyroind disorders')	Thyroid
Multiple sclerosis (see the chapter 'Neurodegenerative disorders')	Brain, optic nerves, spinal cord
Systemic lupus erythematosus	Skin, joints, kidneys, heart, brain

Table 7.5 Some associations between HLA genes and autoimmune disease

Autoimmune disease	HLA genes
Type 1 diabetes mellitus	*DR3, DR4*
Rheumatoid arthritis	*DR1, DR4*
Ankylosing spondylitis	*B27, B51*
Hashimoto's thyroiditis	*DR2, DR5*

There is an association between the presence of particular **human leukocyte antigen (HLA)** genes, also known as major *histocompatibility complex (MHC) genes*, and an increased risk of developing autoimmune disease. Strong associations with a range of autoimmune diseases have been found for the *D2*, *D3*, *D4*, *D5* and *B27* HLA genes (see Table 7.5).

IMMUNODEFICIENCY

Immunodeficient disorders are commonly characterised by impairments affecting antibody activity, lymphocyte function (i.e. T and B cells), phagocytosis or a combination of these. The immune system deficiency can be present at birth (*congenital* conditions) or develop later in life (*acquired* conditions). An **immunodeficiency** can be further classified as either a primary or a secondary condition. A *primary immunodeficiency* chiefly affects the immune system, whereas a *secondary condition* affects immune function as a consequence of its effects elsewhere in the body (e.g. drug treatment with either antimicrobials or glucocorticoids, or a state of malnutrition). A number of immunodeficient disorders are inheritable conditions strongly associated with chromosomal abnormalities, both autosomal and sex-linked.

People with immunodeficiencies might be expected to have more severe COVID-19 infections. However, the evidence is not clear due to the relatively recent appearance of the virus and limited literature available investigating this.

PRIMARY IMMUNODEFICIENCIES

LEARNING OBJECTIVE 4

Describe the characteristics of the main types of primary immunodeficiencies, and provide examples of specific conditions.

Categories of primary immunodeficiency are described in this section, and common examples of disorders from each category are outlined. The main categories discussed are humoral, cellular and combined immunodeficiencies. These conditions can affect the numbers of cells and/or their function.

Humoral immunodeficiencies

Humoral immunodeficiencies usually affect antibody production from **B cells**, but can affect B cell numbers. These disorders can affect the production of one, some or all antibody classes.

Selective IgA deficiency

Aetiology and pathophysiology Selective IgA deficiency is considered the most common primary immunodeficiency. As indicated in Table 7.1, IgA offers local immunity associated with the mucous membranes of the gastrointestinal, respiratory and genitourinary tracts. Forms of this condition have been linked to either an autosomal dominant or recessive inheritance pattern.

There is an increased risk of autoimmune conditions and allergy in people with this immunodeficiency. It has been proposed—and there is some supportive evidence—that IgA may exert a protective role against autoimmunity.

Epidemiology Reported prevalence rates for this condition have been derived from blood donor data, and range between 0.03% and 0.3%. The incidence in Australia has been reported at 0.23%. Interestingly, a strong positive correlation has been found for the frequency of selective IgA deficiency and the prevalence of COVID-19 infection per population.

Clinical manifestations An increased incidence of autoimmune disorders such as arthritis, haemolytic anaemia, inflammatory bowel disease, systemic lupus erythematosus, coeliac disease and type 1 diabetes mellitus is associated with this condition. An increased susceptibility to infection may also be observed in some people.

People with an absolute deficiency in IgA may develop severe hypersensitivity reactions when administered blood products containing this immunoglobulin. Repeated exposure to such blood products in these people leads to the formation of IgA antibodies.

When infections develop, they tend to affect the respiratory, reproductive, urinary and gastrointestinal systems. Sinusitis and urinary tract infections are common. Older people with the condition may be at a higher risk of pneumonia and other respiratory infections, as well as autoimmune disorders.

Clinical diagnosis and management The diagnosis is made on the basis of a history of recurrent infections, hypersensitivity reactions and autoimmune episodes. The diagnosis can be confirmed through the measurement of IgA levels.

No specific treatments are associated with this condition. Infections are managed with the appropriate antimicrobial drug therapy. Autoimmune disorders and hypersensitivity reactions are managed in accordance with the specific type of condition that manifests.

People with IgA antibody titres can receive blood products that do not contain IgA antibodies.

Common variable immunodeficiency

Aetiology and pathophysiology Common variable immunodeficiency (CVID) comprises a group of heterogeneous conditions that tend to manifest in early adulthood and are characterised by a significant decrease in IgG and IgA levels with or without low IgM levels. Autoimmune and inflammatory states are associated with this condition. The aetiology remains unclear, but is considered to have a genetic component.

Epidemiology CVID is considered the second most common primary immunodeficiency. The estimated prevalence in Europe in 2011 was around 0.1 per 100,000 people. It affects both males and females, with the average age of diagnosis around 26 years old. However, around 20% of affected people have symptoms in childhood.

Clinical manifestations Common manifestations involve recurrent respiratory tract infections, which can involve the nasal sinuses, throat, ears, bronchi and lungs. Gastrointestinal infection or inflammation may be apparent. Enlarged lymph nodes in the neck, chest and abdomen can be present, and splenomegaly is common.

Autoimmune manifestations may include haemolytic anaemia and immune thrombocytopenia. Granulomas may occur in CVID, and may involve the lungs, liver or spleen.

Clinical diagnosis and management In addition to the decreased levels of immunoglobulins, the diagnosis should satisfy the following criteria: a poor antibody response to vaccines, B cell numbers and function, T cell numbers and function (no evidence of profound deficiency) and exclusion of secondary causes of hypogammaglobulinaemia.

Treatment options include the replacement of affected immunoglobulins, antimicrobial drug therapy for infections, management of inflammatory conditions and corticosteroid therapy for autoimmune manifestations.

Bruton's agammaglobulinaemia

Aetiology and pathophysiology Bruton's agammaglobulinaemia results from a congenital defect in the synthesis of tyrosine kinase, which is essential in normal B cell development. The condition has been shown to have an X-linked recessive inheritance pattern. A deficiency in B cell numbers results, affecting the production of all antibody classes.

Epidemiology The global prevalence rate of Bruton's agammaglobulinaemia is estimated to be between 1 in 250,000 and 1 in 400,000 people. As it is an X-linked condition, it mainly affects males.

Clinical manifestations Affected children appear to be particularly vulnerable to infections by *Haemophilus influenzae*, as well as *Streptococcus pneumoniae* and *Staphylococcus* species. Frequent and recurrent middle ear infection (otitis media), bronchitis, diarrhoea, meningitis and pneumonia are common in these children. Sepsis may develop.

Clinical diagnosis and management A history of recurrent infection will initiate investigations as to the possibility of Bruton's agammaglobulinaemia. Circulating B cell counts and a quantitative measurement of immunoglobulin levels will provide confirmation of the condition. Genetic counselling is available to couples with an affected child, and for those with a family history of immunodeficiency disorders. A test is available to determine whether the tyrosine kinase affected in this condition is being expressed.

At this time, there is no cure for children affected by this condition. The provision of life-long passive **immunity** by a regular injection of human immunoglobulin is the primary therapy. When infections occur, they require the appropriate antimicrobial drug therapy.

Gene therapy offers significant potential for the treatment and possible cure of X-linked immunodeficiencies. See the section on the management of severe combined immunodeficiency (later in this chapter) for a discussion of gene therapy in this context.

Cellular immunodeficiencies

Cellular immunodeficiencies primarily affect **T cells**, which have roles in direct cellular immune attack and as key facilitators of the general immune response. They can activate B cells and greatly influence antibody production. Frequent opportunistic fungal infection is usually seen as an indicator of poor T cell responsiveness. The site of the impairment can be the T cell itself, or within the tissues responsible for T cell maturation or activation, such as the thymus.

DiGeorge syndrome

Aetiology and pathophysiology DiGeorge syndrome is a clinically important immunodeficiency disorder associated with poor T cell function. This congenital genetic disorder is associated with a deletion of part of chromosome 22 (see Figure 4.13). It is characterised by various degrees of poor development of body structures, such as the heart, vasculature, oesophagus, thymus, parathyroid, face and genitals.

The immune component of this disorder occurs as a consequence of hypoplasia of the thymus gland. Immune dysfunction will depend on the degree of thymus function. In its severest form, the thymus gland is absent (thymic aplasia), leading to negligible levels of T cell maturation. Autoimmune disorders have been observed in a small percentage of people with DiGeorge syndrome.

Epidemiology The prevalence rate of DiGeorge syndrome is estimated at 1 in 3,000–6,000 live births. In Australia, the prevalence appears to be lower than in many other countries, with an estimate of about 1 in 66,000 live births. There do not appear to be any differences in incidence between males and females, or between racial groups.

Clinical manifestations As immune function may be greatly impaired in severely affected children, frequent opportunistic infection by microbes such as *Candida albicans*, cytomegalovirus and *Pneumocystis jiroveci* occur. Thrush, pneumonia, diarrhoea and ear infections are common. Sepsis may also develop. These infections can be severe and may even be life-threatening.

Other common clinical manifestations include congenital heart defects, palate dysfunction leading to feeding difficulties, characteristic abnormal facial features, learning disabilities, mental illness, hypocalcaemia from hypoparathyroidism (which may result in seizures) and renal impairment. For those people with DiGeorge syndrome and congenital heart defects who developed COVID-19 infections, moderate to severe COVID symptoms were reported. Autoimmune manifestations observed in this condition include haemolytic anaemia, immune thrombocytopenia, autoimmune arthritis, autoimmune hepatitis and inflammatory bowel disease.

The mnemonic *CATCH-22* may be used to summarise the characteristics of this disorder: *c*ongenital heart disease, *a*bnormal facies, *t*hymic aplasia, *c*left palate, *h*ypocalcaemia, and a deletion in chromosome *22*.

Clinical diagnosis and management Physical examination, laboratory testing and medical imaging will reveal the characteristic clinical presentation of the condition. Confirmation of the chromosomal abnormality can be achieved through the testing of a blood sample. Prenatal testing for families with affected children is available.

Surgery will be required to correct defects in the heart and palate. Parathyroid impairment can be managed by long-term vitamin D and calcium supplementation. Infections can be managed by the appropriate antimicrobial therapy. The normal childhood immunisation schedule may be possible in children with some thymus function. In severe cases, transplantation of thymus tissue has been used to lessen thymic impairment.

Early intervention programs in occupational and speech therapy are important in order to improve the cognitive, language and social skills in affected children. Where mental illnesses manifest, it is necessary to seek the assistance of psychiatric services.

Combined immunodeficiencies

Defects in the development of lymphoid stem cells affect the differentiation of both T and B lymphocyte subpopulations. This defect will affect the numbers and/or functions of the lymphocytes. Cell-mediated responses, cytokine communication and antibody production will be affected, but to varying degrees, depending on the specific condition and its pattern of inheritance.

Severe combined immunodeficiency (SCID)

Aetiology and pathophysiology Severe combined immunodeficiency (SCID) is an important clinical condition representing a combined disorder of lymphocyte subpopulations. Antibody production and T cell and natural killer cell numbers are greatly decreased or absent; B cell numbers may be reduced, normal or increased.

There are multiple forms of SCID, but the most well-known one, which is the more common type, is the X-linked recessive type. Other forms are associated with single gene mutations that result in congenital enzyme deficiencies. An example of this is a deficiency of adenosine deaminase.

Historically, an affected child was referred to as 'a boy in a bubble' (as it more commonly manifests in boys). This is because such children needed to live in a sterile environment partitioned from the outside world in order to reduce the risk of infection. However, urgent *haematopoietic stem cell transplant (HSCT)* significantly improves their chances of surviving past their first year, and enjoying a more fulsome quality of life.

Autoimmunity can develop in affected children. When first considered, autoimmune manifestations appear paradoxical, as the child's immune function is profoundly deficient. However, the explanation for this is that the development of immune tolerance has been greatly disrupted, allowing the existence of autoreactive T cells.

Epidemiology In Australia, the estimated prevalence of SCID is 0.15 case per 100,000 people. The X-linked form is the most common type of SCID reported, and affects males. The remaining forms are relatively evenly distributed across both sexes. There do not appear to be differences in incidence across race and ethnicity.

Clinical manifestations Babies with SCID commonly have recurrent infections, failure to thrive and frequent diarrhoea. A child with this condition is profoundly susceptible to infection. If acquired, an infection would most likely be fatal. Infections such as thrush (caused by C. *albicans*), *P. jiroveci* pneumonia, measles, otitis media and diarrhoea are common. Sepsis may develop in these children. Without definitive treatment, SCID is fatal within the first two years of life.

Clinical diagnosis and management Babies with SCID may present with fever and an active infection. Being a genetic disorder, assessment of the family history is important. Diagnosis may occur after 2 months of age, but if there is no previous family history it may not occur until approximately 6 months of age. Haematology results will normally show low levels of T lymphocytes and very low gammaglobulin or immunoglobulin levels once the maternal antibodies have gone.

An immunology consultant should be a principal member of the care team. Intravenous immunoglobulin is the first line of treatment. Infection prevention practices include single-room isolation protocols with HEPA-filtered rooms where available, exclusion of staff and family members infected with upper respiratory tract infections or active cold sores, antimicrobial prophylaxis with cotrimoxazole against *P. jirovecii*, and immunoglobulin replacement therapy (IRT) will be required monthly until transplant. Urgent HSCT should be performed early, when the child has no active infection.

Haematopoietic stem cell transplant is considered curative with an extremely high success rate (> 90%). Following the HSCT, immune function is gradually restored, and by approximately one year the child is considered free from danger of serious infections. Currently, gene therapy is not an option in Australia or New Zealand.

SECONDARY IMMUNODEFICIENCIES

LEARNING OBJECTIVE 5

Identify the main environmental circumstances that can lead to secondary immunodeficiencies.

Secondary immunodeficiencies are usually the consequence of *environmental circumstances*, such as severe or prolonged stress, a poor level of nutrition, drug treatment, infection or myeloid cancers, rather than developmental defects. The relationships between immunity and these environmental interactions are explored in this section.

Severe or prolonged stress

The relationship between severe stress and immune function has been described in the chapter 'Stress and its role in disease'. In the exhaustion stage of the stress response, hypertrophy of the adrenal glands occurs, with increased corticosteroid release. High circulating levels of corticosteroids suppress immune processes. Deteriorating immune function is further evidenced by the atrophy of lymphoid tissue and an increased susceptibility to infection.

Poor nutrition

A state of malnutrition will lead to immunodeficiency, as the proteins used to make antibodies or produce chemical mediators undergo catabolism in order to produce adenosine triphosphate (ATP). Furthermore, when nutrition is poor, vitamins A, B, C and E, as well as minerals, such as zinc and iron, which are strongly implicated in normal immunity, may not be available.

Drug treatment

A number of medicines are **immunosuppressants**, either by design or as a side-effect of their action. Drugs can affect immune responsiveness by either inhibiting immune cell proliferation or the production of immune or inflammatory mediators, or altering the balance between normal flora and opportunistic pathogens. Common drug groups that may cause immunosuppression include corticosteroids such as cortisol, prednisone and dexamethasone, non-steroidal anti-inflammatory drugs (NSAIDs) such as ibuprofen and aspirin, antimicrobials and anticancer drugs.

Infection

An important characteristic of pathogenic microbes is that once they enter our bodies they must have a mechanism to evade or disrupt immune attack; either way, the human host's immune system becomes incapable of responding. This mechanism is known as *immune escape or evasion*. This can be achieved by the release of microbial enzymes that neutralise antibody or complement interactions, or impair phagocyte lysosomal enzyme action. Some microbes evade recognition by the immune system and continue to remain viable or proliferate inside cells.

Examples of this are the malaria-causing *Plasmodium* species, which live undetected in erythrocytes, or the tuberculosis microbe *Mycobacterium tuberculosis*, which remains viable inside macrophages after being engulfed.

Many viruses underlying human infection are particularly effective in inducing immune escape. Multiple factors may determine immune escape, including modulation of innate immune responses and high rates of viral mutation. The SARS-CoV-2 virus underlying COVID-19 infection has maintained its effectiveness in inducing immune escape through such means as impaired antigen presentation, monocyte response modulation and decreased interferon secretion. In addition, high mutation rates of viral structural elements, such as spike proteins, can also make a contribution.

Infection with the human immunodeficiency virus (HIV), and the progression to acquired immune deficiency syndrome (AIDS), is an important type of secondary immunodeficiency disorder. This condition is described in detail in a separate section.

Cancer

Cancers that affect lymphoid and myeloid tissues, such as lymphomas and leukaemias, disrupt immune function. The lineage and differentiation of white blood cells is affected in these cancers, affecting the availability and/or function of lymphocyte subpopulations. Cellular and humoral immune responses can become limited under these conditions.

HIV/AIDS

LEARNING OBJECTIVE 6

Describe the epidemiology, pathophysiology and complications associated with HIV/AIDS.

Aetiology and pathophysiology

One of the most virulent forms of immune disruption is associated with the **human immunodeficiency virus (HIV)**, the causative agent in **acquired immune deficiency syndrome (AIDS)**. The major routes of transmission from an HIV-infected person are through unprotected sex, from mother to baby across the placenta, and via contact with blood, contaminated needles, syringes and scalpels, or blood products. There is no evidence to indicate that infection can occur through contact with other body fluids, such as saliva, respiratory aerosols, cerebrospinal fluid, urine or tears.

HIV targets helper T (Th) cells (bearing CD4 surface receptors, and otherwise known as CD41$^+$ T cells), which have a key role to play in normal immune responsiveness. Other cells bearing CD4$^+$ receptors, such as macrophages and dendritic cells, also become infected by HIV. Attachment to the CD4$^+$ receptor and a co-receptor of the integral membrane protein family, called C-chemokine receptor 5 (CCR5), is the means by which the virus infects cells.

After infection, cellular and humoral immune processes become progressively weakened, leaving the affected person vulnerable to opportunistic infections, which, if left untreated, can lead to death.

Historically, the view has been that HIV directly destroys CD4$^+$ cells and impedes the replacement of these cells. This was seen as the cause of the T cell depletion and the immune-deficient state. It is now proposed that HIV infection actually triggers chronic immune activation, T cell proliferation and shorter cell lifespans, which leads to the immune-deficient state. This hypothesis correlates well with the experimental and clinical data associated with HIV infection progression and observed non-AIDS comorbidities (see Table 7.6). The non-AIDS comorbidities (listed in the 'Clinical manifestations' section) are associated with premature ageing in HIV-infected people, and are believed to be linked to the chronic antiviral drug treatment and the consequences of chronic immune activation.

Common opportunistic infections and causative agents associated with HIV/AIDS include infection by *C. albicans*, toxoplasmosis, tuberculosis, forms of bacterial meningitis, cytomegalovirus and *P. jiroveci* pneumonia. Affected people are also susceptible to cancer, particularly a form of skin cancer

Table 7.6 Characteristics of immune activation in HIV infection

Specific example of immune activation	Correlation to disease state
CD4$^+$ cells more activated in HIV infection; proliferate rapidly and have shorter cell lifespan	CD4$^+$ cell depletion and immune deficiency
Cytotoxic T cells (CD8$^+$ cells) activated; proliferate rapidly and have shorter cell lifespan	Marker of HIV progression
Increased expression of inflammatory cytokines TNF-α and interleukins	Marker of HIV progression
Immune activation lower in HIV-2 compared to HIV-1 infection	Slower disease progression rate in HIV-2
Endothelial cell activation, increased endothelial cell division, increased endothelial permeability	Might be linked to the development of non-AIDS-linked comorbidities
Activation of coagulation system	Might be linked to the development of non-AIDS-linked comorbidities

called Kaposi's sarcoma, but also to myeloid or oropharyngeal cancers. These conditions, which are closely associated with AIDS, are known as *AIDS-defining illnesses*.

Epidemiology

Based on recent statistics, over 36,000 Australians and more than 4300 New Zealanders have been diagnosed with HIV infection since the epidemic began in 1984–85. The incidence of AIDS in Australia and New Zealand is very low. Data from 2021 indicates that 30,000 Australians and 3,600 New Zealanders are living with HIV infection, as part of 38.4 million people worldwide.

Clinical manifestations

The course of AIDS and the specific manifestations can vary greatly from person to person, and are dependent on the stage of infection. Common clinical manifestations associated with the early stages of infection include fever, rash, swollen lymph nodes and sore throat. Infected people can then move on to experience an asymptomatic period, depending on the degree of immunocompetence. They may develop mild chronic infections and show weight loss, fever, diarrhoea and swollen lymph nodes.

If AIDS develops, a person will become susceptible to a number of opportunistic AIDS-defining illnesses. Clinical manifestations can include weight loss, persistent fatigue, chronic diarrhoea, cough, headaches, skin rashes, night sweats, fever and the presence of oral lesions.

Non-AIDS comorbidities can include atherosclerosis, increased risk of myocardial infarction, osteoporosis, neurocognitive disorders, metabolic syndrome, frailty and kidney failure.

Clinical diagnosis and management

Diagnosis Assessment of the person's history (including sexual history, blood transfusions, exposure to contaminated syringes, needles or scalpels, the social context and comorbidities) is important in the initial evaluation. Rapid HIV antibody tests at sexual health clinics, other screening opportunities, or testing at home, can take as little as 20 minutes. However, a positive result on this type of test must be confirmed by a traditional serology test, which can take several days to come back. Baseline serology for other viruses should also be taken. A chest X-ray will quantify the person's respiratory health and rule out other thoracic issues that may be present. A Mantoux test should also be performed for tuberculosis, and a Pap smear is indicated for females, as immunodeficiency increases the risk of developing other infections. Incidence of co-infection with tuberculosis or the human papilloma virus is higher in people with HIV.

HIV infection is confirmed by the presence of HIV antibodies, but seroconversion can take anywhere from a couple of weeks to over a year. This is accompanied by acute flu-like symptoms. Initially, in this primary infection stage, the Th cell count drops but then rises back towards normal (normal count => 500 cells/mm^3). There is a period of latency associated with the progression from chronic HIV infection to AIDS. Without treatment, Th cell counts decrease over time. The diagnosis of AIDS is based on a Th cell count lower than 200 cells/mm^3 and the confirmation of one or more AIDS-defining illness.

Management Management principles are based on promoting maximum health to support immunocompetence. Combination antiretroviral drugs are important to control the increasing viral load and to maintain immune function. Significantly, this treatment has transformed HIV/AIDS from a fatal disease into a manageable chronic illness. However, this treatment can be problematic due to the adverse-effect profile of combination therapy and the risk of developing antimicrobial resistance.

Good nutrition and healthy lifestyle choices should be encouraged. In those who have not developed too much immunosuppression, vaccinations against hepatitis A virus, hepatitis B virus and seasonal influenza should be considered. Antibiotics and antifungal agents may be considered for prophylaxis for herpes simplex virus, tuberculosis, *P. jiroveci* pneumonia and candidiasis, depending on individual assessment.

Although HIV infection is a communicable disease, the success in managing the condition has led to it no longer being regarded as a notifiable disease in this region. Figure 7.2 explores the common clinical manifestations and management of HIV infection.

Immune overactivity

HYPERSENSITIVITY REACTIONS

LEARNING OBJECTIVE 7

Identify the four types of hypersensitivity reactions, and give examples of specific conditions associated with these reactions.

A **hypersensitivity reaction** is an *excessive immune response* that induces an *inflammatory response* that can lead to extensive damage to normal tissues, chronic disability and, in some cases, death. There are four types of hypersensitivity reaction, each indicated by a roman numeral: types I to IV. The reactions are differentiated from each other by the speed of onset, whether the response is mediated by antibody or direct immune cell attack, the type of antibody concerned, and the involvement of complement in the reaction. Figure 7.3 explores the common clinical manifestations and management of hypersensitivities.

Hypersensitivity reactions have been implicated in the pathogenesis of autoimmunity (see Table 7.7).

Table 7.7 Hypersensitivity reactions involved in autoimmunity

Hypersensitivity reaction	Autoimmune disorder
Type I	Hashimoto's thyroiditis
Type II	Goodpasture's disease; Graves' disease; Myasthenia gravis
Type III	Systemic lupus erythematosus
Type IV	Type 1 diabetes mellitus

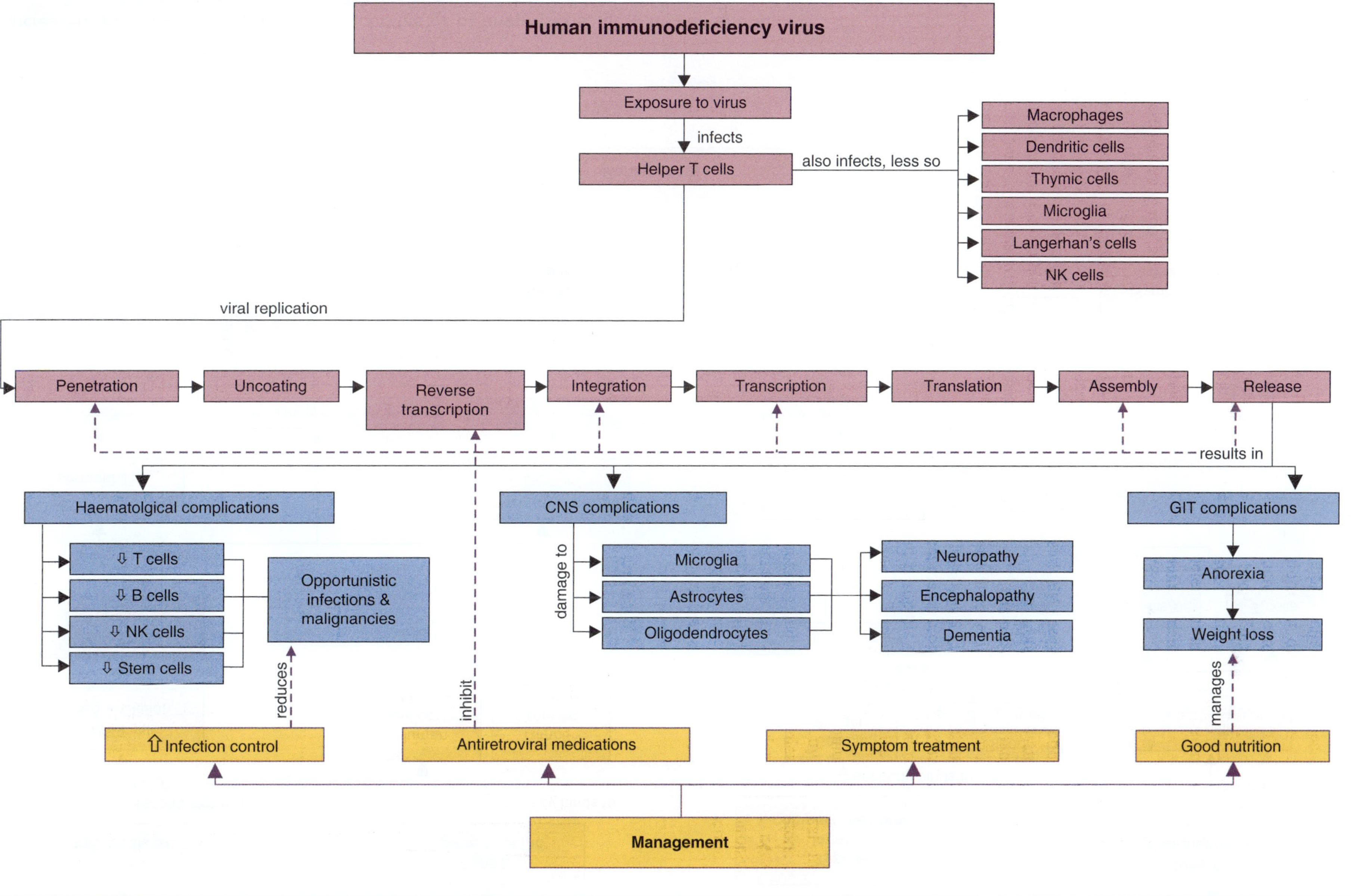

Figure 7.2

Clinical snapshot: Human immunodeficiency virus (HIV)

↓ = decreased; ↑ = increased; CNS = central nervous system; GIT = gastrointestinal tract; NK cells = natural killer cells.

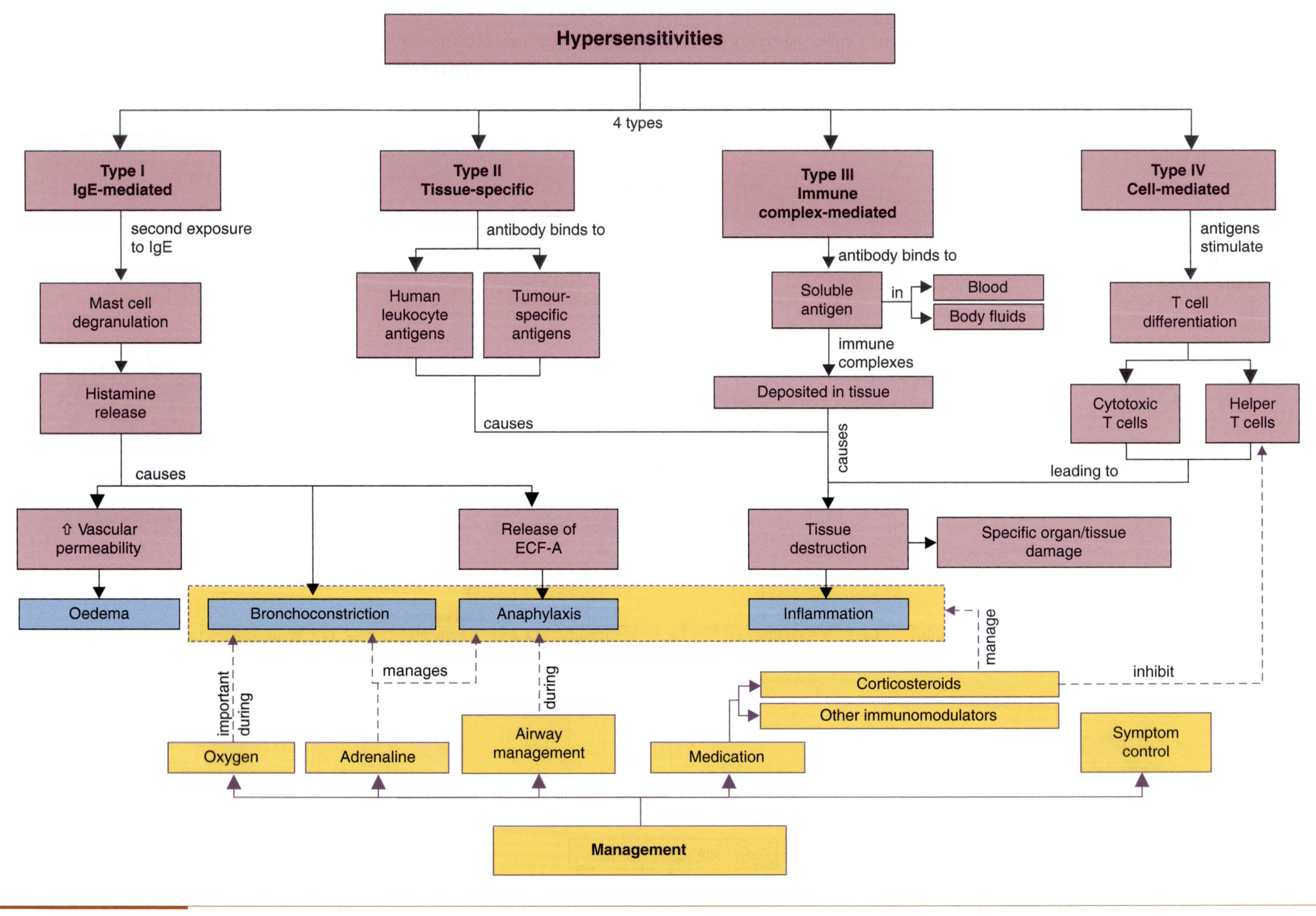

Figure 7.3

Clinical snapshot: Hypersensitivities

↑ increased; ECF-A = eosinophil-chemotactic factor of anaphylaxis; IgE = immunoglobulin E.

LEARNING OBJECTIVE 8

Compare and contrast the characteristics of the hypersensitivity reactions.

Type I hypersensitivity reactions

Aetiology and pathophysiology Type I hypersensitivity is known by a variety of terms, such as an *allergic reaction, atopy, immediate hypersensitivity* and, in its severest form, *anaphylaxis*. When a susceptible person is exposed to a particular antigen, such as certain medicines, foods (such as peanuts), environmental chemicals or pollens, IgE antibodies will be manufactured as a part of the immune response. During the initial exposure, the antigen is neutralised and excess IgE antibodies will bind to mast cells in tissues and basophils in the blood. The cytoplasm of these immune cells is rich in *inflammatory mediators* such as histamine. Mast cells are concentrated in tissues that represent the first line of body defence, such as skin, airways and the gastrointestinal tract.

Upon a subsequent immune challenge, this antigen interacts with the IgE bound to the surface of the mast cell or basophil, triggering the rupture of the cell membrane and the release of inflammatory mediators into the tissue. Histamine and other mediators induce vasodilation, increased capillary permeability and tissue oedema—all features of the inflammatory response—as well as abdominal cramping and bronchoconstriction (see the chapter 'Inflammation and healing'). The pathophysiology of this reaction is represented in Figure 7.4.

The inflammatory response may be *localised*, affecting only the skin (as in a rash), the airways (as in hay fever or asthma) or the gastrointestinal tract (as in abdominal cramping), depending on the route of entry of the antigen. The response can also be *systemic*, developing in the bloodstream in response to administration of a medicine or the presence of a blood-borne infection, manifesting as an anaphylactic reaction. The systemic inflammatory response can lead to a significant drop in blood pressure and a shift in fluid from the blood to the tissues, resulting in shock, which, if not treated promptly and appropriately, may result in death.

Clinical diagnosis and management It is unusual to run investigative tests for type I hypersensitivity reactions. Management is based on a clinical history and symptom control. In the less severe local inflammatory reactions, management with topical corticosteroid medications or intranasal antihistamine administration may be sufficient to control the symptoms. In the more severe type resulting in anaphylaxis, treatment of the symptoms is the mainstay of management. In the event of bronchoconstriction, angioedema and shock symptoms, airway management and administration of adrenaline and fluid support are required. Intravenous hydrocortisone and, later, mast cell stabilisers may be considered, and allergen desensitisation may be a possibility, too. The most important management principle for type I hypersensitivity reactions is to educate the person to avoid, where possible, exposure to the causative allergens.

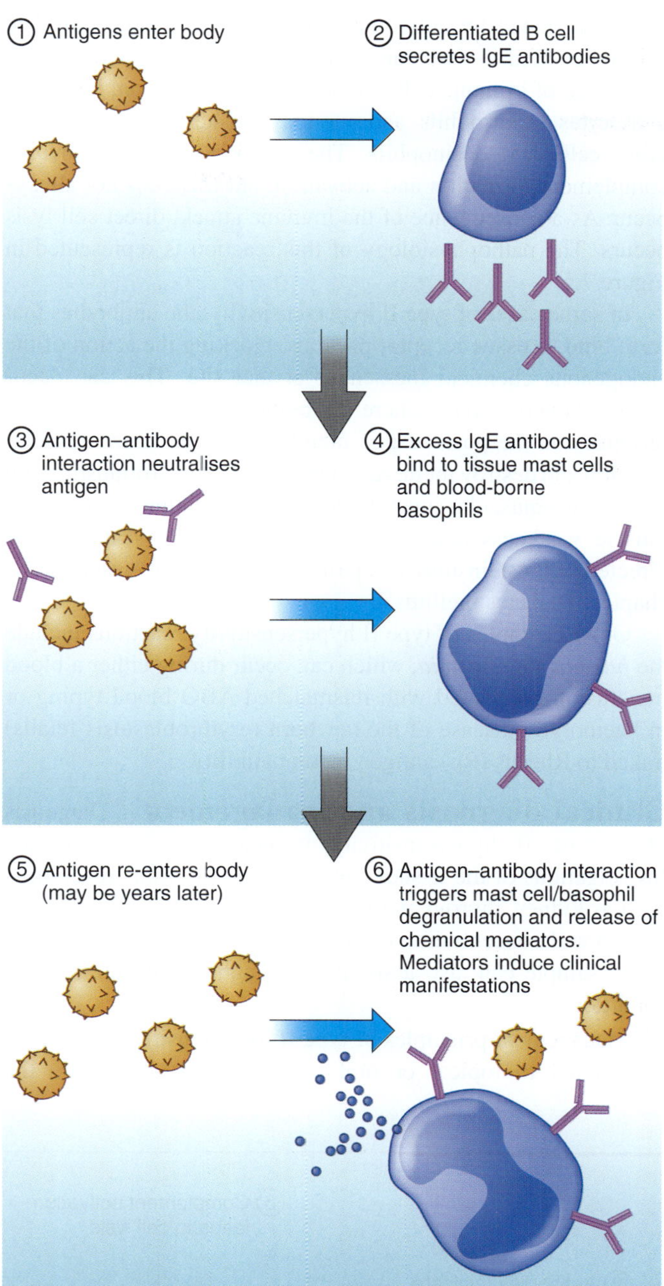

Figure 7.4

Type I hypersensitivity reactions

Source: Adapted from Bullock & Manias (2022), Figure 18.2, p. 178.

Type II hypersensitivity reactions

Aetiology and pathophysiology Type II hypersensitivity reactions involve immune responses directed *against body cells or tissue components*. This gives rise to another common name—*cytotoxic hypersensitivity reactions*.

In this form of hypersensitivity reaction, the response is usually immediate, but can persist over a longer time period, and is mediated by antibodies, in this case IgG or IgM. The antibodies bind to tissue antigens and facilitate the recruitment of a range of immune cells to the site of the reaction, including **phagocytes** (neutrophils and monocyte/macrophages), natural killer cells and eosinophils. The reaction may also involve complement formation and activation, but this does not always occur. As a consequence of the immune attack, direct cell lysis occurs. The pathophysiology of this reaction is represented in Figure 7.5.

In some cases of type II hypersensitivity, the antibodies that form bind to tissue receptor proteins, blocking the action of the endogenous chemical messenger at that site. This can occur in *myasthenia gravis*, where antibodies bind to acetylcholine receptors on the postsynaptic membrane of the neuromuscular junction and destroy them. As a result, normal neurotransmission at the neuromuscular junction is disrupted, leading to profound muscle weakness and paralysis. Autoantibodies can also be directed against insulin receptors in type 2 diabetes (see the chapter 'Diabetes mellitus').

Other examples of type II hypersensitivity reactions include the *haemolytic anaemia*, which can occur during either a blood transfusion associated with mismatched ABO blood typing or in haemolytic disease of the newborn (erythroblastosis fetalis) linked to Rhesus (Rh) antigen incompatibility.

Clinical diagnosis and management Diagnosis of a type II hypersensitivity is generally tissue-specific. Investigations of the tissues usually involved in this reaction—such as kidney, thyroid and liver function—may be useful. The pattern and concentration of antinuclear antibodies (ANA) in a blood sample can also assist in the diagnosis of autoimmune conditions.

Management principles of type II hypersensitivity reactions are related to topical or oral corticosteroids to reduce the inappropriate immune response. The use of plasmapheresis may be beneficial to reduce the circulating autoantibodies, and, depending on the person's presentation, Intragam (an immunoglobulin infusion) may be required to assist with an appropriate immune response. Sometimes, other immunomodulating drugs may be used, but care is necessary as these chemotherapeutic agents can cause significant and concerning adverse reactions.

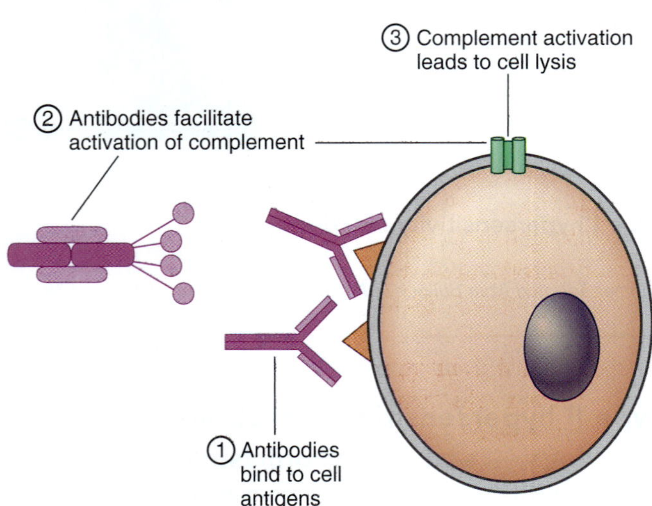

Figure 7.5

Type II hypersensitivity reactions

Source: Adapted from Bullock & Manias (2022), Figure 18.3, p. 178.

Type III hypersensitivity

Aetiology and pathophysiology Type III hypersensitivity is mediated by IgG antibodies. Antigens circulating within the bloodstream bind to antibodies, *forming relatively small complexes* that are not easily removed by phagocytosis and eventually are deposited in tissues (e.g. blood vessels, joints or kidneys), precipitating an inflammatory response involving neutrophils and complement activation. In particular, the neutrophils release digestive enzymes that damage the normal surrounding tissues. Antigens from the environment may also be inhaled into the lungs, where immune complexes are formed and lodge in the walls of the air sacs, which become the site of the immune response. Type III hypersensitivity reactions are not considered immediate; rather they are of an ongoing nature. The condition is also known as *immune complex disease*. The pathophysiology of this reaction is represented in Figure 7.6.

Type III hypersensitivity reactions can occur locally or systemically. An example of a localised response is the *Arthus reaction*. Antigen is introduced locally into the skin. Within hours, antibodies bind with the antigen to form complexes in the tissue blood vessels and trigger an inflammatory reaction called *vasculitis*, which results in tissue necrosis. Systemic reactions develop after the antigen is introduced into the bloodstream, forming immune complexes that are widely deposited into a variety of tissues. A common cause of this kind of systemic reaction in the past has been associated with the intravenous administration of antisera from animal sources, such as horses or rabbits, in the treatment of infection or snake bite (see the chapter 'Bites and stings'). The reaction developed about a week after therapy. The condition is known as *serum sickness*.

Clinical diagnosis and management Type III hypersensitivity reactions can be diagnosed after considering the person's relevant history and presentation. Generic blood tests of haematology and biochemistry can be used to rule out other causes. Management consists of symptom relief. Corticosteroids are administered to reduce the inappropriate immune response, and other immunomodifying agents may be used if symptoms become too severe.

Type IV hypersensitivity reactions

Type IV hypersensitivity reactions are mediated by T lymphocytes, mainly helper T cells (Th or $CD4^+$ cells), that are sensitised to antigens rather than antibodies; they are known as *cell-mediated hypersensitivity.* Examples of type IV hypersensitivity reactions include contact dermatitis, delayed type hypersensitivity and chronic graft rejection.

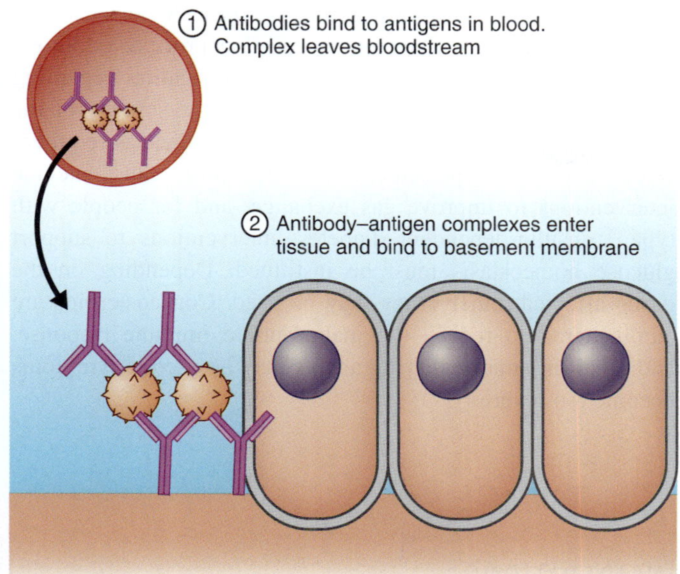

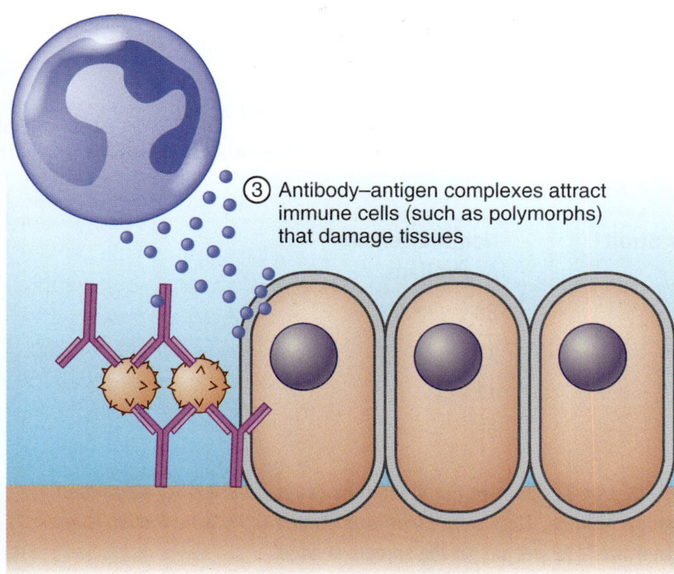

Figure 7.6

Type III hypersensitivity reactions

Source: Adapted from Bullock & Manias (2022), Figure 18.4, p. 179.

In *contact dermatitis*, a novel antigen, such as a plant component, environmental chemical or medicine, enters the skin layers and binds to proteins located there. Like type I hypersensitivity reactions, this initial encounter is resolved with little incident, but memory of the interaction is instilled in Th cells. A subsequent episode, or chronic exposure, triggers the sensitised lymphocytes to release chemical mediators, which attract phagocytes to the area, inducing a localised inflammatory response in the skin. This response is less immediate than other hypersensitivity reactions, and may be delayed for up to a few days following antigen re-exposure. The pathophysiology of this reaction is represented in Figure 7.7.

Delayed type hypersensitivity (DTH) reactions follow a similar course to contact dermatitis, except that the inflammation can develop within tissues other than the skin. A common cause of DTH reactions is through contact with an infectious microbe. This reaction can be put to good clinical use diagnostically in the case of the Mantoux test for tuberculosis. Injection of a purified tuberculin protein (BCG) into the skin indicates exposure to the causative infectious organism, *M. tuberculosis*, although the test does not discriminate between direct infection or contact with an infected person.

Granulomatous disease is also associated with type IV hypersensitivity reactions. This condition arises when a mass of inflammatory cells, mainly macrophages, occupies a spheroid tissue lesion known as a *granuloma*. The macrophages, and derivative cells called epithelioid and giant cells, phagocytose an antigen but are unable to neutralise it. Over time the granuloma becomes fibrotic and calcified, leading to necrosis of the cells inside through a lack of diffusion of nutrients and oxygen (see Figure 7.8). Leprosy and tuberculosis are examples of granulomatous diseases.

Clinical diagnosis and management Type IV hypersensitivity reactions can be diagnosed after considering the person's relevant history and presentation. Generic blood tests of haematology and biochemistry can be used to rule out other causes.

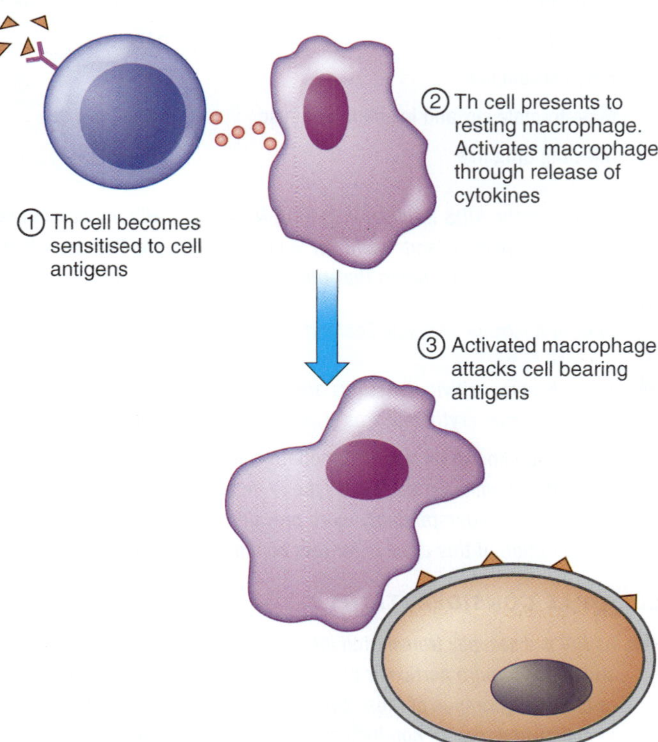

Figure 7.7

Type IV hypersensitivity reactions

Source: Adapted from Bullock & Manias (2022), Figure 18.5, p. 179.

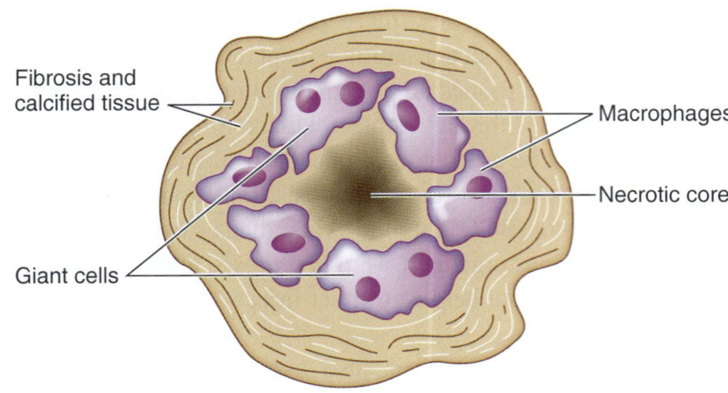

Figure 7.8

Structure of a granuloma

Management principles surrounding type IV hypersensitivity reactions differ depending on the disease process exhibited. For issues such as contact dermatitis, education regarding allergen avoidance is critical. However, as the severity of the disease increases, different symptom management is required. Issues such as hypersensitivity pneumonitis must include interventions to improve gas exchange, and for people with type 1 insulin-dependent diabetes, interventions to support glucose homeostasis must be instituted. Depending on the tissue affected, other drugs may be used. Corticosteroids are administered to reduce the inappropriate immune response, and other immunomodifying agents may be used if symptoms become too severe.

INDIGENOUS HEALTH FAST FACTS AND CULTURAL CONSIDERATIONS

FAST FACTS

- *Recent data from the Kirby Institute indicates that the HIV notification rate for Aborginal and Torres Strait Islander peoples in 2020 was 2.2 per 100,000 people.*
- *In 2019, the age-standardised HIV notification rate among males was 5.1 per 100,000, and among women was 3.1 per 100,000.*
- *A comparison of statistics between Aboriginal and Torres Strait Islander peoples and non-Indigenous Australians with newly diagnosed HIV infection in 2016–20 were as follows:*

Transmission	Aboriginal and Torres Strait Islander peoples	Non-Indigenous Australians
Male-to-male sex	51%	58
Heterosexual sex	21%	18%
Male-to-male sex and injecting drug use	18%	11%
Injecting drug use	7%	5%

- *Data from the AIDS Epidemiology Unit NZ shows a HIV notification rate for 2021 of 37.5% male European New Zealanders, 12.5% Māori men and 8.9% Pacific Islands men. For women, 5.4% were European New Zealander women, 1.8% were Māori women and 0.9% were Pacific Islands women. It should be noted that the total number of notifications for that year was 112 people, so the sample is small.*
- *In both Australia and New Zealand, Indigenous people present later with HIV infection than non-Indigenous people.*
- *Type I hypersensitivity reactions are less common in Aboriginal and Torres Strait Island peoples than in non-Indigenous Australians; however, systemic lupus erythematosus (type III hypersensitivity) rates appear to be between 2.1 and 3.8 times higher for Indigenous Australians.*
- *A condition known as 'kava dermopathy', which can occur in up to 70% of very heavy users of kava, affects Indigenous Australian kava-consuming communities. It is a type IV delayed hypersensitivity reaction, and can result in an ichthyosiform eruption (dry, thickened and scaly skin). This is understandably more prevalent in Aboriginal and Torres Strait Islander peoples than non-Indigenous Australians, because consumption of this drink is far less common among non-Indigenous Australians.*

CULTURAL CONSIDERATIONS

- *As HIV is a sexually transmitted infection, it is important to understand that in Aboriginal and Torres Strait Islander culture, sexual-health-related conditions require particular care and consideration in relation to the concepts of 'shame', 'men's business' and 'women's business'. Inexperience or cultural ignorance of these concepts may impede obtaining and assessing a comprehensive health history and cause undue distress, resulting in diminished trust of non-Indigenous healthcare workers or facilities, and ultimately leading to catastrophic effects, such as late diagnosis and subsequent increased morbidity and mortality. Methods to reduce barriers may include the provision of healthcare professionals care services of the same sex as the person accessing health, adequate cultural competence to enhance communication through non-judgmental attitudes, respecting long silences to encourage adequate time for response, mindfulness of culturally appropriate eye contact, asking permission to discuss sensitive topics, and potentially even becoming familiar with local-language words specific to the sexual health issue.*

Sources: Data from Australian Indigenous HealthInfoNet (2022); Kirby Institute (2021); New Zealand AIDS Epidemiology Group (2022).

CHILDREN AND ADOLESCENTS

- Thirty-five Australian children ($<$ 15 years old) were diagnosed with HIV between the years 2011 and 2020.
- Of all babies born in Australia between 2016 and 2020, 1.5% were born HIV-positive.
- Ten per cent of babies ($\leq$ 12 months) in Australia have an IgE-mediated food allergy.
- Most ($>$ 90%) food hypersensitivities in children are related to egg, milk, peanut, wheat, soy and fish.
- Almost 70% of children outgrow their egg and milk allergies by the age of 16 years.
- Approximately 20% of children outgrow their peanut, tree nut or seafood allergies by the age of 16 years.
- Active exposure to allergenic food (including peanuts) is highly recommended in the first year of life (but not before 4 months of age), as it can reduce the incidence of hypersensitivity among high-risk children (those with eczema or egg allergy) by 80%.

OLDER ADULTS

- In 2016, 43% of people living with HIV were $\geq$ 50 years of age.
- An age-induced reduction in IgE appears to occur in people with allergic rhinitis, asthma and insect allergy, but not in those with atopic dermatitis.

Sources: Data from Australian Indigenous HealthInfoNet (2022); Joshi & Frith (2017); Kirby Institute (2021).

KEY CLINICAL ISSUES

- People living with HIV may have different clinical outcomes. Fewer people now die of HIV/AIDS than in the past, due to the effectiveness of the chronic antiviral drug therapies available. It is important to encourage a focus on wellness, and on lifestyle and nutrition choices that promote health, instead of on a 'diagnosis of HIV'.
- Infection control is paramount to reducing exposure to opportunistic infections in immunocompromised individuals. Education for the affected person, and their carers and those around them, is important to ensure consistent practices promoting the best environment for maintaining health.
- When caring for people living with HIV, as with any chronic disease, significant psychological and emotional support is required to manage the stressors of the diagnosis and its ultimate clinical progression.
- When caring for people with hypersensitivity reactions, identification and avoidance of triggers is critical to the prevention of allergic reactions. In the context of anaphylaxis, if triggers cannot be avoided entirely, the person (and their carers and those around them) should be taught how to use a prefilled automatically injecting syringe of adrenaline.
- Food allergies are common today; it is important to document food allergies appropriately so as to reduce the risk of exposure in healthcare facilities.
- All healthcare professionals should be familiar with basic life support and first aid principles. All staff should be familiar with emergency codes and phone numbers so they can assist in the management of someone experiencing a hypersensitivity reaction.

CHAPTER REVIEW

- The primary function of the immune system is to provide body defence. Immunity can be both cellular and humoral. *Cellular immunity* is provided by a range of immune cells such as lymphocytes, macrophages, neutrophils, eosinophils and basophils. *Humoral immunity* occurs through the action of antibodies and other protein-based systems, such as complement.
- *Immune dysfunction* can manifest as either deficient states or hyperreactive activity.
- Immunodeficiency can exist as either a *congenital* or an *acquired* condition, and be further classified as a primary or secondary disorder. A *primary disorder* mainly affects the immune system, whereas a *secondary disorder* affects the immune system as a consequence of other circumstances, such as severe/prolonged stress, poor nutrition, drug therapy, infection or cancer.
- Some microbes, such as the SARS-CoV-2 virus, can evade or disrupt normal immune responses. This is known as *immune escape or evasion*.
- The primary immunodeficiencies can be classified by whether they affect humoral, cellular or a combination of humoral and cellular immunity.
- *Human immunodeficiency virus (HIV)* is the causative agent in *acquired immune deficiency syndrome (AIDS)*. HIV targets immune cells bearing $CD4^+$ surface receptors, particularly Th cells, as a means to infect cells. Immunity becomes compromised through chronic immune activation, leaving the affected person vulnerable to opportunistic infections that eventually lead to death. AIDS is based on a low Th cell count and the presence of one or more opportunistic infections. The major routes of HIV transmission are by unprotected sex, maternal transfer in utero, and contact with blood products or contaminated needles, syringes or scalpels.
- *Hypersensitivity reactions* are excessive immune responses that lead to tissue damage, chronic disability and, sometimes, death. They are classified as *type I (allergic or anaphylactic), type II (cytotoxic), type III (immune complex disease)* and *type IV (cell-mediated)* hypersensitivity.
- *Type I* hypersensitivity reactions are characterised by immediate antibody-mediated inflammatory responses associated with IgE bound to mast cells and basophils.

- *Type II* hypersensitivity reactions are also immediate, antibody-mediated responses, but involve IgG or IgM. The antibody–antigen interaction induces immune cell action and may also involve complement.
- *Type III* hypersensitivity reactions are IgG-mediated, leading to the formation of antigen–antibody complexes that lodge in tissues and induce a damaging inflammatory response. The reaction is ongoing rather than immediate.
- *Type IV* hypersensitivity reactions are mediated by sensitised T cells rather than antibodies. The response is delayed compared to the other forms of hypersensitivity.
- Autoimmune disease is associated with the *loss of tolerance to self-antigens*. Loss of tolerance can develop when the suppression of sensitised T cells is disrupted, immune cells enter a 'privileged' body site, or antigens on microbes closely resemble self-antigens on tissues, leading to immune cross-reactivity. As a consequence, immune processes are directed towards normal body tissues and chronic inflammatory states ensue.
- The incidence of autoimmune diseases has been linked to hypersensitivity reactions and the presence of particular human leukocyte antigen (HLA) genes. There is a tendency for the incidence of these conditions to be greater in women.

REVIEW QUESTIONS

1 Describe the immune roles of the following leukocyte subtypes:
   a basophils
   b macrophages
   c B cells
   d T cells

2 Briefly outline the roles of the following antibody classes:
   a IgG
   b IgA
   c IgM
   d IgE

3 What are the roles of the following chemical mediators in immunity?
   a tumour necrosis factor-α
   b interleukins

4 Outline the consequences of having an immunodeficiency disorder that primarily targets cellular cells.

5 Compare and contrast the characteristics of DiGeorge syndrome, selective IgA deficiency and severe combined immunodeficiency.

6 Describe how each of the following conditions can lead to an immunodeficient state:
   a prolonged stress
   b corticosteroid therapy
   c leukaemia

7 Describe the pathophysiology of HIV/AIDS.

8 Which of the four types of hypersensitivity reactions matches each of the following clinical conditions?
   a an allergic reaction to peanuts
   b a form of dermatitis that develops a few days after brushing against a plant in the bush
   c a reaction to a blood transfusion
   d the development of a lung granuloma
   e myasthenia gravis

9 A 4-month-old baby boy is admitted to hospital for pneumonia. Over the past two months he has had frequent middle ear infections, thrush and a couple of bouts of diarrhoea.
   a Circle the correct options in this sentence: The child is likely to have a primary/secondary, congenital/acquired immunodeficiency disorder.
   b To what diagnostic tests would the baby be subjected?
   c If the disorder was found to affect lymphocytes, which possible sites of impairment are associated with the development or activation of these cells as a result of this disorder?
   d How would he be managed?

HEALTH PROFESSIONAL CONNECTIONS

Nutritionists/Dieticians Disorders and medications causing immunosuppression can also cause anorexia. Increased metabolic requirements occur in those who develop infections. Adjustments to caloric intake may be required to accommodate a person's nutritional state. Methods to encourage oral intake may be needed, as may a focus on making food appealing. Failing to secure adequate nutrition may result in the need for supplementation, nasogastric tube feeding or total parenteral nutrition.

Social workers Illness as a result of immunosuppression is generally chronic. Immense stress may be placed on the immunosuppressed person or their families when such an admission is required. Support may be needed to arrange accommodation, transport or financial assistance during an admission. Arrangements for end-of-life care may be necessary in conditions with a poor prognosis.

All allied professionals Interactions with people experiencing communicable diseases can be challenging, and personal feelings of concern can be transmitted to the affected individuals, causing a negative psychological impact. In accordance with the principles of psychoneuroimmunology, poor emotional health will directly affect a person's immune system response. Although the appropriate use of personal protective equipment and standard precautions should always be adhered to, care must be taken to ensure that behaviours or actions do not negatively affect the person for whom you are caring. The disease process is challenging enough—adding to their anxiety by negative communications or interactions will not help their recovery, nor help stall disease progression. Healthcare professionals who are having difficulty caring for those with communicable disease due to challenges to their own beliefs or health concerns should speak with their supervisor or institution counsellor to seek assistance, so that a negative impact is not caused for those in their care. Healthcare professionals have a right to their own values and beliefs, but everyone has a right to expert, appropriate, holistic Healthcare.

CASE STUDY

Mr Harry Anderson is a 40-year-old man living with a diagnosis of AIDS (UR number 640642). Mr Anderson is gay and has been in a committed relationship with his partner for the past 11 years. His partner does not have HIV, and the pair have practised safe sex from the time Mr Anderson received his diagnosis. Over the past three years he has struggled with opportunistic infections and persistently low CD41^{+} T cell counts. Two weeks ago Mr Anderson was admitted, and his condition is deteriorating rapidly as he has advanced HIV disease. His treatment regimen includes dolutegravir, abacavir, lamivudine and nystatin.

Mr Anderson is very confused, his Glasgow coma scale is 11, and he is incontinent of both urine and faeces. He has numerous Kaposi's sarcomas, HIV encephalopathy and AIDS dementia complex. He also has oral candidiasis and generalised lymphadenopathy. Mr Anderson has very severe spasticity and requires q2h pressure area care. He requires full nursing cares, and has a lorazepam, phenytoin and levetiracetam regimen (for seizures). His partner is with him for many hours, most days. Mr Anderson's observations are as follows:

Temperature	Heart rate	Respiration rate	Blood pressure	SpO_2
37°C	74	14	100/52	96% (RA*)

*RA = room air.

CRITICAL THINKING

1. Consider Mr Anderson's history. Identify all of the opportunistic infections and diseases. Explain the mechanism of their development.
2. Identify the components of standard and transmission-based precautions. What type of precautions does a healthcare professional require when caring for Mr Anderson?
3. Make a list of the drugs being used. Record their mechanism of action, precautions and adverse reactions.
4. What are T cells? What is the significance of a low CD4^{+} T cell count in relation to HIV infection and AIDS?
5. Identify and explain interventions important for Mr Anderson's care. Ensure that you take into account the range of biopsychosocial needs.

BIBLIOGRAPHY

Australian Health Ministers' Advisory Council's National and Aboriginal and Torres Strait Islander Health Standing Committee (2017). *Cultural respect framework 2016–2026: for Aboriginal and Torres Strait Islander health—a national approach to building a culturally respectful health system*. Canberra: Australian Government Department of Health. https://nacchocommunique.files.wordpress.com/2016/12/cultural_respect_framework_1december2016_1.pdf.

Australian Indigenous Health*Info*Net (2022). *Overview of Aboriginal and Torres Strait Islander health status, 2021.* Perth, WA: Australian Indigenous Health*Info*Net. https://healthinfonet.ecu.edu.au/learn/health-facts/overview-aboriginal-torres-strait-islander-health-status/.

Australian Institute of Health and Welfare (2022). *Australia's health, 2022*. Australia's Health series No. 18. Canberra: AIHW. https://www.aihw.gov.au/reports-data/australias-health.

Bauldoff, G., Gubrud-Howe, P.M., Carno, M.-A., Levett-Jones, T., Hales, M., Berry, K., ... Stanley, D. (2020). *LeMone and Burke's medical–surgical nursing: critical thinking for person-centred care* (4th [Australian] edn). Sydney: Pearson Australia.

Bullock, S. & Manias, E. (2022). *Fundamentals of pharmacology* (9th edn). Sydney: Pearson Australia.

Chakraborty, C., Sharma, A.R., Bhattacharya, M. & Lee, S.-S. (2022). A detailed overview of immune escape, antibody escape, partial vaccine escape of SARS-CoV-2 and their emerging variants with escape mutations. *Frontiers in Immunology* 13:801522. https://doi.org/10.3389/fimmu.2022.801522.

Gilroy, S.A. & Faragon, J.J. (2021). HIV infection and AIDS. *Emedicine*. https://emedicine.medscape.com/article/211316-overview.

Heimall, J. (2022). Severe combined immunodeficiency (SCID): an overview. *UpToDate.* https://www.uptodate.com/contents/3955#!.

Hernandez-Ilizaliturri, F.J., Christ, M.M. & Makhoul, I. (2020). Severe combined immunodeficiency (SCID). *Emedicine*. https://emedicine.medscape.com/article/210249-overview.

Joshi, P. & Frith, K. (2017). Assessing and managing IgE-mediated food allergies in children. *MedicineToday* 18(3):37–43. https://medicinetoday.com.au/sites/default/files/cpd/MT2017-03-037-JOSHI.pdf.

Kirby Institute (2021). *HIV, viral hepatitis and sexually transmissible infections in Australia: annual surveillance report 2021*. Sydney: Kirby Institute, UNSW Sydney. https://kirby.unsw.edu.au/report/asr2021.

Lachowsky, N.J., Saxton, P.J.W., Dickson, N.P., Hughes, A.J., Summerlee, A.J.S. & Dewey, C.E. (2020). National trends in sexual health indicators among gay and bisexual men disaggregated by ethnicity: repeated cross-sectional behavioural surveillance in New Zealand. *BMJ Open* 10(11):e039896. https://doi.org/10.1136/bmjopen-2020-039896.

Liu, B., Shao, Y., & Fu, R. (2021). Current research status of HLA in immune–related diseases. *Immunity, Inflammation and Disease* 9(2):340–50. https://doi.org/10.1002/iid3.416.

Marieb, E.N. & Hoehn, K. (2019). *Human anatomy and physiology* (11th edn). San Francisco, CA: Pearson Benjamin Cummings.

Naito, Y., Takagi, T., Yamamoto, T. & Watanabe, S. (2020) Association between selective IgA deficiency and COVID-19. *Journal of Clinical Biochemistry and Nutrition* 67(2):122–25. https://doi.org/10.3164/jcbn.20-102.

New Zealand AIDS Epidemiology Group (2022). *AIDS—New Zealand Newsletter* 81. Dunedin: Department of Preventive and Social Medicine, Dunedin School of Medicine, University of Otago. https://www.otago.ac.nz/aidsepigroup/otago840423.pdf.

Weifenbach, N., Schneckenberger, A.A.C. & Lotters, S. (2020). Global distribution of common variable immunodeficiency (CVID) in the light of the UNDP human development index (HDI): a preliminary perspective of a rare disease. *Journal of Immunology Research* 2020:8416124. https://doi.org/10.1155/2020/8416124.

Woods, R. (2019). *HIV and Ageing in Australia—The New Frontier.* Newtown, NSW: National Association of People with HIV Australia. https://napwha.org.au/wp-content/uploads/2019/04/HIV-and-Ageing-in-Australia-New-Frontier-April19.pdf.

Infection

8

LEARNING OBJECTIVES

After completing this chapter, you should be able to:

1 Outline the general characteristics of the major groups of infectious organisms.

2 Define the terms 'colonisation', 'pathogenicity', 'virulence' and 'sepsis'.

3 Describe the chain of transmission of infection.

4 Describe the ways in which the chain of transmission can be broken as a means of controlling infection.

5 Discuss the factors that influence a person's susceptibility to infection.

6 Outline the general mechanism of action of antimicrobial drugs.

7 Describe the development and prevention of antimicrobial drug resistance.

8 Discuss emerging infectious diseases and the factors that increase the risks of global threat, with particular focus on SARS-CoV-2 virus.

WHAT YOU SHOULD KNOW BEFORE YOU START THIS CHAPTER

Can you describe the basic concepts of microbiology?

Can you describe the cellular response to stress and injury?

Can you state the role of stress in disease?

KEY TERMS

- Antimicrobial drug resistance
- Antimicrobial drugs
- Arthropods
- Bacteria
- Chain of transmission
- Colonisation
- Eukaryotes
- Fungi
- Helminths
- Infectious disease
- Microbes
- Mycosis
- Opportunistic infection
- Parasites
- Pathogenicity
- Prokaryotes
- Protozoa
- Sepsis
- Severe acute respiratory syndrome-associated coronavirus 2 (SARS-CoV-2)
- Virulence
- Viruses

Introduction

Infectious diseases are among the oldest conditions known to afflict humans. Infections have been noted in the earliest of historical writings. There is evidence of tuberculosis, leprosy, plague and malaria dating back to ancient times. There are countless reports of epidemics of infectious diseases through the ages that have killed significant proportions of the population of the known world at that time.

Today, infectious diseases remain a major global health problem. Some infections can be easily treated or prevented by immunisation. However, cholera, influenza, HIV/AIDS, tuberculosis and other serious infections affect millions of people around the world, leaving death and chronic disability in their wake.

In December of 2019, numerous cases of pneumonia with an unknown cause were reported in Wuhan, China. At that time, it was thought that many of the early cases were linked to Huanan Seafood Wholesale Market, promoting fears that a new zoonotic pathogen, **severe acute respiratory syndrome-associated coronavirus 2 (SARS-CoV-2)** was the cause. Over the next three years and foreseeably beyond the date of this publication, the world has been battling the effects and the phenomenal influence the subsequently named COVID-19 global pandemic has had on every country.

The focus of this chapter is to introduce the major terms and concepts associated with infection. The main types of infectious organisms responsible for human diseases will be described, followed by the principles of treatment and infection control. Finally, SARS-Cov-2 is explored to provide an example of the catastrophic consequences and incredible scientific and knowledge advancements associated with a new zoonotic pathogen jumping the species gap into humans with a naive immunity. Although there is still much more to learn about this ever-developing virus and pandemic, an overview of current knowledge and important considerations will be explored.

Infectious organisms

LEARNING OBJECTIVE 1

Outline the general characteristics of the major groups of infectious organisms.

Infectious organisms can be grouped by taxonomy. The main organisms are the **microbes**—bacteria, fungi, protozoa and viruses—as well as the more macroscopic organisms, such as intestinal worms and arthropods. The defining morphological characteristics of these organisms are described below.

BACTERIA

Bacteria are **prokaryotes**, in contrast to human cells, which are **eukaryotes**. The structural organisation of prokaryotic cells is simpler than that of eukaryotic cells (see Figure 8.1). Among the main differences are that prokaryotic cells have no defined nucleus, and they may possess a cell wall in addition to the cell membrane. They reproduce asexually by cell division.

Bacteria can be classified according to their histological staining properties, their shape, whether they can move in tissues (i.e. motility) and whether they predominately use oxygen-dependent (aerobic) metabolism.

In a process known as Gram staining, some bacteria can take a crystal violet stain, whereas others do not. The former group is referred to as *Gram-positive bacteria*, and stain dark blue or violet; the latter group is *Gram-negative bacteria,* and stain red or pink. Another group of bacteria, which takes up the crystal violet stain (or indeed some other histological stains), but does not lose the colour after being rinsed in an acidic alcohol solution, is termed *acid-fast bacteria*.

Bacteria that are spherically shaped are called *cocci*, while those that are of an elongated shape are termed *rods* or *bacilli*; there are also spiral-shaped ones that are called *spirochetes* or *spirilla* (see Figure 8.2).

Table 8.1 lists examples of common bacteria that are classified using this nomenclature. Figure 8.3 explores the common clinical manifestations and management of a bacterial infection.

FUNGI

Fungi are eukaryotic cells that are widely disseminated throughout our environment. Fungal species may reproduce asexually, like bacteria, or reproduce sexually by exchanging genetic material with each other.

Fungi such as *Candida albicans* live as normal flora in and on our bodies. Under certain conditions—such as during antimicrobial therapy for a bacterial infection or treatment with an immunosuppressant such as a corticosteroid—these microbes can show unrestrained proliferation and trigger an opportunistic 'superinfection' of mucous membranes called thrush. Thrush

Figure 8.1

Prokaryotic and eukaryotic cell organisation

(A) Prokaryotic cells.
(B) Eukaryotic cells.

Sources: (A) Roberto Biasini/Alamy Stock Vector; (B) Daniel Cole/Alamy Stock Vector.

A

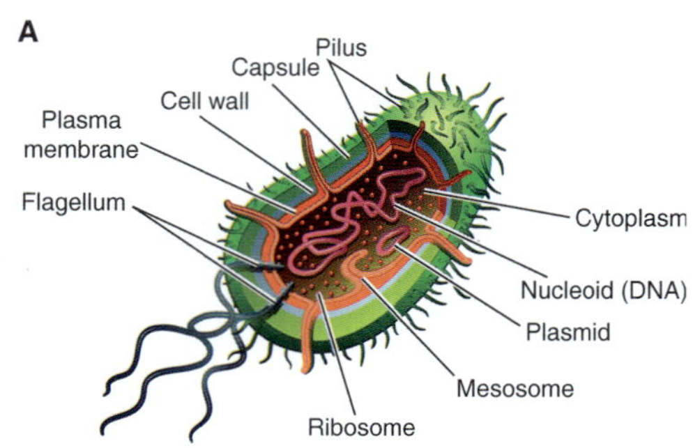

B

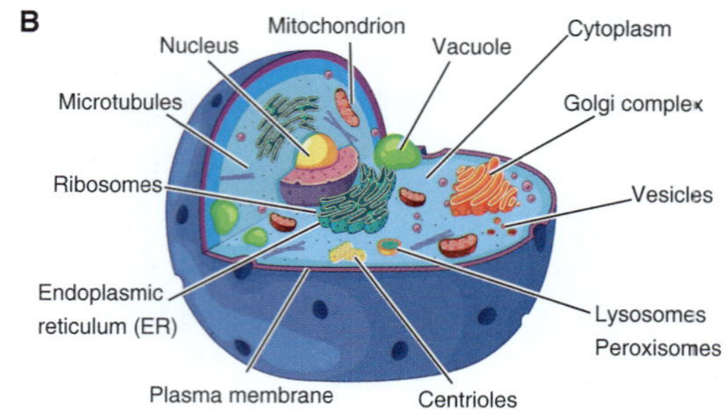

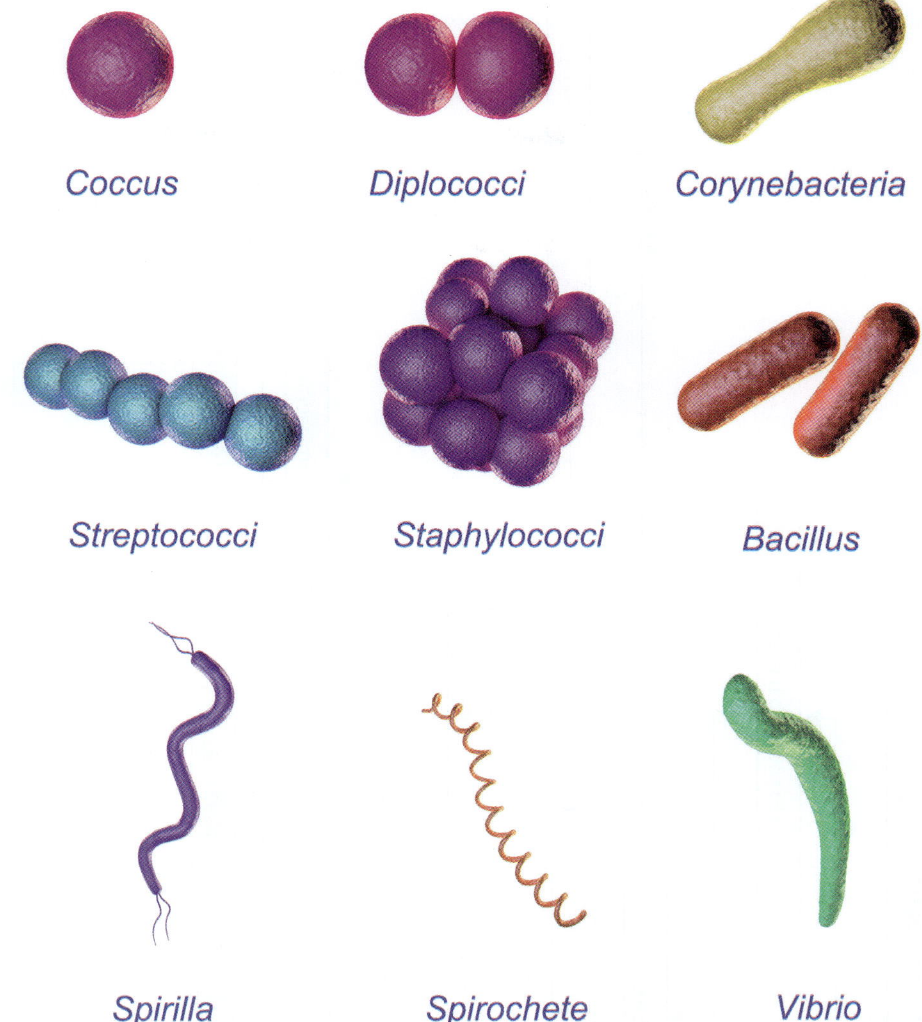

Figure 8.2

Different types of bacteria classified by shape

Source: Andrea Danti/Alamy Stock Photo.

Table 8.1 Examples of the classification of bacteria

Classification	Bacteria genus/species
HISTOLOGICAL STAIN	
Gram-positive	*Staphylococcus* spp.; *Streptococcus* spp.
Gram-negative	*Escherichia coli; Pseudomonas* spp.
Acid-fast	*Mycobacterium tuberculosis*
SHAPE	
Cocci	*Staphylococcus* spp.; *Streptococcus* spp.
Bacilli	*Lactobacillus* spp.
Spirochaetes	*Treponema pallidum; Leptospira* spp.; most rods and spiral bacteria
MOTILITY	
Motile	*Pseudomonas* spp.; *Clostridium* spp.
Non-motile	*Klebsiella* spp.; *Mycobacterium* spp.
TYPE OF METABOLISM	
Aerobes (oxygen-dependent)	*Pseudomonas aeruginosa; Mycobacterium tuberculosis*
Anaerobes	*Clostridium* spp.

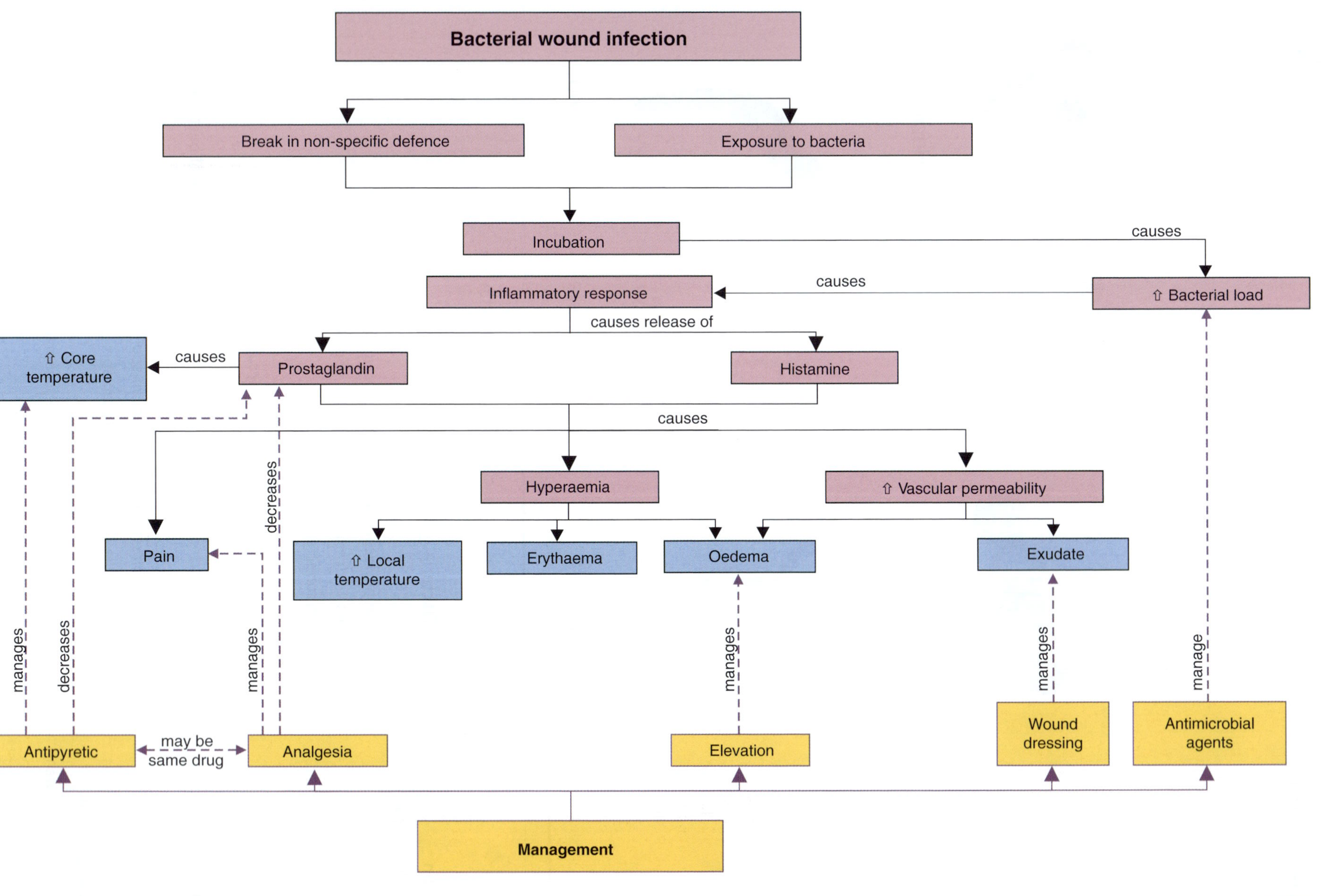

Figure 8.3

Clinical snapshot: Management of bacterial wound infections

↑ = increased.

has a white, crusty appearance on the surface of the mucous membrane, and the most commonly affected body sites are the oral and urogenital regions.

A fungal infection is commonly known as a **mycosis**. Mycoses may be superficial, subcutaneous or systemic. A *superficial mycosis* affects the epidermis and skin appendages (i.e. nails and hair). A *subcutaneous mycosis* occurs when the fungus gains entry to deep tissues through a skin lesion. A *systemic mycosis* is when the fungus gains entry beyond the skin via the lymphatics or is inhaled into the lungs. Systemic and subcutaneous mycoses can be harder to treat, and require systemic antifungal therapy. They may develop into chronic conditions if they do not respond to treatment.

VIRUSES

Viruses are the smallest microorganisms associated with human infections. Their structure is much simpler than that of the prokaryotes; they are little more than nucleic acids contained within a protein capsule. To maintain viability, viruses must enter the host human cells in order to replicate and acquire energy, or, at the very least, be able to inject their nucleic acids directly into the host cell. The viral nucleic acids provide the genetic coding for replicating viral structures. In some viruses the genetic material is DNA, while in others it is RNA. The structures of typical viruses are represented in Figure 8.4.

Viruses can be classified according to their size, the genetic material contained within them, the type of host cell they interact with, how they use the host cell to replicate, and the structural characteristics of the viral capsule. The way in which viruses use the host cell to replicate is an important aspect of virus classification. DNA viruses can be *double-stranded (class I viruses)* or *single-stranded (class II viruses)*. The herpes, pox and hepatitis B viruses are good examples of class I viruses. Parvovirus is an example of a class II virus. Once inside the host cell, the viral DNA leads to the formation of messenger RNA, directing the production of viral structures. RNA viruses can contain *double-stranded RNA (class III viruses)*, the class in which the *rotaviruses* belong. However, the most common RNA viruses contain *single-stranded RNA (class IV and V)*. The RNA viruses use their RNA to direct the host cell to make viral components. Examples of viruses from the latter two groups include the ones that cause mumps, influenza, measles, hepatitis A and C, rabies, rubella, polio, dengue fever and Ross River fever. The last grouping of viruses by this classification system is called the *retroviruses (class VI viruses)*. They contain RNA but use an enzyme called *reverse transcriptase* to convert the viral RNA into double-stranded DNA. This DNA is integrated into the host's DNA so that when the cell replicates, new viruses are also produced. The human immunodeficiency virus (HIV) belongs in this grouping.

PARASITES

The main **parasites** associated with human infectious disease are the **protozoa**, **helminths** (worms) and **arthropods**. Parasitic infections tend to be more common in the developing world compared to in industrialised Western countries. However, certain groups within the industrialised world are particularly vulnerable to parasitic infections—those people receiving immunosuppressant drugs or who have immune deficiencies (e.g. those with HIV/AIDS), and the developing human in utero.

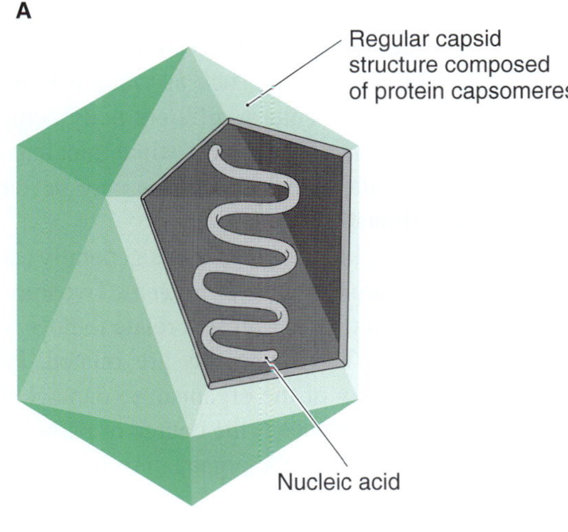

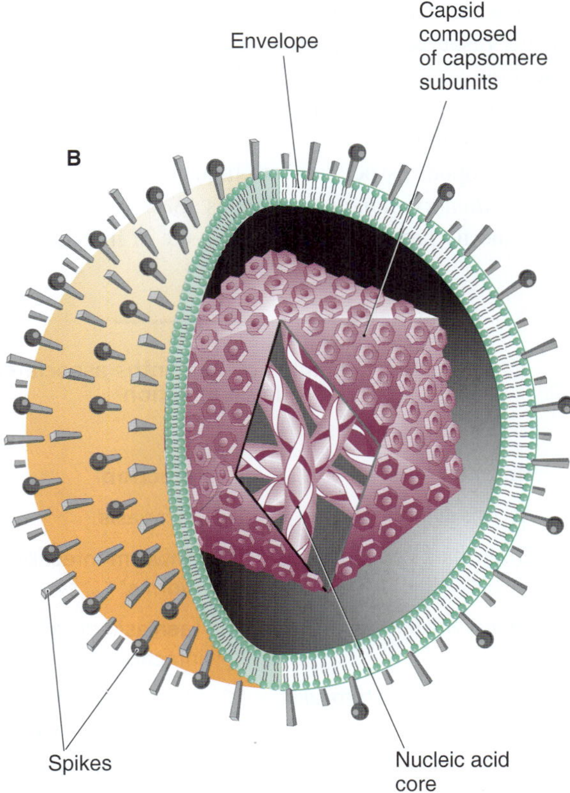

Figure 8.4
Typical viral structures
(A) Naked virus. (B) Enveloped virus.

The protozoa are single-celled organisms that replicate asexually by cell division. The helminths and arthropods are complex multicellular macroscopic animals with organ systems. They have more intricate life cycles than the protozoa, going through stages as eggs, larvae and finally adults. A general characteristic of parasitic infections is that the organism may spend only part of its life cycle in the human body. Parasites enter the human body via either the mouth or through the skin.

There are a number of important protozoan infections, including malaria caused by *Plasmodium* species, amoebic dysentery caused by *Entamoeba histolytica*, traveller's diarrhoea triggered by *Giardia intestinalis* or *Cryptosporidium parvum*, and toxoplasmosis associated with *Toxoplasma gondii* (particularly damaging in utero).

The helminths include flatworms, pinworms, tapeworms, hookworms and roundworms, trematodes (flukes) and cestodes (tapeworms). The reservoir for transmission to humans can be in the soil or in another animal living in close proximity to people. The parasites enter the human body through the skin via penetration or an insect bite, orally after eating poorly cooked meat or fish, or via faecal contamination of food. Common sites of infection include the liver, intestines, gut blood vessels, skin, urinary tract, lymphatics, muscles and eye. In order to show severe symptoms, the parasite density, or burden, must be high. Depending on the site affected, a person will experience symptoms including malnutrition, blindness, weight loss, diarrhoea, abdominal pain, fever, organomegaly, rashes, coughs, muscle pain and anaemia. Common species associated with human infection are listed in Table 8.2.

The group within the community most affected by worm infections is children, and they can experience more than one infection concurrently. While in the body, the worms will feed off nutrients within that compartment, depriving the human of this resource. The gastrointestinal site is a common site of infection and, when the condition is severe, malabsorption, gastrointestinal disturbances, loss of appetite and anaemia are the usual symptoms.

Arthropods associated with human parasitic infestations are lice (*Pediculus humanus*), scabies (*Sarcoptes scabiei*), mites, ticks and fly larvae (maggots). The site of infection is the skin.

Table 8.2 Examples of helminths associated with human infection

Helminth	Infection
Ascaris lumbricoides	Ascariasis
Enterobius vermicularis	Pinworm infection or 'worms'
Taenia solium	Taeniasis or tapeworm infection
Strongyloides steroralis	Strongyloidiasis or threadworm infection
Ancylostoma duodenale	Hookworm infection

Scabies and lice are transmitted from contact with other people or fomites (e.g. combs, brushes and linen). Maggots infect necrotic tissues such as skin ulcers after flies lay eggs on the skin. Ticks are transmitted by contact with grasses or plants, or from pets that have been in such areas. Mite infections are usually obtained through contact with animals. The most common sign of arthropod infestation is pruritus. Ticks and mite infestations can be more problematic. Ticks can cause paralysis when they inoculate the skin with their venom, and the intense itchiness can result in haemorrhagic lesions from scratching the skin.

Types of colonisation by microorganisms

LEARNING OBJECTIVE 2

Define the terms 'colonisation', 'pathogenicity', 'virulence' and 'sepsis'.

The character of the interaction between microbes and people is largely determined by the integrity of our body's defence mechanisms. Microorganisms do inhabit our bodies, and this state, referred to as **colonisation**, can occur in the absence of disease. Some microbes can colonise the skin or our mucous membranes (e.g. nasal and gastrointestinal) without inducing disease; they are called the *normal flora*. They live in a symbiotic, or mutually beneficial, relationship with the human host. The benefit to the microbes is access to nutrients and other resources, while for humans the normal flora control the growth of potential disease-causing organisms through competition for these resources or through the secretion of antimicrobial factors, and contribute to gastrointestinal metabolism through the degradation of indigestible substances and the synthesis of useful compounds, such as vitamin K. However, if the normal flora were to enter a different body compartment, say to move from the skin or gastrointestinal tract into the blood, then tissues may be damaged and illness may develop. This is termed an **opportunistic infection**.

Other kinds of organisms generally associated with inducing disease are known as *pathogens*. Two important terms associated with infectious organisms relate to how pathogenic and virulent they are. The two terms are related. **Pathogenicity** represents the capacity of the organism to damage human cells and cause disease. **Virulence** is the degree of pathogenicity, which is linked to the ability of the organism to induce disease by disabling the host's defence systems.

Virulence depends on the effectiveness of: the organism's ability to enter the body (e.g. gaining access through a tissue lesion, by injecting itself or being injected through the skin in an insect bite); its adherence to a tissue surface that it wants to enter (via the presence of hair-like structures or a glycocalyx on its surface); its invasiveness into surrounding tissues (by releasing proteolytic enzymes that digest collagen, or the fibrin mesh associated with a blood clot); and its ability to encapsulate itself away from, or secrete itself within, immune cells to avoid recognition and attack (see Figure 8.5). A high rate of mutation

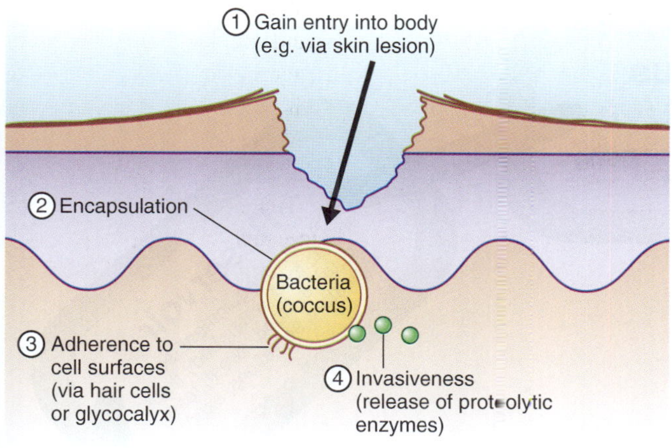

Figure 8.5

Factors affecting an organism's virulence

during mitosis also offers some microbes the opportunity to develop adaptations to human defence mechanisms.

Many microorganisms can enhance their ability to cause human disease through the production of toxins. These toxins can be either exotoxins or endotoxins. *Exotoxins* can be released by the microorganism into the tissue or the systemic circulation, and cause significant damage. These toxins may also be released when the microorganism undergoes cell lysis. *Clostridium botulinum* (associated with botulism) and *Staphylococcus aureus* (golden staph) induce most of their harmful effects on tissues through the release of exotoxins. These toxins disrupt cell signalling or impair cellular metabolic processes, causing widespread deleterious effects. *Endotoxins* are toxins incorporated into the structure of the cell membrane as liposaccharides. These molecules are recognised by the host's immune system, and trigger the release of damaging pro-inflammatory cytokines. Endotoxins are usually associated with Gram-negative bacteria, but there are instances of Gram-positive bacteria with endotoxins.

When microorganisms enter the normally sterile bloodstream, such as in bacteraemia or fungaemia, they can be widely disseminated through the body. Their presence in the blood may induce a systemic inflammatory response. This is referred to as **sepsis**. However, it should be noted that bacteria can be present in the blood without triggering sepsis. Sepsis can lead to a hypotensive state and poor tissue perfusion, with multiple organ dysfunction. This condition is called *septic shock* and is covered in detail in the chapter 'Vascular disorders and circulatory shock'.

Chain of transmission

LEARNING OBJECTIVE 3

Describe the chain of transmission of infection.

The **chain of transmission** associated with human infectious disease is a very useful framework for understanding the infection process. For infection to occur in humans, the chain of transmission cannot be interrupted. Each step in the transmission process represents a link in a chain that, when disrupted, reduces the risk of infection occurring. The main links in the chain of transmission are the establishment of a reservoir of infective organisms, a mode of transmission to humans and a way of entering human bodies (see Figure 8.6). Successful infection once the organism enters humans depends on two factors:

1. the organism's capacity to remain a resident and form colonies
2. the efficacy of the human body's defences in excluding or killing the organism.

The *reservoir of infection* must be a viable environment in close proximity to humans that allows the infectious organism to live in sufficient numbers to infect people. Typical reservoirs include the soil, other humans and non-human animals (e.g. domesticated animals, wild animals and insects).

The *mode of transmission* to humans can be by direct contact with a reservoir, or through indirect contact where the organism has been transferred from the reservoir to an inanimate object (i.e. a fomite) in sufficient numbers. *Direct contact* can be in the form of an insect bite, contact with a pet that has an infection, or the faecal contamination of hands followed by handling food or eating. *Indirect contact* can occur when contaminated wound dressings are used in clinical practice, or there is contact with contaminated clothing or bedding, leading to hand-to-mouth transmission.

Infection can also be transmitted via particles in the air. These particles can be large in size (i.e. droplets) or tiny (i.e. aerosols). *Droplet contact transmission* involves the direct spread to a human nearby via coughing, sneezing or talking. These large droplets cannot travel long distances and tend to lodge on the face, in the mouth and upper respiratory tract, or on the surface of the eye. The droplets quickly dissipate from the air. Measles is an example of an infection transmitted in this way. *Aerosol formation* is also known as *air-borne transmission*. The tiny particles persist in the air, travel long distances and can lodge deep in the lower respiratory tract. The microbes associated with these particles must be resistant to drying out. Tuberculosis, influenza and chickenpox are examples of infectious diseases transmitted by aerosols.

Infectious organisms enter humans via a variety of routes collectively known as *portals of entry*. Common portals of entry are the natural body orifices: the mouth, anus, nose, vagina, urethra and ear canal. Another portal of entry can be through a breach in the skin's integrity, such as a wound, or through injection into the body (e.g. with a needle or via an insect bite).

BREAKING THE CHAIN OF TRANSMISSION

LEARNING OBJECTIVE 4

Describe the ways in which the chain of transmission can be broken as a means of controlling infection.

The main approach in controlling the incidence of infectious diseases in our community is to break the chain of transmission

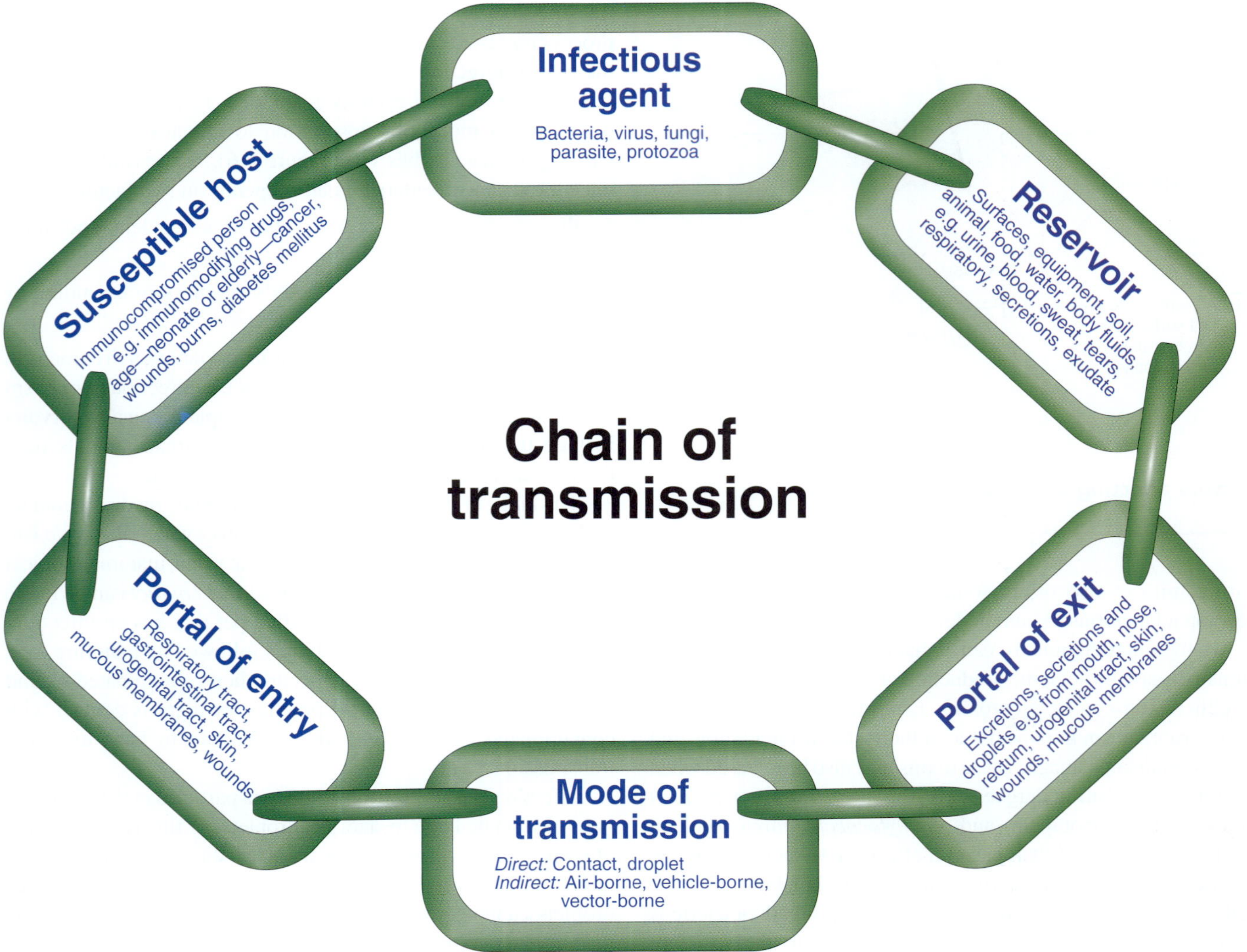

Figure 8.6

Chain of transmission

Sources: Adapted from Pulingam et al. (2022); WHO (2023a, 2023b).

at one or more of its 'links' (see Figure 8.7). This can be achieved by either impeding the establishment or depleting the reservoir of infectious organisms, disrupting the organism's mode of transmission and/or blocking its entry into the human body.

Another important strategy is to inhibit the organism's growth or kill it once it infects our bodies using anti-infective (otherwise known as antimicrobial) drugs. A number of types of anti-infective drugs, such as antibacterial, antiviral, antifungal and antiparasitic agents, are available. An important group of anti-infective agents are known as antibiotics. The term 'antibiotic' is classically defined as anti-infective agents derived from bacterial or fungal sources that selectively target mainly bacterial infections, but can treat some infections caused by other microorganisms. Within this chapter, the authors will not discriminate between antibiotic and non-antibiotic drugs, but will refer to all anti-infectives as antimicrobial agents.

Methods available to deplete the reservoir of infective organisms include using programs that enhance public health, such as improved community sanitation (e.g. systems for clearing rubbish and treating human waste from where people live), access to clean water supplies, eradicating insect-vector breeding grounds (e.g. for mosquitoes that transmit diseases such as malaria, dengue fever and Ross River fever) and immunisation programs for humans and domesticated animals.

The most effective and simplest way to disrupt an organism's mode of transmission is adequate hand-washing before contact with people and after contact with infectious materials. Some highly infectious individuals may have to be managed in clinical areas in isolation from other people in order to minimise cross-infection. Infection control is also facilitated by using *clean* (non-touch, aseptic) techniques in clinical procedures where appropriate, such as the application of wound dressings or *sterile* (microorganism-free) techniques, such as those undertaken for

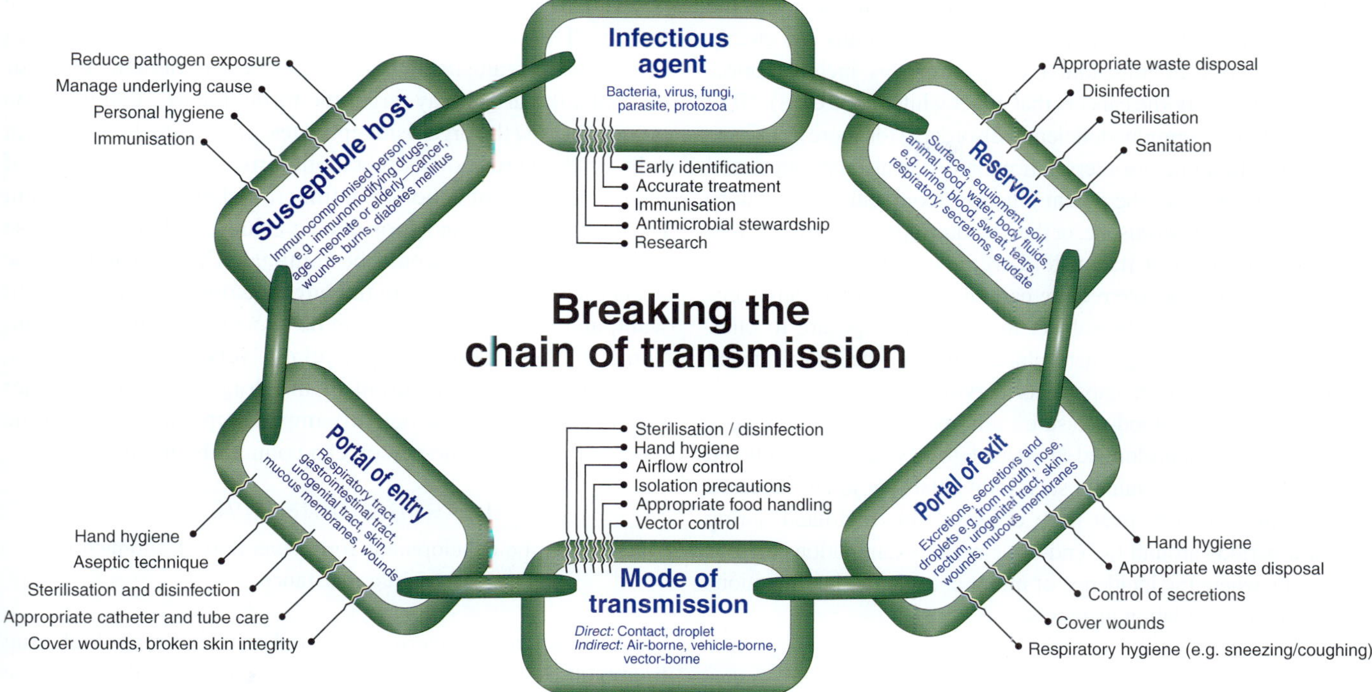

Figure 8.7

Methods to break the chain of transmission

surgical interventions. Eating uncooked meat is an important mode of transmission for a number of infections. This can be addressed by cooking meat thoroughly, not leaving meat at room temperature for a prolonged period, and minimising the contamination of kitchen surfaces and utensils with uncooked meat where other food is being prepared.

A number of strategies are available to block the entry of infectious organisms into humans. Most of these are associated with preventing infections by creating a physical barrier between the organism and the entry portal, such as by wearing gloves and/or face masks when coming into contact with infectious individuals or contaminated material. Asking people with contagious respiratory infections to wear a face mask is also an appropriate way to contain the spread of infection. For sexually transmitted infections, a simple barrier against transmission between partners is provided by wearing a condom.

FACTORS AFFECTING SUSCEPTIBILITY TO INFECTION

LEARNING OBJECTIVE 5

Discuss the factors that influence a person's susceptibility to infection.

People are not equally susceptible to infectious diseases. A number of factors, such as age, current health, levels of nutrition and immune status, can influence the induction and duration of infection.

People at the extremes of the lifespan are more vulnerable to infection. The immune systems of young infants are immature, meaning their immune response to particular organisms may be inadequate. Passive immunity is transmitted to the baby through the transfer of maternal antibodies across the placenta before birth and in breast milk. This transfer is helpful until the production of the full range of antibodies occurs in the child. Immune function in older adults is declining, and so they are particularly susceptible to urinary and respiratory tract infections. Prolonged infection and deaths associated with infection are more common in this age group.

Health status can also influence the onset and development of infectious disease. Poor health due to chronic disease is a major predisposing factor for infection. Chronic conditions such as cardiovascular disease and diabetes mellitus are strongly associated with recurrent, prolonged and potentially fatal infections. Cardiovascular diseases impede the delivery of blood to the sites of infection, leading to a prolongation of the condition or allowing anaerobic organisms to thrive in the oxygen-deprived tissues. Diabetes mellitus is associated with a state of immunosuppression, peripheral neuropathy and altered cardiovascular integrity (see the chapter 'Diabetes mellitus'). Chronically elevated glucose levels affect immune cell function and create a desirable environment for microbial growth in the urinary tract and bloodstream. Some microbes, such as *C. albicans* associated with thrush, can also secrete factors that inhibit the action of phagocytic cells. The sensory nerves involved in nociceptive transmission are damaged, so peripheral tissue injury may not be recognised by the affected person and treated promptly, thus allowing infection to develop. Chronically elevated blood lipid levels in diabetes facilitate the development of atherosclerosis, leading to poor peripheral tissue perfusion.

The level of individual immunity is a key determinant in the susceptibility to infection. Illnesses affecting immunity can greatly increase the risk of infection. Examples of this include cancer (especially blood-borne cancers that affect white blood cells), HIV/AIDS, and other immunodeficiency disorders (for more detail see the chapter 'Immune disorders'). Immunity can also be suppressed during treatment with the potent glucocorticoid anti-inflammatory drugs, such as hydrocortisone, or the immunosuppressant drugs used in the management of rheumatoid arthritis, organ transplantation and cancer. These people require careful monitoring for any signs of infection, and may be subject to restricted exposure to other people and fomites (inanimate objects that can be contaminated with pathogens and are capable of serving as a vehicle for their transmission—e.g. blood-pressure cuffs, pens or a doctor's neck tie). Since severe or prolonged stress leads to elevated glucocorticoid levels that depress immunity, such individuals are at an increased risk of infection. You may have observed this first-hand during stressful periods around the end-of-semester examinations at your university, where the incidence of minor colds and other infections in the student population increases.

Antimicrobial drugs

LEARNING OBJECTIVE 6

Outline the general mechanism of action of antimicrobial drugs.

Antimicrobial drugs can be used to inhibit the growth of or to kill infectious organisms once an infection has developed, or even as a preventive measure in high-risk individuals.

Antimicrobial drugs act by a principle known as *selective toxicity*. They are designed to target the processes or structures of infective organisms that are not present in human cells. For example, the drugs may target the formation of a cell wall, the process of how the organism replicates, how it attaches to human cells or the nature of its metabolic processes. A summary of the mechanisms of action of antimicrobial drugs is provided in Figure 8.8. If such an action can be achieved, then the adverse effects of treatment would be minimal. Unfortunately, these agents are not as specific to the infective organism as we might want, and so human tissues can be damaged during treatment. Some of these drugs are potentially very toxic to humans. Whatever the specific action of the drug, they should either kill the organism or sufficiently impede replication so that the immune system of the person can contain the infection.

LEARNING OBJECTIVE 7

Describe the development and prevention of antimicrobial drug resistance.

A significant concern associated with antimicrobial drug treatment is the development of resistance by the infective organism to the action of the drug being used. This is generally known as **antimicrobial drug resistance**. Antimicrobial drug resistance occurs because microbes develop or acquire biological adaptations that render these drugs ineffective. Adaptations can occur as spontaneous genetic mutations during replication that favour the viability of the organism. The mutation may result in a more effective cellular removal of the drug before toxic intracellular concentrations develop, or

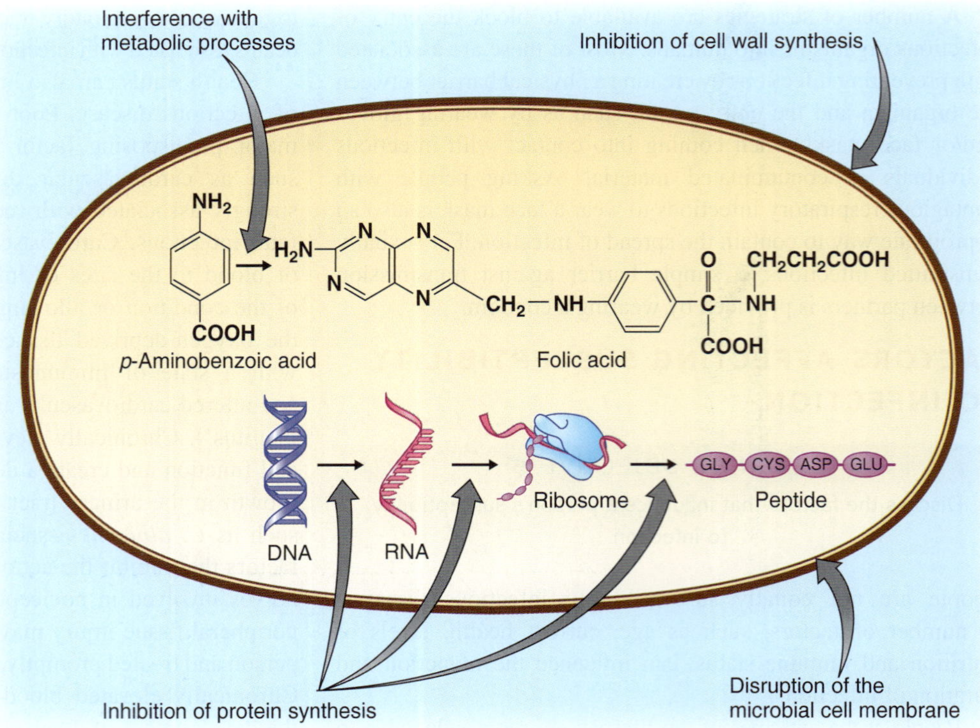

Figure 8.8

General mechanisms of action of antimicrobial drugs

Antimicrobial drugs act by one of four general mechanisms selectively toxic to prokaryotic cells. DNA = deoxyribonucleic acid; RNA = ribonucleic acid

Source: Adapted from Bullock & Manias (2022), Figure 59.1, p. 749.

by bypassing a step in a metabolic pathway that was previously disrupted by the drug. These adaptations can also be acquired by other species of infective organisms through plasmid formation. A *plasmid* is a piece of genetic material containing the adaptation that becomes enclosed in a vesicle, which is exported from the organism to be taken up and incorporated into the genetic material of another organism (see Figure 8.9).

Poor practices by health professionals and the community contribute greatly to the development of antimicrobial drug resistance. A summary of some of these common practices is provided in Figure 8.10. The consequence of antimicrobial drug resistance is that treatment with specific antimicrobial agents becomes ineffective. For some infections, treatment with these drugs is the only way to control the illness. Without this treatment the affected person may die. For some microbes, such as methicillin-resistant or multi-resistant *Staphylococcus aureus* (MRSA) and vancomycin-resistant enterococci (VRE), only one current drug may be effective against infection, and when the organism becomes resistant to it there will be no other treatment options available.

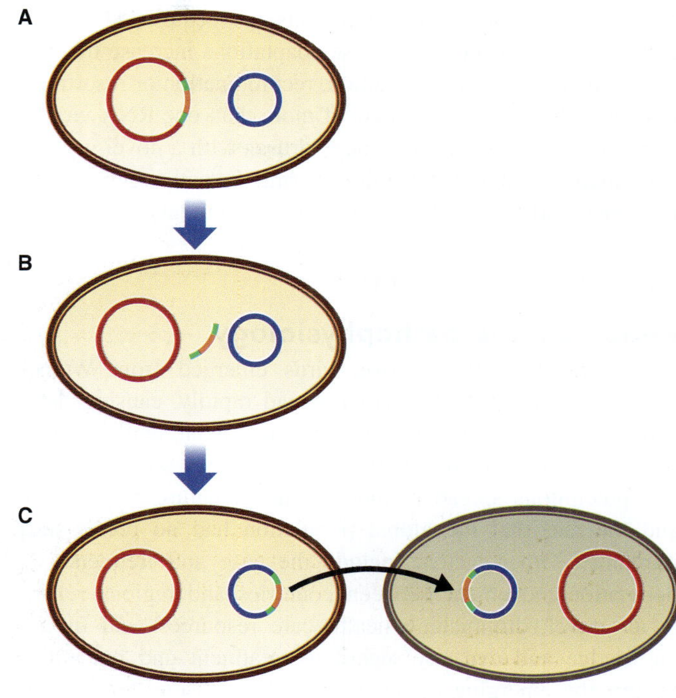

Figure 8.9

Plasmid formation

(A) A gene encodes for an adaptation that impairs the action of an antimicrobial drug.

(B) This gene can be transferred to a plasmid within the microbial cell.

(C) This plasmid can be transferred to another bacterial species, allowing it to acquire the resistance gene.

Emerging infectious diseases

LEARNING OBJECTIVE 8

Discuss emerging infectious diseases and the factors that increase the risks of global threat, with particular focus on SARS-CoV-2 virus.

It is estimated that infectious diseases cause approximately 15 million deaths per year and leave an estimated 1 billion people chronically infected. Some pathogens can spread quickly

Figure 8.10

Factors contributing to antimicrobial drug resistance

Sources: Data from Pulingam et al. (2022); WHO (2023a, 2023b); Zay et al. (2023).

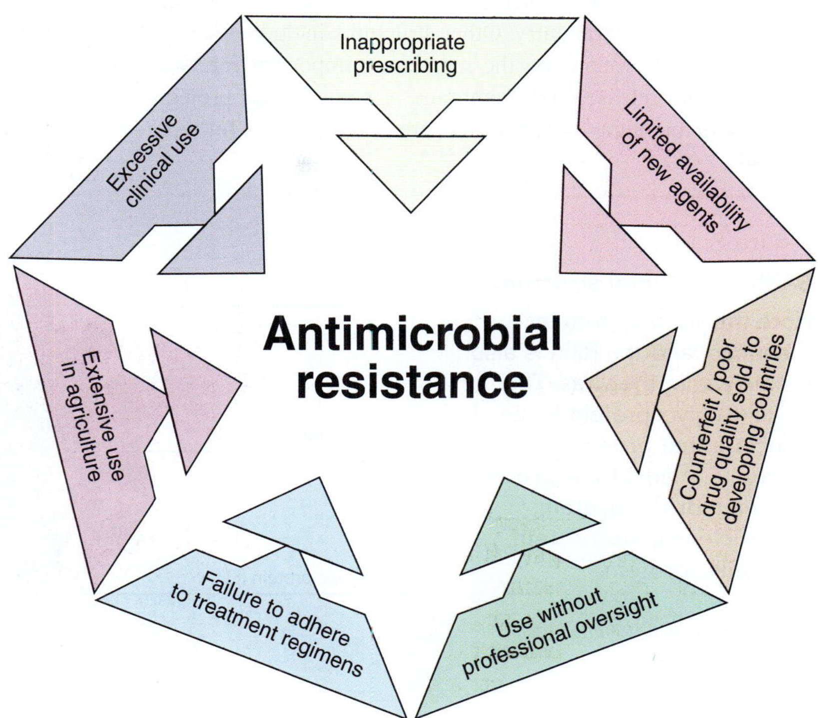

as a result of evolution that permits the acquisition of new pathogenic characteristics. These adaptations increase the ease of the spread by genetic mutation, recombination or resortment (whereby the genetic segments of more than one RNA virus is reshuffled in a host, creating new viruses with a novel genome combination). These new abilities permit the pathogens to infect new hosts and/or survive in different environments.

COVID-19 INFECTION

Aetiology and pathophysiology

In December, 2019, a novel virus emerged from Wuhan, China. The SARS-CoV-2 virus spread rapidly, causing death and significant disruption to health care, social, and economic systems throughout the world. Circumstances contributing to this precipitous spread include the novel nature of the virus and the fact that the global population had no pre-existing immunity. Other factors include the ease and frequency of population movement between countries and regions related to air travel, diminishing health care resources, and limited knowledge and capacity regarding treatment and prevention against the emerging threat. Early variants were complicated by asymptomatic spread (from a long prodromal period with an incubation period of up to 24 days) which resulted in people infecting friends, family and others as they were unaware that they had the virus. Finally, confusion, fear and an increasing number of people choosing to ignore the public health guidelines contributed to the amplification of the crisis.

The SARS-CoV-2 virus is a single-strand RNA virus with a genome of several genes which code for numerous proteins. The virus has a spherical shape and is approximately 60–140 nanometres with a basic structure including spike proteins, which are surface glycoproteins protruding from the surface giving the virus its characteristic 'corona' or crown-like appearance. The spike proteins bind to a receptor on the host cell and facilitate viral entry. Other structures include envelope proteins, small proteins on the membrane important for virus assembly and release, and membrane proteins, larger proteins which help maintain viral shape and are also important for virus assembly and release. The virus contains nucleocapsid proteins, which are proteins that surround and protect the viral RNA, and a number of other non-structural proteins and accessory proteins which are important for replication and virulence (see Figure 8.11).

The SARS-CoV-2 surface proteins are highly variable and can mutate rapidly. This ability to mutate and generate new variants is a leading factor in the ongoing evolution and spread of the pandemic. Mutations in these regions directly influence the development of vaccines and therapeutics.

Transmission and transmissibility

As with many respiratory tract infections, SARS-CoV-2 virus transmission occurs primarily through respiratory droplets that are produced when an infected person talks, coughs or sneezes. These droplets can travel through the air and contact mucous membranes of people nearby (within approximately 2 m). Contact with SARS-CoV-2 virally-contaminated surfaces or fomites (objects) and subsequent contact with respiratory mucosa may also lead to transmission, although this is not a primary mode of transmission. Ineffective hand hygiene, substandard or infrequent surface cleaning, and uncovered rubbish bins can result in microbial contamination and increase the risk of contact spread. Microbial aerosolisation from open-lid toilet flushing or the use of air-forced hand drying systems have also been identified, but not as a significant cause. Faecal–oral transmission is also possible; however, research has only shown a limited number of cases have occurred by this mechanism. Debate still persists regarding the frequency of airborne transmission, with the prevailing opinions considering the likelihood more associated with poorly ventilated, crowded settings. Ultimately, it is probably easiest to consider SARS-CoV-2 is spread along the spectrum across all types of transmission, with the droplet transmission being predominant.

Viral transmission is also influenced by environmental determinants. Factors such as temperature, humidity, pH, salinity, the surface on which the pathogen is located, the presence of ultraviolet radiation and the state of ventilation and airflow can all affect transmission. Interestingly, in the early

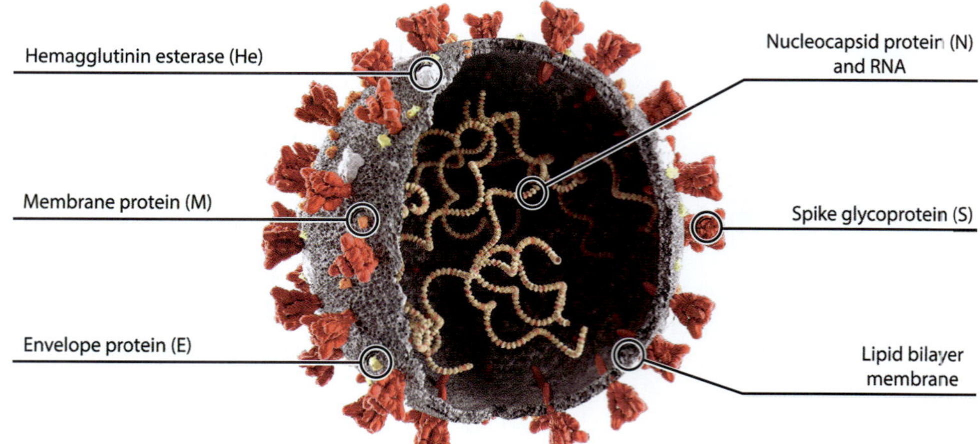

Figure 8.11

SARS-CoV-2 viral structure

Note the various proteins identified, and the RNA is also visible within the virus. The spike (S) glycoprotein is the viral structure that promotes viral uptake. E = envelope protein; M = membrane protein; N = nucleocapsid protein; S = spike protein.

Source: Orpheus FX/Shutterstock.

stages of the pandemic in Australia, several localised outbreaks of SARS CoV-2 implicating airflow and ventilation failures have been attributed to hotels, cruise ships and even aged-care facilities whereby occupants were breathing recirculated, unfiltered, indoor air. Protocols to mitigate the risks associated with environmental determinants of SARS CoV-2 transmission should be instigated to contribute to improved infection control.

The measure of transmissibility is represented by the basic reproduction number (R0—pronounced 'R nought'). It is a mathematical term used to estimate how contagious an infectious disease is by indicating the average number of people who will be infected by one person with the disease in a population which is naïve (has no immunity) to the disease. If R0 is less than 1, every infected person, on average, will transmit the disease to fewer than one other person and the infectious disease will recede as there are too few new people becoming infected to sustain an outbreak. If R0 is greater than 1, every infected person, on average, will transmit the disease to more than one other person. For example, if R0 = 2, every infected person will infect two other people. This will subsequently increase the spread and can potentially cause an epidemic or a pandemic if not controlled. R0 changes over time, across the course of the pandemic, and is influenced by many factors, including disease virulence, the mechanism of transmission and any mitigating factors initiated (and followed) by the involved population. The highest recorded official estimate of the R0 for SARS-CoV-2 was 5.7, based on data from the early stages of the outbreak in Wuhan, China, in around February 2020.

To reduce the rapidly evolving, fast-spreading transmission of SARS-CoV-2, public health guidelines were developed (and in many regions, enforced) to control this respiratory spread. In the first year of the pandemic, there were no vaccines to mitigate the spread, so the use of facemasks and physical distancing were necessary to slow the spread. The use of quarantine and isolation became necessary, and contact tracing (whereby interviews of infected people to determine who else may have been exposed) were employed to help try to control its ever-increasing spread.

Zoonotic risk

The origin of SARS-CoV-2 is yet to be fully determined; however, the current evidence suggests that the virus likely originated in bats and may have been transmitted to humans through an intermediate host such as a pangolin, a member of the anteater family. For a pathogen to successfully infect a new host, the host must have compatible cell receptors. In selected mammals, the SARS-CoV-2 virus can utilise the angiotensin-converting enzyme 2 (ACE-2) receptor to enter host cells. The ACE-2 receptor is found in many locations in humans. Figure 8.12 represents the diversity of ACE-2 receptors throughout the body.

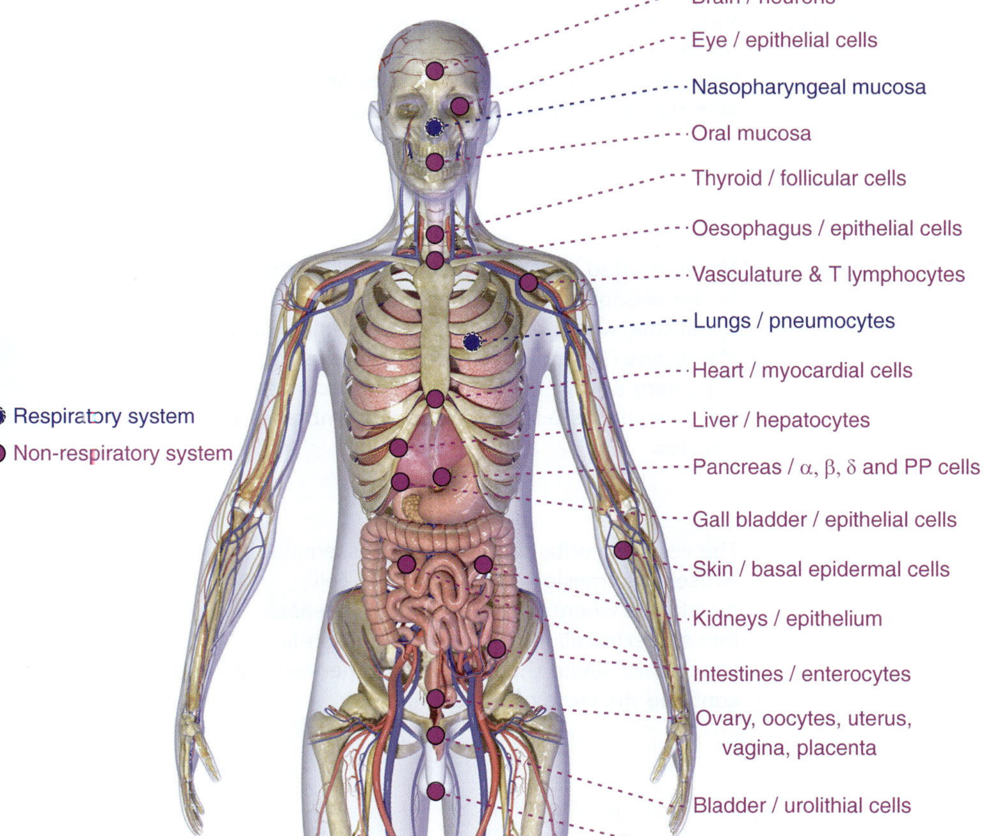

Figure 8.12

Locations of ACE-2 receptors in body structures

Because the ACE-2 receptor is the mechanism by which the SARS-CoV-2 virus enters the cell, any organ with ACE-2 proteins can be the target of direct injury from viral invasion.

Source: Adapted from 7activestudio/123RF.

Viral entry and infection

In the incubation period following entry to the respiratory tract, SARS-CoV-2 will undergo a five-step process to produce the infection of the host cell. Interestingly, the virus appears to be preferentially attracted to ciliated epithelial cells and mucus-producing goblet cells of the upper respiratory tract. However, as previously discussed, the virus can enter cells in any tissue which contain ACE-2 receptors. The five-step process of attachment, penetration, biosynthesis, maturation and release are explained and demonstrated in Table 8.3.

SARS-CoV-2 has a median incubation period of for to five days before symptom onset and causes coronavirus

Table 8.3 The five-step process of viral entry, replication and release

Step	Action	Image
Attachment	SARS-CoV-2 virus spike protein binds to host cells via the ACE-2 receptor (known as *host cell recognition*).	
Penetration	The viral membrane fuses with host cell membrane and endocytosis occurs allowing entry and release of RNA into the cytosol.	
Biosynthesis	Viral genomic RNA replication and transcription occurs in the cytoplasm within double membrane vesicles (DMVs). New viral particles are created with the assistance of the host's own ribosomes.	
Maturation	Newly created viral particles are translocated to the endoplasmic reticulum and the Golgi apparatus, where packaging and assembly occur. Membrane (M) and envelope (E) proteins are important at this stage. Maturation occurs as the new viruses bud off the Golgi membranes in vesicles.	
Release	The vesicles containing the newly assembled viruses are translocated to the host cell membrane where they fuse and are released into the extracellular space through non-lytic exocytosis, where they can infect other cells and continue the cycle of infection.	

Source: Images adapted from designua/123RF.

disease-2019 (COVID-19). A clearer understanding of COVID-19 pathophysiology is developing with evolving clarity around the triggers causing the host's aberrant immune system responses. The current understanding of the disease process can be divided into two distinct mechanisms: the first is a direct invasion of the SARS-CoV-2 virus into particular cells, causing specific tissue damage; and the second mechanism is associated with immune system dysregulation resulting from anomalous responses from the both innate and humoral systems.

As previously discussed, during the initial infection, SARS-CoV-2 uses its spike protein to bind to the ACE-2 receptor on the host cell surface, primarily within the respiratory system. The presence of ACE-2 receptors on the target tissue explains many of the systemic effects, which may encompass almost every organ system. The associated tissue damage will also lead to inflammation and can contribute to further deterioration in a person with more severe disease.

As the *innate immune system* is the first line of defence against pathogens, it is activated soon after the SARS-CoV-2 virus enters the body. Innate immune sensing by multiple host cell pattern recognition receptors promotes activation of a plethora of innate immune cells, such as macrophages, natural killer (NK) cells, neutrophils, dendritic cells, eosinophils, basophils, and innate lymphoid cells (ILCs). This should result in the moderate production of various pro-inflammatory cytokines, type I interferons and chemokines in order to mount a measured response to begin to defeat the invading pathogen. However, in some people—due to comorbidities or immune system dysfunction from disease or drugs—the ability to mount a response is insufficient or aberrant, and the virus is able to replicate rapidly. Subsequently, an excessive and uncontrolled inflammatory response (known as a *cytokine storm*) occurs, which damages tissue through apoptosis causing organ dysfunction and even death. Therefore, innate immune system dysfunction will contribute to a significant amount of tissue damage in people with severe disease.

The *humoral (adaptive) immune system* is critical for defence against respiratory viral infections. Normally, once antigen-presenting cells have interacted with a Th2 cell, they are able to activate B cells and cytotoxic T (Tc) cells. IL-6 and TNF-α are important in this process. Soon, some of these B cells will differentiate into plasma cells and release SARS-CoV-2-specific neutralising antibodies. The Tc cells will begin to identify and destroy infected cells. In some people with COVID-19, humoral immune system dysfunction occurs, resulting in impaired B cell response, potentially due to immunosenescence and 'inflamm-ageing'. Delayed antibody responses due to the virus's influence can then result in a longer time being taken to produce sufficient antibodies. Subsequently, the virus has more time to replicate and increase the viral load. Unfortunately, with some of the evolving mutations, the SARS-CoV-2 virus is developing the capacity to evade antibody recognition. In some people with severe disease, the immune system may become exhausted and less responsive due to excessive cytokines and other factors.

Variants over time

Some of the key variants of SARS-CoV-2 that have emerged over time include Alpha, Beta, Gamma, Delta and Omicron. These variants have different combinations of mutations, which may affect their transmissibility, severity, and resistance to vaccines and treatments. Complicating matters further, there are also subvariants associated with each of these mutations. Examples of changes over time include some mutations in the Delta variant which increase viral transmissibility. Also, at the time of writing, an Omicron subvariant called XBB.1.5, which is spreading through the United States of America, has numerous mutations making it the most transmissible strain yet. Unfortunately, it also has mutations to the ACE-2 receptor, which appears to facilitate immune evasion. As the number and type of mutations continue to expand, vaccine effectiveness and mutation-specific targeted therapeutic agents become less effective.

Epidemiology

In the past two decades, three significant coronavirus outbreaks have emerged. In 2002, the first SARS epidemic resulted in approximately 8,000 cases globally, with a mortality rate of approximately 11%. Then in 2012, Middle East respiratory syndrome (MERS-CoV) spread to 27 countries and resulted in an estimated overall 35% mortality. Finally, the third coronavirus outbreak emerged in 2019, causing the COVID-19 global pandemic. Interestingly, this virus shares 79% nucleotide sequence identity with the virus which caused the 2002 SARS epidemic.

The global mortality rate of the COVID-19 pandemic was estimated at 2.2% in 2020, 2.1% in 2021, and approximately 1.7% in February 2023. However, mortality rates will vary in local regions contingent on factors such as the demographic characteristics, economic capacity, and the prevalence of underlying health conditions in the population. For example, in May 2020, a mortality rate of 4.4% was reported from official data by the Ministry of Health of Ecuador for the city of Guayaquil.

The current COVID-19 pandemic is still evolving, and as of February 2023 the World Health Organization (WHO) reported more than 756 million confirmed cases and more than 6.8 million deaths worldwide. New Zealand has recorded 2,534 deaths and 2.1 million people who have recovered from infection. Australia has recorded 19,168 deaths and 11.34 million people who have recovered from infection.

Clinical manifestations

Pulmonary and extrapulmonary effects COVID-19 disease primarily affects the lungs, but it can also cause a range of extra-pulmonary effects across most body systems. Clinical manifestations can range from mild to severe, with severity correlating to various risk factors and comorbidities. As discussed previously, the organs and tissues affected can be predicted, in part based on the presence or absence of ACE-2 receptors on the surface of the cell membrane.

Pulmonary manifestations can include a dry cough, dyspnoea (especially on exertion), and pleuritic chest pain related to inflamed pleura. Serious pulmonary effects such as pneumonia and acute respiratory distress syndrome are less common (especially with the evolving variants). Severe illness increases the likelihood of requiring mechanical ventilation. People requiring critical care are at significantly increased risk of mortality from the effects of the disease, complications related to comorbidities, and potentially even iatrogenic causes related to effects of drugs or other medical intervention.

Extrapulmonary manifestations include less serious signs and symptoms such as fever, loss of smell (anosmia), loss of taste (dysgeusia), painful joints and muscles (arthralgia and myalgia), sore throat, nausea and vomiting, and headache. The virus presents differently in people, which is likely, at least in part, to be related to the variant, and also the person's own immune system response. Some people may experience rhinorrhea (runny nose), congestion and sputum production, whereas other people experience more gastrointestinal effects and none of the other respiratory disturbances. There is also a subgroup of people who are asymptomatic and only discover they have had a SARS-CoV-2 infection because of serology results.

More serious clinical manifestations affect important organ systems such as the cardiovascular system, with the potential to cause pericarditis or myocarditis, or even thromboembolic events resulting in myocardial infarction, cerebrovascular accident (stroke), pulmonary embolism, or other extremely serious haematological conditions such as microemboli, microangiopathy or disseminated intravascular coagulopathy.

The renal system is populated with ACE-2 receptors, and acute kidney injury is common in severe disease. Unfortunately, some of the drugs and interventions necessary to care for people with severe COVID-19 illness can also be nephrotoxic.

Serious endocrine system effects include direct pancreatic beta-cell damage from viral invasion causing insulin resistance and hyperglycaemia. Even the male and female reproductive systems do not escape damage, with the potential of erectile dysfunction, reduced sperm count, the potential for increased severity and number of premenstrual symptoms and irregular menstruation. Figure 8.13 explores the common clinical manifestations and management of COVID-19.

Risk factors and disease severity

As with most conditions, risk factors can increase the likelihood of experiencing the disease, but there is also often a correlation with disease severity. As such, people who are older (> 65 years of age), or have significant comorbidities—such as cardiac, respiratory, endocrine or immune system dysfunction—are at greater risk of SARS-CoV-2 infection and poorer clinical outcomes from COVID-19 disease.

Other factors which increase risk for COVID-19 disease are: ethnicity, with many Indigenous populations being disproportionately affected; sex, with men at slightly higher risk; and vaccination status, with unvaccinated people at a significantly higher risk for severe illness. Obesity is a risk factor with significant correlation to poor outcomes from severe complications and sequelae. Finally, some viral factors influencing outcomes include viral load and the variant with which the person is infected. As previously discussed, some variants can increase disease severity and influence treatment effectiveness.

Quantifying disease severity is an important consideration as it will help to guide management of the clinical course. The national consensus recommendation for disease severity from the Australian Guidelines for the Clinical Care of People with COVID-19 is represented in Table 8.4.

Long COVID

A post-acute sequelae of SARS-CoV-2 infection (PASC) is a condition also known as 'long COVID', where people continue to experience symptoms related to COVID-19 for weeks or even months following the initial infection. Although many people appear to be symptom-free within four weeks after an infection, a subgroup of people who have had COVID-19 continue to experience multiple, often debilitating symptoms. The literature reports anywhere from 3% to 45% of people still experiencing unresolved symptoms after four months, yet other data record only approximately 7.5% of people experiencing persistent symptoms for three or more months. Because there is little parity in the clinical definition of 'long COVID' within countries or even within regions, the actual prevalence at this time is really unknown.

The clinical course and symptom experience are diverse between those reported to have long COVID. Symptoms which may be considered minor, such as anosmia, dysgeusia, fatigue, myalgia and cough, are reported by some. However, more serious clinical manifestations, such as dyspnoea, cognitive dysfunction, or chest pain and palpitations, are also experienced by people who are often called 'long-haulers'. Long COVID is clearly difficult to formally quantify, as the experiences vary in prevalence and severity and are unique between individuals. Interestingly, there is little correlation between the persistence of long COVID and the severity of the initial disease. The exact mechanism is not yet fully understood; however, it is believed to involve several factors which are most likely related to immune dysregulation in some way. Some mechanisms currently posited include viral persistence and immune response, organ damage, autonomic nervous system dysfunction, microvascular injury, and psychological factors.

In some people, the immune system struggles to clear the infection and the SARS-CoV-2 virus has capacity to continue to replicate and cause tissue damage. As a result of the viral persistence, the inflammatory response continues. The insult from the original infection causing organ damage to multiple systems may have been such that COVID-19 symptoms continue because the tissue has just not yet recovered.

Autonomic nervous system dysfunction may follow COVID-19 infection because of virus- or autoimmune-mediated damage to intrathoracic chemoreceptors and/or mechanoreceptors, resulting in sustained cardiac, respiratory or neurological symptoms.

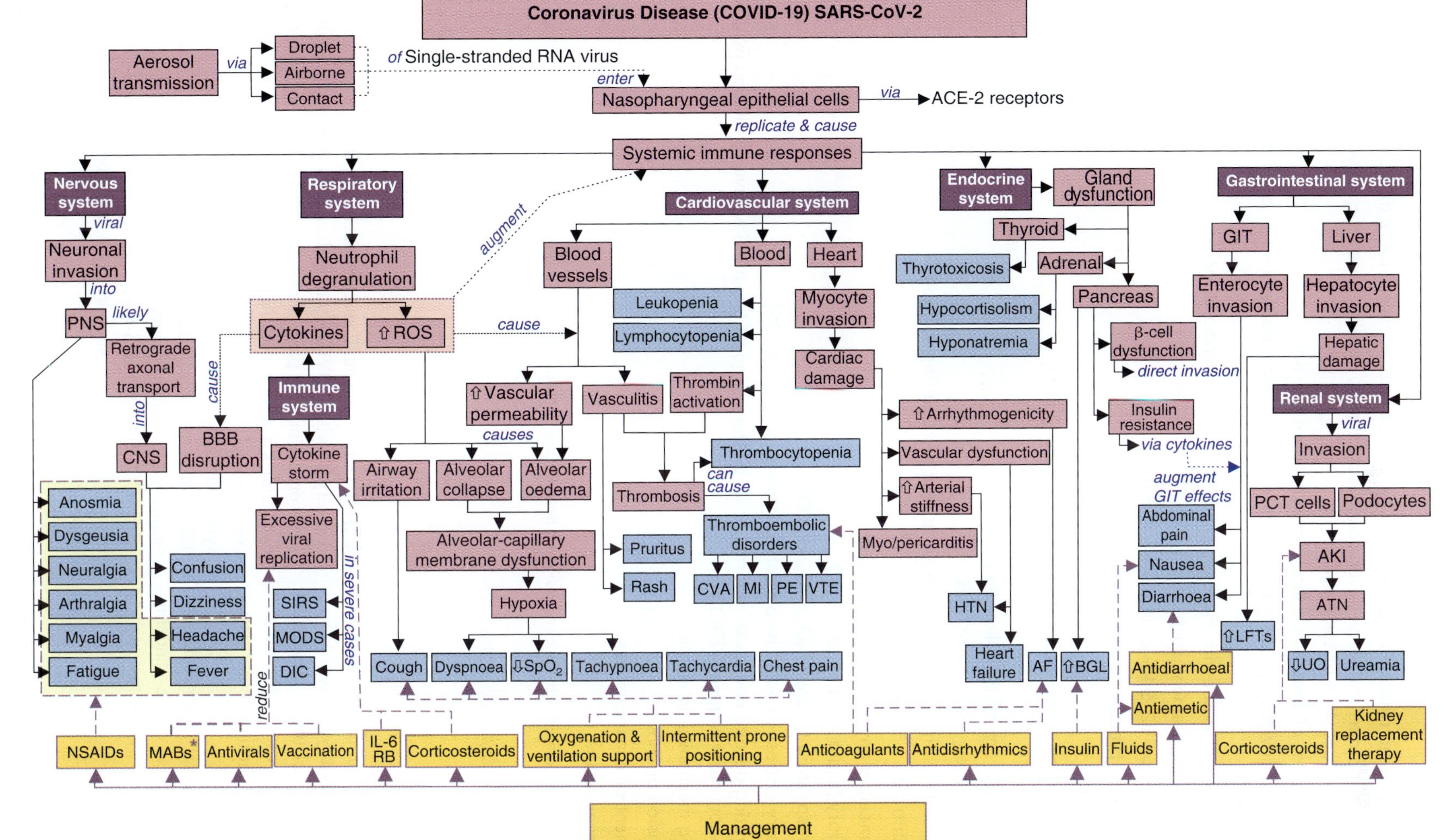

Figure 8.13

Clinical snapshot: Coronavirus disease (COVID-19) from SARS-CoV-2 virus

↓ = decreased; ↑ = increased; β = beta; AF = atrial fibrillation; AKI = acute kidney injury; ATN = acute tubular necrosis; BBB = blood-brain barrier; BGL = blood glucose level; CNS = central nervous system; CVA = cerebrovascular accident; DIC = disseminated intravascular coagulation; GIT = gastrointestinal tract; HTN = hypertension; IL-6 RB = interleukin-6 receptor blocker; LFTs = liver function tests; MI = myocardial infarction; MODS = multi-organ dysfunction syndrome; PCT = proximal convoluted tubule; PE = pulmonary embolism; PNS = peripheral nervous system; ROS = reactive oxygen species; SIRS = systemic inflammatory response syndrome; SpO_2 = oxygen saturations; UO = urine output; VTE = venous thromboembolism.

* = Current monoclonal antibodies (MABs) quickly becoming useless against current variants—new MABs under development.

Table 8.4 COVID-19 disease severity for adults

Severity	Symptom
Mild illness	An individual with no clinical features suggestive of moderate or more severe disease: • mild or no symptoms and signs (fever, cough, sore throat, malaise, headache, muscle pain, nausea, vomiting, diarrhoea, loss of taste and smell) • no new shortness of breath or difficulty breathing on exertion • no evidence of lower respiratory tract disease during clinical assessment or on imaging (if performed)
Moderate illness	A person who is stable but with evidence of lower respiratory tract disease: • during clinical assessment, such as • oxygen saturation 92–94% on room air at rest • desaturation or breathlessness with mild exertion • or on imaging
Severe illness	A person with signs of moderate disease who is deteriorating OR A person meeting any of the following criteria: • respiratory rate $\geq$ 30 breaths/min • oxygen saturation $<$ 92% on room air at rest or requiring oxygen • lung infiltrates $>$ 50%
Critical illness	A person meeting any of the following criteria: • Respiratory failure (defined as any of) • severe respiratory failure ($PaO_2/FiO_2 < 200$) • respiratory distress or acute respiratory distress syndrome (ARDS) • deteriorating despite non-invasive forms of respiratory support (i.e. non-invasive ventilation [NIV], or high-flow nasal oxygen [HFNO]) • requiring mechanical ventilation • hypotension or shock • impairment of consciousness • other organ failure

Definition of disease severity for children and adolescents are not considered here. Further information can be found in the Australian Guidelines for the Clinical Care of People with COVID-19.

Source: National Clinical Evidence Taskforce—COVID-19 (2023), p. 128.

ACE-2 receptors are prolific in endothelial cells and cardiomyocytes, therefore microvascular injury or direct damage by viral invasion into heart or blood vessel tissue may result. Some clinical manifestations may also be caused by resulting oxygen and nutrient delivery deficits to cardiovascular tissues secondary to the direct, original insult.

Finally, psychological and environmental factors related to experiencing a severe illness, and the stress of the pandemic, may contribute to ongoing psychological symptoms such as anxiety and depression.

Special populations

Special populations may require considerations relating to their care. These populations include children, pregnant women, people who are immunocompromised, and those of older age.

Children A small percentage of children who become severely ill with COVID-19 may develop a condition resulting in fever, abdominal pain, shock and rash. There are currently two names for this condition: in the United Kingdom this condition is called 'paediatric inflammatory multisystem syndrome temporally associated with SARS-CoV-2 (PIMS-TS)', while in America and according to the WHO it is termed 'multisystem inflammatory syndrome in children associated with COVID-19 (MIS-C)'. These children will require intensive care and support and appropriate management informed by evidence.

Pregnant women and new mothers Pregnant women, and those who are $<$14 days post-partum, who are COVID-19 positive are at increased risk for venous thrombosis, and so prophylactic anticoagulation should be considered for at least 14 days. Women at risk of preterm birth or pre-eclampsia may be given magnesium sulfate, as there is clear evidence that it provides fetal neuroprotection. Women who are COVID-19 positive who give birth do not need to be separated from their newborn; however, they should be encouraged to undertake good hand hygiene, mask wearing, and, where possible, physical distance from the newborn when not feeding or caring for them.

Immunocompromised people A person with immunocompromise is more likely to develop COVID-19 disease, and is also at risk of developing more severe complications, such as pneumonia, acute respiratory distress syndrome (ARDS) and/or sepsis if they are infected. They are potentially more susceptible to co-infections with other viruses, bacteria or fungi. Depending on their underlying condition (or the immunomodulating drugs they are taking), their immune system may not be capable of mounting a sufficient immune response, or, conversely, they may develop a more aberrant response resulting in significant cytokine release syndrome, thrombosis and hyperinflammation. They may require more doses of antiviral medication. In relation to prevention, an immunocompromised person may require more vaccine doses, or may not even seroconvert. These people must rely on extreme prevention and hygiene practices and also on herd immunity to attempt to keep them safe from SARS-CoV-2 infection.

Older people Age is a critical factor for poor outcomes in SARS-CoV-2 infection. In Australia, until January 2023, 88% of all COVID deaths occurred in people over 70 years of age. Contributing factors to this increased risk include immunosenescence resulting in the decreased production and function of immune cells, and the likelihood of pre-existing conditions and other comorbidities. An older person's respiratory function also declines with age, which can complicate the course of their disease and increase the likelihood of pneumonia and acute respiratory distress syndrome (ARDS). COVID-19 outbreaks have been seen in aged-care facilities. During 2022–23, in Australia, 6.2% of all deaths occurred in aged-care facilities. The Australian Defence Force and a number of private nursing supply companies assisted in supporting workforce deficits in such facilities as local staff tested COVID-19 positive. Vaccination rollouts occurred in aged-care facilities to mitigate the risk, with 85.5% of all residents having received their fourth dose by February 2023. Finally, the Australian government also supplied antivirals such as molnupiravir and the combination drug nirmatrelvir and ritonavir.

Clinical diagnosis and management

Diagnosis There are generally three methods used to diagnose SARS-CoV-2. These include polymerase chain reaction (PCR), rapid antigen test (RAT) and antibody testing.

Polymerase chain reaction (PCR) is considered the gold standard for detecting viral RNA from SARS-CoV-2. It is highly accurate; however, it can take several hours to process the sample in a laboratory. Some more rapid, point-of-care PCR testing processes are becoming available, which can return PCR results in approximately 20 minutes. As technology and knowledge grows, it is likely that even more rapid results will be possible.

Although not available at the beginning of the pandemic, rapid antigen tests are a quick and easy method of detecting nucleocapsid (N) proteins on the surface of the SARS-CoV-2 virus in a sample taken from a person's respiratory tract. Nasopharyngeal, nasal or saliva samples may be used depending on the manufacturer's instructions. These tests can produce results within 15–30 minutes, but are less sensitive and accurate than a PCR. They are less reliable in low disease prevalence settings, especially if used to screen asymptomatic people, as they may return false negative or false positive results. However, because they can be undertaken at home without the assistance of a healthcare professional, their utility is beneficial. Although expensive and difficult to acquire upon their introduction into Australia, these kits are now widely available and less costly, assisting people and businesses to determine their infection status.

Serology antibody tests are used to detect the presence of IgM and/or IgG antibodies against SARS-CoV-2 from a blood sample. Results may be obtained within 15–30 minutes. This test is not useful for identifying active infection, as it does not detect active viral shedding and is ineffective in determining if a person is infectious. Its utility exists in being able to determine a person's past viral exposure.

Management

Prevention Because this communicable disease can be potentially dangerous, it is better to attempt to prevent infection. Interventions such as vaccination, social distancing, frequent, effective hand hygiene, staying home when ill, and improving indoor ventilation are beneficial in preventing COVID-19 disease. Other measures such as wearing a mask and avoiding large crowds might be necessary in the context of immunocompromise or increased local prevalence of the virus.

In order to prevent future zoonotic outbreaks, it is important to recognise the factors that contribute to their emergence such as changes in land use, deforestation, habitat destruction, and wildlife trade. Additionally, the increasing globalisation of travel and trade means that diseases can spread rapidly across borders. Preventing future zoonotic outbreaks requires a multidisciplinary approach that includes surveillance of animal populations, rapid detection and response to new diseases, improved regulation of the wildlife trade, and addressing the root causes of habitat destruction and other drivers of disease emergence.

Treatment The Australian Guidelines for the Clinical Care of People with COVID-19 considers the person's disease severity, comorbidities and risk factors. Non-pharmacological supportive care may include ensuring adequate nutrition and hydration is achieved. Depending on the person's clinical needs, oxygen therapy, ventilation support, and prone positioning may also be required. Pharmacological options are evolving across time as evidence for success or failure of an intervention is understood. Current treatment options include anti-inflammatory drugs, antivirals, monoclonal antibodies, and immunomodulators such as inhaled and parenteral corticosteroids.

Supportive care, such as hydration, fever management with non-steroidal anti-inflammatory drugs and analgesics, can help alleviate symptoms and improve outcomes for people with COVID-19 disease. As gastrointestinal (GIT) effects of COVID-19 are common, and also some COVID-19 chemotherapeutic agents such as antivirals and monoclonal antibodies also contribute to GIT effects, people may struggle to manage sufficient nutrition or hydration needs. If standard oral intake and rehydration with water, isotonic sports drinks or other fluid and electrolyte replacements are impeded, antiemetics and antidiarrhoeals may be beneficial for symptomatic relief. However, it is important to note that antidiarrhoeals or antimotility medications should be considered with caution as they have occasionally been associated with the development of toxic megacolon. There is no current evidence for the use of pro-biotics. If signs of dehydration continue, the person may require hospitalisation to avoid severe dehydration and shock.

Oxygen therapy is recommended in people with COVID-19 disease who are experiencing respiratory distress. Oxygen saturations should be maintained at least 92% SpO_2 in individuals without chronic hypercapnia, and between 88% and 92% in people with hypoxic drive. Nasal prongs or a mask may be used; however, in severe hypoxaemia, continuous positive airway pressure (CPAP) or even mechanical ventilation may be necessary to maintain or improve oxygenation. Intermittent prone positioning in people with COVID-19 disease who are mechanically ventilated has been found to decrease mortality and improve oxygenation.

Antivirals such as nirmatrelvir and ritonavir may be considered in people with less than five days of COVID-19 infection in those who do not require oxygen, and have one or more risk factors of disease progression. Molnuporavir is recommended if the nirmatrelvir and ritonavir combination is considered unsuitable. Nirmatrelvir and molnuporavir act by inhibiting the processing of precursors required for viral replication; and when ritonavir is co-administered, it acts to decrease the CYP3A-mediated metabolism of nirmatrelvir to increase plasma concentrations of nirmatrelvir to therapeutic levels. As with many drugs, efficacy is changing rapidly, in a large part related to the mutations of the SARS-CoV-2 variant which is circulating. Therefore, it is critical to remain up-to-date with local protocols and procedures.

Monoclonal antibodies (MABs) which directly target the SARS-CoV-2 proteins have been previously beneficial in chemoprophylaxis and treatment of COVID-19 disease; however, with the current variants circulating, there are presently no MABs with sufficient efficacy to outweigh the risk and costs associated with their use. There are, however, more drugs in development which may hopefully assist with reducing morbidity and/or mortality associated with immunocompromise or severe infection. However, IL-6 inhibitors such as tocilizumab have been shown to decrease hospitalisation, mechanical ventilation and mortality risk. This group of MABs blocks the interleukin-6 receptor expressed on hepatocytes and some leukocyte subpopulations, which is thought to subsequently interrupt the inflammatory cascade. IL-6 inhibitors are recommended for use in people who are taking corticosteroids and are at risk of, or require, mechanical ventilation.

Corticosteroids are an important contributor to a decrease in all-cause mortality and disease progression. Inhaled corticosteroids are recommended within 14 days of symptom onset for adults and children with COVID-19 disease who do not require oxygen but have one or more risk factors for disease progression. Systemic (oral or parenteral) corticosteroids are recommended for up to 10 days for adults and children who require oxygen (whether or not they are mechanically ventilated). Corticosteroids activate anti-inflammatory mediators and inhibit inflammatory mediators. They ultimately reduce the promotion of cytokine storms and lessen the risk of multi-organ damage. Although corticosteroids reduce viral clearance, their benefits are mostly considered to outweigh their risks. It is important that clinical decisions are personalised to the requirements of the affected person.

Other immunomodulating medications, such as the biological disease-modifying antirheumatic drug (bDMARD) abatacept, block cytokines and efficiently modulate T-cell activation and neutralise the inflammatory factors involved in cytokine release syndrome (CRS) or cytokine storm. As this is an antirheumatic drug which has been repurposed, the exact mechanism contributing to its COVID-19 efficacy requires further investigation. Another immunomodulating agent baricitinib is a Janus kinase (JAK) inhibitor, a subgroup of tyrosine kinase inhibitors. It impedes cytokine-mediated signalling and is thought to interfere with intracellular entry and assembly of the SARS-CoV-2 virus. Current guidelines recommend its concomitant use with corticosteroids in hospitalised people with COVID-19 who require supplemental oxygen and/or non-invasive ventilation. It is important to note that, although both baricitinib and tocilizumab are recommended, only one of these agents should be used, as dual use may increase the risk of opportunistic infections.

People with SARS-CoV-2 infections are at increased risk of venous thromboembolism (VTE). Use of VTE prophylaxis is recommended in those with moderate, severe or critical COVID-19. Low-molecular-weight heparins or unfractionated heparins should be chosen, depending on individualised clinical indications. Unless otherwise clinically indicated, it is not recommended to discharge a person on apixaban for VTE prophylaxis unless they have developed a VTE event in hospital.

Finally, it is important to note that there are some substances which people were taking (with or without medical guidance), which through research and evidence-based medicine have been identified as ineffectual, exceeding reasonable risk–benefit ratios, or in some situations dangerous. Drugs such as ivermectin, hydroxychloroquine, azithromycin, colchicine and convalescent plasma are some agents that should not be used for COVID-19 disease.

Other interventions, once beneficial, are also now not recommended, such as the antivirals favipiravir and lopinavir-ritonavir, and previously used monoclonal antibodies such as tixagevimab plus cilgavimab (Evusheld) for prophylaxis (unless in exceptional circumstances in individuals who are severely compromised). Interferon β_{1a}, with or without antivirals, is also not recommended. Finally, aspirin is not recommended except in children with PIMS-TS who are treated with IVIg, corticosteroids, or biological agents such as anti IL-6 or anti-TNF.

The future

The WHO identifies 'priority' pathogens as those that require immediate attention, because they potentially possess the capacity to cause severe outbreaks for which we currently have few to no medical countermeasures. Other conditions are designated as having an epidemic potential, but are not considered as much of a priority as there are currently significant disease control efforts and research networks (see Table 8.5). These diseases are reviewed annually, and the list is adjusted accordingly.

As of November 2022, in Australia, *Japanese encephalitis virus (JEV)* has been identified as a 'communicable disease incident of national significance' with 46 cases since January, 2021. Although case numbers are low, 19% of the laboratory-confirmed cases have died. Surveillance will continue and reporting will occur through the National Notifiable Diseases Surveillance System.

Mpox (formally known as 'monkeypox') is another zoonosis which has been recently declared a communicable disease incident of national significance in Australia. Mpox was found in 1958 in laboratory monkeys in Denmark, and in 1970 was reported to have jumped the species gap with the first human infection reported in a person in the Democratic Republic of Congo. It was considered endemic only in Central and West Africa, with numerous outbreaks up until 2003, when sporadic outbreaks began in other countries. Recently, it has become a concern with larger outbreaks occurring in non-endemic countries. In July 2022, Mpox was identified as a 'public health emergency of international concern (PHEIC)' by the WHO. By the end of 2022 there were more than 81,000 laboratory-confirmed cases spanning 110 countries; however, in Australia there were only 144 cases. Public health preparations are detailed in National Guidelines, outlining comprehensive principle protection methods for public health units and health care facilities, and the government has secured a vaccine stockpile.

Table 8.5 WHO current and emerging infectious disease priorities

COVID-19
Crimean-Congo haemorrhagic fever
Ebola virus disease and Marburg virus disease
Lassa fever
Middle East respiratory syndrome coronavirus (MERS-CoV)
Severe acute respiratory syndrome (SARS)
Nipah and henipaviral diseases
Rift Valley fever
Zika
'Disease X'*

* Disease X represents the knowledge that a serious international epidemic could be caused by a pathogen currently unknown to cause human disease. The R&D Blueprint explicitly seeks to enable early cross-cutting R&D preparedness that is also relevant for an unknown 'Disease X'.

Source: Data from World Health Organization (2023a).

As in the case of COVID-19, various factors have contributed to the spread of infection, including population density, increased speed of travel, pathogen virulence, poor living standards, natural disasters, deforestation, changes in agricultural practices, and interaction and/or consumption with wild animals. Challenges to defeat these pathogens are multifaceted; however, with improved surveillance, increased research and development on antimicrobial resistance, and the identification and correction of the factors contributing to increased spread, we can prevail.

INDIGENOUS HEALTH FAST FACTS AND CULTURAL CONSIDERATIONS

FAST FACTS

- *Aboriginal and Torres Strait Islander peoples are 8 times more likely than non-Indigenous Australians to develop and be hospitalised for a skin infection resulting in Group A streptococcal bacteraemia.*
- *The incidence of blood-borne viruses and sexually transmitted infections is significantly higher in Aboriginal and Torres Strait Islander peoples compared to non-Indigenous Australians: chlamydia (2.8:1), gonorrhoea (6.9:1), infectious syphilis (5.8:1), newly diagnosed hepatitis B (1.3:1) and hepatitis C (4.5:1).*
- *As a result of the lockdowns that occurred due to COVID-19 infection control measures, STIs notifications reduced significantly. However, Māori and Pacific Islands people are still over-represented in blood-borne and sexually transmitted infection statistics compared to European New Zealanders. It is important to note that sexually transmitted infections do not require mandatory notification in New Zealand, and so these figures are based on the voluntary provision of data from sexual health clinics and positive laboratory surveillance data findings from participating laboratories. These factors contribute to an overall underestimation of the burden of the problem for all ethnicities.*

CULTURAL CONSIDERATIONS

- *Overall, morbidity and mortality rates related to infection in Aboriginal and Torres Strait Islander peoples are significantly higher compared to non-Indigenous Australians. Factors contributing to the increased risk of infection include environmental health factors, such as inadequate infrastructure, overcrowding and reduced access to tradespeople for repairs, which is often exacerbated by the remoteness of communities. Nutritional influences include reduced access to and consumption of fruit and vegetables, and, most importantly, reduced*

breastfeeding rates. Aboriginal and Torres Strait Island babies are more than 2 times less likely than non-Indigenous Australian babies to have been breastfed, or have been breastfed for less than one month. Interestingly, this rate is seemingly not influenced by geographical remoteness. Alongside the need for increased access to services that can improve infrastructure, and provide appropriate accommodation and access to fresh food, it is clear that the development of culturally appropriate, community-centred education regarding the importance of breast milk in a child's development and for the reduction of infection rates will be critical to begin to reduce the health disparities for Aboriginal and Torres Strait Islander peoples.

Sources: Data from AIHW(2023); New Zealand Ministry of Health (2018, 2021); Nguyen et al. (2022); Springall et al. (2022).

CHILDREN AND ADOLESCENTS

- Common childhood infections include viruses such as respiratory syncytial virus (RSV), chickenpox (varicella) and rotavirus. Common acute bacterial infections can cause gastroenteritis and urinary tract, skin and upper respiratory tract infections. *Streptococcal* infections are commonly associated with sore throats, but can also cause any number of other infections. Highly infectious diseases such as pertussis (whooping cough) are spread by the vaccine-preventable *Bordetella pertussis*, which can cause severe respiratory symptoms in children under 5 years of age.
- Middle-ear infections are common in children, and can cause earache or even deafness. Otitis externa can be caused by bacteria or a fungus, and is common in children who swim a lot. Otitis media can be caused by a virus or bacteria, and result in such significant increases in pressure that the tympanic membrane may perforate.

OLDER ADULTS

- Infections in the older person are generally more frequent and more severe compared with those in younger adults.
- Increased infections in older adults may be related to immunosenescence, poorer nutrition and decreasing first-line defences, such as poorer skin integrity, reduced mucociliary clearance, and reduced cough and swallow reflexes.

KEY CLINICAL ISSUES

- Interrupting the chain of transmission of infection at any step will reduce infection rates. An understanding of how the components of the chain can be manipulated will provide a health care professional with powerful tools to improve infection control.
- Age, chronic illness and some pharmacological agents can cause a person to become immunocompromised. Working with individuals who have altered immune defences requires even more care and attention to the principles of infection control.
- Basic hand-washing significantly reduces the transmission of pathogens to individuals, fomites and the environment.
- Antimicrobial resistance is developing for numerous reasons. Ensure that education regarding the importance of completing an antimicrobial course is included as part of the teaching undertaken prior to discharge.
- Several opportunities for antimicrobial spillage into the environment can occur when reconstituting, drawing up, administering and discarding equipment used in the delivery of intravenous antimicrobials. Follow best practice principles to reduce the risk of extending antimicrobial resistance.
- Treatment of the whole family should be undertaken when an individual presents with a helminthic infection.
- Some helminthic, protozoal and parasitic infections may require the rigorous cleaning of bed linen, clothes and the environment to achieve total eradication.

CHAPTER REVIEW

- *Bacteria* are *prokaryotic* cells that are classified by their staining properties, motility, shape and whether they use oxygen-dependent metabolic processes.
- *Fungi* are *eukaryotic* cells. A fungal infection is called a *mycosis*, and can be superficial, subcutaneous or systemic.
- *Viruses* are the smallest infective organisms. They consist of nucleic acids, either DNA or RNA, contained within a protein capsule.

- *Parasitic* infections are caused by protozoa, helminths (worms) or arthropods. Parasitic infections are generally more common in the developing world.
- The *chain of transmission* is a framework for understanding infection. The three main components are a *reservoir of infective organisms*, the *mode of transmission to humans* and a *way of entering the human body*.
- Typical reservoirs of infection include soil, other humans and non-human animals.
- The mode of transmission can be via *direct* contact with a reservoir, or through *indirect* contact with a contaminated inanimate object—a *fomite*.
- Infective organisms enter human bodies through *portals of entry*—natural body orifices or a breach in the skin.
- Some microbes colonise our bodies without inducing disease. These organisms are called the *natural flora*.
- *Pathogenicity* is the capacity of an organism to damage cells and induce human disease.
- *Virulence* is the degree of pathogenicity of an infective organism, and is linked to its ability to induce disease. Virulence depends on a number of factors, such as the ability to enter the body, to adhere to tissue surfaces, to invade surrounding tissues and to hide from immune cells.
- Factors that influence the onset and duration of infection include age, health, nutrition and immune status.
- The main approach in controlling infection is to *break the chain* of transmission. This involves depleting the reservoir of infection, creating barriers to disrupt transmission and preventing entry into our bodies.
- Antimicrobials are useful in treating or preventing infection. The principle of *selective toxicity* guides their mechanism of action. The drugs target structures and processes that are not present or work differently in humans.
- Antimicrobial *resistance* is a major concern. Resistance to an antimicrobial drug's action develops spontaneously or is acquired from other microbes. Poor practices associated with their use contribute to its spread in the community.
- COVID-19 pandemic started in late 2019, and is still continuing globally in 2023 (three years later). The continued pursuit for knowledge and critical understanding of infection control, public health, and emerging communicable threats may help regions, countries and the globe reduce the catastrophic influence of future pandemics.

REVIEW QUESTIONS

1. Outline the chain of transmission for infectious diseases.
2. Define the following terms:
   a. opportunistic infection
   b. virulence
   c. normal flora
   d. pathogenicity
   e. sepsis
3. Outline how age and health status can affect the susceptibility of a person to an infection.
4. State ways in which we can disrupt an infectious organism's mode of transmission to humans.
5. Describe four general mechanisms of action of antimicrobials.
6. State three ways that antimicrobial resistance can develop.
7. State three ways in which antimicrobial resistance can be spread through the community.
8. Outline the defining characteristics of the following infective organisms:
   a. fungi
   b. viruses
   c. bacteria
9. Using malaria as an example, outline the chain of transmission, and indicate ways that the chain can be broken for this particular disease.
10. Describe at least 10 methods to reduce the risk of pathological transmission that individuals and communities can employ to mitigate future pandemics.

HEALTH PROFESSIONAL CONNECTIONS

Midwives Apart from the obvious body fluid risks to which midwives are exposed, neonates can become infected by a mother. Infection may occur in utero, or even as late as exposure to sexually transmitted infections when delivery occurs through a normal vaginal delivery. Ensure that you maintain appropriate standard precautions when caring for both the mother and the newborn.

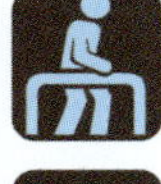

Physiotherapists/Exercise scientists When working with individuals requiring rehabilitation for mobility issues, always monitor for bone pain, especially if the client has experienced an active infection during the recovery. Bone does not need to be injured for osteomyelitis to occur. Haematogenous osteomyelitis is possible where the infection is spread to the bone via the blood.

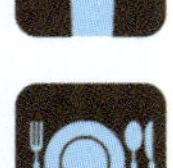

Nutritionists/Dieticians Individuals with active infections have excessive metabolic needs and require increased nutritional and caloric support. Individuals with poor nutrition have an increased risk of infection. Appropriate assessment and planning is crucial to promote (or maintain) optimal nutrition in order to assist in the combat of infection or decrease the risk.

All allied professionals Infection control principles and standard precautions should always be practised. Standard precautions protect health care workers from an increased risk of exposure to pathogens. However, knowledge of a client's 'infection status' will not protect you. In fact, your perceived knowledge about a person's infection status may lead you to become complacent with appropriate infection control practices. Irrespective of what is documented, no one will necessarily know exactly what infections an individual has—potentially not even the affected person.

CASE STUDY

Mr James Gunning, who is 21 years of age (UR number 478002), presented two weeks ago with an accidental self-inflicted gunshot wound to his right upper leg. He underwent a surgical exploration of the wound, haemostasis was achieved, the entry and exit wounds were cleaned and dressed, and a backslab cast was placed on his leg. Both the X-ray and the open inspection confirmed a small fracture on the medial aspect of the right femur from the bullet. Mr Gunning was discharged two days later with oral antimicrobials and crutches. Yesterday, he presented to the emergency department with a painful, red and swollen thigh, with a malodorous, green-coloured purulent exudate from both the entry and exit wounds. Further investigation revealed osteomyelitis. He is booked for surgical debridement this morning. His observations were as follows:

Temperature	Heart rate	Respiration rate	Blood pressure	SpO_2
39.2°C	98	22	138/80	98% (RA*)

*RA = room air.

His haematology and microbiology results have returned as follows:

HAEMATOLOGY

Patient location:	Ward 3	**UR:**	478002		
Consultant:	Smith	**NAME:**	Gunning		
		Given name:	James	**Sex:**	M
		DOB:	27/08/XX	**Age:**	21

Time collected	09:30
Date collected	XX/XX
Year	XXXX
Lab #	46565465

FULL BLOOD COUNT		UNITS	REFERENCE RANGE
Haemoglobin	145	g/L	115–160
White cell count	13.2	$\times 10^9$/L	4.0–11.0
Platelets	220	$\times 10^9$/L	140–400
Haematocrit	0.42		0.33–0.47
Red cell count	3.89	$\times 10^{12}$/L	3.80–5.20
Reticulocyte count	2.8	%	0.2–2.0
MCV	93	fL	80–100
Neutrophils	9.2	$\times 10^9$/L	2.00–8.00
Lymphocytes	2.71	$\times 10^9$/L	1.00–4.00
Monocytes	0.42	$\times 10^9$/L	0.10–1.00
Eosinophils	0.41	$\times 10^9$/L	< 0.60
Basophils	0.08	$\times 10^9$/L	< 0.20
ESR	11	mm/h	< 12

MICROBIOLOGY

Patient location:	Ward 3	**UR:**	478002		
Consultant:	Smith	**NAME:**	Gunning		
		Given name:	James	**Sex:**	M
		DOB:	27/08/XX	**Age:**	21

Time collected	18:10	**Organisms**	**1.** *Staphylococcus aureus*
Date collected	XX/XX	**Isolated**	**2.** *Pseudomonas aeruginosa*
Year	XXXX		
Lab #	15698656		

Specimen site	Entry wound R)leg	**Antimicrobial sensitivities S = Sensitive R = Resistant**					
Leukocytes	++	Organism	1	2	Organism	1	2
Erythrocytes	trace	Ampicillin	R	R	Flucloxacillin	R	R
Proteins	++	Amoxicillin	R	R	Gentamicin	S	S
		Cefotaxime			Rifampicin		
		Ceftriaxone		R	Sodium fusidate	S	S
		Cephalothin	R	R	Ticarcillin		
		Chloramphenicol			Timentin	S	S
		Cotrimoxazole	R	S	Trimethoprim	S	S
		Erythromycin	S	S	Vancomycin		
Gram stain	**Gram-negative**	✓					
	Gram-positive	✓					
	Bacilli	✓					
	Cocci	✓					
	Other						

CRITICAL THINKING

1. Observe the pathology results for Mr Gunning. What pathogen/s has/have caused the osteomyelitis? What are the characteristics of this/these pathogen/s?
2. Using your knowledge of the chain of infection and the history provided, identify how this infection could have occurred. Relate your answer back to each step of the chain. Explore each parameter fully.
3. Using the history and observations provided, identify and explain all of the data that demonstrate that an infective process has occurred.
4. Apart from surgical debridement, what other management options should/will be undertaken? Explain the mechanism of each of these management options.
5. Explore the microbiology report with a specific focus on the sensitivity and resistance testing. Explain how sensitivity and resistance testing is undertaken. What antimicrobials are appropriate for Mr Gunning? Why? Which antimicrobials are inappropriate for Mr Gunning? Why?

BIBLIOGRAPHY

Australian Bureau of Statistics (ABS) (2022). *Causes of death, Australia, 2022.* Canberra: ABS. http://www.abs.gov.au/statistics/health/causes-death.

Australian Bureau of Statistics (ABS) (2023). *COVID-19 mortality in Australia: deaths registered until 31 January 2023.* Canberra: ABS. https://www.abs.gov.au/articles/covid-19-mortality-australia-deaths-registered-until-31-january-2023.

Australian Institute of Health and Welfare (2020). *Aboriginal and Torres Strait Islander Health Performance Framework 2020 report.* Canberra: Australian Government Department of Health. https://www.indigenoushpf.gov.au/publications/hpf-summary-2020.

Australian Institute of Health and Welfare (AIHW) (2020). *Australia's children.* Cat. No. CWS 69. Canberra: AIHW. https://www.aihw.gov.au/getmedia/6af928d6-692e-4449-b915-cf2ca946982f/aihw-cws-69-print-report.pdf.

Australian Institute of Health and Welfare (AIHW) (2022). *Australia's health 2022: data insights.* Australia's Health series No. 18. Cat. No. AUS 240, Canberra: AIHW. https://www.aihw.gov.au/reports/australias-health/australias-health-2022-data-insights/about.

Australian Institute of Health and Welfare (AIHW) (2022). *Principal diagnosis data cubes: separation statistics by principal diagnosis (ICD-10-AM 11th edition), Australia, 2020–21.* Canberra: AIHW. https://www.aihw.gov.au/reports/hospitals/principal-diagnosis-data-cubes/contents/data-cubes.

Australian Institute of Health and Welfare (AIHW) (2023). *Aboriginal and Torres Strait Islander Health Performance Framework: summary report 2023.* Canberra: AIHW. https://www.indigenoushpf.gov.au/Report-overview/Overview/Summary-Report.

Bauldoff, G., Gubrud-Howe, P.M., Carno, M.-A., Levett-Jones, T., Hales, M., Berry, K., … Stanley, D. (2020). *LeMone and Burke's medical–surgical nursing: critical thinking for person-centred care* (4th [Australian] edn). Sydney: Pearson Australia.

Bergman, S.J., Cennimo, D.J., Miller, M.M. & Olsen, K.M. (2023). COVID-19 treatment: investigational drugs and other therapies. *Emedicine.* https://emedicine.medscape.com/article/2500116-overview.

Best, O. & Fredericks, B. (2021). *Yatdjuligin: Aboriginal and Torres Strait Islander nursing and midwifery care.* (3rd edn). Port Melbourne, VIC: Cambridge University Press.

Borczuk, A.C. & Yantiss, R.K. (2022). The pathogenesis of coronavirus-19 disease. *Journal of Biomedical Science* 29:87. https://doi.org/10.1186/s12929-022-00872-5.

Bullock, S. & Manias, E. (2022). *Fundamentals of pharmacology* (9th edn). Sydney: Pearson Australia.

Castanares-Zapatero, D., Chalon, P., Kohn, L., Dauvrin, M., Detollenaere, J., Maertens de Noordhout, C., … Van den Heede, K. (2022). Pathophysiology and mechanism of long COVID: a comprehensive review. *Annals of Medicine (Helsinki)* 54(1):1473–87. https://doi.org/10.1080/07853890.2022.2076901.

Cennimo, D., Bergman, S.J. & Olsen, K.M. (2023). Coronavirus disease 2019 (COVID-19). *Emedicine.* https://emedicine.medscape.com/article/2500114-overview.

Clarke, S.A., Abbara, A. & Dhillo, W.S. (2022). Impact of COVID-19 on the endocrine system: a mini-review. *Endocrinology* 163(1): article bqab203. https://doi.org/10.1210/endocr/bqab203.

Davis, H.E., McCorkell, L., Vogel, J.M. & Topol, E.J. (2023). Long COVID: major findings, mechanisms and recommendations. *Nature Reviews Microbiology* 21(3):133–46. https://doi.org/10.1038/s41579-022-00846-2.

Davis, J.S., Jones, C.A., Cheng, A.C. & Howden, B.P. (2019). Australia's response to the global threat of antimicrobial resistance: past, present and future. *Medical Journal of Australia* 211(3):106–108.e1. https://doi.org/10.5694/mja2.50264.

de Andrade, S.A., de Souza, D.A., Torres, A.L., de Lima, C.F.G., Ebram, M.C., Celano, R.M.G., … Chudzinski-Tavassi, A.M. (2022). Pathophysiology of COVID-19: critical role of hemostasis. *Frontiers in Cellular and Infection Microbiology* 12:896972. https://doi.org/10.3389/fcimb.2022.896972.

Department of Health and Aged Care (2020). *National review of hotel quarantine*. Canberra: Department of Health and Aged Care. https://www.health.gov.au/resources/publications/national-review-of-hotel-quarantine?language=en.

Department of Health and Aged Care (2022). *Monkeypox virus infection: CDNA National Guidelines for Public Health Units.* Canberra: Department of Health and Aged Care. https://www.health.gov.au/sites/default/files/2022-12/monkeypox-virus-infection-cdna-national-guidelines-for-public-health-units.pdf.

Department of Health and Aged Care (2023a). COVID-19 outbreaks in Australian residential aged care facilities: National snapshot. Canberra: Department of Health and Aged Care. https://www.health.gov.au/sites/default/files/2023-03/covid-19-outbreaks-in-australian-residential-aged-care-facilities-3-march-2023_0.pdf.

Department of Health and Aged Care (2023b). *Health alerts: Japanese encephalitis virus (JEV).* Canberra: Department of Health and Aged Care. https://www.health.gov.au/health-alerts/japanese-encephalitis-virus-jev/japanese-encephalitis-virus-jev.

Department of Health and Aged Care (2023c). *National Notifiable Disease Surveillance System.* Canberra: Department of Health and Aged Care. https://www.health.gov.au/resources/publications/national-notifiable-diseases-surveillance-system-nndss-fortnightly-reports-23-january-2023-to-5-february-2023?language=en.

El-Saber Batiha, G., Al-Gareeb, A.I., Saad, H.M., & Al-Kuraishy, H.M. (2022). COVID-19 and corticosteroids: a narrative review. *Inflammopharmacology* 30(4):1189–1205. https://doi.org/10.1007/s10787-022-00987-z.

Gandhi P.A., Patro, S.K., Sandeep, M., Satapathy, P., Shamim, M.A., Kumar, V., … Sah, R. (2023). Oral manifestation of the monkeypox virus: a systematic review and meta-analysis. *eClinicalMedicine* 56:101817. https://doi.org/10.1016/j.eclinm.2022.101817.

Groff, A., Kavanaugh, M., Ramgobin, D., McClafferty, B., Aggarwal, C.S., Golamari, R. & Jain, R. (2021). Gastrointestinal manifestations of COVID-19: a review of what we know. *Ochsner Journal* 21(2):177–80. https://doi.org/10.31486/toj.20.0086.

Jackson, C.B., Farzan, M., Chen, B. & Choe, H. (2022). Mechanisms of SARS-CoV-2 entry into cells. *Nature Reviews Molecular Cell Biology* 23(1):3–20. https://doi.org/10.1038/s41580-021-00418-x.

Lamers, M.M. & Haagmans, B.L. (2022). SARS-CoV-2 pathogenesis. *Nature Reviews Microbiology* 20:270–84. https://doi.org/10.1038/s41579-022-00713-0.

Lu, R., Zhao, X., Li, J., Niu, P., Yang, B., Wu, H., … Tan, W. (2020). Genomic characterisation and epidemiology of 2019 novel coronavirus: implications for virus origins and receptor binding. *The Lancet* 395(10224):565–74. https://doi.org/10.1016/S0140-6736(20)30251-8.

Lumlertgul, N., Baker, E., Pearson, E., Dalrymple, K.V., Pan, J., Jheeta, A., … Ostermann, M. (2022). Changing epidemiology of acute kidney injury in critically ill patients with COVID-19: a prospective cohort. *Annals of Intensive Care* 12(1):118. https://doi.org/10.1186/s13613-022-01094-6.

Marieb, E.N. & Hoehn, K. (2019). *Human anatomy and physiology* (11th edn). San Francisco, CA: Pearson Benjamin Cummings.

Martínez-Baz, I., Miqueleiz, A., Egüés, N., Casado, I., Burgui, C., Echeverría, A., … Castilla, J. (2023). Effect of COVID-19 vaccination on the SARS-CoV-2 transmission among social and household close contacts: a cohort study. *Journal of Infection and Public Health* 16(3):410–17. https://doi.org/10.1016/j.jiph.2023.01.017.

Mesquita, J. (2021). Emerging and re-emerging diseases: novel challenges in today's world. *Animals* 11(8):2383. https://doi.org/10.3390/ani11082382.

Murray, P.R., Rosenthal, K.S., & Pfaller, M.A. (2021). *Medical microbiology* (9th edn). Philadelphia, PA: Elsevier.

National Clinical Evidence Taskforce—COVID-19 (2023). *Australian guidelines for the clinical care of people with COVID-19.* https://files.magicapp.org/guideline/8b6f065b-814f-41f0-a1a5-70279b722e19/published_guideline_4346-12_0.pdf.

New Zealand Ministry of Health (2018). Infectious disease. *Tatau kahukura—Māori health statistics: ngā mana hauora tūohu—health status indicators.* Wellington: Ministry of Health. https://www.health.govt.nz/our-work/populations/maori-health/tatau-kahukura-maori-health-statistics/nga-mana-hauora-tutohu-health-status-indicators/infectious-disease.

New Zealand Ministry of Health (2021). *Sexually transmitted infections in New Zealand: Supplementary annual surveillance report 2021.* Wellington: Ministry of Health. https://surv.esr.cri.nz/PDF_surveillance/STISurvRpt/2021/FINAL_STI_supplementaryreport_2021.pdf.

New Zealand Ministry of Health (2023). *COVID-19: current cases.* Wellington: Ministry of Health. https://www.health.govt.nz/covid-19-novel-coronavirus/covid-19-data-and-statistics/covid-19-current-cases.

Nguyen, A.D.K., Smith, S., Davis, T.J., Yarwood, T. & Hanson, J. (2022). The efficacy and safety of a shortened duration of antimicrobial therapy for group A *Streptococcus* bacteremia. *International Journal of Infectious Diseases* 128:11–19. https://doi.org/10.1016/j.ijid.2022.12.015.

Nitan, P., Nandhakumar, R., Vidyhra, B., Rajesh, S. & Sakunthala, A. (2022). COVID-19: invasion, pathogenesis and possible cure—a review. *Journal of Virological Methods* 300:114434. https://doi.org/10.1016/j.jviromet.2021.114434.

Office of the Prime Minister's Chief Science Advisor (2021). *Kotahitanga: Uniting Aotearoa against infectious disease and antimicrobial resistance.* Auckland: Office of the Prime Minister's Chief Science Advisor. https://cpb-ap-se2.wpmucdn.com/blogs.auckland.ac.nz/dist/f/688/files/2022/06/OPMCSA-AMR-Full-report-FINAL-V3-PDF.pdf.

Parasher, A. (2021). COVID-19: current understanding of its pathophysiology, clinical presentation and treatment. *Postgraduate Medical Journal* 97(1147):312–20. https://doi.org/10.1136/postgradmedj-2020-138577.

Pereira, A.A., de Oliveira Andrade, A., de Andrade Palis, A., Cabral, A.M., Barreto, C.G.L., de Souza, D.B., … da Conceição Lima, V. (2022). Non-pharmacological treatments for COVID-19: current status and consensus. *Research on Biomedical Engineering* 38(1):193–208. https://doi.org/10.1007/s42600-020-00116-1.

Pulingam, T., Parumasivam, T., Gazzali, A.M., Sulaiman, A.M., Chee, J.Y., Lakshmanan, M., … Sudesh, K. (2022). Antimicrobial resistance: prevalence, economic burden, mechanisms of resistance and strategies to overcome. *European Journal of Pharmaceutical Sciences* 170:106103. https://doi.org/10.1016/j.ejps.2021.106103.

Rahmati, M., Koyanagi, A., Banitalebi, E., Yon, D.K., Lee, S.W., Il Shin, J. & Smith, L. (2023). The effect of SARS-CoV-2 infection on cardiac function in post-COVID-19 survivors: a systematic review and meta-analysis. *Journal of Medical Virology* 95(1):e28325. https://doi.org/10.1002/jmv.28325.

Salamanna, F., Maglio, M., Landini, M.P. & Fini, M. (2020). Body localization of ACE-2: on the trail of the keyhole of SARS-CoV-2. *Frontiers in Medicine* 7:594495. https://doi.org/10.3389/fmed.2020.594495.

Springall, T.L., McLachlan, H.L., Forster, D.A., Browne, J. & Chamberlain, C. (2022). Breastfeeding rates of Aboriginal and Torres Strait Islander women in Australia: a systematic review and narrative analysis. *Women and Birth* 35(6):e624–e638. https://doi.org/10.1016/j.wombi.2022.02.011.

Tan, C.C.S., Lam, S.D., Richard, D., Owen, C.J., Berchtold, D., Orengo, C., … Balloux, F. (2022). Transmission of SARS-CoV-2 from humans to animals and potential host adaptation. *Nature Communications* 13(1):1–13. https://doi.org/10.1038/s41467-022-30698-6.

Tortora. G.J., Derrickson, B., Burkett, B., Peoples, G., Dye, D., Cooke, J., … Green, H. (2022). *Principles of anatomy and physiology* (3rd Asia-Pacific edn). Milton, QLD: John Wiley and Sons.

Tudoran, C., Bende, F., Bende, R., Giurgi-Oncu, C., Dumache, R., & Tudoran, M. (2023). Correspondence between aortic and arterial stiffness, and diastolic dysfunction in apparently healthy female patients with post-acute COVID-19 syndrome. *Biomedicines* 11(2):492. http://dx.doi.org/10.3390/biomedicines11020492.

vanMeter, K., & Hubert, R. (2021). *Microbiology for the healthcare professional* (3rd edn). St Louis, MO: Elsevier

Wang, W.-H., Thitithanyanont, A., Urbina, A.N. & Wang, S.-F. (2021). Emerging and re-emerging diseases. *Pathogens* 10(7):827. https://doi.org/10.3390/pathogens10070827.

World Health Organization (WHO) (2023). *Coronavirus—Australia.* https://covid19.who.int/region/wpro/country/au.

World Health Organization (WHO) (2023). *Prioritizing diseases for research and development in emergency contexts.* https://www.who.int/activities/prioritizing-diseases-for-research-and-development-in-emergency-contexts.

Zay Ya, K., Win, P.T.N., Bielicki, J., Lambiris, M., & Fink, G. (2023). Association between antimicrobial stewardship programs and antibiotic use globally: a systematic review and meta-analysis. *JAMA Network Open* 6(2):e2253806. https://doi.org/10.1001/jamanetworkopen.2022.53806.

PART 3

Nervous system pathophysiology

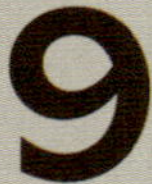

Brain and spinal cord dysfunction

KEY TERMS

Aneurysm
Arteriovenous malformation (AVM)
Ataxia
Athetosis
AVPU scale
Brain abscess
Cerebral infarction
Cerebral ischaemia
Cerebral palsy
Cerebrovascular accident (CVA, or stroke)
Consciousness
Encephalitis
Glasgow coma scale (GCS)
Guillain–Barré syndrome
Hydrocephalus
Meningitis
Meningocele
Myelomeningocele
Neural tube defects
Reticular activating system (RAS)
Spina bifida
Stroke
Transient ischaemic attack (TIA)

LEARNING OBJECTIVES

After completing this chapter, you should be able to:

1. Discuss the different definitions of consciousness.
2. Describe the key brain regions involved in the control of consciousness.
3. Name the acute and chronic levels of altered consciousness, and briefly define them.
4. Name the clinical tests used to assess consciousness.
5. Define a 'cerebrovascular accident', state the main types, identify the key risk factors and outline the pathophysiology of this condition.
6. Describe the clinical manifestations, diagnosis and clinical management of cerebrovascular accidents.
7. Define the main kinds of CNS infection, and the pathogens associated with both mild and severe infections.
8. Outline the pathophysiology, clinical manifestations, clinical diagnosis and management of CNS infections.
9. Outline the pathophysiology, clinical manifestations, clinical diagnosis and management of Guillain–Barré syndrome.
10. State the causes, pathophysiology, clinical manifestations, diagnosis and management of hydrocephalus.
11. Compare and contrast the characteristics of hydrocephalus in adults and infants.
12. Define 'cerebral palsy', and outline the clinical manifestations, diagnosis and management of this condition.
13. Outline the role of the cerebellum, and the likely clinical manifestations of cerebellar disorders in general.
14. Define the neural tube defect 'spina bifida', and outline the clinical manifestations, diagnosis and management of this condition.
15. Compare and contrast spina bifida and anencephaly.

WHAT YOU SHOULD KNOW BEFORE YOU START THIS CHAPTER

Can you describe the types of cellular adaptation?

Can you describe the mechanisms of cellular injury?

Can you describe cerebrospinal fluid dynamics?

Can you outline the major steps in the process of neurotransmission?

Can you outline the organisation of the cerebral vasculature?

Can you outline the anatomical organisation of the central nervous system?

Introduction

In this chapter, you will examine a number of important acute and chronic conditions affecting the *central nervous system (CNS)*. Cerebrovascular accidents, CNS infections, Guillain–Barré syndrome, hydrocephalus, cerebellar disorders and the neural tube defect called spina bifida will be described.

These conditions are associated with a range of causes, including trauma, infection, inheritance, tumours and congenital malformations. When the nervous system is compromised, the effects on the affected person may be life-threatening, and the care required can be intensive and prolonged.

Consciousness

LEARNING OBJECTIVE 1

Discuss the different definitions of consciousness.

Consciousness is an essential part of the human experience, but the term itself is ambiguous. Consciousness can refer equally to the waking state, a state of being 'self-aware', or the possessing of a unique record of past experience (which is referred to as the 'autobiographical self'). A person who is fully conscious is *awake and alert*, responsive to stimuli and aware of their surroundings and responses. At one level this is called *self-awareness*, but at another level it can also be taken to mean that a person is *'aware that they are aware'*. This higher-level cognition is closely linked to the functioning of the human mind, which is not well understood.

THE NEUROPHYSIOLOGY OF CONSCIOUSNESS

LEARNING OBJECTIVE 2

Describe the key brain regions involved in the control of consciousness.

The **reticular activating system (RAS)** plays a key role in the control of consciousness, in terms of maintaining arousal and the waking state. The RAS consists of most of the brainstem and the thalamus. It also has projections from the posterior hypothalamus, which is involved in the control of the sleep–wake cycle. The influences of the RAS descend to the spinal cord and ascend to the cerebral cortex (see Figure 9.1). The RAS has also been implicated in the control of mood, attention, motivation, learning, memory and skeletal muscle movement. A number of neurotransmitters contribute to its function, including acetylcholine, noradrenaline, gamma-aminobutyric acid (GABA), histamine, dopamine and serotonin.

The RAS receives motor information from higher brain regions on its way down to skeletal muscles, and makes a valuable contribution to the control of muscle tone. It also receives a variety of sensory inputs from the periphery, and relays them up to the cerebral cortex. A rise in the activity in the RAS can occur as a result of increased sensory stimulation (visual, auditory, gustatory, tactile or nociceptive inputs) and/or skeletal muscle activity (which increases proprioceptive input). Enhanced RAS activation heightens cortical activity, resulting in increased arousal. An example of this is when you find yourself sitting in a boring lecture and you feel yourself dozing off; by wriggling your toes, stretching your legs or scratching your head you can often keep yourself awake.

ALTERATIONS IN THE LEVEL OF CONSCIOUSNESS

LEARNING OBJECTIVE 3

Name the acute and chronic levels of altered consciousness, and briefly define them.

Altered states of consciousness develop when the activity of the RAS becomes greatly diminished. Cortical neurons are very susceptible to insult, and decreased cortical activity can rapidly lead to changes in consciousness. Alterations in cognition and memory are usually apparent early as consciousness changes, giving rise to disorientation to time, place and person. There are seven acute levels of consciousness that primarily relate to changes in the waking state. In order from the highest to the lowest level, they are: fully conscious, confusion, delirium, lethargy, obtundation, stupor and coma. A standard definition of each level is provided in Table 9.1.

Figure 9.1

The reticular activating system

Sensory information entering the reticular formation can lead to widespread activation of the cortex, raising levels of arousal and wakefulness. Motor information also passes through the reticular formation as it descends towards spinal pathways.

Source: Marieb, E.N. et al., Human anatomy and physiology *(11th edn, Global Edition), © 2019, Figure 12.18, p. 453. Reprinted by permission of Pearson Education Limited.*

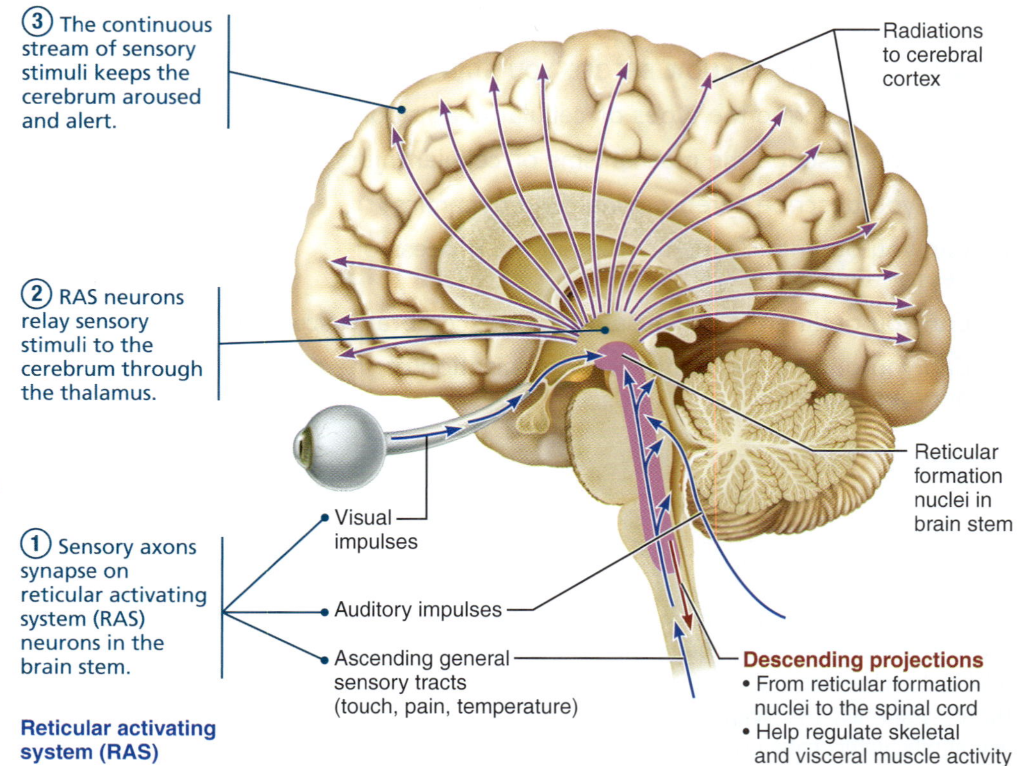

Table 9.1 Levels of consciousness

Level	Description
Fully conscious	The state of being awake and alert: aware of one's environment, and capable of responding to it appropriately
Confusion	The affected person is disoriented to time and place; they have difficulty following instructions
Delirium	The affected person experiences disorientation and mental confusion as a result of hallucinations and delusions
Lethargy	The affected person is drowsy, but can be aroused by moderate stimuli
Obtundation	The affected person is more drowsy than in lethargy, with less interest in their environment and slowed responses when roused
Stupor	The affected person can be aroused only by vigorous stimulation, and immediately lapses into their previously unresponsive state
Coma	The affected person is unresponsive and cannot be aroused from this state

Many pathologies can result in *alterations in the level of consciousness (ALOC)*. One method of organising possible causes of ALOC is by dividing them into intracranial and extracranial causes (see Table 9.2). *Intracranial causes* are related to the direct impact on anatomical structures, whereas *extracranial causes* are those related to secondary insult from issues originating outside the cranial vault. Chronic pathological alterations in consciousness can develop following a brain insult, including persistent coma, the 'locked-in' syndrome and a vegetative state.

Table 9.2 Common causes of altered level of consciousness (ALOC)

Intracranial causes	Extracranial causes
• Head injury • Haemorrhage • Degenerative conditions • Space-occupying lesions (SOL) • Increased intracranial pressure • Vasospasm of cerebral vasculature • Seizures	• Hypoxia • Hypertension • Profound hypotension • Systemic infection • Hepatic or renal dysfunction • Hypo- or hyperglycaemia • Electrolyte imbalance • pH imbalance • Drugs, particularly in overdose

Persistent coma involves unconsciousness and an absence of the sleep–wake cycle. However, the level of responsiveness observed in an affected person can be quite variable. Persistent coma usually involves diffuse injury at the level of the cerebral hemispheres, or more focal damage at the brainstem thalamic level. The *'locked-in' syndrome* involves a brainstem injury that disrupts the transmission of motor function. The affected person appears to be in a coma and cannot respond to stimuli, but has awareness of their surroundings. They have difficulty in expressing this awareness because of the absence of motor function, but may be able to communicate through eye movements. In a *vegetative state*, the affected person shows normal sleep–wake cycles and can be roused by stimuli, but there is no apparent awareness of their surroundings or other signs of cognition. Vegetative states arise from diffuse cortical injury or thalamic necrosis.

ASSESSING CONSCIOUSNESS

LEARNING OBJECTIVE 4

Name the clinical tests used to assess consciousness.

From a clinical perspective, determining the level of consciousness is essential to any assessment of neurological function. Elements of the stages of consciousness form a standardised and reliable test called the **Glasgow coma scale (GCS)**. In this test, verbal, eye and motor responses are given numerical values in order to reflect the level of consciousness (see Table 9.3). Verbal responses indicate how awake the affected person is, and the level of awareness of their surroundings. Eye and motor responses on both sides of the body are scored, as contralateral responses can vary according to the side (or sides) of the brain where the injury or insult occurred.

If required, further information about neurological status can be obtained by an assessment of the functioning of a number of cranial nerves and brainstem nuclei involved in pupil, corneal and oculovestibular *reflexes*. Eye movements and pupil responses to light indicate the integrity of function of cranial nerves II, III, IV and VI. The speed and shape of pupil responses in both eyes, the position of the eyes relative to each other and whether the movement of the eyes are conjugate or synchronised can indicate the location and degree of brain insult.

The absence of the corneal reflex is used to indicate impairment of brain function (the normal response is to elicit a reflex blink when the cornea is touched with a piece of cotton thread). The two oculovestibular reflexes used to assess damage to the brainstem are the doll's eye test and the caloric test. The reflexes are associated with maintaining gaze during head movements. In the *doll's eye test*, the person's eyes are held open and their head is turned from side to side. If the eyes turn in the opposite direction to the head (just as observed when a doll's head is turned), the reflex is normal. In the *caloric test*, cold water is instilled into one ear with a syringe. The normal response is that the eyes will move towards the ear being syringed. In both tests, if the eyes do not move or the relative movement of the eyes is asymmetrical, then damage to the brainstem can be inferred (see Figure 9.2).

Table 9.3 Glasgow coma scale

Measure	Responses	Score
Eye opening	Spontaneous	4
	To speech	3
	To pain	2
	No response	1
Verbal responses	Orientated	5
	Confused	4
	Inappropriate	3
	Incomprehensible	2
	No response	1
Motor movement	Obeys commands	6
	Localises to pain	5
	Withdraws from pain	4
	Flexion to pain	3
	Extension to pain	2
	No response	1
Maximum score achievable		**15**

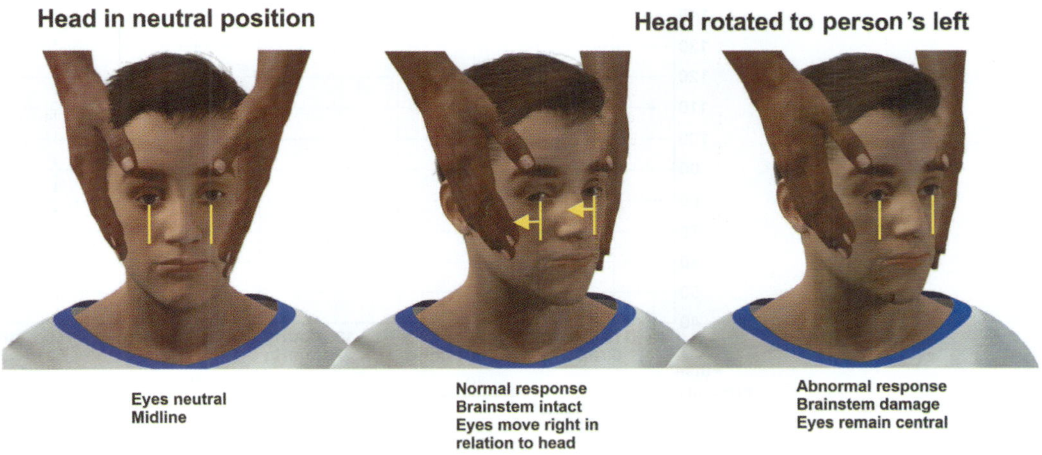

Figure 9.2
Oculocephalic reflex
Also known as the 'doll's eye test'.

Source: Sciencopia.

CLINICAL DIAGNOSIS AND MANAGEMENT

Diagnosis

Initial rapid neurological assessment can be achieved by using the AVPU scale (see Clinical Box 9.1), whose name is an abbreviation of the scale's parameters. In a most basic form, assessment by the **AVPU scale** (**A**lert, **V**oice, **P**ain, **U**nconscious) is a rapid and simple method to determine the gross level of consciousness. If the person is not alert, assessment is made by determining whether they respond to a voice, have poor arousal to someone speaking to them, and altered response to pain/noxious stimuli. Pain/noxious stimulus is assessed by observing for a reaction to a trapezius squeeze or supraorbital pressure. If there is no response to noxious stimuli, they are deemed unresponsive. The AVPU scale is not considered a comprehensive assessment, but it is beneficial in its simplicity and is used in many clinical situations, including prehospital. Basic life support should be ongoing. A GCS should be undertaken as part of the secondary survey in a comprehensive assessment.

Methods to determine the cause of ALOC will be directed at the most obvious considerations based on the available history. Failing this, investigations should be aimed at common causes first (see Table 9.2).

It is critical that airway, breathing and circulation are managed as investigations continue. A head-to-toe assessment is undertaken to identify signs of trauma. The GCS score should be assessed, as this will provide a more accurate account of changes in consciousness. When taken in the first hours of injury, the GCS score can also accurately predict probable outcomes.

A full set of observations are taken, with attention to blood pressure and temperature as possible causes. Widening pulse pressure may suggest increasing intracranial pressure (see Clinical Box 9.2). Hypothermia and hyperthermia can both influence levels of consciousness. Changes in respirations (rate, depth or rhythm) may imply injury and dysfunction to the respiratory centres in the pons (apneustic or pneumotaxic areas). Blood should be drawn for testing glucose, electrolyte and pH imbalance, as well as drug panels for commonly overdosed agents.

Pupillary response and size should be assessed. Both a direct response (shining the light into the pupil and watching that pupil's response) and a consensual response (e.g. shining the light into the left pupil and watching the right pupil's response, and vice versa) should be assessed, as this will give an impression of the cranial nerve III function (oculomotor). Depending on levels of consciousness, motor and sensory limb assessments may be carried out to determine motor cortex function.

Imaging investigations will generally include a computed tomographic (CT) scan to determine the presence of any space-occupying lesion, such as a tumour, or an abscess. Other pathology visible on a CT may include haemorrhage, hydrocephalus, oedema or infarction.

CLINICAL BOX 9.1

AVPU scale

A–Alert
V–Voice
P–Pain
U–Unconscious

CLINICAL BOX 9.2

Calculating pulse pressure

To calculate pulse pressure, take the diastolic value from the systolic value.

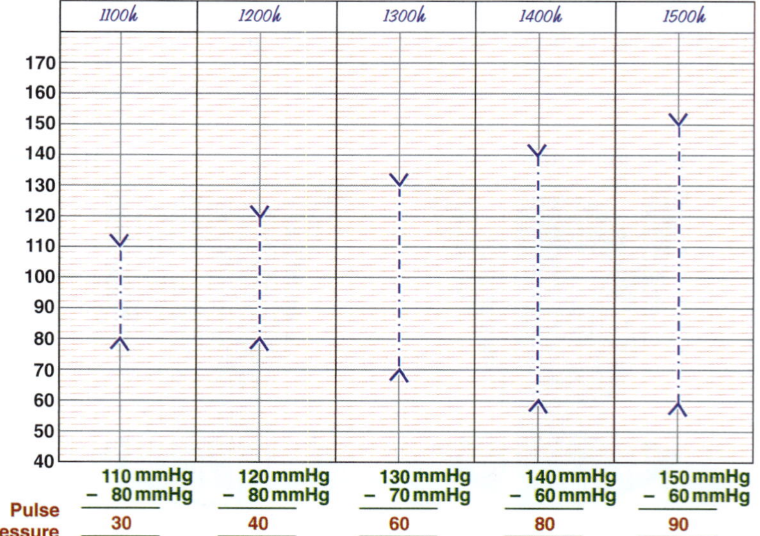

One measure of pulse pressure has little significance. The value comes from observing a trend.
Widening pulse pressure can be a sign of increasing intracranial pressure and should be monitored closely.

Depending on the presentation, a lumbar puncture may be performed if meningitis, encephalitis or subarachnoid haemorrhage is suspected. However, there are many contraindications to lumbar puncture, in which case other methods may be employed instead.

Management

A person who is breathing spontaneously but has an ALOC should be placed in the recovery position. Airway management equipment such as a Guedel's airway (oropharyngeal airway—OP) can be inserted. If someone tolerates the Guedel's airway, then they need it! However, if they are able to remove the equipment with their tongue, they have sufficient control to maintain their own airway. Suction equipment should always be available. More invasive devices, such as laryngeal mask airways or endotracheal intubation, may be required for those who do not have sufficient respiratory effort or who have oxygenation issues.

Safety is the major concern in those with an ALOC. Bed rails and other devices to ensure safety should be instigated. Maintenance of inserted tubes and devices can become complex in a someone who is confused. Depending on the level of agitation, it may be safer to sedate and paralyse them. This decision will have logistical, personnel, equipment and outcome implications. In this event, mechanical ventilation must be initiated and maintained by appropriately trained personnel. Sedating or anaesthetising someone with an ALOC can often complicate their care as it affects neurological assessment. At some stage, they will need to be 'woken' and neurological assessment will need to continue.

Management of the factors contributing to the alterations in level of consciousness is necessary to reverse the effects (where possible). Once the cause has been determined, an appropriate management plan can be formulated.

Cerebrovascular accidents

LEARNING OBJECTIVE 5

Define a 'cerebrovascular accident', state the main types, identify the key risk factors and outline the pathophysiology of this condition.

LEARNING OBJECTIVE 6

Describe the clinical manifestations, diagnosis and clinical management of cerebrovascular accidents.

A **cerebrovascular accident (CVA)**, or as it is more commonly known, a **stroke**, is a localised vascular lesion that develops suddenly within the cerebral circulation where the vessel becomes blocked or bleeds. This results in a **cerebral infarction**, where the neurons in the affected area die. The *primary infarction zone* will be repaired, but the neurons will be irreversibly injured because they do not regenerate. A *secondary infarction zone* involves the area immediately around the primary zone, where cells have been injured but may recover if blood flow can be restored relatively quickly (see Figure 9.3). The consequences will be either a permanent or a temporary loss of brain function associated with the areas affected. Depending on the site of damage, alterations in brain function may consist of sensory dysfunction, visual disturbances, cognitive and/or language impairment, and disturbances in motor control and balance.

AETIOLOGY AND PATHOPHYSIOLOGY

There are two types of stroke—*ischaemic* and *haemorrhagic*. Ischaemic stroke is the more common form. Generally, the rate of secondary injury and degree of morbidity, as well as the death rate, tend to be higher in haemorrhagic stroke. Figure 9.4 outlines the common clinical manifestations and the management of cerebrovascular accident.

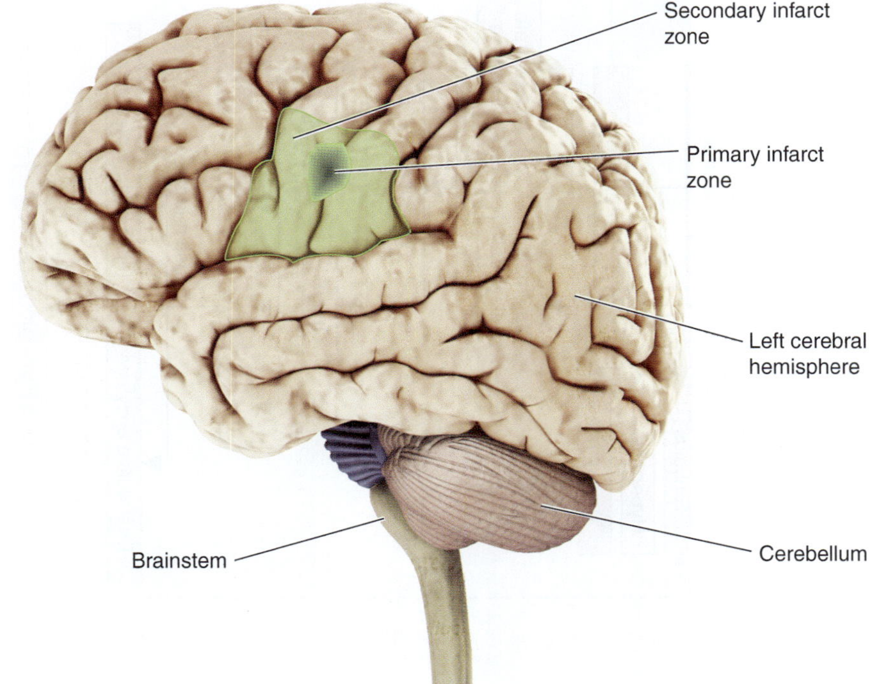

Figure 9.3

Primary and secondary infarction zones

This image represents primary and secondary infarction zones. The primary zone consists of irreversibly damaged neurons that die and are replaced by scar tissue. The secondary infarction zone contains neurons that may recover from injury if blood flow is restored quickly.

Source: © Dorling Kindersley/Getty Images.

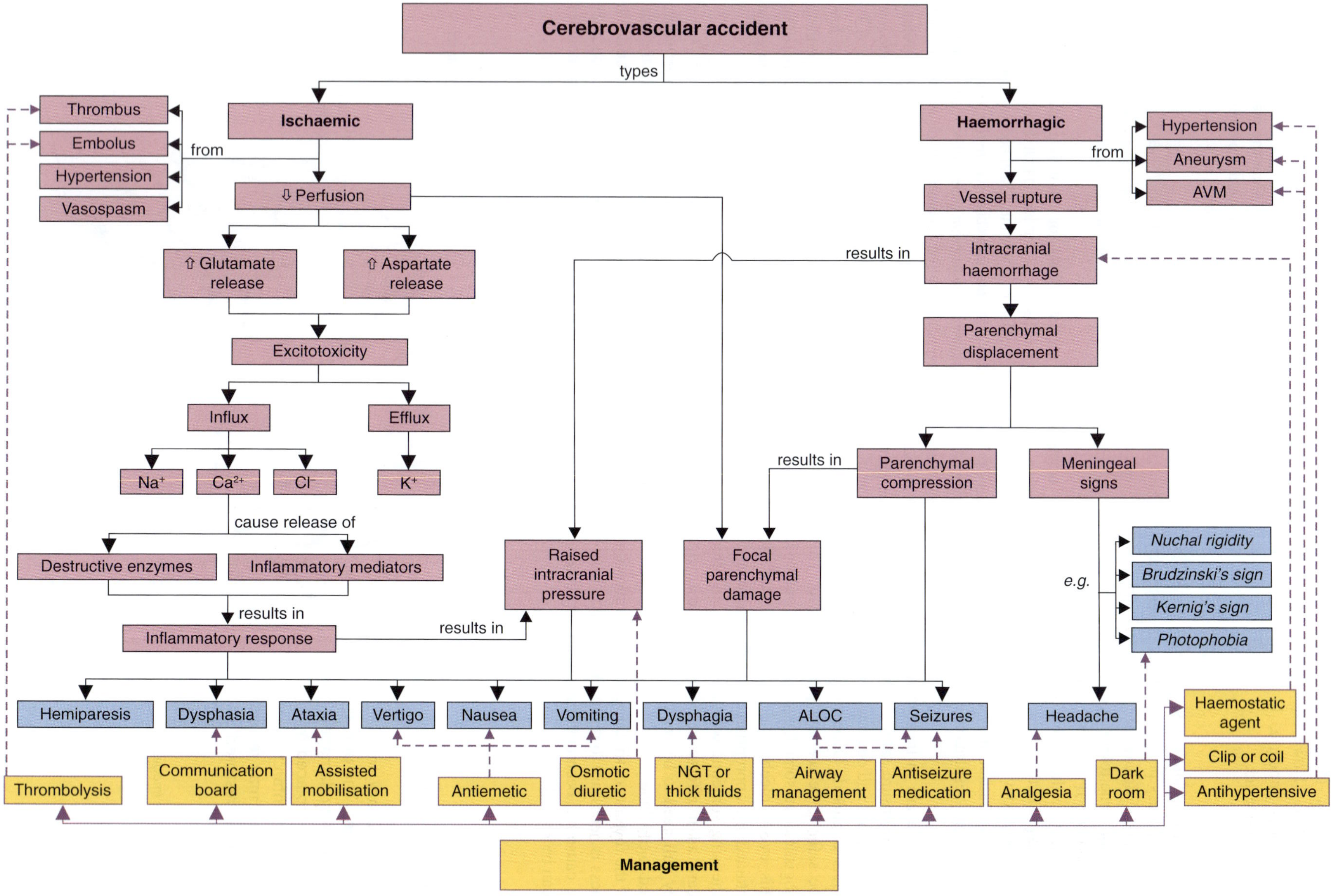

Figure 9.4

Clinical snapshot: Cerebrovascular accidents

↓ = decreased; ↑ = increased; ALOC = altered level of consciousness; AVM = arteriovenous malformation; Ca^{2+} = calcium ion; Cl^{-} = chloride ion; K^{+} = potassium ion; Na^{+} = sodium ion; NGT = nasogastric tube.

The consequences of a stroke depend on the brain region affected by the alteration in cerebral blood flow. Recall the nature of the cerebral circulation and the brain regions served by the principal cerebral arteries. This information will be useful when you link the affected brain regions to the deficits that result. The major cerebral arteries supplying the left and right sides of the brain originate at the base of the brain. They are uniquely linked together by connecting arteries that form a circle around the pituitary gland, known as the *circle of Willis*, which is also connected to the internal carotid and basilar arteries bringing blood up to the head (see Figure 9.5). The anterior cerebral arteries feed the frontal lobes, the middle cerebral arteries supply the lateral hemispheres and the basal ganglia, while the posterior cerebral arteries supply the occipital lobe, temporal lobes and thalamus. The basilar and vertebral arteries feed the cerebellum and brainstem.

Ischaemic strokes

Ischaemic stroke occurs as a result of a sudden obstruction to a cerebral artery. The brain region supplied by this artery becomes ischaemic, and if the situation does not improve quickly an infarct will occur. Due to the high metabolic demands of brain tissue, irreversible damage can develop within minutes of the ischaemia.

The obstruction is due to a *thrombus* or an *embolism* (see Figure 9.6). Thrombosis is usually associated with the formation of *atherosclerotic plaque* within the wall of the arteries supplying the brain, or under conditions when the blood becomes hypercoaguable. Thrombi can easily grow on the surface of an atherosclerotic lesion within the cerebral circulation or in the carotid arteries. Blood *hypercoagulability* is associated with prolonged immobility, such as when a person is bedridden for a period or frequently travels on long-haul international flights. Blood clots can also form within a heart chamber when the pumping ability of the heart becomes impaired and areas of blood stasis develop, such as in *atrial fibrillation* (see the chapter 'Dysrhythmias'), or on *heart valve flaps*. Fragments of thrombi within the heart or in the carotid arteries, or whole clots, may become dislodged and travel up into cerebral circulation, where they block cerebral blood flow and cause ischaemia.

Some people experience episodes of **cerebral ischaemia** that induce neurological deficits, but these symptoms completely resolve within around 24 hours. Such an episode is called a **transient ischaemic attack (TIA)**. The person may experience only one TIA or a series of episodes. Usually, a TIA is an indicator of underlying thrombotic disease, and is a warning to the person that they are at high risk of stroke. The timely commencement of drug therapy will lower the chances of CVA.

Haemorrhagic stroke

Haemorrhagic stroke occurs when a *cerebral artery ruptures* and there is a bleed into the brain tissue, in addition to the loss of blood supply to the areas served by the vessel. The risk of haemorrhagic stroke is strongly associated with chronic hypertension, as the degree of pressure on the artery walls is a contributing factor to their rupture, as well as the presence of structural weaknesses, such as an **aneurysm** or **arteriovenous malformation (AVM)**, within blood vessel walls. Common sites of haemorrhagic stroke are the subcortical regions, such as the thalamus and the basal ganglia.

A significantly higher degree of morbidity and death is associated with this type of stroke, as the haemorrhage can greatly displace brain tissue. This can result in the compression of brain tissue locally in the areas of the bleed, and a profound shift of the brain laterally or inferiorly, affecting functions at other regions some distance from the rupture (see Figure 9.7). Parts of the brain may even become herniated between meningeal compartments.

Aneurysms and arteriovenous malformations are vascular lesions where the blood vessel wall becomes weakened.

Figure 9.5

The circle of Willis

Source: hfsimaging/123RF.

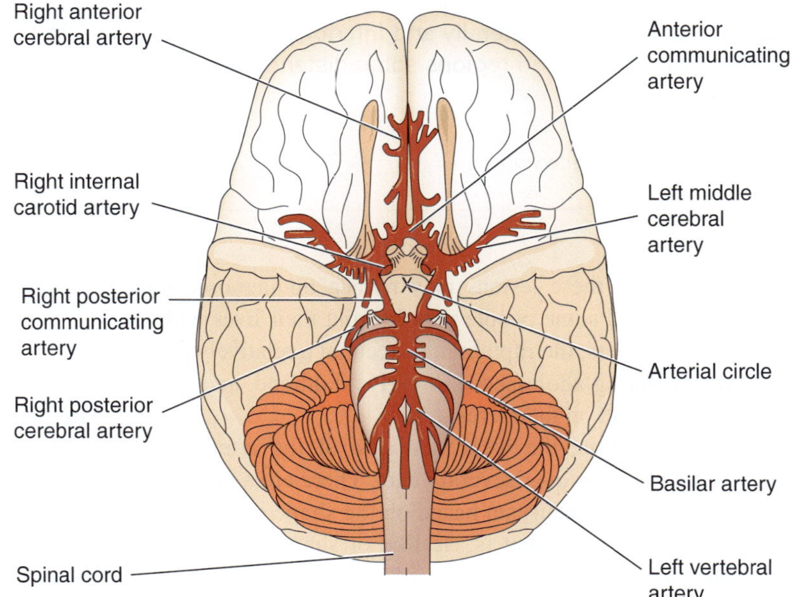

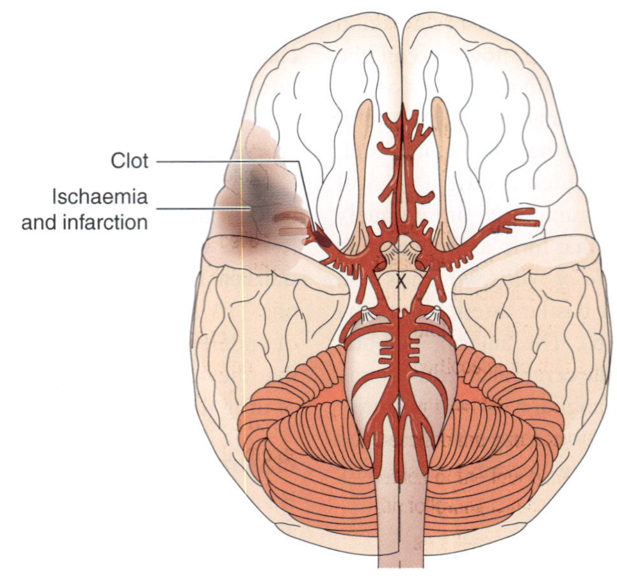

Figure 9.6

Ischaemic stroke

Source: Adapted from hfsimaging/123RF.

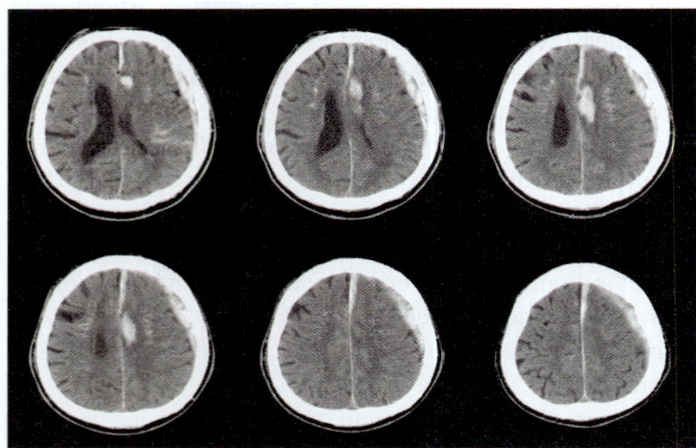

Figure 9.7

Brain displacement in haemorrhagic stroke

Following a haemorrhagic stroke, accumulated blood can displace the brain laterally and inferiorly, and cause altered brain function in regions some distance from the primary lesion.

Source: MossStudio/Shutterstock.

The presence of these lesions may remain undiagnosed until one ruptures, and some people may live out their lives without incident. For others, the rupture may occur at a relatively young age, maybe during adolescence or early adulthood, and have a catastrophic effect on their lives.

In an *aneurysm*, the weakened area of the arterial wall dilates and balloons over several years. There are a number of different forms of aneurysm based on the shape of the lesion, such as an outgrowth that is sac-like or shaped like a berry (*saccular or berry*), or a dilation of the segment of affected vessel wall (*fusiform*) (see Figure 9.8). A useful analogy is a bicycle tyre with a weakened segment of wall. With repeated inflation and under increased tyre pressure, the region can balloon out and burst. As the lesion develops in arteries, the bleed can lead to a significant and rapid accumulation of blood in the tissue. It is likely that if a person develops a brain aneurysm, they will have more than one present in the cerebral circulation. Most cerebral aneurysms occur in the circle of Willis.

In an *arteriovenous malformation*, the normal development of the capillaries between the arterioles and venules does not occur, so the arterioles connect directly with the venules. The relatively higher blood pressure in the arterioles enters directly into the venules, and over time the venules enlarge and congested flow develops. Eventually, the congested flow backs up into the arterioles, causing them to enlarge, too. The enlarged vessel walls become weakened and prone to rupture (see Figure 9.9). Arteriovenous malformations occur during the in-utero development of the vasculature. These malformations can be found throughout the brain and meninges, and are predominantly congenital, although dural arteriovenous malformations can be acquired. Classification of cerebral arteriovenous malformations is based on the *Spetzler–Martin grading system*, in which size, eloquence of adjacent brain and pattern of venous drainage are graded. Arteriovenous malformations are covered in more detail in the chapter 'Vascular disorders and circulatory shock'.

EPIDEMIOLOGY AND RISK FACTORS

In 2018, there were an estimated 387,000 Australians aged 15 and over who had experienced a stroke sometime in their lives. In 2020–21, 49,658 people were admitted to Australian public hospitals experiencing a stroke event. In New Zealand there are around 9,500 stroke events per year. More than 70% of people who have strokes are 65 years of age or older. In Australia, the

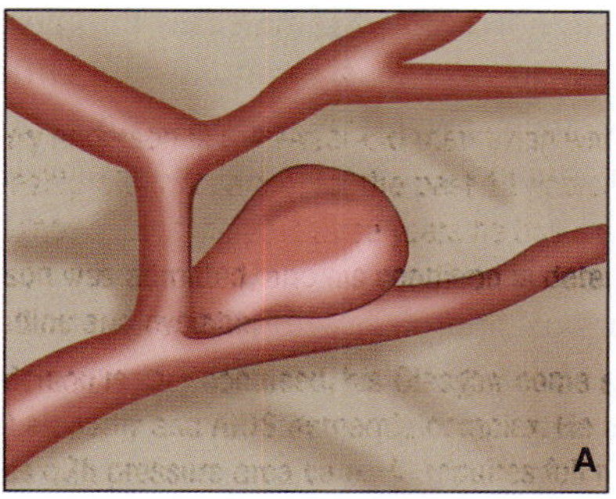

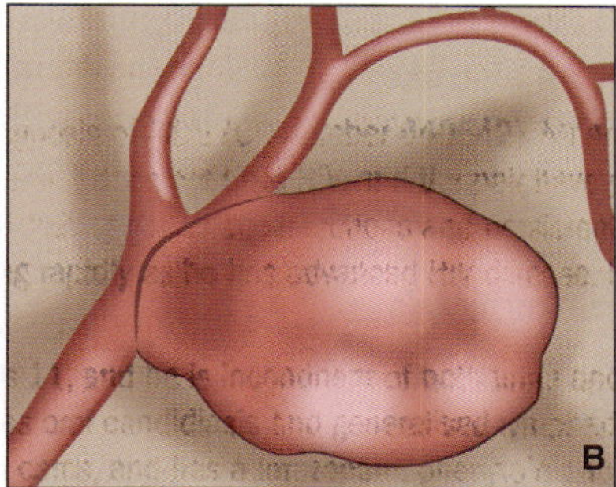

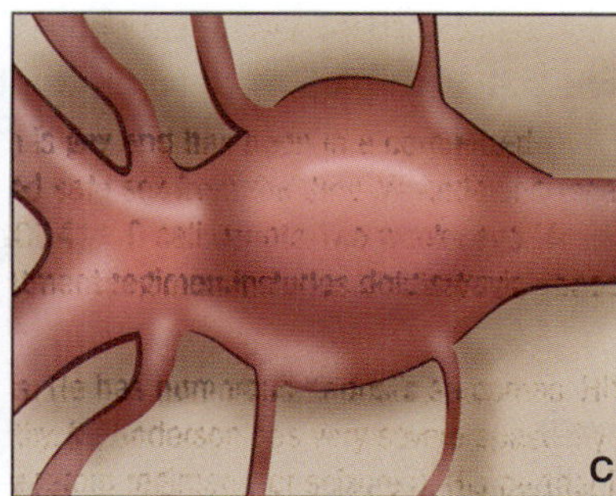

Figure 9.8

Saccule, giant and fusiform aneurysms

(A) Saccular berry aneurysm. (B) Giant aneurysm. (C) Fusiform aneurysm.

Source: © Sciencopia.

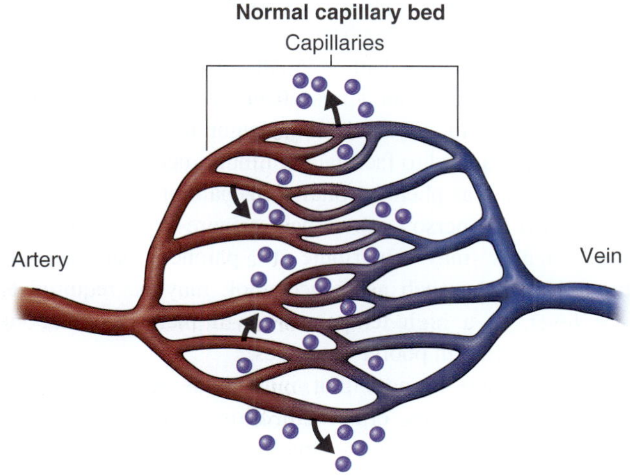

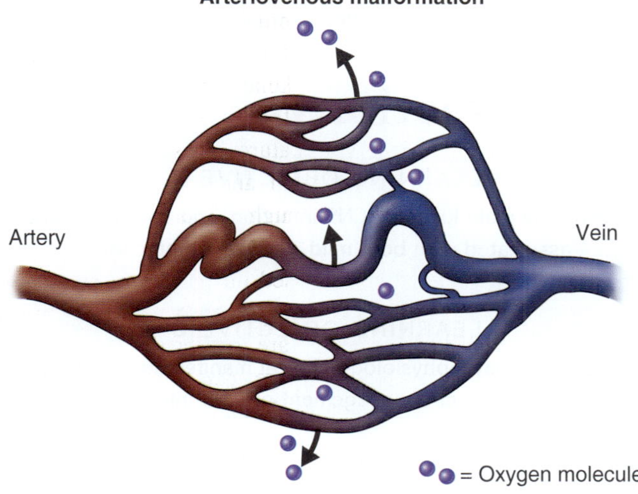

Figure 9.9

Arteriovenous malformation

In arteriovenous malformation during in-utero development of the vasculature, relatively higher pressures of the arterioles cause the venules to dilate. In time, back pressure will cause the arterioles to dilate, too.

rate of stroke had fallen by 25% over the period from 2001 to 2018; however, since the COVID-19 pandemic, there has been a clear increase in stroke statistics. The reasons for this are still under investigation. The prevalence of stroke in Australia is 1.6% for males and 1.1% for females. Around half of stroke hospitalisations (49%) occur for people over 75 years old, and the rates are 1.5 times higher in men.

Stroke is a leading cause of death in Australia and New Zealand, accounting for 5% of all deaths, and is considered a leading cause of disability. Stroke death rates for males and females are similar, but, as there is a higher proportion of older women, more women die from stroke. In New Zealand, the death rates associated with this condition are higher in people of European heritage compared to those in other ethnic groups.

The prevalence of cerebrovascular disease in Indigenous Australians is 1.5 times greater than in non-Indigenous Australians (1.7 times greater for women, 1.3 times greater for men), and they experience this condition at a younger age.

The major *risk factors* for stroke are hypertension, diabetes mellitus, hyperlipidaemia, smoking, age, family history, alcohol consumption and heart disease. The incidence of arteriovenous malformations is estimated at 3 cases per 10,000 people.

CLINICAL MANIFESTATIONS

Brain dysfunction arising from a stroke can involve motor, sensory, language and cognitive deficits. The clinical manifestations associated with a particular stroke depend on the site within the cerebral circulation that the lesion occurs and the extent of disruption. The middle cerebral arteries are most commonly occluded in ischaemic strokes. Table 9.4 summarises the general deficits resulting from a stroke and the likely brain region damaged.

CLINICAL DIAGNOSIS AND MANAGEMENT

Diagnosis

Determining whether the cause of a cerebrovascular accident is ischaemic or haemorrhagic is imperative to the appropriate management. Treating a haemorrhagic stroke in the same way

Table 9.4 Examples of deficits resulting from a stroke and the likely brain region damaged

Function	Brain region
Language	Broca's area, Wernicke's area
Speech	Broca's area
Voluntary movement, muscle weakness	Frontal lobe, brainstem
Vision	Occipital lobe, brainstem
Confusion, disorientation	Frontal lobe
Balance, disequilibrium	Brainstem, cerebellum
Eye movements	Brainstem
Altered coordination and gait	Cerebellum

as an ischaemic stroke (i.e. thrombolysis) can result in death. Physical assessment should include a full set of observations, a neurological assessment, including pupillary response, and a motor and sensory assessment. Identifying the time of the insult is also important, and will direct the type of intervention possible. Obtaining a history is important, and this will hopefully include an estimated or actual time of insult.

Other investigations include haematology and biochemistry blood tests. Although pathology results will not diagnose a cerebrovascular accident, they can rule in or out other causes of ALOC. A coagulation profile can be beneficial for identifying coagulopathies and the risks associated with thrombolysis.

A CT scan is one of the most common imaging investigations; magnetic resonance imaging (MRI) and angiography are often done also. A carotid duplex scan may also be performed to assist with determining the cause, and potentially identify other urgent and necessary interventions. Occasionally, a lumbar puncture may be performed where there is the suspicion of meningitis or subarachnoid haemorrhage; however, this is not common.

The *National Institutes of Health Stroke Scale (NIHSS)* is an evaluation tool used to quantify the severity of stroke. The NIHSS stroke scale includes 15 parameters, such as level of consciousness, facial palsy, motor function, language and visual field involvement. Scores can range from 0 to 42, and the higher the score, the worse the prognosis. Use of this tool is becoming more common in Australia, and many protocols include it as an indicator to assist in the decision to use thrombolytic therapy.

Management

If the cause of the cerebrovascular accident is determined to be ischaemic, treatment with a thrombolytic agent within the first 90 minutes is ideal; however, in some cases thrombolysis has been attempted up to six hours from insult. Different institutions will have their own protocols. In thrombolytic therapy, shorter 'door-to-needle' time results in an increase in favourable outcomes.

If the cause of the cerebrovascular accident is determined to be haemorrhagic, a surgical approach with clot evacuation via a craniotomy, or endovascular embolisation, may be considered. Other options include surgical clipping of aneurysms or other vascular pathologies. In individuals with increased intracranial pressure, osmotic diuretics may be necessary. Ventriculostomy may be necessary to reduce intracranial pressure as a result of obstructive hydrocephalus.

Irrespective of the cause, some basic interventions should be a part of the management plan. Airway support and control of blood pressure, glucose level, seizure activity and temperature are important. Antihypertensives may be required to reduce blood pressure. Alternatively, sympathomimetics and inotropes may be required to support blood pressure. Cerebral perfusion pressures are lost in individuals who have experienced cerebrovascular accidents, because cerebral autoregulation is affected. Therefore, normotensive ranges of blood pressure are most beneficial. Either insulin to reduce glucose levels or glucagon to increase glucose levels may be required to facilitate optimum metabolic function. Medications such as phenobarbital, diazepam or phenytoin may be required if the person experiences seizure activity. Hypoxia during seizures may contribute to parenchymal damage. Antipyretic agents, such as paracetamol, may be required to reduce fever, as a high temperature will increase metabolic processes, resulting in poorer outcomes.

It is important to note that individuals with an ALOC should not receive any oral medications. All drugs should be administered parenterally until the person's level of consciousness and swallow reflex have returned. Intravenous, rectal or nasogastric administration will reduce the risk of developing respiratory complications from aspiration.

CNS infections

LEARNING OBJECTIVE 7

Define the main kinds of CNS infection, and the pathogens associated with both mild and severe infections.

LEARNING OBJECTIVE 8

Outline the pathophysiology, clinical manifestations, clinical diagnosis and management of CNS infections.

This section will focus on the clinically important CNS infections—meningitis, encephalitis and brain abscesses. **Meningitis** is an infection of the membranes surrounding the brain and spinal cord. **Encephalitis** is an infection of the brain tissue (or *parenchyma*). A **brain abscess** is an accumulation of infective purulent material within the brain, or is associated with the CNS membranes.

Meningitis, encephalitis and brain abscesses can be caused by a range of microbes—bacteria, viruses, fungi and parasites. However, the severest types of meningitis and abscesses are related to bacterial infection, while the most serious form of encephalitis is associated with viral infection. A number of these organisms, such as the fungi, are opportunistic and cause CNS infection because they were directly introduced into the CNS through injury or during a clinical procedure, or the affected person has a severe immunodeficiency (e.g. HIV/AIDS).

The *chain of transmission* (see the chapter 'Infectious disease') dictates whether CNS infections will occur. A viable infection depends on the organism's capacity to *remain a resident* in the body and *form colonies*, and on the *efficacy of body defences* to exclude or kill the organism. Factors such as the close proximity to a reservoir of infection, an effective mode of infection, and an available portal, usually through a breach in the natural barriers (e.g. through head trauma, sepsis, neurosurgery or access from craniofacial structures such as the paranasal sinuses or the ear), determine whether infection occurs. The ability of the person to kill the organism depends on factors such as nutritional status, the presence of pre-existing disease and immunodeficiency (either through disease or treatment).

MENINGITIS

Aetiology and pathophysiology

The majority of *bacterial meningitis infections* are caused by *Streptococcus pneumoniae* or *Neisseria meningitides*. Up until recently, *Haemophilus influenzae* type b (*Hib*) was also an important causative organism. However, effective childhood Hib immunisation programs in developed nations have virtually eradicated this form of the condition from these countries.

These organisms usually reside in the nasopharyngeal region. They gain access to the bloodstream by disabling cilia and the mucosal IgA-mediated immune protection in this region. As the two key bacterial species associated with this infection are encapsulated, it is harder for the immune system to recognise them, and so only a weak complement response is provoked. They then cross the blood–brain barrier and colonise the tissue. Damage to CNS structures in this infection is mediated by the release of bacterial toxins. The resultant inflammatory response also makes a significant secondary contribution to the injury. Inflammation induces a vascular response that leads to cerebral oedema. The oedema causes a rise in intracranial pressure, and can cause compression, herniation and ischaemia.

Risk factors for poor outcomes of bacterial meningitis are advanced age, the presence of osteitis/sinusitis, a low GCS score on admission, tachycardia, positive blood culture, elevated erythrocyte sedimentation rate, thrombocytopenia and low cerebrospinal fluid (CSF) white cell count.

Viral meningitis is a much milder, short-lived and self-limiting infection. Causative organisms include the enteroviruses, herpes simplex virus, cytomegalovirus (CMV), the adenoviruses and the arboviruses. The affected person will recover completely from the infection. Most cases are seen in summer, and may be associated with swimming. Figure 9.10 explores the common clinical manifestations and management of meningitis.

Clinical manifestations

Important clinical manifestations of bacterial meningitis are fever, nuchal rigidity (stiff neck) and an altered mental state. These are known as the *classic triad*. The onset of the classic triad is common, but is not always present. At least one manifestation will always be present in this condition. Other manifestations include headache, photophobia, lethargy, vomiting, purpural or petechial rash, and seizures.

Complications of bacterial meningitis are classified as acute and delayed. *Acute complications* can include circulatory shock, coma, seizures and death. *Delayed complications* also include seizures and death, but can consist of sensory and cognitive deficits. Infants may present with a bulging fontanelle, hypotonia and a high-pitched scream.

ENCEPHALITIS

Aetiology and pathophysiology

Causative viruses in encephalitis include herpes simplex virus, herpes zoster virus, the lyssaviruses (e.g. the rabies and Hendra viruses), Epstein–Barr virus, CMV, the enteroviruses and the arboviruses. The arboviruses that are associated with encephalitis are mostly mosquito-borne (e.g. West Nile virus, Eastern and Western equine viruses, and flavivirus). Encephalitis can also be caused by some bacteria and the parasite *Toxoplasma gondii*.

As the reservoirs for many of these viruses are wild animals, such as birds and bats, and domestic animals, such as horses and pigs, there is great potential for the development of epidemics within human communities. Biosecurity and public health protocols have been developed to prevent and contain outbreaks of these infections.

The viruses gain access to the CNS via a number of possible routes:

- the bloodstream
- by direct entry from neighbouring structures (transmission of infections from the paranasal sinuses or the middle ear into the CNS)
- retroaxonally from peripheral nerve endings.

The viruses primarily infect nerve cells, and the damage is mediated by viral cytotoxicity, as well as immune and inflammatory processes. The damage may also involve the meningeal membranes and cerebral blood vessels, leading to concurrent meningitis and vasculitis.

Clinical manifestations

Common clinical manifestations include fever, an ALOC and cerebral dysfunction (e.g. memory loss, cognitive deficits,

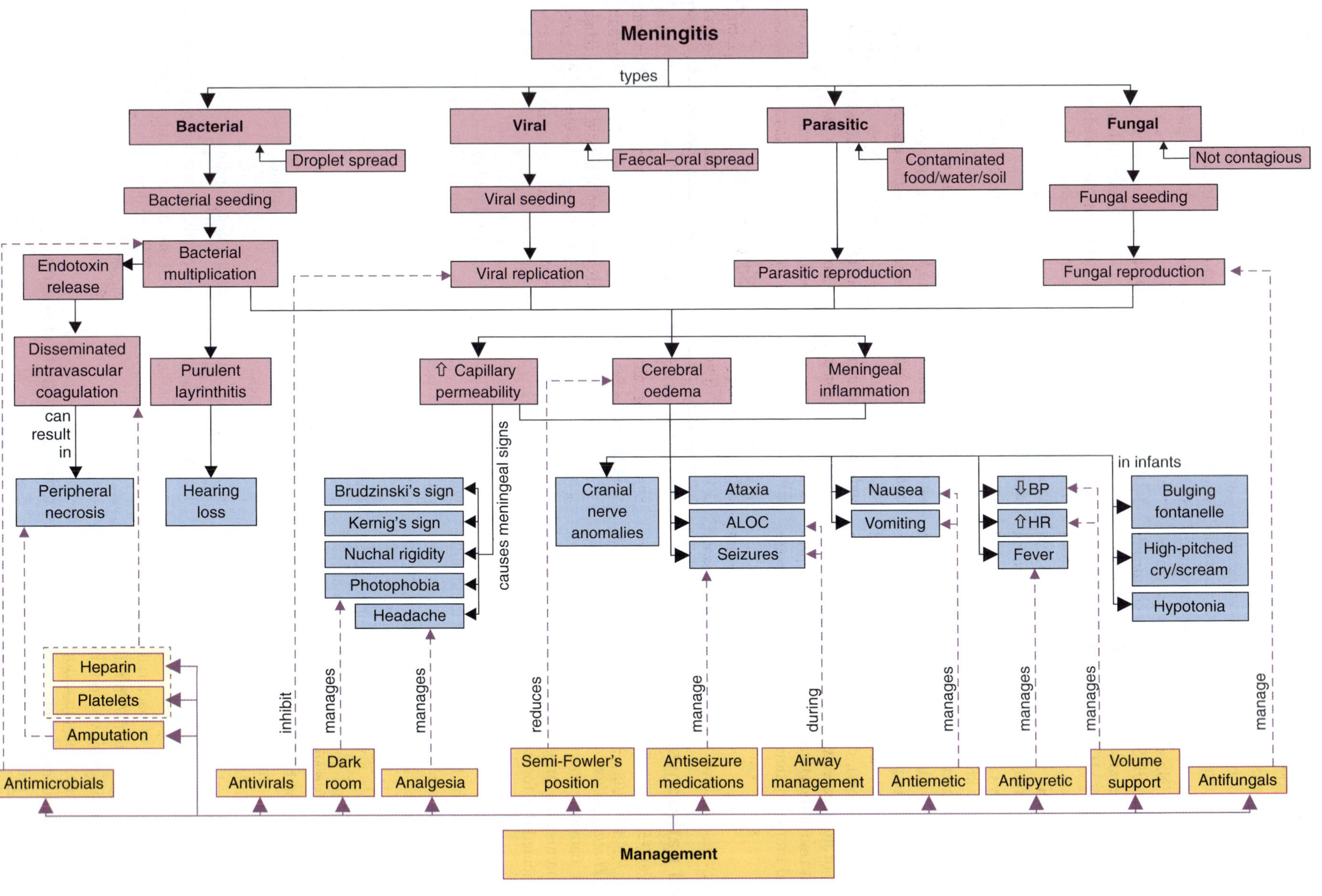

Figure 9.10

Clinical snapshot: Meningitis

↓ = decreased; ↑ = increased; ALOC = altered level of consciousness; BP = blood pressure; HR = heart rate.

changes in personality and hallucinations). Seizures, headache, myalgia, muscle weakness or paralysis and mild respiratory infection may also be seen. The mortality rate is high for some of these forms of viral encephalitis, and those people who survive face long-term neurological disability.

BRAIN ABSCESSES

Aetiology and pathophysiology

Brain abscesses are *purulent infections* that develop focally at either epidural or subdural locations. They can be quite serious and potentially life-threatening infections, and tend to affect more men than women. The most common causative bacterial species are streptococci. However, a number of other bacteria, such as staphylococci, Gram-negative organisms, and anaerobes such as *Propionibacterium acnes*, are associated with this condition. Parasites, such as *T. gondii* and *Entamoeba histolytica*, and cryptococcal fungal species can also cause brain abscesses, but these are more likely to occur in those who are severely immunocompromised.

Generally, brain abscesses arise from infections elsewhere in the body that gain access to the brain either via the bloodstream (in association with endocarditis, pulmonary infection or intravenous drug use) or from nearby regions of the head, such as the teeth, ear, paranasal sinuses or mastoid bone. In cases of head trauma or neurosurgery, the infective organism can be introduced directly into the brain.

An epidural abscess occurs in the potential space between the skull bones and the dura mater. The attachment of the dura to the skull limits the spread of the infection. A subdural abscess develops within the dura and the arachnoid membrane. In this space, the spread of pus is more likely, and can lead to more widespread inflammation, oedema, elevated intracranial pressure and thrombophlebitis (see Figure 9.11).

Clinical manifestations

Neurological manifestations are common, and are dependent on the location of the abscess with respect to the brain region affected; they can include motor impairment or aphasia. Signs of increased intracranial pressure may develop—papilloedema

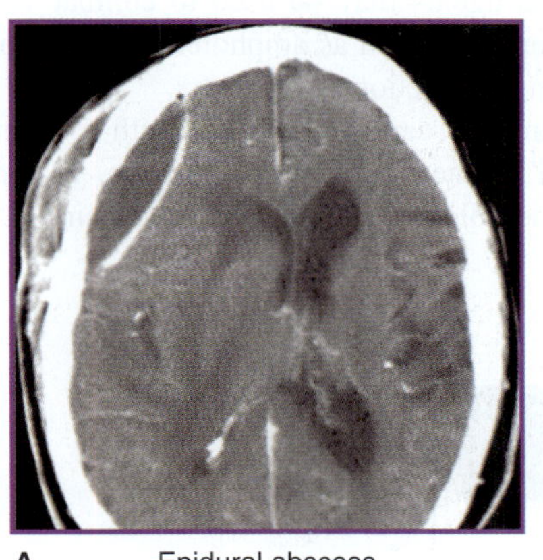

A Epidural abscess

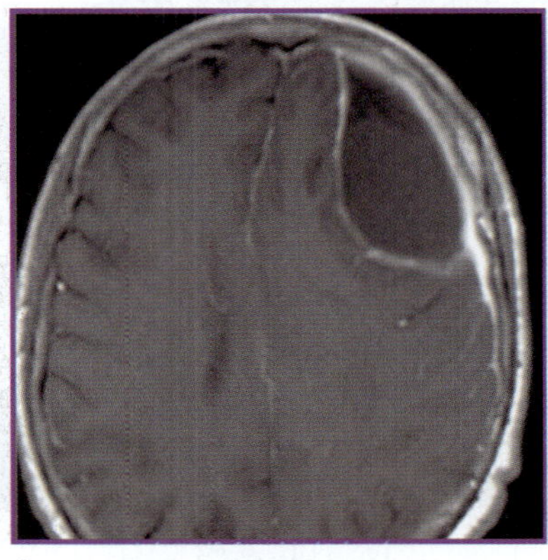

B Subdural abscess

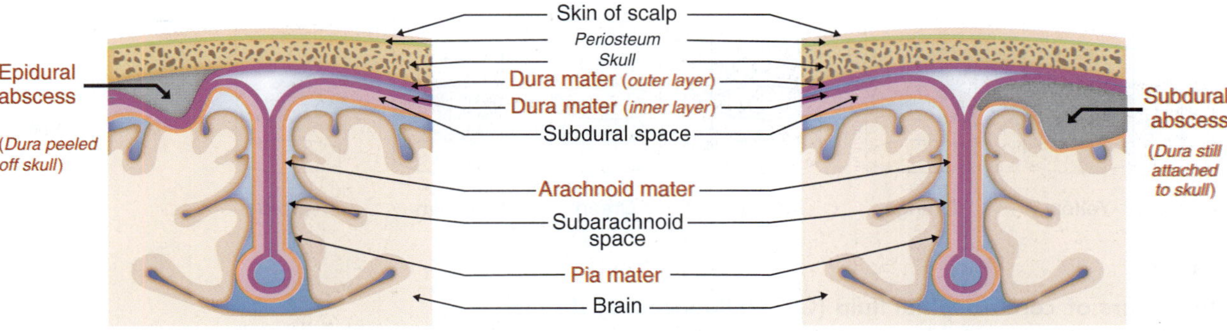

Figure 9.11

Epidural and subdural abscesses

Brain abscesses can develop when CNS infections occur. (A) In an epidural abscess, pus accumulates external to the dura mater. (B) In a subdural collection and extradural empyema, fluid accumulates underneath the dura mater.

Sources: Photographs © Radiology Key; illustration © Sciencopia.

(optic disc swelling) is often present in this CNS infection, but not in others. Fever and seizures are present in about half of the cases.

CLINICAL DIAGNOSIS AND MANAGEMENT OF CNS INFECTIONS

Diagnosis

Physical assessment demonstrating nuchal rigidity, headache, fever and an ALOC should initiate rapid investigation, considering meningitis or encephalitis. Other signs on examination may include positive *Kernig's sign* (pain from flexing the hip 90 degrees, then extending the knee) or *Brudzinski's sign* (hip and knee flexion caused by flexing the person's neck). Papilloedema, photophobia, and nausea and vomiting may also be present on examination.

Lumbar puncture and an assessment of the CSF may reveal the presence of the causative organism, leukocytes, the presence of protein, increased pressure and changes in glucose levels. The CSF should be clear, but the colour may vary in the presence of pathology (see Figure 9.12). Blood may be sampled for full blood count, electrolyte levels and blood cultures. These results will not diagnose meningitis or encephalitis, but may rule in or out other issues that need to be addressed.

Imaging investigations, such as a brain CT scan, may be beneficial and demonstrate changes to ventricular morphology, as well as sulcal effacement (the loss of definition of the sulci, often due to oedema). Many clinicians feel that because of the possible severity of meningitis or encephalitis, treatment should be started before the CT scan is performed; otherwise, treatment may be delayed for too long.

Diagnosis of a brain abscess is achieved through a physical assessment and radiological confirmation. Individuals often present with headache and neurological deficit correlating to the location of the lesion. Imaging investigations, such as CT, are beneficial for identifying and locating a brain abscess. It may present as a well-defined lesion that does not change with the use of intravenous contrast, yet improves with antimicrobial treatment.

Management

Treatment will depend on the causative organism. Bacterial infections causing meningitis, encephalitis or brain abscess will be treated with antibacterials. Other interventions to support oxygenation or circulation may be required. Supplementary oxygen and crystalloid fluid resuscitation (see the chapter 'Fluid imbalances') may be necessary for hypoxic and hypotensive individuals. Reducing oedema with corticosteroids is still under investigation, and, even though some studies have suggested a decrease in antimicrobial action, there are indications that reducing inflammation may result in more favourable outcomes.

Other organisms can cause CNS infections. Antiviral and antiretroviral agents may be used to combat viral meningitis, and antimicrobials such as amphotericin or fluconazole can be used for fungal infections.

Managing the care of someone with a brain abscess will be directed by their clinical presentation. In a person who is seriously neurologically compromised, airway support and

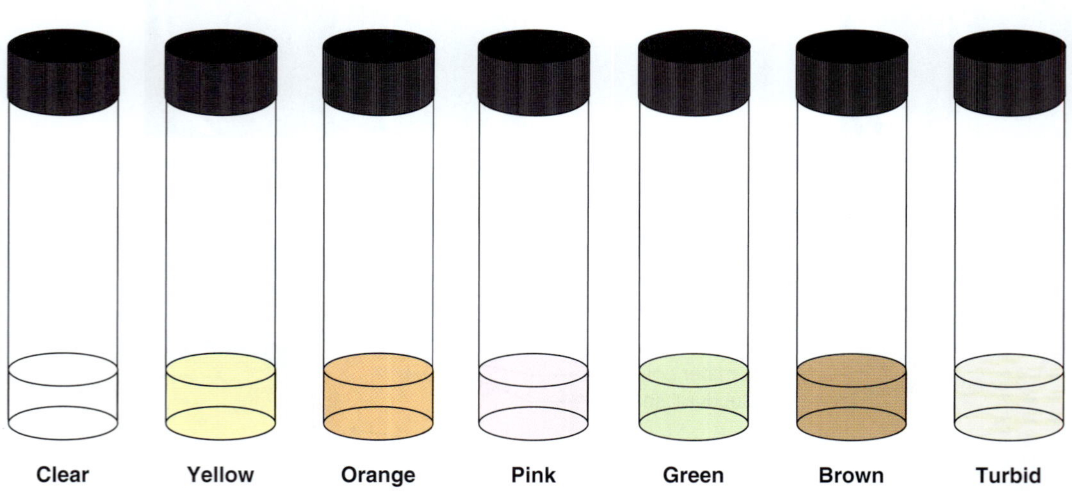

Figure 9.12

Possible colours of cerebrospinal fluid (CSF) influenced by disease

CSF colour:

clear—normal

yellow— ⇑ bilirubin or ⇑ protein

orange—haemolysis or ⇑ carotene ingestion

pink—haemolysis

green—purulent or ⇑ bilirubin

brown—haemolysis or meningeal melanomatosis

turbid—meningitis

seizure management may be necessary; in those presenting with headache, pain relief may be one of the priorities. Pharmacological management is complicated by the presence of the blood–brain barrier. Antimicrobial agents that can penetrate CNS barriers are necessary. Surgical drainage may be necessary with larger lesions.

Guillain–Barré syndrome

LEARNING OBJECTIVE 9

Outline the pathophysiology, clinical manifestations, clinical diagnosis and management of Guillain–Barré syndrome.

Guillain–Barré syndrome is a form of acute peripheral neuropathy, and consists of a number of subtypes. Guillain–Barré syndrome can develop at any age from infancy to old age, and affects both males and females, although some studies have found a slight predominance in males.

AETIOLOGY AND PATHOPHYSIOLOGY

The prevailing pathophysiological view is that Guillain–Barré syndrome is an *autoimmune disorder* where constituents of the immune system, either activated T cells or antibodies, are directed *against peripheral nerve components*. In 50–75% of cases, the condition is regarded as a *post-infection immune-mediated disorder*, where the autoimmune attack is linked to a recent infection, which is usually resolved before the symptoms of Guillain–Barré syndrome occur. Having said this, *non-infectious factors* have been reported.

It is thought that characteristics of the preceding infective organism lead to immune cross-reactivity or molecular mimicry directed against the components of the peripheral nerve. Not everyone exposed to the infectious organism develops Guillain–Barré syndrome, so susceptibility to this condition must be due to an interplay between host and organism factors. The preceding infection may be of a viral or a bacterial origin, and is usually either an upper respiratory tract or gastrointestinal infection. CMV, Epstein–Barr virus, measles, influenza A, *Campylobacter jejuni*, *Mycoplasma pneumonia*, Zika virus or enterovirus D68 infections have been implicated in the aetiology. Guillain–Barré syndrome has also been linked to surgery, and as a rare reaction to vaccines for rabies, influenza A, rubella, cholera and typhoid.

The annual incidence of Guillain–Barré syndrome is 0.5–2 cases per 100,000 people, and is slightly more common in men. The mortality rate is around 3–7%. Guillain–Barré syndrome can develop at any age, but increased incidence is associated with age. It is rare in children under 2 years old. The elderly experience a more severe disease and a poorer prognosis. This is due to an increased risk of pneumonia with hyponatraemia.

CLINICAL MANIFESTATIONS

The major clinical manifestations of Guillain–Barré syndrome fall into the categories of *motor*, *sensory and autonomic dysfunctions*. Symptoms can develop within a few days or weeks of the preceding event in someone who is otherwise healthy. The first symptoms are usually muscle weakness and paraesthesias, such as numbness and tingling. These symptoms usually occur bilaterally, start distally and evolve proximally. Muscle weakness can affect all limbs and the facial muscles. A loss of motor coordination (**ataxia**) can develop. The condition progresses for up to six weeks after the first onset.

Once the manifestations occur, they can progress to their most intense within hours or up to four weeks later. Muscle weakness can progress to paralysis, affecting chewing, speech, swallowing and respiratory functions. Respiratory arrest will lead to death if external ventilation is not commenced. Muscular and neuropathic pain occurs in a significant number of affected people. This pain may be severe, and it is not uncommon for it to be worse at night. Autonomic dysfunctions include heart rate and blood pressure alterations from lower than normal to higher.

CLINICAL DIAGNOSIS AND MANAGEMENT

Diagnosis

No single investigation will enable the diagnosis of Guillain–Barré syndrome. Following a physical assessment (which includes neurological assessment, nerve conduction and reflex testing to identify neurological dysfunction), a full blood count and electrolyte level testing may be performed. Laboratory tests may not show any aberrant values, but can be beneficial to identify other potential causes of neurological dysfunction. Other blood tests, such as folic acid and vitamin B_{12} levels, may exclude other neuropathies. Ganglioside autoantibodies are found in 50% of patients.

Imaging studies such as brain CT and MRI may be undertaken; MRI scans of peripheral nerve roots and cauda equina. However, imaging may be more beneficial for exclusionary reasons than for diagnosis. A lumbar puncture will generally demonstrate a normal cell count, but an increase in protein in the CSF.

Management

Unfortunately, there is no cure for Guillain–Barré syndrome. Management plans include airway management and support, provision of nutrition, prevention of complications related to immobility (e.g. pressure areas, osteoporosis, deep vein thrombosis and pulmonary embolus), appropriate pain relief, control of autonomic dysfunction (particularly bowel and bladder problems) and psychosocial support.

Autoimmunity is managed using immunomodulating medicines that induce targeted B cell depletion, such as cyclophosphamide, rituximab, eculizumab and interferon-β. Plasmapheresis has been used to reduce the severity and duration of the episode; however, its mechanism in Guillain–Barré syndrome is not clear.

Hydrocephalus

AETIOLOGY AND PATHOPHYSIOLOGY

LEARNING OBJECTIVE 10

State the causes, pathophysiology, clinical manifestations, diagnosis and management of hydrocephalus.

LEARNING OBJECTIVE 11

Compare and contrast the characteristics of hydrocephalus in adults and infants.

Hydrocephalus is an *accumulation of CSF within the cranium*. For most of the lifespan the cranium is a rigid encasement around the brain, so any increase in CSF volume exerts an intracranial pressure that will compress the delicate CNS tissues and cause neurological dysfunction without causing external changes to the shape and size of the head. However, in young infants the cranial sutures are yet to fuse, so with increasing CSF volume their heads can characteristically become enlarged, with bulging fontanelles and relatively small faces.

Hydrocephalus can be acquired through trauma, tumour development, cerebral bleeding or infection. There are two types of hydrocephalus: obstructive and communicating. In *obstructive hydrocephalus* there is a blockage that impedes the flow of CSF within or around the brain. The most common site of obstruction is in the cerebral aqueduct leading into the fourth ventricle. It can also be associated with protrusion of the cerebellum below the foramen magnum, which is a form of Chiari malformation. In *communicating hydrocephalus*, there is no obstruction of CSF flow, but its reabsorption is inadequate. Alterations in CSF absorption can arise at the point of absorption when the arachnoid villi become scarred or are malformed, or when a thrombosis develops in the venous sinuses of the brain.

Hydrocephalus may occur sometime prior to, or around the time of, birth, as a consequence of a *developmental defect* (e.g. spina bifida), resulting in congenital hydrocephalus, or it may be acquired later in life. A rare, inheritable, sex-linked form of the condition is called X-linked hydrocephalus. This form has been linked to other symptomology, such as thumb adduction deformity and poor intellectual outcomes. The prevalence of *congenital hydrocephalus* in Australia is 1 in every 1,000 births, but this does not take into account those people who acquire the condition after birth.

The *development of hydrocephalus* depends on an *alteration of CSF dynamics*. Changes occur in the flow of CSF around the CNS and/or its reabsorption back into the general circulation (see Figure 9.13). In rare cases, an increase in CSF production may underlie the condition, and this is associated with cancerous involvement of the choroid plexuses.

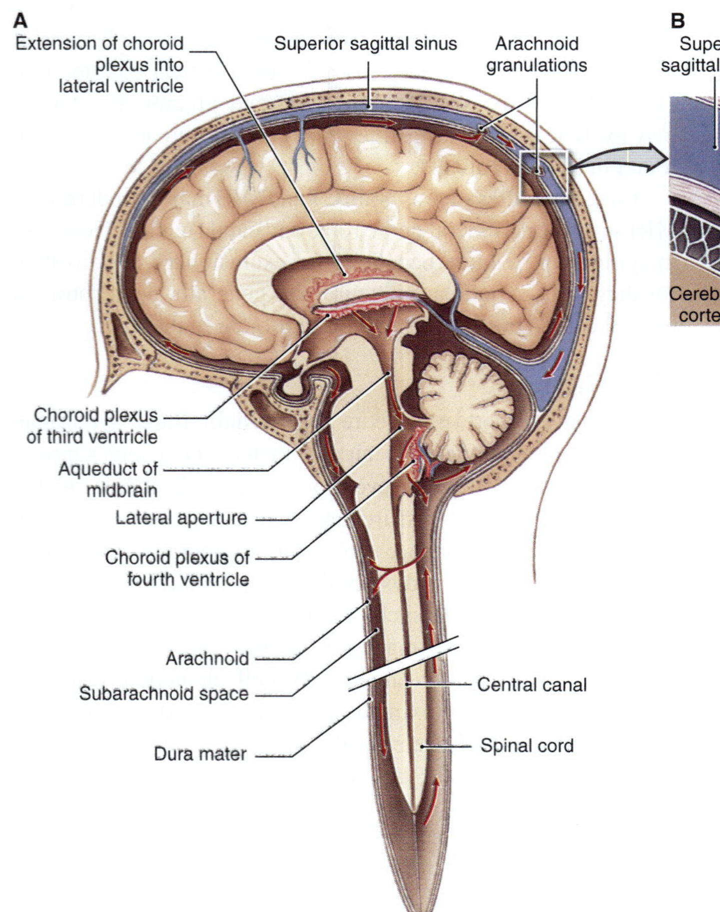

Figure 9.13

Cerebrospinal fluid (CSF) formation and flow

(A) CSF is formed in choroid plexuses in the ventricles. From the fourth ventricle it circulates posteriorly around the cerebellum and posterior cerebrum, as well as around the spinal cord and then up around the anterior cerebrum. It is reabsorbed back into the circulation through arachnoid villi.

(B) A representation of a choroid plexus, where plasma leaking from the capillaries is processed by the ependymal cells to form CSF.

Source: Martini, F.H. et al., Essentials of anatomy and physiology *(5th edn), p. 270. © 2010. Reprinted by permission of Pearson Education, Inc.*

Alterations in the flow of CSF can develop in the cerebral or spinal regions. Scarring due to trauma or infection, or tumour growth, obstructs the normal CSF flow through the subarachnoid space, the cerebral aqueduct and/or the ventricles.

When hydrocephalus develops in adults in the absence of other causes, it usually manifests as a syndrome involving gait disturbances, cognitive deficits, bladder detrusor muscle overactivity and enlarged ventricles. The condition is known as *normal pressure hydrocephalus* or *idiopathic adult hydrocephalus syndrome*. It may be linked to the typical acquired aetiologies stated above, and has been strongly linked to hypertension.

CLINICAL MANIFESTATIONS

The clinical manifestations of hydrocephalus vary across the lifespan, but the most common are headache, nausea and vomiting. Confusion, loss of concentration, seizures and loss of motor coordination can also occur. Visual disturbances, including double vision, strabismus and nystagmus, may also be noted.

In infants, changes in head growth, poor feeding, uncoordinated eye movements and drowsiness are to be expected.

CLINICAL DIAGNOSIS AND MANAGEMENT

Diagnosis

Although in children with unfused sutures the effects of hydrocephalus can be quite visible, imaging investigations such as CT and MRI are the cornerstone to diagnosis of hydrocephalus for all ages to measure ventricular size and brain anatomy, as well as lumbar puncture. In hydrocephalus, there can be increased CSF pressure and enlarged ventricles.

Management

Although diuretic agents (e.g. the carbonic anhydrase inhibitor acetazolamide and the loop diuretic furosemide) can reduce choroid plexus secretion of CSF, surgery is usually necessary. Different surgical interventions are considered, depending on the cause. For the long-term control of hydrocephalus, placement of a shunt will drain excess CSF and reduce intracranial pressure. Although the ventriculoperitoneal (VP) shunt was the most common shunt some years ago, different types of shunts are now inserted (see Table 9.5). More recent shunts can be programmed, enabling an increase or decrease in the volume of CSF permitted to drain through the valve. Other surgical options may include endoscopic third ventriculostomy (ETV), cerebral aqueductoplasty or choroid plexectomy.

Postoperative care includes observation for neurological compromise. Wound management and pain relief are important. Postoperative prophylactic antimicrobials may be ordered. Excessive drainage can result in insufficient CSF volume and cause postural headaches (worse when upright). Frequent medical review is required, especially if the shunt is programmable. Magnets, various toys and some other devices may influence the shunt setting. Long-term monitoring for infection is important, and parents or carers should be taught the signs of raised intracranial pressure. The individual should avoid contact sports, and be carefully observed for neurological signs in the event of head trauma. They may also need education to avoid wearing heavy bags on the insertion side of the shunt, so as not to damage or kink the shunt tubing.

Cerebral palsy

AETIOLOGY AND PATHOPHYSIOLOGY

LEARNING OBJECTIVE 12

Define 'cerebral palsy', and outline the clinical manifestations, diagnosis and management of this condition.

According to the International Working Group on Definition and Classification of Cerebral Palsy, **cerebral palsy** is defined as a group of permanent *disorders of the development of posture and movement, causing activity limitation associated with non-progressive disturbances in the developing fetal or infant brain.* Diagnosis is primarily attributed to motor dysfunction, but this is usually accompanied by alterations in cognitive, sensory and endocrine functioning.

A strong association has been made between the development of cerebral palsy and low birth weight. Other risk factors have been implicated in congenital cerebral palsy, and have been categorised according to when their effect occurred—prenatally, perinatally and postnatally. Intrauterine infection is an important prenatal risk factor. Perinatal risk factors include instrument delivery, neonatal jaundice, birth asphyxia, neonatal convulsions, antepartum bleeding and neonatal infection.

Table 9.5 Different types of CSF shunts

Shunt type	Shunt location
Ventriculoperitoneal (VP) shunt	Between the ventricle and the peritoneum
Ventriculopleural (VPL) shunt	Between the ventricle and the pleural cavity
Ventriculoatrial (VA) shunt	Between the ventricle and the atria
Lumboperitoneal (LP) shunt	Between the subarachnoid cavity in the lumbar region and the peritoneum
Ventriculosubgaleal (VSG) shunt—temporary	Between the ventricle and the subgaleal area (between the scalp and the skull)

Note: Ventricular catheters can be placed to drain outside the cranium for pressure measurement, drainage and sampling.

Interestingly, the role of birth asphyxia in the development of cerebral palsy is controversial and, as yet, remains unresolved. The prevalence of cerebral palsy in Australia has decreased slightly from 1996–97 to 2013–14 from 1.8 cases per 1,000 live births to 1.2 per 1,000 live births.

CLINICAL MANIFESTATIONS

The motor disturbances associated with cerebral palsy consist of *spasticity* (increased muscle tone and increased resistance to stretch), *dystonia* (altered muscle tone; particularly affecting the head, upper back, neck and tongue), *ataxia* (a loss of coordination, with altered posture and staggering gait) and **athetosis** (slow, writhing involuntary movements of the extremities). Spasticity can affect all four limbs (*quadriplegia* or *tetraplegia*), mostly the legs (*diplegia*), or be limited to one side of the body (*hemiplegia*). The degree of impairment is classified according to *severity* and *developmental age*. There are currently four classification systems describing various functional capacity in cerebral palsy (see Table 9.6). Each of these systems has five levels of function, and focuses on different functional aspects. Physical fatigue is a common symptom in adults with cerebral palsy. Epilepsy is also common in children with cerebral palsy. All forms of epilepsy have been observed, with the prevalence greater in people who are more severely disabled.

Children with cerebral palsy may experience some degree of cognitive and behavioural impairment. These include poor visuospatial ability, memory loss, fear of novel situations, hyperactivity, dependency and mental retardation.

Speech can also be affected due to motor impairment (dysarthria), or at a level where language is processed (aphasia). Some severely disabled individuals may not speak at all.

Sensory dysfunction is also associated with cerebral palsy. Common alterations include impairments in two-point discrimination, stereognosis and proprioception. Visual problems can also occur. These can have their origin in the eye or in the cerebral visual centres. Poor visual acuity, strabismus (misalignment of one or both eyes) and retinopathy have been reported. Chronic pain is also reported, but may vary according to the distribution of the spasticity. This pain may be located in the lower back, foot, ankle, knee, neck or shoulder. It may also manifest as a headache.

Other problems affecting the urinary, musculoskeletal and gastrointestinal systems can occur in a significant proportion of children with cerebral palsy. Impairments in sucking and swallowing, micturition, linear growth and bone density have been reported.

CLINICAL DIAGNOSIS AND MANAGEMENT

Diagnosis

Cerebral palsy is generally diagnosed through a physical examination and a consideration of history, especially in the context of some type of insult such as hypoxia, anoxia or infection events that can occur around birth. Laboratory tests and imaging studies are only of benefit to identify other causes of neurological dysfunction.

Table 9.6 Comparison of the four instruments currently used to classify functional ability of individuals with cerebral palsy

	GMFCS *Focus: mobility*	MACS *Focus: interaction with objects*	CFCS *Focus: communication*	EDACS *Focus: eating and drinking*
I	Walks without limitation	Handles objects easily and successfully	Effective sender and receiver	Eats and drinks safely and efficiently
II	Walks with limitations (no mobility aid by age 4)	Handles most objects with reduced speed/quality	Effective but slow-paced sender and receiver	Eats and drinks safely, but with some limitations to efficiency
III	Walks with hand-held mobility device	Handles objects with difficulty, requires help to prepare or modify activity	Effective sender and receiver with familiar partners	Eats and drinks with some limitations to safety; there may also be limitations to efficiency
IV	Self-mobility with limitations, may use power	Handles limited number of objects in adapted setting	Inconsistent sender and receiver with familiar partners	Eats and drinks with significant limitations to safety
V	Transported in manual wheelchair	Does not handle objects	Seldom effective sender and receiver with familiar partners	Unable to eat or drink safely, consider feeding tube

CFCS = Communication, Function Classification System; EDACS = Eating and Drinking Ability Classification System; GMFCS = Gross Motor Functional Classification System; MACS = Manual Ability Classification System.

Sources: Adapted from Palisano et al. (1997); Paulson & Vargus-Adams (2017).

Management

The management plan for individuals with cerebral palsy includes supportive measures. Damage occurs with the initial insult, but as cerebral palsy is non-progressive once the initial injury occurs, there is no continuation or advancement of any 'disease'. However, a person with cerebral palsy is, at some stage, likely to develop complications of infection, seizure or immobility that impair their health and complicate their care.

Common issues that require management include reduction of hypertonia causing spasticity, and contractures if appropriate physiotherapy and limb management are not undertaken. Intramuscular botulinum toxin has been used with success to reduce limb hypertonia. Spasticity and dystonia may be lessened through the intrathecal administration of the muscle relaxant baclofen, as well as through splinting and range-of-movement exercises. Many children with cerebral palsy require treatment with antiseizure agents, assistance with communication, and support with swallowing and nutrition. Depending on the degree of oromotor function, caloric support may need to be achieved with permanent feeding tubes into the stomach (gastrostomy) or jejunum (jejunostomy).

Stem cell transplantation in cerebral palsy is a plausible management strategy, but its usefulness is yet to be proven.

Cerebellar disorders

LEARNING OBJECTIVE 13

Outline the role of the cerebellum, and the likely clinical manifestations of cerebellar disorders in general.

The cerebellum plays a key role in motor function. It is involved in motor coordination, balance and equilibrium, the control of muscle tone, posture, rapid limb movements (particularly the arms) and motor learning. The cerebellum may also contribute to normal cognition and memory.

AETIOLOGY AND PATHOPHYSIOLOGY

Cerebellar disorders can be inheritable, acquired or occur as a result of a congenital malformation. Acquired forms can be associated with tumours, stroke, neurodegenerative disorders and exposure to chemicals (e.g. environmental toxins, medicines and recreational substances like alcohol).

Cerebellar dysfunction usually involves ataxia, affecting the way the person stands and moves, leading to a clumsy and unsteady appearance. The person may appear to be drunk when no alcohol has been consumed. Other clinical manifestations of cerebellar disorders include the loss of sequencing of fine movements, impaired control of the range of movement, poor muscle tone, nystagmus, altered speech patterns, loss of ability to make rapid alternating movements, and tremor during movement (intention tremor).

INHERITABLE ATAXIA

There are a number of inheritable ataxias, of which *Friedreich's ataxia* is relatively common. It is an autosomal recessive degenerative disorder that usually manifests around puberty, but can occur as young as 2 years old or after 25 years of age. The genetic mutation is associated with the expression of a protein called *frataxin* in the nervous system and heart, which is available at lower than normal levels. Frataxin is necessary for normal mitochondrial function.

The ataxia is usually the first symptom diagnosed, and it leads to a progressive deterioration in gait, with a loss of ability to walk or stand without support. Severely affected individuals become wheelchair-bound. Foot deformities and scoliosis (curvature of the spine) usually develop. Other cerebellar manifestations, such as nystagmus and altered speech, may also be observed. Sensory losses accompany this condition, involving an impaired sense of proprioception and vibration, as well as losses in special senses. A hypertrophic cardiomyopathy also develops in about two-thirds of affected people.

Neural tube defects

AETIOLOGY AND PATHOPHYSIOLOGY

LEARNING OBJECTIVE 14

Define the neural tube defect 'spina bifida', and outline the clinical manifestations, diagnosis and management of this condition.

LEARNING OBJECTIVE 15

Compare and contrast spina bifida and anencephaly.

The neural tube is the structure from which the CNS and its bony protections develop. The formation of the neural tube during embryonic development can become disrupted, leading to a situation where it fails to close somewhere along its length.

When the defect occurs at the *caudal end* of the tube, the condition is referred to as **spina bifida**. If the defect is at the *cephalic end*, the cerebral hemispheres will not develop, leading to a condition known as *anencephaly* (see Figure 9.14).

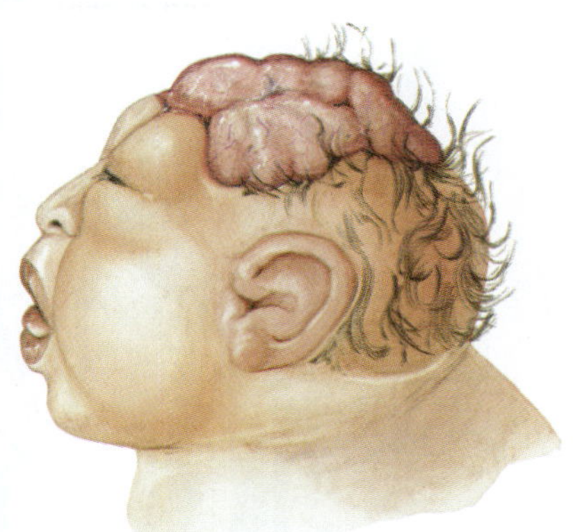

Figure 9.14
Anencephaly

Source: Medical Art Inc/Shutterstock.

In anencephaly, the skull does not form properly either, and the overlying skin may be absent, leaving the underlying brain tissue exposed externally. This condition is not compatible with life, and the child succumbs antenatally or shortly after birth.

The risk factors for spina bifida are associated with an interplay between genetic predisposition for the condition and environmental factors. In terms of genetics, the risk is increased slightly for a couple who have already had a child with spina bifida, or when a first-degree relative has a child with the condition. A chromosomal abnormality, trisomy 18, is also associated with an increased risk of **neural tube defects**. Maternal environmental factors include obesity, diabetes mellitus, the use of certain antiseizure medications, a deficiency in folate or vitamin B_{12}, and hyperhomocystinaemia. In Australia, there has been a significant decrease since the mid-1990s, when the rate was 20 cases per 10,000 births. This decline is thought to be associated with prophylactic therapy with folate. In Australia, in 2016 the prevalence rate was 4 cases per 10,000 births.

In spina bifida, the neural tube fails to close along its length in what will become the spinal column, creating an opening, or cleft, that may expose the underlying spinal cord. Indeed, the translation of spina bifida is 'spinal cleft'.

The severity of spina bifida is dependent on the degree of malformation in the affected region. At one level, one or more vertebrae may be malformed, without much involvement of the underlying tissues, and the skin tissue remains intact above the region. This is referred to *spina bifida occulta* ('occulta' meaning 'hidden'). Increasing severity is associated with the degree of meningeal and cord involvement. The meningeal membranes can protrude through the opening in the spinal column and remain hidden under the skin, or protrude to such a degree as to be visible on the external surface of the body. This is called a **meningocele** (*-cele* meaning 'swelling' or 'hernia'). The most severe form is when the cord tissue also protrudes through the opening along with the meninges. This is referred to as a **myelomeningocele** (see Figure 9.15).

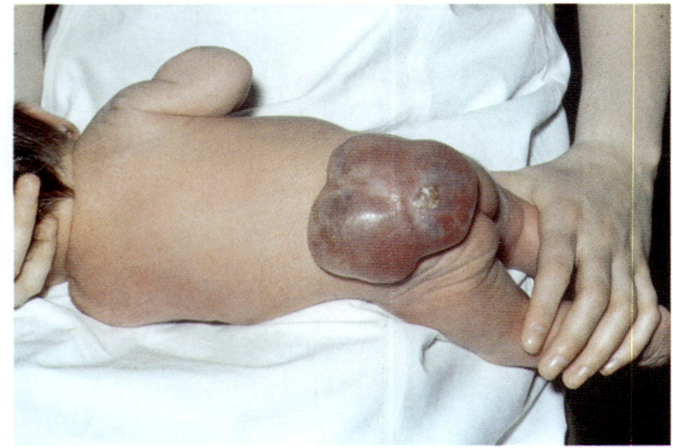

Figure 9.15

A neonate with a lumbar myelomeningocele

Source: Biophoto Associates/Getty Images.

CLINICAL MANIFESTATIONS

In its mildest form, spina bifida does not produce any clinical manifestations. When it does produce symptoms, there are degrees of disability associated with the severity of the underlying defect. The condition can affect autonomic function, resulting in urinary, bladder and bowel dysfunction. Spina bifida also affects motor function below the site of the lesion, resulting in partial or complete paralysis, as well as loss of sensation. Myelomeningocele can also lead to meningitis, which can be life-threatening (see the earlier section in this chapter).

An important complication associated with spina bifida is called *Arnold–Chiari (or Chiari II) malformation*. This occurs as the affected child grows and the lower and rear portion of the brain is pulled downwards, compressing the cord. This leads to dysfunction in feeding and swallowing, as well as postural control.

CLINICAL DIAGNOSIS AND MANAGEMENT

Diagnosis

An antenatal screening test measuring α-fetoprotein (AFP) can be undertaken on maternal serum in the second trimester, or on amniotic fluid via an amniocentesis. If high levels of AFP are identified, there is an increased risk that the fetus has a neural tube defect. Spina bifida occulta may be detected or even accidentally discovered by routine X-ray. However, meningocele and myelomeningocele are both very visible on physical examination. Imaging studies such as CT or MRI may quantify the spinal levels involved and the degree of spinal defect.

Management

Prevention through the adequate intake of folate antenatally and during pregnancy has significantly reduced the incidence of neural tube defects in Australia and New Zealand. However, spina bifida still exists in our society.

Management plans for individuals with neural tube defects are dependent on the type and level of the lesion. People with spina bifida occulta may have little to no neurological deficit. If there are no obvious external signs or neurological deficit, some individuals may not even know that they have a mild case of spina bifida. However, the higher the lesion and the more nerves that are externalised, the greater the neurological deficit. Supportive care initially focusing on closure of the externalised sac, stabilising the deformity and controlling hydrocephalus is the priority. Once the surgical team has succeeded in closing the skin and reducing the risk of further neurological injury, cord tethering and infection, the priority becomes promoting function, increasing mobility and reducing the effects of immobility.

Physiotherapy, splinting and increasing upper body strength may be central to supportive care as the child gets older. Teaching and implementing methods to reduce the risk of osteoporosis, deep vein thrombosis, pulmonary embolism and pressure areas are critical for those who are wheelchair-bound. Individualised management plans are necessary, as each person presents with differing levels of neurological deficit. Emphasis should be on working towards maximising independence.

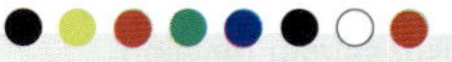

INDIGENOUS HEALTH FAST FACTS AND CULTURAL CONSIDERATIONS

FAST FACTS

- *The notification rate for meningococcal disease in Aboriginal and Torres Strait Islander children is 6 times higher than that for non-Indigenous children.*
- *The notification rate for meningococcal disease in Aboriginal and Torres Strait Islander populations is 3 times as many times as non-Indigenous populations.*
- *Meningococcal disease is more common in Māori and Pacific Islands people than in European New Zealanders.*
- *The rate for cerebral palsy is more common in Aboriginal and Torres Strait Islander children, estimated to be at 50% higher than for non-Indigenous children.*
- *The rate of neural tube defects in Aboriginal and Torres Strait Islander peoples has dropped since the fortification of food with folic acid and iodine in 2009, but is still higher than that of non-Indigenous people.*
- *Aboriginal and Torres Strait Islander peoples are 1.5 times more likely than non-Indigenous Australians to die of stroke.*
- *Death from stroke is approximately 1.5 times more common in Māori than in non-Māori New Zealanders.*
- *Māori are twice as likely as non-Māori New Zealanders to be hospitalised for stroke.*

CULTURAL CONSIDERATIONS

- *An Aboriginal and Torres Strait Islander person's connections to family, community and culture are critical for their well-being. Those who are experiencing a profound disability are at even more risk of social isolation and activity restriction, and have poorer outcomes overall. The additional complication of disability compounds the difficulties experienced by Aboriginal and Torres Strait Islander peoples, leading to lower rates of employment, poorer educational attainment and, ultimately, lower life satisfaction rates.*
- *In attempts to close the gap, there have been significant and various approaches, including movement towards programs that focus on services supporting the mother's and baby's health. It is well understood that investments in health from pre-conception to early childhood can have beneficial effects, as a developing brain has achieved approximately 90% of its adult size by 3 years of age. Many primary health initiatives, such as those resulting in folic acid fortification, have begun to address some of the root causes of disability from neurological conditions. Other approaches include Aboriginal and Torres Strait Islander Engagement Strategies, which come under the National Disability Insurance Scheme, and are responsible for supporting providers to build culturally appropriate skills in communities, enabling engagement in a culturally responsive manner.*

Sources: Data from Australian Institute of Health and Welfare (2018, 2021); Australian Indigenous HealthInfoNet (2022); D'Antoine & Bower (2019); Luke et al. (2022); Marshall (2021); New Zealand Ministry of Health (2021).

CHILDREN AND ADOLESCENTS

- The presence of unfused sutures in a neonate's brain is somewhat protective against raised intracranial pressure in the context of hydrocephalus. Older children with fused sutures may experience brain damage more quickly.
- Neuroplasticity in a child's brain is significantly greater than that in an adult's brain; therefore, learning is achieved more rapidly.
- Appropriate stimulation must occur for a baby's brain to develop. Although brain development occurs at different rates, there is a general and loose consensus about developed function at certain stages. Neurological milestones should be assessed periodically, so that the tracking of growth can lead to the provision of assistance where necessary.
- Stroke can occur in children, and is among the top 10 causes of death within the first 12 months of life.
- The most common cause of stroke in children is related to vascular pathology. About one-quarter of the causes of stroke in children result from ischaemic events from emboli.

OLDER ADULTS

- In an older person, investigations leading to the diagnosis of a brain tumour may not occur because the presenting clinical picture may resemble dementia.
- In adults over 60 years of age, Purkinje cell numbers in the cerebellum decrease significantly, resulting in diminishing movement coordination, visuo-vestibular adaptability and an increase in dizziness.
- Plasticity in an older person's brain is significantly less than that in a child's or a young adult's brain, so learning is achieved less rapidly; however, it is still possible. Continued stimulation is known to delay the effects of neurological dysfunction.

KEY CLINICAL ISSUES

- Airway safety is paramount when caring for individuals with an altered level of consciousness. Always have airway equipment, suction and oxygen available. People with an altered level of consciousness may deteriorate or improve rapidly. Continual observation and frequent assessment are necessary to ensure interventions appropriate for changes to the clinical situation.
- People who cannot maintain their own airway need immediate intervention and review to ensure their safety.
- Knowledge and understanding of the Glasgow coma scale is paramount in assessing and caring for those with neurological deficits.
- Individuals with a cerebrovascular accident may have communication problems in expression and/or reception. Ensure that everything is explained as clearly as possible, and allow time for them to process information. Communication boards may facilitate improved interactions. The use of closed questions may be beneficial for important communications.
- People who have experienced a cerebrovascular accident may unintentionally neglect their affected arm or leg, causing injury. Methods and interventions to reduce limb neglect should be reinforced to the person frequently.
- Rapid diagnosis and management of central nervous system infections are imperative to reduce the risk of mortality in people presenting with signs and symptoms of neurological infection.
- Measuring blood pressure is important in those with neurological deficits. Widening pulse pressure can be a sign of raised intracranial pressure.
- Reducing the volume of cerebrospinal fluid will reduce increased intracranial pressure.
- People with myelomeningocele may have abnormal kinaesthesia in the hands, even though the arms are above the level of the lesion. Therefore, exercise and physiotherapy are important to promote strength and function in their upper body.

CHAPTER REVIEW

- A fully conscious person is awake and alert, responsive to stimuli and aware of their surroundings and responses.
- The *reticular activating system (RAS)* plays a key role in the control of consciousness—in maintaining arousal and the waking state. The RAS has also been implicated in the control of mood, attention, motivation, learning, memory and skeletal muscle movement. The RAS consists of most of the brainstem areas and the thalamus. It also has projections from the posterior hypothalamus. The influences of the RAS descend to the spinal cord and up to the cerebral cortex.
- The RAS receives motor information from higher brain regions on its way down to skeletal muscles, and also receives a variety of sensory inputs from the periphery and relays them up to the cerebral cortex.
- Altered states of consciousness develop when the activity of the RAS becomes greatly diminished. Alterations in cognition and memory are usually apparent early as consciousness changes, giving rise to disorientation to time, place and person.
- There are seven acute levels of consciousness that primarily relate to changes in the waking state. In order from the highest to lowest level, they are: *fully conscious, confusion, delirium, lethargy, obtundation, stupor* and *coma*.
- Chronic pathological alterations in consciousness can develop following a brain insult, including persistent coma, the 'locked-in' syndrome and a vegetative state.
- The *Glasgow coma scale* is a reliable test to assess consciousness. It rates verbal, eye and motor responses on a numerical scale. Pupil, corneal and oculovestibular reflex status also provide information about neurological status.
- A *cerebrovascular accident*, or *stroke*, is a localised vascular lesion that develops suddenly within the cerebral circulation, where the vessel becomes blocked or bleeds, resulting in a cerebellar infarction. Depending on the site of damage, alterations in brain function may consist of sensory dysfunction, visual disturbances, cognitive and/or language impairment and disturbances in motor control and balance.
- There are two types of stroke—ischaemic and haemorrhagic. *Ischaemic strokes* are associated with cerebral thromboembolism, whereas *haemorrhagic stroke* results from a rupture in a cerebral blood vessel wall.
- The clinically important central nervous system (CNS) infections are meningitis, encephalitis and brain abscesses. *Meningitis* is an infection of the membranes surrounding the brain and spinal cord, *encephalitis* is an infection of the brain tissue (or parenchyma), and *brain abscesses* are accumulations of infective purulent material within the brain or associated with the CNS membranes.
- The severest types of meningitis and abscesses are related to bacterial infection, whereas the most serious form of encephalitis is associated with viral infection.
- *Guillain-Barré syndrome* is a form of acute peripheral neuropathy, which is considered to be an autoimmune disorder. Guillain-Barré syndrome can develop at any age from infancy to old age, and appears to affect slightly more males.
- *Hydrocephalus* is an accumulation of cerebrospinal fluid (CSF) within the cranium. In adults, the increase in CSF volume exerts an intracranial pressure that will compress the delicate CNS tissues and cause neurological dysfunction without causing external changes to the shape and size of the head. In young infants, the cranial sutures are yet to fuse, so with increasing CSF volume their heads can characteristically become enlarged, with bulging fontanelles and relatively small faces.
- The development of hydrocephalus depends on an alteration of CSF dynamics. Changes occur in the flow of CSF around the CNS (*obstructive*) and/or its reabsorption back into the general circulation (*communicating*). In rare cases, an increase in CSF production may underlie the condition, and this is associated with cancerous involvement of the choroid plexuses.
- *Cerebral palsy* is defined as a group of permanent disorders of the development of posture and movement, causing activity limitation associated with non-progressive disturbances in the developing fetal or infant brain. Diagnosis is primarily attributed to motor dysfunction, but this is usually accompanied by alterations in cognitive, sensory and endocrine functioning. The motor disturbances associated with cerebral palsy consist of spasticity, dystonia, ataxia and athetosis.
- Cerebellar disorders can be inheritable, acquired or occur as a result of a congenital malformation. *Cerebellar dysfunction* usually involves ataxia, affecting the way the person stands and moves, leading to a clumsy and unsteady appearance. The person may appear to be drunk when no alcohol has been consumed. Other clinical manifestations of cerebellar disorders include the loss of sequencing of fine movements, impaired control of the range of movement, poor muscle tone, nystagmus, altered speech patterns, loss of ability to make rapid alternating movements and tremor during movement (intention tremor).

- *Spina bifida* is a defect in the formation of the neural tube during embryonic development at the caudal end of the tube. If the defect is at the cephalic end, the cerebral hemispheres will not develop, leading to a condition known as *anencephaly*.
- The severity of spina bifida is dependent on the degree of malformation in the affected region. *Spina bifida occulta* is when one or more vertebrae may be malformed, without much involvement of the underlying tissues. Increasing severity is associated with the degree of meningeal and cord involvement. When the meningeal membranes protrude through the opening in the spinal column, it is called a *meningocele*. When the cord tissue also protrudes through the opening along with the meninges, it is referred to as a *myelomeningocele*.

REVIEW QUESTIONS

1 Define the following alterations in consciousness:
   a lethargy
   b vegetative state
   c obtundation
   d coma
   e locked-in syndrome
2 Score the following patients on the Glasgow coma scale.
   a A person appears asleep. In response to speech they open their eyes, but their verbal responses are confused. They demonstrate a withdrawal response to a noxious stimulus.
   b A person is sitting with their eyes open. Their verbal responses are confused, but they are capable of localising a noxious stimulus.
3 Compare and contrast the characteristics of an ischaemic stroke with those of a haemorrhagic stroke.
4 Which cerebral artery (and on which side of the body) would most likely be affected in each of the following examples of stroke?
   a Right-sided muscle weakness and sensory loss, and impaired speech
   b Loss of left side of visual field
5 Compare and contrast the characteristics of encephalitis and meningitis.
6 Compare and contrast the characteristics of an epidural and subdural brain abscess.
7 Outline the general pathophysiology of Guillain-Barré syndrome.
8 Outline the three alterations in CSF dynamics that can lead to hydrocephalus.
9 Compare and contrast the characteristics of hydrocephalus in an adult and an infant.
10 What are the main clinical manifestations of cerebral palsy?
11 What are the main general manifestations of cerebellar disorders?
12 Outline the pathophysiology of neural tube defects.

HEALTH PROFESSIONAL CONNECTIONS

Midwives When counselling women about folate consumption to prevent spina bifida, it is important to ensure that they understand that adequate folate intake is most beneficial before pregnancy is planned. Development of the nervous system occurs early in the pregnancy, and brain and spinal cord formation are well underway before a woman generally knows that she is pregnant. Therefore, when working with women who are planning to conceive, understanding and institution of appropriate nutrition is essential before conception.

Physiotherapists Physiotherapists provide much of the rehabilitation and training for individuals with nervous system insults such as stroke, nervous system infection or even cerebral palsy. Understanding the sensorimotor deficits incurred, remaining intellectual and cognitive functioning, the skills and tasks necessary, the processes required to relearn tasks, and the relationship between the person and physiotherapist will improve the outcomes. Ensuring rehabilitation tasks are meaningful and providing real-time feedback can enable the person to gauge progress, whereas requiring tasks without tangible feedback (e.g. shifting weight compared with reaching for an object) may have less of an effect on the person's enthusiasm for the rehabilitation process.

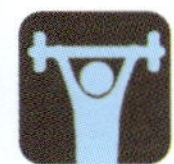

Exercise scientists Neurorehabilitation is a developing area in exercise science for those who have experienced cerebrovascular accidents. Exercise programming focusing on task-specific outcomes is becoming increasingly important. Exercises with high repetition, aerobic exercise and devices to assist with bilateral synchronisation of movement may improve brain plasticity. It is generally accepted that sensorimotor cortical areas representing specific anatomy enlarge or diminish depending on the volume and repetition of use. This capacity for adaptation can be harnessed for rehabilitation practices in stroke-injured clients. Much research is still required in this emerging area of exercise science.

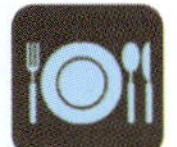

Nutritionists/Dieticians Working with people who have mobility issues as a result of nervous system trauma from cerebrovascular insult, spina bifida or nervous system infection can be difficult as mobility issues result in an increased incidence of obesity. Although the standard nutrient requirements in the food pyramid still apply, people with decreased mobility generally require fewer calories. Other issues related to immobility include constipation. Education to increase the amount of fibre and water is important. Prevention of osteoporosis through the appropriate intake of calcium and vitamin D is important. Reducing the risk of pressure areas is achieved through appropriate nutrition; however, increasing protein, preventing dehydration and ensuring the recommended daily intake of vitamins A and C and zinc is also important. Nutrition plays a major role in the prevention of neural tube disorders, simply by increasing the amount of folic acid in a woman's diet pre-conception.

CASE STUDY

Mr Sam Kwon is a 74-year-old man (UR number 684421). He was brought in by paramedics with right-sided hemiparalysis, aphasia and facial drooping. He has a history of hypertension, congestive heart failure and type 2 diabetes mellitus. He takes oral hypoglycaemic agents. He has also smoked a pack of cigarettes a day for approximately 40 years. His observations were as follows:

Temperature	Heart rate	Respiration rate	Blood pressure	SpO_2
36.8°C	98	24	140/105	96% (RA*)

*RA = room air.

A CT scan without contrast suggested a probable left cerebrovascular accident, with increased density in the left middle and cerebral artery, and possible early signs of oedema. From these results, it is expected that Mr Kwon may also be experiencing homonymous hemianopia, but communication is difficult at this stage. As he is aphasic, he requires a communication board, but he can answer with a head nod to closed questions. Mr Kwon's blood glucose level is 9.4 mmol/L, he has bibasal crackles and has been placed on oxygen via nasal prongs at 2 L/min. A swallowing review has been booked for today; meanwhile he remains nil by mouth. The time of the insult is currently unknown, as his family had been out since early morning and had not found him until later last night. The team was unable to lyse the clot. Mr Kwon requires q2h turns, he has an intravenous catheter in situ and is receiving crystalloid fluids. He also requires q2h blood glucose tests at this stage for review later today.

HAEMATOLOGY

Patient location:	Ward 3	**UR:**	684421		
Consultant:	Smith	**NAME:**	Kwon		
		Given name:	Sam	**Sex:**	M
		DOB:	01/10/XX	**Age:**	74

Time collected	22.30
Date collected	XX/XX
Year	XXXX
Lab #	4325433

FULL BLOOD COUNT		UNITS	REFERENCE RANGE
Haemoglobin	158	g/L	115–160
White cell count	6.4	$\times 10^9$/L	4.0–11.0
Platelets	382	$\times 10^9$/L	140–400
Haematocrit	0.46		0.33–0.47
Red cell count	5.10	$\times 10^{12}$/L	3.80–5.20
Reticulocyte count	0.7	%	0.2–2.0
MCV	93	fL	80–100
Neutrophils	4.82	$\times 10^9$/L	2.00–8.00
Lymphocytes	2.03	$\times 10^9$/L	1.00–4.00
Monocytes	0.46	$\times 10^9$/L	0.10–1.00
Eosinophils	0.34	$\times 10^9$/L	< 0.60
Basophils	0.12	$\times 10^9$/L	< 0.20
ESR	11	mm/h	< 12
COAGULATION PROFILE			
aPTT	38	secs	24–40
PT	17	secs	11–17

BIOCHEMISTRY

Patient location:	Ward 3	**UR:**	684421		
Consultant:	Smith	**NAME:**	Kwon		
		Given name:	Sam	**Sex:**	M
		DOB:	01/10/XX	**Age:**	74

Time collected	22:30
Date collected	XX/XX
Year	XXXX
Lab #	3455645

ELECTROLYTES		UNITS	REFERENCE RANGE
Sodium	136	mmol/L	135–145
Potassium	3.6	mmol/L	3.5–5.2
Chloride	98	mmol/L	95–110
Bicarbonate	23	mmol/L	22–32
Glucose	10.5	mmol/L	3.5–5.4

CRITICAL THINKING

1. Consider Mr Kwon's history. What factors put him at risk of a cerebrovascular accident? Identify and explain each of these factors.
2. What type of stroke do you think Mr Kwon has had (ischaemic or haemorrhagic)? Identify the factors that you have considered in order to justify your answer. Draw up a table with 'Ischaemic' in one column and 'Haemorrhagic' in the other. Draw up two rows, one labelled 'Mr Kwon's signs and symptoms' and the other labelled 'Other possible signs and symptoms'. Complete this table, identifying which factors reported are more likely to be experienced by someone having an ischaemic or a haemorrhagic stroke. This will assist you to justify your answer. Then, complete the remaining boxes, identifying other possible signs or symptoms for either type.
3. Now you have predicted which type of cerebrovascular accident that Mr Kwon has experienced, add a row to your table titled 'Treatment'. Contrast the medical, surgical and pharmacological interventions necessary to manage both types of stroke.
4. Observe Mr Kwon's pathology results. Is there anything of value identified in these results? Explain. What other haematological or biochemical changes might be seen in someone who has had a cerebrovascular accident?
5. What interventions are required to assist Mr Kwon? (Consider all possible interventions, including actions to assist with communication, oxygenation, activities of daily living, circulation, skin integrity and so on.)
6. The team thinks that Mr Kwon may be experiencing homonymous hemianopia. What is this, and why would Mr Kwon be at greater risk of experiencing this? (*Hint:* Think about the lesion location.)

BIBLIOGRAPHY

Australian Health Ministers' Advisory Council's National and Aboriginal and Torres Strait Islander Health Standing Committee (2017). *Cultural respect framework 2016–2026: for Aboriginal and Torres Strait Islander health—a national approach to building a culturally respectful health system*. Canberra: Australian Government Department of Health. https://nacchocommunique.files.wordpress.com/2016/12/cultural_respect_framework_1december2016_1.pdf.

Australian Indigenous Health*Info*Net (2022). *Overview of Aboriginal and Torres Strait Islander health status, 2021* Perth, WA: Australian Indigenous Health*Info*Net. https://healthinfonet.ecu.edu.au/learn/health-facts/overview-aboriginal-torres-strait-islander-health-status/.

Australian Institute of Health and Welfare (AIHW) (2018). *Vaccine preventable disease among Aboriginal and Torres Strait Islander people.* Canberra: AIHW. https://www.aihw.gov.au/getmedia/2fca3ed6-d242-4454-a00f-e298dd120ccb/aihw-phe-236_ATSI.pdf.aspx.

Australian Institute of Health and Welfare (AIHW) (2021). *Heart, stroke and vascular disease—Australian facts*. Canberra: AIHW. https://www.aihw.gov.au/reports/heart-stroke-vascular-diseases/hsvd-facts/contents/summary-of-coronary-heart-disease-and-stroke/coronary-heart-disease.

Bauldoff, G., Gubrud-Howe, P.M., Carno, M.-A., Levett-Jones, T., Hales, M., Berry, K.,... Stanley, D. (2020). *LeMone and Burke's medical-surgical nursing: critical thinking for person-centred care* (4th [Australian] edn). Sydney: Pearson Australia.

Bullock, S. & Manias, E. (2022). *Fundamentals of pharmacology* (9th edn). Sydney: Pearson Australia.

D'Antoine, H. & Bower, C. (2019). Folate status and neural tube defects in Aboriginal Australians: the success of mandatory fortification in reducing a health disparity. *Current Developments in Nutrition* 3(8):nzz071. https://www.doi.org/10.1093/cdn/nzz071.

Engelhard, H.H., Sahrakar, K. & Pang, D. (2020). Neurosurgery for hydrocephalus. *Emedicine.* https://emedicine.medscape.com/article/247387-overview.

Jauch, E.C., Al Kasab, S. & Stettler, B. (2022). Ischemic stroke. *Emedicine*. https://emedicine.medscape.com/article/1916852-overview.

Liebeskind, D.S. (2019). Hemorrhagic stroke. *Emedicine*. https://emedicine.medscape.com/article/1916662-overview.

Luke, C.R., Benfer, K., Mick-Ramsamy, L., Ware, R.S., Reid, N., Bos, A.F.,... Boyd, R.N. (2022). Early detection of Australian Aboriginal and Torres Strait Islander infants at high risk of adverse neurodevelopmental outcomes at 12 months corrected age: LEAP-CP prospective cohort study protocol. *BMJ Open* 12(1):e053646. https://doi.org/10.1136/ bmjopen-2021-053646.

Marieb, E.N. & Hoehn, K. (2019). *Human anatomy and physiology* (11th edn, Global Edition). San Francisco, CA: Pearson Benjamin Cummings.

Marshall, H.S. (2021). Meningococcal surveillance in Southeast Asia and the Pacific. *Microbiology Australia* 42(4):178–81. https://doi.org/10.1071/MA21050.

Martini, F.H. & Bartholomew, E.F. (2020). *Essentials of anatomy and physiology* (5th edn). San Francisco: Pearson.

New Zealand Ministry of Health (2021). *Annual update of key results 2020/2021New Zealand Health Survey*. Wellington: Ministry of Health. https://www.health.govt.nz/publication/annual-update-key-results-2020-21-new-zealand-health-survey.

Palisano, R., Rosenbaum, P., Walter, S., Russell, D., Wood, E. & Galuppi, B. (1997). Development and reliability of a system to classify gross motor function in children with cerebral palsy. *Developmental Medicine and Child Neurology* 39(4):214–23. https://doi.org/10.1111/j.1469-8749.1997.tb07414.x.

Paulson, A. & Vargus-Adams, J. (2017). Overview of four functional classification systems commonly used in cerebral palsy. *Children* 4(4):30. https://doi.org/10.3390/children4040030.

Vasudeva, S.S. (2022). Meningitis treatment and management. *Emedicine*. https://emedicine.medscape.com/article/232915-treatment.

Neurodegenerative disorders

10

LEARNING OBJECTIVES

After completing this chapter, you should be able to:

1. Identify the common pathophysiological mechanisms involved in the neurodegenerative disorders.
2. Describe the aetiology, pathophysiology, epidemiology, clinical manifestations, diagnosis and clinical management of each of the neurodegenerative disorders.
3. Compare and contrast the primary brain regions/tissues affected and the pathophysiologies of the neurodegenerative disorders.
4. Outline, where possible, the common features of the neurodegenerative disorders.

WHAT YOU SHOULD KNOW BEFORE YOU START THIS CHAPTER

Can you identify the main parts of the brain, and outline their functions?

Can you distinguish between autosomal dominant and recessive genetic diseases?

Can you describe the main phases of inflammation?

Can you distinguish between reversible and irreversible cell injury?

KEY TERMS

Alzheimer's disease (AD)
Dementia
Excitotoxicity
Huntington's disease
Lou Gehrig's disease
Motor neurone disease
Multiple sclerosis (MS)
Neuroinflammation
Oxidative stress
Parkinson's disease
Parkinsonism
Plaque
Protein aggregates

Introduction

Neurodegenerative disorders are conditions that induce progressive chronic deterioration in central nervous system (CNS) function, resulting from characteristic changes in the structure of the brain and the spinal cord. The disorders described in this chapter are Parkinson's disease, Alzheimer's disease, Huntington's disease, multiple sclerosis and motor neurone disease.

Common pathophysiological processes implicated in neurodegeneration

LEARNING OBJECTIVE 1

Identify the common pathophysiological mechanisms involved in the neurodegenerative disorders.

Currently it is the accepted view that the pathophysiological processes underlying neurodegenerative disorders—in particular Alzheimer's disease, Parkinson's disease, Huntington's disease and motor neurone disease—have more in common than not.

Common pathophysiological processes that have been proposed include intracellular protein aggregation, oxidative stress and mitochondrial dysfunction. Other mechanisms thought to play significant roles include excitotoxicity, neuroinflammation and apoptosis. It may be that no single mechanism is considered the leading cause. Indeed, different mechanisms may well occur simultaneously or lead into each other sequentially during the course of these diseases. Figure 10.1 provides a visual summary of these processes and their interactions. A brief outline of these mechanisms is provided later.

OXIDATIVE STRESS

Reactive oxygen species (ROS), such as hydrogen peroxide, hydroxyl and superoxide radicals, are formed as a consequence of aerobic metabolism. The consequences of excessive ROS activity can be irreversible cell damage (see the chapter 'Pathophysiological terminology, cellular adaptation and injury' for more details). The brain has a high demand for

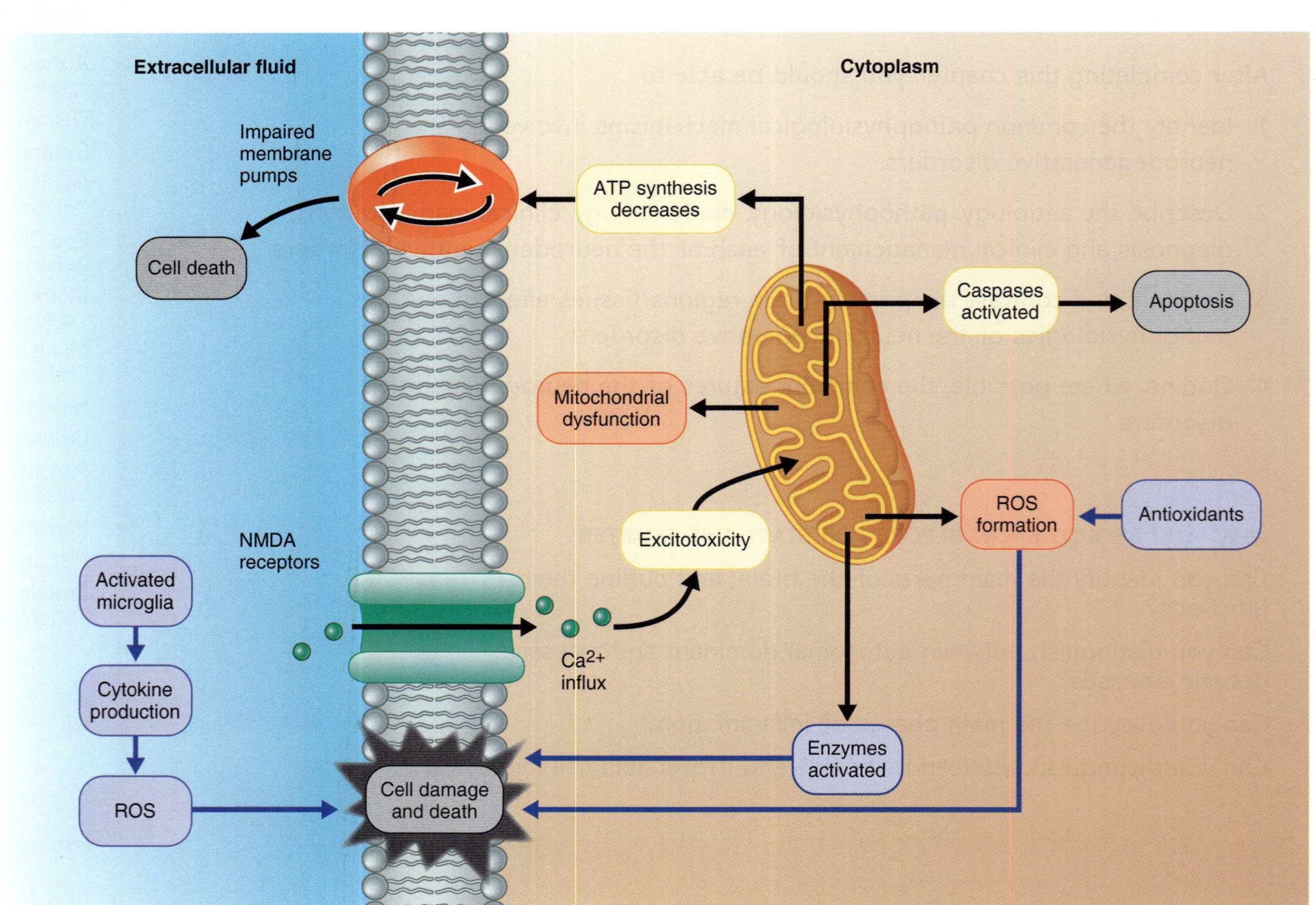

Figure 10.1

Common pathophysiological processes implicated in neurodegenerative disorders

ATP = adenosine triphosphate;
Ca^{2+} = calcium ion;
NMDA = N-methyl-D-aspartate;
ROS = reactive oxygen species.

oxygen, and as such undergoes extensive rates of aerobic metabolism. This makes brain cells particularly vulnerable to ROS production.

As a counter-regulatory mechanism, *antioxidant molecules*, such as superoxide dismutase (SOD) and glutathione, are formed within tissues to mop up and neutralise ROS before they induce cytotoxicity. For example, SOD converts (dismutates or detoxifies) any harmful superoxide particles formed during respiratory processes to hydrogen peroxide or water. The accepted view at this time is that as we age or suffer ill health, antioxidant production is out of balance with that of oxidants, leading to excessive tissue levels of ROS and a risk of neuronal damage.

A lot of research is being done to identify the biomarkers of oxidative stress in the blood, erythrocytes, cerebrospinal fluid, saliva and urine, to aid clinicians in making earlier and more certain diagnoses of neurodegenerative disease.

MITOCHONDRIAL DYSFUNCTION

An impairment of the mitochondrial electron transport chain within neurons derails cellular adenosine triphosphate (ATP) synthesis (which affects the function of the membrane sodium pump— Na^+/K^+-ATPase; see the chapter 'Pathophysiological terminology, cellular adaptation and injury') and promotes **oxidative stress**. These changes may also facilitate the processes of excitotoxicity and apoptosis.

EXCITOTOXICITY

It has been proposed that excessive activation of *N*-methyl-D-aspartate (NMDA) and/or alpha-amino-3-hydroxy-5-methyl-4-isoxazolepropionic acid (AMPA) glutamate receptors—referred to as **excitotoxicity**—may also contribute to neurodegeneration. These receptors are associated with calcium ion influx, where calcium induces increased activity in intracellular enzymes (e.g. proteases, nitric oxide synthase and phospholipases), which are capable of triggering cell death (see the chapter 'Pathophysiological terminology, cellular adaptation and injury').

NEUROINFLAMMATION

In **neuroinflammation**, activated microglial cells accumulate locally in response to cell injury and to the entry of foreign cells or organisms into the brain. Their activation can result in either *neuroprotection* or *neurotoxicity*, depending on the conditions. Activated microglia promote neuroprotection by reducing inflammation and stimulating tissue repair through the release of anti-inflammatory mediators and neurotrophic factors. They have also been implicated in neurotoxicity in neurodegenerative diseases. The mechanisms by which they can induce neuronal death are thought to involve oxidative stress and the release of proteolytic enzymes and pro-inflammatory cytokines.

APOPTOSIS

Apoptotic cell death (see the chapter 'Pathophysiological terminology, cellular adaptation and injury') may also be involved in the neurodegenerative process. It has been suggested that apoptosis occurs as one of the end points of the other pathophysiological processes of oxidative stress, excitotoxicity and neuroinflammation.

LEARNING OBJECTIVE 2

Describe the aetiology, pathophysiology, epidemiology, clinical manifestations, diagnosis and clinical management of each of the neurodegenerative disorders.

LEARNING OBJECTIVE 3

Compare and contrast the primary brain regions/tissues affected and the pathophysiologies of the neurodegenerative disorders.

LEARNING OBJECTIVE 4

Outline, where possible, the common features of the neurodegenerative disorders.

Parkinson's disease

Parkinson's disease (PD) is a common idiopathic neurodegenerative disorder that primarily causes motor impairment. As it advances, there may also be changes in sensory, cognitive and emotional processing.

Parkinsonism is a broad term used to encompass all of the conditions related to Parkinson's disease that have a similar pathology but have different aetiologies and clinical presentations. Parkinsonism can develop as a consequence of brain damage from a variety of causes, such as head trauma, the presence of a tumour growing in a particular brain region or after exposure to certain neurotoxic chemicals.

AETIOLOGY AND PATHOPHYSIOLOGY

The primary pathophysiology of parkinsonism is the *degeneration of the dopaminergic nigrostriatal pathway* in the brain. This pathway is a part of a complex processing loop involving parts of the cerebral cortex, basal ganglia and thalamus. The loop is a part of the *extrapyramidal modulatory system* that modifies the main outputs from the primary motor cortex along the pyramidal pathway through the brain and the spinal cord to skeletal muscles. The extrapyramidal pathways ensure that voluntary movements are efficient and effective by maintaining correct muscle tone, produce smooth and coordinated movement, and add subconscious elements to the movements (e.g. swinging your arms) to support appropriate posture and balance.

The *nigrostriatal pathway*, a component of the basal ganglia, feeds from the substantia nigra of the midbrain (literally meaning 'black substance', and referring to the pigmentation of the nucleus) to the subcortical corpus striatum. At the corpus striatum it interacts with cholinergic neurons, and modulates their transmission to other regions of the corpus striatum, such as the putamen and globus pallidus (see Figure 10.2). The net result of this modulation is activation of the appropriate motor regions of the cortex in the planning and execution of efficient and effective voluntary movements. The loss of dopaminergic input into this particular part of the corpus striatum leads to a localised chemical

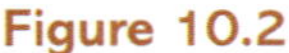

Figure 10.2

The nigrostriatal pathway and its role in motor control

The nigrostriatal pathway is part of a complex motor loop from the frontal cortex through the corpus striatum and thalamus to the supplementary and premotor cortical areas, which are involved in the planning and execution of voluntary movements.

imbalance (a functional dominance of cholinergic transmission even though the levels of synaptic acetylcholine are normal), which results in a loss of control of voluntary movement, which is the characteristic symptomology of the condition. Compensatory mechanisms within the brain are such that neuronal loss within the nigrostriatal pathway must reach 70% of normal before the condition manifests clinically. Thus, the pathophysiological process usually develops over many years, perhaps decades, before the condition becomes apparent and treatment is required.

Another characteristic of parkinsonism is that **protein aggregates** accumulate within the surviving nerve cells in the affected pathway and, to a lesser extent, in other brain regions. The primary protein involved is alpha-synuclein, but another significant component is ubiquitin. The proteins accumulate within discrete, well-defined cytoplasmic structures called *Lewy bodies* (see Figure 10.3), which displace other cellular components. Lewy body formation is common in parkinsonism, but is not present in every form, and is not a pathological change exclusive to this disease. For example, Lewy bodies have also been detected within the cerebral cortex in some forms of dementia.

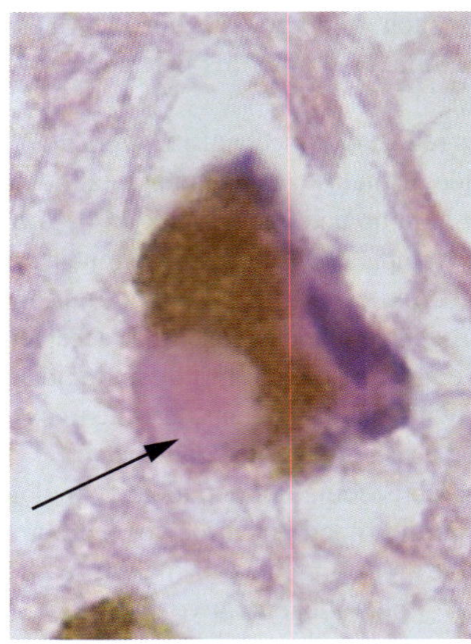

Figure 10.3

A histological sample of a neuron from the neocortex with the Lewy body marked by an arrow

(Haematoxylin/Eosin stain, 500x.)

Source: © Werner et al. (2008); licensee BioMed Central Ltd. Licensed under a Creative Commons Attribution License. http://creativecommons.org/licenses/by/2.0.

The cause of the deterioration of the nigrostriatal pathway in parkinsonism remains unclear. An impairment of the mitochondrial electron transport chain within neural tissue has been strongly implicated in the pathophysiology of Parkinson's disease, as has oxidative stress and excitotoxicity. In the early stages of the pathogenesis, the nigrostriatal pathway is particularly vulnerable to ROS formation. There is evidence that some metabolites of dopamine's degradation can be toxic at high levels, promoting ROS formation. Moreover, there is a high concentration of reactive iron within the substantia nigra, which facilitates toxic hydroxyl radical production from hydrogen peroxide, resulting in lipid peroxidation.

Activated microglial cells, as part of a neuroinflammatory response, have been implicated in neuronal death in the substantia nigra of people with Parkinson's disease, and, as further evidence, pro-inflammatory cytokines, such as tumour necrosis factor-alpha and a number of interleukins, have been detected in the striatum and cerebrospinal fluid of people with the disease.

A number of genetic mutations have been implicated in the pathophysiology of the familial types of parkinsonism. About 13 relevant monogenetic mutations have been identified and have been termed the *PARK* series or loci. Some of these mutations, *PARK1/PARK4 (SNCA)*, can be demonstrably linked to nigrostriatal degeneration, with or without Lewy body formation. It has been proposed that *SNCA* leads to an increased tendency to form intracellular alpha-synuclein aggregates. *PARK8 (LRRK2)* and *SNCA* are associated with autosomal dominant forms of the disease, while *PARK2 (Parkin), PARK6 (PINK1)* and *PARK8 (DJ-1)* are linked to the autosomal recessive form. *LRRK2* has been linked to cognitive decline, while *Parkin* and *DJ-1* are associated with motor impairment. It is hoped that further research into these mutations will provide useful information as to the mechanism of dopaminergic cell degeneration in both familial and sporadic parkinsonism.

Risk factors that have been linked to parkinsonism include age, sex, inheritance, head injury and exposure to chemicals. The condition is more common in older adults, and affects more men than women. A close relative with the sporadic form of Parkinson's disease can marginally increase a person's risk of developing the disease.

Retrospective studies have shown that pesticide and herbicide exposure may be an important risk factor, with a higher incidence in farm workers. Indeed, a pesticide called rotenone is used to induce parkinsonism in an animal model of the disease. The presence of toxic contaminants in illicit drug preparations has also been shown to induce parkinsonism in drug users.

EPIDEMIOLOGY

Parkinson's disease affects 0.1–0.2% of the general population. This rises to 1% in people over 60 years of age. According to recent Australian Bureau of Statistics data, there are approximately 219,000 people with the condition in Australia, a significant rise on that recorded in 2015. According to the Australian Institute of Health and Welfare, in 2020–21, more than 140,000 people were admitted to Australian hospitals for a Parkinson's disease-related cause. This represents 41% of all nervous system disease hospitalisations, and 1.2% of all hospitalisations in that period. This increase is considered to be related to the rise in the ageing population and the increased longevity of people affected due to better management. In New Zealand in 2020, about 11,000 people were affected.

Typically, the distribution within the population is sporadic, with most people being diagnosed between 50 and 75 years of age (although 20% cases occur in people under 50 years old), and the progression is relatively slow. There are also relatively rarer forms that are inheritable. These are grouped under the general heading of *familial parkinsonism*, and account for about 10–15% of cases. These disorders exist as single-gene disorders of either an autosomal dominant or autosomal recessive origin. Some of these forms occur at an earlier age, about 25–40 years of age, and progress very rapidly, while others show a similar age of onset and progression to the sporadic form.

CLINICAL MANIFESTATIONS

The cardinal signs of Parkinson's disease are *t*remor at rest, *r*igidity, *a*kinesia (an absence of spontaneous movement) or bradykinesia (slowed movement), and *p*ostural instability (see Figure 10.4). This is known by the acronym of TRAP. The tremors are unilateral, and do not occur during sleep or motor action. Tremors usually involve the hands (characteristically known as 'pill-rolling' tremors), lips, chin, jaw and legs. There is a postural component to the tremor, which is worse while standing compared to sitting, and sitting on a stool compared to sitting in a chair. The rigidity is described as 'cogwheel', because as a limb is moved through its passive range it rapidly alternates between free and impeded motion, like the turning of a cogwheel. Postural instability occurs late in the disease, and involves an impairment in the integration of visual, vestibular and proprioceptive information. It is a major cause of falls in people with this condition.

Other common features are a flexed posture (which occurs late in the disease), neck and spinal flexion, freezing, loss of facial expression and blinking, monotone voice, impaired swallowing and consequent drooling, dystonia, decreased arm swinging, shuffling gait and small handwriting. Non-motor symptoms include autonomic dysfunction (orthostatic hypotension, constipation, abnormal sweating, sexual impairment and urinary sphincter problems), sleep disorders, sensory dysfunction (poor olfaction, paraesthesias, akathisia, oral and/or genital pain), as well as cognitive and behavioural abnormalities (confusion, memory loss, insecurity, dementia, depression, apathy, anxiety, and obsessive–compulsive or impulsive behaviours). Figure 10.5 explores the common clinical manifestations and management of Parkinson's disease.

Recently, there has been discussion as to whether a *prodromal state* associated with Parkinson's disease exists prior to the onset of motor disturbances. If it does, then people in this phase could be treated at an earlier stage of neurodegeneration, halting the progress of the disease. Proponents believe that the prodromal phase is characterised by olfactory, sleep, bowel and mood dysfunction.

Figure 10.4
Cardinal signs of Parkinson's disease

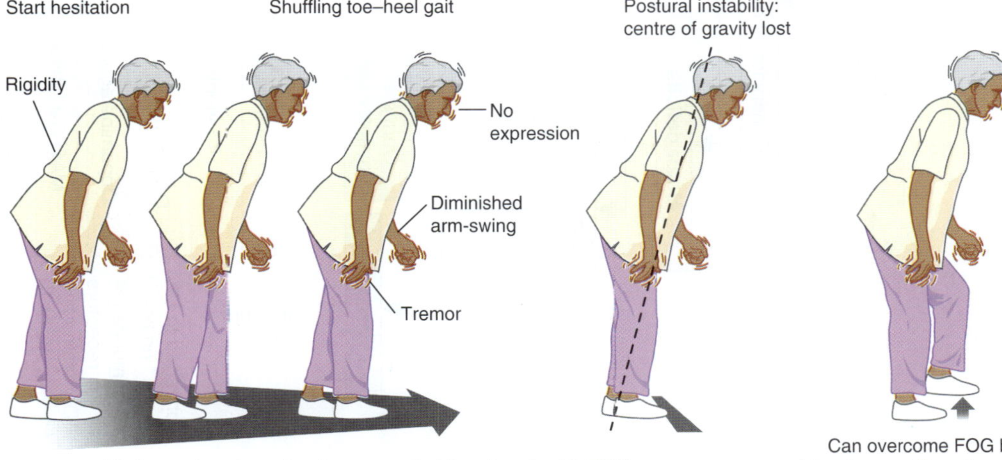

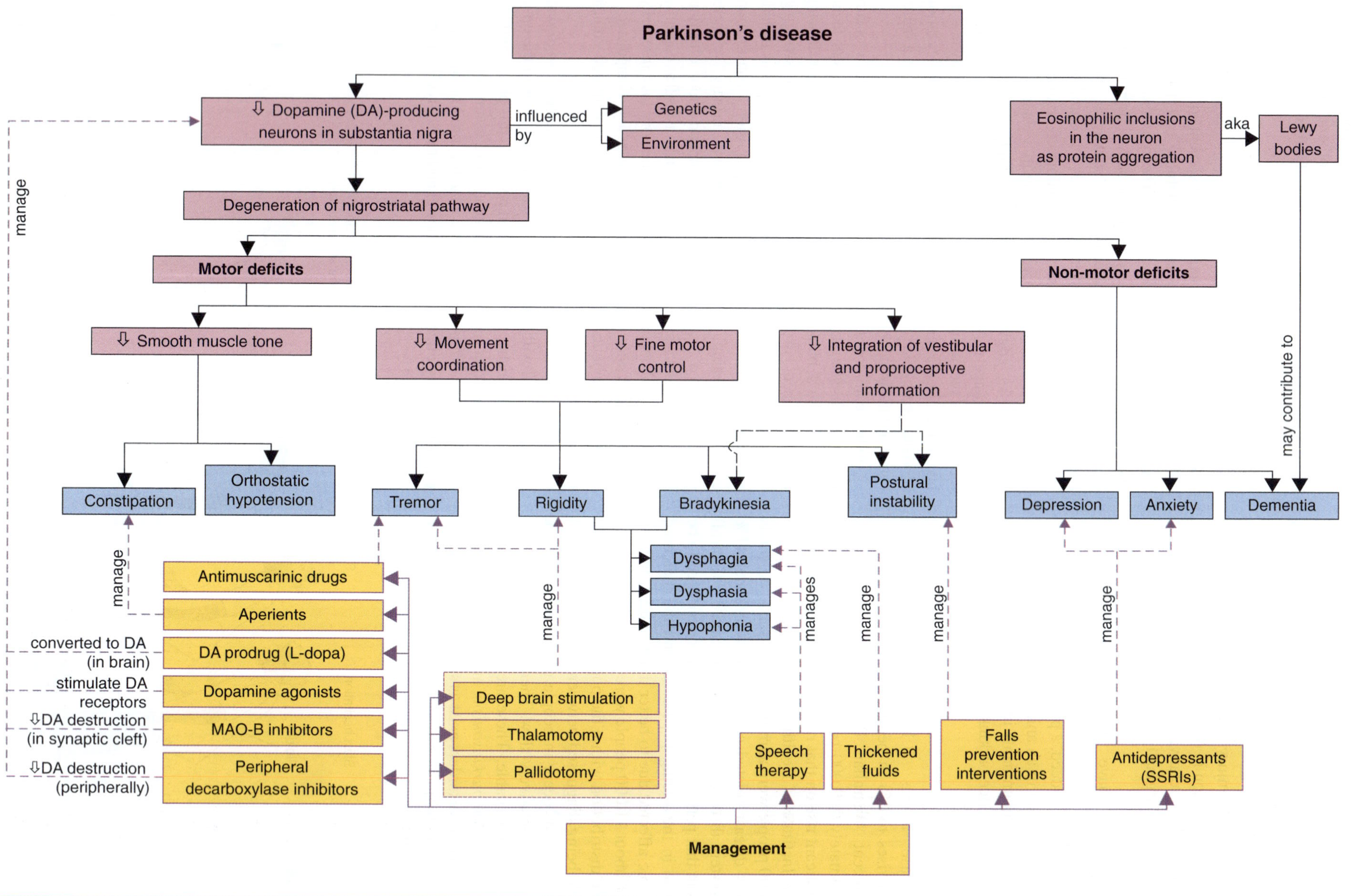

Figure 10.5

Clinical snapshot: Parkinson's disease

↓ = decreased; DA = dopamine; MAO-B = monoamine oxidase B; SSRI = selective serotonin reuptake inhibitor.

CLINICAL DIAGNOSIS AND MANAGEMENT

Diagnosis

Haematology and biochemistry tests are of little benefit in the diagnosis of Parkinson's disease, other than to rule out other organic causes of movement, behavioural or cognitive changes. However, these blood tests may also identify concomitant issues that require management.

Neuroimaging studies cannot be used to diagnose Parkinson's disease either. However, they may identify space-occupying lesions or anatomical issues. The diagnosis of Parkinson's disease relies on the consideration of the clinical picture and an assessment of neurological and psychological signs and symptoms.

Research on the identification of clinical, biochemical, genetic and imaging biomarkers to improve the early diagnosis of parkinsonism is progressing. The presence of alpha-synuclein in body fluids is a particular focus.

Management

A person with Parkinson's disease requires a coordinated team of expert health professionals to support the various challenges of the disease. Safety issues—such as the prevention of falls and aspiration pneumonia—are of paramount importance. Assessment and intermittent reassessment for postural instability, orthostatic hypotension and dysphagia are important to ensure that, as the individual's ability to maintain functions deteriorates, strategies such as the installation of rails or the provision of gait assistance devices can be instituted prior to accident or injury from falls. Education about food preparation techniques and fluid-thickening agents will assist with preventing aspiration pneumonia.

Medication plays an integral role in the management of people with Parkinson's disease. The goals include providing symptomatic control and slowing deterioration by increasing the amount of dopamine available. Use of drugs such as *dopamine precursors* (prodrugs; e.g. L-dopa), which are converted to dopamine, combined with peripheral decarboxylase inhibitors, which reduce the inactivation of peripheral L-dopa, increases the amount of drug available for transport into the brain. Dopamine cannot pass through the blood–brain barrier, so any L-dopa that is converted to dopamine by decarboxylase in the peripheral tissues does not penetrate the brain.

Dopamine agonists reduce Parkinson's effects by stimulating dopamine receptors (mostly D2-receptors), which results in reduced tremor and rigidity. The use of dopamine agonists concomitantly with dopamine prodrugs has a synergistic effect, often resulting in the ability to reduce the prodrug dose.

Selective monamine oxidase inhibitors (MAO-B inhibitors) are used to reduce the destruction of dopamine within the synaptic (and neural) cleft, ultimately increasing the volume of neurotransmitter available for binding. An antiviral agent used in influenza prophylaxis called amantadine can increase the synthesis and release of dopamine. It also has some antimuscarinic action.

Muscarinic antagonists (otherwise known as antimuscarinic drugs) that block muscarinic receptors were the first medications to be used for Parkinson's disease. The mechanism specific to Parkinson's disease appears to be related to correcting the imbalance between the dopaminergic and cholinergic motor pathways by reducing the action of acetylcholine. However, although antimuscarinic agents are very effective in the control of tremor, they do not provide any benefit against rigidity or bradykinesia. Antimuscarinic agents have also been associated with worsening confusional states and hallucinations, especially if they are stopped suddenly.

Surgery may be attempted to provide an improved quality of life. In the past, surgeons used to cause a lesion in either the thalamus (thalamotomy) or the globus pallidus (pallidotomy) to control severe and disabling tremors. These procedures are thought to reduce the excessive inhibition of the neurons in the basal ganglia.

Deep brain stimulation is now becoming more favoured, because the procedure does not create a permanent lesion but, rather, provides a stimulation that can be adjusted as necessary. An implanted device, much like a pacemaker, is inserted in the skin of the chest wall and connected to electrodes that have been implanted in the brain through a burr hole. Electrodes may be placed in the thalamus or globus pallidus as in the lesioning surgery or, recently, in the subthalamic nucleus. The leads are threaded down into the chest (underneath the skin) and connected to the implantable pulse generator (stimulation device). The electrodes required for this device can be implanted while the person is awake, so that the correct location and stimulation amplitude is identified. A transcutaneous device can be used to program the device as the person's condition advances.

Other issues requiring management may include depression and anxiety. These are often controlled with *selective serotonin reuptake inhibitor* antidepressants. Because of the hypotonia, constipation may become an issue. Use of aperients and increasing dietary fibre and fluid intake can assist with this issue.

Alzheimer's disease

Dementias are characterised by a progressive deterioration of the cognitive processes affecting memory, the performance of learned skills, thinking, reasoning and judgment. As dementia progresses, there are changes in sensory processing, perception, language, behaviour and emotions.

AETIOLOGY AND PATHOPHYSIOLOGY

The pathophysiology of **Alzheimer's disease (AD)** is associated with neuronal loss in particular areas of the brain, resulting in severe cerebral atrophy (see Figure 10.6). It was once considered simply an acceleration of the normal ageing process within the brain, but evidence indicates that the focus of the cell loss is within different regions of the brain from those seen in normal ageing. The key regions affected in Alzheimer's disease are the *hippocampus, limbic system* and *frontal cortex*. The disease process predominantly *targets cholinergic neurons* in these areas. Excitotoxicity via the overstimulation of glutamatergic NMDA receptors and oxidative stress are believed to make a major contribution to this process.

The diagnostic hallmarks of this disease are histological. There are two characteristic changes in the physical structure of affected brain regions: the development of neurofibrillary tangles and extracellular beta-amyloid (Abeta) **plaque** deposits. *Neurofibrillary tangles* occur when there is a disruption to the structure and stability

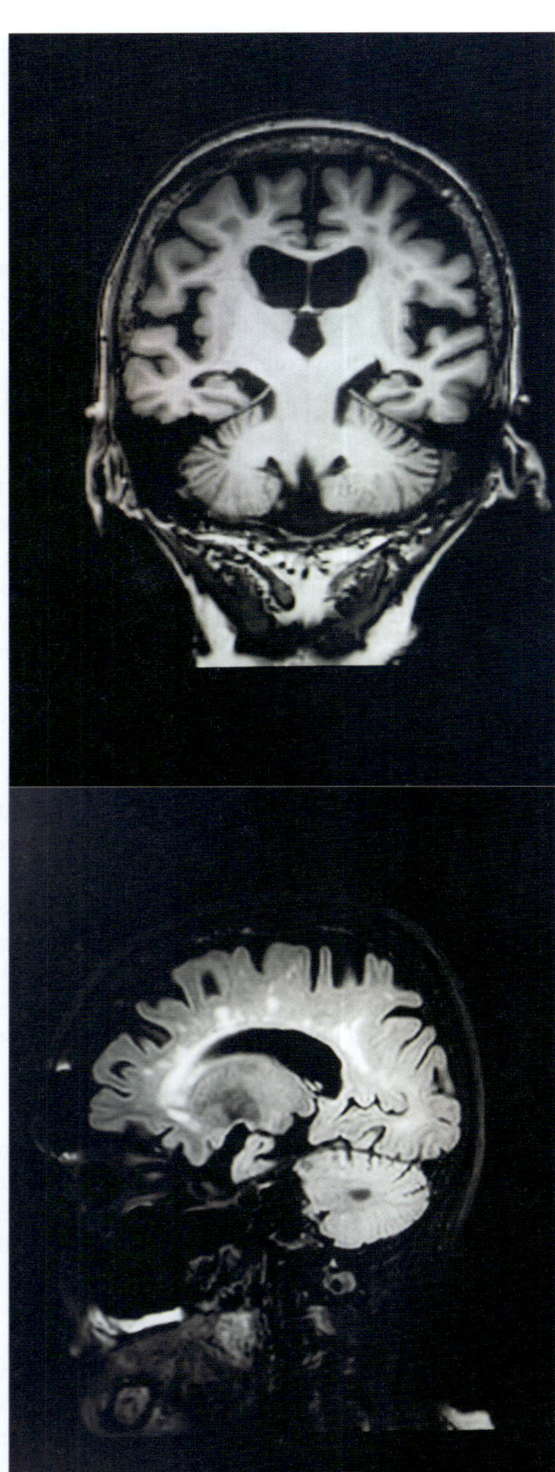

Figure 10.6

MRI showing cerebral atrophy

Cerebral atrophy is indicated by a reduction in the size of the brain, as well as a narrowing of the gyri and a widening of the sulci.

Source: Atthapon Raksthaput/Shutterstock.

of the microtubules that form the cytoskeleton. The microtubules fragment into insoluble intracellular aggregates of phosphorylated tau protein, the neuron's shape collapses (see Figure 10.7) and there is extensive cell loss. *Abeta plaques*, also known as senile plaques, form extracellularly in brain tissue. The Abeta is made from a membrane protein called *amyloid precursor protein (APP)*. A family of enzymes called secretases is responsible for the cleavage of the APP molecule. Importantly, other fragments of APP created by secretase action are not harmful to the brain, and may even perform a role to counteract oxidative stress. The Abeta fragments cannot be easily cleared from the brain and accumulate in the plaques. Apolipoprotein E, which is involved in the transport of cholesterol peripherally, is also involved in the clearance of amyloid fragments from the brain. A mutation in the apolipoprotein E gene (see below) has been implicated in the pathophysiology of Alzheimer's disease. A correlation has been found between the number of senile plaques and the magnitude of cognitive impairment.

Neuroinflammation and oxidative stress are thought to play a key role in the pathophysiology of the disease. As in Parkinson's disease, activated microglia have been implicated in the deposition of protein aggregates into the senile plaques and neuronal loss. Initially these inflammatory processes may actually oppose toxic protein fragment deposition, but over time any neuroprotection is overcome.

One of the earliest theories put forward regarding the pathophysiology of Alzheimer's disease is the *cholinergic hypothesis*, which states that a significant loss of cholinergic nerves in the brain regions to the front and below the corpus striatum is associated with Alzheimer's disease. Further to this, the concentration of the enzyme choline acetyltransferase, responsible for neuronal acetylcholine synthesis, is decreased in the hippocampus and cerebral cortex. According to the hypothesis, these losses are associated with the cognitive impairments symptomatic of the disease.

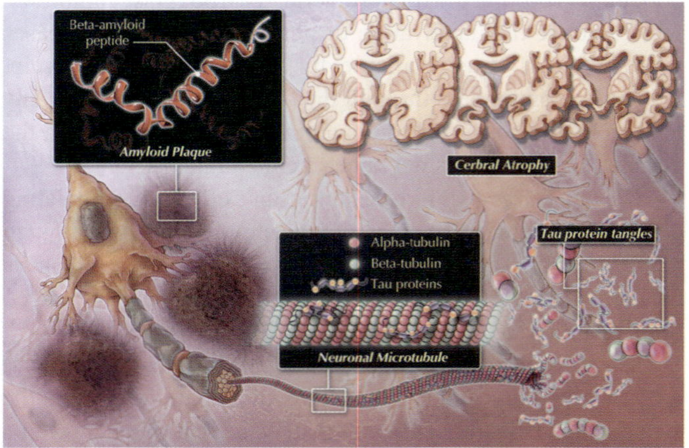

Figure 10.7

Diagnostic hallmarks of Alzheimer's disease—amyloid plaques, neurofibrillary tau protein tangles and cerebral atrophy

Source: Photo Researchers/Science History Images/Alamy Stock Photo.

Age is the most important risk factor for Alzheimer's disease. Another factor is inheritance. An immediate family member with Alzheimer's disease marginally increases a person's risk of developing the condition. Moreover, a further genetic link is the *apolipoprotein E* gene, which has a number of alleles (types 2–4). It has been found that people with at least one copy of the type 4 allele are at greater risk of developing Alzheimer's disease.

Cardiovascular disease increases the risk of developing Alzheimer's disease or other forms of dementia by decreasing cerebral blood flow. By reducing cardiovascular risk factors (e.g. a lack of exercise, poor diet and smoking), the risk of Alzheimer's disease can be lowered. Another risk factor that has been identified is head injury acquired through falls, participation in sport or in military service, or as a result of other trauma.

It has been shown that people who live mentally active lives may have a reduced risk of developing Alzheimer's disease. It appears that those who seek out mental stimulation through such pursuits as reading, further education, puzzle-solving and grammatically rich letter-writing may be at less risk of developing the disease.

EPIDEMIOLOGY

Alzheimer's disease is a common form of dementia, accounting for 50–70% of all dementias. Types of dementia are summarised in Table 10.1. It is estimated that about 390,000 Australians and 70,000 New Zealanders live with some form of dementia. It is estimated that 152.8 million people worldwide will have dementia by 2050. In Australia, the prevalence in women is greater (63%) than in men. The proportion of people affected increases with age, with 25% of people aged 85 years and over showing signs of dementia. Dementia is a leading cause of burden of disease in our community. It is the single greatest cause of disability in older Australians over 65 years, and is the second leading cause of death in Australia per year.

CLINICAL MANIFESTATIONS

The early stages of Alzheimer's disease involve forgetfulness, some impaired recall of new memories and minor losses in the ability to communicate. As the condition progresses, these impairments worsen and are accompanied by confusion, a loss of concentration and disorientation. This is accompanied by irritability, restlessness and agitation. Mood and emotional state alter, leading to mood swings, anxiety and depression. Changes in personality occur.

The cognitive deficits progressively become more severe, affecting problem-solving and judgment. The affected person will go on to show loss of long-term memories to a point where they are unable to recognise immediate family members. They 'unlearn' basic daily motor skills (dyspraxia), such as brushing their teeth and combing their hair, and become totally dependent on care provided by others. Eventually, death ensues within 5–15 years of diagnosis. Figure 10.8 explores the common clinical manifestations and management of Alzheimer's disease.

CLINICAL DIAGNOSIS AND MANAGEMENT

Diagnosis

Alzheimer's disease cannot be confirmed until autopsy. However, the consideration of the clinical presentation and history and various investigations can provide sufficient evidence for a diagnosis of Alzheimer's disease. Investigations to rule out organic causes of confusion, and of behavioural and cognitive changes, are necessary, and may include full blood count, biochemistry, renal and hepatic function tests, and neuroimaging, such as computed tomography (CT) or magnetic resonance imaging (MRI). Lumbar puncture may be used to rule out infective causes. A mini-mental state examination (MMSE) must be undertaken and recorded before some of the pharmacological treatments are authorised.

Table 10.1 Selected types of dementia

Type of dementia	Description
Alzheimer's disease	Most common form of dementia. Affects the structure and function of neurones..
Vascular dementia	The second most common form. Associated with brain damage caused by impaired cerebral circulation by a stroke or vascular disease in small deep blood vessels in the brain.
HIV-associated dementia	This form of dementia occurs in people with advanced stages of HIV/AIDS.
Alcohol-related dementia	Excessive alcohol use can lead to a direct toxic effect or severe deficiency in vitamin B_1 (thiamine). This results in brain damage.
Fronto-temporal dementia	A condition characterised by degeneration of the frontal and/or temporal lobe affecting behaviour, personality, language and movement.
Lewy body disease	Dementia resulting from the degeneration and death of brain cells. Affected cells contain abnormal structures called Lewy bodies. Hard to distinguish from dementia that can occur in Parkinson's disease.

HIV = human immunodeficiency virus.

Source: Dementia Australia, Types of dementia, https://www.dementia.org.au/information/about-dementia/types-of-dementia.

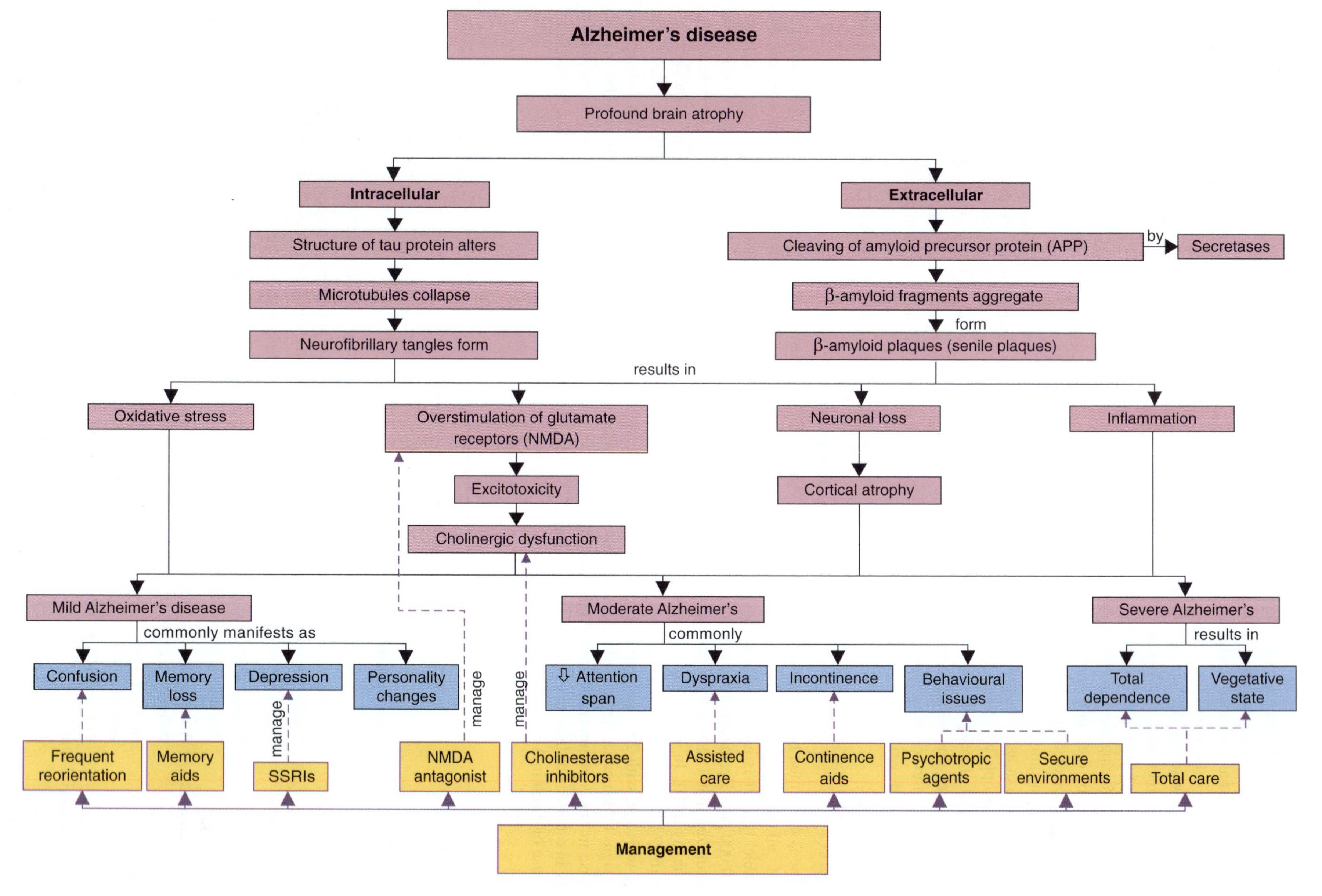

Figure 10.8

Clinical snapshot: Alzheimer's disease

↓ = decreased; β = beta; NMDA = N-methyl-D-aspartate; SSRIs = selective serotonin reuptake inhibitors.

Management

A person who has been diagnosed with Alzheimer's disease will require significant support as their cognitive function declines. Depression will often require management with *selective serotonin reuptake inhibitors*. Caregivers will need to be taught the importance of frequent reorientation and how to deal with the challenges that lie ahead. Loved ones often find that the personality and behavioural changes associated with Alzheimer's disease can be difficult to cope with. Individuals with moderate Alzheimer's disease may require admission to secure healthcare facilities that specialise in the care of people with Alzheimer's disease, because the family members are no longer able to care for their loved ones safely as a result of aggression or wandering behaviours.

It is thought that undertaking frequent mental challenges, such as completing crossword puzzles (or the equivalent), may delay disease progression somewhat or even protect from disease development. However, there is currently no cure for Alzheimer's disease. *Acetylcholinesterase inhibitors* and *NMDA receptor antagonists* may be beneficial to slow down progression. Both of these drugs work by improving acetylcholine levels. Acetylcholinesterase inhibitors reduce the destruction of acetylcholine. NMDA receptor antagonists reduce the overstimulation of glutamate, which ultimately causes excitotoxicity and results in further cholinergic dysfunction.

As a person's health declines, they will become increasingly unresponsive and less capable of participating in any activity. At this stage, they require total care and, in time, will not even appear to be conscious of their surroundings.

Huntington's disease

Huntington's disease—also known as *Huntington's chorea* (due to the characteristic dance-like movements)—is an autosomal dominant genetic disorder involving a mutation in a single gene. This means that if you possess one copy of the mutated gene, even if the other copy is normal, you will develop the disease. It is characterised by progressive dementia and involuntary writhing movements.

AETIOLOGY AND PATHOPHYSIOLOGY

The pathophysiology involves the production of a protein called huntingtin, which is programmed by a gene on chromosome 4. In Huntington's disease, the *huntingtin gene* is corrupted so that the codon for the *amino acid glutamine, CAG, is overexpressed.* Normally, the gene codes for up to 30 CAG codons, but in Huntington's disease there may be up to 125 CAG codons. Therefore, the formed protein contains too many glutamine residues, represented using the abbreviation 'polyQ'. As a consequence, the huntingtin protein folds abnormally and becomes rigid, interacting abnormally with other proteins (e.g. HAP-1). *Protein aggregates* are deposited in the nuclei of neurons within specific brain regions. The activity of a key enzyme involved in the production of gamma-aminobutyric acid (GABA)—glutamic acid decarboxylase—alters so that a *deficiency in GABA signalling* develops. It has been proposed that this, in turn, may facilitate *oxidative stress* with excitotoxic and apoptotic processes that contribute to cell losses. A widespread loss of neurons occurs, particularly in the basal ganglia and cerebral cortex (see Figure 10.9).

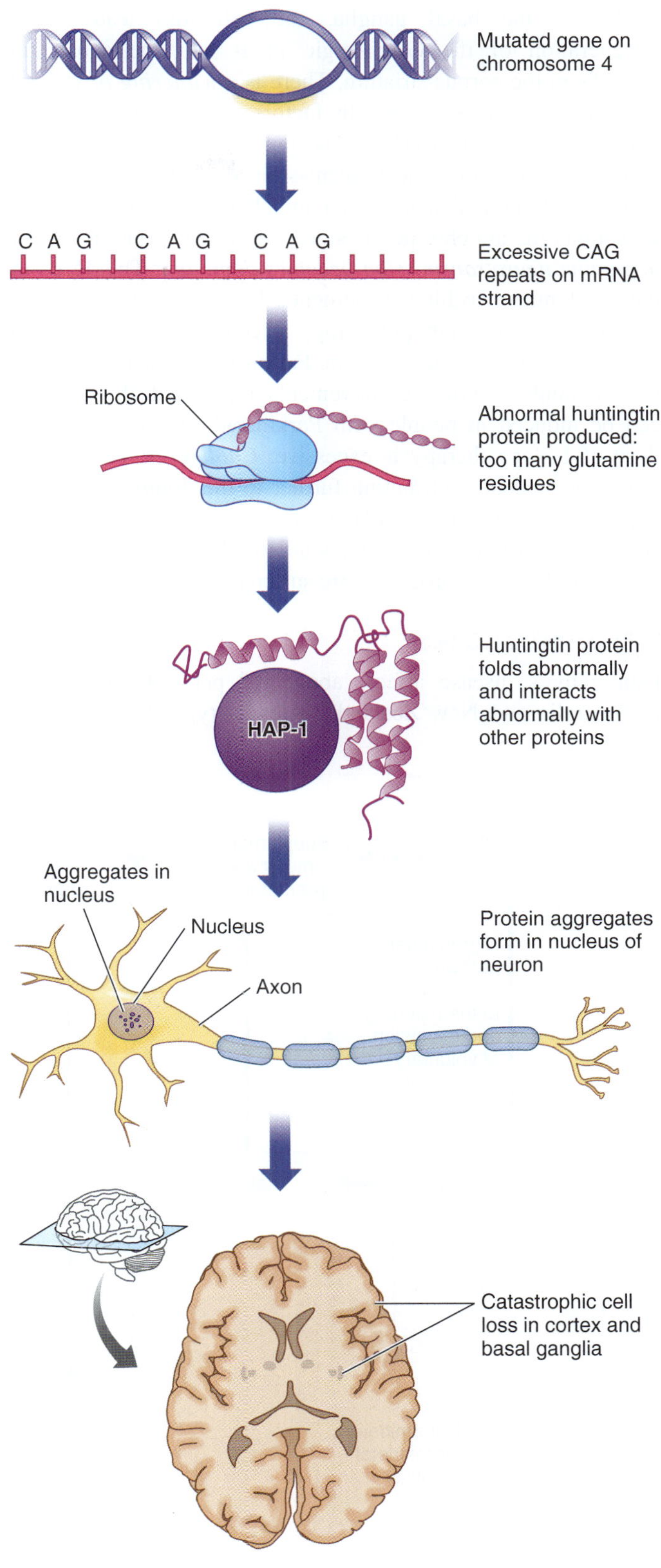

Figure 10.9

Pathophysiology of Huntington's disease

CAG = cytosine–adenine–guanine; HAP-1 = Huntington-associated protein-1; mRNA = messenger RNA.

Source: Adapted from Marieb & Hoehn (2016).

Within the basal ganglia, the cell loss leads to a degeneration of the GABAergic input into the substantia nigra from the corpus striatum. There is a *withering of striatal cells* due to a loss of growth factors such as brain-derived neurotrophic factor (BDNF). The purpose of this pathway is to regulate dopaminergic transmission along the nigrostriatal pathway. Without this input, an imbalance develops between dopaminergic and cholinergic signalling in the striatum so that *dopamine neurotransmission becomes dominant*. This leads to the involuntary writhing movements. It is reasonable, then, to conclude that the pathophysiology affecting the basal ganglia is the opposite of that seen in Parkinson's disease. Indeed, the involuntary writhing movements typical of this disease can be induced in people with Parkinson's disease when the dose of L-dopa therapy is excessive. *Cholinergic cell loss* is also pronounced, contributing further to the dominance of the dopaminergic signalling. At the cortical level, the cholinergic cell loss contributes to the characteristic dementia observed in these people. These processes are summarised in Figure 10.10.

EPIDEMIOLOGY

Huntington's disease affects about 7.5 per 100,000 people in Australia and New Zealand, which is typical of the rates reported for other Western countries. Regional differences have been reported, with the prevalence in Tasmania reported to be as high as 12 people per 100,000. This is thought to be due to a 'founder effect', where an early settler of European origin with the disorder passed on the mutation within this relatively smaller community.

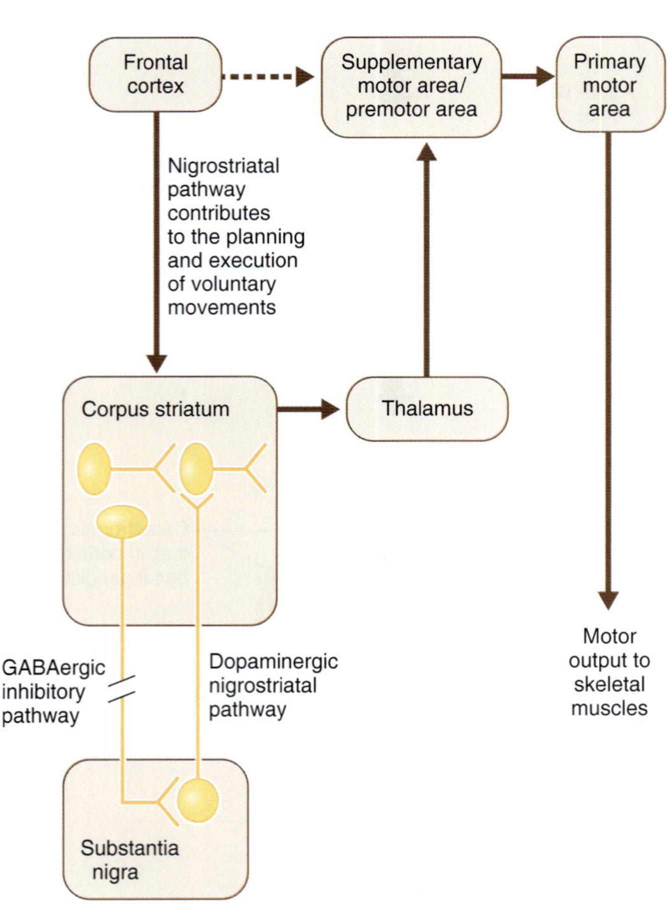

Figure 10.10
Changes in basal ganglia in Huntington's disease

CLINICAL MANIFESTATIONS

The usual onset of Huntington's disease is around 30–50 years old, although there are early-onset forms of the condition. The early manifestations include slight, hyperkinetic involuntary muscle movements, particularly affecting the face and arms (tics and grimacing), as well as a loss in motor coordination leading to clumsiness and stumbling. The early cognitive manifestations affect decision-making and organisational skills, and also include a loss of concentration, forgetfulness and mood swings. As the condition progresses, the motor and cognitive manifestations become more global and severe. The involuntary jerky, ceaseless dance-like movements become more pronounced, affecting the whole body. Movement progressively becomes more hypokinetic and dystonic. A difficulty in speaking and swallowing develops. Cognitive impairments are accompanied by antisocial behaviour (hostility, apathy), psychosis (delusions, paranoia and hallucinations), impulsiveness and depression. A common cause of death in people with Hungtington's disease is pneumonia.

CLINICAL DIAGNOSIS AND MANAGEMENT

Diagnosis

Until recently there were no definitive tests for Huntington's disease. However, genetic testing observing for a CAG repeat in each allele may be available in some facilities. This option may be considered in the event of prenatal testing in a family with a positive history of Huntington's disease. Genetic counselling should be provided to families in this situation, as significant decisions may need to be considered as a consequence of the test result. Other than genetic testing, consideration of the family history and clinical presentation form the basis of the diagnosis.

Investigations to rule out organic causes of motor and cognitive dysfunction are important. Analysis of haematology and biochemistry panels may also identify other issues that need to be addressed. Neuroimaging such as CT or MRI will rule out space-occupying lesions and trauma. They may also be used to identify atrophy of the caudate nuclei. Some studies demonstrate that even someone with early-stage Huntington's disease may present with measurable atrophy. Positron emission tomography (PET) may show the areas involved; however, this information does nothing to guide clinical management, and can be financially burdensome to either the individual or the government's healthcare budget.

Management

Currently there is no cure for Huntington's disease. Tetrabenzine may control the chorea by selectively binding to monoamine transporters and depleting stores of transmitter, thus reducing the action of the dopaminergic neurons in the substantia nigra. Caution should be taken with this drug, though, as it may increase depression, suicidality and confusion.

Depression is common in people with Huntington's disease. Initially, SSRIs and then, if necessary, other antidepressants have been found to be beneficial. Antipsychotic agents may be required if hallucinations and delusions become problematic.

As a person's functional abilities decline, they will require assistance with activities of daily living. In time, they will become totally dependent for all cares. Palliative care services will be required, and they may benefit from admission to a healthcare facility if their loved ones are unable to manage the demands of their care.

Multiple sclerosis

Multiple sclerosis (MS) is a neurodegenerative disorder characterised by sensory, motor, behavioural and emotional dysfunction.

AETIOLOGY AND PATHOPHYSIOLOGY

The focus of the disease process is the *myelin sheath of neurons* and the cells that make it (which are called *oligodendrocytes*) within the brain, spinal cord and optic nerve. The myelin is attacked and damaged. Consequently, the transmission of impulses along myelinated CNS nerves is slowed or blocked completely, leading to significant functional impairments.

The disease is widely considered to be an *autoimmune condition*. Immune cells, particularly T lymphocytes, gain entry to the brain, where they attack the myelin and the oligodendrocytes. Through the action of T cells, cytokines and activated microglia, *oxidative stress* and *chronic neuroinflammation* develop. Excitotoxicity, apoptosis, calcium ion overload, mitochondrial dysfunction and proteolysis (see the chapter 'Pathophysiological terminology, cellular adaptation and injury') occur. The damaged myelin sheaths release iron, which accumulates in the plaques to promote greater levels of oxidative stress and cell loss.

The damaged area heals as a scar or plaque. The hardened non-functional tissue is referred to as an area of *sclerosis* (see Figure 10.11). Functional impairments correlate with the areas of plaque formation, which can form anywhere in the CNS and occur over multiple sites. This process gives rise to the name—multiple sclerosis.

There is much conjecture as to the reason for the autoimmune attack. It may occur because the CNS is usually quarantined from access by the immune system. CNS tissue components such as the myelin may not be recognised as 'self', and may be regarded as antigenic under certain conditions. An unknown event triggers a temporary disruption in the blood–brain barrier, which allows these immune cells to gain entry to the CNS and interact with the myelin. A viral infection has long been touted as a possible initiator of the phenomenon. However, no candidate has yet been clearly identified. It is also possible that such a viral infection changes immune function to heighten reactivity with CNS myelin.

A

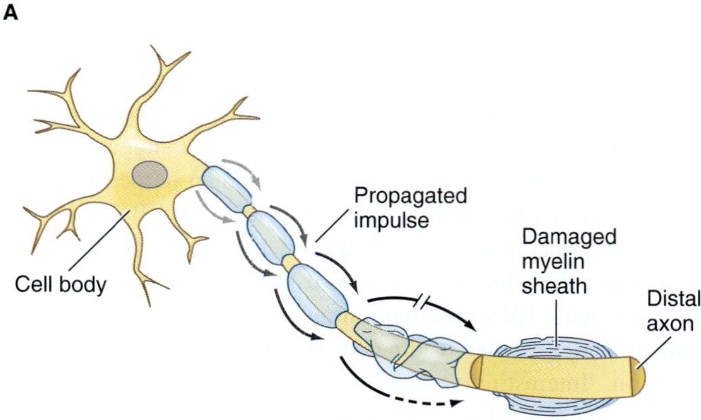

B

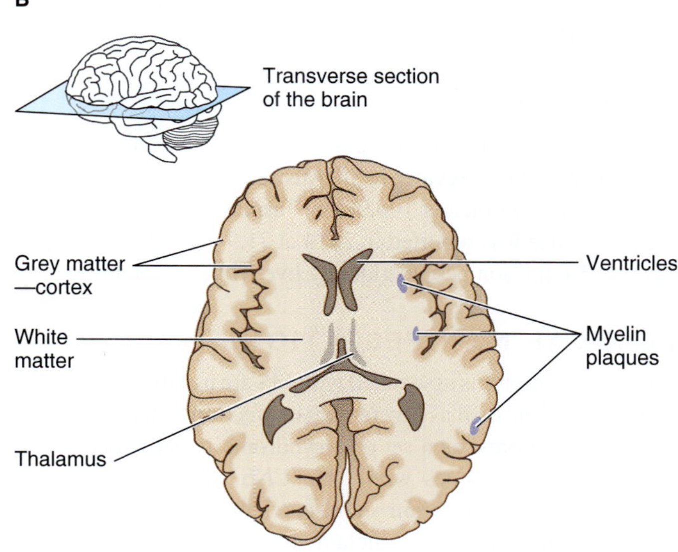

Figure 10.11

Multiple sclerosis

(A) Myelin destruction and plaque formation in multiple sclerosis. (B) Plaque formation within CNS white matter.

Source: Adapted from Marieb & Hoehn (2016).

There are two forms of MS—relapsing–remitting and progressive—which can be differentiated from each other by their rates of progression. In *relapsing–remitting MS*, symptomatic episodes are separated by periods of remission. The degree of degeneration may or may not worsen between episodes. In *progressive MS*, no remission periods occur, and the degeneration progressively worsens over time. Relapsing–remitting MS can become the progressive form.

MS is considered to be caused by an interaction of genetic and environmental factors. An immediate family member with MS increases a person's risk of developing the condition only marginally. This condition appears to predominantly affect people with Northern European or Caucasian heritage, equating to > 97% of all cases. In Australia, women are more likely than men to develop MS, with approximately 75% of all cases.

Environmental risk factors, such as infection and climate, have also been implicated. It has long been thought that certain viral or bacterial infections, such as the Epstein–Barr virus (EBV), may be triggers for the later development of MS. Recently, stronger evidence has resulted in the suggestion of a mechanism whereby an infection with human herpes virus 6A (HHV-6A) in a person previously infected with EBV may lead to a T-cell-mediated autoimmune phenomenon. This appears to occur when the HHV-6A virus induces B cells latently infected with EBV altering immune and glial cell function, and ultimately either leading to or enhancing an autoimmune reaction. Interestingly, people living in temperate climates, such as New Zealand and south-eastern Australia, are more likely to develop MS than those living in tropical climates (such as northern Australia). The same trend is also apparent in the Northern Hemisphere.

EPIDEMIOLOGY

About 25,000 Australians have MS, with the highest prevalence in Tasmania. The prevalence in Australia is 105 per 100,000 people (138.7 people per 100,000 in Tasmania). In New Zealand the prevalence was reported in 2014 at 71.9 per 100,000 people. Around 2.8 million people globally live with the condition.

CLINICAL MANIFESTATIONS

The initial symptoms associated with MS are usually precipitated by some trigger, such as severe stress, infection or fatigue. These symptoms manifest as a set or a syndrome in accordance with the location of plaques within the CNS. The syndromes are referred to as spinal, brain stem, cerebellar and cerebral. The clinical manifestations can include neuropathic pain, paralysis, muscle spasms and optic neuritis.

The *spinal syndrome* is the most common. It affects the upper motor neurons of motor pathways and manifests as spastic paraparesis. Muscle stiffness, slowness and weakness may also be observed. The dorsal column lemniscal ascending pathway may also be affected, manifesting as symmetrical paraesthesias (tingling and numbness) and loss of sensory acuity. These sensory and motor changes tend to be more severe in the lower limbs. Autonomic dysfunction occurs, which affects the gastrointestinal tract and urinary bladder, usually resulting in constipation and urinary incontinence.

The *brain stem syndrome* is associated with lesions to the cranial nerves. This can affect all cranial nerves bar the first two. Common manifestations include visual impairment in coordinating eye movement, blurred vision, eyeball pain, nystagmus, vertigo, tinnitus, facial weakness and impaired facial sensations.

The *cerebellar syndrome* leads to symmetrical gait impairments, ataxia (poor coordination of movements involving loss of speed of movement, an inability to judge distance and alter speed of movement, intention tremor and poor speech articulation), hypotonia and muscle weakness.

The main feature of the *cerebral syndrome* is optic neuritis, which is characterised by a loss of visual acuity, impaired colour perception and a diminished pupil response to light. Intellectual and emotional changes are also a part of this syndrome, with mood swings occurring; a state of depression is very common. Affected people may show altered attention, concentration, memory and judgment.

Over time, a person with MS will show a mixture of syndrome signs and symptoms as more plaques form.

A woman with MS may experience pregnancy-related influences. During the pregnancy there is often a reduction in signs and symptoms; however, approximately three months after the pregnancy a woman with MS may experience exacerbations. Breastfeeding is not possible if the woman is on certain immunomodulating drugs.

CLINICAL DIAGNOSIS AND MANAGEMENT

Diagnosis

A revised *McDonald criteria* is used in the diagnosis of MS. The revisions are thought to simplify the criteria and improve diagnostic specificity and sensitivity. Components of the criteria include objective clinical evidence of lesions and considerations of history of prior attacks. MRI can provide evidence of lesions, and an elevation of immunoglobulin G in the cerebrospinal fluid may also need to be considered, depending on the type of MS suspected. Other investigations should also be undertaken to rule out neurological signs and symptoms, including haematology and biochemistry, and neuroimaging scans. Because the signs and symptoms of MS are so diverse between individuals, physical assessment should include testing cognitive and motor function, the five senses, sensory perception and language functions. It may also be beneficial to test evoked potentials to examine nerve response times for vision, somatosensory or auditory functions in the brain stem.

Significant research is currently being undertaken to identify biomarkers of oxidative stress in body fluids such as blood, cerebrospinal fluid, urine and saliva, which can be used to more accurately diagnose the disease earlier.

Management

The main management principles in caring for someone with MS include symptom relief, delaying disease progression, and reducing the severity and duration of exacerbations. These are generally achieved through the use of pharmacological agents such as corticosteroids and other immunomodulating therapies such as interferon beta, glatiramer and newer monoclonal antibody preparations (natalizamab, ocrelizumab and alemtuzumab). During an exacerbation, the administration of methylprednisolone—an intermediate acting glucocorticoid—can lessen the severity and duration of the attack.

Stress, fatigue, heat and infection can cause MS exacerbations. Interventions to reduce these triggers should be a priority. Frequent rest, good infection control practices and the use of antipyretic agents are important to reduce the episodes of deterioration. Avoidance of hot showers and saunas, using air conditioning on hot days, and dressing appropriately for the weather can also be advantageous in people with MS.

Some people experience urological symptoms. They may need to be taught self-catheterisation in order to prevent urinary retention or infection from urinary stasis. Early intervention with antimicrobials when urinary tract infections occur is important to reduce the duration and intensity of an infection-related exacerbation.

Gastric emptying may be impeded, or the development of constipation could occur in those with MS. Medications to increase gastric emptying and encouragement of taking fluids and increased dietary fibre will be beneficial. As the disease process continues, many individuals will experience dysphagia, so swallowing assessments and speech therapy become important to ensure that sufficient oromotor control exists so as not to develop aspiration pneumonia. As oral nutrition becomes unsafe or unachievable, gastric tube feeding via a nasogastric tube or a percutaneous endoscopic gastric (PEG) tube may need to be commenced.

Physiotherapy and occupational therapy will be required to assist with the control of limb rigidity or spasticity. Occupational therapists can provide devices to promote as much independence as is achievable. Physiotherapists can assist with exercises and rehabilitation to reduce muscle deformities, aid pulmonary hygiene and preserve lung function. Measures to prevent the complications associated with immobility should be instituted. Examples of these include thromboembolic deterrent stockings (TEDS), anticoagulation, passive or active range of movements, and deep breathing and coughing exercises.

Pain is common in those with MS. Tricyclic antidepressants and some anticonvulsants can be used to manage neuropathic pain secondary to demyelination. Musculoskeletal pain can be managed with non-steroidal anti-inflammatory drugs. End-stage management will require palliative care, with significant home or healthcare facility support required.

Motor neurone disease

In its most common form, **motor neurone disease** is associated with a progressive degeneration of the upper and lower motor neurons. It first manifests as muscle weakness; however, deterioration in muscle function is unrelenting, eventually leading to fatal paralysis. This form of the disease is called *amyotrophic lateral sclerosis (ALS)*. In the United States, the condition is commonly referred to as **Lou Gehrig's disease**, named after a famous sportsman who developed the condition. Other types of motor neurone disease affect only upper motor neurons, such as *primary lateral sclerosis* and *progressive bulbar palsy*, or just lower motor neurons, as in *progressive muscular atrophy*.

AETIOLOGY AND PATHOPHYSIOLOGY

The typical onset of ALS is during middle age, usually between 45 and 60 years of age, and it affects more men than women. The prognosis is very poor, with death ensuing between one and five years after diagnosis. The majority of cases are sporadic, occurring without an obvious genetic basis. In about 10% of cases the condition is familial, usually in a dominant inheritance pattern, and manifesting in adulthood (although it has been observed in juveniles). The aetiology of the sporadic form of ALS remains unknown. Risk factors for this disease, other than genetics, are yet to be identified.

The name of the condition is derived from the major features of the pathophysiological process. Amyotrophic refers to *muscle wasting* or *atrophy*. As axons degenerate, demyelination occurs, accompanied by glial cell proliferation. The area becomes scarred and hard, giving rise to the term 'sclerosis'. The corticospinal tract—the primary pathway affected in this condition—extends from the motor cortex to the spinal cord. Nerves in this tract synapse with lower motor neurons in the anterior horn that connect with skeletal muscles. Both upper and lower motor neurons are affected in this condition (see Figure 10.12).

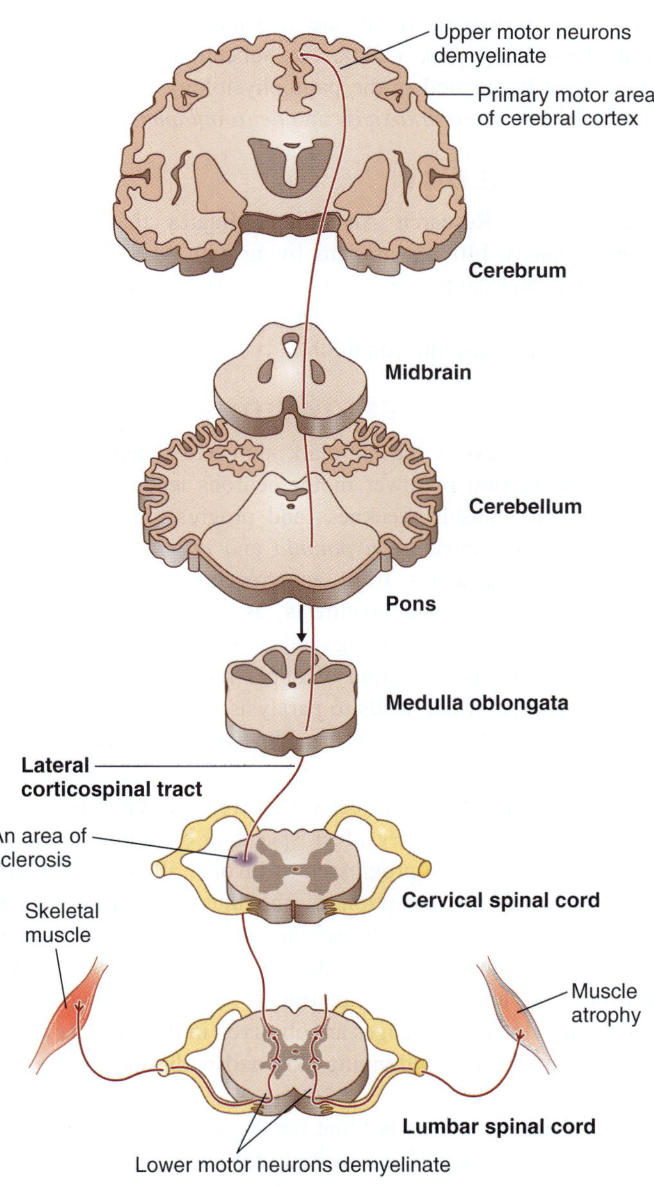

Figure 10.12

Pathophysiology of motor neurone disease

Source: Adapted from Marieb & Hoehn (2016), Figure 12.33a, p. 495.

An understanding of the cellular and molecular pathophysiology of ALS comes from studying the familial form, which is strikingly similar clinically to that of the sporadic form. The most common inherited form shows a genetic mutation in the gene coding for superoxide dismutase (copper/zinc), or *SOD1*. In people with an SOD1 mutation, the SOD1 protein misfolds, leading to the accumulation of protein aggregates, particularly neurofilaments, preferentially in the cytoplasm of motor neurons. While the toxicity of protein aggregates has not been proven, it has been proposed that motor neuron degeneration is due to this phenomenon. Cellular mechanisms by which aggregate toxicity may develop include *deregulation of cytoplasmic organelles* (e.g. Golgi apparatus, endoplasmic reticulum and mitochondria) and *impairment of axonal transport*, which are dependent on neurofilament function. Other toxic cellular or subcellular processes that have been implicated in the pathophysiology of ALS include *oxidative stress, excitotoxicity* and *neuroinflammation*.

EPIDEMIOLOGY

Neuroscience Research Australia estimates that there are approximately 1400 Australians living with ALS. The disease was most prevalent in men (60%) and in people aged 75–84 years. In New Zealand, the latest figures indicate around 1 in 15,000 people have the condition.

CLINICAL MANIFESTATIONS

Muscle weakness is the hallmark sign associated with ALS. The degeneration of lower motor neurons leads to *flaccidity*, starting with muscle weakness and progressing to paralysis. This is accompanied by *hypotonia* and *muscle atrophy*. The muscle atrophy arises from an irreversible denervation of affected muscles, and manifests as muscle fasciculations (muscle twitching or quivering) and cramps. Muscle reflexes are decreased. The degeneration of upper motor neurons induces mild *spasticity*, which leads to paralysis. Deep muscle reflexes are usually heightened in this case. Spasticity and flaccidity can coexist in one muscle.

The muscles initially affected vary from person to person; it can affect hands, arms, legs, feet, speech or breathing. For most people, the condition progresses to involve all of the skeletal muscles, with the exception of the muscles that move the eyeball and form the bladder sphincter. The pathophysiology is specific to voluntary muscles; there are generally no cognitive, sensory or autonomic impairments associated with this condition. However, changes are observed in the integrity of the integument, including thinning skin and body hair, as well as decreased sweating.

As skeletal muscles become paralysed, the affected person becomes wheelchair-bound or bedridden. Speech, swallowing and breathing difficulties worsen. The condition is fatal, with denervation of the respiratory muscles causing respiratory failure.

CLINICAL DIAGNOSIS AND MANAGEMENT

Diagnosis

Consideration of the clinical presentation, history and results of needle electromyography (EMG) will assist in the diagnosis of motor neurone disease. EMG and neurological assessment will demonstrate that sensory function is still intact but motor function is not. Other assessments should be undertaken to rule out other causes of peripheral neuropathy, including biochemistry results (especially glucose levels), haematology results (observing for anaemia) and neuroimaging to eliminate the possibility of space-occupying lesions or trauma.

Management

It is critical to remember that mental functioning is not affected in motor neurone disease, yet the physical effects of the disease are incredibly disabling. Emotional support, informed consent and detailed explanations of the disease process and treatment are important at diagnosis and throughout the progression.

Although there is no cure, riluzole, a drug that disrupts glutamatergic transmission and the activation of voltage-gated sodium channels, may be beneficial to reduce the motor nerve degeneration through the reduction of excitotoxicity. However, this drug requires strict criteria surrounding its authorisation. Proof of respiratory function, age and diagnosis by a neurologist is required for approval on application. As this drug will not necessarily improve symptoms, but, rather, reduce the motor nerve degeneration, education is necessary to ensure compliance. Otherwise, individuals will stop taking the medication when there is no perceived effect.

As with any movement disorder, interventions to reduce the risk of complications associated with immobility are important. Examples of these include the wearing of thromboembolic deterrent stockings (TEDS), anticoagulation, passive or active range of movements, and deep breathing and coughing exercises.

Dysphagia will develop over time, and a change to enteral feeding will be required. Pressure area care, range-of-motion exercises and chest physiotherapy will assist with the preservation of skin integrity and lung function. As the disease progresses, ventilatory support will be required. This is a critical decision that should not be taken lightly. Individuals may choose not to receive this type of therapy. Counselling and support is required regarding this decision, as an election to abstain from mechanical ventilation will result in death as respiratory function declines. If someone with motor neurone disease chooses ventilatory support, even more specialist care and education will be required. People may continue to live in the community, provided the support is sufficient to manage their needs. Failing this, admission to a healthcare facility may be necessary, as total dependence for all cares, and critically for respiratory support, is required.

INDIGENOUS HEALTH FAST FACTS AND CULTURAL CONSIDERATIONS

FAST FACTS

- *No comprehensive national data for Alzheimer's disease, Parkinson's disease or other neurological degenerative disorders currently exist for Aboriginal and Torres Strait Islander peoples.*
- *Parkinson's disease has been reported as the 10th leading cause of burden of disease in Aboriginal and Torres Strait Islander peoples compared to the 6th leading cause for non-Indigenous Australians.*
- *Dementia can be seen as a natural part of ageing within some Aboriginal and Torres Strait Islander communities, and is managed through family and community support rather than medical intervention.*
- *Less than 3% of Aboriginal and Torres Strait Islander peoples with dementia use government community programs focused on aged-care and respite support.*
- *Anecdotal evidence suggests that the incidence of Indigenous people with Alzheimer's disease and Parkinson's disease is increasing, as Aboriginal and Torres Strait Islander peoples are living longer.*
- *The incidence of Parkinson's disease in Māori and Pacific Islands communities is lower than in European New Zealanders—20 per 100,00 people (Māori), 27 per 100,000 people (Pacific Islands people), compared to 33 per 100,000.*
- *A more rapid increase in dementia in Māori and Pacific Islands and Asian peoples over 65 years old compared to European New Zealanders has been forecast.*
- *In 2020, the number of European New Zealanders with dementia is estimated to double by 2050. In the same period, the number of Māori and Pacific Islands and Asian peoples with dementia is expected to triple.*

CULTURAL CONSIDERATIONS

- *Standard tools for cognitive assessment (e.g. mini-mental state examination—MMSE) have been shown to possess cultural, educational and language bias. Use of these tools when assessing an Indigenous person's cognition is therefore likely to cause an erroneous result. Recently, a culturally appropriate tool has been developed and validated for use with people who identify as an Aboriginal or Torres Strait Islander person. The Kimberly Indigenous Cognitive Assessment (KICA) tool assists in not only cognitive assessment, but in behavioural and psychological symptoms, too. Medical history, smoking and alcohol usage are also assessed in this tool.*
- *Other considerations for healthcare professionals undertaking culturally appropriate cognitive assessment include both logistical and physical issues. Logistically, Aboriginal and Torres Strait Islander culture has over 250 spoken languages, and therefore it may be likely that a healthcare professional could be working through an interpreter. It is important to consider the influence that the interpreter has on assessment measures, including response time and accuracy of translation. Physical issues might include the use of tactile measures in place of assessments requiring adequate vision, as there are a significant number of visually impaired Indigenous people because of the high incidence of glaucoma in many communities.*

Sources: Data from Alamri et al. (2020); Australian Indigenous HealthInfoNet (2015); Australian Institute of Health and Welfare (2021); LoGiudice (2016); LoGiudice et al. (2016); Ma'u et al. (2021).

CHILDREN AND ADOLESCENTS

- Neurodegenerative diseases are rare in children. Investigations to identify organic causes to explain declining neurological or motor function are important.
- Early-onset Huntington's disease may develop in children as young as 2 years of age or as old as 20 years of age.
- If a younger child develops symptoms of early-onset Huntington's disease, the progression is generally more rapid.
- If children exhibit symptoms of an inheritable neurodegenerative disorder, such as motor neurone disease, a family may also be coping with the cares of an older family member (e.g. a parent). In this case, support needs for both the child and the family become even more complex.

OLDER ADULTS

- Dementia is not a normal part of ageing.
- Cognitive impairments and changes in behaviour in older adults should be investigated and not just assumed to be the onset of dementia.

- Irrespective of an older person's cognitive function, modification of the environment should occur to reduce falls risk.
- Urinary tract infection (UTI) may cause delirium and confusion in an older adult. Eliminate UTIs as a possible cause of confusion.
- Assessment of pain can be difficult in older people, especially if they have neurodegenerative diseases. Use appropriate pain assessment tools.

KEY CLINICAL ISSUES

- Safety related to mobilisation becomes more challenging in people with declining balance and motor control as a result of neuromuscular diseases. Frequent assessments are required as function declines. The addition of new mobilisation or transfer devices will be necessary.
- Someone with a neuromuscular disease will experience progressive decline in oromotor function. Regular assessments and adjustment to meal protocols will be required to prevent aspiration pneumonia.
- Psychological support, counselling and education are necessary for those who are newly diagnosed with a neurodegenerative disorder. For some disorders that will ultimately compromise respiratory function, decisions need to be made as to how much medical intervention they are willing to accept as their function declines. Significant choices about the use of mechanical ventilators, and the challenges associated with this decision, must be fully understood so that informed consent is possible. A choice not to begin mechanical ventilation will result in death as respiratory muscles become unable to support the oxygen requirements of the body.
- Autonomic dysfunction will interfere with urinary and bowel functions. Interventions to support elimination will be required as function diminishes.
- Pain is common in people with neurodegenerative disorders. Aggressive management of pain is important to reduce suffering and improve quality of life in those parameters that can be influenced.

CHAPTER REVIEW

- A number of pathophysiological processes have been implicated in the development of neurodegenerative disorders, including *mitochondrial dysfunction*, *oxidative stress*, *neuroinflammation*, *excitotoxicity*, *proteolysis*, protein aggregation and *apoptosis*.
- *Parkinson's disease* is associated with the degeneration of the dopaminergic nigrostriatal pathway involved in the planning and execution of voluntary movements. *Lewy body formation* is a common feature of Parkinson's disease.
- *Alzheimer's disease* is associated with neuron loss in the hippocampus, limbic system and frontal cortex. Cholinergic nerves are particularly targeted. The presence of neurofibrillary tangles and beta-amyloid plaques on autopsy are diagnostic hallmarks.
- *Huntington's disease* is an autosomal dominant genetic disorder involving a mutation in the formation of a protein called huntingtin. The protein misfolds, interacts inappropriately with other molecules, and aggregates inside cells. The focus of neuronal cell loss is within the basal ganglia and cerebral cortex.
- In *multiple sclerosis*, CNS myelin and the cells that make it are damaged by an inappropriate immune response. The reaction leads to the formation of multiple plaques in the brain and the spinal cord, which cause profound sensory, motor, cognitive and emotional impairments.
- *Motor neurone disease* is associated with the degeneration of the upper and lower motor neurons. It is a muscle-wasting disorder that initially manifests as muscle weakness and progresses to a fatal paralysis. Axons of affected nerves degenerate, leading to demyelination and glial cell proliferation.

REVIEW QUESTIONS

1. Identify the brain regions/tissues primarily affected in each of the neurodegenerative disorders.
2. What type of protein aggregates are characteristic in each neurodegenerative disorder?
3. Identify the diagnostic hallmarks of each of the disorders.
4. Which of the disorders has/have a strong familial inheritance pattern?
5. Mr Simon Pertwee is a 75-year-old man living in a retirement village. He has been showing signs of confusion and impairment of recent memory. This has led to frustration and agitation. He has indicated to his general practitioner that he does not want his family and friends to visit him, and has withdrawn from social interaction with other residents. Until recently he had shown great care in his appearance and dress, but lately he has demonstrated carelessness in his appearance.
   a. Which degenerative disorder do you think Mr Pertwee has?
   b. What *two* changes characteristically occur in the brains of people affected with this condition?
   c. Which drugs are useful in the management of this condition, and outline their mechanism of action?
6. Ms Fanny Godfrey is a 62-year-old woman whom you are visiting as a community nurse. She has a resting tremor in her hands and head. Her posture is very stooped, she speaks in a monotone whisper and her face is expressionless.
   a. What condition do you think she is probably suffering from?
   b. What is the transmitter imbalance associated with this condition, and in which part of the brain does it occur?
   c. Identify the major drug groups used in the management of this condition, and outline their actions.

HEALTH PROFESSIONAL CONNECTIONS

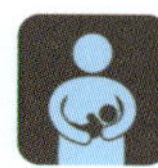

Midwives Couples who have a family history of inheritable neurodegenerative diseases are faced with difficult decisions about whether or not to start a family. During this time, it is important to seek the support of experts such as genetic counsellors, so that all options are identified. During pregnancy, women can undertake genetic testing to determine whether the fetus has the disease; however, prior to undertaking the test they need to determine whether a therapeutic termination is something that they are willing to consider.

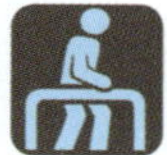

Physiotherapists People experiencing neurodegenerative conditions may present with a range of unique needs depending on their condition and disease progression. Clearly, individualised assessment and treatment plans are required: however, approaches focusing on postural adjustment, safe transfers, gait balance, flexibility and strength may be essentials for many individuals. Rigidity of muscles in both axial and appendicular musculature may develop or, conversely, flaccidity and sensory loss may become the dominant issues. Reduced cardiovascular function is common, and with some conditions (such as Parkinson's disease, where autonomic dysfunction can occur) early evidence suggests that aerobic exercise may improve motor action and reduce the dyskinesia that may develop as a result of the disease or the medications. Further considerations that may be necessary surround the timing of therapy in relation to medication dosing, as in some conditions movement potential may be improved when plasma concentrations are highest, whereas in other conditions medication dosing may be irrelevant to the success of a therapy program.

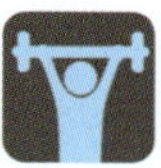

Exercise scientists Providing exercise for people with neurodegenerative disease can assist in slowing the neurological decline; however, because of postural instabilities, loss of motor tone and poorly functioning proprioceptor systems, this can be challenging. Ensure that the physical environment is safe and designed to reduce the risk of falls. Focusing on exercises to improve leg muscle strength and balance can have dramatic effects on reducing the incidence of falls. Also, recent research has identified that exercise may influence dopamine, glutamate and brain-derived neurotrophic factors. Although the effects of exercise on neuroplasticity are not yet fully understood, a sufficient knowledge base exists to support its benefits.

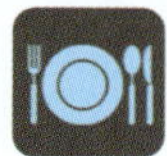

Speech pathologists/Nutritionists/Dieticians Although it is widely established that adequate nutrition can influence brain function, more recent investigations into specific foods to reduce the effects of neurodegenerative disease are suggesting that diets rich in fruit, vegetables and nuts can provide antioxidant and anti-inflammatory actions that may slow decline. Other issues faced by individuals with neurodegenerative disorders include dysphagia and malnutrition. It is important to ensure that individualised nutrition plans take into account the person's oromotor functioning. As this declines, alternative methods to support caloric and nutritional needs must be found. Insertion of enteral feeds via nasogastric or percutaneous endoscopic gastrostomy tubes present different challenges in a person's nutrition management plan.

CASE STUDY

Mr Patrick Drew is a 74-year-old man (UR number 452342). He was referred by his general practitioner to the neurology team for investigation and management of his Parkinson's disease, dysphagia and falls. On assessment he demonstrated bradykinesia, gaze limitations (in all directions), a persistent unilateral tremor in his right arm, and a shuffling gait (with limited arm swing). His limb rigidity is 'lead pipe rigidity', but he also has 'cogwheel rigidity' in his wrists. His wife, Mrs Betty Drew, has described an increasing frequency of choking and coughing during meals. His lung fields are clear, and there are currently no indications of aspiration pneumonia. Mr Drew has right-sided facial bruising, including a large periorbital haematoma, where he fell and hit his head earlier in the week. A CT scan performed to rule out head injury in that episode was unremarkable. His frequency of falls has also increased in the past few months. On arrival to the ward, Mr Drew's observations are as follows:

Temperature	Heart rate	Respiration rate	Blood pressure	SpO_2
36.7°C	64	14	140 / 82	97% (RA*)

* RA = room air.

Speech pathology and a barium swallow have been booked. He still requires a falls risk assessment and Waterlow pressure area assessment. He has been taking Sinemet CR (a combination of levodopa and carbidopa) for three years and, most recently, amantadine has been added to his regimen. His most recent pathology results are:

HAEMATOLOGY

Patient location:	Ward 3	**UR:**	452342		
Consultant:	Smith	**NAME:**	Drew		
		Given name:	Patrick	**Sex:**	M
		DOB:	06/11/XX	**Age:**	74

Time collected	11:30
Date collected	XX/XX
Year	XXXX
Lab #	53453455

FULL BLOOD COUNT		UNITS	REFERENCE RANGE
Haemoglobin	127	g/L	115–160
White cell count	6.2	$\times 10^9$/L	4.0–11.0
Platelets	254	$\times 10^9$/L	140–400
Haematocrit	0.38		0.33–0.47
Red cell count	4.58	$\times 10^{12}$/L	3.80–5.20
Reticulocyte count	1.4	%	0.2–2.0
MCV	92	fL	80–100
COAGULATION PROFILE			
aPTT	38	secs	24–40
PT	15	secs	11–17

BIOCHEMISTRY

Patient location:	Ward 3	**UR:**	452342		
Consultant:	Smith	**NAME:**	Drew		
		Given name:	Patrick	**Sex:**	M
		DOB:	06/11/XX	**Age:**	74

Time collected	11:30
Date collected	XX/XX
Year	XXXX
Lab #	4345454

ELECTROLYTES		UNITS	REFERENCE RANGE
Sodium	141	mmol/L	135–145
Potassium	4.2	mmol/L	3.5–5.2
Chloride	99	mmol/L	95–110
Glucose	5.2	mmol/L	3.5–6.0
RENAL FUNCTION			
Urea	4.2	mmol/L	2.5–7.5
Creatinine	78	µmol/L	30–120

CRITICAL THINKING

1. Consider Mr Drew's assessment data. How does a dopamine deficit cause these movement disorders? Explain.
2. Why were there no observable changes in Mr Drew's CT scan? (Why are CT scans of no benefit to the diagnosis of Parkinson's disease?)
3. Observe Mr Drew's pathology results. Are these of any benefit to assist with a diagnosis?
4. Mr Drew takes a combination of levodopa and carbidopa, as well as amantadine. His problem is related to a deficit of dopamine within the brain. Neither of these drugs is dopamine. Why isn't he given a dopamine infusion? For the combination of the two drugs in one preparation, describe the role that each drug plays in Mr Drew's management.
5. What interventions does Mr Drew require? (Consider all of the elements of his condition.) Draw up a table identifying signs and symptoms, interventions and rationales.
6. Contrast Parkinson's disease with schizophrenia. Draw up a table identifying the neurotransmitter involved and the cause. Can a person with schizophrenia acutely develop symptoms of Parkinson's disease? How? Explain.

BIBLIOGRAPHY

Alamri, Y., Pitcher, T. & Anderson, T.J. (2020). Variations in the patterns of prevalence and therapy in Australasian Parkinson's disease patients of different ethnicities. *BMJ Neurology Open* 2(1):e000033. https://doi:10.1136/bmjno-2019-000033.

Australian Health Ministers' Advisory Council's National and Aboriginal and Torres Strait Islander Health Standing Committee (2017). *Cultural respect framework, 2016–2026: for Aboriginal and Torres Strait Islander health—a national approach to building a culturally respectful health system.* Canberra: Australian Government Department of Health. https://nacchocommunique.files.wordpress.com/2016/12/cultural_respect_framework_1december2016_1.pdf.

Australian Huntington's Disease Associations (2020). *Huntington's disease and residential aged care: submission to the Aged Royal Commission.* https://agedcare.royalcommission.gov.au/system/files/2020-12/AWF.600.01586.0001.pdf.

Australian Indigenous Health*Info*Net (2015). *The Kimberley Indigenous Cognitive Assessment tool (KICA).* Perth, WA: Australian Indigenous Health*Info*Net. https://healthinfonet.ecu.edu.au/key-resources/resources/25256/?title=Kimberley+Indigenous+Cognitive+Assessment+%28KICA%29&contentid=25256_1.

Australian Institute of Health and Welfare (AIHW) (2021a). *Dementia in Australia* Canberra: AIWH. https://www.aihw.gov.au/reports/dementia/dementia-in-aus/contents/summary.

Australian Institute of Health and Welfare (AIHW) (2021b). *Older Australians: older Aboriginal and Torres Strait Islander people.* Canberra: AIWH. https://www.aihw.gov.au/reports/older-people/older-australia-at-a-glance/contents/diverse-groups-of-older-australians/aboriginal-and-torres-strait-islander-people.

Australian Institute of Health and Welfare (AIHW) (2022). *Principal diagnosis data cubes: Separation statistics by principal diagnosis (ICD-10-AM 11th edition), Australia, 2020–21.* Canberra: AIWH. https://www.aihw.gov.au/reports/hospitals/principal-diagnosis-data-cubes/contents/data-cubes.

Ayton, D., Ayton, S., Barker, A.L., Bush, A.I. & Warren, N. (2018). Parkinson's disease prevalence and the association with rurality and agricultural determinants. *Parkinsonism and Related Disorders* 61:198–202. https://doi.org/10.1016/j.parkreldis.2018.10.026.

Bauldoff, G., Gubrud-Howe, P.M., Carno, M.-A., Levett-Jones, T., Hales, M., Berry, K., … Stanley, D. (2020). *LeMone and Burke's medical–surgical nursing: critical thinking for person-centred care* (4th [Australian] edn). Sydney: Pearson Australia.

Bullock, S. & Manias, E. (2022). *Fundamentals of pharmacology* (9th edn). Sydney: Pearson Australia.

Dementia Australia (2022). Types of dementia. https://www.dementia.org.au/information/about-dementia/types-of-dementia.

Dorsey, E.R., Sherer, T., Okun, M.S. & Bloem, B.R. (2018). The emerging evidence of the Parkinson pandemic. *Journal of Parkinson's Disease* 8(s1):S3–S8. https://doi.10.3233/JPD-181474.

GBD 2019 Dementia Forecasting Collaborators (2022). Estimation of the global prevalence of dementia in 2019 and forecasted prevalence in 2050: an analysis for the Global Burden of Disease Study 2019. *Lancet Public Health* 7(2): e105–e125. https://doi.org/10.1016/S2468-2667(21)00249-8.

Hauser, R.A. (2020). Parkinson disease. *Emedicine*. https://emedicine.medscape.com/article/1831191-overview.

LoGiudice, D. (2016). The health of older Aboriginal and Torres Strait Islander peoples. *Australasian Journal on Ageing* 35(2):82–85. https://doi:10.1111/ajag.12332.

LoGiudice, D., Smith, K., Fenner, S., Hyde, Z., Atkinson, D., Skeaf, L., … Flicker, L. (2016). Incidence and predictors of cognitive impairment and dementia in Aboriginal Australians: a follow-up study of 5 years. *Alzheimer's and Dementia* 12(3):252–61. https://doi:10.1016/j.jalz.2015.01.009.

Luzzo, C. (2023). Multiple sclerosis. *Emedicine.* https://emedicine.medscape.com/article/1146199-overview.

Marieb, E.N. & Hoehn, K. (2019). *Human anatomy and physiology* (11th edn). San Francisco, CA: Pearson Benjamin Cummings.

Ma'u, E., Cullum, S., Yates, S., Te Ao, B., Cheung, G., Burholt, V., … Kerse, N. (2021). *Dementia economic impact report 2020.* Auckland: University of Auckland.

MS Research Australia (2022). Implementation Plan for a Roadmap to Defeat Multiple Sclerosis in Australia: 2022-23 Pre-budget Submission. MS Australia. https://treasury.gov.au/sites/default/files/2022-03/258735_multiple_sclerosis_ms_australia.pdf

Neuroscience Research Australia (NeuRA) (2022). *Motor neuron disease: health information.* https://www.neura.edu.au/health/motor-neurone-disease/.

Simpson-Yap, S., Atvars, R., Blizzard L., van der Mei, I. & Taylor, B.V. (2022). Increasing incidence and prevalence of multiple sclerosis in the Greater Hobart cohort of Tasmania, Australia. *Journal of Neurology, Neurosurgery and Psychiatry* 93:723–31. https://doi:10.1136/jnnp-2022-328932.

11 Neurotrauma

KEY TERMS

Acquired brain injury (ABI)
Autonomic dysreflexia
Central cord syndrome
Cerebral blood flow (CBF)
Cerebral perfusion pressure (CPP)
Concussion
Contrecoup contusions
Conus medullaris
Coup contusion
Diffuse axonal injury (DAI)
Extradural haematoma (EDH)
Flaccid paralysis
Intracranial pressure (ICP)
Mean arterial pressure (MAP)
Primary brain injury
Secondary brain injury
Spastic paralysis
Spinal shock
Subdural haematoma (SDH)
Traumatic brain injury (TBI)

LEARNING OBJECTIVES

After completing this chapter, you should be able to:

1 Compare and contrast the pathophysiology of primary and secondary head injury.

2 Explore the relationship of the Monro–Kellie doctrine to traumatic brain injury.

3 Outline the clinical diagnosis and current management for traumatic brain injury.

4 Outline the pathogenesis of spinal cord injury.

5 Identify the common classifications of spinal cord injury.

6 Discuss the characteristics of common spinal cord syndromes.

7 Explore the clinical diagnosis and management of spinal cord injury.

8 Examine the common complications associated with spinal cord injury.

WHAT YOU SHOULD KNOW BEFORE YOU START THIS CHAPTER

Can you name the major anatomical structures of the brain, and explain how they relate to function?

Can you identify the components of the cranial vault, and explain how the Monro–Kellie doctrine dictates management of these components within the skull?

Can you describe how mean arterial pressure influences cerebral perfusion pressure, and what the significance of this is in relation to control of blood pressure?

Can you describe the inflammatory process, and identify the cardinal signs of inflammation?

Can you describe the relationship between the vertebral divisions and the spinal cord in relation to function?

Introduction

A person's brain is the centre of their existence, and their spinal cord is a critical element to facilitate interaction and participation in life. Alterations in brain or cord function can therefore have a devastating effect on a person's abilities and their place in society.

This chapter will focus on the effects of brain and spinal cord injury. *Traumatic brain injury (TBI)* is often devastating, yet it may occur along a spectrum from mild to severe in nature. However, even mild injuries may compromise a person's function or independence with changes in memory, cognition, personality and/or behaviour. Coma and death are significant and severe consequences of TBI. *Spinal cord injury* can also be life-shattering and result in profound disability and loss of independence.

Traumatic brain injury (TBI)

Traumatic brain injury (TBI) is characterised by an alteration of brain function usually caused by an external force. The mechanism can be divided into **primary brain injury**, which is damage occurring at the time of insult as a direct result of tissue loss due to the trauma, and **secondary brain injury**, which is damage occurring post-injury because of other extracranial causes, such as hypoxia, hypotension or hypoglycaemia, or intracranial causes, such as haemorrhage, swelling or infection. Primary and secondary brain injury will be discussed in detail later in this chapter.

Acquired brain injury (ABI) is most commonly associated with the misuse or abuse of drugs and/or alcohol, or other causative agents, including infections, strokes, tumours and a large number of other diseases and disorders. Stroke and CNS infections are covered in the chapter 'Brain and spinal cord dysfunction'.

A TBI results in damage or alteration in brain function as a direct result of injury. Causes can include blunt-force trauma, such as falls, penetrating force where an object such as a knife enters the cranial vault, and acceleration–deceleration injury, which often occurs in motor vehicle accidents and sport. In the latter instance, the injury to the brain occurs when the brain itself moves backwards and forwards with rapid succession. TBI can manifest as confusion, alteration in consciousness level, seizure, coma, autonomic dysfunction and neurological deficit.

EPIDEMIOLOGY

It is estimated that approximately 27 million new, medically-treated TBIs occur each year worldwide, and TBI is a leading cause of post-injury mortality and long-term disability in both industrialised and developing countries. The incidence of TBI in Australia is reported as approximately 275 per 100,000, in New Zealand, 683 per 100,000, and worldwide rates on average 346 per 100,000. Brain Injury Australia states that traumatic brain injury is 10 times more common than spinal injury, causing three times more disability. Almost 30% of hospitalisations for intracranial injury occur between the ages of 10 and 29 years old, with the unequal gender distribution thought to be due to increased risk-taking behaviour by males. TBIs from falls is the cause of 10% of admissions of people over 85 years of age, and this is the only age group where female injury rates exceed male rates. Unfortunately, brain injury in individuals over 85 years of age results in almost 100% mortality. TBI statistics overall are also most likely underestimated, as many people who sustain a mild head injury may never seek medical attention.

It is estimated that within the general population approximately 17% of men and 9% of women have a history of head injury resulting in loss of consciousness; however, interestingly, individuals within the correctional system have significantly higher rates of TBI. Juvenile offenders are approximately three times more likely to have sustained a previous head injury, and in some studies between 34% and 82% of inmates have received a previous TBI.

Falls, transportation-related accidents and assaults are identified as the top three mechanisms of injury contributing to TBI. Alcohol use was reported as an important factor in all cases. Falls caused over two in every five TBIs.

While the majority (70–80%) of primary head injuries are classified as minor, a significant proportion of individuals who sustain minor TBI may continue to experience poor functional outcomes as a result of secondary brain injury, missed injuries and existing comorbidities. Of the 20–30% of people who sustain moderate-to-severe head injury, approximately 10% of these are dead on arrival at the emergency department, while the remainder will require admission to an intensive care unit, with management lasting approximately 7–10 days.

PRIMARY BRAIN INJURY

LEARNING OBJECTIVE 1

Compare and contrast the pathophysiology of primary and secondary head injury.

Aetiology and pathophysiology

The *primary or acute phase* of TBI describes the cellular and structural injury that occurs as a direct result of the force of the injury. The severity of the primary injury is determined by the *extent of neuronal and vascular damage*. Glial injury and loss of axonal integrity result in neuronal cellular leakage and alteration in cell membrane potential. Increased capillary permeability alters vascular homeostasis, especially in relation to solutes (see the chapters 'Pathophysiological terminology, cellular adaptation and injury' and 'Inflammation and healing'). The physical mechanisms of TBI can be classified as impact loading, impulsive loading and static loading.

Physical mechanisms of traumatic brain injury

Impact loading Impact loading causes TBI through a combination of contact and inertial forces. It is defined as a collision of the head with a solid object at a tangible speed. For example, a motorbike rider is travelling at 110 km/h and is thrown from the motor bike. The rider's head strikes the side of a small car, resulting in TBI. Contact or inertial forces may strain the brain beyond its structural and mechanical tolerance. Brain tissue can be deformed by compression forces, which compress tissue and cause damage. Brain tissue can also be deformed by stretching or shearing. Shearing distorts tissues by causing the tissues to slide over each other, resulting in damage.

Impulsive loading Inertial force occurs when the head is set in motion, leading to acceleration-induced TBI. It is defined as sudden motion without significant physical contact. As an example, after failing to stop, a truck collides with the rear of the station wagon and the impact forces the station wagon and the driver forward in a sudden motion. Even though the station wagon driver's head does not physically strike another object, the brain moves within the skull as a result of the force of impulse loading.

Static loading Static loading is rare, and occurs when a slowly moving object traps the person's head against a fixed rigid structure and gradually squeezes the skull, causing numerous fractures, which may result in deformity of the skull and brain. It is defined as a loading in which the effect of speed may not be significant. For example, a worker's head is pinned and crushed between a very large, slow-moving cylinder and the cement floor.

Protective and preventative measures, such as the wearing of helmets, safety equipment and seatbelts, and anti-speeding campaigns are regarded as sound risk-mitigation strategies that can reduce the degree of injury sustained at the time of impact. However, where a TBI has occurred, the mechanism of injury can provide the clinician with some degree of insight into the degree of trauma sustained and the potential site(s) of injury.

Common effects of primary traumatic brain injury

Skull fracture Skull fractures are generally labelled and categorised according to location, pattern and whether they are open or closed. *Closed fractures* do not permit communication with the outside environment, whereas *open fractures* do. A *simple fracture* is defined as having one bone fragment, while a *compound fracture* exists when there are two or more bone fragments.

Linear fractures A linear fracture is a fracture in the line of the skull that passes through its entire thickness (see Figure 11.1A). Linear fractures are generally caused by a significant blow to the head.

Depressed fractures A depressed skull fracture results in bone fragmentation that causes an actual depression in the surface of the skull. Depressed skull fractures are generally the result of a powerful mechanism of injury, and bone fragments may become embedded in underlying brain tissue (see Figure 11.1B).

Base of skull fractures Base of skull (BOS) fractures are fractures that involve the base of the skull and the cribriform plate (see Figure 11.1C). The most common BOS fractures involve the petrous portion of the temporal bone, external auditory canal and the tympanic membrane. BOS fractures are commonly associated with the tearing of the dura mater, resulting in cerebrospinal fluid (CSF) leakage from the ear due to the open conduit with the external environment. Periorbital ecchymosis, also known as raccoon eyes, is a type of intraorbital bleeding usually seen with cribriform plate fracture (see Figure 11.2). Battle's sign (see Figure 11.3), an ecchymosis over the mastoid process, usually occurs 12–24 hours post-injury and also indicates a BOS fracture.

Concussion A **concussion** is a transient alteration in cerebral function without structural defect, which manifests as a loss of consciousness followed by rapid recovery. Concussion is usually caused by an acceleration–deceleration force or blunt-force trauma. The *reticular activating system (RAS)*, which is primarily responsible for maintaining an alert and conscious state, is thought to be disrupted. The concussed person may provide a history of unconsciousness or memory

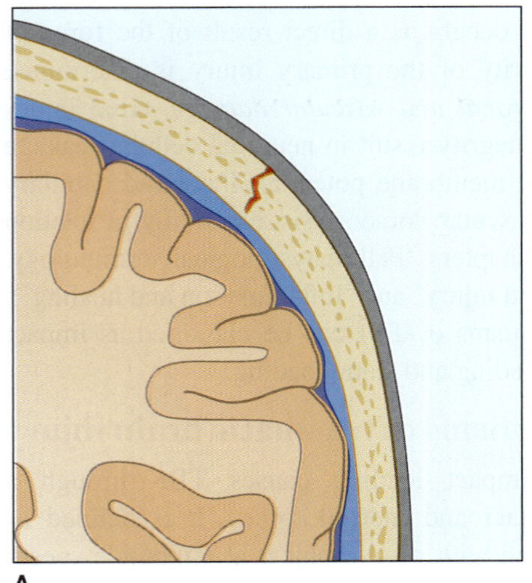

A

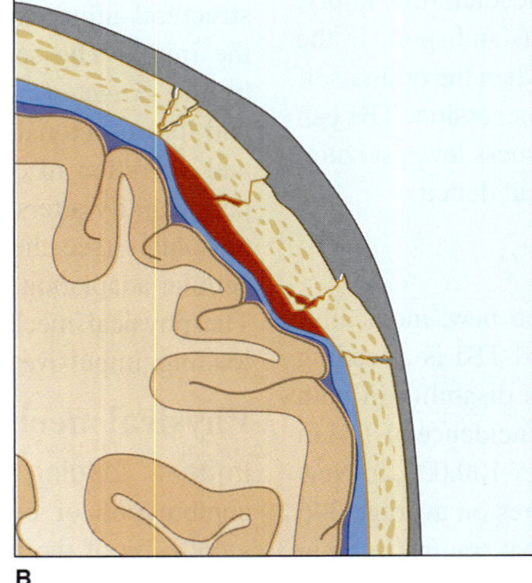

B

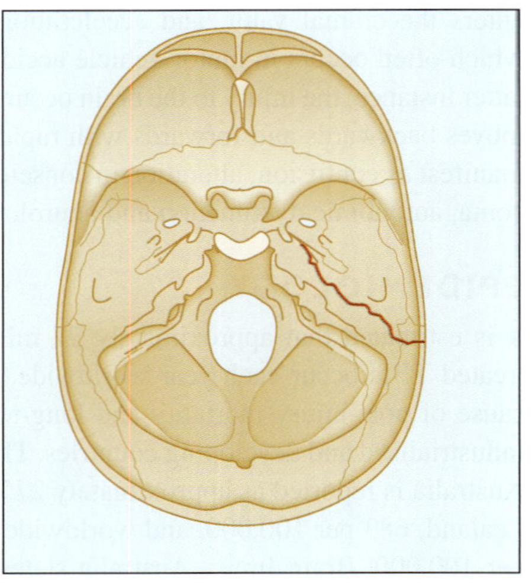

C

Figure 11.1

Skull fractures

(A) Linear skull fracture. (B) Depressed fracture. (C) Base of skull fracture.

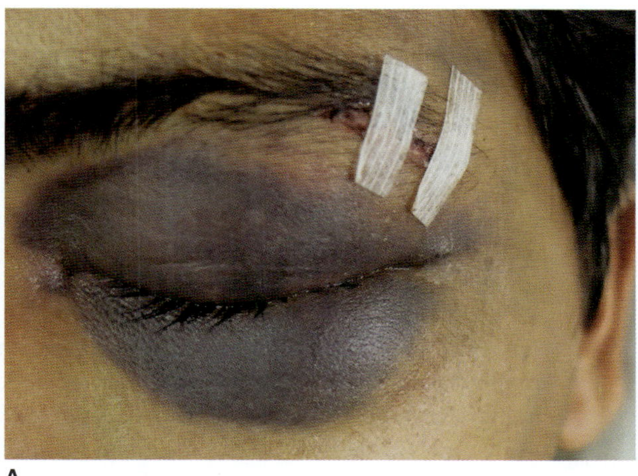

A

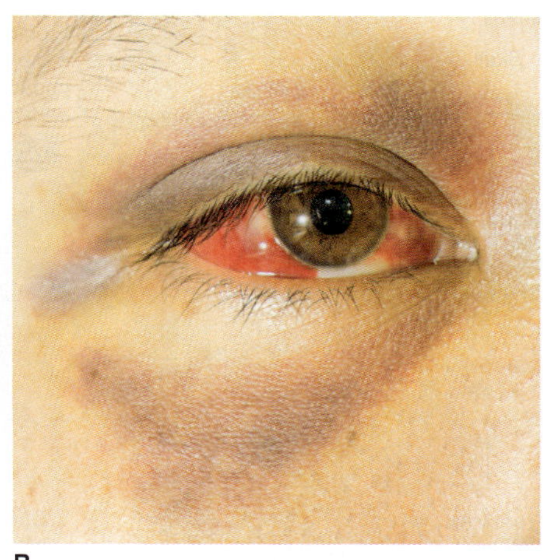

B

Figure 11.2

Racoon eyes, or periorbital ecchymosis

(A) Periorbital ecchymosis with lids almost swollen shut. (B) Periorbital ecchymosis with eyes open and subconjunctival haemorrhage visable.

Source: (A) Casa nayafana/Shutterstock; (B) ARZTSAMUI/Shutterstock.

loss for the event. The period of unconsciousness is usually brief. Concussion can also produce light-headedness, vertigo, headache, nausea, vomiting, photophobia, tinnitus, fatigue and cognitive dysfunction. For many people, concussive symptoms may remain three months post-injury, and, for some, symptoms may remain at one year.

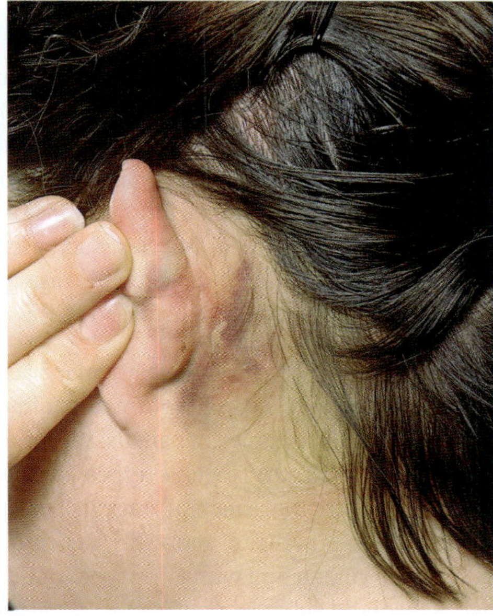

Figure 11.3

Battle's sign

Source: Mediscan/Alamy Stock Photo.

The term *post-concussion syndrome* is used to describe the presence of at least three manifestations (such as headache, fatigue, irritability, dizziness, impaired memory and concentration, photophobia, phonophobia or insomnia) appearing within the week following the concussion. *Persistent post-concussive syndrome (PPCS)* is described as the manifestations continuing for more than three months.

Contusion—coup and contrecoup It must be remembered that the brain is mobile within the cranial vault and, as a result, can sustain multiple injuries. *Cerebral contusion* is bruising to the brain tissue, resulting in an altered consciousness. The most common locations for cerebral contusions are the frontal and temporal lobes. Cerebral contusions occur in 20–30% of cases of severe TBI, and larger contusions can be associated with haematoma formation. Causes include blunt-force trauma and severe acceleration–deceleration forces. **Coup contusions** occur at the site of impact, and occur because of the generation of negative pressure when the skull is distorted and then returns to its normal shape. **Contrecoup contusions** are similar to coup contusions but are located in a brain region opposite the site of impact.

The amount of energy dissipated at the site of direct impact determines the ensuing contusion. For example, the energy impact from a small, hard object will dissipate at the site of impact, resulting in a coup contusion (see Figure 11.4). In contrast, impact from a larger object causes less injury at the impact site as energy is dissipated at the beginning or end of the head motion, leading to a contrecoup contusion (see Figure 11.4).

Intracranial haemorrhage There are many types of intracranial haemorrhage. Some are named according to a description of their anatomical location in relation to the *meninges*, such as *extradural, subdural* and *subarachnoid*

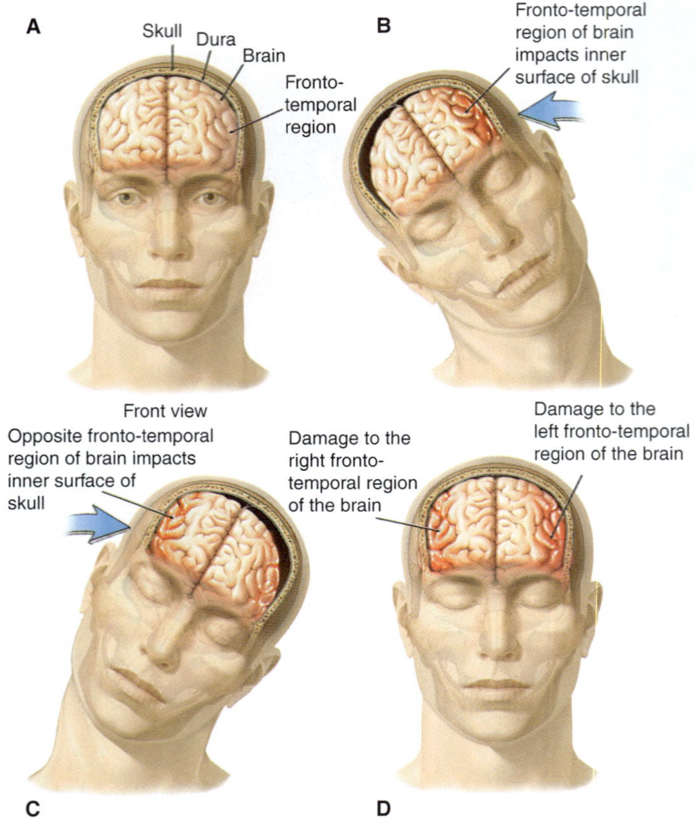

Figure 11.4

Coup and contrecoup contusion

(B) Coup contusion—in this example the temporal lobe injury is sustained from trauma of impacting the windscreen.

(C) Contrecoup contusion—in this example the injury occurs to the occipital lobe as a result of the backward motion of the brain onto the back of the skull.

Source: Nucleus Medical Media Inc/Alamy Stock Photo.

haematomas. *Intracerebral haemorrhages* occur within the brain *parenchyma*. *Intraventricular haemorrhages* occur within the *ventricles* of the brain. Figure 11.5 explores the common clinical manifestations and management of intracranial haemorrhage.

Extradural haematoma An **extradural haematoma (EDH)**, also known as an *epidural haematoma*, occurs from impact loading to the skull with associated *laceration of the dural arteries or veins*. As a result, blood collects in the potential space (the *extradural space*) between the skull and the dura mater (see Figure 11.6). EDHs are relatively rare, and account for about 2% of all TBIs, with the most common presentations in people 20–40 years of age. Typically, EDHs result from blunt-force trauma to the temporal bone and injury to the underlying middle meningeal artery. The principal threat to the brain is from the expanding mass of blood displacing the temporal lobe medially and resulting in herniation. The classic history for EDH presentation is a brief loss of consciousness, followed by an increase in conscious state and then a rapid decline into unconsciousness. The conscious period is known as the *lucent interval*, and during this time the person may appear lethargic, nauseated and confused, and complain of headache. This clinical pattern occurs in a small number of cases, as the majority of individuals either never lose consciousness or never regain consciousness after the initial injury. The mortality rate for EDH is about 20%, but may be greatly reduced with rapid surgical evacuation of the haematoma.

Subdural haematoma A **subdural haematoma (SDH)** is usually caused by the sudden acceleration then deceleration of brain tissue, with subsequent *tearing of the bridging veins*. This results in bleeding between *the dura and the arachnoid layers* of the meninges (see Figure 11.6). SDHs are usually venous in origin and, as a result, blood tends to collect more slowly than in EDHs. However, SDHs are often associated with other brain injuries. SDHs account for 30% of severe TBIs, and result in a high mortality risk (> 50%). SDHs are usually precipitated by moderate-to-severe blunt trauma to the head and a reduction in conscious level. SDHs may be classified as acute, subacute or chronic depending on presentation. *Acute* SDH symptoms generally appear within 14 days post-injury. After two weeks post-injury, SDHs are classified as *subacute* or *chronic*.

Intracerebral haematoma An intracerebral haematoma is associated with haemorrhage in the *brain tissue* itself (see Figure 11.6). It may occur at any location in the brain, but the most common locations are the *temporal and frontal lobes*. The mechanisms of injury include penetrating trauma with resultant laceration, or diffuse injury from blunt-force trauma. Oedema and haemorrhage formation contribute to reduce cerebral blood flow (CBF) and raise intracranial pressure (ICP). Signs, symptoms and prognosis are dependent on the location and size of the bleed.

Subarachnoid haemorrhage A traumatic subarachnoid haemorrhage (SAH) occurs when vessels in the *subarachnoid space*, the space between the arachnoid and pia mater, have been *ruptured* as a direct result of trauma (see Figure 11.6). Subarachnoid haemorrhage is common following major TBI, and may be associated with other focal injuries, such as contusion and lacerations. Hydrocephalus and cerebral vasospasm can develop post-injury and can result in increased ICP.

Intraventricular haemorrhage Intraventricular haemorrhage occurs when *subependymal vessels rupture* and, although it is most common in premature babies, it can also occur as a result of blunt-force trauma. Of the various types of intracranial haemorrhage, intraventricular haemorrhage is less common and is associated with significant mortality and morbidity. It most often occurs in conjunction with other types of intracranial haemorrhage, especially subarachnoid, but it can also occur in isolation. Intraventricular haemorrhage may develop in only one or both of the *lateral ventricles*, but can also develop in the *third and fourth ventricles* independently. Haemorrhage within all ventricles is also possible and presents a very poor prognosis.

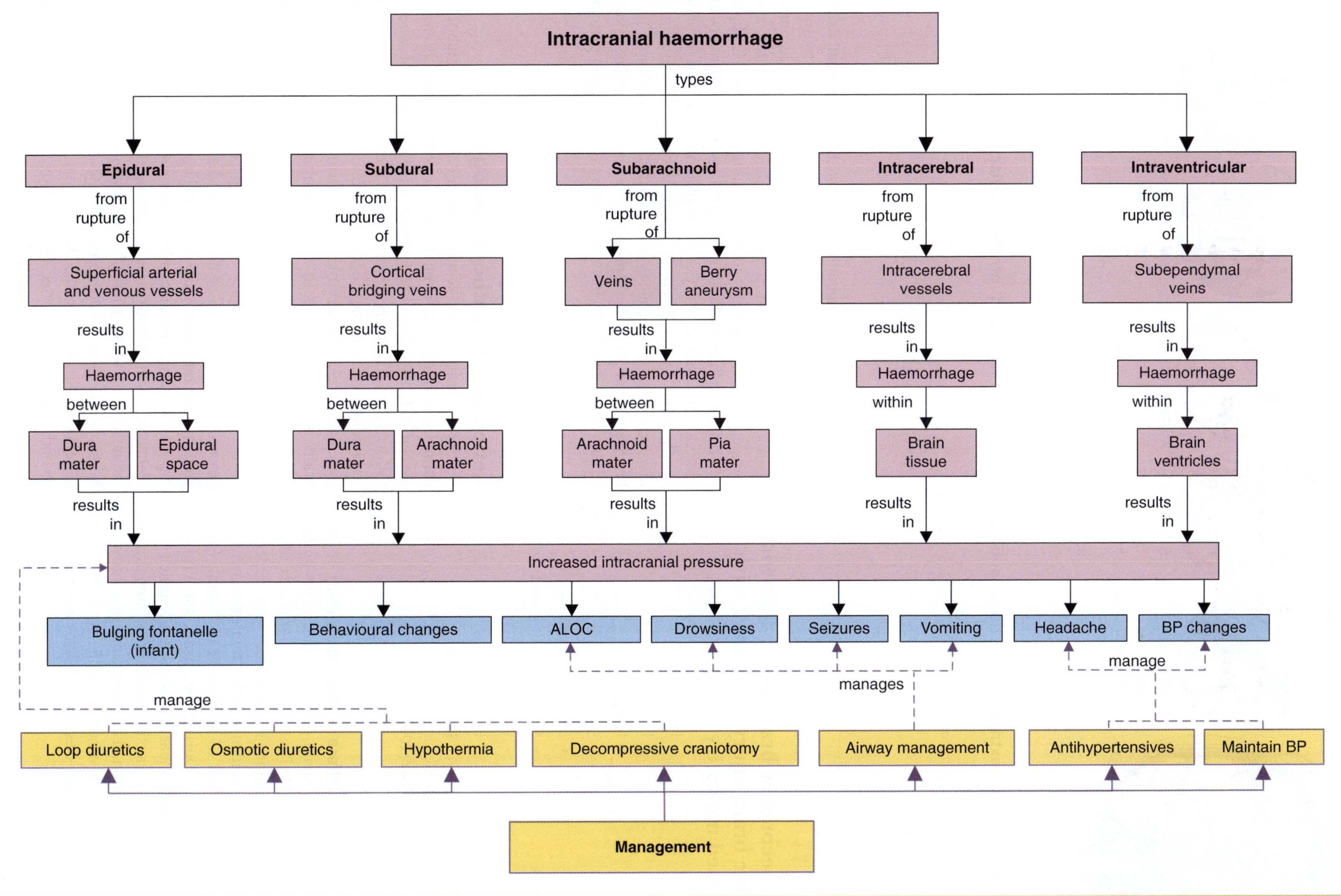

Figure 11.5

Clinical snapshot: Intracranial haemorrhage

ALOC = altered level of consciousness; BP = blood pressure.

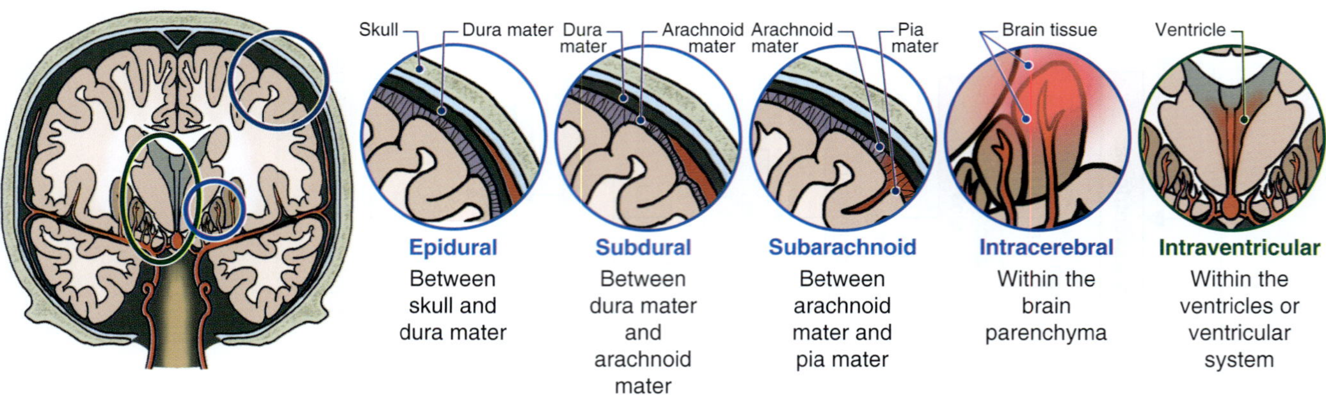

Figure 11.6

Five types of haematoma: extradural, subdural, subarachnoid, intracerebral and intraventricular

Source: Illustration S. Elliott © Sciencopia.

CLINICAL BOX 11.1

Causes of secondary brain injury following traumatic brain injury associated with increased mortality and morbidity

- Hypoxia
- Hypotension
- Hypocapnia
- Hypercapnia
- Hyperthermia
- Hypoglycaemia
- Hyperglycaemia
- Hyperosmolality
- Acidosis
- Hyponatraemia
- Hypernatraemia
- Infection
- Seizure
- Delayed haematoma
- Subarachnoid haemorrhage
- Vasospasm
- Hydrocephalus
- Inflammation

Sources: Data from Bersten & Handy (2018), p. 582; Golman et al. (2022).

Diffuse axonal injury **Diffuse axonal injury (DAI)** is the *tearing or disruption of axonal fibres in the white matter and brainstem.* Generally, DAI is caused by significant blunt-force trauma. This type of injury is commonly seen in people involved in motor vehicle accidents, falls from great heights, assaults and infants subjected to abusive head trauma (such as shaken baby syndrome). During the insult, the brain is subjected to rotational and shearing forces that stretch and rupture the axonal network, causing widespread impairment in the cortex and diencephalon. The axonal network provides the infrastructure for cognitive ability and supports major structural and functional processes. Three forms of DAI exist: mild, moderate and severe.

In *mild DAI*, post-traumatic coma lasts 6–24 hours and death is uncommon. Residual cognitive, psychological and sensory/motor deficits may be ongoing. In *moderate DAI*, widespread neurological impairment is found in the cerebral cortex and diencephalon. Axons are torn and damage occurs in both cerebral hemispheres. Prolonged coma, lasting for 24 hours or more, occurs, and recovery is incomplete in more than 90% of people who survive. *Severe DAI* is produced by severe axonal disruption in the cerebral hemispheres, diencephalon and brainstem, and 30–40% of people who survive a severe injury remain at reduced levels of consciousness for prolonged periods of time.

SECONDARY BRAIN INJURY

Aetiology and pathophysiology

Secondary brain injury occurs when a cascade of metabolic, cellular and molecular events *damage cells that are already susceptible after the initial injury*. In the hours and weeks following the primary injury, tissue ischaemia associated with compressive forces, cerebral oedema or vascular injury can lead to cellular necrosis. Both primary and secondary brain injury contribute to the development of intracranial inflammation and an alteration in the cerebral autoregulatory mechanisms.

Secondary brain injury is a complex pathophysiological process that develops 2–24 hours after the primary injury. The predominant mechanism of secondary head injury is that of *impaired cerebral oxygenation* due to impaired CBF. *Hypotension* (defined as systolic blood pressure < 90 mmHg), *hypoxia* (oxygen saturation $< 90\%$ or $PaO_2 < 50$ mmHg), *hypoglycaemia*, *hyperpyrexia* and *hypocapnia* ($PaCO_2 < 30$ mmHg) are identifiable symptoms in the development and exacerbation of secondary head injury. (See Clinical Box 11.1 for some other causes of secondary brain injury.) Unfortunately, the development of these symptoms can occur during resuscitation, transportation, and surgical and intensive care unit intervention. Any evidence of hypotension and hypoxia has a deleterious effect on the outcome, and contributes to the vicious cycle of insufficient CBF, which in turn can damage susceptible neurons and facilitate the development of secondary brain injury. Figure 11.7 explores the common clinical manifestations and management of secondary head injuries.

Intracranial inflammation Brain injury promotes an inflammatory response and the release of cytokines, free radicals and excitatory amino acids. As with any inflammatory response, when capillary permeability is altered and swelling occurs in this location it involves the blood–brain barrier and glial cells. *Increased blood–brain barrier permeability* may render the brain vulnerable to the effects of pharmacological agents that under normal circumstances cannot cross into the cerebral compartment, such as osmotic diuretics. The degree of inflammation is an important consideration in the management of raised ICP, as the inflammatory response may continue for some time.

LEARNING OBJECTIVE 2

Explore the relationship of the Monro–Kellie doctrine to traumatic brain injury.

Pressure–volume relationship and the Monro–Kellie doctrine Once the fontanelles have fused, usually by 2 years of age, the brain is enclosed in a rigid vault. This means cerebral circulation is vulnerable to conditions that increase intracranial volume. Normal **intracranial pressure (ICP)** is usually less than 15 mmHg and is determined by the volume of the brain parenchyma (~1300 mL in adults), CSF (100–150 mL) and intravascular blood (100–150 mL). The *Monro–Kellie doctrine* notes that an increase in volume of any one of the cerebral components will increase ICP and decrease the volume of other cerebral components. If this compensatory reduction in volume does not occur, then ICP will rise, as volume and pressure are inversely related.

The brain accounts for only 2% of total body weight, but consumes over 20% of the body's total oxygen requirements and 15% of the total cardiac output. The maintenance of cerebral perfusion is therefore critical. **Cerebral perfusion pressure (CPP)** is the difference between outflow and inflow, and is the driving pressure for **cerebral blood flow (CBF)**. Estimates of CPP assume that the relevant inflow pressure is equivalent to the **mean arterial pressure (MAP)** and outflow is related to the ICP. The formula for CPP is:

$$CPP = MAP - ICP$$

Therefore, CPP is used as a measure of CBF. Clinical Box 11.2 outlines the definitions and formulae that relate to cerebral blood pressure and perfusion.

Similarly, any *space-occupying mass* within the cranial vault, such as a haematoma, tumour or oedema, can result in the compression and displacement of the cerebral contents. Initially, circulating CSF and blood volume (principally venous) are reduced, but as the mass size is increased the space-occupying lesion compresses brain tissue and reduces CBF due to increased ICP. As ICP rises outside the normal range, autoregulation is lost, and CBF becomes totally dependent on CPP, which in turn is dependent on systemic blood pressure. Rapid rises in ICP can lead to compression of the brain tissue and herniation, where the brain tissue itself is displaced and moves towards the foramen magnum; also known as 'coning'. The common phenomenon known as the *Cushing reflex*—hypertension, bradycardia and irregular respiration—is a direct result of a rapid rise in ICP.

CLINICAL BOX 11.2

Important formulae relating to cerebral blood pressure and perfusion

Cardiac output (CO):

$$CO = HR \times SV$$

If CO ↓, then heart rate (HR) and/or stroke volume (SV) need to ↑ in order to be able to maintain CO (hence we see the tachycardia).

Blood pressure (BP):

$$BP = PVR \times CO$$

In order to maintain blood pressure (BP), the person's CO will ↑ (as above) and pulmonary vascular resistance (PVR) will also ↑ (tachycardia may be seen with poor distal perfusion as ↑ PVR causes vasoconstriction of peripheral vessels).

Mean arterial pressure (MAP):

$$MAP = \tfrac{1}{3}\ \text{pulse pressure} + dBP$$

As MAP is a measurement of BP, we are able to see the effect of ↓ BP (hypotension) on the brain. (dBP = diastolic blood pressure.)

Cerebral perfusion pressure (CPP):

$$CPP = MAP - ICP$$

CPP is reliant on a balance of MAP (systemic BP) and intracranial blood pressure (ICP). If MAP is ↓ (due to ↓ BP) and ICP is ↑, then autoregulatory mechanisms will try to ↑ BP and HR in order to improve CO.

This autoregulatory mechanism has a small window of time before it becomes inactive. It will not work below a CPP of 50 mmHg.

As MAP and BP both ↓, CPP can only follow this trend. ICP ↑ further, and systemic BP is not able to generate an MAP that is able to overcome the ICP and perfuse the brain. As a result of the poor perfusion, neurons die from hypoxia.

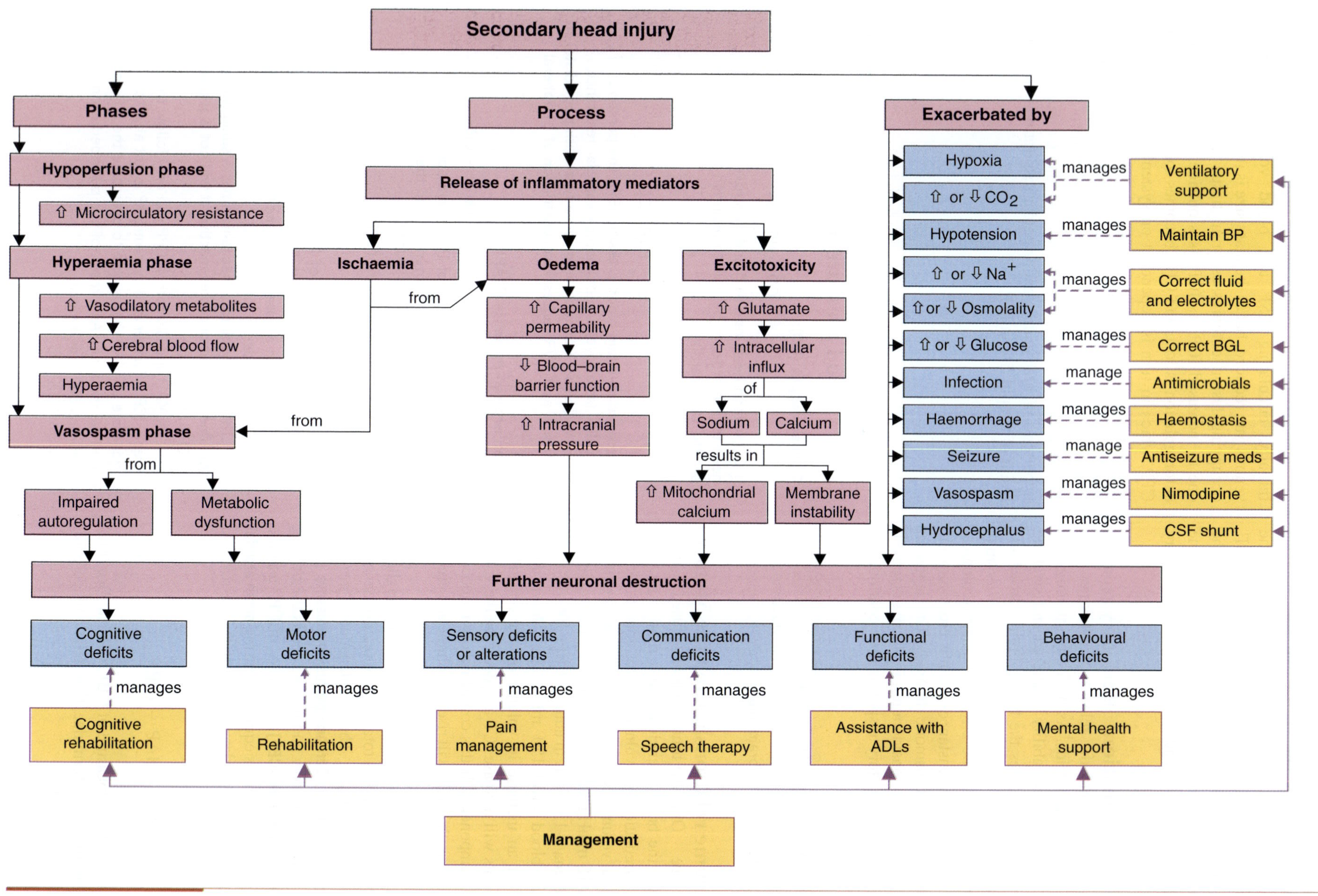

Figure 11.7

Clinical snapshot: Secondary head injury

↓ = decreased; ↑ = increased; ADLs = activities of daily living; BGL = blood glucose level; BP = blood pressure; CO_2 = carbon dioxide; CSF = cerebrospinal fluid; Na^+ = sodium ion.

Under normal circumstances, CBF is maintained by local microcirculation that results from changes in arterial pressure. This is termed *autoregulation*, and ensures that brain tissue is adequately *perfused with oxygen* and that *wastes are removed*. Autoregulation of CBF has a functional CPP range of 65–150 mmHg; outside of these ranges, autoregulation is diminished. Under normal circumstances, a *pressure–volume relationship* exists in the brain vasculature that maintains CPP and CBF. The major regulatory mechanisms for maintaining adequate CBF are the partial pressure of carbon dioxide ($PaCO_2$), blood pressure and blood pH. Alteration in $PaCO_2$, blood pressure or blood pH will result in cerebral vasoconstriction or vasodilation. Hypotension and/or hypoventilation results in an increase in $PaCO_2$ and a decrease in pH (acidosis); as a consequence, cerebral vasodilation occurs in an attempt to increase CBF and deliver more oxygen. Conversely, hypertension, hyperventilation and an increase in pH (alkalosis) can cause cerebral vasoconstriction and a reduction in CBF. Hypocapnia is capable of reducing CBF by 4% for each mmHg change in $PaCO_2$.

Elevated intracranial pressure The Monro–Kellie doctrine provides the framework for understanding the mechanism behind rising ICP. CBF is dependent on autoregulation and CPP. Baroreceptors constantly monitor systemic blood pressure and provide a positive feedback loop. Myogenic regulation of systemic blood pressure is achieved by vasodilation and vasoconstriction, thus altering peripheral vascular resistance in an effort to maintain adequate CPP and blood flow.

Alterations to cerebral perfusion When the homeostatic autoregulation mechanism is impaired, neuronal damage and intracranial inflammation occur.

The hypoperfusion phase Within the first 72 hours following brain injury, CBF is reduced, resulting in cerebral ischaemia. When autoregulation fails, the degree of CBF is directly dependent on systemic blood pressure. The maintenance of systemic blood pressure may require catecholamine infusion and intravenous fluid administration to support the CPP and CBF. Insufficient oxygen delivery renders neurons ischaemic and exacerbates the speed of the inflammatory process, which results in oedema and, in turn, attracts more inflammatory mediators to the injured site. Therefore, oedema and the alteration in cellular permeability increase ICP further. Increased ICP reduces CBF, and this establishes a *cycle of raised ICP and reduced CBF*. Cerebral hypoperfusion is found in most cases where the person has sustained a severe head injury and has a Glasgow coma scale (GCS) score of less than 8.

The hyperaemic phase Improved CBF is the hallmark of the hyperaemic phase, and is due to somewhat *improved autoregulatory mechanisms*. The hyperaemic phase can last for 7–10 days post-injury, and will occur in up to 30% of brain-injured people. While improved CPP and blood flow is a positive development, other management challenges can still exist. Alteration in blood–brain barrier permeability and intracranial inflammation can contribute to *cerebral oedema* (see reperfusion injury in the chapter 'Pathophysiological terminology, cellular adaptation and injury', under ischaemic and hypoxia agents). This oedema may be due to vasospasm caused by *intracranial inflammation*, or by *catecholamine infusion* that has been used to promote and maintain CPPs during the cerebral hypoperfusion phase.

The vasospastic phase The vasospastic phase is characterised by *cerebral hypoperfusion* due to arterial vasospasm, impaired autoregulation and metabolic dysfunction. Typically, this pattern of ischaemia is seen in individuals with severe primary and secondary brain injury and accounts for 10–15% of injuries. Vasospastic-induced reduction to CBF may persist for this group.

Excitotoxicity Following TBI, excessive extracellular cerebral concentrations of *excitatory amino acids (EAA)*, such as glutamate, develop. In the central nervous system (CNS), *glutamate* is the primary excitatory neurotransmitter. However, excessive levels of glutamate can alter cell permeability and result in the release of toxic chemicals—excitotoxicity. Glutamate reacts with sodium and calcium channels, leading to an influx of these cations. Calcium enters damaged neurons and causes the axon to swell and burst. Excessive calcium concentration also activates proteases, such as calpains, which are especially damaging to nerve cells.

Changes in function of two important glutamate receptor subtypes are predominantly involved in excitotoxic responses. These glutamatergic receptors are named according to the agonist substances that activate them: *alpha-amino-3-hydroxyl-5-methyl-4-isoxazole-propionic acid (AMPA)* and *N-methyl-D-aspartic acid (NMDA)*.

AMPA receptor changes post-TBI Post-TBI, cells become more permeable to calcium, a positively charged ion (Ca^{2+}). The *increased intracellular concentration of calcium* leads to a loss of cellular function and integrity. The cell membrane can no longer regulate the influx of calcium, and the cell becomes overstimulated and swollen due to the increased concentration of calcium.

NMDA receptor changes post-TBI A deadly influx of calcium into the cell results when nitric oxide binds with intracellular NMDA receptors. With the increased concentration of intracellular calcium, the cell relocates some of this calcium to its mitochondria in an attempt to restore normal calcium concentrations.

Once inside the mitochondria, the increased calcium concentrations result in increased reactive oxygen species. Subsequent lipid peroxidation contributes to further irreversible damage to cell membranes and DNA fragmentation (see the chapter 'Pathophysiological terminology, cellular adaptation and injury').

Clinical manifestations

A person with TBI can present in various ways. Some factors that may influence the clinical presentation include the force and mechanism of the injury, the developmental age of the skull, and the friability and structure of the vasculature. A person may initially present with no symptoms but deteriorate into unconsciousness, or they may become confused and manifestly neurologically impaired.

Severe TBI is a leading cause of long-term disability in developed countries, particularly in young adults. Examples of long-term disability include motor and sensory impairment, intellectual and cognitive dysfunction, and memory impairment. The financial, social and emotional costs of TBI care are enormous. Depression, mood anxieties and psychiatric disorders can result from TBI, and can hinder recovery, affect relationships and reduce a person's quality of life. Depression is a frequent consequence of TBI, with severe depression more likely in those people in whom mood and anxiety disorders were present before the injury. Major depression is associated with reductions in memory and the inability to perform tasks independently. Children who have sustained TBI are more likely to have cognitive and behavioural impairment, especially if support post-injury is poor.

It is well established that trauma brain injury often results in impaired judgement, increased aggression and impulsivity, and diminished empathy. As such, those with TBI disproportionately interact with the criminal justice system, resulting in estimates of between 40% and 90% of incarcerated offenders in Australia having sustained traumatic brain injury sometime during their life.

Clinical diagnosis and management

LEARNING OBJECTIVE 3

Outline the clinical diagnosis and current management for traumatic brain injury.

Diagnosis Concussion and the duration of concussion are markers for the severity of neurotrauma. Episodes of concussion and a brief loss of consciousness (< 30 minutes) occur in 60% of people who have sustained TBI. TBI cases associated with an intracranial injury (haemorrhage, haematoma) have a higher mortality rate compared to TBI cases without intracranial injury. When evaluating someone with TBI, comprehensive neurological examination is essential. Assessing and monitoring a person's vital signs are essential tools used to ascertain the person's current level of neurological function and the potential for deterioration. Basic vital signs assessments include the *Glasgow coma scale (GCS)* score, heart and respiratory rate and rhythm, blood pressure, pupil response and motor/sensory response.

The GCS is a quick and easy tool for assessing the severity of TBI in the pre-hospital and hospital environments. Individuals are assessed in three areas: *eye (E) opening, motor (M)* and *verbal (V) response* (see Table 11.1). With reference to TBI, a person with a score between 13 and 15 is classified as having a *mild TBI*. A score of between 9 and 12 may indicate a *moderate TBI*. With a score of 8 or less, a *severe TBI* is indicated. The lowest score is 3 ($E = 1; V = 1; M = 1$). The value of the score is dependent on the absence of systemic alterations, such as hypotension, hypoxia, hypothermia and hypoglycaemia, as well as drugs that affect the

Table 11.1 Glasgow coma scale (GCS) for adults and infants

Adults

Eye opening response (E)	Best verbal response (V)	Best motor response (M)
4 Spontaneously	5 Oriented	6 Obeys command
3 To verbal command	4 Confused	5 Localises to pain
2 To pain	3 Inappropriate words	4 Withdraws from pain
1 Nil	2 Incomprehensible sounds	3 Abnormal flexion to pain
	1 Nil	2 Abnormal extension to pain
		1 Nil

Infants

Eye opening response (E)	Best verbal response	Best motor response (M)
4 Spontaneously	5 Coos or babbles	6 Spontaneous or purposeful
3 To speech	4 Irritable	5 Localises to pain
2 To pain	3 Cries to pain	4 Withdraws from pain
1 Nil	2 Moans to pain	3 Abnormal flexion to pain
	1 No verbal response	2 Abnormal extension to pain
		1 Nil

CNS, such as benzodiazepines and alcohol. A slightly varied GCS is used for infants (see Table 11.1). The GCS gives a prognosis for survival rather than for functional outcome.

Post-traumatic amnesia *Post-traumatic amnesia (PTA)* refers to the inability of the brain to form and retain *new continuous day-to-day memory* post-injury. The duration of PTA is the best indicator of the extent of cognitive dysfunction following TBI. In Australia, the most common means of assessing PTA is the *Westmead scale* (developed by a group at the Westmead Hospital in Sydney). During hospital assessment and management, assessment of PTA is often used in conjunction with the GCS in determining the degree of DAI and TBI severity. *Mild* TBI cases are characterised as having a GCS score of 12–15, and a PTA of less than 24 hours. *Moderate* cases of TBI are defined as having a GCS score of 9–11, and a PTA of 1–7 days in duration. *Severe* TBI cases are defined as a GCS score of 3–8, and a PTA lasting more than four weeks in duration.

Classification of neurotrauma severity Neurotrauma severity is classified as follows:

Minimal

- No loss of consciousness, and
- GCS score of 15, and
- Normal alertness and memory, and
- No neurological deficit, and
- No palpable depressed fracture or other sign of skull fracture.

Mild

- Brief (<5 minutes) loss of consciousness, or
- Amnesia for the event, or
- GCS score of 14, or
- Impaired alertness or memory, and
- No palpable depressed fracture or other sign of skull fracture.

Moderate or potentially severe

- Prolonged (>5 minutes) loss of consciousness, or
- Persistent GCS score of <14, or
- Focal neurological deficit, or
- Post-traumatic seizure, or
- Intracranial lesion on computed tomographic (CT) scan, or
- Palpable depressed skull fracture.

The *assessment of pulse pressure* (systolic minus diastolic blood pressure; see Clinical Box 9.3, and the chapter 'Brain and spinal cord dysfunction') is important, as widening pulse pressure can be a sign of increasing ICP. *Pupillary response* can provide insight into some cranial nerve function, and other cranial nerves can be assessed using various techniques to elicit reflexes. Other neurological assessments include motor assessments that test strength and symmetry in both arms and legs.

ICP monitoring devices can be inserted surgically, and this guides decision-making for interventions and management plans. Depending on the person's age and whether their cranial sutures have closed, normal ICP is 1–10 mmHg. ICP exceeding 15 mmHg represents mild intracranial hypertension, above 20 mmHg is moderately high, and above 40 mmHg is severe. If a person is sedated and chemically paralysed, conventional neurological assessments such as the GCS are worthless, yet ICP monitoring will still provide an indication of CPP and enable the informed manipulation of interventions to achieve the most beneficial outcomes.

Other investigations to quantify the extent of a TBI may include *imaging techniques* such as CT, X-ray and magnetic resonance imaging (MRI). Diagnostic imaging permits assessment of bone, soft tissue and the formation of collections such as haematoma. Other important evaluations include the possibility of a brain structure having shifted from midline. These imaging techniques are also beneficial to monitor the progression or resolution of trauma on the contents of the cranial vault. CT and MRI are expensive investigations and may not be used for all people presenting with head injury. Minor injury may be assessed with plain skull films. The mechanism of injury and clinical presentation will inform the team as to whether further, more expensive, invasive investigations are required.

Electroencephalography (EEG) may be used to determine depth of unconsciousness, and predict survival or functional outcomes following TBI. EEG measures the electrical activity of the brain. Cerebral perfusion and metabolic activity to specific brain areas can be inferred. The benefit of EEG is improved when used in conjunction with other imaging techniques and assessment data. EEG can also be useful in tracking progress to recovery when comparing initial results to those obtained during rehabilitation.

Other monitoring techniques employed to assess a person with TBI may include:

- *brain tissue oxygenation* ($PbrO_2$; can be achieved with some ICP catheters)—brain oxygenation can often detect evolving injury in at-risk tissue
- *transcranial Doppler ultrasound (TCD)*—another technique beneficial for its non-invasive capacity to measure flow velocities in basal cerebral arteries, providing information about CBF and vasospasm
- *cerebral microdialysis*—enables assessment of the extracellular environment surrounding at-risk tissue; this technique enables evaluation of brain ischaemia markers, including glutamate, lactate, glucose and glycerol.

Management The management of TBI is dictated by the severity of the injury and the expectation of recovery. Principles of management are focused on stabilising the person and preventing secondary neuronal injury. Priorities of care include preventing hypoxia and hypotension.

Airway management People with severe TBI (GCS score ≤ 8) and people with ventilatory compromise should be intubated and ventilated to maintain optimal oxygenation. The possibility of spinal cord injury (especially cervical spine) should also be considered. Ventilation should be titrated to maintain oxygenation and prevent hypocapnoea. Sedation and chemical paralysis (neuromuscular blockade) may be necessary to reduce ventilator dysynchrony and agitation; however, it interferes with neurological assessment and, if undertaken for long periods, is associated with complications such as reduced CBF and myopathy.

Blood pressure management Fluid volume management is important, the goal of which is to maintain adequate hydration and prevent dehydration or fluid overload, which can exacerbate the risk of poor outcomes. Beta-blockers may be necessary to control excessive sympathetic hyperactivity as a result of cerebral oedema. Vasodilators may be used, but questions remain about their safety in relation to their potential effect on ICP.

Management of intracranial hypertension Brain oedema can be managed with the use of osmotic diuretics, such as mannitol, or loop diuretics, such as furosemide. Reducing cerebral oedema is important in order to promote adequate CBF. Elevating the head of the bed by 15–20 degrees is very beneficial in reducing ICP, but may not be possible for those with other significant orthopaedic trauma. Thermoregulation is important, and fever should be aggressively treated because of its influence on metabolic demand. Induced hypothermia may be used to reduce increased ICP and metabolic demand. However, it is generally used judiciously because it can also be associated with significant complications, such as coagulopathy, immunosuppression and skin necrosis. Antiseizure therapy may be necessary to reduce seizure activity, providing a beneficial effect on the development of ICP. Surgical interventions, such as decompressive craniotomy or the placement of intraventricular drains, may also be necessary in the control and management of intracranial hypertension.

Interventions to reduce the likelihood of requiring the Valsalva manoeuvre—such as the administration of stool softeners, adequate fluid balance and increased fibre—will assist in reducing strain during defecation. Codeine is beneficial in reducing the risk of excessive coughing, which is linked to increased intrathoracic pressures and a subsequent raising of ICP. Antiemetics should be provided to reduce emesis. It is also important to remember the beneficial effects of therapeutic communication, such as an explanation of care to the affected person and their loved ones, which can reduce anxiety-related increased sympathetic nervous system stimulation.

Spinal cord injury

Spinal cord injury can result in devastating disability. It can affect people of any age, culture and socioeconomic status, although there is an inverse relationship between spinal cord injury and education level.

EPIDEMIOLOGY

There are currently more than 20,800 people in Australia living with spinal cord injury, with the addition of approximately 380 more every year. In New Zealand, approximately 200 people are diagnosed with spinal cord injury every year. Most spinal cord injuries are a result of traffic accidents, with falls the next most common cause. Age has a significant influence on the mechanism of a person's injury, with motor vehicle accidents being the most common in the young, and falls the most common in the older adult population.

AETIOLOGY AND PATHOPHYSIOLOGY

LEARNING OBJECTIVE 4

Outline the pathogenesis of spinal cord injury.

Primary injury

The mechanism of the trauma and the severity of insult will significantly influence clinical outcomes. Cellular responses that occur as a result of damage to the spinal cord also contribute to these outcomes. At the time of the initial injury (the mechanisms of which are discussed later in this chapter), damage to the intramedullary blood vessels will result in *haemorrhage*. As there is limited space within the vertebral canal, this haemorrhage may begin to cause compression of the cord and the surrounding blood vessels. Vasospasm may also occur and further impede circulation to the central grey matter, resulting in worsening ischaemia.

Secondary injury

In any injury, an inflammatory process begins (see the chapter 'Inflammation and healing') and triggers *a series of biochemical events that may cause further damage*. As with the secondary process in TBI, a release of inflammatory mediators results in the intracellular accumulation of calcium, eicosanoid production, the release of oxygen free radicals, and the release of excitatory neurotransmitters such as glutamate. Energy depletion also occurs as energy-dependent processes begin to fail due to ischaemia (see the chapter 'Pathophysiological terminology, cellular adaptation and injury'). The subsequent destruction of neurons results from the loss of membrane integrity and cytoskeleton disruption. Further inflammatory mediators are released, increasing oedema and contributing to the loss of spinal cord blood flow. Axonal degeneration may commence, and demyelination may also exacerbate the initial damage. The compression of the affected blood vessels—induced as a result of the swelling and blood in the confined space, or the haemostatic mechanisms from platelet aggregation and fibrin deposition—can stem haemorrhage into the area. Pressures distal to the vascular obstruction increases and causes protein loss into the interstitial space, further increasing the oedema. Figure 11.8 explores the common clinical manifestations and management of spinal cord injury.

Spinal shock Within an hour of spinal cord injury, spinal shock (also known as *spinal cord concussion*) may develop. **Spinal shock** is the transient loss of all reflexive and autonomic function below the level of cord damage. (Spinal shock differs from neurogenic shock; see Clinical Box 11.3.) It is thought to result from an extracellular accumulation of potassium, which interferes with nerve impulse generation. There is debate regarding the definitive resolution of spinal shock, with some

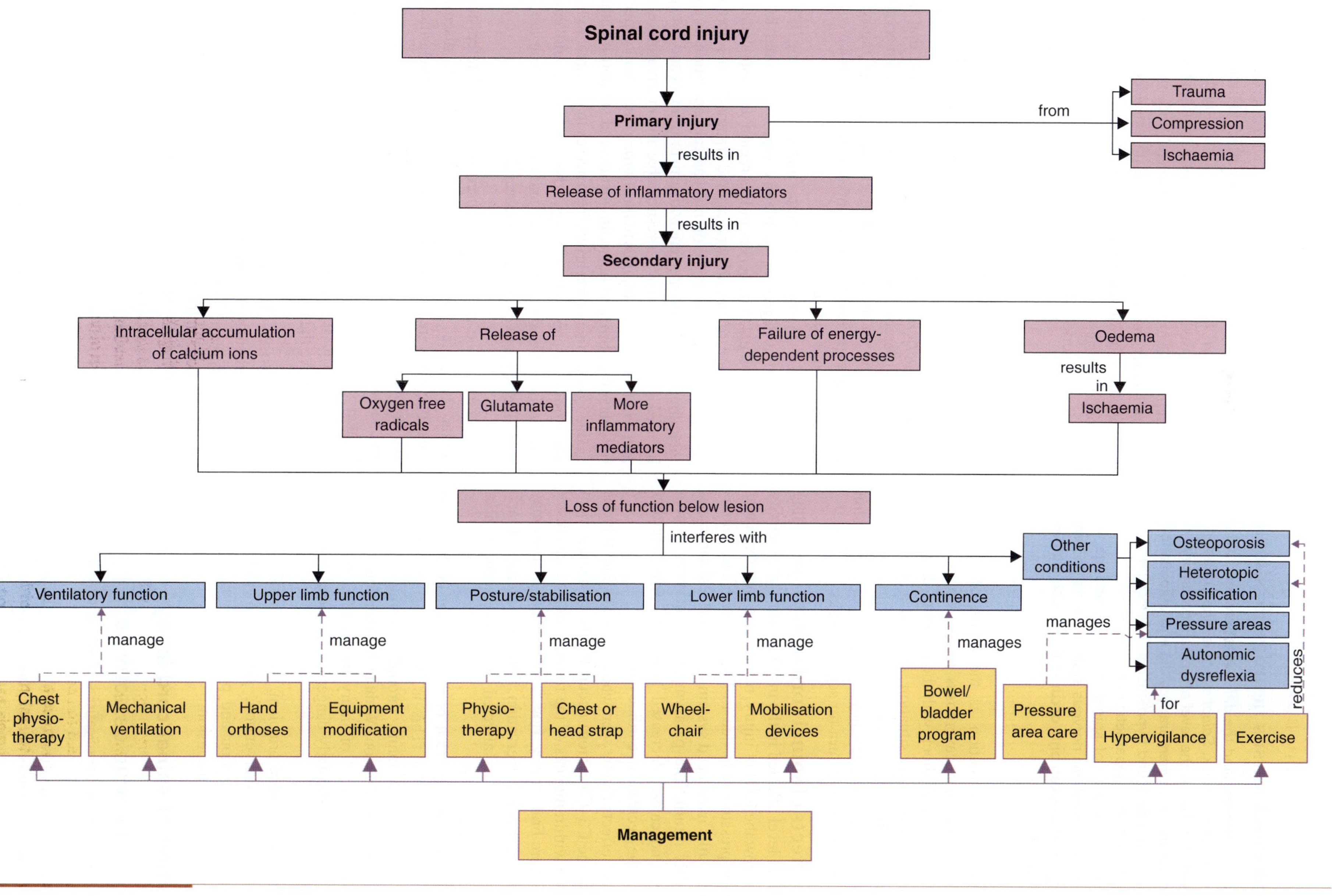

Figure 11.8
Clinical snapshot: Spinal cord injury

CLINICAL BOX 11.3

Spinal shock versus neurogenic shock

It is imperative to understand the difference between spinal shock and neurogenic shock. *Spinal shock* is when reflexes are temporarily lost below the level of spinal cord injury.

Neurogenic shock is when bradycardia and vasodilation occur, resulting in a profound hypotension. This occurs because of the loss of sympathetic nervous system innervation below the level of spinal cord injury and the unopposed parasympathetic nervous system effects on heart rate. Neurogenic shock can only occur in those with injuries above the level of T6.

clinicians suggesting resolution as the return of cutaneous reflexes, such as the bulbocavernosus reflex, whereas others identify the end of spinal shock with the return of deep tendon reflexes. Compounding this situation, there is a disparity in spinal shock resolution by several weeks, as bulbocavernosus reflexes may return within a few days of injury, yet deep tendon reflexes will not generally return for several weeks.

Systemic effects of spinal cord injury Depending on the vertebral level affected in the insult, sympathetic activity may be lost below the level of injury, resulting in cardiovascular effects. Blood pressure falls due to both arterial and venous dilation, and results in reduced systemic vascular resistance and reduced venous return. The parasympathetic nervous system is unopposed and causes decreased heart rate, which further contributes to the decrease in cardiac output.

Respiratory effects can be seen when cervical spine injuries (especially in the C3–C5 region) occur. If airway management is not initiated within minutes of the trauma, apnoea will result in death or severe brain injury. Lower-level spinal injuries may preserve diaphragmatic innervation, but the intercostal and abdominal muscles may be affected and cause reduced tidal volume and hypoventilation.

The loss of thermoregulation below the level of the lesion is known as *poikilothermia*. This is defined as the inability to maintain a core temperature through sweating, shivering, vasodilation or vasoconstriction. Without intervention, the body temperature below the level of injury moves towards ambient temperature. This is particularly dangerous for those with injury above T1.

A male may experience priapism, which generally resolves quickly and without intervention. Both men and women may develop urinary retention and paralytic ileus, which are evidenced by abdominal distension.

Classification of spinal cord injury

LEARNING OBJECTIVE 5

Identify the common classifications of spinal cord injury.

Spinal cord injuries are often classified into *complete* spinal cord injury, where all sensorimotor function beneath the level of injury is lost, and *incomplete* spinal cord injury, where some sensorimotor function remains. However, clinicians prefer not to use the terms 'complete' and 'incomplete' in isolation, because these arbitrary classifications are often difficult to apply, some function may be recovered with time and treatment, and the label itself may erode hope for affected individuals. The *American Spinal Injury Association's (ASIA) impairment scale* is commonly used to grade severity of sensorimotor loss, and, although it still uses the terms 'complete' and 'incomplete', it also uses other parameters to provide an extended assessment and classification of sensory and motor function.

Spinal injuries are commonly classified according to three criteria: the vertebral level, the degree and the mechanism affected.

Vertebral level The classification based on 'vertebral level' refers to the anatomical location, occurring within the cervical, thoracic, lumbar or sacral vertebrae (see Figure 11.9). *The higher the injury, the greater the level of disability experienced.* It is important to understand that there is a slight difference between motor and sensory innervation. So, depending on the vertebral level and degree of injury, the person may experience a motor impairment, but still have some sensation above that level.

In relation to motor function, injuries including C3–C5 will dictate the degree of ventilatory support required by the injured individual. The nerves in this region are responsible for the innervation of the diaphragm, and trauma to this area can result in significant reliance on mechanical ventilation. Injuries including C5–C7 will interfere with arm movement and strength, as nerves in this region are responsible for innervating elbow and wrist movement. Injuries to the *thoracic spine* will generally influence the ability to maintain posture and support breathing, as intercostal innervation arises from nerves in this area. *Lumbar spine* injuries can influence hip, knee and ankle movement. Lower-limb strength, and bowel and bladder function are also controlled by nerves in the lumbosacral regions.

Degree The classification based on 'degree' refers to the terms 'complete' and 'incomplete'. As previously discussed, these two terms are only of some benefit when further clarification can be made. The definition of complete loss of all movement and sensation beneath the level of injury is dependent on time. It takes several weeks before swelling (known as spinal shock; discussed earlier in this chapter) reduces. When this occurs, some function above the initial level of injury may begin to return.

Mechanism The classification based on 'mechanism' is important, and may inform to some extent the clinical outcomes and recovery expectations. Common mechanisms that result in spinal cord injury are flexion, flexion–extension, rotation, compression and hyperextension (see Figure 11.10).

Flexion and *flexion–extension* are commonly caused by acceleration–deceleration situations, such as a car accident. *Rotation* injuries occur commonly in the cervical spine, and may result from diving accidents. *Compression* can occur as a result of the primary injury, but may also be caused by secondary swelling, ruptured intervertebral discs, and pressure from a tumour, or as a result of chronic disease, such as a

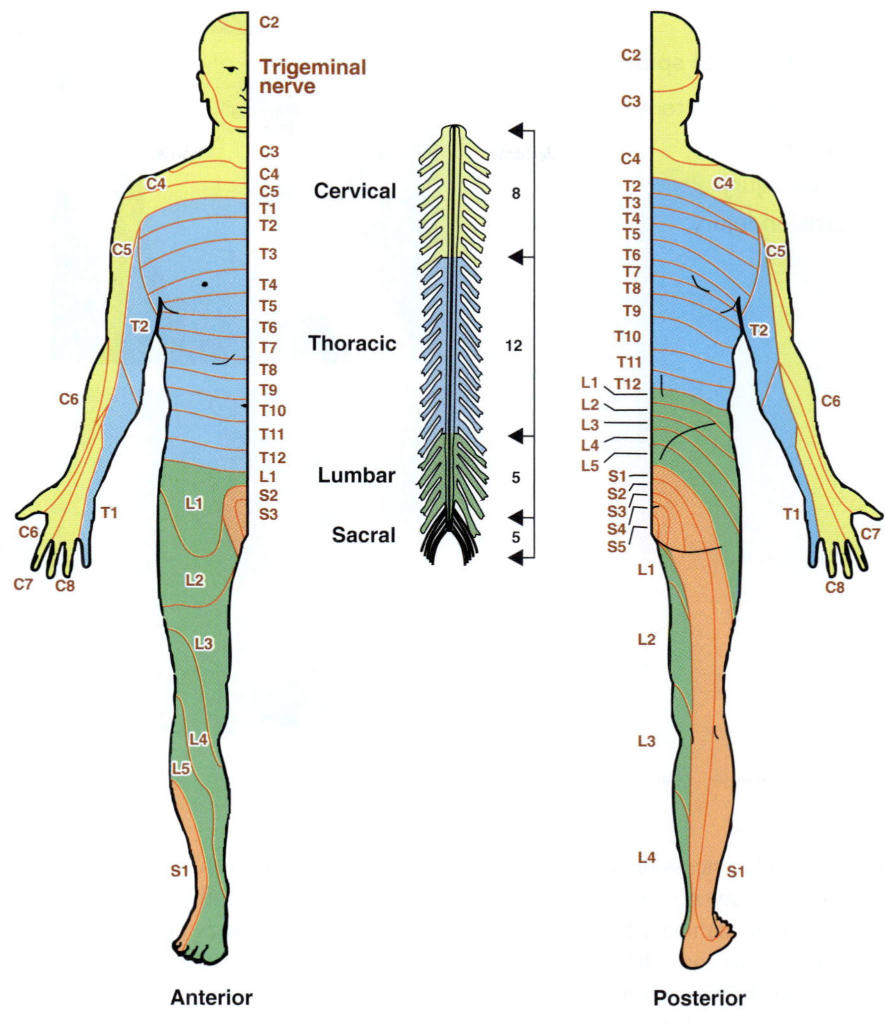

Figure 11.9

Classification of spinal cord injury based on 'vertebral level', demonstrating areas of muscular innervation related to spinal nerve

spondylopathy. *Hyperextension* may occur as a result of falling forward and striking the head, face or chin on a step or other structure, which allows the occipital region of the skull to move forcefully towards the back.

Other descriptive classification terms Other common terminology used in the description of spinal cord injury includes laceration, transection, contusion, compression, distraction and concussion.

Laceration The spinal cord may be partly damaged by a rip or tear from vertebral fractures that have become displaced in the trauma, or by external causes such as a knife or a bullet. A laceration will result in permanent injury, and can be associated with oedema and further cord compression.

Transection The true definition of 'transection' is when the spinal cord is completely severed. This may occur as a result of penetrating trauma or from fragments of fractured vertebrae. Complete transection is less common. Clinicians may also use the terminology 'partial transection' when they are referring to a large laceration (e.g. half the spinal cord).

Contusion Spinal contusion can be caused by falls or acceleration–deceleration injuries. The vessels supplying the spinal cord rupture and a haemorrhage occurs in the spinal cord and the meninges.

Compression Spinal compression occurs as a result of crushing or distorting the spinal cord within the vertebral canal. Cord compression can occur as a result of the primary injury from fragments of fractured vertebrae, or ruptured or dislocated intervertebral disc, and from any number of other non-trauma causes, such as an abscess or a tumour. Cord compression also often occurs as a secondary injury as a result of the inflammatory process and haemorrhage from the primary trauma.

Distraction Distraction is the process of pulling the spinal cord apart. This often occurs as a result of a lap seatbelt and acceleration–deceleration incidents, when motion thrusts the top and bottom half of the body forward with excessive force, but a portion of the thoracolumbar vertebrae is restrained by the lap seatbelt, resulting in a stretching of the soft tissue structures and spinal cord in these areas.

Figure 11.10

Common mechanisms of spinal injury

(A) Flexion and flexion–extension injury.
(B) Rotation injury.
(C) Compression injury.
(D) Hyperextension injury.

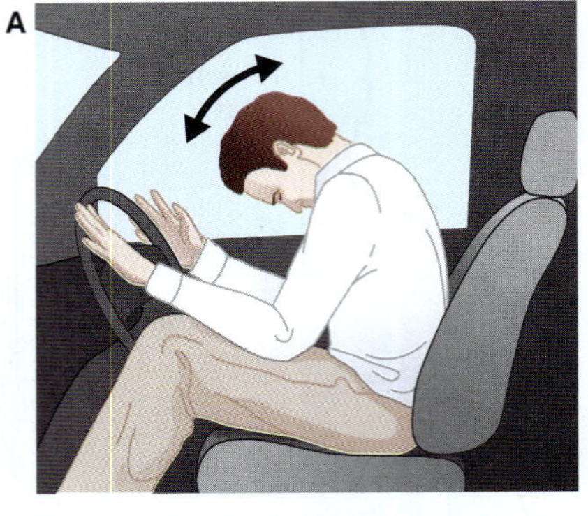

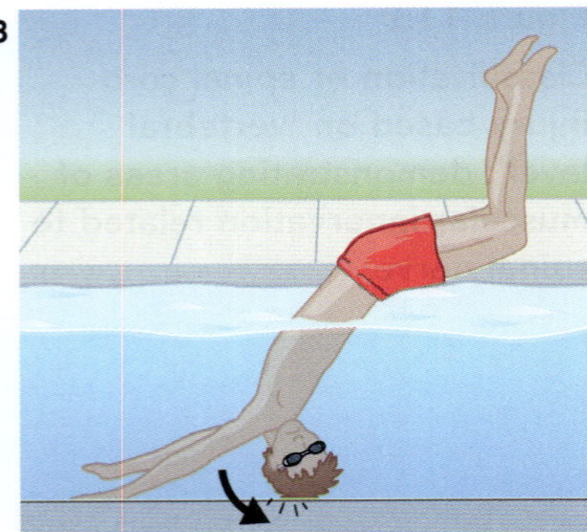

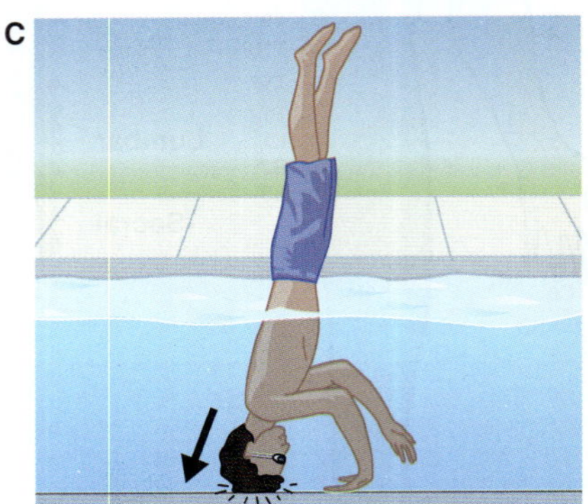

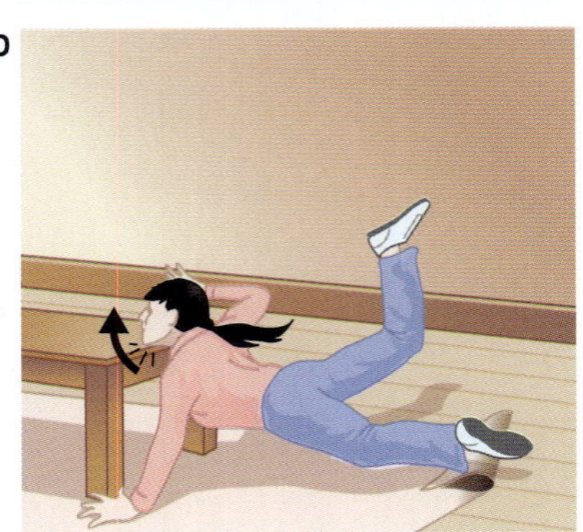

Concussion Spinal concussion can be caused by a violent blow. There may or may not be vertebral damage; however, there is no apparent damage to the cord. Neurologically there are motor and sensory deficits, and spinal shock may occur; however, the deficits subside in a very short period of time (maybe even hours). Most often, there are no residual neurological deficits once recovered.

Complete spinal cord injury Although less common, complete spinal cord injury results in a total absence of function beneath the level of the injury, in the absence of spinal shock. In this type of injury, there is little or no prospect of regaining function (without significant advances in current research). Complete spinal cord injury tends to occur more in the thoracic and lumbar regions, as the relative dimension of the vertebral foramen (the canal for the spinal cord) to the spinal cord width is smaller. As seen in Figure 11.11, the *vertebral canal* varies in size, depending on the vertebral region. A small canal affords less area for mechanical stress and post-injury swelling, and can affect the extent of the damage. Chronic disease can also influence the size of the canal. Vertebral canal stenosis can cause or contribute to spinal cord injury, as can dislocation of the intervertebral discs.

CLINICAL MANIFESTATIONS

As previously discussed, complete spinal injury will result in the loss of all sensory and motor function beneath the level of the injury. Along with the symmetrical sensorimotor deficits dictated by the affected region or vertebral level, systemic effects may also occur (as discussed above).

Incomplete spinal cord injury

It is more common for individuals to experience an incomplete spinal cord injury. Once spinal shock has reduced, the function regained will be dependent on the area of cord damaged. The spinal cord is arranged into both *ascending and descending tracts* that are located in different regions within the spinal cord (see Figure 11.12). The affected regions will influence the

Figure 11.11

Vertebral foramen of various vertebrae

(A) Cervical vertebra.
(B) Thoracic vertebra.
(C) Lumbar vertebra.

Source: © Sciencopia.

A

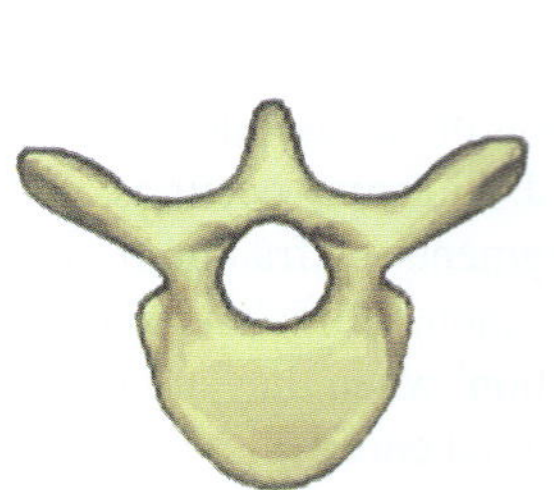

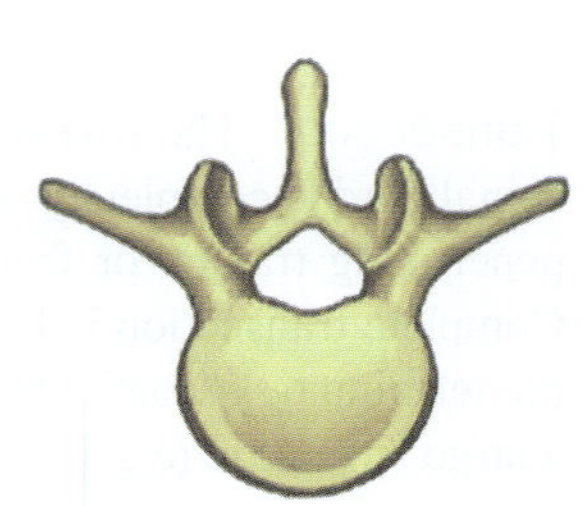

Figure 11.12

Ascending and descending spinal cord tracts

The blue areas of this diagram denote ascending tracts, and the red areas denote descending tracts.

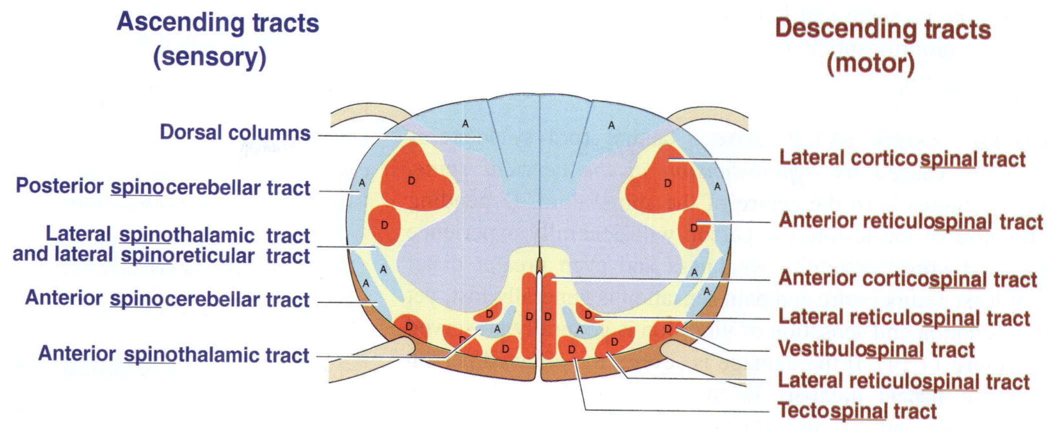

severity of the motor and sensory deficit, and each person will experience gain or retain different function.

The *ascending tracts are sensory tracts*, and tend to have the prefix *spino-* and a suffix pertaining to where the fibres first synapse. An example of this is the *anterior spinocerebellar tract*. This tract is located anteriorly and synapses in the cerebellum. Sensory tracts transmit sensory information from proprioceptors, and cutaneous and visceral receptors. Information such as temperature, pressure, pain and the relative location of body parts is relayed through these fibres.

The *descending tracts are motor tracts* and tend to have a prefix that denotes the brain region from which the fibres begin and the suffix *-spinal*. An example of this is the *anterior corticospinal tract*. This tract is also located anteriorly and carries information from the cerebral cortex. These tracts control visceral and somatic motor activity.

LEARNING OBJECTIVE 6

Discuss the characteristics of common spinal cord syndromes.

Several different types of injuries can occur. Some more common injuries can be classified as anterior cord syndrome, central cord syndrome, Brown-Séquard syndrome and cauda equina syndrome.

Anterior cord syndrome Anterior cord syndrome is commonly caused by *mechanical events*, such as trauma or disc herniation, but can also be caused by *vascular events*. The front of the spinal cord is affected, and therefore the person will often lose distal motor function and some sensory function, such as pain and temperature sensation (see Figure 11.13). Unconscious proprioception (proprioception associated with posture) is also lost. People with anterior cord syndrome may retain the sense

Figure 11.13

Anterior cord syndrome

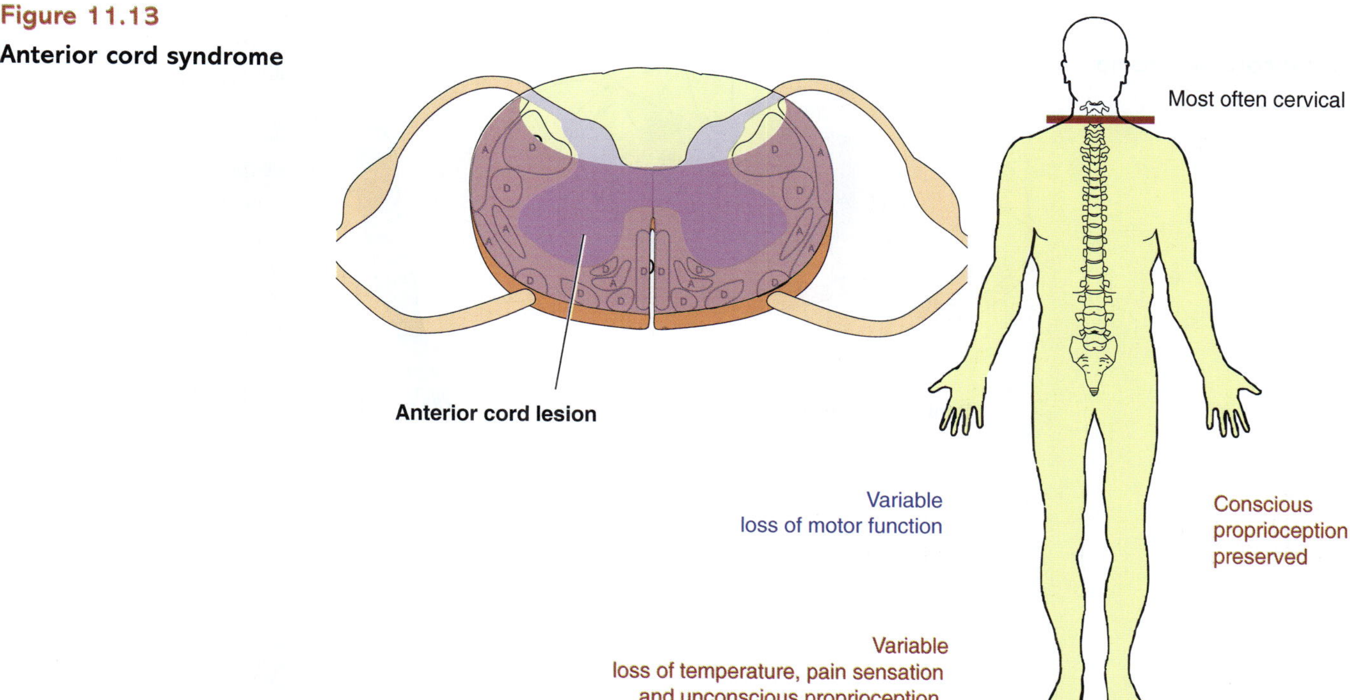

of vibration, pressure and light touch. They will usually retain conscious proprioception (proprioception of limbs, and joint position and range).

Central cord syndrome **Central cord syndrome** is commonly caused by *hyperextension in the cervical spine*, causing contusion to the centre of the spinal cord. Depending on the size of the lesion, the person will generally experience significant upper extremity weakness and even greater distal motor loss. Temperature and pain sensation is generally lost, yet proprioception and sensation of vibration is generally preserved (see Figure 11.14). If the damage is severe, the affected person may have **flaccid paralysis** in the upper limbs and **spastic paralysis** in the lower limbs. They will commonly retain perianal sensation and preserved voluntary anal tone, resulting in faecal continence.

Brown-Séquard syndrome Brown-Séquard syndrome is commonly caused by *penetrating injuries*. Transection occurs across half a section of the spinal cord (*hemi-section*). There is complete loss of motor function on the affected side (*ipsilateral*) but not on the unaffected side (*contralateral*) (see Figure 11.15). Proprioception is lost on the ipsilateral side but not the contralateral side, and other sensory activities, such as pain and temperature, are lost on the contralateral side but not on the ipsilateral side.

Cauda equina syndrome Cauda equina syndrome is commonly caused by *compression or trauma* affecting the *lumbosacral nerve roots* beneath the **conus medullaris** (the base of the spinal cord). There are various causes of cauda equina syndrome, including trauma, tumour or, most commonly, intervertebral disc herniation or rupture (see Figure 11.16). Neurological deficit may be either unilateral or bilateral, but is most often unilateral and asymmetric. Motor deficits include lower extremity weakness and reduced or absent reflexes. Urinary incontinence and constipation or urinary retention are common, and result from both motor and sensory deficits. Lower back and sciatic pain are common.

CLINICAL DIAGNOSIS AND MANAGEMENT

LEARNING OBJECTIVE 7

Explore the clinical diagnosis and management of spinal cord injury.

Initial assessment of neurological function will generally have occurred pre-hospital and, most often, spinal immobilisation will have been applied. Basic life support measures may need to be initiated. If the injury is high in the cervical region, airway support will be required and manual ventilation may also be necessary. Circulatory support may be required for either neurogenic or hypovolaemic shock. Spinal cord injuries are often experienced in the context of multitrauma, so circulatory and orthopaedic stabilisation is necessary before transport.

Diagnosis

In the emergency department, a full primary and secondary assessment should be undertaken, followed by a further, more comprehensive neurological assessment. Motor function is evaluated through muscle strength and rectal tone. Limb muscle strength is graded on a six-point scale, with a score of 0 the

Figure 11.14
Central cord syndrome

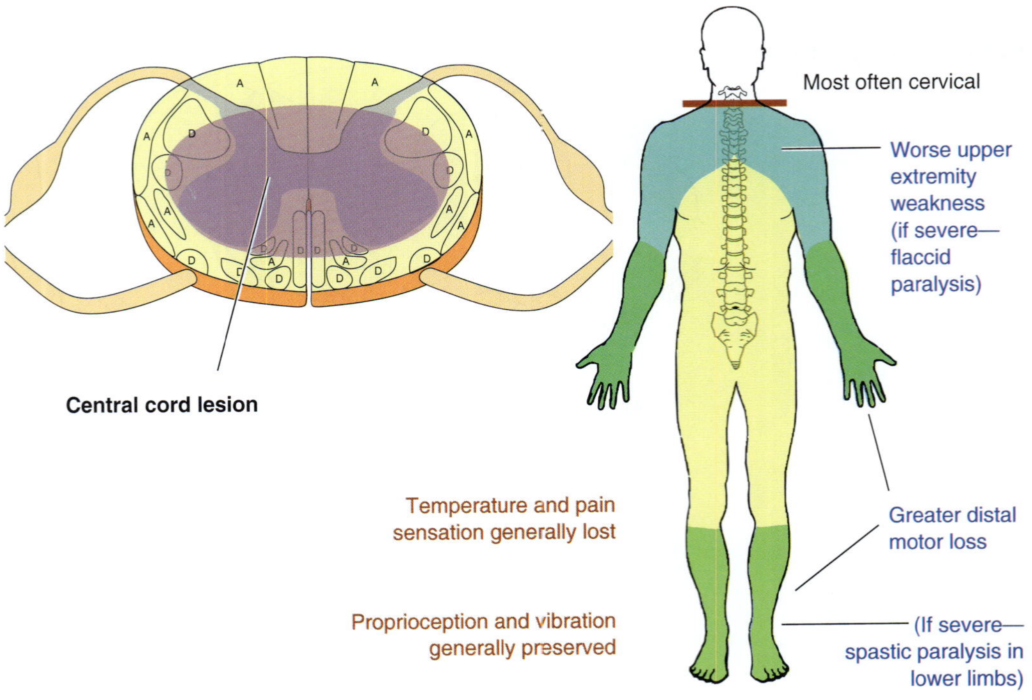

Figure 11.15

Brown-Séquard syndrome

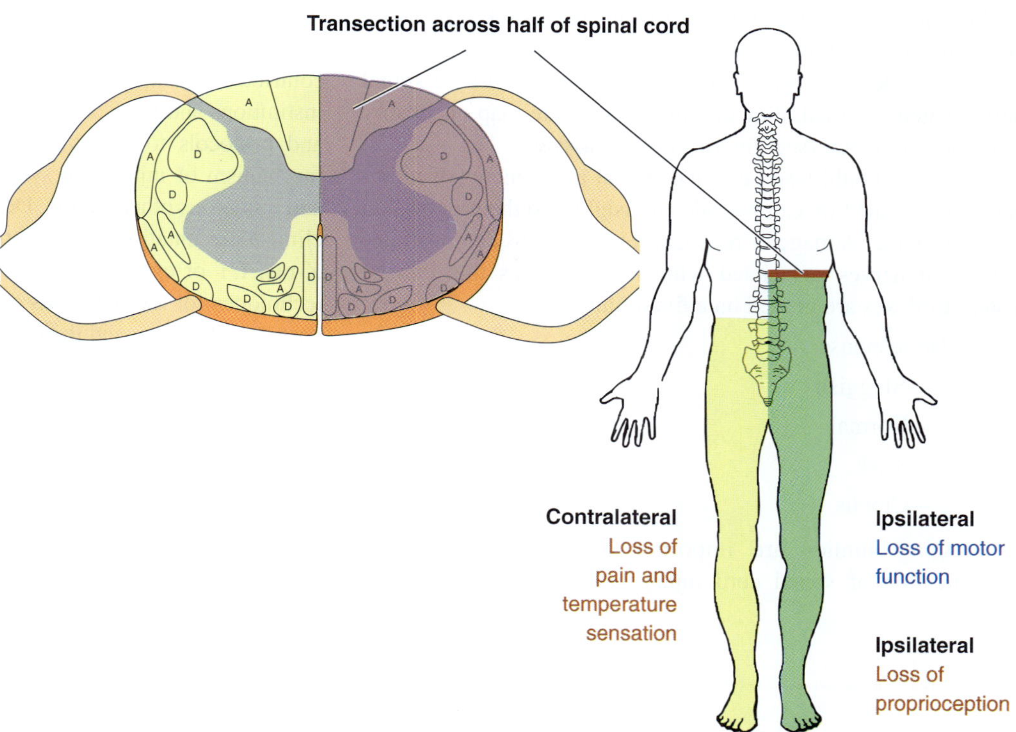

most severe loss and a score of 5 representing no loss of motor function:

0—Total paralysis, no movement

1—Slight contraction assessed visually or by palpation (but no movement)

2—Active movement (no movement against gravity)

3—Active movement (against gravity)

4—Active movement (against some resistance)

5—Active movement (against strong resistance)

Figure 11.16

Cauda equina syndrome

Source: © Sciencopia.

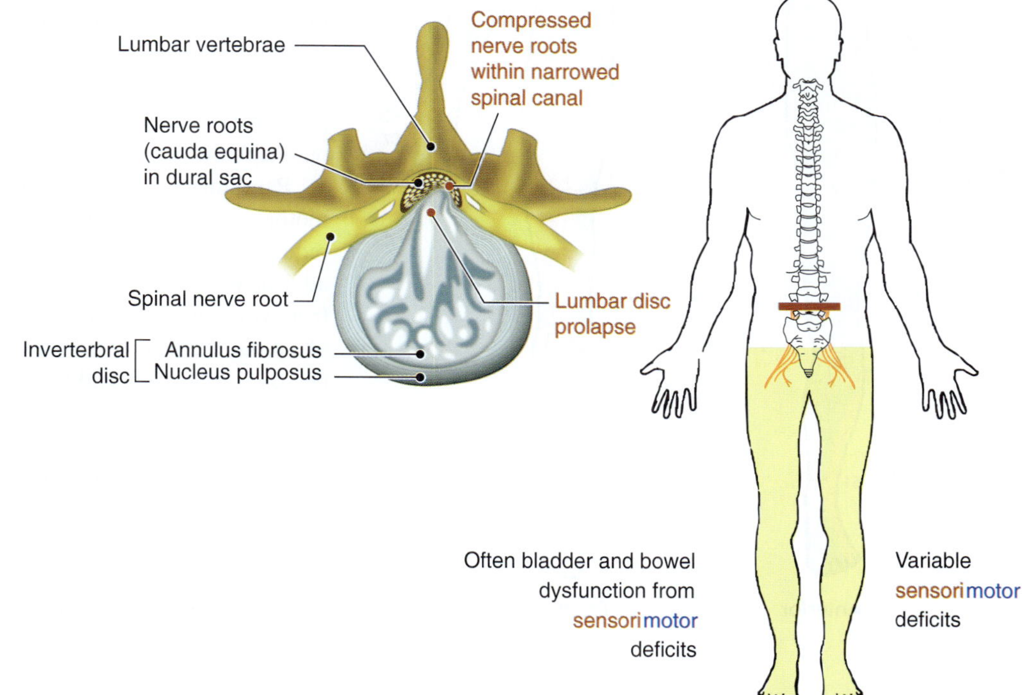

Sensory assessment should be evaluated using light touch and pin-prick responses over *dermatomes* on both sides of the bodies. Dermatomes are areas of skin supplied by a spinal nerve; when assessed, they provide an accurate map of sensory function and deficit (see Figure 11.17).

Reflexes should also be tested. Serial assessments of motor and sensory function can provide an insight into the progression of neurological damage or recovery. Figure 11.18 demonstrates the spinal nerves associated with some reflexes that can be tested. Reflexes are graded on a five-point system.

0—No response

1 + —Sluggish

2 + —Normal

3 + —Brisk

4 + —Clonus

Imaging studies are important in the diagnosis and quantification of spinal cord injury severity. There is debate regarding the best method of spinal cord assessment that is sufficiently capable of demonstrating injury but does not contribute to an unnecessary financial burden. Healthcare institutions and medical professionals have their own procedures and protocols to assess spinal cord injury, depending on the mechanism of injury, the symptomology of the affected person and numerous other factors. Depending on the circumstances and clinical presentation, investigations may include imaging such as X-ray, CT or even MRI. MRI is far superior to other imaging techniques for the diagnosis of spinal cord injury. However, the cost is prohibitive, and the use of the resource is unnecessary for a significant percentage of those who present following minor trauma.

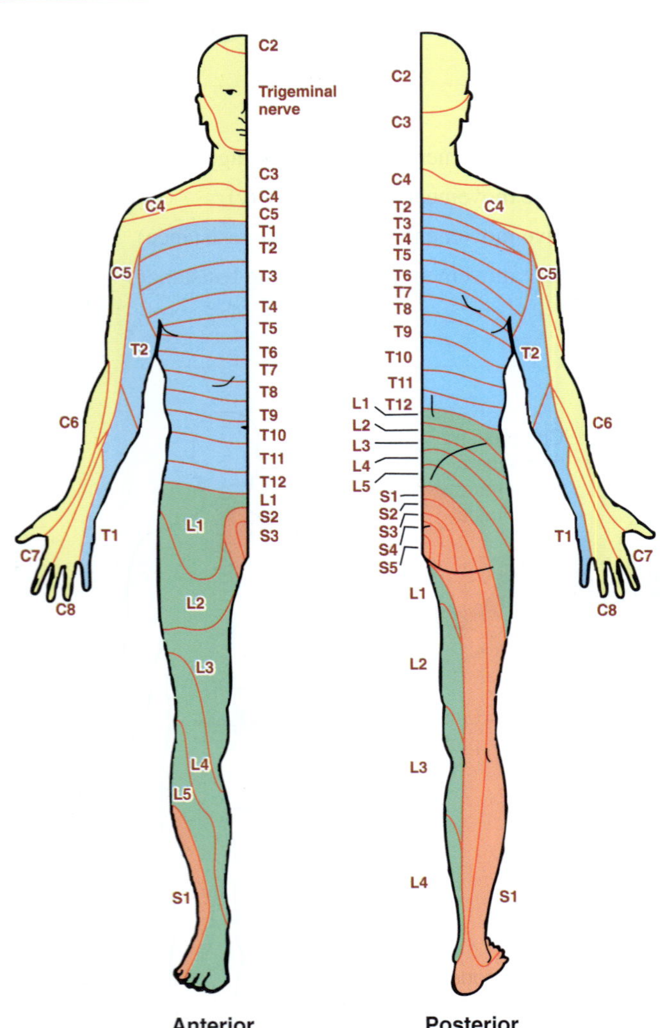

Figure 11.17
Dermatomes

Management

Management of airway, breathing and circulation is the priority in the treatment of spinal cord injuries. Injuries above C5 may require airway support, and mechanical ventilation will be required if hypoventilation or apnoea develops. Intubation is complicated by the necessity to maintain immobilisation in a neutral position, as well as when maxillofacial injuries have occurred as a result of the original trauma. Circulatory support may be necessary in the context of neurogenic shock resulting in hypotension and bradycardia, or from hypovolaemic shock because of significant blood loss from the trauma. Fluid resuscitation with colloid or crystalloid solutions, or blood, may be necessary to establish haemodynamic stability.

Following management of respiratory and cardiovascular issues, an orthosis or rigid collar can be applied to achieve immobilisation, or surgical reduction can provide stabilisation and alignment of vertebrae (see Figure 11.19).

The debate of whether to administer high-dose corticosteroids has been resolved. For many years, methylprednisolone was administered post-spinal-trauma in order to attenuate neuroinflammatory processes causing secondary damage, despite limited, quality evidence supporting the effects. However, more recently, literature reviews and further research have indicated that the risks associated with immunosuppression, metabolic, pulmonary, adrenal and haematological complications far outweigh the possible limited and unproven functional gains.

Pain management is essential, especially in those with motor deficits but intact sensation. Opioid analgesics may be required initially. The administration of an antiemetic agent is advisable to reduce the risk of airway compromise or aspiration from vomiting, especially in the context of the emetic properties of opioid therapy. A nasogastric tube should be inserted if the person is intubated, and it may also be needed in someone who is not intubated to ensure gastric decompression and to manage gastric stasis if it develops.

Other medications that may be required include an anticoagulant to reduce the risk of deep vein thrombosis, and antimicrobial agents to prevent infection if any open fractures or lacerations have occurred as a result of the initial injury.

A urinary catheter will probably be required to manage a neurogenic bladder, but it will also be beneficial to monitor accurate urine output and reduce the risk of movement that may have been necessary to assist with urinary elimination.

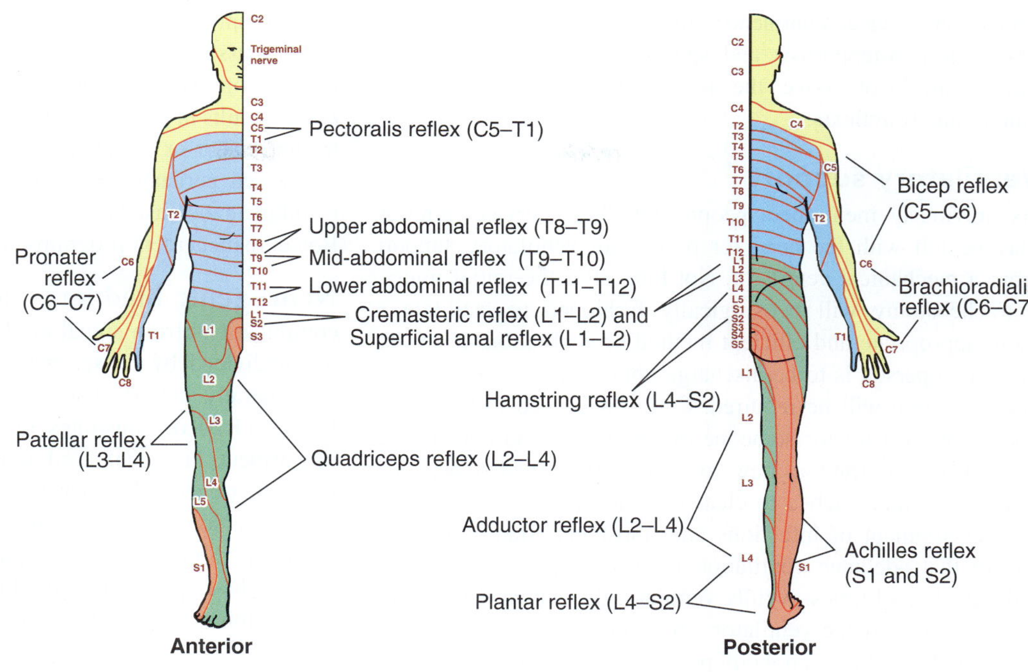

Figure 11.18

Spinal nerves and their associated reflexes

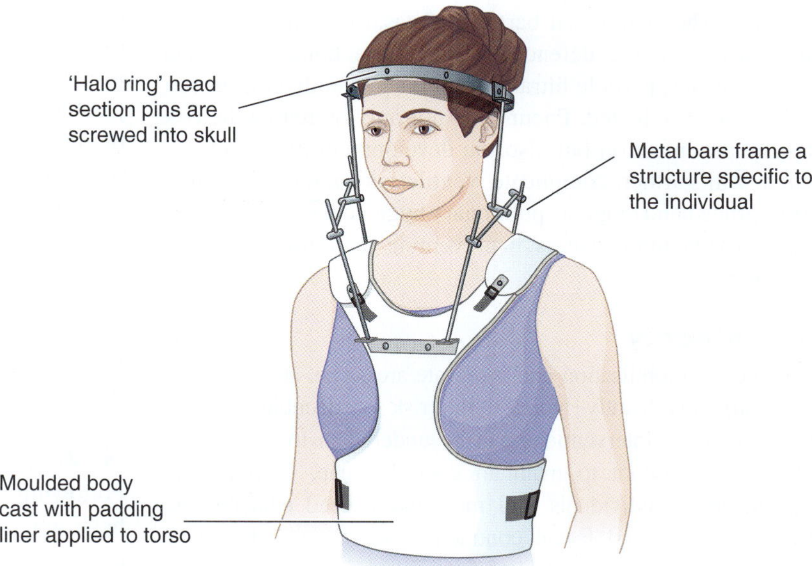

Figure 11.19

Halo-cervical orthosis

Used to stabilise injury yet permit the individual to mobilise or begin rehabilitation earlier, rather than being confined to bed. The halo can reduce the complications associated with total immobility.

Pressure area care is essential to reduce the risk of decubitus ulcers, which can form very rapidly during immobilisation. Removal of the transport backboard should be undertaken as soon as possible. Pressure-relieving equipment should be used, and care should be taken to protect skin integrity. This task becomes easier following spinal stabilisation.

Spinal cord injury may result in significant disability requiring months in hospital and even more time in rehabilitation. Psychological support is paramount to ensuring progress, and assistance from other people with spinal cord injuries may help the person embrace the potential of succeeding in life after a spinal cord injury.

COMPLICATIONS OF SPINAL CORD INJURY

LEARNING OBJECTIVE 8

Examine the common complications associated with spinal cord injury.

Even after the acute trauma has been managed and rehabilitation has begun, many issues may complicate the health of a person with a spinal cord injury. Examples include: the need for ventilatory support; the preservation of skin integrity; the management of urinary and faecal continence; the prevention of heterotopic ossification, osteoporosis and spasticity; and, for those with injuries at T6 or above, the assessment and management of autonomic dysreflexia.

Ventilatory support

As previously mentioned, people with high cervical injuries may be left with the need for permanent ventilatory support from a mechanical ventilator. Not long after the initial injury, a tracheostomy will be surgically fashioned to facilitate a more appropriate and efficient method of ventilation. If a fully ventilated person is to be discharged home, significant support and education will be required. Carers will need to be taught about how to care for someone on ventilation, how to reduce the risk of barotrauma, how to suction the affected person's oropharynx and trachea to clear secretions, how to assess for the development of infections and, most importantly, how to ensure that adequate ventilation is occurring for the apnoeic individual at all times. A fully ventilator-dependent person will die in minutes if the ventilator circuit disconnects or becomes obstructed and there is nobody present to correct the problem.

Ventilatory-associated pneumonia is a concern for those who are dependent on mechanical ventilation. Because of the need for artificial airway placement, respiratory defences are bypassed. The anatomical barriers of nasal hair and the nasal turbinates, reflexive defences such as the cough, gag and sneeze reflexes, particle filtration and the mucociliary transport system are all affected. Pneumonia not only increases the risk of systemic infection but also the development of atelectasis, which will further complicate ventilation and oxygenation. Appropriate hand hygiene, pulmonary hygiene and maintenance of adequate health will assist in preventing ventilator-associated pneumonia.

Skin integrity

Prolonged immobilisation and insensate areas (i.e. areas without sensation) significantly increase the risk of decubitus ulcers. However, many interventions can be undertaken to reduce this risk. It is important to maintain good hygiene, especially in perineal areas. Individuals will most likely need education to promote urinary and faecal continence. Techniques should be employed to reduce the risk of friction when positioning and turning. Pressure-relieving techniques and devices should be used to reduce the risk of prolonged immobilisation. It is important that surfaces and material in contact with insensate areas are flat and free from buttons, plastic or other material that may apply pressure and compromise skin integrity. Maintaining adequate nutrition is also imperative to promote skin integrity and wound healing.

Continence

People with spinal cord injury can develop neurogenic bowel and neurogenic bladder.

Neurogenic bowel One of the determining factors for bowel continence is whether the person develops a spastic (*reflexic*) or a flaccid (*areflexic*) bowel. A *spastic bowel* is when the gastrointestinal muscles still have tone, and the reflex to and from the spinal cord (beneath the level of injury) enables peristalsis and anal sphincter tone. This will occur in cervical or thoracic spine injuries. There may be no sensory perception of a faecal mass in the anus, but through bowel training and regular elimination patterns continence can be achieved. A *flaccid bowel* results in poor or no gastrointestinal muscle tone. Injuries to the lumbar or sacral spine will result in an areflexic bowel. Decreased peristalsis and decreased anal sphincter tone may result in an increased risk of constipation or faecal incontinence. Bowel management programs can assist to some degree.

Neurogenic bladder There are several types of bladder complications from spinal cord injury, and, although they can be subdivided by cause, spinal cord bladder impairment can be generally classified as *storage failure* or *voiding failure*. Figure 11.20 demonstrates the causes of urinary continence impairment in spinal cord injury. The management options for a neurogenic bladder include intermittent or indwelling catheterisation, reflex voiding and the use of α-adrenergic blockers. Some surgical options include urethral stents, transurethral sphincterotomy, bladder augmentation, electrical stimulation or urinary diversion.

Osteoporosis

Loss of bone density in someone with spinal cord injury occurs as a result of changes in bone metabolism due to immobilisation and decreased weight bearing. Although both osteoclast and osteoblast activity increase after spinal cord injury, osteoclast activity exceeds osteoblast activity. Chronic increases in the parathyroid hormone occur, and result in further demineralisation of non-weight-bearing bone. The risk of osteoporosis can be reduced within weeks of injury through the use of supported weight-bearing exercises, functional electrical stimulation, and the administration of bisphosphonate drugs. Newly injured individuals will benefit greatly from these prophylactic measures. However, it is not yet possible to improve bone density in demineralised bone associated with chronic osteoporosis from spinal cord injury, so the management of fractures will still be necessary. Osteoporosis is discussed in detail in the chapter 'Bone and joint disorders'.

Neurogenic heterotopic ossification

Following spinal cord injury, individuals may develop heterotopic ossification, which is the growth of bone in the connective tissue near a joint below the level of injury. Although heterotopic ossification can occur anywhere, common sites of heterotopic ossification include the flexor and adductor areas of the hip, the medial–collateral ligament in the knees, and sometimes in the shoulders and elbows. The mechanism is not well understood, but it is known that deposition of calcium phosphate occurs in affected muscle, which begins to ossify over time by replacement with hydroxyapatite crystals. Individuals with heterotopic ossification may present with peri-articular inflammation or a reduced range of motion. Severe cases may result in ankylosis of peripheral joints. Frequent and regular passive range-of-motion exercises are the best way to prevent heterotopic ossification. Treatment may consist of attempting to block ectopic bone deposition through the administration of bisphosphonates, which are known to play an important role in calcium–phosphate metabolism. Surgical resection of the ossification can result in significant complications, such as infection, excessive bleeding, potential postoperative

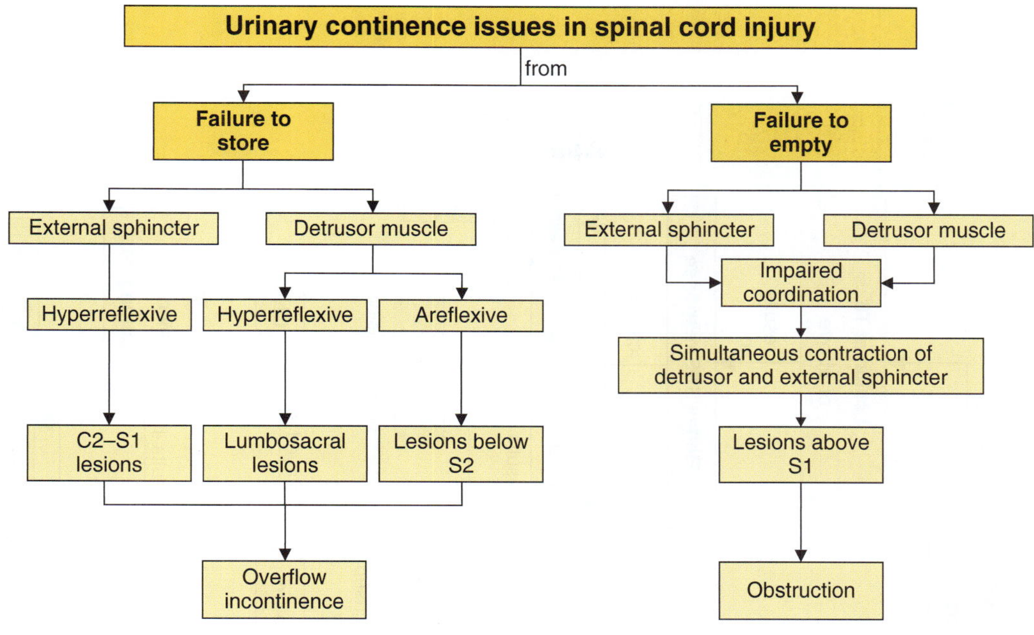

Figure 11.20
Causes of urinary continence issues in spinal cord injury

fracture of severely osteoporotic bone, and recurrence. Surgical resection may benefit individuals whose ossification interferes with positioning to reduce pressure area or muscle spasm.

Spasticity and muscle spasms

Muscle spasms below the level of spinal cord injury occur as a result of uninhibited spinal reflexes. Motor reflexes from noxious stimuli, such as stretching, pressure and inflammation, trigger a muscle contraction, which, in a person with an intact spine, would be blocked by a descending inhibited signal. In someone with spinal cord injury, structural damage to the cord prevents an inhibitory signal and a spasm occurs. There are some benefits of muscle spasm, so it is generally not treated unless it interferes with activities of daily living. Spasms can also, to a small extent, decrease disuse osteoporosis, because a limb in spasm applies some stress to the bone, which may retard osteoclast and stimulate osteoblast activity. In addition, the muscle contraction occurring in a spasm provides a small amount of work to the muscle groups involved, which may reduce the speed of disuse atrophy development.

The presence of spasm and spasticity in a person with insensate areas can signify a problem that needs to be found and rectified (e.g. infection or malpositioning).

Management options include the use of medications such as the muscle relaxant baclofen. Baclofen is a gamma-aminobutyric acid (GABA) derivative that acts on the presynaptic GABA receptors to inhibit excitatory neurotransmitters (glutamate and aspartic acid), reducing reflex activity. This drug can be administered systemically or via an intrathecal pump. Muscle relaxants such as benzodiazepines may also be used. Therapeutic botulinum toxin may be used to reduce tone and spasticity for three to four months. Severe spasticity may be managed by an aggressive surgical intervention called a radiofrequency rhizotomy, which destroys the nerve innervating the affected joints.

Autonomic dysreflexia

Autonomic dysreflexia is a medical emergency that can occur in individuals with a spinal cord injury at T6 or higher. An exaggerated and uninhibited autonomic nervous system response to a noxious stimulus beneath the spinal cord lesion results in a reflex sympathetic outflow, causing vasoconstriction. The profound vasoconstriction causes severe hypertension and results in a reflexive parasympathetic nervous system response causing bradycardia (see Figure 11.21).

Immediate identification of the noxious stimulus is imperative. The most common causes of autonomic dysreflexia include irritation or obstruction in the bladder or bowel, a pressure area or wound infection, or fracture beneath the spinal cord lesion. Once the cause has been identified, immediate interventions to rectify the problem should be undertaken. If the individual has a urinary catheter, it should be checked for kinks, obstructions or infections. The catheter may need to be flushed or replaced, and antimicrobial agents commenced. Faecal impaction can cause autonomic dysreflexia. The use of enemas or manual evacuation may be necessary to resolve the issue. Checking for creases, buttons or other materials that could cause pressure areas is important, and the assessment of skin integrity may reveal a pressure area. Repositioning and relief from the causative agent may begin to resolve the situation.

The most critical observation in autonomic dysreflexia is blood pressure. Profound hypertension may exceed a systolic volume of 250 mmHg and significantly increase the risk of haemorrhage from vessel failure in the brain, kidney or eyes, or may result in myocardial infarction or seizure. Antihypertensive drugs may be required immediately, especially if there is some difficulty in isolating the cause. Due to the life-threatening potential of autonomic dysreflexia, prevention is a priority. Bowel and bladder management programs, appropriate and frequent pressure area care, and hypervigilance for events or phenomena that may cause autonomic dysreflexia should be undertaken to ensure that it does not develop.

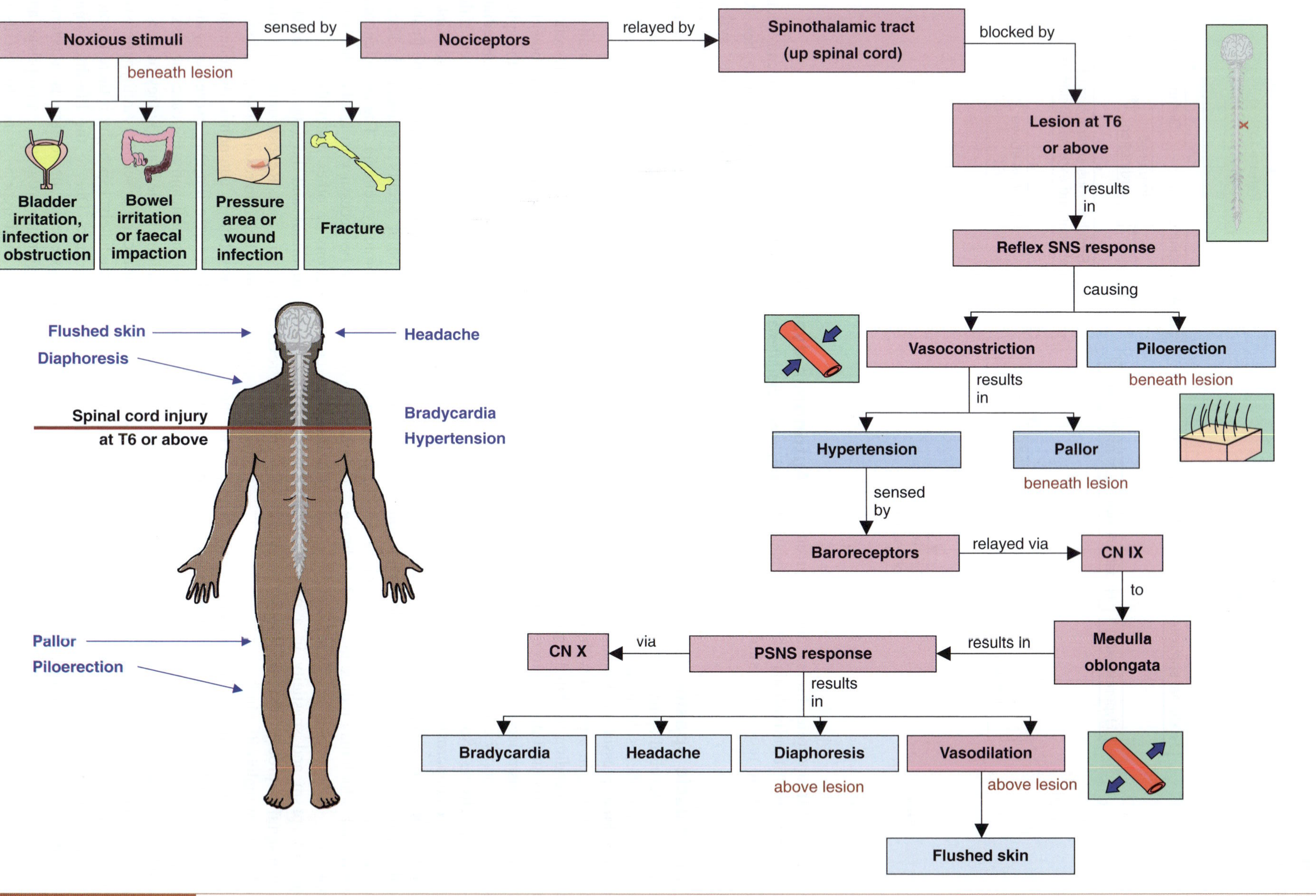

Figure 11.21

Autonomic dysreflexia

CN = cranial nerve; PSNS = parasympathetic nervous system; SNS = sympathetic nervous system.

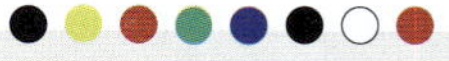

INDIGENOUS HEALTH FAST FACTS AND CULTURAL CONSIDERATIONS

FAST FACTS

- *Aboriginal and Torres Strait Islander women are 12 times more likely than non-Indigenous Australian women to experience a traumatic brain injury (TBI) from assault.*
- *Aboriginal and Torres Strait Islander men are between 25 and 44 times more likely than non-Indigenous Australian men (of the same age) to experience a TBI from assault.*
- *Aboriginal and Torres Strait Islander peoples are admitted with injuries to their head and neck 2.4 times more often than non-Indigenous Australians. Statistics on spinal cord injuries in Aboriginal and Torres Strait Islander peoples are difficult to locate; however, anecdotal evidence suggests that Indigenous Australians are over-represented in relation to admission for secondary complications.*
- *Māori males in the age groups between 0–4 and 15–34 years are significantly overrepresented in hospitalisations for TBI compared to their European New Zealander counterparts.*
- *Pacific Islands people are 1.4 times more likely than European New Zealanders to experience TBI.*
- *Māori are 1.5 times more likely than European New Zealanders to experience spinal cord injury.*
- *Pacific Islands people are 2.4 times more likely than European New Zealanders to experience spinal cord injury.*

CULTURAL CONSIDERATIONS

- *Apart from the mobility and access difficulties experienced by all individuals with brain or spinal injury, which are often exacerbated in rural and regional areas, Aboriginal and Torres Strait Islander peoples experience additional challenges.*
- *A particular difficulty exists in the cultural limitations of the psychometric tools used to assess intellectual function and behavioural changes following TBI. Many neuropsychological testing tools have significant limitations or are inappropriate in the assessment of Aboriginal and Torres Strait Islander peoples. The tests are often culturally deficient, undertaken in English, and rely on written responses and the need to answer many questions. Most psychometric instruments have not been validated for their use in Indigenous Australian populations. Healthcare professionals need to understand that in some cultures it is rude to ask numerous questions, maintain eye contact or even discuss some issues if the assessor is of a different gender. Reliance on unmodified tests that do not take into account a person's history, culture, language, customs or life experiences will result in inaccurate measurement. Choice of assessment tools such as the Kimberley Indigenous Cognitive Assessment (KICA-Cog), the Westmead Post Traumatic Amnesia Test, or Cogstate are likely to be the most appropriate.*

Sources: Data from Australian Institute of Health and Welfare (2022b); Bentley et al. (2022); Fitts et al. (2022); New Zealand Trauma Registry & National Trauma Network (2021); van den Heuvel et al. (2017).

CHILDREN AND ADOLESCENTS

- If a child develops a spinal cord injury before the adolescent growth spurt, they are most likely to develop scoliosis.
- Babies and young children have a large head-to-body ratio and relatively weak cervical musculature, which increases the risk of cervical spine injuries because of a higher fulcrum of motion. (A baby's head is approximately 25% of their body mass, whereas an adult's head is approximately 10% of their body mass.)
- Children under 8 years of age are most at risk of developing spinal cord injury without radiographic abnormality, because of immature bone and lax ligaments, which permit excessive compression or distraction of the spinal cord.

OLDER ADULTS

- Older adults over 65 years of age are at an increased risk of cervical spine injury from falls and osteoporotic changes contributing to spinal cord injury.
- Many spinal cord injuries in older adults result in central cord syndrome due to falls, resulting in neck hyperextension.

KEY CLINICAL ISSUES

- Airway management is imperative for someone with either traumatic brain injury or spinal cord injury. The mechanism causing the injury may also result in anatomical deformity, and airway obstruction or oxygenation and ventilation may be compromised because of a neurological cause.
- Airway management using airway devices and manual or mechanical ventilation may be necessary to support oxygenation and ventilation in a person with neurotrauma.
- When undertaking airway management in someone with trauma or an altered level of consciousness, always consider the probability of cervical spine damage.
- Cardiovascular instability is common in traumatic brain injury as a result of raised intracranial pressure. It is also common in spinal cord injury because of neurogenic shock or even hypovolaemic shock from the soft tissue or orthopaedic damage that caused the spinal trauma.
- Depending on the cause, fluid volume support, vasopressors or inotropes may be required to manage hypotension in individuals with neurotrauma. Hypotension will interfere with cerebral perfusion pressure, and can exacerbate the damage in traumatic brain injury and spinal cord injury.
- Profound hypertension may occur in the context of raised intracranial pressure or in spinal cord injury in the context of autonomic dysreflexia. β-Blockers or nitrates may be required to manage hypertension to prevent a cerebrovascular accident.
- The Glasgow coma scale is important in the initial and continuing assessment of a person who has experienced neurotrauma.
- Those with spinal cord injury may have a disparity in motor and sensory function. Never assume that paralysis means that they cannot feel the area involved. Both motor and sensory assessments are necessary to gauge the exact deficits occurring. Assessments should also be repeated as necessary to monitor clinical changes.
- Many complications associated with spinal cord injury are preventable. Maintenance of skin integrity is achieved with good pressure area care and hygiene; continence issues can be managed with bowel and bladder programs; and osteoporosis, spasticity and muscle spasm can be assisted with range-of-movement and weight-bearing exercises.
- Individuals and carers of people with spinal cord injury above T6 must be hypervigilant for the life-threatening development of autonomic dysreflexia. Severe headache, flushed skin and profound sweating above the lesion, coupled with pallor and piloerection below the injury, are classic signs. Assessment to determine the cause must be undertaken immediately.

CHAPTER REVIEW

- *Traumatic brain injury (TBI)* is caused by traumatic forces that are applied to the skull and brain. The mechanisms of injury include blunt and penetrating force trauma and acceleration–deceleration injuries.
- TBI results in an alteration in brain function evidenced by *cognitive dysfunction* and *alteration in conscious level*.
- The demographic trend for TBI demonstrates that males are more than twice as likely as females to suffer death and disability from TBI.
- Adults over 75 years of age have the highest rate of TBI-related hospitalisation and death.
- Falls, transportation (motor vehicle accidents) and assault are the primary precipitating factors in TBI death and disability.
- The *Glasgow coma scale* and *post-traumatic amnesia tools* are used to assess functionality and cognitive impairment.
- *Primary brain injury* occurs at the time of impact, whereas *secondary brain injury* occurs post-injury.
- *Cerebral blood flow (CBF)* relies on adequate *cerebral perfusion pressure (CPP)* and is closely autoregulated.
- *Autoregulation* of CBF occurs with a CPP of 50–150 mmHg. Outside this range, autoregulation is lost and CBF is dependent upon systemic blood pressure
- The *Monro–Kellie doctrine* provides the framework for understanding the mechanism involved in rising *intracranial pressure (ICP)*. Cerebral components include cerebral spinal fluid (CSF), blood and brain tissue. An increase in one component will elevate pressure and decrease the volume of the other components. Any space-occupying mass, such as a haematoma or oedema, has the potential to also increase ICP.
- Compliance of brain tissue is poor and, if compensatory reduction in volume does not occur, then ICP will rise, as pressure and volume are inversely related. Compression and displacement of cerebral contents can occur due to raised ICP.
- As ICP rises, autoregulation is lost and CBF is reduced. Ischaemia and infarction of cerebral tissue ensues.
- *Concussion* is a transient alteration in cerebral structure, and is thought to be due to disruption of the *reticular activating system (RAS)*.
- *Contusion* is bruising to brain tissue and can include *coup* and *contrecoup injuries*.
- *Brain haemorrhage* can include extradural, subdural, intracerebral and subarachnoid haemorrhage.
- *Diffuse axonal injury* is caused by significant blunt-force trauma, and results in the tearing of axonal fibres in the white matter and the brainstem.
- *Secondary brain injury* develops post-injury. Inflammation, elevated ICP, ischaemia and excitotoxicity are all mechanisms of injury.
- *Primary spinal cord injury* occurs directly to the tissue at the time of the initial injury and cannot be reversed.
- *Secondary spinal cord injury* occurs as a result of haemorrhage, oedema and ischaemia, and results in further destruction of neurons.
- *Spinal shock* is a transient loss of reflexive and autonomic function below the spinal cord lesion, and resolves in days to weeks.
- Spinal cord injuries can be classified in a number of different ways, including by *vertebral level, degree or mechanism*.
- *Complete spinal cord injuries* result in the total loss of all function beneath the lesion, and are less common than incomplete spinal cord injuries.
- Many common *incomplete spinal cord injuries* can be classed into spinal syndromes, such as anterior cord syndrome, central cord syndrome, Brown-Séquard syndrome and cauda equina syndrome.
- Spinal cord injuries can result in significant and various *complications*, such as the need for ventilatory assistance, breaks in skin integrity, issues with maintaining continence, the development of osteoporosis, neurogenic heterotopic ossification, muscle spasms and spasticity.
- *Autonomic dysreflexia* is a complex, life-threatening complication of spinal cord injury above the level of T6. It results in severe hypertension and bradycardia because of the failure of the autonomic nervous system control as a result of a spinal cord lesion.

REVIEW QUESTIONS

1. Compare and contrast the major characteristics of primary and secondary brain injury.
2. What are the mechanisms of injury that cause primary and secondary brain injury?
3. From an epidemiological perspective, who is most at risk of sustaining a TBI?
4. A man has fallen from a horse. His conscious level is reduced, and he withdraws, grunts and opens his eyes to pain. What is his Glasgow coma scale (GCS) score?
5. Differentiate between extradural and subdural haematomas. Why are older adults more at risk of suffering subdural haematomas?
6. Outline normal brain physiology, and utilise the terms CBF, CPP, MAP and ICP in your answer.
7. How does the Monro–Kellie doctrine help to explain the Cushing reflex?
8. Compare and contrast coup and contrecoup contusion injuries.
9. If a person has a blood pressure of 90/45 mmHg, what is their MAP? Is this sufficient to maintain CBF?
10. Jane is a 35-year-old woman who has been injured while playing hockey. The hockey ball has struck the right temporal region of her skull. She has had a period of brief unconsciousness and now is conscious. Her GCS score is 14 (E = 4, V = 4, M = 6), blood pressure (BP) is 140/90 mmHg, and heart rate (HR) is 110 beats per minute (bpm) (sinus tachycardia). She does not want an ambulance to attend or to go to hospital. She convinces her friends to take her home. What injuries could Jane have sustained, and what are the risks in non-assessment and treatment?
11. A short period of time has passed and Jane is now very unwell. She has a GCS score of 7 (E = 2, V = 2, M = 3), BP of 95/45 mmHg and HR of 160 bpm (sinus tachycardia). Explain how rising intracranial pressure reduces cerebral blood flow, and relate this to Jane's case.
12. With relation to spinal cord injury, define:
    a. spinal shock
    b. neurogenic shock
    c. transection
    d. compression injury
13. What is the difference between complete and incomplete spinal injuries?
14. What is the difference between all of the different types of spinal cord syndrome in incomplete spinal injury?
15. What complications can occur as a result of spinal cord injury? Explain the mechanism.
16. What are the signs and symptoms of autonomic dysreflexia? How should it be managed?

HEALTH PROFESSIONAL CONNECTIONS

Midwives Midwives must be able to identify neonatal spinal cord injury. Although rare, neonatal spinal cord injury can occur as a result of delivery, or it may occur in utero. Intrapartum manipulation, such as traction or rotation, increases the risk of spinal cord injury; however, spinal cord injury may also occur as a result of situations causing cord compression or ischaemia. In-utero malposition, vascular insults and prenatal ischaemia can result in cord injury. Post-delivery procedures, such as lumbar puncture, umbilical arterial cannulation and the placement of a central venous catheter, have also, on rare occasions, resulted in spinal cord injury. If assessment of a newborn indicates respiratory compromise and profound hypotonia, spinal cord injury should be considered.

Physiotherapists Physiotherapists provide critical support to individuals following traumatic brain injury or spinal cord injury. Significant rehabilitation programs must be designed to facilitate maximum function. Programs are generally several months in duration and focus on specific goals, depending on the predicted function. In caring for someone with spinal cord injury, there are two distinct phases in therapy plans. Initially, in the acute stages, management of respiratory function, positioning, stretching and range-of-movement exercises are a priority. Depending on the level of injury, a physiotherapist may assist individuals with breathing and coughing techniques, as well as with pulmonary hygiene, such as suctioning. Maintenance of joint range of movement with passive exercises for paralysed limbs and active exercises for non-paralysed limbs will also form an important component of the role of a physiotherapist in the acute stages of spinal injury. As the rehabilitation commences—a less acute phase—the focus is on increasing sitting endurance, strengthening active muscles groups and working towards achieving some degree of functional mobility, depending on the level of injury. Also, as physiotherapists spend so much time with individuals who have experienced spinal cord injury, it is imperative to understand the causes and management of autonomic dysreflexia.

Nutritionists/Dieticians Because individuals with spinal cord injury have a lower resting metabolic rate and often reduced activity levels, their energy requirements are lower than in active, able-bodied individuals. Obesity can become a problem and complicate physiotherapy, transfers and activities of daily living. Considerations of activity factor should be made in the estimation of caloric intake requirements. The activity factor may differ depending on the vertebral level of the lesion, because this can influence the activity level. Vertebral level will also influence gastric emptying and bowel motility. Important nutrition and dietary considerations for individuals with spinal cord injury must include bowel function. An increase in fibre and adequate hydration are necessary to reduce the risk of constipation. Excessive consumption of caffeine, fruit and spicy foods may result in diarrhoea. Cardiovascular disease is common in people with spinal cord injury, so common sense and healthy eating, avoiding foods high in fat, salt and sugar, will be beneficial. It is important to ensure adequate protein, vitamins and minerals to facilitate wound healing, especially in the context of pressure area sores. Avoidance of carbonated drinks and citrus juices can reduce the risk of urinary tract infection, as they can influence urinary pH to become too alkaline.

Occupational therapists Occupational therapists are responsible for maximising an individual's capacity to perform activities of daily living. A critical factor in understanding the potential function of an individual with spinal cord injury is to recognise the deficits caused by injuries at specific vertebral levels. It is also important to be cognisant of the remaining motor and sensory function following the trauma, as this will influence a person's capacity to perform certain tasks. Occupational therapists are also responsible for designing and often constructing splints to maintain optimal function. Organisation of adaptive equipment, such as devices to assist with mobility, eating, grooming or writing, will be necessary and dictated by the injured person's functional capacity.

CASE STUDY

Ms Tonya Walton was a passenger in a motor vehicle accident where the 25-year-old male driver died. She is 29 years of age (UR number 276984), and was brought in by the paramedics with a Glasgow coma scale (GCS) score recorded as $E = 2, V = 3, M = 6$. All of the occupants of the car tested positive for drugs and alcohol. Ms Walton was not wearing a seatbelt, and hit her forehead on the windscreen during the accident. Although she had no skull fracture, she developed a subdural haematoma and had a craniotomy five days ago. Apart from some minor skin abrasions, Ms Walton had no other injuries. Upon return to the ward after two days in intensive care, her GCS score was recorded as $E = 4, V = 4, M = 6$. She demonstrated moderate weakness in her right grip but equal strength in her legs.

At the start of this shift, her blood pressure was 140/100 mmHg, her pain was recorded as 2/10 (headache) and her GCS score was recorded as $E = 4, V = 5, M = 6$. Her other neurological assessments included slight weakness in her right hand and normal strength in both legs. Her pupils were equal and reacting to light. She had both direct and consensual reactions.

Her most recent observations (5 minutes ago) are as follows:

Temperature	Heart rate	Respiration rate	Blood pressure	SpO_2
36.5°C	84	18	175/115	98% (RA*)

*RA = room air.

Her pain is 7/10 (headache) and her GCS score is $E = 4, V = 4, M = 6$. Her other neurological assessments include moderate weakness in her right hand and normal strength in both legs. Her pupils are equal and reacting to light, but sluggish. This morning's pathology results are as follows.

HAEMATOLOGY

Patient location:	Ward 3	**UR:**	276984		
Consultant:	Smith	**NAME:**	Walton		
		Given name:	Tonya	**Sex:**	F
		DOB:	08/05/XX	**Age:**	29

Time collected	08:30
Date collected	XX/XX
Year	XXXX
Lab #	2345434

FULL BLOOD COUNT		UNITS	REFERENCE RANGE
Haemoglobin	132	g/L	115–160
White cell count	5.3	$\times 10^9$/L	4.0–11.0
Platelets	204	$\times 10^9$/L	140–400
Haematocrit	0.44		0.33–0.47
Red cell count	4.12	$\times 10^{12}$/L	3.80–5.20
Reticulocyte count	1.5	%	0.2–2.0%
MCV	89	fL	80–100
Neutrophils	3.12	$\times 10^9$/L	2.00–8.00
Lymphocytes	3.13	$\times 10^9$/L	1.00–4.00
Monocytes	0.28	$\times 10^9$/L	0.10–1.00
Eosinophils	0.29	$\times 10^9$/L	< 0.60
Basophils	0.08	$\times 10^9$/L	< 0.20
ESR	9	mm/h	< 12
COAGULATION PROFILE			
aPTT	32	secs	24–40
PT	15	secs	11–17

BIOCHEMISTRY

Patient location:	Ward 3	**UR:**	276984		
Consultant:	Smith	**NAME:**	Walton		
		Given name:	Tonya	**Sex:**	F
		DOB:	08/05/XX	**Age:**	29

Time collected	08:30
Date collected	XX/XX
Year	XXXX
Lab #	345655

ELECTROLYTES		UNITS	REFERENCE RANGE
Sodium	138	mmol/L	135–145
Potassium	4.4	mmol/L	3.5–5.2
Chloride	102	mmol/L	95–110
Bicarbonate	24	mmol/L	22–32
Glucose	5.8	mmol/L	3.0–7.7

CRITICAL THINKING

1. Considering Ms Walton's demographic information and the cause of her injury, how does this compare with the epidemiology of traumatic brain injury?
2. What was Miss Walton's initial GCS score? What type of traumatic brain injury does this signify? What is the significance of the initial GCS score in relation to potential neurological outcome?
3. Consider Ms Walton's most recent observations. What neurological changes has she experienced? Make a list of all of the significant observations.
4. What could be causing this change in neurological status? Observe the pathology results. Are these of any benefit in determining what might be occurring? (*Hint:* Is there any significance in observing the coagulation profile? Can it add any important information to the clinical picture?)
5. What interventions are required to assist Ms Walton immediately? What are the immediate dangers in relation to Ms Walton's change in neurological status? If her neurological status deteriorates further, what new dangers may present?
6. Review Ms Walton's most recent GCS score. What parameter suggests that assessment might be becoming complicated? (*Hint:* Think 'V'.) What other assessments can be used in evaluating a person's neurological status?

BIBLIOGRAPHY

Abrams, G.M. & Wakasa, M. (2020). Chronic complications of spinal cord injury and disease. *UpToDate*. https://www.uptodate.com/contents/chronic-complications-of-spinal-cord-injury-and-disease.

Ainsworth, C.R. & Brown, G.S. (2021). Head trauma. *Emedicine*. https://emedicine.medscape.com/article/433855-overview.

AlphaBeta Australia for SpinalCure Australia & Insurance and Care NSW (icare) (2020). *Spinal cord injury in Australia: the case for investing in new treatments*. https://www.spinalcure.org.au/wp-content/uploads/2020/12/SCI-in-Australia-SpinalCure-20201209-.pdf.

American Spinal Injury Association (2019). *International Standards for Neurological Classification of Spinal Cord Injury (ISNCSCI)* (rev.). Atlanta, GA: American Spinal Injury Association.

Australian Institute of Health and Welfare (AIHW) (2019). *The health of Australia's prisoners, 2018*. Cat. No. PHE 246. Canberra: AIHW. https://www.aihw.gov.au/getmedia/2e92f007-453d-48a1-9c6b-4c9531cf0371/aihw-phe-246.pdf.aspx?inline=true.

Australian Institute of Health and Welfare (AIHW) (2022a). *Australia's health, 2022*. Australia's Health series No. 18. Canberra: AIHW. https://www.aihw.gov.au/reports-data/australias-health.

Australian Institute of Health and Welfare (AIHW) (2022b). Tier 1—Health status and outcomes. 1.03 Injury and poisoning. *Aboriginal and Torres Strait Islander Health Performance Framework*. Canberra: AIHW. https://www.indigenoushpf.gov.au/measures/1-03-injury-poisoning.

Babl, F.E., Tavender, E., Dalziel, S., on behalf of the Guideline Working Group for the Paediatric Research in Emergency Departments International Collaborative (PREDICT) (2021). *Australian and New Zealand Guideline for Mild to Moderate Head injuries in Children—Full Guideline.* Melbourne, VIC: PREDICT. file:///C:/Users/User/Downloads/PREDICT-Head-Injury-Guideline-_Full-guideline-V1-29.1.21-.pdf.

Bauldoff, G., Gubrud-Howe, P.M., Carno, M.-A., Levett-Jones, T., Hales, M., Berry, K., ... Stanley, D. (2020). *LeMone and Burke's medical–surgical nursing: critical thinking for person-centred care* (4th [Australian] edn). Sydney: Pearson Australia.

Bentley, M., Singhal, P., Christey, G. & Amey, J. (2022). Characteristics of patients hospitalised with traumatic brain injuries. *New Zealand Medical Journal* 135(1550):111–20. https://journal.nzma.org.nz/journal-articles/characteristics-of-patients-hospitalised-with-traumatic-brain-injuries-open-access.

Bernard, F. (2023). Neurotrauma and intracranial pressure management. *Critical Care Clinics* 39(1):103–21. https://doi.org/10.1016/j.ccc.2022.08.002.

Bersten, A. & Handy, J.M. (2018). *Oh's intensive care manual* (8th edn). Edinburgh: Elsevier.

Best, O. & Fredericks, B. (2021). *Yatdjuligin: Aboriginal and Torres Strait Islander nursing and midwifery care* (3rd edn). Port Melbourne, VIC: Cambridge University Press.

Bullen, J., Hill-Wall, T., Thomas, E., Norman, R. & Cowen, G. (2022). Concussion in Aboriginal and Torres Strait Islander peoples: what is the true epidemiology? *Medical Journal of Australia* 216(6):271–72. https://doi.org/10.5694/mja2.51457.

Bullock, S. & Manias, E. (2022). *Fundamentals of pharmacology* (9th edn). Sydney: Pearson Australia.

Chin, L.S., Mesfin, F.B. & Dawodu, S.T. (2018). Spinal cord injuries. *Emedicine*. https://emedicine.medscape.com/article/793582-overview.

Christensen, B. (2019). ASIA Impairment Scale. *Emedicine*. https://emedicine.medscape.com/article/2172437-overview.

Curtis, K., Gabbe, B., Shaban, R.Z., Nahidi, S., Pollard, C., Vallmuur, K., ... Christey, G. (2020). Priorities for trauma quality improvement and registry use in Australia and New Zealand. *Injury* 51(1):84–90. https://doi.org/10.1016/j.injury.2019.09.033.

Dawodu, S.T. (2021). Traumatic brain injury (TBI): definition, epidemiology, pathophysiology. *Emedicine.* https://emedicine.medscape.com/article/326510-overview.

Fitts, M.S., Cullen, J., Kingston, G., Wills, E. & Soldatic, K. (2022). 'I don't think it's on anyone's radar': the workforce and system barriers to healthcare for Indigenous women following a traumatic brain injury acquired through violence in remote Australia. *International Journal of Environmental Research and Public Health* 19(22):14744. https://doi.org/10.3390/ijerph192214744.

Gilmore, N., Katz, D.I. & Kiran, S. (2021). Acquired brain injury in adults: a review of pathophysiology, recovery, and rehabilitation. *Perspectives of the ASHA Special Interest Groups* 6(4):714–27. https://doi.org/10.1044/2021_PERSP-21-00013.

Goldman, L., Siddiqui, E.M., Khan, A., Jahan, S., Rehman, M.U., ... Vaibhav, K. (2022). Understanding acquired brain injury: a review. *Biomedicines* 10(9):2167.https://doi.org/10.3390/biomedicines10092167.

Gupta, G. & Roychowdhury, S. (2018). Intracranial pressure monitoring. *Emedicine*. https://emedicine.medscape.com/article/1829950-overview.

Lin, C.-L., Dumont, A.S., Zhang, J.H., Zuccarello, M. & Chen, C.-H. (2017). Improving and predicting outcomes of traumatic brain injury: neuroplasticity, imaging modalities, and perspective therapy. *Neural Plasticity* 2017:4752546. https://doi.org/10.1155/2017/4752546.

Maas, A.I.R., Menon, D.K., Manley, G.T., Abrams, M., Åkerlund, C., Andelic, N., ... Zemek, R. for the InTBIR Participants and Investigators (2022). Traumatic brain injury: progress and challenges in prevention, clinical care, and research. *Lancet Neurology* 21(11):1004–60. https://doi.org/10.1016/S1474-4422 (22)00309-X.

Marieb, E.N. & Hoehn, K. (2019). *Human anatomy and physiology* (10th edn). San Francisco, CA: Pearson Benjamin Cummings.

National Academies of Sciences, Engineering, and Medicine (2022). *Traumatic brain injury: a roadmap for accelerating progress.* Washington, DC: The National Academies Press. https://doi.org/10.17226/25394.

New Zealand Spinal Cord Injury Registry (2022). *New Zealand Spinal Cord Injury Registry annual summary report 2021.* https://spinalsupport.nz/2022/11/21/nzcir-annual-report-2021/.

New Zealand Trauma Registry & National Trauma Network (2021). *Annual report 2020/21.* https://www.majortrauma.nz/assets/Publication-Resources/Annual-reports/National-Trauma-Network-Annual-report-2020-2021.pdf.

Pangillinan, P.H., Kelly, B.M. & Hornyak, J.E. (2022). Classification and complications of traumatic brain injury. *Emedicine.* https://emedicine.medscape.com/article/326643-overview.

Quatman-Yates, C.C., Hunter-Giordano, A., Shimamura, K.K., Landel, R., Alsalaheen, B.A., Hanke, T. A., ... Silverberg, N. (2020). Physical therapy evaluation and treatment after concussion/mild traumatic brain injury. *Journal of Orthopaedic and Sports Physical Therapy* 50(4):CPG1–CPG73. https://doi.org/10.2519/jospt.2020.0301.

Ropper, A.E. & Ropper, A.H. (2017). Acute spinal cord compression. *New England Journal of Medicine* 376(14):1358–69. https://doi.org/10.1056/NEJMra1516539.

Rupp, R., Biering-Sørensen, F., Burns, S.P., Graves, D.E., Guest, J., Jones, L., ... Kirshblum, S. (2021). International Standards for Neurological Classification of Spinal Cord Injury. *Topics in Spinal Cord Injury Rehabilitation* 27(2):1–22. https://doi.org/10.46292/sci2702-1.

Sandean, D. (2020). Management of acute spinal cord injury: a summary of the evidence pertaining to the acute management, operative and non-operative management. *World Journal of Orthopedics* 11(12):573–83. https://doi.org/10.5312/wjo.v11.i12.573.

Soufineyestani, M., Dowling, D. & Khan, A. (2020). Electroencephalography (EEG) technology applications and available devices. *Applied Sciences* 10(21):7453.https://doi.org/10.3390/app10217453.

SpinalCure Australia (SCA) (2020). *SCI facts.* Woolloomooloo, NSW: SCA. https://www.spinalcure.org.au.

van den Heuvel, M., Jansz, L., Xiong, X. & Singhal, B. (2017). People with spinal cord injury in New Zealand. *American Journal of Physical Medicine and Rehabilitation* 96(2 Suppl 1):S96–S98. https://pubmed.ncbi.nlm.nih.gov/28059890/.

Weber, C., Andreassen, J.S., Isles, S., Thorsen, K., McBride, P., Søreide, K. & Civil, I. (2022). Incidence, mechanisms of injury and mortality of severe traumatic brain injury: an observational population-based cohort study from New Zealand and Norway. *World Journal of Surgery* 46(12):2850–57. https://doi.org/10.1007/s00268-022-06721-8.

Weiss, D. (2021). Osteoporosis and spinal cord injury. *Emedicine.* https://emedicine.medscape.com/article/322204-overview.

Seizures and epilepsy

12

LEARNING OBJECTIVES

After completing this chapter, you should be able to:

1 Differentiate between a seizure and epilepsy.

2 Outline the characteristics of an epileptic focus.

3 Describe the electrical changes that contribute to a neuron's hyperexcitable state.

4 Define the terms 'focal onset' and 'generalised onset' as they are used in the ILAE classification of seizure types.

5 Discuss the challenges associated with a diagnosis of temporal lobe epilepsy.

6 Explore the characteristics, dangers and management of status epilepticus.

WHAT YOU SHOULD KNOW BEFORE YOU START THIS CHAPTER

Can you identify the major parts of the brain and their functions?

Can you describe the process of neurotransmission?

Can you describe the mechanisms involved in maintaining the resting membrane potential?

Can you outline the process of generating a neuronal action potential?

KEY TERMS

Absence seizure
Aura
Electroencephalography (EEG)
Epilepsy
Epileptic focus
Epileptogenic
Focal cortical dysplasia
Focal seizure
Generalised seizure
Malformations of cortical development
Myoclonic seizure
Periventricular heterotopia
Polymicrogyria
Post-ictal period
Seizure
Status epilepticus
Temporal lobe epilepsy
Tonic–clonic seizure

Introduction

Epilepsy is a common nervous system disorder that still carries a stigma in some cultures, even though individuals with epilepsy have been revered in other cultures. In ancient Egypt, a person with epilepsy was considered to be in verbal contact with the gods, and the hieroglyph denoting epilepsy is the same one meaning 'fortunate person'.

The hallmark of epilepsy is the inappropriate, episodic, spontaneous electrical activity of a cluster of cells within the cortex, called the **epileptic focus**. The physical manifestations of an epileptic seizure will depend entirely on the location of the cells that constitute the focus and the networks that they activate. Foci located in the motor cortex or connected to it will manifest as muscle movement, such as the convulsing which most people associate with an epileptic seizure. However, those located in the prefrontal or temporal cortices will manifest as behavioural changes that might involve personality changes, hallucinations, paranoia or violence. For this reason, some forms of epilepsy will be missed, as the physical symptoms will either be too subtle to make an impact (e.g. a twitching thumb) or be misinterpreted/misdiagnosed as another condition, such as an anxiety condition or schizophrenia.

Although research has identified the underlying reason for a small number of epilepsy causes, the overwhelming majority have no identifiable cause and are therefore considered idiopathic. If the epileptic focus is identifiable it may sometimes be surgically removed, often leaving the person epilepsy-free, but the excised tissue appears to be perfectly normal on examination in the laboratory.

Seizures

LEARNING OBJECTIVE 1

Differentiate between a seizure and epilepsy.

A **seizure** is defined as *an episode of inappropriate electrical discharge resulting in disordered brain activity*. A surprising number of factors can trigger a one-off seizure, including bacterial or viral infections, alcohol, caffeine, a blow to the head, prescription (and illicit) drugs, fever, electrolyte disturbances and certain diseases. Most commonly, once the trigger has been removed the seizures stop. Ten per cent of Australians will have a seizure in their life, but only 3–3.5% will be diagnosed with epilepsy. It is important to recognise that one seizure does not constitute epilepsy.

By contrast, **epilepsy** is a condition in which there are *repetitive but largely unpredictable episodes of seizure activity*. This activity may be preceded by an **aura**—a set of symptoms such as a taste, smell, visual disturbance or sound, or a combination of these, which gives the affected person a warning that the seizure is about to commence, and in the case of more severe seizures allows them to prepare. Interestingly, some people have epilepsy that comprises only the aura portion of the activity, and therefore auras are generally considered to be a separate seizure. Having said that, there is some debate on this issue, since most migraine sufferers have an aura that is as consistent and has the same type of symptoms as those experienced by those with epilepsy, but they do not appear to be having seizures.

LEARNING OBJECTIVE 2

Outline the characteristics of an epileptic focus.

A majority of those with epilepsy, although certainly not all, have an identifiable *epileptic focus*. This focus constitutes a group of cells located somewhere in the cortex that are responsible for the seizure activity, and, by their nature, are hyperexcitable. In individuals with severe conditions in which their seizures occur multiple times in an hour and severely disrupt their lives, the ability to locate this epileptic focus may qualify them for the surgical removal of the offending cells. However, not all of those with epilepsy have a definable focus, seriously hampering efforts to surgically intervene when their condition becomes severe or life-threatening.

AETIOLOGY AND PATHOPHYSIOLOGY

LEARNING OBJECTIVE 3

Describe the electrical changes that contribute to a neuron's hyperexcitable state.

The cells of the epileptic focus have certain characteristics that mark them as different from their neighbours and contribute to their *hyperexcitability*. First, the membrane potential of such cells is less negative than normal cells, which means that the cells' membrane potential is closer to threshold, and therefore *more easily activated by incidental electrical signals*. An excellent example of this is that many of those with epilepsy will experience a seizure if exposed to strobe lights. In fact, a strobe light is often used to help diagnose epilepsy. A type of reflex seizure known as *photosensitive epilepsy*, can be elicited by television or video games, especially in the deep red band wavelength (680–700 nm) at a rate of approximately 15–25 flashes per second. In 1997, 67 people in Japan were taken to hospital with seizure activity from viewing a Pokemon cartoon episode. Approximately 10% of people with seizure disorders are thought to experience seizures induced by photic stimulation.

A second feature of the cells of the epileptic focus is that they are *very sensitive to small changes in local ion availability*. Once the initial action potential is triggered, the cells of the epileptic focus demonstrate a third characteristic; namely, they experience a *repetitive signalling that most closely resembles re-entry*, a mechanism by which the majority of tachycardias occur (see the chapter 'Dysrthymias'). Interestingly, ion channel mutations have been identified as being responsible for a small proportion of both tachycardias and epilepsies, and often the same or similar ion channels. As a final characteristic, after the seizure is finished the cells of the epileptic focus are now further from threshold and much less sensitive to ion levels. This **post-ictal** (post-seizure) period may last from minutes to hours.

Some types of epilepsy are due to structural changes within the brain that may or may not resolve as the child matures. Of these, a small subset has been identified and constitutes the types most likely to be intractable to medication (can't be completely controlled by drugs). Improvements in medical imaging have allowed surgeons to precisely locate the source of the altered cells and remove them. This subset of epilepsies is grouped as **malformations of cortical development (MCD)**. Of these, three have been fairly well studied: focal cortical dysplasia, periventricular heterotopia and polymicrogyria.

Focal cortical dysplasia involves pockets of neuronal cells that are either malformed or in the wrong position. Remember that in the formation of the brain, fledgling neurons must migrate to the appropriate position and finish their differentiation before sending out their axons to make the appropriate connection. Therefore, if these neurons fail to finish differentiating, their characteristics will be wrong for their location (i.e. they might express the wrong receptors or ion channels), or they might not migrate to the correct location, and therefore they are not the right type of cell for their location.

Periventricular heterotopia broken down as: *peri* = 'near' or 'around', *ventricular* = 'ventricles of the brain', *hetero* = 'different', *topia* = 'place'. In other words, these are clusters of cells that are found around the ventricles of the brain, which is the wrong place for them because they failed to migrate from this location during development. Because of this, these cells are inappropriately sensitive to the local environment. The cells of theses nodules are often spontaneously active (**epileptogenic**), not unlike the cells of the sinoatrial node in the heart.

Polymicrogyria is another potentially problematic word that is easily broken down: *poly* = 'many', *micro* = 'small', *gyria* = 'the hills' of the folds of the surface of the cortex. In this condition, the cortical surface has an excess number of tiny invaginations. The outermost cortical layer fuses to give an inappropriately smooth brain surface in that region, with the multitude of tiny gyri immediately under the surface. Although the exact mechanism by which polymicrogyria contributes to epilepsy is unknown, the cells of that region appear to be destabilised and interact inappropriately with the surrounding cortical cells. Interestingly, surgical resection of the region that encompasses the polymicrogyria rarely resolves the epilepsy, which implies a critical role for the surrounding apparently normal tissue. Further complicating matters, not all of those with identified polymicrogyria have epilepsy.

In addition to physical anomalies of brain formation, a number of *gene mutations* have been associated with epilepsy. Despite the rather surprising number of genes found, however, this still represents only a tiny proportion of the total number of cases of epilepsy. The list of the genes is often quite logical in retrospect, including faults in the ion channels that control cell excitability (e.g. Na^+, K^+, Ca^{2+}), receptors that regulate brain excitability (e.g. gamma-aminobutyric acid [GABA], glutamate), enzymes that control neuronal function (e.g. glutamic acid decarboxylase, which is responsible for GABA synthesis, and protein L-isoaspartate-(D-aspartate)-O-methyltransferase, a protein repair enzyme), a number of proteins involved in neurotransmitter release (e.g. synapsin 1 and 2) and other proteins associated with normal brain function (e.g. amyloid precursor protein, brain-derived neurotrophic factor and Huntington's amino-terminal polyglutamine sequence), as well as more generic cell proteins (e.g. the transcription factor c-Fos and the cytokine interleukin-6).

In 1881, Sir William Gowers observed that 'seizures beget seizures', by which he meant that a person who has one untreated epileptic seizure becomes more likely to have a subsequent seizure, and that the subsequent seizure is more likely to be worse than the previous one. Evidence from animal studies has shown that the inhibitory neurons in the hippocampus that use GABA as a neurotransmitter (referred to as *GABAergic neurons*) are more sensitive to seizure-mediated cell death, whereas the excitatory neurons that use glutamate (*glutamatergic neurons*) are somewhat resistant to destruction. Death of the GABAergic neurons causes the glutamatergic neurons to invade the space left empty due to the loss of these GABAergic neurons. Note that these are not new glutamatergic neurons, but rather extensions of existing neurons. The loss of GABAergic neurons and the outgrowth of the glutamatergic neurons then tips the regulatory balance in the region, making the cells not only more excitable but less controlled, because the primary role of the GABAergic neurons is to inhibit excitability. Further, some of the extensions from the glutamatergic neurons were found to synapse back onto themselves, creating a form of self-perpetuating loop that enhances the excitability of this region. How this correlates to the human brain remains to be seen.

Unfortunately, given the dearth of knowledge about epilepsy, the only risk factors that are relevant are those associated with individual seizures and acquired epilepsy. Head injury is a primary risk factor, and the at-risk population is young men between 18 and 34 years of age, as they are the ones most likely to engage in activities that are commonly associated with head trauma. Fevers in very young children can cause individual seizures, and damage secondary to these seizures can leave the child with an ongoing epilepsy, although while the risk of a single seizure is high, the risk of epilepsy is low. Alcohol abuse, excess caffeine consumption and prescription drug use and abuse are all risk factors for seizures, but do not appear to be linked to epilepsy.

EPIDEMIOLOGY

It is estimated that 50 million people worldwide have epilepsy, with approximately 80% of them living in low- and middle-income countries. The World Health Organization has identified epilepsy as the most common serious brain disorder worldwide, and estimates that up to 70% of people could live seizure-free if they were given the opportunity to be properly diagnosed and appropriately medically managed. In Australia, approximately 0.6% of people have been diagnosed with epilepsy, with an even distribution of prevalence between males and females; although, males are more likely to die as a result of epilepsy than females. Fortunately, in the past 20 to 30 years, there has been a steady decline of epilepsy-related deaths in Australia.

Aboriginal and Torres Strait Islander peoples are almost twice as likely to have epilepsy than non-Indigenous Australians, and three times more likely to be hospitalised. New Zealand reports incidence as approximately half of Australian epilepsy rates; and Māori and Pacific Islands children are less likely to experience epilepsy than European New Zealanders.

Epilepsy is second only to stroke as the most common serious neurological disorder, although this incidence is considered to be an underestimate, as some people with epilepsy either are not diagnosed or are misdiagnosed. Further, in some cultures there is a resistance to treatment based on cultural perceptions about the condition.

Generally, the condition manifests before the individual is 20 years of age, and is most frequently diagnosed in the first year of life. Epilepsy can be an acquired condition, such as after a head injury or viral infection, but is more commonly idiopathic. To date, at least 40 seizure types have been identified, with approximately one-third demonstrated to be associated with an underlying genetic predisposition. Genes have been identified for more than 35 inherited epilepsies, but this represents only a very tiny fraction ($< 0.1\%$) of all epilepsies.

CLINICAL MANIFESTATIONS

LEARNING OBJECTIVE 4

Define the terms 'focal onset' and 'generalised onset' as they are used in the ILAE classification of seizure types.

Clinical manifestations vary depending on the type of seizure. Familiarity with seizure classifications will assist in understanding symptomology.

As several classification systems are used to diagnose and describe epilepsy, confusion surrounding the identification and

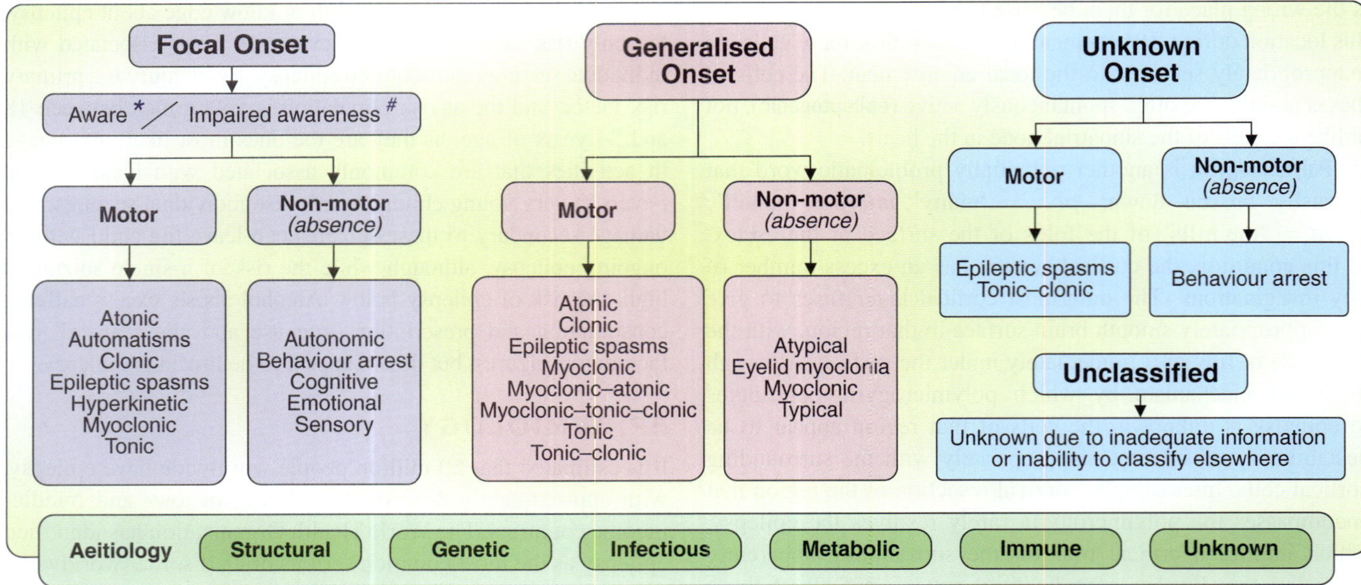

Figure 12.1

2017 International League Against Epilepsy (ILAE) Operational Seizure Classification

* = 'focal aware' previously known as 'simple partial'; # = 'focal impaired' previously known as 'complex partial'.

Sources: Data from and based on Fisher et al. (2017); Scheffer et al. (2017).

management of the condition is not unexpected. However, in April 2017 the International League Against Epilepsy (ILAE) published a new classification system that attempts to be more inclusive and better organise seizure activity into easily definable categories. The new system considers three parameters: *onset, motor activity* and *awareness*. Figure 12.1 describes the 2017 *ILAE system of classifying seizures*.

There is a significant amount of specialised terminology involved in describing seizure activity. Table 12.1 defines some important taxonomy surrounding epilepsy and seizures.

Electroencephalography (EEG) is one of the most beneficial diagnostic tests for epilepsy during a seizure. The different types of brain wave activity that can be detected by EEG are outlined in Clinical Box 12.1.

Table 12.1 Important epilepsy-associated terminology

Terminology	Description
Absence seizure	Short, loss of awareness and cessation of all activity, commonly assumes a blank stare commonly lasting < 10 seconds. May involve ocular manifestations, including eyelid flutter or eye-roll.
Atonic seizure	Sudden, brief loss of muscle tone of head, trunk or limbs.
Atypical absence seizure	Similar to absence seizures, but may be able to respond a little.
Automatisms	Purposeless, repetitive movements associated with impaired awareness.
Autonomic manifestations	SNS or PSNS activity caused by activation of the ANS may be cardiovascular, respiratory, GIT, urinary, cutaneous, pupillary or genital/sexual manifestations.
Behaviour arrest	Cessation of talking and/or moving, displaying a blank stare.
Clonic seizure	Rapid paroxysms of limb muscles resulting in stiffening and relaxing, causing jerking movements. May be associated with altered awareness.
Cognitive manifestations	Confusion, difficulty talking or understanding, and/or slowed thinking.
Emotional manifestations	Sensation of fear, dread, anxiety or pleasure associated with seizure activity.
Epileptic spasms	Bilateral or unilateral flexion, extension or mixed flexion–extension of the proximal and truncal muscles lasting approximately 1–2 seconds, which often occur on waking.
Eyelid myoclonia	Involuntary eye closure lasting < 6 seconds, may be associated with absences.
Febrile seizure	A convulsion in children < 6 years old occurring with a temperature > 38°C.

Table 12.1 Important epilepsy-associated terminology (*continued*)

Terminology	Description
Hyperkinetic seizure	Irregular, sequential, ballistic movements in the axial or proximal limb muscles, which may recur repeatedly after a few second intervals. Often occurring during sleep.
Myoclonic seizure	Brief shock-like jerks of one or many muscle groups often lasting < 2 seconds; rarely associated with altered awareness.
Myoclonic–tonic–clonic seizure	Begins with myoclonic jerks (rapid, brief shock-like jerks) followed by tonic–clonic activity of increased tone and sustained, rhythmic jerking of muscles, especially in the limbs, lasting seconds to minutes.
Sensory manifestations	Sensations of heat, cold, pain, tingling, numbness, movement or agnosia (inability to recognise objects, people, sounds, shapes or smells).
SUDEP	Acronym for *S*udden *U*nexplained *D*eath in *E*pilepsy.
Tonic seizure	Results in the stiffening of the major muscle groups (symmetric or asymmetric), often lasting < 20 seconds, and may be associated with slight altered awareness.
Tonic–clonic seizure	First, results in the tonic phase with the stiffening of muscles, loss of awareness and sometimes a groan-like vocalisation, as the contracted diaphragm forces air through vocal cords, followed by the clonic phase, where rapid paroxysms of the limb muscles result in stiffening and relaxing, causing jerking movements.

ANS = autonomic nervous system; GIT = gastrointestinal tract; PSNS = parasympathetic nervous system; SNS = sympathetic nervous system.

CLINICAL BOX 12.1

Electroencephalography

Electroencephalography (EEG) is used to quantify the electrical changes that occur within the brain. In this procedure, electrodes are attached to various areas of a person's head (see Figure 12.2). Different types of brain activity can be organised into four common waves. *Alpha waves* are characterised by activity that has approximately 8–13 cycles per second and may have an amplitude of 20–200 μV (see Figure 12.3A). This wave is generally associated with an adult in a state of relaxation who is mentally alert; alpha waves become higher in amplitude when the person's eyes are closed. *Beta waves* are characterised by activity that has approximately 14–35 cycles per second and an amplitude of 5–10 μV (see Figure 12.3B). This wave is generally associated with rapid eye movement (REM) sleep; however, paradoxically, it is also associated with mental alertness. *Theta waves* are characterised by activity that has approximately 4–7 cycles per second and an amplitude of 10–100 μV (see Figure 12.3C). This wave occurs more commonly in children, but can also be found in drowsy adults. *Delta waves* are characterised by activity that has approximately 1–4 cycles per second and an amplitude of 20–200 μV (see Figure 12.3D). This wave is common in someone who is asleep (including as a result of an anaesthetic agent). If this wave is present when a person is awake, it can indicate brain damage.

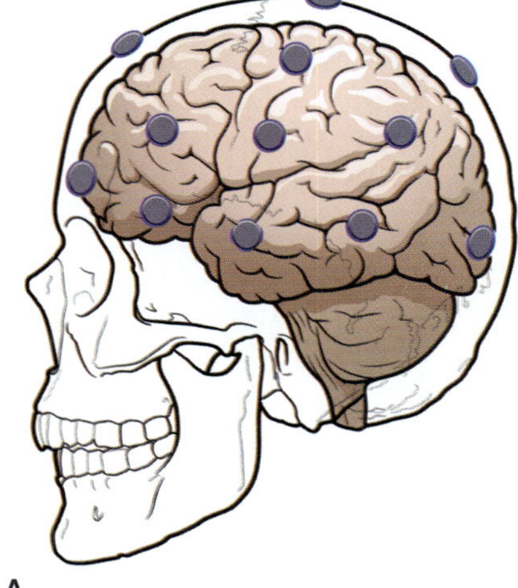

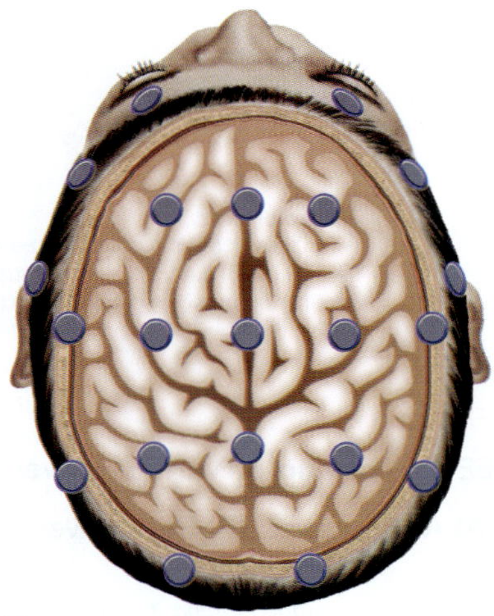

Figure 12.2

Placement of EEG electrodes on the head

(A) Schematic placement of EEG electrodes (lateral view).
(B) Schematic placement of EEG electrodes (top view).

Sources: (A) Adapted from Bill Fehr/Shutterstock; (B) Sciencopia; (C) & (D) Photographs courtesy of E. Hales.

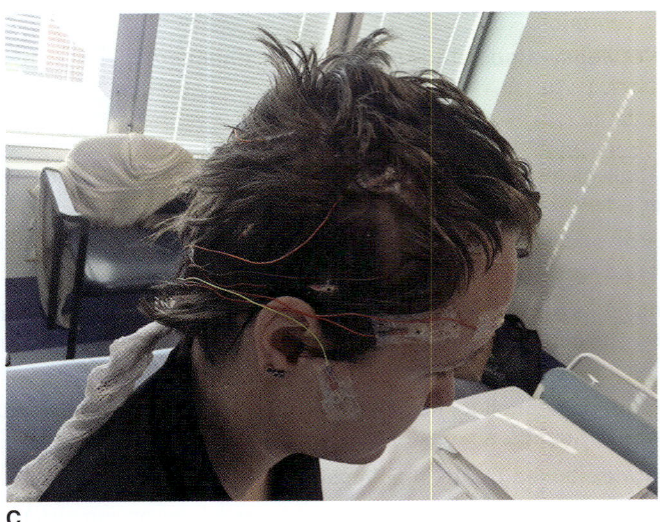
C

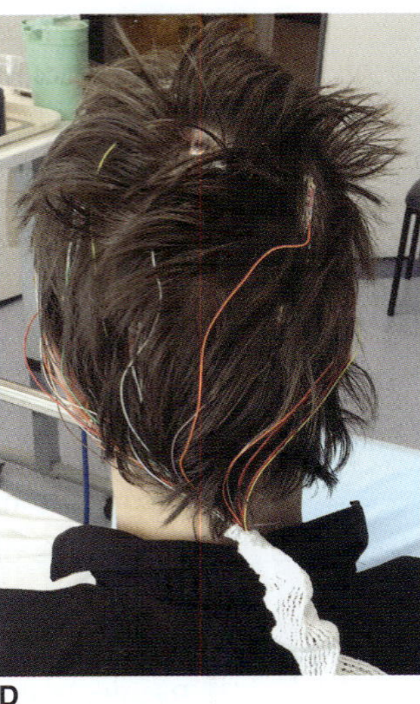
D

Figure 12.2

Placement of EEG electrodes on the head (continued)

(C) Person undergoing a continuous EEG (lateral view).
(D) Posterior view showing how electrode wires are contained and secured. This investigation may continue for as long as 1–2 weeks, with continuous monitoring.
EEG = electroencephalography.

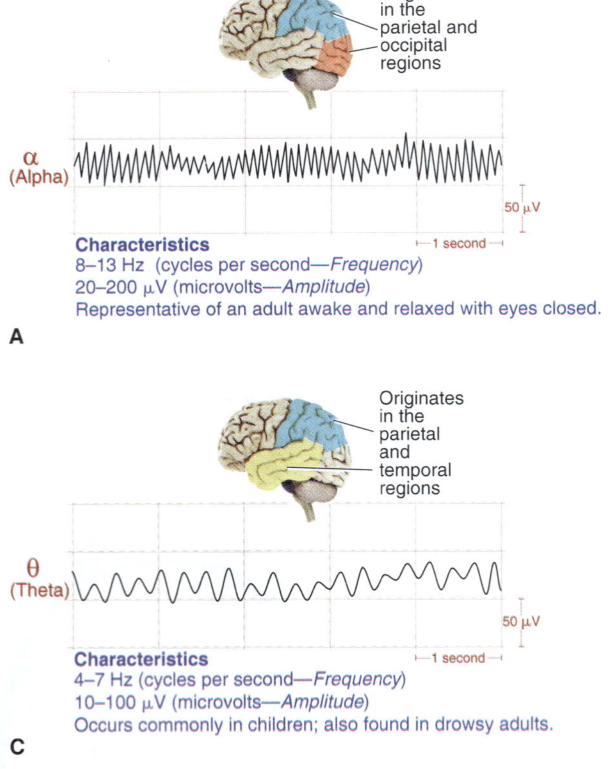

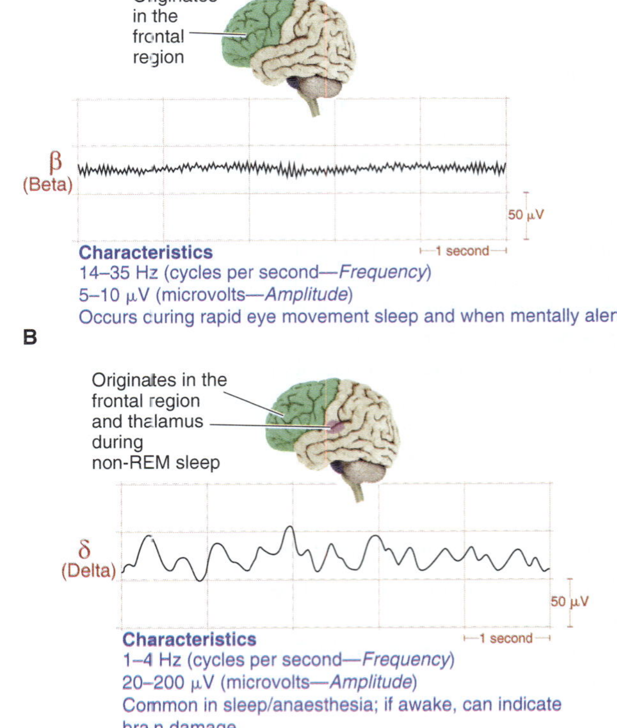

Figure 12.3

EEG recording of various waves

(A) Alpha waves. (B) Beta waves. (C) Theta waves. (D) Delta waves.

Source: Brain image Dorling Kindersley/Getty Images.

A **focal seizure** is one in which the electrical activity stays localised to a specific area (see Figure 12.4). By contrast, a **generalised seizure** shows activity throughout the forebrain, and may spread within a single hemisphere or may encompass both hemispheres. If it is a *focal aware* seizure, then consciousness is maintained, whereas a *focal impaired* seizure results in either altered consciousness or altered cognitive ability. Awareness is the key which differentiates between the two types of focal seizures. In a focal aware seizure the person remains conscious, but the other manifestations of the event are defined by the location of the focus, and may include such things as muscle 'tics' or small muscle movements that last for 20–60 seconds. By contrast, a focal impaired awareness seizure may include purposeless movements, such as hand wringing, a pill-rolling motion, hand flapping or face washing, and during which time the person is either unconscious or unaware of their actions. These movements may last for 30 seconds to 2 minutes.

Other terms are often used in this classification system, such as **myoclonic seizures**. This form of epilepsy involves brief but marked muscle contractions that might involve a specific muscle group or an entire limb. **Tonic–clonic seizures**, formerly known as *grand mal seizures* ('big bad' or 'big sick'), involve several phases: a tonic phase during which there is marked tension within the muscles of the body, a clonic phase marked by rhythmic convulsing of the muscles, and then a post-ictal coma (see Figure 12.5). Individuals with tonic–clonic type seizures are almost always unconscious or semi-conscious, but occasionally they may be awake and alert but unable to control the seizure. Incontinence is common in this type of seizure.

Absence seizures are a form of generalised seizure in which the person loses awareness of their surroundings and seems to freeze or stare off into space. Some people will experience small behaviours, such as lip-smacking or eye-rolling, but generally there is no other activity. The person has no sense of the loss of time, and in fact will usually rejoin a sentence exactly where they left off. The change in electrical activity in the brain resembles an electrical storm or a wave of static that consumes the brain; this is propagated throughout the brain with the cooperation of the thalamus (see Figure 12.6). These seizures usually last less than 30 seconds, but some people can have dozens of these seizures every hour. For the most part, absence seizures are the ones previously called *petit mal seizures*, but some allied health professionals use the phrase 'petit mal' to refer to any seizure that is not a tonic–clonic (grand mal) seizure.

LEARNING OBJECTIVE 5

Discuss the challenges associated with a diagnosis of temporal lobe epilepsy.

The final group of seizures that we will consider are the temporal lobe epilepsies; these are fraught with controversy as they are behavioural seizures. Some people manifest with automaticity, in which they continue with whatever they were doing when the seizure occurred but do so without any conscious awareness.

Figure 12.4

EEG recording of a focal seizure

In this example, only three EEG electrodes are placed on each side of the skull—at the frontal (first two traces), temporal (middle two traces) and occipital (last two traces) lobes—and electrical activity in the brain is recorded. The constant activity in the occipital lobes reflects the fact that the individual is lying on a bed with their eyes scanning the room. The trace shows seizure activity in the left frontal and temporal lobes.

Source: Based on Beniczky & Schomer (2020). Brain image Dorling Kindersley/Getty Images.

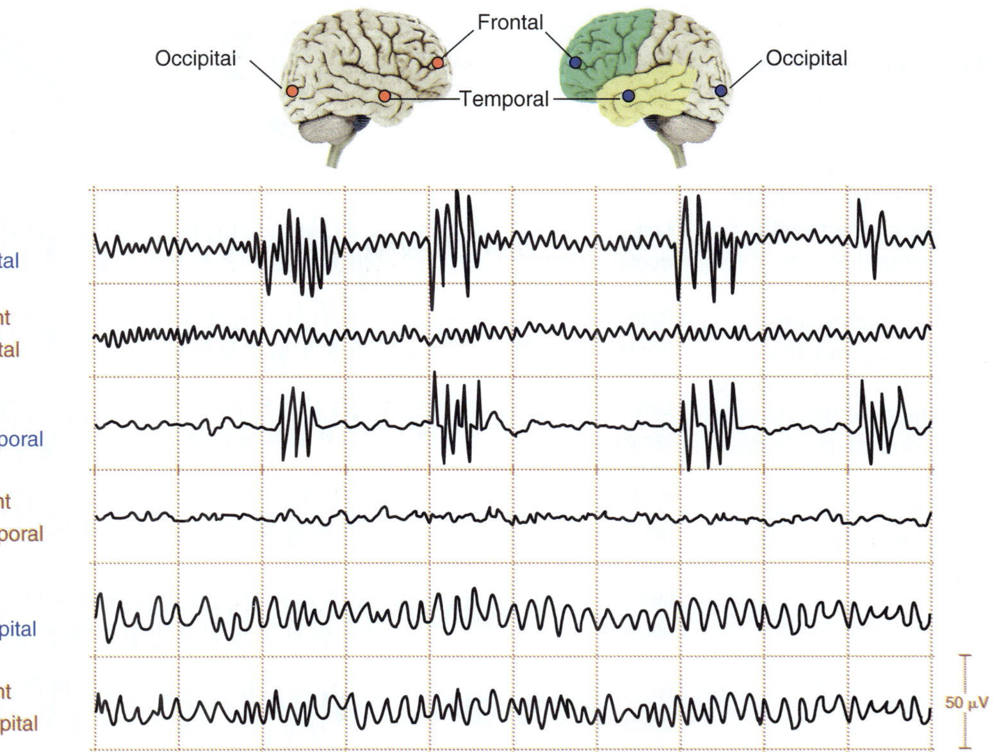

Figure 12.5

EEG recording of a tonic–clonic seizure

In phase 1 of a tonic–clonic seizure, the person is at rest; it is during this phase that they would experience an aura if they have one. The tonic phase (phase 2) is marked by tension and rigidity in the muscles of the body. This is followed by the rhythmic convulsing of the muscles, which is the hallmark of the clonic phase (phase 3). The individual then goes into a post-ictal coma (phase 4). Note that all of the electrodes show the same activity.

Source: Based on Beniczky & Schomer (2020). Brain image Dorling Kindersley/Getty Images.

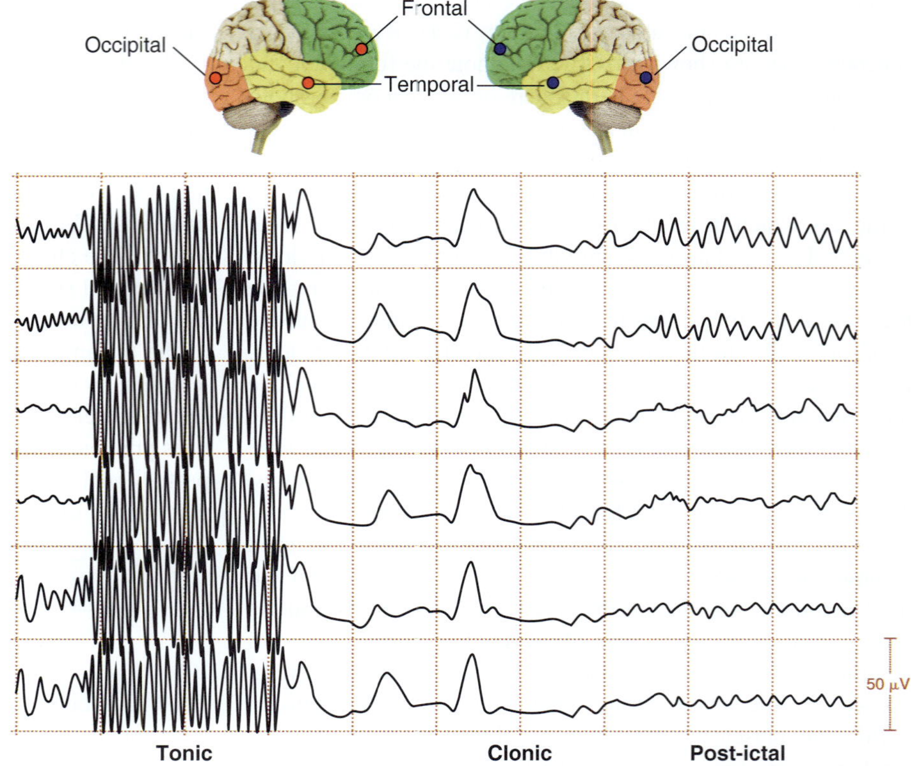

Figure 12.6

EEG recording of an absence seizure

The absence seizure, previously known as a 'petit mal seizure'. Note how the characteristic waveforms that are the hallmark of an absence seizure are seen throughout the brain. During this seizure the individual has no knowledge of the loss of time, and after the seizure may pick up exactly where they left off.

Source: Based on Beniczky & Schomer (2020). Brain image Dorling Kindersley/ Getty Images.

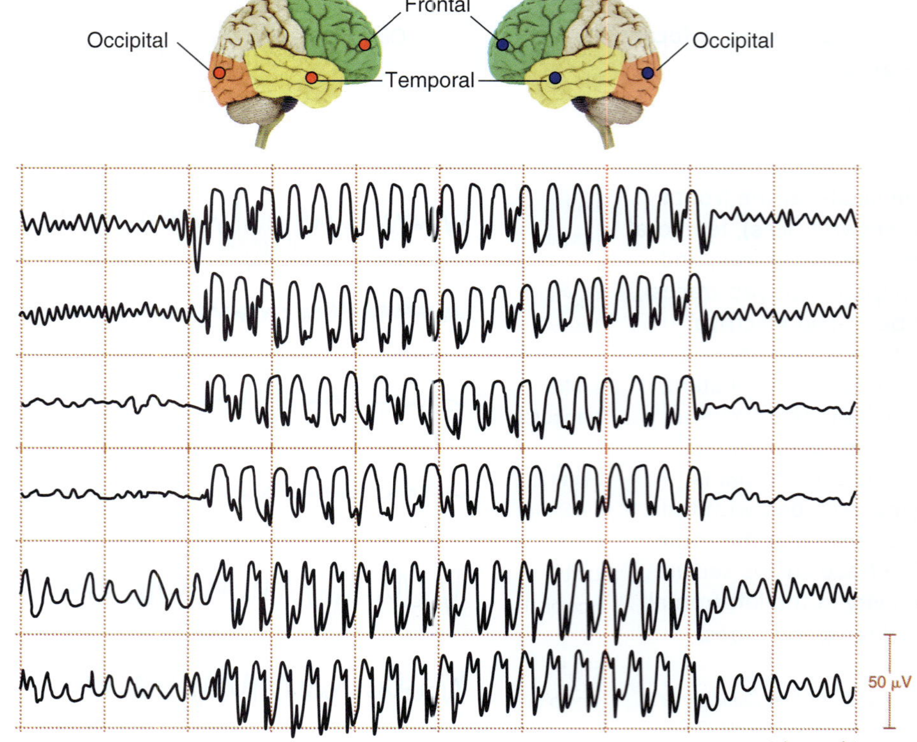

For example, if they are driving a car when their seizure occurs, they will continue to drive the car but will do so on autopilot. Other people experience violent or aggressive behaviour, sexually inappropriate behaviour or religiosity. Still others will relive (not remember) a memory, which will consume their awareness. Not all of those with **temporal lobe epilepsy** experience altered consciousness. Some people will experience hallucinations (which may be visual, olfactory, gustatory or a combination), alterations to their perception or changes to their personality. This family of epilepsies are often misdiagnosed or missed entirely, as most people do not associate changes in behaviour with epilepsy. The well-known author Karen Armstrong, who writes about comparative religions, was in her 30s before she learnt that she had been experiencing temporal lobe seizures for most of her life. She had just assumed that everyone found themselves in strange places without knowing how they got there.

LEARNING OBJECTIVE 6

Explore the characteristics, dangers and management of status epilepticus.

The primary complication of epilepsy is **status epilepticus**, a condition in which either the epileptic seizure does not stop spontaneously, or subsequent seizures follow so closely on from the first seizure as to leave virtually no recovery time. Usually, for most types of epilepsy other than temporal lobe epilepsy, the person is defined as being in status epilepticus if the seizure activity has lasted for more than five minutes. Given the unusual nature of temporal lobe epilepsy and the fact that a standard seizure might last significantly longer than five minutes, the definition of status epilepticus will vary from individual to individual. Every type of epilepsy has a form of status epilepticus associated with it. Status epilepticus constitutes a medical emergency due to the risk of brain damage and even death. Children and the elderly are the most susceptible to status epilepticus, with the elderly more likely to die as the consequence of this unrestrained electrical activity.

Figure 12.7 explores the common clinical manifestations and management of epilepsy.

Sudden unexpected death in epilepsy (SUDEP) may occur, yet at post-mortem a cause cannot be determined (exclusive of status epilepticus). Some risk factors include early-onset and poorly controlled epilepsy. Other risks include the presence of tonic–clonic seizures and an increased number of seizures.

CLINICAL DIAGNOSIS AND MANAGEMENT

Diagnosis

It is critical to eliminate all other causes of seizure before the diagnosis of epilepsy is confirmed. Laboratory tests for drug toxicity, metabolic disorders, trauma or other seizure-causing triggers should be eliminated first. One of the most beneficial diagnostic tests for epilepsy during a seizure is an EEG. Attempts to induce a seizure through sleep deprivation or photostimulation are sometimes used in someone with epilepsy, as a neurological investigation will generally be normal when they are seizure-free. If a seizure event can be recorded, the location and the type of epilepsy can be determined. An EEG can be combined with video monitoring to enable the observation and interpretation of seizure behaviours.

Several neuroimaging studies may be undertaken. Either computer tomography (CT) or magnetic resonance imaging (MRI) should be used to eliminate other causes of seizure, including trauma or space-occupying lesions.

Management

Once a diagnosis of epilepsy has been confirmed (generally after more than one seizure), anticonvulsant (antiseizure) medication may be commenced. A wide range of antiseizure medications, each with different mechanisms of action, are now available on the market (see Figure 12.8).

Appropriate care of a person experiencing a generalised seizure is critical to ensure their safety. Follow the basic principles of first aid—*DRABC*:

- ***D***anger: The immediate area should be cleared of anything that may cause the person injury. Try to cushion their head. Do not hold them down or try to put anything in their mouth.
- ***R***esponse: Stay with them until they recover.
- ***A***irway and ***B***reathing: Once their seizure has stopped, they should be placed in the recovery position until they become conscious. During this post-ictal time, they may rouse but still be confused. They may also vomit, so basic airway management procedures apply.
- ***C***irculation: Control any bleeding that has occurred as a result of the seizure. Document a description of the seizure, including length and characteristics, such as what body parts were moving, how they were moving, the presence of cyanosis, incontinence or any injury sustained. Support and reorientate them following the event.

Care of someone experiencing a focal seizure involves the same principles of basic first aid. However, depending on the type of seizure, the person may remain conscious. Common sense should prevail, as it is not possible to identify all of the variations of behaviour that may occur. Ensure the environment is safe, observe and document the characteristics, and support and reorientate the person after the episode.

Seizures may occur in infants and young children as a result of fever. A febrile seizure most commonly occurs in infants 8–20 months of age. Prevention of fever can be achieved with the use of an antipyretic agent such as paracetamol.

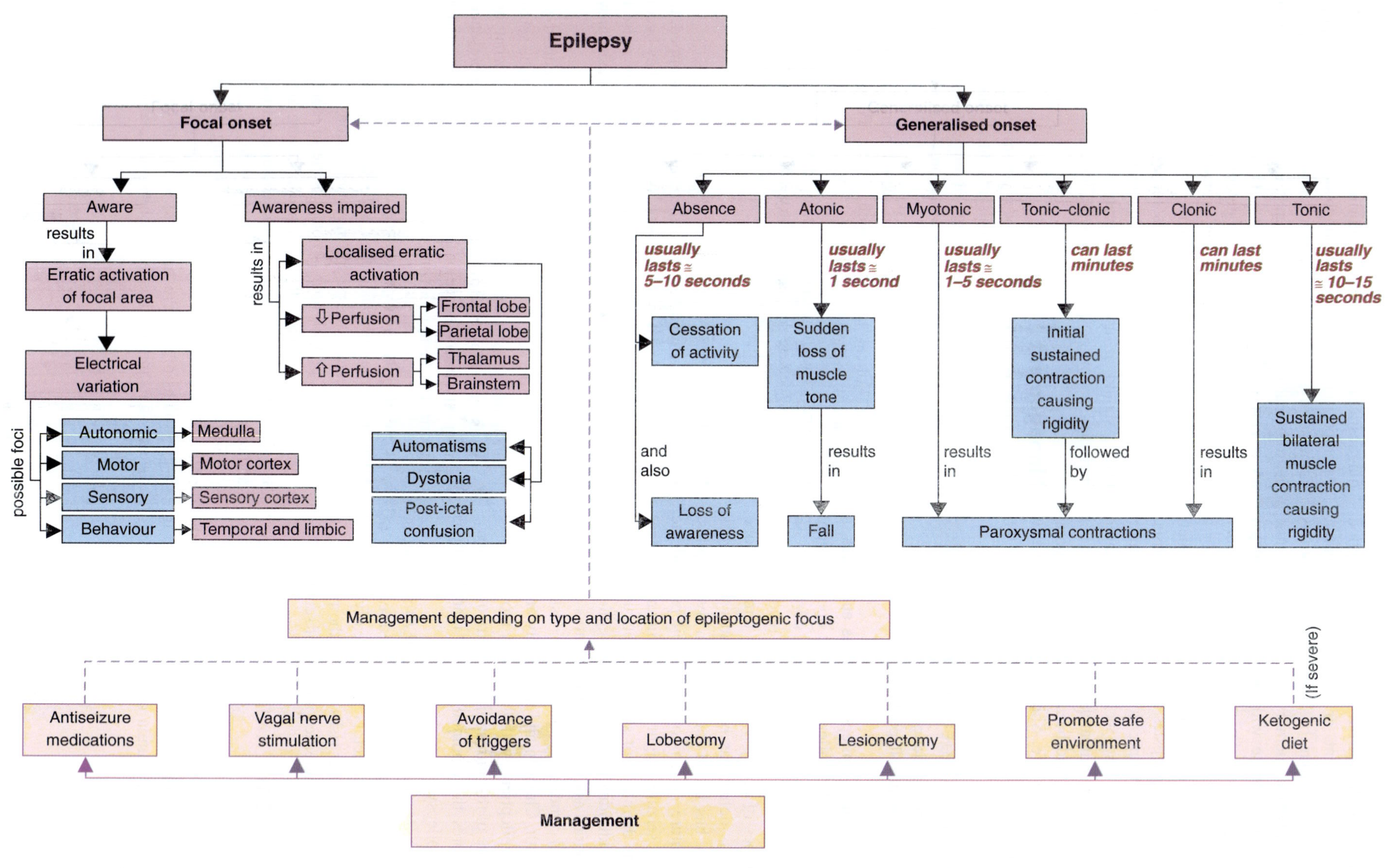

Figure 12.7
Clinical snapshot: Epilepsy
↓ = decreased; ↑ = increased.

	Gated ion channel modulation			GABA enhancers			Glutamate blockers	Regulation of NT release
	Na^+ channel antagonist	Ca^{2+} channel antagonist	K^+ channel enhancer	GABA receptor agonist	GABA reuptake inhibitor	GABA transaminase inhibitors	AMPA/NDMA Glutamate antagonist	Alter NT release
Carbemazepine	✓							
Lamotrogine	✓	✓						
Oxcarbazepine	✓		✓					
Phenytoin	✓							
Sodium valproate	✓	✓		✓			✓	
Topiramate	✓	✓		✓				
Zonisamide	✓	✓		✓				
Ethosuximide		✓						
Gabapentin			✓					✓
Benzodiazepines				✓				
Phenobarbital				✓				
Tiagibine					✓			
Vigabatrin						✓		
Perampanel							✓	
Brivaracetam								✓
Levetiracetam								✓
Pregabalin								✓

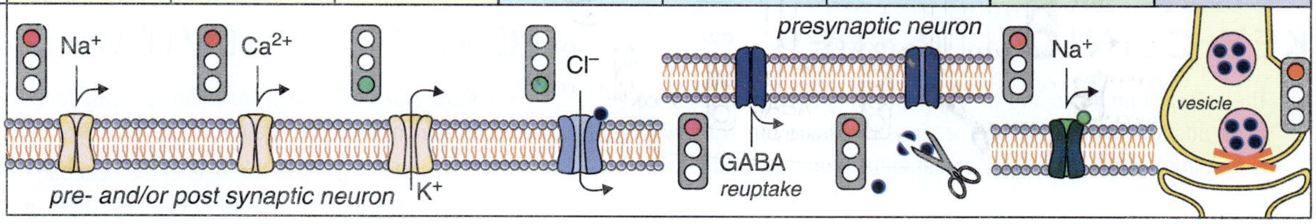

Na^+ Ca^{2+} K^+ Cl^- presynaptic neuron GABA reuptake Na^+ vesicle pre- and/or post synaptic neuron

Figure 12.8

Mechanism of action for common antiseizure drugs

AMPA = alpha-amino-3-hydroxy-5-methyl-4-isoxazolepropionic acid; Ca^{2+} = calcium ion; K^+ = potassium ion; GABA = gamma-aminobutyric acid; Na^+ = sodium ion; NMDA = N-methyl-D-aspartic acid; NT = neurotransmitter.

Sources: Developed using information from Ochoa & Riche (2022); Bullock & Manias (2022).

INDIGENOUS HEALTH FAST FACTS AND CULTURAL CONSIDERATIONS

FAST FACTS

- *Aboriginal and Torres Strait Islander peoples are almost twice as likely to have epilepsy as non-Indigenous Australians, and three times more likely to be hospitalised.*
- *Status epilepticus is more than twice as common in Aboriginal and Torres Strait Islander peoples than in non-Indigenous Australians.*
- *Māori and Pacific Islands children are less likely to experience epilepsy than European New Zealand Children.*

CULTURAL CONSIDERATIONS

- *Recent socioeconomic data suggests that management of Aboriginal and Torres Strait Islander peoples' epilepsy treatment is largely limited to crisis care, because of geographical challenges, cultural challenges and, most importantly, a lack of funding, which has resulted in insufficient education and support in Aboriginal and Torres Strait Islander communities.*
- *Education for healthcare workers and culturally appropriate programs for communities regarding the causes, consequences, safety considerations and management of epilepsy are critical, as in some communities seizure activity is still seen as spiritual possession.*

Sources: Data from Ali et al. (2021); Australian Institute of Health and Welfare (2022a); Australian Institute of Health and Welfare (2022b).

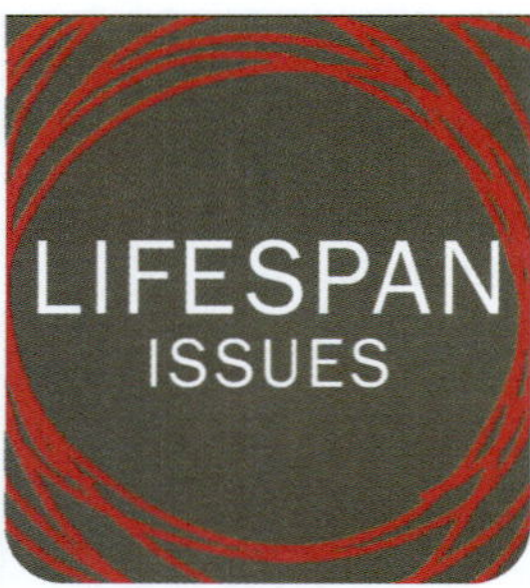

CHILDREN AND ADOLESCENTS

- Febrile seizures occur most commonly in infants and young children aged 8–20 months.
- A diagnosis of epilepsy can be challenging for teenagers, especially as they near ages associated with activities that represent the common 'rite of passage to adulthood', such as learning to drive and sexual activity.
- Compliance with medications and an increased risk of trigger exposure can become complex as an adolescent begins to experiment with alcohol, drugs and environments with strobe-type lighting.

OLDER ADULTS

- The incidence of seizure can increase after the age of 60 years.
- Cerebrovascular disease and head trauma can contribute to an increasing incidence of seizure in the older adult.
- The administration of antiseizure medication can be complex in an older adult, because of the increased potential for polypharmacy and drug interactions, the changes in gastrointestinal absorption and the risk of cognitive side-effects.

KEY CLINICAL ISSUES

- The safety of an individual with epilepsy is of critical importance. In an unstable individual, interventions to ensure that the environment is free from sharp or dangerous elements should be a priority of care.
- Airway management of someone with epilepsy can be challenging. A person experiencing a tonic–clonic seizure may have a period of hypoxia and can become cyanotic. Always ensure that airway equipment and oxygen are within reach.
- If a person has an endotracheal tube in situ, they can bite on the tube and obstruct the artificial airway. In someone with an altered level of consciousness, the insertion of an oropharyngeal airway or a bite block (when they are not fitting) will be beneficial to maintain an airway during a myotonic or tonic–clonic seizure.
- Individuals who experience atonic seizures may injure themselves as they briefly lose tone and/or consciousness during the drop attack. Although difficult, interventions to reduce the potential injuries in an unstable individual should be considered.
- Thermoregulation techniques should be instigated and maintained in neonates, infants and children to avoid febrile seizures. Manipulation of the environment and the use of antipyretics can reduce the risk of febrile seizure.
- There are many causes of seizure. In someone who is being investigated for a seizure event, possible causes, such as brain trauma or tumour, chemical imbalance, medicines or environmental factors such as toxic chemical exposure, should be investigated before any consideration of the diagnosis of epilepsy is applied.
- Some antiseizure drugs can cause renal or hepatic issues. Appropriate dosing should be considered in the context of severity, refractoriness and the potential to use more than one therapy at lower levels to avoid nephrotoxicity or hepatotoxicity.

CHAPTER REVIEW

- Most types of epilepsy have an *epileptic focus*, which is a group of cells in the cortex of the brain that are *hyperexcitable*.
- The characteristics of the cells of the epileptic focus are: resting membrane potential closer to threshold than normal (i.e. less negative); sensitivity to small fluctuations in local ion concentrations; capacity for repetitive action potentials after the initial depolarisation; and a post-ictal state that is hyperpolarised and relatively insensitive to ion fluctuations.
- A small proportion of epilepsies are the consequence of *structural malformation of the cortex*. These conditions are more likely to be intractable to pharmacological intervention and, provided that a focus can be identified, qualify for surgical intervention.
- A number of classification systems are used for the diagnosis and description of the different types of epilepsy, but as yet there is no one comprehensive system. The International League Against Epilepsy (ILAE) classifies seizures around three considerations: *onset, motor activity* and *awareness*.
- Seizure taxonomy is changing to improve clarity and include more types of seizure activity. The term *partial* has been replaced with *focal, simple* to *aware*, and *complex* to a state of *impaired awareness*.

REVIEW QUESTIONS

1 What is an epileptic focus?
2 Describe the characteristics of the cells of an epileptic focus.
3 What potential role might the balance between GABA and glutamate activity in the brain play in the development of status epilepticus?
4 Gowers argued that 'seizures beget seizures'. What did he mean by that?
5 Differentiate between the terms 'focal' and 'generalised' as they relate to the classification of epileptic seizures.

HEALTH PROFESSIONAL CONNECTIONS

Midwives Managing the care of a pregnant woman with epilepsy can be complex because of the potential teratogenic properties of some antiseizure medications. Sodium valproate has been linked with fetal malformations, and there are suggestions that phenytoin and phenobarbital may cause reduced cognitive capacity in the baby. However, if antiseizure medication is reduced, the risk of hypoxia from maternal seizure can also cause fetal trauma. If a pregnancy is unplanned and the woman was taking a known teratogenic agent, consultations with medical and gynaecological teams will be necessary so that investigations can determine any significant congenital malformation. Depending on the clinical picture, a woman may require medically prescribed, high-dose folate and/or vitamin K supplementation as a result of some antiseizure medications interfering with their metabolism. A multidisciplinary team approach is necessary in the care of a pregnant woman with epilepsy.

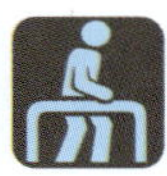

Physiotherapists Most people with epilepsy do not require physiotherapy; however, some with epilepsy may develop movement or coordination issues, or, if they are admitted to the intensive care unit for status epilepticus, may have periods of prolonged immobility. Treatment plans may involve activities to improve core strength, balance and motor control, strengthen major muscle groups or prevent atrophy during prolonged periods of immobility.

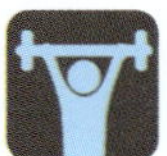

Exercise scientists For many years, an overprotective attitude has been taken towards people with epilepsy, because of the risk of potentially exacerbating the seizure disorder or because of a fear of an increased risk of injury as a result of seizure during activity. However, these opinions appear to be based on sparse anecdotal evidence, as no prospective, well-designed study has supported the position that exercise increases the risk of seizure. Some believe that exercise decreases seizure activity through the generation of exercise-induced metabolic acidosis, which reduces cortical irritability and influences GABA metabolism or concentration. Other theories include inhibition of seizure activity by endorphins, or through the need for intensified sensorimotor processing as a result of increased movement, sensation and proprioception. In the absence of exercise, hyperventilation can be epileptogenic; however, during effort, the respiratory alkalosis is thought to be offset by the lactic acid production, so that hyperventilation in exercise does not appear to trigger seizures. There are instances of individuals having exercise-induced epilepsy; however, these are exceedingly rare. Therefore, as with anyone else, development of an exercise program should be individualised and focused on the desired outcomes. Careful consideration should be given to activities such as scuba diving, solo aerial sports and motor sports, and to high-altitude activities such as mountain climbing, as they may be too risky in a person with poorly controlled seizures. Understanding the pathophysiology of epilepsy and having an awareness of the epilepsy type and triggers of the presenting individual is imperative in the design of a safe and effective exercise program.

Nutritionists/Dieticians Occasionally, someone with medically unresponsive epilepsy may be placed on a ketogenic diet, causing a shift from glycolysis to fatty acid oxidation to reduce seizure activity. A ketogenic diet includes high-fat and low-carbohydrate and low-protein intake, and results in the creation of ketone bodies. Under strict medical supervision, this type of diet may benefit individuals with intractable epilepsy. It is thought that children respond better to this diet than adults, but this may be related to compliance and the fact that a child's meals are generally prepared for them, whereas an adult has more freedom to eat foods that are not part of the incredibly limiting diet. This intervention generally commences in an inpatient episode and is closely monitored. A nutrition professional will play a pivotal role in the programming and education associated with this diet.

CASE STUDY

Bradley Jackson is a 5-year-old boy (UR number 948492). He has been admitted for the investigation and management of seizures. Over the past four months, Bradley has had several witnessed tonic–clonic-type seizures, involving mainly the left side of his body with loss of consciousness and occasional incontinence. Three days ago, he was brought in by paramedics in status epilepticus, having sequential seizure episodes, each lasting approximately 1.5 minutes despite treatment with the benzodiazepine midazolam. Neurologically, he did not recover to a Glasgow coma scale score of 15 between seizures. Following stabilisation in the emergency department, a CT scan and transfer to the paediatric intensive care unit, he became seizure-free within 16 hours. He had an intravenous cannula inserted and blood taken for analysis. He has now been transferred to a neurology ward and is undergoing continuous EEG for the next 24 hours. On arrival to the ward, his observations were as follows:

Temperature	Heart rate	Respiration rate	Blood pressure	SpO_2	Glasgow coma scale
37.1°C	98	22	110/58	98% (RA*)	15

*RA = room air.

Bradley's CT scan results were unremarkable, with no abnormalities detected. Since transfer to the ward, he has been seizure-free. He has been commenced on oral sodium valproate, and is to have any seizure activity documented. The pathology results taken in the emergency department are as follows:

HAEMATOLOGY

Patient location:	Emergency Dep.	**UR:**	948492		
Consultant:	Johnson	**NAME:**	Jackson		
		Given name:	Bradley	**Sex:**	M
		DOB:	04/02/XX	**Age:**	5

Time collected	12.30
Date collected	XX/XX
Year	XXXX
Lab #	345435334

FULL BLOOD COUNT		UNITS	REFERENCE RANGE
Haemoglobin	122	g/L	115–160
White cell count	6.4	$\times 10^9$/L	4.0–11.0
Platelets	323	$\times 10^9$/L	140–400
Haematocrit	0.39		0.33–0.47
Red cell count	4.61	$\times 10^{12}$/L	3.80–5.20
Reticulocyte count	1.6	%	0.2–2.0
MCV	95	fL	80–100
COAGULATION PROFILE			
aPTT	31	secs	24–40
PT	14	secs	11–17

BIOCHEMISTRY

Patient location:	Emergency Dep.	**UR:**	948492		
Consultant:	Johnson	**NAME:**	Jackson		
		Given name:	Bradley	**Sex:**	M
		DOB:	04/02/XX	**Age:**	5

Time collected	12:30
Date collected	XX/XX
Year	XXXX
Lab #	4345454

ELECTROLYTES		UNITS	REFERENCE RANGE
Sodium	135	mmol/L	135–145
Potassium	4.4	mmol/L	3.5–5.2
Chloride	102	mmol/L	95–110
Glucose	4.6	mmol/	3.5–5.4
Renal function			
Urea	3.7	mmol/L	2.5–7.5
Creatinine	92	μmol/L	30–120

CRITICAL THINKING

1 Consider Bradley's assessment data. Are his observations appropriate for a child of his age?
2 Why were there no observable changes to Bradley's CT scan? Observe his pathology results. Are these of any benefit to assist with a diagnosis? (*Hint:* Think of other causes of seizure.)
3 Bradley has been ordered sodium valproate. What is the mechanism of action of this drug? What are the precautions and potential side-effects associated with this drug?
4 What interventions does Bradley require? Consider all of the elements of his condition (especially safety). Draw up a table identifying actual or potential problems, interventions and their rationale.
5 Observing the duration and characteristics of a seizure episode can enable a clinician to develop some understanding of the possible areas involved. Explain. What were the characteristics of Bradley's seizure event that resulted in his admission? What can be determined from this information?

BIBLIOGRAPHY

Ali, S., Stanley, J., Davis, S., Keenan, N., Scheffer, I.E. & Sadleir, L.G. (2021). Epidemiology of treated epilepsy in New Zealand children: a focus on ethnicity. *Neurology* 97(19):E1933–E1941. https://doi.org/10.1212/WNL.0000000000012784.

Australian Institute of Health and Welfare (2022a). *Epilepsy in Australia*. Cat No. NEU 1. Canberra: AIHW. https://www.aihw.gov.au/getmedia/04ec4cc1-71ba-423e-96db-78ba3f495f1b/Epilepsy-in-Australia.pdf.aspx?inline=true.

Australian Institute of Health and Welfare (2022b). *Epilepsy in Australia: Fact sheet*. Canberra: AIHW. https://www.aihw.gov.au/reports/chronic-disease/epilepsy-in-australia/related-material.

Australian Institute of Health and Welfare (AIHW) & Pointer, S. (2016). *Hospitalised injury in Aboriginal and Torres Strait Islander children and young people, 2011–13*. Injury Research and Statistics series no. 96. Cat. No. INJCAT 172. Canberra: AIHW. https://www.aihw.gov.au/getmedia/ef9ac10c-7f72-4332-af8d-c0ac25c47d85/19575.pdf.aspx?inline=true.

Bauldoff, G., Gubrud-Howe, P.M., Carno, M.-A., Levett-Jones, T., Hales, M., Berry, K., ... Stanley, D. (2020). *LeMone and Burke's medical–surgical nursing: critical thinking for person-centred care* (4th [Australian] edn). Sydney: Pearson Australia.

Beniczky, S. & Schomer, D.L. (2020). Electroencephalography: basic biophysical and technological aspects important for clinical applications. *Epileptic Disorders* 22(6):697–715. https://doi.org/10.1684/epd.2020.1217.

Bullock, S. & Manias, E. (2022). *Fundamentals of pharmacology* (9th edn). Sydney: Pearson Australia.

Carroll, E. & Benbadis, S.R. (2021). Complex partial seizures. *Emedicine.* https://emedicine.medscape.com/article/1183962-overview.

Crunelli, V., Lőrincz, M.L., McCafferty, C., Lambert, R.C., Leresche, N., Di Giovanni, G. & David, F. (2020). Clinical and experimental insight into pathophysiology, comorbidity and therapy of absence seizures. *Brain* 143(8):2341–68. https://doi.org/10.1093/brain/awaa072.

Epilepsy Action Australia (2020). *Facts and statistics about epilepsy*. Epping, NSW: Epilepsy Action Australia. https://www.epilepsy.org.au/about-epilepsy/facts-and-statistics/.

Gonzalez-Viana, E., Sen, A., Bonnon, A. & Cross, J.H. (2022). Epilepsies in children, young people, and adults: summary of updated NICE guidance. *BMJ* 378:o1446. https://doi.org/10.1136/bmj.o1446.

Hanif, S. & Musick, S.T. (2021). Reflex epilepsy. *Aging and Disease* 12(4):1010–20. https://doi.org/10.14336/AD.2021.0216.

International League Against Epilepsy (ILAE) (2022). *Epilepsy Diagnostic Manual*. https://www.epilepsydiagnosis.org/

Jaffer, M.H. & Benbadis, S.R. (2022). Focal (partial) epilepsy. *Emedicine*. https://emedicine.medscape.com/article/1186635-overview.

Ko, D.Y. (2022a). Epilepsy and seizures. *Emedicine*. https://emedicine.medscape.com/article/1184846-overview.

Ko, D.Y. & Sahai-Srivastava, S. (2022b). Generalized tonic–clonic seizures. *Emedicine.* https://emedicine.medscape.com/article/1184608-overview.

Marieb, E.N. & Hoehn, K. (2019). *Human anatomy and physiology* (11th edn). San Francisco, CA: Pearson Benjamin Cummings.

National Institute for Health and Clinical Excellence (NICE) (2022). Epilepsies in children, young people and adults. Manchester & London: NIHCE. https://www.nice.org.uk/guidance/ng217.

New Zealand Ministry of Health (2021). *Annual update of key results 2020/2021: New Zealand Health Survey.* Wellington: Ministry of Health. https://www.health.govt.nz/publication/annual-update-key-results-2020-21-new-zealand-health-survey.

Nouri, S. (2020). Sudden unexpected death in epilepsy. *Emedicine*. https://emedicine.medscape.com/article/1187111-overview.

Ochoa, J.G. & Riche, W. (2022). Antiepileptic drugs. *Emedicine*. https://emedicine.medscape.com/article/1187334-overview.

Pressler, R.M., Cilio, M.R., Mizrahi, E.M., Moshé, S.L., Nunes, M.L., Plouin, P., ... Zuberi, S.M. (2021). The ILAE classification of seizures and the epilepsies: modification for seizures in the neonate: position paper by the ILAE Task Force on Neonatal Seizures. *Epilepsia* 62(3), 615–28. https://doi.org/10.1111/epi.16815.

Segan, S. (2018). Absence seizures. *Emedicine.* https://reference.medscape.com/article/1183858-overview.

Specchio, N., Wirrell, E.C., Scheffer, I., Nabbout, R., Riney, K., Samia, P., ... Auvin, S. (2022). International League Against Epilepsy classification and definition of epilepsy syndromes with onset in childhood: position paper by the ILAE Task Force on Nosology and Definitions. *Epilepsia* 63(6), 1398–442. https://doi.org/10.1111/epi.17241.

Wang, G., Wu, W., Xu, Y., Yang, Z., Xiao, B. & Long, L. (2022). Imaging genetics in epilepsy: current knowledge and new perspectives. *Frontiers in Molecular Neuroscience* 15:891621. https://doi.org/10.3389/fnmol.2022.891621.

World Health Organization (WHO) (2022). *Epilepsy*. Geneva: WHO. https://www.who.int/news-room/fact-sheets/detail/epilepsy.

Zonnoor, B. & Diaz, M.E. (2022). Seizure assessment in the emergency department. *Emedicine*. https://emedicine.medscape.com/article/1609294-overview.

Zuberi, S.M., Wirrell, E., Yozawitz, E., Wilmshurst, J.M., Specchio, N., Riney, K., ... Nabbout, R. (2022). ILAE classification and definition of epilepsy syndromes with onset in neonates and infants: position statement by the ILAE Task Force on Nosology and Definitions. *Epilepsia* 63(6), 1349–97. https://doi.org/10.1111/epi.17239.

Nociception and pain

13

LEARNING OBJECTIVES

After completing this chapter, you should be able to:

1. Differentiate between Aδ- and C-fibres.
2. Differentiate between nociception and pain.
3. Outline the physiological characteristics of itching.
4. Outline the role of the change in threshold of nociceptive neurons.
5. Describe hyperalgesia and allodynia, and the role they are thought to play in normal nociceptive signalling.
6. Differentiate between productive and non-productive pain.
7. Explain why pain is described as a subjective sensation.
8. Describe the pain gate mechanism, and the role played by the substantia gelatinosa in this process.
9. Describe how neuropathic pain differs from chronic pain.
10. Explain the principle of wind-up, and the role it is thought to play in the development of neuropathic pain.

WHAT YOU SHOULD KNOW BEFORE YOU START THIS CHAPTER

Can you identify the major parts of the brain and their functions?

Can you describe the process of neurotransmission?

Can you describe the processes involved in inflammation and healing?

Can you describe the role of stress in disease?

KEY TERMS

Aβ-fibre
Aδ-fibre
Allodynia
Analgesic
Bradykinin
C-fibre
Descending inhibitory pathway
Hyperalgesia
Neospinothalamic tract
Neuropathic pain
Nociception
Nociceptive neurons
Non-productive pain
Pain
Pain Gate Theory
Palaeospinothalamic tract
Phantom limb pain
Productive pain
Prostaglandins
Spinoreticular tract
Spinothalamic tract
Substance P
Substantia gelatinosa
Sympathetic causalgia
Trigeminal neuralgia
Wind-up

Introduction

A primary reason for people seeking medical care is unmanageable pain, which can be one of the most difficult conditions to treat. **Pain** is the sensation perceived that is triggered by noxious stimuli. Pain itself is a *subjective sensation* that involves multiple brain regions and depends on the decision-making processes of the brain. The pain experience is therefore highly variable and individual. Variability in response can even occur in one individual for separate episodes of the same type of injury. Pain cannot be quantified, and will be influenced by such things as circumstances and emotional context. By contrast, the neuronal signals that alert the brain to an injury, called **nociception**, are readily quantifiable.

Pain can be classified in many ways according to its character. Factors such as duration, localisability, the type of structure affected and the nature of the pain trigger are used in the classification. The major types of pain are described in Table 13.1.

Epidemiology of pain

It can be difficult to discuss the epidemiology of pain, as statistics are not often kept, and the condition can go under-recognised, misdiagnosed or under-reported. According to data released by the Australian Institute of Health and Welfare, 1 in 5 Australians over the age of 45 live with persistent, ongoing pain. Women are more likely to experience chronic pain than men, as are older people.

Furthermore, the prevalence of neuropathic pain is estimated at 7–10% of the population. Common causes of neuropathic pain are diabetic neuropathy and shingles.

Nociception and pain

LEARNING OBJECTIVE 1

Differentiate between Aδ- and C-fibres.

LEARNING OBJECTIVE 2

Differentiate between nociception and pain.

LEARNING OBJECTIVE 3

Outline the physiological characteristics of itching.

Nociception comes from the Latin *nocere*, meaning 'to harm', and represents the signal that is sent to the brain in recognition of an injury. Noxious stimuli are detected by tissue nociceptors, usually free nerve endings that convert the information into nerve impulses. Two types of **nociceptive neurons** —the **Aδ-fibre** and the **C-fibre**, each associated with different types of pain—transmit these signals. The signals from the myelinated Aδ-fibres are interpreted as sharp, well-localised pain, whereas the unmyelinated C-fibre inputs are linked to sensations of dull, aching pain that are difficult to pinpoint. Nociceptors respond to a variety of triggers, such as temperature (hot or cold), mechanical (tearing, slicing, ripping) and chemical (acid, base) information, but, under normal physiological conditions, are considered *high-threshold* cells. This means that only actual tissue damage can elicit a signal of sufficient intensity to activate these neurons. By contrast, the highly sensitive nerve fibres associated with mechanoreceptor responses (**Aβ-fibres**) in your fingertips are *low-threshold* neurons, allowing fine discrimination.

Table 13.1 Types of pain

Type	Characteristics
Fast	Sharp, highly localised pain. Rapid perception.
Slow	Diffuse, dull pain. Hard to localise. Includes aching, throbbing pain. Delayed perception, but can increase over time.
Acute	Pain lasting less than 6 months.
Chronic	Pain lasting longer than 6 months.
Productive	Correlated to tissue damage. Serves a purpose as a warning of injury. Wanes as damage resolves. Accompanied by sympathetic nervous system responses.
Non-productive	Does not serve as a warning of injury. Cause of pain may be difficult to identify. Often accompanied by stress and depression.
Somatic	Pain arising from somatic structures.
Visceral	Pain arising from organs and involuntary body structures.
Inflammatory	Pain in the presence of inflammation.
Neuropathic	Pain associated with damage to or disease of the somatosensory system.

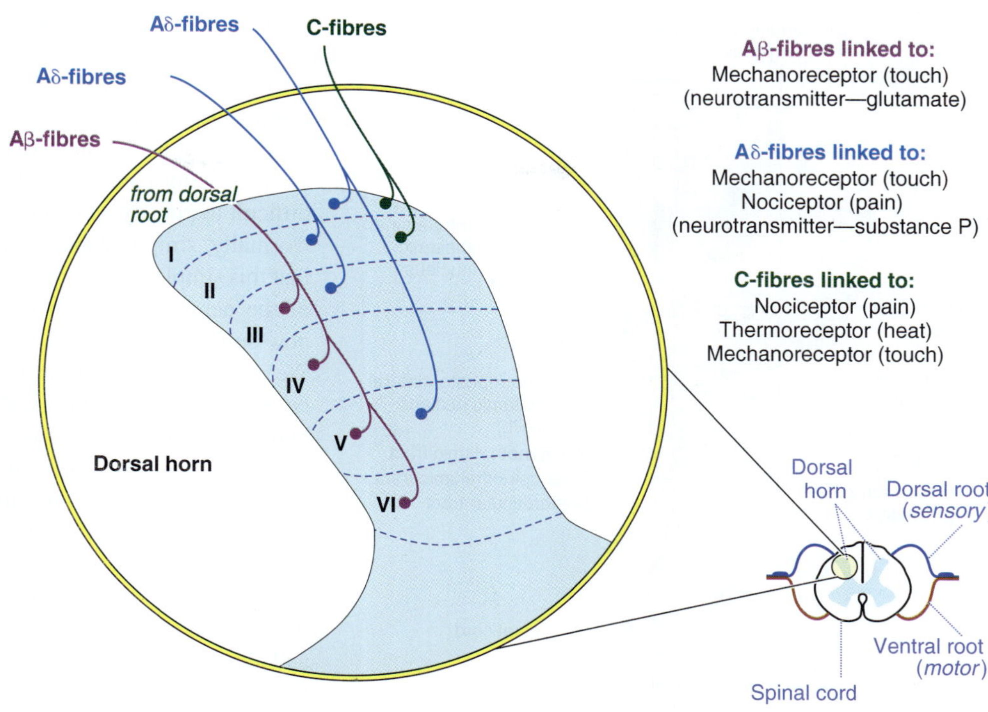

Figure 13.1

Pathway of *A*δ-, *A*β- and C-fibres from the periphery to the dorsal horn

Incoming neurons synapse onto ascending fibres in different layers (lamina) of the dorsal horn of the spinal cord. This spatial pattern is used by the brain to locate the injury within the body, while the difference in timing of the incoming signals (temporal pattern) is interpreted by the brain as the nature of the pain, such as whether it is dull and achy or sharp and well-localised.

The Aδ- and C-fibres travel from the target tissue in the periphery, past the cell bodies in the dorsal root ganglia, to the dorsal horn of the spinal cord, where they synapse in specific layers (*lamina*) onto ascending fibres (see Figure 13.1), travelling primarily to the thalamus, but also to structures in the brainstem, via the **spinothalamic tract** and **spinoreticular tract**, respectively (see Figure 13.2). The spinothalamic tract is actually comprised of two tracts terminating in different parts of the thalamus; namely, the **palaeospinothalamic tract** and the **neospinothalamic tract**. The two primary neurotransmitters in these pathways are substance P and glutamate. Interestingly, unlike most other types of neurons, the nociceptive neurons employ more than one neurotransmitter. A number of compounds, known as *neuromodulators*, act like the fine control on a microscope, and are responsible for the finetuning of the synaptic activity—they either increase or decrease nociceptive transmission. In addition, nociceptive neurons are able to release neurotransmitter from both ends of the neuron: namely, the peripheral end that was initially triggered, and the synaptic end in the dorsal horn.

Nociceptive signals along the neospinothalamic tract mainly terminate within the thalamus, and synapse with ascending neurons that connect to the somatosensory cortex. Pain perception and localisation occurs here. Nociceptive signals from the palaeospinothalamic tract are directed to various lower brain regions, primarily the brainstem and midbrain, as well as the thalamus. From these regions, connections are made to the hypothalamus and limbic system, where the emotional, behavioural and visceral characteristics of the pain experience are initiated. In the context of nociception, the spinoreticular tract terminates in the reticular formation, so that information related to pain increases arousal and wakefulness.

A discussion of nociception and pain is often linked to the processing of another sensation, the itch. This is not surprising, as there are a number of similarities. *Puritoceptive itch* is the most common form of itch that is generated in the skin when there is inflammation or in response to tissue damage. Like productive pain, puritoceptive itch is associated with protection and avoidance of noxious stimuli. It is transmitted along C-fibres to the brain after the activation of free nerve endings along the contralateral spinothalamic tract. Activation of this pathway is set at a *low threshold*. Other types of itch include *neurogenic itch* (secondary to organ diseases like renal or liver disorders), *psychogenic itch* (associated with mental health illnesses) and *neuropathic itch* (resulting from central or peripheral nervous system dysfunction in the absence of physiological stimuli).

PAIN SENSITISATION AND INFLAMMATION

In the periphery, the release of neurotransmitters helps to sensitise the neuron, *converting this high-threshold cell into a low-threshold one* that is much more easily activated. One driver for this effect is **substance P**, which is a peptide neurotransmitter. In addition, the neuron will be sensitised by the inflammatory mediators released at the site of injury, and by compounds such as adenosine triphosphate (ATP) and protons (H^+), which are disgorged into the surrounding environment when cells are injured or die (see Figure 13.3). Key *inflammatory mediators* of this sensitisation are the **prostaglandins**, which are unable to activate the cells themselves, but can change the threshold for activation of the neurons and promote the release of a potent activator of nociceptive cells called **bradykinin**. This increased sensitivity of the nociceptive neurons at the site of injury will persist through the healing process, reversing as healing nears completion.

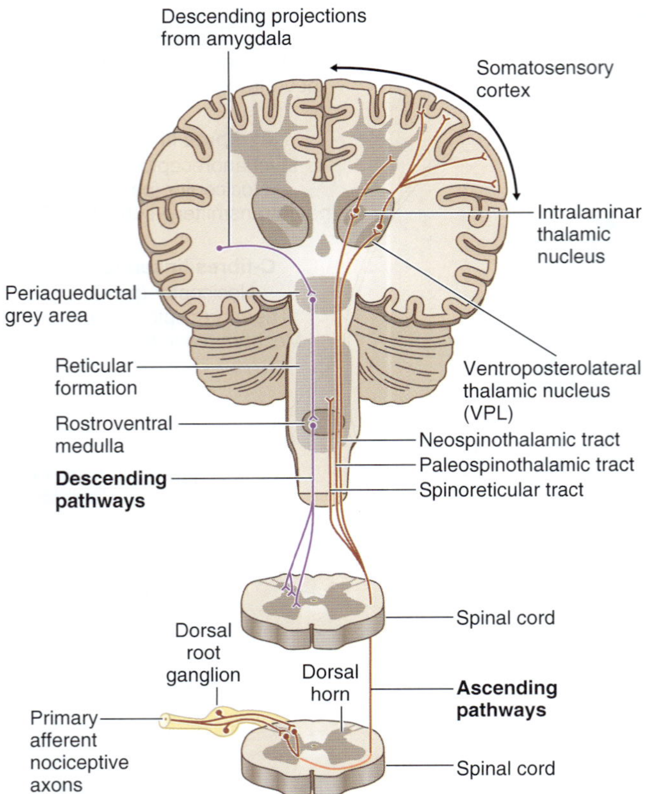

Figure 13.2

Ascending nociceptive pathways

The incoming nociceptive Aδ- and C-fibres synapse onto ascending fibres at the dorsal horn. There are three main ascending pathways: the neospinothalamic, palaeospinothalamic and spinoreticular tracts. From the thalamus, the two pathways that comprise the spinothalamic tract can synapse onto neurons that carry the incoming information to the cortex for processing and interpretation.

Source: Adapted from Nestler et al. (2015), Figure 11.1, p. 271.

LEARNING OBJECTIVE 4

Outline the role of the change in threshold of nociceptive neurons.

LEARNING OBJECTIVE 5

Describe hyperalgesia and allodynia, and the role they are thought to play in normal nociceptive signalling.

LEARNING OBJECTIVE 6

Differentiate between productive and non-productive pain.

In order to understand the potential value of this type of sensitisation, consider what happens when someone sprains their ankle. The immediate pain associated with the injury is referred to as **productive pain**, and is a near-direct correlate of the fact that tissue has been damaged. Once the injury is over and the healing begins, the ongoing pain experience is referred to as **non-productive pain**, as it is not the injury that is responsible for the pain, but the ongoing changes at and around the neurons that are producing pain. After the initial injury, the person finds it difficult to put any weight onto the foot because it is too painful. Normally, simply standing should not cause pain, but the fact that this simple action now causes pain means that the sensitivity of the neurons has been changed; a low-intensity stimulus is now sufficient to activate the formerly high-threshold neurons. We refer to this situation, in which something that should not be painful causes pain, as **allodynia**. The injured ankle is now hypersensitive to even minor injury. For example, if you were to knock the ankle against a chair leg, normally this would cause a small discomfort, but when the ankle is already sprained, this small injury takes on greater proportions, a process referred to as **hyperalgesia**.

In practice, hyperalgesia and allodynia are thought to involve changes in the periphery, the spinal cord (dorsal horn) and the brain, restricting use of the injured limb in order to facilitate healing and prevent re-injury. As the wound heals, the mechanisms that led to the hyperalgesia and allodynia should reverse, restoring the high-threshold character of the nociceptive neurons. An inability to reverse these processes is thought to contribute to the development of neuropathic pain, which is discussed in more detail later in this chapter.

Figure 13.4 describes the characteristics of selected types of pain, including stimulus, receptors, site, cause, threshold activation and function.

ASSESSING THE CHARACTERISTICS OF PAIN

Once the nociceptive signals synapse in the dorsal horn, their identity as either C- or Aδ-fibre signals is lost. The question then arises: How does the brain know what type of injury has occurred, and therefore what type of pain to experience? The *arrangement* (spatial pattern) of these synapses within the lamina (layers) of the dorsal horn is mirrored in the thalamus, providing the brain with both *positional information*, which is used to locate the injury, and *qualitative information* to assess its nature. The answer also lies in the speed of the different signals and the pattern that they create in the brain. You can think of the Aδ- and C-fibres as the equivalent of Morse code: Aδ-fibres convey abbreviated jolts of information delivered in rapid succession, resembling the dots of the code, while the dashes are the C-fibre signals that arrive at the synapse (and therefore the brain) at some delay after the Aδ signals, and are of a diffuse character. Therefore, the brain interprets the *temporal pattern* of the signals along with their *spatial pattern* to determine the characteristics of the pain from that injury.

LEARNING OBJECTIVE 7

Explain why pain is described as a subjective sensation.

However, this is not the only information that the brain uses to determine the nature of pain, or in fact whether pain

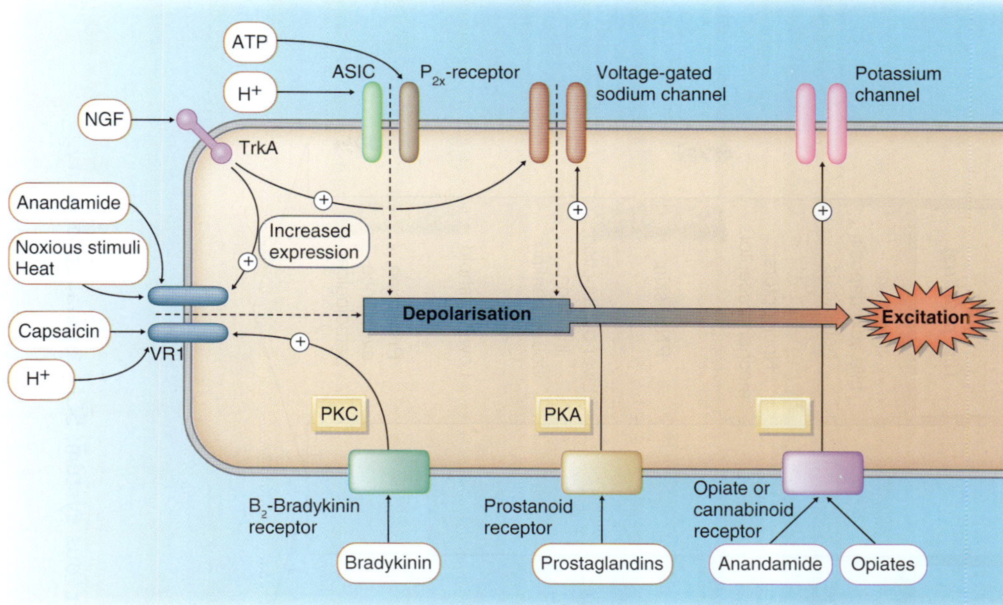

Figure 13.3

Compounds that sensitise peripheral nociceptive neurons

In addition to the release of neurotransmitters from the peripheral ends of the nociceptive neurons, a number of local mediators will sensitise the cells, converting the high threshold of activation to a low threshold. This state will persist during the healing process, decreasing as the tissue heals. Mediators such as adenosine triphosphate (ATP) and protons (H^+) are available due to cell damage and death subsequent to injury. Other compounds are derived from the inflammatory process, such as nerve growth factor (NGF), prostaglandins and bradykinin. Activation of opioid and cannabinoid receptors will attempt to counteract this sensitisation. Anandamide is an endogenous cannabinoid transmitter.

ASIC = acid-sensing ion channels; ATP = adenosine triphosphate; B_2 = bradykinin type 2; H^+ = hydrogen ion; NGF = nerve growth factor; P_{2X} = ATP-sensitive channels; PKA = protein kinase A; PKC = protein kinase C; TrkA = tyrosine kinase A; VR1 = vanilloid receptor type 1.

Source: Adapted from Rang et al. (2016), Figure 42.5, p. 514.

is experienced at all. The incoming nociceptive information is generally a priority because of its links with survival. People with diabetes who suffer diabetic neuropathy experience severe nerve injury that results in a lack of awareness of injury, leading to infection of the injured tissue, gangrene and the necessity for amputation. In a more extreme example, those with an inherited condition in which they are born without C-fibres, known as *congenital insensitivity to pain*, will usually die young as a result of injuries and infections that escape notice.

On the other hand, ignoring the injury if the circumstances are equally life-threatening (e.g. needing to escape a burning building with a sprained ankle) will necessitate a reconsideration of the injury in the light of this context. Therefore, when the nociceptive information is received by the brain, an assessment of other potentially pertinent information is undertaken. The sensory cortex will be accessed to determine the *circumstances* surrounding the injury, as will brain structures associated with the processing of emotions, such as the amygdala and cingulate gyrus. Memory stores, which are linked to the hippocampus and distributed around the cerebral cortex, will be tapped to determine whether this situation has occurred before and what the outcome was at that time. Indeed, *memory and emotional information* will combine to provide an assessment of the person's emotional context, such as whether they are socially isolated, have experienced major loss or trauma recently, or are part of a supportive network of family and friends. The status of the body will be determined using information from the hypothalamus and cerebellum to ascertain whether homeostasis is intact, whether the person is highly stressed or whether something about their posture and/or position is relevant, such as whether they are upside down, having difficulty breathing or immersed in water. All of this information is then summed along with the nociceptive signals, allowing the brain to make an informed decision as to how to proceed.

If circumstances allow, some degree of pain will be experienced and the degree of pain will be completely unique to the individual and their circumstances. Generally, a person

	Productive pain	Inflammatory pain	Neuropathic pain	Itch (*i.e. pruritus*)
Stimulus	Noxious	Inflammation, infection	Nerve damage, chemotherapy, ectopic discharge	Infection, bile acid deposit, botanicals
Receptors	Nociceptors, mechanoreceptors	Nociceptors, mechanoreceptors	Nociceptors	Nociceptors, mechanoreceptors
Site	PNS, muscle, bone, viscera, skin	PNS, CNS, muscle, bone, viscera, skin	PNS, CNS	PNS, skin
Cause	Acute trauma	Acute trauma, arthritis, surgery	PNS or CNS lesion, chemotherapy, DM, MS, SCI	Liver dysfunction, infection, wound healing
Threshold activation	High threshold	Low threshold	Low threshold	Low threshold
Function	Protection, avoidance	Wound healing, repair, pathological	Pathological	Protection, avoidance, pathological

Figure 13.4

Characteristics of selected types of pain

CNS = central nervous system; DM = diabetes mellitus; MS = multiple sclerosis; PNS = peripheral nervous system; SCI = spinal cord injury.

Source: Adapted from Veldhuis et al. (2015), Figure 1, p. 39.

who has a strong support network, has not recently experienced trauma or loss, is not depressed and is not in a highly stressful situation may report less pain than someone who is socially isolated, traumatised, dejected, fearful, sleep-deprived and/or stressed. However, such generalisations must always be made cautiously about someone's pain experience. By contrast, if the circumstances necessitate that the experience of pain be *postponed* (e.g. in cases of emergencies when escape is a priority, or when there is a powerful emotional context, such as an injured loved one taking priority over one's own injury), a system is available to temporarily reduce nociceptive signalling until such time as it is considered *safe* to be aware of the experience. This system is known as the descending inhibitory pathways.

DESCENDING INHIBITORY PATHWAYS

Originating in the brain, the purpose of the **descending inhibitory pathway** is to *terminate nociceptive signalling* in the dorsal horn of the spinal cord, allowing the brain to conduct necessary activities in the absence of the pain, which are normally integral to survival, and therefore prioritised over other activities (see Figure 13.5). If the evaluation outlined in the previous section leads to a decision to suspend recognition of the injury, a structure known as the *periaqueductal grey (PAG)* is activated, triggering a chain reaction that sees the activation of two secondary structures, the *nucleus raphe magnus (NRM)* in the rostroventral medulla and the *locus coeruleus (LC)* in the dorsolateral pontine tegmentum.

Each of these structures sends axons down the spinal cord to the dorsal horn, where they will terminate in two locations: onto the synapses between the incoming C- and Aδ-fibres and the ascending spinothalamic and spinoreticular neurons; and onto the interneurons of the substantia gelatinosa, which is the regulatory region, named for its resemblance to jelly (**substantia gelatinosa** means 'jelly-like substance'), located at the top of the dorsal horn (see Figure 13.6), which controls nociceptive signalling. *Inhibitory interneurons* in this area are important in modulating the transmission of ascending nociceptive neurons.

A balance between ascending nociceptive signalling and inhibitory modulation provided by the descending pathways and the interneurons at the level of the dorsal horn is required for normal physiological pain responsiveness.

The pathways from the NRM use *enkephalins* (one group of the body's natural opioid peptides) and *serotonin* as neurotransmitters, while LC neurons use *noradrenaline*. The interneurons of the substantia gelatinosa will use *enkephalins*, *dynorphins* (another group of endogenous opioid peptides), *gamma-aminobutyric acid (GABA)* and *cholecystokinin (CCK)* to further inhibit the nociceptive synapses. Receptors for opioids and noradrenaline on the presynaptic cell inhibit the release of neurotransmitters from the Aδ- and C-fibres, while opioid, noradrenaline, GABA, cholecystokinin and serotonin receptors on the postsynaptic cells hyperpolarise the neuron, driving them away from threshold and preventing activation. Temporary suspension of this signalling allows the brain to undertake other activities that are considered a more pressing priority. Figure 13.7 explores the common clinical manifestations and management of pain.

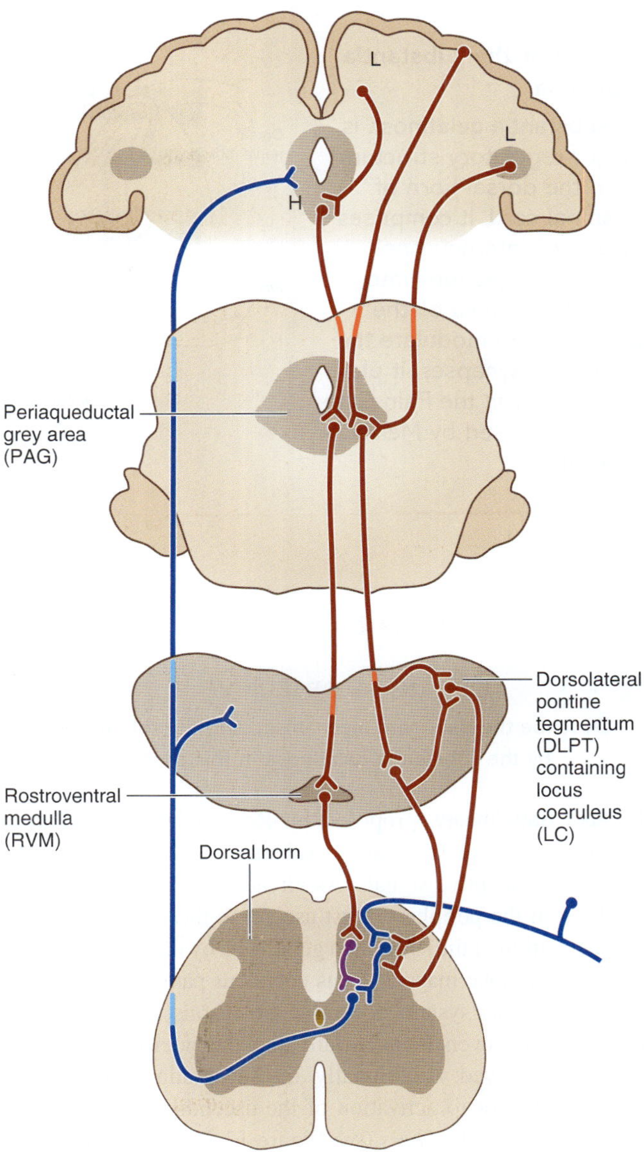

Figure 13.5

Descending inhibitory pathways

Once a decision has been made to suspend nociceptive signalling, neurons from various cortical structures will activate the periaqueductal grey area (PAG) of the midbrain. This activation involves the inhibition of the tonically active gamma-aminobutyric acid (GABA) neurons to allow output from the PAG to the nucleus raphe magnus (NRM) located in the rostroventral medulla (RVM), and to the locus coeruleus (LC) in the dorsolateral pontine tegmentum (DLPT). The NRM and LC then send projections to the dorsal horn of the spinal cord to activate the interneurons of the substantia gelatinosa, and to directly inhibit the synapses between the incoming nociceptive fibres and the ascending spinothalamic and spinoreticular tract neurons.

H = hypothalamus; L = limbic system.

Source: Adapted from McMahon et al. (2013).

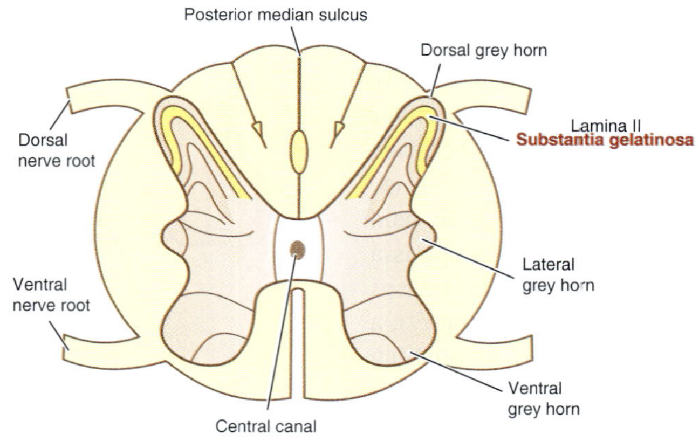

Figure 13.6

Location of the substantia gelatinosa

The substantia gelatinosa is a major regulatory structure within the dorsal horn of the spinal cord. It comprises a group of interneurons that send projections into the various lamina of the dorsal horn to modulate the nociceptive synapses. It plays a critical role in the Pain Gate Theory proposed by Melzack and Wall.

PAIN GATE THEORY

LEARNING OBJECTIVE 8

Describe the pain gate mechanism, and the role played by the substantia gelatinosa in this process.

The **Pain Gate Theory**, proposed by Ron Melzack and Patrick Wall in 1965, proposes that the substantia gelatinosa regulates incoming nociceptive signals. As already outlined, a few initial signals from the periphery must ascend to the brain in order to allow activation of the substantia gelatinosa by the periaqueductal grey–nucleus raphe magnus–locus coeruleus pathways. Generally, activation of this system occurs at an unconscious level, with the person not even being aware that the nociceptive signals have been received. Additionally, the substantia gelatinosa can be triggered prior to activation of the ascending fibres through competition from *Aβ-fibres* (see Figure 13.8). The incoming Aβ signals activate the substantia gelatinosa directly, competing with branches of the incoming nociceptive fibres, which endeavour to turn off the regulatory influence of the substantia gelatinosa. If the Aβ signal is sufficient, it will overcome the Aδ-/C-fibre input, ensuring activation of the interneurons and suppression of nociceptive signalling. If you have ever subconsciously rubbed part of your body that you have just injured, such as a knee that you banged against a desk, you are activating this system: the Aβ-fibres triggered by massaging your knee will compete with the incoming nociceptive fibres in the dorsal horn. As you know, most people will feel some degree of relief from this action, generally when the injury is relatively minor. However, this provides a physiological basis for the value of massage therapy in more noteworthy pain.

Pain assessment

Accurate assessment of a person's pain is vital to ensuring appropriate therapeutic management of their condition. Although a proportion of health professionals are averse to the use of drugs like morphine, due to concern that the recipient will become addicted, the evidence argues strongly that if the analgesic matches a properly assessed report of pain, addiction is not an issue, with an analgesic step-down procedure critical to acute pain management with opioids. Therefore, it is essential to be diligent in the evaluation of the person's pain prior to the initiation of treatment, and a number of tools are available to facilitate this assessment.

An example of the most simplistic of these tools is the *Wong–Baker FACES® Pain Rating Scale* (see Figure 13.9), which is often used with children and those for whom English is not their first language. This simple, straightforward scale uses a series of cartoon faces to denote pain on a scale from 0 (no hurt; happy face) to 10 (hurts worst; excruciating, extreme grimace on crying face). Note that people often respond better to scales that use ethnically appropriate photographs rather than a cartoon scale, and this appears to be particularly true with children.

By contrast, a more comprehensive, if markedly more complex, tool is the *McGill pain questionnaire*, which ranks 78 adjectives on a scale of 0 to 5. The evaluation of the results relies on groups of adjectives that correspond to and self-correct for different aspects of pain. Unfortunately, given the subtle differences between some of the adjectives, high-level language skills are a major advantage in those with whom this scale is used.

While valuable for an initial report, any assessment scale should be used as part of a more *holistic pain interview* that determines the person's social, emotional and physical context, evaluating such parameters as social isolation, social withdrawal, support networks, recent trauma, the ability to sleep and the ability to eat. It is well recognised that mood and social status have a marked influence on a person's self-report of pain, and therefore such scales as those described above should not be used in isolation.

Frequent *re-evaluation of pain* is very important to clinical management, particularly in the control of acute pain. As mentioned, a step-down procedure when using opioid analgesics is important to prevent addiction to these powerful drugs. In a *step-down plan*, the person's pain is assessed at the outset and appropriate **analgesics** are prescribed. The person is then

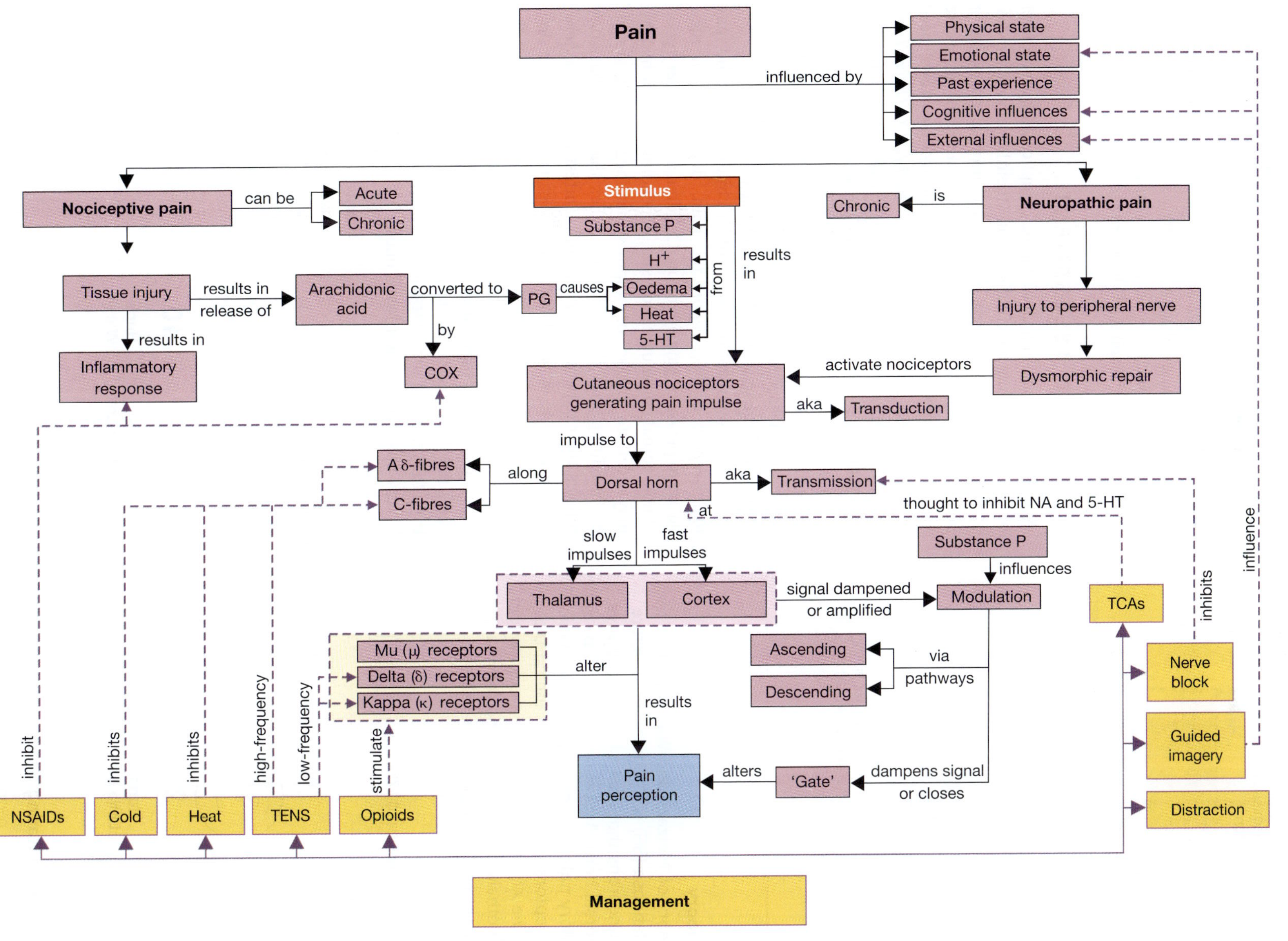

Figure 13.7

Clinical snapshot: Pain

COX = cyclo-oxygenase; 5-HT = serotonin; H^+ = protons; NA = noradrenaline; NSAIDs = non-steroidal anti-inflammatory drugs; PG = prostaglandins; TCAs = tricyclic antidepressants; TENS = transcutaneous electrical nerve stimulation.

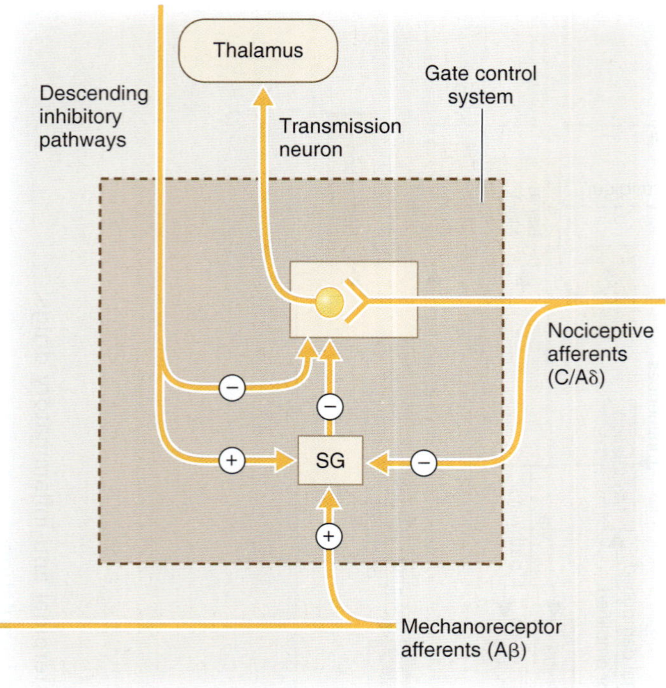

Figure 13.8

The Pain Gate Theory

The Pain Gate Theory of Melzack and Wall proposes that the substantia gelatinosa (SG) is a regulatory structure comprised of interneurons that control the nociceptive synapses in the dorsal horn. Activation of the SG by either descending inhibitory pathways or incoming mechanical fibres (mechanoreceptors, $A\beta$) will, in turn, inhibit the synapse between the $A\delta$ and C nociceptive neurons and the ascending spinothalamic and spinoreticular neurons. This theory is thought to contribute to the value of massage in the management of pain.

Source: Adapted from Veizi & Hayek (2017).

re-evaluated at regular intervals, with a plan to reduce the efficacy and type of analgesics used over time as the injury heals, with the expectation that the person will be drug-free within a defined interval. By engaging them in this process, particularly reinforcing the notion that healing should necessitate a reduced reliance on analgesics, the person is empowered, and their awareness and self-report of pain are improved. This approach is in keeping with the recommendations of the US Agency for Health Care Policy and Research, which are used at key institutions, such as the Royal Children's Hospital in Melbourne (see Table 13.2).

PAEDIATRIC ASSESSMENT

Assessment of pain in a child can be complicated by a number of factors, including the child's age and their life circumstances.

When assessing children, particularly a neonate, pre-verbal or non-verbal child, a combination of *physical cues*, such as posture and facial expression, as well as *parent/caregiver reports* will need to be evaluated. Rating scales, such as the *FLACC (Face, Legs, Activity, Cry, Consolability) scale* from the University of Michigan (see Table 13.3), are available for this purpose. It is important to use age-appropriate approaches, including the use of dolls and toys, which may have the added benefit of allowing the child to create some distance between themselves and the pain when there are personal circumstances that complicate the situation.

In the assessment of pain in older children, the child may *under-report* or *over-report* the pain, depending on their desire to please or gain attention. Children are often very good at non-verbal communication and, depending on their history, may seek to please or impress healthcare professionals by providing the 'right' answer rather than one that truly reflects their experience. This can manifest as either a *hero-like behaviour*, in which attention is gained for being stoic or denying pain, or a desire to *fulfil the expectations* of the healthcare professional as a way of gaining approval. In other instances, most notably in children with long-standing cancer pain, the child may seek to *protect their parents/caregivers* from the reality of their experience, knowing that the situation is very upsetting to their loved ones.

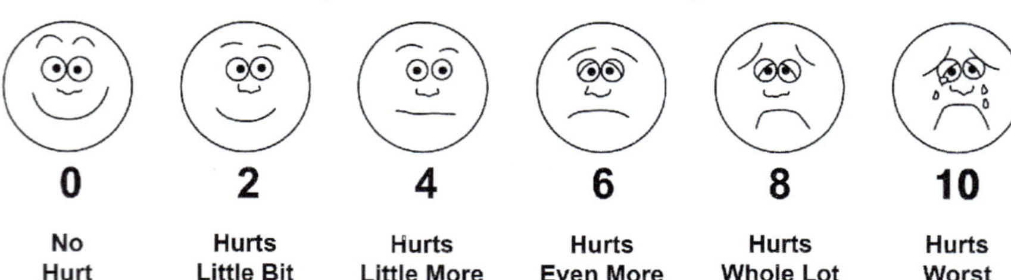

Figure 13.9

Wong-Baker FACES® Pain Rating Scale

Using a series of cartoons to represent a rating from 0 (no hurt) to 5 (hurts worse), the Wong–Baker face scale for pain is a simple, easy-to-use way of assessing pain. This scale should be used in conjunction with a pain assessment interview to determine the social, emotional and physical contexts associated with the person's pain experience.

Source: © 1983 Wong-Baker FACES Foundation. www.WongBakerFACES.org. Used with permission. Originally published in Whaley & Wong's Nursing Care of Infants and Children. © Elsevier Inc.

Table 13.2 The ABCs of pain management*

A	*Ask* about pain regularly. *Assess* pain systematically.
B	*Believe* the person and their family about reports of pain and what relieves it.
C	*Choose* pain control options appropriate for the person, family and setting.
D	*Deliver* interventions in a timely, logical and coordinated fashion.
E	*Empower* individuals and their families. *Enable* them to control their course to the greatest extent possible.

*These guidelines are taken from the US Agency for Health Care Policy and Research, as outlined by the Children's Pain Management Service of the Royal Children's Hospital in Melbourne, Australia.

For children experiencing domestic trauma, a desire for attention can skew their self-report of pain, with some children trapped in a situation where the only attention that they obtain from their parents or guardians is when they are in physical distress, causing some of these children to over-report their pain in order to obtain the love and attention they would not receive otherwise. Conversely, the child may deny pain in order to prevent being perceived as a problem. Additionally, it is not unusual for parents and/or caregivers to dismiss children's self-report of pain, particularly when there is no obvious injury. Unfortunately, all of these circumstances will markedly impede attempts to obtain an accurate picture of the child's pain.

PAIN AND MENTAL HEALTH

People with mental health conditions, such as schizophrenia or dementia, can be equally difficult to assess, as their perception of their situation and ability to report pain can be markedly impaired. They might not be able to articulate their experience, may be unable to report accurately on their experience due to memory lapses, or might confuse events that were painful in the past with current events. Although a number of tools are available to attempt to evaluate the pain experience, as yet there is no consensus on the approach to be taken or the reliability of any given tool over the others.

Table 13.3 The FLACC scale*

FLACC Scale	
FACE	
0	No particular expression or smile
1	Occasional grimace or frown, withdrawn, disinterested
2	Frequent to constant frown, clenching jaw, quivering chin
LEGS	
0	Normal position or relaxed
1	Uneasy, restless, tense
2	Kicking or legs drawn up
ACTIVITY	
0	Lying quietly, normal position, moves easily
1	Squirming, shifting back and forth, tense
2	Arched, rigid or jerking
CRY	
0	No cry (awake or asleep)
1	Moans or whimpers, occasional complaints
2	Crying steadily, screams or sobs, frequent complaints
CONSOLABILITY	
0	Content, relaxed
1	Reassured by occasional touching, hugging or 'talking to', distractable
2	Difficult to console or comfort

*This scale, developed by the University of Michigan Health System, makes use of both physical signs and behaviour to assist in the assessment of a child's pain.

Neuropathic pain

LEARNING OBJECTIVE 9

Describe how neuropathic pain differs from chronic pain.

The current widely accepted definition of **neuropathic pain** is pain initiated or caused by a *primary lesion or dysfunction in the somatosensory system*. Neuropathic pain can be generalised and symmetrical, or localised. Common conditions associated with neuropathic pain include post-herpetic neuralgia (i.e. shingles), trigeminal neuralgia, diabetic neuropathy, HIV infection, leprosy, amputation and stroke. Importantly, not all those who experience somatosensory nerve injury or dysfunction manifest this form of pain.

Neuropathic pain is not the same as other forms of chronic pain, such as that associated with chronic inflammation. Neuropathic pain is often described as burning or electrical-like in character, and non-painful stimuli, such as a light touch, can trigger it. As it persists, neuropathic pain responds less to conventional analgesics. As a result, the quality of life with neuropathic pain is more impaired than for those with other forms of pain.

Characteristically, there is an alteration of the electrical properties of somatosensory neurons. An imbalance between the inhibitory and excitatory transmission of nociceptive impulses develops, so that the descending and interneuronal inhibitory pathways decrease their capacity for pain modulation. Excitatory nociceptive signalling, particularly involving dorsal horn neurons and/or C-fibres, shows a gain in function. Nociceptive signalling becomes hyperexcitable. Alterations in sodium, calcium and potassium ion channels have been reported, with a loss of function of potassium channels and a gain in function of calcium and sodium channels. Imbalances in GABA (inhibitory) and glutamate (excitatory) have also been implicated.

The development of neuropathic pain has been linked to structural changes resulting from injury where signalling changes are induced by altered pathways and the establishment of inappropriate synapses. An example of this is the formation of ectopically active neuromas after injury or amputation. Unlike the central nervous system, the peripheral nervous system is capable of a degree of self-repair. The repair is effected by the creation of sprouts off the damaged neuron, which seek out and re-establish connection with the intended target tissue. Excess sprouts are then trimmed, and the myelin sheath is restored. Unfortunately, unconnected sprouts are not always eliminated, particularly when the target tissue is lost, such as in amputations. They can then establish synapses onto themselves, creating structures known as *neuromas*. Although some neuromas are benign, others will be altered in such a way as to send out spontaneous, regular action potentials known as *ectopic signals*, generally due to either instability in the membranes or changes in the structure or functioning of ion channels and receptors on the cell surface. If these neurons are C- or Aδ-fibres, the brain will interpret these signals as pain, and the person will experience an ongoing pain syndrome that is independent of any actual injury.

Attempts to reconnect a neuron with its target can also occur at the level of the dorsal horn. An injury to an incoming compound nerve can lead to loss of innervation from a nociceptive neuron like a C-fibre, and its replacement with a mechanical (Aβ) fibre (see Figure 13.10). The same form of sprouting can occur as seen with neuromas, but in this case the Aβ-fibre not only re-establishes its original connections, but a sprout will travel into the adjacent lamina to synapse inappropriately onto the ascending spinothalamic/spinoreticular neurons with which the C-fibres normally synapse. This will mean that all incoming mechanical signals from these Aβ-fibres will be interpreted in the brain as nociception, because it is the pattern from the lamina that is interpreted, not the identity of the peripheral neuron.

LEARNING OBJECTIVE 10

Explain the principle of wind-up, and the role it is thought to play in the development of neuropathic pain.

As mentioned previously, hyperalgesia and allodynia are a normal part of the non-productive pain process, and generally reverse as an injury heals. As part of the establishment of these states, a process called **wind-up** will occur in the spinal cord, and this has also been shown to occur in the brain. When the initial nociceptive signals access the synapses of the dorsal horn, the neurons are in what might be considered their natural state. As the number of signals through the synapses increases owing to the ongoing inflammatory and neurotransmitter-mediated increase in the sensitivity of the nociceptive neurons, a learning-like process occurs in the dorsal horn.

During the process of short-term memory formation, a synapse begins to change (remodel) in a process that strengthens the connection between two neurons. The repetitive signals through the presynaptic neuron trigger reciprocal changes in the two cells, increasing the ease with which the synapse can be activated. In wind-up, a similar process is thought to occur. The two cells involved in the synapse change the number and identity of the proteins at the synaptic cleft, increasing the *ease* with which the signals are transmitted and the *strength* of those signals at the postsynaptic cell. It is generally accepted that these changes can occur both at the level of the dorsal horn and in the brain, and that they should reverse once the injury has healed and the pressure on the cell to maintain the altered state is lost as the number of signals falls. In some forms of neuropathic pain, it appears that the wind-up becomes a permanent state, not unlike a short-term memory becoming a long-term memory. In this case, the pressure on the synapse to maintain the altered state is lost, but the alterations do not reverse, including a lowered threshold for activation, an increased number of receptors and/or ion channels, and a change in the identity of the protein complement of the cells.

PHANTOM LIMB PAIN

Phantom limb pain is *pain attributed to the missing limb*, usually in the most distal structures (e.g. fingers, toes), generally described as shooting, stabbing, pricking, boring, squeezing, throbbing and/or burning pain. The phantom limb experience is more likely to occur if there was pain in the tissues prior to amputation, and the phenomenon has been attributed to the sort of remodelling commonly associated with neuropathic pain; namely, changes in nerve threshold and the expression of different sodium channels that are either *more easily activated* or are *leak channels*. Sodium leak channels do not respond to changes in voltage like typical sodium channels. Their purpose is to maintain the resting membrane potential, and so the signal for firing is not an external environmental change, but rather is intrinsic to the channel's conformation. If they behave normally they can alter the nerve threshold for the firing of an action potential.

Interestingly, there is significant debate on the role of remodelling, as some evidence shows that the changes are in the brain and not in the periphery, with the thalamus and cortical structures more likely to be implicated. However, there is evidence for changes in the responsiveness of *N*-methyl-D-aspartate (NMDA) glutamate channels in the spinal cord as well. Many amputees are known to have temperature intolerances, depending on whether the C- or Aδ-fibres are responsible for the additional discharges that are linked to their pain experience.

SYMPATHETIC CAUSALGIA

Sympathetic causalgia is a condition of *burning pain* associated with changes in sympathetic signalling. Normally, sympathetic nerve activity has little or no effect on nociceptive signalling. However, a condition of altered responsiveness can occur, which appears due, at least in part, to the *sprouting of sympathetic fibres* at the site of injury, particularly in the dorsal root ganglia and in partially denervated skin. This response appears to be mediated primarily by α_2-adrenergic receptors on injured sensory neurons, leading to activation of these neurons by sympathetic activity to initiate ectopic firing. The ability of sympathetic signalling to trigger nociception and pain is in direct contrast to normal signalling, as spinally injected adrenergic agonists have an analgesic effect. Normally, adrenergic agonists synergise with the opioid agonist to provide a profound analgesic effect, and the descending inhibitory pathways from the locus coeruleus use noradrenaline as a neurotransmitter.

TRIGEMINAL NEURALGIA

Trigeminal neuralgia is a syndrome marked by *episodic unilateral facial pain* that is excruciating and characterised by piercing or

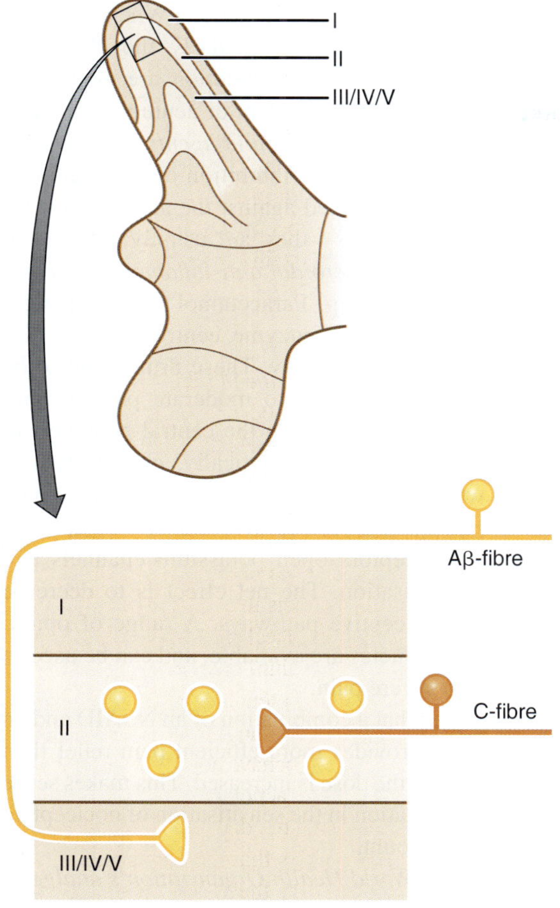

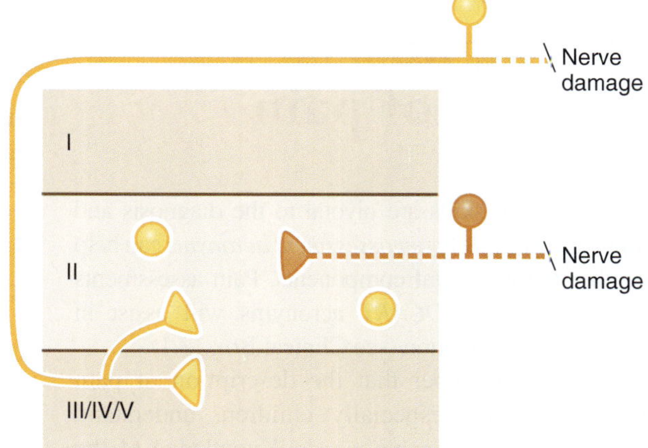

Normal arrangement
Dorsal horn
Normal termination pattern

Hypersensitive arrangement
C-fibre terminal atrophy
Aδ-fibre sprouting
Interneuron degeneration

Figure 13.10

Inappropriate synapse formation in the dorsal horn subsequent to nerve injury

Injury to a compound nerve can lead to reconnection of only some neurons within that nerve and, hence, inappropriate synapse formation. As seen here, injury to a compound nerve can result in failure of the C-fibre to re-establish connection with its ascending fibres, while the mechanical Aβ-fibre might not only reconnect with its ascending fibre but also infiltrate the space left by the C-fibre, resulting in an inappropriate synapse with the ascending fibres from lamina II. In this case, the mechanical information from the Aβ-fibre will now be interpreted by the brain as pain, because the brain relies on the pattern from the dorsal horn and not the identity of the peripheral neurons per se to identify the nature of the incoming signals.

Source: Adapted from McMahon et al. (2013).

stabbing sensations, although bilateral conditions have been reported. The frequency of episodes varies widely from a few seconds occasionally to hundreds of attacks each day, with normal daily tasks such as smiling, chewing, teeth-brushing and shaving acting as triggers. While the underlying cause is unknown, there is evidence for *focal demyelination of the trigeminal nerve root*, allowing cross-talk between axons and, therefore, ectopic activity. Vascular compression of the nerve has been shown to trigger demyelination, while viral infections have been implicated based on comparison with pain syndromes secondary to herpes zoster (shingles) infections.

It is important to note that demyelination is not the only cause associated with trigeminal neuralgia. *Other factors* include infiltration by amyloid, arteriovenous malformations, bony compression and small infarcts in the pons and medulla. The statistics are skewed, with females more likely than males to experience this condition (ratio of 1.5:1), with a peak incidence of between 60 and 70 years of age, although cases in significantly younger people have been reported. Those with hypertension are more likely to experience trigeminal neuralgia than those with normotensive blood pressure.

CLINICAL BOX 13.1

Pain assessment acronyms

PQRST	OLDCART
P—Provokes (or Palliates)	O— Onset
Q—Quality	L—Location
R—Region (or Radiation)	D—Duration
S—Severity	C—Characteristics
T—Timing	A—Aggravating factors (or Associated factors)
	R—Relieving factors
	T—Treatment

Clinical diagnosis and management of pain

DIAGNOSIS

Thorough pain assessment skills are pivotal to the diagnosis and management of pain. The use of *pain assessment acronyms* can help someone remember the important components. Pain assessments using the *PQRST* or the *OLDCART* acronyms will assist in gathering the necessary information (see Clinical Box 13.1).

It is important to remember that the description of pain is very *subjective*. People, especially children, understand or associate pain with very *specific words*. Knowledge of the various ways pain can be described is beneficial to truly assess a person's pain, as they may deny pain, but, when questioned specifically, they might agree that they have discomfort, burning or tightness, for example. This subjective description may mask a physiological issue needing intervention.

During pain assessment, providing words to help the person explain their pain may be beneficial. Some examples of words used to describe a sensation that may be understood by health professionals as pain include:

- aching
- burning
- cold
- cramping
- crushing
- discomfort
- dull
- gnawing
- hurting
- intense
- numb
- pinching
- pressure
- pulsing
- radiating
- searing
- sharp
- shooting
- smarting
- sore
- stabbing
- stinging
- tender
- throbbing
- tightness
- uncomfortable
- wrenching.

MANAGEMENT

The key to pain management is evaluation. When *the pain report is matched to treatment*, particularly the choice of analgesic drugs, problems such as addiction are negligible. Standard drugs used in the management of acute pain include non-opoid and opioid agents. *Non-opioid agents* act to reduce nociceptive signalling through the inhibition of prostaglandin synthesis. Their action is directed against the action of cyclo-oxygenase (COX) isoenzymes—they are usually referred to as *COX inhibitors*. The *non-steroidal anti-inflammatory drugs (NSAIDs)* belong to this group. Paracetamol is also thought to act by inhibiting a COX isoenzyme centrally, but it has negligible anti-inflammatory activity. These drugs tend to be used in the management of mild to moderate pain. *Opioid drugs*, act on opioid mu-receptors in the central pathways to alter the perception of pain. Presynatically, opioids reduce c-AMP levels which inhibit the opening voltage-gated calcium channels that would lead to neurotransmitter release. Postsynaptically mu-receptors open potassium channels and cause nerve hyperpolarisation. The net effect is to decrease transmission along nociceptive pathways. A range of opioid drugs with different potencies are available, and can be used to alleviate moderate to severe pain.

It is well recognised that a combination of an NSAID and an opioid analgesic often provides more efficient pain relief than either drug alone, even if the dose is increased. This makes sense when the role of inflammation in the sensitisation of nociceptive neurons is taken into account.

For cancer pain, the *World Health Organization's analgesic ladder* (see Figure 13.11) is valuable.

Neuropathic pain is notoriously difficult to treat, largely because this type of pain tends to be intractable to opioid analgesics and NSAIDs. First-line adjuvant therapies include antidepressants and antiseizure medications. These medications are believed to improve the balance between the inhibitory and excitatory nociceptive pathways. Antidepressants and related agents alter the central nervous system's availability of the monamines, serotonin and noradrenaline, to enhance the descending inhibitory modulation from the brainstem. The antiseizure drugs can alter the responsiveness of ion channels, GABA and glutamate availability.

Pain can also be managed non-pharmacologically with heat, cold, electrical stimulation, bracing and positioning, or interventions such as providing distraction, music or guided imagery. Helping someone with relaxation techniques may also be beneficial. Exercise can also be considered a *non-pharmacological intervention*.

The use of *thermal modalities* such as the application of heat or cold have various influences. Topical heat can help reduce the impulse speed of nerve fibres, promote muscle relaxation, and increase blood vessel diameter to facilitate interstitial drainage and 'wash out' the damaged region of inflammatory mediators. The application of cold can result in vasoconstriction, which can reduce haemorrhage, the accumulation of inflammatory mediators and swelling. Cold can also influence the speed of nerve conduction.

Transcutaneous electrical nerve stimulation (TENS) is thought to affect nociception through the inhibition of impulse propagation along C-fibres, effectively 'shutting the gate' at the presynaptic level in the dorsal horn. TENS can also result in the release of some endogenous analgesic agents, such as endorphins and enkephalin.

Exercise can also cause the release of endorphins, although some studies have demonstrated no correlation between pain control and the amount of pain reported. The other mechanism by which exercise may inhibit pain is through activation of large afferent fibres 'closing the gate' and inhibiting afferent pain impulses.

In the early stages of an injury, *bracing and positioning* can help to support the affected area and reduce inflammation, which will ultimately reduce pain. However, immobilisation should not continue for too long, as muscle atrophy and other orthopaedic effects may actually exacerbate injury and delay recovery.

The *neuropsychological influences of pain modulation* can be powerful if practised and psychologically accepted by the person in pain. Distraction, guided imagery and music can reduce a person's focus and attention on the pain. As previously discussed, pain modulation occurs within the thalamic and hypothalamic regions and limbic systems. Nociceptive input must be processed as pain; influence over this area's function can assist the emotional and behavioural components of pain perception.

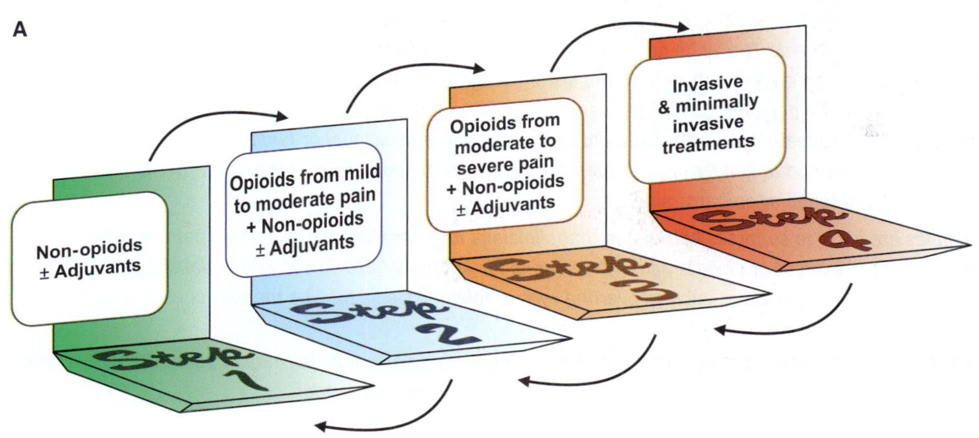

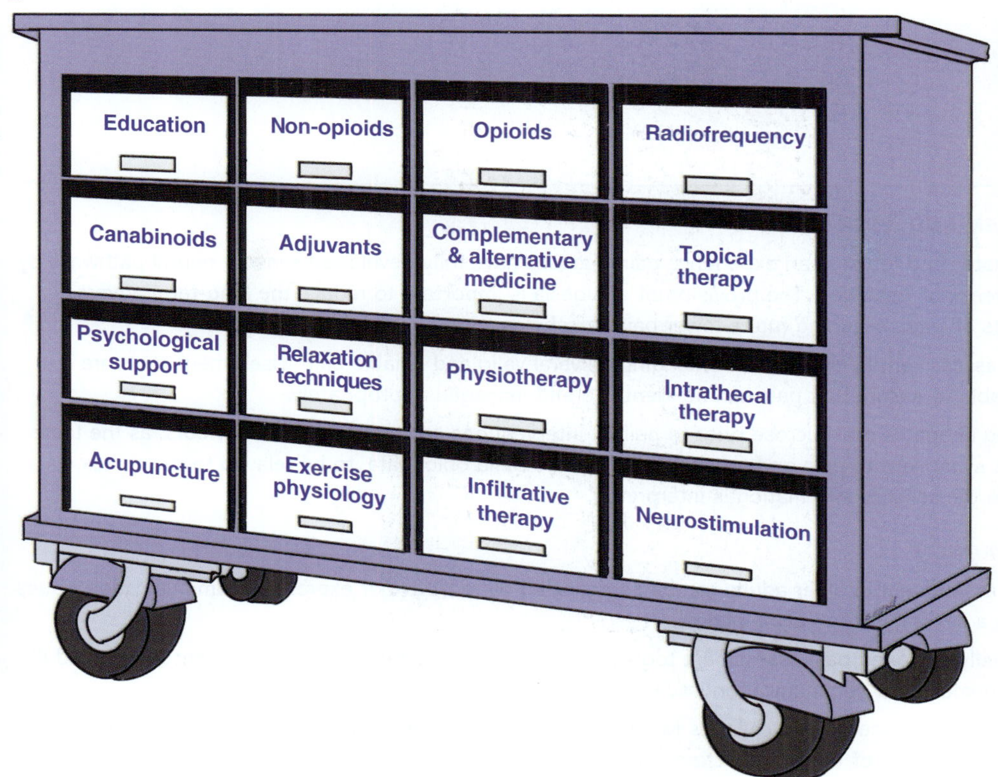

Figure 13.11

(A) Modified WHO analgesic ladder; and (B) analgesic trolley for pain management

The use of the World Health Organization's (WHO) analgesic ladder begins with the evaluation of the pain experience. The choice of analgesic is then based on the level at which the person is experiencing pain, with step 1 representing mild pain, step 2 mild to moderate pain, and step 3 moderate to severe pain. The lowest dose of the relevant analgesics for that step are then used, and the dose titrated until satisfactory analgesia is achieved. More recently, a fourth step has been suggested when analgesia cannot be achieved. It involves minimally invasive and invasive treatments, including epidural or intrathecal analgesic, local anaesthetics or even neurosurgical procedures such as cordotomy, nerve blocks or ablative procedures. This second model suggests an analgesic trolley model for pain management.

Sources: Adapted from Anekar & Cascella (2022); Cuomo et al. (2019).

INDIGENOUS HEALTH FAST FACTS AND CULTURAL CONSIDERATIONS

FAST FACTS

- *Statistics on pain are difficult to obtain. However, it is reported that Aboriginal and Torres Strait Islander peoples experience painful, long-term musculoskeletal diseases such as back pain, osteoarthritis and rheumatoid arthritis 1.2–1.5 times more than non-Indigenous Australians.*
- *Aboriginal and Torres Strait Islander women are slightly less likely than non-Indigenous women to receive pain relief during labour. Indigenous mothers have fewer interventions than non-Indigenous mothers, and are 14 times more likely to live in a remote or very remote area. 'Birthing on Country' rates are increasing and have been shown to be a positive experience for mothers and babies.*
- *Māori women are less likely non-Māori New Zealand women to be given analgesia for childbirth.*
- *Some disparities appear to affect access to pain medicines for Māori compared to non-Māori New Zealanders with lung cancer in palliative care. Access to these medicines for the former was more likely two weeks before death, and less likely more than 24 weeks prior to death.*

CULTURAL CONSIDERATIONS

- *There are many languages in Aboriginal and Torres Strait Islander cultures. Some words for pain include pika, kwarneme, badarratjun and utyene. Sharp pain may be known as wakani or antantheme. It may be necessary and beneficial to utilise the services of professional interpreters. However, an understanding that, due to the diverse cultural and linguistic backgrounds and relationships between communities, there is potential for distrust between the person requiring care and the professional interpreter. Issues of health professionals listening carefully and showing respect greatly influence treatment outcomes. Non-professional or family interpreters may be helpful; however, there may be some health topics related to gender or age differences between the person requiring care and the interpreting family member that may be considered taboo or embarrassing.*
- *Aboriginal and Torres Strait Islander peoples are likely to suppress behaviours that clinicians may normally use to identify pain, making pain assessment difficult. They may be reluctant to express or discuss pain. When caring for Aboriginal and Torres Strait Islander peoples, astute observation for culturally specific pain behaviour nuances, such as averting eyes or feigning sleep, may be the only cues to assist in pain assessment.*

  It is important to be aware that the protocols surrounding 'men's and women's business' may present as barriers to pain assessment, and it is important to ask whether a person would prefer to speak with a healthcare professional of their own gender.

Sources: Data from Arthur & Rolan (2019); Australian Indigenous HealthInfoNet (2021; Australian Institute of Health and Welfare (2020a); Gurney et al. (2021); New Zealand Ministry of Health (2016); O'Brien et al. (2020); Queensland Health (2015).

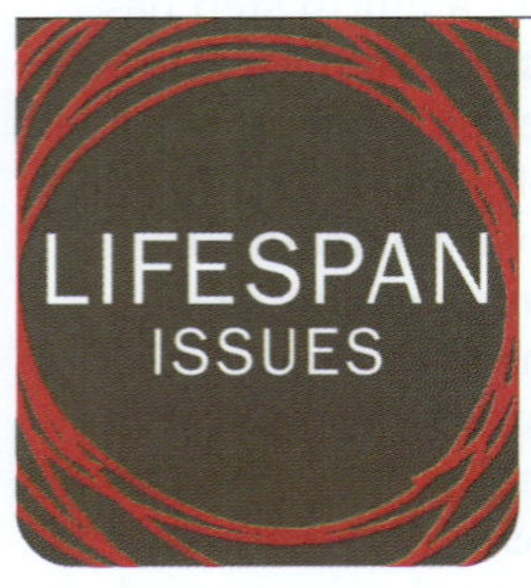

CHILDREN AND ADOLESCENTS

- Neonates and fetuses can experience pain. Fetuses have fully developed sensory neural pathways by 22 weeks of gestation. The provision of analgesia is important to reduce the long-term adverse effects of pain, including future lower pain thresholds.
- Pain assessment in children is challenging. Several valid and reliable pain assessment tools are available to ensure that pain can be identified and managed appropriately.
- Giving neonates oral sucrose prior to painful interventions can reduce pain behaviours, as the taste fibres synapse with pain and touch fibres in the medulla oblongata, to be relayed to the cortex, where the sensory information is interpreted.

OLDER ADULTS

- Pain assessment in older adults can be complicated by receptive or expressive communication issues or by a decline in cognitive function.
- Specially designed pain assessment tools are available to assist with pain assessment in older adults with dementia or communication issues.
- Polypharmacy, age-related changes to pharmacokinetics, and environmental issues can result in a higher incidence of adverse reactions or even toxicity with pain medication.

KEY CLINICAL ISSUES

- Pain is what the individual says it is. As pain is subjective and no specific objective indicators may occur when someone is experiencing pain, the clinician should, in most circumstances, assume that the person is expressing a legitimate experience.
- People from different cultures may have culture-specific needs for assessment and management; however, all individuals experience pain in their own way, irrespective of cultural stereotypes.
- Special populations make the assessment of pain more complex. People with communication, cognitive decline and mental health issues require special attention to detail and the use of appropriate pain assessment tools. Neonates, children and adolescents also present unique difficulties in the assessment of pain.
- Analgesia must be provided to reduce or relieve pain as soon as possible. Prolonged pain can cause adverse physical, psychological, emotional and social effects.
- Various methods of pain relief exist in not only pharmacological agents but also non-pharmacological methods of pain relief, such as position, heat, cold, pressure and transcutaneous electrical nerve stimulation, and adjuvant drugs, such as tricyclic antidepressants and some serotonin-reuptake inhibitors.

CHAPTER REVIEW

- Pain fibres travel from the periphery to the dorsal horn of the spinal cord and via *ascending (afferent) fibres* through the *spinothalamic and spinoreticular tracts* to the brainstem.
- *Substance P* and *glutamate* are two important *neurotransmitters* associated with nociception.
- *Descending inhibitory pathways* and *interneurons* within the dorsal horn can modulate pain signals.
- *Endogenous opioid peptides* can also influence pain signals.
- The *Pain Gate Theory* proposes that incoming nociceptive signals on Aδ- and C-fibres can be blocked by signals on Aβ-fibres.
- *Pressure and massage* can initiate signals on Aβ-fibres.
- *Age-appropriate pain assessment* is important to ensure that accurate judgments are made and interventions enacted.
- *Neuropathic pain* is caused by somatosensory nerves that have incompletely or incorrectly healed.
- *Trigeminal neuralgia* causes piercing or stabbing facial pain. Trigeminal neuralgia is usually unilateral.
- The World Health Organization has developed an *analgesia ladder* to guide the management of mild through to severe pain.

REVIEW QUESTIONS

1. What is the difference between Aδ-, Aβ- and C-fibres? Create a table with a column for each fibre type. Describe the speed of transmission, whether it is myelinated or unmyelinated, and whether it has a large or small axon.
2. What is the difference between nociception and pain?
3. What does hyperalgesia mean? Give an example.
4. What does allodynia mean? Give an example.
5. How do hyperalgesia and allodynia play a role in nociceptive signalling?
6. What is the difference between productive and non-productive pain?
7. How can knowledge of the Pain Gate Theory influence clinical pain management practices?
8. Which pain management interventions/equipment utilise the principles from the Pain Gate Theory?
9. What are the major differences between neuropathic pain and other chronic pain?
10. Briefly outline the pathogenesis of neuropathic pain.
11. In relation to neuropathic pain, what is the principle of wind-up? Explain.

HEALTH PROFESSIONAL CONNECTIONS

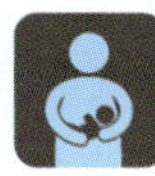

Midwives Pain associated with the first stages of labour is generally as a result of lower uterine segment distension, dilation of the cervix and uterine contraction. This pain is associated with sympathetic nerve fibres in spinal segments T10–L1, and is thought to be carried by the unmyelinated C-fibres. Pain in the second stage of labour results from pressure and traction on the muscles of the pelvic floor, as well as the uterus, bladder, rectum and peritoneum. Myelinated Aδ-fibres transmit this impulse rapidly along the pudendal nerve through nerve fibres in spinal segments S2–S4. Analgesia for labour pain may include inhaled agents, opioid agents, transcutaneous electrical nerve stimulation or blocks. Depending on the route and the agent, transplacental transfer of most analgesic agents is possible. It is important to observe for neonatal respiratory depression where appropriate.

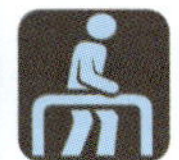

Physiotherapists Physiotherapists can play a pivotal role in the management of pain, especially when the underlying cause of the pain is musculoskeletal. An important principle when working with people who have chronic pain includes going *low and slow*. Gradual increases in load, duration and intensity can reduce the risk of exacerbating pain conditions. Some therapies may include posture awareness and body mechanics education, strengthening and flexibility exercises, and potentially even manual therapy and massage. The use of ultrasound, heat/cold therapy, and even electrical simulation using transcutaneous electrical nerve stimulation (TENS) may be beneficial. It is important to educate the person regarding the potential for some increased pain at the beginning of the process, and the importance of being able to differentiate the type and quality of their own pain to help guide the physiotherapist's understanding so that modifications can be made as necessary.

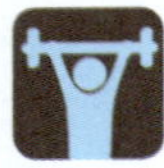

Exercise scientists Some people believe that excessive pain is required to achieve physical advantage. The phrase 'No pain, no gain' can be very dangerous in the exercise and rehabilitation environment. Exercise professionals need to ensure that those with whom they work understand that many factors will influence the amount of discomfort that an individual will experience when undertaking a training or rehabilitation program. Pain may take many forms, including discomfort from stretching, delayed-onset muscle soreness, discomfort caused from aerobic exercise, or even pain caused by injury. It is important to ensure that communication between the client and the exercise or rehabilitation professional provides opportunities to distinguish between the identification of necessary discomfort and the prevention of pain and injury. Discuss measures to reduce intra- and post-exercise discomfort, and ensure that unexpected, severe or chronic pain is investigated further by people who are appropriately qualified. Exercise can reduce pain and improve health, so it is important that people don't have experiences that may prevent them from wanting to undertake an appropriately planned and executed training or rehabilitation program.

Nutritionists/Dieticians The relationship between pain and nutrition is complex, inter-related and powerful. When someone experiences injury or pain, they usually become anorexic, yet in such times the body requires good nutrition to promote healing and reduce stress. A few essential fatty acids are known to be effective in reducing inflammation and maintaining nerve fibres. Essential nutrients refer to nutrients that must be consumed in the diet as they cannot be produced in the body. Omega-3 fatty acids are found in fish oils, and are known to reduce inflammation and influence the progression of cardiovascular and joint diseases. Omega-6 fatty acids are found in soy, canola and sunflower oils, and are known to reduce diabetic neuropathy and inflammation from joint disorders. Antioxidants to reduce oxidative stress and inflammation and pain are found in fruit and vegetables high in vitamins C, E and beta-carotene.

CASE STUDY

Mr Daniel Jenkins (UR number 459135) is an 86-year-old man presenting with herpes zoster and post-herpetic neuralgia (PHN). He was admitted four days ago with severe pain uncontrolled by simple analgesic agents. His most recent observations are as follows:

Temperature	Heart rate	Respiration rate	Blood pressure	SpO_2
37.2°C	88	26	158/90	96% (RA*)

*RA = room air.

On assessment, Mr Jenkins has several erythematous vesicular lesions on his left torso running down along the dermatomes on his chest. He also has some smaller lesions on his neck. His pathology results are as follows:

HAEMATOLOGY

Patient location:	Ward 3	**UR:**	459135		
Consultant:	Smith	**NAME:**	Jenkins		
		Given name:	Daniel	**Sex:**	M
		DOB:	12/12/XX	**Age:**	86

Time collected	09:30
Date collected	XX/XX
Year	XXXX
Lab #	67636546

FULL BLOOD COUNT		UNITS	REFERENCE RANGE
Haemoglobin	143	g/L	115–160
White cell count	17.3	$\times 10^9$/L	4.0–11.0
Platelets	289	$\times 10^9$/L	140–400

Haematocrit	0.41		0.33–0.47
Red cell count	4.23	$\times 10^{12}$/L	3.80–5.20
Reticulocyte count	1.8	%	0.2–2.0
MCV	88	fL	80–100
Neutrophils	10.1	$\times 10^{9}$/L	2.00–8.00
Lymphocytes	2.96	$\times 10^{9}$/L	1.00–4.00
Monocytes	0.38	$\times 10^{9}$/L	0.10–1.00
Eosinophils	0.28	$\times 10^{9}$/L	< 0.60
Basophils	0.09	$\times 10^{9}$/L	< 0.20
ESR	13	mm/h	< 12

BIOCHEMISTRY

Patient location:	Ward 3	**UR:**	459135		
Consultant:	Smith	**NAME:**	Jenkins		
		Given name:	Daniel	**Sex:**	M
		DOB:	12/12/XX	**Age:**	86

Time collected	09:30
Date collected	XX/XX
Year	XXXX
Lab #	3453453

ELECTROLYTES		UNITS	REFERENCE RANGE
Sodium	136	mmol/L	135–145
Potassium	3.9	mmol/L	3.5–5.2
Chloride	99	mmol/L	95–110
Bicarbonate	24	mmol/L	22–32
Glucose	5.3	mmol/L	3.5–5

CRITICAL THINKING

1. How did Mr Jenkins's post-herpetic neuralgia (PHN) start? Explain the mechanism for the development of PHN.
2. Mr Jenkins's pain is not controlled with simple analgesia. Using the World Health Organization's analgesic ladder, identify the next options, and describe the mechanism of action for each of the options identified.
3. Look at Mr Jenkins's observations. Are these observations to be expected in someone with pain? Compare and contrast the effects of pain on the physical observations. Should a clinician rely solely on physical observations to determine whether a person is reporting the pain truthfully? Discuss.
4. If Mr Jenkins was taking the beta-blocker metoprolol for hypertension, would this influence his physical observations? Identify and explain the mechanism of at least four different types of medications that may influence physical observations and therefore complicate pain assessment.
5. What further interventions may assist Mr Jenkins? (Consider all aspects of his presentation and the disease process. Extend your response beyond pharmacological agents.)

BIBLIOGRAPHY

Anekar, A.A. & Cascella, M. (2022). WHO Analgesic Ladder. *StatPearls*. https://www.ncbi.nlm.nih. gov/books/NBK554435/.

Arthur, L. & Rolan, P. (2019). A systematic review of western medicine's understanding of pain experience, expression, assessment, and management for Australian Aboriginal and Torres Strait Islander people. *Pain Reports* 4(6):e764. http://dx.doi.org/10.1097/PR9.0000000000000764.

Australian Commission on Safety and Quality in Health Care (ACSQHC) (2022). Opioid analgesic stewardship in acute pain clinical care standard. Sydney: ACSQHC. https://www.safetyandquality.gov.au/standards/clinical-care-standards/opioid-analgesic-stewardship-acute-pain-clinical-care-standard.

Australian Health Ministers' Advisory Council's National and Aboriginal and Torres Strait Islander Health Standing Committee (2017). *Cultural respect framework 2016–2026: for Aboriginal and Torres Strait Islander health—a national approach to building a culturally respectful health system*. Canberra: Australian Government Department of Health. https://nacchocommunique.files.wordpress.com/2016/12/cultural_respect_framework_1december2016_1.pdf.

Australian Indigenous Health*Info*Net (2022). *Overview of Aboriginal and Torres Strait Islander health status, 2021*. Perth, WA: Australian Indigenous Health*Info*Net. https://healthinfonet.ecu.edu.au/learn/health-facts/overview-aboriginal-torres-strait-islander-health-status.

Australian Institute of Health and Welfare (AIHW) (2020a). *Australia's mothers and babies, 2018: in brief.* Perinatal Statistics series No. 36. Cat. No. PER 108. Canberra: AIHW. https://www.aihw.gov.au/getmedia/aa54e74a-bda7-4497-93ce-e0010cb66231/aihw-per-108.pdf.aspx?inline=true.

Australian Institute of Health and Welfare (AIHW) (2020b). *Chronic pain in Australia.* Cat. No. PHE 267. Canberra: AIHW. https://www.aihw.gov.au/getmedia/10434b6f-2147-46ab-b654-a90f05592d35/aihw-phe-267.pdf.aspx?inline=true.

Bauldoff, G., Gubrud-Howe, P.M., Carno, M.-A., Levett-Jones, T., Hales, M., Berry, K.,… LeMone, P. (2020). *LeMone and Burke's medical–surgical nursing: critical thinking for person-centred care* (4th [Australian] edn). Sydney: Pearson Australia.

Best, O. & Fredericks, B. (2021). *Yatdjuligin: Aboriginal and Torres Strait Islander nursing and midwifery care* (3rd edn). Port Melbourne, VIC: Cambridge University Press.

Bullock, S. & Manias, E. (2022). *Fundamentals of pharmacology* (9th edn). Sydney: Pearson Australia.

Cuomo, A., Bimonte, S., Forte, C.A., Botti, G. & Cascella, M. (2019). Multimodal approaches and tailored therapies for pain management: the trolley analgesic model. *Journal of Pain Research* 12:711–14. https://doi.org/10.2147/JPR.S178910.

Gurney, J.K., Stanley, J., Adler, J., McLeod, H., Atkinson, J. & Sarfati, D. (2021). National study of pain medicine access among Māori and non-Māori patients with lung cancer in New Zealand. *JCO Global Oncology* 7:1276–85. https://doi.org/10.1200/GO.21.00141.

Marieb, E.N. & Hoehn, K. (2019). *Human anatomy and physiology* (11th edn). San Francisco, CA: Pearson Benjamin Cummings.

McMahon, S.B., Koltzenburg, M., Tracey, I. & Turk, D.C. (2013). *Wall and Melzack's textbook of pain*. Philadelphia, PA: Elsevier Saunders.

Morgan, K.J. & Anghelescu, D.L. (2017). A review of adult and pediatric neuropathic pain assessment tools. *Clinical Journal of Pain* 33(9):844–52. https://doi.org/10.1097/AJP.0000000000000476.

Nestler, E.J., Hyman, S.E., Holtzman, D.M. & Malenka, R.C. (2015). *Molecular neuropharmacology: a foundation for clinical neuroscience* (3rd edn). NewYork: McGraw Hill.

New Zealand Ministry of Health (2016). *Health loss in New Zealand 1990–2013: A report from the New Zealand Burden of Diseases, Injuries and Risk Factors Study*. Wellington: Ministry of Health. https://www.health.govt.nz/system/files/documents/publications/health-loss-in-new-zealand-1990-2013-aug16.pdf.

O'Brien, P., Bunzli, S., Lin, I., Gunatillake, T., Bessarab, D., Coffin, J., … Choong, P. (2020). Tackling the burden of osteoarthritis as a health care opportunity in Indigenous communities—a call to action (editorial). *Journal of Clinical Medicine* 9(8):2393. https://doi.org/10.3390/jcm9082393.

Queensland Health (2015). *Sad news, sorry business: guidelines for caring for Aboriginal and Torres Strait Islander people through death and dying.* Brisbane: Queensland Health. https://www.health.qld.gov.au/__data/assets/pdf_file/0023/151736/sorry_business.pdf.

Rang, H.P., Ritter, J.M., Flower, R.J. & Henderson, G. (2016). *Rang and Dale's pharmacology* (8th edn) Edinburgh: Churchill Livingstone.

Veizi, E. & Hayek, S.M. (2017). Chapter 71: spinal cord stimulation: implantation techniques. *Anesthesia Key*. https://aneskey.com/spinal-cord-stimulation-implantation-techniques-2/.

Wong-Baker FACES Foundation (2018). *Wong-Baker FACES® Pain Rating Scale*. http://www.WongBakerFACES.org.

Yang, J., Bauer, B.A., Wahner-Roedler, D.L., Chon, T.Y. & Xiao, L. (2020). The modified WHO analgesic ladder: is it appropriate for chronic non-cancer pain? *Journal of Pain Research* 13:411–417. https://doi.org/10.2147/JPR.S244173.

14 Disorders of the special senses

LEARNING OBJECTIVES

After completing this chapter, you should be able to:

1 Discuss the various causes of vision impairment.

2 Differentiate between myopia and hyperopia.

3 Explore the pathophysiology, manifestations and management of common vision disorders, including cataracts, glaucoma, maculopathy, diabetic retinopathy and colour blindness.

4 Describe the pathophysiology, manifestations and management of conjunctivitis.

5 Briefly discuss the most common causes of acquired hearing loss.

6 Explore some congenital causes of hearing loss.

7 Analyse the association between hearing and balance.

KEY TERMS

Age-related maculopathy
Cataracts
Colour blindness
Conjunctivitis
Diabetic retinopathy
Glaucoma
Hyperopia
Intraocular pressure
Labyrinthitis
Myopia
Presbycusis
Tinnitus

WHAT YOU SHOULD KNOW BEFORE YOU START THIS CHAPTER

Can you identify the major parts of the eye, and describe their functions?

Can you describe how a visual image is converted into a representation that can be interpreted by the cortex?

Can you identify the major parts of the ear, and describe their functions?

Can you name the components of conduction, and those of neural transmission of sound?

Can you outline how balance is achieved by the nervous system?

Can you identify the structures and describe the mechanisms that contribute to balance?

Introduction

The *sensory system* is responsible for monitoring our environment, both internal and external, and detecting change. The special senses we refer to here are vision, hearing and equilibrium. The receptor systems for the special senses are distinctive because they are localised to the head and are relatively complex structures. Our perception of the world is greatly influenced by the information provided by these senses. Impairments of these senses, especially vision and hearing, can have a significant effect on a person's quality of life.

In this chapter, common disorders affecting the special senses are described, with a focus on vision, hearing and equilibrium.

Vision impairment

LEARNING OBJECTIVE 1

Discuss the various causes of vision impairment.

The eye is the receptor system involved in the processing of visual information. The function of the eye is to bend the light entering it so that it can be focused on the neural layer—the retina—on its posterior wall. Photoreceptors incorporated into the structure of the retina convert the light received into the language of the nervous system—nerve impulses. The impulses are transmitted along visual pathways into the cerebral cortex of the occipital lobe. Here the information is interpreted, reference is made to past visual experience, and an appropriate set of responses is activated. Figure 14.1 explores the common clinical manifestations and management of visual pathologies. In Figure 14.2, the effects of various common visual impairments are demonstrated using the same image.

In this section, the discussion is restricted to common disorders affecting the eye itself, including myopia and hyperopia, cataracts, glaucoma, age-related maculopathy, diabetic retinopathy, colour blindness and conjunctivitis. Almost 54% of Australians have one or more conditions affecting their eyesight: 28% have hyperopia, 25% have myopia, 2% are colour-blind. In Australians 65 years and older, 9.1% have cataracts, 3.6% have glaucoma, and 4.5% have macular degeneration. Figure 14.2 represents the effect that some of these conditions can have on vision and acuity.

MYOPIA AND HYPEROPIA

LEARNING OBJECTIVE 2

Differentiate between myopia and hyperopia.

Aetiology and pathophysiology

Myopia and hyperopia are vision disorders characterised by a refractive error as to where the eye focuses light in relation to the retina (see Figure 14.3). In **myopia**, or near-sightedness, the focal point is in front of the plane of the retina, causing an object in the distance to be out of focus. However, near objects appear in focus. In **hyperopia** (far-sightedness, long-sightedness or hypermetropia), the focal point is behind the plane of the retina so that a near object is viewed out of focus. Generally, far objects appear in focus, but this is not always the case.

Abnormal focal length can be due to an error in the refractive surfaces of the eye, particularly the cornea and lens, or in the length of the eyeball along its long axis (axial length). The *axial length* is increased in myopia and decreased in hyperopia. The degree of error is measured in units known as *diopters*, which are a measure of the reciprocal length of the focal length in metres. In myopia, the more negative the diopters, the more severe the degree of short-sightedness. In hyperopia, the more severe condition is measured in positive diopter units. Both myopia and hyperopia are classified in terms of severity: a low, medium or high degree of *refractive error*.

Clinical manifestations

Common clinical manifestations of hyperopia include blurred or dim vision, poor accommodation, eye strain and squinting. Myopia is characterised by blurred distance vision, but good near vision (see Figure 14.2B).

Diagnosis and management

The diagnosis of refractive errors is determined by eye examination. Each eye may have a different degree of refractive capacity, so both eyes are tested for visual acuity, accommodative function, curvature of eye structures and the reflection of light off the retina. Refractive errors in vision are treated by the wearing of corrective lenses (see Figure 14.3), such as eyeglasses or contact lenses, and/or by refractive surgery. The lenses are individually manufactured according to a prescription to suit the degree of refractive error in the person's eye/s.

Refractive surgery is directed at reshaping the surface of the cornea, usually with a laser, to correct the error. An example of this form of surgery is the laser-assisted sub-epithelial keratomileusis (LASEK) procedure.

CATARACT

LEARNING OBJECTIVE 3

Explore the pathophysiology, manifestations and management of common vision disorders, including cataracts, glaucoma, maculopathy, diabetic retinopathy and colour blindness.

Aetiology and pathophysiology

Cataracts are associated with an increasing *opacity*, or clouding, of the lens (see Figure 14.4A). Cataract development causes vision impairment, which can eventually lead to blindness. The condition may develop as a result of the ageing process, exposure to drugs or radiation, traumatic injury (e.g. blunt trauma, a penetrating eye injury or even eye surgery), or it can arise congenitally. Cataracts can also develop secondary to another disease, such as diabetes mellitus, hypothyroidism or glaucoma.

The structure of the lens is organised into a *lens fibre layer*, an *anterior epithelial layer* and an *outer capsule*. The lens epithelial cells have a homeostatic function. They lie between the lens fibres and capsule, and synthesise the other two layers. The capsule surrounds the lens and consists of collagen and

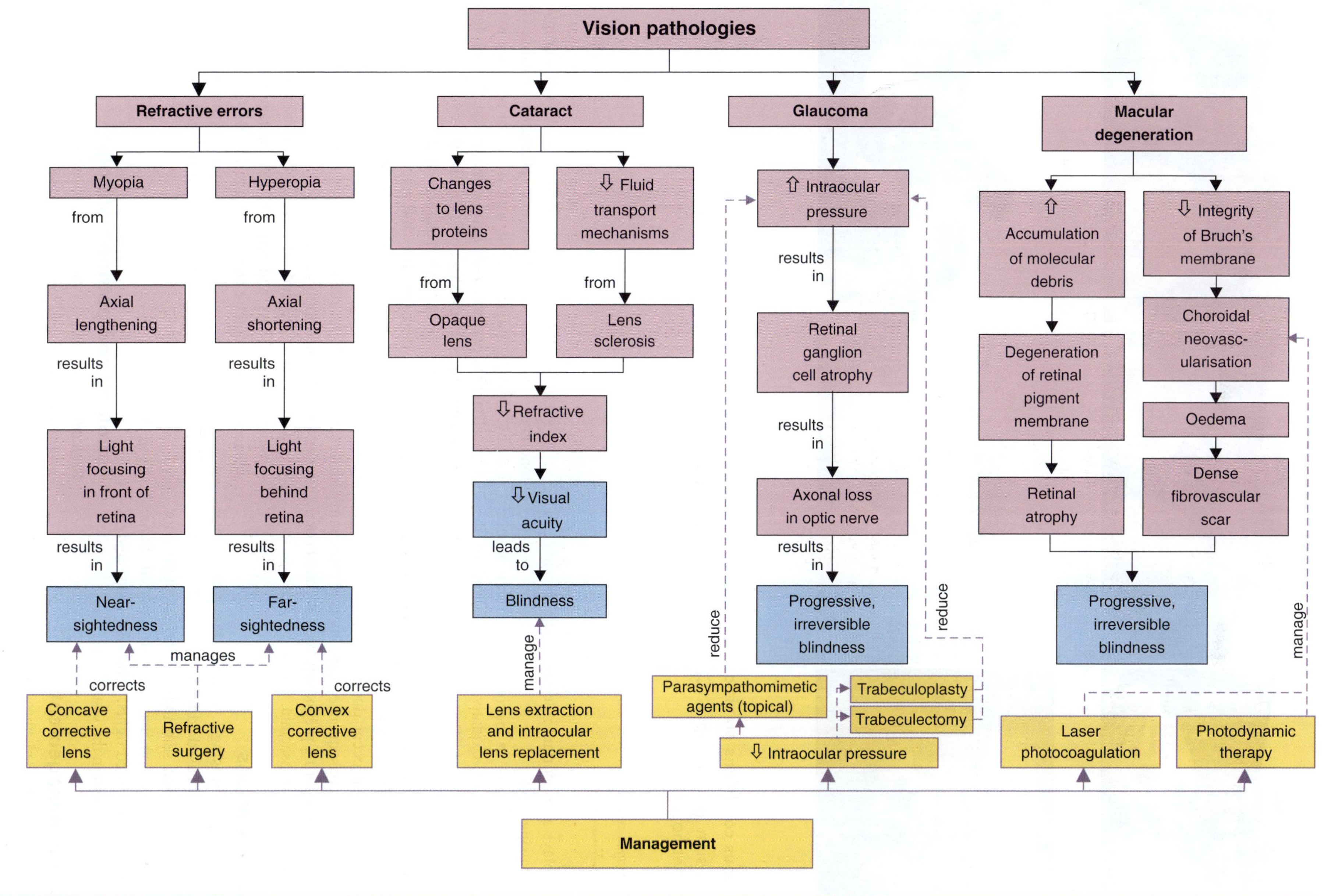

Figure 14.1

Clinical snapshot: Vision pathologies

↓ = decreased; ↑ = increased.

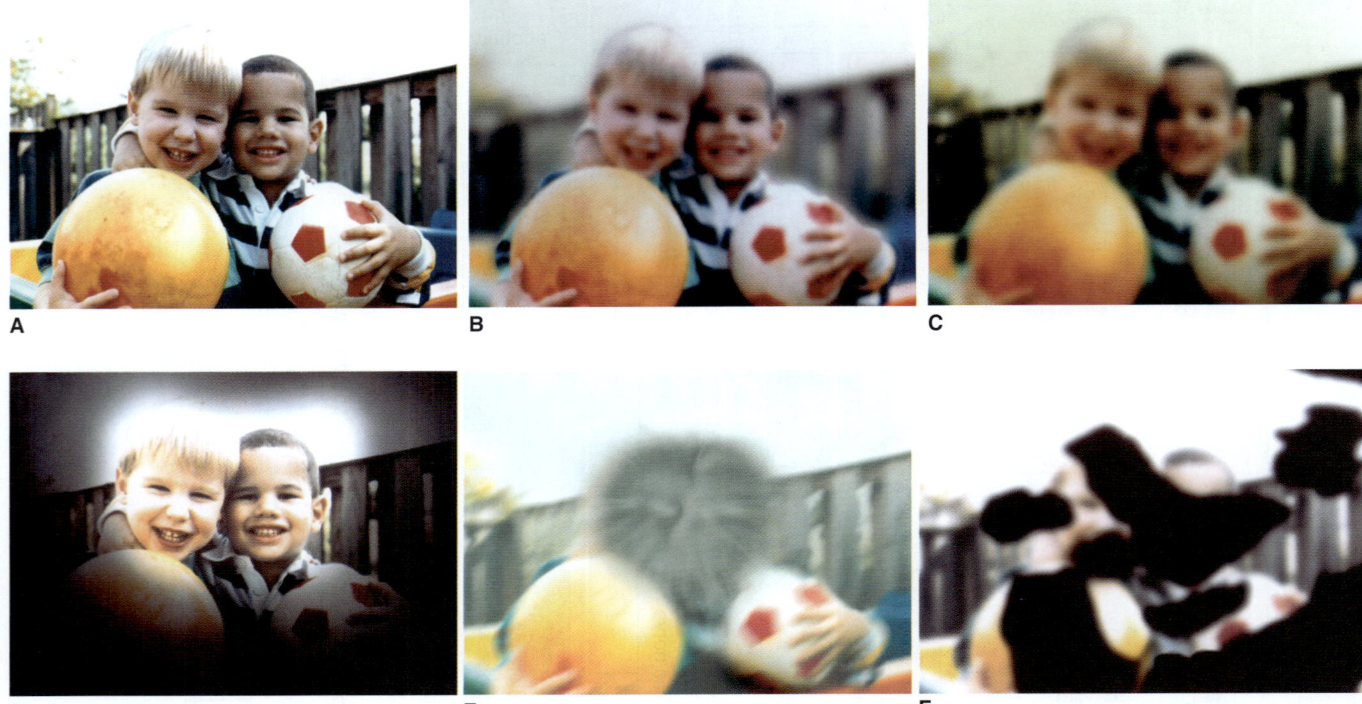

Figure 14.2

Effects of various conditions on vision using the same image

(A) = Normal vision. (B) = Myopia. (C) = Cataract. (D) = Glaucoma. (E) = Age-related macular degeneration. (F) = Diabetic retinopathy.

Source: Modified images courtesy of National Eye Institute, National Institutes of Health.

elastic fibres. It plays an important role in altering the shape of the lens when focusing light.

Cataracts cause the lens to become stiffer and opaque through processes involving oxidative stress, failure of the sodium–potassium (Na^+/K^+-ATPase) pump and/or increases in membrane permeability of the lens. Cataracts can also develop after exposure to radiation, drugs (such as glucocorticoids and the phenothiazine antipsychotic agents) or trauma.

Congenital cataracts can occur due to the presence of an inheritable disorder or as a consequence of an illness or infection that the mother developed during pregnancy, such as rubella or a metabolic disorder like galactosaemia.

Clinical manifestations

As the lens becomes increasingly opaque, the person may experience decreased, unfocused, dim or 'foggy' vision (see Figure 14.2C), An increased sensitivity to bright light, poor night vision, and double vision may also be reported. Some people see halos around viewed lights, yellowish vision and, in other cases, brown spots within the visual field.

Diagnosis and management

Cataract diagnosis is achieved through testing vision and undertaking an eye examination. These tests provide information on visual acuity and the health of the eye structures.

A suitably qualified health professional will complete tonometry to check the **intraocular pressure**, visualise the lens by inducing pupil dilation with a muscarinic antagonist medication, and perform a slit lamp examination. The slit lamp instrument shines a thin sheet of light into the eye; this enables the magnification of the eye structures at the front of the eye: eyelids, cornea, sclera, iris, lens and anterior cavity.

Cataract development can be prevented by reducing exposure to known risk factors through wearing sunglasses when in direct bright sunlight, reducing alcohol consumption, smoking cessation and maintaining euglycaemia.

Cataract surgery is indicated when the person experiences significant vision loss and requires the damaged lens to be replaced with a synthetic one (see Figure 14.4B). Complications of cataract surgery include inflammation, posterior capsular cataract development, infection and retinal detachment.

GLAUCOMA

Aetiology and pathophysiology

Glaucoma is a group of ocular neuropathies characterised by *progressive visual field loss* and *irreversible damage to the optic nerve*. Retinal ganglion cells and axons within the retinal nerve fibre layer are damaged. The most common forms are open-angle glaucoma and angle-closure glaucoma. *Open-angle glaucoma*

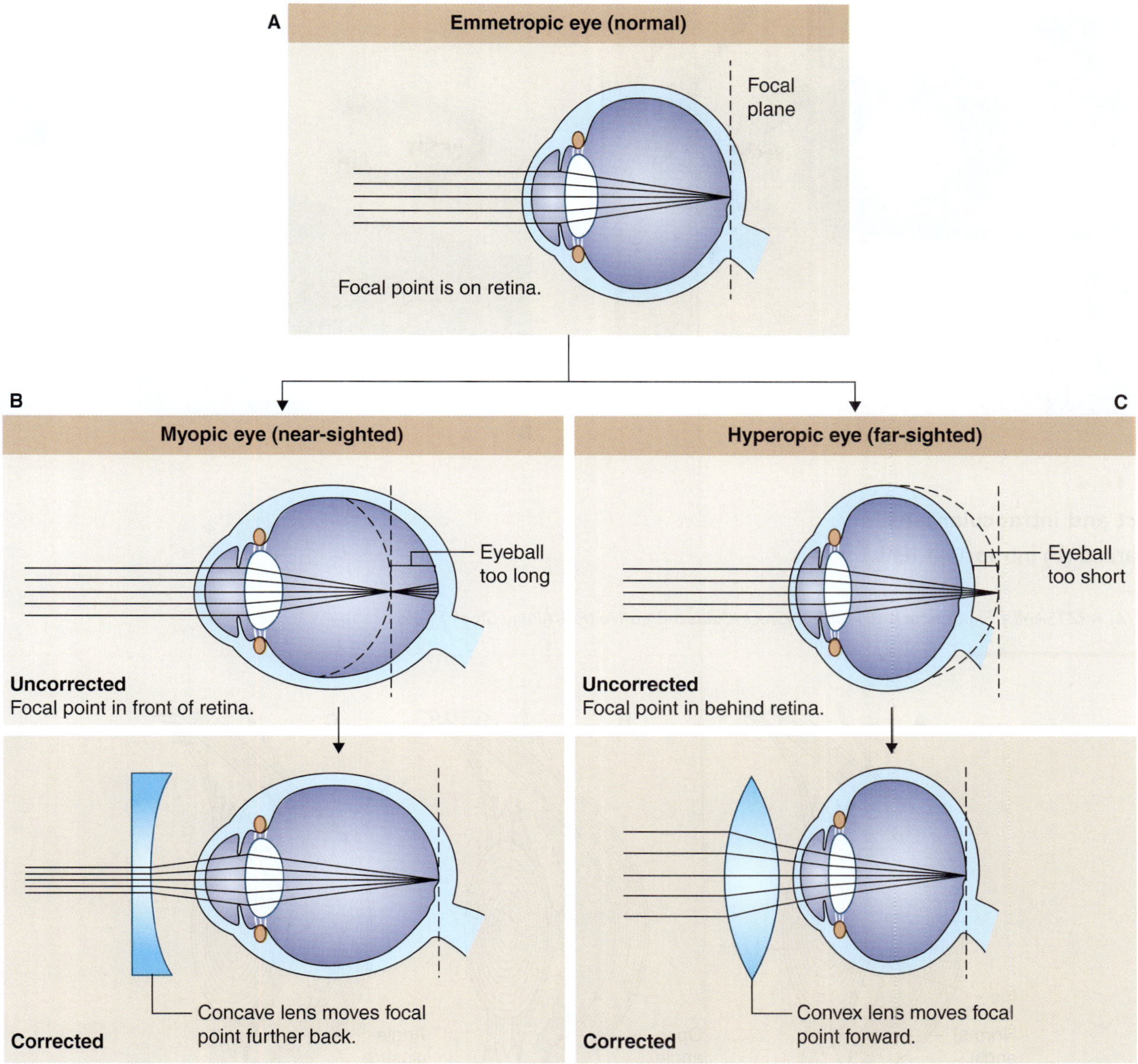

A
Emmetropic eye (normal)
Focal plane
Focal point is on retina.

B
Myopic eye (near-sighted)
Eyeball too long
Uncorrected
Focal point in front of retina.
Concave lens moves focal point further back.
Corrected

C
Hyperopic eye (far-sighted)
Eyeball too short
Uncorrected
Focal point in behind retina.
Convex lens moves focal point forward.
Corrected

Figure 14.3

Vision disorders of the eye

(A) Normal vision = Emmetropia. (B) Myopia is corrected by a concave lens. (C) Hyperopia is corrected by a convex lens.

Source: Adapted from Marieb & Hoehn (2019), Figure 15.14, p. 598.

results in a reduced outflow of fluid; however, the drainage canal is not anatomically blocked. Increased pressure over time results in damage to the optic nerve and is painless. *Angle-closure glaucoma* results in a narrowed outflow tract and a significant risk of acute blockage (constituting an eye emergency), causing pain, headache and vision disturbances. The pathophysiological characteristics of the two types are shown in Figure 14.5.

Clinical manifestations

As symptoms are slow and insidious, they are not readily noticeable until irreversible optic nerve damage has occurred. A person may notice difficulty focusing, trouble adjusting to dark rooms, dry eyes or excessively watery eyes. Peripheral vison is gradually lost (see Figure 14.2D).

People with open-angle glaucoma can remain asymptomatic until late in the progression of the disease. When symptoms do appear, the affected person reports a severe central vision impairment in one or both eyes that may be irreversible.

In angle-closure glaucoma, sudden eye pain and vision loss are typical symptoms. Other clinical manifestations include seeing a halo around bright light, red eye, high intraocular pressure, nausea, vomiting and a fixed, mid-dilated pupil.

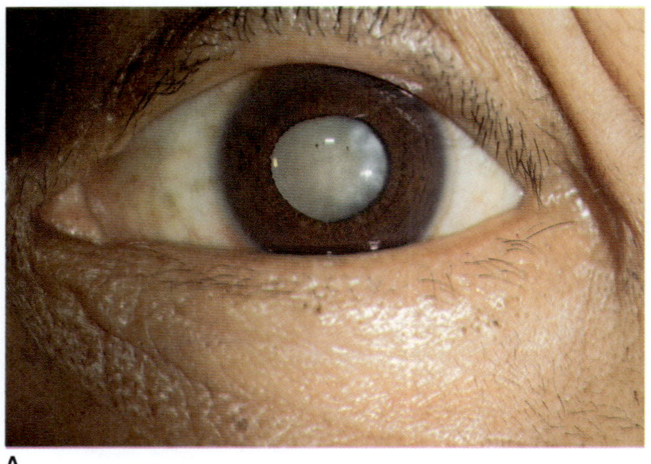

A

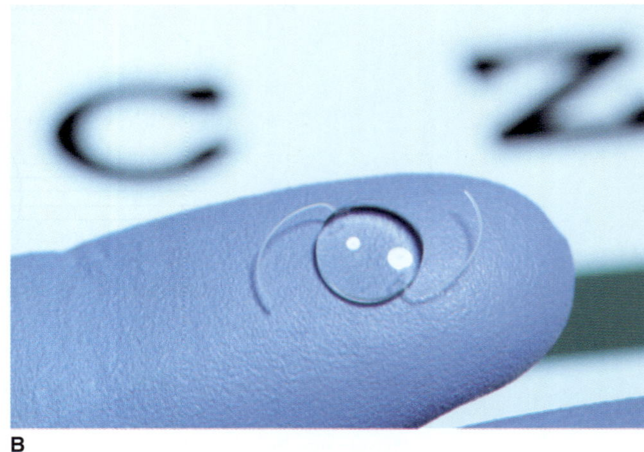

B

Figure 14.4

Cataract and intraocular lens

(A) Cataract. (B) Intraocular lens.

Sources: (A) ARZTSAMUI/Shutterstock. (B) GIPhotoStock/Cultura Creative (RF)/Alamy Stock Photo.

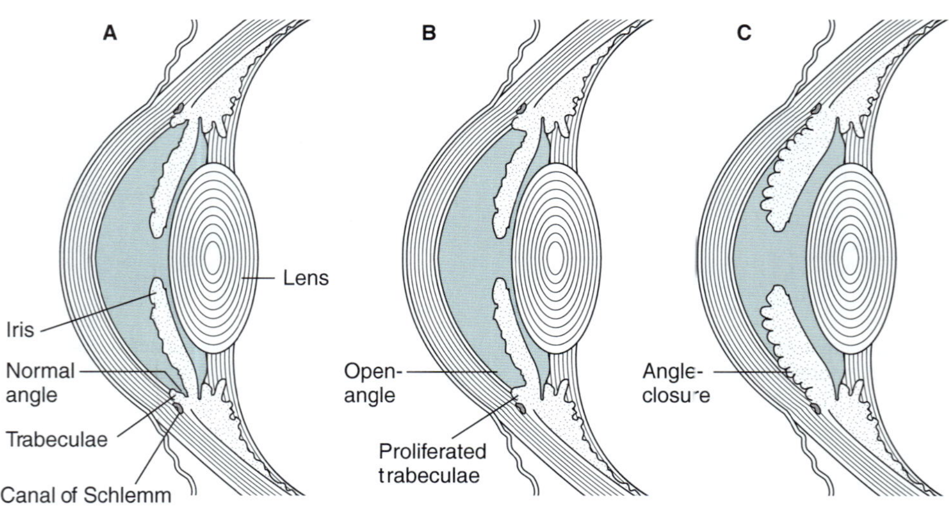

Figure 14.5

Types of glaucoma

(A) Normal. (B) Open-angle glaucoma. (C) Angle-closure glaucoma.

Source: Bullock & Manias (2022), Figure 66.2, p. 862.

Diagnosis and management

An eye examination observing the size and/or shape of each eye, retinal exam, tonometry, and visual field assessments are standard. Gonioscopy is also undertaken to measure the anatomical angle between the cornea and iris, in order to classify the type of glaucoma.

In open-angle glaucoma, the aim of treatment is to halt further losses in vision by reducing intraocular pressure with either drug therapy or surgery. Five classes of medications can be used to lower intraocular pressure: muscarinic agonists (miotics), β-adrenergic antagonists, α_2-adrenergic agonists, carbonic anhydrase inhibitors (a form of diuretic), prostaglandin analogues and prostamides. The characteristic profiles of each of these classes are summarised in Table 14.1.

The surgical approach involves facilitating drainage of the aqueous humour through the obstructed trabecular meshwork. This can be achieved with an argon laser or incision though the meshwork.

Table 14.1 Profiles of drug classes used in the treatment of glaucoma

Drug class	Example generics	Mechanism of action	Common adverse effects
β-Blockers(antagonists)	Betaxolol	Decreased aqueous humour production	Eye irritation, dry eyes, blurred vision, bronchospasm (in susceptible people), bradycardia
Muscarinic agonists/ Parasympathomimietics (miotics)	Pilocarpine	Increased drainage of aqueous humour	Headache, pupil constriction, myopia, loss of visual acuity, ocular hyperaemia (engorged blood vessels)
α_2-Agonists	Apraclonidine	Decreased aqueous humour production and increased drainage of aqueous humour	Headache, stinging sensation, pupil dilation, blurred vision
Carbonic anhydrase inhibitors	Acetazolamide, brinzolamide	Decreased aqueous humour production	Skin rashes, nausea and vomiting, blurred vision, eye irritation
Prostaglandins ($PGF_{2\alpha}$)	Latanoprost	Increased drainage of aqueous humour	Prostaglandins: eye irritation, blurred vision, increased eyelash growth
Prostamides	Bimatoprost	Increased drainage of aqueous humour	Prostamides: increased eyelash growth, increased iris/eyelid pigmentation, itching, ocular hyperaemia

AGE-RELATED MACULOPATHY

Aetiology and pathophysiology

Age-related maculopathy (ARM) is a progressive degenerative disease affecting the central retina. It is classified into two types: the early and late forms. The late form is also known as *age-related macular degeneration (AMD).*

The *early form of ARM* is associated with the accumulation of protein aggregates (*drusen*) between the retinal pigment epithelium and the underlying Bruch's membrane. Local inflammatory responses and ocular ischaemia have been proposed as major pathophysiological processes leading to choroid and choriocapillary atrophy, impaired retinal pigment epithelial function and a thickening of Bruch's membrane. These changes result in impaired diffusion of oxygen and other substances to the neuroretina, and subsequent hypoxia and late AMD.

Late AMD is classified as either dry or wet. *Dry AMD*, also known as *geographic atrophy*, is characterised by a distinct area of hypopigmentation due to the atrophy of the retinal pigment epithelium. *Wet AMD* can manifest as detachment of the retinal pigment epithelium or neovascularisation of the choroid and retina. Chronic hypoxia leads to an up-regulation of vascular endothelium growth factor (VEGF), which leads to neovascularisation of the choroid and retina. The new vessels are fragile and easily damaged. Their growth increases vascular permeability and produces macular oedema, inflammation, fibrosis and scarring. The retinal pigment epithelium may become detached as a result of the oedema and inflammation, causing a loss of central vision.

Clinical manifestations

Symptoms involve changes to central vision (see Figure 14.2E). In dry AMD, the affected person usually experiences blurred vision. In wet AMD, straight lines may appear crooked as the macular oedema lifts the macula and distorts the image.

Irrespective of the type, as the condition becomes more advanced a blind spot in central vision develops that progressively grows over time.

Diagnosis and management

Diagnosis is achieved through testing vision by eye examination, and tonometry in order to measure intraocular pressure. The health of the retina will be determined using ophthalmoscopy, where differentiation between wet and dry is possible. Drusen deposits, neovascularisation or submacular haemorrhages may be observed (see Figure 14.6). Other tests for AMD include viewing an Amsler grid, in order to check the image processing of straight lines within the central visual field, and undertaking a retinal angiogram.

Management No conventional therapies are available for the management of dry AMD. In wet AMD, the aim of treatment is to target the neovascularisation process. Argon laser therapy can be used to destroy new blood vessels within the lesion. However, it lacks specificity and can damage healthy retinal tissue. The photosensitiser verteporfin, which is available in Australia and New Zealand, can also target the neovascularisation process, and is more specific than laser surgery. When infused intravenously, it is preferentially taken up by the neovasculature of the choroid, and, when exposed to

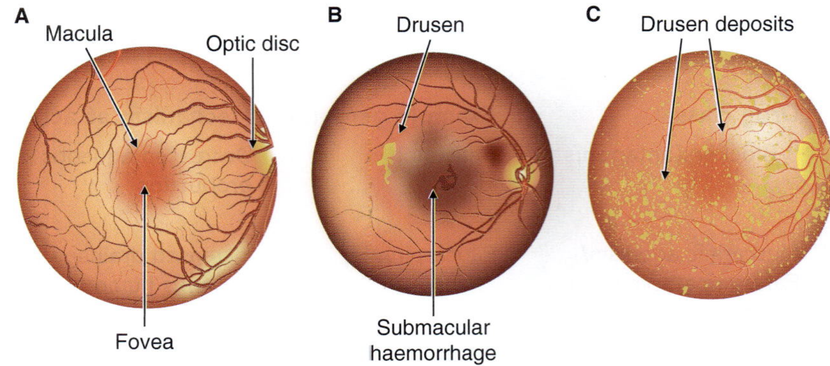

Figure 14.6

Fundoscopic changes from age-related macular degeneration

(A) Normal retina. (B) Wet AMD with haemorrhage from ruptured neovascularisation. (C) Dry AMD with drusen deposits.

Source: Adapted images courtesy of National Eye Institute, National Institutes of Health.

a particular wavelength of red light, this tissue is destroyed. The medication is well tolerated, but it can cause an inflammatory reaction at the injection site and photosensitivity to bright light for about 48 hours post-administration.

A more novel therapeutic approach is to target the growth factor VEGF, a key mediator in the neovascularisation process. Two anti-VEGF agents are available in Australia and New Zealand, the monoclonal antibody ranibizumab and fusion protein aflibercept, and are indicated in AMD. Their actions are directed against the effects of VEGF. These medications are not without serious adverse effects, however. They can induce conjunctival and retinal haemorrhage, and ocular pain and irritation, as well as retinal detachment.

DIABETIC RETINOPATHY

Aetiology and pathophysiology

Diabetic retinopathy is one of the chronic complications associated with the microvascular damage that can occur in diabetes mellitus (see the chapter 'Diabetes mellitus'). Retinal tissue has a high metabolic demand, and damage can be significant if blood flow becomes severely compromised. Consistent with this view, retinal arteriolar dilation is associated with diabetic retinopathy, and may represent an early marker of microvascular impairment. Chronic hyperglycaemia, hypertension and hyperlipidaemia set in motion changes to biochemical processes that lead to vascular impairment and retinal dysfunction.

It appears that the two key pathophysiological processes in diabetic retinopathy are heightened enzyme activity of intracellular protein kinase C and the binding of glucose to protein side chains, which leads to the formation of *advanced glycation end products (AGEs)*. An inability to maintain a euglycaemic state increases the amount of AGEs formed. An increase in protein kinase C affects the retinal vasculature, leading to increased permeability, retinal ischaemia and the release of VEGF. VEGF induces ocular neovascularisation, which actually worsens the ischaemic state. AGEs are strongly linked to microaneurysm development.

Other pathophysiological mechanisms thought to contribute to diabetic retinopathy are inflammation, up-regulation of the renin–angiotensin system (which is thought to increase VEGF release), oxidative stress and intracellular polyol accumulation due to the activity of an enzyme called aldose reductase. Oxidative stress is associated with the formation of oxygen free radicals that can damage the retinal vasculature. Hyperglycaemia leads to an increased intracellular accumulation of the polyol sorbitol, which exerts a strong osmotic pressure on the retinal vasculature (see the chapter 'Diabetes mellitus').

Clinical manifestations

Diabetic retinopathy is characterised by the presence of microaneurysms that can rupture the retinal vasculature, leading to haemorrhage. The appearance of these haemorrhages varies according to the depth of the retina in which they occur. Small dots or blot haemorrhages occur deeper within the densely arranged layers, whereas more superficial ones appear as flame- or flare-shaped. Increased vascular permeability leads to the formation of a yellowish, hard and waxy exudate rich in lipid around the leaking capillaries. The exudates can greatly affect vision, especially in the macula. In this stage, dead white patches in the retina can be visualised (called 'cotton wool spots'). This is considered to be the *non-proliferative stage*.

With worsening ischaemia, neovascularisation occurs. The new blood vessels that form are fragile and easily damaged. The blood vessels form at the edge of the retina and extend into the vitreous humour. This stage is considered to be the *proliferative phase*. In the *advanced stage*, retinal detachment, vitreous haemorrhages and neovascular glaucoma can lead to significant vision loss and total blindness (see Figure 14.2F).

Diagnosis and management

The diagnosis involves standard evaluation with vision acuity, and eye examination. Other techniques involve stereoscopic fundus photography, angiography and retinal imaging viewed through dilated pupils to determine changes in the thickness of the retina, microaneurysms, haemorrhages and cotton wool spots (see Figure 14.7). Cotton wool spots are thought to be intra-axonal accumulations of from interrupted axoplasmic flow through the new fibre caused by ischaemia from diabetic changes.

The focus of management is preventative—to stop the development or the progression of the retinopathy. Studies have

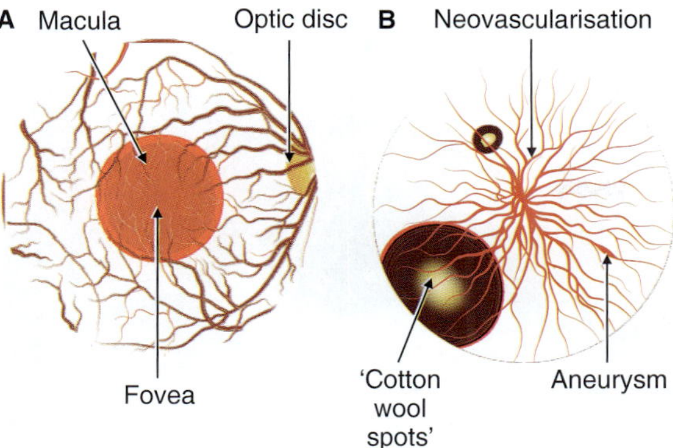

Figure 14.7

Diabetic retinopathy

(A) Normal retina. (B) Diabetic retinopathy showing neovascularisation, 'cotton wool spots' and aneurysm.

Source: Adapted images courtesy of National Eye Institute, National Institutes of Health.

shown that good glycaemic control can achieve both of these preventative aims. Control of hypertension and blood lipid levels also have beneficial effects. First-line therapy with an angiotensin-converting enzyme (ACE) inhibitor for the control of hypertension, and a statin for the control of lipid levels, have produced reasonable results.

Surgical interventions have also been found to be useful in the management of diabetic retinopathy. The exposure of argon laser light on neovascularised tissue has been found to enhance vision in cases of proliferative retinopathy. In cases of vitreous haemorrhage, conventional laser treatment has also been demonstrated to be of assistance.

COLOUR BLINDNESS

Aetiology and pathophysiology

Deficiencies in colour vision, or **colour blindness**, are relatively common vision disorders that can be classified as either *congenital* or *acquired.* Congenital colour vision dysfunction is associated with genetic errors that disrupt the complete expression of all the cone photoreceptors. Generally, colour blindness is an *X-linked* condition, and the most common forms are X-linked recessive. The incidence of this condition is, therefore, higher in males than females.

The three main forms of colour blindness—anomalous trichromacy, dichromacy and monochromacy—range in severity. *Anomalous trichromacy* is the mildest of the three forms. All three photoreceptors are present, but one type has impaired function, resulting in an abnormal mixing of colours. In *dichromacy*, colour discrimination is greatly reduced, and in *monochromacy*, colour discrimination is virtually absent.

The most common form of colour blindness affects red–green colour vision, and can occur in trichromacy and dichromacy. In total colour blindness, an affected person cannot distinguish colours from grey, which literally results in a black and white view of the world.

Acquired forms of colour blindness can occur as a result of neurotrauma, retinal injury, exposure to excessive sunlight or, rarely, during treatment with some medications.

Clinical manifestations

The common clinical manifestations of colour blindness include an inability to discriminate between certain colours, and between shades of the same colour or similar colours. The brightness of colours may also be impeded. In severe forms of colour blindness, the affected person may experience photophobia, poor vision and nystagmus.

Diagnosis and management

Testing with the Ishihara colour charts is the quickest and most effective way to detect colour blindness (see Figure 14.8). Numerals and wiggly lines are formed through the arrangement of differently coloured dots. People with normal vision can see these figures, which are not recognisable by affected individuals. Discrimination between different types of colour blindness is possible using this test.

Colour blindness cannot be cured. However, improvements in colour discrimination are reported through the use of tinted

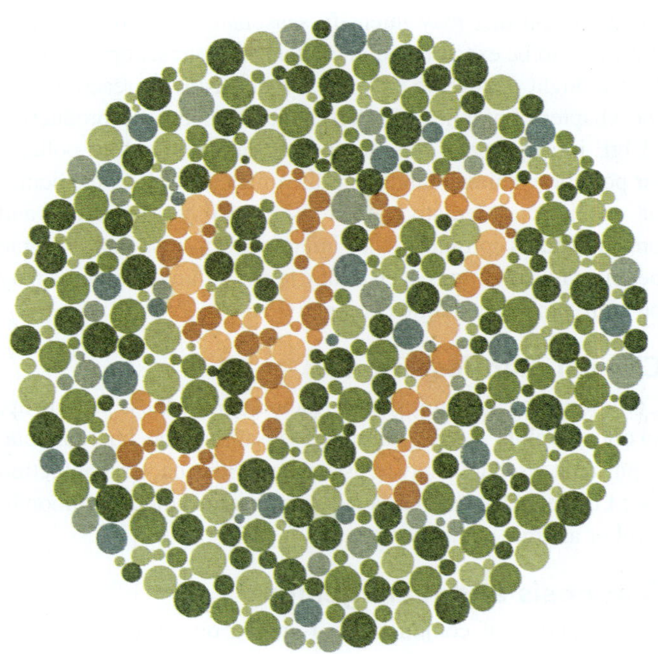

Figure 14.8

Example plate from the Ishihara charts

In a person with colour vision, the number '97' is visible; however, it is not visible to a person with red–green colour blindness.

Source: Eight Ishihara charts for testing colour blindness, Europe, 1917–1959. Science Museum, London. Attribution 4.0 International (CC BY 4.0) https://creativecommons.org/licenses/by/4.0.

contact lenses and filters. Such filters may be worn monocularly or binocularly. Monocular filters induce contrasting inputs that may provide a surrogate for colour vision.

CONJUNCTIVITIS

LEARNING OBJECTIVE 4

Describe the pathophysiology, manifestations and management of conjunctivitis.

Aetiology and pathophysiology

Conjunctivitis is an *inflammation of the conjunctival membrane* that covers and protects the ocular surface. The condition (also known as '*pink eye*') is common, and may develop in an acute or a chronic form. Conjunctivitis may involve other neighbouring structures, giving rise to *keratoconjunctivitis* (involving the cornea), *blepharoconjunctivitis* (involving the eyelids) and *dermoconjunctivitis* (involving neighbouring skin).

Acute conjunctivitis may be due to a microbial infection (viral or bacterial), an allergic reaction, or exposure to a chemical or medication. The most common form of viral conjunctivitis is due to infection by an adenovirus. However, conjunctival infection with herpes simplex virus and *Chlamydia trachomatis* are clinically important.

Allergic conjunctivitis is a common form of *chronic conjunctivitis*, and is generally associated with chronic allergic inflammation that may intensify seasonally (mainly in spring, but can also be exacerbated in winter) or be present perennially. It is thought to involve a type I hypersensitivity reaction (see the chapter 'Immune disorders') mediated by the production of IgE in response to the presence of antigens such as pollens, air pollution, animal dander or dust mites, as well as medicines or cosmetics. Mediators such as cytokines, histamine and prostaglandins promote the inflammatory response. Atopic people with conditions such as hay fever, asthma or eczema may be more prone to allergic conjunctivitis.

Clinical manifestations

Common clinical manifestations include eye redness, tearing up, swollen eyelids, itching, burning sensations and photophobia. A purulent discharge may be associated with a bacterial infection (see Figure 14.9), whereas a clear discharge is more common in viral or allergic conjunctivitis.

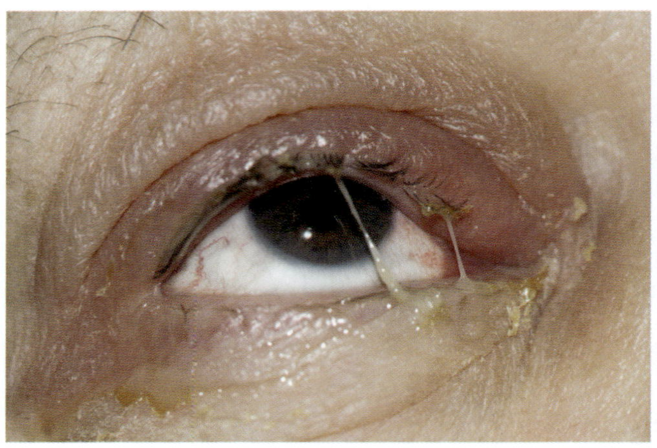

Figure 14.9

Conjunctivitis

Note the redness and discharge present. Bacterial conjunctivitis is commonly caused by Staphylococcus aureus, Streptococcus pneumonia and Haemophilus influenzae.

Source: Zoonar GmbH/Adelheid Möller/Alamy Stock Photo.

Diagnosis and management

The diagnosis of conjunctivitis is based on an assessment of the person's history and an eye examination. The eyes should be examined for evidence of papules, ulcerations, crusting, discharge, papillae, subconjuctival bleeding and enlarged regional lymph nodes.

Most acute conjunctivitis will resolve with limited intervention within a week or so. Supportive measures—such as the application of cold compresses, eye baths, the administration of artificial tears and topical antihistamine preparations where itching is problematic—may be beneficial. Topical antimicrobial therapy is indicated in the management of bacterial conjunctivitis; however, it is often difficult to ascertain the cause.

A variety of topical eye medications can reduce the symptoms of inflammation and irritation of chronic allergic conjunctivitis. Antihistamine preparations, ocular decongestants and mast cell stabilisers (e.g. sodium cromoglycate) may relieve itching and redness. Glucocorticoid preparations may be useful in severe forms of allergic conjunctivitis; however, immunosuppression and superinfection are a significant risk of these medications.

Hearing impairment

LEARNING OBJECTIVE 5

Briefly discuss the most common causes of acquired hearing loss.

Hearing impairment can be categorised in many ways. Hearing loss can be temporary or permanent; it can be congenital or acquired. It can occur before language has developed (prelingual) or after someone has learnt to speak (postlingual). However, the most common way to categorise hearing loss is using terms that describe the anatomical location associated with the deficiency. *Conductive hearing loss* refers to a cause in the outer or middle ear, such as blockage of the ear canal, infection, a perforated ear drum or otosclerosis. *Sensorineural hearing loss* refers to a cause involving the inner ear, such as the cochlear or the vestibulocochlear nerve (cranial nerve VIII), and is associated with ageing, noise-induced hearing loss, acoustic neuroma, Ménière's disease, viral infections, ototoxic drugs, head injuries or a number of congenital causes.

The World Health Organization's grades of hearing impairment indicate an audiometry value of 26–40 dB as slight impairment, 41–60dB as moderate, 61–80 dB as severe, and over 81 dB as profound. In Australia, one in three people have some degree of noise-related ear damage. Nationally, the most common causes of hearing loss are ageing and excessive exposure to loud noises. In New Zealand, almost one in six people have some degree of hearing loss.

CONDUCTIVE HEARING LOSS

There are many causes of conductive hearing loss, including the blockage of the external auditory canal or eustachian tube, infection, a perforated ear drum or otosclerosis.

Blockage of canal

The *external canal* can be obstructed by *cerumen* (earwax), *foreign bodies* such as small toys, or even by *congenital defects* where the morphology of the ear canal impedes the passage of the sound towards the tympanic membrane. If a foreign object is involved, it may be removed by irrigation, suction or manipulation with instruments. The management of congenital defects depends on the anatomical deformities, and may include either medical management with the use of hearing aids, or surgical options involving repair of the canal or the implantation of bone-anchored hearing aids.

Infection

Ear infections can develop in the external auditory canal (*otitis externa*) or in the eustachian tube in the middle ear (*otitis media*). Otitis externa is also known as 'swimmer's ear', and can induce temporary hearing impairment as a result of swelling of the canal.

There are many forms of otitis media (also known as 'glue ear'). Five types of otitis media include: *acute otitis media (AOM), recurrent acute otitis media (rAOM), otitis media with effusion (OME), chronic otitis media with effusion (COME)* and *chronic suppurative otitis media (CSOM)*. Otitis media results in hearing impairment from a complex and multifaceted process. Figure 14.10 explores the common clinical manifestations and management of ear infections.

Aetiology and pathophysiology Research suggests that almost every child will experience at least one episode of *otitis media* before they turn 3 years of age. The causative bacteria are most commonly *Staphylococcus*, *Streptococcus* and *Pseudomonas* species. Common viral infections associated with both otitis externa and otitis media include respiratory syncytial virus, influenza A and adenovirus.

Otitis externa (also known as 'swimmer's ear') can occur when someone with excess cerumen is also exposed to conditions resulting in excessive water; the canal may begin to macerate and a localised infection can develop. Other causes of otitis externa can include irritation of the sensitive epidermal layer within the ear canal through the use of objects for cleaning, hair products and chemicals, or skin conditions with an inflammatory component, such as dermatitis or eczema.

Otitis media is a general term describing inflammation of the middle ear. The various forms of otitis media present a different clinical picture and outcomes. AOM is described as an active inflammation or infection of the middle ear that is usually accompanied by ear pain and a bulging, red, opaque tympanic membrane. Fever may be present, and perforation of the tympanic membrane may also occur. Obstruction of the eustachian tube by allergic or inflammatory conditions or as a result of an upper respiratory tract infection can contribute to the environmental conditions that promote AOM. When obstruction occurs, substances cannot drain into the pharynx, and pressure changes within the middle ear occur. Stasis augments bacterial colonisation in what should be a sterile space. Bacteria implicated in the majority of AOM infections include *Streptococcus pneumoniae, Moraxella catarrhalis* and *Haemophilus influenzae*. rAOM is described as three or more episodes of AOM within six months, or four or more episodes in 12 months. OME is described as mucoid or serous fluid (non-purulent) in the middle ear without inflammation of the tympanic membrane. COME is otits media with effusion that remains for long periods of time and is associated with greater hearing deficits. CSOM is a recurrent form and is caused by a bacterial infection that quickly develops antibacterial drug resistance. It is often associated with a fungal co-infection. These various types of otitis associated with infection are summarised in Figure 14.10.

Hearing loss associated with otitis media can occur as a result of numerous issues. A ruptured/perforated tympanic membrane can interfere with sound transmission, as the damage reduces the capacity of the membrane to transmit vibrations through the chain of ossicles to the cochlea. The bacterial infection can cause conduction deafness by interfering with the ossicular chain, causing bony erosions and destruction or ankylosis (stiffness) of the ossicles. Otorrhoea also contributes to obstruction of the ear canal. Sensorineural deafness may occur if the infection penetrates the inner ear and damages the hair cells. Although classed as a conduction problem, severe otitis media may result in a mixed hearing loss (both conduction and sensorineural).

Tinnitus is the perception of sound that does not originate from a source outside the body; that is, intermittent or persistent tones, clicks, buzzes or ringing perceived within a person's head. Many diseases of the ear can cause tinnitus, as can otitis media. In some cases, the sound may be caused by physical or mechanical mechanisms, such as a clicking jaw or the sound of turbulence from vascular anomalies being transmitted through central auditory pathways. Although the cause is understood, the sound is still most often unwanted. However, typically no physical basis for tinnitus may be found. The pathophysiology of this type of tinnitus is unknown, and may be as a result of damage to any number of sites in the ear or the brain.

Diagnosis and management As with all ear pathologies, visual examination with an otoscope is the most appropriate method to perform an assessment. Sampling of exudate for culture and sensitivity can be undertaken during the

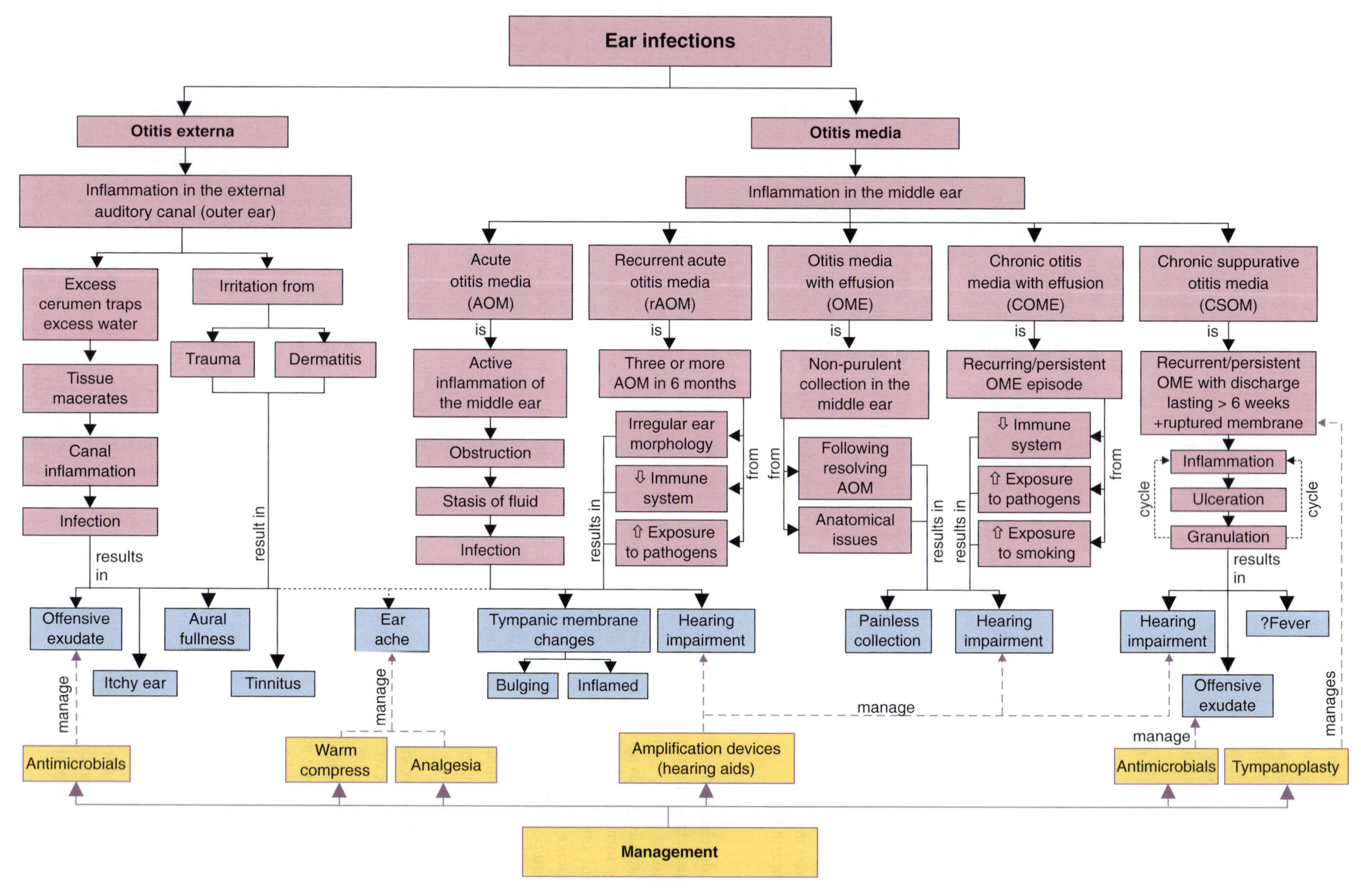

Figure 14.10

Clinical snapshot: Ear infections

↓ = decreased; ↑ = increased; ? = possible.

assessment. Audiology testing may be necessary, especially in the presence of more chronic episodes of either otitis externa or media.

Otitis externa can be treated with topical antibacterial or antifungal preparations. A sample should be collected for culture and sensitivity so that the exact causative organism can be identified.

In recent years, a change in the management practices of otitis media has resulted in the use of antimicrobials for suppurative AOM, in the presence of systemic symptoms only, or in children younger than 6 months of age (with or without systemic symptoms). It is suggested that there is little benefit from anitmicrobials in non-suppurative AOM, and, in keeping with the principles of antimicrobial stewardship, reduction of unnecessary use is an important step in reducing resistance.

Aural hygiene practices should be discussed with the affected person or their carer. If recurrent episodes occur, the insertion of a grommet (tympanoplasty tube) into the tympanic membrane can assist with drainage and ventilation of the eustachian tube, enabling the elimination or reduction of recurrent episodes.

Prophylactic antimicrobial treatments may be necessary to prevent or control more chronic episodes. Alteration of the management plan should occur as directed by culture and sensitivity reports.

Ototoxic antimicrobials (such as aminoglycosides) should be used with caution and under strict supervision. Hearing impairment can occur as a result of the disease process; however, iatrogenic hearing loss should be prevented.

Perforated tympanic membrane

A perforated eardrum (tympanic membrane) can occur as a result of trauma or infection. A rupture results in failure of the membrane separating the external auditory canal and the eustachian tube. The ossicular chain is then disrupted and the process of hearing is compromised. Common causes of a ruptured tympanic membrane include trauma from excessive noise (acoustic trauma), external pressure (barotrauma), penetration (such as a cotton bud), otitis media (where there is pressure from exudate trapped within the middle ear), or from traumatic perforation (such as a blow to the ear or a head injury). Perforated tympanic membrane can be asymptomatic; or the person may complain of hearing impairment, a large amount of exudate coming from their ear, and/or an audible whistling sound occurring when sneezing or blowing their nose.

In trauma, *viscous serosanguinous fluid* may come from the ear (otorrhoea), and is a sign of a fracture to the base of the skull. This fluid is most likely to be a cerebrospinal fluid leak, and indicates severe injury that requires immediate investigation and management.

A small, uncomplicated tympanic membrane perforation will generally heal on its own over a few months. Perforations caused by infections should be treated with appropriate topical and systemic antimicrobials following the collection of an exudate sample for culture and sensitivity. Simple analgesia may be necessary to manage discomfort. Depending on the severity and cause, surgical intervention (tympanoplasty) may be necessary.

Otosclerosis

Otosclerosis is a disease of the middle ear resulting in the interference of the ossicular chain from fixation of the stapes, thus reducing sound transmission. Women are twice as likely to develop otosclerosis, often during their 20s, and the disease is generally bilateral. The pathogenesis is not well understood, although it is clearly linked to endocrine factors, as hearing impairment rapidly progresses during pregnancy, and oestrogen is known to influence bone metabolism. Hearing impairment is the principal manifestation, although tinnitus may also be reported. There is generally no pain involved. Medical management of otosclerosis consists of the supply of hearing aids, and the surgical option of a stapedectomy (or stapedotomy) may be necessary.

SENSORINEURAL HEARING LOSS

Sensorineural hearing loss may be either acquired or congenital. The eighth cranial nerve, or *vestibulocochlear nerve (CN VIII)*, is divided into two and has two sensory functions. The *vestibular nerve* is responsible for detecting the movement of the head and body motion. This is discussed in the 'Balance' section of this chapter. The *cochlear nerve* is responsible for detecting sound. *Acquired issues* affecting the cochlear nerve include ageing (presbycusis), noise-induced hearing loss, tumours (particularly acoustic neuroma), Ménière's disease, viral infections, ototoxic drugs and head injuries. *Congenital causes* (those present at birth) of sensorineural hearing loss include inherited causes, such as when deafness is passed on because of genetic factors. Congenital hearing loss can also occur because of illness, such as intrauterine infections (from viruses such as cytomegalovirus and rubella), hypoxic episodes, prematurity and jaundice.

Age-related hearing loss (presbycusis)

Presbycusis is an acquired sensorineural hearing loss as a result of the cumulative effects of ageing on the structures associated with hearing. The majority of adults over 70 years of age have age-related hearing loss. A person may complain of difficulty discriminating conversation when ambient noise increases, and family members and others may also complain of the affected individual withdrawing from group conversation. The person may also complain of hearing loss of high frequencies. There is no cure for presbycusis, so management may consist of the use of amplification devices, such as hearing aids.

Noise-induced hearing loss

Any environment resulting in excessive noise can cause sensorineural hearing loss. If the environment is related to employment, the resulting hearing impairment is called *occupational noise-induced hearing loss*. If the environment is not related to employment, it is called *socioacusis*. Hearing impairment causing sensorineural hearing loss from a single exposure to an intense sound exceeding 130 dB can be called *acoustic trauma*. In both Australia and New Zealand, the standard for exposure to occupational noise is an average of 85 dB. Exposure above this level constitutes an unacceptable risk to hearing.

Permanent noise-induced hearing loss occurs because of irreversible damage to the *stereocilia* of the hair cells within the cochlear. The intensity and duration of exposure determines the deficit, which is generally bilateral. Once the cause is removed, the progress of the hearing loss should also cease; however, the deficit will not improve in permanent noise-induced hearing loss. There is no cure for noise-induced hearing loss; however, it is easily prevented with the consistent use of hearing protection devices for occupational and domestic exposure to loud noises.

Acoustic neuroma

Acoustic neuroma is a benign tumour that grows from the Schwann cell of the vestibular portion of *cranial nerve VIII (vestibulocochlear)*; it is also known as a *vestibular schwannoma*. As there is limited space in the internal auditory canal, vestibular schwannomas most often compress the cochlear nerve, and therefore tinnitus and hearing loss are generally the first symptoms noticed. It is thought to be associated with a defective suppressor gene function, and can cause sensorineural hearing loss, tinnitus and balance issues. In some people, the sensation of vertigo or spinning can be very disabling. If the tumour encroaches on the trigeminal nerve, unilateral facial paraesthesias can develop. Larger tumours that begin to compress the cerebellum, pons and the fifth cranial nerve will cause more substantial issues, including serious gait disturbance and ataxia. Obstruction of the cerebrospinal fluid pathways may develop in significant growths, and will result in hydrocephalus and, potentially, death.

There are a few management choices for people with acoustic neuromas. 'Watchful waiting' with imaging investigations done every six months may be considered for small tumours; however, surgery may be necessary, and often results in total hearing loss on the affected side. The person may also develop either transient or permanent facial paralysis, dysphagia, tinnitus or vertigo.

Ménière's disease

Ménière's disease is an idiopathic disorder of the inner ear that results in an acquired sensorineural hearing loss. It appears to be an issue with the regulation of fluid (endolymph) within the inner ear. In Ménière's disease, an *excess of endolymph* from increased secretion or impaired removal causes an increased pressure within the labyrinth, and causes mechanical damage to the auditory and otolithic organs. Tinnitus, vertigo and disequilibrium and hearing loss will occur. Episodic attacks may occur frequently for several years, with symptoms resolving between episodes; however, as the disease progresses, tinnitus and hearing loss may become permanent.

Some people can develop a type of Ménière's disease that causes 'drop attacks' (*otolithic crisis of Tumarkin*), which result in a sudden, overwhelming sensation of rotational vertigo, with the person falling to the ground; it resolves within seconds to minutes, and is usually accompanied by vomiting. This manifestation is particularly dangerous for older adults, as the fall (although not caused by unconsciousness) is uncontrollable and can result in severe trauma.

Medical management of Ménière's disease includes restriction of sodium intake, as well as the administration of diuretics and vestibular suppressant drugs. Low-sodium diets and diuretic therapy are aimed at managing the cause of the vertigo by decreasing intravascular volume to reduce the accumulation of fluid within the inner ear. Surgical options are generally reserved for severe or refractory cases, and can be divided into those that preserve residual hearing (*non-destructive*) and those that do not (*destructive*). The use of *transtympanic micropressure therapy* with a hand-held pump-like pressure generator to reduce the volume of endolymph within the inner ear has proven to be beneficial.

Ototoxic drugs

Even though medications are administered to relieve suffering or manage an illness, many drugs have the capacity to damage structures within the inner ear. Ototoxicity is the ability of a chemical to damage internal auditory and vestibular structures and cause hearing deficits, tinnitus, balance issues and/or dizziness. Although hundreds of drugs can cause hearing loss, there are some common classes of drugs that are frequently used. Drugs such as aminoglycosides, diuretics, antineoplastic, anti-inflammatory and antidepressant drugs are renowned for their ototoxicity.

Mechanisms for ototoxicity differ between chemicals. Aminoglycosides, such as gentamicin, irreversibly damage the hair cells in the organ of Corti and produce hearing deficits in high frequencies. Loop diuretics, such as furosemide, affect the gradient between the perilymph and endolymph, causing epithelial oedema in the stria vascularis. Antineoplastic agents cause irreversible, progressive damage to hair cells from free-radical-mediated cell death. NSAIDs such as aspirin (salicylates) cause metabolic changes, resulting in mild to moderate hearing loss, and tinnitus is common with salicylates, occurring at a high frequency. Antidepressant drugs can cause or exacerbate tinnitus and affect balance. Although there is debate about whether these classes are ototoxic, several can certainly influence vestibulocochlear function. As some ototoxic medications cause irreversible damage, avoiding their use is the best option. Administration of parenteral ototoxic drugs over a longer duration and in a lesser concentration may reduce some degree of ototoxicity.

Congenital causes of hearing loss

LEARNING OBJECTIVE 6

Explore some congenital causes of hearing loss.

Congenital causes of hearing loss can be organised into inherited or prenatal (non-inherited) factors. *Inherited factors* are varied, complex and can involve autosomal recessive, autosomal dominant, X-linked or even mitochondrial factors. *Non-inherited factors* include intrauterine or fetal infections of herpes, rubella or cytomegalovirus. Other factors can include jaundice, prematurity and hypoxia or anoxia.

Aetiology and pathophysiology Congenital sensorineural hearing loss can be further subdivided into syndromic and non-syndromic factors. *Syndromic genetic factors* refer to hearing loss associated with other clinical factors, and *non-syndromic factors* refer to hearing loss not associated with other clinical factors (see Figure 14.11).

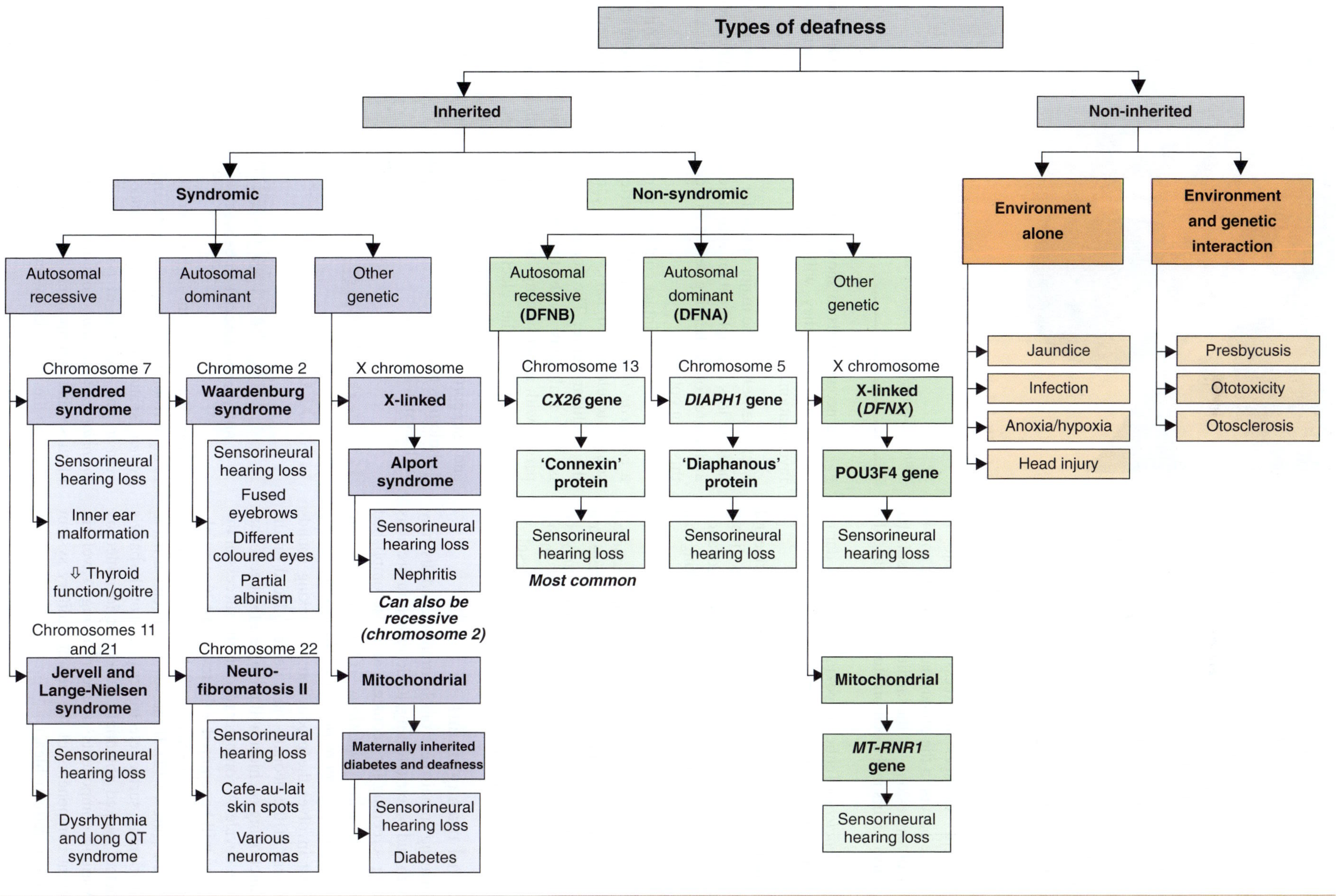

Figure 14.11

Types of congenital deafness

↓ = decreased.

Infection-related congenital sensorineural hearing loss can occur from intrauterine exposure to any number of viruses, including herpes, rubella or cytomegalovirus; however, the most common virus causing infection related to hearing loss is cytomegalovirus (CMV). *Congenital CMV infection* may demonstrate no apparent clinical manifestations, or the neonate may develop petechiae, hepatosplenomegaly and/or neurological deficits. Sensorineural hearing loss is common. The mechanism by which viral infections cause sensorineural hearing loss is unclear; however, damage to the stria vascularis has been found on autopsy. The characteristics of the hearing loss are variable, have no standard audiometric configuration, and can occur quickly or many years later, making diagnosis difficult.

Jaundice-related hearing loss results from *kernicterus*. Because the blood–brain barrier of a neonate is not sufficiently developed to prevent 'spillage' of excess bilirubin into the brain tissue, damage occurs in the globus pallidus of the corpus striatum and involves lesions in the auditory and vestibular nuclei. Damage also occurs in the oculomotor structures and the cerebellum.

Fetal oxygen deficiency (either hypoxia or anoxia) during delivery may result in damage to auditory pathways, haemorrhage involving the labyrinth or atrophy of the organ of Corti.

Prematurity also results in an increased risk of sensorineural hearing loss, because a premature neonate is more likely than a full-term neonate to develop kernicterus. Oxygenation problems are also common in premature neonates, resulting in a multifactorial cause.

Clinical manifestations The primary clinical manifestation is hearing impairment; however, if there are syndromic congenital factors, other clinical signs may be present, depending on the genetic syndrome involved in the sensorineural hearing loss. Over 390 syndromes can result in some degree of sensorineural hearing loss.

Diagnosis and management

Diagnosis Hearing impairment of children and adults may be identified with audiometric testing, as described in previous sections. Hearing screening for neonates can be accomplished with painless *otoacoustic emissions (OAE) testing* and *automated auditory brainstem response (AABR) testing*.

The OAE test involves the production of clicking sounds played into the ear of the neonate via a device placed on the baby's ear. A functioning cochlear will produce a faint echo that is detected by the device. A computer records the success of the test; further testing will be required if the test is not successful.

The AABR test uses a device to play clicking sounds into the neonate's ear (see Figure 14.12). If the vestibulocochlear nerve (CN VIII) is functioning, surface electrodes placed on the baby's scalp should detect evoked potentials, which are identified by a computer. Various components of the resulting waveform represent different components of the neural auditory system beyond the cochlear (retrocochlear).

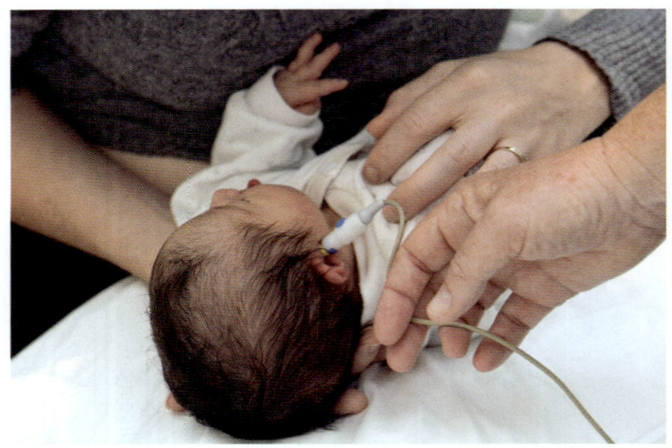

Figure 14.12
Baby undergoing AABR screening

Source: ChameleonsEye/Shutterstock.

If a neonate fails to show responses to both the OAE and the AABR tests, they will require further assessment and investigation.

Management The major option for those with sensorineural hearing loss is amplification with a hearing device. The cause and degree of the hearing deficit will determine whether or not this is an option.

Those with an intact cochlear nerve may be able to have a *cochlear implant* surgically inserted. This device converts sounds to electric signals, which can then be interpreted by the cochlear nerve. The sound that is heard by the person is not analogous with the normal sound heard by a person with intact hearing; however, with training, the person learns to interpret the 'electronically generated' sounds.

Those without an intact cochlear nerve will need education and support, and assistance from speech and language pathologists to assist with alternative means of communication, such as sign language.

Balance and vestibular disorders

LEARNING OBJECTIVE 7

Analyse the association between hearing and balance.

Balance is achieved through muscular adjustment in response to input from three sensory systems: image cues from the *visual system*; spatial orientation and balance cues from the *vestibular system*; and the state of posture and joint location from the *proprioceptive system*. Loss of balance can occur when any one of these three components is dysfunctional. This section will focus on the vestibular system and its control over balance.

As previously discussed, part of the eighth cranial nerve is the vestibular nerve, which plays an important role in the maintenance of balance. Several disorders can cause issues with balance, including labyrinthitis. **Labyrinthitis** is an inflammation of the inner ear (labyrinth) that results in a transient inability to maintain balance, and also often causes either temporary or permanent hearing impairment in the frequencies around 2000 Hz.

Although people experience vertigo and dizziness, these are not diseases but actual clinical manifestations. *Vertigo* is the sensation of dizziness where the person feels as though they are in motion when they are actually stationary. *Dizziness* is a sense of light-headedness, and is also often used to describe loss of balance and unsteadiness.

LABYRINTHITIS, VERTIGO AND DIZZINESS

Aetiology and pathophysiology

Labyrinthitis occurs as a result of *bacterial or viral infection* or from an autoimmune process causing *localised inflammation*. It can develop bilaterally or only in one ear. Bacterial infection may occur secondary to otitis media or meningitis. Translocation of the bacteria may occur through the semicircular canal, internal auditory canal or even from the cerebral spinal fluid. Other pathogens that may contribute to labyrinthitis include cytomegalovirus infection, rubella, measles, mumps or herpes. Sudden vertigo can be so severe that even the slightest movement can exacerbate the dizzy sensation. Hearing loss can also occur suddenly. The symptoms can reduce in days to weeks; however, they may not fully resolve for several months.

Vertigo can be a symptom of many diseases, disorders and imbalances; however, it is most often associated with *inner ear issues*. Any damage to structures in the vestibular system, such as the labyrinth, vestibular nerve or vestibular nuclei within the brain, can cause vertigo.

Dizziness (presyncope) can occur for many reasons, including low blood pressure, cardiac dysrhythmia, hypoxia, hypocapnia, hypoglycaemia and anaemia, and also from vestibular pathologies.

Clinical manifestations

People reporting issues with balance or vertigo may also experience nausea and vomiting. If the vestibular system is involved, it is also not uncommon to report tinnitus, hearing deficits or aural fullness. The person may present with a fever if the cause is related to infection.

Diagnosis and management

Diagnosis Collection of a thorough history is important, and should include recent and past medical history. If there is an infectious component to the balance issues, a full blood count and blood cultures may be beneficial to note the white cell count and potentially identify a causative organism. Microscopy, culture and sensitivity testing of any aural exudate would assist with the selection of an appropriate antimicrobial regimen.

A lumbar puncture may be indicated to rule out meningitis, and imaging studies (e.g. computed tomography [CT] or magnetic resonance imaging [MRI]) may be beneficial to rule out space-occupying lesions or other causes of vertigo and disequilibrium.

The characteristics of the vertigo may give some indication of the structures involved. The fluid-filled semicircular canals sense angular motion and can produce a sensation of rotational movement, whereas the otolith organs (utricle and saccule) sense linear motion and can produce a sensation of floating or tipping.

Vestibular testing can be undertaken to determine whether there are vestibular nerve issues. Electronystagmography can be divided into four separate tests. The calibration test examines rapid eye movements; the tracking test examines the ability of the eyes to follow a target; the positional test examines head movement associated with dizziness; and the caloric test measures the reflex to cold and warm temperatures within the external auditory canal, which will cause a nystagmus and ipsilateral or contralateral eye movement depending on the functioning of the vestibular nerve.

Audiometry may be necessary to evaluate persistent hearing loss in order to develop a management plan.

Management Management plans are developed depending on the cause. Bacterial infections can be treated with antimicrobials, and autoimmune labyrinthitis can be managed with corticosteroids. Corticosteroids may also be used in viral labyrinthitis. Vomiting and fluid deficits can be managed with intravenous fluids and antiemetic medications. Antiemetic medications will also assist with the vertigo and dizziness, as they can be vestibular suppressants. Benzodiazepines may also be used as vestibular suppressants.

Surgical interventions may be necessary, with the placement of a grommet (ventilation tube) in the context of labyrinthitis caused by otitis media. This can assist with reducing the size of the effusion.

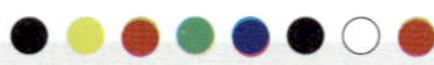

INDIGENOUS HEALTH FAST FACTS

FAST FACTS

- *Aboriginal and Torres Strait Islander peoples are 1.7 times more likely to develop cataracts, 2.83 times more likely to experience vision loss, and 2.4 times more likely to report blindness when compared to non-Indigenous Australians.*
- *Aboriginal and Torres Strait Islander peoples are 3.6 times more likely than non-Indigenous Australians to develop hearing loss.*
- *The burden of otitis media in Aboriginal and Torres Strait Islander children under 15 years of age is 3.5 times higher than that of non-Indigenous Australian children. media.*
- *The incidence of hearing impairment in Māori children is almost two times that of non-Māori children.*
- *As a result of the pneumococcal vaccination rollout between 2006 and 2015, otitis media rates in Māori children decreased by 51%, and Māori children are now only 1.2 times more likely to experience otitis media than non-Māori children.*
- *Pacific Islands children are 1.5 times more likely to experience otitis media than non-Pacific Islands children.*

CULTURAL CONSIDERATIONS

Environment and nutrition play a significant role in the risk factors for ear and eye infections. Seventy-two per cent of Aboriginal and Torres Strait Islander peoples self-report that they live in housing of acceptable standard (i.e. structurally safe with functioning shower and toilet facilities). However, a significant number of Aboriginal and Torres Strait Islander peoples living in remote and very remote areas report that they live in unacceptable dwellings. More than 93% of Aboriginal and Torres Strait Islander peoples report that they do not eat the recommended servings of fruit and vegetables every day. Culturally appropriate, community-driven support to improve living standards, and education regarding the benefits of, and access to, improved nutrition can have a positive influence in reducing the risk factors associated with conditions that may compromise a person's hearing or vision.

There is much evidence that of the 25,000 Australian native species of flora, several possess significant health-enhancing properties as foods (bush foods). Working with communities to identify, embrace and capitalise on the benefits of traditional natural sources to improve the nutrition, health and prosperity of the community may strengthen resilience against health challenges.

Sources: Data from Australian Indigenous HealthInfoNet (2022a, 2022b); Australian Institute of Health and Welfare (2022a); Digby et al. (2021).

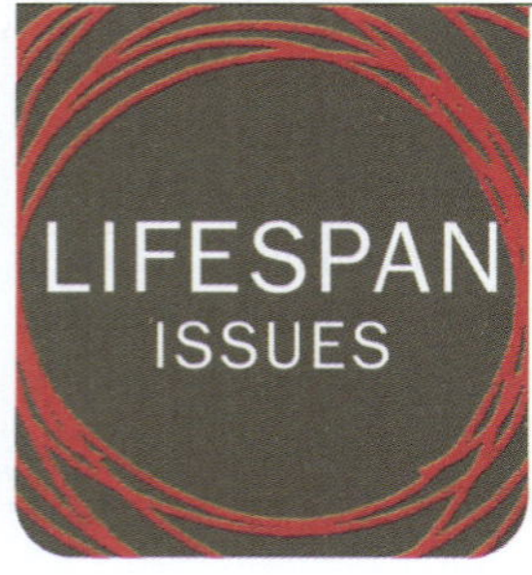

CHILDREN AND ADOLESCENTS

- Four per cent of children under 14 years of age are myopic.
- Three and a half per cent of children under 14 years of age are hyperopic.
- Severe vision loss in children is more commonly associated with developmental delay, cerebral palsy or hearing loss.
- Hearing loss in children is associated with poorer education outcomes when not identified and managed early.

OLDER ADULTS

- More than half of older adults (over 65 years of age) have hyperopia.
- More than one-third of older adults (over 65 years of age) have myopia.
- More than half of older adults (60–70 years of age) and more than two-thirds of adults over 70 years of age have hearing impairment or loss.

KEY CLINICAL ISSUES

- When caring for someone with vision impairment, knowledge of the specific disease process or mechanism of their vision loss is important to understand whether the vision loss will progress or remain stable.
- Implications for unilateral vision loss are important in the perception of depth. Any vision impairment increases the risk of falls.
- The need to explain activities and environmental noise is even more important when caring for a person with vision loss. Among some of the safety considerations in caring for someone with vision impairment, care with self-administered medications, trip hazards and burn prevention are important elements to consider when developing a management plan.
- When caring for those with hearing impairment, it is important not to cover your mouth when speaking, to face the person and to avoid speaking too rapidly. Conversation in quiet environments may make understanding easier.
- Chronic ear infections can lead to profound hearing loss. Aggressive management of chronic ear infections is important.
- If the administration of ototoxic drugs is necessary, consider reconstituting to a less concentrated solution and administering it over a longer period of time. Determination of serum drug levels may be valuable when using some drugs, such as aminoglycosides.

CHAPTER REVIEW

- Myopia and hyperopia are caused by refractive errors in the focusing of light on the retina. In *myopia* (near-sightedness or short-sightedness), the focal point is in front of the plane of the retina, causing an object in the distance to be out of focus. However, near objects appear in focus. In *hyperopia* (far-sightedness, long-sightedness or hypermetropia), the focal point is behind the plane of the retina such that a near object is viewed out of focus. These conditions can usually be treated using corrective lenses, such as contact lenses or eyeglasses.
- *Cataracts* are due to clouding of the lens. Cataracts reduce visual acuity and can lead to blindness. They develop as a result of ageing, exposure to chemicals or radiation, eye injury or secondary to disease. The three main types of age-related cataract are *cortical*, *nuclear* and *posterior subcapsular*. Prevention of their development is the best management strategy; however, cataract surgery can be very effective in improving vision.
- Common causes of hearing impairment include *conductive causes*, such as infection or otosclerosis, and *sensorineural causes*, such as presbycusis or noise-induced hearing loss.
- *Prevention* is critical in maintaining hearing, because, although alternative methods and equipment can be used to assist people's hearing, hearing loss is incurable.
- *Balance disorders* significantly increase the risk of falling. Use of medication and methods to reduce falls risk should be considered in people with vestibular issues.

REVIEW QUESTIONS

1. What are the most common conditions causing low vision and blindness in this region of the world?
2. Identify the three main types of cataract, and the distinguishing characteristics of each.
3. In what ways are age-related maculopathy and diabetic retinopathy similar, and in what ways are they different?
4. Differentiate between the two main forms of glaucoma.
5. Which drug classes can be used in the treatment of glaucoma? Briefly describe their mechanisms of action.
6. What colours are commonly confused in people with colour blindness?
7. What are some causes of conjunctivitis?
8. What are some causes of conductive hearing loss?
9. What are some causes of sensorineural hearing loss?
10. How does a chronic ear infection result in hearing loss?
11. What is the relationship between balance and hearing?
12. What interventions can reduce the risk of falls in a person with a vestibular disorder?

HEALTH PROFESSIONAL CONNECTIONS

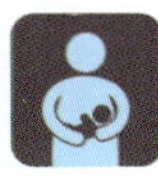

Midwives Hearing is critical for appropriate language development, and so the sooner an hearing impairment is detected, the less negative impact it will have in developmental milestones. Some midwives are being trained in the use of hearing screening equipment so that they can assess a newborn's hearing at 1–2 days old. If an issue is identified, babies should be referred to an audiologist within one month, so that further assessment can be undertaken.

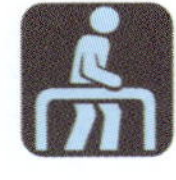

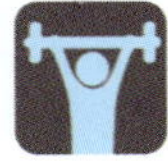

Physiotherapists/Exercise scientists Physiotherapists and exercise scientists must assess a person's falls risk as part of the process of developing an exercise prescription or rehabilitation program. Many conditions can increase the risk of falls. Assessment of an individual's risk is not only beneficial for duty of care and injury prevention, it also provides an opportunity to program appropriate exercises so as to reduce the likelihood of a fall. It is critical for exercise and rehabilitation professionals to understand the mechanisms that contribute to increased falls risk and that challenge balance recovery, including neurological and biomechanical influences.

Balance testing may include the reach test, one-leg-stand and sit-to-stand tests in the assessment phase. Balance training and falls prevention programs may include both static and dynamic balance exercises. Other components may include the stretching of calf, hamstring and hip flexor muscles; the strengthening of stabilising structures, such as the quadriceps, gluteal and dorsiflexor muscles; and posture and functional strength training. Progressing through graduated stages, including with eyes open and with eyes closed, is important for development.

Education regarding the identification of home hazards may be required. Referral for further medical assessments may also be required when it is considered that the instability is related to an acute medical condition.

CASE STUDY

Ms Mia Thomas (UR number 765564) is a shy, quiet 3-year-old girl who lives in a remote Aboriginal community. Mia lives with her mother, two aunties and seven other children in a small three-bedroom house. All three adults and one older child in the household smoke cigarettes. Mia shares a bed with two other children. As part of an otitis media screening and management program, an Aboriginal Health Worker visited the community and observed that four children in Mia's household had otitis media (including the other two children who shared her bed). However, Mia's condition was the worst, as she has chronic suppurative otitis media; bilateral, moderate-grade ruptured tympanic membranes; and an aural discharge her mother said has been constant for about three weeks. Mia's mum thought that Mia was getting better, because about a month ago she was really 'playing-up', crying and pulling at her ears all the time, but then a few weeks ago that behaviour stopped. Mrs Thomas also said that Mia has had 'deadly ears' almost ever since she was born. Mia's observations are as follows.

Temperature	Heart rate	Respiration rate	Blood pressure	SpO_2
37.3°C	106	26	104/55	98% (RA*)

*RA = room air.

The healthcare worker sampled the exudate in both of Mia's ears and sent it off for microscopy, culture and sensitivity testing. After consultation and video otoscopy, images were sent via a telehealth system (computer) to an ear, nose and throat specialist, and Mia (and the three other children) were commenced on treatment. Mia's treatment consisted of ototopical administration of the antimicrobial agent ciprofloxacin twice a day, and gentle ear cleaning with a povidone-iodine antiseptic solution (before drops) to remove the purulent material. The healthcare worker stayed at this location for a fortnight, and so was able to assist with the cleaning and ototopical treatment regimen. Before the screening and management program team left, they performed audiometry on Mia and found that she has a 54 dB hearing impairment in her left ear and a 63 dB hearing impairment in her right ear.

Her microbiology results came back later, showing:

MICROBIOLOGY (LEFT EAR)

Patient location:	Outpatient	**UR:**	765564		
Consultant:	Smith	**NAME:**	Thomas		
		Given name:	Mia	**Sex:**	F
		DOB:	21/06/XX	**Age:**	3
Time collected	12:10	**Organisms**	**1.** *Pseudomonas aeruginosa*		
Date collected	XX/XX	**Isolated**	**2.**		
Year	XXXX				
Lab #	456354644				

Specimen site	L) Ear	**Antimicrobial sensitivities S = Sensitive R = Resistant**			
Leukocytes	++	Organism	1 2 3	Organism	1 2 3
Erythrocytes	+	Ampicillin	R	Flucloxacillin	R
Proteins	trace	Amoxicillin	R	Gentamicin	S
		Ciprofloxacin	S	Rifampicin	
		Ceftriaxone	R	Sodium fusidate	S
		Cephalothin	R	Ticarcillin	
		Chloramphenicol	S	Timentin	S
		Cotrimoxazole	S	Trimethoprim	S
		Erythromycin		Vancomycin	
Gram	**Gram negative**	✔			
stain	**Gram positive**	✗			
	Bacilli	✗			
	Cocci	✗			
	Other	rod			

MICROBIOLOGY (RIGHT EAR)

Patient location:	Outpatient	**UR:**	765564		
Consultant:	Smith	**NAME:**	Thomas		
		Given name:	Mia	**Sex:**	F
		DOB:	21/06/XX	**Age:**	3
Time collected	12:10	**Organisms**	**1.** *Pseudomonas aeruginosa*		
Date collected	XX/XX	**Isolated**	**2.**		
Year	XXXX				
Lab #	456354645				

Specimen site	L) Ear	**Antimicrobial sensitivities S = Sensitive R = Resistant**			
Leukocytes	+ +	Organism	1 2 3	Organism	1 2 3
Erythrocytes	+	Ampicillin	R	Flucloxacillin	R
Proteins	trace	Amoxicillin	R	Gentamicin	S
		Ciprofloxacin	S	Rifampicin	
		Ceftriaxone	R	Sodium fusidate	S
		Cephalothin	R	Ticarcillin	
		Chloramphenicol	S	Timentin	
		Cotrimoxazole	S	Trimethoprim	S
		Erythromycin		Vancomycin	S
Gram	**Gram negative**	✔			
stain	**Gram positive**	✗			
	Bacilli	✗			
	Cocci	✗			
	Other	**rod**			

CRITICAL THINKING

1. What risk factors does Mia have for the development of chronic suppurative otitis media? List them all, and explain how each factor contributes to an increased risk.
2. A statement in the case study suggests that 'Mia's mum thought that Mia was getting better'. Why would Mia's mum think that? What may have occurred three weeks ago that resulted in a change in Mia's behaviour? (*Hint:* Think about anatomical issues.)
3. Observe the microbiology results. What organism/s has/have caused Mia's chronic suppurative otitis media? Is/Are this/these organism/s different from the common pathogens responsible for acute otitis media? Is the antimicrobial likely to work? Explain.
4. Mia had an audiometry assessment. What is the significance of her results? What does this mean for Mia's development and future schooling? What considerations need to be undertaken in the light of these results? (*Hint:* How do Mia's results compare to the grades on the World Health Organization hearing impairment scale? What is the association between language development and hearing?) Given the history provided, is it likely that the hearing impairment has already had an impact on her development?
5. Analysing the risk factors you have identified earlier, what interventions will be necessary to prevent the otitis media from affecting this family in the future?

BIBLIOGRAPHY

Australian Health Ministers' Advisory Council's National and Aboriginal and Torres Strait Islander Health Standing Committee (2017). *Cultural respect framework 2016–2026: for Aboriginal and Torres Strait Islander health—a national approach to building a culturally respectful health system.* https://nacchocommunique.files.wordpress.com/2016/12/cultural_respect_framework_1december2016_1.pdf.

Australian Indigenous HealthInfoNet (2022a). *Overview of Aboriginal and Torres Strait Islander health status, 2021.* Perth, WA: Australian Indigenous HealthInfoNet. https://healthinfonet.ecu.edu.au/learn/health-facts/overview-aboriginal-torres-strait-islander-health-status.

Australian Indigenous Health*Info*Net (2022b). *Summary of Aboriginal and Torres Strait Islander health status—selected topics 2021.* Perth, WA: Australian Indigenous Health*Info*Net. https://apo.org.au/sites/default/files/resource-files/2022-03/apo-nid317082_0.pdf.

Australian Institute of Health and Welfare (AIHW) (2020). *Aboriginal and Torres Strait Islander Health Performance Framework 2020.* Cat. No. IHPF 2. Canberra: AIHW. https://www.indigenoushpf.gov.au/publications/hpf-summary-2020.

Australian Institute of Health and Welfare (AIHW) (2021a). *Indigenous eye health measures 2021.* Cat. No. IHW 261. Canberra: AIHW. https://www.aihw.gov.au/getmedia/8cbb0723-1623-4b97-99f6-179c9d420f63/aihw-ihw-261.pdf.aspx?inline=true.

Australian Institute of Health and Welfare (AIHW) (2021b). *Queensland's Deadly Ears Program: Indigenous children receiving services for ear disease and hearing loss 2007–2019.* Cat. No. IHW 249. Canberra: AIHW. https://www.aihw.gov.au/getmedia/122ae9b5-2a08-4375-8e19-f2543c080dfc/aihw-ihw-249.pdf.aspx?inline=true.

Australian Institute of Health and Welfare (AIHW) (2022a). *Ear and hearing health of Aboriginal and Torres Strait Islander people 2021*. Cat. No. IHW 262. https://www.aihw.gov.au/getmedia/557cc818-3c84-4138-b8a5-daf1b35f28ba/aihw-ihw-262.pdf.aspx?inline=true.

Australian Institute of Health and Welfare (AIHW) (2022b). *Eye health*. Cat. No. PHE 260. Canberra: AIHW. https://www.aihw.gov.au/getmedia/12000df9-44cd-40ef-8d71-ea8117792ee4/Eye-health.pdf.aspx?inline=true.

Australian Institute of Health and Welfare (AIHW) (2022c). *Hearing health outreach services to Aboriginal and Torres Strait Islander children and young people in the Northern Territory: July 2012 to December 2021.* Cat. No. IHW 266. Canberra: AIHW. https://www.aihw.gov.au/getmedia/4aed9af4-0ded-4260-aabb-959bef2968c2/aihw-ihw-266.pdf.aspx?inline=true.

Bashour, M., Menassa, J. & Gerontis, C.C. (2018). Congenital cataract. *Emedicine*. https://emedicine.medscape.com/article/1210837-overview.

Bauldoff, G., Gubrud-Howe, P.M., Carno, M.-A., Levett-Jones, T., Hales, M., Berry, K., ... Stanley, D. (2020). *LeMone and Burke's medical–surgical nursing: critical thinking for person-centred care* (4th [Australian] edn). Sydney: Pearson Australia.

Best, O. & Fredericks, B. (2021). *Yatdjuligin: Aboriginal and Torres Strait Islander nursing and midwifery care* (3rd edn). Port Melbourne, VIC: Cambridge University Press.

Best Practice Advocacy Centre New Zealand (BPAC NZ) (2022). *Otitis media: A common childhood illness.* Dunedin: BPAC NZ. https://bpac.org.nz/2022/otitis-media.aspx.

Bloomenstein, M. (2016). An atlas of conjunctival and scleral anomalies. *Review of Optometry.* https://www.reviewofoptometry.com/article/an-atlas-of-conjunctival-and-scleral-anomalies.

Bullock, S. & Manias, E. (2022). *Fundamentals of pharmacology* (9th edn). Sydney: Pearson Australia.

Casani, A.P., Gufoni, M. & Capobianco, S. (2021). Current insights into treating vertigo in older adults. *Drugs and Aging* 38(8):655–70. https://doi.org/10.1007/s40266-021-00877-z.

Centre for Eye Research Australia and Vision (2020). *The National Eye Health Survey 2016.* https://www.vision2020australia.org.au/wp-content/uploads/2019/06/National-Eye-Health-Survey_Full-Report_FINAL.pdf.

Centre for Genetics Education (2019). *Fact sheet 63: deafness and hearing loss.* St Leonards, NSW: Centre for Genetics Education. https://www.genetics.edu.au/PDF/Deafness_and_hearing_loss_fact_sheet-CGE.pdf.

Digby, J.E., Purdy, S.C. & Kelly, A.S. (2021). *Deafness notification report (2020): hearing loss (not remediable by grommets) in New Zealanders under the age of 19.* Auckland: New Zealand Audiological Society. https://audiology.org.nz/assets/Uploads/DND/Deafness-Notification-Database-2020-Report.pdf.

Higgins, T.S. (2022). Otitis media with effusion. *Emedicine*. https://emedicine.medscape.com/article/858990-overview.

Kesser, B.W. (2022). Aural atresia. *Emedicine*. https://emedicine.medscape.com/article/878218-overview.

Li, J.C. (2020). Ménière's disease (idiopathic endolymphatic hydrops). *Emedicine*. https://emedicine.medscape.com/article/1159069-overview.

Mantooth, R. (2021). Ear foreign body removal in emergency medicine. *Emedicine*. https://emedicine.medscape.com/article/763712-overview.

Marieb, E.N. & Hoehn, K. (2019). *Human anatomy and physiology* (11th edn). San Francisco, CA: Pearson Benjamin Cummings.

Mathur, N.J. (2022). Noise-induced hearing loss. *Emedicine.* https://emedicine.medscape.com/article/857813-overview.

McCreery, K.M. (2022). Cataract in children. *UpToDate*. https://www.uptodate.com/contents/cataract-in-children.

Mudd, P.A., Jones, J.W., Glatz, F.R., Campbell, K.C.M. & Rybak, L.P. (2021). Ototoxicity. *Emedicine.* https://emedicine.medscape.com/article/857679-overview.

Ocampo, V.V.D. & Foster, C.S. (2021). Senile cataract (age-related cataract). *Emedicine.* https://emedicine.medscape.com/article/1210914-overview.

Saadi, R.A. & Isildak, H. (2021). Presbycusis. *Emedicine.* https://reference.medscape.com/article/855989-overview.

Shohet, J.A. (2021). Otosclerosis. *Emedicine.* https://emedicine.medscape.com/article/859760-overview.

Varughese, D. & Ying, Y.-I.M. (2021). Chronic suppurative otitis media. *Emedicine.* https://emedicine.medscape.com/article/859501-overview.

Waitzman, A.A. (2022). Otitis externa. *Emedicine.* https://emedicine.medscape.com/article/994550-overview.

Walker, R.E., Bartley, J, Flint, D., Thompson, J.M.D. & Mitchell, E.A. (2017). Determinants of chronic otitis media with effusion in preschool children: a case-control study. *BMC Pediatrics* 17(2017):4. https://doi.org/10.1186/s12887-016-0767-7.

Mental health disorders

15

LEARNING OBJECTIVES

After completing this chapter, you should be able to:

1. Discuss mental health and the factors influencing affect, cognition and behaviour.
2. Describe the pathophysiology, clinical manifestations, diagnosis and management of common affective disorders, such as depression, mania and bipolar disorder.
3. Explore the pathophysiology, clinical manifestations and management of anxiety disorders.
4. Describe the influence of gut dysbiosis on mental health and illness.
5. Explore the complexities of schizophrenia, including its clinical manifestations, diagnosis and management.
6. Discuss the complexities of substance dependence and behavioural addictions.
7. Review the significance of dual diagnosis in relation to mental health disorders.

WHAT YOU SHOULD KNOW BEFORE YOU START THIS CHAPTER

Can you describe the process of neurotransmission?

Can you identify key neurotransmitters within the central nervous system?

Can you identify the principal parts and regions of the brain, and state their functions?

KEY TERMS

Anxiety
Behavioural addiction
Bipolar disorder
Depression
Dopamine (DA)
Dual diagnosis
Gamma-aminobutyric acid (GABA)
Harm minimisation
Mania
Noradrenaline (NA)
Obsessive–compulsive disorder (OCD)
Post-traumatic stress disorder
Psychosis
Schizophrenia
Serotonin (5-HT)
Substance dependence

Introduction

In this chapter, mental health disorders concerned with abnormal affect (emotions), behaviour and thought processes will be examined. As there are over 300 conditions that can influence cognitive function, affect and/or behaviour, this chapter will only deal with selected conditions that are more prevalent or particularly disabling. Specific focus will target affective disorders that primarily relate to conditions influencing mood and emotional state (e.g. depression and mania); anxiety disorders that influence emotions, behaviour and motor function; psychoses (e.g. thought disorders) associated with alterations in cognition and behaviour;

and addiction. These disorders present with varying degrees of severity that can result in profound and chronic disability, requiring complex management needs and, sometimes, there may be limited successful treatment options. Moreover, these conditions are associated with high rates of comorbid substance misuse, suicide attempts and relationship breakdowns.

Factors influencing mental health and wellness

LEARNING OBJECTIVE 1

Discuss mental health and the factors influencing affect, cognition and behaviour.

A good way to begin to recognise the depth and breadth of defined mental health issues is through observing how they are classified and organised in systems such as ICD-10. Although not specific to mental health, the classification system provides a practical method through which to organise conditions affecting a person's mental health (see Figure 15.1). It is important to note that, although not discussed in this text, the *Diagnostic and Statistical Manual of Mental Disorders, Fifth Edition, Text Revision (DSM-5-TR)* is the comprehensive clinical resource for mental health professionals.

Research into factors influencing mental health and wellness is prolific and ever-evolving. Some common overarching themes include biological, nutritional, environmental and sociocultural influences, and drug exposure. Figure 15.2 demonstrates the complexity of the various influences affecting mental health and wellness along a relative continuum, beginning with early developmental considerations and progressing through early and later exposures.

Brain regions involved in affect, cognition and behaviour

A number of brain regions have been implicated in normal affect, cognition and behaviour. These regions include areas within the cerebrum, diencephalon and brainstem. Historically, these areas have been grouped together into a regional network called the *limbic system*. While the concept that normal brain function requires successful communication across networks of brain regions is still accepted, the contributions of some areas of the so-called limbic system as it was originally conceived are now considered to be less important than once thought. The major brain areas include the prefrontal area, anterior cingulate gyrus, amygdala, basal ganglia, hippocampus, hypothalamus and brainstem. Each of these brain areas contributes to the processing of emotions, cognition and behaviour (see Figure 15.3).

Currently, the pathophysiology of affective and thought disorders is believed to involve an impairment in one or more of these brain areas that results in disruptions to communication through this network. However, as a greater understanding of more complex physiology develops, new and emerging considerations regarding other types of influence of seemingly disparate systems may hold more keys to explain significant gaps in our knowledge regarding mental health conditions. One example is the research on the influence of gut micro-organisms on health, mood and behaviour.

Affective disorders

LEARNING OBJECTIVE 2

Describe the pathophysiology, clinical manifestations, diagnosis and management of common affective disorders, such as depression, mania and bipolar disorder.

Mood disorders involve extremes of affect—at one end depression and at the other end mania. Some people experience only one of these states, while others cycle from one state to the other. The latter condition is referred to as bipolar disorder.

DEPRESSION

Depression is characterised as a state of profound sadness. It is also variously known as *melancholia*, 'the blues' or living with/having 'the black dog'. Depression can develop across the lifespan—from childhood to old age. The degree or intensity of the condition also varies greatly from person to person, manifesting as a mild, moderate or severe (major) disorder.

Depression is now considered one of the most important causes of non-fatal disease burden worldwide, a burden considered to be greater than that of having arthritis, asthma, diabetes or angina. In part, the greater burden is believed to be accounted for by the relatively poorer clinical management of depression compared to these other conditions. Indeed, it is highly likely that people with these other chronic diseases will have comorbid depression.

Aetiology and pathophysiology

The two main types of depression are reactive and endogenous. *Reactive depression* develops in response to an external trigger, such as the death of a family member or a friend, the breakdown of a close relationship, difficulties at work or in education, or upon hearing bad news. This form of depression usually does not require long-term therapy, and most people can overcome this state with good support from family and friends. *Endogenous depression* manifests without a recognisable external trigger, and can be very debilitating. This form usually requires longer-term clinical management to help normalise the affected person's state of mind.

A long-held view on the pathophysiology of depression is that there is a chemical imbalance in the brain associated with decreases in the synaptic levels of the biogenic amine neurotransmitters **serotonin (5-HT)** (5-hydroxytryptamine) and **noradrenaline (NA)** in the pathways controlling mood. This is referred to as the *biogenic amine theory of depression* (also known as the *biogenic amine hypothesis*). Serotonin is considered to be more strongly implicated in motor activity, which also changes in this condition. Another biogenic amine transmitter, **dopamine (DA)**,

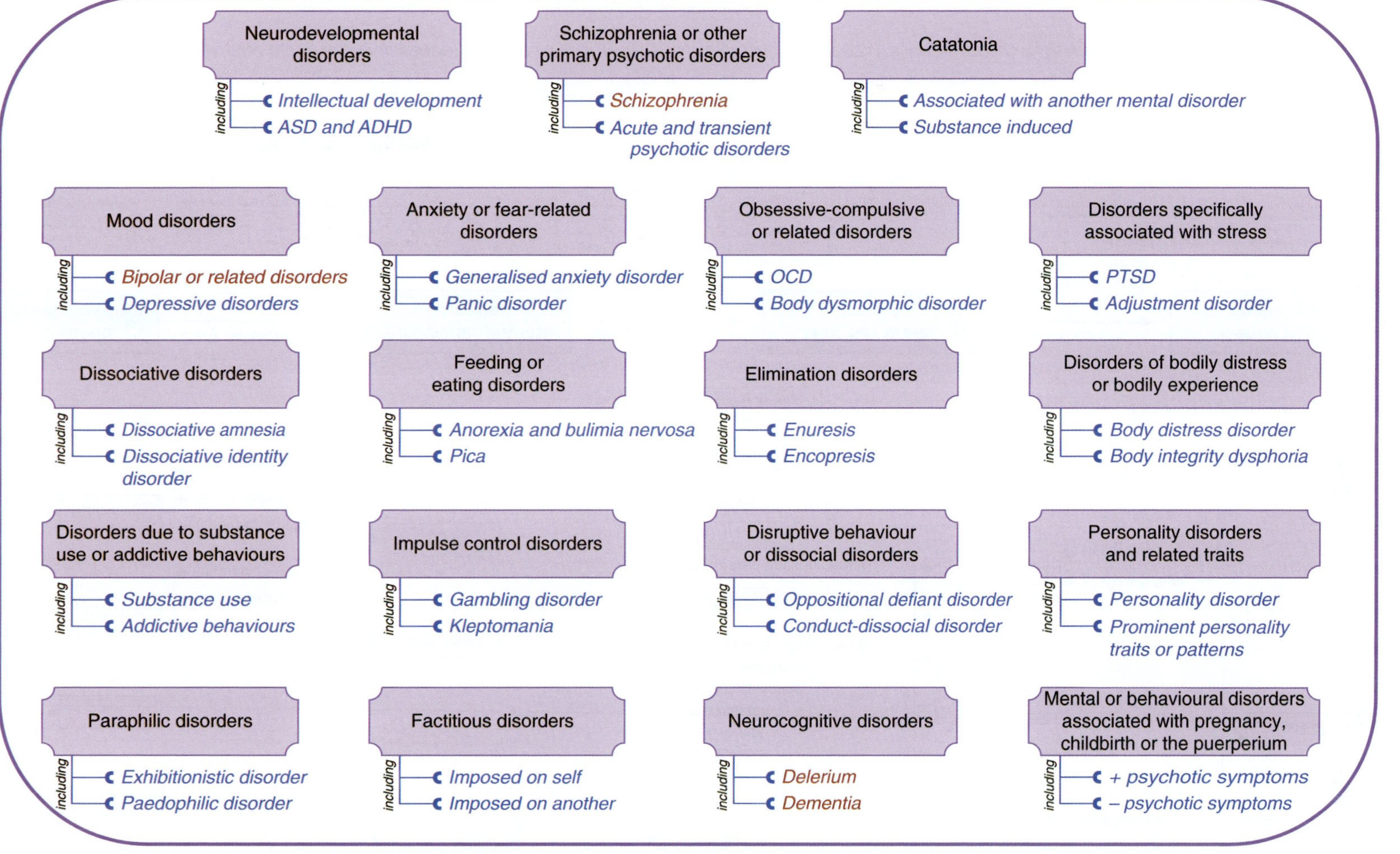

Figure 15.1

Selected mental health disorders organised by ICD-11 classification

+ = with; – = without; ADHD = attention deficit hyperactivity disorder; ASD = autism spectrum disorder; IQ = intelligence quotient; OCD = obsessive-compulsive disorder; PTSD = post-traumatic stress disorder.

Items in red are conditions discussed in depth in this chapter.

Source: Data from the World Health Organization (2022a).

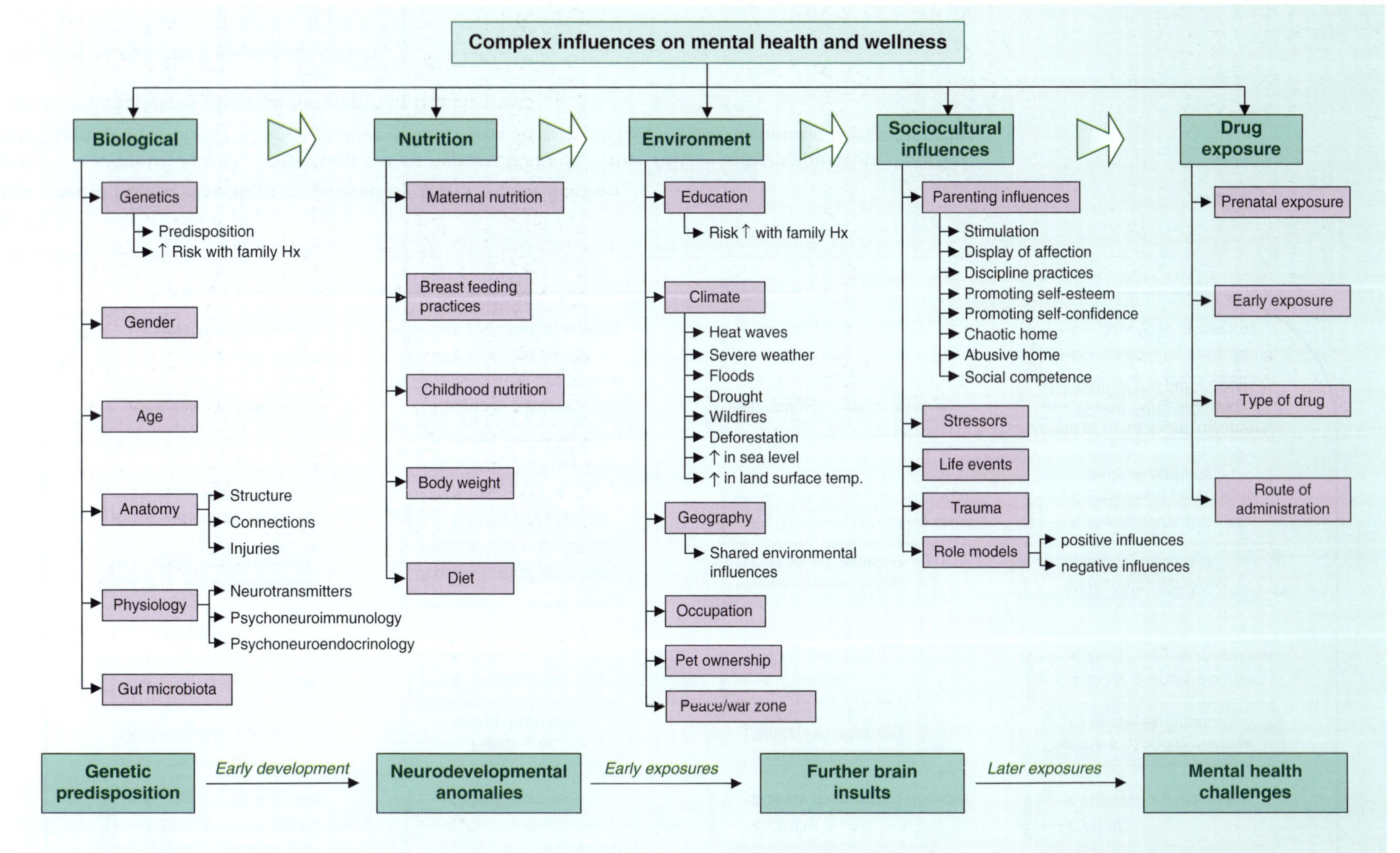

Figure 15.2

Common influences on mental health and wellness

↑ = increased; Hx = history.

Sources: Data from Cortes-Albornoz et al. (2021); Hui Gan et al. (2020); Hungerford et al. (2021); Mac Giollabhui et al (2021); Sui et al. (2022); Toso et al. (2020); Uher & Zwicker (2017); Wang et al. (2017).

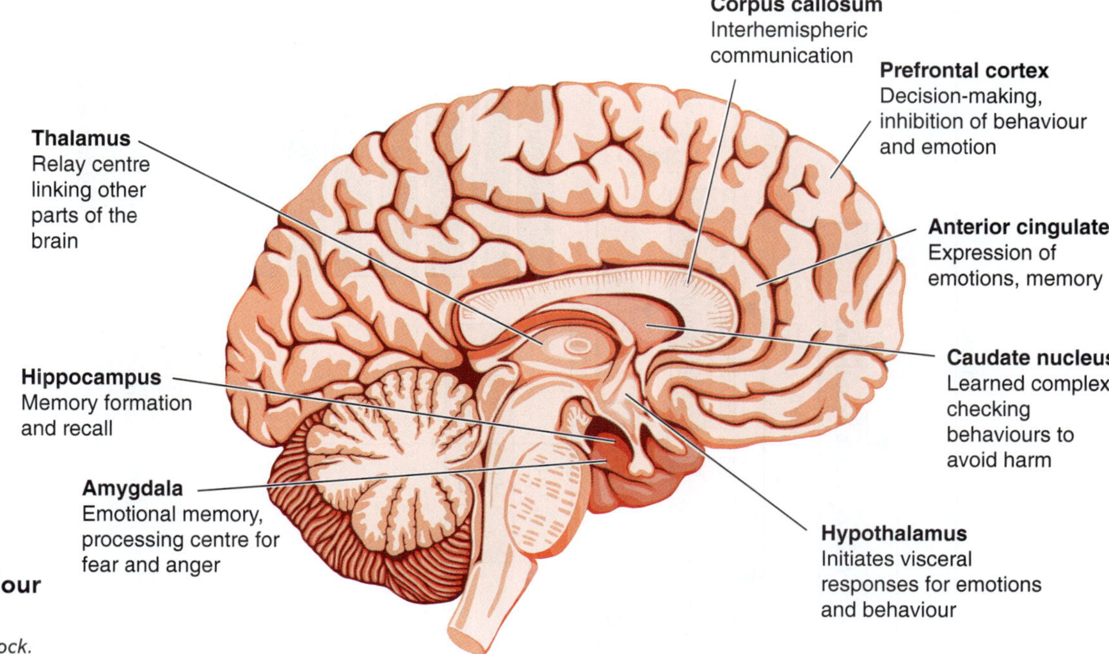

Figure 15.3

Major brain areas involved in affect, cognition and behaviour

Source: Soul wind/Shutterstock.

may also be involved in the pathophysiology, but its specific role in the dysfunction remains relatively less clear. In support of this view, antidepressant drug treatments that raise the synaptic levels of serotonin and/or noradrenaline in the brain can induce clinical improvement in people with depressive illness.

This theory, however, does not reflect the full picture of the pathophysiological processes underlying depression. Acute elevations of synaptic transmitter levels are not sufficient to improve mood, as it takes two to six weeks of therapy before clinical benefits are observed. Therefore, long-term antidepressant drug treatment is required for the relief of depression. Further to this, drugs that antagonise the central serotonin receptors do not induce depression. This has led to a change in the pathophysiological perspective in more recent years. It is now argued that *the way the brain is wired changes in depressive illness*. There is evidence that connections between neurons, connections between each brain region and the size of brain regions change in depression. In depression, the availability of certain neuronal growth factors, such as *brain-derived neurotrophic factor (BDNF)*, may be deficient. In chronic severe depression, the *hypothalamic hormone corticotropic-releasing factor* is elevated, which in turn induces cortisol secretion from the adrenal gland. Changes in the levels of these hormones correlate with a decrease in the size of the hippocampus, which is involved in the formation of long-term memories and contributes to the control of emotions.

Long-term antidepressant therapy is believed to assist in the normalisation of these connections, which is why it takes weeks before clinical improvement takes place. Indeed, this process may well be influenced by an increased availability of factors such as BDNF being triggered by drug treatment.

Epidemiology

Approximately 38% of all general practitioner (GP) encounters in 2022 were related to mental health conditions, and 38% of those presentations were for depression. Antidepressant medications were prescribed 29% of the time, and women were almost twice as likely to present compared to men. The 2021 National Survey of Mental Health and Wellbeing estimates that 44% of people aged between 16 and 85 years old have experienced a mental health disorder in their lifetime. Approximately 44% of Australians surveyed reported that they had experienced symptoms of mental illness, and about 5% have a severe episodic or persistent illness. In New Zealand, approximately 22% of people report poor mental wellbeing. From puberty onwards, Australian and New Zealand women are twice as likely to experience depression and report it compared to men from these countries. Older adults are particularly susceptible to depression as a result of circumstances such as chronic disease, chronic pain, isolation and bereavement.

Clinical manifestations

Accompanying the profound feelings of sadness, a person with depression will also experience other symptoms, including loss of interest in their appearance, anhedonia (absence of pleasure), apathy, fatigue, insomnia, loss of appetite, changes in body weight, psychomotor agitation, feelings of worthlessness and suicidal intent. Figure 15.4 explores the common clinical manifestations and management of depression.

Clinical diagnosis and management

Diagnosis As with all mental health issues, organic causes of behavioural change must be ruled out. Measurement of full blood count and vitamin B_{12} (for anaemia), thyroid function (for hypothyroidism), and liver and kidney function (for hepatic or renal disorders) should be performed. A magnetic resonance imaging (MRI) or computed tomography (CT) scan should be performed if bizarre or atypical behaviours are reported. However, the primary diagnostic tools for depression include a review of the presenting history and a mental status assessment.

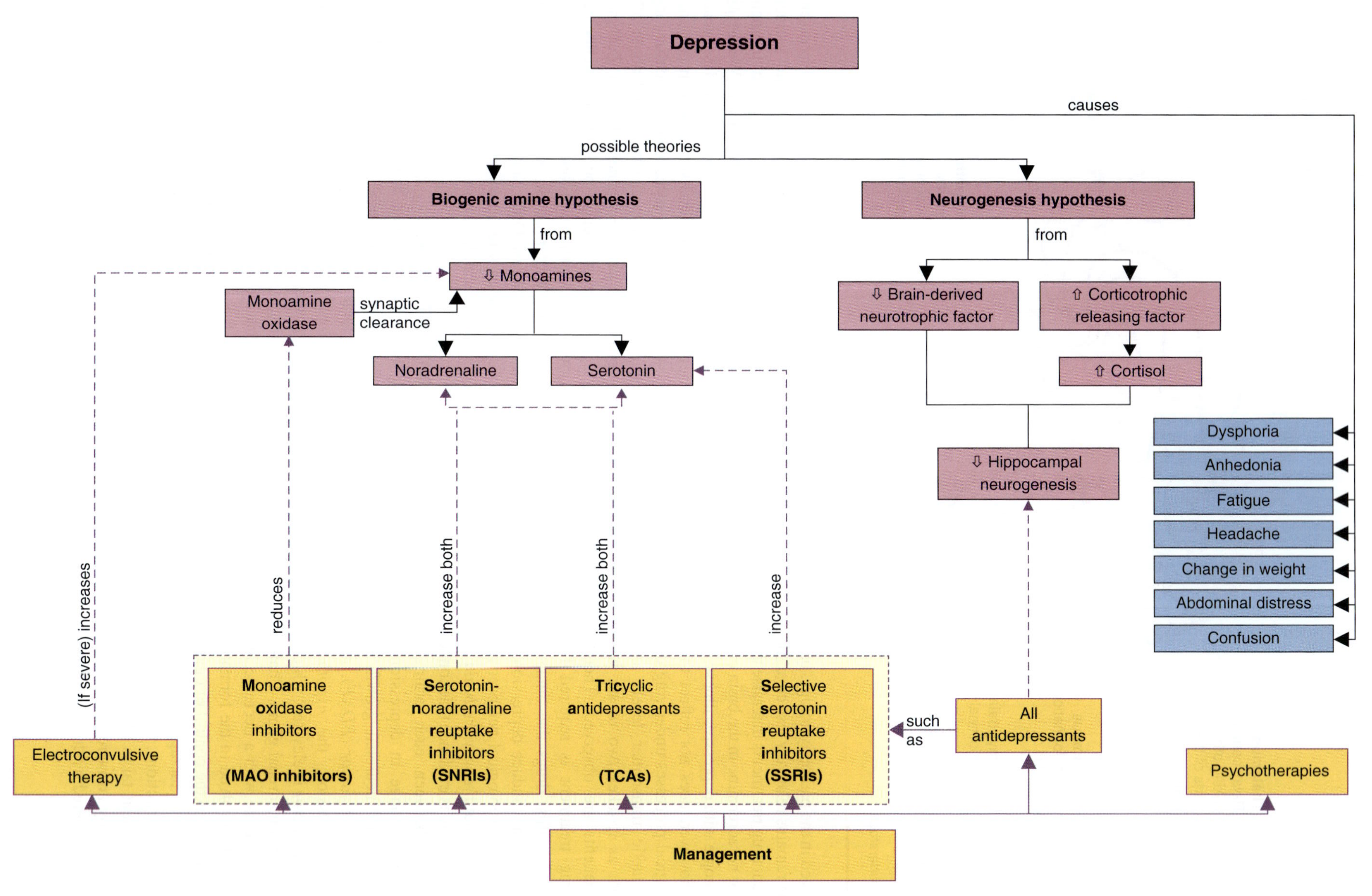

Figure 15.4
Clinical snapshot: Depression
↓ = decreased; ↑ = increased.

Specific discussion surrounding perceived causes may be beneficial, especially in the context of reactive depression.

Management The best management of depression includes a combination of psychotherapy, exercise, good nutrition and antidepressant therapy. Although there is a shift in theories related to the pathophysiology of depression, the manipulation of the neurotransmitters serotonin and noradrenaline with antidepressant medications still remains the most common intervention. Several different types of antidepressants are available, each having their own benefits, limitations and side-effects (see Figure 15.5). Medication adherence can be an issue in the management of people with depression. Antidepressant treatment may take a few weeks to reach therapeutic levels, delaying an appreciable gain by the affected person. This issue must be clearly explained to the individual and to their significant others in order to improve the chances of success.

People who are refractory to antidepressant therapy (when therapeutic levels are established) and become significantly disabled by overwhelming depression or catatonia may benefit from electroconvulsive therapy (ECT).

BIPOLAR DISORDER

In **bipolar disorder**, a person's mood swings between the extremes—from depression to mania. Until relatively recently, this condition was known as *manic–depressive disease*. **Mania** is characterised by a heightened mood state and increased activity. The two main forms of bipolar disorder are called type I and type II. *Type I* is characterised by longer, more severe manic episodes and the person may show psychosis. *Type II* is milder, with shorter episodes and no psychosis.

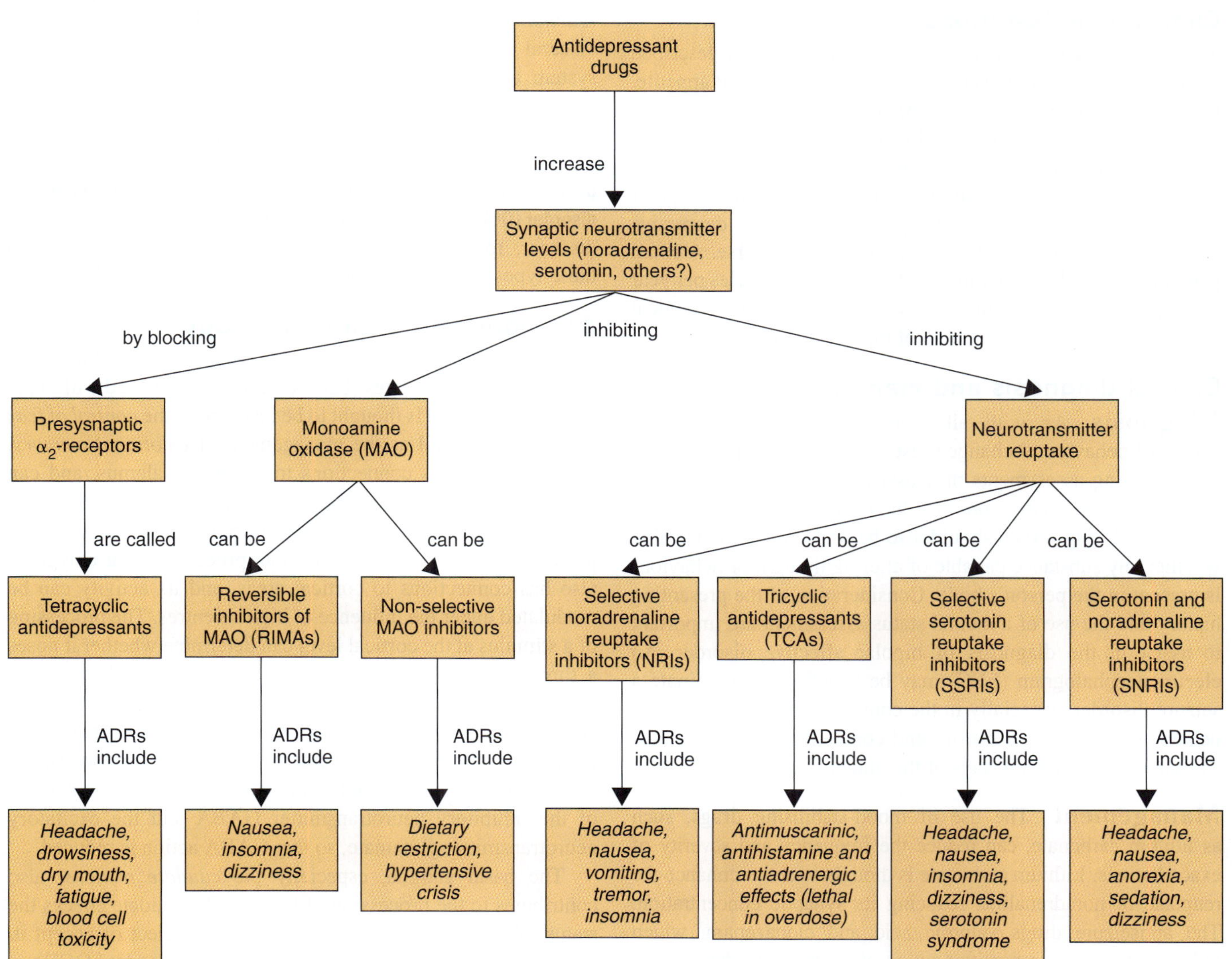

Figure 15.5

Antidepressant drugs and their profiles

ADR = adverse drug reaction.

Source: Bullock & Manias (2022), Figure 24.3, p. 273.

Aetiology and pathophysiology

According to the biogenic amine theory, mania is associated with an elevation in the synaptic levels of noradrenaline and serotonin. It has been suggested that synaptic transmitter levels are *labile* in bipolar disorder. It is thought that as the synaptic transmitter levels change, there is an attempt to shift them back in the direction of normal, but they overshoot the normal range and move towards the other extreme. A correction then sends the synaptic levels too far the other way.

Epidemiology

As a result of the COVID-19 pandemic, the World Health Organization suggests that the prevalence of anxiety and depression has increased by 25%. When compared to people with depression, people with bipolar disorder show higher rates of substance misuse, greater disability and increased suicide attempts.

Clinical manifestations

The clinical manifestations of depression have been described earlier. The manifestations of mania include decreased appetite, talkativeness (pressure of speech), grandiose ideas, insomnia, racing thoughts, euphoria, irritability, impulsiveness, increased sex drive and being easily distracted.

There is a lot of variability in the way in which bipolar disorder manifests. Some people show more depressive episodes than mania, while for others it is the reverse. A small percentage will show only mania. The number of cycles per year can also vary greatly. Figure 15.6 explores the common clinical manifestations and management of bipolar disorder.

Clinical diagnosis and management

Diagnosis As with all mental health issues, organic causes of behavioural change must be ruled out. Pathology and neuroimaging assessments may assist in ruling out an organic cause (see the section on the diagnosis of depression). An alcohol and drug screen should also be performed to determine whether any substance capable of altering thought or behaviour is present in the person's body. Consideration of the presenting history and the use of a mental status assessment are important to assist in the diagnosis of bipolar affective disorder. An electroencephalogram (EEG) may be beneficial to eliminate a seizure disorder, especially in the context of bizarre or atypical behaviour. Obtaining a history and conducting a mental status assessment are the mainstays of the diagnosis.

Management The use of mood-stabilising drugs, such as lithium carbonate, can reduce the frequency and severity of exacerbations. Lithium carbonate is thought to act to enhance the reuptake of noradrenaline, reducing its synaptic concentration. The antiseizure drugs valproic acid and clonazepam, which influence the neurotransmitter action of **gamma-aminobutyric acid (GABA)** in the brain, are considered beneficial when the affected person is unresponsive to lithium or cycles rapidly between the two extremes of mood. Some atypical (second-generation) antipsychotics can be useful during both the manic and the depressive phases of the disorder. During the depressive phase, a person may require antidepressant medications, or even ECT in severe episodes. In the manic phase of the disorder, first- and/or second-generation antipsychotics may be required. There is no one protocol beneficial for everyone, as the severity of disease and the effect of therapy, metabolism and environment are all different. Unfortunately, trialling different drug regimens is really the only method to find the individualised ideal dose titration.

Anxiety disorders

LEARNING OBJECTIVE 3

Explore the pathophysiology, clinical manifestations and management of anxiety disorders.

Anxiety is associated with circumstances in which a person *perceives a stimulus as a threat*, irrespective of whether or not it may actually be threatening. The stimulus *evokes a patterned reaction* involving cognitive, emotional, behavioural, motor and visceral responses. The responses include sympathetic nervous system activation, alterations in attention and concentration, sleep disturbances, ritualised behaviour and changes in motor responsiveness. There are a number of types of anxiety disorder, including *generalised anxiety disorder, phobias, panic attacks,* **post-traumatic stress disorder (PTSD)** and **obsessive-compulsive disorder (OCD)**. The most common of these is generalised anxiety disorder, followed by the phobias. The differences between these types of anxiety disorders are summarised in Table 15.1.

Aetiology and pathophysiology

Evidence indicates that the *amygdala* is the key area of the brain involved in anxiety states. This brain region is located within the temporal lobe, and is thought to be involved in the *control of fear and anger*, as well as the management of *emotional memory*. The amygdala has connections to the hypothalamus, and can activate the visceral and behavioural responses associated with emotional states. These responses can be rapidly activated in the presence of a threat without conscious processing. The amygdala also has connections to cortical areas, and its activity can be modulated under the influence of higher centres. The processing of a stimulus at the cortical level can determine whether it poses a threat and whether the visceral and behavioural responses activated by the amygdala should be heightened or inhibited. A *distortion in the interaction* between these brain regions is thought to underlie the development of these anxiety states, and is believed to be linked to the balance between the activity of the inhibitory neurotransmitter GABA and the excitatory neurotransmitter glutamate, so that GABA action is reduced.

The basal ganglia, especially the *caudate nucleus*, also contributes to the processing of threats. The caudate checks the status of the threat and decides whether to reject or accept it. In disorders such as obsessive–compulsive disorder (OCD), it has been proposed the caudate becomes 'stuck' in one position, maintaining the threat status rather than rejecting it. This leads to repetitive ritualised behaviours by the person to cope with the threat, such as washing their hands or opening a door a set number of times.

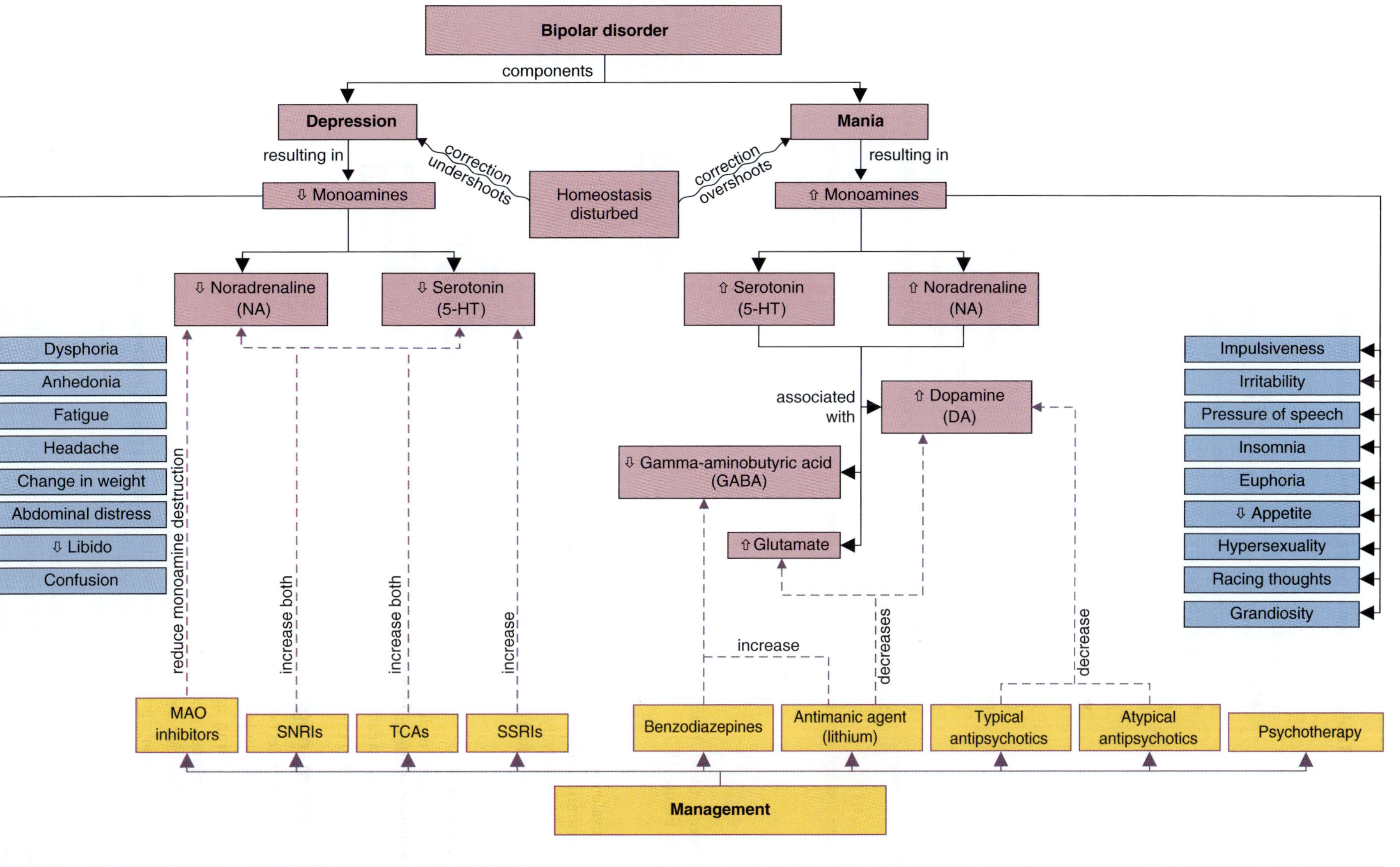

Figure 15.6

Clinical snapshot: Bipolar disorder

↓ = decreased; ↑ = increased; atypical antipsychotics = second-generation antipsychotics; typical antipsychotics = first-generation antipsychotics; MAO inhibitors = monoamine inhibitors; SNRIs = selective noradrenaline reuptake inhibitors; SSRIs = selective serotonin reuptake inhibitors; TCAs = tricyclic antidepressants.

Table 15.1 Some types of common anxiety disorders

Disorder	Features
Panic attack	A short-lived period of intense fear and discomfort.
Generalised anxiety disorder	Excessive anxiety over a number of events, occurring on more days than not for at least 6 months.
Agoraphobia	Fear of being trapped in places or situations where escape or help might not be possible.
Post-traumatic stress disorder (PTSD)	Anxiety associated with exposure to a traumatic event where the person was confronted by death or serious injury and their response involved fear, helplessness or horror.
Obsessive–compulsive disorder (OCD)	Anxiety or distress associated with recurrent and persistent thoughts, experienced as intrusive and inappropriate, which are products of the person's own mind. The person engages in repetitive, ritualised behaviours in order to reduce anxiety.
Social phobias	Fear of social situations where the person is exposed to unfamiliar people or scrutiny by others and where they believe they will act in an embarrassing manner.
Specific phobias	Unreasonable and persistent fear triggered by the presence or anticipation of specific situations or objects.

Source: Data from Diagnostic and Statistical Manual of Mental Disorders *(5th edn, Text Revision), http://www.psychiatryonline.com/.*

The interaction between these brain regions in anxiety disorders is represented in Figure 15.7.

Epidemiology

The pooled lifetime prevalence of any anxiety disorders worldwide (including Australia and New Zealand) has been estimated at 17% and 15%, respectively. Anxiety disorders can manifest at any age, but they tend to first occur during childhood or in early adulthood.

Clinical manifestations

Common manifestations of anxiety include sleep disturbances, irritability and agitation, tiredness, restlessness, poor concentration, tightness in the chest, dyspnoea, sweating, tachycardia, light-headedness, tremors and feelings of apprehension.

Clinical diagnosis and management

Diagnosis Investigations to rule out any organic reasons for behavioural changes should be undertaken (see the section on the diagnosis of depression). Drug and alcohol screening should be undertaken to determine whether any substance capable of altering thought or behaviour is present in the person's body. Illicit drug and alcohol use can significantly increase the chances of developing anxiety disorders. Obtaining a history and conducting a mental status assessment will assist in the diagnosis.

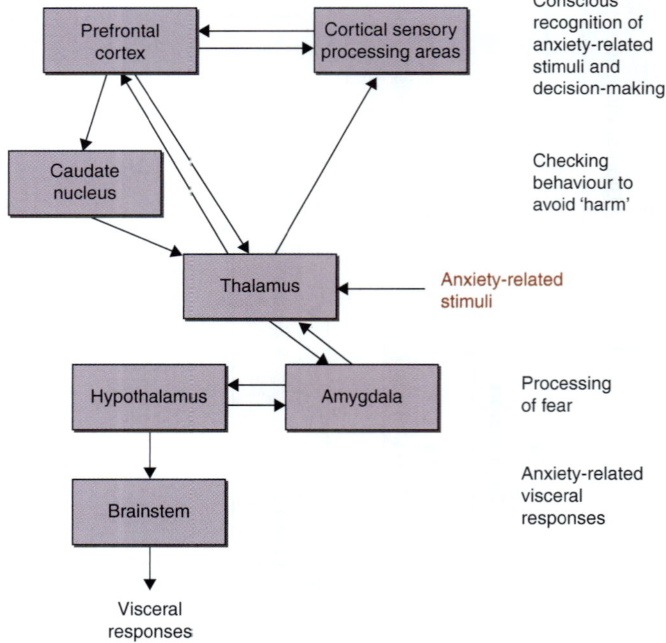

Figure 15.7

Interactions between brain regions in anxiety disorders

Management Many agents have anxiolytic properties. Antidepressants (in particular, the selective serotonin reuptake inhibitors or SSRIs), antiseizure agents and benzodiazepines can have a role in the management of people with anxiety disorders. The benzodiazepines act to enhance the action of the neurotransmitter GABA on its receptors in the central nervous system (CNS). Specific benzodiazepines that are commonly used as anxiolytics in acute anxiety states include alprazolam, bromazepam, clobazam, diazepam, lorazepam and oxazepam.

It is important that psychotherapy is made a central component of the management plan; otherwise deterioration and/or dependence may develop, complicating care.

Microbiome–gut–brain axis

Humans have a symbiotic relationship with the microorganisms colonising the gastrointestinal tract (GIT). This dynamic and complex population, once called *gut flora*, is now more commonly known as *gut microbiota*. Estimations of ratios of bacterial cell to human cell counts vary from 100:1 (in the 1980s) to as many as 1:1 (depending on the definition of 'cells' and inclusion criteria for the count). However, irrespective of the ratio, the sheer number of microorganisms inhabiting the GIT contributes to between 100 and 300 times more genomic content (microbiome) than the human genome. Some biologists refer to this collective entity as a *superorganism*.

Although there is a core presence of microorganisms with the two major phyla, consisting of the Gram-positive *Firmicutes* and the Gram-negative *Bacteroidetes* (approximately 75%), many factors influence the composition of a person's microbiota. The method of birth delivery (vaginal or caesarean section) will commence the differentiation, with vaginally delivered babies having a microbial load significantly more similar to their mother than that of a baby delivered via caesarean section. Other differences occur with gender, age and genetics, and also from variations in diet (including breastfed versus bottle-fed), the environment, activity levels and socioeconomic influences.

In recent years, knowledge of the role of the gut microbiota has expanded from simply assisting with harvesting energy, through to more complex interactions such as immunomodulation, protection against GIT invasion by pathogens, and maintenance of the gut mucosal barrier. It is becoming clearer that the role of microbiota may be even more significant in relation to mood, affect and behaviour as numerous complex methods of communication between these entities are revealed. Figure 15.8 demonstrates established bidirectional relationships between a person's microbiota, GIT and brain. This series of connections has come to be known as the *microbiota–gut–brain axis*.

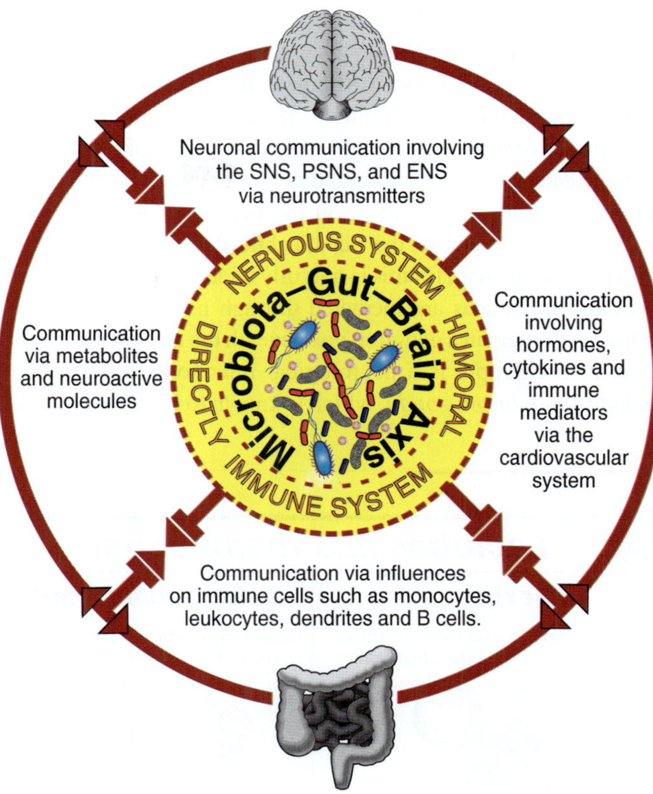

Figure 15.8

A simplified model of the microbiota–gut–brain axis

There is bidirectional communication between the brain, the gastrointestinal tract and the microorganisms within the GIT, via nerves, hormones and the immune system, and also from cytokines, metabolites and neuroactive molecules.

ENS = enteric nervous system; PSNS = parasympathetic nervous system; SNS = sympathetic nervous system.

GUT DYSBIOSIS AND MENTAL HEALTH

LEARNING OBJECTIVE 4

Describe the influence of gut dysbiosis on mental health and illness.

With this new knowledge comes an appreciation of the gastrointestinal microbiota's role in health and illness. The term *dysbiosis* refers to the alteration in the composition of one's microbiota resulting in the imbalance of a previously balanced gut ecology. It can be categorised into three different types: (1) loss of beneficial microorganisms; (2) loss of microbial diversity; and (3) excessive growth of potentially harmful microorganisms. Gut dysbiosis is being linked to numerous conditions such as irritable bowel syndrome, obesity, diabetes mellitus and colorectal cancers. Recent research is focusing on the influence of gut microbiota on mood, behaviour and mental health.

Animal research is beginning to demonstrate that certain microorganisms may change mood and/or behaviour. Gastrointestinal colonisation by the bacteria *Lactobacillus rhamnosus* is known to modulate mood and anxiety in rats through its effects on the inhibitory neurotransmitter GABA. Distinct and isolated brain regions are affected, resulting in decreased GABA receptor expression in the amygdala and hippocampus, and increased GABA receptor expression in the prelimbic and cingulate regions, resulting in a blunted stress response and a down-regulation of the hypothalamus–pituitary–adrenal axis (HPA).

An example of parasite manipulation of host behaviour occurs in crickets infected with the hairworm *Paragordius tricuspidatus*. Once the hairworm has reached reproductive maturity, the cricket is compelled by neuromodulating molecules released by the parasite to jump into a large body of water. This action enables the large hairworm to exit the cricket and continue with its life cycle. The proteins released by the parasite have been shown to influence the development of a cricket's CNS. There also appears to be changes to nocturnal behaviours, visual processes and circadian rhythm.

Another example of the manipulation of animal behaviour by host–parasite interaction is when ants infected with the fluke *Dicrocoelium dendriticum* participate in contrary behaviours, which increase the susceptibility to predation by compelling the ant to stray from their nest at night and climb a blade of grass where it can be eaten by a grazing animal the next day. This enables the fluke to continue its life cycle in the herbivore, where it exits the ant and migrates to the hepatic bile duct and gallbladder. While the mechanism for this is not fully understood, it is believed that these influences are mediated through neuromodulators or neurotransmitters in a ganglion just beneath the ant's oesophagus.

A final example is a neurological infection caused by the parasite *Toxoplasma gondii*, which is known to have behavioural influences on chronically infected rodents, resulting in a shift from fear of cat odour to one of attraction. *T. gondii* exerts neurophysiological changes on the host rat directly through chemicals secreted by the parasite, and indirectly through modulation of immune responses with an increase in tumour necrosis factor-α (TNF-α) and specific interleukins, and through hormonal manipulation via the HPA and altered testosterone. Collectively, the host experiences numerous biochemical and neurotransmitter effects, including a decrease in serotonin, noradrenaline and dysregulated glutamate signalling, and an increase in dopamine. Figure 15.9 illustrates situations where the effect of interactions between microbes and parasites on animal mood and behaviour has been clearly demonstrated.

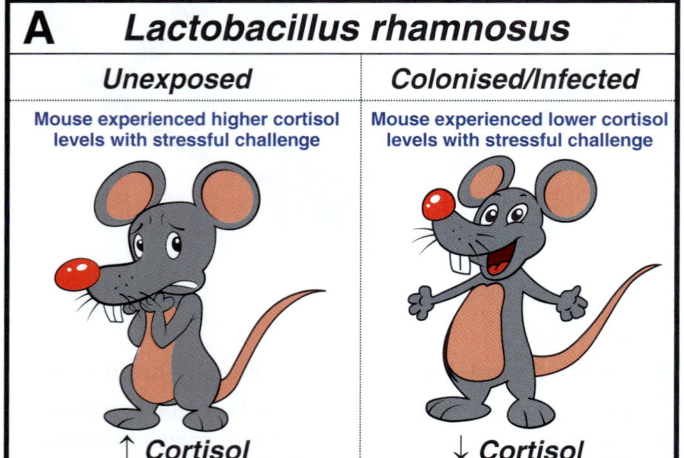

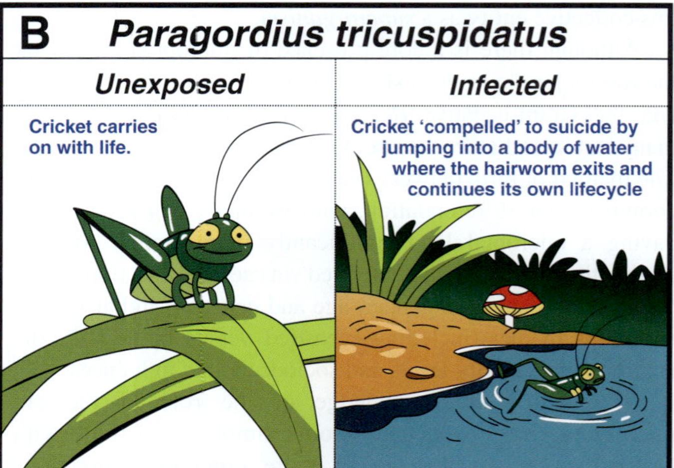

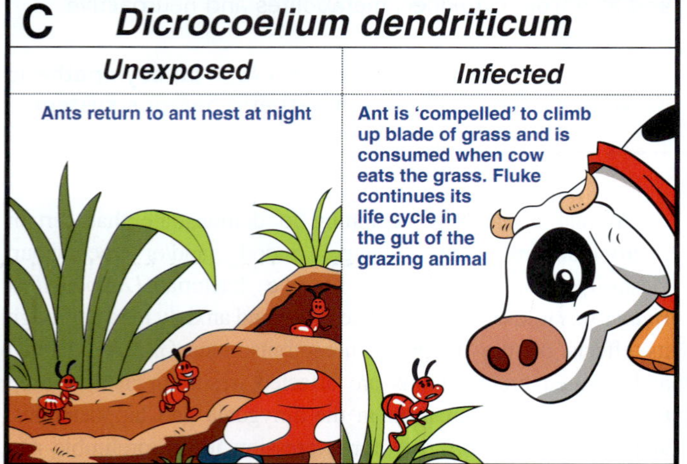

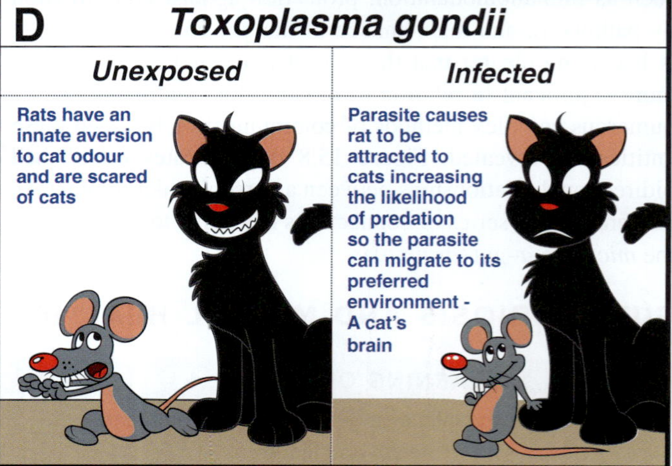

Figure 15.9

The effect of interactions between microbes and parasites on animal mood and behaviour

(A) When mice are colonised with the bacteria Lactobacillus rhamnosus, they demonstrate fewer depressive and anxiety behaviours, and lower cortisol levels when exposed to stressful situations. (B) When crickets are infected with the hairworm Paragordius tricuspidatus, they are compelled to suicide by jumping into a large body of water so that the parasite can continue its life cycle. (C) When ants are infected with the fluke Dicrocoelium dendriticum, they are compelled to climb blades of grass where they can be eaten by ruminant animals. (D) The intracellular protozoan Toxoplasma gondii changes the behaviour of chronically infected rats, inducing attraction to instead of fear of cats.

Sources: Developed using data from Dash et al. (2022); da Silva Soares et al. (2022); Lucius (2022); Zhao et al. (2022); Zhou et al. (2022).

This area of research is relatively new in comparison to other neurological and mental health studies. While these examples have focused on animals and not humans, the potential for microorganisms to contribute to, or manipulate, our affect, cognition and behaviour is fascinating and worthy of further exploration. Figure 15.10 describes some established interactions between a person's gut microbiota and multiple body systems. These interactions are complex and may contribute to alterations to a person's mental health.

A The *hypothalamus–pituitary–adrenal gland axis* becomes dysregulated in those with depression, anxiety and psychosis. Normally, increased catecholamines (such as adrenaline and noradrenaline) and cortisol are released in times of stress. This response enables physiological changes that help the person deal with the stressor. Cortisol levels may be high or low in depression, depending on numerous factors. High cortisol levels are negatively correlated with cognitive performance, and hypercortisolaemia is found in more than 50% of people with depression. Interestingly, one would assume that if cortisol levels were high, there should be an associated reduction in inflammation; however, it appears that, for many, the HPA dysregulation evident in mental health conditions also results in cortisol receptor desensitisation. The microbiota appears to influence the HPA through the release of pro-inflammatory cytokines and other neuroactive peptides. The complex interactions between the gut microbiota and the nervous, immune and endocrine systems have yet to be fully elucidated; however, Figure 15.10 explores some generally accepted relationships and influences currently supported by a sufficient volume of evidence.

B The *enteric nervous system* contains the most neurons of any body structure outside the brain, and 95% of all the body's serotonin is produced by the enteric nervous system. There is a bidirectional relationship between the brain and the GIT via the enteric and autonomic nervous systems. Recently, it has been demonstrated that gut microbiota produce neurotransmitters, including 5-HT, DA, NA, GABA, glutamate and histamine. It is also known that different bacteria produce different neurotransmitters. The microbiota may also generate neuroactive metabolites such as tryptophan, which is the precursor to serotonin synthesis. These molecules can influence enteric neurons after entry through spaces between the epithelial cells, because of increased permeability (known as 'leaky-gut syndrome'). Another potential mechanism of communication between the gut and the brain involves stimulation of the enterochromaffin cells by the neuroactive neuropeptides. As enteric neurons also interact with immune system tissue, bacterial-derived products are thought to influence the immune system of the gut. Many people with inflammatory gastrointestinal conditions such as irritable bowel syndrome also present with mental health conditions such as depression and anxiety.

C The concept of *psychoneuroimmunology* is long established, linking immune system function and mental health. A pattern of immune system dysregulation is being linked to people experiencing depression and psychosis. The gut microbiota have an indirect action on the immune system via enteric neurons. In addition, the innate and adaptive immune system can be influenced directly by the organisms within the GIT. Seventy per cent of immune system components are found in the GIT within the gut-associated lymphoid tissue (GALT), which contains numerous immune cells, including B cells, T cells, dendritic cells and macrophages. As the adaptive immune system is sampling the microorganisms, it determines whether the bacteria will be tolerated or targeted. If the microorganism is to be targeted, antibodies, pro-inflammatory cytokines and neurotoxic metabolites will be produced that may enter the bloodstream and set up a state of chronic inflammation, contributing to pathological changes throughout the body, and possibly the brain. Coupled with alterations to neurotransmitter volumes and types, these changes can interfere with neuron formation, the growth of new dendrites and synapses, and neuroplasticity.

D The *endocrine system* is affected by not only the direct action of the autonomic nervous system (ANS) and the immune system, but also by bacterial-derived metabolites that can cause the enterochromaffin cells to produce and release neuropeptides and neuroactive gut hormones (such as peptide YY, neuropeptide Y, cholecystokinin, substance P, and glucagon-like peptide-1 and -2—GLP-1 and GLP-2). Many of these substances are likely to play a role in bidirectional gut–brain communication. Once in the blood, they can influence the enteric nervous system, the brain (including the HPA axis), other endocrine glands, metabolism and/or the gut microbiota. Depending on the neuropeptides, neuroactive hormone, location and receptors, these substances may augment or reduce depression- or psychosis-related effects. As a result of the 'leaky-gut' from inflammatory mediators causing increased gut wall permeability, bacterial migration may also occur.

E The *blood–brain barrier* may also be manipulated by products from the GIT that would normally be prevented from entry across a healthy intestinal epithelium. Bacterial-derived lipopolysaccharides (LPS—from Gram-negative organisms such as *E. coli*) are pro-inflammatory endotoxins and can mediate in immune responses. They have been linked to processes causing inflammatory neurodegeneration, and are known to increase blood–brain barrier permeability. Conversely, short-chain fatty acids (SCFA), such as butyrate, are produced by gut microbiota from fermenting carbohydrate in a high-fibre diet, and are known to decrease blood–brain barrier permeability. The action of LPSs and SCFAs demonstrates that gut microbiota can influence access of blood-borne substances to the brain. These SCFAs are emerging as products critical for neuroplasticity, with probable links to enhancing learning and memory, and reducing depression and cognitive decline.

The cumulative physiological effects of these interactions may result in chronic neuroinflammation, altered microglial function, and an influence on neurodevelopmental and neurodegenerative processes. Ultimately, evidence is growing that the microorganisms within the gut appear to exert more influence over neurological function than previously considered.

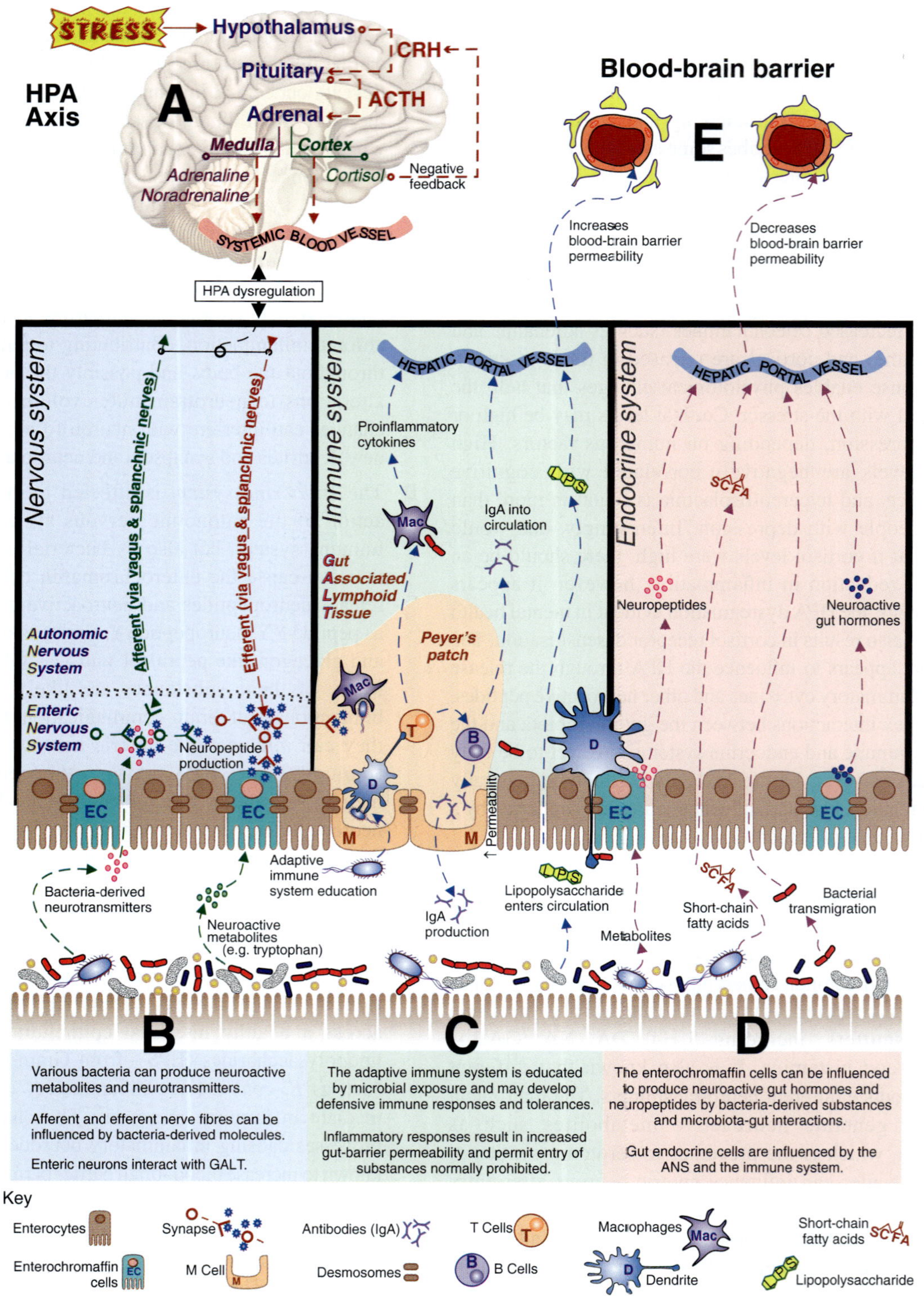

Figure 15.10

Gut dysbiosis and mental health and illness

Gut dysbiosis can result in: (A) dysregulation of the HPA axis; (B) manipulation of nervous system response; (C) modifications to non-specific and specific immune responses; (D) changes to the endocrine system; and (E) alterations to blood–brain barrier permeability.

ACTH = adrenocorticotropic hormone; ANS = autonomic nervous system; CRH = corticotropin-releasing hormone; CRH = corticotropin-releasing hormone; EC = enterochromaffin (cell); ENS = enteric nervous system; GALT = gut-associated lymphoid tissue; HPA = hypothalamus-pituitary-adrenal; IgA = immunoglobulin A; LPS = lipopolysaccharide; SCFA = short-chain fatty acids.

Sources: Data from Almeida et al. (2020); Bashir & Khan (2022); Bolek (2022); Jacobson et al. (2021); Nikolova et al. (2021); Queiroz et al. (2022); Zhou (2022). Brain image adapted from Alexilusmedical/Shutterstock.com.

Psychosis

LEARNING OBJECTIVE 5

Explore the complexities of schizophrenia, including its clinical manifestations, diagnosis and management.

Psychosis is a thought disorder associated with a loss of contact with reality. It is characterised by abnormal behaviour and perceptual distortion. **Schizophrenia** is a common form of chronic psychosis where the affected person shows disordered and disorganised thoughts, unusual behaviour, abnormal speech and altered emotions. The prevalence of schizophrenia is about 0.5%–1.5%, with a slightly increased prevalence for males. Approximately 2,000 Australians are diagnosed with schizophrenia each year. The first episode of schizophrenia tends to occur in adolescence or young adulthood.

AETIOLOGY AND PATHOPHYSIOLOGY

A chemical transmitter imbalance within certain regions of the brain is useful to explain the pathophysiology of schizophrenia. The imbalance involves synaptic dopamine neurotransmission, and is commonly referred to as the *dopamine hypothesis of schizophrenia*. It is proposed that a key brain pathway associated with the control of emotions and behaviour, called the *mesocorticolimbic pathway*, shows heightened dopaminergic activity. This pathway begins in the midbrain (part of the mesencephalon) and connects to areas of the limbic system and cerebral cortex. It has connections to the amygdala, hippocampus, caudate nucleus, anterior cingulate gyrus and prefrontal cortex (see Figure 15.11). Overactivity of this pathway is thought to underlie the disordered thought, emotions and behaviour.

The excessive activation of D_2-dopamine receptors within this pathway has been implicated in the pathophysiology. D_4-dopamine receptors may also play a role, to a lesser extent. Other cerebral neurotransmitter systems such as serotonin (at $5HT_2$-receptors) and GABA have also been implicated in the pathophysiology of schizophrenia, but this may be due to their ability to modulate dopaminergic neurotransmission in these brain regions.

Improvements in medical imaging technology have allowed us to investigate the possibility of structural changes in the brain associated with schizophrenia. Consistent alterations in brain structure have been found in the brains of people with schizophrenia, including an enlargement of the cerebral ventricles and reductions in the size of the whole brain, as well as similar decreases in the size of the limbic, thalamic and cortical regions.

Research into schizophrenia indicates that the onset of the illness involves an interaction between genetic, environmental and developmental factors. A family history of schizophrenia is an important risk factor, but does not guarantee its onset. The possibility of injury to the brain of the fetus during pregnancy or at the time of birth has also been implicated as a risk factor, due to conditions such as an in-utero viral infection (e.g. influenza), vitamin D deficiency, malnutrition or birth trauma.

The use of some drugs, such as the CNS stimulant cocaine, can induce an acute psychotic state. Drug use cannot cause schizophrenia, but recreational use of cannabis or amphetamines can provide the trigger to transform a subclinical psychosis into a clinical condition.

CLINICAL MANIFESTATIONS

The clinical manifestations of schizophrenia are grouped into two categories—positive and negative symptoms. *Positive symptoms* are manifestations not usually seen in the normal population, and include hallucinations, delusions, paranoia, unusual behaviour and altered speech. These symptoms are particularly prominent during the acute phase of the illness. *Negative symptoms* are manifestations that, compared to the normal population, are diminished or absent in people with schizophrenia, and include social withdrawal, apathy, flat affect, alogia (an inability to speak), avolition (lack of motivation) and anhedonia. These symptoms are characteristic of the chronic phase of the illness, and can be more resistant to drug treatment. Figure 15.12 explores the common clinical manifestations and management of schizophrenia.

CLINICAL DIAGNOSIS AND MANAGEMENT

Diagnosis

No tests will diagnose schizophrenia. As with all mental health issues, investigations that rule out other organic pathologies should be undertaken (see the section on the diagnosis of depression earlier

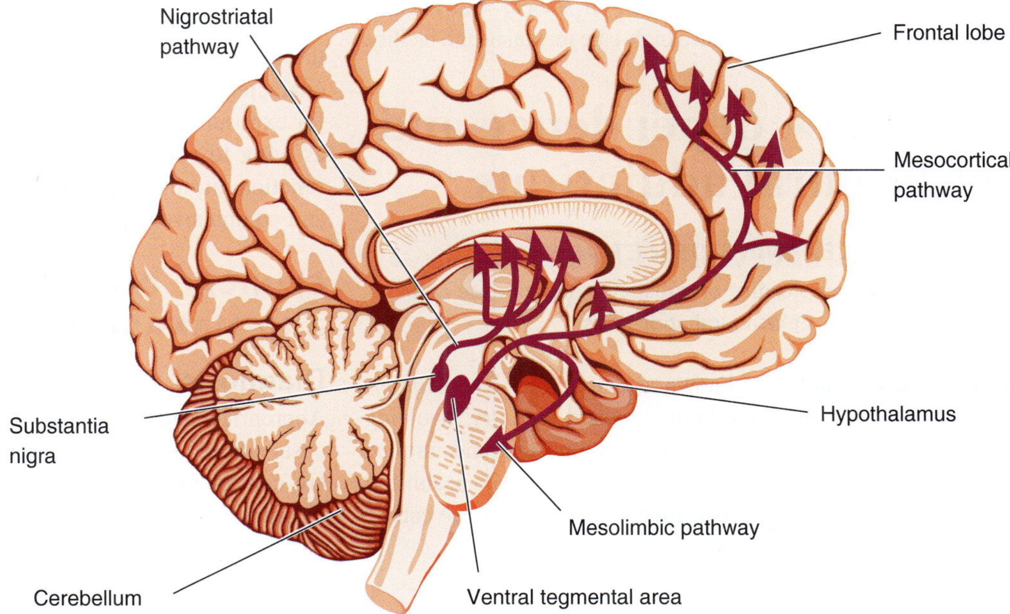

Figure 15.11
The mesocorticolimbic pathway

Source: Image adapted from Soul wind/Shutterstock.

in this chapter). It is important to obtain an alcohol and drug screen to determine whether any substance capable of altering thought or behaviour is present in the person's body. However, a positive drug screen does not rule out schizophrenia, especially if signs and symptoms continue once the drugs have been eliminated from the person's body. Recent history, presentation observations and a mental status assessment are pivotal in determining a diagnosis.

Management

If acute, rapid control of a psychotic episode is required, chemical restraint with benzodiazepines or butyrophenones (a class of first-generation antipsychotics e.g. haloperidol or droperidol) should be used. Physical restraint may be required for administration until sedation begins to take effect. If possible, de-escalation techniques should be attempted. However, the most important consideration in this situation is the safety of the staff and the person involved.

Long-term control of the effects of schizophrenia may be achieved through treatment with antipsychotic agents. There are two broad categories of antipsychotic drugs: first-generation or *typical antipsychotics* (also known as *classic antipsychotics*) and second-generation or *atypical antipsychotics*. The first-generation antipsychotics antagonise central D_2-dopamine receptors in the brain regions associated with behaviour and affect. The second-generation drugs are believed to have a different profile of receptor affinities, acting on a range of serotonin (particularly antagonism at $5HT_2$-receptors) and dopamine receptor subtypes. The first-generation antipsychotics are more prone to producing debilitating adverse reactions. The second-generation antipsychotics can be less problematic, but monitoring serum levels to ensure that therapeutic concentrations are developed is still important for many agents. Antimuscarinic (muscarinic receptor antagonist) agents may be used concomitantly in an attempt to reduce extrapyramidal effects (side-effects caused by dopamine antagonism resulting in parkinsonian symptoms, dystonia, akathisia or tardive dyskinesia). However, these, too, can produce side-effects that some people may find intolerable.

A lack of medication adherence can complicate the care of people with schizophrenia. Even when compliance is achieved, a small percentage of individuals may be refractory to treatment. These individuals require intensive care and support. However, the affected person's needs can exceed the capacity of community services. They often do not cope well in society and become incarcerated or institutionalised in a high-care mental health facility.

Substance dependence and behavioural addictions

LEARNING OBJECTIVE 6

Discuss the complexities of substance dependence and behavioural addictions.

Substance dependence, also known as a *substance-use disorder*, is a chronic condition of the brain's reward circuitry involving motivation and memory centres. It causes compulsive, uncontrolled use of one or more chemicals, which ultimately impairs health and can significantly influence social function. Substance use can be categorised as *harmful use* or *dependence*. **Behavioural addiction** is a disorder where activities are excessively and compulsively undertaken despite the negative consequences of participation. Common behavioural addictions include gambling, shopping, eating, sex, or watching the internet or television.

AETIOLOGY AND PATHOPHYSIOLOGY

The exact process of substance-use disorder is not entirely understood; however, there is a strong body of evidence implicating numerous neurotransmitters, such as dopamine, serotonin and noradrenaline. Alterations in dopamine levels in the nucleus accumbens and orbitofrontal cortex are associated with reward-seeking; decreased serotonin is associated with impulsivity, sensation and pleasure; and increased noradrenaline signalling appears to be involved in the hedonic effects associated with all addiction experiences.

Exposure to 'rewarding effects' results in positive reinforcement and contributes to the frequent or repetitive use of the substance. Substance-use disorder can be divided into three stages, with the first stage being *binge/intoxication*, resulting in overstimulation of the reward circuit and a reduction in the person's ability to resist the impulse. The second stage is known as *withdrawal/negative mood*, where exposure to the addictive substances or behaviours has altered the number of dopamine receptors in the nucleus accumbens, and changes in the amygdala cause anxiety, stress and irritability in the absence of the substance or behaviour. This is followed by the *preoccupation/anticipation* stage, where changes to the frontal lobe modify the person's control over thoughts and actions, and alter the hippocampus's ability to consolidate memories. The accumulation of the volume and distribution of these changes results in overwhelming desire despite the presence of negative consequences. Figure 15.13 illustrates the neurobiological basis of substance-use disorder.

CLINICAL MANIFESTATIONS

Signs and symptoms of substance dependence and behavioural addiction can be specific to the substance or behaviour involved. However, there are some common traits, including preoccupation with the behaviour or substance, diminished control over it, development of withdrawal symptoms, including anxiety, depression or cardiovascular effects representing activation of the sympathetic nervous system. Tolerance is also a common characteristic, so that as time passes there is an increasing need for exposure to the substance or behaviour. Other signs—such as lying to conceal the activity, and changes in relationships, functionality or financial stressors brought about by excessive and compulsive exposure—are also common.

CLINICAL DIAGNOSIS AND MANAGEMENT

Diagnosis

Appropriate and detailed assessment of the person's history and observations for responses to denial of the substance or behaviour are central to identifying the presence of this mental health disorder.

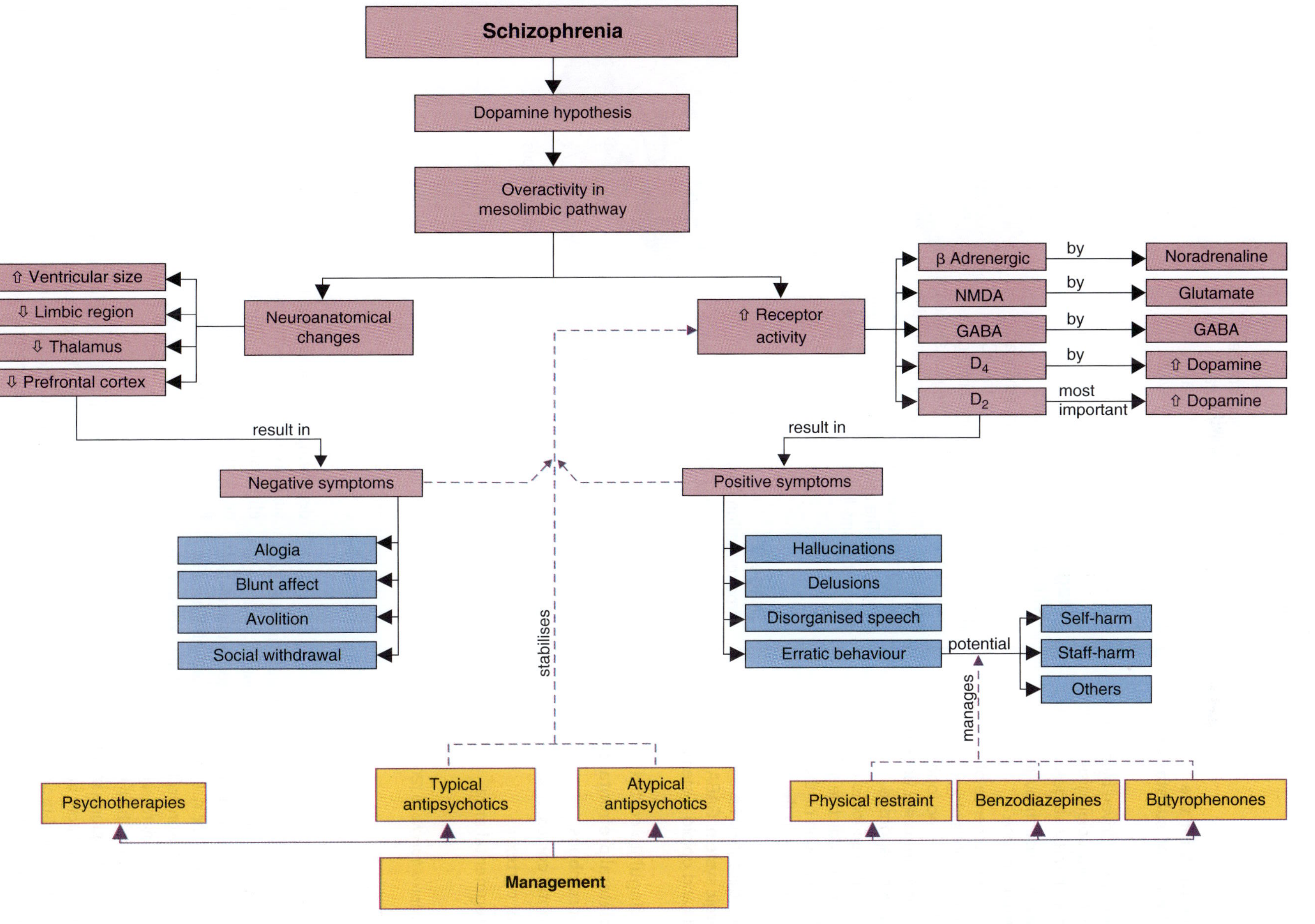

Figure 15.12

Clinical snapshot: Schizophrenia

↓ = decreased; ↑ = increased; atypical antipsychotics = second-generation antipsychotics; D_2 = D_2-dopamine receptor; D_4 = D_4-dopamine receptor; GABA = gamma-aminobutyric acid; NMDA = N-methyl-D-aspartate; typical antipsychotics = first-generation antipsychotics.

Stage 1
Binge / intoxication
The ventral tegmental area (VTA) and nucleus accumbens (NAc) circuit of the mesolimbic system is the key reward pathway, with the NAc providing a **dopamine surge,** resulting in reward from the addiction stimuli.

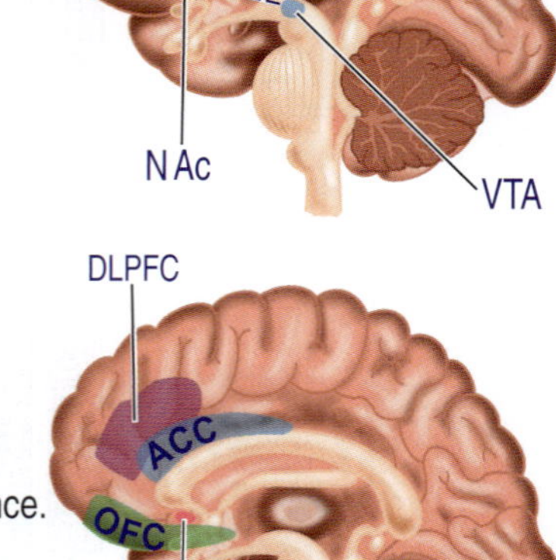

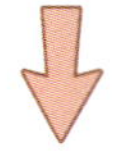

Stage 2
Withdrawal / negative affect
Poor decision-making and impulsivity are associated with the DLPFC and the ACC, while the OFC results in overestimating reward value and underestimating consequence. Withdrawal of the stimuli results in **reduced** NAc **dopamine** causing dysphoria, depression and craving. The amygdala is associated with stress symptoms like anxiety and restlessness.

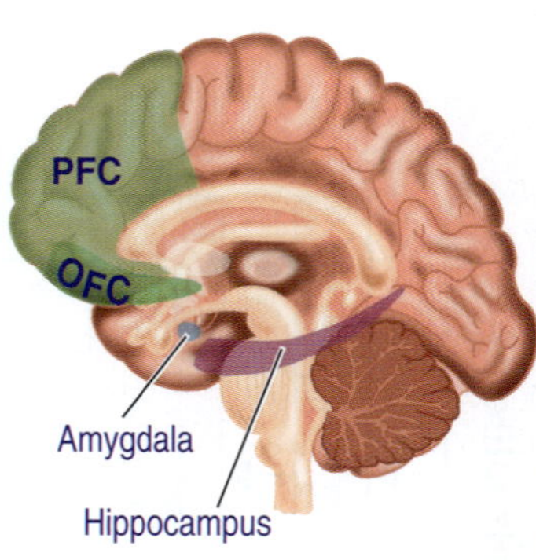

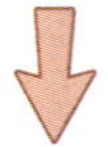

Stage 3
Preoccupation / Anticipation
The prefrontal cortex (PFC) and OFC are associated with impaired decision-making and fixation on drug-related cues. Stress responses involve the hypothalamus and the hippocampus retrieves stimuli-associated memories which reinforce cravings and uncomfortable physiological responses driving the desire for the addictive stimuli.

PFC
OFC
Amygdala
Hippocampus

Figure 15.13

Conceptual framework for the neurobiological basis of substance-use disorder

Substance-use disorder is driven by a complex interplay of neurobiological processes occurring in three stages.

Stage 1 reinforces drug use through heightened dopamine release.

Stage 2 results in the emergence of negative emotional and physiological symptoms when the drug is no longer available. This results in impaired decision-making, anxiety-driven responses.

Stage 3 involves an intense focus on obtaining and using the addictive substance. The cravings and anticipation of the rewarding effects can result in the cycle feeding back to stage 1.

Although the focus described here is on the dopaminergic system, GABA, endocannabinoids and opioid systems also play a role.

ACC = anterior cingulate cortex;
DLPFC = dorsolateral prefrontal cortex;
NAc = nucleus accumbens;
OFC = orbitofrontal cortex;
PFC = prefrontal cortex;
VTA = ventral tegmental area.

Sources: Concepts adapted from Koob (2021), Figure 1, p. 166; brain image by S. Elliott, Sciencopia.

Management

Public health action includes prevention and early intervention programs. Harm minimisation is also important to protect the community from the damage that is often associated with addiction and substance-use disorder. The risks associated are influenced by the type of substance-use disorder, but may include exposure to blood-borne infections, or increased crime from those who are financially unable to support their habit so resort to offences in order to fund their needs. Programs may include needle exchanges, diversionary programs, mandatory treatment and decriminalisation for drug possession of personal-use volumes.

How to assist someone with substance-use disorder and behavioural addiction depends on the addiction. The use of antagonists, drugs that may reduce cravings, or agents for detoxification and abstinence may form part of the management plan for a person with substance dependence. However, depending on the addiction, total avoidance may not be possible, such as if the person is addicted to overeating. They cannot eliminate food from their life. Cognitive behavioural therapy, counselling, residential programs and group support may all form part of the management plan.

TOBACCO, ALCOHOL AND OTHER DRUGS

The Australian Institute of Health and Welfare (AIHW) estimates that tobacco is the leading cause of preventable death, resulting in an 8.6% of the burden of disease. Fortunately, tobacco smoking rates are falling; however, 12% of males and 10% of females over 14 years of age consider themselves daily smokers.

Alcohol consumption rates are also falling, with recent data recording approximately 17% of Australians over 14 years of age consuming alcohol. However, 25% of people over 14 years

Table 15.2 Burden of non-fatal drug-related disease and injury

Drug	Non-fatal burden	Explanation
Tobacco smoking	9%	80% of lung cancer 75% of chronic obstructive pulmonary disease
Alcohol *(ethanol—the psychoactive constituent of alcohol)*	5.1%	28% of road traffic injuries 24% of chronic liver disease 23% of suicide and self-inflicted injuries 19% of stroke
Illicit drug use	1.8%	0.6% of infectious disease *Also* management of poisoning, overdose and dependence

Sources: Data from Australian Institute of Health and Welfare (2016c, 2017a, 2017c).

of age exceed safe consumption guidelines at least monthly. This behaviour results in alcohol being the highest cause of drug-related ambulance attendances.

In relation to illicit drugs, almost 12% of the population use marijuana/cannabis, 4.2% use cocaine, 3% use ecstasy and 1.4% use meth/amphetamines. In the two decades since 2000, the death rate from methamphetamine and other stimulants has increased four times. Table 15.2 shows some important Australian statistics related to non-fatal drug-related disease and injury, and therefore economic burden.

The AIHW survey found that 43% of Australians had tried an illicit drug at least once in their life, and 16.4% of the population had used an illicit drug in 2019. Interestingly, it is estimated that 4.2% of the population regularly misuse prescription pharmaceuticals, with 2.7% misusing prescription analgesics and opioids, which is decreased from 2016. Forty per cent of people who misuse prescription pharmaceuticals also misuse illicit drugs. Figure 15.14 explores selected drugs of dependence within various drug classes.

As discussed, addiction results in stimulation of the reward pathway through increased dopamine in the *nucleus accumbens (NAcc)*, otherwise known as the *pleasure centre*. The NAcc plays a major role in emotion, and interfaces with the corpus striatum, which is involved in the initiation and control of movement. The NAcc is responsible for processing the emotion and translating the stimulus into a behaviour (such as seeking the repeated sensation). Whether the addiction is substance- or behaviour-based, the repetitive conditioning of the 'reward pathway' ultimately cultivates the addiction.

Route of administration

As with any drug, the route of administration will be an important factor in the absorption time and concentration. Common routes of illicit drug use include *parenteral routes* such as inhaling or snorting (insufflation), and injecting (either subcutaneously, intramuscularly or intravenously). Insufflation is common for drugs such as tobacco, cocaine, heroin, ecstasy and amphetamines. Intravenous drug use is rapid with almost immediate effects, and greater dosage, as, like all parenteral routes, it bypasses the first-pass effect. Heroin is the most commonly injected drug; however, any water-soluble drug can be injected, including amphetamines, buprenorphine, benzodiazepines, barbiturates, cocaine and methamphetamines. This route is commonly associated with the most risk of spreading blood-borne diseases such as hepatitis and HIV. *Oral (enteral) routes* are common with drugs of abuse that commonly come in tablet or other palatable formulation, such as marijuana, ecstasy (MDMA) and gamma hydroxybutyrate (GHB), opium, amphetamines, lysergic acid diethylamide (LSD) and psilocybin (magic mushrooms). Another route of administration is called 'plugging', where the illicit drug is inserted into the rectum. Again, this results in a parenteral delivery, fast absorption and a higher concentration of drug getting into the system quickly.

Apart from the obvious dangers of the illicit drugs—the increased risk of infectious disease when injecting, risk of overdose, and the social, financial, emotional and mental health burden of illicit drug use—it is also important to note that there can be serious tissue damage to the body part constantly receiving the illicit drugs. For example, plugging can cause destruction of the mucosal tissue, leading to serious issues such as perforating the lower colon and subsequent death. Insufflation can cause damage to the nasal mucosa, and even erode the cartilage which forms the septum. Although the oral route possesses less risk for damage of the gastric mucosa, people with an altered level of consciousness who vomit may aspirate that vomitus into the airway. This becomes a significant short-term risk for airway obstruction, and longer-term risk for aspiration pneumonia.

MATERNAL USE OF, AND FETAL EXPOSURE TO, SELECTED DRUGS

When examining substance-use disorder, it is also appropriate to consider the effects of maternal substance misuse on intrauterine growth. Birth weight is dependent on two factors: the rate of fetal growth during the pregnancy, and the gestational age at time of delivery. As can be seen by Figure 15.15, all of the drugs

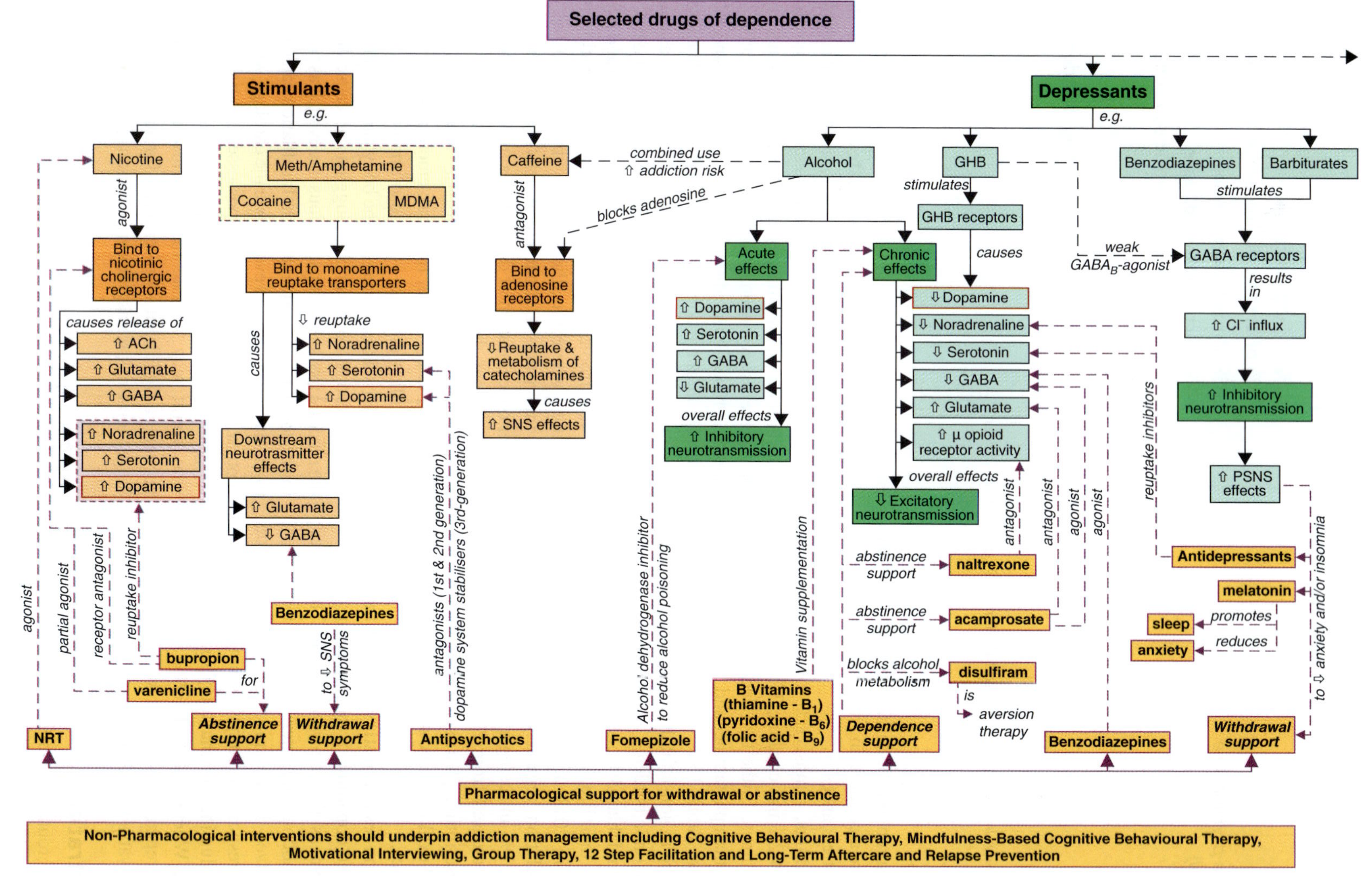

Figure 15.14

Selected drugs of dependence

It is important to note that although the mechanisms of these selected drugs have been briefly described independently, it is more common for individuals to have many substances in the bloodstream at the same time. The risks of polypharmacy often complicate the clinical management of an individual with a substance use disorder.

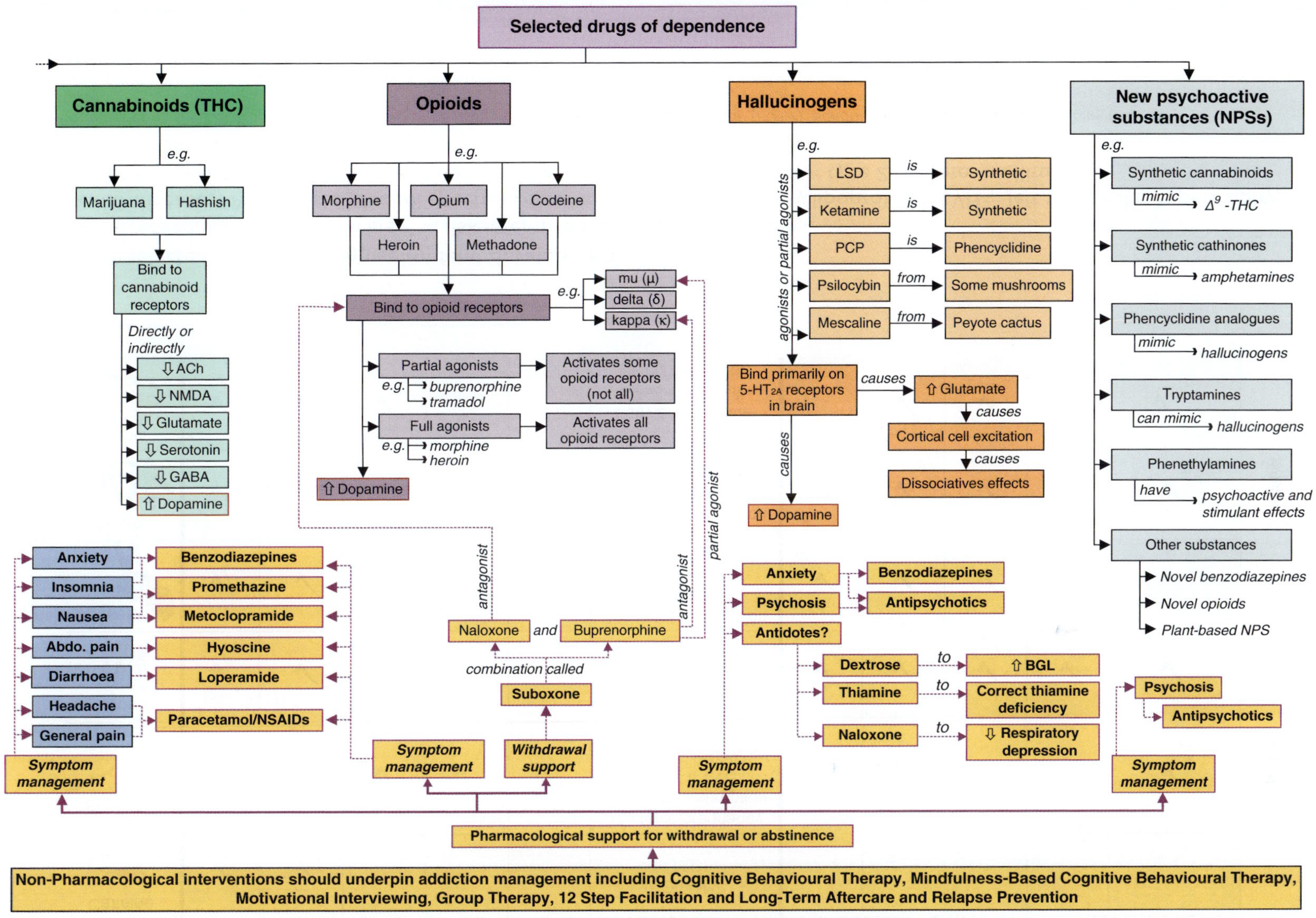

Selected drugs of dependence

Cannabinoids (THC)
e.g.
Marijuana
Hashish
Bind to cannabinoid receptors
Directly or indirectly
⇩ ACh
⇩ NMDA
⇩ Glutamate
⇩ Serotonin
⇩ GABA
⇧ Dopamine

Opioids
e.g.
Morphine
Opium
Codeine
Heroin
Methadone
Bind to opioid receptors
e.g.
mu (μ)
delta (δ)
kappa (κ)
Partial agonists
e.g. buprenorphine, tramadol
Activates some opioid receptors (not all)
Full agonists
e.g. morphine, heroin
Activates all opioid receptors
⇧ Dopamine

Hallucinogens
e.g.
agonists or partial agonists
LSD is Synthetic
Ketamine is Synthetic
PCP is Phencyclidine
Psilocybin from Some mushrooms
Mescaline from Peyote cactus
Bind primarily on 5-HT_{2A} receptors in brain
causes ⇧ Glutamate
causes Cortical cell excitation
causes Dissociatives effects
causes ⇧ Dopamine

New psychoactive substances (NPSs)
e.g.
Synthetic cannabinoids
mimic Δ^9-THC
Synthetic cathinones
mimic amphetamines
Phencyclidine analogues
mimic hallucinogens
Tryptamines
can mimic hallucinogens
Phenethylamines
have psychoactive and stimulant effects
Other substances
Novel benzodiazepines
Novel opioids
Plant-based NPS

Anxiety – Benzodiazepines
Insomnia – Promethazine
Nausea – Metoclopramide
Abdo. pain – Hyoscine
Diarrhoea – Loperamide
Headache – Paracetamol/NSAIDs
General pain
Symptom management

antagonist
Naloxone and Buprenorphine
antagonist
partial agonist
combination called
Suboxone
Symptom management
Withdrawal support

Anxiety – Benzodiazepines
Psychosis – Antipsychotics
Antidotes?
Dextrose to ⇧ BGL
Thiamine to Correct thiamine deficiency
Naloxone to ⇩ Respiratory depression
Symptom management

Psychosis
Antipsychotics
Symptom management

Pharmacological support for withdrawal or abstinence

Non-Pharmacological interventions should underpin addiction management including Cognitive Behavioural Therapy, Mindfulness-Based Cognitive Behavioural Therapy, Motivational Interviewing, Group Therapy, 12 Step Facilitation and Long-Term Aftercare and Relapse Prevention

FIGURE 15.14 Selected drugs of dependence (continued)

↓ = decreased; ↑ = increased; 5-HT = serotonin; abdo. = abdomen; ACh = acetylcholine; BGL = blood glucose level; BP = blood pressure; Cl^- = chloride ion; e.g. = for example; GABA = gamma aminobutyric acid; GHB = gamma hydroxybutyrate; HR 5 heart rate; LSD = lysergic acid diethylamide; MDMA = 3,4-methylenedioxy-methamphetamine (aka 'ecstasy'); NMDA = N-methyl-D-aspartate; NPSs = new psychoactive substances; NRT = nicotine replacement therapy; NSAIDs = non-steroidal anti-inflammatory drugs; PCP = phencyclidine; PSNS = parasympathetic nervous system; SNS = sympathetic nervous system; Δ^9-THC = Δ^9-tetrahydrocannabinol.

Sources: Data from Chawla (2018); Volkow et al. (2016); Volkow et al. (2017); Yang et al. (2022). © Sciencopia.

	Physical developmental risks						Neurological developmental risks*				
	Prematurity	Intrauterine growth restriction	Cardiac effects	Respiratory effects	Immunological effects	Other effects	⇩ Cognition & executive function	⇩ Attention	⇩ Memory	Hyperactivity	Aggression, defiance &/or behavioural issues
Caffeine	✓	✓				⇧ Obesity* ⇧ T2D*					
Smoking	✓	✓	✓	✓	✓	⇧ Ectopic pregnancy ⇧ Placental abruption ⇧ BP#, ⇧ LVH* ⇧ LDLs*, ⇧ CVD* ⇧ Obesity#*	✓	✓		✓	✓
Alcohol	✓	✓	✓			⇧ FASD# ⇧ Ethanol abuse*	✓	✓	✓	✓	✓
Opiates	✓	✓	✓	✓		⇧ Placental abruption ⇧ NAS# ⇧ NOWS# ⇧ Obesity*	✓	✓	✓	✓	✓
Cannabinoids	✓	✓				⇧ Placental abruption Early marijuana experimentation#	✓	✓	✓	✓	✓
Psychostimulants	✓	✓	✓			⇧ Placental abruption Early onset sexual behaviour & risk-taking behaviour#		✓	✓	✓	✓

Figure 15.15

Risks associated with selected maternal drug use on fetal development

↓ = decreased; ↑ = increased; # = risk early in life; * = risk later in life; BP = blood pressure; CVD = cardiovascular disease; FASD = fetal alcohol spectrum disorder; LDLs = low-density lipoproteins; LVH = left ventricular hypertrophy; NAS = neonatal abstinence syndrome; NOWS = neonatal opioid withdrawal syndrome; T2D = type 2 diabetes mellitus.

Sources: Data from Baranger et al. (2022); Gupta (2017); Popova et al. (2017); Qian et al. (2020); Sabra et al. (2017); Sanou et al. (2017); Stankovic & Colak (2022); Vaux & Chanbers (2023).

of addiction listed result in an increased risk of prematurity and *intrauterine growth restriction (IUGR)*. It is important to note that fetal growth restriction is a major contributor to perinatal morbidity and mortality. IUGR is associated with intrauterine death, premature birth and hypoxic brain injury.

Clearly, avoiding substances with such a profound effect on fetal development is critical for the health and safety of both the mother and the developing child. In 2021, more than 26,000 neonates were treated in public hospitals across Australia with disorders of gestation and fetal growth, although it is not known what percentage was related to maternal drug use. During the same period, nearly 285 babies were treated for neonatal withdrawal symptoms from maternal use of drugs of substance use disorder. All of these statistics demonstrate the need for better health education to ensure that women understand the effects that drug use during pregnancy may have on their developing baby.

Caffeine

Caffeine has stimulatory effects through antagonism at adenosine receptors. Adenosine is a major neuromodulator that can inhibit overactive excitatory neurotransmitters. Therefore, antagonising adenosine results in caffeine's well renowned stimulatory effects. Caffeine easily crosses the placenta. The half-life of caffeine is prolonged in a pregnant woman (~15 hours) compared to a non-pregnant woman (~4 hours). This is caused by ion trapping once it has diffused across the placenta. The more acidic environment of the fetal blood makes it more difficult for the caffeine to return from the fetal side of the placenta. Fetal effects of caffeine include reduced bone mass, low birth weight, growth retardation, and increased risk of obesity and type 2 diabetes in later life. The threshold of toxicity appears to be approximately 300 mg of caffeine per day. Less than this dose is associated with a clinically insignificant reduction in birth weight. Maternal caffeine doses higher than 300 mg per day increase the risk of adverse fetal effects.

Cigarette smoking

Cigarette smoking exposes the fetus to an extreme mutagen with absorption of over 4,000 chemicals, of which almost half are considered to be toxic or carcinogenic. Its effects are varied and span several different mechanisms. Nicotine, carbon monoxide and myriad other toxic components cross the placental barrier and compromise the developing fetus. Carbon monoxide induces a state of hypoxia through its greater affinity to haemoglobin than oxygen, resulting in reduced oxygen binding. Nicotine causes vasoconstriction, and reduces placental development and function through delayed maternal–fetal circulation, decreased placentation, decreased cytotrophoblasts and a thickening of the villous membrane. Cumulatively, these changes all contribute to reduced nutrient diffusion through the placenta, and subsequent intrauterine growth restriction.

Multiple organs are affected by perinatal maternal smoking exposure, including cardiovascular effects such as endothelial dysfunction from the cadmium, lead and mercury in cigarettes, altered platelet-vessel wall interactions from impaired prostacyclin production, and an increased risk of cardiovascular disease later in life. Overall organ size is also reduced in the fetuses of pregnant women who smoke. Lung volumes are reduced, parenchymal maturity is often delayed, and the likelihood of premature delivery increased, all of which can contribute to an increased risk of infant respiratory distress syndrome. The immune and endocrine systems are also affected, with increased inflammatory mediator release and subsequent glucocorticoid hypersecretion resulting in reduced maternal immune responses. Other changes to hormone balance can be seen with the reduced secretion of oestradiol, human chorionic gonadotropin hormone (hCG), progesterone and human placental lactogen (hPL). Finally, the direct neurotransmitter action of nicotine on acetylcholine receptors can result in the increased release of other neurotransmitters, such as glutamate, serotonin, dopamine and even acetylcholine. This nicotine–receptor interaction can also cause an increased release of catecholamines, adrenocorticotropic hormone (ACTH) and growth hormones.

Cigarette smoking appears to be dose-dependent, with an approximate 27 g reduction in birth weight for every cigarette smoked per day in the third trimester. As smoking cigarettes during pregnancy is associated with increased risks of spontaneous abortion, reduced intrauterine growth, prematurity and sudden infant death syndrome, it is highly recommended that women do not smoke during pregnancy or in the postnatal period.

Alcohol

Alcohol consumed during pregnancy is associated with: alterations to facial morphology (see Figure 15.16); CNS involvement; and intrauterine growth restriction with

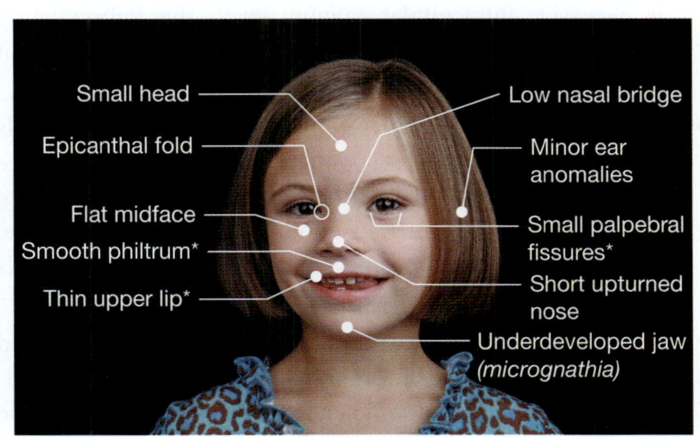

Figure 15.16

Five-year-old with the facial features indicative of fetal alcohol syndrome

Although there are numerous facial features associated with fetal alcohol syndrome, there are three diagnostic features (*), all of which must be present—a short palpebral fissure, a smooth philtrum (a vertical groove between the nose and upper lip), and a thin upper lip.

Source: Adapted from Rick's Photography/Shutterstock.

subsequent poor childhood growth, continuing as failure to thrive and limited growth catch-up. The term encompassing the range of effects along a continuum is *fetal alcohol spectrum disorder (FASD)*, with *fetal alcohol syndrome (FAS)* being the most severe example along this spectrum. The development of FASD is complex, with timing, duration, the amount of alcohol consumed, genetic factors, maternal nutritional status and body mass index all having an influence on the degree of alcohol teratogenicity. Both alcohol (ethanol) and its metabolite (acetaldehyde) are teratogens, and can pass freely across the placenta in a bidirectional fashion. Ethanol and acetaldehyde can cause significant issues through a number of mechanisms, including:

- *Nutrient disruption* to the developing fetus, through interference of placental amino acid, glucose, folic acid and zinc transfer, resulting in fetal nutrient deprivation and intrauterine growth restriction.
- *Oxidative stress* via two different mechanisms, causing a double insult. First, through the production of oxygen free radicals as a by-product of ethanol metabolism, and, secondly, through ethanol-mediated antioxidant suppression resulting in reduced oxygen free radical elimination.
- *Neurotransmitter consequences* through the alterations in levels of serotonin, glutamate and GABA. During the early development of the CNS, these three neurotransmitters are thought to play an important role in the migration and organisation of neurons. Serotonin regulates cortical growth and development, and glutamate is thought to have a critical role in stabilising the neurons. Ethanol exposure can reduce these neurotransmitters. Conversely, rapid withdrawal in the context of chronic alcohol misuse may also cause fetal neurotransmitter chaos, such as a significant increase in glutamate-*N*-methyl-D-aspartate receptor binding, resulting in excessive intracellular calcium levels that subsequently cause excitotoxicity, leading to necrosis and/or apoptosis of the fetus's neurons.
- *Altered migration and cell adhesion* from radial glial cells converting to astrocytes prematurely. In an ethanol-free developing brain, radial glial cells guide the developing neurons to their correct location. With ethanol exposure, neurons are often misplaced because the glial cells inappropriately convert to astrocytes.
- *Reduced retinoic acid* production from ethanol-exposed radial glial cells results in craniofacial features. In an ethanol-free developing brain, sufficient levels of vitamin A provide the source of radial glial cell-derived retinoic acid critical for the normal development of various tissues.

The regions of the brain affected include the basal ganglia, corpus callosum, cerebellum and hippocampus. These regions play roles in motor, cognitive, memory, learning and executive functions. Often, all of these important neurological functions are compromised in a child affected by FAS. Nonetheless, it is important to note that different tissues are affected at different rates and to varying degrees. Neurons are most easily affected by ethanol exposure, and it is possible for children to have neurological issues without the characteristic craniofacial anomalies. However, alcohol effects extend beyond neurological and craniofacial compromise. Other organs and systems may be malformed as well. Commonly, cardiac, renal, skeletal, ocular and auditory effects can occur in alcohol-related birth defects. The fetus relies on maternal detoxification of alcohol, and no amount of alcohol is considered safe for consumption at any stage of pregnancy.

Opioids

Opioids such as morphine, heroin, methadone, buprenorphine, tramadol, oxycodone and fentanyl misused during pregnancy can enter fetal tissue within an hour, and can have numerous effects on a developing brain. Immediately, on delivery, the newborn may experience respiratory depression and hypotonia. In a newborn whose mother received excessive opioids to manage the acute pain of labour, it may be necessary to administer naloxone (an opioid antagonist) as part of the resuscitation efforts. However, when managing hypoventilation and poor response to stimuli in a newborn from a mother with chronic opioid misuse, naloxone should be avoided, as it may result in symptoms of acute withdrawal for the neonate. These may manifest as life-threatening issues such as cardiac dysrhythmias, hypertension and even potentially seizure. Assisted ventilation is the priority in neonates of suspected or known chronic maternal opioid users.

Although opioids appear to be associated with less structural congenital abnormalities compared to other drugs of substance-use disorder, there are clearly physiological issues, such as alterations in neurotransmitter levels. There is an increased risk of spontaneous abortion, intrauterine growth restriction, premature rupture of the membranes or antepartum haemorrhage. With chronic maternal drug use, neonates born to addicted mothers often develop *neonatal abstinence syndrome (NAS)*. NAS results in irritability, temperature dysregulation, poor sucking and ultimately failure to thrive. However, abrupt withdrawal may result in even more physical effects as a result of neurotransmitter disarray (see Figure 15.17). Effects requiring intensive medical management may continue for many months following birth. Pregnant women addicted to opioids may benefit from opioid maintenance therapies, as untreated illicit drug use may result in poorer obstetric care and outcomes.

Cannabinoids

Although tetrahydrocannabinol (THC) can cross the placenta, the placental barrier appears to be somewhat more effective as fetal concentrations are lower than maternal concentrations. Apart from intrauterine growth restriction and an increased risk of premature birth, there are mixed results reported in the literature regarding whether THC causes developmental issues. Infants prenatally exposed to marijuana often exhibit

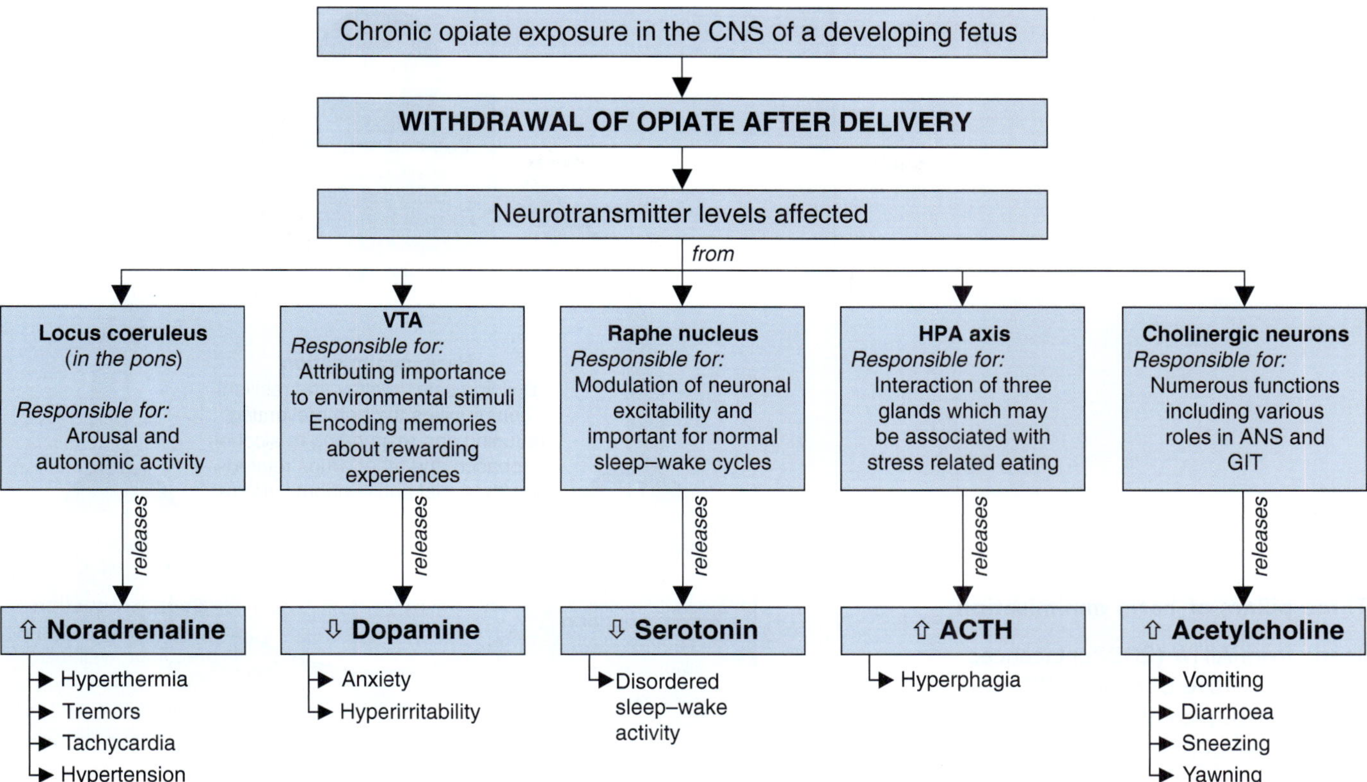

Figure 15.17

Mechanism of neonatal opioid withdrawal—neonatal abstinence syndrome

Chronic opiate use during pregnancy affects the release of numerous neurotransmitters. Acute withdrawal of opiates, which occurs soon after the neonate is born, results in further significant neurotransmitter derangement, leading to the common manifestations of neonatal opiate withdrawal.

↓ = decreased; ↑ = increased; ACTH = adrenocorticotropic hormone; ANS = autonomic nervous system; CNS = central nervous system; GIT = gastrointestinal tract; HPA = hypothalamus-pituitary-adrenal; VTA = ventral tegmental area.

sleep disturbances, increased startles and altered responses to visual stimuli. Interestingly, there are a number of studies that demonstrate few effects in infants aged 1–3 years in lower-use maternal cohorts, but in higher-use maternal cohorts poorer cognitive development, short-term memory, and decreased visual and verbal skills are demonstrated. Interestingly, by ages 5–6, a number of studies report that previously undetected attention deficits, impulsivity and hyperactivity may develop. Older adolescents and young adults who were prenatally exposed to marijuana demonstrate an increased risk of neuropsychiatric disorders, including conduct issues and depression, and are at greater risk of experimentation with marijuana at an early age. It is likely that THC influences alterations to neurotransmitter systems, as documented increases in dopamine receptor (D_2) activity has been seen in the amygdala, and decreased D_2 activity in the nucleus accumbens of fetuses exposed to THC.

Psychostimulants

Psychostimulants such as cocaine, amphetamine, methamphetamine and 3,4-methylenedioxymethamphetamine (MDMA, or ecstasy) used during pregnancy can cause maternal hypertension, uteroplacental vasoconstriction and subsequent fetal hypoxia. Chronic intrauterine exposure to psychostimulants appears to interfere with the developing monoamine neurotransmitter systems, and disrupts the balance between the dopaminergic and noradrenergic systems. All psychostimulants block the reuptake of monoamines back into the presynaptic neuron, causing a significant increase in the amount of neurotransmitter at the synapse. However, methamphetamine also appears to increase dopamine release from the presynaptic neuron as well. There are conflicting impressions about the teratogenicity of cocaine; however, it is commonly reported that it alters dopamine, noradrenaline and serotonin levels in the striatum, hippocampus, frontal cortex

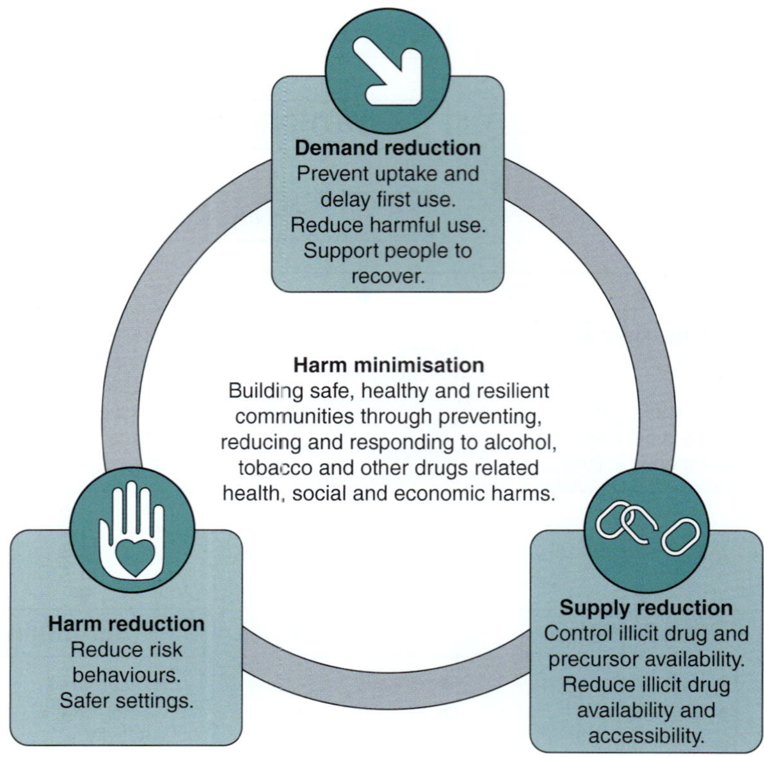

Figure 15.18

Three pillars of harm minimisation

Image from AIHW (2022c) Licenced under a Creative Commons BY 4.0 licence, https://creativecommons.org/licenses/by/4.0/.

and cingulate cortex. There are less common reports of potential optic nerve demyelination resulting in visual defects, and potentially other anomalies such as heart defects.

As expected, liver function in a fetus is immature, and systems such as the cytochrome P450 family of liver enzymes are only produced in small volumes during the first trimester. This system develops gradually throughout gestation and is barely functional until the postnatal period. Interestingly, with intrauterine exposure to amphetamine, methamphetamine and MDMA, this immaturity appears to paradoxically protect the fetus's brain somewhat, because it is the metabolites of this system's interaction with the psychostimulants that are thought to cause the neurotoxicity. It is clear that just as with most drugs of addition, the dose, duration and time of exposure play a role in the severity of impairment. Apart from intrauterine growth restriction and prematurity, fetal exposure may result in an increased risk of behavioural, attention, spacial, memory and motor difficulties.

HARM MINIMISATION

Harm minimisation is a strategy to prevent and reduce the risk and detrimental effects of alcohol and other drugs, not only for that person, but also the community. Figure 15.18 illustrates the three pillars of harm minimisation. The pillars focus on reducing uptake or delaying first use, reducing supply through various means, and harm reduction to reduce the effects on a community. Primary health strategies such as education programs that prevent uptake or delay the first use of a drug have significant benefits. Prevention or delay is medically, socially and economically more cost-effective than managing the drug-related consequences of established addiction.

Dual diagnosis

LEARNING OBJECTIVE 7

Review the significance of dual diagnosis in relation to mental health disorders.

Dual diagnosis is the presence of a mental illness and a concomitant substance misuse problem. It is very common, and increases the complexity and risks, and complicates the development of a management plan. The prevalence of dual diagnosis is thought to be as high as 50%. Figure 15.19 quantifies dual diagnosis across severity of mental illness and substance misuse of alcohol, tobacco and other drugs.

People may resort to misuse of a substance in an attempt to medicate themselves and reduce or relieve the unwanted effects of their condition, reality or medication. The success of managing dual diagnosis is influenced by age, gender, culture, education, peer group and social settings.

Young people are at particular risk, because of their neurological, psychological and physical development. Those who are older are also at greater risk, because of their ageing physiology, potential concomitant medical conditions, and, for some, their reduced social inclusion.

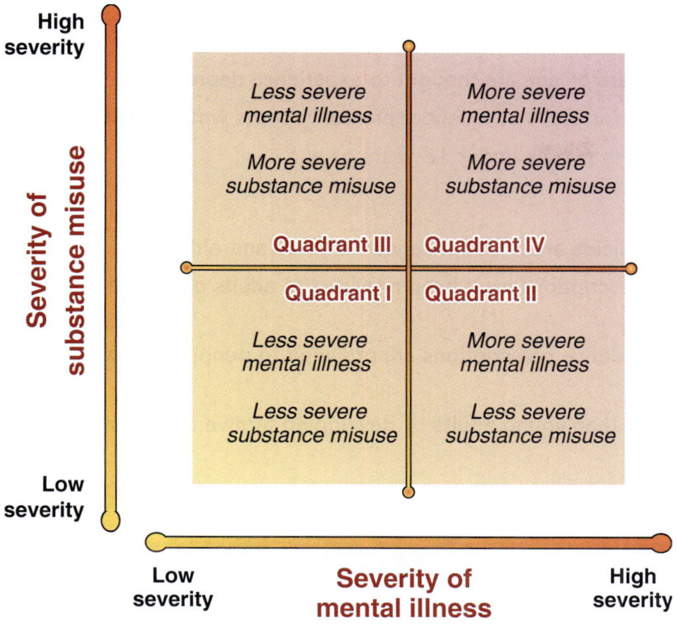

Figure 15.19

Representing the interaction between mental health and substance misuse (alcohol, tobacco and other drugs)

Each quadrant represents the varying degrees of severity of either substance misuse or mental illness. This model may be used in various ways, including determination and referral to the most appropriate services. For example, a person experiencing issues that lie within quadrant I may need the least support services, and be coordinated by their general practitioner and potentially supported by community health services or private providers, whereas those experiencing issues that lie within quadrant IV may require maximum support with potential admission to inpatient services for assistance with withdrawal management, and specialist assessments and multiple services co-management plans.

Source: Adapted from Queensland Health (2021), Appendix A, p. 9.

INDIGENOUS HEALTH FAST FACTS AND CULTURAL CONSIDERATIONS

FAST FACTS

- *Hospitalisations for intentional self-harm are 3 times higher in Aboriginal and Torres Strait Islander peoples than non-Indigenous Australians, having risen 60% since 2008.*
- *Aboriginal and Torres Strait Islander peoples are 2.3 times more likely than non-Indigenous Australians to die from intentional self-harm (suicide).*
- *Aboriginal and Torres Strait Islander peoples received community mental healthcare services 3 times more frequently than non-Indigenous Australians.*
- *Illicit drug use is 1.4 times higher in Aboriginal and Torres Strait Islander peoples than in non-Indigenous Australian people.*
- *Drug-related deaths are three times higher in Māori than Pacific Islands people or European New Zealanders.*
- *Māori women are 3.6 times more likely to smoke than non-Māori women.*
- *Māori are subjected to compulsory community treatment orders for mental health issues 4.1 times more than non-Māori.*
- *Rates for psychological distress are higher in Māori (1.7%) and Pacific Islands New Zealanders (1.5%) than in European New Zealanders.*
- *Pacific Islands New Zealanders and Māori are 1.3 times less likely than European New Zealanders to access healthcare for mental health issues.*

CULTURAL CONSIDERATIONS

- *There is anthropological and ethnographical evidence that severe mental illness was rare in traditional Aboriginal societies prior to colonisation. However, every year the statistical gap separating the social and emotional well-being of Aboriginal and Torres Strait Islander peoples from non-Indigenous Australians is widening.*
- *The historical discrimination, racism and violence against Indigenous Australians, and the introduction of psychoactive substances, have had a profound impact on the mental health of Australia's Aboriginal and Torres Strait Islander peoples. Healthcare professionals need to understand the factors that can enhance social and emotional well-being and contribute to culturally acceptable actions that have a positive influence on this unacceptable disparity. These factors include the importance of community, the connection to country, and spirituality. Other important elements include self-determination and community governance. Embracing and understanding these concepts will help to reduce distress, and subsequently reduce mental health conditions exacerbated by stress.*

Sources: Data from AIHW (2022a); AIHW (2022b), AIHW (2022e); New Zealand Drug Foundation (2022); New Zealand Mental Health and Wellbeing Commission (2022).

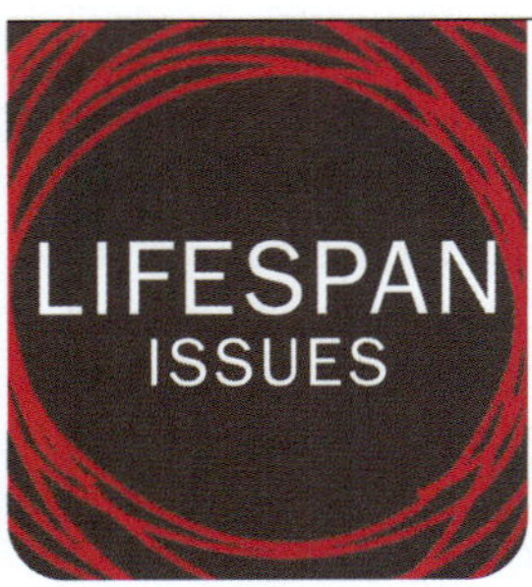

CHILDREN AND ADOLESCENTS

- Approximately 14% of children 4–17 years of age are thought to experience depression.
- People under 18 years of age accounted for 3.9% of all antidepressant scripts written Australia.
- Approximately 34% of all suicides occur in people under 18 years of age.

OLDER ADULTS

- Approximately 14% of all deaths from suicide are in people aged 70 years and older.
- In Australia, 13.7% of antidepressant prescriptions have been provided to adults older than 75 years of age.
- In Australia,48.5% of all hypnotic and sedative prescriptions are provided to people 65 years and older.
- Older adults are at significantly more risk than young adults of developing tardive dyskinesia when treated with antipsychotic agents.

KEY CLINICAL ISSUES

- Determining suicidal ideation is important in the context of providing pharmacological support for people with mental health issues. Antidepressants and hypnotic agents are commonly used in suicide attempts.
- A significant number of people with mental health issues have 'dual diagnosis'. This refers to the combination of a mental health disorder and a substance use problem.
- Proficiency in performing mental status and psychosocial assessments is imperative to ensure that important clinical assessments are observed, documented and considered in the context of a person's presentation and ongoing care.
- A knowledge of drug mechanisms, and observations for signs of toxicity and side-effects, will reduce the significant risks associated with psychotropic drugs. Extrapyramidal effects can be disabling and even life-threatening.
- Observations for prodromal or early signs of psychosis may enable early recognition and treatment. Monitoring for signs of decreased motivation, irritability, alterations in sleep or concentration, or erratic behaviour can facilitate early management and promote better long-term outcomes.
- Legal parameters must be observed in the context of physical or chemical restraint. Ultimately, interventions to promote the safety of someone with mental health issues and the staff involved in their care are a priority. However, this challenge is often difficult to achieve.

CHAPTER REVIEW

- *Mental health illnesses* (e.g. depression, bipolar disorder, psychosis and anxiety disorders) affect mood, emotions, thoughts and behaviour. They can produce severe, chronic disability, and are related to high rates of *substance use, suicide attempts* and *relationship breakdowns*. These conditions can occur alone, concurrently with each other, or in association with other chronic diseases, such as diabetes, cancer and cardiovascular disease.
- The *interaction of gut microbiota and the brain* is an emerging source of describing potential mechanisms for the development of mental health conditions.
- *Depression* is characterised as a state of profound sadness.
- The pathophysiology of depression has traditionally been explained as a chemical imbalance in the brain pathways controlling mood. It has been argued that depression is related to a synaptic deficiency in serotonin and/or noradrenaline. This is known as the *biogenic theory of depression*. The pathophysiology of depression now incorporates changes in neuronal connectivity and the size of brain regions triggered by alterations in the availability of neurotrophic factors and glucocorticoid secretion.
- *Bipolar disorder* is characterised by mood swings between depression and mania. The biogenic theory has been applied in the pathophysiology of mania. It proposed that there is an *overcorrection* from deficient synaptic levels of noradrenaline and serotonin to one where the synaptic levels of these transmitters are excessive.
- *Psychosis* is associated with a loss of contact with reality characterised by disordered thoughts, speech and behaviour. *Schizophrenia* is a common form of psychosis.
- The theory that has proposed for the pathophysiology of schizophrenia is called the *dopamine hypothesis of schizophrenia*. The activity of the dopaminergic mesocorticolimbic pathway, a key pathway in the control of emotions and behaviour, is thought to be excessive. D_2-dopamine receptor involvement in this overactive state has been strongly implicated, along with other transmitters, such as GABA and serotonin. Consistent reductions in the size of the cortical, thalamic and limbic regions in schizophrenia are considered characteristic of this condition.
- The onset of schizophrenia has been linked to an *interplay between genes, the environment and brain development*. Family history of schizophrenia is an important risk factor, and the possibility of brain injury in utero or at birth is also being considered.
- *Anxiety* is associated with cognitive, emotional, behavioural, motor and visceral reactions in response to a stimulus perceived as threatening. Common anxiety disorders include generalised anxiety disorder, phobias, obsessive-compulsive disorder, panic attacks and post-traumatic stress disorder.
- The activity of the *amygdala* is strongly implicated in the pathophysiology of anxiety disorders. Interactions of the amygdala with other brain areas, such as the cortex, basal ganglia and hypothalamus, are thought to give rise to anxiety disorders. An imbalance in the neurotransmitter actions of GABA and glutamate in these brain areas has been linked to anxiety states.

- It is critical to understand the anatomical and physiological *effects of drugs on the developing fetus*.
- *Harm minimisation strategies* are an important primary health undertaking.

REVIEW QUESTIONS

1 Define the following terms:
 a bipolar disorder
 b schizophrenia
 c phobias

2 Name the brain regions or pathways that have been implicated in pathophysiology of each of the following conditions:
 a schizophrenia
 b anxiety disorders

3 Name the chemical imbalances that have been proposed to explain the pathophysiology of each of the following conditions:
 a mania
 b schizophrenia

4 Name the condition associated with each of the following sets of clinical manifestations:
 a talkativeness, racing thoughts, impulsiveness and grandiose ideas
 b tachycardia, poor concentration, tightness in the chest, tremors and feelings of apprehension
 c insomnia, loss of appetite, psychomotor agitation, fatigue, feelings of worthlessness and suicidal intent

5 Mr Craig Pterovsky is a 22-year-old man studying at university. After being absent from university for a few days and not answering calls on his mobile phone, a couple of his close friends go looking for him at his apartment. Recently, he had been boasting to his friends that he had started to smoke pot with a new group of friends. They find Mr Pterovsky at home in an agitated state. The apartment is a mess. He has not eaten for a day and, when pressed by his friends, Mr Pterovsky says 'the voices' told him not to eat because the food was poisoned.
 a What is the most likely condition underlying this episode?
 b Outline the pathophysiology of this condition.
 c How does drug use contribute to the development of this condition?
 d What type of medications would be used to manage this condition, and what are their mechanisms of action?

HEALTH PROFESSIONAL CONNECTIONS

Midwives Women can experience mood disturbances during pregnancy (antenatal depression) and also following delivery (postnatal depression). Postnatal depression is indistinguishable from normal depression; however, it generally occurs within the first three months following delivery. Signs and symptoms may include anhedonia, suicidal ideation, appetite disturbances, insomnia or overwhelming fatigue. A small percentage of women may even experience a more severe psychiatric illness—postnatal psychosis. Postnatal psychosis resembles mania, and may include irritability, erratic or disorganised behaviour, euphoria and insomnia. Hallucinations may also occur. This situation is serious and presents a significant mortality risk for either the baby (infanticide) or the mother (suicide). Observations of behaviour and mental status assessments should be performed to enable the early identification of mood disorders or psychosis.

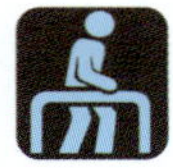

Physiotherapists/Exercise scientists It is well established that exercise reduces the duration and severity of episodes that result in mood alterations. Several theories exist on the mechanism. The monoamine hypothesis suggests that exercise promotes the release of serotonin, noradrenaline and dopamine neurotransmitters. This theory is supported by measurable increases in plasma concentrations of monoamine metabolites following exercise. Other theories focus more on behaviours, such as the positive effects of achieving personal goals. Others suggest that frequent and repeated exposure to anxiety-producing experiences, such as exercise, can result in sensitisation and ultimately control over unpleasant emotions. Exercise prescription for people experiencing mood disorders should embrace the basic concepts of starting slowly and building up. Exercises with rhythmic or repetitive actions, such as swimming, walking or dancing, may be more beneficial. Participation in competitive sports may not be advisable early in the program, as competition stressors may worsen anxiety disorders.

Nutritionists/Dieticians Adequate nutrition can assist with mood disorders; increasing various vitamins and nutrients may decrease the severity or duration of a depressive episode. Eating foods with a low glycaemic index (GI) will assist in keeping blood glucose levels higher for longer. Low blood glucose levels can reduce mood. Omega-3 fatty acids are essential fatty acids, and are pivotal to neuronal membrane structure. Omega-3 fatty acids may also influence serotonin levels. An increase in the consumption of fish, beans and eggs may therefore result in increased serotonin levels. B-group vitamins are important for neurological function and to reduce the risk of certain types of anaemia. Fruit and vegetables are high in vitamins. A balanced diet will assist with mood stabilisation; however, unfortunately, nutrition is often one of the first casualties in a person with mood disorders, anxiety or psychosis. Novel and interesting approaches may need to be found to help them with making good nutrition choices during their illness.

CASE STUDY

Mr Paul Gregs is a 47-year-old man (UR number 891143) who was brought in 10 days ago by paramedics, after having been found in his car, unconscious from an acute alcohol overdose. On admission, his blood alcohol level was 0.45 g/dL. Mr Gregs was intubated and transferred to the intensive care unit for airway management and supportive care. A head CT demonstrated some cortical atrophy but no lesions. He was extubated on day 2 and transferred to the drug and alcohol rehabilitation centre as an inpatient. His most recent observations are as follows:

Temperature	Heart rate	Respiration rate	Blood pressure	SpO_2
36.2°C	92	22	150/80	99% (RA*)

*RA = room air.

To reduce the effects of alcohol withdrawal, Mr Gregs completed a reducing regimen of therapy with the benzodiazepine diazepam. Currently, he is ordered 5 mg of diazepam q12h prn. He is to continue on alcohol withdrawal observations q4h (while awake) until further review. Mr Gregs has become increasingly depressed over the past few days, and has revealed that he has been taking the selective serotonin reuptake inhibitor sertraline 'on and off' for a year or so. He also stated that he 'ends up not taking it because it doesn't do anything'. When asked about what originally made him depressed, he replied that he didn't know, he 'just started to feel down and everything went downhill from there'. Mr Gregs stated that he also has severe episodes of anxiety. They are often worse after he 'comes off a bender' (i.e. an episode of binge-drinking alcohol). His most recent pathology results are:

HAEMATOLOGY

Patient location:	D&A Rehab.	**UR:**	891143		
Consultant:	Devon	**NAME:**	Gregs		
		Given name:	Paul	**Sex:**	M
		DOB:	16/10/XX	**Age:**	47
Time collected	22.30				
Date collected	XX/XX				
Year	XXXX				
Lab #	4325433				

FULL BLOOD COUNT		UNITS	REFERENCE RANGE
Haemoglobin	114	g/L	115–160
White cell count	4.1	$\times10^9$/L	4.0–11.0
Platelets	138	$\times10^9$/L	140–400
Haematocrit	0.34		0.33–0.47
Red cell count	3.78	$\times10^{12}$/L	3.80–5.20
Reticulocyte count	0.9	%	0.2–2.0
MCV	108	fL	80–100
COAGULATION PROFILE			
aPTT	45	secs	24–40
PT	22	secs	11–17
Thiamine	56	nmol/L	70–200

BIOCHEMISTRY

Patient location:	D&A Rehab.	**UR:**	891143		
Consultant:	Devon	**NAME:**	Gregs		
		Given name:	Paul	**Sex:**	M
		DOB:	16/10/XX	**Age:**	47
Time collected	22:30				
Date collected	XX/XX				
Year	XXXX				
Lab #	3455645				

ELECTROLYTES		UNITS	REFERENCE RANGE
Sodium	135	mmol/L	135–145
Potassium	3.3	mmol/L	3.5–5.2
Chloride	98	mmol/L	95–110
Glucose	9.9	mmol/L	3.5–6.0
Vitamin B_{12}	89	pmol/L	120–780
LIVER FUNCTION TESTS			
Alanine aminotransferase	68	U/L	5–40
Aspartate aminotransferase	39	U/L	5–35
Alkaline phosphatase	59	U/L	30–110
Gamma glutamyltransferase	78	U/L	5–50
Bilirubin (total)	18	μmol/L	< 20
LIPID STUDIES			
Total lipids	8.6	g/L	4.0–8.0
Triglycerides	5.9	mmol/L	0.2–4.8
Total cholesterol	7.87	mmol/L	4.45–7.69
HDL cholesterol	2.05	mmol/L	0.98–2.38
LDL cholesterol	5.87	mmol/L	2.59–5.80
RENAL FUNCTION			
Urea	6.8	mmol/L	2.5–7.5
Creatinine	118	μmol/L	30–120

CRITICAL THINKING

1. Given Mr Gregs' history, what type of depression does he have? (*Hint:* Endogenous or reactive?) Explain. What is the difference?
2. Observe Mr Gregs' pathology results. Specifically observe his liver function test results, coagulation profile, thiamine, vitamin B_{12} and red blood cell profile. What clinical effects could be seen as a result of these aberrant parameters? Do any of these measures provide/imply information about Mr Gregs' nutrition? How might depression factor into these observations?
3. Mr Gregs stated that he had been taking sertraline 'on and off' for a year or so. What is the mechanism of action of sertraline? How does it reduce depression? Why should someone remain on sertraline for an extended period? When sertraline is prescribed, what advice is necessary in relation to alcohol?
4. Mr Gregs was commenced on a diazepam regimen to reduce the effects of alcohol withdrawal. What is the mechanism of this drug in relation to its effects on withdrawal? How will this drug influence depression?
5. Consider Mr Gregs' history. Is there a relationship between excessive alcohol consumption, anxiety and depression? If so, what is it?
6. What interventions are required to assist Mr Gregs? (Consider all possible interventions, including actions to assist with depression, nutrition, alcohol use disorder, coagulation profile, liver function tests, etc.)

BIBLIOGRAPHY

Alcohol and Drug Foundation (2021). *Understanding drug and alcohol addiction (dependence).* https://adf.org.au/insights/understanding-aod-dependence/.

Almeida, C., Oliveira, R., Soares, R. & Barata, P. (2020). Influence of gut microbiota dysbiosis on brain function: a systematic review. *Porto Biomedical Journal* 5(2):1–8. https://doi.org/10.1097/j.pbj.0000000000000059.

American Psychiatric Association (APA) (2022). *Diagnostic and statistical manual of mental disorders.* (5th edn, Text Revision; *DSM-5-TR*). Washington DC: APA. https://www.psychiatry.org/psychiatrists/practice/dsm.

Australian Institute of Health and Welfare (AIHW) (2020). *National Drug Strategy Household Survey 2019.* Drug Statistics series No. 32. PHE 270. Canberra AIHW. https://www.aihw.gov.au/getmedia/77dbea6e-f071-495c-b71e-3a632237269d/aihw-phe-270.pdf.aspx?inline=true.

Australian Institute of Health and Welfare (AIHW) (2022a). *Alcohol, tobacco and other drugs in Australia.* Cat. No. PHE 221. Canberra: AIHW. https://www.aihw.gov.au/reports/alcohol/alcohol-tobacco-other-drugs-australia/contents/about.

Australian Institute of Health and Welfare (AIHW) (2022b). *Australia's health 2022: data insights.* Australia's Health series No. 18. Cat. No. AUS 240. Canberra: AIHW. https://www.aihw.gov.au/reports/australias-health/australias-health-2022-data-insights/about.

Australian Institute of Health and Welfare (AIHW) (2022c). *Mental health: Data tables*. Canberra: AIHW. https://www.aihw.gov.au/mental-health/resources/data-tables.

Australian Institute of Health and Welfare (AIHW) (2022d). *Mental health services in Australia: Mental health: prevalence and impact.* Canberra: AIHW. https://www.aihw.gov.au/reports/mental-health-services/mental-health.

Australian Institute of Health and Welfare (AIHW) (2022e). Suicide and self-harm monitoring: people & age groups—data. AIHW, Australian Government https://www.aihw.gov.au/suicide-self-harm-monitoring/data/populations-age-groups.

Baranger, D.A.A., Paul, S.E., Colbert, S.M.C., Karcher, N.R., Johnson, E.C., Hatoum, A.S. & Bogdan, R. (2022). Association of mental health burden with prenatal cannabis exposure from childhood to early adolescence: longitudinal findings from the Adolescent Brain Cognitive Development (ABCD) Study. *JAMA Pediatrics* 176(12):1261–65. https://doi.org/10.1001/jamapediatrics.2022.3191.

Bashir, Y. & Khan, A.U. (2022). The interplay between the gut-brain axis and the microbiome: a perspective on psychiatric and neurodegenerative disorders. *Frontiers in Neuroscience* 16:1030694. https://doi.org/10.3389/fnins.2022.1030694.

Best, O. & Fredericks, B. (2021). *Yatdjuligin: Aboriginal and Torres Strait Islander nursing and midwifery care* (3rd edn). Port Melbourne, VIC: Cambridge University Press.

Bhatt, N.V., Baker, M.J. & Jain, V.B. (2019). Anxiety disorders. *Emedicine*. https://emedicine.medscape.com/article/286227-overview.

Boere, K., Lloyd, K., Binsted, G. & Krigolson, O.E. (2023). Exercising is good for the brain but exercising outside is potentially better. *Scientific Reports* 13:1140. https://doi.org/10.1038/s41598-022-26093-2.

Bolek, M.G. (2022). Parasites in the driver's seat: understanding parasite natural history when the parasites lead us in asking the questions. *Journal of Parasitology* 108(6):648–660. https://doi.org/10.1645/22-89.

Bullock, S. & Manias, E. (2022). *Fundamentals of pharmacology* (9th edn). Sydney: Pearson Australia.

Chawla, J. & Suleman, A. (2018). Neurologic effects of caffeine. *Emedicine*. https://emedicine.medscape.com/article/1182710-overview.

Cianconi, P., Betrò, S. & Janiri, L. (2020). The impact of climate change on mental health: a systematic descriptive review. *Frontiers in Psychiatry* 11:74. https://doi.org/10.3389/fpsyt.2020.00074.

Commonwealth of Australia—Department of the Prime Minister and Cabinet (DPMC) (2017). *Closing the Gap: prime minister's report 2017.* Canberra: DPMC. https://www.niaa.gov.au/sites/default/files/reports/closing-the-gap-2017/sites/default/files/ctg-report-2017.pdf.

Cortés-Albornoz, M.C., Garcia-Guáqueta, D.P., Velez-van-Meerbeke, A. & Talero-Gutiérrez, C. (2021). Maternal nutrition and neurodevelopment: a scoping review. *Nutrients* 13(10):3530. https://doi.org/10.3390/nu13103530.

Dash, S. Syed, Y.M. & Khan, M.R. (2022). Understanding the role of the gut microbiome in brain development and its association with neurodevelopmental psychiatric disorders. *Frontiers in Cell and Developmental Biology* 10. https://doi.org/10.3389/fcell.2022.880544.

da Silva Soares, G.L., de Leão, E.R.L.P., Freitas, S. F., Alves, R. M. C., Tavares, N. P., Costa, M. V. N.,... Diniz, C. W. P. (2022). Behavioral and neuropathological changes after *Toxoplasma gondii* ocular conjunctival infection in BALB/c mice. *Frontiers in Cellular and Infection Microbiology* 12:812152. https://doi.org/10.3389/fcimb.2022.812152.

DeGruttola, A.K., Low, D., Mizoguchi, A. & Mizoguchi, E. (2016). Current understanding of dysbiosis in disease in human and animal models. *Inflammatory Bowel Diseases* 22(5):1137–50. https://doi.org/10.1097/MIB.0000000000000750.

Department of Health (2017). *National drug strategy 2017–2026*. Pub. No. 11814. Canberra: Department of Health. https://www.health.gov.au/sites/default/files/national-drug-strategy-2017-2026.pdf.

Fisher, A., Rochesson, S.E.D., Mills, K. & Marel, C. (2022). Guiding principles for managing co-occurring alcohol/other drug and mental health conditions: a scoping review. *International Journal of Mental Health and Addiction*. https://doi.org/10.1007/s11469-022-00926-7.

Forray, A. (2016). Substance use during pregnancy. *F1000 Research (F1000 Faculty Review* 5):887. https://www.doi.org/10.12688/f1000research.7645.1.

Frankenburg, F.R. (2017). Schizophrenia. *Emedicine*. https://emedicine.medscape.com/article/288259-overview.

Gupta, R.C. (ed.) (2017). *Reproductive and developmental toxicology* (2nd edn). San Diego: Elsevier Science.

Headspace—National Youth Mental Health Foundation (2017). Understanding bipolar disorder—for health professionals. *Headspace*. https://headspace.org.au/.

Hui Gan, G.Z., Hill, A.-M., Yeung, P., Keesing, S. & Netto, J.A. (2020). Pet ownership and its influence on mental health in older adults. *Aging and Mental Health* 24(10):1605–12. https://doi.org/10.1080/13607863.2019.1633620.

Hungerford, C., Hodgson, D., Clancy, R., Murphy, G. & Doyle, A.K. (2021). *Mental health care: an introduction for health professionals* (4th edn). Milton, QLD: John Wiley and Sons.

Jacobson, A., Yang, D., Vella, M. & Chiu, I.M. (2021). The intestinal neuro-immune axis: crosstalk between neurons, immune cells, and microbes. *Mucosal Immunology* 14(3):555–65. https://doi.org/10.1038/s41385-020-00368-1. https://www.sciencedirect.com/science/article/pii/S193302192200157X.

Koob, G.F. (2021). Drug addiction: hyperkatifeia/negative reinforcement as a framework for medications development. *Pharmacological Reviews* 73(1):163–201. https://doi.org/10.1124/pharmrev.120.000083.

Kourrich, S., Calu, D.J. & Bonci, A. (2015). Intrinsic plasticity: an emerging player in addiction. *Nature Reviews Neuroscience* 16(3):173–84. hhttps://www/doi.org/10.1038/nrn3877.

Kramer, P. & Bressan, P. (2015). Humans as superorganisms: how microbes, viruses, imprinted genes, and other selfish entities shape our behavior. *Perspectives on Psychological Science* 10(4):464–81. https://doi.org/10.1177/1745691615583131.

Lucius, R. (2022). *Dicrocoelium dendriticum*. *Trends in Parasitology* 38(12):1089–1090. https://doi.org/10.1016/j.pt.2022.09.002.

Mac Giollabhui, N., Ng, T.H., Ellman, L.M. & Alloy, L.B. (2021). The longitudinal associations of inflammatory biomarkers and depression revisited: systematic review, meta-analysis, and meta-regression. *Molecular Psychiatry* 26(7):3302–14. https://doi.org/10.1038/s41380-020-00867-4.

Malhi, G.S., Acar, M., Kouhkamari, M.H., Chien, T.H., Juneja, P., Siva, S. & Baune, B.T. (2022). Antidepressant prescribing patterns in Australia. *BJPsych Open* 8(4):e120. https://doi.org/10.1192/bjo.2022.522.

Marieb, E.N. & Hoehn, K. (2019). *Human anatomy and physiology* (11th edn). San Francisco, CA: Pearson Benjamin Cummings.

Munro, M. (2015). The hijacked brain. *Nature* 522:S46–S47. https://doi.org:10.1038/522S46a.

Nikolova, V.L., Smith, M.R.B., Hall, L.J., Cleare, A.J., Stone, J.M. & Young, A.H. (2021). Perturbations in gut microbiota composition in psychiatric disorders: a review and meta-analysis. *JAMA Psychiatry* 78(12):1343–1354. https://doi.org/10.1001/jamapsychiatry.2021.2573.

Queiroz, S.A.L., Ton, A.M.M., Pereira, T.M.C., Campagnaro, B.P., Martinelli, L., Picos, A.,... Vasquez, E. C. (2022). The gut microbiota–brain axis: a new frontier on neuropsychiatric disorders. *Frontiers in Psychiatry* 13:872594. https://doi.org/10.3389/fpsyt.2022.872594.

New South Wales Ministry of Health (2015). *Effective models of care for comorbid mental illness and illicit substance use: evidence check review.* North Sydney: NSW Ministry of Health. https://www.health.nsw.gov.au/mentalhealth/resources/Publications/comorbid-mental-care-review.pdf.

New Zealand Drug Foundation (NZDF) (2022). *State of the nation 2022: a stocktake of how New Zealand is dealing with drug use and drug harm.* Wellington: NZDF. https://www.drugfoundation.org.nz/policy-and-advocacy/state-of-the-nation-2022/.

New Zealand Mental Health Foundation (NZMHF) (2014). *Quick facts and stats: mental disorders and psychological distress.* Auckland: NZMHF. https://www.kelmarnagardens.nz/uploads/6/0/1/1/60114025/mhf-quick-facts-and-stats-final-2016.pdf.

New Zealand Mental Health and Wellbeing Commission (NZMHWC) (2022). *Te huringa: change and transformation. Mental Health Service and Addiction Service monitoring report 2022.* Wellington: NZMHWC. https://www.mhwc.govt.nz/assets/Te-Huringa/FINAL-MHWC-Te-Huringa-Service-Monitoring-Report.pdf.

New Zealand Ministry of Health (2015). *Tatau kahukura: Māori health chart book 2015* (3rd edn). Wellington: Ministry of Health. https://www.health.govt.nz/publication/tatau-kahukura-maori-health-chart-book-2015-3rd-edition.

Obata, Y. & Pachnis, V. (2016). The effect of microbiota and the immune system on the development and organization of the enteric nervous system. *Gastroenterology* 151(5):836–44. https://doi.org/10.1053/j.gastro.2016.07.044.

Oberbarnscheidt, T. & Miller, N. S. (2017). Pharmacology of marijuana. *Journal of Addiction Research and Therapy* S11:012. doi:10.4172/2155-6105.1000S11-012.

Popova, S., Lange, S., Probst, C., Gmel, G. & Rehm, J. (2017). Estimation of national, regional, and global prevalence of alcohol use during pregnancy and fetal alcohol syndrome: a systematic review and meta-analysis, *Lancet Global Health* 5(3):e290–e299. https://doi.org/10.1016/S2214-109X(17)30021-9.

Qian, J., Chen, Q., Ward, S.M., Duan, E. & Zhang, Y. (2020). Impacts of caffeine during pregnancy. *Trends in Endocrinology and Metabolism* 31(3):218–27. https://doi.org/10.1016/j.tem.2019.11.004.

Queensland Health (2021). *Co-occurring substance use disorders and other mental health disorders: policy position statement for Mental Health Alcohol and Other Drugs Services 2021*. Queensland Health Guideline: QH-GDL-964:2021. https://www.health.qld.gov.au/__data/assets/pdf_file/0023/1118246/qh-gdl-964.pdf.

Royal Australian College of General Practitioners (RACGP) (2022). General practice: health of the nation 2022. Melbourne: RACGP. https://www.racgp.org.au/getmedia/80c8bdc9-8886-4055-8a8d-ea793b088e5a/Health-of-the-Nation.pdf.aspx.

Sabra, S., Gratacós, E. & Gómez Roig, M.D. (2017). Smoking-induced changes in the maternal immune, endocrine, and metabolic pathways and their impact on fetal growth: a topical review. *Fetal Diagnosis and Therapy* 41(4):241–250. https://doi.org/10.1159/000457123.

Sanou, A.S., Diallo, A.H., Holding, P., Nankabirwa, V., Engebretsen, I.M.S., Ndeezi, G.,… Kashala-Abotnes, E. (2017). Maternal alcohol consumption during pregnancy and child's cognitive performance at 6–8 years of age in rural Burkina Faso: an observational study. *PeerJ* 5:e3507. https://doi.org/10.7717/peerj.3507.

Soreff, S. (2022). Bipolar affective disorder. *Emedicine*. https://emedicine.medscape.com/article/286342-overview.

Stankovic, I.N. & Colak, D. (2022). Prenatal drugs and their effects on the developing brain: insights from three-dimensional human organoids. *Frontiers in Neuroscience* 16:848648. <https://doi.org/10.3389/fnins.2022.848648>

Sui, Y., Ettema, D. & Helbich, M. (2022). Longitudinal associations between the neighborhood social, natural, and built environment and mental health: a systematic review with meta-analyses. *Health and Place* 77:102893. https://doi.org/10.1016/j.healthplace.2022.102893.

Toso, K., Cock, P. & Leavey, G. (2020). Maternal exposure to violence and offspring neurodevelopment: a systematic review. *Paediatric and Perinatal Epidemiology* 34(2):190–203. https://doi.org/10.1111/ppe.12651.

Uher, R. & Zwicker, A. (2017). Etiology in psychiatry: embracing the reality of poly-gene–environmental causation of mental illness. *World Psychiatry* 16(2):121–29. http://doi.org/10.1002/wps.20436.

Vaux, K.K., & Chambers, C. (2023). Fetal alcohol syndrome. *Emedicine*. https://emedicine.medscape.com/article/974016-overview.

Volkow, N.D., Koob, G.F. & McLellan, A.T. (2016). Neurobiologic advances from the brain disease model of addiction. *New England Journal of Medicine* 374(4):363–71. https://doi.org/10.1056/NEJMra1511480.

Volkow, N.D., Wiers, C.E., Shokri-Kojori, E., Tomasi, D., Wang, G.-J. & Baler. R. (2017). Neurochemical and metabolic effects of acute and chronic alcohol in the human brain: studies with positron emission tomography. *Neuropharmacology* 122:175–88. https://doi.org/10.1016/j.neuropharm.2017.01.012.

Wang, R.A.H., Davis, O.S.P., Wootton, R.E., Mottershaw, A. & Haworth, C.M.A. (2017). Social support and mental health in late adolescence are correlated for genetic, as well as environmental, reasons. *Scientific Reports* 7(1):13088. doi: 10.1038/s41598-017-13449-2.

World Health Organization (WHO) (2022a). Chapter 6: mental and behavioural disorders. *International statistical classification of diseases and related health problems* (11th rev). Geneva: WHO. https://www.who.int/standards/classifications/classification-of-diseases.

World Health Organization (WHO) (2022b). COVID-19 pandemic triggers 25% increase in prevalence of anxiety and depression worldwide. https://www.who.int/news/item/02-03-2022-covid-19-pandemic-triggers-25-increase-in-prevalence-of-anxiety-and-depression-worldwide#:~:text=Wake%2Dup%20call%20to%20all,mental%20health%20services%20and%20support&text=In%20the%20first%20year%20of,Health%20Organization%20(WHO)%20today.

Yang, W., Singla, R., Maheshwari, O., Fontaine, C.J. & Gil-Mohapel, J. (2022). Alcohol use disorder: neurobiology and therapeutics. *Biomedicines* 10(5):1192. https://doi.org/10.3390/biomedicines10051192.

Yew, D. (2022). Caffeine toxicity. *Emedicine.* https://emedicine.medscape.com/article/821863-overview.

Zhao, N.O., Topolski, N., Tusconi, M., Salarda, E.M., Busby, C.W., Lima, C.N.N.C.,… Fries, G.R. (2022). Blood–brain barrier dysfunction in bipolar disorder: molecular mechanisms and clinical implications. *Brain, Behavior, and Immunity. Health* 21:100441. https://doi.org/10.1016/j.bbih.2022.100441.

Zhou, B., Jin, G., Pang, X., Mo, Q., Bao, J., Liu, T.,… Cao, H. (2022). *Lactobacillus rhamnosus* GG colonization in early life regulates gut-brain axis and relieves anxiety-like behavior in adulthood. *Pharmacological Research* 177:106090. https://doi.org/10.1016/j.phrs.2022.106090.

PART

4

Endocrine pathophysiology

16 Concepts of endocrine dysfunction

KEY TERMS

Ectopic hormone secretion
Hormone hypersecretion
Hormone hyposecretion
Target tissue responsiveness

LEARNING OBJECTIVES

After completing this chapter, you should be able to:

1 Define 'hormone hyposecretion', and indicate some common causes.
2 Define 'hormone hypersecretion', and indicate some common causes.
3 Briefly describe some common causes of extraglandular disturbances affecting endocrine function.
4 Define the term 'altered target tissue responsiveness'.
5 Differentiate between poor tissue responsiveness and hormone hyposecretion.
6 Outline the principles of drug treatment associated with endocrine dysfunction.

WHAT YOU SHOULD KNOW BEFORE YOU START THIS CHAPTER

Can you identify the main components of the endocrine system?

Can you compare and contrast the characteristics of endocrine and nervous body control?

Can you outline the principles associated with autoimmunity?

Can you describe the major concepts of neoplasia?

Introduction

The endocrine system and the nervous system act together to coordinate and regulate normal body function. The endocrine system is involved in many body processes, including fluid balance, electrolyte homeostasis (particularly sodium, potassium and calcium), metabolism, cell growth and the development of body systems, glucose homeostasis, gastrointestinal and cardiovascular functions, body responses to stress, as well as lactation and reproduction. When the endocrine system is disrupted, serious, even life-threatening, effects can occur.

An overview of the main concepts related to endocrine pathophysiology will help you to develop a framework for understanding the specific disease states covered in this part of the book. First, a brief overview of the importance of endocrine feedback is provided. The common mechanisms underlying endocrine disease processes are then discussed, followed by the principles associated with diagnostic testing and the treatment of endocrine diseases.

The importance of endocrine feedback mechanisms

Hormone secretion from endocrine glands tends to fluctuate depending on the time of day, the sex of the person, individual variability and age. Generally, the degree of fluctuation is kept under tight control between normal upper and lower circulating levels through a system of integrated feedback mechanisms. A sound knowledge of these mechanisms is important in understanding why specific dynamic tests are used to diagnose endocrine disorders and the symptoms they produce.

Hormone levels provide feedback to their secreting gland to maintain normal endocrine function. The feedback acts to inhibit or stimulate the release of other hormones. Hormone secretion is generally under the control of one or more of the following processes:

- *The hormone itself.* For example, glucocorticoids provide feedback to the hypothalamus and pituitary to cause it to release corticotropin-releasing hormone (CRH) and adrenocorticotropic hormone (ACTH).
- *Other hormones.* As an example, somatostatin regulates the release of insulin and glucagon from the beta and alpha cells of the pancreas, respectively, leading to an alteration in blood glucose levels. The thyroid hormones and several other hormones also play a role in glucose homeostasis (see the chapters 'Thyroid and parathyroid disorders', 'Adrenal gland disorders' and 'Diabetes mellitus').
- *Internal and/or external stimuli.* Examples of such stimuli are fear (in respect to the stress response) and starvation.
- *The end effect or end product of the hormone action.* The end product can be changes in ion, metabolite or body fluid levels. For example, the electrolyte calcium regulates parathyroid hormone (PTH) secretion; the metabolite glucose regulates insulin and glucagon secretion; and extracellular fluid volume (serum osmolality) regulates vasopressin, renin and aldosterone secretion.

Forms of endocrine feedback are summarised in Figure 16.1. Endocrine function is controlled by the hypothalamic–pituitary axis or by freestanding endocrine glands.

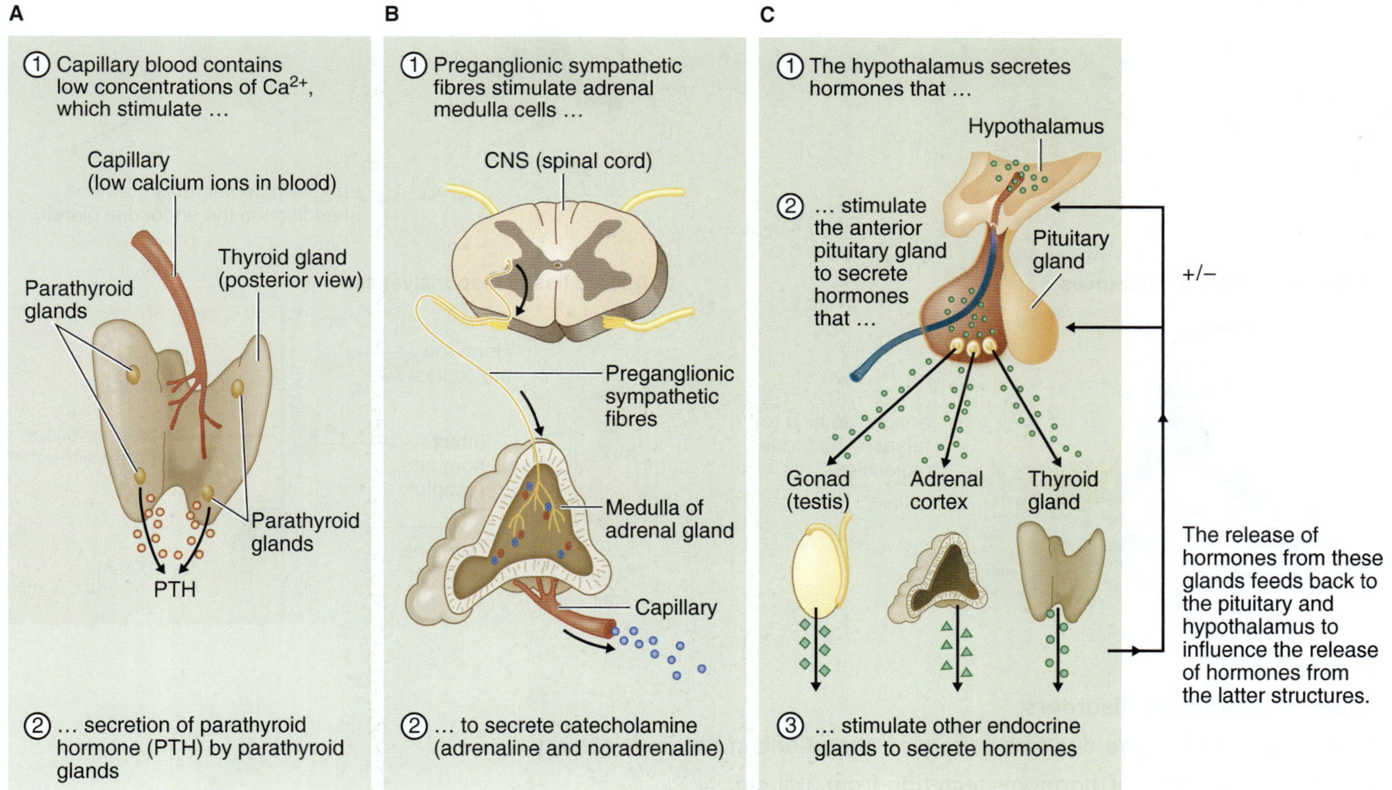

Figure 16.1

Endocrine feedback mechanisms

(A) Humoral stimulus.
(B) Neural stimulus.
(C) Hormonal stimulus.

Ca^{2+} = calcium ion; CNS = central nervous system.

Source: Adapted from Marieb & Hoehn (2019), Figure 16.4, p. 639.

Types of pathophysiological mechanisms

Endocrine disorders can be classified according to the following pathophysiological processes: hormone hyposecretion, hormone hypersecretion, extraglandular disturbances or altered tissue responsiveness (see Figure 16.2). In some endocrine diseases only one process is responsible, whereas in others a combination of processes may be occurring.

Figure 16.3 is a concept map exploring the mechanisms and management principles of endocrine dysfunction. The pink shaded boxes represent the pathophysiological characteristics, the blue shaded boxes represent the clinical manifestations, and the yellow shaded boxes represent the management principles for each of the conditions.

HORMONE HYPOSECRETION

LEARNING OBJECTIVE 1

Define 'hormone hyposecretion', and indicate some common causes.

Hormone hyposecretion is characterised by insufficient hormone production to meet the body's requirements. It can occur when glandular cells are injured or destroyed by pathophysiological processes. Such processes include autoimmune attack, invasive tumour growth, infections or chronic inflammation. Examples of specific endocrine disorders associated with these processes are listed in Table 16.1.

A. Normal state

B. Hormone hyposecretion

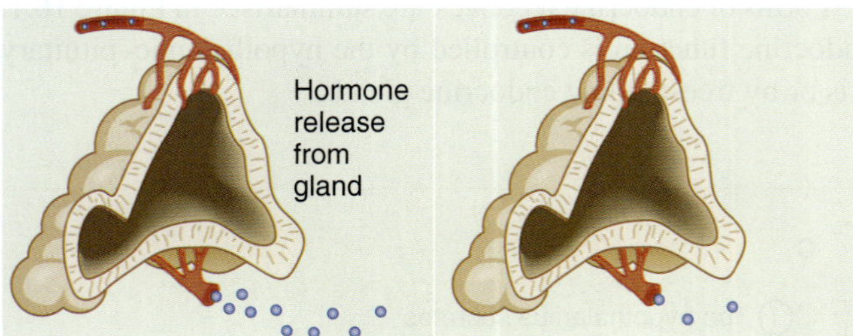

C. Hormone hypersecretion

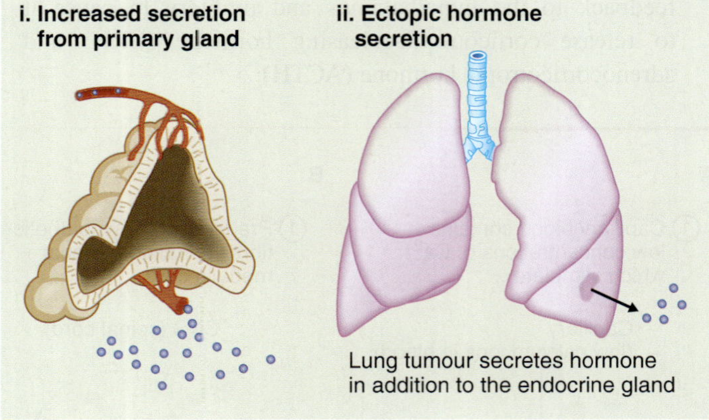

D. Extraglandular disturbances

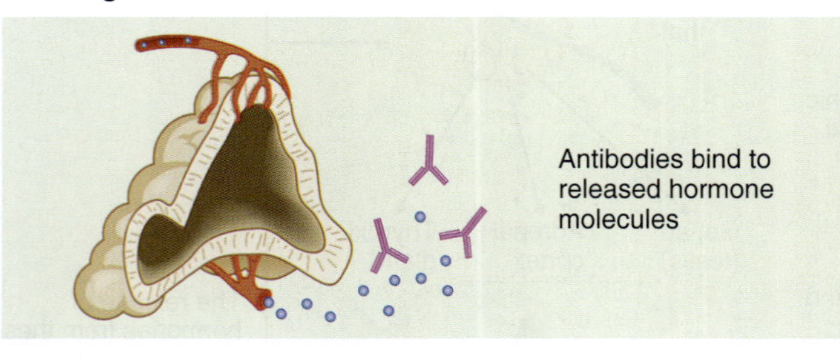

E. Altered tissue responsiveness

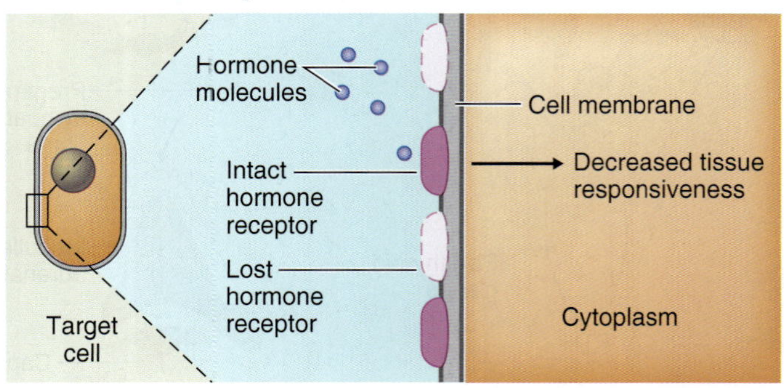

Figure 16.2

Types of endocrine disorders

Endocrine disorders are due to a variety of alterations in hormone activity.

(A) The normal state of hormone secretion from a gland.

(B) Hormone hyposecretion: the levels of hormone secretion from the gland are insufficient.

(C) Hormone hypersecretion: this may be due to either (i) a marked increase in glandular secretion, or (ii) ectopic hormone secretion associated with the presence of a tumour in addition to glandular secretion.

(D) In extraglandular disturbances, glandular hormone secretion is normal, but the levels of circulating hormone are abnormal due to excessive breakdown by autoantibodies or altered liver metabolism.

(E) The target cell's responsiveness to the hormone is altered by changes in the number of hormone receptors or in their sensitivity.

Source: Adapted from Marieb & Hoehn (2019), Figure 16.4, p. 639.

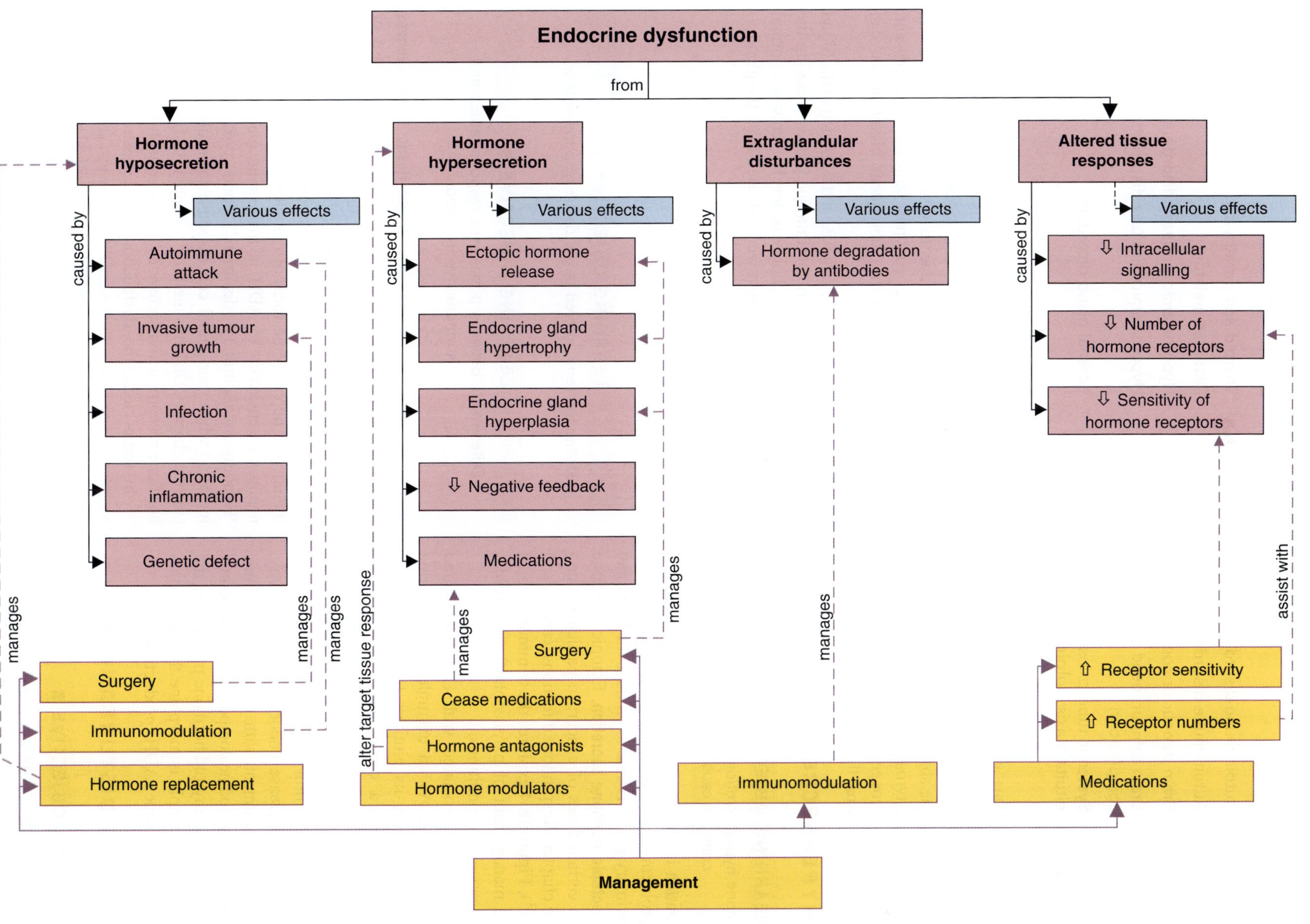

Figure 16.3

Clinical snapshot: Endocrine dysfunction

↓ = decreased; ↑ = increased.

Table 16.1 Endocrine disorders associated with hormone hyposecretion

Disorder	Causes	Chapter reference
Hashimoto's thyroiditis	Autoimmune disorder	'Thyroid and parathyroid disorders'
Type 1 diabetes mellitus	Autoimmune disorder	'Diabetes mellitus'
Pituitary dwarfism	Brain tumour or congenital malformation	'Hypothalamic–pituitary disorders'
Diabetes insipidus	Brain tumour; head trauma; tumour surgery complication	'Hypothalamic–pituitary disorders'
Addison's disease	Systemic tuberculosis; failure of hypothalamic–pituitary axis; autoimmune disorder; trauma	'Adrenal gland disorders'

Insufficient hormone production may also be related to glandular cells being unable to synthesise the appropriate endocrine product. This might be due to a genetic defect affecting enzyme availability within the synthetic pathway, or the absence of a specific precursor substance (e.g. the amino acid tyrosine) required to make the hormone. For example, 10% of congenital hypothyroid disorders are associated with defects in normal thyroid hormone synthesis.

HORMONE HYPERSECRETION

LEARNING OBJECTIVE 2

Define 'hormone hypersecretion', and indicate some common causes.

Hormone hypersecretion is characterised by *excessive hormone production*. The problem may develop because another tissue, in addition to the primary gland, is able to produce the hormone. This is known as **ectopic hormone secretion**. Ectopic hormone secretion occurs in certain types of cancer; in particular, lung carcinomas (see the chapter 'Respiratory infections, cancers and vascular conditions'). Figure 16.4 explores the common clinical manifestations and management of paraneoplastic syndromes that can develop in cancerous conditions.

Hypersecretion can be associated with *endocrine gland hypertrophy and hyperplasia*. As an example, an endocrine gland that is *overstimulated* by its pituitary tropic factor can undergo enlargement and, as a consequence, its hormonal output can rise dramatically. Gland hypersecretion may also be due to an *impairment of negative feedback*, such as rising blood hormone levels being unable to limit its secretion.

Certain medicines also increase endocrine gland activity. A case in point is during treatment with the antidysrhythmic agent amiodarone, which has an iodine component to its structure, and hence can cause increased thyroid hormone production and hyperthyroidism. Another example is morphine therapy, which can increase antidiuretic hormone (ADH) production.

EXTRAGLANDULAR DISTURBANCES

LEARNING OBJECTIVE 3

Briefly describe some common causes of extraglandular disturbances affecting endocrine function.

The blood levels of a particular hormone can also be influenced by *extraglandular processes* that occur between glandular release and hormonal interaction with the target tissue. Depending on the circumstances, this can lead to increased or decreased circulating hormone levels. When the liver is damaged or malfunctioning due to disease, or when genetic defects that affect hepatic enzyme structure are present, hormone metabolism, and the subsequent blood levels, can change dramatically.

The hormone may also be attacked and degraded in the blood by antibodies as a part of an autoimmune process, leaving the person with lower circulating hormone levels even when normal amounts of the hormonal agent were released from the gland.

ALTERED TARGET TISSUE RESPONSIVENESS

LEARNING OBJECTIVE 4

Define the term 'altered target tissue responsiveness'.

LEARNING OBJECTIVE 5

Differentiate between poor tissue responsiveness and hormone hyposecretion.

In some endocrine disorders, the **target tissue responsiveness** to normal levels of the hormone can markedly increase or decrease. This is generally thought to be associated with a change in the *number and/or sensitivity of cellular hormone receptors*. Disorders characterised by poor tissue responsiveness include the nephrogenic form of diabetes insipidus, where the nephron's sensitivity to ADH is inadequate (see the chapter 'Hypothalamic–pituitary disorders'), and type 2 diabetes mellitus, where peripheral cell response to insulin is reduced (see the chapter 'Diabetes mellitus'). There is also evidence that hormone receptor activity changes in cancerous tumours.

In some cases, the dysfunction lies downstream from the receptor, where intracellular signalling pathways are abnormal. A G-protein or second messenger linked to a particular receptor may not be formed in adequate amounts, or an inappropriate chemical can be substituted for the functional second messenger. A condition called *pseudoparathyroidism* is a good example of this kind of dysfunction. The affected person shows resistance to the action of parathormone in one or more of its target tissues. The disorder arises because of mutations in the G-protein linked to the receptor.

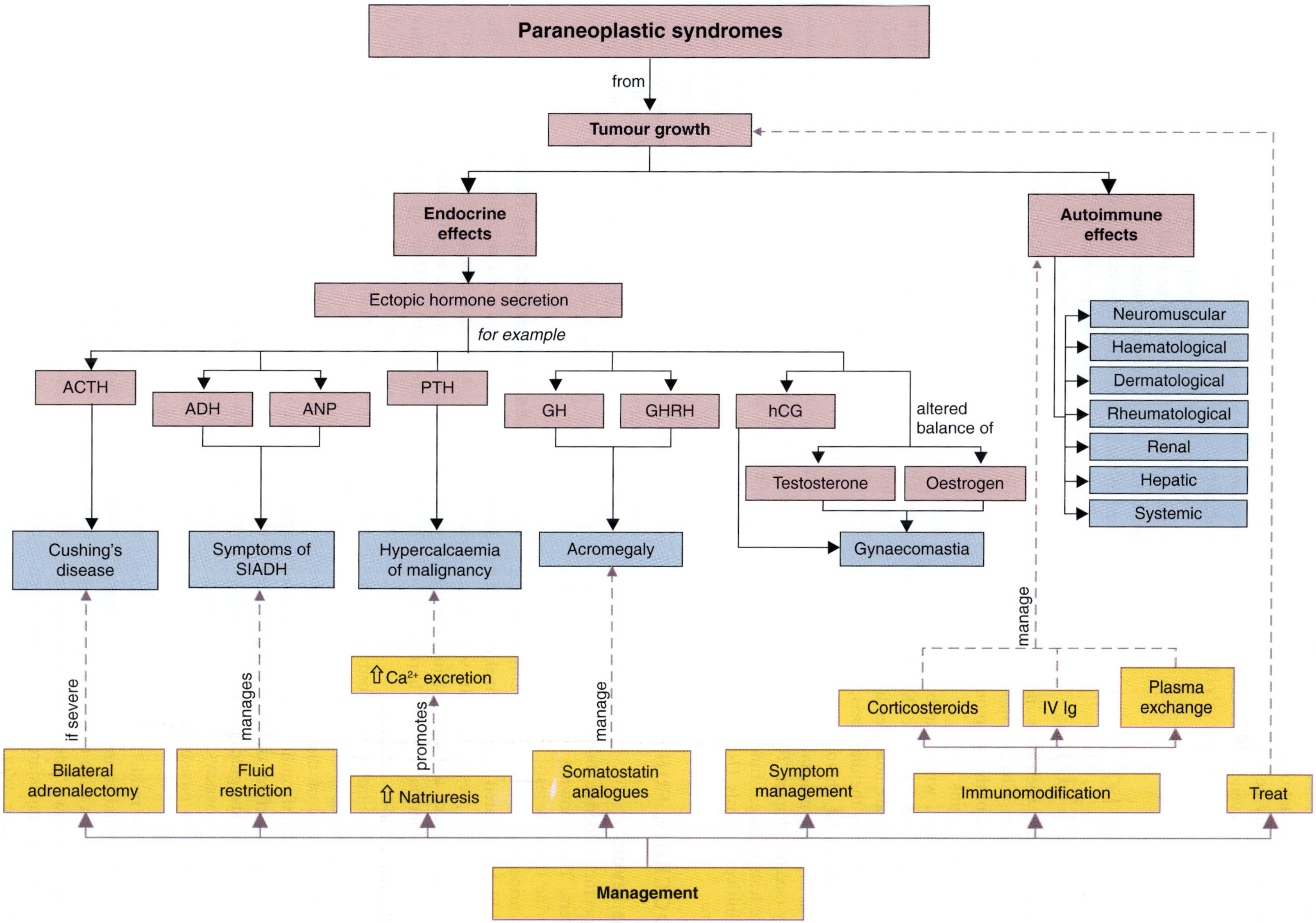

Figure 16.4

Clinical snapshot: Paraneoplastic syndromes

↑ = increased; ACTH = adrenocorticotropic hormone; ADH = antidiuretic hormone; ANP = atrial natriuretic peptide; Ca^{2+} = calcium ion; GH = growth hormone; GHRH = growth-hormone-releasing hormone; hCG = human chorionic gonadotropin; IV Ig = intravenous immunoglobulin; PTH = parathyroid hormone; SIADH = syndrome of inappropriate antidiuretic hormone secretion.

An endocrine condition characterised by poor tissue responsiveness to its hormone will show a set of clinical manifestations similar to that of hormone hyposecretion. A way of differentiating the two aetiologies, especially in the early stages of the disorder, may be the levels of circulating hormone. Poor tissue responsiveness can develop in the presence of normal, or near normal, blood levels of a particular hormone.

Methods used to assess endocrine function

Two important issues to consider when assessing the endocrine system are *structure* and *function*. Changes in structure and/or function are responsible for most of the symptoms of endocrine disorders. The assessment begins with a comprehensive history and physical examination, which can be suggestive of an endocrine disease but are not diagnostic. Many signs and symptoms of endocrine diseases are non-specific and can have multiple causes, which can delay the diagnosis, often until the disease is well advanced. Serial photographs from previous years can be helpful in depicting gradual physical changes; for example, acromegaly (see the chapter 'Hypothalamic–pituitary disorders'). Objective tests to assess function and structure are needed to make a definitive diagnosis. Usually, function is tested first and then structure.

TESTING ENDOCRINE FUNCTION

Basal hormone levels

Function tests for specific endocrine diseases are discussed in the next four chapters. The following information generally applies to all endocrine function tests. *Basal hormone levels* in the blood and/or urine are measured to establish whether the levels are low or high compared to the normal range, and are consistent with the clinical presentation. In some cases, this is all that is needed to make a diagnosis; for example, hypothyroidism. However, a normal random hormone level does not exclude endocrine disease.

Blood hormone levels provide important information about the function of particular endocrine glands (e.g. gland hypo- or hypersecretion) and the location of the abnormality/disease. Blood tests are also used to identify antibodies such as thyroid antibodies, or to determine the effect of a hormone on other substances; for example, insulin and glucagon on blood glucose levels. Sometimes radioimmunoassays, using radioisotope-labelled antigens, are needed to measure hormones or other substances.

If the endocrine disease is mild, it can be difficult to distinguish normal from abnormal hormone levels using basal hormone tests, because there is a wide degree of 'normal'. In addition, individuals have their own 'normal hormone ranges', whereas the accepted normal ranges are based on population data. Likewise, hormones have very short half-lives and are often secreted intermittently (in short bursts) and/or in a diurnal rhythm (peaks and troughs). Thus, blood may be taken during a trough and the hormone level may be below the normal range, or during a burst and the hormone level may be within the normal range. *Measuring serial hormone changes over time* may be more useful, and is usual in addition to basal sampling.

A number of hormones circulate in the blood in bound and unbound states (free). The free molecules of the hormone are physiologically active and important, but the levels are often hard to measure or there may be no test to measure it. Most hormone function tests involve measuring the active hormone levels, but sometimes they measure the precursor (e.g. serum 25-hydroxy vitamin D to detect vitamin D deficiency) and/or the hormone metabolite (e.g. urine catecholamine levels to detect an adrenal medullary tumour).

Another important consideration in regard to endocrine testing is *normal variation*. For example, the normal ranges for some hormones differ between men and women (e.g. testosterone and oestrogen). Furthermore, hormone levels in any individual can vary at different life stages and at different times of the day.

Urine tests are needed to measure the free hormone and hormone metabolite levels secreted by the kidneys. Sometimes a single urine specimen is collected, or urine is collected for 24 hours to measure the urine levels of free hormones; for example, catecholamines, to detect a tumour in the adrenal medulla. Sometimes blood and urine tests are performed simultaneously during dynamic endocrine function tests; for example, serum sodium, potassium, osmolality and urine osmolality to diagnose diabetes insipidus (see the chapter 'Hypothalamic–pituitary disorders').

Dynamic tests of endocrine function

Ideally, it would be useful to measure the *action* of the hormone, which results in the organ response and symptoms of endocrine disease. However, very few accurate measures of hormone action are available. Thus, dynamic endocrine tests are used based on current knowledge of the physiological actions and feedback mechanisms that *reflect* hormone actions.

Dynamic endocrine tests involve collecting blood at specific time points according to evidence-based protocols, and are best performed under supervision in an endocrine department. The blood must be collected in the appropriate tube and labelled appropriately with the time the sample was collected, as well as whether it is the basal sample (0) or the appropriate number in the sequence. Some hormones and/or their metabolites degrade quickly; therefore, many blood samples for hormone estimations need to be placed on ice and sent to the laboratory quickly. Not all laboratories are equipped to measure hormones or their metabolites, so it often takes time for the results of hormone tests to become available. These tests are designed to account for normal hormone peaks and troughs and diurnal variations. Usually, basal levels of the hormone/s of interest are measured in blood and sometimes urine samples. After the basal samples are collected, a stimulatory or suppressor hormone is administered and serial blood/urine samples are collected at set time points, sometimes over several hours or days.

Dynamic endocrine tests fall into two categories: *stimulation tests*, which are performed when hyposecretion is suspected; and *suppression tests*, which are performed when hypersecretion is suspected. Suppression tests are designed to differentiate hypersecretion from a hormone-secreting tumour.

Endocrine imaging

Endocrine imaging consists of general radiology procedures (e.g. computed tomography [CT] scans, magnetic resonance imaging [MRI] and ultrasound scans) to assess structure, and specific imaging techniques to assess function and differentiate among the possible causes of endocrine diseases. For example, radioactive iodine is used to determine the specific cause of hyperthyroidism (see the chapter 'Thyroid and parathyroid disorders').

Structural imaging is usually used to *confirm* the presence of an endocrine tumour after the diagnosis is made biochemically using dynamic endocrine tests. Structural imaging also provides important information about the size, location and state of the tumour and surrounding tissues, and helps the endocrinologist, surgeon or radiation oncologist plan the management strategy best suited to the individual person.

Structural imaging can also help the clinician assess the structural damage to surrounding tissues in contact with the tumour; for example, the effects of a pituitary tumour on the sella and optic chiasm. Bone densitometry may also be indicated to detect osteoporosis caused by a parathyroid adenoma secreting PTH (see the chapter 'Thyroid and parathyroid disorders').

Principles of treatment

LEARNING OBJECTIVE 6

Outline the principles of drug treatment associated with endocrine dysfunction.

MANAGING HORMONE-HYPOSECRETORY STATES AND POOR TISSUE RESPONSIVENESS

In general, the rationale in hormone hyposecretion is replacement therapy with the deficient hormone. For a number of endocrine disorders, the specific hormone is available for therapeutic purposes. In the past, these substances were obtained from *animal sources* wherever the structures of the animal and human hormone were similar. Hormones such as insulin were originally sourced from cattle and pig pancreases, whereas calcitonin can be obtained from salmon. While some of these animal forms of hormones are still available, they are no longer commonly used in clinical practice. A major problem associated with hormones sourced from animal tissue is that these substances are foreign proteins and can induce allergic reactions in hypersensitive people.

Hormones can also be extracted from *human sources*, such as from urine or cadaverous tissues, but in the latter case it is possible to transfer infectious organisms into those who are receiving treatment; for example, a significant number of people who received human growth hormone from cadaverous pituitaries became infected with a type of prion that causes a degenerative brain disease called Creutzfeldt–Jakob disease.

Over the past decade or so, human hormones have been obtained for therapeutic purposes through *recombinant DNA technology*. The process involves the insertion of a human gene for a hormone, say insulin, into a microbe such as *Escherichia coli* or *Saccaromyces cerevisiae* (brewer's yeast) and, as it proliferates in culture, all progeny contain the insulin gene. Human insulin is synthesised by the microbial colony, and is readily extracted and prepared for clinical use.

Importantly, hormone replacement therapy may not be useful in the management of a disorder characterised by poor tissue responsiveness. The provision of more circulating hormone in itself does not resolve the dysfunction if the tissues cannot respond to the chemical stimulus. In these situations, the therapy is directed towards enhancing the sensitivity of the tissue to the endogenous hormone. Drug treatment may help to achieve this aim; for example, the oral hypoglycaemic medicine metformin, used to manage type 2 diabetes mellitus (see the chapter 'Diabetes mellitus').

MANAGING HORMONE HYPERSECRETION STATES

Drug treatment can be used in excessive hormone states to relieve the clinical manifestations of the condition. However, generally this approach is not curative. The best way of resolving the hormone hypersecretion is to address the underlying pathology, such as removing a tumour that is causing increased hormone production.

Pharmacological therapy can be geared towards introducing a hormonal antagonist that directly prevents hormone stimulation of the target tissue, inhibiting hormone synthesis or stopping target tissue responses by blocking a different type of receptor linked to the observed effects (see Figure 16.5). Surgical removal or chemical ablation of the affected endocrine gland may also be an option. This approach has been used successfully in the management of the hyperthyroid condition (see the chapter 'Thyroid and parathyroid disorders').

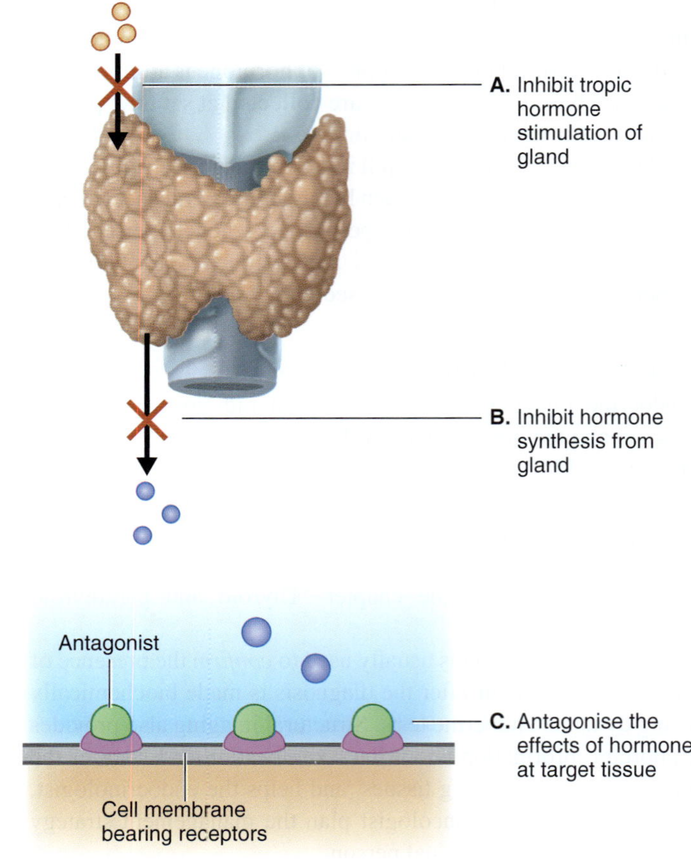

Figure 16.5

Drug treatment approaches in hormone hypersecretion states

(A) Inhibition of tropic hormone stimulation of the affected gland will decrease the output of hormone.

(B) The affected gland's hormone synthesis and/or secretion can be targeted directly.

(C) The function of the hormone's target cells can be altered by blocking the hormone's receptors directly or by blocking other transmitter receptors that induce similar responses (e.g. blocking beta receptors on heart muscle in hyperthyroid states).

CHILDREN AND ADOLESCENTS

- Although, statistically, approximately half of all child and adolescent presentations for endocrine disorders are for type 1 diabetes mellitus (although the incidence of type 2 diabetes is increasing in adolescents), other endocrine disorders include issues relating to growth and puberty.
- Precocious puberty or late puberty are generally caused by endocrine disorders. Consideration of the age of pubertal onset, duration, bone growth and secondary sex characteristics are all important factors in identifying puberty-related issues.

OLDER ADULTS

- Endocrine gland atrophy as a direct result of senescence can cause changes to the function of the endocrine system.
- Age-related decreases in aldosterone production may result in reduced blood pressure, contributing to an increased risk of falls. Other hormones that are frequently reduced with age include calcitonin, growth hormone and renin, testosterone (men), and prolactin and oestrogen (women). Various effects can be seen as a result of these changes.
- Age-related increases in noradrenaline may occur because of declining adrenoreceptor activity, and increases in parathyroid hormone can contribute to the development of osteoporosis.

KEY CLINICAL ISSUES

- Endocrine dysfunction generally results as a consequence of the under- or overproduction of a hormone.
- Underproduction of hormone can often be aided by the administration of exogenous hormone. However, overproduction often requires surgical resection of the structure involved.
- A comprehensive history and assessment is an important diagnostic process. It is usually followed by hormone stimulation tests if hyposecretion is suspected, or suppression tests if hypersecretion is suspected, in addition to imaging.
- Management depends on the findings, but includes medicines to stimulate or suppress abnormal endocrine gland function and/or surgery. If surgery is required, hormone replacement therapy is required for life. Thus, endocrine disease could be considered to be a chronic disease.
- Endocrine dysfunction causes significant psychological distress and affects quality of life even when a therapeutic cure is achieved. These issues must be considered as part of the management plan.

CHAPTER REVIEW

- Hormone *hyposecretion* is characterised by an insufficient production of hormone. It can occur when glandular cells are injured or destroyed by *pathophysiological processes*. It may also be related to glandular cells being *unable to synthesise* the appropriate endocrine product.
- *Hormone hypersecretion* is characterised by *excessive hormone production*. It can develop as a result of *ectopic hormone secretion*, where another tissue produces and releases the hormone in addition to the primary gland. Hypersecretion can be associated with both *endocrine gland hypertrophy and hyperplasia*.
- *Extraglandular processes* can also influence blood levels of a particular hormone. Depending on the circumstances, this can lead to either higher or lower circulating hormone levels. Circulating hormone levels can change as a result of altered metabolism of the hormone, or autoimmune destruction of the endocrine product.
- A target tissue's chronic responsiveness to normal levels of the hormone can markedly increase or decrease. This is generally thought to be associated with a change in the number and/or the sensitivity of cellular hormone receptors. *Altered responsiveness* may also be due to changes in intracellular signalling downstream of the receptor.
- A way of differentiating between poor tissue responsiveness and hormone hyposecretion may be the *levels of circulating hormone*. Poor tissue responsiveness can develop in the presence of normal, or near normal, blood levels of a particular hormone.
- In general, the rationale in hormone hyposecretion is *replacement therapy* with the hormone that is underproduced. In states of poor target tissue responsiveness, the therapy is directed towards *enhancing the sensitivity* of the tissue to the endogenous hormone.
- In excessive hormone states, drug therapy is geared towards introducing a *hormonal antagonist* that directly prevents hormone stimulation of the target tissue, inhibiting hormone synthesis or stopping target tissue responses by blocking a different type of receptor linked to the observed effects. *Surgical removal or chemical ablation* of the affected endocrine gland may also be an option.

REVIEW QUESTIONS

1. Name the four types of pathophysiological mechanisms underlying endocrine diseases.
2. Identify some specific causes of endocrine dysfunction that could lead to a state of either hormone hyposecretion or hormone hypersecretion. Briefly explain why, for each cause identified.
3. State one drug treatment approach for each of the following forms of endocrine dysfunction:
   - a hormone hypersecretion
   - b poor tissue responsiveness
   - c hormone hyposecretion
4. A 57-year-old man with renal disease is showing clinical manifestations of low circulating ADH levels, but tests indicate acceptable pituitary function with respect to the release of this hormone. Account for this man's condition.
5. List three types of investigative processes used to diagnose endocrine disorders.

HEALTH PROFESSIONAL CONNECTIONS

See the chapters 'Hypothalamic-pituitary disorders', 'Thyroid and parathyroid disorders', 'Adrenal gland disorders' and 'Diabetes mellitus' for relevant health professional connections.

CASE STUDY

Mr Graham Donovan is a 66-year-old man (UR number 727340) admitted for investigation of suspected paraneoplastic syndrome and hypercalcaemia from a non-small-cell lung cancer (NSCLC). A squamous cell carcinoma was confirmed by fine-needle aspiration biopsy yesterday. On admission he was dyspnoeic and had haemoptysis. Mr Donovan complained of fatigue, anorexia and polyuria. He appeared dehydrated. His observations were as follows:

Temperature	Heart rate	Respiration rate	Blood pressure	SpO_2
36.7°C	52	12	98/52	92% (RA*)

*RA = room air.

Mr Donovan was ordered intravenous sodium chloride 0.9%, 1000 mL q5h, for review after 2 L. His pathology results were as follows:

HAEMATOLOGY

Patient location:	Ward 3	**UR:**	727340		
Consultant:	Smith	**NAME:**	Donovan		
		Given name:	Graham	**Sex:**	M
		DOB:	03/07/XX	**Age:**	66

Time collected	11:22
Date collected	XX/XX
Year	XXXX
Lab #	45345354

FULL BLOOD COUNT		UNITS	REFERENCE RANGE
Haemoglobin	121	g/L	115–160
White cell count	7.1	$\times 10^9$/L	4.0–11.0
Platelets	180	$\times 10^9$/L	140–400
Haematocrit	0.38		0.33–0.47
Red cell count	4.1	$\times 10^{12}$/L	3.80–5.20
Reticulocyte count	0.8	%	0.2–2.0
MCV	95	fL	80–100
Neutrophils	4.8	$\times 10^9$/L	2.00–8.00
Lymphocytes	2.01	$\times 10^9$/L	1.00–4.00
Monocytes	0.33	$\times 10^9$/L	0.10–1.00
Eosinophils	0.32	$\times 10^9$/L	< 0.60
Basophils	0.11	$\times 10^9$/L	< 0.20
ESR	9	mm/h	< 12

BIOCHEMISTRY

Patient location:	Ward 3	**UR:**	727340		
Consultant:	Smith	**NAME:**	Donovan		
		Given name:	Graham	**Sex:**	M
		DOB:	03/07/XX	**Age:**	66

Time collected	11:22
Date collected	XX/XX
Year	XXXX
Lab #	45345354

ELECTROLYTES		UNITS	REFERENCE RANGE
Sodium	136	mmol/L	135–145
Potassium	3.5	mmol/L	3.5–5.2
Chloride	99	mmol/L	95–110
Calcium	3.61	mmol/L	2.1–2.6
Phosphate	0.65	mmol/L	0.75–1.5
25-hydroxy vitamin D	23	nmol/L	50–125
Bicarbonate	25	mmol/L	22–32
Glucose (random)	3.9	mmol/L	3.5–5.4
Iron	19	μmol/L	11–30
PTH	0.8	pmol/L	1.0–5.5
PTH-related peptide	24.3	pmol/L	0–2

CRITICAL THINKING

1 Consider Mr Donovan's clinical picture. What electrolyte imbalances would be related to which signs and symptoms? Create a table listing the abnormal electrolytes in one column, and the signs and symptoms relating to the abnormality in a second column.

2 How does the parathyroid-hormone-related peptide influence calcium and phosphate levels? Trace the mechanism of this interaction.

3 Mr Donovan was ordered a significant intravenous fluid volume, which was to be reviewed in 10 hours. What was this order attempting to achieve? How will you know that this has been achieved? What adverse reactions should you be observing for? How will you know when these are developing?

4 One controversial pharmacological intervention for individuals with hypercalcaemia is the administration of loop diuretics. Why may these not have been instituted in the first instance?

5 Examine all of Mr Donovan's presenting signs and symptoms. Identify all of the non-pharmacological interventions that should be initiated to manage Mr Donovan's problems.

BIBLIOGRAPHY

Australian Institute of Health and Welfare (AIHW) (2022). *Australia's health 2022: data insights.* Australia's Health series No. 18. Cat No. 240. Canberra: AIHW. https://www.aihw.gov.au/reports/australias-health/australias-health-2022-data-insights/about.

Bauldoff, G., Gubrud-Howe, P.M., Carno, M.-A., Levett-Jones, T., Hales, M., Berry, K., ... Stanley. D. (2020). *LeMone and Burke's medical–surgical nursing: critical thinking for person-centred care* (4th [Australian] edn). Sydney: Pearson Australia.

Best, O. & Fredericks, B. (2021). *Yatdjuligin: Aboriginal and Torres Strait Islander nursing and midwifery care* (3rd edn). Port Melbourne, VIC: Cambridge University Press.

Bullock, S. & Manias, E. (2022). *Fundamentals of pharmacology* (9th edn). Sydney: Pearson Australia.

Marieb, E.N. & Hoehn, K. (2019). *Human anatomy and physiology* (11th edn). San Francisco, CA: Pearson Benjamin Cummings.

New Zealand Ministry of Health (2021). *Annual update of key results 2020/2021: New Zealand Health Survey.* Wellington: Ministry of Health. https://www.health.govt.nz/publication/annual-update-key-results-2020-21-new-zealand-health-survey.

Rang, H.P., Ritter, J.M., Flower, R.J. & Henderson, G. (2016). *Rang & Dale's Pharmacology* (8th edn). Harlow, Essex: Elsevier.

Stats New Zealand (2021). *National and subnational period life tables: 2017-2019.* Wellington: Stats New Zealand. https://www.stats.govt.nz/information-releases/national-and-subnational-period-life-tables-2017-2019.

Hypothalamic–pituitary disorders

17

LEARNING OBJECTIVES

After completing this chapter, you should be able to:

1 Outline the relationship between the hypothalamus and the pituitary gland with respect to neuroendocrine regulation.

2 Identify the pituitary hormones associated with endocrine disorders.

3 Describe the pathophysiological mechanisms and epidemiology involved in each of the pituitary endocrine disorders.

4 Describe the clinical manifestations, diagnosis and clinical management of each of the pituitary disorders.

WHAT YOU SHOULD KNOW BEFORE YOU START THIS CHAPTER

Can you identify the main components of the endocrine system?

Can you describe the anatomical and physiological relationship between the hypothalamus and the pituitary?

Can you identify the hormones of the pituitary, and their functions?

Can you outline the effects associated with body fluid excess and deficiency?

Can you outline the effects of body sodium ion excess and deficiency?

KEY TERMS

Acromegaly
Antidiuretic hormone (ADH)
Diabetes insipidus (DI)
Gigantism
Growth hormone (GH)
Hypernatraemia
Hyperprolactinaemia
Hyponatraemia
Hypothalamus
Pituitary dwarfism
Pituitary gland
Prolactin (PRL)
Syndrome of inappropriate ADH secretion (SIADH)

Introduction

LEARNING OBJECTIVE 1

Outline the relationship between the hypothalamus and the pituitary gland with respect to neuroendocrine regulation.

LEARNING OBJECTIVE 2

Identify the pituitary hormones associated with endocrine disorders.

The **hypothalamus** and **pituitary gland** represent a key *interface between the nervous and endocrine systems* in the regulation and coordination of body function. Figure 17.1 depicts the pituitary gland, its lobes and its relationship to the brain. The hormones released by these structures influence normal growth and development, homeostasis, metabolism, reproductive function and the body's response to stress. Figure 17.2 lists the anterior and posterior pituitary hormones and their major physiological effects. When the pituitary or the hypothalamic–pituitary axis is disrupted, one or more of these functions will be profoundly altered.

Disruption of the *hypothalamic–pituitary axis* can occur through under-secretion (i.e. hyposecretion) or over-secretion (i.e. hypersecretion) of the hormones produced, or released, by

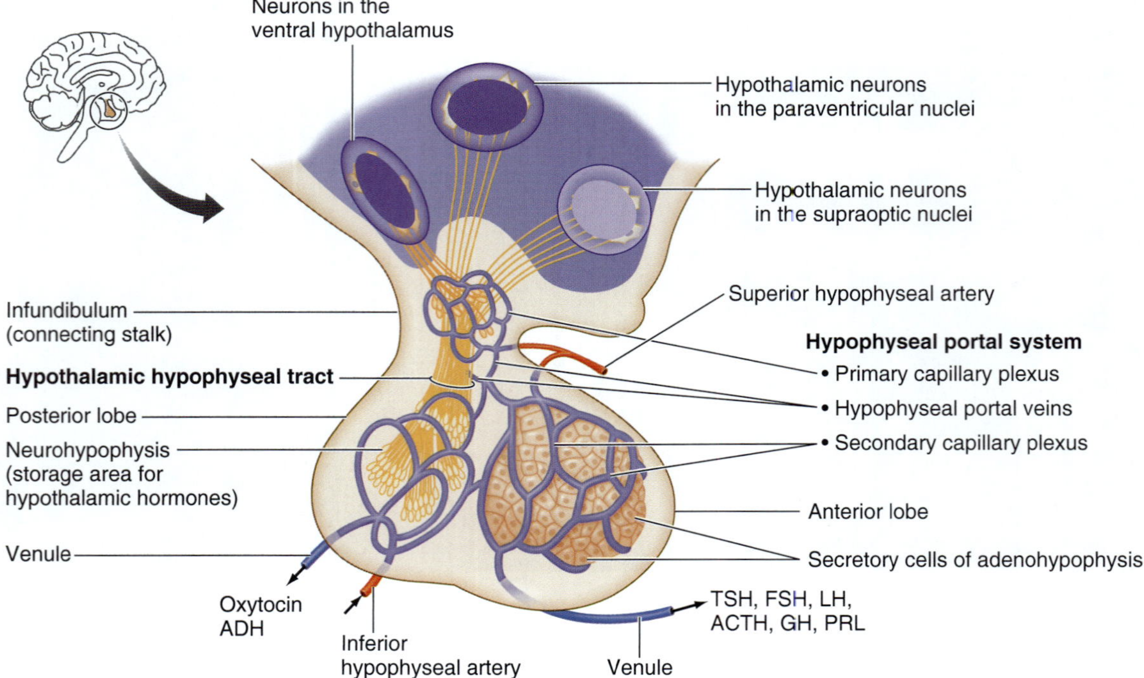

Figure 17.1

The pituitary gland and its relationship to the brain

ACTH = adrenocorticotropic hormone; ADH = antidiuretic hormone; FSH = follicle-stimulating hormone; GH = growth hormone; LH = luteinising hormone; PRL = prolactin; TSH = thyroid-stimulating hormone.

Source: Adapted from Marieb & Hoehn (2019), Figure 16.1, pp. 642–3.

the hypothalamus and pituitary gland. This can affect growth (through changes in *growth hormone [GH]* activity) and fluid balance (through changes in *antidiuretic hormone [ADH]* activity), as well as the functioning of the thyroid, adrenal glands and gonads. Here, the focus is on disorders affecting the activity of GH, ADH and prolactin.

Disorders affecting the thyroid, adrenals and gonads are covered in the chapters 'Thyroid and parathyroid disorders', 'Adrenal gland disorders', 'Female reproductive disorders' and 'Male reproductive disorders', respectively.

Abnormalities can occur in the anterior and posterior pituitary gland independently of each other. Hormone hypersecretion often involves *adrenocorticotropic hormone (ACTH)*, resulting in Cushing's disease (see the chapter 'Adrenal gland disorders'), or GH, resulting in acromegaly in adults or gigantism in children. Hormone hyposecretion of pituitary hormones can involve all of the anterior pituitary hormones, and is referred to as *panhypopituitarism*. Panhypopituitarism is a serious condition and leads to shrinkage and poor functioning of target organs, such as the thyroid and the adrenal glands, due to a lack of stimulation by the relevant stimulating hormones.

A common cause of these imbalances is the presence of space-occupying lesions, such as tumours. Such tumours tend to be slow-growing, and are more likely to occur in older adults. Many of these tumours go undetected, particularly if they do not exert an altered secretory pattern. Studies have shown that 10–25% of autopsies and 10% of brain imaging scans for another purpose reveal undiagnosed pituitary tumours. The signs and symptoms of pituitary disease are due to the destruction/compression of the pituitary and surrounding tissues, in combination with altered hormone production and its consequent effects. Figure 17.3 explores the common clinical manifestations and management of pituitary gland disorders associated with hormone deficiency, and Figure 17.4 explores the common clinical manifestations and management of pituitary gland disorders associated with hormone excess.

Growth hormone

LEARNING OBJECTIVE 3

Describe the pathophysiological mechanisms and epidemiology involved in each of the pituitary endocrine disorders.

LEARNING OBJECTIVE 4

Describe the clinical manifestations, diagnosis and clinical management of each of the pituitary disorders.

Growth hormone (GH) release promotes normal body cell growth (especially connective tissue) and facilitates the development

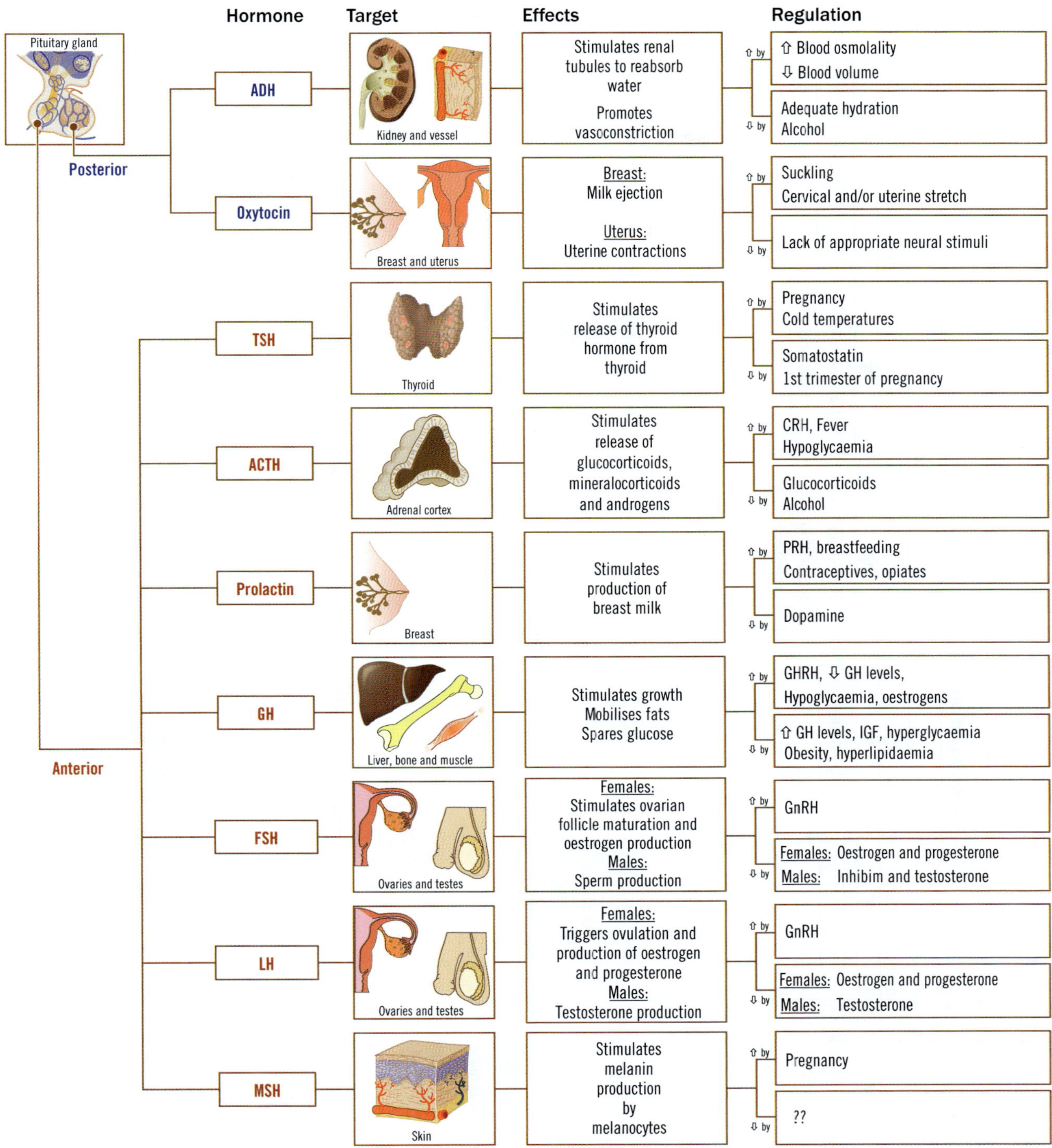

Figure 17.2

Pitutary hormones and their functions

↑ by = stimulated by; ↓ by = inhibited by; ACTH = adrenocorticotropic hormone; ADH = antidiuretic hormone; CRH = corticotropin-releasing hormone; FSH = follicle-stimulating hormone; GH = growth hormone; GHRH = growth-hormone-releasing hormone; GnRH = gonadotropin-releasing hormone; IGF = insulin-like growth factor; LH = luteinising hormone; PRH = prolactin-releasing hormone; TSH = thyroid-stimulating hormone; MSH = melanocyte-stimulating hormone.

of the musculoskeletal system. It also acts as an anabolic agent, stimulating cellular protein synthesis. It does this through the secretion and subsequent action of intermediary substances released from the liver and other tissues. The main intermediary is called *insulin-like growth factor-1 (IGF-1)*, or *somatomedin*, which actually interacts with body tissues. It also has direct anti-insulin activity on the liver and peripheral tissues, triggering a rise in blood glucose levels and increased lipolysis (see Figure 17.5).

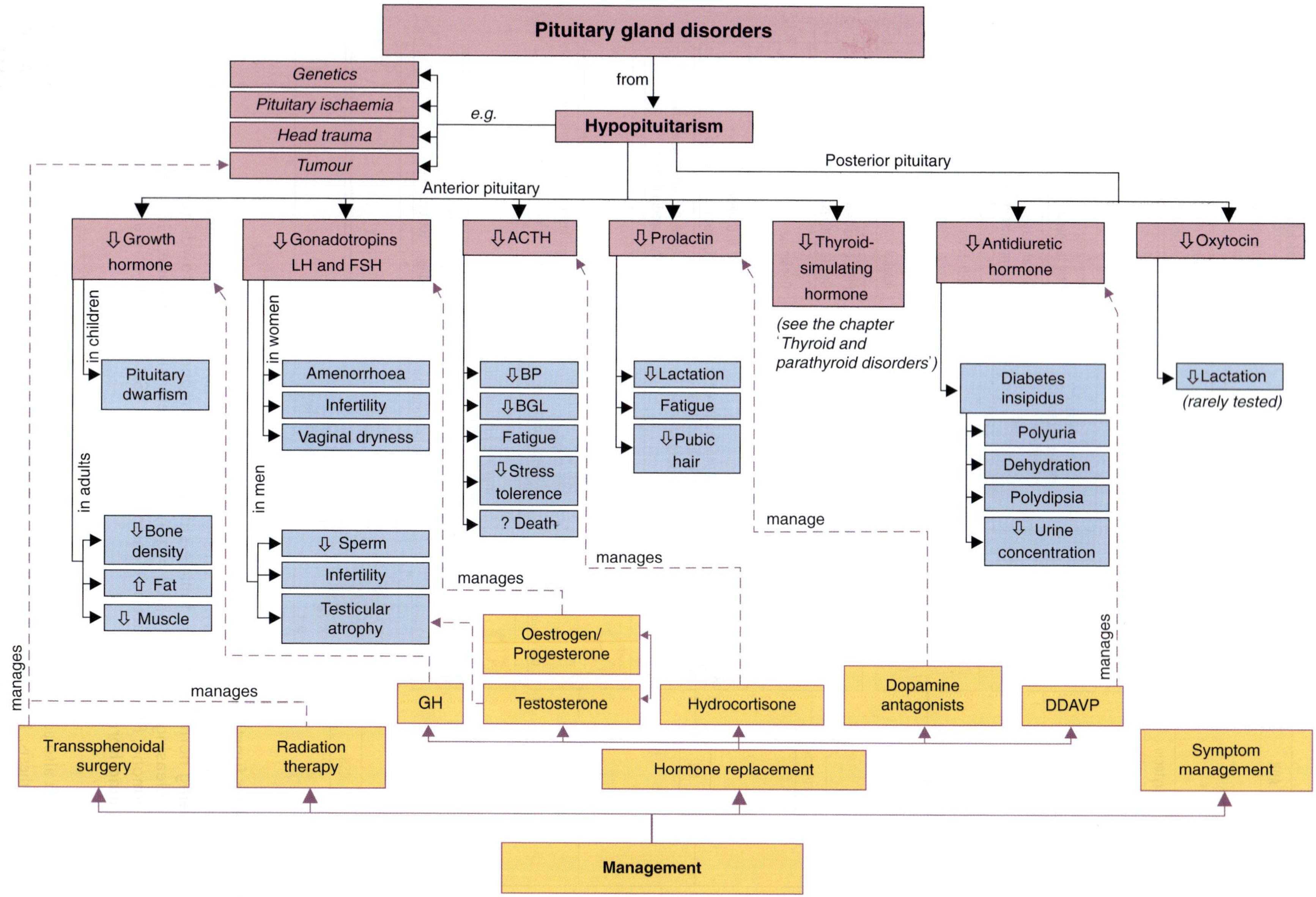

Figure 17.3

Clinical snapshot: Pituitary gland hyposecretory disorders

↓ = decreased; ↑ = increased; ACTH = adrenocorticotropic hormone; BGL = blood glucose level; BP = blood pressure; DDAVP = 1-desamino-8-d-arginine vasopressin (vasopressin); FSH = follicle-stimulating hormone; GH = growth hormone; LH = luteinising hormone.

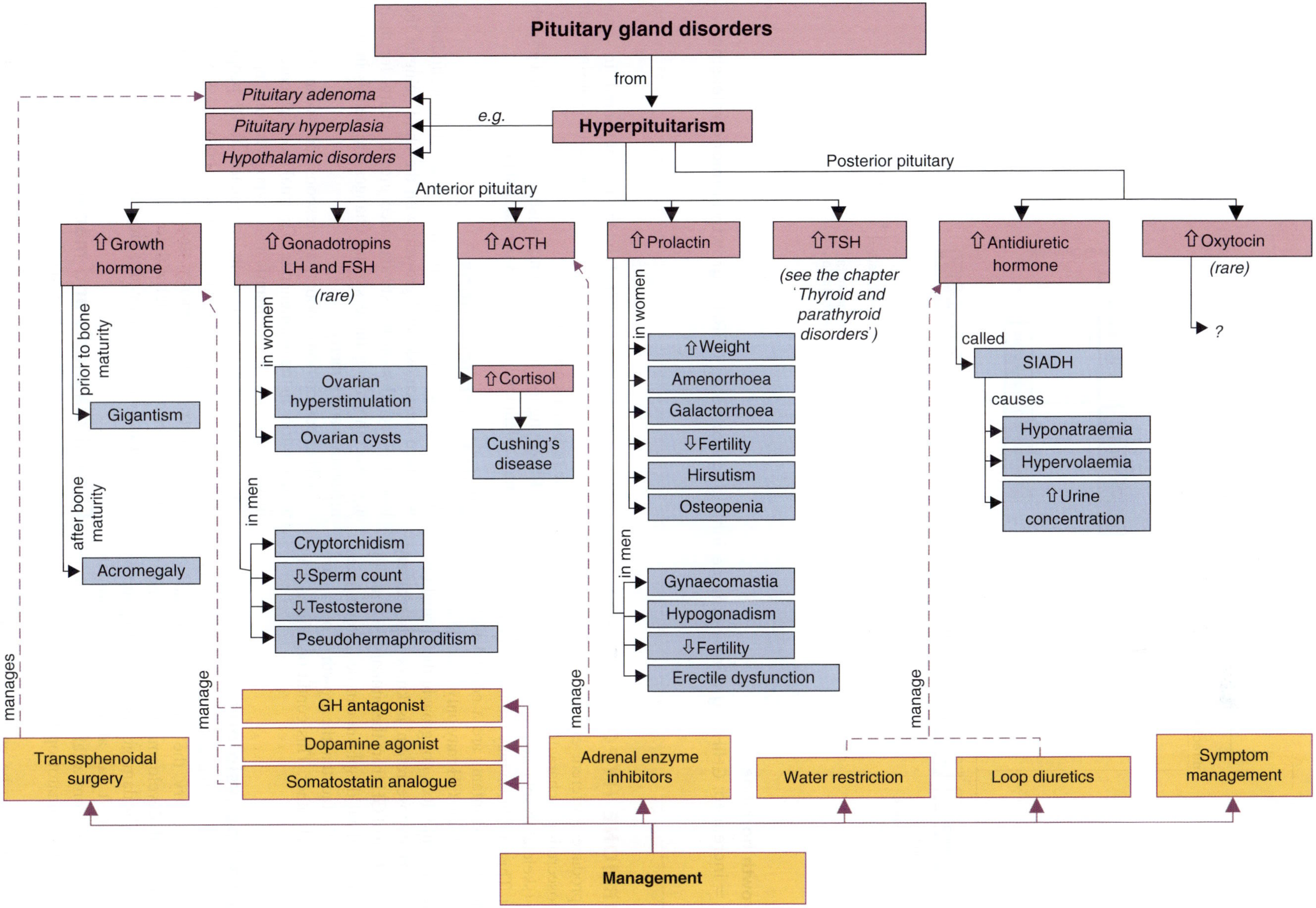

Figure 17.4

Clinical snapshot: Pituitary gland hypersecretory disorders

↓ = decreased; ↑ = increased; ACTH = adrenocorticotropic hormone; FSH = follicle-stimulating hormone; GH = growth hormone; LH = luteinising hormone; SIADH = syndrome of inappropriate antidiuretic hormone; TSH = thyroid-stimulating hormone.

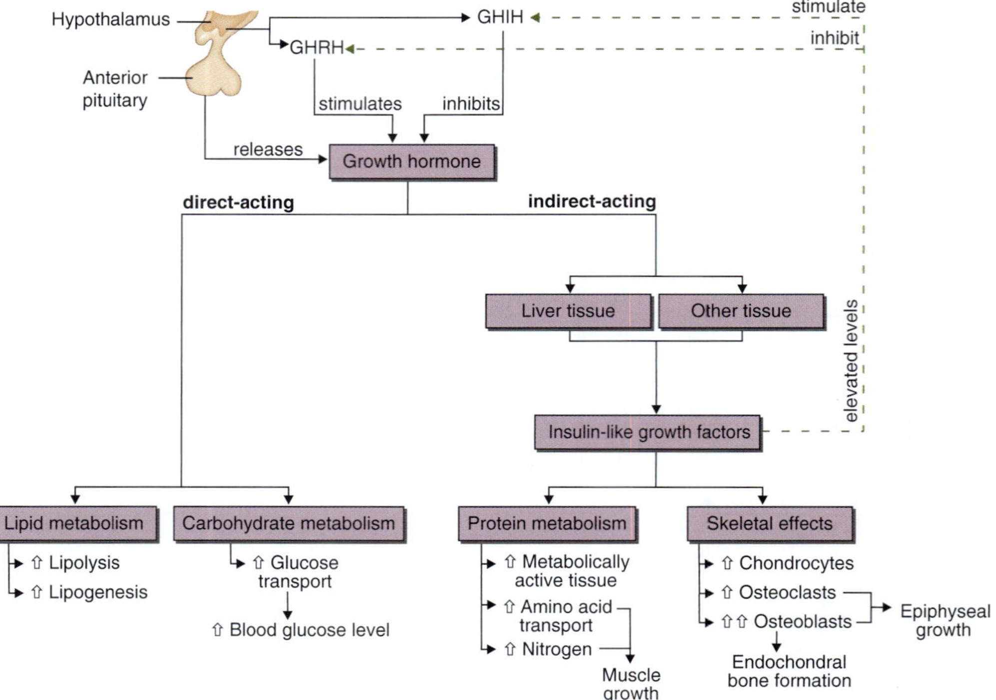

Figure 17.5

The actions of growth hormone

↓ = decreased; ↑ = increased; GHIH = growth-hormone-inhibiting hormone; GHRH = growth-hormone-releasing hormone.

GROWTH HORMONE HYPOSECRETION

GH hyposecretion produces different effects at different ages. Classically, GH hyposecretion is characterised by stunted growth in affected children (skeletal dysplasias), when musculoskeletal growth is prominent. This condition may not be detected at birth because most of the affected infants are a normal weight and length at birth. The effect of low GH may only become apparent at an older age when the child does not grow at the normal rate. The classic form of GH hyposecretion is known as **pituitary dwarfism**, when the secretion of GH from the pituitary is primarily impaired. This form of skeletal dysplasia can be differentiated from genetic aetiologies by the fact that the growth of body parts remains proportional to each other. This condition affects 1 in 25,000 children in Australia.

Aetiology and pathophysiology

GH hyposecretion occurs when the cells responsible for GH synthesis in the anterior pituitary, the *somatotrophes*, do not form properly during fetal development or are irreversibly damaged during childhood. The damage may be due to pituitary infarction or a brain tumour. It can also occur in traumatic brain injury (TBI) resulting from a fall, violence, at work or during sport. It appears that somatotrophes are commonly lost after a TBI.

The somatotrophes may also be unable to respond to the hypothalamic factor signalling mechanisms, or in certain types of liver disorders where IGF-1 synthesis is impaired. In some cases the target cell GH receptor may be defective, causing poor tissue responsiveness to GH.

Recent figures from Hormones Australia indicate that growth hormone deficiency affects 2–3 per 10,000 people.

Clinical manifestations

A major clinical manifestation of GH hyposecretion in childhood is stunted musculoskeletal growth, with the child being in the lowest percentiles on the standardised growth charts for their age. Accompanying these system changes are delays in teeth maturation and puberty.

GH hyposecretion or poor tissue responsiveness can also lead to disruptions in the maintenance of normal blood glucose levels in neonates, which can manifest as hypoglycaemic episodes. This condition is rare in adults (estimated at 10 people per million) and often presents as loss of lean body mass, reduced bone density, reduced energy and psychological symptoms, such as poor memory, social withdrawal and depression. Often, other hormone disorders are also present.

Clinical diagnosis and management

Diagnosis A careful history and physical examination is important in both children and adults. Short stature can be part of non-endocrine disease processes, such as kidney disease, malnutrition, gastrointestinal disease and chronic respiratory disease. Endocrine causes only account for 10–15% of cases. In children, height alone is not the best predictor for a definitive diagnosis.

Where a GH deficiency in a child is suspected, the assessment and diagnostic testing should be undertaken by a paediatric endocrinologist. Complete GH deficiency in children usually presents before 3 years of age. Lesser degrees of GH deficiency present later. Thus, serial growth charts are important to plot the child's growth pattern. Children below the first percentile for their age and gender are considered to be abnormally short.

Infants of non-diabetic mothers who develop hypoglycaemia early may have hypopituitarism. Male infants so affected often have micropenis as a result of the condition. In situations when hypopituitarism is suspected, children must be carefully assessed because untreated GH deficiency in childhood is associated with increased morbidity from conditions such as cardiac disease.

Blood hormone levels are also measured in children and adults. These include GH, *thyroid-stimulating hormone (TSH)*, ACTH, *luteinising hormone (LH)* and *follicle-stimulating hormone (FSH)*. Serial measurements are usually preferred, and sometimes overnight GH tests are needed. Bone density studies are useful in both children and adults.

Management GH hormone replacement is the medical treatment of choice for hypopituitary disorders. Guidelines for GH replacement are available from the Pharmaceutical Benefits branch of the Australian Government Department of Health and Ageing. Generally, serial height measurement to determine growth velocity is required on three to four occasions at least three months apart, over 12 months. If the guideline criteria are met, GH replacement with a synthetic GH analogue (somatropin) by subcutaneous injection can be used in children for the following conditions: idiopathic GH deficiency, retarded growth secondary to an intracranial lesion or irradiation, risk of hypoglycaemia secondary to GH deficiency in neonates, Turner's syndrome and growth failure associated with chronic renal failure.

Some experts have suggested that recombinant synthetic GH may have beneficial effects on body composition and well-being, and might reduce cardiovascular risk in adults with proven GH deficiency.

GROWTH HORMONE HYPERSECRETION

The names of conditions associated with excessive GH secretion depend on whether it occurs in adulthood or childhood. In adults, excess GH production is referred to as **acromegaly**. In children and adolescents, it is called **gigantism** (otherwise known as *giantism*). As expected, the condition is characterised by excessive skeletal growth.

Aetiology and pathophysiology

The most common cause of an overproduction of GH (in 70% cases) is a benign, slow-growing pituitary tumour that affects the somatotrophes. This tumour is referred to as a *macroadenoma*. This can occur in adults or in children. The altered hormone levels result in overstimulation of cell growth, particularly affecting connective tissues. Associated with this condition are metabolic, skeletal, cardiovascular, cerebrovascular and respiratory comorbidities. These comorbidities reduce life expectancy.

Epidemiology

These conditions are relatively rare. The incidence of acromegaly worldwide is considered to be 50 affected people per million people. Recent Australian statistics indicate that between 750 and 3,500 Australians live with this condition.

Clinical manifestations

All affected people are characteristically taller, well above average height. The major difference in the manifestations of this condition between adults and children is that the accelerated body growth due to excessive hormone action is more harmonious with the accelerated growth that normally occurs in childhood. As a consequence, the excessive skeletal growth is more in proportion than that seen in affected adults. In adults, hands and feet become enlarged, and the lower jaw protrudes. Bony regions, such as the facial ridges and the forehead, tend to be more prominent and result in a coarser facial appearance. Spinal disorders may develop due to periosteal vertebral growth. These alterations in bone growth can also alter the calcium–phosphate balance, resulting in a mild form of hyperphosphataemia (see the chapter 'Electrolyte imbalances') and an increased risk of vertebral fractures. Osteoarthralgia is commonly reported.

Consistent with the proliferative stimulus of GH on connective tissue in affected adults, the tongue tends to be enlarged, skin and hair tend to become coarser and the skin may become thickened. The affected person may experience weight gain. The thyroid gland and the heart may increase in size; the former change may result in goitre, while the latter change can lead to chronic cardiovascular problems. Tissue oedema may develop. Joints may become enlarged, leading to joint pain and mobility difficulties.

Interestingly, sweat glands undergo hypertrophy, leading to increased perspiration. The increased activity of these glands may result in the person experiencing a problem associated with a strong body odour.

The anti-insulin action of excessive GH secretion can lead to insulin resistance, which manifests as hyperglycaemia. Blood glucose levels need to be monitored because there is an increased risk of the development of diabetes mellitus and dyslipidaemia.

Excessive GH secretion can induce hypertension. Sodium retention, vasomotor dysfunction and endothelial disruption have been implicated in the development of this state.

Other common manifestations include headache, paraesthesias and fatigue.

Clinical diagnosis and management

Diagnosis All of the pituitary hormones should be assessed because of the wide-ranging effects on the endocrine system. GH is secreted in pulses, and the concentration in the blood can vary, making random and basal samples not specific enough to make a definitive diagnosis. Thus, GH must be measured at intervals; for example, at time 0, 15 and 30 minutes to detect peak and trough variations. In many cases, a three-hour *oral glucose tolerance test (OGTT)* is performed, because consuming 75–100 g of glucose normally suppresses serum GH to less than 1 ng/mL in one to two hours in healthy people.

The diagnosis of acromegaly is made on the basis of elevated GH and IGF-1 levels, which are not suppressed during an OGTT. The procedure for performing an OGTT is the same as that used to diagnose diabetes mellitus, except that it is usually a three-hour test, and GH as well as glucose is measured.

IGF-1 levels are more stable during the day than GH, and are a practical and reliable screening measure. If the IGF-1 level is high, it usually means that the person has acromegaly. The exceptions are during pregnancy (as IGF-1 is usually two to three times higher than normal), during puberty, in people with liver or kidney disease, during hyperglycaemia or in people with diabetes mellitus, and in people with anorexia nervosa.

Once acromegaly is diagnosed, a magnetic resonance imaging (MRI) scan of the head is performed to determine the presence, size and location of the pituitary tumour. Computed tomography (CT) can be used if MRI is contraindicated (e.g. in people with pacemakers, or implants containing metal). If a tumour is not detected on a head scan, the person should have a CT scan to detect an ectopic tumour in the chest, pelvis or abdomen, and have serum *growth-hormone-releasing hormone (GHRH)* measured.

Management The primary aims of management are the normalisation of both GH and IGF-1 secretion, the control of tumour growth and enhanced life expectancy.

Surgical management Management in adults consists of surgically removing the tumour, usually transsphenoidally (through the nose and sphenoid bone, the latter being located at the base of the skull). The overall surgical success rate is determined by the normalisation of GH and IGF-1 levels. In around 50% of people, there can be persistence of elevated GH secretion.

If the GH and IGF-1 levels remain high after surgery, radiation therapy or a treatment with a somatostatin analogue (see the following section) may be indicated to shrink the tumour and reduce GH and IGF-1 levels. Sometimes these treatments are used preoperatively if the tumour is very large or where surgery is contraindicated. Life-long hormone replacement is often necessary, as already indicated.

Medical management *Somatostatin analogues* (also known as *somatostatin receptor ligands*) prevent GH production and reduce GH and IGF-1 levels in 50–70% of affected people, as well as slightly reducing tumour size. This treatment needs to be individualised. Somatostatin analogues include subcutaneous octreotide 12-hourly until GH secretion is controlled, at which time deep intramuscular injections of modified-release octreotide can be administered monthly. Alternatively, deep intramuscular injections of another somatostatin analogue, lanreotide, can be given every 14 days or, in some cases, every 7 or 10 days if higher doses are required. Relatives can be taught to administer these medicines, but usually the affected person attends an endocrine outpatient service or their general practitioner to have the injection administered.

Side-effects of somatostatin analogues include loose bowel motions, flatulence, cholelithiasis (which is often asymptomatic and does not require treatment), abdominal pain, diarrhoea and sometimes diabetes mellitus.

The dopamine agonist bromocriptine is indicated in some people with tumours that secrete prolactin as well as GH. Paradoxically, unlike normal somatotrophes, somatotrophic tumour cells express dopaminergic receptor subtypes (D_2-receptors) that suppress GH secretion. The commencing dose is usually given at night and is gradually increased.

Prolactin hypersecretion

Prolactin (PRL) is synthesised by a group of cells in the pituitary gland known as *lactotrophes*. PRL plays a key role in the development of breast tissue in preparation for lactation. In animals, evidence suggests that PRL may facilitate bonding with the new offspring, and this may also be the case for humans. At high levels, PRL can also affect reproductive function. It is normally produced in low amounts in males, but its role is unknown. Importantly, the inhibition of PRL release by lactotrophes is due to dopaminergic receptor stimulation from the hypothalamus. PRL hypersecretion is known as **hyperprolactinaemia**.

AETIOLOGY AND PATHOPHYSIOLOGY

The most common cause of hyperprolactinaemia is a benign tumour in the anterior pituitary involving the lactotrophes. Damage to the hypothalamic dopaminergic neurons or masses that compress the pituitary stalk can also induce this condition. Other conditions that can be associated with hyperprolactinaemia include primary hypothyroidism, adrenocortical insufficiency, hepatic cirrhosis, renal failure, polycystic ovary syndrome and some forms of lung cancer.

High PRL levels stimulate the mammary glands of the breast to induce lactation and breast enlargement. Excessive PRL levels inhibit gonadotropin secretion and alter the responsiveness of the reproductive tissues to oestrogen and progesterone. As a result, the menstrual and ovarian cycles are greatly disrupted.

Hyperprolactinaemia can be induced during treatment with antipsychotic or some antidepressant drugs that act to block central dopamine receptors located in the hypothalamus that control PRL release. Excess PRL can lead to gynaecomastia (increased breast development) in males.

CLINICAL MANIFESTATIONS

The typical clinical manifestations of hyperprolactinaemia in women are breast enlargement and galactorrhoea, weight gain, absence of menstruation (amenorrhoea), anovulatory cycles and infertility. Lower oestrogen levels can lead to an increased risk of osteoporosis and atherosclerosis. In men, common manifestations include impotence, loss of libido and galactorrhoea.

In both sexes, the growth of the tumour can lead to increased intracranial pressure and visual defects.

CLINICAL DIAGNOSIS AND MANAGEMENT

Diagnosis

Diagnosis is based on the clinical findings, especially galactorrhoea both in women and men, and sometimes other hormone abnormalities. Blood hormone levels are measured; PRL levels in particular need to be assessed, but the levels of the other pituitary hormones and the thyroid and adrenal hormones are also taken. Investigations should occur to exclude kidney, lung or liver disease. In order to determine the size of the tumour and the extent of damage to any surrounding tissue, MRI and CT scans are performed.

Management

The aims of management are to normalise PRL levels, restore normal gonadal function, reduce or stabilise the size of the pituitary tumour and manage concomitant abnormalities, such as sexual dysfunction and visual defects.

Small glandular tumours, or microadenomas, can usually be monitored by regularly estimating serum PRL levels combined with yearly MRI imaging. Treatment, usually with medicines, is indicated if there are significant effects from the tumour. The PRL level returns to normal quickly, usually within days or weeks of starting treatment, and gonadal function returns to near normal. Menstruation recommences within a few weeks. Therefore, contraceptive advice might be required.

Macroadenomas require treatment. Management usually consists of treatment with dopamine receptor agonists, like cabergoline or bromocriptine. Drug doses start low and are gradually increased. Subsequent dose increases are made on the basis of the clinical response, serum PRL levels and pituitary imaging.

Approximately 20% of those treated with bromocriptine experience side-effects, such as nausea, abdominal pain, postural dizziness, orthostatic hypotension, headache and fatigue. These side-effects usually resolve, but dose reductions may be needed. Cabergoline causes fewer side-effects than bromocriptine, but can cause nausea, headache and postural hypotension.

Like other pituitary tumours, prolactinomas often increase in size during pregnancy up to ten-fold. Preconception risk assessment and close monitoring of the tumour size and function is essential during pregnancy. As they increase, they can cause local pressure symptoms and, of these, 4–7% require surgery with or without radiation. Bromocriptine is usually continued during pregnancy, but there are concerns related to the safety of injected bromocriptine during pregnancy. Information about cabergoline is sparse, but it also appears to be safe during pregnancy.

PRL levels normalise with treatment in 85–90% of people. Medical treatment with or without surgery is very effective; radiation treatment is seldom required. Regular symptom and PRL monitoring, as well as radiological imaging, is needed. The preferred surgical procedure is transsphenoidal pituitary adenectomy.

Antidiuretic hormone

Antidiuretic hormone (ADH) facilitates the reabsorption of water from the distal tubule and collecting ducts of the nephron. It plays a key role in fluid balance through determining urine concentration under normal circumstances and in response to changing environmental conditions. It can also reduce fluid loss through the sweat glands and by stimulating vasoconstriction of peripheral arterioles during haemorrhage (hence its alternative name, *vasopressin*). ADH is synthesised in the hypothalamus and transported to the posterior pituitary for storage until release.

ANTIDIURETIC HORMONE HYPOSECRETION OR POOR TISSUES RESPONSIVENESS

ADH hyposecretion or poor tissue responsiveness involves a partial or complete inability to concentrate the urine, and results in excessive water loss from the body. The condition is also known as **diabetes insipidus (DI)**, meaning the production of weak or dilute urine.

Aetiology and pathophysiology

DI is a disorder associated with poor ADH activity. Without the appropriate activation of the vasopressin (V_2) receptors on nephron cells, fewer water pores (aquaporins) can be established in the distal tubules and collecting duct walls. As a consequence, facilitatory water reabsorption cannot occur, leading to excessive water loss and the production of a large volume of dilute urine. Within a short period the excessive water loss will lead to a state of dehydration and **hypernatraemia**. Hypernatraemic dehydration can lead to brain damage. The alteration in urine formation can dilate the urinary tract.

The most significant presenting symptoms are polyuria with very large volumes of dilute urine and polydipsia. The specific gravity (SG) of the urine is often 1.001–1.005, but the urine does not contain abnormal substances. Fluid intake is excessive, up to 20 L per day, and people have been known to drink from the toilet if they are deprived of fluid. Restricting fluid intake can lead to dehydration, hypernatraemia and severe dehydration. The onset in adults can be abrupt (e.g. following pituitary surgery) or more insidious.

All four types of DI—neurogenic, nephrogenic, polydipsic and gestational—are associated with abnormal water diuresis. *Neurogenic DI*, sometimes known as *central DI*, occurs as a result of pituitary ADH hyposecretion. Common causes are either *acquired* (e.g. brain tumours, head trauma, granulomatous diseases, autoimmune disorders and idiopathic disorders) or *inherited* (e.g. autosomal dominant or mutation in the ADH gene).

Nephrogenic DI occurs because the kidney tissue is unable to respond to the ADH signal. In nephrogenic DI, circulating ADH levels are adequate, but the target cells of the nephron do not respond, due to a loss of V_2-receptors on these cells, a decrease in their sensitivity to the hormone or a combination of both. Nephrogenic DI may occur in chronic renal failure or during treatment with lithium carbonate for bipolar disorder. This is a case of altered tissue responsiveness to the hormone (see the chapter 'Concepts of endocrine dysfunction'). Nephrogenic DI is treated differently from DI associated with pituitary disease; thus, it is important to determine the cause of DI.

Nephrogenic DI often occurs at birth. It may be acquired transiently during hypokalaemic or hypercalcaemic states, in obstructive uropathy or it can be inherited. The inherited forms can be associated with an X-linked recessive mutation in the ADH receptor or, alternatively, an autosomal recessive or dominant mutation in the aquaporin molecule. The inherited forms tend to mostly affect males.

Primary polydipsic DI occurs as a result of suppression of ADH by excessive fluid intake. The most common causes are idiopathic, chronic meningitis, granulomatous diseases, multiple sclerosis or other brain disease that causes diffuse pathology and psychiatric illness. It may be due to a high fluid intake in response to excessive thirst, psychological or emotional disturbances or an inaccurate belief that high fluid intake is beneficial.

Gestational DI occurs during pregnancy, and is due to excessive destruction of ADH by aplacental enzyme.

Clinical manifestations

The clinical manifestations of DI include increased frequency of urination (polyuria), increased thirst, increased drinking of fluid (polydipsia), the production of urine with a low specific gravity, low urine osmolality and high plasma osmolality. The clinical manifestations of the dehydrated state include poor tissue turgor, darkened eye sockets, altered consciousness and seizures. The clinical manifestations of hypernatraemia are summarised in the chapter 'Electrolyte imbalances' (see Clinical Box 31.2).

Clinical diagnosis and management

Diagnosis

Diabetes mellitus also causes polydipsia and polyuria, and must be distinguished from DI because the treatment of the two diseases is very different. A significant difference is that DI is an abnormal state of *water* diuresis, whereas diuresis associated with diabetes mellitus is *osmotic* diuresis. Backed by a careful history review, normal blood glucose levels and the absence of glucose in the urine usually rules out diabetes mellitus.

Twenty-four hour urine collection can be undertaken to screen for DI. A total volume greater than 40 mL/kg body weight per day, osmolality less than 300 mOsm/kg H_2O and an SG less than 1.010 indicate that further testing is required. Young children who are not toilet-trained and who drink more than 100 mL/kg body weight per day may require investigation, especially if they cry frequently and have cool, dry skin, fever and failure to thrive. The serum sodium level is usually above the normal range despite urine osmolality being less than 300 mOsm/kg H_2O.

DDAVP challenge test

A challenge test using the ADH analogue 1-desamino-8-D-arginine vasopressin (DDAVP or desmopressin) is also used. This test will differentiate between the neurogenic and nephrogenic forms. The test involves measuring urine osmolality followed by a subcutaneous injection of DDAVP, where the dose depends on the individual's age and body weight, then measuring urine osmolality after one to two hours or in the next voided sample. Neurogenic DI is confirmed if the urine osmolality rises by greater than or equal to 50%. Increases in urine osmolality of less than 50% may indicate nephrogenic DI. If the serum sodium level is normal and urine osmolality is less than 300 mOsm/kg H_2O, then a water deprivation test is required to make a definitive diagnosis.

Water deprivation test

Water deprivation is undertaken to distinguish between the major forms of DI and whether the person is capable of concentrating urine, which would be evident by an increase in SG. Inability to concentrate urine, continued excretion of large volumes of dilute urine, rising serum osmolality and elevated serum sodium levels, low urine SG and weight loss greater than 5% of initial weight are indicative of DI. The serum osmolality and ADH should be measured on blood collected in heparinised tubes. The test should be performed only if the basal serum potassium level is within the normal range. If it is outside the normal range and urine osmolality is less than 300 mOsm/kg H_2O, a water deprivation test is unnecessary and could lead to adverse events. A DDAVP challenge test may be indicated. Water deprivation is also contraindicated in those with renal failure, uncontrolled diabetes mellitus, hypovolaemia and uncorrected adrenal or thyroid hormone deficiency.

The procedure for conducting a water deprivation test during pregnancy is the same as for other affected people, except blood must be collected in tubes containing an enzyme inhibitor to prevent ADH being degraded by placental vasopressinase, which is present in maternal plasma.

Other diagnostic tests

The DDAVP challenge test has already been described, but sometimes therapeutic doses of DDAVP are administered for one to two days to determine the effect on thirst, fluid intake and output, osmolality, body weight and serum sodium. This test must be undertaken in hospital because of the risk of water intoxication.

Other less common diagnostic tests are used to distinguish between neurogenic and nephrogenic DI, such as a hypertonic saline infusion and MRI of the brain to identify the normal pituitary 'bright spot'. If the spot is clearly visible, the most likely diagnosis is primary polydipsia. If it is small or absent, the person has either neurogenic or nephrogenic DI.

Management

Once the diagnosis is made, the cause needs to be determined and treated. In the case of hereditary DI, other family members may need to be tested and counselled. Treatment aims are to control the fluid imbalance and replace ADH, if indicated, which is usually for the long term. Hypernatraemia is managed by fluid replacement therapy. Patient education about how to administer DDAVP and monitor the response is important. The dose is adjusted according to clinical need.

Synthetic DDAVP limits water loss in the urine to maintain the water–sodium balance and prevent hypernatraemia and its potential consequences—seizures and, in extreme cases, death. Synthetic DDAVP does not have the vascular effects that ADH exhibits. The dose is administered intranasally, but can also be administered in an oral form.

Thiazide diuretics are sometimes used in cases of mild DI, because these medicines potentiate the action of ADH. The thiazides help to increase urine osmolarity and facilitate sodium excretion. Treatment of nephrogenic DI consists of thiazide diuretics, mild sodium depletion and non-steroidal anti-inflammatory drugs (NSAIDs), such as indomethacin, ibuprofen and aspirin. NSAIDs act to reduce water diuresis.

ANTIDIURETIC HORMONE HYPERSECRETION

As expected, an overproduction of ADH results in excessive water reabsorption. It is also known by the rather cumbersome name of the **syndrome of inappropriate ADH secretion (SIADH)**.

Aetiology and pathophysiology

Common causes of SIADH involve ectopic secretion of ADH by a tissue other than the pituitary and during certain drug treatments. Ectopic ADH secretion results in unregulated ADH secretion, and is associated with some cancers, such as those involving the lung (i.e. small-cell carcinomas). A number of common drug therapies can increase the sensitivity of V_2-receptors to endogenous ADH. Examples include the tricyclic antidepressants, the selective serotonin reuptake inhibitor paroxetine, the antipsychotic agent haloperidol, morphine, the anti-seizure drug carbamazepine, and the thiazide diuretics.

The excessive water reabsorption that characterises this condition leads to a slight expansion of blood volume and a dilution of the extracellular fluid compartment. Sodium is the most abundant electrolyte in the extracellular fluid, so this expansion of the extracellular compartment greatly lowers the sodium concentration. A key fact to note here is that ADH does not directly affect the reabsorption of salts like sodium from the nephron, just water. As the extracellular fluid expands, there is no stimulus for aldosterone secretion, which is activated as a part of the renin–angiotensin system when renal blood pressure drops. As aldosterone facilitates sodium and water reabsorption, more sodium will be lost in the urine. The net effect of these changes is that a euvolaemic **hyponatraemia** will develop as a consequence of SIADH.

Clinical manifestations

With the expansion of the extracellular fluid, the hallmark signs of SIADH are hyponatraemia and a decrease in serum osmolality. The urine produced by affected individuals is highly concentrated and will have a high osmolality. The clinical manifestations of hyponatraemia are summarised in the chapter 'Electrolyte imbalances' (see Clinical Box 31.1).

Clinical diagnosis and management

Diagnosis There is no single laboratory test to diagnose SIADH. Differential diagnoses include adrenal insufficiency, hyponatraemia and hypothyroidism. The classic findings needed to make a diagnosis are summarised in Table 17.1.

Thyroid and adrenal function tests are also performed. The results are usually within the normal range. A brain MRI and/or CT scan might be indicated if signs of cerebral oedema are present, but this is rare.

Management The treatment depends on the symptoms and the severity and duration of the hyponatraemia. Generally, transient or drug-induced forms are readily treated. Those who are asymptomatic are usually managed with water restriction. Those with central nervous system symptoms usually require more rapid correction of the hyponatraemia. Treatment of chronic SIADH is not necessary and can have adverse consequences.

Table 17.1 Clinical findings used to diagnose syndrome of inappropriate ADH secretion (SIADH)

Clinical diagnostic feature	Characteristics
Electrolytes	• Hyponatraemia and corresponding serum hypo-osmolality. • Serum bicarbonate and potassium are usually within the normal range. • The anion gap is reduced secondary to equal dilution of the electrolytes, especially sodium and chloride. • The blood urea nitrogen (BUN) is usually low (< 10 mg/dL).
Urine	• Urine is not maximally diluted. • Urine osmolality must be inappropriately elevated, but not necessarily higher than the corresponding serum osmolality. • Low urine output. • Increased glomerular filtration rate (GFR).
Skin	• No evidence of volume depletion: skin turgor is normal and blood pressure is within the normal range.
Uric acid levels	• Hypouricaemia is often present during hyponatraemia as a result of volume expansion and reduced distal tubular reabsorption. However, hypouricaemia occurs in any state where volume expansion occurs and lacks sensitivity and specificity for SIADH.
Plasma ADH levels	• Elevated.
Other features	• No other causes of hyponatraemia present.

Water restriction reverses hyponatraemia, volume expansion and sodium depletion. Restrictions usually consist of less than 75% of maintenance level (1000 mL/m^2/day), which enables the excess fluid to be slowly excreted and urinary sodium to fall. The person needs to be monitored during the initial fluid restrictions, and the amount of restriction needs to be re-evaluated and restrictions increased or reduced if indicated.

Sodium restriction is not usually necessary. If intravenous (IV) fluids are needed, 5% dextrose in 0.45 isotonic sodium chloride or 5% dextrose in Ringer's lactate solution is used. Surgery is indicated for malignant ADH-secreting tumours. Loop diuretics are indicated in some cases. Lithium carbonate, an important drug in the management of bipolar disorder, is sometimes used in children with chronic SIADH. The V_2-receptor antagonist tolvaptan can be used in the management of hypovolaemia. Tolvaptan opposes the effects of ADH on the nephron. The tetracycline antibacterial agent democycline has V_2-receptor antagonist activity and can also be used. Democycline's usefulness is limited by significant nephrotoxic and phototoxic skin reactions. Patient and family/carer education is important. They need to closely monitor fluid balance (input and output), serum electrolyte status and neurological status.

Transient DI is a common consequence of pituitary surgery, other brain surgery or trauma, and must be distinguished from hypothalamic/pituitary causes. This form generally requires no treatment.

Multi-hormone pituitary disruptions

In some cases the disruption is focused on the pituitary itself, but in other cases the damage may be superior to this gland. It may be that the functioning of the hypothalamus has changed or that the connecting stalk, the *infundibulum*, has been cut (see Figure 17.6). Normal endocrine function is greatly dependent on an intact and normally functioning hypothalamic–pituitary axis. Through the secretion of a number of releasing and inhibiting factors, the hypothalamus determines the function of the pituitary. Multi-hormone pituitary disruptions can be associated with either hypoactivity or hyperactivity.

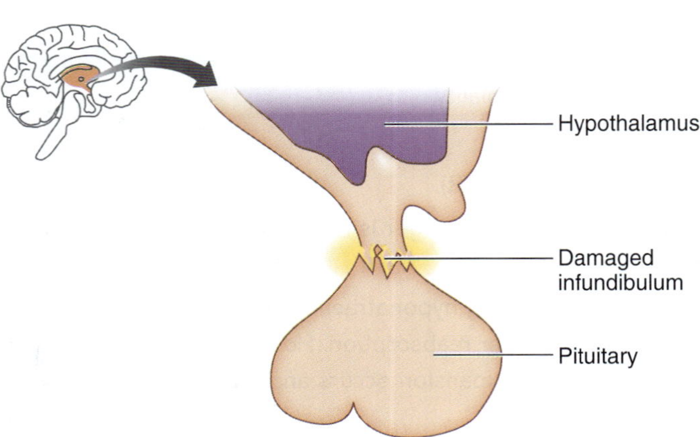

Figure 17.6
A lesion of the infundibulum

HYPOPITUITARISM

Hypopituitarism can lead to either partial or complete failure of pituitary function.

Aetiology and pathophysiology

The most common causes of hypopituitarism involve pituitary infarction, brain infections, head injury and neurosurgical damage. These can occur in adults and in children. The alteration in pituitary activity can result in deficient thyroid and reproductive function, growth and fluid balance, as the secretion of TSH, the gonadotropins, PRL, GH and ADH is affected.

Hypopituitarism can occur as a result of hypothalamic or pituitary gland dysfunction. It can present acutely or as a chronic disease, which is more difficult to diagnose. It may be due to destruction of the anterior pituitary lobe for a number of reasons, including a complication of radiation to the head and neck area, trauma, vascular lesions in the pituitary gland, pituitary tumours (usually benign, but their location and the type of tumour affects hormone production and the presenting symptoms) and lymphocytic hypophysitis (a rare autoimmune disorder that occurs in late pregnancy or within the first postnatal year).

Sheehan's syndrome is a rare condition associated with hypopituitarism. The syndrome consists of pituitary infarction in peripartum women who have severe blood loss, hypovolaemia and hypotension. Simmonds' disease, which is also a rare form of hypopituitarism, is characterised by a loss of body hair, premature ageing and progressive wasting of the body.

Loss of pituitary function means normal stimulation of the thyroid (see the chapter 'Thyroid and parathyroid disorders') and adrenal glands (see the chapter 'Adrenal gland disorders'), as well as the gonads, does not occur. Thus, cortisol, ACTH, TSH and ADH are often low or absent.

The World Health Organization's (WHO) *Classification of tumours affecting the central nervous system* describes 14 pituitary tumour subtypes, and classifies them according to the clinical presentation, serum hormone levels and tumour size, extension and invasiveness, histopathology and the specific features of the tumour cells. Of particular interest in this discussion is that small pituitary adenomas affect about 7% of the population; most of these do not cause symptoms or excess hormone secretion. Approximately 50% of pituitary tumours are inactive, in that they do not secrete hormones, while the other 50% are associated with hormone secretion.

Clinical manifestations

The resultant acute clinical manifestations depend on the specific cause of the problem, and include headache, altered mental state, postural hypotension, hyponatraemia, hypoglycaemia and visual field defects due to local pressure from the tumour on the optic nerve and optic chiasm. Intercurrent illnesses, especially those that cause infection, vomiting, dehydration and trauma, can precipitate acute hypopituitarism in people with undiagnosed pituitary disease or can exacerbate treated hypopituitarism.

Chronic hypopituitarism can be difficult to diagnose. Blood tests for hormone levels usually show low oestrogen and androgen levels without a concomitant increase in LH and FSH, and there is no elevation of TSH. The preceding signs and symptoms may be present, as well as weight loss, atrophy of the other endocrine glands and organs, hair loss, dry, soft skin, low body temperature, obesity, loss of libido, erectile dysfunction, testicular atrophy, amenorrhoea, hypometabolism, cold intolerance and delayed reflexes. The individual, or a close relative or associate, may report descriptions of symptoms suggestive of hypoglycaemia or hypotension.

Chronic growth retardation and delayed puberty can develop in children and is the most striking feature. However, physical growth retardation needs to be distinguished from familial short stature, constitutional delay in growth and maturation (occurring more commonly in boys), Turner's syndrome (the most frequent cause of short stature in girls) or some part of another disease process.

The diversity of these signs and symptoms reflects the significance of the hypothalamus and pituitary gland to life. In fact, if therapy is not commenced quickly in those with hypopituitarism, coma and death occur.

Clinical diagnosis and management

Diagnosis A careful assessment and a physical examination are necessary, including examination of the visual fields, and CT and MRI to determine the presence and size of the pituitary tumour. Blood levels of the pituitary hormones are measured, as are the hormones produced by the target organs—the thyroid and adrenal glands and the gonads. Approximately 8–12% of all brain tumours are due to pituitary tumours, which can be functioning and cause hormone abnormalities and their consequences, or non-functioning, causing local effects, such as visual defects and headache.

Management

Surgery Surgical removal of the tumour (hypophysectomy) is the usual treatment, with the exception of some microadenomas and very large prolactinomas, because these tumours often shrink dramatically in response to treatment with the first-line drugs, dopamine agonists such as cabergoline and bromocriptine. Surgical approaches include transfrontal, subcranial and oronasal–transsphenoidal surgery, the last being the least invasive and preferred approach. Sometimes, octreotide is used preoperatively to shrink large tumours. Conventional or stereotactic radiation therapy may be indicated.

Hormone replacement therapy Generally, hormone replacement therapy is needed after surgical treatment, and is required for the rest of the person's life. Therefore, educating them about how to monitor their medicine doses, the importance of adhering to the treatment and what to do if another illness develops is essential. It is usually necessary to double the dose. Generally, the hormones of the three target glands—glucocorticoids, thyroxine, testosterone and oestrogen/progesterone—are replaced rather than the pituitary hormones. GH replacement therapy in hypopituitarism is controversial in adults, but is often necessary in children (for more information, refer to the section on growth hormone hypoactivity). Gonadotropin therapy is required if a woman wants to become pregnant. However, the person's age, lifestyle, risk factors and bone density need to be considered when replacing gonadal hormones. Table 17.2 shows the medicines commonly used to manage pituitary-deficient states.

Glucocorticoids are usually replaced with cortisone acetate or hydrocortisone, which is usually given in divided doses—two-thirds in the morning and one-third in the afternoon—to reflect the normal diurnal rhythm of cortisol secretion. Sometimes glucocorticoid medicines are alternated (e.g. the intermediate-acting prednisolone and the long-acting dexamethasone as maintenance therapy), but most experts do not recommend this practice, and it is confusing for those taking the medicines, and increases the risk of non-adherence. Dexamethasone is not recommended for children; it has a long half-life and may retard growth. Hormone dose adjustments are made on the basis of the clinical response as well as hormone levels, and depend on the duration of action of the medicines used. It is not usually necessary to replace mineralocorticoid hormones.

Thyroid hormone is replaced using oral thyroxine, gradually increasing the dose over three to six months to achieve normal serum-free thyroxine levels. A lower starting dose is used in older people and those with coronary artery disease, to reduce the risk of acute myocardial infarction or worsening angina. The

Table 17.2 Commonly used pituitary medicines as hormone replacement therapy, the available dose forms and pituitary-related indications for use

Medicine and dose form	Pituitary-related indications for use
ANTERIOR PITUITARY REPLACEMENT	
Tetracosactrin (Synacthen) IM, IV	Diagnose ACTH deficiency
Cortisol (Prednisone, Hydrocortisone), IM, IV	Diagnose ACTH deficiency Replace ACTH
Somatropin (Recombinant hGH), IM, subcutaneous	Treat GH deficiency in children in the long term
POSTERIOR PITUITARY REPLACEMENT	
Desmopressin, intranasal	Treat central DI
Vasopressin, IM, subcutaneous	Treat neurogenic DI
Vasopressin tannate in oil, IM	DI

ACTH = adrenocorticotropic hormone; DI = diabetes insipidus; hGH = human growth hormone; IM = intramuscular; IV = intravenous.

dose is adjusted according to clinical symptoms and serum free thyroxine levels.

A number of important management issues need to be considered during thyroid hormone therapy. Replacing thyroxine without replacing glucocorticoid hormones can precipitate adrenal insufficiency (see the chapter 'Adrenal gland disorders') in those with impaired glucocorticoid reserve. Furthermore, serum TSH is not a reliable indicator of thyroid hormone replacement requirements in people with hypopituitarism. Finally, glucocorticoid and thyroid hormone replacement therapy coupled with under-treated endocrine diseases can predispose the individual to osteoporosis, fractures and pain.

Pituitary deficiency in those treated for hypopituitarism

Acute pituitary deficiency in treated individuals is usually a result of under-treatment with glucocorticoids, non-adherence to the hormone replacement regimen, abnormal fluid loss from vomiting, and the person and/or the health professionals not understanding the need to increase glucocorticoid replacement doses during acute illness, stress, surgery and trauma. Signs of glucocorticoid deficiency can occur rapidly over 8–24 hours. These include vomiting, altered conscious state, abdominal pain, hypotension and circulatory collapse.

Glucocorticoid replacement with the short-acting hydrocortisone intravenously is usually necessary until oral doses are tolerated, and is usually commenced on the basis of symptoms while waiting for the results of serum hormone and other relevant tests. Intravenous fluid replacement with glucose saline to maintain blood glucose levels and prevent hyponatraemia is usually also necessary. Once the person stabilises, the glucocorticoid dose is gradually reduced to maintenance level over two to three days.

HYPERPITUITARISM

Conditions characterised by an increase in the secretion of two or more pituitary hormones are termed *hyperpituitarism.*

Aetiology and pathophysiology

The most common cause of hyperpituitarism is slow-growing benign tumours of the pituitary involving different populations of hormone-secreting cells. The profile of the condition in each individual will depend on which hormones are involved. Sometimes, the tumour may apply pressure to other regions of the anterior pituitary, which results in reductions in the secretion of particular pituitary hormones, leaving the person showing a blend of hypo- and hyperpituitarism. For some people, the presence of the tumour remains asymptomatic.

Depending on the site of the tumour, its position may exert some compression on nearby brain regions and cranial nerves. If present, the pressure can lead to alterations in cranial nerve functions and other neural effects.

Clinical manifestations

Common endocrine clinical manifestations are summarised in Table 17.3 in relation to specific pituitary hormones: PRL, GH and the glucocorticoids are usually affected. The neural clinical manifestations that may develop include visual disturbances, cranial nerve palsies and headaches.

Table 17.3 Common endocrine clinical manifestations of hyperpituitarism

Hormone affected by increased secretion	Common clinical manifestations
Growth hormone	Increased height, bony prominences become more prominent, enlarged hands and feet, mild hyperphosphataemia
Prolactin	In women: breast enlargement and non-gestational lactation, weight gain and absence of menstruation (amenorrhoea) In men: increased breast development (gynaecomastia)
Glucocorticoids (through elevated ACTH)	Increased blood pressure, fluid retention, euphoria, increased susceptibility to infection, 'moon-faced', 'buffalo hump', osteoporosis, muscle atrophy, paper-thin skin, poor wound healing, skin easily bruised

ACTH = adrenocorticotropic hormone.

Clinical diagnosis

The diagnosis depends on determining the underlying cause or causes. A number of diagnostic tests are performed, and imaging studies, including MRI, are also undertaken. The diagnostic tests are outlined below.

PRL levels A single PRL measurement may be sufficient to diagnose a prolactinoma if the value is greater than 200 ng/mL; however, PRL is secreted in a pulsatile fashion, and so a single sample may not detect mildly increased levels. Therefore, morning samples obtained on three separate days are required to diagnose prolactinoma.

Thyrotropin-releasing hormone (TRH) stimulation test

Normally, intravenous TRH causes a fast rise in serum PRL in 15–30 minutes, and peak levels are at least twice the baseline level. Those with PRL-secreting tumours usually show little or no rise in PRL levels in response to TRH.

Adrenocorticotropic-hormone-releasing adenoma *Urinary free cortisol (UFC)* excretion directly measures unbound cortisol (not bound to plasma protein) and is the most reliable and useful test for assessing the cortisol secretion rate. Several 24-hour UFC measurements are usually obtained, and UFC values need to be corrected to take account of the body surface area in children. Daily UFC excretion in excess of 70 μg over 24 consecutive hours suggests hypercortisolism.

Plasma cortisol levels Normally, plasma cortisol levels are highest from 6 am to 8 am, and then the level declines during the day to less than 50–80% of the morning level from 8 pm to midnight. The diurnal variation in plasma cortisol levels typically occurs in Cushing's disease. Blood samples for cortisol should be collected at 30-minute intervals from 6 am to 8 am and from 8 pm to midnight.

Dexamethasone suppression testing Dexamethasone is often used to screen for hypercortisolism. If present, dexamethasone does not suppress the cortisol level. The test involves administering 0.3–0.5 mg/m^2 of dexamethasone at 11 pm to suppress the 8 am plasma cortisol level to less than 5 μg/dL. If the 24-hour UFC excretion is suppressed by more than 50% using high-dose dexamethasone (120 μg/kg/day divided into qid doses) but not by using low-dose dexamethasone (30 μg/kg/d divided qid), it suggests that the person has a primary hypothalamic–pituitary disorder. If the UFC is not suppressed, an adrenal tumour or ectopic ACTH secretion may be the cause.

Plasma ACTH levels If hypercortisolism is present and the plasma ACTH levels are high or high-normal, it suggests that the excess ACTH secretion comes from a pituitary or non-pituitary origin. If the ACTH is suppressed, the primary disorder is most likely in the adrenal glands.

Corticotropin-releasing hormone (CRH) stimulation testing

Ectopic ACTH production and hypercortisolism secondary to an adrenal tumour generally produce a flat response in ACTH and cortisol, but both hormone responses remain intact in Cushing's disease.

Inferior petrosal sinus sampling (IPSS) IPSS is performed to lateralise the tumour to the right or left side of the pituitary gland, and can help minimise pituitary manipulation during surgery. It is helpful because small microadenomas may not be visible on MRI. IPSS should only be performed in centres with experienced radiographers.

Growth-hormone-releasing adenoma Insulin-like growth factor-1 (IGF-1) is a useful screening test for acromegaly. IGF-1 levels closely correlate with the mean 24-hour GH level. If the IGF-1 level is elevated and the person also has the relevant clinical signs, they most likely have GH excess. Note the previous comment that a single GH level is inadequate because GH is secreted in pulses.

An inability to suppress serum GH levels during an OGTT (see the chapter 'Adrenal gland disorders') indicates that the negative feedback by IGF-1 on GH secretion is lost. Glucose induces insulin secretion, which suppresses the release of hepatic IGF-1 binding protein (IGFBP-1), the carrier protein for IGF-1 in the blood. This change increases free IGF-1, which suppresses pituitary secretion of GH. However, if the person has diabetes the findings can be misleading.

INDIGENOUS HEALTH FAST FACTS AND CULTURAL CONSIDERATIONS

FAST FACTS

- ***The mortality of Aboriginal and Torres Strait Islander peoples with brain cancers is 2.7 per 100,000 people compared to 5.1 per 100,000 people for non-Indigenous Australians, but experience a rate of 27% acute brain injury compared to 18% for non-Indigenous people.***
- ***There is a disparity of 40% higher mortality between Māori and European New Zealanders with respect to selected central nervous system (CNS) cancers for the period 2007–16.***

CULTURAL CONSIDERATIONS

- ***The transgenerational trauma experienced by Aboriginal and Torres Strait Islander peoples can have an impact on the development and function of a person's endocrine system. Increased life stressors can contribute to changes in the hypothalamus–pituitary–adrenal (HPA axis), intensifying the release of corticotrophin-releasing factor (CRF), adrenocorticotrophin hormone (ACTH), and the stress hormones noradrenaline and cortisol. Coupled with amplified amygdala activation and reduced cortical blood flow, chronic stress responses and increased survival behaviours are perpetuated. Provision of culturally appropriate, comprehensive support for children, the family unit and the community, with a focus on creating a safe, reassuring environment, may reduce the severity of conditions also influencing the HPA axis.***

Sources: Data from Australian Institute of Health and Welfare (AIHW) & Pointer (2019); Garmston (2016); National Cancer Control Indicators (2022); Te Aho o Te Kahu (2021).

CHILDREN AND ADOLESCENTS

- Synthetic growth hormone is now administered to children with pituitary pathologies resulting in growth hormone deficiency.
- Exogenous growth hormone is associated with several side-effects, including an increased risk of intracranial hypertension and scoliosis. Children having treatment with growth hormone are also monitored for cancers, as the influence on cell growth may also be influencing growth in neoplastic cells.

OLDER ADULTS

- Research into the use of growth hormone to reduce senescence and age-associated changes to body composition is demonstrating benefits such as increased muscle mass and decreased fat mass. However, serious side-effects, such as oedema and impaired glucose regulation, are also common. Other issues include the development of carpel tunnel syndrome and gynaecomastia. Also, the potential for an increased risk of cancer has not yet been eliminated.

KEY CLINICAL ISSUES

- The psychological consequences of endocrine disorders, such as body image, depression and mood changes, need to be considered as well as the physical changes.
- Investigations need to be interpreted according to the age and gender of the individual, and considering any other disease processes present.
- Endocrine tests must be carried out under supervision and in accordance with relevant protocols.

CHAPTER REVIEW

- The *hypothalamic-pituitary axis* is a key part of neuroendocrine control. It influences a broad spectrum of body functions, including daily homeostasis, normal growth and development, metabolism, reproductive function and the body's response to stress.
- *Primary pituitary disruptions* that lead to human illnesses are associated with imbalances in the following hormones: growth hormone (GH), antidiuretic hormone (ADH) and prolactin (PRL). Illnesses may arise in the form of an excess or a deficiency for ADH and GH, whereas only an excess of PRL manifests as a clinical disorder.
- *GH hyposecretion* can be caused by impaired secretion of releasing factors from the hypothalamus, of GH from the pituitary or of insulin-like growth factor-1 from the liver. A clinical condition may also arise from poor target tissue responsiveness to GH. It is characterised by stunted musculoskeletal growth, delayed puberty and, in some cases, hypoglycaemic episodes.
- *GH hypersecretion* can occur in adults (acromegaly) or in children (gigantism or giantism). A common cause is a benign pituitary tumour, which is characterised by excessive linear growth in children. In adults, through its effects on the connective tissues, multisystem changes affecting the bones, heart, thyroid, joints, skin and metabolism can be induced.
- *PRL hypersecretion* is usually caused by a pituitary tumour, but can also be induced by antipsychotic drug therapy. In affected women, it induces breast enlargement, galactorrhoea, weight gain, infertility and amenorrhoea.
- *ADH deficiency* is also known as *diabetes insipidus*. It may be associated with impaired release from the pituitary (neurogenic) or poor tissue responsiveness (nephrogenic). It is characterised by impaired water reabsorption from the kidneys and a deficiency in urine-concentrating ability. Diabetes insipidus leads to polyuria, polydipsia, dehydration and hypernatraemia.
- *ADH hypersecretion* is also known as the *syndrome of inappropriate ADH secretion (SIADH)*. It is usually associated with ectopic ADH secretion. SIADH induces hyponatraemia and decreases serum osmolality.
- *Hypopituitarism* is associated with a deficiency in more than one pituitary hormone. The most common causes of hypopituitarism involve pituitary infarction, brain infections, head injury and neurosurgical damage. Hypopituitarism can occur in adults and in children.
- *Hyperpituitarism* is characterised by an increase in the secretion of two or more pituitary hormones. The most common cause of hyperpituitarism is slow-growing, benign tumours of the pituitary involving different populations of hormone-secreting cells. The tumour's location may exert some compression on nearby brain regions and cranial nerves. This can lead to alterations in cranial nerve functions and other neural effects.

REVIEW QUESTIONS

1. a What is the hypothalamic-pituitary axis?
   b What endocrine structures are directly influenced by the hypothalamic-pituitary axis?
2. Name two consequences of disruption of the hypothalamic-pituitary axis.
3. What are the most common pituitary conditions that involve hormone hyposecretion?
4. What are the most common pituitary conditions that involve hormone hypersecretion?
5. What is the most common pituitary endocrine disorder?
6. Given the following sets of clinical manifestations, indicate the most likely pituitary disorder:
   a delayed linear growth, hypoglycaemic episodes and delayed puberty
   b polyuria, polydipsia and hypernatraemia

c galactorrhoea, weight gain and amenorrhoea in a non-pregnant woman

d coarse facial features, goitre, cardiovascular impairment, large hands and feet

7 What clinical manifestations would you expect in a woman if thyroid-stimulating hormone and gonadotropin secretion were impaired in hypopituitarism?

8 A 7-year-old boy recently suffered a closed head injury after a bike accident. Following hospitalisation he appeared to recover fully. Sometime later he started to experience continuous thirst and drank copious amounts of fluid during the day. He urinated frequently and observed that his urine is 'like water' because it is clear in colour. Urinalysis revealed urine with a low specific gravity and low osmolarity. He also showed a slow heart rate, constipation, cold intolerance and had put on some weight even though his appetite had decreased. What is the most likely pituitary condition affecting this boy?

HEALTH PROFESSIONAL CONNECTIONS

Midwives The hypothalamic–pituitary axis will not only affect a woman during the course of pregnancy, but a disorder in this axis can also cause infertility. Midwives should be aware of the effects of hormonal changes related to disorders of the hypothalamic–pituitary axis on perinatal mood disorders, as well as the metabolic disorders that can affect reproduction.

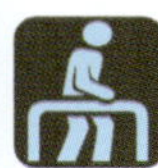

Physiotherapists Following injury, the hypothalamic–pituitary axis will drive the stress response, causing a significant influence on metabolism and wound healing. Rehabilitation programs need to take into account the influence of the endocrine system on healing. Increased cortisol levels can cause reduced bone density, and protein catabolism may increase. Developmental age and gender can influence the degree of metabolic influence on an individual. Even without endocrine pathology, the hypothalamic–pituitary axis can modify an individual's rehabilitation significantly.

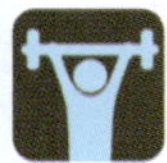

Exercise scientists The hypothalamic–pituitary axis can influence an athlete's performance, not only in disease, but also in health. Exercise scientists should understand the effects of hormonal pulses, as well as other endocrine principles, in order to assist an athlete to improve their performance, or adjust a training regimen in relation to the hormonal influences of their endocrine system. An understanding of the hormonal effects of pregnancy on strength, flexibility and joint laxity are important considerations in relation to exercise prescription. The growth and development of the child athlete in relation to puberty is an important aspect, especially in relation to strength, conditioning and epiphyseal closure.

Nutritionists/Dieticians During injury, the hypothalamic–pituitary axis will be influenced by the sympathetic nervous system, and a stress response will increase metabolic demands and can decrease immune system function. Protein catabolism can occur, and can be exacerbated by low carbohydrate states. Pathology affecting the hypothalamic–pituitary axis can influence fluid and electrolyte balance. During healing, or while a metabolic disorder is affecting an individual's metabolic requirements, caloric, carbohydrate, protein and micronutrient adjustment may be required. Manipulation will differ depending on the disorder, and effective communication within the healthcare team can improve an individual's outcome.

CASE STUDY

Mr Brian Rite is a 56-year-old man (UR number 298471) presenting after a closed head injury four days ago when he fell off a ladder. On admission, his Glasgow coma scale score was 13 and his neurological examination was unremarkable. The CT scan showed a fractured base of the skull. During the next 24 hours he started to develop polydipsia and polyuria. Last night he drank in excess of 2 L of fluid overnight, and was awake, voiding almost every two hours. He is in a negative fluid balance from the previous day. Mr Rite is being investigated for diabetes insipidus. He is currently undergoing a 24-hour urine collection, and has a DDAVP challenge booked for later today. His observations were as follows:

Temperature	Heart rate	Respiration rate	Blood pressure	SpO_2
37.7°C	98	14	114/84	99% (RA*)

*RA = room air.

Mr Rite requires a strict fluid balance chart and is ordered IV sodium chloride 0.9%, 1000 mL q8h. His pathology results were as follows.

HAEMATOLOGY

Patient location:	Ward 3	**UR:**	298471		
Consultant:	Smith	**NAME:**	Rite		
		Given name:	Brian	**Sex:**	M
		DOB:	06/03/XX	**Age:**	56

Time collected	10.12
Date collected	XX/XX
Year	XXXX
Lab #	87665775

FULL BLOOD COUNT		UNITS	REFERENCE RANGE
Haemoglobin	164	g/L	115–160
White cell count	6.1	$\times 10^9/L$	4.0–11.0
Platelets	320	$\times 10^9/L$	140–400
Haematocrit	0.48		0.33–0.47
Red cell count	4.8	$\times 10^{12}/L$	3.80–5.20
Reticulocyte count	0.7	%	0.2–2.0
MCV	92	fL	80–100
Neutrophils	4.3	$\times 10^9/L$	2.00–8.00
Lymphocytes	2.22	$\times 10^9/L$	1.00–4.00
Monocytes	0.37	$\times 10^9/L$	0.10–1.00
Eosinophils	0.28	$\times 10^9/L$	< 0.60
Basophils	0.09	$\times 10^9/L$	< 0.20
ESR	10	mm/h	< 12

BIOCHEMISTRY

Patient location:	Ward 3	**UR:**	298471		
Consultant:	Smith	**NAME:**	Rite		
		Given name:	Brian	**Sex:**	M
		DOB:	06/03/XX	**Age:**	56

Time collected	10:12
Date collected	XX/XX
Year	XXXX
Lab #	4543545

ELECTROLYTES		UNITS	REFERENCE RANGE
Sodium	143	mmol/L	135–145
Potassium	3.5	mmol/L	3.5–5.2
Chloride	108	mmol/L	96–109
Bicarbonate	25	mmol/L	22–26
Glucose (random)	4.9	mmol/L	3.5–8.0
Iron	18	μmol/L	7–29
ADH	0.8	pg/mL	2–8

FLUID BALANCE CHART

	Previous 24-hour intake: 2300 mL			Previous 24-hour output: 2950 mL			
	INTAKE			OUTPUT			
Time	IV1	IV2	Oral	Urine	Vomit/ aspirate	Other sites	Bowels
0100	0.9% NS (600) 100		500 mL H_2O	350			
0200	100						
0300	100		250 mL H_2O	450			
0400	100			350			
0500	100						
0600	100		375 mL Coke	300			
0700	0.9% NS (1000) 100						BO
0800	100		275 mL Tea				
0900	100		275 mL Orange juice	350			
1000	100						
1100	100		375 mL Coke	350			
1200							
Subtotal							

BO = bowels opened; NS = normal saline.

CRITICAL THINKING

1. Consider Mr Rite's clinical picture. Observe his fluid intake and output. What risks should be considered in relation to Mr Rite's fluid consumption and elimination?
2. If Mr Rite was unable to access sufficient fluid replacement, what clinical manifestations may occur? How would this be assessed? What would be observed?
3. What is the mechanism of Mr Rite's diabetes insipidus? Is it central or nephrogenic? Explain.
4. What medication will be ordered? How is it administered? What client education will be required in relation to Mr Rite's management plans?
5. What non-pharmacological interventions should be initiated to manage Mr Rite's diabetes insipidus?

BIBLIOGRAPHY

Australian Institute of Health and Welfare (AIHW) (2022). *Australia's health, 2022*. Australia's health 202: data insights. Australia's Health series No. 18. Cat. No. AUS 240. Canberra: AIHW. https://www.aihw.gov.au/reports/australias-health/australias-health-2022-data-insights/about.

Australian Institute of Health and Welfare (AIHW) & Pointer, S.C. (2016). *Hospitalised injury among Aboriginal and Torres Strait Islander people, 2011–12 to 2015–16.* Injury Research and Statistics series No. 118. Cat. No. INJCAT 198. Canberra: AIHW. https://www.aihw.gov.au/getmedia/89ae4b17-ad35-42da-958f-5c48ee209cf3/aihw-injcat-198.pdf.aspx?inline=true.

Bauldoff, G., Gubrud-Howe, P.M., Carno, M.-A., Levett-Jones, T., Hales, M., Berry, K., … Stanley, D. (2020). *LeMone and Burke's medical–surgical nursing: critical thinking for person-centred care* (4th [Australian] edn). Sydney: Pearson Australia.

Best, O. & Fredericks, B. (2021). *Yatdjuligin: Aboriginal and Torres Strait Islander nursing and midwifery care* (3rd edn). Port Melbourne, VIC: Cambridge University Press.

Bullock, S. & Manias, E. (2022). *Fundamentals of pharmacology* (9th edn). Sydney: Pearson Australia.

Garmston, C. (2016). Transgenerational trauma: development of a neurobiological therapeutic tool. *Neuropsychotherapy* 35:7–13. http://www.mediros.com.au/e-journal.

Khardori, R. (2022). Diabetes insipidus. *Emedicine.* https://emedicine.medscape.com/article/117648-overview.

Marieb, E.N. & Hoehn, K. (2019). *Human anatomy and physiology* (11th edn). San Francisco, CA: Pearson Benjamin Cummings.

National Cancer Control Indicators (2022). 5-year relative survival from diagnosis. https://ncci.canceraustralia.gov.au/outcomes/relative-survival-rate/5-year-relative-survival-diagnosis.

Te Aho o Te Kahu | Cancer Control Agency (2021). *He pūrongo mate pukupuku o Aotearoa 2020 | The state of cancer in New Zealand 2020.* Wellington: Te Aho o Te Kahu | Cancer Control Agency. www.teaho.govt.nz/reports/cancer-state.

Thyroid and parathyroid disorders

18

LEARNING OBJECTIVES

After completing this chapter, you should be able to:

1 Identify the hormones produced by the thyroid and their functions.

2 Identify the hormone produced by the parathyroid gland and its function.

3 Describe the pathophysiological mechanisms and epidemiology involved in each of the thyroid endocrine disorders.

4 Define 'goitre', and outline its relationship with thyroid disorders.

5 Describe the diagnostic procedures used for thyroid disorders.

6 Describe the pathophysiological mechanisms, clinical manifestations and clinical management of various thyroid disorders.

7 Describe the pathophysiological mechanisms and epidemiology involved in each of the parathyroid disorders.

8 Describe the clinical manifestations, diagnosis and clinical management of each of the parathyroid disorders.

WHAT YOU SHOULD KNOW BEFORE YOU START THIS CHAPTER

Can you state where the thyroid and parathyroid glands are located?

Can you describe the functions of the thyroid?

Can you describe the function of the parathyroid glands?

Can you outline the mechanisms involved in calcium homeostasis?

Can you describe the process of thyroid hormone synthesis?

Can you outline the processes involved in cellular metabolism and energy production?

Can you state the key concepts associated with endocrine dysfunction?

KEY TERMS

Calcitonin
Congenital or neonatal hypothyroidism
Goitre
Graves' disease
Hypercalcaemia
Hypercalciuria
Hyperparathyroidism
Hyperphosphataemia
Hyperthyroidism
Hypocalcaemia
Hypoparathyroidism
Hypophosphataemia
Hypothyroidism
Multiple endocrine neoplasia (MEN)
Myxoedema
Parathormone/ parathyroid hormone (PTH)
Parathyroid gland
Thyroid gland
Thyroid-stimulating hormone (TSH)
Thyrotoxicosis
Thyroxine (T_4)
Triiodothyronine (T_3)

Introduction

LEARNING OBJECTIVE 1

Identify the hormones produced by the thyroid and their functions.

The **thyroid gland** plays a key role in endocrine function, and is located in the anterior neck region, immediately inferior to the larynx. Embedded on the posterior surface are three or four nodes of quite different endocrine cells that comprise the **parathyroid glands**. The anatomical relationship between these separate glands is shown in Figure 18.1.

Three hormones are secreted by the thyroid glands—**thyroxine (T_4)**, **triiodothyronine (T_3)** and **calcitonin**. Thyroxine and triiodothyronine set the basal metabolic rate, and are essential for the normal maturation of the brain, musculoskeletal and reproductive systems, and are involved in the maintenance of some body systems in adulthood. The effects are summarised in Table 18.1. It is common practice to refer to T_3 and T_4 as the *thyroid hormones*. Calcitonin is involved in calcium ion balance.

LEARNING OBJECTIVE 2

Identify the hormone produced by the parathyroid gland and its function.

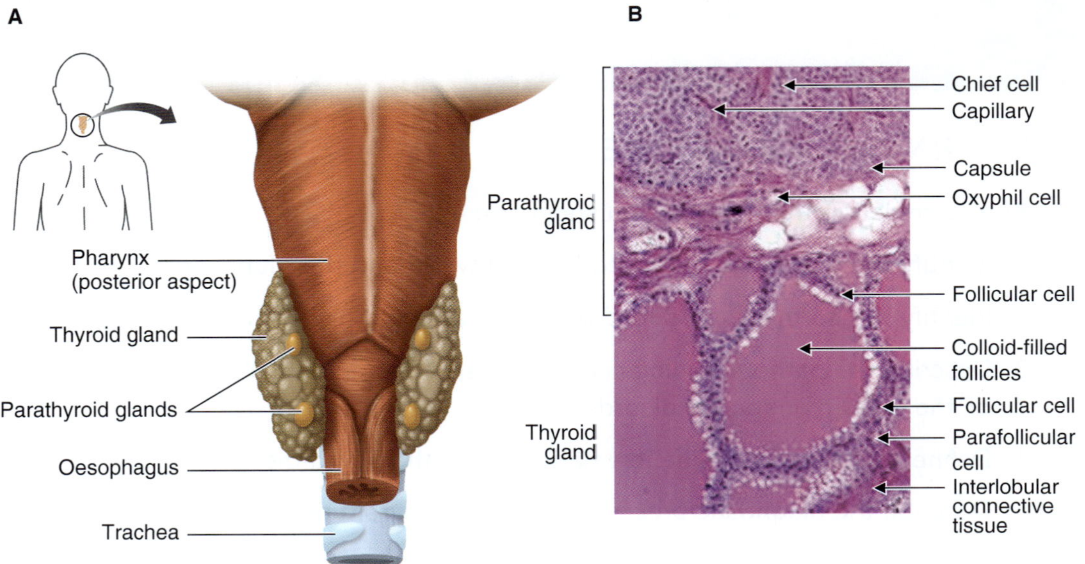

Figure 18.1

Anatomical relationship between the thyroid and the parathyroid glands

(A) Gross anatomy demonstrating the relationship between the thyroid gland and the parathyroid gland.

(B) Microscopic view of thyroid and parathyroid tissue.

Source: (A) Based on Marieb & Hoehn (2019), Figure 16.11, p. 653. (B) Adapted from Michael Ross/Science Source/Getty Images.

Table 18.1 The effects of thyroid hormones on the body

Process or system affected	Normal physiological effects
Basal metabolic rate (BMR)/temperature regulation	Promotes normal oxygen use and BMR; calorigenesis; enhances effects of sympathetic nervous system
Carbohydrate/lipid/protein metabolism	Promotes glucose catabolism; mobilises fats; essential for protein synthesis; enhances liver synthesis of cholesterol
Nervous system	Promotes normal development of the nervous system in the fetus and infant; promotes normal adult nervous system function
Cardiovascular system	Promotes normal functioning of the heart
Muscular system	Promotes normal muscular development and function
Skeletal system	Promotes normal growth and maturation of the skeleton
Gastrointestinal (GI) system	Promotes normal GI motility and tone; increases secretion of digestive juices
Reproductive system	Promotes normal female reproductive ability and lactation
Integumentary system	Promotes normal hydration and secretory activity of the skin

Source: Adapted from Marieb & Hoehn (2019), Table 16.4, p. 650.

The parathyroid gland secretes only one hormone, which is called **parathormone** or **parathyroid hormone (PTH)**. PTH is the major regulator of calcium balance. Calcitonin and parathormone are physiological antagonists: calcitonin lowers blood calcium levels and PTH raises them.

Alterations in the synthesis and release of the hormones from these glands can lead to profound disruptions in metabolism, body system function and calcium balance.

Thyroid disorders

LEARNING OBJECTIVE 3

Describe the pathophysiological mechanisms and epidemiology involved in each of the thyroid endocrine disorders.

AETIOLOGY AND PATHOGENESIS

Imbalances in thyroid function can manifest as either a hyperactive state—**hyperthyroidism**—or a hypoactive state—**hypothyroidism**. Dysfunction of calcitonin secretion can sometimes occur, but rarely manifests as a clinical disorder, because the influence of parathormone is much more significant in calcium ion homeostasis. Hence, the focus of this section is on the thyroid hormones, T_4 and T_3.

EPIDEMIOLOGY

The prevalence of thyroid disease in the Australian and New Zealand populations is not readily known. The rates are expected to be similar to that of the United States. Hypothyroidism is more common than hyperthyroidism, with the former being the second most prevalent endocrine disorder after diabetes mellitus. The prevalence rate is estimated to be at 0.5% clinical cases, and up to 5% for subclinical cases. For hyperthyroidism, the prevalence rate is 0.5% clinical cases and 1% subclinical cases. It is estimated that around 1 million people are living with undiagnosed thyroid disease.

Figure 18.2 explores the common clinical manifestations and management of thyroid disorders.

GOITRE

LEARNING OBJECTIVE 4

Define 'goitre', and outline its relationship with thyroid disorders.

The thyroid gland can enlarge in both hypothyroid and hyperthyroid states. This is known as **goitre**. An enlarged thyroid can be easily identified by palpation and, in some cases, by visual observation.

In hypothyroidism, the levels of **thyroid-stimulating hormone (TSH)** released from the pituitary increase in an attempt to boost thyroid hormone production by the thyroid gland. The gland increases in size in response to the extra signalling. This is a compensatory mechanism. An example of a pronounced goitre is shown in Figure 18.3. However, as the primary problem is that thyroid functioning has failed, the compensation is usually ineffective and leads to gland exhaustion. In hyperthyroidism, gland enlargement is part of the pathophysiology, and results in increased thyroid hormone production.

Goitre can be classified as non-toxic or toxic, and diffuse or nodular. *Non-toxic goitre* is when the gland is enlarged but there are no clinical manifestations. A *toxic goitre* is when clinical manifestations of thyroid dysfunction occur. A *diffuse goitre* is when the whole gland is enlarged, whereas a *nodular goitre* is when one or more parts of the gland are enlarged. These categories can be combined in order to complete the classification of a particular goitre, such as a 'toxic nodular goitre'.

DIAGNOSIS OF THYROID DYSFUNCTION

LEARNING OBJECTIVE 5

Describe the diagnostic procedures used for thyroid disorders.

The diagnostic procedures used in assessing thyroid dysfunction are the same no matter which thyroid imbalance has developed. These procedures are summarised here:

Physical examination Physical examination of the thyroid gland is undertaken to detect any swelling or asymmetry, and to determine the size and shape, consistency and presence of any nodules or tenderness.

Thyroid function tests Tests include laboratory measurements of relevant hormones to determine thyroid function, particularly radioimmunoassay levels of TSH and free thyroxine (FT_4).

TSH assay is the best screening test for thyroid dysfunction. TSH tests have greater than 95% sensitivity and specificity in the assessment of thyroid function. Serum TSH is also used to differentiate between thyroid and pituitary or hypothalamic disorders, as well as to monitor thyroid hormone replacement therapy in those people who are being treated.

FT_4 correlates well with metabolic status. It is elevated in hyperthyroidism and reduced in hypothyroidism.

Serum T_4 and T_3 levels Total T_4 and T_3 levels include protein-bound and free hormone, which are stimulated by TSH. Eighty per cent of T_4 is bound to thyroxine-binding globulin. T_3 is less tightly bound. The percentage of unbound hormone is low for both T_4 (0.03%) and T_3 (0.3%). Usually T_4 and T_3 rise and fall simultaneously, but in hyperthyroidism there tends to be a greater increase in T_3 (normal range: 4.0–8.0 pmol/L). Anything that affects hormone binding can influence the serum levels; for example, serious systemic disease, low serum proteins or protein loss in kidney disease, medicines such as oral contraceptives, corticosteroids, the antiseizure agent phenytoin, salicylates and androgen therapy.

Thyroid antibodies Antithyroid antibodies are present in 10–20% of the general population. Antithyroid antibodies, especially antimicrosomal antibodies, suggest that autoimmune thyroid disease—either hypothyroidism or hyperthyroidism—is present. The types of antithyroid antibodies of clinical significance are anti-thyroperoxidase (anti-TpOAb), anti-thyroglobulin (anti-TgAb) antibodies and anti-TSH antibodies. These

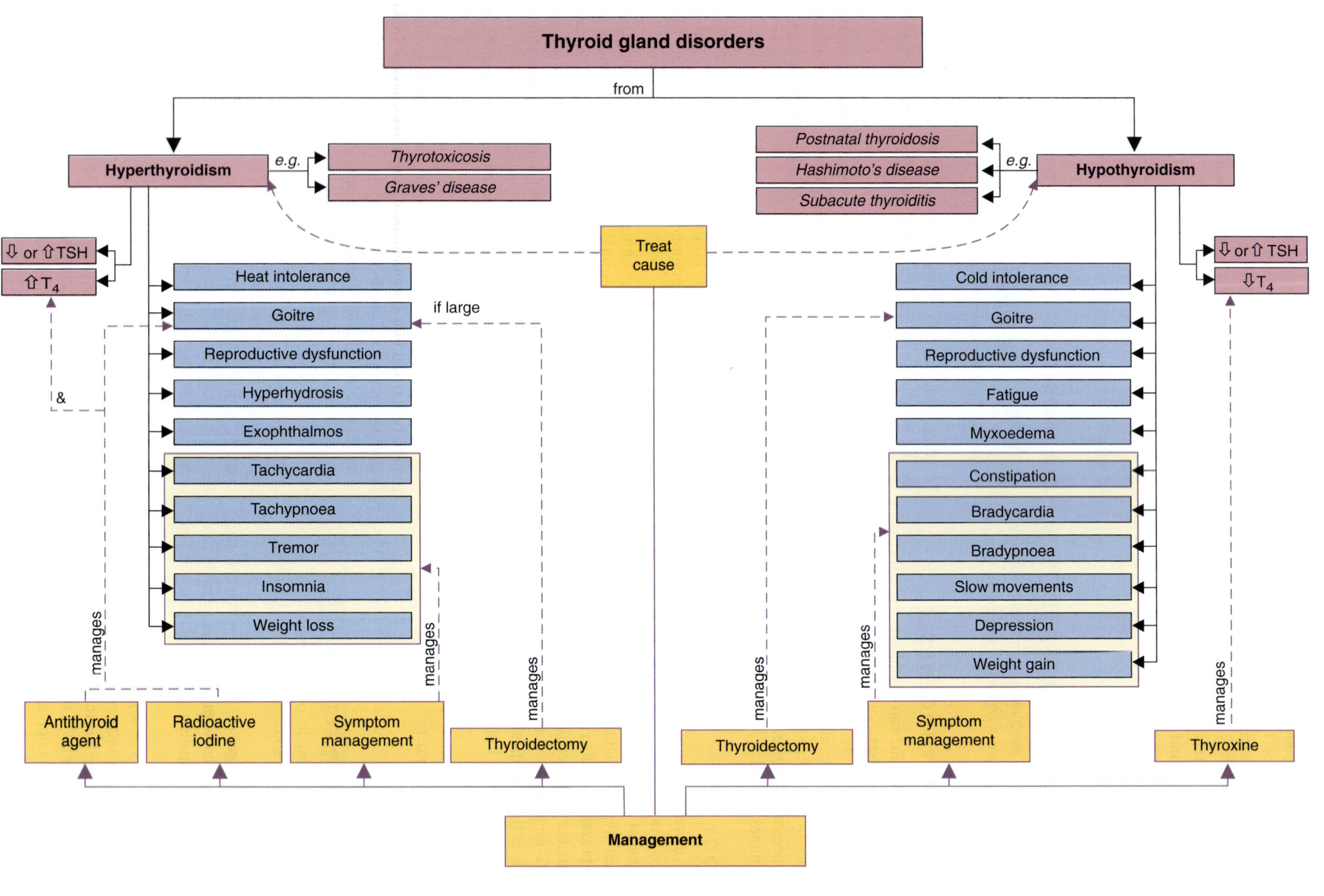

Figure 18.2

Clinical snapshot: Thyroid gland disorders

↓ = decreased; ↑ = increased; T_4 = thyroxine; TSH = thyroid-stimulating hormone.

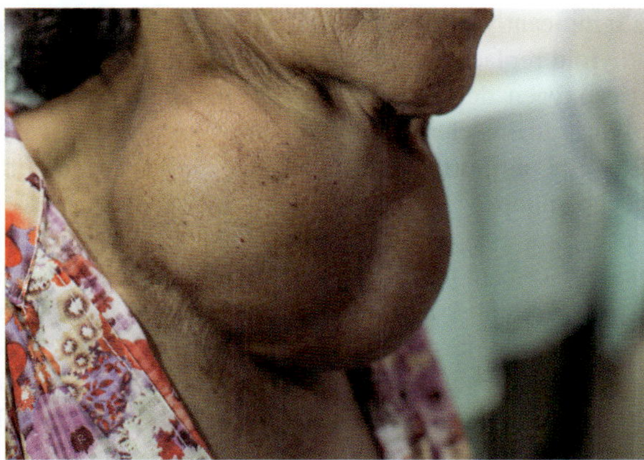

Figure 18.3

Close-up lateral view of a woman with significant thyroid gland enlargement.

Source: Karan Bunjean/Shutterstock.

antibodies can be detected using immunoassay testing, and tests are positive in 90% of cases of autoimmune thyroid disease, such as Hashimoto's thyroiditis (100% positive) and Graves' disease (80% positive), as well as in other organ-specific autoimmune diseases, such as rheumatoid arthritis. If thyroid autoantibodies are present, the person should be assessed and regularly monitored for other autoimmune diseases, such as type 1 diabetes.

Radioactive iodine uptake Radioactive iodine (I^{123}) uptake is measured to detect hypo- or hyperthyroidism, and to determine the dose needed to treat hyperthyroidism once the diagnosis is made. Normal uptake varies among geographical regions, and is affected by iodine intake or exogenous thyroid medications. Uptake is as high as 90% in hyperthyroidism, and is low in hypothyroid states.

Fine-needle biopsy Fine-needle biopsy is indicated if thyroid malignancy is suspected, and may be undertaken as an initial screening test if a thyroid mass is detected.

Thyroid scans A range of radioactive isotopes are used to determine the shape, location and size of the thyroid gland, and are particularly helpful for assessing large thyroid masses that extend into the sub-sternal area.

Ultrasounds, computed tomography (CT) scans and magnetic resonance imaging (MRI) are also used, usually in addition to one or more of the tests described.

LEARNING OBJECTIVE 6

Describe the pathophysiological mechanisms, clinical manifestations and clinical management of various thyroid disorders.

HYPOTHYROIDISM

Hypothyroidism can develop prior to or shortly after birth (**congenital or neonatal hypothyroidism**) or in a previously euthyroid adult or child (*acquired hypothyroidism*). In the past, congenital or neonatal hypothyroidism was known as *cretinism*, a term no longer preferred. When the acquired form of hypothyroidism is particularly severe or persistent, it is usually called **myxoedema**. When myxoedema develops acutely and severely, such that the affected person deteriorates quickly, it is termed *myxoedema coma* and can be life-threatening.

There are a number of causes of *primary hypothyroidism*. The thyroid gland may not develop normally in utero, or it can be damaged by some pathological process, such as chronic inflammation or an autoimmune process, as in Hashimoto's thyroiditis. Those with Hashimoto's thyroiditis have a higher risk of developing other autoimmune conditions such as coeliac disease or vitamin B_{12} deficiency. Thyroid hormone production is determined by the availability of iodine in the diet, so a dietary deficiency in iodine can result in hypothyroidism. *Dietary iodine deficiency* is common in the developing world. Interestingly, recent studies have suggested that Australian and New Zealand diets may be low in iodine. A return to iodine supplementation, such as iodised table salt or by fortifying bread with iodised salt, has been advocated as a way of addressing this problem. People who require thyroidectomy due to cancer or hyperthyroidism can also become hypothyroid. In primary hypothyroidism, TSH levels rise initially, with a decline in T_4/T_3 levels developing later and more slowly.

Hypothyroidism can also develop as a consequence of inadequate communication along the hypothalamic–pituitary–thyroid axis. Inadequate release of TSH is regarded as *secondary hypothyroidism*, while inadequate secretion of thyrotropin-releasing factor from the hypothalamus is a form of *tertiary hypothyroidism*. It can be hard to discriminate between the secondary and tertiary forms clinically.

Factors that can contribute to poor thyroid function include trauma, stress, infection, radiation exposure, medications, toxins and autoimmune conditions such as coeliac disease.

Mild hypothyroidism may also develop in the absence of frank pathology as a part of the normal ageing process. This occurs as a result of a decreasing efficiency in thyroid function.

Subclinical hypothyroidism is characterised by dysfunction of thyroid function without clinical manifestations. This disorder requires clinical management as it is associated with an increased risk of coronary heart disease, heart failure, cognitive impairment, depression and fractures. Around 8% of Australian women and 3% of Australian men have this condition.

Congenital/neonatal hypothyroidism

The thyroid dysfunction characterising these forms of hypothyroidism develops in utero or shortly after birth during the neonatal period. It is usually the thyroid gland itself that is affected. The most common cause is thyroid dysgenesis, but it can be due to ectopic causes such as maternal TSH autoantibodies crossing into the fetal circulation or a maternal iodine deficiency. Technetium scans may be indicated to determine the cause. The condition will have profound effects on early brain and musculoskeletal development, leading to retarded growth. Thyroid function in utero may not be affected if circulating maternal thyroid hormones are available to the developing child, but may manifest in the neonatal period.

Low-birth-weight preterm infants can also develop a transient hypothyroxaemia and need to be monitored closely.

Congenital/neonatal hypothyroidism occurs in around 1 in 2,000 births. The rate appears to be rising, though, which may be due to more screening in the perinatal period and increasing survival of preterm neonates who are at risk of the disorder. The condition can be treated with thyroid hormone supplements soon after the child is born, usually within the first two weeks after birth.

Myxoedema

Myxoedema gets its name from the accumulation of mucopolysaccharides within the interstitial fluid (i.e. mucoid oedema). With a lowered metabolic rate, the breakdown of these compounds decreases. As these substances accumulate, a thicker, gel-like fluid develops in the tissues in contrast to the watery quality of typical oedematous states.

Clinical manifestations

The key physiological alteration associated with hypothyroidism is a decreased metabolic rate. All of the clinical manifestations are derived from this alteration, especially in regard to the functioning of the brain, heart and gastrointestinal tract. The range of clinical manifestations includes bradycardia, constipation, loss of appetite, lethargy, slowed mental function, hyporeflexia, fatigue, muscle weakness, cold intolerance and weight gain.

The mucoid oedema leads to a thickening of the skin and tongue. An affected person's facial features will alter as their nose and lips thicken, and the skin around their eyes becomes puffy. Goitre may be present. The skin becomes dry and coarse, and their hair may be brittle and thin out, leaving bald patches. In women, menstrual dysfunction involving heavy periods may occur. Infertility is also associated with hypothyroidism.

In children, normal growth is impaired, leading to delays in skeletal development and the onset of puberty. Without intervention, permanent mental retardation will develop in infants with the congenital and neonatal forms.

Clinical management

Management depends on the underlying cause. Pituitary and hypothalamic disease is discussed in the chapter 'Hypothalamic–pituitary disorders'. Primary hypothyroidism usually responds to thyroid hormone replacement, commonly with synthetic levothyroxine (L-thyroxine). The aim of treatment is to restore normal thyroid functioning; therefore, the dose is based on serum TSH levels. In some cases, combination therapy of levothyroxine and triiodothyronine has been used, particularly where there is persistence of psychological manifestations using thyroxine monotherapy despite normal TSH levels.

Existing disease processes, such as cardiovascular disease, also need to be managed carefully with appropriate medications, as well as diet and exercise. Rapid or excessive thyroid hormone replacement can precipitate cardiac ischaemia, and over the long term treatment can have adverse effects on cardiac function and bone, leading to osteoporosis. Medicines that affect absorption of oral thyroxine may need to be ceased or alternative dose forms used. Significantly, angina and cardiac dysrhythmias often occur after thyroid replacement therapy improves the metabolic rate, because oxygen demand increases in the cardiac muscle but underlying atherosclerosis compromises oxygen delivery. In addition, thyroid hormone enhances the cardiovascular effects of catecholamines.

Since most people with hypothyroidism are older adults, thyroid replacement is often started at a low dose and gradually increased to minimise the cardiovascular effects. Those younger than 60 years with no underlying cardiovascular disease are usually commenced on daily oral thyroxine, gradually increasing the dose over three to six months to reach a TSH level of 0.5–2 mU/L. It should be noted that the normal range of TSH levels varies across the population and is influenced by age, pregnancy and ethnicity. Treatment needs to be titrated according to the clinical response. If the person is older than 60 years and has underlying cardiac disease, the commencing dose is lower. Treatment is usually required for life. Evaluation of mental status is also warranted once therapy improves cognitive functioning. Persistent elevation of TSH levels is most commonly due to non-adherence to treatment, drug interactions, or thyroid hormone malabsorption associated with gastrointestinal disease as the pituitary gland is attempting to signal the thyroid gland to increase T_4 secretion.

Myxoedema coma is a serious emergency, and fluid replacement, monitoring electrolyte balance and conserving body temperature are essential, in addition to thyroid hormone replacement. Initial management usually consists of thyroxine administration.

Thyroxine doses progressively increase by 20–40% during pregnancy, because the placenta metabolises T_4. Normal thyroid hormone levels (0.4–4.0 mU/L) are important for fetal brain development in the first trimester. Thus, TSH should be measured early in the pregnancy and then in each trimester to determine replacement doses. Doses are usually reduced again postnatally.

In congenital or neonatal hypothyroidism, oral thyroxine replacement doses are usually higher than those used in adults on a weight basis, and are titrated according to the response and free T_4 and TSH levels every three months. Physical and mental development must be monitored. Timely normalisation of thyroid function leads to the best cognitive outcomes for these children.

Medicine clearance rates in hypothyroidism

As a result of the decreased metabolic rate in hypothyroid states, medicine clearance rates are often reduced. Medicines such as oral anticoagulants, sedatives, hypnotics, analgesics, anaesthetics and digoxin may need to be reduced to avoid overdose.

HYPERTHYROIDISM

The most common cause of hyperthyroidism has an autoimmune basis, and is known as **Graves' disease**. Autoantibodies are formed that can stimulate TSH receptors on the thyroid gland, leading to hyperactivity of the follicular cells (see Figure 18.4). The incidence of Graves' disease is higher in women and can follow a familial inheritance pattern. Interestingly, the onset of the clinical condition in women tends to be associated with

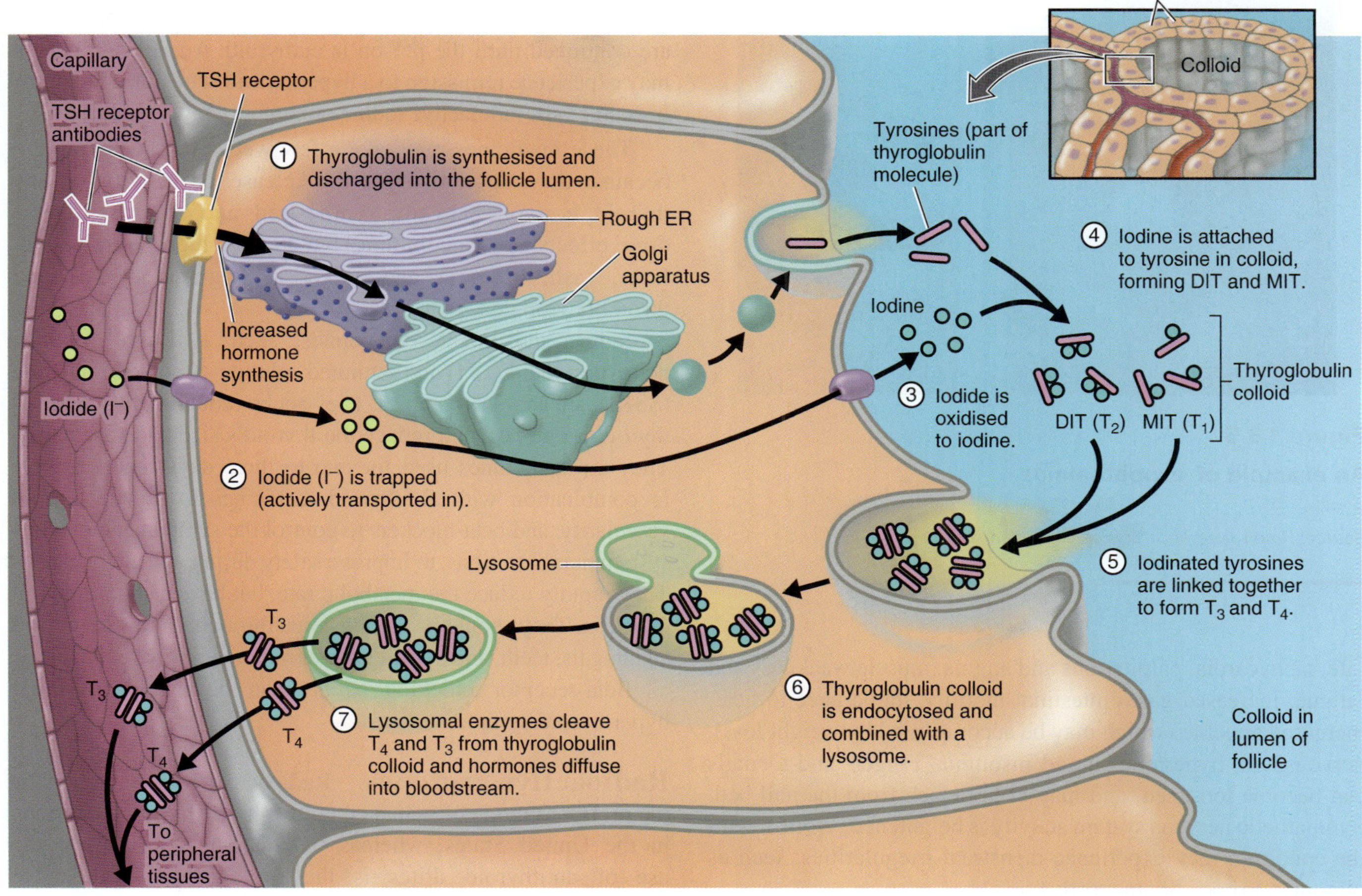

Figure 18.4

The action of autoantibodies on thyroid follicles

DIT (T_2) = di-iodinated tyrosine; ER = endoplasmic reticulum; MIT (T_1) = mono-iodinated tyrosine; T_3 = triiodothyronine; T_4 = thyroxine; TSH = thyroid-stimulating hormone.

Source: Adapted from Marieb & Hoehn (2019), Figure 16.9, p. 651.

major life changes—menopause, pregnancy or menarche. For men, it usually develops in maturity.

Graves' disease has been linked to bacterial infections caused by *Yersinia enterocolitica*, which is thought to be due to TSH receptor mimicry, as well as to vitamin D deficiency.

Thyrotoxicosis is synonymous with hyperthyroidism, and these terms are often used interchangeably to reflect an increase in the synthesis and secretion of thyroid hormones. In primary hyperthyroidism, TSH levels decline in response to the elevation in T_4/T_3 levels. Other causes of hyperthyroidism include tumour development, usually a pituitary tumour that increases TSH secretion. In some cases, a thyroid tumour itself can overproduce thyroid hormones. Some medications—such as the antidysrhythmic agent amiodarone—contain iodine, and prolonged therapy with these drugs can lead to excessive iodine availability, facilitating increased thyroid hormone production. This can also occur when food that is fortified with iodine is ingested in significant amounts.

The thyroid is capable of storing large amounts of preformed thyroid hormone, a supply that can last a number of months. Chronic inflammatory conditions affecting the thyroid (i.e. thyroiditis) can trigger a significant release of these stores in the early stages of the condition and induce a hyperthyroid state. When the stores are exhausted and the glandular tissue is damaged by the inflammatory process, the affected person usually becomes hypothyroid.

A life-threatening form of thyrotoxicosis, called a *thyroid storm*, can develop quickly, and is usually precipitated by stresses such as intercurrent illnesses, pregnancy, surgery and reducing or stopping antithyroid medications. People presenting with thyroid storm are acutely ill. Thyroid storm is relatively uncommon today, because of accurate methods of diagnosis, treating and monitoring of thyroid status.

Clinical manifestations

The clinical manifestations of hyperthyroidism, or thyrotoxicosis, are characterised by a significantly increased metabolic

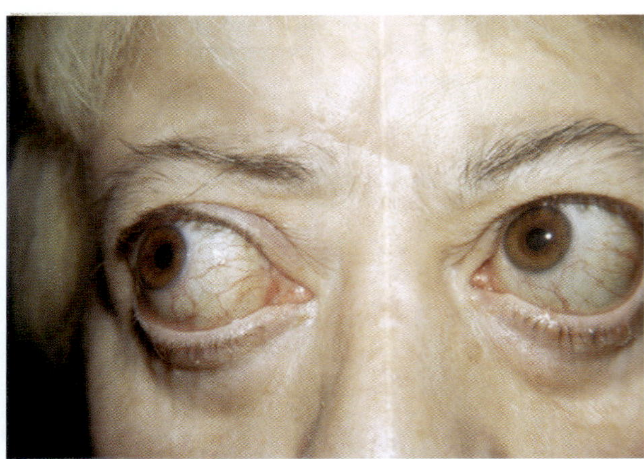

Figure 18.5

An example of exophthalmos

Source: Ralph Jr/Science Source/Getty Images.

rate: tachycardia, palpitations and angina, muscle weakness and fatigue, increased gastrointestinal motility, intolerance to heat, increased appetite (which may be accompanied by weight loss), nervousness, hyperreflexia and insomnia. Finger- and toenails can become loosened, and may even detach from the nail bed. Sympathetic nervous system activity is heightened. Women with the condition may experience menstrual irregularities, such as oligomenorrhoea or amenorrhoea.

Another clinical manifestation that characterises Graves' disease is exophthalmos. In *exophthalmos*, the eyeballs bulge forward because there is a localised autoantibody-induced inflammation and increased development of connective tissue in the socket behind the eyes. With bulging eyeballs, the eyelids close more slowly, leading to the manifestation of lid lag, accompanied by staring and lid tremor. The eye is more exposed to the air and, as a consequence, there is tearing-up and a burning sensation associated with less lubrication. Exophthalmos is shown in Figure 18.5.

The clinical manifestations of thyroid storm include hyperpyrexia (high fever), tachycardia (greater than 130 beats per minute [bpm]), hyperthyroid symptoms as above, and evidence that one or more major body systems are compromised. For example, cardiovascular compromise is indicated by oedema, chest pain, dyspnoea and palpitations, neurological symptoms such as delirium, extreme lethargy, psychosis or coma.

Clinical management

The aim of thyroid treatment is to control the symptoms and normalise the thyroid hormone level. The underlying cause also needs to be investigated and managed. Three main management options are available—antithyroid medicines, radioactive isotopes and surgery—and they are often used in combination.

Antithyroid medicines These medicines affect hormone synthesis or release by blocking iodine utilisation during thyroid hormone synthesis. They also block conversion of T_4 to T_3 outside the thyroid gland. Commonly used medicines are the thionamides, propylthiouracil (PTU) and carbimazole, which are continued until the person is euthyroid. An affected person may experience remission to a hyperthyroid state during therapy. In such cases, radioactive iodine or surgery may be indicated.

These medicines may take a few weeks to have an effect, because they do not affect the release or activity of any thyroid hormone already synthesised and stored. Adverse drug effects are uncommon, but can include sensitisation, fever, rash, urticaria and sometimes agranulocytosis and thrombocytopenia.

Iodine and iodine compounds, such as Lugol's iodine, potassium iodide (KI) and saturated solution of potassium iodide (SSKI), are adjunct therapies. They act by reducing the release of thyroid hormones, and reduce the thyroid's size and vascularity. They are sometimes used for two to three days preoperatively in combination with antithyroid medicines to reduce thyroid vascularity, and beta-blockers to control the sympathetic nervous system manifestations, to improve safety during and after surgery. They rapidly reduce the metabolic rate, but have a short duration of action. They should be administered through a straw to prevent staining the teeth, and in fruit juice or milk to improve palatability.

Beta-receptor blocking agents can be useful in initial hyperthyroid symptom control.

Radioactive isotopes Radioactive iodine therapy is the preferred mode of management for hyperthyroid conditions in the United States, whereas in Australia and Europe the use of antithyroid drugs is the first choice. Radioactive isotopes of iodine, I^{123} or I^{131}, are used to treat toxic thyroid adenomas, multinodular goitre and relapsed Graves' disease. This treatment is the most common choice for older people with hyperthyroidism. Treatment with radioactive isotopes is contraindicated during pregnancy and breastfeeding, because the radioactive iodine crosses the placenta and is secreted in breast milk, and so can affect the baby's thyroid gland. It is also not suitable for young children or in the presence of Graves' ophthalmopathy, which can worsen after the administration of radioactive iodine, especially in smokers.

Irradiating the thyroid gland with radioactive iodine destroys the thyroid tissue. Most of the dose of the radioactive isotope concentrates in the thyroid gland; thus, thyroid cells are destroyed over a period of time but other body cells are preserved. A single oral dose based on the estimated weight of the thyroid gland is used. Most people (approximately 80%) are cured with a single dose. Sometimes a second dose is required, and, on rare occasions, a third dose.

The person must be closely monitored for signs of thyroid storm, and until symptoms subside and the person becomes euthyroid. Hypothyroidism is the major side-effect of thyroid irradiation, which can occur in 90% of people up to 10 years after irradiation, in which case thyroid hormone replacement is then needed (see hypothyroidism).

Surgery Surgery is not the treatment of choice, but is still indicated during pregnancy, for women who are allergic (or develop serious adverse drug effects) to antithyroid medicines, in those with very large goitres that affect local structures and cause obstructive symptoms, in severe exophthalmos, and in remission to the hyperthyroid state during thionamide therapy. Usually, surgery is delayed until thyroid function is normalised with antithyroid medicines.

The main consequence of any of these three management methods is hypothyroidism or recurrent hyperthyroidism. The occurrence rate of recurrent hyperthyroidism depends on the initial severity of the disease and the dose used. People who receive lower doses of radioactive iodine are more likely to require subsequent treatment than those receiving high doses, but the latter are more at risk of hypothyroidism. Relapse following subtotal thyroidectomy occurs in about 19% of people, and about 25% of people develop hypothyroidism 18 months after surgery.

Thyrotoxicosis in pregnancy Thyrotoxicosis occurs in approximately 0.2% of pregnancies, and 90% of cases are due to Graves' disease. Other causes include *hyperemesis gravidarum* (morning sickness of pregnancy). The clinical manifestations are similar to those of hyperthyroidism already described. Serum T_3 usually remains within the normal range, and TSH falls in the first trimester. Pregnancy may aggravate symptoms in women with existing thyrotoxicosis. Both PTU and carbimazole can be used, with dose adjustments according to hormone changes during each trimester and postnatally. Radioactive iodine therapy is contraindicated in pregnancy. Thyroidectomy is considered if medication therapy fails.

Thyrotoxicosis in children Thyrotoxicosis is rare in children, especially before the age of 5 years. Clinical manifestations include behavioural changes such as hyperactivity, declining performance at school, and the signs and symptoms already described. The child may be above the height percentile for their age. The cause is nearly always autoimmune, and treatment is with carbimazole rather than PTU, which can be hepatotoxic.

Management of thyroid storm The aims of management are to reverse the thyrotoxicosis and manage the symptoms. The approaches used consist of temperature reduction, oxygen therapy, monitoring arterial blood gases and pharmacological therapy.

The temperature can be reduced by placing the person in a cool environment, cool sponging and/or using medicines such as paracetamol. Salicylate non-steroidal anti-inflammatory drugs (NSAIDs) are contraindicated because they displace thyroid hormone from plasma proteins and worsen the hypermetabolism. Intravenous dextrose is administered to supplement endogenous glycogen stores, which are depleted in hypermetabolic states.

A number of drugs are administered to control the condition. Hydrocortisone is given to manage shock and adrenal insufficiency, which often occurs concomitantly. PTU is administered six-hourly via nasogastric tube to block conversion of T_4 to T_3 and to reduce thyroid hormone synthesis. Iodine can be used to reduce T_4 release from the thyroid gland. Other medicines may be administered to manage major system symptoms, such as atrial fibrillation and agitation. Agitation can lead to high fever, because it inhibits central thermoregulation.

Once the major crisis resolves, ongoing management is determined, as discussed in the preceding section.

Parathyroid disorders

LEARNING OBJECTIVE 7

Describe the pathophysiological mechanisms and epidemiology involved in each of the parathyroid disorders.

Parathyroid hormone (PTH), or *parathormone*, is the key regulator of body calcium levels. Its secretion facilitates increased blood levels of calcium ions. It does this through three major actions: *enhancement of bone resorption; inhibition of calcium ion excretion via the kidneys*; and *increasing calcium absorption from the gastrointestinal tract*. In humans, endocrine disorders can be associated with either deficient or excessive parathormone secretion.

LEARNING OBJECTIVE 8

Describe the clinical manifestations, diagnosis and clinical management of each of the parathyroid disorders.

HYPOPARATHYROIDISM

Hypoparathyroidism is characterised by low blood calcium levels—**hypocalcaemia**. The pathophysiological consequences of this electrolyte imbalance are covered in detail in the chapter 'Electrolyte imbalances'. Importantly, the alteration in calcium availability leads to changes in nerve and muscle excitability so that the nerves become more easily excited and the force of muscle contraction is lessened.

Hypoparathyroidism can be a *permanent condition*, with a prevalence rate of 0.9–1.6%, or more commonly as a *transient condition*, which has a prevalence rate of 6.9–46%. Magnesium has an important role in the activation of the parathyroid receptors and the secretion of PTH. Transient hypoparathyroidism can develop in hypomagnesaemia associated with renal disease, alcoholism or malnutrition. It can also occur in hypermagnesaemia. A common permanent cause of hypoparathyroidism is neck surgery or in thyroidectomy, which may be undertaken for thyroid cancer or hyperthyroidism. In Australia, recent data indicates that thyroid cancer is the ninth most commonly diagnosed cancer.

As a result of this surgery, the blood supply to the glands can be disrupted, or there may be surgically related damage or fibrosis that affects the parathyroid glands. Hypoparathyroidism is associated with congenitally malformed parathyroid glands (such as in DiGeorge syndrome) or when the glands are subjected to autoimmune-initiated damage. Hypoparathyroidism can also arise as a result of peripheral resistance to PTH due to a change in PTH receptor sensitivity. Figure 18.6 explores the common clinical manifestations and management of parathyroid disorders.

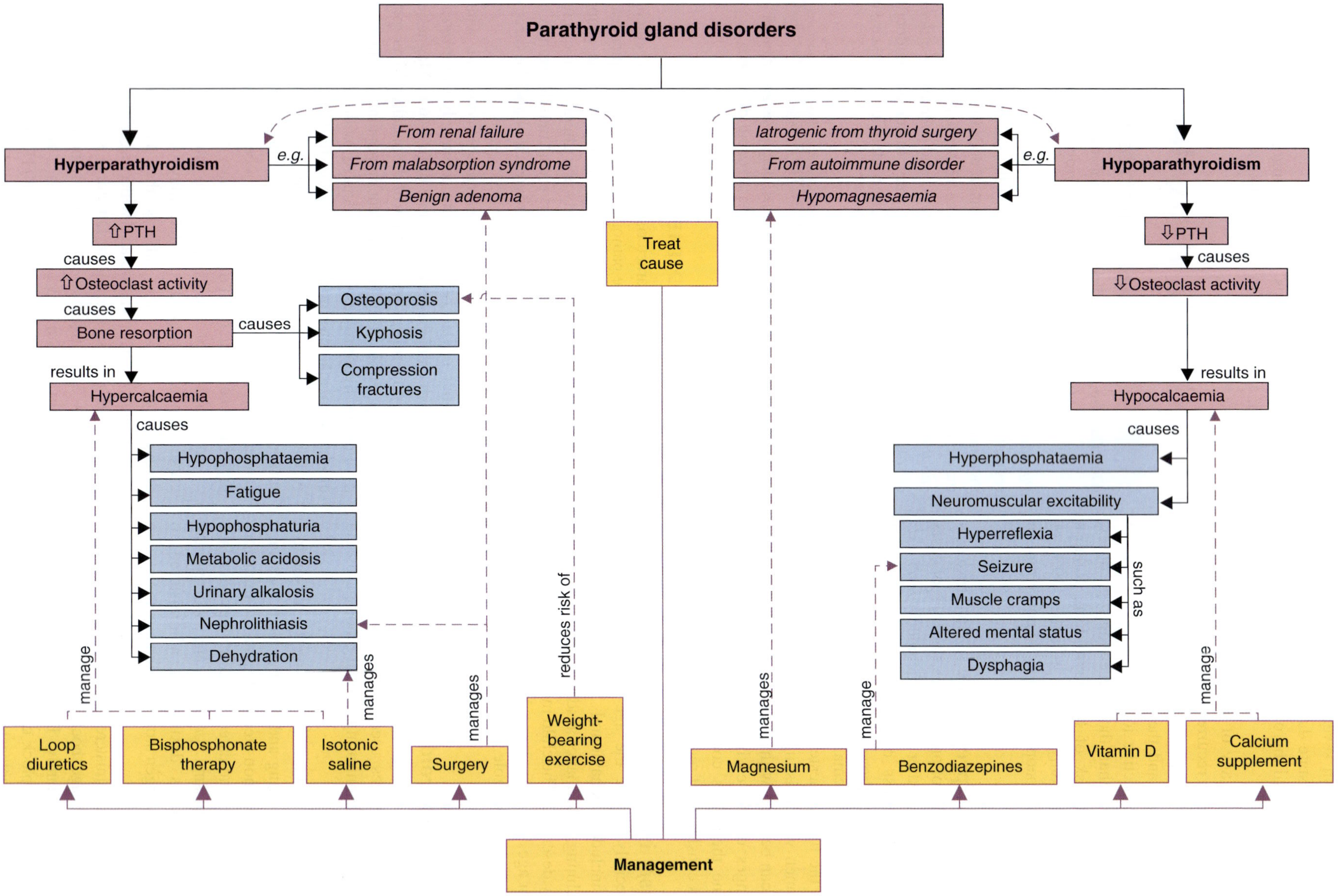

Figure 18.6

Clinical snapshot: Parathyroid gland disorders

↓ = decreased; ↑ = increased; PTH = parathyroid hormone.

Clinical manifestations

The clinical manifestations of hypoparathyroidism are linked to a decrease in calcium availability, and include muscle twitches and spasms, paraesthesias, fatigue, changes in emotional and mood state, and cardiac dysrhythmias. Mild **hyperphosphataemia** can occur (see the chapter 'Electrolyte imbalances' for more detail). In severe hypocalcaemia, laryngeal spasms, tetany and seizures may occur.

Clinical diagnosis and management

Diagnosis Laboratory tests include serum calcium, which is usually less than 1.2–1.5 mmol/L, and phosphate, which is usually elevated. X-rays and bone densitometry show increased bone density and calcification in particular body regions. Vitamin D and serum magnesium levels should also be measured to rule out other causes.

Tetany occurs when the serum calcium is low, and can be detected on a positive Chvostek's sign (where tapping over the facial nerve in front of the parotid gland anterior to the ear causes the mouth, nose and eye to twitch/spasm). Likewise, Trousseau's sign is also usually positive—occluding the blood flow in the arm by inflating a blood pressure cuff for three minutes induces carpopedal spasm (see the chapter 'Electrolyte imbalances' for more details).

Management The aim of therapy is to raise the serum calcium to the normal level and eliminate the signs and symptoms. The treatment regimen is determined after serum calcium levels are available. If hypocalcaemia and tetany occur after thyroid surgery, intravenous (IV) calcium gluconate is used. Sedatives may be required to manage neuromuscular irritability and seizures, if they occur.

Parenterally administered synthetic PTH may be indicated to manage acute hypoparathyroidism and tetany. However, allergic reactions are common to injected PTH, and so the person must be closely monitored to quickly detect allergic reactions. Serum calcium levels also need to be closely monitored. Intubation and bronchodilator medications might be indicated if the person develops respiratory distress. The environment should be quiet and free from bright lights and sudden movements to reduce the seizure risk.

The diet should generally be high in calcium and low in phosphate. Milk, milk products and egg yolk are high in both calcium and phosphate, and are usually restricted because of the latter. Spinach is also restricted because it contains high levels of oxylate, which can form insoluble calcium substances.

Oral calcium gluconate supplements may be needed. Oral magnesium supplements are indicated if hypomagnesaemia is present. Various calcium preparations are used, including Citracal (calcium citrate) and Oscal (calcium carbonate), to minimise gastrointestinal symptoms such as constipation. Sometimes two different types of calcium are prescribed. Vitamin D supplementation is also usually required. Vitamin D preparations (ergocalciferol or cholecalciferol) are usually needed to enhance calcium absorption from the gastrointestinal tract. Aluminium hydroxide gel is used to bind phosphate and promote excretion through the gastrointestinal tract.

Daily injections of teriparatide, a synthetic form of PTH, may be indicated to treat osteoporosis. This increases bone formation and inhibits bone reabsorption.

Parathyroid gland autotransplantations are sometimes performed in secondary hypoparathyroidism due to renal failure or dialysis. The glands are transplanted into muscles, such as those in the forearm.

HYPERPARATHYROIDISM

Hyperparathyroidism is characterised by elevated blood calcium levels—**hypercalcaemia**—in response to excessive bone resorption, increased gastrointestinal absorption of calcium and less calcium excretion. The prevalence rate for this condition is estimated at around 1%, up to 1.5% in older populations. It is more common in women, and those of Black or Asian ethnicity, and its peak age range for diagnosis is 50–60 years old.

Common causes are a benign adenoma of the parathyroid tissue, or glandular hyperplasia. Some carcinomas in other tissues may secrete PTH. Another important cause is chronic renal failure in association with imbalances in calcium and phosphate levels. There may also be an increased risk of hyperparathyroidism associated with radiotherapy to the head or neck.

Clinical manifestations

The main clinical manifestations are associated with hypercalcaemia. Affected individuals may experience fatigue, depression and poor concentration. Excessive bone resorption and demineralisation leads to pathological fractures, particularly affecting the long bones, the hips and the spine. Increased renal excretion of calcium—**hypercalciuria**—can result in renal calculi (renal stones), as the higher concentrations of calcium in the urine lead to decreased water solubility. **Hypophosphataemia** may also develop (see the chapter 'Electrolyte imbalances' for more details). If the degree of hypercalcaemia is severe, then gastrointestinal disturbances (e.g. anorexia, abdominal pain, constipation, nausea and vomiting), polyuria and dehydration, as well as cardiac dysrhythmias, can arise.

Clinical diagnosis and management

Diagnosis Persistently elevated serum calcium levels and high PTH levels confirm the diagnosis of hyperparathyroidism. Elevated serum calcium levels alone are not diagnostic, because these can be affected by diet, some medicines, and renal and bone diseases.

Radioimmunoassays are undertaken to differentiate primary hyperparathyroidism and elevated PTH levels from other causes. High-frequency ultrasound in combination with ultrasound-guided fine-needle aspiration and PTH washings are used to confirm which gland/s is/are abnormal.

If the serum calcium level does not drop, multiple parathyroid glands are likely to be involved, and a thallium isotope or sestamibi (a radiopharmaceutical coupled with a technetium radioisotope) scan is undertaken to localise the adenoma. Sometimes the sestamibi scans enable three-dimensional pictures of the parathyroid glands to be obtained. If a sestamibi scan fails to localise the tumour, surgical neck exploration might be needed. MRI scans rarely provide enough detailed information. CT scans can sometimes be helpful, but are not used as frequently if sestamibi scans are available. Sometimes inactive adenomas are detected in the absence of calcium imbalance when ultrasound scans are performed for other reasons; these are called *parathyroid incidentalomas*.

X-rays and bone densitometry may be indicated to detect abnormalities that could signify compromised growth in children and adolescents, and fracture risk in older people (see the chapters 'Musculoskeletal trauma and muscle disorders' and 'Bone and joint disorders').

Management Surgical removal of the relevant parathyroid gland or glands is the preferred treatment. This should be undertaken by a skilled thyroid surgeon to minimise damage to important structures and nerves in the neck. Cure rates in the hands of skilled surgeons are greater than 93%. The glands are easily missed during neck surgery involving the thyroid gland. The surgeon must identify all four parathyroid glands and remove the adenomatous gland. All four parathyroid glands are adenomatous in 4–5% of affected people (*parathyroid hyperplasia*), in which case the surgeon would remove three or three and a half glands, leaving some parathyroid tissue behind to function normally in the future.

Minimally invasive parathyroid surgery is the treatment of choice. Calcium levels begin to fall after surgery. If only one gland was involved, it may take a few weeks for the remaining underactive glands to begin to function normally again. Therefore, most people will initially be prescribed calcium. The need for continued supplements is determined after recovery.

Medical management consists of encouraging the person to have a high fluid intake to help prevent renal calculi (renal stones), constipation and dehydration. The latter can precipitate a hypercalcaemic crisis. Renal calculi may require hospital admission if severe. Cranberry juice lowers the urinary pH and is sometimes used. Oral phosphates lower serum calcium levels, but are not recommended for long-term use.

Treatment with bisphosphonates can be helpful. Thiazide diuretics elevate serum calcium levels and are generally contraindicated in this condition. Calcium intake may need to be restricted. Antacids may be needed to manage associated gastrointestinal symptoms. Prune juice and stool softeners may be needed to manage constipation. The person should be encouraged to be active, to reduce loss of calcium from bones and the risk of renal calculi.

Hypercalcaemic crisis Acute hypercalcaemic crisis with extremely high serum calcium levels ($>$ 3.5 mmol/L) causes neurological and cardiovascular symptoms, and can result in death if it is not corrected. Treatment includes IV rehydration, diuretics to promote renal calcium excretion, and phosphate to correct hypophosphataemia, promote calcium deposition in bone and reduce absorption of calcium from the intestine. In emergency situations, calcitonin, corticosteroids, bisphosphonates or cytotoxic agents, or a combination of these medicines, may be indicated.

MULTIPLE ENDOCRINE NEOPLASIA

Multiple endocrine neoplasia (MEN) is an autosomal dominant genetic disease where an affected person is at risk of developing enlargement and hyperactivity of some endocrine glands. The condition is associated with dysfunction of a protein called *menin*, which is involved in cell proliferation and DNA maintenance. As a result, cell proliferation becomes unregulated and DNA repair declines in selected endocrine tissues. The parathyroid, pancreas and pituitary glands are the most common glands affected. Several glands may be affected simultaneously or at separate times. Two types of MEN occur: MEN 1 and MEN 2. Different genes are associated with MEN 1 and MEN 2.

MEN 1 is also known as *multiple endocrine adenomatosis type 1 (MEA 1)* or *Wermer's syndrome*. MEN 1 is a rare disease, occurring in fewer than 1 in 20,000 people. Men and women are equally likely to inherit MEN 1, and it occurs in all racial groups. Almost everybody who develops MEN 1 develops hyperparathyroidism at some stage in their life, and usually hyperactivity in more than one endocrine gland. Endocrine gland hyperactivity is rare before 10 years of age, and the likelihood increases with increasing age. By 30 years of age most people who are genetically predisposed to MEN 1 will have some endocrine gland hyperactivity. Malignant adenomas are rare, but, if present, are likely to be in the pancreas or thymus. Regular testing is important to detect malignancy early.

MEN 2, also called *Schmidt's syndrome*, usually affects young adults. Features include hypothyroidism, delayed sexual development and diabetes mellitus. Approximately 10% of those with MEN 2 have the chronic skin condition vitilago, which is associated with loss of skin pigmentation.

Clinical manifestations

MEN 1 occurs in children. People who develop MEN 1 will develop the symptoms associated with the affected gland or glands; commonly, hyperparathyroidism, hyperpituitarism (discussed in the chapter 'Hypothalamic–pituitary disorders'), delayed sexual development, pernicious anaemia, chronic *Candida albicans* infection, chronic active hepatitis and sometimes hair loss.

Overproduction of pancreatic hormones is the second most common endocrine abnormality associated with MEN 1. Certain types of pancreatic adenoma are more likely to be associated with MEN 1: *Zollinger–Ellison syndrome* (*gastrinoma*) and *insulinoma* (see the following section). The pancreas produces several hormones, and thus the signs and symptoms vary. They include gastric ulcers and diarrhoea due to the overproduction of gastrin, and hypoglycaemia due to hyperinsulinaemia. Both manifestations are more common before the age of 30 years.

Diagnosis and management

Diagnosis Two diagnostic tests are important in this condition: testing for the MEN genes and testing endocrine function. All people who are at risk of this condition should be genetically screened for the MEN gene even though they feel well, as symptoms are rare before the age of 30 years. DNA testing can be performed on a blood sample. People who test positive should be evaluated regularly for endocrine hyperactivity, through monitoring serum hormones and taking the relevant scans and ultrasounds.

Testing endocrine function to detect hyperactivity early is important, as many symptoms are vague and non-specific, and may be due to a range of aetiologies in addition to endocrine disease. Blood tests include serum ionised calcium levels, because hyperparathyroidism is the most common abnormality associated with MEN 1. Serum prolactin levels are also taken, because prolactinomas and somatotropinomas are the most frequently reported pituitary diseases related to MEN 1. Other hormone tests include insulin-like growth factor (IGF-1), cortisol, thyroid hormones, gastrin and insulin.

Management Management consists of regular monitoring and treating the underlying glandular abnormality, as described elsewhere.

INDIGENOUS HEALTH FAST FACTS AND CULTURAL CONSIDERATIONS

FAST FACTS

- *Iodine levels in Aboriginal and Torres Strait Islander peoples are within acceptable levels, and are generally higher than those in non-Indigenous Australians.*
- *The prevalence of vitamin D deficiency is equal in Aboriginal and Torres Strait Islander adults to the general Australian adult population (23%). It is more prevalent in remote areas (39%) and in older adults.*
- *Thyroid cancer rates are slightly lower in Indigenous Australians compared to non-Indigenous Australians (5-year prevalence ratio is 0.8).*
- *There is a higher incidence of thyroid cancers for Māori women (1.6:1) and Māori men (1.5:1) compared to European New Zealanders.*
- *There is a higher incidence of thyroid cancers for Pacific Islands women (3.6:1) and Pacific Islands men (1.2:1) compared to European New Zealanders.*

CULTURAL CONSIDERATIONS

- *Aboriginal and Torres Strait Islander peoples living in remote areas have higher levels of iodine yet lower levels of vitamin D than those living in non-remote areas. This suggests a difference in environmental and/or nutritional experiences between the communities of the two regions. Data suggest that Aboriginal and Torres Strait Islander peoples living in remote areas consumed, on average, less iodine than those living in non-remote areas, and also less than non-Indigenous people. Yet both remote and non-remote Indigenous people had, on average, higher serum or urine iodine concentrations than non-Indigenous people. Disparities in iodine levels between people of the two regions also appear to be more complex than just dietary-related factors alone.*
- *In relation to vitamin D levels, data suggest that Aboriginal and Torres Strait Islander peoples living in remote areas consumed, on average, less vitamin D than those living in non-remote areas. It is also understood that obesity levels can influence vitamin D absorption, as excess body fat can interfere with vitamin D absorption. This is supported by the data that demonstrated that obese Aboriginal and Torres Strait Islander peoples were twice as likely as non-obese Indigenous Australians to have a vitamin D deficiency. Although it is known that darker skin pigmentation influences vitamin D levels (i.e. light-skinned people synthesise six times the amount of vitamin D than dark-skinned people do), paradoxically, individuals with darker skin most often have higher intestinal calcium absorption, higher levels of cholecalciferol, and increased bone density. Is there a difference in average skin tone or sun exposure between Aboriginal and Torres Strait Islander peoples living in remote and non-remote areas? At this stage, it is clear that we do not completely understand the complexities of ethnicity and remoteness for some important biomarkers.*

Source: Data from Australian Indigenous HealthInfoNet (2022); Black et al. (2021); Haigh et al. (2018); Meredith et al. (2014).

CHILDREN AND ADOLESCENTS

- In Australia, only 10% of children 2–3 years of age and 6% of children 5–11 years of age are mildly iodine deficient.
- Iodine deficiency in New Zealand children is less common (5% had urinary iodine concentration of < 50 µg/L[WHO recommends < 20%] and 39% had urinary iodine concentration of < 100 µg/L [WHO recommends < 50%]) since the mandatory fortification of bread with iodised salt in 2009.
- In 1920, 61% of children had enlarged thyroids, and today the incidence of goitre in children in Australia and New Zealand is virtually non-existent.

OLDER ADULTS

- Hypothyroidism is more common in the older population than in younger adults, potentially as a result of poor dietary habits, autoimmune disease, previous treatment for hyperthyroidism, and increased consumption of drugs that can alter thyroid function.
- Hyperthyroidism is less common in the older population than in younger adults.

Source: Australian Bureau of Statistics (2015).

KEY CLINICAL ISSUES

- The signs and symptoms of thyroid and parathyroid diseases can be vague and mimic other disease processes, including the ageing process. Health professionals are in an ideal position to observe and document subtle signs to help make an early diagnosis.
- Iodine deficiencies are common in developing countries, and can be present in refugees and migrants from these countries to Australia and New Zealand.
- Medicines are frequently needed to manage the symptoms associated with thyroid disease, such as tachycardia, atrial fibrillation, heart failure, eye symptoms and skin manifestations.

CHAPTER REVIEW

- The thyroid and parathyroid glands are located in the neck. The *thyroid* produces *thyroxine* and *triiodothyronine*, known as the 'thyroid hormones', as well as *calcitonin*. The thyroid hormones set the basal metabolic rate, as well as influence the maturation and maintenance of the brain, musculoskeletal system, cardiovascular system and reproductive system. Calcitonin is involved in calcium balance.
- The *parathyroid gland* produces *parathormone*, or *parathyroid hormone (PTH)*, which is a primary regulator of body calcium levels.
- *Goitre* is defined as an enlargement of the thyroid gland. It can develop in hypothyroidism as a compensatory mechanism, and in hyperthyroidism as part of the primary pathophysiological process.
- *Hypothyroidism* can occur congenitally or in the neonatal period. It may also be acquired in both children and adults. When the acquired form is prolonged, it is known as *myxoedema*.
- *Congenital hypothyroidism* can lead to permanent delayed development of the brain and major body systems. *Acquired hypothyroidism* can be caused by autoimmune attack, chronic inflammation, deficient dietary iodine intake, thyroidectomy or a disruption to the hypothalamic–pituitary–thyroid axis.
- Clinical manifestations of hypothyroidism include bradycardia, constipation, loss of appetite, lethargy, slowed mental function, hyporeflexia, fatigue, muscle weakness, cold intolerance and weight gain. The skin becomes thickened, dry and coarse, and hair may become brittle and thin out.
- *Hyperthyroidism*, also known as *thyrotoxicosis*, can be caused by a *tumour* growing in the thyroid or pituitary; it can also be *induced by some medications* that contain iodine, such as the antidysrhythmic agent amiodarone.
- The most common form of hyperthyroidism is *Graves' disease*. This is an autoimmune condition where autoantibodies mimic thyroid-stimulating hormone (TSH) at its receptors on the thyroid, leading to the increased production of thyroid hormones. A defining characteristic that can help to differentiate Graves' disease from other forms of hyperthyroidism is *exophthalmos* (i.e. bulging eyes).
- Clinical manifestations of hyperthyroidism include tachycardia, palpitations and angina, muscle weakness and fatigue, increased gastrointestinal motility, intolerance to heat, increased appetite (which may be accompanied by weight loss), nervousness, hyperreflexia and insomnia. Fingernails and toenails can become loosened, and may even detach from the nail bed.
- *Hypoparathyroidism* is characterised by *hypocalcaemia*. Hypoparathyroidism is associated with thyroidectomy, congenital malformation or autoimmune attack.
- Clinical manifestations of hypoparathyroidism include muscle twitches and spasms, paraesthesias, fatigue, changes in emotional and mood state, and cardiac dysrhythmias. Mild hyperphosphataemia can occur. In severe hypocalcaemia, laryngeal spasms, tetany and seizures may occur.
- *Hyperparathyroidism* is characterised by *hypercalcaemia*. Common causes include tumours in parathyroid tissue or carcinoma in other tissues. Another important cause is chronic renal failure.
- Clinical manifestations of hyperparathyroidism include pathological fractures, particularly affecting the long bones, the hips and the spine, renal stones and hypophosphataemia. If the degree of hypercalcaemia is severe, then gastrointestinal disturbances (e.g. anorexia, constipation, nausea and vomiting), polyuria and dehydration, as well as cardiac dysrhythmias, can arise.

REVIEW QUESTIONS

1 What are the names and main functions of the hormones produced by the thyroid and parathyroid glands?

2 a What is a goitre?
  b Under what circumstances does a goitre form?
  b Differentiate between a toxic and a non-toxic goitre.

3 What is the main change in body function associated with the following endocrine disorders?
  a hyperparathyroidism
  b hypothyroidism

4 Differentiate between congenital hypothyroidism and myxoedema.

5 Differentiate between thyrotoxicosis and Graves' disease.

6 Attempt to identify the correct endocrine disorder from the set of clinical manifestations provided:
  a muscle twitches, paraesthesias, cardiac dysrhythmias and fatigue
  b tachycardia, fatigue, increased gastrointestinal motility, intolerance to heat, increased appetite and weight loss
  c kidney stones, pathological fractures and gastrointestinal disturbances
  d thickened tongue, mental retardation, dry and coarse skin, and delayed skeletal growth

7 A man has recently had thyroid surgery for hyperthyroidism. He visits his doctor to have his blood pressure checked. After having the cuff applied to his arm and partially inflating it, the man's wrist and hand muscles spasm. The doctor lightly taps the man's face in front of his earlobe, and this induces a twitch of his facial muscles. A subsequent blood test shows low serum calcium and high phosphate levels.
  a Which endocrine disorder do you think this man is experiencing?
  b How has it developed?
  c What are the names of the two tests that the doctor has used to reveal the clinical manifestations of the condition?

HEALTH PROFESSIONAL CONNECTIONS

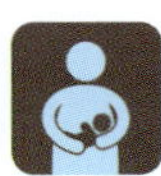

Midwives Thyroid and parathyroid disorders can contribute to fertility issues through influences on ovulation. Women who are having difficulty conceiving or are experiencing ectopic or failed pregnancies should have investigations for issues relating to endocrine function. During pregnancy, the thyroid gland undergoes a degree of hyperplasia. Women with low dietary iodine should be educated about the risks of neurological impairment for the developing fetus. Hyperthyroidism in pregnancy is common, and can be as serious as causing abortion or neonatal thyrotoxicosis. Postnatal hyperthyroidism should be considered in women with goitre. The maternal and fetal effects of parathyroid pathology are related largely to calcium homeostasis. Endocrinologists should be part of the team caring for women with thyroid or parathyroid disorders during pregnancy.

Physiotherapists Individuals undergoing a thyroidectomy will require neck and shoulder range-of-movement exercises to assist rehabilitation. When working with clients experiencing thyroid and parathyroid disorders, bone density should be considered, especially as gait instability and ataxia can result.

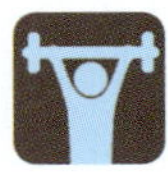

Exercise scientists Fatigue and lethargy are common with hypothyroidism, and hypermetabolism and weight loss are common with hyperthyroidism. When working with a client experiencing endocrine disorders, consultation with the endocrinologist is important to ensure that the most appropriate exercise regimens can be developed. Calcium issues, especially those resulting in reduced bone mineral density, are a significant issue with hyperparathyroidism. Exercise stimulates osteoblast activity, and will therefore assist in reducing the effects of bone-leaching conditions.

Nutritionists/Dieticians Depending on the deficiency or excess, and whether the affected gland is the thyroid or parathyroid, vitamin and mineral considerations are paramount. Vitamin D, calcium and magnesium levels may be affected. Specific vitamin-rich foods or supplements may be required. Consultation with other members of the healthcare team will be important to ensure that the nutritional needs are being modified based on the pathology results.

CASE STUDY

Mrs Sandra Barns is a 42-year-old woman (UR number 821746) presenting for investigation of Hashimoto's disease. She has a large goitre, dysphagia, sleep apnoea and a hoarse voice. Mrs Barns also complains of fatigue and cold intolerance. On her neurological examination she demonstrates memory loss, ataxia and peripheral neuropathy. She is clinically depressed. Her observations were as follows:

Temperature	Heart rate	Respiration rate	Blood pressure	SpO_2
35.2°C	54	12	100/75	98% (RA*)

*RA = room air.

Mrs Barns also presents with menorrhagia. She has been married for three years and has been unable to conceive. A barium swallow and a fine-needle aspiration biopsy of her goitre have been booked. Her pathology results were as follows:

HAEMATOLOGY

Patient location:	Ward 3	**UR:**	821746		
Consultant:	Smith	**NAME:**	Barns		
		Given name:	Sandra	**Sex:**	F
		DOB:	02/03/XX	**Age:**	42

Time collected	13:30
Date collected	XX/XX
Year	XXXX
Lab #	75838294

FULL BLOOD COUNT		UNITS	REFERENCE RANGE
Haemoglobin	98	g/L	115–160
White cell count	6.1	$\times 10^9$/L	4.0–11.0
Platelets	310	$\times 10^9$/L	140–400
Haematocrit	0.33		0.33–0.47
Red cell count	3.45	$\times 10^{12}$/L	3.80–5.20
Reticulocyte count	1.8	%	0.2–2.0
MCV	82	fL	80–100
Neutrophils	4.5	$\times 10^9$/L	2.00–8.00
Lymphocytes	3.12	$\times 10^9$/L	1.00–4.00
Monocytes	0.45	$\times 10^9$/L	0.10–1.00
Eosinophils	0.35	$\times 10^9$/L	< 0.60
Basophils	0.14	$\times 10^9$/L	< 0.20
ESR	7	mm/h	< 12
COAGULATION PROFILE			
aPTT	32	secs	24–40
PT	14	secs	11–17

BIOCHEMISTRY

Patient location:	Ward 3	**UR:**	821746		
Consultant:	Smith	**NAME:**	Barns		
		Given name:	Sandra	**Sex:**	F
		DOB:	02/03/XX	**Age:**	42

Time collected 13:30
Date collected XX/XX
Year XXXX
Lab # 4543545

ELECTROLYTES		UNITS	REFERENCE RANGE
Sodium	146	mmol/L	135–145
Potassium	4.4	mmol/L	3.5–5.2
Chloride	98	mmol/L	95–110
Bicarbonate	24	mmol/L	22–32
Glucose	4.6	mmol/L	3.5–6.0
Iron	6	μmol/L	11–30
THYROID FUNCTION TESTS			
TSH	7.3	mIU/L	0.3–5
FT3	2.4	mIU/L	2.5–7.5
FT4	11	mIU/L	12–22
Anti-TpOAb	High		
Anti-TgAb	Present		
Cholesterol	8.2	mmol/L	3.6–6.9
Triglycerides (fasting)	2.5	mmol/L	0.3–2.3

CRITICAL THINKING

1 Consider Mrs Barns's signs, symptoms and observations (not pathology results). Draw up a table, listing these in one column (one sign, symptom or observation per row). Explain the mechanism for each sign, symptom or observation in the adjacent column.

2 Observe the pathology results. Many parameters are outside their reference range. Extend your table to include a new column for the pathology tests, comprising each outlying parameter from the pathology results, and outline what it means.

3 Hashimoto's thyroiditis can be considered an autoimmune disorder. Explore the concepts of this autoimmune disorder, relating your answer back to the presence of anti-thyroperoxidase (anti-TpOAb) and anti-thyroglobulin (anti-TgAb) antibodies.

4 Add a third column to the table you have constructed. Title this column 'Intervention'. Explore the interventions required to assist Mrs Barns. Add these to the third column.

5 Individuals experiencing hypothyroidism can develop myxoedema coma. What observations could alert you to the development of this life-threatening condition? How should it be managed?

BIBLIOGRAPHY

Australian Bureau of Statistics (ABS) (2015). Iodine. *Australian Health Survey: usual nutrient intakes, 2011–12.* Canberra: ABS. https://www.abs.gov.au/statistics/health/health-conditions-and-risks/australian-health-survey-usual-nutrient-intakes/latest-release.

Australian Indigenous Health*Info*Net (2022). *Overview of Aboriginal and Torres Strait Islander health status, 2021.* Perth, WA: Australian Indigenous Health*Info*Net. https://healthinfonet.ecu.edu.au/learn/health-facts/overview-aboriginal-torres-strait-islander-health-status/.

Australian Institute of Health and Welfare (AIHW) (2021). *Cancer in Australia, 2021.* Cancer series No. 133. Cat. No. CAN 144. Canberra: AIHW. https://www.aihw.gov.au/reports/cancer/cancer-in-australia-2021/summary.

Australian Institute of Health and Welfare (2022). *Australia's health 2022: in brief.* Australia's Health series No. 18. Cat. No. AUS 241. Canberra: AIHW. Retrieved from https://www.aihw.gov.au/getmedia/c6c5dda9-4020-43b0-8ed6-a567cd660eaa/aihw-aus-241.pdf.aspx?inline=true.

Bauldoff, G., Gubrud-Howe, P.M., Carno, M.-A., Levett-Jones, T., Hales, M., Berry, K., ... Stanley, D. (2020). *LeMone and Burke's medical–surgical nursing: critical thinking for person-centred care* (4th [Australian] edn). Sydney: Pearson Australia.

Best, O. & Fredericks, B. (2021). *Yatdjuligin: Aboriginal and Torres Strait Islander nursing and midwifery care* (3rd edn). Port Melbourne, VIC: Cambridge University Press.

Black, L., Dunlop, E., Lucas, R., Pearson, G., Farrant, B. & Shepherd, C. (2021). Prevalence and predictors of vitamin D deficiency in a nationally representative sample of Australian Aboriginal and Torres Strait Islander adults. *British Journal of Nutrition* 126(1):101–9. http://doi:10.1017/S0007114520003931.

Bullock, S. & Manias, E. (2022). *Fundamentals of pharmacology* (9th edn). Sydney: Pearson Australia.

Eastman, C.J. & Zimmerman, M.B. (2014). The iodine deficiency disorders. *Thyroid Disease Manager.* http://www.thyroidmanager.org.

Haigh, M., Burns, J., Potter, C., Elwell, M., Hollows, M., Mundy, J., ... Thompson, S. (2018). Review of cancer among Aboriginal and Torres Strait Islander people. *Australian Indigenous Health*Bulletin 18(3). https://healthbulletin.org.au/wp-content/uploads/2018/09/cancer-review-2018-web.pdf.

Kim, L. (2022). Hyperparathyroidism. *Emedicine.* https://emedicine.medscape.com/article/127351-overview.

Lee, S.Y. & Pearce, E.N. (2022). Assessment and treatment of thyroid disorders in pregnancy and the postpartum period. *Nature Reviews Endocrinology* 18(3):158–71. https://doi.org/10.1038/s41574-021-00604-z.

Marieb, E.N. & Hoehn, K. (2019). *Human anatomy and physiology* (11th edn). San Francisco, CA: Pearson Benjamin Cummings.

Meredith, I., Sarfati, D., Atkinson, J. & Blakely, T. (2014). Thyroid cancer in Pacific women in New Zealand. *New Zealand Medical Journal* 127(1395):52–62. https://pubmed.ncbi.nlm.nih.gov/24929693/.

Orlander, P.R. (2022). Hypothyroidism. *Emedicine.* https://emedicine.medscape.com/article/122393-overview.

Schraga, E.D. (2022). Hyperthyroidism, thyroid storm, and Graves disease. *Emedicine.* https://emedicine.medscape.com/article/767130-overview.

Singh, G.R., Davison, B., Ma, G.Y., Eastman, C.J. & Mackerras, D.E.M. (2019). Iodine status of Indigenous and non-Indigenous young adults in the Top End, before and after mandatory fortification. *Medical Journal of Australia* 210(3):121–25. https://doi.org/10.5694/mja2.12031.

19 Adrenal gland disorders

KEY TERMS

Addison's disease
Adrenal cortex
Adrenal insufficiency
Adrenal medulla
Aldosterone
Androgens
Congenital adrenal hyperplasia (CAH)
Conn's disease
Corticosteroids
Cortisol
Cushing's disease
Glucocorticoids
Gonadocorticoids
Mineralocorticoid
Sex hormones

LEARNING OBJECTIVES

After completing this chapter, you should be able to:

1. Identify the hormones produced by the adrenal glands and their functions.
2. Outline the pathophysiological mechanisms associated with adrenal gland dysfunction.
3. Describe the clinical manifestations, diagnosis and clinical management of adrenal insufficiency.
4. Describe the clinical manifestations, diagnosis and clinical management of endocrine disorders characterised by imbalances in glucocorticoid secretion.
5. Describe the pathophysiological mechanisms and epidemiology involved in endocrine disorders characterised by imbalances in mineralocorticoid secretion.
6. Describe the clinical manifestations, diagnosis and clinical management of endocrine disorders characterised by imbalances in mineralocorticoid secretion.
7. Describe the pathophysiological mechanisms and epidemiology involved in endocrine disorders characterised by imbalances in gonadocorticoid secretion.
8. Describe the clinical manifestations, diagnosis and clinical management of endocrine disorders characterised by imbalances in gonadocorticoid secretion.
9. Describe the pathophysiological mechanisms and epidemiology involved in the endocrine disorder characterised by an imbalance in adrenal medullary hormone secretion.
10. Describe the clinical manifestations, diagnosis and clinical management of the endocrine disorder characterised by an imbalance in adrenal medullary hormone secretion.

WHAT YOU SHOULD KNOW BEFORE YOU START THIS CHAPTER

Can you identify the main components of the endocrine system?

Can you describe the anatomical and physiological relationship between the hypothalamus, the pituitary and the adrenal glands?

Can you identify the hormones of the adrenal glands and their functions?

Can you outline the effects of altered sodium levels?

Can you outline the effects of altered potassium levels?

Introduction

LEARNING OBJECTIVE 1

Identify the hormones produced by the adrenal glands and their functions.

The main functions of the adrenal glands can be summarised by the '4S' principle: the glands are involved in *s*tress responsiveness, *s*ugar (glucose) availability, *s*alt balance, as well as *s*exual development and maintenance. Anatomically, the glands are divided into two main regions: the *outer cortex* and the *inner medulla*.

The hormones secreted by the **adrenal cortex** are called the **corticosteroids**, because they are all steroids that are produced from the precursor substance cholesterol, which makes them highly fat-soluble. The cortex secretes **glucocorticoids**, the main one being **cortisol** (otherwise known as *hydrocortisone*), the **mineralocorticoid aldosterone**, and the **gonadocorticoids** or **sex hormones** (predominantly **androgens**, as well as *oestrogens* and *progesterone*). Their functions are summarised in Figure 19.1.

The **adrenal medulla** is part of the *sympathetic nervous system (SNS)* and, when stimulated, releases *adrenaline* and *noradrenaline*, which enhances its activity. A common link between the cortex and the medulla is their involvement in the *stress response* (see the chapter 'Stress and its role is disease' for further details). A distinctive difference between the two regions is that the glucocorticoids are involved in the regulation of intermediate to longer-term stress, while adrenal medullary hormone release is directed towards controlling short-term stress.

When the function of the adrenal glands is impaired, the ability to maintain normal homeostasis and adapt to stressors can be severely compromised and may lead to a life-threatening situation.

Disorders of the adrenal cortex

LEARNING OBJECTIVE 2

Outline the pathophysiological mechanisms associated with adrenal gland dysfunction.

A number of clinical conditions are associated with imbalances in corticosteroid hormone secretion, involving both hyperactive and hypoactive states. This is the case with the synthesis of glucocorticoids and mineralocorticoids. Only hypersecretion of gonadocorticoids manifests as a human clinical disorder.

Secretion of the adrenocortical hormones is controlled by the *hypothalamic–pituitary axis*. The hypothalamus discharges releasing hormones, which stimulates the pituitary to secrete *adrenocorticotropic hormone (ACTH)*. If dysfunction arises from the adrenal glands, it is regarded as a *primary disorder*. If the problem lies in the pituitary, it is known as a *secondary disorder*, and if it has its origins in the hypothalamus, it is a *tertiary disorder* (see Figure 19.2).

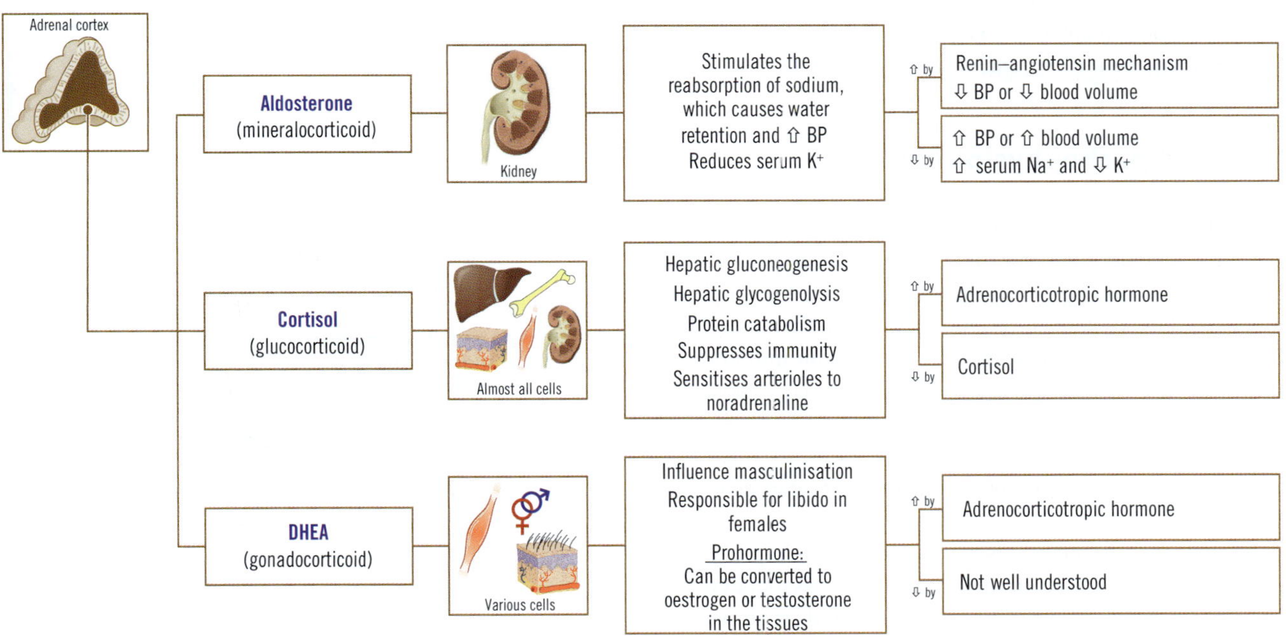

Figure 19.1

Adrenal cortex hormones and their functions

↑ by = stimulated by; ↓ by = inhibited by; BP = blood pressure; DHEA = dehydroepiandrosterone; K^+ = potassium ion; Na^+ sodium ion.

Source: Images adapted from Marieb & Hoehn (2019), Chapter 16.

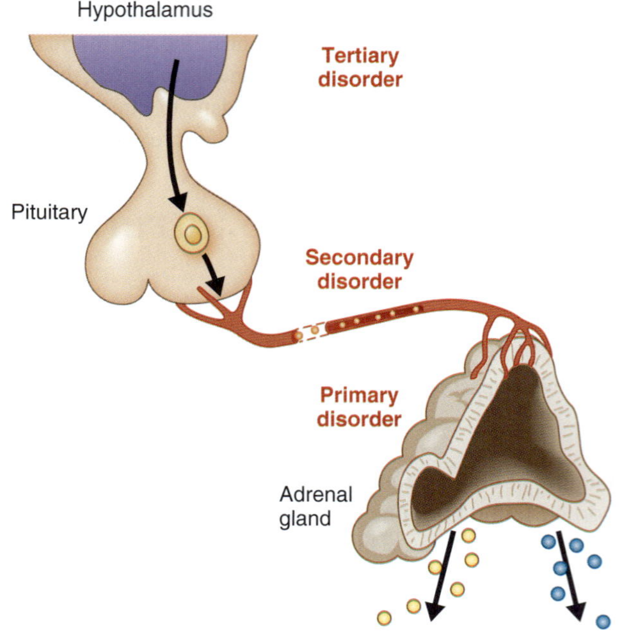

Figure 19.2

Levels of adrenal gland dysfunction

Source: Adapted from Marieb & Hoehn (2016).

ADRENAL INSUFFICIENCY

LEARNING OBJECTIVE 3

Describe the clinical manifestations, diagnosis and clinical management of adrenal insufficiency.

Aetiology and pathophysiology

A severe deficiency in adrenocortical function is referred to as **adrenal insufficiency**. In this condition, the secretion of all cortical hormones is affected: glucocorticoids (resulting in *hypocortisolism*), mineralocorticoids (resulting in *hypoaldosteronism*) and gonadocorticoids. Primary adrenal insufficiency, generally referred to as **Addison's disease**, can arise as a result of autoimmune attack (known as *autoimmune adrenalitis*) and represents about 70% of all cases. The antibodies are directed against an enzyme involved in adrenal steroidogenesis called *21-beta-hydroxylase*. Other common causes involve chronic inflammation, cancer or congenital malformation.

When adrenal insufficiency is severe or develops rapidly, it is a life-threatening state. In this state, it is associated with very poor responsiveness to stressors, and requires urgent treatment. In Western countries, systemic tuberculosis infection accounts for a significant proportion of adrenal insufficiency cases.

A form of hypocortisolism can develop as a secondary endocrine disorder when pituitary secretion of ACTH is deficient. Another common cause of this form occurs after prolonged and/or high-dose therapy with a glucocorticoid medication, such as hydrocortisone, dexamethasone or prednisolone. The glucocorticoid medication acts to suppress the hypothalamic–pituitary–adrenal (HPA) axis through negative feedback mechanisms. When the medication is stopped, the axis may remain suppressed for a period and induce an endogenous glucocorticoid deficiency (see Figure 19.3).

Epidemiology

Addison's disease is quite rare, with statistics from Western countries indicating prevalence of 10–14 person in 100,000. It generally strikes people in adulthood, usually between the ages of 30 and 60 years.

Clinical manifestations

The clinical manifestations of Addison's disease result from deficiencies in cortisol, aldosterone and androgens, and include poor responsiveness to stress, hypoglycaemia, sparse body hair, fatigue, anorexia and weight loss, chronic hypotension, decreased heart size, muscle weakness, depressed mood, hyponatraemia and hyperkalaemia. Skin pigmentation can darken in pale-skinned individuals, conferring a generalised tanned appearance. The alteration in skin pigmentation is particularly noticeable in palmar creases, the buccal mucosa, lips, nipples and around scars. The pigmented changes are due to significant elevation of ACTH, which, at this level, acts like melanin-stimulating hormone on skin cells.

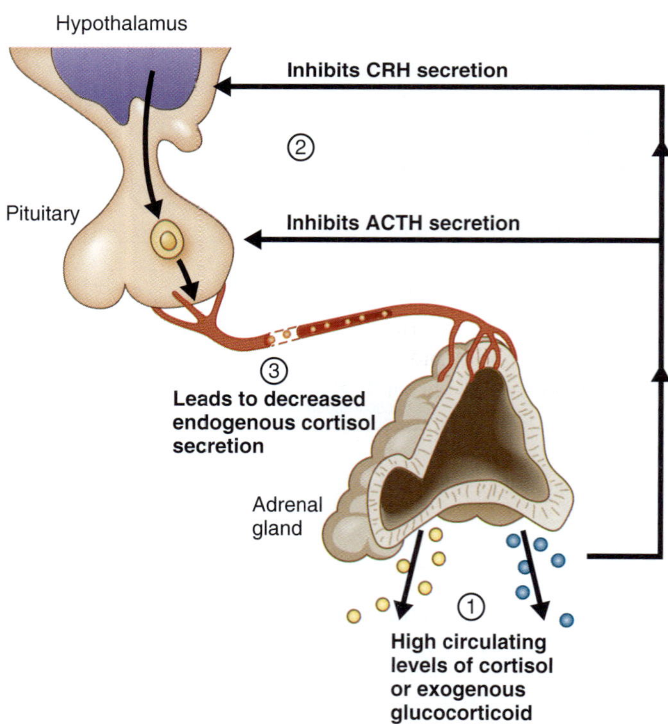

Figure 19.3

Mechanism of suppression of the hypothalamic–pituitary–adrenal axis

ACTH = adrenocorticotropic hormone;
CRH = corticotropin-releasing hormone.

Addisonian crisis If the hypoadrenal state is not detected and treated, the disease can progress and the person may present in an Addisonian crisis, which is characterised by acute hypotension, cyanosis, circulatory shock, apprehension, tachycardia, weak pulse, tachypnoea, headache, nausea, confusion and restlessness.

Addisonian crisis can be precipitated by exertion, exposure to cold, acute infections and reduced salt intake. In addition, fasting for diagnostic endocrine tests and procedures can precipitate a crisis. Addisonian crisis can occur in treated people with Addison's disease if they do not manage their medicines appropriately during illness, stress and surgery. Thyroid hormone therapy in people with undiagnosed Addison's disease can induce an Addisonian crisis.

Clinical diagnosis and management

Diagnosis The symptoms listed are suggestive of Addison's disease, but it can be difficult to diagnose in the early stages. The diagnosis is made on laboratory tests of serum and urine cortisol, aldosterone and other hormone levels, such as ACTH. Undetectable serum cortisol is diagnostic, but the basal cortisol may be within the normal range. Measuring cortisol and ACTH at 9 am is a sensitive test for Addison's disease: the ACTH level is elevated for the corresponding cortisol level.

ACTH stimulation test The short *synacthen test* is the specific test used to diagnose Addison's disease. If relevant, the person must be weaned off corticosteroid medicines before undertaking synacthen testing. Synacthen is a form of ACTH, and is administered intravenously (IV) or intramuscularly (IM). Normally, synacthen causes a rise in serum cortisol levels.

If the response is inconclusive, a long synacthen test may be performed to confirm secondary adrenal insufficiency, but the response may be within the normal range if the secondary adrenal failure commenced within the preceding two weeks. Normally, serum cortisol rises to higher levels than for the short synacthen test.

If the adrenal cortex is destroyed, baseline synacthen does not induce the rise in serum cortisol and urinary 17-hydroxycorticosteroids that it normally would. If the adrenal glands are normal but are not stimulated by the pituitary gland, the response to synacthen is normal but no ACTH response occurs following administration of metyrapone, a drug that stimulates the pituitary to release ACTH; this indicates secondary adrenal insufficiency.

Insulin tolerance test (ITT) The insulin tolerance test (ITT) is used to determine how the pituitary and hypothalamus respond to stress. The aim of the ITT is to induce hypoglycaemia (for the purposes of the ITT, this refers to a blood glucose level of 2 mmol/L) by administering a dose of insulin IV. Normally, the blood glucose falls and cortisol rises. IV dextrose is administered after blood is collected during the hypoglycaemic episode.

Other tests Other tests include measuring 21-beta-hydroxylase antibodies, a screening test for infection, X-rays of the adrenal and pituitary glands to detect calcification that could indicate tuberculosis (if calcification is present, a tuberculin test is indicated), and measuring plasma renin levels to assess mineralocorticoid status (elevated renin is one of the earliest indications of Addison's disease). The levels of other hormones, such as thyroid hormone, progesterone, luteinising hormone (LH) and dehydroepiandrosterone (DHEA, an adrenal steroid hormone intermediate) can also be assessed, as can be enzymes such as 21-beta-hydroxylase. People with 21-beta-hydroxylase deficiencies cannot produce steroid hormones such as aldosterone and cortisol from cholesterol (see the section on congenital adrenal hyperplasia).

Computed tomography (CT) of the abdomen may show adrenal gland enlargement or calcification, which might indicate tuberculosis, infiltration by metastatic disease, or small atrophic glands indicative of autoimmune adrenalitis. CT and/or magnetic resonance imaging (MRI) scans may also be indicated to determine the size and shape of the pituitary gland if secondary adrenal insufficiency is suspected.

Management Management of Addison's disease consists of replacing the hormones that are lacking, usually cortisol. This is achieved with daily or twice-daily doses of oral hydrocortisone. The intermediate-acting corticosteroid prednisolone, or occasionally the long-acting dexamethasone, may be used if pigmentation is severe and if the morning ACTH level is elevated. Glucocorticoid stress-dosing is important during illness or when the person requires a surgical procedure, including endoscopy.

If aldosterone is also lacking, oral mineralocorticoid medicines, such as daily fludrocortisone acetate, are needed (see the section on hypoaldosteronism). The doses of medicines are adjusted according to individual need. If aldosterone replacement is required, salt replacement might also be necessary. People with secondary adrenal insufficiency do not usually require aldosterone replacement, because they usually continue to produce normal amounts of this hormone. Androgen replacement therapy is not required in adult males, as the testes produce sufficient androgen for normal reproductive function. DHEA supplementation may be useful in women with Addison's disease, as adrenal androgens play a role in reproductive function and have been shown to improve well-being.

People with Addison's disease requiring anaesthesia and surgery for any reason will require IV hydrocortisone and saline, preferably commenced the day before surgery and continued until the person is stable postoperatively, after which the dose is gradually reduced to a maintenance dose.

Pregnant women with Addison's disease continue their usual replacement medicines, but replacement may need to be by injection if nausea and vomiting prevent oral dosing and compromise medicine absorption from the gastrointestinal tract. During delivery, treatment is similar to that for those undergoing surgery. The dose is usually gradually reduced after delivery to a maintenance dose.

Patient education is essential. People with Addison's disease must carry identification, such as a medical alert device, that includes their condition, treatment and doctor's name and contact details, for emergencies. They should know how to increase their medicine doses during periods of illnesses and severe stress.

In Addisonian crisis, urgent fluid resuscitation is needed to manage shock and restore the circulation to prevent death, even when a definitive diagnosis of Addison's disease has not been made. Serum cortisol and other relevant hormones should be measured before IV hydrocortisone is commenced to make the diagnosis. Management consists of IV hydrocortisone followed by 5% dextrose in normal saline. Once they can tolerate oral fluids and medicines, the hydrocortisone dose is gradually reduced until a maintenance dose is achieved. Fludrocortisone acetate replacement will also be needed if aldosterone levels are low. Vasopressor medicines may be required if this treatment does not correct hypotension. Oral fluids are introduced when the person stabilises. Antibiotics may be required if infection precipitated the crisis. It is essential that the person and their relatives receive education about managing their medicines. Once they recover, and medication has ceased, definitive synacthen testing is usually delayed for up to one month to obtain an accurate diagnosis.

Secondary adrenal insufficiency Secondary adrenal insufficiency is most commonly due to pituitary disease resulting in inadequate ACTH production, such as pituitary tumours, infection or loss of blood flow to the glands, leading to pituitary atrophy. Pituitary atrophy can occur following radiation treatment of pituitary tumours, surgical removal of parts of the hypothalamus or the pituitary gland during neurosurgery, or pituitary apoplexy (see the chapter 'Hypothalamic–pituitary disorders').

Secondary adrenal insufficiency can also occur after the removal of benign ACTH-producing tumours (where the source of ACTH is suddenly removed, and replacement ACTH and cortisol are required either temporarily or permanently), or when corticosteroid medications are used to control other disease processes (which may be temporary or long-term, depending on the doses, the particular dose formulation used and the duration of treatment). Glucocorticoids block the release of the hypothalamic-releasing hormone called corticotropin-releasing hormone (CRH) and ACTH, which in turn affect cortisol output by the adrenal glands.

Corticosteroid medicines Corticosteroid medicines are used extensively as anti-inflammatory and immune-suppressing agents to treat a range of health conditions. These medications are available in a variety of formulations: topical (e.g. applied to the skin or inhaled into the lungs), oral and parenteral forms. They can suppress ACTH and endogenous glucocorticoid hormone production because they have a negative feedback effect on the hypothalamic–pituitary axis, which suppresses CRH and ACTH, leading to atrophy of the adrenal cortex. Short-term treatment (less than three weeks) does not usually have a significant effect on adrenal function, except in people with existing adrenocortical insufficiency.

However, the person may still be at risk of adrenal insufficiency within a week of stopping corticosteroid medicines if they are subject to stress states such as infection, trauma and surgery or illness, and will require corticosteroid medicines to reduce the risk of adrenal crisis. High-dose corticosteroids enable the person to tolerate significant stress by their action in maintaining blood pressure, glucose homeostasis and other important effects. People who have been on glucocorticoid medicines in the previous 12 months may have degrees of adrenal insufficiency and may require corticosteroid replacement during stress states. Long-term use, systemic administration and high-dose therapy are more likely to suppress adrenal function than short-term use, low-dose therapy or topical courses.

If exogenous corticosteroids are stopped suddenly, the cortex cannot respond and the person rapidly becomes acutely ill. Thus, steroid doses need to be reduced gradually, rather than stopped suddenly, to enable normal adrenal function to return. Table 19.1 shows the main glucocorticoid preparations and their glucocorticoid potency and mineralocorticoid effects.

Table 19.1 The properties of some glucocorticoid agents

Corticosteroid	Duration	Anti-inflammatory activity	Mineralocorticoid activity
Hydrocortisone	Short	1	1
Cortisone	Short	0.8	1
Methylprednisolone	Intermediate	3.3–7.5	–
Prednisone	Intermediate	4	0.3–0.8
Prednisolone	Intermediate	4.2–5	0.3–0.8
Triamcinolone	Intermediate	5	–
Fluocortolone	Long	5	–
Budesonide	Short	17–20	–
Dexamethasone	Long	25–30	–
Betamethasone	Long	25–40	–
Fludrocortisone	Short	10	250

Note: – No activity.

Source: Bullock & Manias (2022), Table 54.2, p. 697

Corticosteroid treatment side-effects The most significant side-effect is relative *insulin resistance syndrome (IRS)*, which leads to hyperglycaemia. This may be new in onset, or become worse in people with an established diagnosis of diabetes mellitus. In this case, it may precipitate *hyperglycaemic hyperosmolar non-ketotic states (HONK)* (see the chapter 'Diabetes mellitus').

IRS causes post-prandial hyperglycaemia, and occurs because the glucocorticoid steroids down-regulate the glucose transporter GLUT-4 in muscles, so that more insulin is required to facilitate glucose uptake in cells, promote gluconeogenesis in the liver, reduce insulin binding to insulin receptors, and reduce insulin secretion from the pancreatic beta cells.

In addition, corticosteroid medicines can: suppress pituitary, adrenal and central nervous system (CNS) function even with short-term dosing; cause cardiovascular effects (e.g. hypertension, thrombophlebitis, thromboembolism and atherosclerosis); suppress the immune system, predisposing the individual to infection and delaying healing after surgery or wounds; cause glaucoma and cataracts; lead to muscle wasting and weakness; contribute to osteoporosis (and the consequent risk of spontaneous fractures and aseptic necrosis of the head of the femur); cause physical changes (e.g. moon face, buffalo hump, thin skin, striae, acne, thin hair); and induce mood changes.

Serious adverse effects are more likely to be associated with systemic rather than topical administration.

GLUCOCORTICOID IMBALANCES

LEARNING OBJECTIVE 4

Describe the clinical manifestations, diagnosis and clinical management of endocrine disorders characterised by imbalances in glucocorticoid secretion.

Hypercortisolism

Aetiology and pathophysiology

Hypercortisolism is characterised by *excessive cortisol secretion*. It is also known as **Cushing's disease**. Like hypocortisolism, it is classified as a rare condition, affecting 10–15 individuals per million people. It is commonly associated with a tumour that either secretes cortisol or stimulates cortisol production through excessive ACTH production. The tumour may be growing within the pituitary (representing 70–80% of all cases), the adrenal cortex itself or within another tissue not normally associated with the synthesis of these hormones (accounting for about 17% of cases), such as the lungs, thyroid, pancreas or thymus. Interestingly, ACTH-releasing pituitary tumours appear to be more common in young to middle-aged adults, and affect more women. ACTH-releasing ectopic tumours are more common in older men. Rarely, corticotropin-releasing hormone-secreting tumours are a cause of hypercortisolism through the stimulation of ACTH from the pituitary. They can arise within the thyroid, adrenal medulla and in neuroendocrine tumours.

Cushing's syndrome, another form of hypercortisolism, may also be seen in people during prolonged or high-dose glucocorticoid drug treatments. A dysfunctional state induced by drug therapy is known as an *iatrogenic condition*. We note that the terms 'Cushing's syndrome' and 'Cushing's disease' appear to be used interchangeably.

Clinical manifestations

Clinical manifestations of hypercortisolism involve a redistribution of subcutaneous fat, accumulating in three characteristic sites: the face, the abdomen (causing truncal obesity) and the upper thoracic region of the back. The lay terms for these distinctive signs involving the face and the back are 'moon face' and 'buffalo hump', respectively.

There may be weight gain, partly associated with sodium and water retention, due to the excessive glucocorticoid molecules interacting with aldosterone receptors. Blood pressure becomes elevated, to a degree due to water retention, and also associated with increased adrenergic receptor numbers on the vasculature, inducing a stronger vasoconstrictive response in response to SNS activation.

Increased gluconeogenesis and glycogenesis lead to the development of insulin resistance. Glucose intolerance may develop, which can deteriorate into diabetes mellitus in some people. The rate of protein catabolism is increased in order for more gluconeogenesis to take place. This can lead to peripheral muscle atrophy. Collagen synthesis is inhibited, leading to thin skin, which is easily bruised and, in combination with the increased protein catabolism, results in paper-thin skin and poor wound healing.

Glucocorticoids stimulate the increased loss of calcium ions into the forming urine (hypercalcaemia), which creates the ideal environment for kidney stone formation. The loss of calcium and protein from bones can induce a state of osteoporosis.

As glucocorticoids have a major modulating influence on immunity, immune suppression is an important consequence of hypercortisolism. Helper T (Th) cells are particularly vulnerable to this suppression, and, as they are key cells in promoting the immune response, the effect is significant. Glucocorticoid excess also inhibits pro-inflammatory chemical mediator production. Immune suppression makes the affected person susceptible to microbial infection: bacterial, viral and, in particular, *Candida albicans* infection. A focus of healthcare for these individuals must be to reduce the risk of infection wherever possible.

Glucocorticoids cross the blood–brain barrier, and in high concentrations can affect brain function. Irritability, psychotic behaviour and depression alternating with euphoria can occur. Excess glucocorticoid levels can induce androgen-like effects, leading to increased body hair, acne and oligomenorrhoea.

Clinical diagnosis and management

Diagnosis An initial 24-hour screening test to measure urinary free cortisol is the first test to be performed, but, as it has a 5–10% false negative rate, it is usually combined with other tests, such as an overnight dexamethasone suppression test. If both of these tests are within the normal range, Cushing's disease is unlikely.

Dexamethasone suppression test An overnight dexamethasone suppression test is performed to differentiate between pituitary-dependent and adrenal Cushing's disease. Dexamethasone is a long-acting glucocorticoid medication, which suppresses ACTH secretion but does not cross the blood–brain barrier; this enables the affected part of the HPA axis to be identified. Normally, cortisol levels are suppressed. If the HPA axis is functioning normally, cortisol production will be suppressed.

The test results need to be interpreted in light of a thorough history and assessment, because obesity, depression, stress and some medicines, such as antiseizure (anticonvulsant) medicines and oestrogen, can lead to elevated cortisol levels.

Once the diagnosis is established, high- or low-dose dexamethasone suppression testing may be needed to distinguish pituitary tumours from ectopic causes. These tests are similar to the overnight suppression test, but the dexamethasone dose and the sample collection times are different.

Other tests A low-dose dexamethasone suppression test can also be used where the drug is given every six hours for 48 hours (9 am, 3 pm, 9 pm, 3 am), which should suppress cortisol levels. Serum cortisol is measured at baseline and on day two.

Midnight cortisol levels can be used to determine loss of circadian rhythm, which is usually the case in Cushing's syndrome. The person must be asleep. Midnight is the normal cortisol nadir and the level is usually low. Those with pseudo-Cushing's syndrome also lose the normal cortisol diurnal rhythm, so an ITT might be performed.

Other hormones are usually measured as a part of this diagnostic phase, including thyroid hormone, growth hormone, thyroid-stimulating hormone, gonadotropins and androgens. CT, ultrasound or MRI scans of the adrenal glands and/or pituitary gland can be used in combination with the administration of the ferrometallic metal element gadolinium to localise the tumour.

Management Management depends on the cause. In the case of pituitary-dependent Cushing's disease, surgical removal of the tumour by transsphenoidal surgery is usual, and results in a successful cure in 90% of cases (see the chapter 'Hypothalamic–pituitary disorders'). Hydrocortisone is usually administered preoperatively on the assumption that the person will become cortisol-deficient postoperatively. The dose is gradually reduced postoperatively, and cortisol levels monitored.

Radiation therapy of the pituitary gland can be undertaken, but it takes longer than surgery to control the symptoms. Sometimes medicines and/or radiation are used to shrink pituitary tumours prior to surgery or following unsuccessful surgery, but it takes a long time to control the dysfunction. Radiotherapy also reduces the possibility of Nelson's syndrome occurring following adrenalectomy. Nelson's syndrome is where a pituitary tumour enlarges rapidly after adrenalectomy. Adrenalectomy is the treatment of choice in people with adrenal hyperplasia.

Symptoms of adrenal insufficiency occur after surgery when the ACTH and cortisol levels drop, usually within 12–48 hours. Hydrocortisone replacement therapy may be required for several months until normal adrenal function returns. However, replacement therapy will be required permanently if both adrenal glands are removed.

If surgery is contraindicated, an adrenal steroidogenesis inhibitor, such as metyrapone, can be used to treat ectopic ACTH or cortisol-producing tumours if they cannot be treated in any other way (surgery or chemotherapy). Metyrapone can lead to adrenal insufficiency; therefore, close monitored is required.

Treatment of Cushing's syndrome consists of reducing the dose gradually, if possible, so as to avoid the development of adrenal insufficiency. If not, alternate-day dosing reduces the symptoms and allows the adrenal glands to recover and respond normally to ACTH. Figure 19.4 explores the common clinical manifestations and management of adrenal cortical pathology related to cortisol.

MINERALOCORTICOID IMBALANCES

LEARNING OBJECTIVE 5

Describe the pathophysiological mechanisms and epidemiology involved in endocrine disorders characterised by imbalances in mineralocorticoid secretion.

The main stimulus for the release of the mineralocorticoid aldosterone is the renin–angiotensin system. However, activation of the HPA axis will, in addition to the release of cortisol, also trigger the secretion of aldosterone.

LEARNING OBJECTIVE 6

Describe the clinical manifestations, diagnosis and clinical management of endocrine disorders characterised by imbalances in mineralocorticoid secretion.

Hypoaldosteronism

Aetiology and pathophysiology The most common cause of primary hypoaldosteronism, unaccompanied by changes in glucocorticoid levels, is renal disease in which renin synthesis and release is impaired. The renin–angiotensin system (see Figure 19.5) is a major trigger for aldosterone secretion. As a part of its action, aldosterone facilitates the action of the sodium–potassium pump on the distal convoluted tubule cells to retain sodium ions in the blood and excrete potassium ions. Water molecules passively follow sodium back into the blood (see Figure 19.6).

Primary hypoaldosteronism may be seen in Addison's disease (see the previous section), and is also a consequence of congenital adrenal hyperplasia (see the following section). Hypoaldosteronism can develop in individuals with high, normal or low renin levels, but the latter state is more common, and is termed *hyporeninemic hypoaldosteronism*. Hypoaldosteronism can be induced by some commonly used medicines. Non-steroidal anti-inflammatory drugs (NSAIDs) can induce prostaglandin deficiency, and have been shown to be a reversible cause of hypoaldosteronism. Heparin, angiotensin-converting enzyme (ACE) inhibitors, angiotensin II receptor antagonists, aldosterone antagonists, calcium channel blockers and beta-adrenergic blockers can exacerbate hypoaldosteronism.

Clinical manifestations Hypoaldosteronism leads to increased sodium and water excretion accompanied by potassium retention. As a consequence, the clinical manifestations of this condition include hypotension, metabolic acidosis, hyponatraemia and hyperkalaemia. The effects of these electrolyte imbalances are outlined in the chapter 'Electrolyte imbalances'.

Clinical diagnosis and management Idiopathic hypoaldosteronism typically shows low levels of plasma and urine aldosterone and increased plasma renin. Management usually consists of therapy with the aldosterone-like corticosteroid fludrocortisone, and a liberal salt intake.

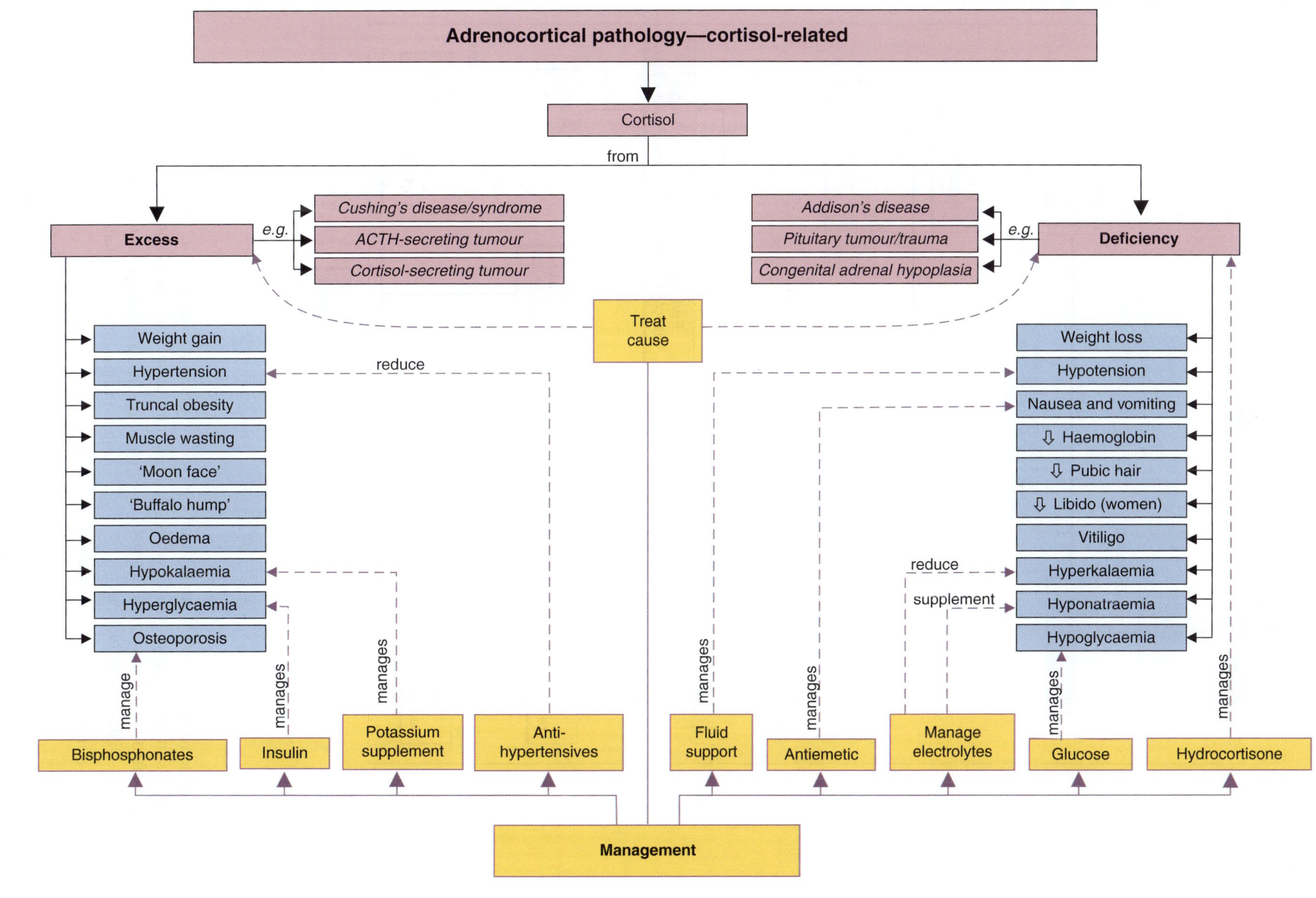

Figure 19.4

Clinical snapshot: Adrenocortical pathology—cortisol-related

↓ = decreased; ACTH = adrenocorticotropic hormone.

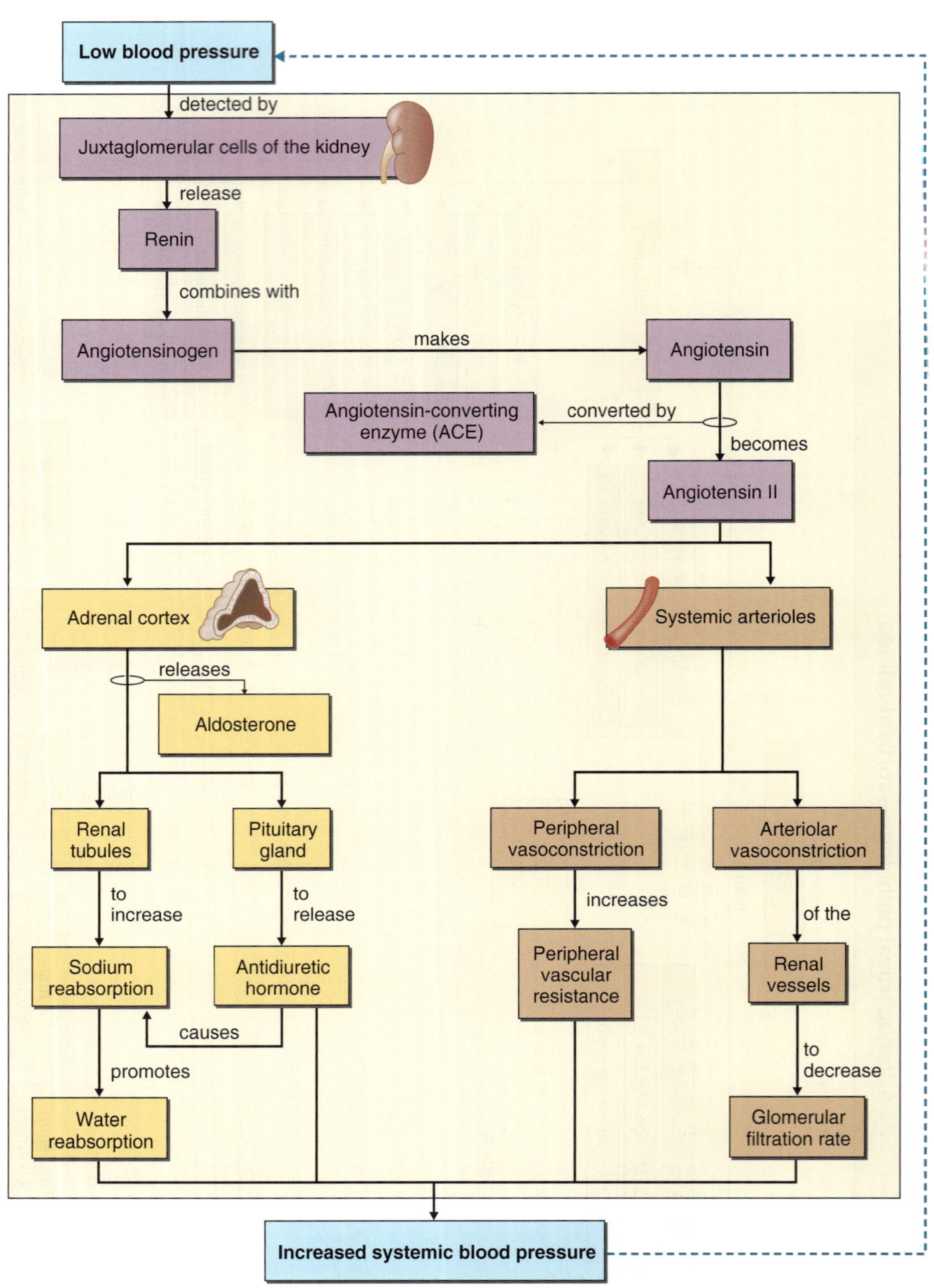

Figure 19.5
Renin–angiotensin system

Hyporeninemic hypoaldosteronism is often mild and undiagnosed. It usually presents in people aged over 45 years, and those with the condition often have chronic renal disease, including diabetic renal disease. Diagnostic features are:

- unexplained hyperkalaemia—a mild non-anion gap metabolic acidosis may be present
- low plasma aldosterone in the presence of hyperkalaemia—the ratio of aldosterone to renin tends to be in the normal range
- no significant increase in renin or aldosterone on administration of oral or IV furosemide
- the peak aldosterone response to ACTH is less than 16 ng/dL despite the prevailing hyperkalaemia.

Management consists of correcting the acidosis and liberalising sodium intake. Fludrocortisone therapy may be needed to control potassium levels without inducing congestive heart failure.

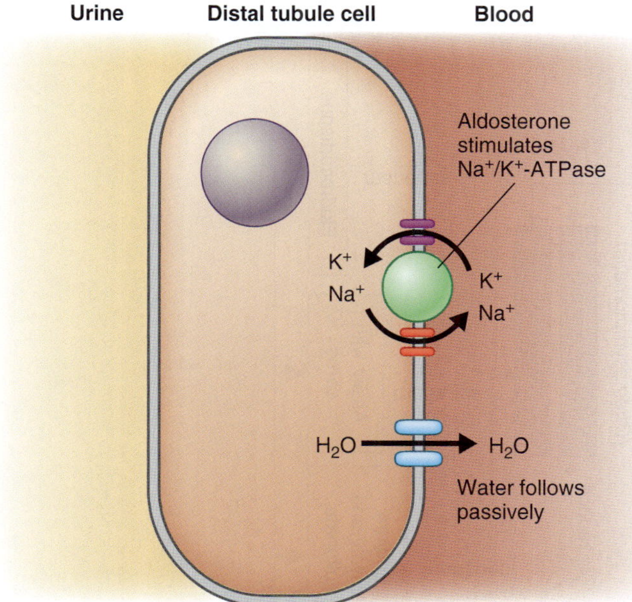

Figure 19.6

Cellular action of aldosterone

H_2O = water;
Na^+/K^+ ATPase = sodium–potassium pump.

A careful medication review is important to determine whether medicines are contributing causes. If that is the case, the medicine regimen will need to be revised.

If diabetes is a contributing cause, achieving optimal blood glucose levels will be important.

Hyperaldosteronism

The primary form of excessive aldosterone secretion is commonly associated with adrenal gland tumours or gland hyperplasia. It is also known as **Conn's disease**. Secondary hyperaldosteronism can develop in heart failure, kidney disease and cirrhosis of the liver as a result of significant disturbances in fluid homeostasis.

Clinical manifestations Excessive aldosterone secretion induces significant sodium and water retention in the blood, as well as undue potassium excretion. Therefore, the hallmark clinical manifestations of hyperaldosteronism are hypertension and hypokalaemia. The hypokalaemic state induces a number of manifestations, including muscle weakness, cardiac dysrhythmias, metabolic alkalosis and polyuria (see the chapter 'Electrolyte imbalances' for more detail). The alkolotic state affects calcium availability, leading to altered excitability in nerves and muscle. This manifests as tetany and paraesthesias.

Clinical diagnosis and management

Diagnosis Careful preparation is important before undertaking diagnostic investigations. If the serum potassium level is less than 3 mmol/L, it should be corrected. Angiotensin-converting enzyme (ACE) inhibitors and angiotensin II antagonists, diuretics, spironolactone, beta-blockers and calcium channel blockers can affect the test results, and so, if possible, the taking of these medicines should be ceased at least two to four weeks prior to testing. α-Adrenergic blockers can be used if necessary. Sometimes, a salt-loading diet is needed because a low-salt diet can mask hypokalaemia.

Diagnostic tests for hyperaldosteronism include serum potassium levels. Diuretic therapy may need to be ceased before collecting the urine because it can affect the results.

Plasma renin levels also need to be assessed, because renin is suppressed in primary hyperaldosteronism (which is also the case in one-third of people with essential hypertension). Importantly, antihypertensive medication and salt intake can affect the results of these tests. The ratio of aldosterone to renin can be a valuable indicator. The higher the ratio, the more likely the person has primary hyperaldosteronism. However, factors such as the time of the test, posture, antihypertensive medicines, especially beta-blockers and diuretics, and chronic renal failure (false negative) affect the results.

Other tests include an oral salt-loading diet, in which 120 mmol sodium/day is given for three days, which usually precipitates hypokalaemia. The dexamethasone suppression test, as already described, can be used. Aldosterone and blood pressure fall if the underlying cause of the hyperaldosteronism is Conn's syndrome, adrenal hyperplasia or *glucocorticoid-suppressible hyperaldosteronism (GSH*, a rare form of systemic hypertension). CT and/or MRI can also be used to determine the size, location and character of the adenoma.

A radiolabelled idocholesterol scan can be used to visualise adrenal adenomas. Dexamethasone is administered for three days prior to administering the isotope, and is continued for a week after the scan. Adenomas are visible before the fifth day of isotope treatment, whereas normal adrenal glands are seen after the fifth day.

Management Laparoscopic adrenalectomy is the treatment of choice for aldosterone-secreting adenomas. Fluids, corticosteroids and other medicines to maintain the blood pressure during surgery are imperative to prevent intra- and postoperative complications. Corticosteroid replacement is required temporarily, or permanently if a bilateral adrenalectomy is performed. Over 50% of people become normotensive within a month, and 70% within a year after surgery.

Medical management is sometimes successful; for example, angiotensin II-responsive adenomas might respond to ACE inhibitor therapy. Spironolactone, an aldosterone antagonist, can be used to treat hypertension and hypokalaemia associated with bilateral adrenal hyperplasia and idiopathic hyperaldosteronism, which do not respond well to surgery. Other antihypertensive agents, such ACE inhibitors and calcium channel blockers, are often needed. Potassium-sparing diuretics, such as amiloride and triamterene, are also used. The carbonic anhydrase inhibitor acetazolamide is useful in managing metabolic alkalosis.

GSH can be treated using low-dose dexamethasone twice a day. Spironolactone may be preferred, however, because of the side-effects of dexamethasone. Figure 19.7 explores the common clinical manifestations and management of adrenocortical pathology related to aldosterone.

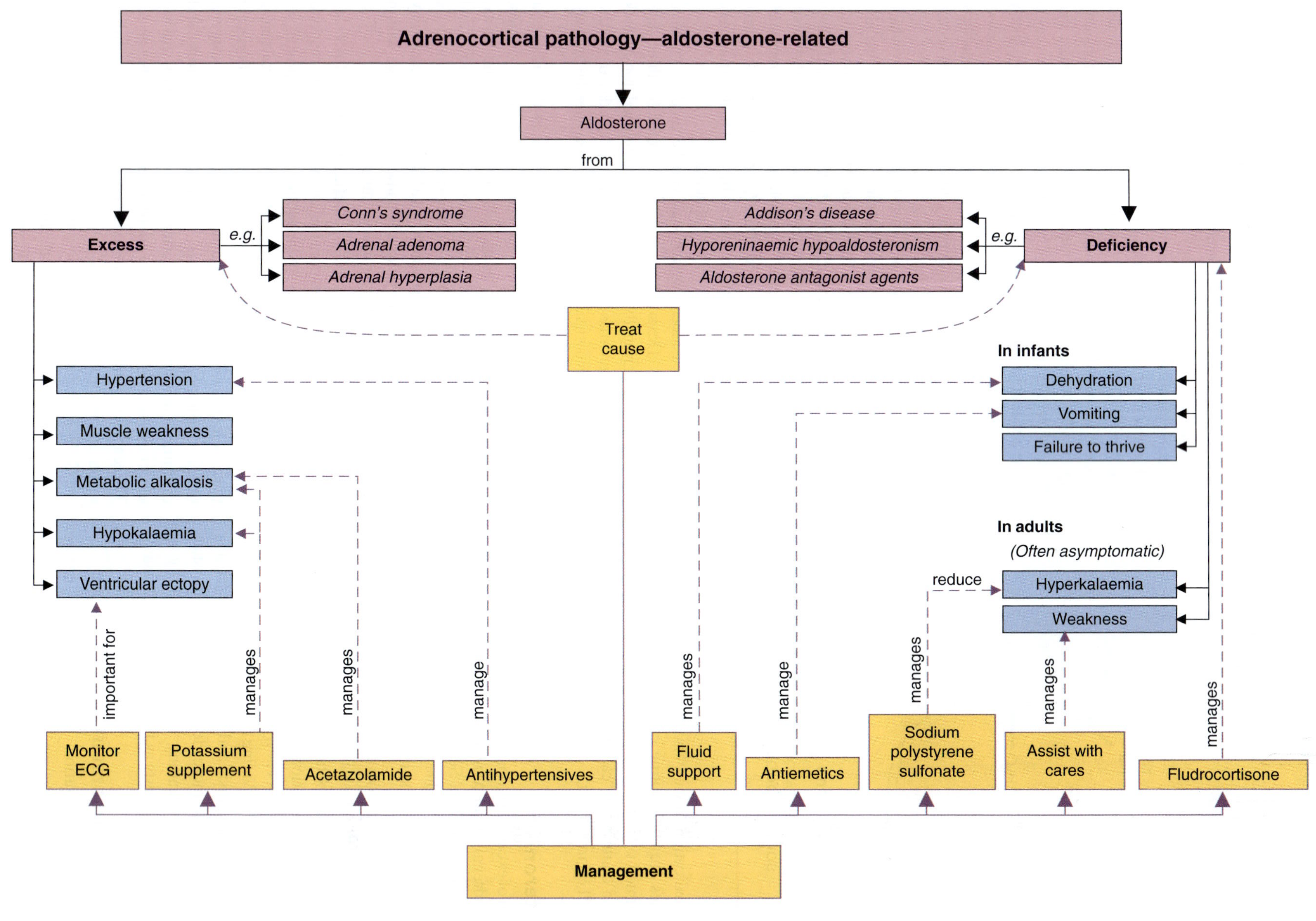

Figure 19.7

Clinical snapshot: Adrenocortical pathology—aldosterone-related

ECG = electrocardiogram.

GONADOCORTICOID IMBALANCES

LEARNING OBJECTIVE 7

Describe the pathophysiological mechanisms and epidemiology involved in endocrine disorders characterised by imbalances in gonadocorticoid secretion.

Excessive gonadocorticoid production is the only clinical disorder associated with a gonadocorticoid imbalance.

Hypersecretion of adrenal sex hormones

LEARNING OBJECTIVE 8

Describe the clinical manifestations, diagnosis and clinical management of endocrine disorders characterised by imbalances in gonadocorticoid secretion.

Aetiology and pathophysiology Hypersecretion of adrenal sex hormones may be seen in Cushing's disease or as a result of a tumour growing in the adrenal cortex. It also develops in a condition known as **congenital adrenal hyperplasia (CAH)**. As the terminology indicates, affected individuals are born with the disorder, although it may not be diagnosed until later in childhood. Australian and New Zealand statistics indicate an incidence of 1 affected baby in 15,000–20,000 births. In certain ethnic groups, such as Ashkenazi Jews and Hispanics, the incidence can be as high as 1 in 5,000.

In CAH, the most common form is an autosomal recessive condition involving a deficiency in the key enzyme in the corticosteroid biosynthetic pathway, 21-β-hydroxylase. In rarer forms, different enzymes in the pathway (3-β-hydroxysteroid dehydrogenase or 11-β-hydroxylase) will be affected. The corticosteroid pathway is shown in Figure 19.8, highlighting the role of 21-β-hydroxylase. There is a breakdown in the cortisol negative feedback system, leading to elevated corticotropin-releasing hormone and ACTH levels. The pathway for cortisol, corticosterone and aldosterone synthesis is disrupted, resulting in an accumulation of intermediate substances at the point of the blocked pathway. The only synthetic pathway that remains intact is the one to the gonadocorticoids, so production of these hormones is increased. In effect, hypersecretion of gonadocorticoids occurs at the cost of normal glucocorticoid and mineralocorticoid production. In affected persons, severe adrenal insufficiency is a medical emergency and can be life-threatening. This state can also affect adrenomedullary development, leading to adrenaline deficiency.

There are three main forms of the condition: *salt-losing, virilising* and *mild forms*. The first two forms are grouped as *classic CAH*. The mild form is referred to as *non-classic CAH*.

Clinical manifestations Severely affected infants will show signs of adrenal insufficiency: hyperkalaemia, elevated renin levels, hyponatraemia, hypovolaemia and shock.

In the mild form, the condition may not be detected for some years. The first evidence may well manifest as precocious puberty, where the child shows enhanced development of secondary sex characteristics at around 8–9 years old, such as the presence of pubic and axillary hair, accelerated skeletal maturation and linear growth.

In female infants the presence of ambiguous male-like genitalia would be readily detected. For male infants, there may be hyperpigmentation of the external genitalia, but otherwise it will appear normal.

In adolescents and adults, CAH is easier to recognise in females. Common manifestations include hirsutism, irregular menses, acne and infertility.

Clinical diagnosis and management Diagnosis is made on the basis of sex hormone levels and their precursor steroids, such as 17-hydroxyprogesterone (17-OHP), and levels of the enzyme 21-β-hydroxylase. However, 17-OHP can be

Figure 19.8
Simplified corticosteroid biosynthetic pathway

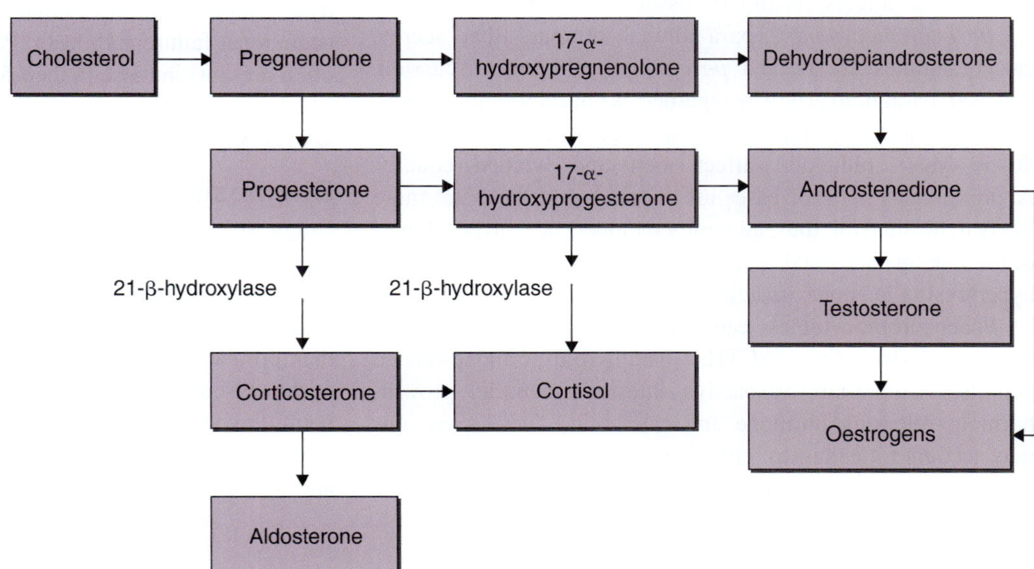

normal in babies who are deficient in 21-β-hydroxylase and in the presence of interfering substances, such as residual steroids from the mother. Gas chromatography and mass spectrometry can be used to measure 15 urinary steroids and their metabolites, and have recently been shown to improve the diagnosis.

Prenatally, amniotic fluid tests for 17-OHP and testosterone can be performed. Management depends on correctly assigning the child to the gender they are most closely orientated towards. This involves careful explanations and counselling for the family to help them decide on management.

Management options include sex hormone therapy and/or genital surgical correction, followed by regular physical and emotional follow-up. Fludrocortisone is used in mineralocorticoid replacement therapy. The choice of glucocorticoid therapy depends on the age of the individual. Hydrocortisone is preferred in infants and children; prednisolone or dexamethasone is used in the management of adolescents and adults. Stress dosing with glucocorticoids is required during illness or at times of stress. Antiandrogen treatment is useful in women with severe acne and hirsutism.

Disorders of the adrenal medulla

AETIOLOGY AND PATHOPHYSIOLOGY

LEARNING OBJECTIVE 9

Describe the pathophysiological mechanisms and epidemiology involved in the endocrine disorder characterised by an imbalance in adrenal medullary hormone secretion.

Only one endocrine disorder affecting the adrenal medulla manifests as a human clinical condition. This disorder involves hypersecretion of the catecholamine hormones, adrenaline and noradrenaline. These hormones are a normal part of the short-term stress response, enhancing SNS activation. In excess, the affected person experiences overstimulation of SNS effects.

The most common cause of this state is a benign adrenal tumour that affects medullary tissue. This tumour is called a *phaeochromocytoma*. Extra-adrenal tumours that secrete catecholamines are termed *paragliomas*. In this discussion, however, paragliomas will be regarded as phaeochromocytomas.

Phaeochromocytomas tend to occur in middle age, 40–50 years old, and affect men and women equally. Approximately 10% of cases are familial, and these are more likely to be bilateral; thus, all family members need to be advised of the risk and screened. Such a tumour is the cause of chronic hypertension in approximately 1 in 1,000 people.

Phaeochromocytomas can co-secrete a range of other hormones, including ACTH, parathyroid-hormone-related peptide, vasopressin, vasoactive intestinal peptide, growth-hormone-releasing hormone and calcitonin. These secretions may account for a range of clinical manifestations separate from those related to catecholamine action.

LEARNING OBJECTIVE 10

Describe the clinical manifestations, diagnosis and clinical management of the endocrine disorder characterised by an imbalance in adrenal medullary hormone secretion.

CLINICAL MANIFESTATIONS

The specific symptoms and their severity are influenced by the proportion of adrenaline and noradrenaline the tumour produces. Typical symptoms include the coexistence of the 'five Hs', which occurs in 94% of those presenting and has a diagnostic sensitivity of 90%. The five Hs are *h*ypertension, *h*eadache, *h*yperglycaemia, *h*ypermetabolism and *h*yperhydrosis. Hypertension can be sustained or episodic, and is often resistant to antihypertensive medicines. Phaeochromocytoma is a rare underlying cause of new diagnosis of hypertension (0.2%). If it is not detected and treated, it can be fatal. Hypertension can be paroxysmal or present all of the time, when it can be difficult to distinguish from other more common causes of hypertension. Postural hypertension is present in approximately 70% of those with the condition. Phaeochromocytoma should be considered if significant hypertension is occurring in association with signs of SNS overactivity.

Other symptoms include cardiovascular symptoms, gastrointestinal symptoms, heat intolerance, tremor, flushing and anxiety.

A significant concern associated with this state is that if is not treated it will lead to long-term complications such as cardiac and kidney disease, visual impairment and stroke. Phaeochromocytoma sometimes presents as part of multiple endocrine neoplasia type 2 (MEN 2), and this association should be considered in those who present with thyroid carcinoma or parathyroid hyperplasia (see the chapter 'Thyroid and parathyroid disorders').

Symptoms often occur in paroxysms of varying duration, from seconds to several hours. People report a variety of symptoms during these paroxysms, such as anxiety or a feeling of impending doom, weakness, headache, dizziness, visual changes, polysuria, gastrointestinal symptoms, dyspnoea and hunger. Blood pressure may be dangerously high during a paroxysm, and predispose the individual to cardiac dysrhythmias, cerebrovascular events, dissecting aneurysm, and acute renal failure and death. Paroxysmal phaeochromocytoma often presents in those in their 50s.

CLINICAL DIAGNOSIS AND MANAGEMENT

Diagnosis

Diagnosis consists of a careful history to elicit symptoms. Twenty-four hour urine is collected in bottles containing acid as an initial screening test to determine urinary free catecholamines and/or their metabolites. Catecholamine levels will be higher than normal. Twenty-four hour collections are needed because of the episodic nature of catecholamine secretion. It can also be helpful to collect urine during a symptomatic episode.

Some medicines and foods can affect the results of these tests, and so the person needs written instructions about preparing for

Table 19.2 Examples of foods, medicines and activities that can affect urine and serum catecholamine (adrenaline and noradrenaline) levels

Foods	Medicines that can increase catecholamine output	Medicines that can decrease catecholamine output	Other
Coffee	Aspirin	Clonidine	Smoking
Tea	Caffeine	Disulfiram	Stress
Coca-Cola	Paracetamol	Imipramine	Trauma
Bananas	Levodopa	MAO inhibitors	Surgery
Vanilla	Tetracyclines	Phenothiazines	Infection
Chocolate	Glyceryl trinitrate	Salicylates	
Blue vein cheese	Decongestants		
	Tricyclic antidepressants		

MAO = monoamine oxidase.
Physical and emotional stress also cause the release of the catecholamine hormones as part of the normal stress response. These factors must be controlled as much as possible when undertaking diagnostic testing for phaeochromocytoma.

the test and how to collect their urine. Substances and activities that can affect the test results are shown in Table 19.2.

Levels significantly higher than the normal range are diagnostic of phaeochromocytoma, but further testing might be needed if the level is not significantly above normal and unexplained sympathetic symptoms are present. The types of diagnostic tests are described below.

Clonidine suppression test Blood is collected at baseline and then 120 and 180 minutes after an oral dose of clonidine is administered. Clonidine is a centrally acting antiadrenergic agent, which suppresses catecholamine release mediated by the SNS. Normally, the total serum catecholamine level falls by about 40% from baseline within two to three hours. In phaeochromocytoma, catecholamine levels increase because excess catecholamine hormones bypass the usual storage and releasing mechanisms and diffuse into the circulation; this process is not suppressed by clonidine. False positive results can occur in those with primary hypertension.

Pentolinium suppression test In this test, a basal blood sample is collected, then a dose of pentolinium is administered IV, and a second blood sample is collected after 30 minutes to measure plasma catecholamine levels.

Glucagon test This test is rarely used because it can provoke a crisis, and α- and β-receptor blockade is needed before the test is performed. An IV dose of glucagon is administered after collecting a basal blood sample, followed by sampling at 2, 4, 6, 8 and 10 minutes to measure plasma catecholamine levels.

Scans CT, MRI and ultrasound scans are used to detect and localise the phaeochromocytoma.

Other blood tests Serum levels of other endocrine hormones are performed to detect any concomitant hormone abnormalities. Serum calcium and calcitonin testing might also be indicated if MEN 2 is likely (see the chapter 'Thyroid and parathyroid disorders').

Adrenal vein sampling is sometimes used to localise the tumour if CT and other imaging techniques are not helpful. Full α- and β-receptor blockade before the procedure is necessary. Venous drainage of both adrenal glands is via the central vein. Catecholamines are measured in each adrenal vein, as well as from a peripheral vein. A higher noradrenaline than adrenaline ratio is suggestive of a phaeochromocytoma.

Management

Surgical removal of the phaeochromocytoma is the usual treatment, but medical management is needed to manage paroxysms and prepare the person for surgery.

Medical management Medical management consists of managing hypertensive paroxysms by bed rest, with the head of the bed elevated, and managing the associated anxiety and emotional distress. Careful preoperative blood pressure control over 7–10 days is imperative to ensure the blood pressure will remain stable during anaesthesia and surgery. The medicine doses and the person's response must be monitored very carefully, because those with phaeochromocytomas can be very sensitive to these agents. Cardiac monitoring is indicated, and α- and β-adrenoreceptor blockade is needed.

α-Adrenergic blockade using phenoxybenzamine is commenced as soon as the diagnosis is made. Beta blockade follows after 48–72 hours using propranolol. Vasodilators such as sodium nitroprusside may be required to lower the blood pressure and prevent cardio- and cerebrovascular events.

Other medicines that inhibit catecholamine synthesis (e.g. metyrosine) are sometimes used. In addition, the person needs to be well hydrated before surgery.

Surgical management Adrenalectomy to remove the tumour is the most effective treatment. Exploration of other potential tumour sites is sometimes indicated to ensure all of the tumour tissue is removed. Bilateral adrenalectomy will be necessary if bilateral tumours are present. The blood pressure must be closely monitored during surgery, because manipulation of the tumour can precipitate the release of stored catecholamines. Surgical stress contributes to the risk of intraoperative hypertension.

Postoperatively, corticosteroid replacement therapy is usual in the first few days or weeks, and will be necessary long term if bilateral adrenalectomy was performed. Hypotension and hypoglycaemia can occur postoperatively due to the sudden drop in catecholamine levels. Figure 19.9 explores the common clinical manifestations and management of phaeochromocytoma.

INDIGENOUS HEALTH FAST FACTS AND CULTURAL CONSIDERATIONS

FAST FACTS

- *Aboriginal and Torres Strait Islander peoples are more likely than non-Indigenous Australians to experience high levels of stress and have a higher incidence of mental health disorders.*
- *In 2018–19, 31% of Aboriginal adults and 23% of Torres Strait Islander adults reported high to very high levels of psychological distress.*
- *In a small laboratory-based study, cortisol awakening response was found to be blunted in Indigenous Australian participants compared to non-Indigenous peers, correlating to higher levels of chronic stress. No difference was found in cortisol excretion in response to acute psychosocial stress.*
- *On average, Māori and Pacific Islands people are 1.5 times more likely than European New Zealanders to experience high or very high levels of stress, and Māori males are two times more likely to experience high or very high levels of stress. This potentially accounts for some of the reasons for increased levels of cortisol in this population.*

CULTURAL CONSIDERATIONS

- *As discussed in 'Cultural considerations' in the chapter 'Hypothalamic–pituitary disorders', dysregulation of stress hormones resulting from experiences of transgenerational trauma can have a critical influence in the development and function of an Aboriginal and Torres Strait Islander person's endocrine system. The adrenal gland produces noradrenaline and cortisol. Alterations in secretion of these hormones can contribute to many pathological conditions. Self-determination is seen as a powerful means to mitigate psychological distress.*

Source: Data from Australian Indigenous HealthInfoNet (2022); Berger et al. (2017); New Zealand Ministry of Health (2015).

CHILDREN AND ADOLESCENTS

- The incidence of congenital adrenal hyperplasia (CAH) is monitored by the Australian Paediatric Surveillance Unit, and is determined to be around 1 in 15,000 births. A screening program for CAH was recommended in 2020.
- New Zealand introduced congenital adrenal hyperplasia screening for newborns in the 1980s, and reports an incidence of approximately 1 in 20,000 births.

OLDER ADULTS

- Adrenal gland function changes with ageing. Cortical senescence and potentially compensatory hyperplasia (as a consequence of an inability to replace lost tissue) result in increased glucocorticoid secretion and decreased androgen secretion.
- Ageing causes dehydroepiandrosterone (DHEA) levels to decrease to approximately 20% of maximal levels, decreasing immune function, and contributing to atherosclerosis and osteoporosis.

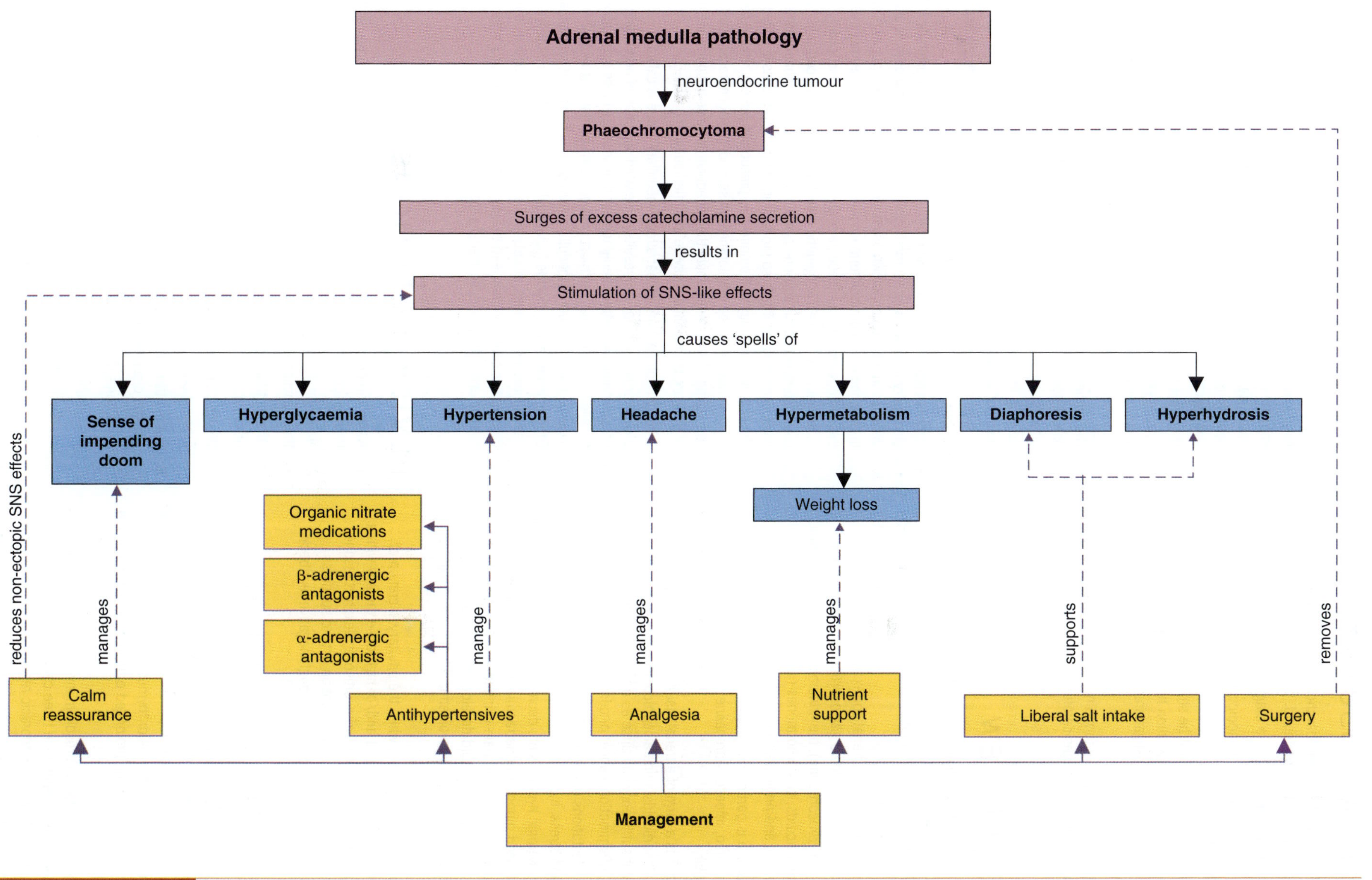

Figure 19.9

Clinical snapshot: Phaeochromocytoma

α = alpha; β = beta; SNS = sympathetic nervous system.

KEY CLINICAL ISSUES

- Body image and the emotional and psychological consequences of adrenal gland disorders can be profound.
- Life-long monitoring is needed once a diagnosis is made.
- Patient education about managing medicines, including during acute illnesses, is important.
- Corticosteroid medicines should not be stopped suddenly. Therefore, it is essential that those with the condition have written instructions for managing these medicines if investigations and surgery are required for another reason.
- Effective nursing care is necessary to maintain skin integrity, reduce infection risk and monitor vital signs carefully.

CHAPTER REVIEW

- The *adrenal glands* are involved in stress responsiveness, sugar availability and salt balance, as well as sexual development and maintenance. The glands are divided into two main regions: the *outer cortex* and the *inner medulla*.
- The hormones secreted by the adrenal cortex are called the *corticosteroids*. The cortex secretes *glucocorticoids*, the main one being *cortisol* (or *hydrocortisone*), the *mineralocorticoid aldosterone*, and the *gonadocorticoids*, or sex hormones (predominantly *androgens*, but also *oestrogens* and *progesterone*).
- The adrenal medulla is part of the *sympathetic nervous system* and, when stimulated, releases *adrenaline* and *noradrenaline*, which enhance its activity.
- *Addison's disease* is a form of adrenal insufficiency, which affects the secretion of glucocorticoids, mineralocorticoids and gonadocorticoids. Primary adrenal insufficiency can arise as a result of autoimmune attack, chronic inflammation, cancer or congenital malformation.
- The clinical manifestations of *adrenal insufficiency* include poor responsiveness to stress, hypoglycaemia, sparse body hair, anorexia and weight loss, chronic hypotension, decreased heart size, muscle weakness, depressed mood, hyponatraemia and hyperkalaemia. Skin pigmentation can darken in pale-skinned individuals to confer a tanned appearance. Severe or rapid development of this condition can be life-threatening, resulting in hypovolaemia, electrolyte imbalances and shock.
- *Secondary hypocortisolism* occurs when the pituitary secretion of ACTH is deficient, or after prolonged and/or high-dose therapy with a glucocorticoid medication, such as hydrocortisone, dexamethasone or prednisolone. The glucocorticoid medication acts to suppress the hypothalamic–pituitary–adrenal axis through negative feedback mechanisms.
- Hypercortisolism is also known as *Cushing's disease or Cushing's syndrome*. It is commonly associated with a tumour that either secretes cortisol or stimulates cortisol production through excessive ACTH production. The tumour may be growing within the pituitary or the adrenal cortex itself, or be due to ectopic secretion from another tissue, such as the lungs, thyroid, pancreas or thymus. Cushing's syndrome may be seen in people receiving prolonged or high-dose glucocorticoid drug treatments.
- Clinical manifestations of hypercortisolism involve a redistribution of subcutaneous fat, accumulating in three characteristic sites: the face, the abdomen and the upper thoracic region of the back. Weight gain, hypertension and glucose intolerance may develop, as well as peripheral muscle atrophy, skin that is easily bruised and becomes paper-thin, poor wound healing, hypercalcaemia and osteoporosis. As glucocorticoids have a major modulating influence on immunity, immune suppression is an important consequence of hypercortisolism. Irritability, depression alternating with euphoria, and psychotic behaviour can occur. Excess glucocorticoid levels can induce androgen-like effects, leading to increased body hair, acne and oligomenorrhoea.
- The most common cause of *hypoaldosteronism*, unaccompanied by changes in glucocorticoid levels, is *renal disease* in which renin synthesis and release is impaired. The clinical manifestations of this condition include hypotension, hyponatraemia and hyperkalaemia.
- The primary form of *excessive aldosterone secretion* is commonly associated with adrenal gland tumours or *gland hyperplasia*. It is also known as *Conn's disease. Secondary hyperaldosteronism* can develop in heart failure, kidney disease and cirrhosis of the liver as a result of significant disturbances in fluid homeostasis. The hallmark clinical manifestations of hyperaldosteronism are hypertension and hypokalaemia.
- Hypersecretion of adrenal sex hormones may be seen in Cushing's disease or as a result of a tumour growing in the adrenal cortex. It also develops in a condition known as *congenital adrenal hyperplasia (CAH)*. In CAH, the most common form involves a deficiency in a key enzyme in the corticosteroid biosynthetic pathway, *21-beta-hydroxylase*, due to an autosomal recessive genetic defect. The pathway for cortisol, corticosterone and aldosterone synthesis is blocked, but gonadocorticoid production remains intact, so production of these hormones is increased. The first evidence may well manifest as precocious puberty, where the child shows enhanced development of secondary sex characteristics at a very young age. In cases where the gonadocorticoid secretion is untypical of that sex, the condition may be identified early.
- A benign adrenal tumour that affects medullary tissue is called a *phaeochromocytoma*, and results in elevated secretion of adrenaline and noradrenaline. An extra-adrenal tumour that secretes these substances is called a *paraglioma*. The most common clinical manifestation of hypersecretion of adrenal medullary hormones is persistent hypertension. Other manifestations include facial flushing, tachycardia, palpitations, headaches, nervousness, anxiety and a state of hypermetabolism. If not treated, this condition may lead to long-term complications, such as cardiac and kidney disease, visual impairment and stroke.

REVIEW QUESTIONS

1. Name the hormones that are synthesised by the adrenal cortex, and their functions.
2. Name the hormones that are synthesised by the adrenal medulla, and their functions.
3. Differentiate between a primary, secondary and tertiary endocrine disorder.
4. Why is it important to gradually reduce the dose of corticosteroid medications?
5. Outline the main causes and clinical manifestations of the following adrenal disorders:
   - a Conn's disease
   - b Addison's disease
   - c Cushing's disease
   - d congenital adrenal hyperplasia

6 What are the warning signs of an Addisonian crisis?

7 What are the consequences of hypersecretion of adrenal medullary hormones?

8 A 55-year-old man with kidney disease goes to his doctor complaining of weakness in the muscles of his arm, and that he seems to be going to the toilet to urinate more frequently during the day. He has observed that his urine is very dilute in appearance. The doctor does some tests on the man, and determines that his blood pressure is elevated and that his blood potassium levels are low. Which adrenal disorder is this man experiencing?

9 A woman in her 50s has been having trouble with weight gain and hypertension for some months. Her family thinks that her face is getting fatter, and she has noticed that she is getting a 'fat tummy'. She observes more facial hair growing, but dismisses it as being postmenopausal. She appears to catch every minor respiratory infection that is going around and gets frequent bouts of thrush. Small wounds tend to take longer to heal. Her family also thinks that over this time she has been experiencing mood swings, going from a bit depressed to almost euphoric. There is evidence of some muscle wasting of the extremities. A bone scan shows that she has a decreased bone density.

a Which endocrine disorder do you think she is experiencing?

b State two possible causes of this condition.

HEALTH PROFESSIONAL CONNECTIONS

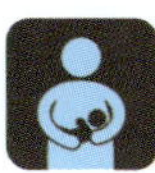

Midwives Pregnancy can have a significant effect on adrenal metabolism and function. The maternal and fetal pituitary–adrenal axes are also modified. Adrenocorticotropic hormone levels increase, and plasma cortisol levels peak during labour. A midwife should understand these significant adrenal changes so as to predict potential clinical sequelae. Also, delivery of any neonate with indeterminate genitalia should be investigated for possible causes. Adrenal disorders can cause very serious fluid and electrolyte disturbances. Neonates have very few compensatory mechanisms and no reserve, and, as such, can deteriorate rapidly. Frequent and appropriate observations for dehydration are important.

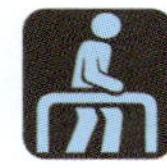

Physiotherapists Working with clients experiencing issues with adrenal pathology can complicate rehabilitation and exercise tolerance. Sodium retention can cause fluid overload and add significant volume to circulation or even into the interstitium. Fluid overload on the cardiac and respiratory system may interfere with oxygenation and impede efforts to promote mobility. Physiotherapists should report new observations of dyspnoea, or declining exercise tolerance. This information will be beneficial for understanding changes to the person's progress.

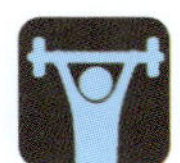

Exercise scientists Pathology affecting the function of the adrenal gland can have a significant influence on sodium and water balance. Exercise scientists should know and observe for the signs and symptoms of fluid or sodium excess or deficiency. Strenuous activity/exercise can exacerbate electrolyte imbalances.

Nutritionists/Dieticians People with adrenal pathology will experience issues with electrolytes. They may require dietary restrictions or supplements for sodium and potassium. Electrolyte balance can change rapidly, and modifications may be necessary as the individual's condition progresses or improves. Communication within the healthcare team is important to ensure that appropriate dietary modifications are occurring to best support the person's clinical status.

CASE STUDY

Baby Alicia Johnson is a 4-day-old old girl born at term following an uncomplicated labour and birth. On physical examination she had ambiguous genitalia. She has vomiting, dehydration and poor feeding. She has been diagnosed with congenital adrenal hyperplasia (CAH). Her observations were as follows:

Temperature	Heart rate	Respiration rate	Blood pressure	SpO_2
36.2°C	146	32	52/34	99% (RA*)

* RA = room air.

Baby Alicia's pathology results were as follows:

HAEMATOLOGY

Patient location:	Ward 3	**UR:**	824245		
Consultant:	Jones	**NAME:**	Johnson		
		Given name:	Alicia	**Sex:**	F
		DOB:	04/05/XX	**Age**	4d

Time collected	08:35
Date collected	XX/XX
Year	XXXX
Lab #	7866586

FULL BLOOD COUNT		UNITS	REFERENCE RANGE
Haemoglobin	115	g/L	115–160
White cell count	5.3	$\times 10^9$/L	4.0–11.0
Platelets	320	$\times 10^9$/L	140–400
Haematocrit	0.35		0.33–0.47
Red cell count	4.45	$\times 10^{12}$/L	3.80–5.20
Reticulocyte count	1.1	%	0.2–2.0
MCV	92	fL	80–100
Neutrophils	3.23	$\times 10^9$/L	2.00–8.00
Lymphocytes	2.12	$\times 10^9$/L	1.00–4.00
Monocytes	0.41	$\times 10^9$/L	0.10–1.00
Eosinophils	0.34	$\times 10^9$/L	< 0.60
Basophils	0.11	$\times 10^9$/L	< 0.20
ESR	5	mm/h	< 12

BIOCHEMISTRY

Patient location:	Ward 3	**UR:**	824245		
Consultant:	Jones	**NAME:**	Johnson		
		Given name:	Alicia	**Sex:**	F
		DOB:	04/05/XX	**Age:**	4d

Time collected	08:3
Date collected	XX/XX
Year	XXXX
Lab #	6865987

ELECTROLYTES		UNITS	REFERENCE RANGE
Sodium	129	mmol/L	132–147
Potassium	5.7	mmol/L	3.8–6.5
Chloride	96	mmol/L	98–115
Bicarbonate	21	mmol/L	15–28
Glucose	7.9	mmol/L	3.5–5.4
Iron	21	μmol/L	11–30

CRITICAL THINKING

1 Interpret baby Alicia's observations. Do they fall within appropriate ranges for a neonate? If not, identify any outlying observations, and explain their occurrence.

2 Observe baby Alicia's biochemistry results. Identify any parameter outside the reference range, and explain the pathophysiological reason for the change in relation to CAH.

3 What observations and physical assessments would you see in a neonate with dehydration?

4 Does the clinical presentation of a female neonate with CAH differ from that of a male neonate with CAH? Explain.

5 What interventions will be required to assist baby Alicia with her current clinical issues? Create a table identifying all of the outlying assessments and clinical data. List the symptoms in one column, and the interventions to manage each symptom in the other column.

BIBLIOGRAPHY

Australian Indigenous Health*Info*Net (2022). *Overview of Aboriginal and Torres Strait Islander health status, 2021.* Perth, WA: Australian Indigenous Health*Info*Net. https://healthinfonet.ecu.edu.au/learn/health-facts/overview-aboriginal-torres-strait-islander-health-status/.

Australian Institute of Health and Welfare (AIHW) (2022). *Australia's health, 2022*. Australia's Health series No. 15. Cat. No. AUS 241. Canberra: AIHW. https://www.aihw.gov.au/reports-data/australias-health.

Barthel, A., Benker, G., Berens, K., Diederich, S., Manfras, B., Gruber, M., ... Bornstein, S.R. (2019). An update on Addison's disease. *Experimental and Clinical Endocrinology and Diabetes* 127(02/03):165–75. https://doi.org/10.1055/a-0804-2715.

Bauldoff, G., Gubrud-Howe, P.M., Carno, M.-A., Levett-Jones, T., Hales, M., Berry, K., ... Stanley, D. (2020). *LeMone and Burke's medical–surgical nursing critical thinking for person-centred care* (4th [Australian] edn). Sydney: Pearson Australia.

Berger, M., Leicht, A., Slatcher, A., Kraeuter, A.K., Ketheesan, S., Larkins, S. & Sarnyai, Z. (2017). Cortisol awakening response and acute stress reactivity in First Nations people. *Scientific Reports* 7:41760. https://doi.org/10.1038/srep41760.

Best, O. & Fredericks, B. (2021). *Yatdjuligin: Aboriginal and Torres Strait Islander nursing and midwifery care* (3rd edn). Port Melbourne, VIC: Cambridge University Press.

Bornstein, S.R., Allolio, B., Arlt, W., Barthel, A., Don-Wauchope, A., Hammer, G.D., ... Torpy, D.J. (2016). Diagnosis and treatment of primary adrenal insufficiency: an Endocrine Society Clinical Practice Guideline. *Journal of Clinical Endocrinology and Metabolism* 101(2):364–89. https://doi.org/10.1210/jc.2015-1710.

Blake, M.A. (2021). Pheochromocytoma. *Emedicine*. https://emedicine.medscape.com/article/124059-overview.

Bullock, S. & Manias, E. (2022). *Fundamentals of pharmacology* (9th edn). Sydney: Pearson Australia.

Griffing, G.T. (2022). Addison disease. *Emedicine*. https://emedicine.medscape.com/article/116467-overview.

Marieb, E.N. & Hoehn, K. (2016). *Human anatomy and physiology* (10th edn). San Francisco, CA: Pearson Benjamin Cummings.

Marieb, E.N. & Hoehn, K. (2019). *Human anatomy and physiology* (11th edn). San Francisco, CA: Pearson Benjamin Cummings.

New Zealand Ministry of Health (2015). *Tatau kahukura: Māori health chart book 2015* (3rd edn). Wellington: Ministry of Health. http://www.health.govt.nz.

Nguyen, H.C.T. (2022). Endogenous Cushing syndrome. *Emedicine.* https://emedicine.medscape.com/article/2233083-overview.

Stats New Zealand (2021). *New Zealand period life tables: 2017–19.* Wellington: Stats New Zealand. https://datainfoplus.stats.govt.nz/item/nz.govt.stats/6e1b4ccb-d27b-415c-91c6-f9df3cb64484/2.

Wilson, T.A. (2022). Congenital adrenal hyperplasia. *Emedicine*. https://emedicine.medscape.com/article/919218-overview.

20 Diabetes mellitus

KEY TERMS

Diabetes mellitus
Diabetic ketoacidosis (DKA)
Hyperglycaemia
Hypoglycaemia
Kussmaul breathing
Macrovascular disease
Metabolic syndrome
Microvascular disease
Neuropathies
Non-ketotic hyperosmolar coma

LEARNING OBJECTIVES

After completing this chapter, you should be able to:

1 Define 'diabetes mellitus', and differentiate it from diabetes insipidus.

2 Describe and contrast the pathophysiologies of type 1, type 2 and gestational diabetes mellitus.

3 Outline the defining characteristics of each type of diabetes mellitus.

4 Define 'metabolic syndrome'.

5 Describe the acute complications of diabetes mellitus, and indicate which types are more likely to show each complication.

6 Outline the ways in which a diagnosis of diabetes mellitus is determined.

7 State the chronic complications of diabetes mellitus, and the pathophysiology of each.

8 Outline the ways in which types 1 and 2 diabetes mellitus are monitored and managed.

WHAT YOU SHOULD KNOW BEFORE YOU START THIS CHAPTER

Can you describe the endocrine functions of the pancreas?

Can you outline how the blood glucose level is normally controlled?

Can you describe the processes involved in cellular metabolism and energy production?

Can you define the term 'osmosis'?

Can you identify the important determinants of fluid movement between body compartments?

Can you outline the key concepts associated with endocrine dysfunction?

Introduction

LEARNING OBJECTIVE 1

Define 'diabetes mellitus', and differentiate it from diabetes insipidus.

Diabetes mellitus is a metabolic disorder characterised by the abnormal secretion and/or action of the pancreatic hormone insulin, which is essential for the cellular uptake of glucose. As a consequence, blood glucose levels rise and **hyperglycaemia**—the defining feature of this disorder—develops. Diabetes mellitus should not be confused with *diabetes insipidus*, which is characterised by the deficient secretion or action of the pituitary hormone, antidiuretic hormone (ADH) (see the chapter 'Hypothalamic–pituitary disorders').

Diabetes mellitus is not regarded as one single disease; instead, it is a group of quite separate diseases with different causes, genetic patterns, epidemiology and pathophysiologies that share the common feature of insulin dysfunction and hyperglycaemia. However, the boundaries separating the different diseases in this group are somewhat blurred. Some people with diabetes mellitus can show a combination of the features of two or more of the different forms, and in some instances move from one type to another. Still, in the long term, sufferers of the various forms of diabetes mellitus frequently end up with a severe imbalance between the supply of insulin and its demand. This imbalance has a similar effect on metabolism, and results in a suite of comparable complications.

Diabetes is a global health problem with a staggering increase in the number of people affected over the past decade or so. Recent statistics from 2021 estimate the global prevalence in adults to be 536.6 million people. By 2045, this figure is expected to increase by 46%. Globally, an estimated 108,300 children under 15 years old were diagnosed with diabetes in 2021. The Australian Bureau of Statistics' 2020–21 National Health Survey has revealed that 1.3 million Australians have diabetes mellitus, representing 5.3% of the population. Up to 500,000 more are believed to have silent, undiagnosed diabetes. The prevalence is similar in males (5.7%) and females (4.9%). In people 75 years and over, the prevalence increases to 19.2%. In New Zealand, it is estimated that more than 250,000 people have the disorder, with an overall prevalence of 6.2%.

Diabetes mellitus is associated with significant morbidity, disability and premature death, and, according to the Australian Institute of Health Welfare, it accounted for about 6% of the overall disease burden in Australia in 2018. People with diabetes mellitus frequently go on to develop chronic cardiovascular, renal, visual and nervous system impairments.

This chapter will focus on three main forms of diabetes: type 1, type 2 and gestational diabetes mellitus.

LEARNING OBJECTIVE 2

Describe and contrast the pathophysiologies of type 1, type 2 and gestational diabetes mellitus.

LEARNING OBJECTIVE 3

Outline the defining characteristics of each type of diabetes mellitus.

Type 1 diabetes mellitus

AETIOLOGY AND PATHOPHYSIOLOGY

Type 1 diabetes mellitus (T1D or T1DM) is characterised by extensive damage to the pancreatic islet-beta cells that synthesise and release insulin. The damage is induced by the person's own immune system via an autoimmune attack. This attack comprises both humoral and cellular processes; however, T cells are the dominant immune cell within the lesion site. Autoantibodies are produced against insulin, proinsulin, cellular zinc transporters and other beta pancreatic cell proteins. However, these autoantibodies are not sufficient for clinical development. In some people, autoantibodies are present but the person does not manifest clinical diabetes.

In time, the islet-beta cell population will become decimated. Insulin production and release decreases to a point where the hormone deficiency that arises becomes absolute (see Figure 20.1). The condition can develop slowly over a number of years (indeed,

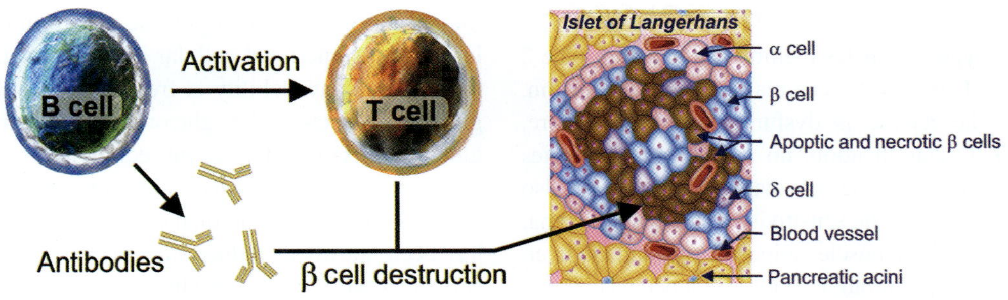

Figure 20.1

Pathophysiology of autoimmune type 1 diabetes mellitus

After plasma B cells produce antibodies and activate T cells, pancreatic beta cells begin to be destroyed. α = alpha; β = beta; δ = delta.

a person can show islet cell autoantibodies in the blood long before the condition manifests) or relatively rapidly. It is possible for an affected person's body to compensate physiologically up until 80–90% of their beta pancreatic cells are destroyed.

The cause of this autoimmune attack is unclear. The current view is that some people are genetically predisposed to such a response, and, when exposed to a suitable environmental trigger, the process is activated. Possible triggers include viral infection, dietary proteins (e.g. A1 beta-casein), stress, increased hygiene altering the maturation of the immune system, and an increased insulin demand brought about by rapid body growth (e.g. during puberty). Research also suggests that an alteration in the gut's normal flora composition (i.e. the microbiome) might change metabolic and immune signalling to the pancreas, resulting in a pancreatic autoimmune attack.

Interestingly, an association between other autoimmune diseases and T1D has been found, as conditions such as coeliac disease or autoimmune thyroiditis may be present, either at a clinical or subclinical level, in those affected. Genetic predisposition to these conditions can be predicted by the presence of a particular set of genetic markers called *human leukocyte antigens (HLAs)* (see the chapter 'Immune disorders'). T1D may also arise secondary to another disease, such as pancreatitis.

EPIDEMIOLOGY

The incidence of T1D is 10–13 new cases per 100,000 people with diabetes in Australia, and accounts for 10% of all diabetes cases. T1D can develop at any age, but the peak age of diagnosis is 10–19 years old, with people under 25 years old accounting for 63% of new diagnoses. This is not surprising, as the metabolic demands of an older child or adolescent with this condition start to exceed the supply of insulin, revealing the dysfunction clinically. The incidence rate is higher in males across most age groups. The International Diabetes Foundation (IDF) Diabetes Atlas 2021 estimates that globally 1,211,900 children and adolescents under the age of 20 have T1D.

Figure 20.2 explores the common clinical manifestations and management of T1D.

Type 2 diabetes mellitus

AETIOLOGY AND PATHOPHYSIOLOGY

Unlike people with type 1 diabetes mellitus, people with type 2 diabetes mellitus (T2D or T2DM) can make and release insulin, but the nature of the release is dysfunctional. Furthermore, according to the T2D classification, no insulin autoantibodies should be present at the time of diagnosis. T2D is also characterised by a change in the sensitivity to the insulin signal of peripheral tissues, such as muscle, adipose tissue and the liver. This change in sensitivity is thought to involve a decrease in the number of insulin receptors (called *receptor down-regulation*), a *derangement in the intracellular signalling cascades* following receptor activation, or a combination of the two. This phenomenon is referred to as *cellular insulin resistance*. Transient insulin resistance can occur normally during our lives, at times such as puberty and/or pregnancy. The insulin resistance that occurs under these conditions is due, at least in part, to the increased secretion of growth hormone and other substances that have an anti-insulin action. Normally, compensatory processes are activated regarding pancreatic insulin secretion. As insulin sensitivity decreases, insulin release increases in order to maintain glucose homeostasis (see Figure 20.3).

In T2D, the pancreatic beta cells cannot compensate for this loss of sensitivity, and become dysfunctional as a result of persistent stimulation. *Hyperglycaemia* (a high blood glucose level) develops. Indeed, in people with T2D, a compensatory hyperinsulinaemia can occur at the early stages of the disease, particularly in the pre-clinical phase, providing a functional reserve of insulin secretion. The degree of insulin resistance usually worsens over time, leading to progressive beta cell dysfunction, loss of functional reserve, cell loss and, ultimately, exhaustion. A lack of insulin triggers higher glucagon levels, contributing to further elevations in blood glucose levels.

There is evidence that the stressed islet-beta cell stimulates a local inflammatory response which may contribute to cell loss. Vitamin D deficiency has also been linked to the development of insulin resistance and hyperinsulinaemia. Vitamin D has a role in the normal release of insulin from the pancreas. Excessive insulin release triggers intracellular calcium overload and the formation of reactive oxygen species (see the chapter 'Pathophysiological terminology, cellular adaptation and injury'). Vitamin D may have a role in mediating hyperinsulinaemia and helping to reduce inflammation, intracellular calcium release and free radical formation.

Importantly, insulin resistance is associated with premorbid states, such as obesity, and in disorders such as polycystic ovary syndrome (see the chapter 'Female reproductive disorders'), but beta cell dysfunction and failure are the defining characteristics of T2D.

Genetic predisposition and lifestyle factors, such as diet and activity levels, do interact to induce and advance T2D. The condition shows a clear-cut familial inheritance pattern, where the offspring and siblings of an affected person have a greatly increased risk of developing this type of diabetes, especially in Indigenous families (see the 'Indigenous health fast facts' section).

T2D is strongly associated with *obesity*, especially when there are excess central (abdominal) fat deposits. There are a number of reasons for this. Insulin resistance has been found to be strongly linked to obesity, whether diabetes is present or not. Fat accumulation within the liver and muscle in obese people impairs insulin-mediated glucose uptake into these tissues and leads to dysfunctional cellular insulin signalling. Excess body fat boosts the availability of free fatty acids, increasing hepatic glucose production (i.e. gluconeogenesis) and inhibiting both glucose utilisation and insulin secretion.

Certain types of fatty acids appear to produce stronger effects on insulin action than others. Release of free fatty acids has been shown to induce *insulin resistance* and impair beta cell function. Peptides produced by fat cells also play a very important role in regulating metabolism and immune function. One of these peptides, adiponectin, has been shown to increase the sensitivity of peripheral cells to insulin. Low adiponectin levels correlate with insulin resistance, beta cell dysfunction and increased abdominal fat deposits. Indeed, adiponectin levels have been found to be low in people with T2D and in those with insulin resistance.

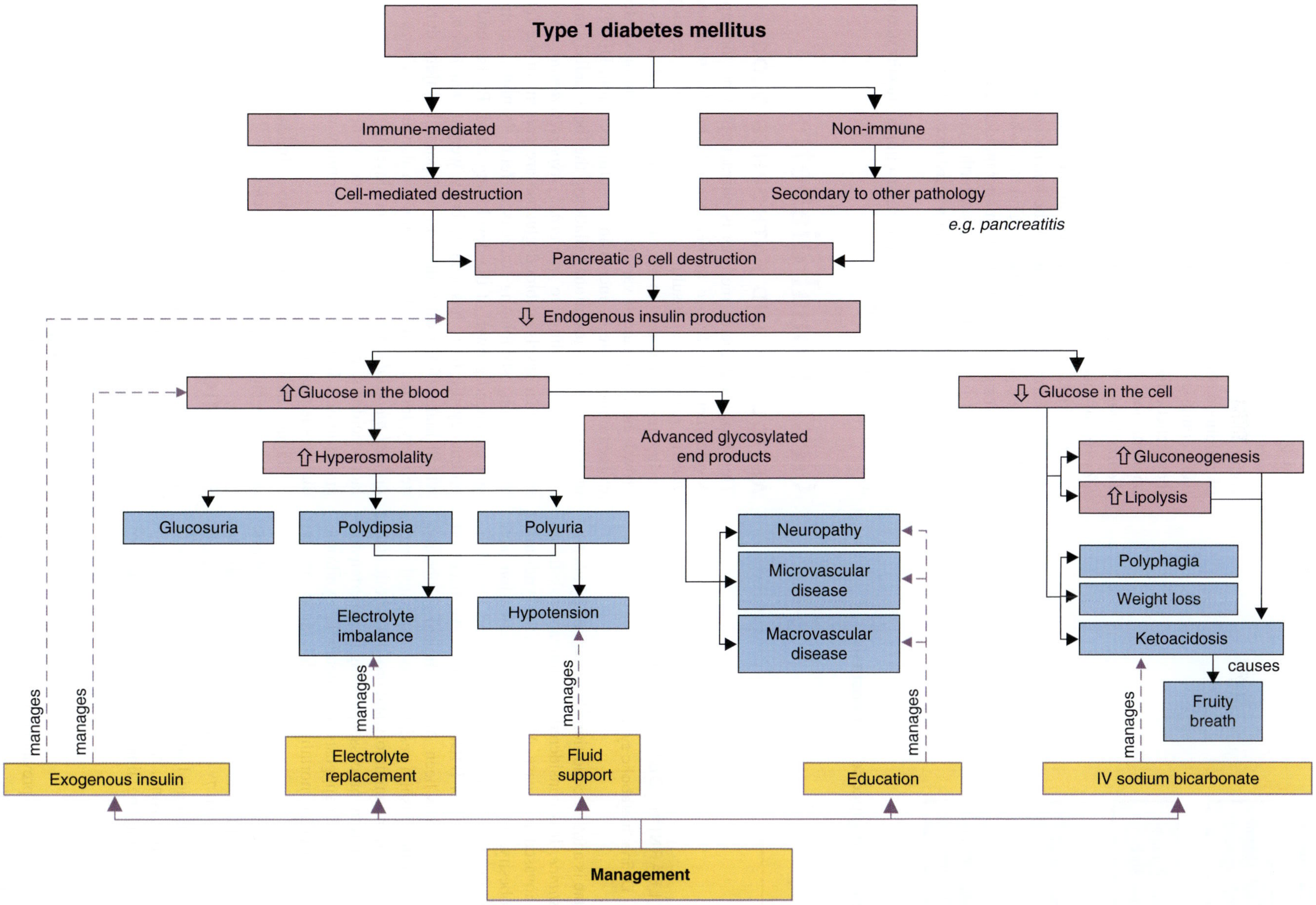

Type 1 diabetes mellitus
Immune-mediated
Non-immune
Cell-mediated destruction
Secondary to other pathology
e.g. pancreatitis
Pancreatic β cell destruction
⇩ Endogenous insulin production
⇧ Glucose in the blood
Advanced glycosylated end products
⇩ Glucose in the cell
⇧ Hyperosmolality
⇧ Gluconeogenesis
⇧ Lipolysis
Glucosuria
Polydipsia
Polyuria
Neuropathy
Microvascular disease
Macrovascular disease
Polyphagia
Weight loss
Ketoacidosis
causes
Fruity breath
Electrolyte imbalance
Hypotension
manages
manages
manages
manages
manages
manages
Exogenous insulin
Electrolyte replacement
Fluid support
Education
IV sodium bicarbonate
Management

Figure 20.2

Common clinical manifestations and management of type 1 diabetes mellitus (T1D)

↓ = decreased; ↑ = increased; β = beta; IV = intravenous.

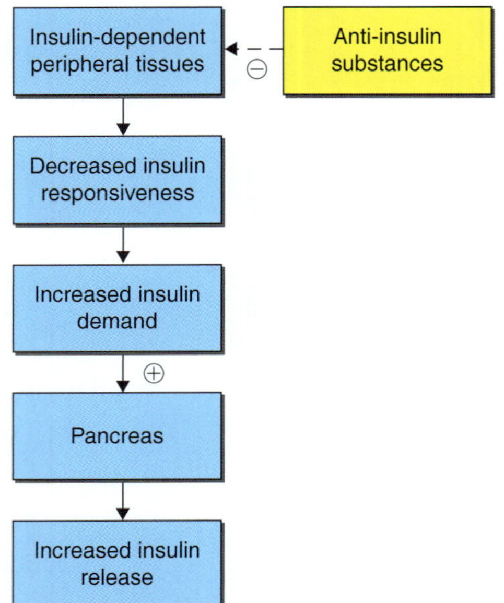

Figure 20.3

Insulin resistance and glucose homeostasis

⊖ = inhibits
⊕ = stimulates

LEARNING OBJECTIVE 4

Define 'metabolic syndrome'.

Metabolic syndrome is another condition characterised by *obesity* and *insulin resistance*. It is considered a significant risk factor for T2D and cardiovascular disease. A person with the syndrome shows central obesity, insulin resistance, hypertension and dyslipidaemia (high plasma triglyceride levels and low high-density lipoprotein cholesterol [HDL-C] levels). As discussed above, insulin resistance has been strongly linked to obesity. Research has shown that insulin resistance is associated with the development of a pro-inflammatory and pro-thrombotic state that promotes atherosclerotic processes, leading to hypertension and heart disease. Research suggests that metabolic syndrome may increase cardiovascular mortality in middle-aged men by up to 60%.

Recent studies indicate that the onset of metabolic syndrome starts in childhood. Interestingly, one study by De Long and Holloway (2017) posits that exposure in early childhood or in utero to chemical contaminants associated with food production and processing, as well as in the manufacture of household goods, may be linked to the development of metabolic syndrome.

EPIDEMIOLOGY

Type 2 diabetes is far more prevalent in the community than other forms of diabetes mellitus; around 87–90% of people with diabetes have this type. The incidence rate in 2020 was 172 new cases per 100,000 population, which is a decline on the rate in 2008 (336 cases per 100,000 population).

In Western industrialised nations such as Australia and New Zealand, the incidence in T2D in children and adolescents is increasing alarmingly, particularly in First Nations communities. This has been linked to an increased prevalence of childhood obesity, which has developed over a short period in these countries. Given the short timeline, environmental rather than genetic factors are considered to have contributed to this phenomenon. The key environmental factors implicated are *dietary habits* that promote an energy surplus and the *sedentary lifestyles* of this age group.

Other risk factors implicated in the development of the childhood form of T2D relate to the *nutritional and metabolic status during fetal development*. Children whose mothers had diabetes during pregnancy show a higher incidence of childhood obesity and diabetes. Conversely, low birth weight has also been linked to the development of insulin resistance, which may lead to T2D.

Figure 20.4 explores the common clinical manifestations and management of T2D.

Gestational diabetes

AETIOLOGY AND PATHOPHYSIOLOGY

This form of diabetes mellitus is characterised by the rapid development of *glucose intolerance and insulin resistance during pregnancy*. Insulin resistance normally develops during pregnancy due to the actions of increased levels of growth hormone and a variety of placental hormones. Most women compensate by increasing insulin secretion. However, in women with gestational diabetes the beta cells cannot compensate, leading to *maternal hyperglycaemia*. As a result, higher levels of blood glucose are present in the fetal bloodstream, stimulating increased fetal insulin secretion and enhanced growth of the developing child. By the end of pregnancy the fetus has a large body weight (*macrosomia*), which makes for a difficult birth and possible injury during delivery. Increased insulin secretion can also lead to *alterations in fetal metabolism*, resulting in the development of hypoxia, lactic acidosis, cardiac dysfunction, neonatal hypoglycaemia and jaundice. In utero death is a possibility when gestational diabetes is present.

Figure 20.5 explores the common clinical manifestations and management of gestational diabetes.

EPIDEMIOLOGY

According to the Australian Institute of Health and Welfare National Hospital Morbidity Database, in 2019–20, 1 in every 7 women aged 15–49 who gave birth in hospital was diagnosed with gestational diabetes. Between 2000–01 and 2019–20, the incidence rates of gestational diabetes have increased from 5.2% to 16.7% (noting, however, that the diagnostic guidelines were changed during this time). The pooled global standardised prevalence of gestational diabetes was reported at 14% by the IDF Diabetes Atlas in 2021.

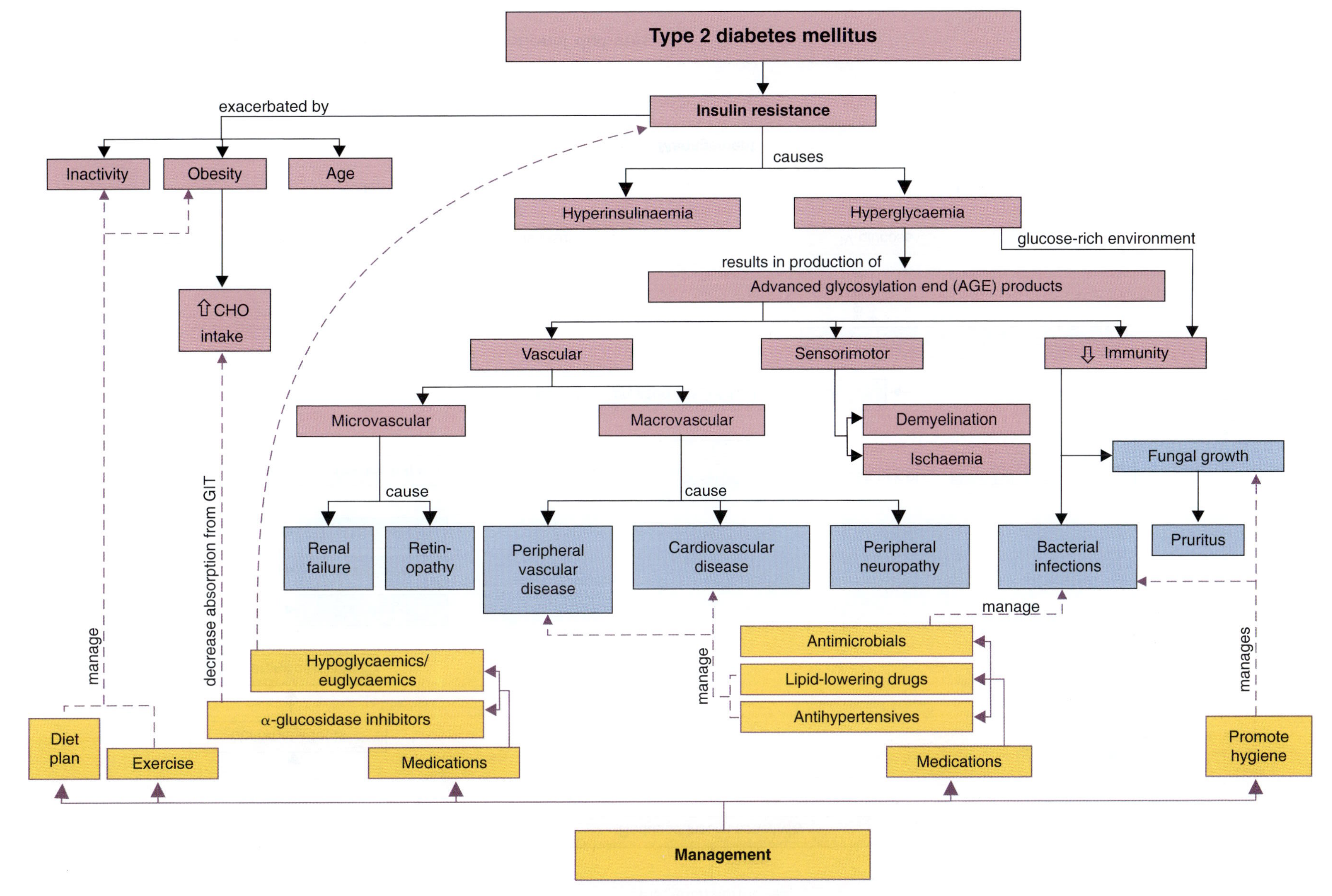

Figure 20.4

Common clinical manifestations and management of type 2 diabetes mellitus (T2D)

↓ = decreased; ↑ = increased; α = alpha; CHO = carbohydrate; GIT = gastrointestinal tract.

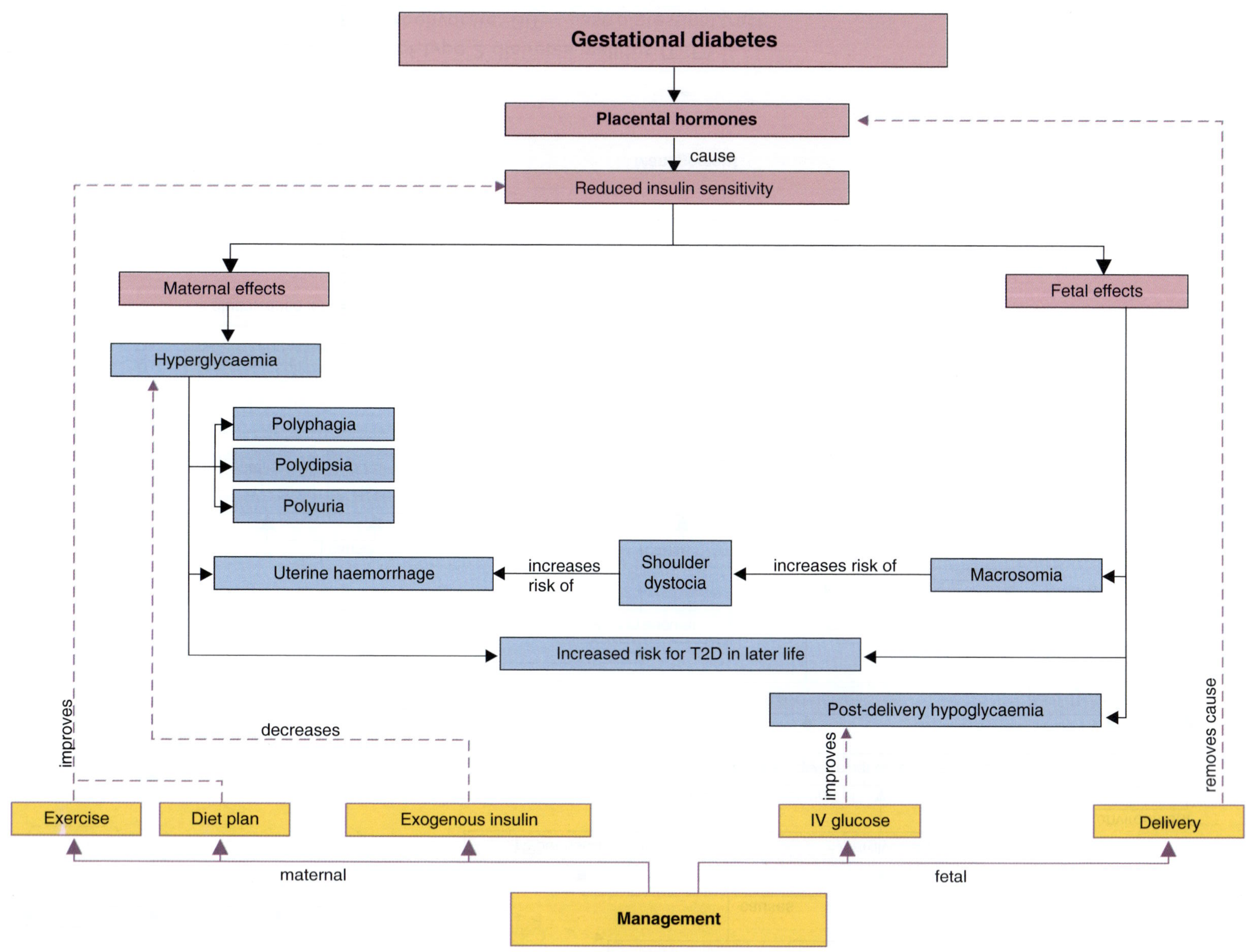

Figure 20.5

Common clinical manifestations and management of gestational diabetes

T2D = type 2 diabetes mellitus IV = intravenous.

Glucose homeostasis returns to normal after the pregnancy has ended, but the condition can occur again during later pregnancies. The recurrence rate for subsequent pregnancies is 30–69%. Women diagnosed with this condition have not been diagnosed with other types of diabetes mellitus previously.

Women who are older or obese at the time of pregnancy are at a greater risk of developing this form of diabetes. Gestational diabetes most resembles T2D. Indeed, studies have shown that about 50% of women who have the gestational form develop T2D later in life. Other risk factors for gestational diabetes include a family history of diabetes mellitus, ethnic background (gestational diabetes is more prevalent in Indigenous Australian, Melanesian/Polynesian, Chinese and Indian populations), a history of previous fetal death, and previous occurrence of macrosomic infant delivery. Vitamin D deficiency has also been implicated.

Clinical manifestations and complications of diabetes

ACUTE COMPLICATIONS

LEARNING OBJECTIVE 5

Describe the acute complications of diabetes mellitus, and indicate which types are more likely to show each complication.

LEARNING OBJECTIVE 6

Outline the ways in which a diagnosis of diabetes mellitus is determined.

The acute complications of diabetes mellitus arise because of the *disruptions to glucose homeostasis*. The normal range for blood glucose levels is 4–8 mmol/L. Depending on a person's physiological state, blood glucose levels can fluctuate dramatically between excessive (hyperglycaemia—11 mmol/L or greater after meals) and deficient (hypoglycaemia—less than 3 mmol/L).

Hyperglycaemia

One of the major consequences of hyperglycaemia is that the high plasma concentration of glucose exerts a strong influence on *blood osmotic pressure*. When high blood glucose levels develop, fluid is osmotically drawn from the interstitial compartment into the bloodstream, where the concentration of water is relatively lower. In turn, the intracellular fluid levels become depleted as the osmotic pressure of the interstitial compartment increases. As a consequence, *cellular dehydration* develops (see Figure 20.6). A greater degree of cell dehydration is associated with a higher level of blood glucose. The function of cells, particularly neurons, can become severely compromised, leading to nervous system dysfunction. Rapid fluctuations in blood glucose levels can lead to significant fluid shifts between the interstitium and the blood in an attempt to counteract changing compartment osmotic pressures. When this happens, tissues can rapidly change from a dehydrated state to an *oedematous* one. Again, such shifts in fluid can profoundly affect brain function and vision.

The affected person will experience thirst, and attempt to compensate for the dehydration by increasing their fluid intake. This is manifested as *polydipsia* (increased drinking). The increased blood volume, resulting from the shift in fluid from the interstitial and intracellular compartments, leads to increased urine production. This manifests as frequent micturition (*polyuria*). This loss of fluid from the body further contributes to the dehydration (see Figure 20.7). Normally, any glucose in the filtrate is reabsorbed back into the bloodstream. In hyperglycaemia, glucose transport across the nephron wall becomes oversaturated; excess glucose is excreted in the urine, which can be detected by urinalysis.

The hyperglycaemic state can sometimes develop slowly and insidiously, such that clinical manifestations may not occur until blood glucose levels become very high (about six to seven times normal). Under these circumstances, the dehydration is extreme. Within the brain, such a degree of dehydration leads to slurred speech, losses of sensory function on one side of the body (hemiparesis), seizures, coma and death. This complication is called **non-ketotic hyperosmolar coma (NKHC)** and is associated with T2D.

In people with gross destruction or failure of beta pancreatic cells where insulin secretion is negligible, peripheral tissues (e.g. muscle) become starved because glucose uptake into these tissues is dependent on the action of insulin. Glucose is the preferred energy source of these tissues. And this is the cruel irony of diabetes—there is actually a 'feast' of glucose present in the blood, but insulin-dependent peripheral tissues are in a functional state of 'famine'. Importantly, the brain does not require insulin for glucose uptake into cells, so its energy production is not directly compromised by decreased insulin action or availability. As a result of peripheral cell starvation, the affected person may display hunger and increased eating (*polyphagia*). In this state, peripheral cells, especially muscle cells, switch to the mobilisation of fats in order to produce energy.

Free fatty acids are metabolised into intermediate substances called *ketone bodies*, which can enter the Kreb's cycle to make energy. A good example of a ketone is acetone, which is a common solvent and is widely available as nail-polish remover. Ketone bodies are acids. During fasting or starvation, the synthesis of ketone bodies increases dramatically and can induce a state of metabolic acidosis.

The metabolic acidosis that develops in sufferers of diabetes during hyperglycaemia is called **diabetic ketoacidosis (DKA)**. In this state, nervous system function is impaired. In the early stages, vascular tone decreases, resulting in peripheral vasodilation. The skin may feel warm to touch. Neural impairment can progress to coma and death. In DKA, ketone bodies are excreted in the urine and on the breath. They can be detected by urinalysis, and are sometimes smelt on the breath as a 'fruity' odour. As a compensatory mechanism, a person with DKA will attempt to remove carbon dioxide from the blood via deep, laboured respirations (**Kussmaul breathing**) (see Figure 20.8). DKA is more likely to occur in T1D. In T2D, it occurs more rarely, because the affected person usually has sufficient circulating insulin to avoid cellular starvation.

A. Normal

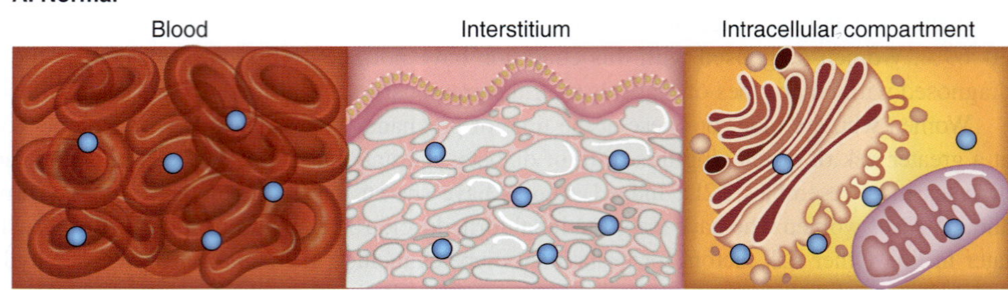

B. Hyperglycaemia

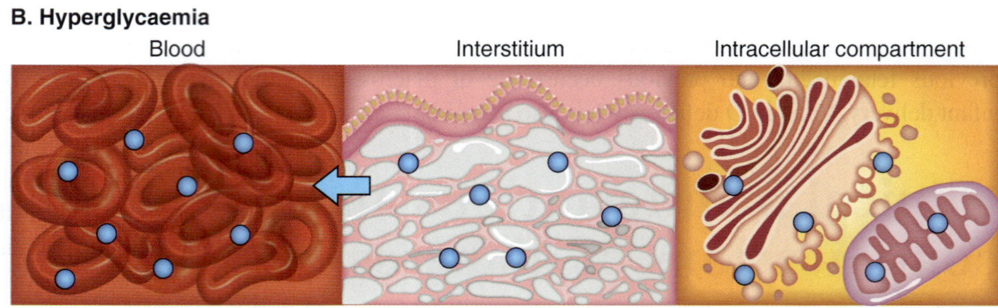

C. Prolonged hyperglycaemia

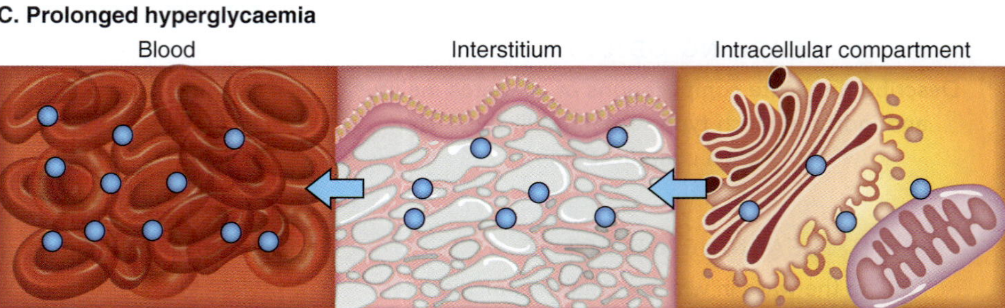

Figure 20.6

Hyperglycaemia and osmotic pressure

(A) In the normal state, there is no net movement between compartments.

(B) In hyperglycaemia, the increase in glucose molecules draws fluid from the interstitium, leading to polyuria and dehydration.

(C) In prolonged hyperglycaemia, the loss of water from the interstitium promotes an osmotic imbalance between it and the intracellular compartment. Fluid is drawn from the intracellular compartment, causing more severe cellular dehydration.

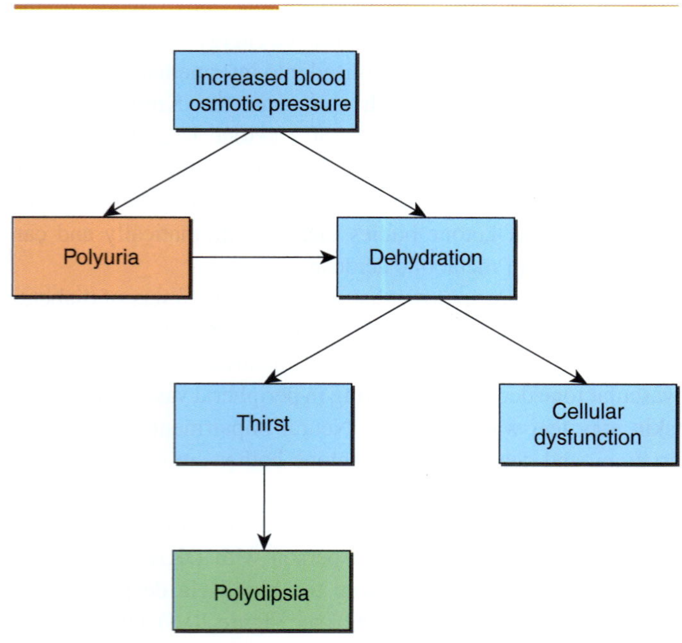

Figure 20.7

Dehydration and clinical manifestations

Hypoglycaemia

Blood glucose levels can drop below normal when there is an imbalance between eating, activity levels and the dose of drugs used to manage hyperglycaemia. The combination of missing a meal, excessive exercise and the mistiming or overdose of a diabetes medication can combine to create the hypoglycaemic state.

In **hypoglycaemia**, brain function is particularly disrupted, because glucose is its preferred energy source. The condition develops rapidly, with impaired brain function triggering activation of the sympathetic nervous system. At first, an affected person will show lapses in concentration, headaches and irritability. Fine tremors of the hands develop, the skin becomes pale, cool and clammy, and there are changes in heart rate and blood pressure. Seizures, coma and death may ensue in advanced hypoglycaemia (see Figure 20.9).

CHRONIC COMPLICATIONS

LEARNING OBJECTIVE 7

State the chronic complications of diabetes mellitus, and the pathophysiology of each.

As a long-term consequence of poor blood glucose control and chronic hyperglycaemia, the function of the cardiovascular, renal, nervous and visual systems will deteriorate. These

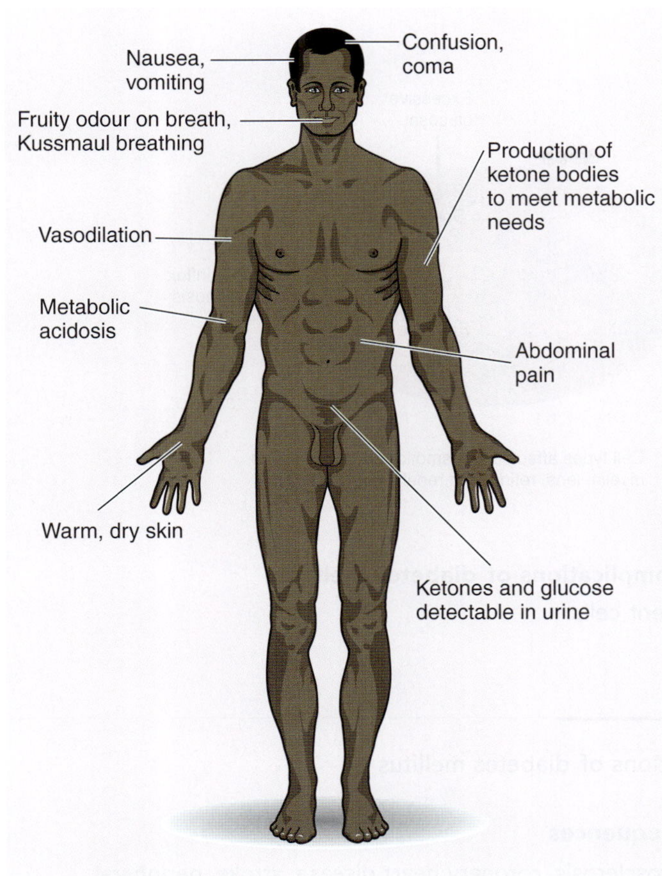

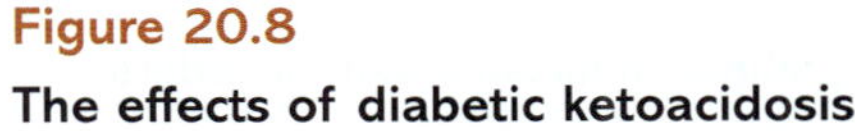

Figure 20.8

The effects of diabetic ketoacidosis

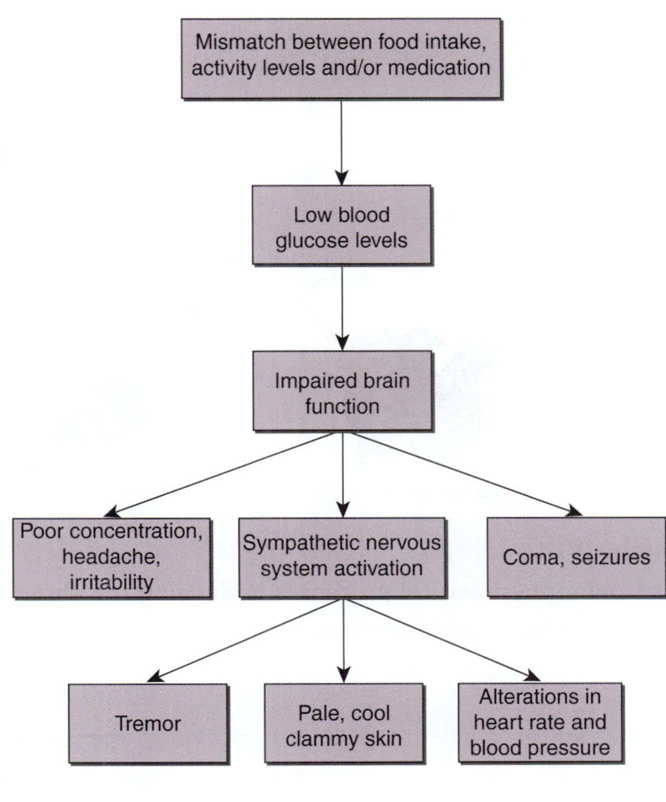

Figure 20.9

The effects of hypoglycaemia

impairments fall into three broad pathophysiological categories—**macrovascular disease**, **microvascular disease** and **neuropathies**—and are the major causes of poor health and death in people with diabetes. The specific chronic problems that can develop include hypertension, coronary heart disease (CHD), stroke, peripheral vascular disease, renal impairment and failure, autonomic nervous system impairments, poor peripheral sensory function, erectile dysfunction, cataracts, blindness and alterations in skin integrity.

Underlying these conditions are two main pathophysiological processes—glycosylation and altered intracellular glucose metabolism leading to osmotic cell injury (see Figure 20.10). *Glycosylation* involves the binding of glucose to protein; the more glucose present in the blood, the greater the degree of glycosylation. The products of this reaction, called *advanced glycosylation end (AGE) products*, accumulate within tissues and blood vessel walls, damaging these structures and leading to macrovascular diseases, such as atherosclerosis, CHD, stroke and peripheral vascular disease.

Within cells that are not insulin-dependent, increased glucose levels are subjected to alternative metabolic pathways, leading to the production of *sorbitol* (belonging to a group of chemicals called *polyols*), which is converted into *fructose*. These substances exert an increased intracellular osmotic pressure, which eventually damages the cells. These changes *damage the myelin* on peripheral nerves (disrupting nerve impulse transmission) and the lens of the eye (causing cataracts), as well as causing *microvascular problems* that affect renal and retinal blood vessels (the latter leading to retinal microaneurysms). A summary of the chronic complications of diabetes mellitus and the underlying pathophysiological process is provided in Table 20.1.

Microvascular disorders are characterised by a thickening of the basement membrane of small blood vessels, and an alteration in *vascular permeability*. In the kidneys, this thickening greatly affects the glomerulus, the site of filtration. Normal glomerular function becomes disrupted. As kidney function deteriorates, proteins such as *albumin* will appear in the filtrate and be detectable in urine—small amounts at first (*microalbuminuria*) and then later much larger amounts (*macroalbuminuria*). The presence of glucose in urine also provides a suitable medium for bacterial growth, so recurrent urinary tract infections can occur, which can ascend to the kidneys and cause further damage. Progressive renal impairment leads to renal failure and the need for dialysis and transplantation. High glucose

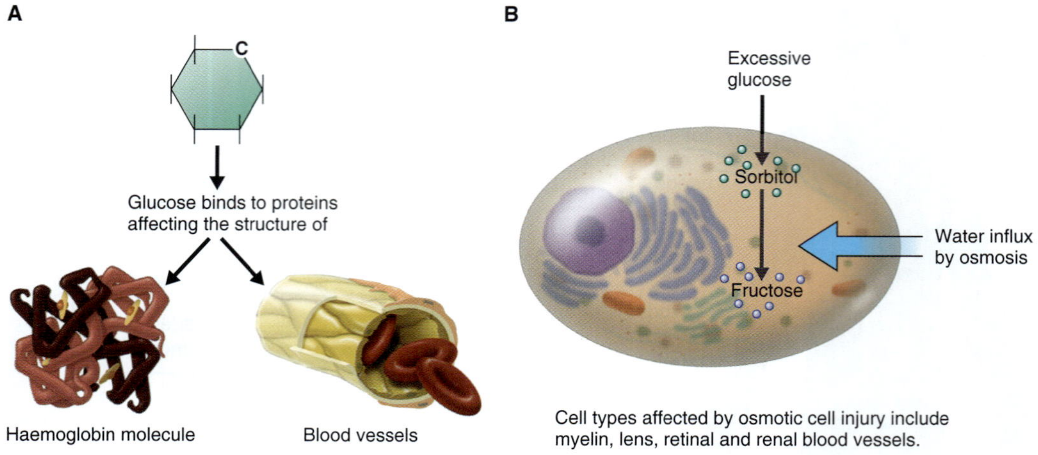

A

C

Glucose binds to proteins affecting the structure of

Haemoglobin molecule

Blood vessels

B

Excessive glucose

Sorbitol

Fructose

Water influx by osmosis

Cell types affected by osmotic cell injury include myelin, lens, retinal and renal blood vessels.

Figure 20.10

The pathophysiological processes underlying the chronic complications of diabetes mellitus

(A) Glycosylation. (B) Osmotic cell injury in non-insulin-dependent cells.

Table 20.1 Chronic complications of diabetes mellitus

Complication	Pathophysiological process	Consequences
Macrovascular disease	Glycosylation	Atherosclerosis, coronary heart disease, stroke, peripheral vascular disease
Microvascular disease	Osmotic cell injury	Renal impairment, cataracts, retinal aneurysms, skin disorders
Neuropathy	Osmotic cell injury	Sensory and motor impairments

concentrations inhibit immune cell function, increasing the risk of *Candida albicans* infections of the skin and mucous membranes.

The combination of *peripheral neuropathy* and *peripheral vascular disease* is very problematic for people with diabetes mellitus. The damage to myelin leads to impaired transmission of sensory information, including pain, from peripheral regions, especially the feet. Foot injury can occur without the accompanying pain signalling and conscious awareness of the damage. Impaired circulation results in poor healing processes, compounded by impaired immune processes. Small wounds can ulcerate and become infected, and may become gangrenous. The gangrenous area will eventually require amputation and result in further disability.

Chronic alterations in skin integrity can also develop. The two most common non-infectious changes are xanthomas and shin spots. *Xanthomas* are raised skin nodules that comprise a lipid core. They have a reddish zone around the nodule and are often itchy. Xanthomas tend to develop on the limbs and buttocks. *Shin spots* are characteristic round, brownish scaly lesions that are seen on the lower legs. They are associated with alterations in blood flow to the skin due to microvascular disease.

Clinical diagnosis and management of diabetes mellitus

LEARNING OBJECTIVE 8

Outline the ways in which types 1 and 2 diabetes mellitus are monitored and managed.

DIAGNOSIS

Diabetes mellitus is diagnosed using a combination of clinical manifestations, medical history and blood glucose testing (Figure 20.11).

As discussed, increased thirst and urination are strongly associated with dehydration due to osmotic diuresis for all types of diabetes. Other clinical signs include headache, weakness, fatigue and blurred vision. In T1D, the affected person will show a significant weight loss and hunger as energy stores are depleted. Acute illness may occur as DKA develops, manifesting as nausea, vomiting and abdominal pain. As this state worsens, acidosis, confusion and coma can ensue. Some

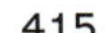

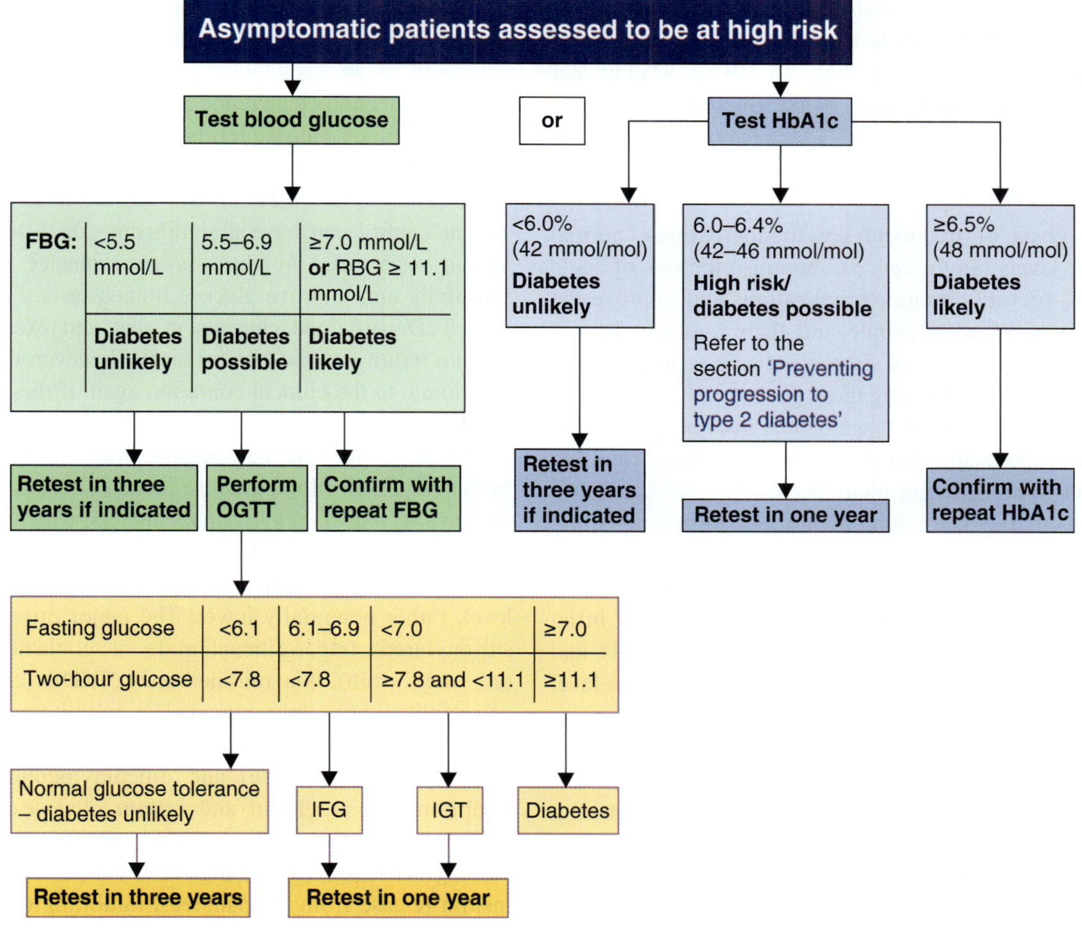

Figure 20.11

Screening and diagnosing type 2 diabetes mellitus in asymptomatic people.

FBG = fasting blood glucose; HbA_{1c} = glycated haemoglobin; IFG = impaired fasting glucose; IGT = impaired glucose tolerance; OGTT = oral glucose tolerance test; RBG = random blood glucose.

Source: Royal Australian College of General Practitioners (RACGP) (2020). Management of type 2 diabetes: A handbook for general practice. *East Melbourne, VIC: RACGP, Figure 1, p. 7.*

people with T2D can show DKA on first presentation. People with T2D can also present with chronic skin infection, recurrent urinary tract infection, thrush or pruritus.

A family history of diabetes and ethnicity can also be useful when making a diagnosis. As obesity is strongly associated with T2D, a measure of body fat content may be helpful in assessing risk or making a diagnosis of this type of diabetes. The *body mass index (BMI)* is considered a useful substitute for a measure of body fat percentage. The BMI is a ratio of weight to height, and is represented by the formula:

$$\text{BMI} = \frac{\text{Weight (kg)}}{\text{Height (m}^2\text{)}}$$

The *normal range* for BMI is 20–25. A person with a BMI greater than 25 is considered *overweight*, while a person with a BMI of greater than 30 is considered *obese*.

A significant number of affected people remain asymptomatic, and are diagnosed as part of a medical examination for another condition or during regular health check-ups.

Blood glucose testing can occur randomly or during fasting. Normal fasting blood glucose levels should be 4–6 mmol/L. An important diagnostic test is the oral glucose tolerance test (OGTT). After fasting overnight, the person taking an OGTT is usually given a 75g glucose solution to drink, and blood glucose samples are taken up to two hours later. A fasting blood glucose reading of greater than or equal to 7 mmol/L, or random blood glucose test of greater than or equal to 11 mmol/L, suggests impaired glucose tolerance.

Another important measure in diabetes mellitus diagnosis and management is the level of *glycosylated haemoglobin (HbA_{1c})* in the blood. The abbreviation 'HbA_{1c}' reflects the part of the haemoglobin molecule where glycosylation takes place. Remember, glycosylation occurs as a result of chronic hyperglycaemia. Normally, glycosylated haemoglobin represents less than

6% of blood haemoglobin. It is useful as a measure of longer-term blood glucose control over six to eight weeks, compared to the acute situation by blood glucose testing. An HbA_{1c} level greater than or equal to 8% reflects poor blood glucose control over this period.

MANAGEMENT

The general goals of treatment are to approximate normal blood glucose levels (*euglycaemia*), minimise the risk of acute complications, prevent chronic complications and improve the quality of life of affected people and their families. Patient education regarding the risk factors, disease process and management is vital in achieving these goals.

In T1D, the mainstay of management is *insulin replacement therapy*. Insulin and insulin-like drugs are available as a number of preparations with differing pharmacokinetic profiles. Ultra-rapid, short-, intermediate-, long-acting and ultra-long-acting preparations are designed to meet the different metabolic needs of people over the day and across the lifespan. Good meal planning and activity levels (particularly exercise) will bring into line the relationship between blood glucose levels and insulin action. Abnormal fluctuations in the blood glucose level can arise when these elements are not matched.

Invariably, a person with T1D will experience hypoglycaemia (BGL < 3.5 mmol/L) from either too much insulin or not enough carbohydrate. Hypoglycaemia can be life-threatening and must be managed quickly. Symptoms of hypoglycaemia include sweating, restlessness, confusion or headache. In severe hypoglycaemia, a person may become unconscious. If the person is conscious, they should consume 15 g of carbohydrate immediately; this may be five to six jellybeans, three squares of glucose tablets, or three heaped teaspoons of sugar or other quickly absorbed glucose. This should be repeated if the symptoms have not diminished in 10 minutes. This should be followed by consumption of a carbohydrate with a lower glycaemic index (which will be metabolised more slowly), such as a sandwich or a piece of fruit. If the person is unconscious, they should be positioned in the lateral position and glucagon should be administered intramuscularly or intravenously. Glucagon is an exogenous polypeptide hormone equivalent to the endogenous pancreatic glucagon that is responsible for increasing blood glucose levels.

In T2D, diet and activity are major factors in the control of blood glucose levels. For those who are overweight or obese, weight control can have a significant effect on the degree of insulin resistance. Weight loss can enhance cellular insulin sensitivity and improve glucose homeostasis. For some people with T2D, sustained changes in diet and exercise alone can effect a return to a pre-clinical state. However, these people can deteriorate to the clinical condition again if they lose control of bodyweight.

Some people with T2D require drug therapy to assist them in the control of blood glucose levels. These drugs are termed *oral hypoglycaemic/euglycaemic agents*, which, unlike insulin, can be taken by mouth. The term 'eugylcaemic' indicates that the drug treatment lowers to the normal blood glucose level, rather potentially lower. The major drug groups are the sulfonylureas (e.g. glibenclamide or gliclazide), biguanides (e.g. metformin), thiazolidinediones (TZDs) (e.g. pioglitazone or rosiglitazone), alpha-glucosidase inhibitors (e.g. acarbose), incretin-enhancing agents made up of the subgroups of incretin agonists (e.g. exenatide) and dipepidylpeptidase-4 (DPP-4) inhibitors (e.g. sitagliptin) and sodium–glucose co-transporter-2 inhibitors (e.g. dapagliflozin). These drug groups act to lower blood glucose levels by a range of effects, including stimulating insulin release from the pancreas, inhibiting the conversion of fats and proteins into glucose in the liver (gluconeogenesis), slowing the absorption of glucose from the gastrointestinal tract into the bloodstream, increasing the cellular glucose uptake, enhancing intracellular utilisation of glucose or reducing renal glucose reabsorption (see Table 20.2).

Some people with T2D go on to develop elements of T1D as well. They may require insulin therapy to control blood glucose levels in addition to their oral hypoglycaemic medications.

Table 20.2 Oral hypoglycaemic/euglycaemic agents and their actions

Drug group	Main actions
Sulfonylureas	Stimulate release of insulin from pancreas Enhance cellular glucose uptake
Biguanides	Inhibit hepatic gluconeogenesis Slow glucose absorption from gut Enhance cellular glucose utilisation
Alpha-glucosidase inhibitors	Slow glucose absorption from gut
Thiazolidinediones (TZDs)	Insulin sensitisers Enhance cellular glucose utilisation
Incretin-enhancing agents (Incretin agonists and dipepidylpeptidase-4 [DPP-4] inhibitors)	Enhance sensitivity of beta-pancreatic cell glucose sensor to increase insulin secretion
Sodium–glucose co-transporter-2 inhibitors	Reduce renal reabsorption of filtered glucose to reduce blood glucose levels

INDIGENOUS HEALTH FAST FACTS AND CULTURAL CONSIDERATIONS

FAST FACTS

Diabetes-related statistics for Australian and New Zealand Indigenous peoples and selected ethnic groups compared to non-Indigenous peoples.

	Aboriginal and Torres Strait Islander peoples compared to non-Indigenous Australians	Māori compared to European New Zealanders	Pacific Islands people compared to European New Zealanders
Diabetes mellitus	3.0 × ↑	2 × ↑	2.8 × ↑
Type 1 diabetes	0	1.03 × ↓	1.06 × ↓
Type 2 diabetes	3 × ↑	1.7 × ↑	~3 × ↑
Gestational diabetes	1.3 × ↑	1.3 × ↑	2.7 × ↑
Mortality	Overall: 4.7 × ↑ ♂ age 45–54: 12 × ↑ ♀ age 45–54: 20.2 × ↑	4.9 × ↑	9.3 × ↑
Hospitalisations	3.8 × ↑	1.6–3 × ↑ (depending on age)	1.7 × ↑
Limb amputation	3.8 × ↑	3.4 × ↑	1.25 × ↓
Renal complications/ chronic kidney disease	5 × ↑	2.8 × ↑	3.9 × ↑

× ↑ = times higher; × ↓ = times lower; ♂ = male; ♀ = female.

CULTURAL CONSIDERATIONS

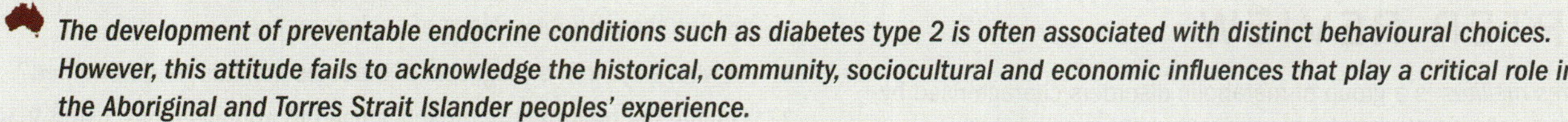

- ***The development of preventable endocrine conditions such as diabetes type 2 is often associated with distinct behavioural choices. However, this attitude fails to acknowledge the historical, community, sociocultural and economic influences that play a critical role in the Aboriginal and Torres Strait Islander peoples' experience.***
- ***Pre-colonisation Indigenous Australians were lean and fit, and did not appear to demonstrate the metabolic conditions that now affect their health and well-being. The contemporary changes in physical activity, nutrition and economic opportunities contribute strongly to determinants of health. As a result, the introduction of multiple risk factors, including reduced levels of fitness, poor nutrition, and alcohol and tobacco consumption, can be considered key targets for culturally appropriate, community-centred programs to contribute to closing the health equality gap.***

Sources: Data from Australian Bureau of Statistics (2018); Australian Indigenous HealthInfoNet (2022); Australian Institute of Health and Welfare (2017, 2020, 2022); New Zealand Ministry of Health (2018).

CHILDREN AND ADOLESCENTS

- Children are more likely to develop type 1 diabetes mellitus than type 2 diabetes mellitus.
- The increase in the prevalence of type 2 diabetes in children is associated with the increasing issue of childhood obesity.

OLDER ADULTS

- Insulin sensitivity commonly reduces as people age.
- Insulin resistance can increase as a direct result of increasing body fat and abdominal adiposity.
- When long-lasting relationships terminate as a result of the death of a spouse (especially if the deceased was the one normally responsible for food preparation), nutrition challenges and inactivity may develop in the remaining spouse.
- Age-related glucose intolerance is not limited to obesity. Glucose intolerance related to beta cell dysfunction, and insulin resistance also occurs.

KEY CLINICAL ISSUES

- The long-term effects of diabetes mellitus are devastating. If clinicians can reduce the risk of someone developing diabetes they will significantly influence the physical, emotional and financial burden of this disease. Assessing people and implementing management plans in those who have pre-diabetes will reduce this burden for the individual and the country.
- People with type 1 diabetes mellitus (T1D) will need to modify their entire lifestyle to manage their T1D successfully. Regular glucometry and insulin administration are the mainstay of T1D management. Long-term adherence to monitoring and insulin regimens can be analysed with the measurement of glycosylated haemoglobin (HbA_{1c}). This serum value will inform clinicians of the previous three months of a person's glucose control. Irrespective of self-reported success, the HbA_{1c} level is definitive and will provide insight into their disease management.
- Insulin resistance is exacerbated by obesity. Assisting the person with a management plan that includes exercise and good nutritional choices will reduce the risk of T2D. Generally, as weight is lost, insulin resistance decreases. In some instances, oral glucose-lowering agents can be ceased as insulin resistance normalises.
- The mechanism (placental hormones) causing gestational diabetes is resolved when the baby is delivered. However, women who experience gestational diabetes are at risk of developing T2D in the future.
- Understanding the action of insulin and glucagon is imperative in the safe and appropriate management of people with diabetes. Rapid intervention for hyper- or hypoglycaemia is critical. Administration of insulin for hyperglycaemia, and glucose or glucagon for hypoglycaemia, may be necessary to ensure a person's survival.

CHAPTER REVIEW

- *Diabetes mellitus* is a group of metabolic disorders characterised by an *abnormal secretion and/or action of insulin*. A severe imbalance between the supply of and the demand for insulin develops.
- *Type 1 diabetes mellitus (T1D)* develops as a result of extensive damage to the pancreatic beta cells that make and release insulin. The damage is induced by an *autoimmune attack*.
- T1D can occur at any age, but is more commonly diagnosed in children and adolescents aged 10–19 years.
- *Type 2 diabetes mellitus (T2D)* is the more prevalent form of diabetes. Affected people can synthesise and release insulin, but the sensitivity of insulin-dependent peripheral tissues is altered. This alteration is called *cellular insulin resistance*.
- Inheritance and obesity are strongly associated with T2D.
- *Gestational diabetes mellitus* occurs when elevated blood glucose levels occur in pregnancy. Alterations in fetal metabolism that result from this state can lead to high birth weight, hypoxia, lactic acidosis, cardiac dysfunction and jaundice. The affected fetus is at risk of in-utero death or possible injury during birth.
- Acute alterations in blood glucose levels can lead to hyperglycaemic or hypoglycaemic states. *Hyperglycaemia* induces significant changes in blood osmotic pressure, leading to cellular dehydration. It may also induce alterations in blood pH, resulting in acidosis. These states have profound effects on body function. *Hypoglycaemia* primarily disrupts the delivery of glucose to the brain, resulting in brain dysfunction and activation of the sympathetic nervous system.
- *Chronic complications* of diabetes mellitus include hypertension, coronary heart disease, stroke, peripheral vascular disease, renal impairment, neuropathies, blindness and alterations in skin integrity.
- *Diagnosis* involves observed clinical manifestations, patient history and blood glucose testing.
- *Treatment* of diabetes mellitus is directed towards approximating normal blood glucose levels, preventing or minimising complications, and improving the person's quality of life. A combination of *diet* and *activity management, drug treatment* and *education* is used to achieve these aims.

REVIEW QUESTIONS

1. Compare and contrast the major characteristics of type 1, type 2 and gestational diabetes mellitus.
2. What are the possible consequences of having gestational diabetes?
3. What are the characteristics that differentiate diabetic ketoacidosis, hypoglycaemia and non-ketotic hyperosmolar coma from each other?
4. Define 'metabolic syndrome'.
5. Describe each of the chronic complications of diabetes mellitus, and outline the pathophysiology of each complication.
6. In what ways can a diagnosis of diabetes mellitus be determined?
7. Outline the treatment approaches used to manage types 1 and 2 diabetes mellitus.
8. Sophie Chartre is a 5-year-old girl who is brought in to her local general practitioner's clinic by her mother. Sophie has experienced significant weight loss over the past couple of months. Her mother says that Sophie is drinking a lot of fluids and is going to the toilet frequently during the day. The doctor performs a urinalysis on a sample provided by Sophie; it is positive for glucose but negative for proteins and ketones. There is no family history of diabetes. Which form of diabetes mellitus could be suggested by this scenario? Provide your reasons.
9. Alfie Pravastrian is 17 years old and has recently been diagnosed with type 1 diabetes mellitus. While at school one day he experiences nausea and some abdominal pain. This progresses to confusion and lethargy. His skin is warm and dry, and his breathing becomes laboured. What complication of diabetes could Alfie be experiencing? Briefly explain why it is happening.

HEALTH PROFESSIONAL CONNECTIONS

Midwives Assessment and monitoring for gestational diabetes is important to reduce health risks during pregnancy. A woman who is over 30 years, has had gestational diabetes during a previous pregnancy and is overweight is at greater risk. Neonatal complications, such as macrosomia, shoulder dystocia and post-delivery neonatal hypoglycaemia, are significant complications of pregnancy affected by maternal hyperglycaemia. Another consideration for caring for women who have pre-existing type 2 diabetes mellitus is that most of the oral hypoglycaemic/euglycaemic agents are contraindicated during pregnancy. Hyperglycaemic mothers may be placed on insulin for the duration of the pregnancy. Although, more recently, metformin is used throughout pregnancy, despite its 'C' pregnancy category.

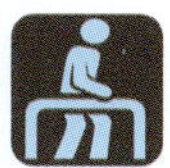

Physiotherapists The microvascular changes resulting in visual problems and the neuropathies experienced by some people with diabetes may interfere with the person's ability or confidence to engage in exercise/rehabilitation programs. Ensure that you are fully aware of the degree of disability caused by diabetes, and modify your plan to accommodate these limitations. Also, if working with heat as a therapy, be hypervigilant to avoid burning the person, as they may not be able to perceive the initial stages of heat injury.

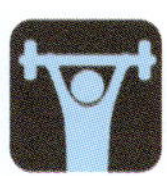

Exercise scientists Exercise for those with type 2 diabetes will significantly reduce the insulin resistance. Depending on diet (and other factors), exercise and weight loss may actually reduce the need for pharmacological intervention for glycaemic control. However, exercise prescription for people with type 1 diabetes can be difficult. Open lines of communication should be kept with the person's endocrinologist and healthcare team. In those with type 1 diabetes, the blood glucose level will generally rise dramatically as a result of strenuous exercise. Consultation with the diabetes care team is important to program the insulin doses in relation to the type and time of exercise undertaken.

Nutritionists/Dieticians Teaching someone with newly diagnosed diabetes about carbohydrate exchange and low glycaemic index (GI) foods can be very difficult. Anyone who has just been given a diagnosis will progress through a period of grief. The speed of acceptance and the reaction to this new challenge will be different for everyone; however, understanding the concepts around nutrition and appropriate food selection is critical to the successful management of diabetes. Ensure that you tailor your education program to the needs, learning capacity and style of each individual. They will probably need many sessions with you before the content makes sense.

CASE STUDY

Mr Bob Lewis is a 70-year-old Aboriginal man (UR number 954002). He was admitted through community health referral for investigation of polyuria, polydipsia and fatigue. He was newly diagnosed with diabetes mellitus type 2. His weight is 103 kg and his height is 170 cm. He retired from truck driving nine months ago, and since his retirement he has gained 14 kg. He has been complaining of visual changes. His observations were as follows:

Temperature	Heart rate	Respiration rate	Blood pressure	SpO_2
37°C	88	20	150/90	98% (RA*)

* RA = room air.

On the neurovascular assessment his dorsalis pedis and posterior tibial pulses were significantly reduced. His capillary refill was sluggish, both feet were cool to touch, and a sensory deficit was present. His lower legs also had very little hair, and he denied shaving them. His biochemistry and renal function test results were as follows:

BIOCHEMISTRY

Patient location:	Ward 3	**UR:**	954002		
Consultant:	Smith	**NAME:**	Lewis		
		Given name:	Robert	**Sex:**	M
		DOB:	16/10/XX	**Age:**	70

Time collected	09:21
Date collected	XX/XX
Year	XXXX
Lab #	8767869

ELECTROLYTES		UNITS	REFERENCE RANGES
Sodium	136	mmol/L	135–145
Potassium	5.4	mmol/L	3.5–5.2
Chloride	97	mmol/L	95–110
Bicarbonate	23	mmol/L	22–32
Glucose	14.2	mmol/L	3.5–5.4
Iron	16	μmol/L	11–30
HbA_{1c}	9.6	%	3–6
Urea	9.4	mmol/L	2.5–7.5
Creatinine	135	μmol/L	30–120

CRITICAL THINKING

1. Calculate Mr Lewis's body mass index (BMI). What is an appropriate BMI? In what range does Mr Lewis's BMI fall? How does this data influence a clinician's understanding of insulin resistance? (If you are having trouble with the calculation, BMI calculators are easily found on the internet.)
2. Observe the history and other assessment data. What data inform you of neuropathy, microvascular and macrovascular changes? Explain your response to each of these parameters.
3. What is HbA_{1c}? Explain fully. Although Mr Lewis is newly diagnosed, what information does the HbA_{1c} tell you about the duration of his disease process?
4. Explain the pathophysiology relating to Mr Lewis's experience of polyuria and polydipsia. How might this affect his biochemistry levels?
5. What interventions are required to assist Mr Lewis? (Consider all aspects of his presentation and the disease process.)

BIBLIOGRAPHY

Australian Bureau of Statistics (ABS) (2018). *National Health Survey: first results, 2017–18*. Canberra: ABS. https://www.abs.gov.au/statistics/health/health-conditions-and-risks/national-health-survey-first-results/latest-release.

Australian Health Ministers' Advisory Council's National and Aboriginal and Torres Strait Islander Health Standing Committee (2017). *Cultural respect framework, 2016–2026: for Aboriginal and Torres Strait Islander health—a national approach to building a culturally respectful health system*. Canberra: Australian Government Department of Health. https://nacchocommunique.files.wordpress.com/2016/12/cultural_respect_framework_1december2016_1.pdf.

Australian Indigenous Health*Info*Net (2022). *Overview of Aboriginal and Torres Strait Islander health status, 2021*. Perth, WA: Australian Indigenous Health*Info*Net. https://healthinfonet.ecu.edu.au/learn/health-facts/overview-aboriginal-torres-strait-islander-health-status/.

Australian Institute of Health and Welfare (AIHW) (2017). Burden of lower limb amputations due to diabetes in Australia. In *Australia: Australian Burden of Disease Study, 2011*. Australian Burden of Disease Study series No. 10. Cat. No. BOD 11. Canberra: AIHW. https://www.aihw.gov.au/getmedia/9292ab2b-4dbb-44ca-846f-832d02db7220/20681.pdf.aspx?inline=true.

Australian Institute of Health and Welfare (AIHW) (2021). *Australian Burden of Disease Study: impact and causes of illness and death in Australia 2018*. Australian Burden of Disease Study series No. 23. Cat. No. BOD 29. Canberra: AIHW. https://www.aihw.gov.au/reports/burden-of-disease/abds-impact-and-causes-of-illness-and-death-in-aus/summary.

Australian Institute of Health and Welfare (AIHW) (2022). *Australia's health, 2022*. Canberra: AIHW. https://www.aihw.gov.au/reports-data/australias-health.

Australian Institute of Health and Welfare (AIHW) (2023). *Diabetes: Australian facts*. https://www.aihw.gov.au/reports/diabetes/diabetes/contents/how-common-is-diabetes/all-diabetes.

Bauldoff, G., Gubrud-Howe, P.M., Carno, M.-A., Levett-Jones, T., Hales, M., Berry, K., … Stanley, D. (2020). *LeMone and Burke's medical–surgical nursing: critical thinking for person-centred care* (4th [Australian] edn). Sydney: Pearson Australia.

Best, O. & Fredericks, B. (2021). *Yatdjuligin: Aboriginal and Torres Strait Islander nursing and midwifery care* (3rd edn). Port Melbourne, VIC: Cambridge University Press.

Bullock, S. & Manias, E. (2022). *Fundamentals of pharmacology* (9th edn). Sydney: Pearson Australia.

De Long, N.E. & Holloway, A.C. (2017). Early life chemical exposures and risk of metabolic syndrome. *Diabetes, Metabolic Syndrome and Obesity: Targets and Therapy* 10:101–9. https://doi.org/10.2147/DMSO.S95296.

Golden, T. N. & Simmons, R. A. (2021). Immune dysfunction in developmental programming of type 2 diabetes mellitus. *Nature Reviews Endocrinology* 17(4):235–45. https://doi.org/10.1038/s41574-020-00464-z.

Haynes, A., Bulsara, M.K., Bergman, P., Cameron, F., Couper, J., Craig, M.E., … Davis, E.A. (2020). Incidence of type 1 diabetes in 0 to 14 year olds in Australia from 2002 to 2017. *Pediatric Diabetes* 21(5):707–12. https://doi.org/10.1111/pedi.13025.

Hirsch, I.B. (2022). Pathogenesis of type 1 diabetes mellitus. *UpToDate*. https://www.uptodate.com/contents/pathogenesis-of-type-1-diabetes-mellitus.

Khardori, R. (2022a). Type 1 diabetes mellitus. *Emedicine*. https://emedicine.medscape.com/article/117739-overview.

Khardori, R. (2022b). Type 2 diabetes mellitus. *Emedicine*. https://emedicine.medscape.com/article/117853-overview.

Marieb, E.N. & Hoehn, K. (2019). *Human anatomy and physiology* (11th edn). San Francisco, CA: Pearson Benjamin Cummings.

New Zealand Ministry of Health (2018). Diabetes indicators. In *Tatau kahukura: Māori health statistics*. Wellington: Ministry of Health. https://www.health.govt.nz/our-work/populations/maori-health/tatau-kahukura-maori-health-statistics/nga-mana-hauora-tutohu-health-status-indicators/diabetes.

Ogle, G.D., James, S., Dabelea, D., Pihoker, C., Svennson, J., Maniam, J., … Patterson, C.C. (2022). Global estimates of incidence of type 1 diabetes in children and adolescents: results from the International Diabetes Federation Atlas, 10th edition. *Diabetes Research and Clinical Practice* 183:109083. https://doi.org/10.1016/j.diabres.2021.109083.

Robertson, R.P. & Udler, M.S. (2021). Pathogenesis of type 2 diabetes mellitus. *UpToDate*. https://www.uptodate.com/contents/pathogenesis-of-type-2-diabetes-mellitus/.

Royal Australian College of General Practitioners (RACGP) (2020). Management of type 2 diabetes: A handbook for general practice. East Melbourne, VIC: RACGP. https://www.racgp.org.au/getattachment/41fee8dc-7f97-4f87-9d90-b7af337af778/Management-of-type-2-diabetes-A-handbook-for-general-practice.aspx.

Sun, H., Saeedi, P., Karuranga, S., Pinkepank, M., Ogurtsova, K., Duncan, B.B., … Magliano, D.J. (2022). IDF Diabetes Atlas: global, regional and country-level diabetes prevalence estimates for 2021 and projections for 2045. *Diabetes Research and Clinical Practice* 183:109119. https://doi.org/10.1016/j.diabres.2021.109119.

Tandon, S., Ayis, S., Hopkins, D., Harding, S. & Stadler, M. (2021). The impact of pharmacological and lifestyle interventions on body weight in people with type 1 diabetes: a systematic review and meta-analysis. *Diabetes, Obesity and Metabolism* 23(2):350–62. https://doi.org/10.1111/dom.14221.

Wang, H., Li, N., Chivese, T., Werfalli, M., Sun, H., Yuen, L., … IDF Diabetes Atlas Committee Hyperglycaemia in Pregnancy Special Interest Group (2022). IDF Diabetes Atlas: estimation of global and regional gestational diabetes mellitus prevalence for 2021 by International Association of Diabetes in Pregnancy Study Group's criteria. *Diabetes Research and Clinical Practice* 183:109050. https://doi.org/10.1016/j.diabres.2021.109050.

PART 5

Cardiovascular pathophysiology

21 Blood disorders

KEY TERMS

Acute lymphoblastic leukaemia (ALL)
Acute myelogenous leukaemia (AML)
Agranulocytosis
Anaemia
Chronic lymphocytic leukaemia (CLL)
Chronic myelogenous leukaemia (CML)
Haemolytic anaemia
Haemophilia
Hodgkin lymphoma (HL)
Leukaemia
Leukopenia
Lymphoma
Multiple myeloma
Neutropenia
Non-Hodgkin lymphoma (NHL)
Pernicious anaemia
Polycythaemias
Sickle cell anaemia
Thalassaemia
Thrombocytopenia
von Willebrand disease

LEARNING OBJECTIVES

After completing this chapter, you should be able to:

1 Compare and contrast the various types of anaemia and their management.

2 Outline the factors that are believed to contribute to polycythaemia and its management.

3 Differentiate between the main types of haemophilia and von Willebrand disease.

4 Explain the prevention, pathophysiology and management of thrombocytopenia.

5 Discuss the various conditions caused by changes to white blood cell function, including leukaemia, lymphoma, myeloma and agranulocytosis.

WHAT YOU SHOULD KNOW BEFORE YOU START THIS CHAPTER

Can you outline the composition of blood?

Can you identify the main blood cell types, and outline their functions?

Can you identify the structure of haemoglobin, and outline its functions?

Can you describe the process of blood cell formation?

Introduction

Blood disorders commonly occur as a result of an imbalance between blood cell production, use and/or destruction. They may involve incorrectly formed cells (see Figure 21.1).

Haematological conditions may be inherited or acquired through nutritional deficiencies or exposures to drugs or toxins. Generally, these conditions are grouped as *erythrocyte disorders* (anaemias), *white blood cell disorders* (leukocyte and lymphocyte disorders such as leukaemias and lymphomas), *platelet disorders* and *haematological function disorders* (thalassaemias, haemophilias, sickle cell disease), although some boundaries are crossed when classified in this manner.

Anaemias

LEARNING OBJECTIVE 1

Compare and contrast the various types of anaemia and their management.

As a group, **anaemia** refers to disorders that involve a reduction in the number of erythrocytes, and include both inherited and acquired disorders. As a general rule, anaemias are the result of altered production of red cells, loss of blood volume, increased erythrocyte destruction or a combination of these. The most common classification system used to define anaemias focuses on the physical characteristics of the erythrocytes; namely, size and haemoglobin content. If there is a change in cell *size*, the suffix *-cytic* is used (e.g. normocytic, macrocytic, microcytic), whereas if there is an alteration in *haemoglobin content*, the suffix *-chromic* is used (e.g. normochromic, hyperchromic, hypochromic). Macrocytic disorders include pernicious and folate-deficiency anaemias, while microcytic disorders are iron-deficiency anaemias and thalassaemias. Aplastic, haemolytic and sickle cell anaemias are normocytic disorders (see Table 21.1). Anaemias can also be classified by their aetiology (see Figure 21.2).

CLINICAL MANIFESTATIONS

All anaemias, irrespective of the cause, result in reduced oxygen-carrying capacity, with the degree and duration relating directly to the cause. Early symptoms are easily missed or misinterpreted, and commonly include fatigue, weakness, dyspnoea, headaches and irritability. The signs of anaemia commonly become more apparent once the haemoglobin levels decline to 70–80 g/L. The conjunctiva may appear pale, as will extremities such as earlobes and the palms of the hands. As the condition worsens, impaired capillary circulation may lead to brittle, ridged, thin, spoon-shaped fingernails, tingling numbness, neuromuscular changes and vasomotor disturbances. Papillae atrophy can lead to a sore, red, painful tongue. Other oral manifestations include hyposalivation, resulting in difficulty swallowing, and angular stomatitis (damage to epithelium at the corner of the mouth). Finally, manifestations associated with signs of sympathetic nervous system compensation, such as tachycardia and tachypnoea, may occur, depending on the severity of the condition.

Decreased production of erythrocytes

Anaemias caused by a decreased production of erythrocytes include megalobastic, iron deficiency, and aplastic anaemias and thalassaemia. Anaemia can also be caused by chronic kidney disease and endocrine dysfunction. In 2020–21, over 140,800 people were admitted to Australian hospitals with anaemia as their principal diagnosis. Nutritional anaemias accounted for the majority (55%) of all admissions. Ninety-eight per cent of all nutritional anaemias were due to iron deficiency, with the remaining due to folate (1%) and vitamin B_{12} (1%) deficiency. Women accounted for 65% of all admissions.

IRON-DEFICIENCY ANAEMIA

Aetiology and pathophysiology

As the name suggests, a deficiency in iron is the cause of this anaemia, often secondary to dietary deficiencies. Dietary iron is found in both plant and animal sources, with non-haem plants containing an estimated 90–95% of dietary iron, of which only 2–10% is absorbed. By contrast, animal tissue contains 5–10% of dietary iron, of which 25% is absorbed. Simultaneous consumption of vitamin C facilitates the absorption of dietary iron. A standard Western diet contains very close to the recommended daily requirement for iron, rather than an excess, and consequently people on kilojoule-reduced diets or those who are inattentive to a vegetarian or vegan lifestyle will

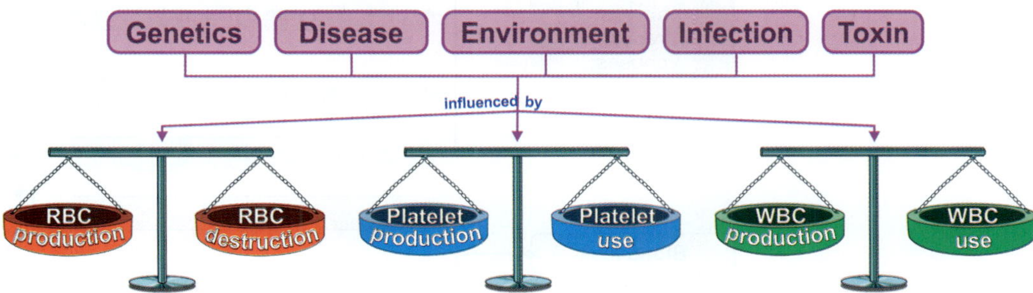

Figure 21.1
Balance of blood cell production, use and destruction

RBC = red blood cell; WBC = white blood cell.

Table 21.1 Types of anaemia by cell characteristics

Microcytic anaemia	Macrocytic anaemia	Normocytic anaemia
• Iron-deficiency anaemia • Thalassaemia	• Vitamin B_{12} deficiency anaemia • Pernicious anaemia • Leukaemias	• Anaemia from haemorrhage • Chronic renal failure associated anaemia • Haemolytic anaemia
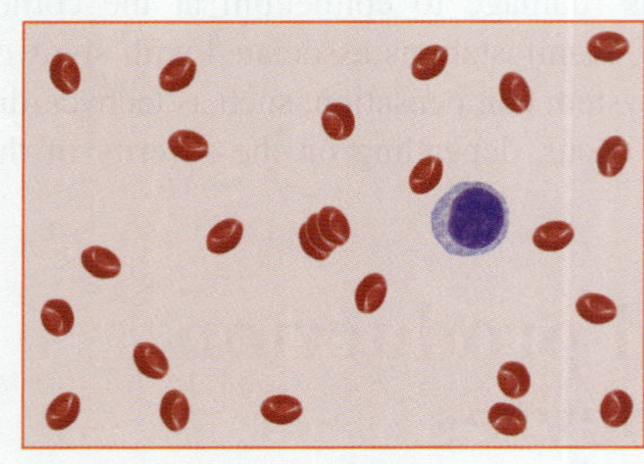	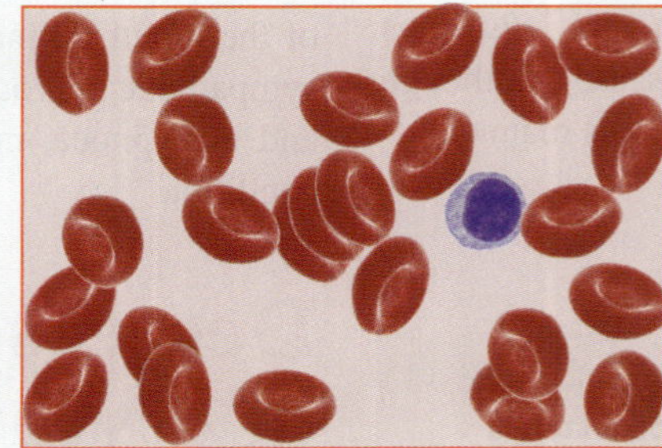	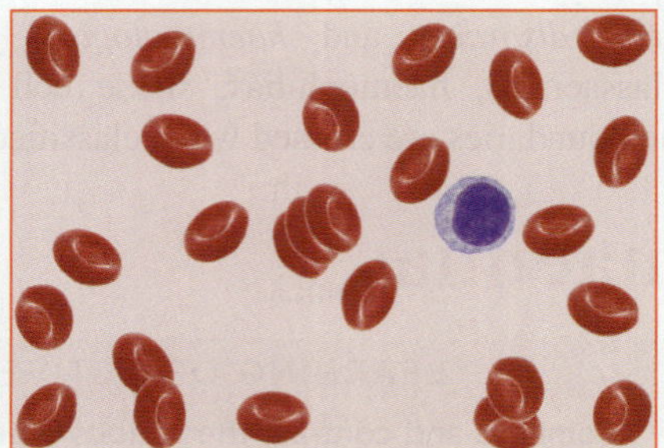

Source: Illustrations adapted from joshya/Shutterstock.

Figure 21.2

Classification of anaemias by aetiology

↓ = decreased; ↑ = increased; CKD = chronic kidney disease; DNA = deoxyribonucleic acid; *E. coli* = *Echerichia coli*; GIT = gastrointestinal-tract; G6PD = glucose-6-phosphate dehydrogenase; Hb = haemoglobin; PNH = paroxysmal nocturnal haemoglobinuria; r/t = related to.

Sources: Based on Braunstein (2022); Keohane et al. (2019).

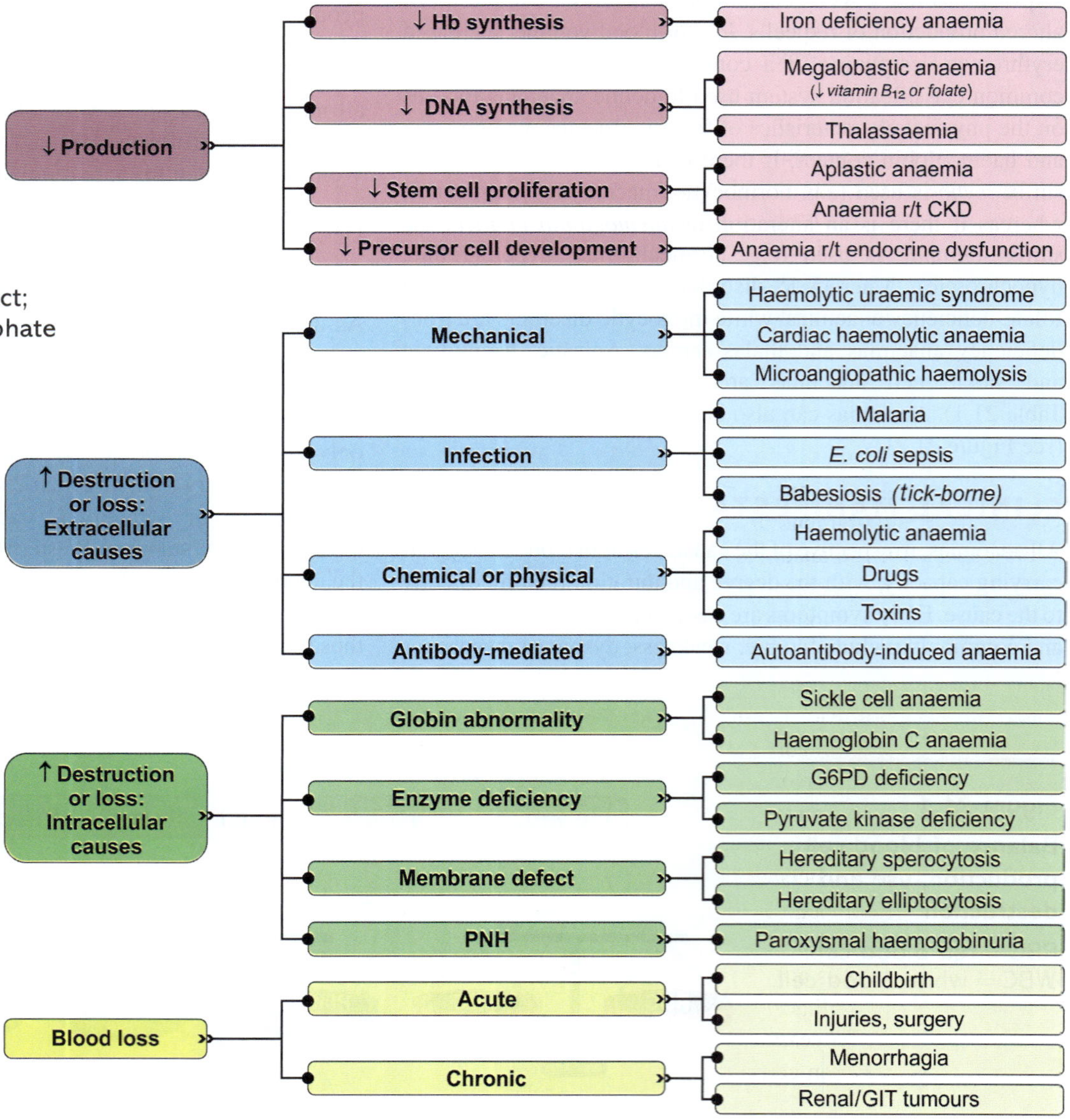

- ↓ Production
  - ↓ Hb synthesis
    - Iron deficiency anaemia
  - ↓ DNA synthesis
    - Megalobastic anaemia (↓ *vitamin B_{12} or folate*)
    - Thalassaemia
  - ↓ Stem cell proliferation
    - Aplastic anaemia
    - Anaemia r/t CKD
  - ↓ Precursor cell development
    - Anaemia r/t endocrine dysfunction
- ↑ Destruction or loss: Extracellular causes
  - Mechanical
    - Haemolytic uraemic syndrome
    - Cardiac haemolytic anaemia
    - Microangiopathic haemolysis
  - Infection
    - Malaria
    - *E. coli* sepsis
    - Babesiosis *(tick-borne)*
  - Chemical or physical
    - Haemolytic anaemia
    - Drugs
    - Toxins
  - Antibody-mediated
    - Autoantibody-induced anaemia
- ↑ Destruction or loss: Intracellular causes
  - Globin abnormality
    - Sickle cell anaemia
    - Haemoglobin C anaemia
  - Enzyme deficiency
    - G6PD deficiency
    - Pyruvate kinase deficiency
  - Membrane defect
    - Hereditary sperocytosis
    - Hereditary elliptocytosis
  - PNH
    - Paroxysmal haemogobinuria
- Blood loss
  - Acute
    - Childbirth
    - Injuries, surgery
  - Chronic
    - Menorrhagia
    - Renal/GIT tumours

rapidly develop an iron deficiency unless supplements are taken. Generally, people living in chronic poverty, pregnant women, and people with ulcers or conditions associated with blood loss, including menorrhagia, are susceptible to iron-deficiency anaemia.

Chronic blood loss, associated with bleeding lesions within the gastrointestinal tract, can occur for several months before the person seeks assistance for their symptoms. This form of haemorrhage can lead to a depletion in body iron stores that results in iron-deficiency anaemia.

Clinical manifestations

People with iron-deficiency anaemia may experience a loss of platelets, leading to thrombocytopenia and inappropriate bleeding. At its worst, iron-deficiency anaemia can be associated with malignancies of the epithelium, particularly in the gastrointestinal tract.

Clinical diagnosis and management

Diagnosis Diagnosis requires blood tests to determine serum ferritin levels, transferrin saturation or total iron-binding capacity, and may include a biopsy of bone marrow to determine iron stores.

Management Management will begin with an evaluation of the situation to determine whether the iron deficiency is due to blood loss, diet or, more rarely, a transferring receptor deficiency. Iron replacement therapy can usually be undertaken using oral preparations, but the iron can also be administered intramuscularly or intravenously. Ferrous iron is preferred to ferric iron, as the former is more easily absorbed into the system. Co-administration of oral vitamin C supplements will also improve iron absorption. Figure 21.3 explores the common clinical manifestations and management of iron-deficiency anaemia.

MEGALOBLASTIC ANAEMIA

Aetiology and pathophysiology

Pernicious anaemia, the most common cause of megaloblastic anaemia, is an autoimmune disease of the gastric parietal cells, leading to macrocytic anaemia, atrophy of the gastric mucosa, the presence of megaloblasts in the bone marrow, **leukopenia**, thrombocytopenia and potentially psychiatric and neurological disease. One underlying reason for this condition is an antibody attack on, and destruction of, parietal cells, decreasing the availability of intrinsic factor, thereby markedly reducing vitamin B_{12} (cobalamin) absorption.

Alternatively, the person may have a congenital deficiency of intrinsic factor secretion, secretion of a defective intrinsic factor, or failure of vitamin B_{12} absorption due to gastrectomy or gastric atrophy associated with chronic gastritis. In rare cases, nutritional deficiencies secondary to chronic poverty or a poorly maintained vegan or vegetarian lifestyle can manifest symptoms of pernicious anaemia. Interestingly, because of liver stores of cobalamin, clinical signs of pernicious anaemia may not manifest for 5–10 years after the onset of the parietal cell loss. The other common cause of pernicious anaemia is folate deficiency due to malnutrition, chronic alcohol abuse, increased metabolic need (e.g. infancy, pregnancy) or drug treatment. The loss of folate leads to impaired DNA synthesis and the subsequent transformation of red blood cells.

Clinical manifestations

Symptoms develop slowly with pernicious anaemia, and early signs are easily missed or misinterpreted. Many of the common manifestations will reverse with treatment; of serious concern are the irreversible neurological changes that can result secondary to a vitamin B_{12} deficiency, such as nerve demyelination and neuronal destruction. By contrast, the behavioural changes, such as short-term memory loss, changes in personality, depression and even psychosis do appear to respond well to treatment.

Clinical diagnosis and management

Diagnosis Vitamin B_{12} and folic acid blood levels will generally be low, and homocysteine will often be high. Antibodies for intrinsic factor or parietal cell bodies may be present.

Management Treatment generally involves intramuscular injections of vitamin B_{12}, to avoid the loss/dysfunction of parietal cells, or through dietary supplementation taken orally. Figure 21.4 explores the common clinical manifestations and management of pernicious anaemia.

THALASSAEMIA

Aetiology and pathophysiology

Thalassaemias are inherited mutations of haemoglobin molecules that cause a reduction in the synthesis of, and possibly complete absence of, one of the polypeptide, or globin, chains that combine to form haemoglobin. Thalassaemia may result from a defect in either the *α- or β-globin chain* (see Figure 21.5). Geographical and cultural influences affect the distribution of this genetic disorder. In South-East Asian and Chinese populations, α-thalassaemia is more common; however, in people from a Mediterranean heritage, β-thalassaemia is more common. Thalassaemia is also more common in people of African or Middle Eastern heritage than in Caucasians. Interestingly, thalassaemia is more common in regions where malaria is endemic, and appears to provide improved immune clearance and reduced erythrocyte invasion from the malarial parasite.

Thalassaemia results in an *imbalance in the number of globin chains* through reduced, defective or the absence of specific globin chain synthesis. This imbalance causes erythrocyte destruction, which may ultimately result in haemolytic anaemia and iron overload. Iron deposition creates a risk of diabetes, cardiomyopathy, liver fibrosis and cirrhosis. Ineffective erythropoiesis also results in hypochromic and microcytic red blood cells.

Since α-globin production begins in utero, and all forms of haemoglobin require this polypeptide, symptoms of *α-thalassaemia* can manifest in either the fetus or the child after birth. The severity of the condition depends on the nature of the

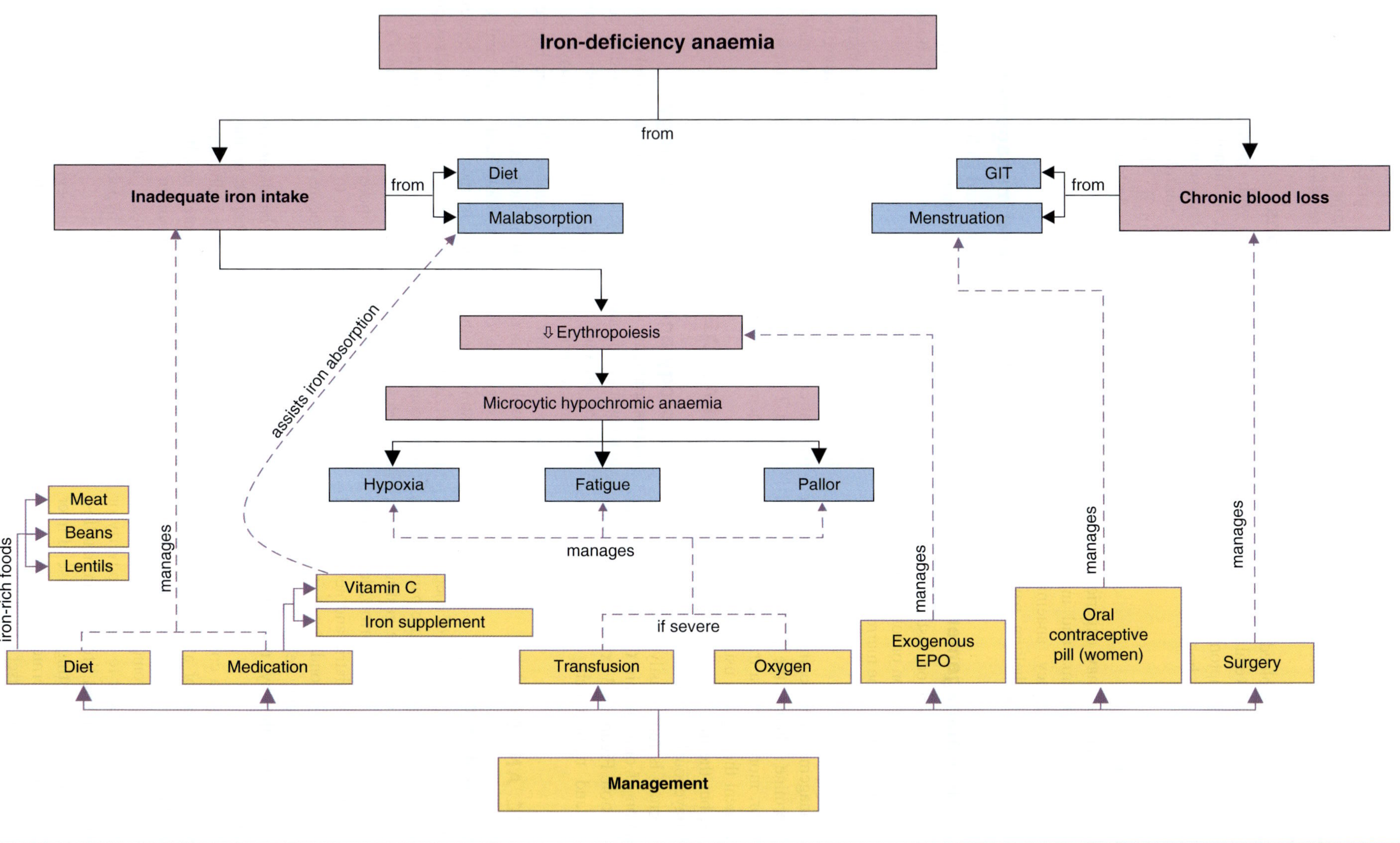

Figure 21.3

Clinical snapshot: Iron-deficiency anaemia

↓ = decreased; EPO = erythropoietin; GIT = gastrointestinal tract.

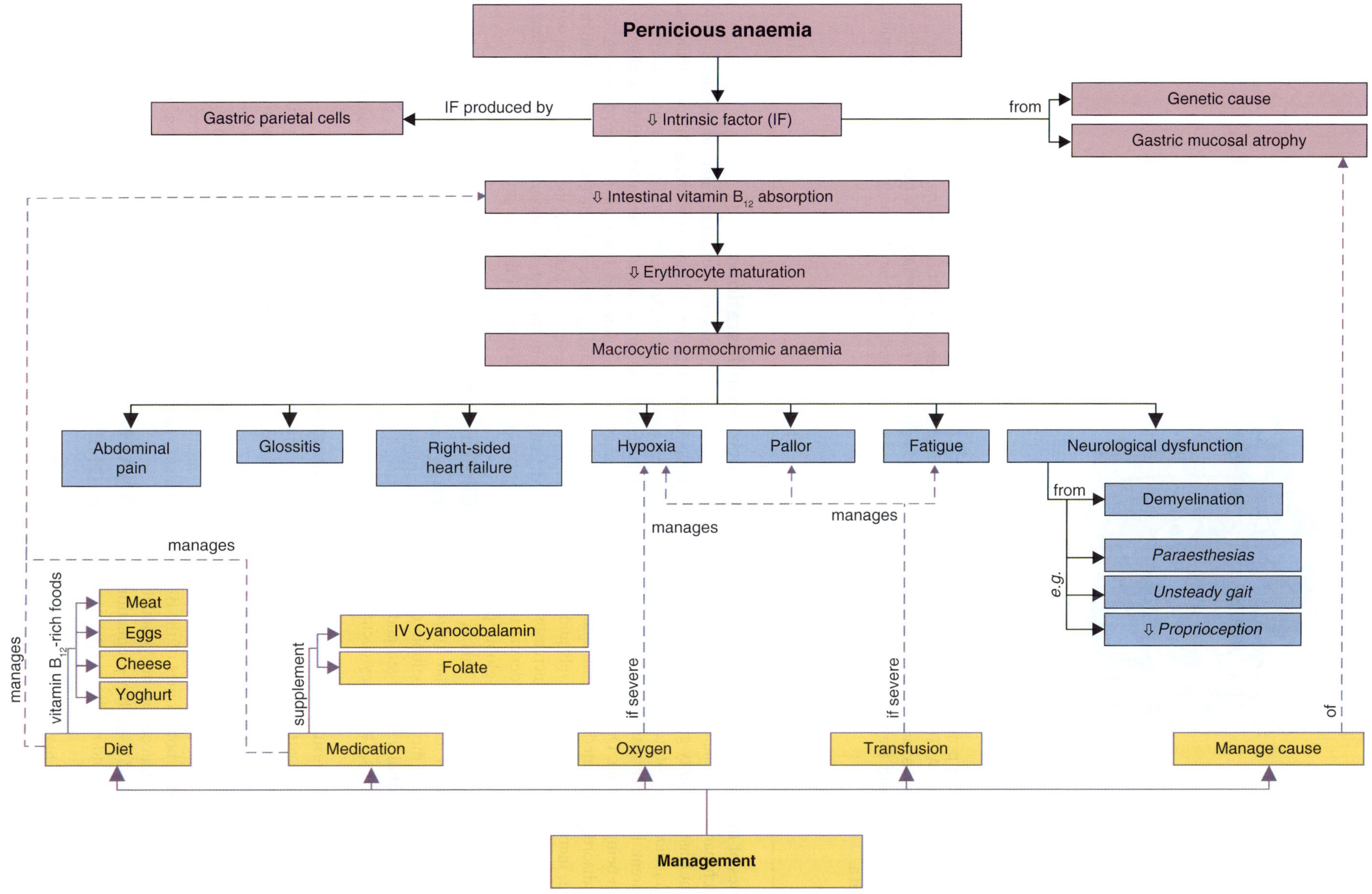

Figure 21.4

Clinical snapshot: Pernicious anaemia

↓ = decreased; IF = intrinsic factor; IV = intravenous.

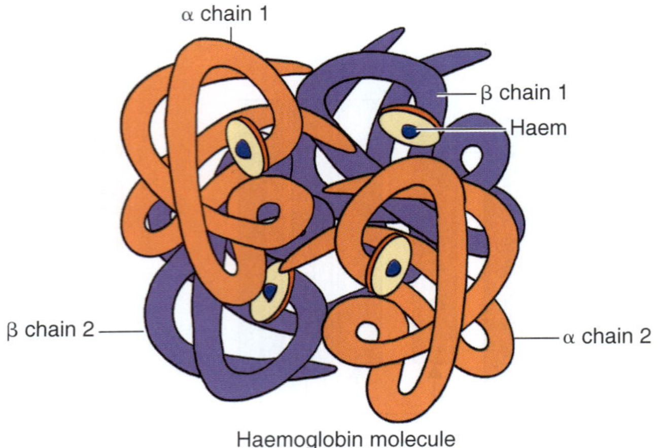

Figure 21.5

Normal haemoglobin

Haemoglobin is made up of four polypeptide subunits called globin. Each haemoglobin molecule contains two α-globin chains and two β-globin chains. A -Thalassaemia results from an impaired synthesis of α-globin chains, and an increase in the γ-globin chains in the fetus, and β-globin chains in children and adults. β-Thalassaemia results from an impaired synthesis of β-globin chains, and an increase in the γ-globin chains in the fetus, and α -globin chains in children and adults. α = alpha; β = beta.

Source: Sciencopia.

mutation. Two copies of the α-globin gene on chromosome 16 are provided by each parent. As thalassaemia is an autosomal recessive disorder, at least one faulty gene is required from both parents. *α-Thalassaemia minor* occurs if only one defective gene from one parent has been passed on. This generally results in the person being a carrier. Occasionally a person may present with a mild disorder associated with mild anaemia, bone marrow hyperplasia, increased serum iron levels and moderate splenomegaly. The severity of symptoms increases with the number of alleles affected. If the genetic disorder causes a defect in both α-globin chains, compete loss of α-globin production and a relative increase in β-globin occurs. This is known as *haemoglobin Bart's*, which results in the fatal *hydrops fetalis* (or *α-thalassaemia major*), where the haemoglobin consists of four γ-globins, has increased affinity of oxygen and therefore little oxygen delivery to the tissues. Death may occur before or at birth.

β-Thalassaemia occurs as a result of a defect in at least one β-globin. *β-Thalassaemia minor* occurs when one β-globin gene on chromosome 11 is defective and results in the production of approximately 50% less β-globin protein. People with β-thalassaemia minor are carriers, but may experience some mild anaemia. People with *β-thalassaemia major* have a defect or deletion in both copies of the β-globin genes, resulting in severely reduced or no production of β-globin and a relative excess of α-globin production. This is also called *Cooley's anaemia* and results in severe, chronic anaemia, beginning within months after birth and requiring life-long treatment. Fragile haemoglobin, inadequate erythropoiesis and bone marrow hyperplasia develop, and extramedullary haematopoiesis results in hepatomegaly and splenomegaly.

Clinical manifestations

Clinical manifestations of β-thalassaemia major are usually apparent within the first 6–12 months of life, and include lethargy, poor appetite, failure to thrive, irritability, developmental delay and haemolytic anaemia. Growth retardation with bone changes, particularly of the spine and bones of the face, fractures, leg ulcers, bronze colouring of the skin and enlargement of both the spleen and liver are seen in childhood, the severity of which will be directly related to the type of gene mutation and whether a single copy or both copies of the gene are affected.

Clinical diagnosis and management

Diagnosis Diagnosis of thalassaemia will depend on a family history, a clinical evaluation of symptoms and blood tests to identify the species of haemoglobin present. Prenatal screening using amniocentesis can identify hydrops fetalis.

Management

While individuals with thalassaemia minor will have few symptoms, other people will be treated with blood transfusions to return haematocrit levels to near normal, iron chelation to reduce organ damage, and splenectomy to reduce the need for transfusions, prolonging erythrocyte survival. Figure 21.6 explores the common clinical manifestations and management of thalassaemia.

ANAEMIA RELATED TO CHRONIC KIDNEY DISEASE

Aetiology and pathophysiology

Chronic kidney disease is covered in detail in the chapter 'Acute kidney injury and chronic kidney disease'. Anaemia of chronic kidney disease is caused by a combination of the increased

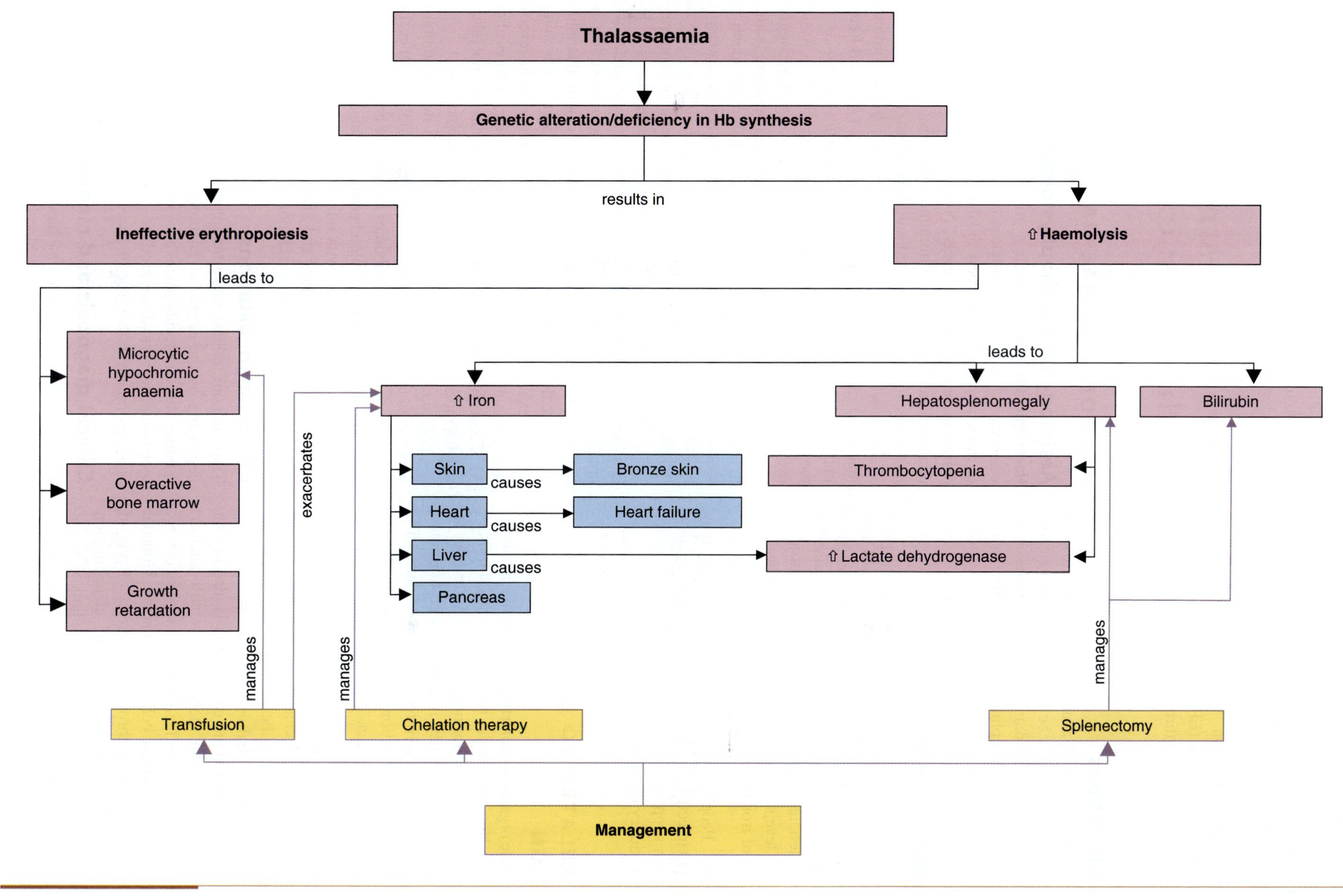

Figure 21.6

Clinical snapshot: Thalassaemia

↑ = increased; Hb = haemoglobin.

destruction of and the decreased production of red blood cells. Several mechanisms can cause the destruction of red blood cells: turbulence and trauma to the erythrocytes from haemodialysis results in a shortened red blood cell survival; and the exposure of erythrocytes to highly ureamic conditions may also result in premature red blood cell destruction. A decrease in production is caused by reduced erythropoietin (EPO) availability. In people with uraemia, the induction of erythropoiesis from hypoxaemia appears to be blunted.

Clinical manifestations

Along with the common signs of anaemia, signs of orthostatic hypotension (e.g. presyncope) may be observed. Neurologically, an inability to concentrate and decreased cognitive abilities may be reported. They may also complain of non-specific issues, such as cold intolerance and sleep disturbances.

Clinical diagnosis and management

Diagnosis Serum EPO can be measured, and will most often be low. Haemoglobin and red blood cell counts will also be low. Investigations for chronic kidney disease can assist in the diagnosis. It is also important that other causes of anaemia are ruled out. Iron-deficiency tests, such as transferrin saturation and serum ferritin levels, should be undertaken to assess the presence or degree of iron deficiency.

Management People with chronic kidney disease may require regular EPO injections to stimulate the production of new red blood cells. Iron supplementation may also be necessary for those with chronic kidney disease in the context of anaemia.

ANAEMIA RELATED TO ENDOCRINE DYSFUNCTION

Numerous endocrine organs can contribute to anaemia; however, many of the mechanisms are not yet fully established. Pituitary gland deficiencies can result in normochromic and normocytic anemias when there is a deficiency in anterior lobe hormones (such as thyroid-stimulating hormone) that modulate EPO production. Thyroid gland dysfunction may result in normocytic, microcytic or macrocytic anaemia, possibly related to iron, vitamin B_{12} or folic acid deficiencies. Thyroxine appears to potentiate the effect of EPO. There is also some suggestion that rates of intrinsic factor deficiency are higher in people with hypothyroidism, which may be related to autoantibodies cross-reacting against thyroglobulins and intrinsic factor or gastric parietal cells. Adrenal gland dysfunction is also known to cause anaemia; however, the mechanism is still unclear. Possible suggestions include an influence of adrenocorticotropic hormone on EPO or erythropoietic cells in the marrow. Gonadal dysfunction can cause anaemia through the direct effects of androgens on the production of EPO, and the augmentation of its effects on bone marrow. However, although large doses of oestrogen appear to be able to cause an iron-deficiency anaemia, by which mechanism this occurs is unknown. Finally, anaemia is not uncommon in pregnancy, and is thought to be caused by a combination of haemodilution (from increased circulating plasma volume), dietary restriction and potentially even folic acid deficiency.

Increased destruction of erythrocytes: extracellular causes

HAEMOLYTIC ANAEMIA

Aetiology and pathophysiology

Haemolytic anaemia represents a group of disorders that occur when there is an early destruction of erythrocytes, leading to a mismatch between production and destruction, and a consequent deficit in red blood cell levels. Numerous causes have been identified, and include autoimmune reactions, drugs, trauma, infections, toxins and inherited mutations of enzymes.

Immunohaemolytic anaemias are due to autoimmune reactions, and each is the responsibility of a different immunoglobulin. *Western antibody haemolytic anaemia* is the most common of these disorders, primarily affecting women over 40 years of age. Immunoglobulin G (IgG) recognises erythrocyte antigens, binding best at body temperature, leading to intravascular haemolysis. Approximately half of the identified cases are idiopathic, while the remainder are secondary to conditions such as lymphomas, leukaemias (e.g. chronic lymphocytic leukaemia), systemic lupus erythematosus or drugs.

Cold agglutination immune haemolytic anaemia is a less common disorder affecting older women, and is associated with optimal antibody–erythrocyte binding at temperatures near freezing (i.e. 0–4°C). In this condition, red cells form clumps that inhibit the proper flow of blood, causing tissue ischaemia. Such clumps are characteristic of *Raynaud's disease*. Symptoms can be reversed with warming, as the antibody binds poorly at temperatures above 31°C, but antibodies already bound to erythrocytes may not release as the temperature increases, and can trigger haemolysis.

Cold haemolysis haemolytic anaemia is a rare condition in which cold temperatures trigger profound haemolysis rather than aggregate formation. The antibodies responsible are IgG in origin, and are directed against the P blood group antigen. This disease has been found to be associated with infections such as mycoplasmal pneumonia, measles, mumps and various cold viruses. Syphilis appears to be responsible for a chronic form of the condition.

Clinical manifestations

The common clinical manifestations are present, with the severity depending on the degree of haemolysis. Lysis of a significant number of erythrocytes places excessive demands on the liver to metabolise the breakdown products. As a consequence, jaundice is also common in this type of anaemia.

Clinical diagnosis and management

Diagnosis Diagnosis is based on symptoms, history, bone marrow evaluation and blood tests. Premature release of erythrocytes occurs secondarily to the loss of red blood cells from circulation, and this is associated with an increased number of erythroid stem cells in the marrow.

Management Acquired haemolytic anaemias are managed with treatment of the precipitating condition, while inherited conditions are managed with steroids, transfusions and splenectomy.

HAEMOLYTIC DISEASE OF THE NEWBORN

Aetiology and pathophysiology

Incompatibility between the maternal and fetal Rh factor is the most recognised underlying cause of *haemolytic disease of the newborn (HDN)*, although blood antigens of the ABO blood group are more commonly responsible (see Figure 21.7).

Almost one-quarter of pregnancies involve an ABO incompatibility, with an estimated 10% leading to haemolytic disease of the newborn. By contrast, Rh incompatibility occurs in less than 10% of all pregnancies, and while it does not affect the first pregnancy, it will sensitise the maternal system, leading to HDN in about one in three cases.

Clinical manifestations

In mild cases, the newborn will appear healthy, though somewhat pale, with only a small increase in the size of the liver and spleen. Marked pallor, splenomegaly and hepatomegaly are signs of severe anaemia and can lead to heart failure and shock.

Erythrocyte destruction proceeds after birth due to the persistence of maternal antibodies in the newborn's circulation. This leads to neonatal jaundice and possible bilirubin deposition in the brain, causing brain damage, mental retardation, cerebral palsy, high-frequency deafness and possibly death. Figure 21.8A shows the cutaneous effects of anaemia and jaundice on a neonate.

Figure 21.9 explores the common clinical manifestations and management of HDN.

Clinical diagnosis and management

Diagnosis Diagnosis is made via blood tests. If a Coombs test is performed, a positive result will produce agglutination of red blood cells. An indirect Coombs test is performed on the maternal antenatal antibodies, and a direct Coombs test is performed on the newborn, identifying antibodies or complement proteins. Neonatal bilirubin can rapidly increase and remain elevated. Anaemia will develop, and reticulocyte counts will rise. **Neutropenia** (i.e. a decreased number of neutrophils) and thrombocytopenia may develop.

Management Management may differ between pregnancies. *Alloimmunisation*, the sensitisation of the immune system to foreign erythrocyte surface antigens, is more likely to have occurred during the second pregnancy unless the mother has been exposed to previous transfusions. Prevention

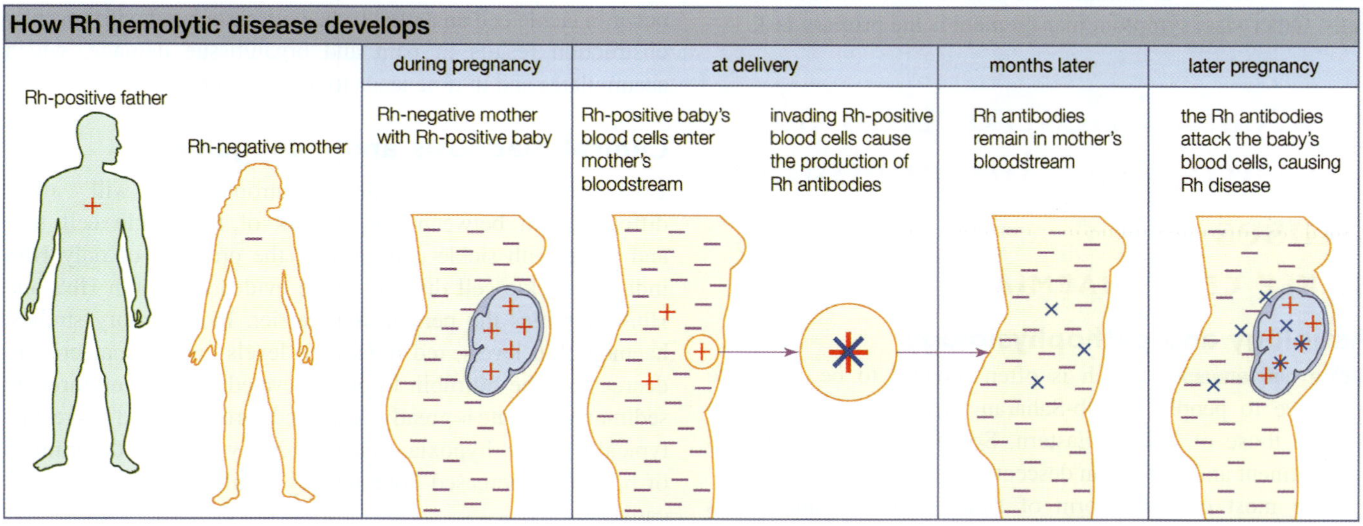

Figure 21.7

Rh factors in pregnancy

If a Rh^- mother is exposed to Rh^+ blood from the fetus in her first pregnancy, maternal antibodies will be produced which can result in haemolysis of fetal erythrocytes in subsequent pregnancies.

Source: Encyclopaedia Britannica/Universal Images Group North America LLC/Alamy Stock Photo.

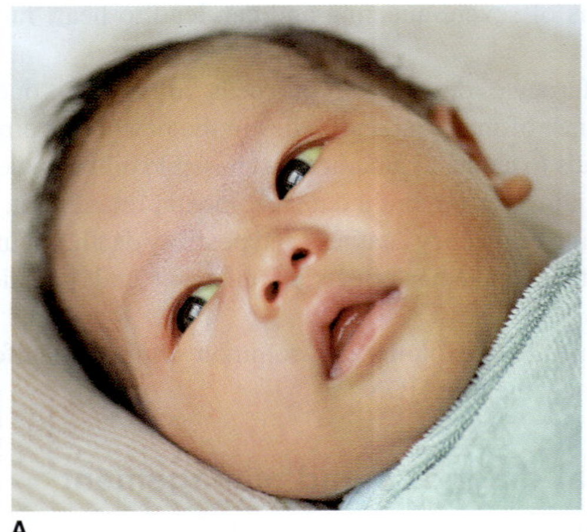

A

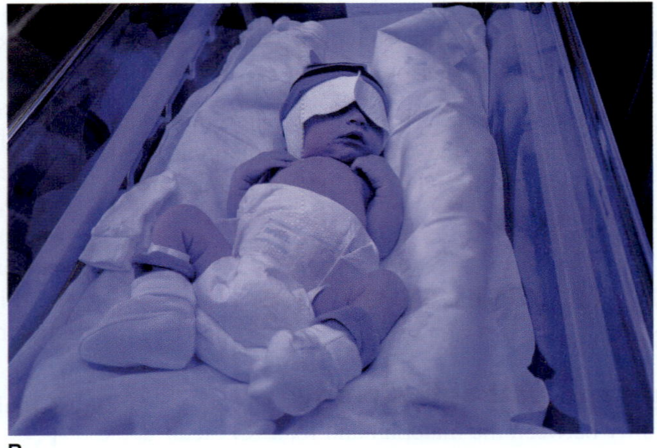

B

Figure 21.8

Haemolytic disease of the newborn (HDN)

(A) Neonate with hyperbilirubinaemia. Note the yellow sclera. (B) Phototherapy to reduce jaundice.

Source: (A) GOLFX/Shutterstock. (B) Chris James/Alamy Stock Photo.

is better than cure, and maternal serology can be sent for testing. Maternal anti-D antibody testing will help determine the appropriate management, which may include the administration of intravenous immunoglobulin (IV IgG) in an attempt to reduce the transport of antibodies to the fetus. Intrauterine transfusion may be required if the HDN is severe. Hyperbilirubinaemia is managed with phototherapy to reduce the risk of kernicterus (Figure 21.8B). Other treatments may include the administration of exogenous EPO to stimulate the production of more red blood cells. Otherwise, symptom management is the primary task.

Increased destruction of erythrocytes: intracellular causes

SICKLE CELL ANAEMIA

Aetiology and pathophysiology

Sickle cell anaemia, which is often thought to be a disease exclusive to people of sub-Saharan African descent, is also seen in those of Middle Eastern, Southern European, Indian subcontinent and Caribbean descent.

The most common form of sickle cell anaemia results from a glutamate-to-valine mutation in the β-globin chain, creating a *variant haemoglobin* to the normal form (HbA) known as *haemoglobin S (HbS)*, which causes the erythrocyte to adopt the characteristic sickle shape in response to repeated deoxygenation and dehydration (see Figure 21.10). The gene mutation is autosomal recessive, and carriers are not only free of symptoms but are, ironically, at an advantage, as their mixed blood phenotype gives them a degree of resistance to malaria. Because the altered erythrocyte shape prevents the normally flexible erythrocyte from navigating capillary beds, the person experiences repeated blood flow obstructions, leading to ischaemia of the affected tissue or organ.

Clinical manifestations

The usual clinical manifestations associated with anaemia occur in sickle cell anaemia. Ischaemia associated with vascular obstruction results in pain and organ/tissue damage, which accumulates and in time leads to organ failure.

Clinical diagnosis and management

Diagnosis Haemoglobin electrophoresis will allow differentiation between the carriers of the sickle cell trait and those with sickle cell disease; the presence of only HbS indicates sickle cell disease, while evidence of both HbS and HbA identifies the person as a carrier. In laboratory studies, haemoglobin levels, red blood cell levels and haematocrit are decreased. The bilirubin level is elevated, and the erythrocyte sedimentation rate is greatly decreased. Arterial blood gas results typically show hypoxia. Skeletal X-ray reveals deformities of bone and increased bone density, while chest X-ray shows cardiomegaly.

Management Management goals for sickle cell anaemia should focus on the relief of pain, prevention of infection and stroke, and the management of complications, including anaemia, organ damage and pulmonary hypertension. Interventions may include the administration of oxygen

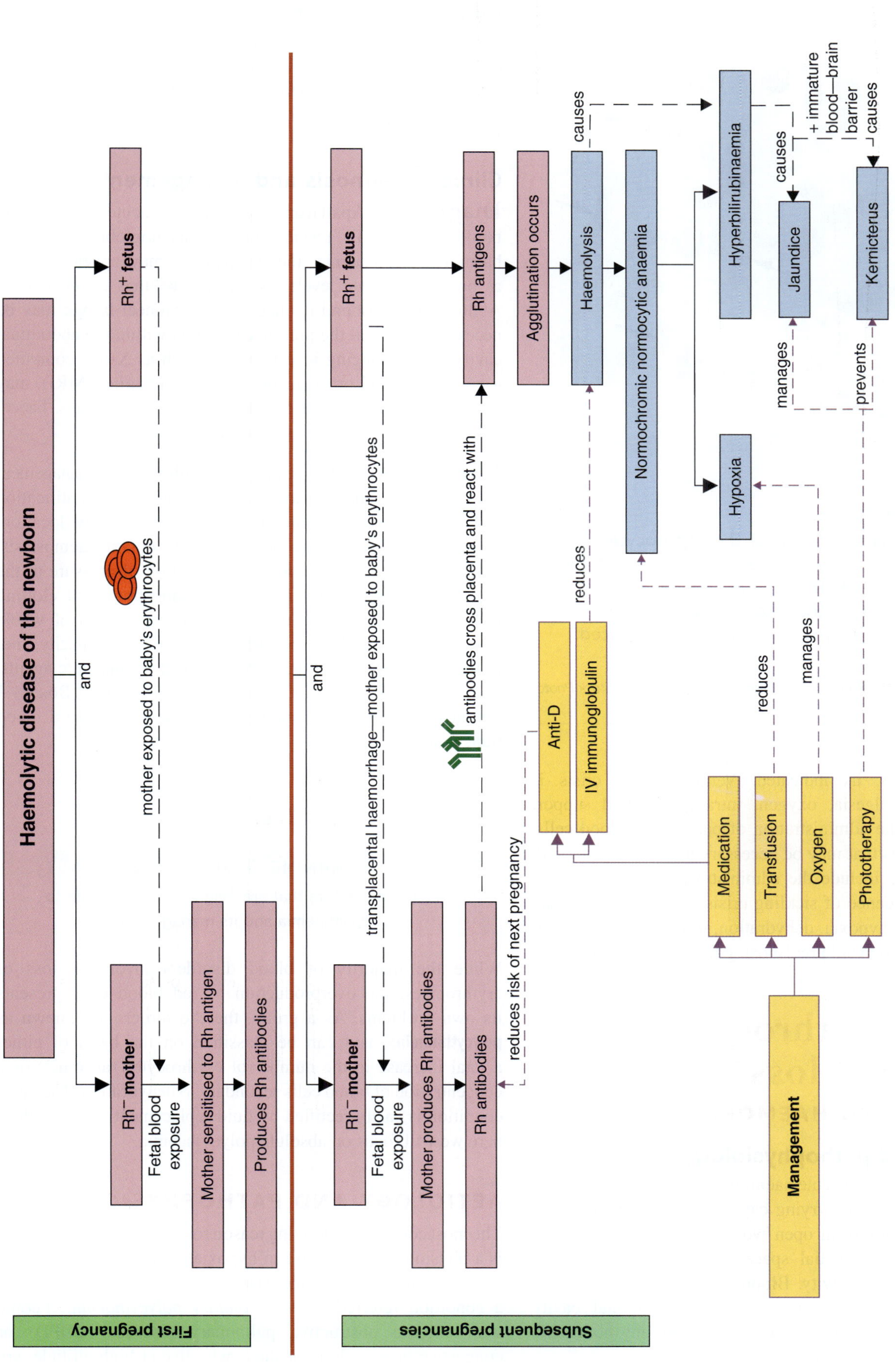

Figure 21.9

Clinical snapshot: Haemolytic disease of the newborn

IV = intravenous; Rh = rhesus.

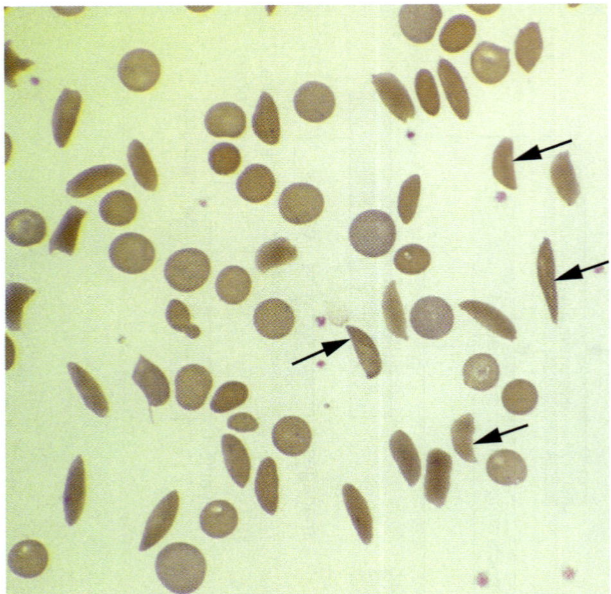

Figure 21.10

Sickle cell anaemia

Note the sickle shape of many of the erythrocytes (marked by arrows). These affected cells are rigid, fragile and prone to breakage. They can impede blood flow, which results in tissue ischaemia or infarction. Their oxygen-carrying capacity is also significantly reduced.

Source: SIU School of Medicine/Avalon/Bruce Coleman Inc/Alamy Stock Photo.

and antimicrobials, as indicated. Veno-occlusive crisis is managed with analgesia, oxygen, intravenous fluid support and, potentially, the administration of packed red blood cells. Other interventions that may be necessary to assist people with sickle cell disease include the administration of hydroxyurea to reduce the incidence of sickling crisis. An acute crisis may be precipitated by hypoxia, dehydration, infection or the use of sedatives, so care to avoid predisposing factors should be taken.

Loss of erythrocytes from blood loss

SECONDARY TO HAEMORRHAGE

Aetiology and pathophysiology

Red blood cell loss from acute haemorrhage or chronic bleeding will reduce the oxygen-carrying capacity of the blood. Blood loss may be obvious from open wounds, or it may be occult haemorrhage into interstitial spaces, such as the abdomen, pelvic region or chest cavity. Blood lost into the abdomen is particularly difficult to visualise, as the abdominal cavity can hold a significant amount of blood before any noticeable increase in girth is observed.

Clinical manifestations

The signs and symptoms of the anaemic state may well be obscured by the clinical manifestations of the haemorrhage. Sympathetic nervous system activation in compensation for the loss of blood volume can lead to pallor, sweating and tachycardia. If severe enough, the haemorrhage may lead to circulatory shock.

Clinical diagnosis and management

Diagnosis Apart from observations for acute haemorrhage, blood testing will reveal reduced haemoglobin levels. In haemorrhagic anaemia, the haematocrit may appear normal, as both erythrocyte levels and plasma volume are decreased. Abdominal ultrasound or diagnostic peritoneal lavage may be necessary to reveal the presence of blood within the abdominal cavity. Other imaging investigations, such as X-ray, computed tomography (CT) or magnetic resonance imaging (MRI), may also reveal collections of blood within various cavities. Faecal testing for occult blood may also be informative.

Management The primary imperative for the management of anaemia secondary to acute haemorrhage is the identification and control of the acute blood loss. Depending on the location, surgical intervention may be required to obtain haemostasis. Other interventions may include application of pressure to the area (either directly or indirectly), administration of clotting factors or platelets to control bleeding, transfusion of whole blood or packed cells to support oxygen-carrying capacity, and/or the administration of antifibrinolytics or haemostatic agents, such as aproptinin or ε-amino-caproic acid. Clinical Box 21.1 outlines the issues surrounding refusal to consent to a blood transfusion.

Polycythaemias

LEARNING OBJECTIVE 2

Outline the factors that are believed to contribute to polycythaemia and its management.

While the majority of blood disorders involve a loss of erythrocytes, the overproduction of red blood cells presents its own problems. As a group, these disorders are known as **polycythaemias**, and can be classified on the basis of either a total increase in the number of erythrocytes (absolute) or a concentration of blood cells secondary to dehydration. The latter condition is easily rectified by fluid replacement, and therefore here we will focus on absolute polycythaemia.

AETIOLOGY AND PATHOPHYSIOLOGY

The most common underlying reason for *absolute polycythaemia* is a physiological response to hypoxia, which causes secretion of EPO, and therefore increased production of erythrocytes, a condition referred to as *secondary polycythaemia*. People with chronic obstructive pulmonary disorder (COPD) or congestive heart failure, or those who live at high altitude, are

CLINICAL BOX 21.1

Refusal to consent to blood transfusion, and alternatives available

People may refuse blood transfusions for fear of infection, religious beliefs or any number of other reasons. Alternative therapies are available for people who do not wish to receive homologous blood transfusions; however, these options may be less efficient at replacing the required red blood cells necessary to sustain sufficient oxygenation. A full explanation of the risks, including risk of death, should be discussed, so that those concerned may make informed decisions. Ultimately, it is the individual's choice. Alternatives to red blood cell transfusion may include the use of:

- antifibrinolytic therapy
- autologous transfusion
- cell salvage
- desmopressin
- erythropoietin
- euvolaemic haemodilution
- hypotensive anaesthesia
- iron-replacement therapy
- recombinant factors VIIa or IX
- topical haemostatic agents
- vitamin K
- volume expanders.

the most likely to develop this condition. People with abnormal haemoglobin may also develop secondary polycythaemia, as may those with renal cell carcinoma, hepatoma and cerebellar haemangioblastomas, as each of these tumours is associated with inappropriate EPO secretion.

Primary polycythaemia, also known as *polycythaemia vera* or *polycythaemia rubra vera*, is a rare condition marked by increased erythrocyte, white cell and platelet production, as well as splenomegaly. This condition has an age of onset of approximately 55–60 years of age, although earlier onsets have been reported. The disorder is associated with changes in the bone marrow, with hyperplasia of the myeloid, erythroid and megakaryocyte precursor cells. Although the aetiology is not fully understood, the majority of cases are associated with the *JAK2 V617F* mutation of the *Janus kinase 2* gene, which encodes a tyrosine kinase involved in erythropoiesis.

CLINICAL MANIFESTATIONS

The greatest concern associated with the polycythaemias is increased blood viscosity and an increase in incidental thrombus formation, leading to the occlusion of blood vessels of virtually all sizes, and marked tissue and organ ischaemia and, ultimately, infarction. In association with the change in blood viscosity, blood flow becomes sluggish, and the person affected will manifest signs such as plethora and engorgement of retinal and cerebral vessels.

Symptoms include headache, drowsiness, delirium, changes to vision, chorea and behaviour alterations, including delirium, mania and psychotic depression. Although death due to cerebral thrombosis is more common in polycythaemia, there are remarkably few cardiovascular disturbances, and myocardial infarctions are relatively rare. An additional and interesting symptom is extreme, painful itching skin that is exacerbated by heat or water. Figure 21.11 explores the common clinical manifestations and management of polycythaemia.

CLINICAL DIAGNOSIS AND MANAGEMENT

Diagnosis

Determination of haematocrit and red cell count, as well as total blood volume, is the mainstay of diagnosis of polycythaemias.

As polycythaemia is the increase in circulating red blood cells (and therefore an increase in the amount of haemoglobin), it will have a negative effect on the veracity of oximetry measurements (see Clinical Box 21.2).

Management

The primary treatment goal for those at low risk is to reduce erythrocyte production and the increase in blood volume using regular phlebotomy, initially two to three times per week and then every three to four months to maintain near-normal haematocrit levels.

In addition, low-dose aspirin treatment can be used to reduce the incidence of incidental thrombus formation. Routine venesection can trigger an increase in thrombosis; therefore, care should be taken to monitor for this during treatment. Those at high risk require intervention with cytotoxic agents. Use of radioactive phosphorous (P^{32}) suppresses increased erythrocyte production and has lasting effects subsequent to a single exposure, with an effective period of 12–18 months. Treatment is well-tolerated with few side-effects, although acute leukaemia is a possible side-effect of treatment. More commonly, hydroxyurea, a highly effective non-radioactive myelosuppressive agent, is used, and is associated with lower risks of thrombosis and leukaemia. Some people are either tolerant or resistant to hydroxyurea, in which case the use of interferon-α or anagrelide, which suppresses platelet production, may be indicated, although interferon-α has a high degree of toxicity. Despite a link to the presence of mast cells in the skin, antihistamines provide little relief.

Prompt treatment provides a therapeutic remission, extending the person's life by 10–15 years. By contrast, those who do not receive appropriate treatment in the early stages of their illness generally die within two years of symptom onset.

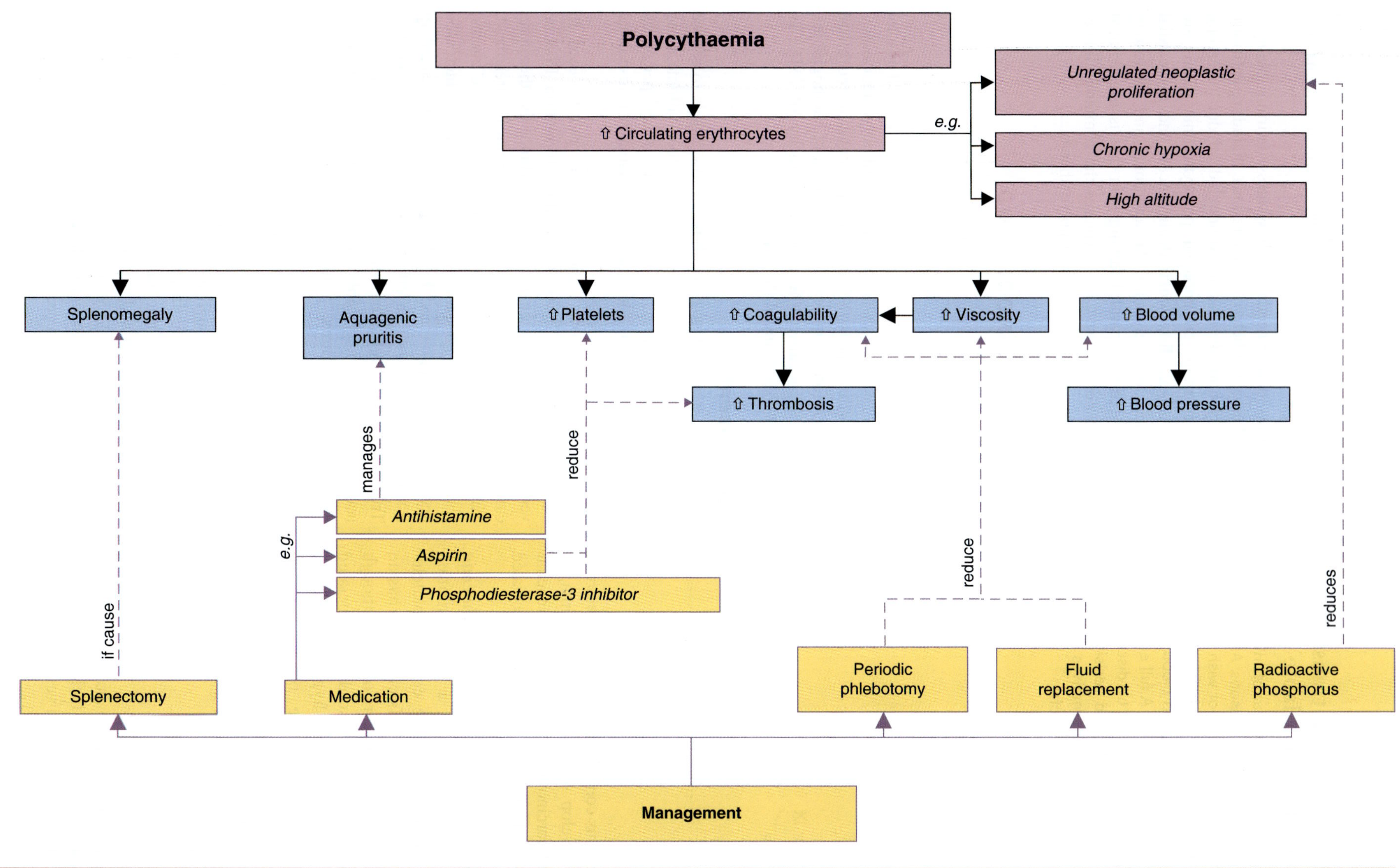

Figure 21.11
Clinical snapshot: Polycythaemia
↑ = increased.

CLINICAL BOX 21.2

Erythrocytes and oximetry

Any pathology that reduces the amount of haemoglobin or number of circulating red blood cells will cause errors in oximetry measurements that may confuse the clinical picture. Oximetry measures the percentage of oxygenated haemoglobin. If haemoglobin levels are appropriate and oxygen levels are reduced, the percentage of haemoglobin bound with oxygen will be reduced. Therefore, lower oxygen saturations will be accurately represented by the oximeter. However, when haemoglobin levels are low, all haemoglobin may be bound with oxygen (even if oxygen levels are low), and therefore the oximeter will falsely display high oxygen saturation. Clinically, the person may be hypoxic at the cellular level; however, the pulse oximeter may show acceptable oxygen saturations. Before placing confidence in the pulse oximetry measurement, determine that the person is not anaemic (see Figure 21.12).

Haemophilias

LEARNING OBJECTIVE 3

Differentiate between the main types of haemophilia and von Willebrand disease.

The three types of **haemophilia** are now known as *A*, *B* and *C*, but were previously known as *classic haemophilia*, *Christmas disease* (named for the surname of the first individual identified with the disorder) and *factor XI deficiency*, respectively. A fourth disorder, **von Willebrand disease (VWD)**, is actually a group of disorders with a secondary reduction in factor VIII levels.

AETIOLOGY AND PATHOPHYSIOLOGY

Haemophilias are bleeding disorders that result from the absence of a key clotting factor required for normal coagulation. The coagulation pathway is represented in Figure 21.13.

Haemophilia A is associated with an X-linked factor VIII deficiency, *haemophilia B* with an X-linked factor IX deficiency and *haemophilia C* with an autosomal recessive loss of factor XI. Haemophilia A is best known for its association with the descendants of Queen Victoria, culminating in Alexis, son of Nicholas, the Tsar of Russia, being affected.

Von Willebrand disease is actually a group of six disorders associated either with quantitative (types 1 and 3) or qualitative (the type 2 group) mutations of the *von Willebrand factor (VWF) gene*. Most people with von Willebrand disease only have a mild bleeding disorder, in contrast to those with classic haemophilia. The glycoprotein known as von Willebrand factor creates a link between platelets and collagen. It also acts as a carrier protein for factor VIII, and prevents its degradation; hence, the early belief that von Willebrand disease represented another form of factor VIII deficiency.

CLINICAL MANIFESTATIONS

The severity of the bleeding disorder will depend on the extent of the deficit of the clotting factor in question. In mild cases (5–35% of normal), bleeding is only an issue after major trauma or surgery, whereas in moderate disorders (1–5% of normal), bleeding results from more general trauma. In people with a severe reduction in clotting factor levels (< 1% of normal), bleeding is spontaneous rather than event-mediated. Excessive bleeding will lead to joint malformation, crippling and death if left untreated.

Figure 21.12

The effect of erythrocyte levels on oximetry accuracy

Both anaemia and polycythaemia can cause inaccuracies in oxygen saturation levels.

Oxygen level	Haemoglobin level	Oximeter reading	Actual clinical situation
Normal	Normal	✓ Potentially accurate	Oxygen demand equals oxygen supply
	Low (e.g. anaemia)	✗ Inaccurately high	Potential cellular hypoxia
	High (e.g. polycythaemia)	✗ Inaccurately low	Oxygen demand equals oxygen supply
Low	Normal	✓ Potentially accurate	Potential cellular hypoxia
	Low (e.g. anaemia)	✗ Inaccurately high	Potential cellular hypoxia
	High (e.g. polycythaemia)	✗ Inaccurately low	Potential cellular hypoxia

Figure 21.13

Coagulation pathway

Intrinsic, extrinsic and common pathways of the coagulation cascade.

Ca^{2+} = calcium ion.

Source: Marieb, E.N. et al., Human anatomy and physiology *(11th edn, Global Edition), Figure 17.14, p. 691.© 2019. Reprinted by permission of Pearson Education Limited.*

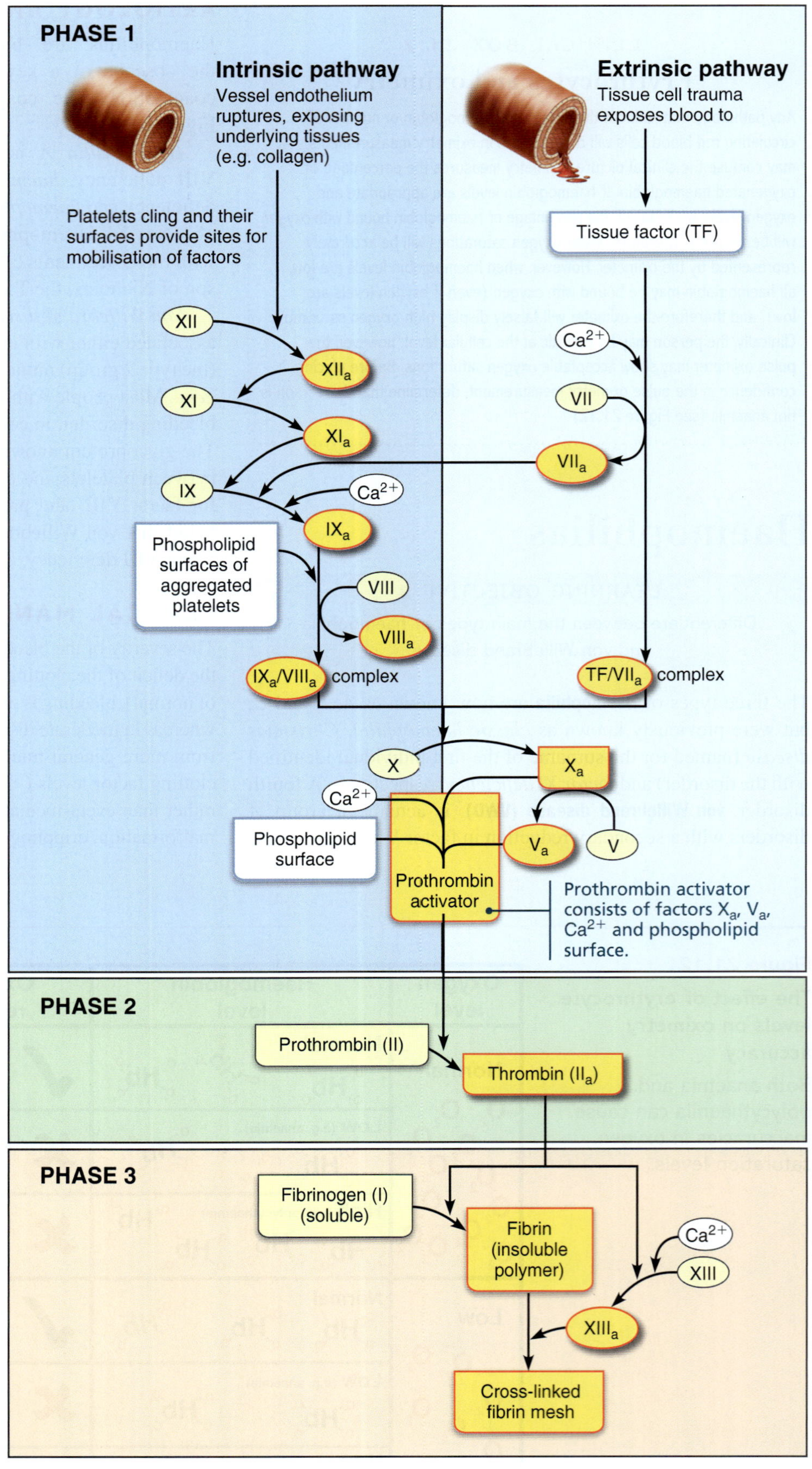

CLINICAL DIAGNOSIS AND MANAGEMENT

Diagnosis

Diagnosis is based on history, physical symptoms and determination of the three phases of coagulation; namely, the activated partial thrombin time, prothrombin time and thrombin time.

Management

The development of techniques to produce clotting-factor-rich cryoprecipitates in the early 1960s revolutionised the treatment of people with haemophilia, although the rise of viral diseases such as human immunodeficiency virus (HIV) and hepatitis caused a crisis in management in the 1980s. Improved screening methods for blood donation have reduced the risk of the transmission of viral diseases, but it remains a possibility of treatment. Since a significant proportion of children have their first episode of bleeding before 1 year of age, treatment begins early and continues until 18 years of age to ensure proper joint formation.

People with von Willebrand disease require supplementation with von Willebrand factor as well as factor VIII. However, long-term prophylaxis in people with von Willebrand disease is less common than in those with haemophilia.

Thrombocytopenia

LEARNING OBJECTIVE 4

Explain the prevention, pathophysiology and management of thrombocytopenia.

AETIOLOGY AND PATHOPHYSIOLOGY

Thrombocytopenia is a condition marked by a *loss of platelets*, and is therefore regarded as a bleeding disorder. The degree of platelet loss determines whether the bleeding is associated with trauma or is spontaneous. The condition may be secondary to another condition such as a congenital condition (e.g. Wiskott–Aldrich syndrome); viral infections such as HIV or rubella; nutritional deficiencies such as vitamin B_{12}, folate or iron; bone marrow replacement; and chemotherapy or other drug therapies. In fact, heparin treatment is a common cause of thrombocytopenia, with an estimated 2–15% of people treated with heparin demonstrating reduced platelet levels, although the advent of the disorder begins 5–10 days after the initiation of heparin treatment. The heparin-mediated destruction of platelets is due to the formation of an immunogenic complex comprised of platelet factor 4 (PF4) and heparin sulfate, and an IgG-mediated immune reaction to this complex.

The primary disorder associated with increased platelet destruction is *immune thrombocytopenic purpura*, which is also known as *idiopathic or primary thrombocytopenic purpura*. In this condition, the surface of platelets becomes antigenic, triggering an IgG-mediated immune response that targets either glycoprotein IIb/IIIa or glycoprotein Ib/IX. Immune thrombocytopenic purpura is more common in women than men, and its incidence is highest in those between 20 and 40 years of age. An acute form of the disease is seen in children subsequent to viral infections, and usually lasts one to two months, but can persist for up to six months before resolving, while up to about one-quarter of affected children will develop a chronic condition.

CLINICAL MANIFESTATIONS

Abnormal bleeding is the main manifestation of this condition. In the early stages, people with immune thrombocytopenic purpura manifest with petechial haemorrhages and purpura, and progress to serious haemorrhages from mucosa or due to menorrhagia, bleeding gums and haematuria.

CLINICAL DIAGNOSIS AND MANAGEMENT

Diagnosis

Diagnosis is based on a history of bleeding and associated symptoms, such as weight loss, fever and headache, as well as a complete blood count and a peripheral blood smear.

CLINICAL BOX 21.3

COVID-19 and thrombocytopenia

Thrombocytopenia has also been associated with infection by the severe acute respiratory syndrome coronavirus 2 (SARS-CoV-2—also known as COVID-19), and also as a rare result of vaccination against COVID-19. The thrombocytopenia associated with the virus is known as idiopathic thrombocytopenic purpura (ITP) and the one associated with the vaccine is called vaccine-induced thrombotic thrombocytopenia (VITT) or thrombosis with thrombocytopenia syndrome (TTS).

The incidence of thrombotic complications associated with COVID-19 is reported in up to 69% of people in intensive care, and a mild thrombocytopenia is detected in up to 95% of people with severe illness. Although many of these events are most likely related to venous thromboembolism (VTE) (see the chapter 'Vascular disorders and circulatory shock'), immune-mediated thrombocytopenia is a well known complication of viral infection.

Some possible mechanisms resulting in COVID-associated ITP include inflammation-induced changes in megakaryocyte differentiation, changes to the bone marrow microenvironment, and possibly reduced hepatic thrombopoietin.

The incidence of COVID-19 vaccine-induced thrombocytopenia is estimated to be approximately 1 in 263,000 people. VITT/TTS appears to occur when antibodies formed as a result of vaccination (associated mostly with the Oxford/AstraZeneca and the Janssen/Johnson & Johnson vaccines) recognise platelet factor 4 and initiate platelet activation. Although through a similar autoimmune process to heparin-induced thrombocytopenia (HIT), the platelet region associated with VITT is different to the platelet region associated to HIT.

Management

Standard treatment provides symptom control, and includes the use of glucocorticoids to prevent the sequestration and destruction of platelets, splenectomy, immunoglobulins and vinca alkaloids. Second-generation thrombopoietin receptor agonists such as eltrombopag are now available in Australia and New Zealand, and are proving efficacious in inducing the proliferation and differentiation of megakaryocytes to enable improved platelet production. Figure 21.14 explores the common clinical manifestations and management of thrombocytopenia.

LEARNING OBJECTIVE 5

Discuss the various conditions caused by changes to white blood cell function, including leukaemia, lymphoma, myeloma and agranulocytosis.

Leukaemia and lymphoma

Neoplastic diseases of the white blood cells fall into two broad categories: lymphoid and myeloid. Nomenclature is somewhat problematic, as a disorder can be described as a lymphocytic leukaemia, making it difficult to differentiate between a leukaemia and a lymphoma.

Leukaemia refers to *malignant disorders of the bone marrow* involving the blocked or impaired differentiation of haematopoietic stem cells, leading to the presence of numerous tumour cells in circulating blood. By contrast, **lymphoma** is generally considered to refer to *malignancies of lymphoid cells* and their progenitor cells that do not include bone marrow, and are characterised by the marked proliferation of these cells. An *acute leukaemia* has a rapid onset and generally an abbreviated survival time, with undifferentiated or immature cells. By contrast, a *chronic leukaemia* is characterised by poorly functioning mature cells, a gradual onset of the disease and a longer survival time.

The 2021 revision of the World Health Organization's (WHO) classification of lymphoid neoplasms includes a list of more than 100 distinct disorders reordered into a slightly modified nomenclature. In the interests of brevity, we will address leukaemias, with attention to a few examples, as well as Hodgkin and non-Hodgkin lymphoma.

TYPES OF LEUKAEMIA

Aetiology and pathophysiology

Of the various leukaemias identified, the ages of onset and pathophysiological underpinnings can be wide-ranging. Remember that in the process of haematopoiesis (blood cell formation) the pluripotent stem cell (the cells from which all blood cells originate) may divide down a myeloid pathway or lymphoid pathway. When myeloid cells are affected, myeloid or myelogenous leukaemia develops. When myeloid cells are affected, lymphocytic leukaemia develops.

Acute myelogenous leukaemia (AML) is a group of white blood cell cancers with approximately eight subtypes. It is characterised by the uncontrolled proliferation of myeloblasts (myeloid precursor cells), which can crowd out other cells and interfere with haematopoiesis in the bone marrow. As with other leukaemias, it can result in anaemia (from the effects on red blood cell production), thrombocytopenia (from the effects on platelet production), and interference with body defences (related to white blood cell effects). There appears to be a wide variety of genetic mutations leading to AML, resulting in some cytogenetic changes that respond well to current treatments, and others with poorer prognosis. Clinically, it is identified as AML when myeloblasts make up to 20% or more of the leukocytes (in the bone and the peripheral blood). It is more common in people over 60 years of age.

Chronic myelogenous leukaemia (CML) represents a group of white blood cell cancers that develop gradually and often progress slowly over months. It is characterised by the uncontrolled proliferation of granulocytes. The most common type of CML results from a genetic abnormality involving chromosome 22, in which a translocation of part of chromosome 9 is transferred to it. The resulting mutation is called the *Philadelphia chromosome*, and induces physiological disruption, destabilises the genome and triggers resistance to apoptosis (programmed cell death). The majority of people with CML are over 50 years of age.

Generally, lymphoblastic leukaemias are subdivided based on the maturity of B and/or T cells. **Acute lymphoblastic leukaemia (ALL)**, for example, represents a group of conditions associated with plentiful *immature B or T cells*. The majority of conditions involving B cells present in childhood, usually about the age of 4 years. By contrast, ALL conditions involving T cells and the thymus are more appropriately referred to as *acute lymphoblastic lymphomas*, and are seen in adolescent boys. While a small subset of ALL cases is associated with an inherited disease, the overwhelming majority have no known cause. Greatly elevated blood leukocyte counts are associated with poorer outcomes. ALL is the most common childhood leukaemia.

By contrast, **chronic lymphocytic leukaemia (CLL)** is considered a disorder of older people, with the majority of people diagnosed after the age of 60 years. Lymphocytes escape programmed cell death, and accumulate in a number of reservoirs, including blood, bone marrow and lymph nodes. An absolute lymphocyte count greater than 5×10^9 cells/L is considered the primary sign of CLL, but identification of recognised surface proteins will confirm the diagnosis. Diagnosis is made using routine blood tests, and remarkably the majority of people will be asymptomatic at this time. Approximately one-third of people with CLL will never require treatment, dying of unrelated causes, while a further third will require treatment at some stage of their disease, with the remaining people requiring immediate intervention.

Clinical manifestations

Most people with leukaemia will experience symptoms based on the changes occurring in the blood, such as fatigue due to anaemia, fevers secondary to infections, as well as bleeding into tissues such as the gums, gastrointestinal tract and mucous membranes from thrombocytopenia. They often

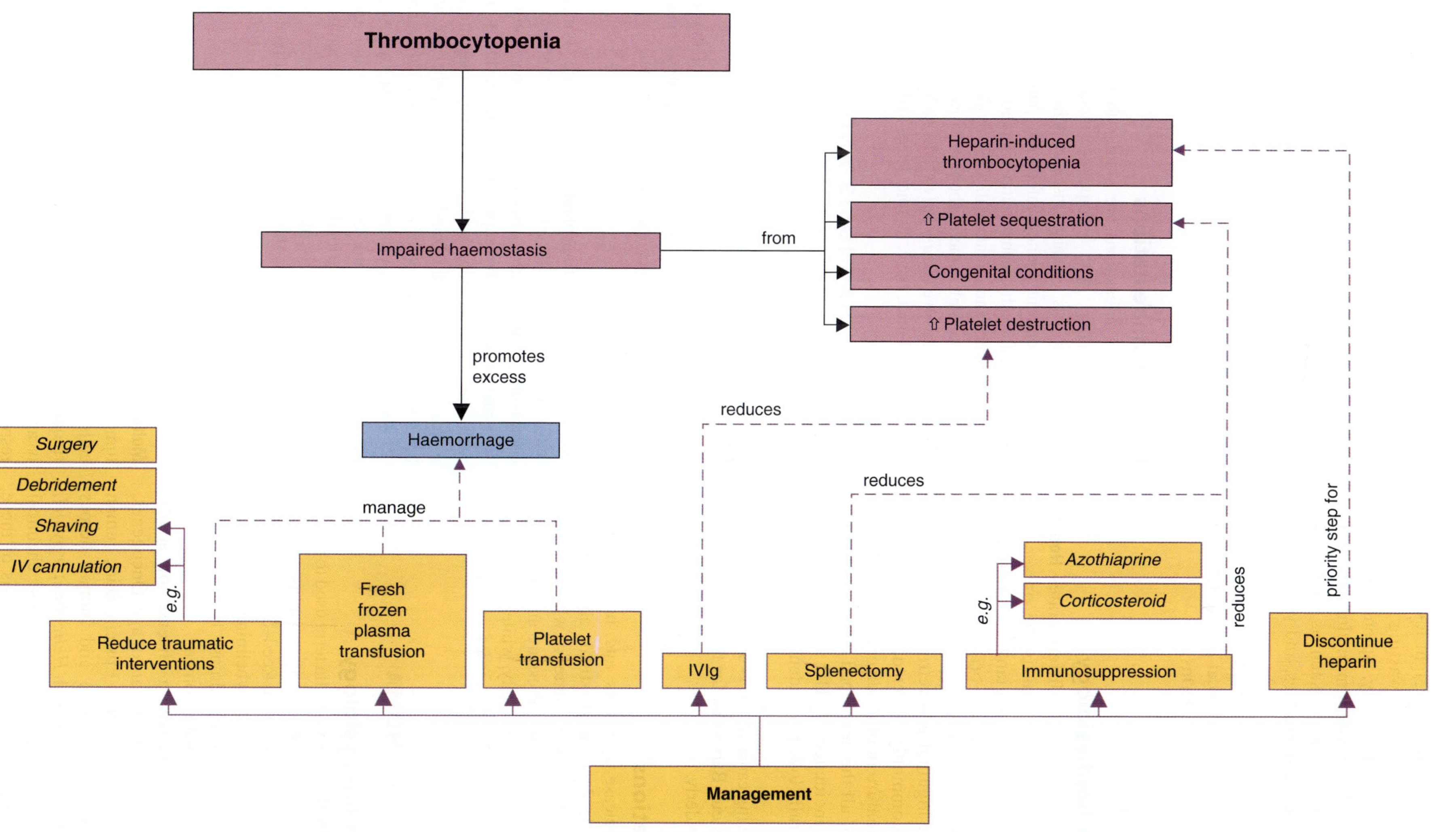

Figure 21.14

Clinical snapshot: Thrombocytopenia

↑ = increased; IV = intravenous; IVIg = intravenous immunoglobulin.

experience anorexia and consequent weight loss, loss of the ability to taste sweet and sour, muscle wasting and difficulty swallowing, as well as heaptomegaly, splenomegaly and lymph node enlargement. Other symptoms include abdominal pain and neurological disturbances, such as facial palsy, blurred vision and auditory disturbances, and vomiting.

In addition, some will experience night sweats, fatigue and fever. A small subset may develop autoimmune complications. Figure 21.15 explores the common clinical manifestations and management of leukaemia (in general terms).

HODGKIN LYMPHOMA

Aetiology and pathophysiology

The key distinguishing feature that differentiates **Hodgkin lymphoma (HL)** from other lymphomas is the presence of *Reed–Sternberg cells*, multinucleated giant cells that precede malignant transformation. The disease originates in a single lymph node or chain of nodes, spreading to adjoining nodes, with cervical, axillary, inguinal and retroperitoneal lymph nodes being the most commonly affected. Although Reed–Sternberg cells might feature in other disorders, this finding is rare. Interestingly, of all the developed nations, Australia has one of the lowest incidences of HL, while developing nations have an overall lower incidence than Western nations.

Although the underlying cause of HL is unknown, a link has been proposed with Epstein–Barr virus for the development of HL in children and the elderly.

Clinical manifestations

The malignant cells release cytokines and haematopoietic growth factors, which leads to mediastinal, abdominal and large, painless masses in the neck, the latter of which represent a common initial sign of the disease. Pressure and obstruction will lead to adenopathy and splenomegaly, while fever, weight loss, night sweats and pruritus are symptoms associated with B cells.

NON-HODGKIN LYMPHOMA

Aetiology and pathophysiology

Non-Hodgkin lymphoma (NHL) is an umbrella term used to refer to a series of conditions in which there is malignant transformation of T or B cells without involvement of Reed–Sternberg cells. These conditions make up the overwhelming majority of malignant lymphoma cases, and are almost 1.5 times more likely to occur in men compared with women.

Unlike HL, NHL is primarily a disease of adults, particularly those between 50 and 70 years of age. Oncogenes, immunoglobulin genes, viruses such as Epstein–Barr, human T cell lymphotropic virus (HTLV-1) and human herpes virus-8 (HHV-8), bacterial infection with *Helicobacter pylori*, and environmental factors such as radiation and chemical exposure have been implicated in the pathogenesis of these disorders.

Unlike HL, NHL has a *multifocal origin* that involves discontinuous lymph nodes. The initial presenting symptom is often non-tender lymph node enlargement, marked by architectural changes to the nodes, which has lasted for more than two weeks. Classification of this disorder is primarily by cell type—namely, precursor B cells, peripheral B cells, precursor T cells and peripheral T and NK cells—but includes determination of whether the infiltration of the nodes is follicular (germinal), interfollicular, within the mantle or medullary.

Clinical manifestations

The clinical manifestations are similar to those in HL, with people presenting with symptoms including fever, night sweats, weight loss, malaise, visceral pain, abdominal masses, back pain, recurrent kidney infections, pain and/or bleeding, peripheral neuropathy, behavioural alterations and leg swelling. Haematological examination will show lymphocytopenia as the sole characteristic unless there is bone marrow involvement. Unlike HL, NHL can involve *extranodal tissues*, such as the nasopharynx, gastrointestinal tract, bone, thyroid, testes and soft tissues.

CLINICAL DIAGNOSIS AND MANAGEMENT OF LEUKAEMIAS AND LYMPHOMAS

Diagnosis

Diagnosis is dependent on the identification of the leukaemic lymphoblasts, which is undertaken using flow cytometry to separate and immunotype the cells in the plasma.

Management

Allogenic stem-cell transplantation in acute lymphoblastic leukaemia is the most intense form of therapy, although contrasting this with chemotherapy does not clearly delineate which is the superior treatment. Daily treatment with the antimetabolite anticancer drugs methotrexate and mercaptopurine form the backbone of chemotherapy, which will be continued for a period of two to two and a half years.

Therapeutic management of CLL employs such drugs as alkylating agents, nucleoside analogues and monoclonal antibodies, such as rituximab or alemtuzamab. Careful monitoring of side-effects, particularly bone marrow suppression and infections, is vital in those undergoing treatment.

Multiple myeloma

AETIOLOGY AND PATHOPHYSIOLOGY

Multiple myeloma, also known as *plasma cell neoplasms*, is a tumour of B cells marked by the slow growth of bone marrow cells, and affects adults of any age. Men are slightly more frequently affected than women, and the mean age at diagnosis is approximately 65–70 years of age. Although people often respond well to therapy in the early stages, the average survival is only 24–36 months after diagnosis.

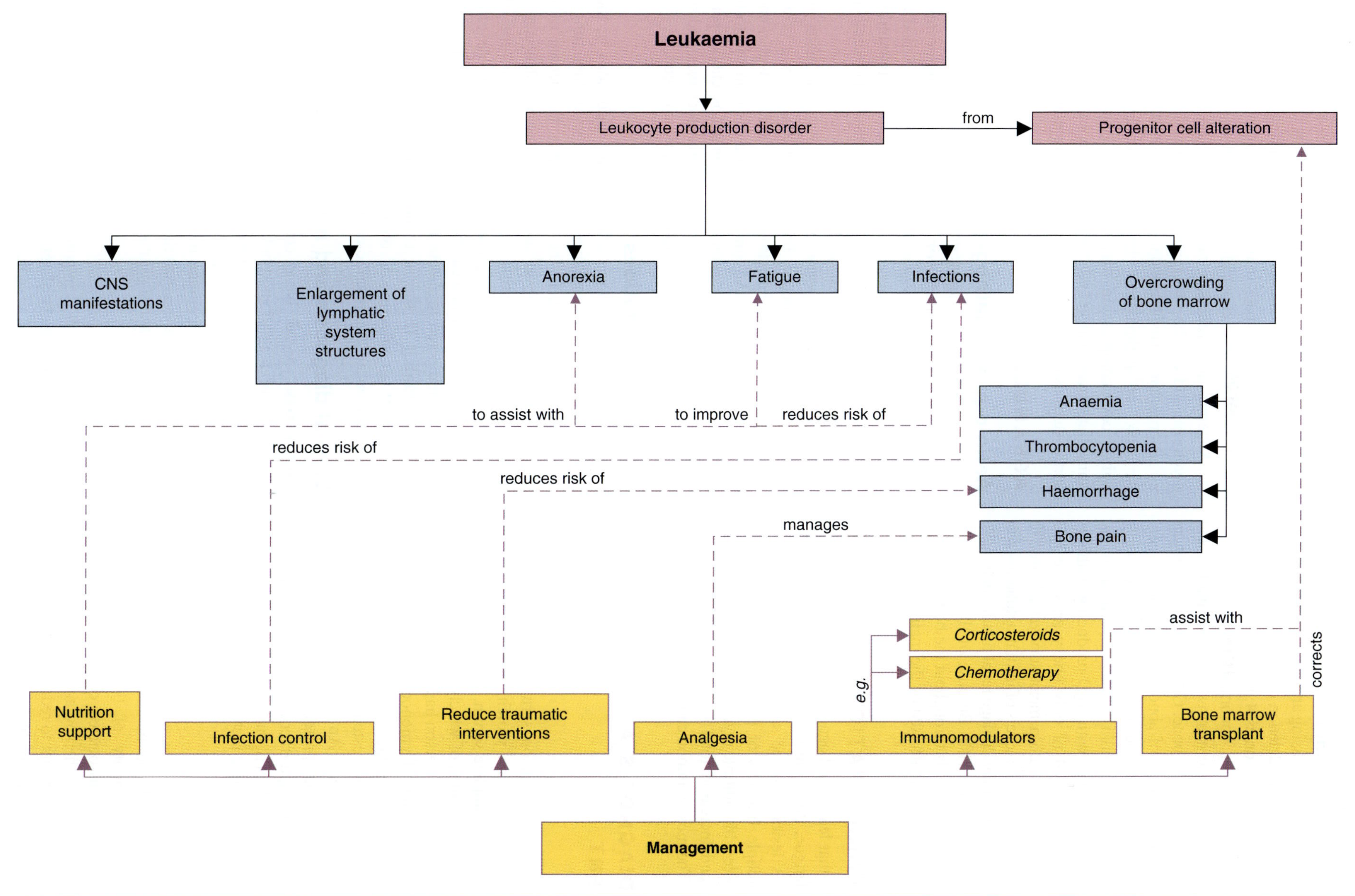

Figure 21.15

Clinical snapshot: Leukaemia

CNS = central nervous system.

While the underlying cause of this disease is unknown, there is evidence for an association with increasing age, radiation, regular exposure to herbicides, food-processing and agricultural products, and genetic mutations, such as a deletion on chromosome 13 and a translocation between chromosomes 4 and 14. The malignant cells produce vast quantities of abnormal immunoglobulins, leading to infiltration of the bone marrow and bone matrix, and ultimately lesions that destroy the bone. Generally, the malignant cells will produce only one type of abnormal immunoglobulin, and the tumour can be characterised on that basis. Interestingly, the identity of the immunoglobulin species is linked to the aggressiveness of the tumour, with IgD-producing tumours associated with a mean survival of only one year, while IgG myelomas are less aggressive with a mean survival of three to four years. The markedly elevated levels of immunoglobulins will increase blood viscosity, and may damage renal tubules and make thromboembolism a significant risk. Because of the ubiquitous nature of the movement of B cells throughout the body, virtually all tissues will be infiltrated and affected by the malignant cells.

CLINICAL MANIFESTATIONS

Initial complaints that lead to a diagnosis are back or bone pain associated with fatigue, due to lesions of the bone that can be seen on X-ray. As lesions can be sufficiently plentiful, there is the risk of multiple fractures of the pelvis and femur. On investigation, people with multiple myeloma often have anaemia, hypercalcaemia, and increased total serum protein and serum creatinine levels. The most common cause of death is infection.

CLINICAL DIAGNOSIS AND MANAGEMENT

Diagnosis

Use of protein electrophoresis on serum and urine samples determines whether a monoclonal protein is being expressed. If such a protein is found, complete serum, urine and radiological testing is undertaken, the results of which will determine which of the six disorder subtypes the person has developed. While it is vital to determine the presence of a monoclonal protein, it is also important to determine the presence of vitamin deficiencies or changes to bone marrow, as suggested by macrocytic anaemia, leukopenia or thrombocytopenia. An analysis of the metabolic function will determine the presence of hypercalcaemia, hyperuricaemia or renal impairment. Multiple myeloma is associated with elevated levels of β_2-microglobulin, interleukin-6 and serum albumin, making these factors useful in the diagnosis of the condition.

Management

Multiple myeloma is incurable, but monitoring and manipulating disease progression is a priority of the management plan. Interventions to assist with associated complications are also important. Chemotherapy, radiotherapy and immunosuppression will generally be used in an attempt to reduce the tumour burden. Autologous stem-cell transplantation (using the person's own cells) may be attempted for some people. These cells, once removed, are heavily irradiated or subjected to intense doses of chemotherapy far in excess of that which could be tolerated if they were inside the person. Once the treatment on the cells is completed, they are reinfused and migrate back to the bone. Bisphosphonates may be used to control bony complications of multiple myeloma.

Anaemia and infection can be associated with multiple myeloma, and can be managed with EPO and antimicrobials as appropriate. Bisphosphonates can assist in reducing the risk of pathological fractures and hypercalcaemia. Spinal cord compression may occur and require rapid and immediate investigation and management, including the use of corticosteroids to reduce the inflammatory response.

AGRANULOCYTOSIS

Aetiology and pathogenesis

Agranulocytosis is a *significantly decreased number of neutrophils, eosinophils or basophils (granulocytes)*. Agranulocytosis suggests that the bone marrow has failed to produce sufficient numbers to provide adequate immunity. There are several causes of agranulocytosis, including a *congenital form* and several acquired forms.

An *autoimmune response* can cause the neutrophils to become significantly reduced. Infections arise as a result of an increased consumption of neutrophils, and treatment with some chemotherapeutic agents. An important cause of agranulocytosis is *clozapine*. This common second-generation antipsychotic agent has been linked with an increased risk of agranulocytosis, and so frequent monitoring is required when clozapine is ordered.

Clinical manifestations

People with agranulocytosis often develop infections in the oral cavity mucous membranes and skin. Secondary fungal infections may develop. In the early stages, the person may present with malaise, fever and an oral or oropharyngeal infection, such as stomatitis, periodontitis or pharyngitis. If treatment is not instituted, severe agranulocytosis may develop and result in sepsis, which can be life-threatening. If a fever is present, the temperature may be high (> 40°C) and associated with tachycardia. If sepsis is developing, hypotension is observed. If an infection is obvious, purulent discharge is uncommon because of insufficient neutrophils to generate pus.

Clinical diagnosis and management

Diagnosis A full blood count will be beneficial for the observation of platelet morphology and the differentiation of leukocytes. An absence or significant decrease in neutrophils is indicative of agranulocytosis. Serum antineutrophil antibodies may suggest an autoimmune neutropenia if an obvious cause of agranulocytosis is evasive. Sampling of wound exudate for microscopy, culture and sensitivity is indicated in a person with a fever.

Management It is important to cease drugs that may be causing the development of agranulocytosis, so a complete and thorough collection of a medication history will be beneficial to guide management plan decisions. Antimicrobials may manage the infection if it is caused by bacteria, and, in severe cases, recombinant human granulocyte colony stimulating factors may assist in increasing neutrophil numbers.

Symptom relief of the stomatitis, gingival and perioral infections can be achieved with improved mouth hygiene and the administration of local anaesthetic gels and rinses. People who are immunocompromised should have foods that are very thoroughly cooked to ensure that they are free of bacterial contamination.

INDIGENOUS HEALTH FAST FACTS AND CULTURAL CONSIDERATIONS

FAST FACTS

- *Aboriginal and Torres Strait Islander peoples are 1.9 times more likely than non-Indigenous Australians to have anaemia.*
- *Iron deficiency rates as high as 52% have been recorded in some Aboriginal and Torres Strait Islander school-aged children in some Northern Territory communities, which is more than 10 times the significant rates identified by the World Health Organization (WHO).*
- *Indigenous Australians are less likely to develop leukaemia and lymphoma; however, when they are diagnosed it is more likely to be at an advanced stage, and subsequently their survival rate is 20% lower than that for non-Indigenous Australians.*
- *Pacific Islands New Zealanders are 2.1 times more likely than Māori and European New Zealanders to develop leukaemia.*
- *Pacific Islands New Zealanders and Māori are less likely than European New Zealanders to develop lymphoma.*
- *Thalassaemia is more common in Māori and Pacific Islands New Zealanders than in European New Zealanders.*

CULTURAL CONSIDERATIONS

- *Aboriginal and Torres Strait Islander Australians are significantly more at risk of anaemia caused by nutritional deficiencies when they live in rural and remote areas. Geographical challenges and the tyranny of distance complicate food availability and increase the cost of even basic food requirements. In one survey, in the previous 12 months almost one-third of Aboriginal and Torres Strait Islander Australians in remote areas had not had enough money to buy food, or had run out of food because of access issues. This should not be one of the challenges that people in Australia in the 21st century have to deal with. Programs to help ensure readily available, iron-rich, nutritionally appropriate food are critical to reduce anaemia in Indigenous Australians. Potentially, more research, education and development surrounding traditional foods (bush tucker) may begin to assist the problem, as there are many sources of bush tucker known to be high in iron and vitamin C (which helps absorb the iron).*

Sources: Data from Antenor (2022); Australian Bureau of Statistics (2022); Australian Institute of Health and Welfare (2022a); Health New Zealand (2022); Moore et al. (2022); Royal Australian College of General Practitioners (2018); Sherriff et al. (2022).

CHILDREN AND ADOLESCENTS

- Neonates are born with a special type of haemoglobin—fetal haemoglobin. Fetal haemoglobin has a greater affinity to oxygen, because the oxygen concentration in the uterus is far below that of a functioning lung. A baby's fetal haemoglobin is replaced by mature haemoglobin by about 6 months of age.
- Haemolysis in a neonate is a significant problem, and can result in jaundice and anaemia. Haemolytic disease of the newborn results when the immune system of the mother attacks the red blood cells of the neonate because of an Rh incompatibility.
- Vertical transmission of blood-borne infections can occur from the mother to the child if there is trauma or placental rupture, resulting in the mixing of the blood of the neonate and the mother. However, in uncomplicated births, mixing of the mother's and the neonate's blood does not occur.

OLDER ADULTS

- Ageing reduces bone marrow function, and causes a slight decrease in formed elements as the years advance.
- The volume of cells is generally sufficient to maintain relatively normal function. However, reduced red cell numbers prove problematic when an older person sustains blood loss.
- A decrease in the number and function of white blood cells results in an overall reduction of immune system function, and a slightly increased risk of infection is experienced.
- Immunosurveillance is compromised and cancer risk increases.

KEY CLINICAL ISSUES

- Anaemia is a common condition experienced by people in healthcare facilities and within the community.
- Surveillance for the signs and symptoms of anaemia will enable earlier detection.
- Both anaemia and polycythaemia artefactually influence peripheral oxygen saturation monitoring.
- Anaemia negatively influences cellular oxygenation. Those who are anaemic will benefit from supplemental oxygenation.
- Anaemias require differing interventions due to the different nature of the causes.
- Neonates may become anaemic as a result of an immune system reaction. Observe for haemolytic disease of the newborn in Rh^{+} babies whose mother is Rh^{-}.
- Polycythaemia increases the risk of clotting from increased viscosity. Observe for the signs and symptoms of coagulopathy.
- Haemophilia can cause haemorrhage. Educate people with haemophilia (and their carers) in the signs and symptoms of occult bleeding. Ensure that a management plan explicitly identifies methods to reduce the risk of bleeding.
- Thrombocytopenia increases bleeding risks. Educate those affected how to identify and manage bleeding risks.
- Terminology describing oxygenation is complex. Ensure that the correct acronyms are used, as incorrect documentation may influence clinical outcomes.
- People with leukaemia will generally have a poorly functioning immune system. Appropriate infection control measures will decrease the risks of negative outcomes related to infection.
- People with leukaemia may be at an increased risk of bleeding. Educate them and their significant others in the identification and management of occult haemorrhage.
- Lymphomas often cause swelling of the lymph nodes. Identify and report all observations related to lymph node enlargement.
- Back or bone pain are common in multiple myeloma. Perform thorough pain assessments and report all observations of bone pain.
- Agranulocytosis can be associated with the antipsychotic medication clozapine. Always ensure that haematological studies are occurring regularly in people taking clozapine. Observe for signs of agranulocytosis in those on this antipsychotic medication.

CHAPTER REVIEW

- *Thalassaemias* are inherited mutations of haemoglobin polypeptides that will result in an altered haemoglobin profile and anaemias of varying severity.
- *Iron-deficiency anaemia* is often the result of a dietary deficiency in iron, and is frequently missed or misdiagnosed, as initial symptoms such as fatigue are uninformative. Generally this form of anaemia responds well to dietary supplements and education.
- *Pernicious anaemia* results from a *deficiency of either vitamin* B_{12} *or folate*. A loss of parietal cell function or a loss of intrinsic factor causes an inability to absorb vitamin B_{12} from the diet. Because of stores in the liver, this disorder has a slow, insidious onset that can take 5–10 years for symptoms to manifest. By contrast, folate deficiencies are associated with acquired conditions such as malnutrition, poor diet and alcoholism. Regular injection of supplements overcomes the problem in most instances.
- *Haemolytic anaemia* is the result of the early destruction of erythrocytes. Numerous causes have been identified, including autoimmune reactions, drugs, trauma, infections, toxins and inherited mutations of enzymes.
- *Sickle cell anaemia* is the consequence of a single amino acid substitution in the β- polypeptide chain of haemoglobin, which leads to a malformation of erythrocytes into the characteristic sickle shape. These abnormal erythrocytes cannot transit capillary beds, and therefore create obstructions that lead to organ damage and, ultimately, failure.
- *Haemolytic disease of the newborn (HDN)* occurs when there is a maternal–fetal incompatibility in blood antigens. The best known of these involves Rh incompatibility, but mismatched ABO antigens are more common causes. Early recognition and intervention is necessary to prevent damage to the brain, which could lead to cerebral palsy, deafness, mental retardation and possibly death.
- *Polycythaemias* result from an overproduction of red cells, leading to a marked increase in blood viscosity and a greatly increased risk of cerebral thromboembolism.
- *Haemophilias* are bleeding disorders that result from a deficiency in a member of the clotting cascade; namely, factors VIII (haemophilia A), IX (haemophilia B) and XI (haemophilia C). Identification of the factor that is missing, and the immediate initiation of treatment with factor replacement, are vital to prevent joint damage and the risk of haemorrhage.
- *Von Willebrand disease* is a group of six disorders involving mutations of either the quantity or quality of *von Willebrand factor (VWF)*, which is required to maintain the integrity of factor VIII in the clotting cascade. Treatment requires supplementation of both VWF and factor VIII.
- *Thrombocytopenia* is the name given to a group of bleeding disorders characterised by a loss of platelets. The primary disorder in this group is *immune thrombocytopenic purpura*, which results from an IgG-mediated immune attack on surface antigens on platelets. The condition generally affects those between 20 and 40 years of age. Acute conditions are usually secondary to viral infections in children, and generally resolve within one to two months, although in a small proportion of cases, they will become chronic conditions.
- *Leukaemias* are malignant bone marrow neoplasms that arise as the consequence of blocked or impaired differentiation of haematopoietic stem cells, leading to an accumulation of tumour cells in the circulating blood. By contrast, *lymphomas* are malignancies of the lymphoid cells and their progenitor cells that do not include bone marrow, and are characterised by a marked proliferation of these cells. Unfortunately, a lymphoma can progress to include bone marrow involvement, seeming to convert to a leukaemia.
- *Multiple myelomas* are B cell tumours marked by damage to, and lesions of, bone that occur secondary to the overproduction of immunoglobulins and increased blood viscosity.

REVIEW QUESTIONS

1. What mechanisms are thought to underlie acquired anaemias, as compared to those that are inherited?
2. What is the difference between anaemias and polycythaemias? How do they both influence peripheral pulse oximetry measurements? Is this situation a risk when using an arterial sample to determine oxygen saturation measurements?
3. Haemophilia A (classic haemophilia) and von Willebrand disease both result from a loss of the coagulation factor, factor VIII. What is the difference between these two disorders? Ensure that your answer discusses the underlying reasons for the loss of factor VIII and their prognosis.
4. Bleeding disorders can arise from a variety of blood cell deficits. What are the main types of bleeding disorders? In your answer, pay particular attention to the nature of the inherited changes.
5. What risks are associated with neutropenia?
6. How does lymphoma influence the immune system?

HEALTH PROFESSIONAL CONNECTIONS

Midwives Haemolytic disease of the newborn (HDN) is a preventable condition. In-depth history-taking, knowledge of the woman's (and their partner's) blood type, and a general understanding of the factors contributing to alloimmunisation in pregnancy are critical for a midwife. Although the risks are high on the second pregnancy, the woman may not know what blood exposure they have had previously, so care must be taken with any Rh^- pregnant woman.

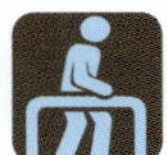

Physiotherapists Considerations for healthcare professionals providing rehabilitation to those with blood disorders goes beyond understanding the increased risk of bleeding, and reduced cardiac function and oxygen-carrying capacity. People with anaemia may fatigue quickly, have a more profound increase in heart rate, and possibly even have chest pain. Shortness of breath and dizziness should also be monitored during sessions. However, the physiotherapist may play a role in less obvious treatments, such as assisting with jaw range of motion and strength in those with periodontal issues and painful mastication related to aplastic anaemia in preparation for and following periodontal surgery. Commonly, people with blood conditions resulting in vaso-occlusive events may experience strokes or even more localised loss of function from ischaemic events. Individualised, person-centric programs must be designed to not only assist with any new strength, mobility or circulation issues, but also take into account the persistent condition that caused the ischaemia in the first instance.

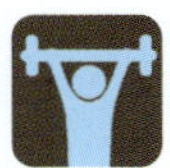

Exercise scientists Athletes who train at higher altitudes will effectively expose their body to a lower oxygen state, causing an increase in erythropoiesis. If timed appropriately, this polycythaemic state increases the oxygen-carrying capacity of the blood. Sports relying on aerobic capacity may benefit from this type of training; however, dangers exist with this practice. An increase in red blood cells increases the viscosity and can cause hypercoagulability and influence stasis. These physiological changes can result in thrombosis. Blood doping—when a person has their own blood taken and stored, so that when a sporting competition comes, their circulating erythrocyte levels have increased since the venesection, and they are given back their own blood so as to increase their oxygen-carrying capacity—is not permitted in athletes because of the risk of polycythaemia. High-altitude training produces similar increases in erythrocyte production.

Nutritionists/Dieticians Leukaemias (especially acute types of leukaemias) commonly cause anorexia and changes in taste. Poor nutrition can result in an increase in infections. People with leukaemia are already immunocompromised. They also have increased nutrient needs to cope with the disease process and with treatment regimens.

CASE STUDY

Mrs Janet Simpson is a 45-year-old woman (UR number 568712) who presented with abdominal pain and frequent diarrhoea, with frank blood in her stools. Her observations were as follows:

Temperature	Heart rate	Respiration rate	Blood pressure	SpO_2
36°C	72	20	104/72	98% (RA*)

*RA = room air.

Mrs Simpson's skin was described as pale, and her peripheries were cool. Her admission pathology results have returned as follows. She had a colonoscopy that showed ulcerative colitis, inflammation, pus, abscesses and bleeding.

HAEMATOLOGY

Patient location:	Ward 3	**UR:**	568217		
Consultant:	Smith	**NAME:**	Simpson		
		Given name:	Janet	**Sex:**	F
		DOB:	21/08/XX	**Age:**	45

Time collected	15:30
Date collected	XX/XX
Year	XXXX
Lab #	6658602

FULL BLOOD COUNT		UNITS	REFERENCE RANGE
Haemoglobin	73	g/L	115–160
White cell count	10.9	$\times 10^9$/L	4.0–11.0
Platelets	296	$\times 10^9$/L	140–400
Haematocrit	0.23		0.33–0.47
Red cell count	4.72	$\times 10^{12}$/L	3.80–5.20
Reticulocyte count	1.8	%	0.2–2.0
MCV	90	fL	80–100
Neutrophils	7.87	$\times 10^9$/L	2.00–8.00
Lymphocytes	2.06	$\times 10^9$/L	1.00–4.00
Monocytes	0.43	$\times 10^9$/L	0.10–1.00
Eosinophils	0.19	$\times 10^9$/L	< 0.60
Basophils	0.04	$\times 10^9$/L	< 0.20
ESR	2	mm/h	< 12
COAGULATION PROFILE			
aPTT	22	secs	24–40
PT	13	secs	11–17
ABG			
pH			7.35–7.45
$PaCO_2$	–	mmHg	35–45
PaO_2	–	mmHg	> 80
HCO_3^-	–	mmHg	22–32
Oxygen saturations	–	%	> 95

BIOCHEMISTRY

Patient location:	Ward 3	**UR:**	568217		
Consultant:	Smith	**NAME:**	Simpson		
		Given name:	Janet	**Sex:**	F
		DOB:	21/08/XX	**Age:**	45

Time collected 15:30
Date collected XX/XX
Year XXXX
Lab # 6658602

ELECTROLYTES		UNITS	REFERENCE RANGE
Sodium	133	mmol/L	135–145
Potassium	3.4	mmol/L	3.5–5.2
Chloride	96	mmol/L	95–110
Bicarbonate	22	mmol/L	22–32
Glucose	5.2	mmol/L	3.5–6.0
Iron	5.4	µmol/L	11–30

CRITICAL THINKING

1. Observe the haematology results for Mrs Simpson. Identify parameters that would influence your understanding of Mrs Simpson's oxygen-carrying capacity.
2. Are these parameters within normal limits? Explain.
3. Observe Mrs Simpson's biochemistry results. Why are the sodium, potassium and chloride levels decreased?
4. Relate the result for the iron in the biochemistry report to parameters in the haematology report. How will this situation affect Mrs Simpson clinically? (Confine your answers to matters of haematology.)
5. What nursing interventions are required to assist Mrs Simpson? (Consider oxygenation, activities of daily living and circulation.)
6. How would Mrs Simpson's current clinical situation impact on the interpretation of her oxygen saturation when using a saturation probe placed on a digit?

BIBLIOGRAPHY

Advani, P. (2022). Beta thalassemia. *Emedicine.* https://emedicine.medscape.com/article/206490-overview.

Alaggio, R., Amador, C., Anagnostopoulos, I., Attygalle, A.D., Araújo, I.B.O., Berti, E., ... Xiao, W. (2022). The 5th edition of the World Health Organization Classification of Haematolymphoid Tumours: lymphoid neoplasms. *Leukemia* 36(7):1720–48. https://doi.org/10.1038/s41375-022-01620-2.

Alharbi, M.G., Alanazi, N., Yousef, A., Alanazi, N., Alotaibi, B., Aljurf, M. & El Fakih, R. (2022). COVID-19 associated with immune thrombocytopenia: a systematic review and meta-analysis. *Expert Review of Hematology* 15(2):157–66. https://doi.org/10.1080/17474086.2022.2029699.

Antenor, L. (2022). *Leukaemia Foundation stands with First Nations communities living with blood cancer.* https://www.leukaemia.org.au/media/leukaemia-foundation-stands-with-first-nations-communities-living-with-blood-cancer/.

Australian Bureau of Statistics (ABS) (2022). *Estimates of Aboriginal and Torres Strait Islander Australians.* Canberra: ABS. https://www.abs.gov.au/statistics/people/aboriginal-and-torres-strait-islander-peoples/estimates-aboriginal-and-torres-strait-islander-australians/latest-release.

Australian Health Ministers' Advisory Council's National and Aboriginal and Torres Strait Islander Health Standing Committee (2017). *Cultural respect framework 2016–2026: for Aboriginal and Torres Strait Islander health— a national approach to building a culturally respectful health system.* Canberra: Australian Government Department of Health. https://nacchocommunique.com/wp-content/uploads/2016/12/cultural_respect_framework_1december2016_1.pdf.

Australian Indigenous Health*Info*Net (2020). *Summary of cancer among Aboriginal and Torres Strait Islander people.* Perth, WA. Australian Indigenous Health*Info*Net. https://healthinfonet.ecu.edu.au/cancer.

Australian Institute of Health and Welfare (AIHW) (2021). *Australian Cancer Incidence and Mortality (ACIM) books: data by cancer type.* Canberra: AIHW. https://www.aihw.gov.au/getmedia/b1f82a73-cc49-4bfe-bbe7-1d71e2002617/AIHW-CAN-122-ACIM_pancreas.xlsx.aspx.

Australian Institute of Health and Welfare (AIHW) (2022a). Data insights. *Australia's health, 2022.* Australia's Health series No. 18. Cat. No. AUS 240. Canberra: AIHW. https://www.aihw.gov.au/reports/australias-health/australias-health-2022-data-insights/summary.

Australian Institute of Health and Welfare (AIHW) (2022b). *Principal diagnosis data cubes: separation statistics by principal diagnosis (ICD-10-AM 11th edition), Australia, 2020–21.* Canberra: AIHW. https://www.aihw.gov.au/reports/hospitals/principal-diagnosis-data-cubes/contents/data-cubes.

Australian Institute of Health and Welfare (AIHW) (2023). *Aboriginal and Torres Strait Islander Health Performance Framework: summary report 2023.* Canberra: AIHW. https://www.indigenoushpf.gov.au/Report-overview/Overview/Summary-Report.

Australian Institute of Health and Welfare (AIHW) & National Indigenous Australians Agency (2023). Tier 1—Health status and outcomes. 1.08 Cancer. Data tables. *Aboriginal and Torres Strait Islander: Health Performance Framework.* Canberra: AIHW. https://www.indigenoushpf.gov.au/measures/1-08-cancer.

Bauldoff, G., Gubrud-Howe, P.M., Carno, M.-A., Levett-Jones, T., Hales, M., Berry, K., ... LeMone, P. (2020). *LeMone and Burke's medical–surgical nursing: critical thinking for person-centred care* (4th [Australian] edn). Sydney: Pearson Australia.

Best, O. & Fredericks, B. (2021). *Yatdjuligin: Aboriginal and Torres Strait Islander nursing and midwifery care* (3rd edn). Port Melbourne, VIC: Cambridge University Press.

Braunstein, E.M. (2022). Etiology of anemia. *Merck Manual*s. https://www.msdmanuals.com/en-nz/professional/hematology-and-oncology/approach-to-the-patient-with-anemia/etiology-of-anemia.

Bullock, S. & Manias, E. (2022). *Fundamentals of pharmacology* (9th edn). Sydney: Pearson.

Carr, J.H. (2021). *Clinical hematology atlas* (6th edn). St Louis, MO: Elsevier Saunders.

Carter, E., Lane, K., Ryan, E. & Jayaratnam, S. (2022). Incidence of iron deficiency Anaemia during pregnancy in Far North Queensland. *The Australian Journal of Rural Health* 31(1):124–31. https://www.doi.org/10.1111/ajr.12929.

Colbert, G.B., Lerma, E.V. & Stein, R. (2023). Anemia of chronic disease and renal failure. *Emedicine.* https://emedicine.medscape.com/article/1389854-overview.

Health New Zealand | Te Whatau Ora (2022). *Historical cancer data.* https://www.tewhatuora.govt.nz/our-health-system/data-and-statistics/historical-cancer/.

Keohane, E., Otto, C.N. & Walenga, J. (2019). *Rodak's hematology: clinical principles and applications* (6th edn). St Louis, MO: Elsevier Saunders.

Maarkaron, J., Taher, A.T. & Conrad, M.E. (2021). Anemia. *Emedicine*. https://emedicine.medscape.com/article/198475-overview.

Maarkaron, J.E. & Taher, A.T. (2022). Sickle cell disease (SCD). *Emedicine*. https://emedicine.medscape.com/article/205926-overview.

Marieb, E.N. & Hoehn, K. (2019). *Human anatomy and physiology* (11th edn, Global Edition). San Francisco, CA: Pearson Benjamin Cummings.

Martini, F.H. & Nath, J.L. (2009). *Fundamentals of anatomy and physiology* (8th edn). New York: Benjamin Cummings.

Moore, E.M., Blacklock, H., Wellard, C., Spearing, R., Merriman, L., Poplar, S., … MRDR investigators (2022). Māori and Pacific peoples with multiple myeloma in New Zealand are younger and have inferior survival compared to other ethnicities: a study from the Australian and New Zealand Myeloma and Related Diseases Registry (MRDR). *Clinical Lymphoma, Myeloma and Leukemia* 22(8):e762–e769. https://doi.org/10.1016/j.clml.2022.04.004.

Nagalla, S. & Besa, E.C. (2022). Polycythemia vera. *Emedicine*. https://emedicine.medscape.com/article/205114-overview.

Nagalla, S. & Kim, S. (2022). Pernicious anemia. *Emedicine*. https://emedicine.medscape.com/article/204930-overview.

Pollack, E.S. (2021). von Willebrand disease. *Emedicine*. https://emedicine.medscape.com/article/206996-overview.

Royal Australian College of General Practitioners (RACGP) (2018). Chapter 3. Child health: Anaemia. *National Guide to a Preventive Health Assessment for Aboriginal and Torres Strait Islander People*. Melbourne: RACGP. https://www.racgp.org.au/clinical-resources/clinical-guidelines/key-racgp-guidelines/view-all-racgp-guidelines/national-guide/chapter-3-child-health/anaemia /.

Royal Children's Hospital Melbourne (RCHM) (2019). *Clinical practice guidelines: anaemia guideline*. Melbourne: RCHM. https://www.rch.org.au/clinicalguide/guideline_index/Anaemia/.

Shah, D. & Seiter, K. (2023). Multiple myeloma. *Emedicine*. https://emedicine.medscape.com/article/204369-overview.

Sherriff, S., Kalucy, D., Tong, A., Naqvi, N., Nixon, J., Eades, S., … Muthayya, S. (2022). *Murradambirra Dhangaang* (make food secure): Aboriginal community and stakeholder perspectives on food insecurity in urban and regional Australia. *BMC Public Health* 22(1066). https://doi.org/10.1186/s12889-022-13202-z.

Southern Cross Healthcare Group (SCHG) (2019). *Iron deficiency anaemia*. Auckland: SCHG. https://www.southerncross.co.nz/medical-library/blood-and-blood-vessel-conditions/iron-deficiency-anaemia-symptoms-causes-and-treatment#.ZAF4P3ZByUk.

Tortora, G.J., Derrickson, B., Burkett, B., Peoples, G., Dye, D., Cooke, J., … Green, H. (2022). *Principles of anatomy and physiology* (3rd Asia-Pacific edn). Milton, QLD: John Wiley and Sons.

van der Geest, B.A.M., de Mol, M.J.S., Barendse, I.S.A., de Graaf, J.P., Bertens, L.C.M., Poley, M.J., … Starship Study Group (2022). Assessment, management, and incidence of neonatal jaundice in healthy neonates cared for in primary care: a prospective cohort study. *Scientific Reports* 12:14385. https://doi.org/10.1038/s41598-022-17933-2.

Wang, H., Fu, B.-b., Gale, R. & Liang, Y. (2021). NK-/T-cell lymphomas. *Leukemia* 35:2460–68. https://doi.org/10.1038/s41375-021-01313-2.

Warkentin, T.E. & Cuker, A. (2023). COVID-19: Vaccine-induced immune thrombotic thrombocytopenia (VITT). *UpToDate*. https://www.uptodate.com/contents/covid-19-vaccine-induced-immune-thrombotic-thrombocytopenia-vitt.

Wool, G.D. & Miller, J.L. (2021). The impact of COVID-19 disease on platelets and coagulation. *Pathobiology* 88(1):15–27. https://doi.org/10.1159/000512007.

Yaish, H.M. (2022). Pediatric thalassemia. *Emedicine.* https://emedicine.medscape.com/article/958850-overview.

Zidan, A., Noureldin, A., Kumar, S.A., Elsebaie, A. & Othman, M. (2023). COVID-19 vaccine-associated immune thrombosis and thrombocytopenia (VITT): diagnostic discrepancies and global implications. *Seminars in Thrombosis and Hemostasis* 49(1):9–14. https://doi.org/10.1055/s-0042-1759684.

Vascular disorders and circulatory shock

22

LEARNING OBJECTIVES

After completing this chapter, you should be able to:

1. Discuss the causes and management of hypertension.
2. Differentiate between the types of peripheral vascular disease.
3. Identify the various types of aneurysm and their distinguishing features.
4. Discuss the significance, effects and management of arteriovenous malformation.
5. Outline the pathophysiology and management of Raynaud's syndrome.
6. Describe the aetiology and management of varicose veins.
7. Differentiate between thrombophlebitis and phlebothrombosis.
8. Outline the pathophysiology and management of circulatory shock.

WHAT YOU SHOULD KNOW BEFORE YOU START THIS CHAPTER

Can you describe the structure of a blood vessel wall?

Can you identify the types of blood vessels?

Can you contrast the structural and functional characteristics of the types of blood vessels?

Can you define 'blood pressure'?

Can you state the factors that determine blood pressure, blood flow and tissue perfusion?

Can you describe the regulation of blood pressure and tissue perfusion?

KEY TERMS

Arteriovenous malformation (AVM)
Circulatory shock
Claudication
Deep vein thrombosis (DVT)
Dissecting aneurysm
Fistula
Hyperaemia
Hypertension
Peripheral arterial disease (PAD)
Peripheral vascular disease (PVD)
Phlebothrombosis
Post-thrombotic syndrome (PTS)
Pre-eclampsia
Raynaud's syndrome
Thromboangiitis obliterans
Thrombophlebitis
True aneurysm
Varicose veins
Venous thromboembolism (VTE)

Introduction

Many health conditions influence vascular health. One of the most clinically important disorders to understand is hypertension. It is not only multifactorial and exceedingly complex in its development, but it also represents a substantial disease burden through its contribution as a risk factor to many other conditions. Other conditions outlined in this chapter include peripheral vascular disease, varicose veins and thrombophlebitis. Other vascular issues such as Raynaud's syndrome, aneurysm and arteriovenous malformations are addressed. Finally, the various types, pathophysiology and management of circulatory shock will be examined.

Hypertension

LEARNING OBJECTIVE 1

Discuss the causes and management of hypertension.

Hypertension is the foremost preventable contributor to cardiovascular disease, with an estimated 1.28 billion people worldwide affected by hypertension, with at least 46% of them unaware they have the condition. The World Health Organization estimates that hypertension contributes to 10 million deaths worldwide every year. The average blood pressure considered normal is 120/80 mmHg. By definition, **hypertension** is a consistently elevated blood pressure at or above 140 mmHg (systolic), at or above 90 mmHg (diastolic), or at or above both of these pressures in at least two consecutive clinical visits. Interestingly, an elevated diastolic pressure is more commonly seen in people younger than 45 years of age, while older people are more likely to have an elevated systolic pressure independent of the diastolic pressure. Unfortunately, identification of affected individuals is hampered by the fact that the disorder is largely asymptomatic, and as a consequence it is estimated that almost half of hypertensive individuals remain undiagnosed.

AETIOLOGY AND PATHOPHYSIOLOGY

The system of classification of hypertension currently used in Australia and New Zealand is given in Table 22.1. Globally, changes to the classification of hypertension have been evolving for the past decade. Mild hypertension is considered to start at 140/90 mmHg. Hypertension does not require a change in both systolic and diastolic pressures.

It is important to acknowledge that numerous foods and drugs may influence blood pressure, and so comprehensive history-taking skills may identify those foods or substances that may be contributing to a person's blood pressure changes.

Although there are different types of hypertension, most individuals have *essential hypertension,* also known as *primary or idiopathic hypertension* (*idios*, Greek, meaning 'one's own'), a condition for which there is no identifiable underlying cause. *Secondary hypertension* is the result of an underlying condition, such as kidney disease, renovascular disease or alcoholism. Once the underlying condition is adequately managed, the blood pressure may reduce to near-normal levels.

Gestational hypertension (also known as hypertension secondary to pregnancy, or *pregnancy-induced hypertension*) is a concern for gravid women. If the increase in blood pressure affects other organs (such as the kidneys) it is known as **pre-eclampsia**. Elevated blood pressure resulting in proteinuria affects up to 20% of pregnant women in Western countries, and more in the developing world. In Australia in 2020, over 7,300 women experienced gestational-induced hypertension, and more than 4,000 women experienced pre-eclampsia. Pre-eclampsia is a leading cause of both maternal and fetal morbidity and mortality, and a major contributing factor in the development of this condition is an immune system maladaptation linked to placenta development.

Table 22.1 Heart Foundation of Australia's classification of hypertension

National Heart Foundation Blood Pressure Guidelines are consistent with the current European Society of Cardiology/European Society of Hypertension Guidelines, but vary slightly from the current American College of Cardiology/American Heart Association Guidelines.

Category	Systolic (mmHg)	Diastolic (mmHg)
Optimal	< 120	< 80
Normal	120–129	80–84
High–normal	130–139	85–89
Stage 1 (mild hypertension)	140–159	90–99
Stage 2 (moderate hypertension)	160–179	100–109
Stage 3 (severe hypertension)	≥ 180	≥ 110
Isolated systolic hypertension	≥ 140	< 90

Source: Adapted from National Heart Foundation of Australia (2016), Table 2.1, p. 12.

It is estimated that approximately 30–50% of people have a genetic predisposition to hypertension, and recently 107 new genetic regions have been linked to an increased risk of hypertension. Many gene mutations are associated with the renin–angiotensin–aldosterone system, including some regulators of vascular tone (e.g. nitric oxide synthase, adrenergic receptors) and ion transport in the kidneys (e.g. Na^+/H^+ antiporter). Essential hypertension is a multifactorial condition most likely involving numerous genes.

The pathophysiology of hypertension remains obscure; however, what is known appears to involve a self-perpetuating cycle of vessel wall inflammation, vascular smooth muscle hypertrophy and, ultimately, loss of vessel integrity. As with atherosclerosis, some evidence suggests that viral or other infections may trigger the initial inflammation, leading to inappropriate compensation and the cycle of vasoconstriction and wall thickening. In general, however, there are four primary theories for the underlying disease development: excess sympathetic activity, an overactive renin–angiotensin–aldosterone system, altered neurohumoral control, and a metabolic disturbance involving insulin resistance, inadequate dietary electrolytes and endothelial cell dysfunction.

The *sympathetic nervous system (SNS)* controls vascular tone via the vasomotor centre of the medulla. Communication with *α-adrenergic receptors* on the vascular smooth muscle results in constriction sufficient to maintain tissue perfusion. In addition, sympathetic control of the heart regulates cardiac output and, therefore, blood volume. Balance is achieved by local mediators opposing vascular tone and causing vascular smooth muscle relaxation, which results in vasodilation. The most potent local vasodilator is the gas *nitric oxide (NO)*, which is released from endothelial cells. When homeostatic mechanisms are lost, environmental conditions can contribute to deterioration in adequate blood pressure control.

Similarly, the *renin–angiotensin–aldosterone system* controls both vascular tone and blood volume. *Angiotensin II* is one of the most potent *vasoconstrictors* known, and contributes to aldosterone release. Synthesis of angiotensin II by *angiotensin-converting enzyme (ACE)* promotes vasoconstriction, but also causes a concomitant decrease in nitric oxide and prostaglandin levels. This contributes to a loss of local control of vascular tone, leaving the combination of angiotensin II-mediated constriction and centrally mediated sympathetic tone largely unopposed. Further, angiotensin II appears to augment SNS activation, further amplifying the degree of vasoconstriction.

Angiotensin II-triggered aldosterone release promotes sodium and water retention, increasing blood volume, thereby further increasing blood pressure. Additionally, aldosterone promotes myocardial hypertrophy, which will aggravate the burden on the heart in an ongoing hypertensive condition, and can contribute to heart failure.

The *neurohumoral system* generally acts in opposition to the renin–angiotensin–aldosterone system, and comprises such compounds as atrial natriuretic peptide, brain natriuretic peptide and adrenomedullin, all of which are released in response to reduce blood volume and blood pressure. Their role is to promote *sodium excretion (natriuresis)* and mediate vasodilation. *Atrial natriuretic peptide* is primarily released from atrial myocytes in response to stretch of the atrial walls. *B-type natriuretic peptide* (also known as *brain natriuretic peptide*) is primarily released from ventricular myocytes, while *adrenomedullin* is released by the endothelial cells of the cardiovascular, renal, pulmonary, gastrointestinal, cerebral and endocrine tissues, and like NO it acts as a vasodilator. Identification of a subset of specialised neuroendocrine cells in the heart, called *intrinsic adrenergic cells*, which release *noradrenaline* and *adrenaline* as well as a small amount of *dopamine*, makes the possibility of maladaptive neurohumoral regulation all the more intriguing.

Finally, a *generalised metabolic syndrome* associated primarily with *insulin* resistance has been proposed (see the chapter 'Diabetes mellitus'). In this condition, individuals without diabetes but displaying insulin resistance have higher blood pressure than age-matched controls, and their blood pressure is lowered if treated with diabetic drugs. Loss of sensitivity to insulin is associated with increased sympathetic tone, elevated angiotensin II activity, reduced endothelial-cell-mediated vasodilation and altered renal function. Interestingly, just as the therapeutic management of insulin resistance can help reduce blood pressure, the use of ACE inhibitors improves cellular insulin responsiveness by improving post-receptor insulin signalling (increasing glut-4 function), reducing gluconeogenesis, and improving microvascular blood flow.

As can be seen, determining the pathophysiology of hypertension is complicated by the fact that alterations in one part of the complex system involved in the regulation of blood pressure have a 'knock-on' effect on other parts of the system. Since many hypertensive people are not identified early in the development of their condition, it is difficult to ascertain the primary triggering factor/s. Prevention must therefore focus on the risk factors associated with hypertension and early screening to pick up people before their condition becomes complex and involves other organs, particularly the heart and kidneys.

EPIDEMIOLOGY

Almost 34% of adult Australians have hypertension, of which almost 50% are obese or overweight and have a chronic cardiovascular condition. Hypertension affects males more than females, at a rate of 1.2:1, and, in adults 18–34 years of age, men are twice as likely to have uncontrolled hypertension. However, age is the overwhelmingly significant non-modifiable risk factor, with hypertension affecting almost 90% of people 85 years or older.

It is clear that ethnicity plays a role in increased risk of hypertension, although the exact underlying mechanism for this remains obscure. Is there a specific hereditary component, or is it in part a combination of geography, lifestyle, diet, and healthcare education and access that influences the prevalence disparity seen in certain populations? In Oceania, Aboriginal and Torres Strait Islander peoples, Māori and Pacific Islands people are all at increased risk of hypertension.

MODIFIABLE RISK FACTORS

It is well established that by controlling modifiable lifestyle risk factors a person can have a significant effect on their ability to reduce their blood pressure. Figure 22.1 identifies the current Australian guidelines for various modifiable lifestyle risk factors to prevent and reduce hypertension in adults.

The link between hypertension and *sodium intake* is relatively straightforward. In normotensive individuals, as sodium intake increases, blood pressure increases proportionately; however, as homeostatic mechanisms initiate, blood pressure will reach a plateau as sodium excretion results in reduced circulating blood volume and subsequently reduced blood pressure. In hypertensive individuals, homeostatic mechanisms appear to fail, and insufficient sodium excretion results in increasing blood pressure.

Obesity results in a mechanical risk for hypertension largely because of the increased blood vessel length required to maintain the excess body mass. It is estimated that some 20 km of blood vessels are required to sustain every kilogram of additional body weight. However, obesity adds further complications that can also influence blood pressure. Factors associated with obesity—including the extent of atherosclerosis due to poor diet, sedentary lifestyles that change metabolism and venous return, physical stress on the vasculature and the consequent impediment of venous return, the potential for associated hyperinsulinaemia, and/or impaired kidney function—may also play a direct role in the development of hypertension.

Additional risk factors of varying influence include: regular nicotine consumption; reduced dietary intake of potassium, calcium and magnesium; heavy alcohol consumption; and glucose intolerance or diabetes mellitus. For individuals with sensitivity to the effects of nicotine, marked changes in blood pressure, even in young people, can be observed. Generally, if these individuals quit using tobacco products (e.g. cigarettes, cigars, snuff, chewing tobacco, vaping), their blood pressure often

Physical activity
Accumulate
150–300 mins/wk moderate intensity or 75–150 mins/wk vigorous intensity
Dietary modification
Emphasis on
Whole grains
Low-fat dairy
Vegetables (5 serves)
Fruit (2 serves)
Relaxation techniques
Limited evidence as current studies are too heterogenous
Hypothesis
↓SNS = ↓BP
Salt restriction
Reduce salt intake
1° prevention
≤ 6 g/day
2° prevention
≤ 4 g/day
↓Dietary fat
Reduce fat intake
Total fat/day:
20–35% of energy intake
↓Alcohol intake
Reduce alcohol intake
Male:
≤ 2 *drinks/day
Female:
≤ 1 *drink/day
Stop smoking
5 As approach
Ask
Assess
Advise
Assist
Arrange
Weight control
Waist circumference
Male: < 94 cm
Female: < 80 cm
Salt

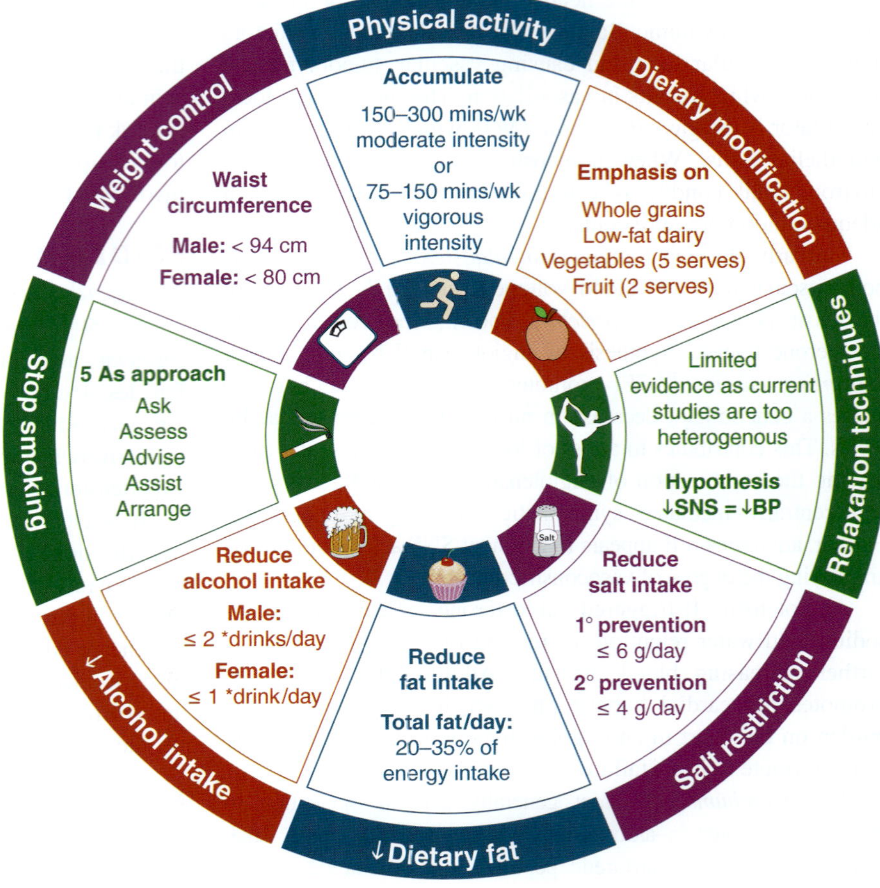

Figure 22.1

Modifiable lifestyle risk factors

* = standard drink (10g of alcohol);
↓ = decreased;
1° = primary;
2° = secondary;
BP = blood pressure;
mins/wk = minutes per week;
SNS = sympathetic nervous system.

Source: Specific guidelines extracted from the National Heart Foundation of Australia (2016).

returns to normal. Alcohol consumption is paradoxical, since people defined as heavy drinkers (those individuals consuming more than three standard drinks per day) are more likely to have hypertension compared with those classed as moderate drinkers (two to four standard drinks per week), who are less likely than either heavy drinkers or abstainers to have hypertension. Figure 22.2 identifies several mechanisms proposed to contribute to hypertension in someone with excessive alcohol intake.

CLINICAL DIAGNOSIS AND MANAGEMENT OF HYPERTENSION

Diagnosis

The Heart Foundation of Australia has released guidelines that advise that blood pressure should be measured on several occasions to gauge the blood pressure parameters of a particular person. If systolic blood pressure is greater than 140 mmHg or diastolic blood pressure is greater than 90 mmHg, further investigations should be initiated, including ambulatory/home monitoring to confirm hypertension.

The calculation of an *absolute cardiovascular risk assessment* using the Framingham risk equation should be used to predict the risk of a cardiovascular event within the next five years in all adults over 45 years of age (or over 35 years of age if the person is of Aboriginal or Torres Strait Islander heritage). This calculation is not necessary if the person has already been diagnosed with cardiovascular disease. A value of < 10% is considered *low risk*, 10–15% is considered *medium risk*, and > 15% is considered *high risk*. Clinical interventions will differ depending on the risk profile, with increased monitoring and intervention required with increasing risk levels. These recommendations are driven by a risk assessment and management algorithm devised by the National Vascular Disease Prevention Alliance (which includes peak bodies such as Diabetes Australia, Kidney Health Australia, the National Heart Foundation of Australia and Stroke Foundation—Australia).

Management

Apart from the lifestyle interventions previously discussed (see Figure 22.1), five medication groups are commonly used to manage hypertension. These are *diuretics, beta-blockers (β-blockers), angiotensin-converting enzyme inhibitors (ACE inhibitors), angiotensin II receptor blockers (ARBs)* and *calcium channel blockers (CCBs)*.

Table 22.2 outlines suggested recommendations related to the pharmacological management of hypertension.

Thiazide diuretics, such as hydrochlorothiazide, block the reabsorption of sodium or water, and therefore remove excess sodium and water from the body. They also cause the excretion of potassium from the body, which can sometimes lead to potassium deficiency. Potassium supplementation is therefore required. Other types of diuretics that can be used to treat hypertension include *aldosterone antagonists*, such as epilerenone, and *potassium-sparing diuretics*, such as amiloride, which produce a weak diuresis without affecting potassium excretion.

Beta-blockers, such as atenolol, metoprolol or propranolol, can be used for hypertension. However, they tend to be less

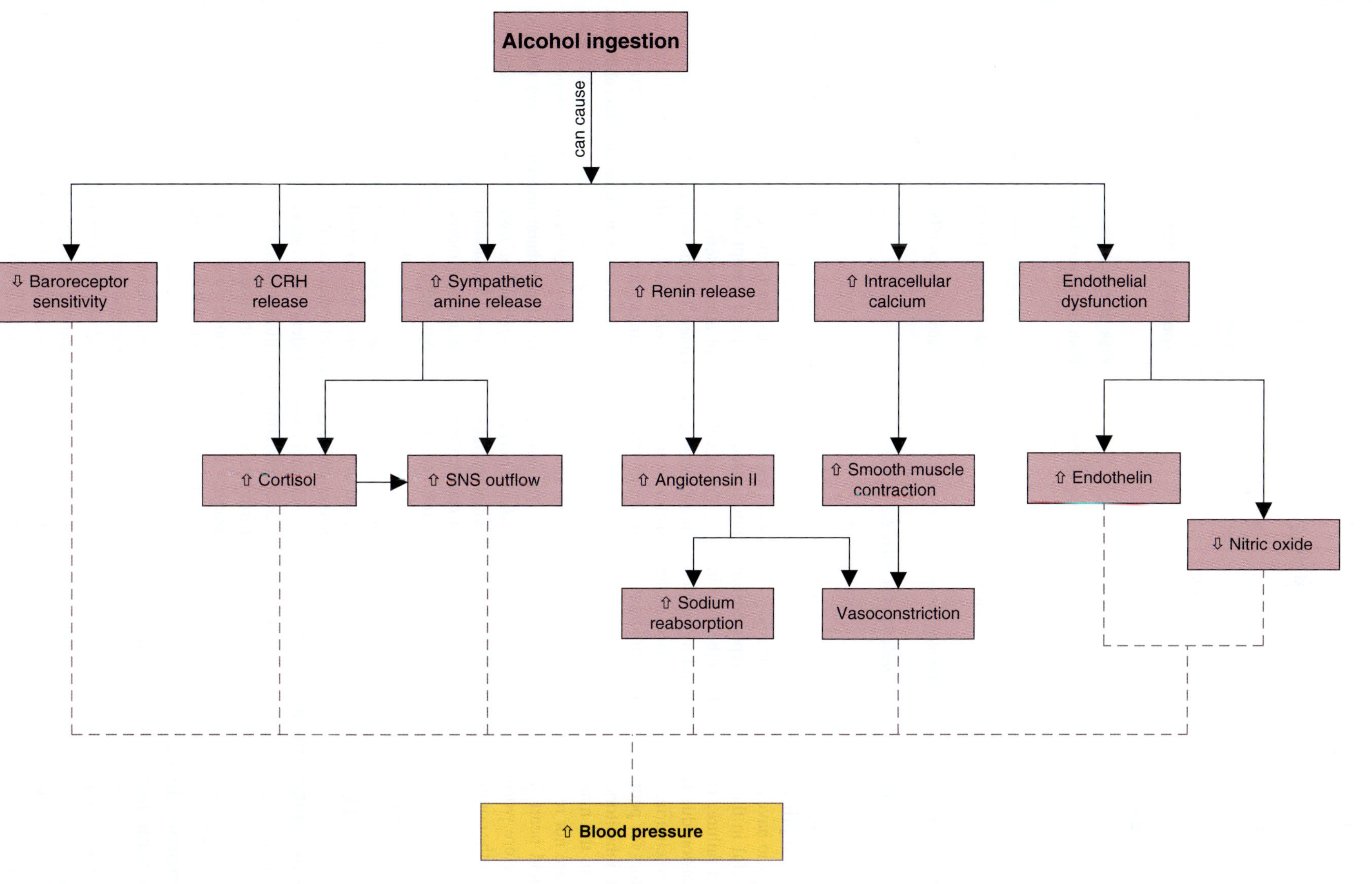

Figure 22.2

Possible mechanisms associated with alcohol-induced hypertension

↑ = increased; ↓ = decreased; CRH = corticotropin-releasing hormone; SNS = sympathetic nervous system.

Source: Image generated using information extracted from Hwang et al. (2022); Puddey (2019).

Table 22.2 Effective drug combinations for hypertension management

First drug		Second drug	Comment
Effective drug combinations			
ACE inhibitor or ARB	*plus*	CCB	Especially in diabetes and/or lipid issues
ACE inhibitor or ARB	*plus*	Thiazide	Especially in heart failure or stroke
ACE inhibitor or ARB	*plus*	β-blocker	Especially in heart failure or MI
Combinations to use with care			
Diltiazem (CCB)	*plus*	β-blocker	Risk of heart block
ACE inhibitor or ARB	*plus*	Potassium-sparing diuretic	Risk of hyperkalaemia
Combinations to avoid			
ACE inhibitor	*plus*	ARB	Risk of renal dysfunction
Verapamil (CCB)	*plus*	β-blocker	Risk of heart block

ACE = angiotensin-converting enzyme; ARB = angiotensin receptor blocker; β = beta; CCB = calcium channel blocker; MI = myocardial infarction.

Source: Adapted from National Heart Foundation of Australia (2016), Table 6.2, p. 37.

effective than thiazides, and are not recommended as first-line therapy in uncomplicated primary hypertension. They are contraindicated in people who have asthma or heart block.

ACE inhibitors are useful in the treatment of hypertension if the person also has heart failure. They should also be used in people who have hypertension due to diabetes and associated micro-albuminuria and proteinuria. *ARBs* can be used as an alternative to ACE inhibitors for people who are not tolerant to the adverse effects of ACE inhibitors.

CCBs are also useful in the management of hypertension. Verapamil and diltiazem are not recommended in people with coexisting hypertension and heart failure, because they slow heart conduction, and therefore worsen the symptoms of heart failure. Figure 22.3 explores the common clinical manifestations and management of hypertension.

Common conditions affecting arteries

LEARNING OBJECTIVE 2

Differentiate between the types of peripheral vascular disease.

PERIPHERAL VASCULAR DISEASE

Aetiology and pathophysiology

The hallmark of **peripheral vascular disease (PVD)** is the *disruption of peripheral perfusion* due to an obstruction of the blood vessels and increased thrombogenesis. The terms *peripheral vascular disease* and *peripheral arterial disease* are often used interchangeably; however, technically, the word 'vascular' pertains to arteries, veins and lymphatic vessels. Disorders affecting veins are most accurately, collectively described as *peripheral venous diseases*, and include conditions such as chronic venous insufficiency, plebothrombosis, and varicose veins. This chapter will focus on the more common vascular conditions that have a higher disease burden.

Peripheral arterial disease is overwhelmingly associated with atherosclerosis and diabetes, but also may be associated with vasospasm, venous insufficiency, embolism, vasculitis, fibromuscular dysplasia and entrapment.

The development of atherosclerotic plaques is discussed in more detail in the chapter 'Coronary artery disease', while the pathophysiology of diabetes is discussed in the chapter 'Diabetes mellitus'. The key issue in the diagnosis of PVD is to identify the underlying cause, as conditions such as **thromboangiitis obliterans** and Raynaud's syndrome can also be classed as PVDs, but occur in the absence of atherosclerosis or excessive thrombogenesis.

The primary feature of **peripheral arterial disease (PAD)** is *reduced perfusion in the peripheral tissues*, leading to ischaemia and potential tissue necrosis. Ischaemia of skeletal muscle leads to **claudication**, wherein affected individuals experience severe, painful cramps in the legs and feet (or arms and hands). As with stable angina, the ischaemia only occurs on exertion, when metabolic requirements are elevated in the face of insufficient blood supply. Eventually, the condition will worsen and the person will experience claudication at rest.

There is some evidence for inadequate regulation of the vasoconstriction–vasodilation balance in the blood vessels, particularly in cells with atherosclerotic plaques, as femoral arteries and calf resistance vessels in people with PAD have reduced endothelium-dependent vasodilation in response to both changes in flow and pharmacological interventions. There is some speculation of an imbalance between local mediators, such as the dilators adenosine and prostacyclin and the constrictors thrombin, serotonin and angiotensin II. Interestingly, there is also evidence for anatomical changes, with people with PAD showing a reduced number of perfused skin capillaries, as well as partial axon denervation in affected skeletal muscle, but the question remains as to whether this is a cause or consequence of PAD progression.

Figure 22.4 explores the common clinical manifestations and management of PVD.

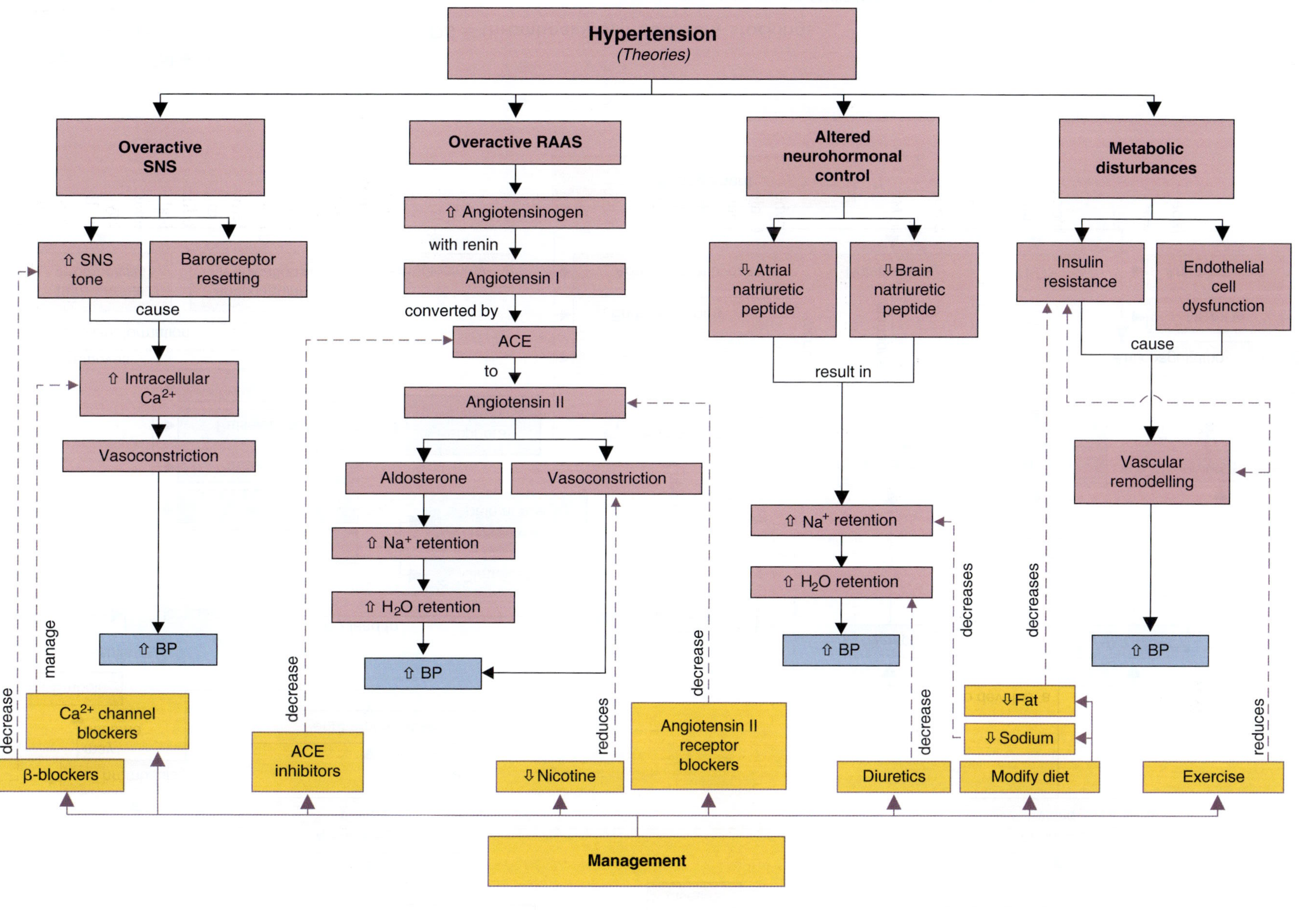

Figure 22.3

Clinical snapshot: Hypertension

↓ = decreased; ↑ = increased; ACE = angiotensin-converting enzyme; β = beta; BP = blood pressure; Ca^{2+} = calcium ion; H_2O = water; Na^+ = sodium ion; RAAS = renin–angiotensin–aldosterone system; SNS = sympathetic nervous system.

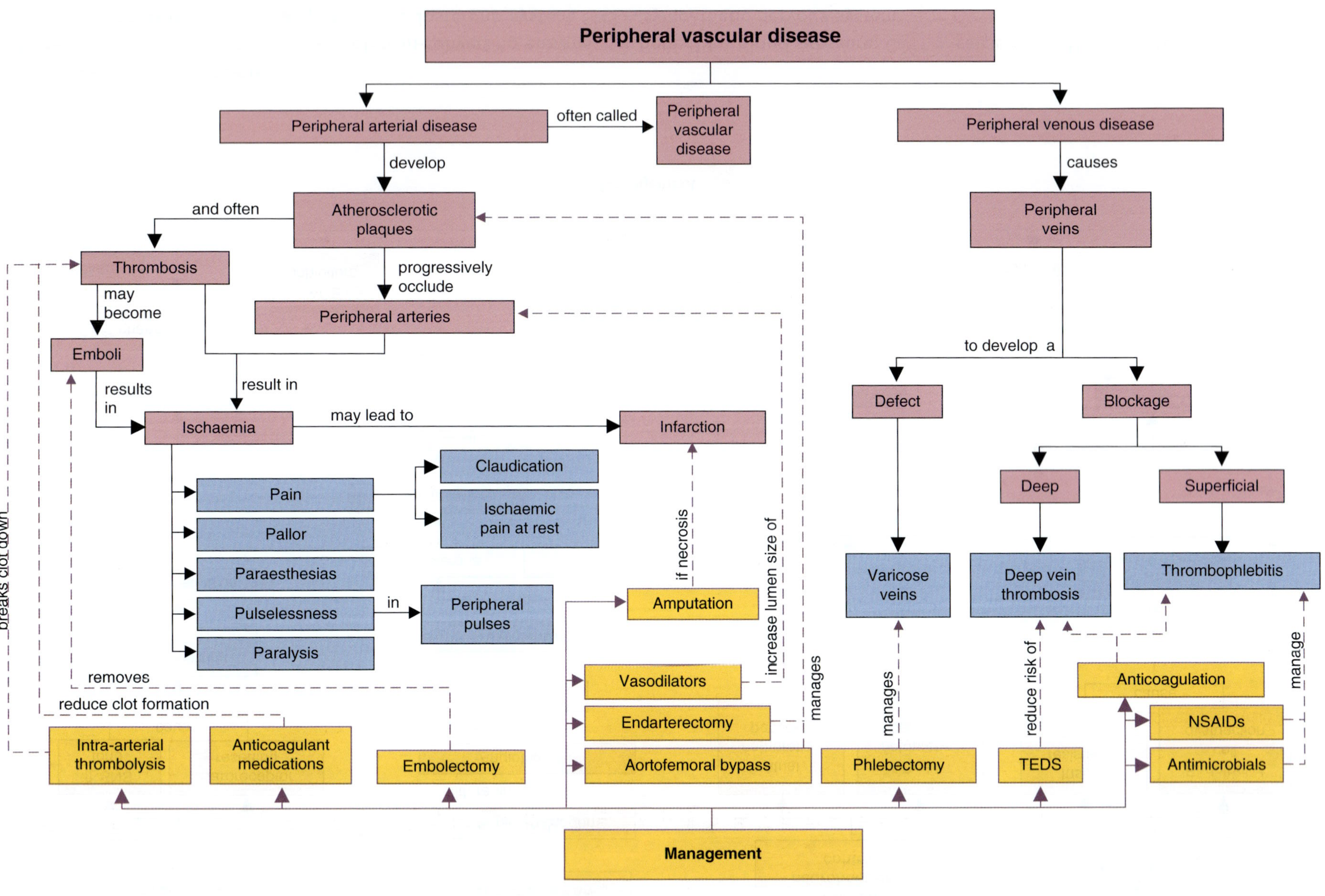

Figure 22.4

Clinical snapshot: Peripheral vascular disease

NSAIDs = non-steroidal anti-inflammatory drugs; TEDS = thromboembolic deterrent stockings.

Epidemiology

The statistics for the incidence of PVD in both Australia and New Zealand are difficult to ascertain, as they are frequently reported as part of cardiovascular disease statistics. PVD commonly occurs secondary to type 2 diabetes or heart disease. The Australian Institute of Health and Welfare estimates that 10% of people in primary care settings experience vascular disease, and 20% of people over 75 years of age.

Clinical diagnosis and management

Diagnosis A goal of diagnosis is to assign classification into one of three categories: (1) asymptomatic disease; (2) the presence of intermittent claudication; or (3) the presence of limb-threatening ischaemia. Blood flow can be evaluated through *Doppler studies* (also known as *ultrasonography*). This is a non-invasive procedure that involves the transmission of sound waves through the skin. These sound waves are reflected from moving blood cells in the underlying blood vessels. Sound waves are recorded through a microphone placed over particular blood vessels. The procedure is used to monitor the vascular networks of the arms and legs, and therefore can be used to determine abnormalities of the arteries and veins outside the heart. Invasive diagnostic investigations, such as angiography and venography, may also be undertaken to determine the extent of vessel disease. An *angiogram* is an investigation where a needle is inserted into the artery, and a *venogram* is where a needle is inserted into a vein. In both tests, radio-opaque dye is injected and X-rays are taken to observe the patency of the blood vessel.

Management Treatment goals involve maintaining or improving circulation in the peripheries, and, where possible, reducing progression of the disease process. In people with intermittent claudication and those with critical limb ischaemia, revascularisation is indicated. *Revascularisation* may occur percutaneously through *endoluminal techniques* using endovascular technologies such as balloons (angioplasty) and drug-eluting stents (a stent coated in a slow-release medicine), or may require *open surgical techniques* such as endarterectomy or bypass grafts. The various sites (aorta, femoral artery, leg vessels, carotid arteries) and the type of lesion (atherosclerotic or nonatherosclerotic), and the degree of disease can all play a significant part in the technique choice and management decisions. *Non-pharmacological measures* that may be used include cessation of smoking, maintaining an exercise program and ensuring a dependent position for the legs (hanging down) to improve peripheral perfusion. Care should be taken to avoid skin trauma, and regular examination of the feet is important to prevent shoe pressure.

Thrombus formation can be reduced by administering platelet inhibitors such as aspirin, or anticoagulant therapy such as oral thrombin inhibitors (e.g. dabigatran). Peripheral vasodilators, such as calcium channel blockers, can assist by enhancing blood flow in the peripheries through the development of a collateral circulation.

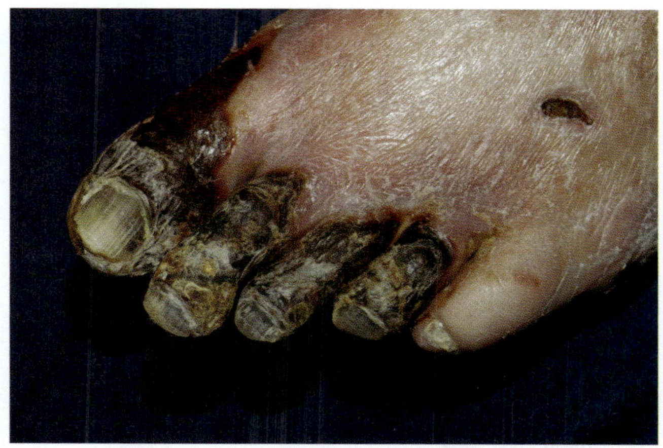

Figure 22.5

Peripheral vascular disease

Necrotic toes in a person with severe peripheral arterial disease secondary to type 2 diabetes.

Source: Scott Camazine/Getty Images.

If *ulcers* develop in association with PVD, the gangrenous area may need to be debrided or eventually amputated, to avoid spreading the disease to the systemic circulation and to alleviate the pain of ischaemia (see Figure 22.5).

Aneurysms

LEARNING OBJECTIVE 3

Identify the various types of aneurysm and their distinguishing features.

AETIOLOGY AND PATHOPHYSIOLOGY

Aneurysms represent a *change in the characteristics and integrity of arterial walls*, leading to either rupture or collapse of the vessel. Aneurysms are commonly associated with atherosclerosis formation, due to the wear and tear on the vessel wall at the edges of a plaque. In this section, the focus is on peripheral aneurysms. Brain aneurysms and their association with cerebrovascular accidents are covered in the chapter 'Brain and spinal cord dysfunction'.

The aorta is particularly vulnerable to aneurysms, due in large part to the force of the ejected blood volume against the aortic walls. An aneurysm may develop anywhere along the aorta from the root to even beyond the artery femoral bifurcation (see Figure 22.6). If the aneurysm is above the diaphragm, it is considered a *thoracic aortic aneurysm (TAA)*, and if it is beneath the diaphragm it is called an *abdominal aortic aneurysm (AAA)*. Aneurysms may also involve the renal arteries. Furthermore, certain conditions, such as *Marfan syndrome*, make the aorta vulnerable to tears, known as *aortic dissection*.

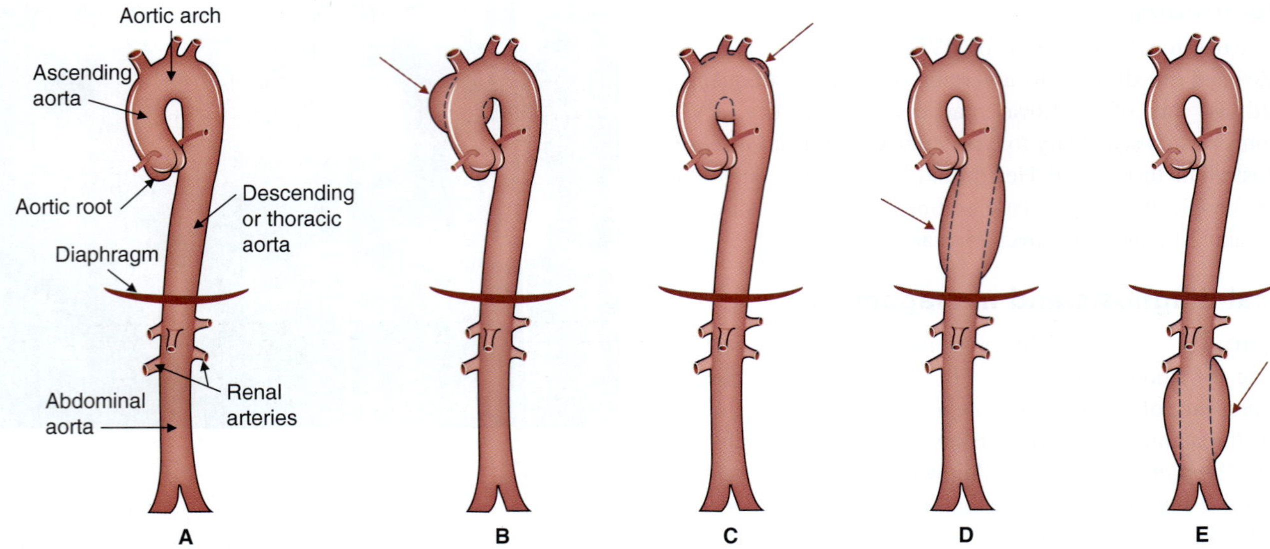

Figure 22.6

Aortic aneurysm locations

(A) Normal aorta; (B) ascending aortic aneurysm; (C) aortic arch aneurysm; (D) thoracic aortic aneurysm (TAA); (E) abdominal aortic aneurysm (AAA).

Source: © *Sciencopia.*

The two primary types of aneurysm are true and dissecting. A **true aneurysm** is associated with weakness of all three layers of the vessel wall, leading to a *ballooning outward* of the wall in response to blood pressure. If this outpouching is present on only one side of the vessel, it is referred to as a *saccular aneurysm* (see Figure 22.7A). If both sides are involved, then it is a *fusiform or circumferential aneurysm* (see Figure 22.7B). Depending on the location of the aneurysm, and the blood pressure in that vessel, the artery may be at risk of rupture. These aneurysms can become quite large and, since they

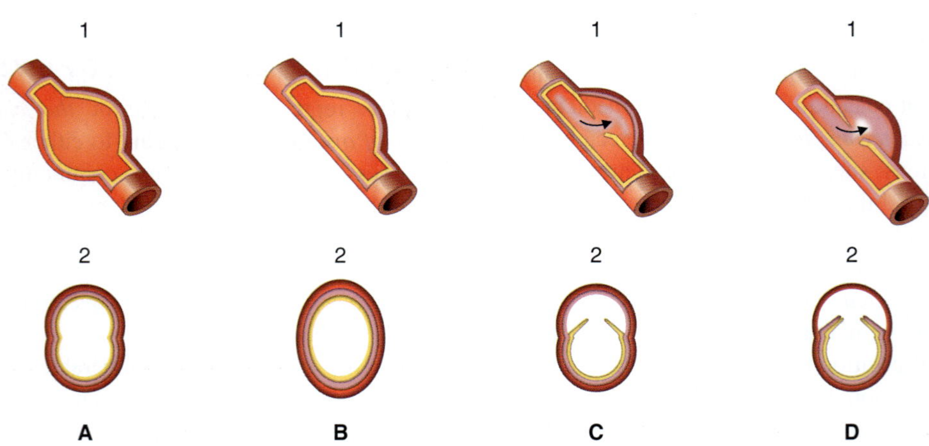

Figure 22.7

Types of aneurysm

(A) 1. Saccular; 2. saccular aneurysm in cross-section. (B) 1. Fusiform; 2. fusiform aneurysm in cross-section. (C) 1. Dissecting; 2. dissecting aneurysm in cross-section. (D) 1. False; 2. false aneurysm in cross-section.

Source: © *Sciencopia.*

are generally asymptomatic, may go undiagnosed until they rupture. An abdominal aneurysm can reduce blood flow to the extremities, resulting in ischaemia.

A **dissecting aneurysm** involves a *tear in the wall* of the vessel either between the tunica intima and tunica media, or through the tunica intima to the tunica adventitia (see Figure 22.7C). In this case, the blood seeps into the wall of the artery. As the blood flows into the false lumen, it may track either up towards the heart or down towards the kidneys or lower. The vessel may rupture or occlude branches (e.g. at the kidneys, resulting in an acute kidney injury). An aortic dissection may also cause pericardial effusion or tamponade, or maybe even result in aortic regurgitation depending on the size and location.

A *false aneurysm*, also known as a *pseudoaneurysm*, is a *tear through all layers* of the blood vessel wall with the formation of a haematoma collecting underneath the periarterial connective tissue, or sometimes by the adventitia (see Figure 22.7D). It is often a pulsatile mass, and can be caused by trauma, vessel injury, inflammatory conditions, or penetrating atherosclerotic ulcers. It can also be caused by iatrogenic mechanisms such as arterial catheterisation, biopsy or surgery.

CLINICAL MANIFESTATIONS

Aneurysms can be dangerous time bombs just waiting to go off. As many aneurysms are *'silent'* (not producing any symptoms), individuals are often oblivious to the fact that they have a blood vessel at considerable risk of rupture. Upon rupture, the manifestations will differ, depending on the location of the aneurysm. Cerebral aneurysms will cause a stroke. Thoracic, abdominal and ventricular aneurysms rupture will generally result in almost immediate death, with little hope of survival, even within a healthcare facility. Aneurysms are commonly found accidently as a result of investigations for other health issues or random screening assessments for insurance or occupational reasons. Non-ruptured abdominal aortic aneurysms will generally present as a pulsatile abdominal mass; however, no other signs or symptoms are obvious.

Figure 22.8 explores the common clinical manifestations and management of aneurysms.

CLINICAL DIAGNOSIS AND MANAGEMENT

Diagnosis

An abnormal chest X-ray reveals a definite increase in the size of the diameter of the aorta and possible calcification of the aortic wall. Abdominal ultrasound and angiography assist in determining the region of the aneurysm. Blood pressure in the upper extremities is often found to be higher than that in the lower extremities.

Management

Usually, surgical treatment is warranted to prevent an aortic aneurysm from becoming very large or rupturing. Prior to surgery, it is important to maintain blood pressure within normal limits. Symptomatic management of blood pressure by alleviating exertion, stress, coughing or constipation is helpful. Surgical repair involves resection of the affected area and replacement with a synthetic graft. However, recently, use of a sheath anchored by stents has revolutionised surgical interventions for some aneurysms (see Figure 22.9).

Arteriovenous malformations

LEARNING OBJECTIVE 4

Discuss the significance, effects and management of arteriovenous malformation.

AETIOLOGY AND PATHOPHYSIOLOGY

An **arteriovenous malformation (AVM)** represents a group of disorders in which two or more arteries drain directly into two or more veins through small openings with the absence of a capillary bed to link the two. AVMs associated with the cerebral circulation are covered in the chapter 'Brain and spinal cord dysfunction', so the focus of this section is on peripheral AVMs.

The centre of the structure is called the *nidus* (Latin, meaning 'nest'), which is the location of the shunting of blood between the vessels, and can involve a number of arteries and veins. Since a **fistula** is defined as a single identified artery connected to a single identified vein, AVMs can be considered to represent a cohort of fistulas. AVMs are part of a larger group of vascular disorders that include cavernous angiomas, telangiectasias and arteriovenous fistulas.

AVMs are referred to as *high-flow lesions*, in which blood flow and velocity increase in both the arteries and the veins that comprise the anomalous structure. The vessels then undergo dilation and morphological alterations, involving a loss of endothelial cells, thickened elastic membranes that are also broken, thin wall muscle, increased fibrous tissue in the wall and the development of a vasovasorum. These changes make the vessels prone to aneurysm, thrombosis and embolism formation. Generally, the venous changes are more marked than those on the arterial side, and if found in the brain, the blood–brain barrier loses integrity.

Interestingly, small AVMs are more likely to rupture than larger ones. Generally, individuals are at risk of bleeds and re-bleeds, and the prognosis depends on the location of the AVM.

CLINICAL DIAGNOSIS AND MANAGEMENT

Diagnosis

The physical findings and clinical course of the condition are rated using either the *Mulliken–Glowacki or the Spetzler–Martin classification systems.* MRI, echocardiography and CT can also be used to localise the lesion and determine the spatial relationships with the surrounding tissues, with MRI recognised as the most informative tool to estimate blood flow within the lesion. Angiography can also be used to identify the individual vessels involved.

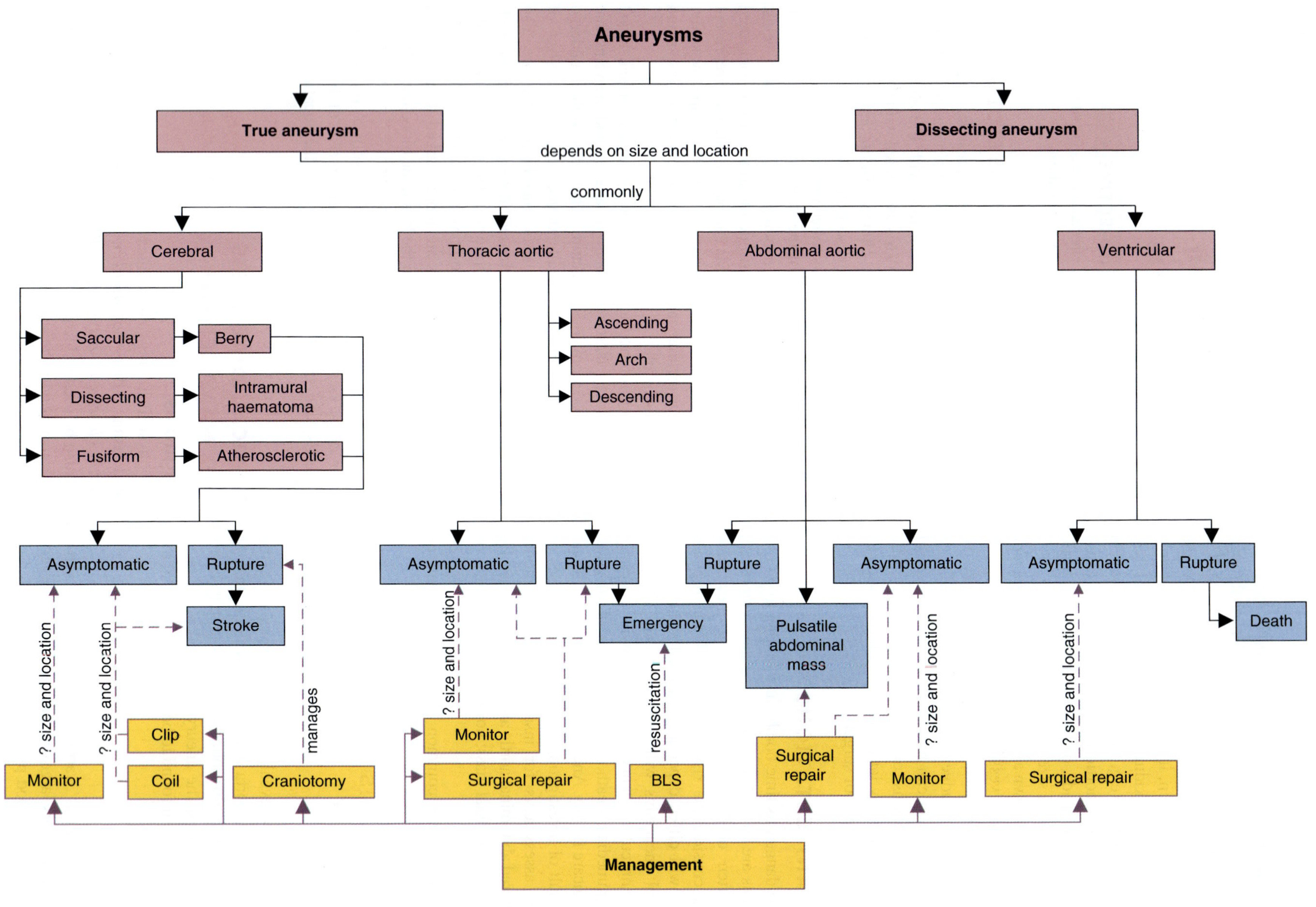

Figure 22.8

Clinical snapshot: Aneurysms

? = depends upon; BLS = basic life support.

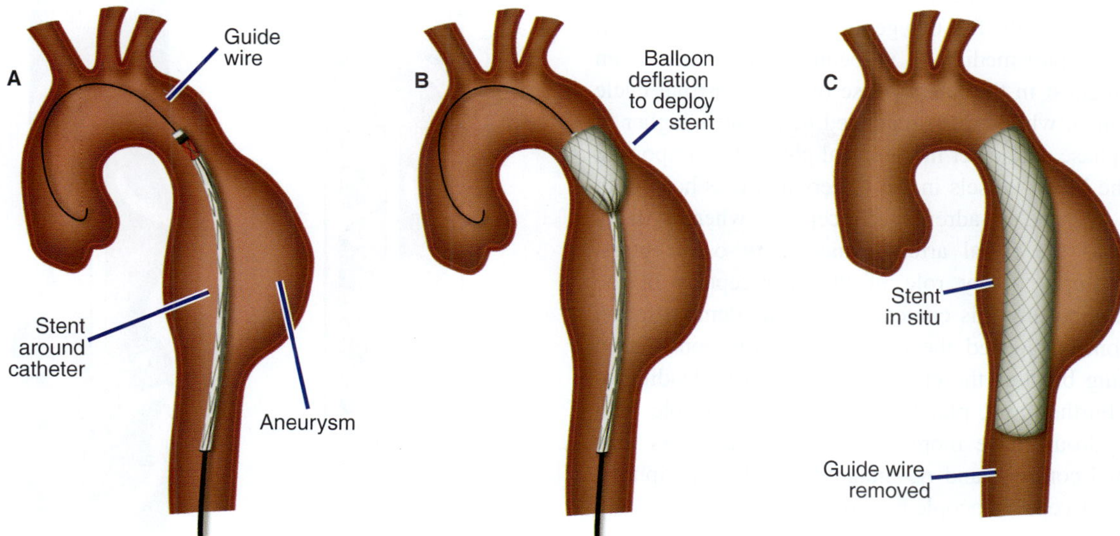

Figure 22.9

Endovascular aneurysm repair

(A) The vessel is accessed, and a sheath and guide wire are placed in the area of the aneurysm. The catheter has radio-opaque markings to enable accurate placement to be monitored via fluoroscopy.

(B) The balloon on the outside of the catheter is inflated and the stent is deployed.

(C) The balloon is deflated and removed. The guide wire, catheter and sheath are also removed. The deployed stent remains in situ to support and strengthen the vessel.

Source: © Sciencopia.

Management

Treatment will depend on the nature and location of the AVM. Cryotherapy, corticosteroids, interferon-α_{2a}, laser therapy, sclerotherapy, surgery and embolisation are all treatment options, and management decisions will be tailored to the person affected. Selective angiography with embolisation provides a valuable presurgical treatment for AVMs.

RAYNAUD'S SYNDROME

LEARNING OBJECTIVE 5

Outline the pathophysiology and management of Raynaud's syndrome.

Aetiology and pathophysiology

The primary hallmark of **Raynaud's syndrome** is a transient episode of reduced blood flow to the hands and feet, as well as to the nose and outer ear structures. An initial vasospasm occurs, leading to reduced blood flow to the tissue, which is associated with white colouration of the hands or feet. The tissue consumes the oxygen in the limited amount of blood trapped in the area, leading to a blue colour. Subsequently, a red phase occurs during which there is **hyperaemia**, as the episode resolves and blood flow is restored. Quite often, pain is associated with the attack, due to sensory nerve ischaemia.

Primary Raynaud's syndrome occurs in the absence of any underlying cause, and generally represents a benign condition, although occasionally small ulcerations might arise on the tips of the fingers and toes. Interestingly, people with primary Raynaud's syndrome can also experience other vascular disorders, such as coronary vasospasm and migraines. No apparent vascular abnormalities have been identified in these people, although microvascular changes have been reported.

By contrast, *secondary Raynaud's syndrome* is a potentially dangerous and life-threatening condition associated with autoimmune disorders, inflammatory conditions, haematopoietic disease or connective tissue conditions, such as scleroderma. Digital gangrene is often associated with this condition, and individuals show both structural changes to the peripheral vasculature and significant alterations to vascular reactivity.

In general, women are more likely than men to experience Raynaud's syndrome, with symptoms beginning after menarche and often ceasing after menopause. Interestingly, baseline cutaneous peripheral blood flow in young women is approximately half of that in age-matched young men when adjusted for body mass. Furthermore, sympathetic control of vascular tone is alleviated by warming the hands, and subsequent blood flow in young women increases over that of similarly treated young men. Since cutaneous flow rates are stable across the menstrual cycle, although hormones are likely to be involved in the process, those hormones that fluctuate throughout the cycle are unlikely to be solely responsible for the gender difference. However, α_1-adrenergic-receptor-mediated vasoconstriction has been shown to be highest in the luteal phase of the menstrual cycle in normal women, while the α_2-mediated response is higher in the follicular phase and lower in the luteal phase. It is important to note that the blood vessels in the fingers and toes have both post synaptic α_1- and α_2-adrenergic receptors, whereas distal vessels, such as the radial arteries, have only α_1-receptors, which would imply a key role of the α_2-receptors in the vasospasms. Supporting this contention was the demonstration that α_2-antagonists blocked the cold-induced vasoconstriction and that cooling blocked the effects of α_1-agonists, leading to vasodilation. Furthermore, platelets isolated from people with Raynaud's syndrome have more α_2-adrenergic receptors than those of normal controls, and α_2-antagonists reduce peripheral vasospasms in susceptible people but do not eliminate them.

Adding to this speculation was the demonstration that people who had their digital sympathetic nerves anaesthetised or who experienced a sympathectomy still experienced vasospastic attacks, implying that a nerve-independent factor was responsible. Other factors that have been implicated include oestrogen, serotonin, endothelin, neurohumoral compounds, such as atrial natriuretic peptide or adrenomedullin, and nitric oxide. In addition, it is common for family members across generations to manifest the condition, indicating a genetic contribution to disease development.

Common conditions affecting veins

LEARNING OBJECTIVE 6

Describe the aetiology and management of varicose veins.

VARICOSE VEINS

Aetiology and pathophysiology

Varicose veins represent a condition in which the superficial veins of the lower legs are abnormally twisted, lengthened and dilated, and often appear raised above the surrounding tissue (*varix*, Latin, meaning 'twisted'). People with this disorder will have an ankle venous pressure of 90–100 mmHg when they are standing.

The two most common underlying contributions to the development of varicose veins are venous valve insufficiency and vessel wall dilation (see Figure 22.10). There is also evidence of leukocyte infiltration of the valve and blood vessel wall, up-regulation of matrix metalloproteinase activity and abnormal collagen production. In addition, it has been demonstrated histologically that a remodelling of the wall of the veins occurs. Interestingly, there is data to suggest that these changes are not restricted to the peripheral veins, but also appear in vessels in other parts of the body. When combined with evidence for a familial link to varicose veins, this suggests for a genetic predisposition to the disorder. Unfortunately, the actual pathophysiology of the condition remains obscure.

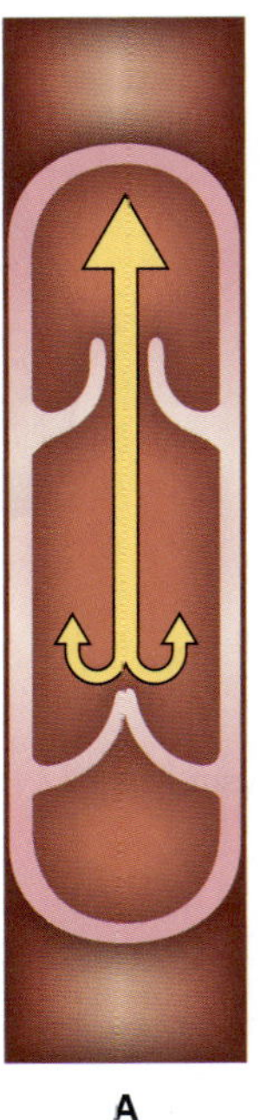
A

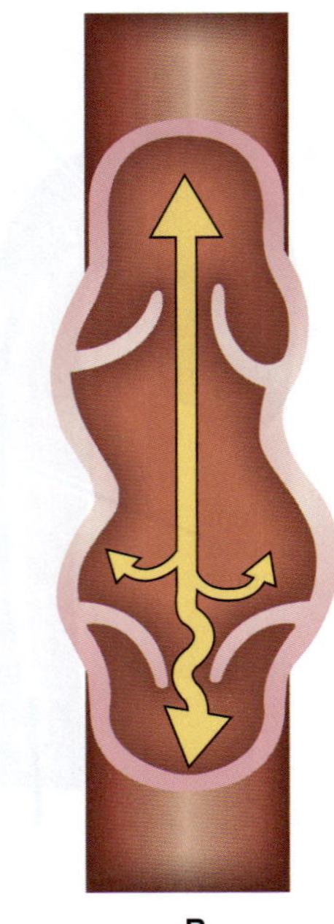
B

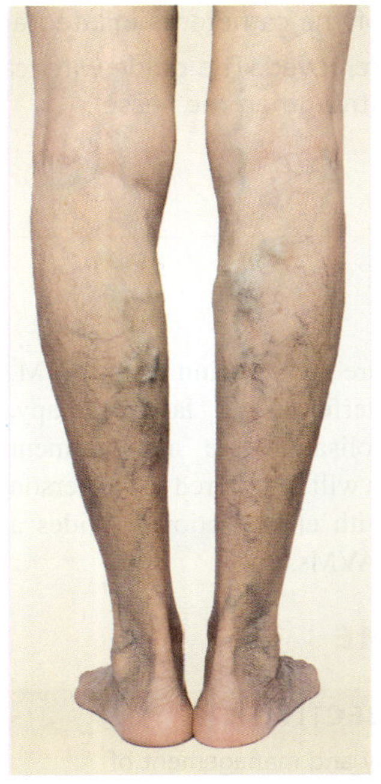
C

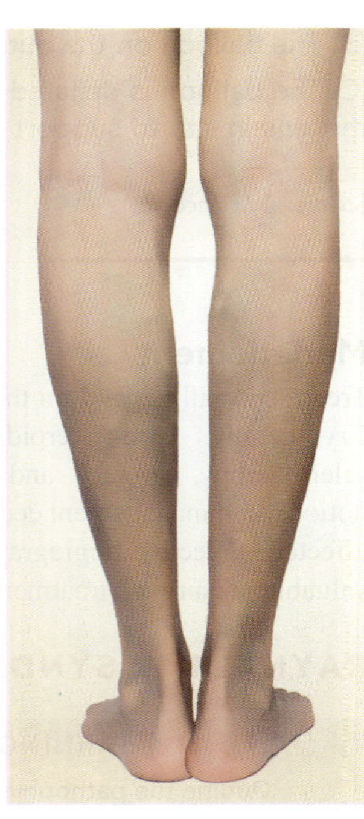
D

Figure 22.10

Varicose veins

(A) Vein with functioning valve. (B) Valvular insufficiency causing reflux, resulting in an increasing loss of valve competence. (C) Varicose veins. (D) No evidence of varicose veins in the same leg following endovenous laser ablation.

Sources: (A) & (B) © Sciencopia; (C) & (D) Solarysys/AlamyStock Photo.

Epidemiology

Over 19,000 people are admitted to Australian hospitals with a principal diagnosis of varicose veins each year. This figure is not even a close estimation of prevalence, as most people do not seek medical attention for varicose veins. Over 60% of people admitted are between 40 and 70 years of age, and 62% of these admissions are women. These statistics reflect the two primary risk factors associated with varicose veins: age and gender. Additional risk factors include pregnancy, oestrogen therapy, obesity, family history, phlebitis and prior leg injury.

Clinical manifestations

Varicose veins appear as *tortuous, superficial vessels*, most often occurring in the legs. Usually varicose veins are painless; however, as they enlarge, they may start to become itchy and cause aching or heavy legs that become worse when standing for long periods. Inadequate management of varicose veins may lead to chronic venous insufficiency, resulting in pain, oedema, erythema, claudication and potentially even skin changes, including ulceration. Varicose veins may also develop in other regions of the body. The effects of portal hypertension can cause varicose veins anywhere in the gastrointestinal tract; however, they commonly occur in the oesophagus, called *oesophageal varices* (see the chapter 'Disorders of the liver, the gall bladder and the pancreas') and the stomach, called *gastric varices*. Distorted vessels may also develop in the scrotum, called *varicocoeles* (see the chapter 'Male reproductive disorders').

Clinical diagnosis and management

Diagnosis

Varicose veins are diagnosed by direct observation of the superficial tortuous vessels, which are often very visible in the legs or groin. They are worse when the person's legs are in the dependent position (hanging down while sitting). An endoscopy can demonstrate oesophageal varices, and an ultrasound or venogram may reveal the extent of varicocoeles, although X-rays are best avoided to reduce radiation exposure to the testis (see Figure 22.11).

Management

Treatment of varicose veins involves keeping the legs elevated as much as possible and wearing graduated support stockings to facilitate venous return. Exercise and weight loss are important elements of management. Any restrictive clothing that concentrates pressure on an isolated area should be avoided, and individuals should avoid crossing their legs. If a person is required to stand for long periods, position changes through the voluntary movement of the feet can help with venous return. Varicose veins associated with pregnancy do not generally require interventions, as they should improve within 12 months of delivery provided the sensible self-care principles identified above are followed. Oesophageal varices may be managed by medications to reduce portal hypertension, or surgical ligation of bleeding varices. Although not always necessary, varicocoeles are primarily managed with surgery when continued pain or concern for fertility is an issue.

For peripheral varicose veins, most surgical interventions work on the principle of directing flow through collateral

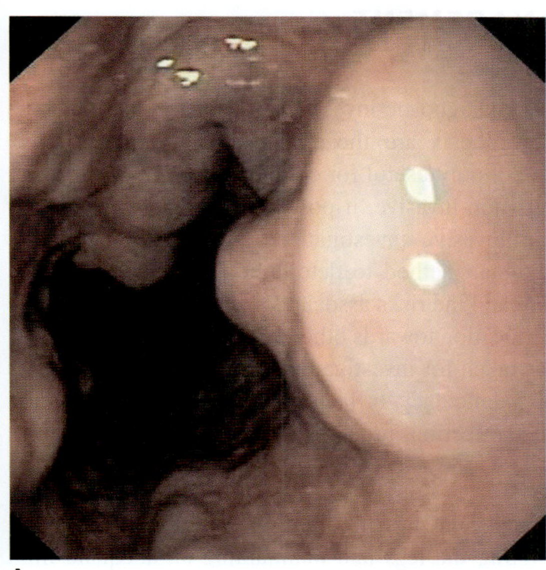

A

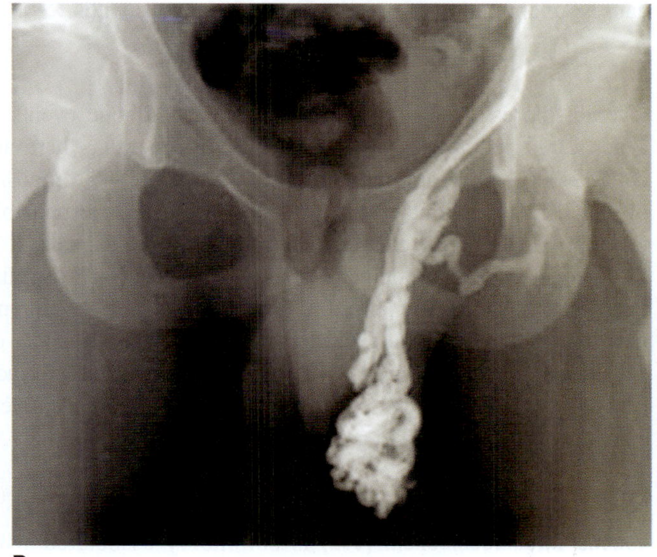

B

Figure 22.11

Alternative sites for varicose veins

(A) Oesophageal varices—an endoscopic image of varicose veins pushing inward, reducing luminal diameter.

(B) Varicocoeles—a venogram demonstrating left-sided scrotal varices.

Sources: (A) Gastrolab/Science Photo Library; (B) Dr Ali Nawaz Khan.

circulation, such as deeper vessels without varicosity. In severe instances of varicose veins, foam sclerotherapy of large veins seals the vessels to facilitate redirection of flow. Laser surgeries may manage smaller vessels and spider veins; catheter-assisted procedures using radiofrequency or laser energy can also seal the affected vessels. Ligation by removing affected vessels through small incisions is also now available in an outpatient setting with minimal visible scarring.

Thrombophlebitis and phlebothrombosis

LEARNING OBJECTIVE 7

Differentiate between thrombophlebitis and phlebothrombosis.

AETIOLOGY AND PATHOPHYSIOLOGY

Thrombophlebitis and phlebothrombosis are both associated with inappropriate thrombus formation, differing only in the location in which those thrombi are found and the conditions under which they arise. **Thrombophlebitis** refers to thrombic events associated with *venous wall inflammation* and can occur in any part of the venous circulation. **Phlebothrombosis** is more commonly known as **deep vein thrombosis (DVT)**, and is defined as *thrombus formation in the deep veins independent of inflammation*. Phlebothrombosis is known as *venous thromboembolism (VTE)*.

Thrombophlebitis is often secondary to other conditions, such as trauma to the veins, thromboangiitis obliterans, infection (e.g. middle ear sepsis, bronchiectasis), and any condition that causes inflammation of or irritation to the venous walls.

EPIDEMIOLOGY

Overall, the estimated incidence for thromboembolic events is 1 per 1,000 people annually worldwide. In Australia, there are over 19,000 people admitted annually with venous thrombosis, of which 62% are female. It is estimated that VTE is responsible for approximately 7% of all deaths in Australian hospitals. It is the second most common cause of maternal death in Australia. People who have experienced VTE are at risk of developing **post-thrombotic syndrome (PTS)**, which develops in 20–50% of people with VTE within one to two years. The risks for VTE include post-surgical immobility, obesity, use of oral contraceptives, existing varicose veins and congestive heart failure.

CLINICAL MANIFESTATIONS

Venous thromboembolism (VTE) is commonly associated with the deep veins in the calf, leading to swelling and oedema, and the leg is often warm to touch. Those affected might experience tenderness or pain in the leg, particularly upon dorsiflexion of the foot, but are largely asymptomatic until the migration of the embolism to the lung triggers noteworthy symptoms. Symptoms of PTS include heaviness in the leg, pain, swelling, itching, cramps, paraesthesia, hyperpigmentation, redness and eczema, and, if severe, lipodermatosclerosis and ulceration.

CLINICAL BOX 22.1

COVID-19 and thrombosis

People who become infected with severe acute respiratory syndrome coronavirus 2 (SARS-CoV-2—also known as COVID-19) have an increased risk of venous thromboembolism (VTE). Approximately 10–31% of all people with serious COVID-19 illness in intensive care develop VTE, with a mortality rate of approximately 12% within 10 days.

Although the mechanisms for VTE associated with COVID-19 infection are not yet fully elucidated, there is some preliminary understanding. This type of VTE is most likely caused by a combination of inflammation with endothelial dysfunction. There appears to be a low-grade disseminated intravascular coagulopathy, with widespread microangiopathy and thrombosis reported within the pulmonary vasculature.

There is currently no consensus with regard to prophylaxis regimens; however, much research continues. Current treatment protocols for VTE in COVID-19 infection include recommendations of full-dose anticoagulation with parenteral anticoagulation with heparin in acutely ill people. However, as knowledge regarding the virus's mechanism improves, interventions targeting the pathological process will most likely improve clinical outcomes.

Figure 22.12 explores the common clinical manifestations and management of venous thrombosis.

CLINICAL DIAGNOSIS AND MANAGEMENT

Diagnosis

The most useful diagnostic investigations for thrombophlebitis and phlebothrombosis are those that view the vasculature. Ultrasound is not only useful for confirming the diagnosis, but, given that it is non-invasive, it poses fewer risks and is better tolerated than invasive investigations. Although venography was the traditional method to determine thrombophlebitis, its invasive nature and the risks associated with the technique have resulted in a transition towards other more advanced modalities. Blood may be taken for investigation of hypercoagulable states (protein C or S deficiency, or factor V Leiden) or identification of an associated infectious process (high white blood cell count).

Management

Preventative management is important, and includes encouraging exercise, elevating the legs and maintaining an adequate fluid intake. People taking long-haul trips or who are immobilised for long periods in bed should be encouraged to wear support stockings and perform leg movement exercises regularly.

For the prevention of venous thromboembolism in moderate risk situations, such as following an acute myocardial infarction, low-dose heparin is usually effective. For high-risk situations, such as following elective hip surgery or a knee replacement, the use of low-molecular-weight heparin (e.g. dalteparin or

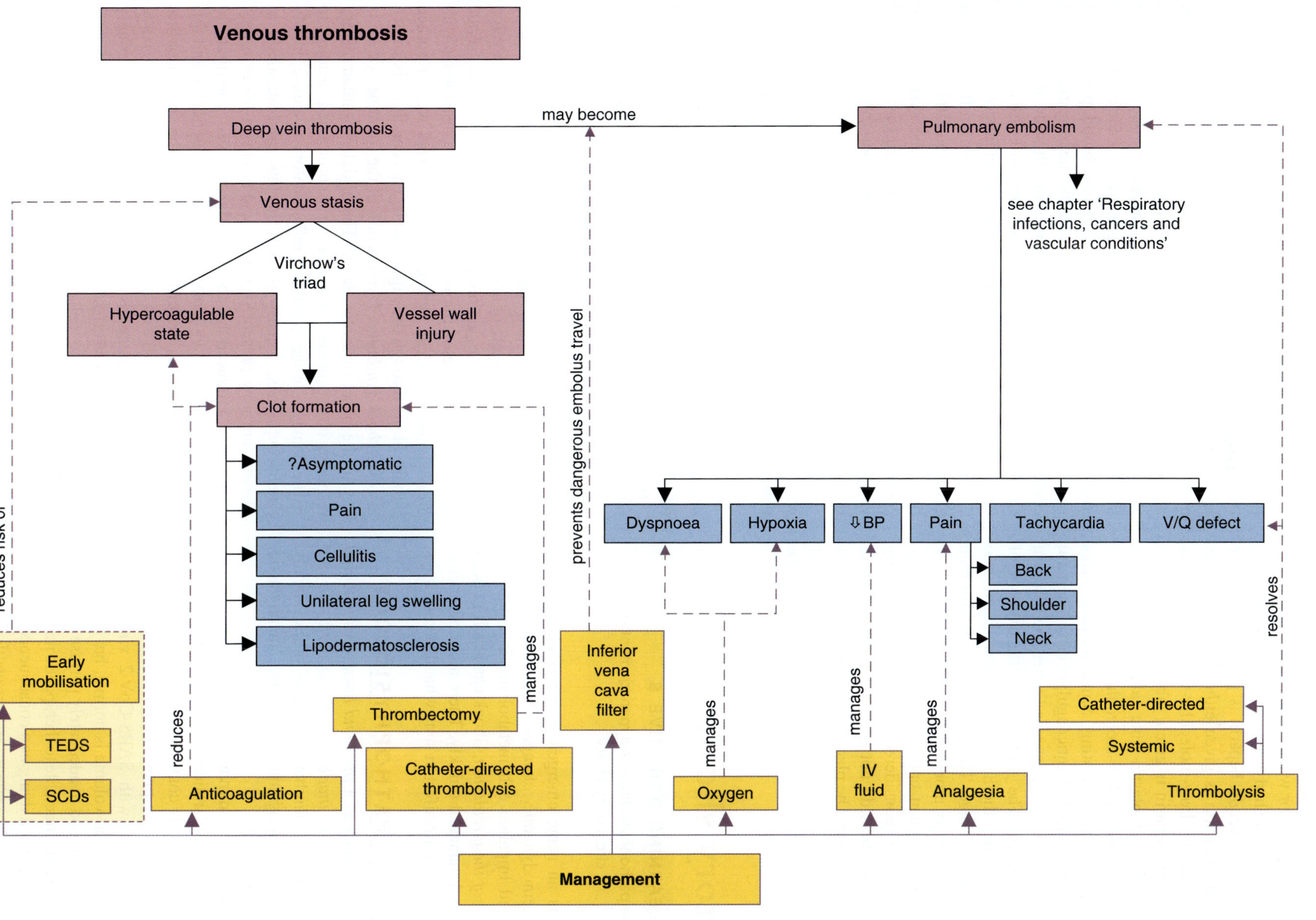

Figure 22.12

Clinical snapshot: Venous thrombosis

? = possibly; BP = blood pressure; IV = intravenous; SCDs = sequential compression devices; TEDS = thromboembolic deterrent stockings; V/Q = ventilation/perfusion.

enoxaparin) is required. Preventative treatment with low-dose heparin or low-molecular-weight heparin is continued for about seven to 10 days after surgery or when the person is mobile.

For treatment of established venous thromboembolism, heparin or low-molecular-weight heparin is given at the same time as oral warfarin. Heparin is given either by intravenous infusion or subcutaneously. Low-molecular-weight heparin is given subcutaneously. If heparin is given, laboratory testing of the activated partial thromboplastin time (aPTT) is required. On the other hand, the use of low-molecular-weight heparin does not require any laboratory testing. Since warfarin takes about five days to establish its full anticoagulant effect, heparin or low-molecular-weight heparin is stopped when the warfarin is therapeutically effective. The therapeutic effectiveness of warfarin is determined when the international normalised ratio (INR) is in the therapeutic range. Treatment with warfarin then usually continues for about six months.

In individuals with frequent episodes of thrombophlebitis, vena caval filters may be considered to prevent pulmonary embolism; however, as filters do not prevent the development of clots, more emphasis should be placed on anticoagulation. As the literature is still weak on the benefits of vena caval filters for thrombophlebitis, placement will continue to be a choice of the management team.

Circulatory shock

LEARNING OBJECTIVE 8

Outline the pathophysiology and management of circulatory shock.

Circulatory shock is an acute emergency that is characterised by significant haemodynamic changes that result in poor tissue perfusion and impaired cell metabolism. In essence, it represents a *failure of the circulation*. Shock can result in death if not recognised and managed quickly. There are a number of types of shock, which can manifest in somewhat different ways.

AETIOLOGY AND PATHOPHYSIOLOGY

Circulatory shock is defined as a *profound haemodynamic and metabolic impairment due to inadequate tissue perfusion and oxygen delivery*. There are a number of types of shock; namely, cardiogenic, neurogenic (vasogenic)/distributive, anaphylactic, hypovolaemic and septic.

Cardiogenic shock is commonly seen as a secondary condition to a myocardial infarction or as the consequence of progressive heart failure, poorly controlled dysrhythmias, angina, pericardial infections or tension pneumothorax. It has also been reported following infection with SARS-CoV-2 virus. In this form of shock, the total blood volume is normal, but the heart is unable to pump sufficient blood to adequately perfuse the organs. Cardiogenic shock is often intractable to therapeutic management, with 50–80% of those affected dying as a consequence.

Neurogenic shock, also known as *vasogenic shock*, is primarily associated with a change in central nervous system (CNS) control of the vasoconstriction–vasodilation balance, leading to widespread vasodilation and, therefore, inadequate organ perfusion. Again, the total blood volume remains normal. Drugs that lower sympathetic activity or enhance parasympathetic activity can trigger neurogenic shock, as the two systems are no longer in balance and vascular tone is lost. Likewise, damage to the spinal cord or brain can also trigger neurogenic shock, as can vasovagal syncope (i.e. fainting), although the latter often represents a transient episode and only rarely progresses to shock. Some sources combine distributive and neurogenic shock into a single group, because both are associated with widespread vasodilation, blood pooling and poor organ perfusion. However, whereas neurogenic shock is commonly associated with generalised vasodilation, *distributive shock* is associated with the altered perfusion of a subset of organs, leading to tissue ischaemia and organ failure.

Anaphylaxis represents an *allergic* reaction, often with an extremely rapid onset, and is more likely to be fatal than other types of shock. The activation of the immune system as the consequence of the response to the allergen triggers widespread vasodilation, loss of vascular integrity and, therefore, peripheral blood pooling, leading to poor tissue perfusion and oedema.

As the name suggests, *hypovolaemic shock* is associated with a reduced blood volume, due to a loss of whole blood, plasma or interstitial fluid. It often involves haemorrhage, but can also occur secondary to serious burns, or to conditions such as diabetes mellitus and diabetes insipidus, where excess urination depletes body fluid levels. In cases in which the patient is bleeding, the problem can be an internal bleed, not just an external bleed. Bleeding into the abdominal cavity or into a large muscle such as the rectus femoris (the muscle at the front of the thigh), or even severe menorrhagia, can also trigger hypovolaemic shock.

Septic shock is a complex form of shock that is due to bacterial infections that invade the normally sterile blood compartment. The state of bacteraemia is most likely to develop from a respiratory or gastrointestinal infection. However, septic shock can also develop through contamination of tampons with *Staphylococcus aureus*, where bacterial toxins were absorbed into the blood through the vaginal wall. This condition is known as *toxic shock syndrome*. Dysfunction of the immune system is key to the onset of septic shock. The initial pro-inflammatory response is considered excessive, or is prolonged, leading to tissue damage. In the initial pro-inflammatory response, highly potent cytokines, usually present in low concentrations in plasma, are now present in excess and result in tissue injury. Endotoxins produced by the bacteria can also contribute to tissue damage. The cytokines are released sequentially, and this process is known as the *cytokine cascade*. The first cytokines to be released are tissue necrosis factor-alpha (TNF-α) and interleukin subpopulations (ILs). Their effects are strongly linked to the clinical effects of septic shock. These mediators activate the immune cells and recruit them to the site of infection. They also produce fever, induce hypotension, depress the myocardium and activate procoagulant processes. Activated neutrophils induce endothelial cell dysfunction, and trigger the release of cytotoxic free radicals. Endothelial dysfunction results in a loss of sensitivity of the vascular smooth muscle to adrenaline and noradrenaline, so as blood pressure drops, vascular tone cannot be maintained. Vasodilation slows blood flow and compromises tissue perfusion.

Initially, mediator release may induce a hyperdynamic state characterised by increased heart rate and cardiac output in order to maintain blood pressure. An increase in cellular metabolism also occurs in response to fever. Eventually, lactic acidosis develops as cellular oxygen delivery fails. Damage to the endothelial cells also leads to capillary leakiness, with a depleted intravascular volume and tissue oedema. The balance between natural procoagulant and anticoagulant mediators is also lost, leading to thrombus formation. A vicious cycle of coagulation and inflammatory responses can develop. In its most severe form, disseminated intravascular coagulation can develop. Septic shock clearly displays elements of distributive shock (through widespread vasodilation) and cardiogenic shock (through myocardial depression).

Irrespective of the cause of circulatory shock, the phases of the condition are similar and are called compensated and non-compensated shock. *Non-progressive (compensated) shock* occurs when compensatory mechanisms provide benefit to the affected person and minimal organ ischaemia occurs. In these cases, the underlying cause is easily determined and corrected, and the situation resolves. In cases such as vasovagal syncope or mild menorrhagia, the situation will resolve itself without intervention, often within a few hours, as the condition is transient.

Progressive (non-compensated) shock occurs when the compensatory mechanisms are inadequate to resolve the problem, and intervention is necessary. Poor tissue perfusion leads to ischaemia and tissue damage. At this point the compensatory mechanisms are terminated. Vasomotor activity ceases due to hypoxia. Blood is diverted away from non-essential organs. Signs of metabolic acidosis are seen, and other organs are compromised. Irreversible shock occurs as systemic acidosis worsens, cardiac function begins to fail markedly, pronounced renal, CNS and pulmonary dysfunction occurs, consciousness is lost, ischaemic cell death becomes widespread and the person in shock becomes comatose. At this stage, the person is generally insensitive to therapeutic intervention and death may result.

Compensatory mechanisms in shock

When blood pressure drops, baroreceptors in the aortic arch, carotid arteries and intestinal aorta signal the loss of stretch to the brainstem. In response, the SNS is activated. The renin–angiotensin–aldosterone system is also activated. These systems attempt to improve cardiac output and vascular tone, and therefore blood pressure. Heart rate and contraction force increase, leading to the racing or pounding heart often experienced by people in circulatory shock. An increase in vascular tone is an attempt to ensure adequate perfusion pressure, even if volume is reduced. The kidneys retain fluid in order to improve arterial blood volume and venous return. If the underlying reason for the shock is transient, these compensatory mechanisms can restore blood pressure and tissue perfusion.

However, if the condition worsens, these compensatory mechanisms will actually aggravate the shock, as the workload of the heart and kidneys, in the absence of adequate blood supply, is excessively increased. This leads to tissue ischaemia and the activation of chemoreceptors. In response to this signalling, and in an attempt to ensure survival, the brain redirects blood to the essential organs and away from non-essential structures. Interestingly, in this response non-essential tissues and organs include fingers, toes, the gastrointestinal system, the cerebral cortex and the lungs. The redirection involves vasoconstriction of the vessels leading to the targeted structures, and vasodilation of those vessels leading to more essential organs. Unfortunately, dilation of the blood vessels can slow the rate of blood flow and, therefore, perfusion pressure, which can actually worsen the ischaemia. Simultaneously, vasoconstriction at target organs can cause pressure-related damage due to the high-pressure jet of the small volumes of blood coming into the structure. At this stage, therapeutic intervention will need to be two-pronged: dilation of constricted vessels, and constriction of dilated vessels. If the condition continues to worsen, the compensatory mechanisms cease and the heart rate, vascular tone and kidney function all slow. This can lead to widespread ischaemia, organ failure and, possibly, death.

CLINICAL MANIFESTATIONS

Early recognition of the clinical manifestations of shock will reduce the mortality and morbidity associated with this condition. Decreases in blood pressure, cardiac output and urination often occur, but may not always be present. Respiration rate is usually increased. Consciousness may also be impaired. Affected people may also speak of not feeling well or that they are feeling nauseous.

Depending on the type of shock, variation in clinical manifestations occurs, such as heart rate, total peripheral resistance and skin characteristics, as well as the presence and location of oedema. These variations are summarised in Table 22.3.

CLINICAL DIAGNOSIS AND MANAGEMENT

Diagnosis

As the clinical manifestations of shock are so profound, frequent observations of heart rate, blood pressure and urine output are crucial to identify, track the progress of, and assess the effectiveness of interventions of ensuing shock. For all types of shock except for neurogenic shock, SNS responses to the cause will result in tachycardia, but blood pressure is generally reduced. Urine output will also decrease, as renal blood flow is compromised and adequate glomerular filtration pressure is lost. Peripheral monitoring of oxygenation is also valuable, but may become difficult as compensatory peripheral vasoconstriction can make monitoring inaccurate or unobtainable. Arterial blood gas results will initially show respiratory alkalosis, which is soon followed by metabolic alkalosis. Hypoxaemia is also usually present. Laboratory results may show an elevated haematocrit due to a low blood volume. If haemorrhage is present, haemoglobin will be decreased. Further diagnostic investigations cannot be attempted until resuscitation and stabilisation are achieved by

Table 22.3 Variation in clinical manifestations in circulatory shock

Clinical manifestation	Cardiogenic shock	Neurogenic shock	Hypovolaemic shock	Anaphylactic shock	Septic shock
Heart rate	↑	↓	↑	↑	↑
Total peripheral resistance	↑	↓	↑	↓	↓
Skin temperature, colour,* turgor and feel	Cool, dusky, normal turgor, clammy	May be warm and pink, normal turgor	Cool, pale, poor turgor and clammy	Cool, pale, normal turgor	Usually hot, pink, normal turgor
Oedema and location	Pulmonary and systemic	Not usually	Not usually	Systemic	Systemic

*Colour change in Caucasians.

fluid and/or inotropic support, haemostasis from pressure or chemicals/blood products, and/or surgical control of blood loss.

Management

The treatment for circulatory shock will depend largely on the type of shock, the state of its progression and the effects on various body systems (see Figure 22.13). Although various types of shock will be managed in different ways, some basic principles exist across all types. A golden rule with conditions that interfere with oxygenation is 'time is tissue'; therefore, promoting oxygenation is a priority. Supplemental oxygen will be necessary from the outset, and, as the person's condition deteriorates, mechanical ventilation may be required in order to maintain adequate oxygenation. Determination of the cause is imperative, as this will direct further management decisions.

As blood pressure is compromised, interventions to support it will be required quickly, and, in most types of shock, intravenous infusions of crystalloid or colloid solution are appropriate. However, in some instances, such as cardiogenic shock, volume support would exacerbate the clinical situation.

In the early stages of shock, adrenaline can be used to improve cardiac contractility (inotropy) and maintain vascular tone. As shock progresses and the heart begins to experience ischaemia, dobutamine may be a better option. Dobutamine is a partial agonist at β-adrenergic receptors and is a good inotrope for shock, as it does not strain an already compromised heart. Dopamine can be used to ensure kidney perfusion as the condition worsens. The effects of dopamine on adrenoreceptors is dose-dependent, and at lower doses it preferentially affects a subset of renal β-receptors. Once a person is in the later stages of non-progressive shock and is moving towards irreversible shock, a combination of prostacyclin (PGI_2) and corticosteroids can be used to try to restore the vasoconstriction–vasodilation balance. PGI_2 will vasodilate the vessels surrounding the non-essential organs, while the corticosteroids will improve vascular tone around essential organs, in each case attempting to correct the perfusion pressure.

Other interventions required may be the administration of antimicrobials to manage infection, corticosteroids to manage inflammation, vasopressors to cause vasoconstriction and support blood pressure, anticoagulants to reduce blood clot formation, platelet infusions to reduce bleeding, and atropine to increase heart rate. All of these interventions are dependent on the type and degree of shock exhibited (see Figure 22.14).

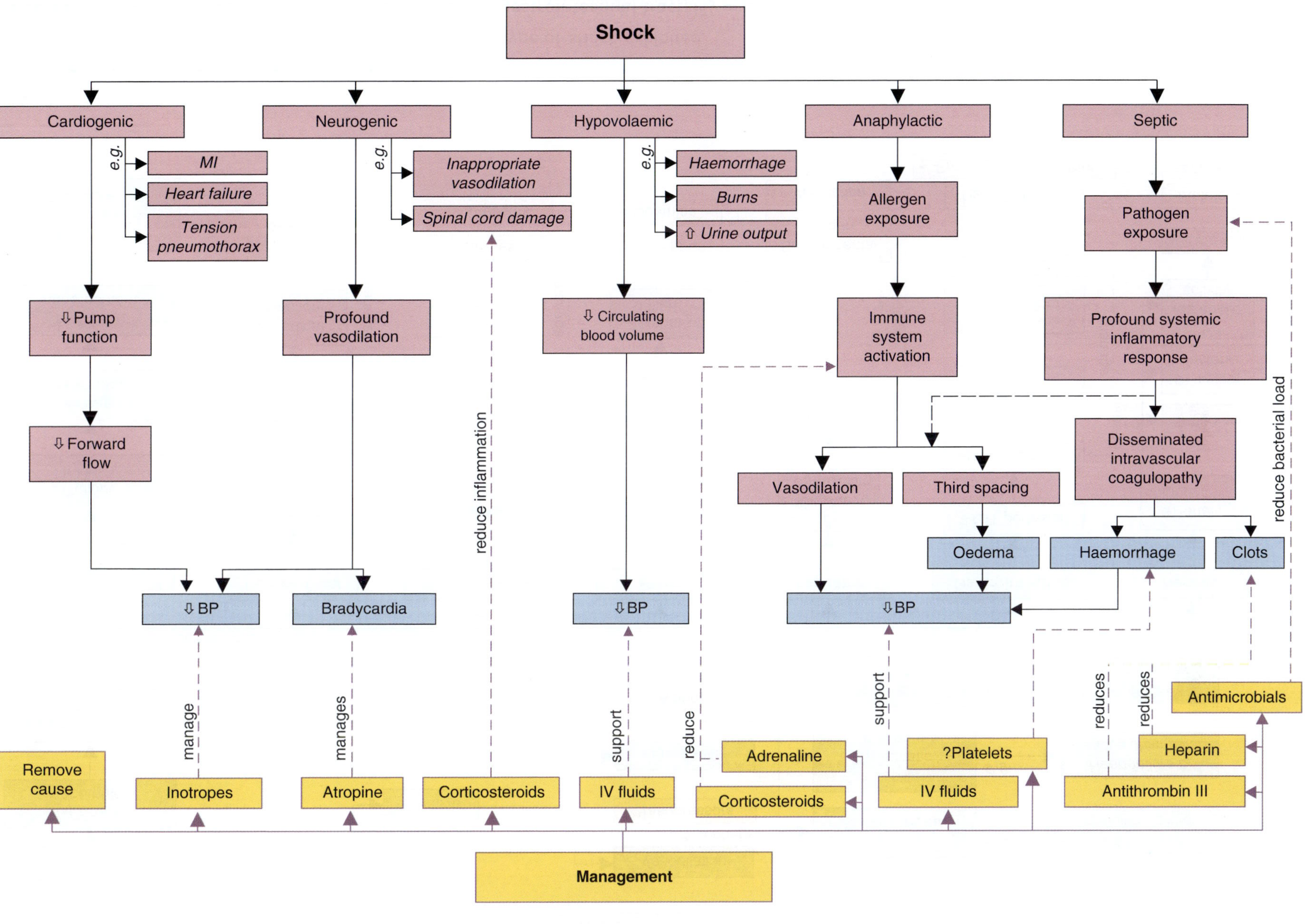

Figure 22.13

Clinical snapshot: Circulatory shock

↓ = decreased; ↑ = increased; ? = possibly; BP = blood pressure; IV = intravenous; MI = myocardial infarction.

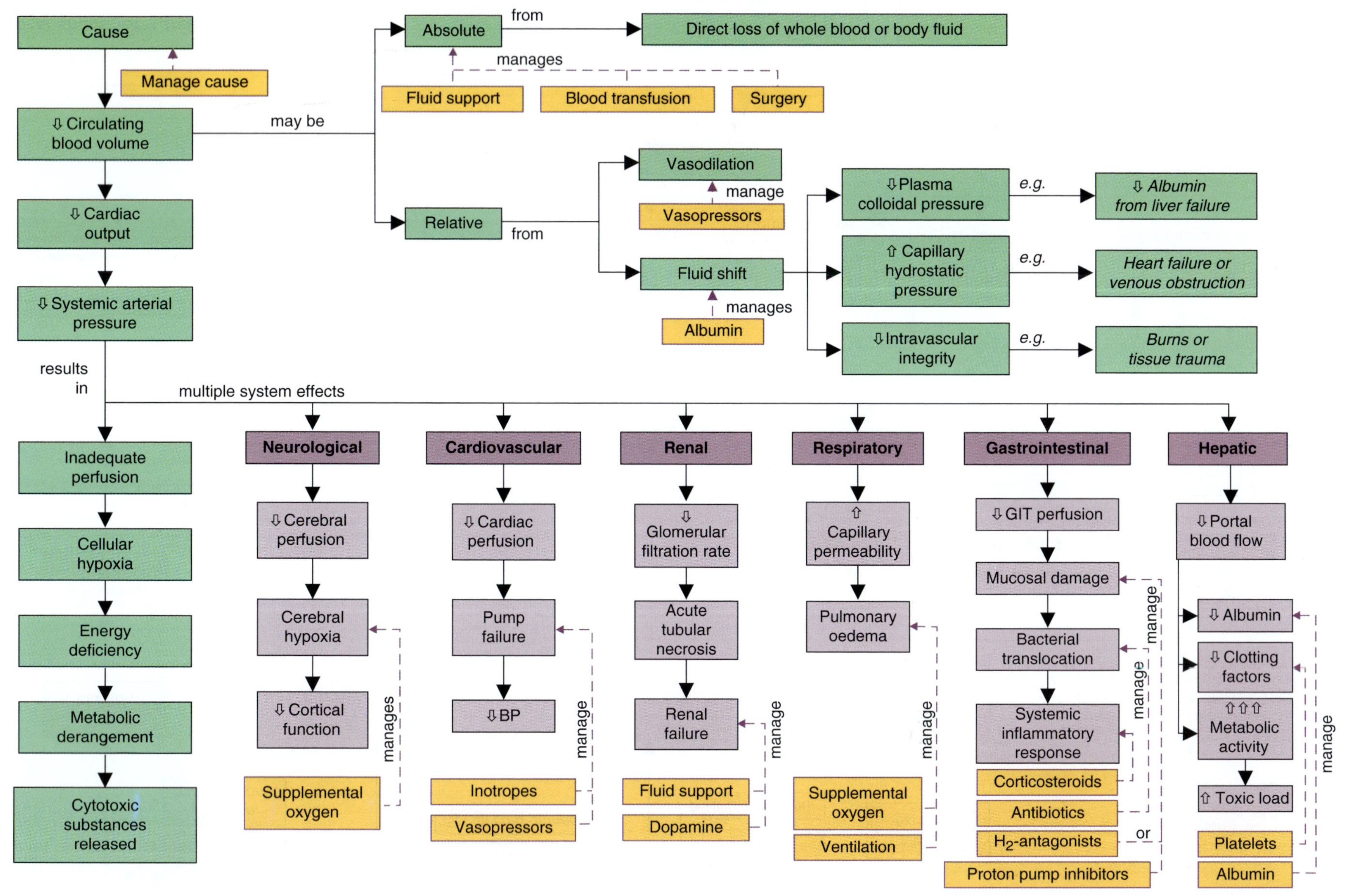

Figure 22.14

Progression of shock and management by systems

Management of shock will differ depending on the stage and type of shock exhibited.

↓ = decreased; ↑ = increased; BP = blood pressure; GIT = gastrointestinal tract; H_2 = histamine-2 receptor.

INDIGENOUS HEALTH FAST FACTS AND CULTURAL CONSIDERATIONS

FAST FACTS

- *Aboriginal or Torres Strait Islander peoples are almost 2.9 times more likely than non-Indigenous Australians to be a daily smoker.*
- *Aboriginal and Torres Strait Islander peoples are 1.5 times more likely than non-Indigenous Australians to die from circulatory system diseases.*
- *Aboriginal and Torres Strait Islander peoples are 2.8 times more likely than non-Indigenous Australians to develop diabetes mellitus.*
- *Aboriginal or Torres Strait Islander peoples are 1.2 times more likely than non-Indigenous Australians to have hypertension (1.2:1).*
- *Smoking and diabetes are significant risk factors for peripheral vascular disease (PVD). As Aboriginal and Torres Strait Islander peoples have an increased incidence of the risk factors for PVD, it can be suggested that they would have a higher incidence of PVD itself.*
- *Māori are 2.3 times more likely, and Pacific Islands people are 2.5 times more likely, than European New Zealanders to have diabetes.*
- *Māori are 1.26 times more likely, and Pacific Islands people are 1.32 times more likely, than European New Zealanders to have hypertension.*
- *Māori are 2.9 times more likely, and Pacific Islands people are 2.3 times more likely, than European New Zealanders to smoke.*
- *As smoking and diabetes are significant risk factors for PVD, it can be suggested that Māori and Pacific Islands people would have an increased risk of PVD.*

CULTURAL CONSIDERATIONS

- *Although Australia's overall cardiovascular burden is reducing, Aboriginal and Torres Strait Islander peoples are still approximately 10 times more likely than non-Indigenous Australians to die from cardiovascular disease. This extreme difference suggests that there is still significant progress to be made. There are still many health services that are not culturally appropriate. Focus should be placed on improving accessibility to healthcare through the provision of affordable, community-centred health promotion campaigns designed specifically for Aboriginal and Torres Strait Islander peoples. An increase in Aboriginal and Torres Strait Islander Health Workers and more provision of services to rural and remote areas are still factors that can be improved.*

Sources: Data from Australian Institute of Health and Welfare (2023); New Zealand Ministry of Health (2023).

CHILDREN AND ADOLESCENTS

- Blood vessels in neonates and infants requiring medical attention are very small and rubbery, making venous access difficult.
- If venous access is required in an emergency and the vasculature cannot be accessed, intraosseous access (into the proximal tibia, femur or iliac crest) can support drug administration and fluid support.
- In neonates, umbilical vessels can be cannulated for venous access as they are larger than peripheral vessels.

OLDER ADULTS

- As people age, the amount of collagen within their vasculature decreases, so structural integrity begins to decline. Arterial wall stiffening can occur as a result of atherosclerotic deposits, and the receptors responsible for vasomotor control (i.e. to vasoconstrict and vasodilate) become less responsive.
- Capillary wall thickening reduces the efficiency of nutrient and waste exchange.
- Baroreceptors within critical vessels are less responsive to position change, resulting in orthostatic hypotension.

KEY CLINICAL ISSUES

- As hypertension is a relatively asymptomatic illness, individuals often cease taking their antihypertensive agents because they do not 'feel sick'.
- The act of measuring someone's blood pressure can make it increase. 'White coat' hypertension is an issue when individuals are so concerned with what their blood pressure is going to be that sympathetic nervous system activation results in vasoconstriction, increased heart rate and, ultimately, in some instances, hypertension.
- Many theories have been suggested for the development of hypertension. Therefore, many factors should be controlled in individuals with hypertension. Short, unsustained management of hypertension can result in rebound hypertension, making treatment and clinical outcomes worse over time.
- Assisting a person to control their anxiety will be beneficial to a blood pressure reading.
- People should be encouraged to eliminate additional salt to food and select low-sodium food options. Reducing salt intake reduces intravascular fluid, which reduces hypertension.
- People with peripheral vascular disease can develop large and poorly healing lesions. These commonly get infected and may not disappear for years. Identifying and managing peripheral vascular disease early reduces the risk of serious complications, such as amputation or death.
- There is a significant difference between peripheral arterial and peripheral venous disease. Ensure familiarity with both issues to be best informed about the identification and management of these peripheral vascular diseases.
- Varicose veins can be unsightly and even painful. Enable individuals to discuss management options regarding varicose veins. This may also reduce the burden of the varicose veins in years to come.
- A distinguishing sign in aortic dissection is a description of a 'ripping feeling in the centre of the chest'. Observation of blood pressures in both arms (one after the other) will assist in gathering information about the potential of an aortic dissection.
- Community members may get confused about the meaning of the word 'shock', mistaking it for meaning 'a terrible surprise'. Circulatory shock refers to an exceedingly low blood pressure as a result of many mechanisms. When dealing with those close to the person affected, ensure an appropriate understanding of this terminology.

CHAPTER REVIEW

- *Hypertension* is defined as an elevated blood pressure above 140 mmHg systolic and/or 90 mmHg diastolic, and constitutes the major preventable risk factor for heart disease, kidney disease and stroke.
- Major risk factors for hypertension include age, race/ethnicity, sodium intake, alcohol consumption, tobacco use, inadequate physical activity and obesity.
- The underlying pathophysiology of hypertension is unknown, but evidence from family studies indicates that those affected have significant differences in their ability to regulate vasoconstriction and fluid balance both locally and globally.
- *Circulatory shock* is a sharp drop in blood pressure and/or distribution of blood, and in many cases constitutes a medical emergency.
- Generally, the compensatory mechanisms activated in shock—namely, the sympathetic nervous system and the renin-angiotensin-aldosterone system—will rectify the problem in non-progressive shock, but can exacerbate progressive shock, worsening tissue ischaemia and necrosis, leading to death.
- *Peripheral arterial disease* is a condition in which there is ischaemia to peripheral tissues. It is commonly associated with atherosclerosis and diabetes, and leads to ischaemia of the peripheral tissues.
- *Aneurysms* occur as the consequence of damage to or weakness of arterial walls. *True aneurysms* result when the weakened vessel wall balloons out from either one or both sides of the affected vessel. By contrast, a *dissecting aneurysm* is associated with a tear in the wall of the artery, which can allow blood to enter into the wall and become trapped there, forming a thrombus that, if it becomes large enough, can collapse the vessel.
- While aneurysms affect arteries, *varicose veins* constitute a loss of integrity of veins. Dilation of the vessel walls that impedes closure of the valves, or damage to the valves themselves, contributes to varicose veins, although there is good histological evidence for changes to the structure of the venous walls. Whether these changes are causative or result from the process that creates varicose veins is unknown.
- *Phlebothrombosis (deep vein thrombosis)* is a condition marked by inappropriate thrombus formation in veins in the absence of inflammation in the vessel walls. Should the thrombus become an embolism, then a common site of complication is the pulmonary system where pulmonary embolisms constitute a serious health risk.
- *Arteriovenous malformations* occur when a set of arteries connect directly to a set of veins without a capillary bed between them. The resulting nest of vessels, known as a *nidus*, is generally under high pressure, and there is a risk of bleeds and ruptures. The symptoms associated with these disorders depend largely on the location of the malformation.

REVIEW QUESTIONS

1. What are the way/s in which the risk factors for hypertension are thought to contribute to the development of the disorder?
2. What is the difference between primary and secondary hypertension? What would be the key difference in the management goals of these two conditions?
3. What are the different types of circulatory shock, and what is the underlying cause of each?
4. What are the three stages of shock? What are the compensatory mechanisms in each?
5. Thromboangiitis obliterans, deep vein thrombosis and thrombophlebitis are all conditions involving inappropriate thrombus formation. What is the difference between them?
6. Aneurysms are often associated with atherosclerosis formation. Given what you know about the types of aneurysms, how might atherosclerosis contribute to aneurysm formation?
7. What is the relationship between arteriovenous malformations and hereditary haemorrhagic telangiectasia?
8. Both aneurysms and varicose veins are associated with changes in vascular walls. What is the difference between these two disorders?

HEALTH PROFESSIONAL CONNECTIONS

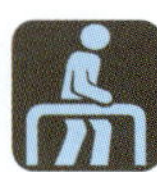

Physiotherapists The skeletal pump can be utilised to improve vascular return through active or passive leg exercises. Deep breathing and coughing will produce intrathoracic pressure changes, and will also have a positive influence on venous return. It is also important to note that leg exercises will not only improve oxygenation, increase venous return and decrease muscle wastage, but they will also reduce the risk of deep vein thrombosis (DVT). Assessment of a client's limbs and observation of colour or size changes, or complaints of pain, should be shared with other members of the healthcare team so that further investigation can commence as necessary.

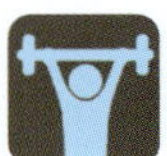

Exercise scientists Exercise scientists should understand the direct relationship between physical activity and control of blood pressure. Exercise prescription for individuals with vascular disorders should reflect considerations of existing vascular health. Medical assessment prior to commencing exercise programs is recommended for individuals with cardiovascular pathology. Both resistance and aerobic training will result in profound increases in blood pressure during the effort. Care must be taken with individuals with friable vessels or aneurysms, as increasing blood pressure can result in vessel rupture. Assessment for symptoms such as claudication, and signs such as colour changes in the peripheries, should be a priority consideration. Insulin resistance will contribute to vascular remodelling; exercise reduces insulin resistance. Generally speaking, increasing physical activity will promote vascular health.

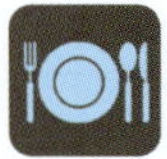

Nutritionists/Dieticians Low-sodium diets will assist in reducing high blood pressures, as the increased sodium promotes water retention, which increases circulating blood volume. In clients with hypertension, unless otherwise indicated, low-sodium diets are necessary to assist with blood pressure control. Excess lipids (especially low-density lipoproteins–LDLs) will contribute to the development of atherosclerosis. Educating clients on appropriate foods and possible substitutes will assist them to make informed decisions about their total fat intake.

All allied professionals When working with people who complain about signs and symptoms suggesting vascular issues (e.g. claudication, paraesthesia, colour changes to the peripheries and poor wound healing in lower limbs), it is important to discuss your assessments with other members of the healthcare team so that investigations into the person's vascular health can occur as required.

CASE STUDY

Mr Robert Tucker is a 65-year-old man (UR number 308469) who was admitted through the emergency department three hours ago with moderate to severe abdominal pain. His observations were as follows:

Temperature	Heart rate	Respiration rate	Blood pressure	SpO_2
36.8°C	92	18	160/90	93% (RA*)

*RA = room air.

Mr Tucker has a pulsating mass (with bruit) in his mid-abdomen. He is being investigated for an abdominal aortic aneurysm (AAA) and will be undergoing a CT scan today. Intravenously administered glyceryl trinitrate (GTN) is infusing, and is to be titrated to obtain a blood pressure of approximately 100 mmHg systolic. He is on telemetry, and is to have frequent non-invasive blood pressure measurement (NIBP) while on the GTN. He has smoked cigarettes for 52 years. He states that he has smoked a pack a day for the past 40 years. Mr Tucker has a history of hypertension. His diet is poor and his BMI is 33.5. He has a positive family history for cardiovascular event. His father died of a ruptured AAA (abdominal aortic aneurysm), and his brother died of a myocardial infarction. His pathology results are as follows:

HAEMATOLOGY

Patient location:	Ward 3	**UR:**	308469		
Consultant:	Smith	**NAME:**	Tucker		
		Given name:	Robert	**Sex:**	M
		DOB:	31/12/XX	**Age:**	65

Time collected	11:30
Date collected	XX/XX
Year	XXXX
Lab #	53534564

FULL BLOOD COUNT		UNITS	REFERENCE RANGE
Haemoglobin	132	g/L	115–160
White cell count	5.2	$\times 10^9$ /L	4.0–11.0
Platelets	280	$\times 10^9$ /L	140–400
Haematocrit	0.42		0.33–0.47
Red cell count	4.13	$\times 10^{12}$ /L	3.80–5.20
Reticulocyte count	1.3	%	0.2–2.0
MCV	94	fL	80–100
Neutrophils	4.13	$\times 10^9$ /L	2.00–8.00
Lymphocytes	2.45	$\times 10^9$ /L	1.00–4.00
Monocytes	0.64	$\times 10^9$ /L	0.10–1.00
Eosinophils	0.35	$\times 10^9$ /L	< 0.60
Basophils	0.11	$\times 10^9$ /L	< 0.20
ESR	8	mm/h	< 12
COAGULATION PROFILE			
aPTT	27	secs	24–40
PT	13	secs	11–17

BIOCHEMISTRY

Patient location:	Ward 3	**UR:**	308469		
Consultant:	Smith	**NAME:**	Tucker		
		Given name:	Robert	**Sex:**	M
		DOB:	31/12/XX	**Age:**	65

Time collected	11:30
Date collected	XX/XX
Year	XXXX
Lab #	73663576

ELECTROLYTES		UNITS	REFERENCE RANGE
Sodium	139	mmol/L	135–145
Potassium	4.5	mmol/L	3.5–5.2
Chloride	101	mmol/L	95–110
Bicarbonate	25	mmol/L	22–32
Glucose (random)	7.2	mmol/L	3.0–7.7
Iron	11	μmol/L	11–30

CRITICAL THINKING

1 Analyse Mr Tucker's history. What factors increase his risk of experiencing vascular disorders? Explain the relationship between cardiovascular risk factors and the development of aortic aneurysms.

2 Most abdominal aortic aneurysms (AAAs) are infrarenal. What other signs or symptoms may Mr Tucker present with if his AAA was suprarenal? Explain.

3 AAAs are frequently known as 'silent time bombs', because they can be asymptomatic. What does this mean? If Mr Tucker's AAA were to rupture, what signs would be observed or symptoms reported? How would this situation be managed?

4 As Mr Tucker has an AAA, what can you infer about the health of the rest of his vascular system? Before the AAA is corrected, what other investigations should take place? Why? (*Hint:* One would be to determine the risk of cerebrovascular accident.)

5 Mr Tucker's father and brother have died of cardiovascular issues. What is the significance of this information? What implications does this information have for the rest of the family?

BIBLIOGRAPHY

Acin, M.T., Rueda, J-R., Saiz, L.C., Parent Mathias, V., Alzueta, N., Solà, I., ... Erviti, J. (2020). Alcohol intake reduction for controlling hypertension. *Cochrane Database of Systematic Reviews* 9:CD010022. https://doi.org/10.1002/14651858.CD010022.pub2.

Alexander, M.R., Madhur, M.S., Harrison, D.G., Dreisbach, A.W. & Riaz, K. (2022). Hypertension. *Emedicine.* https://emedicine.medscape.com/article/241381-overview.

Angelini, D.E., Kaatz, S., Rosovsky, R.P., Zon, R.L., Pillai, S., Robertson, W.E., ... Khorana, A. (2022). COVID-19 and venous thromboembolism: a narrative review. *Research and Practice in Thrombosis and Haemostasis* 6(2):E12666. https://doi.org/10.1002/rth2.12666.

Australian Bureau of Statistics (ABS) (2022). *Causes of death, Australia, 2022.* Canberra: ABS. http://www.abs.gov.au/statistics/health/causes-death.

Australian Commission on Safety and Quality in Health Care (ACSQHC) (2022). *Venous Thromboembolism Prevention Clinical Care Standard.* Sydney: ACSQHC. https://www.safetyandquality.gov.au/standards/clinical-care-standards/venous-thromboembolism-prevention-clinical-care-standard.

Australian Institute of Health and Welfare (AIHW) (2022a). *Australia's health, 2022: data insights*. Australia's Health series No. 18, Cat. No. AUS 240. Canberra: AIHW. https://www.aihw.gov.au/reports/australias-health/australias-health-2022-data-insights/summary.

Australian Institute of Health and Welfare (AIHW) (2022b). *Principal diagnosis data cubes: separation statistics by principal diagnosis (ICD-10-AM 11th edition), Australia, 2020–21.* Canberra: AIHW. https://www.aihw.gov.au/reports/hospitals/principal-diagnosis-data-cubes/contents/data-cubes.

Australian Institute of Health and Welfare (AIHW) (2023a). *Aboriginal and Torres Strait Islander Health Performance Framework: summary report 2023*. Canberra: AIHW. https://www.indigenoushpf.gov.au/Report-overview/Overview/Summary-Report.

Australian Institute of Health and Welfare (AIHW) (2023b). *Heart, stroke and vascular disease: Australian facts*. Web report. Canberra: AIHW. https://www.aihw.gov.au/reports/heart-stroke-vascular-diseases/hsvd-facts/contents/about.

Bauldoff, G., Gubrud-Howe, P.M., Carno, M.-A., Levett-Jones, T., Hales, M., Berry, K., ... LeMone, P. (2020). *LeMone and Burke's medical–surgical nursing: critical thinking for person-centred care* (4th [Australian] edn). Sydney: Pearson Australia.

Best, O. & Fredericks, B. (2021). *Yatdjuligin: Aboriginal and Torres Strait Islander nursing and midwifery care* (3rd edn). Port Melbourne, VIC: Cambridge University Press.

Bullock, S. & Manias, E. (2022). *Fundamentals of pharmacology* (9th edn). Sydney: Pearson Australia.

Department of Health and Aged Care (2022). *Tackling Indigenous smoking (TIS)—national statistics.* Canberra: Department of Health and Aged Care. https://www.health.gov.au/our-work/tackling-indigenous-smoking.

Ehret, G.B. (2022). Genetic factors in the pathogenesis of hypertension. *UpToDate.* https://www.uptodate.com/contents/genetic-factors-in-the-pathogenesis-of-hypertension.

Hillegass, E., Lukaszewicz, K. & Puthoff, M. (2022). Role of physical therapists in the management of individuals at risk for or diagnosed with venous thromboembolism: evidence-based clinical practice guideline 2022. *Physical Therapy* 102(8):pzac057. https://doi.org/10.1093/ptj/pzac057.

Hollenberg, S.M., Safi, L., Parrillo, J.E., Fata, M., Klinkhammer, B., Gayed, N., ... Turi, Z.G. (2021). Hemodynamic profiles of shock in patients with COVID-19. *American Journal of Cardiology* 153:135–39. https://doi.org/10.1016/j.amjcard.2021.05.029.

Hwang, C., Muchira, J., Hibner, B., Phillips, S. & Piano, M. (2022). Alcohol consumption: a new risk factor for arterial stiffness? *Cardiovascular Toxicology* 22:236–45. https://doi.org/10.1007/s12012-022-09728-8.

Ji, L., Tang, N.L.S., Xu, Z. & Xu, J. (2020). Genes regulate blood pressure, but 'environments' cause hypertension. *Frontiers in Genetics* 11:580443. https://doi.org/10.3389/fgene.2020.580443.

Khan, A.N. & Sabih, A. (2021). Esophageal varices imaging and diagnosis. *Emedicine.* https://emedicine.medscape.com/article/367986-overview.

Khilnani, N.M. & Winokur, R.S. (2016). Varicose vein treatment with endovenous laser therapy. *Emedicine*. https://emedicine.medscape.com/article/1815850-overview.

Levy, H.D. (2022). *History of the Framingham Heart Study*. Framingham, MA: National Heart Institute. https://www.framinghamheartstudy.org/fhs-about/history/.

Moss, J.-L., Klok, F.A., Vo, U.G. & Richards, T. (2023). Controversies in the management of proximal deep vein thrombosis. *Medical Journal of Australia* 218(2):61–64. https://doi.org/10.5694/mja2.51796.

National Heart Foundation of Australia (2016). *Guideline for the diagnosis and management of hypertension in adults.* Melbourne: National Heart Foundation of Australia. https://www.heartfoundation.org.au/getmedia/c83511ab-835a-4fcf-96f5-88d770582ddc/PRO-167_Hypertension-guideline-2016_WEB.pdf.

New Zealand Ministry of Health (2023). *Annual update of key results 2021/22: New Zealand Health Survey.* Wellington: Ministry of Health. https://www.health.govt.nz/publication/annual-update-key-results-2021-22-new-zealand-health-survey.

Patel, K. & Chun, L.J. (2019). Deep venous thrombosis (DVT). *Emedicine*. https://emedicine.medscape.com/article/1911303-overview.

Puddey, I.B., Mori, T.A., Barden, A.E. & Beilin, L.J. (2019). Alcohol and hypertension—new insights and lingering controversies. *Current Hypertension Reports* 21(10):79. https://doi.org/10.1007/s11906-019-0984-1.

Queensland Health (2020). *Venous thromboembolism (VTE) prophylaxis in pregnancy and the puerperium*. Queensland Clinical Guidelines. Guideline No. MN20.9-V7-R25. Brisbane: Queensland Health. https://www.health.qld.gov.au/__data/assets/pdf_file/0011/140024/g-vte.pdf.

Queensland Health (2021). *Hypertension and pregnancy*. Queensland Clinical Guidelines. Guideline No. MN15.13-V8-R26. Brisbane: Queensland Health. https://www.health.qld.gov.au/__data/assets/pdf_file/0034/139948/g-hdp.pdf.

Tortora. G.J., Derrickson, B., Burkett, B., Peoples, G., Dye, D., Cooke, J., ... Green, H. (2022). *Principles of anatomy and physiology* (3rd Asia-Pacific edn). Milton, QLD: John Wiley and Sons.

Vacca, A., Bulfone, L., Cicco, S., Brosolo, G., Da Porto, A., Soardo, G., ... Sechi, L.A. (2023). Alcohol intake and arterial hypertension: retelling of a multifaceted story. *Nutrients* 15(4):958. http://dx.doi.org/10.3390/nu15040958.

Weiss, R., Anariba, D.E.I., Lanza, J. & Lessnau, K.-D. (2020). Venous insufficiency. *Emedicine*. https://emedicine.medscape.com/article/1085412-overview.

Whelton, P.K., Carey, R.M., Mancia, G., Kreutz, R., Bundy, J.D. & Williams, B. (2022). Harmonization of the American College of Cardiology/American Heart Association and European Society of Cardiology/European Society of Hypertension blood pressure/hypertension guidelines: comparisons, reflections, and recommendations. *Circulation* 146(11):868–77. https://doi.org/10.1161/CIRCULATIONAHA.121.054602.

White, W.M., Mobley, J.D. & Kim, E.D. (2021). Varicocele. *Emedicine*. https://emedicine.medscape.com/article/438591-overview.

World Health Organization (WHO) (2021a). *Guideline for the pharmacological treatment of hypertension in adults.* Geneva: WHO. https://apps.who.int/iris/bitstream/handle/10665/344424/9789240033986-eng.pdf.

World Health Organization (WHO) (2021b). *Guideline for the pharmacological treatment of hypertension in adults. Web annex A. summary of evidence.* Geneva: WHO. https://www.who.int/publications/i/item/9789240033993.

World Health Organization (WHO) (2022). *Guideline for the pharmacological treatment of hypertension in adults: summary.* Geneva: WHO. https://www.who.int/publications/i/item/9789240050969.

Zhong, L., Chen, W., Wang, T., Zeng, Q., Lai, L., Lai, J., ... Tang, S. (2022). Alcohol and health outcomes: an umbrella review of meta-analyses base on prospective cohort studies. *Frontiers in Public Health* 10:859947. https://doi.org/10.3389/fpubh.2022.859947.

Coronary artery disease

23

LEARNING OBJECTIVES

After completing this chapter, you should be able to:

1 Discuss the epidemiology of cardiovascular disease.

2 Explore the effects of ageing on vascular integrity.

3 Describe the development of atherosclerosis.

4 Identify the risk factors associated with atherosclerosis.

5 Discuss the influence of the immune system on cardiovascular disease.

6 Describe the relationship between gut microbiota and cardiovascular disease.

7 Explain how metabolic syndrome relates to coronary artery disease.

8 Define 'acute coronary syndrome', and describe its various presentations.

9 Discuss the clinical manifestations and management of acute coronary syndrome.

WHAT YOU SHOULD KNOW BEFORE YOU START THIS CHAPTER

Can you name the structures of the heart?

Can you outline the coronary circulation?

Can you describe the structure of the arterial wall and the function of each layer?

Can you describe the cellular effects of hypoxia?

Can you describe the mechanisms involved in reversible and irreversible cell injury?

KEY TERMS

Acute coronary syndrome
Angina pectoris
Atherosclerosis
Cholesterol
Coronary artery disease
High-density lipoprotein (HDL)
Ischaemia
Low-density lipoprotein (LDL)
Myocardial infarction
Triglycerides
Very-low-density lipoprotein (VLDL)

Introduction

Coronary artery disease (also known as *ischaemic heart disease*), is the most common cause of disease and death in the Western world. It results from damage to, and the death of, cells in the heart as a consequence of inadequate blood flow (**ischaemia**) and reduced oxygen delivery (*hypoxia*) to meet the workload of the heart.

Although any organ or tissue can suffer ischaemic damage, the cells of the heart are particularly vulnerable because they lack regenerative ability, and, once damaged, previously functioning muscle is replaced with granulation tissue and eventually non-contractile, fibrous scar tissue. If the initial insults to the myocardium do not result in the person's death, further stressors or subsequent insults can result in continued deterioration, and subsequently the development of heart failure (see the chapter 'Cardic muscle and valve disorders').

The primary underlying cause of this coronary ischaemia is the development of atherosclerosis, a largely reversible condition. Although ischaemia and atherosclerosis are the key features that underlie heart disease, the physiological conditions that result are referred to as **angina pectoris** (or, more simply, *angina*)—where the cells experience a temporary ischaemic state—and **myocardial infarction**—when the cells experience anoxia and subsequently die.

EPIDEMIOLOGY

LEARNING OBJECTIVE 1

Discuss the epidemiology of cardiovascular disease.

Coronary artery disease (CAD) is the leading cause of death in Australia. *Cardiovascular disease* (*CVD*—comprising coronary artery disease and stroke) costs the Australian federal government \$11.7 billion each year (8.7% of total health expenditure), including \$1.8 billion just for the cost of the drugs needed to manage these conditions. Currently, approximately 6.2% of the population over 18 years of age report having one or more CVD. Importantly, as the population ages, the burden of cardiovascular disease increases, and a recent projection forecasts direct healthcare costs for CVD between 2020 and 2029 will surpass \$61.8 billion. Also, in high-income countries with increasing obesity, reducing physical activity and exposure to numerous other risk factors that contribute to coronary artery disease, morbidity and mortality costs are only set to rise. Women are twice as likely to die of cardiovascular disease than they are to die of breast cancer.

VASCULAR CHANGES IN AGEING

LEARNING OBJECTIVE 2

Explore the effects of ageing on vascular integrity.

Coronary artery disease is the leading cause of death in Australia, and on average 74% of all deaths from coronary disease occur in those aged 75 years and older. Interestingly, when analysing mortality data in the context of age there is a significant gender disparity. Male deaths between 45 and 74 years of age are more than three times those of females, yet, after 75 years of age, the disparity reduces to 1.3 times that of females.

The role of endothelial cells

The *endothelium* is the single-cell layer that lines the blood vessel wall. It plays a key role in cardiovascular function. Endothelial cells are involved in: the manipulation of vascular tone (vasodilation and vasoconstriction); the control of vascular permeability; mediation of inflammation; angiogenesis (production of new blood vessels); and haemostasis (blood clotting).

The extent to which a blood vessel is constricted or dilated at any given moment is referred to as the *vascular tone*, and reflects the net balance between the central control exerted by the brainstem and the local responses to metabolic activity of the tissue or organ in which the blood vessels are found. *Systemic vasoconstriction* can be controlled centrally when noradrenaline (released from vasomotor neurons) binds to α-adrenergic receptors. *Local vasoconstriction* is mediated by two key factors: local *oxygen availability* and a compound called *endothelin-1*, which is released by endothelial cells.

Oxygen in the vascular beds of the body acts as a vasoconstrictor (this is not the case in the lungs). Although we require oxygen for survival, high levels of oxygen can lead to cellular damage and even cell death. The primary mediators of these deleterious effects of oxygen are a group of highly reactive and damaging compounds known as *free radicals*, otherwise known as *reactive oxygen species (ROS)* (see the chapter 'Pathophysiological terminology, cellular adaptation and injury'). The body has numerous processes in place to manage these free radicals, including the natural antioxidants, such as vitamin E (alpha-tocopherol), and tight regulation of oxygen availability. The purpose of these antioxidants is to act as sponges to mop up the free radicals both produced by normal metabolic processes (e.g. the use of oxygen by cells) and consumed in our diet (e.g. trace pesticides, charred food). In response to changing levels of metabolites and other compounds in the blood, endothelin-1 causes local vasoconstriction.

Counteracting these vasoconstricting factors, endothelial cells release three key *vasodilatory compounds* that respond to the fluctuations in the metabolic activity of the tissue or organ, providing additional blood flow locally when required. Foremost among these is the most potent vasodilatory substance, *nitric oxide (NO)*. This very small compound (comprised only of a single nitrogen molecule and a single oxygen molecule) is present in the body as a gas, allowing it to travel freely between cells. In response to compounds present in the blood, endothelial cells produce NO, which diffuses to the smooth muscle cells of the blood vessel walls, where it selectively interacts with a key regulatory enzyme, *guanylate cyclase*. Activation of guanylate cyclase causes production of *cyclic guanosine monophosphate (cGMP)*, which, in turn, closes the membrane voltage-gated calcium channels, reduces contractility, and causes the blood vessel to dilate.

A second key vasodilator is *adenosine*. As you will recall, adenosine is the building block of the cell's energy molecule, namely *adenosine triphosphate (ATP)*. When the metabolic rate of a tissue or organ is increased, the rate of ATP breakdown is also increased. This leads to an increase in adenosine availability, some of which passively leaves the cell to act as a local regulator. Adenosine acting on smooth muscle cells activates a group of adenosine receptors called *adenosine A_2-receptors*. This leads to an activation of *adenylate cyclase* and an increase in *cyclic adenosine monophosphate (cAMP)* availability. Like its counterpart cGMP, cAMP can close voltage-gated calcium channels, reducing smooth muscle contraction resulting in vasodilation.

The final group of vasodilators of interest are the *prostaglandins*. This large group of local hormones belongs in the family called *eicosanoids*, and plays a key role in a number of bodily functions, including inflammation, smooth muscle contraction and dilation, glandular secretions, reproduction, lipid metabolism and immune responses. Endothelial cells produce the prostaglandin called *prostacyclin*, opposing the action of thromboxane A_2 (another eicosanoid that promotes platelet aggregation). Consequently, prostacyclin prevents incidental thrombus formation.

In addition, endothelial cells release plasmin to dissolve thrombi that have formed, ensuring that these structures do not persist, and therefore do not become emboli. The various substances capable of influencing vascular diameter are summarised in Figure 23.1.

To protect the endothelial cells, increases in shear stress cause the release of substances (e.g. nitric oxide—NO) to promote vasodilation. Conversely, reduced shear stress will result in the release of substances (e.g. endothelin—ET) to promote vasoconstriction.

The ageing endothelium undergoes many senescent changes, resulting in the reduction of vasodilating molecules and an increase in vasoconstricting molecules. Ultimately, this causes the vessel wall to become stiffer. Other vascular changes of senescence

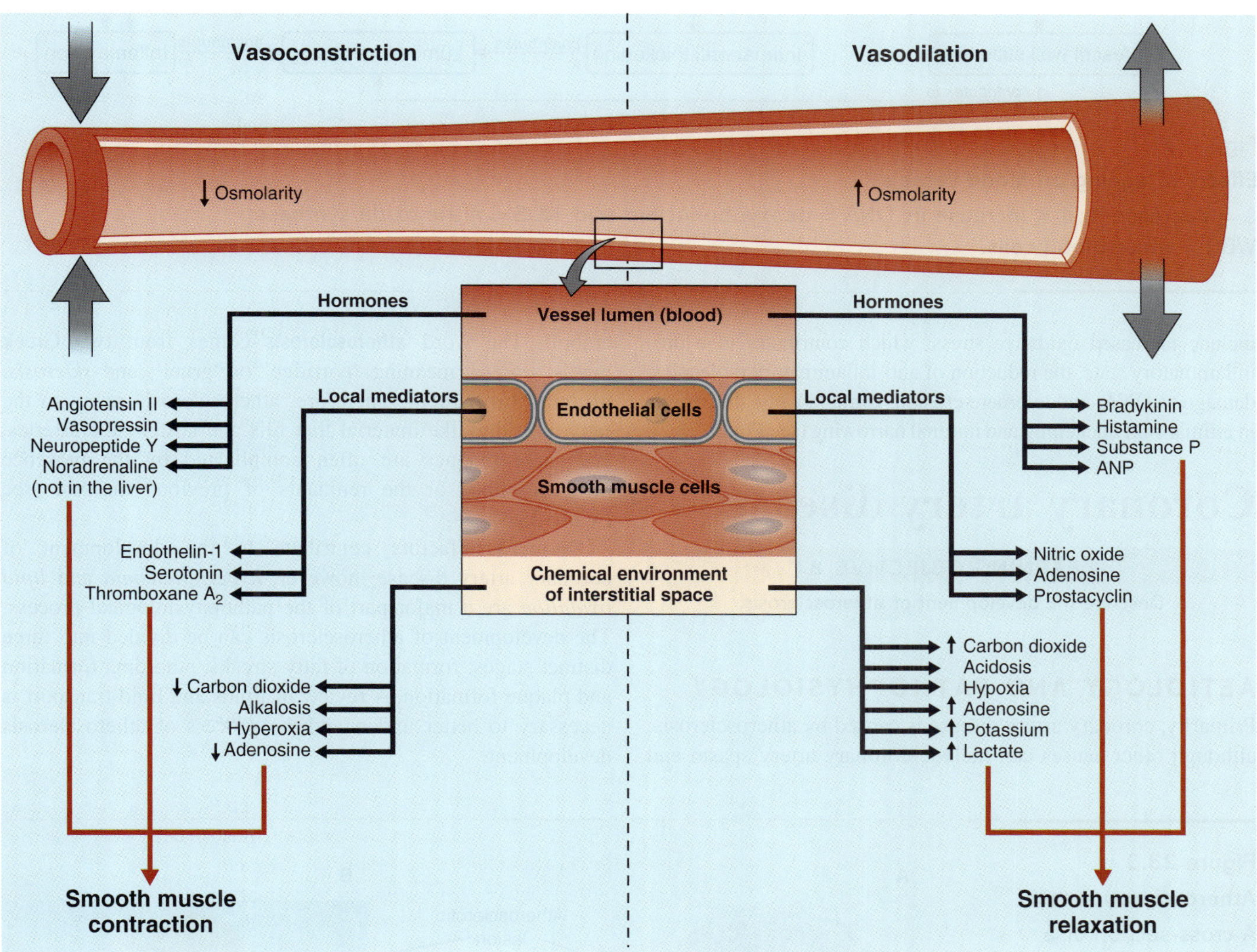

Figure 23.1

Substances capable of exerting local regulation on vascular tone

In response to mediators in the bloodstream and released locally, the endothelial cell controls the local vasodilation–vasoconstriction balance through the availability of nitric oxide, adenosine, prostaglandins and endothelin-1. Atherosclerotic plaques are established between the endothelial cells and the smooth muscle cells, resulting in the loss of this balance, leading to unchecked neuronally-mediated vasoconstriction.

↓ = decrease in; ↑ = increase in; ANP = atrial natriuretic peptide.

Source: Adapted from Lilly (2007), Figure 6.2, p. 146.

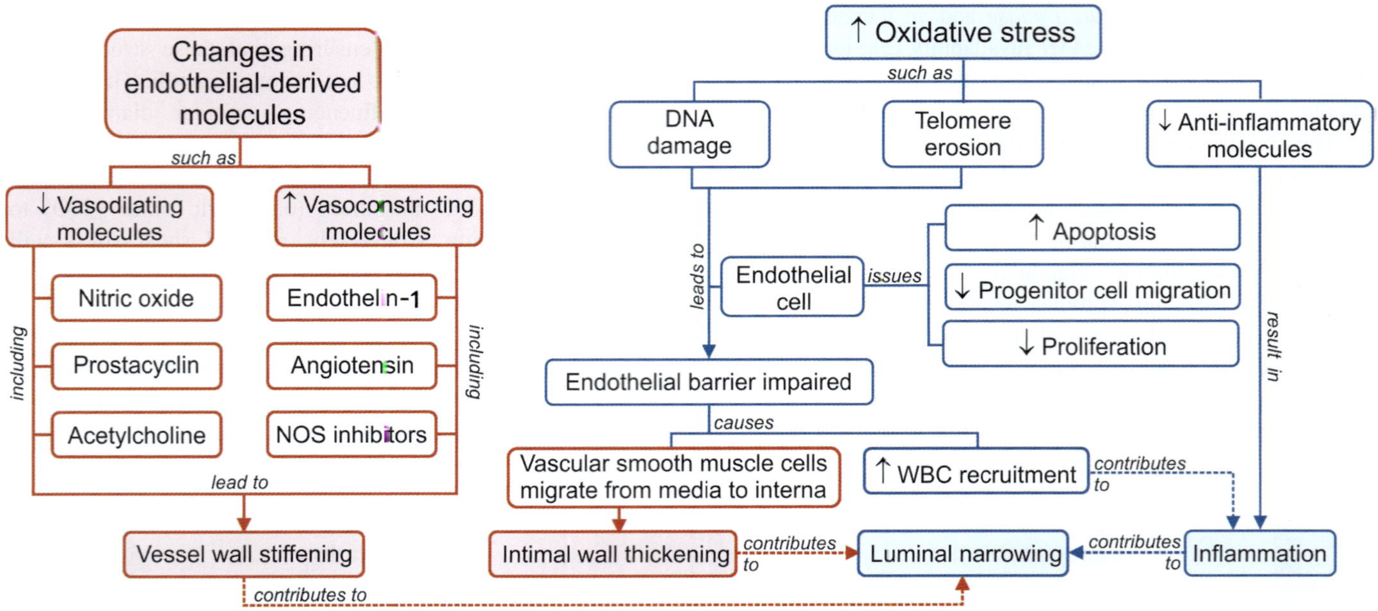

Changes in endothelial-derived molecules
such as
↓ Vasodilating molecules
including
Nitric oxide
Prostacyclin
Acetylcholine
↑ Vasoconstricting molecules
including
Endothelin-1
Angiotensin
NOS inhibitors
lead to
Vessel wall stiffening
contributes to

↑ Oxidative stress
such as
DNA damage
Telomere erosion
↓ Anti-inflammatory molecules
leads to
Endothelial cell
issues
↑ Apoptosis
↓ Progenitor cell migration
↓ Proliferation
Endothelial barrier impaired
causes
Vascular smooth muscle cells migrate from media to interna
↑ WBC recruitment
contributes to
result in
Intimal wall thickening
contributes to
Luminal narrowing
contributes to
Inflammation

Figure 23.2

Effects of ageing on blood vessels

↓ = decrease in; ↑ = increase in; DNA = deoxyribonucleic acid; NOS = nitric oxide synthase; WBC = white blood cells.

include increased oxidative stress, which contributes to a pro-inflammatory state, the reduction of anti-inflammatory molecules, damage to DNA, and telomere erosion. Cumulatively, this results in intimal wall thickening and luminal narrowing (see Figure 23.2).

Coronary artery disease

LEARNING OBJECTIVE 3

Describe the development of atherosclerosis.

AETIOLOGY AND PATHOPHYSIOLOGY

Primarily, coronary artery disease is caused by atherosclerosis, although other causes can include coronary artery spasm and emboli. The word **atherosclerosis** comes from two Greek words: *athera*, meaning ‘porridge’ or ‘gruel’, and *sklerosis*, meaning ‘to harden’. Therefore, atherosclerosis refers to the fatty, porridge-like material that fills and stiffens the arteries, and these plaques are often complicated by the presence of a thrombus or the remnants of previous thrombi (see Figure 23.3).

Numerous factors contribute to the development of coronary artery disease; however, *hyperlipidaemia* and *lipid oxidation* are a major part of the pathophysiological process. The development of atherosclerosis can be divided into three distinct stages: formation of fatty streaks, atheroma formation and plaque formation. A review of lipids and lipid transport is necessary to better understand the process of atherosclerosis development.

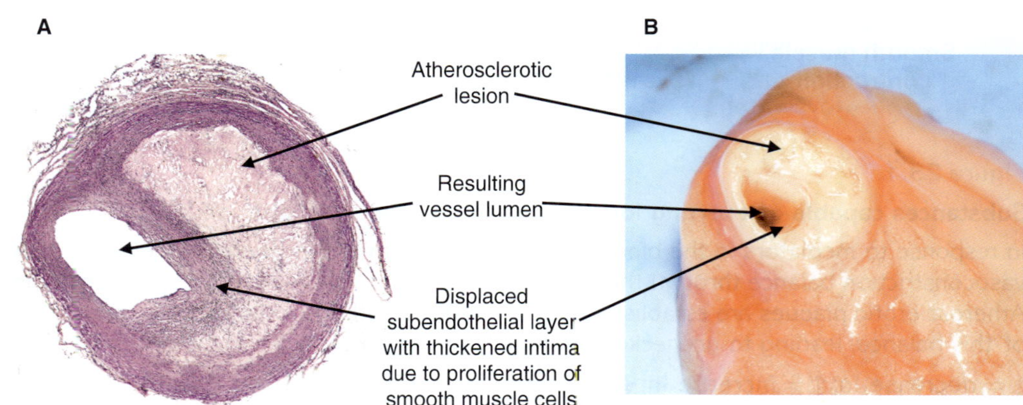

Figure 23.3

Atherosclerotic vessel

A cross-section of a vessel with significant atherosclerosis. Note the resulting vessel lumen size.

Sources: (A) Dr P. Marazzi/Science Photo Library; (B) Jose Luis Calvo/Shutterstock.

Lipids and lipid transport

Lipids need to be transported throughout the circulatory system, as they are necessary for many cellular functions. *Lipoproteins* are structures that package insoluble lipids so that they can be transported in the water-soluble medium of blood. **Triglycerides** and **cholesterol** are two important types of lipid carried by lipoproteins. Triglycerides are a critical energy source, and cholesterol is necessary for the production of cell membranes, steroids and bile acid. Interwoven around and through the structure are *apoplipoproteins*. There are many types of apolipoproteins; however, their functions can be broken into four different categories. Some apopliproteins are responsible for the *assembly of lipoproteins*, some for the *maintenance of structural integrity*, some act as *receptor ligands* and some as *coactivators for enzymes*.

Two types of lipoproteins have gained much media attention. **High-density lipoprotein (HDL)** is responsible for the retrieval of cholesterol from the arterial walls for delivery to, and disposal by, the liver. Because of these functions, HDL is colloquially known as *'good' cholesterol. Serum apolipoprotein A1 (apoA1)* can be used as a measure of HDL. **Low-density lipoprotein (LDL)** is responsible for the deposition of cholesterol to the arterial walls for use or accumulation. However, when there are too many LDLs in the blood, they will accumulate inappropriately in the sub-endothelial space of blood vessel walls. Because of this, LDL is colloquially known as *'bad' cholesterol. Serum apolipoprotein B (apoB)* can be used as a measure of LDL.

Other types of lipoproteins include **very-low-density lipoprotein (VLDL)**, which is responsible for carrying triglycerides to cells for use as energy. Most VLDLs become *IDLs (intermediate-density lipoproteins)*, which ultimately become LDLs as triglyceride is being transferred to the cells. Finally, *chylomicrons* are the largest, least-dense lipoprotein. They transport dietary triglycerides and cholesterol from the intestinal epithelial cells to the liver, skeletal muscle and adipose tissue. Chylomicrons circulate through the intestinal lymphatic system, and also in the blood. Once chylomicrons are depleted, some of their apolipoproteins are transferred to HDLs, while the remaining substances, known as *remnant particles*, are removed by the liver. VLDLs, LDLs, IDLs and chylomicrons are collectively known as *non-HDL cholesterol*. Figure 23.4 illustrates the various types of lipoproteins and their characteristics.

Cells require small amounts of cholesterol and fat in order to maintain cell membranes and skin, to form steroid hormones and to perform basic metabolic functions. Lipoproteins with more protein are more easily transported into the cells of the body, because the elevated protein content increases the probability of cell-receptor recognition. Lipoproteins with less protein can be recognised by fewer cells, and consequently are less likely to be taken up by cells and are more likely to be found freely circulating in the bloodstream. This freely circulating lipoprotein provides the building blocks for atherosclerotic plaque development. The recommended serum levels for cholesterol and triglycerides are given in Clinical Box 23.1.

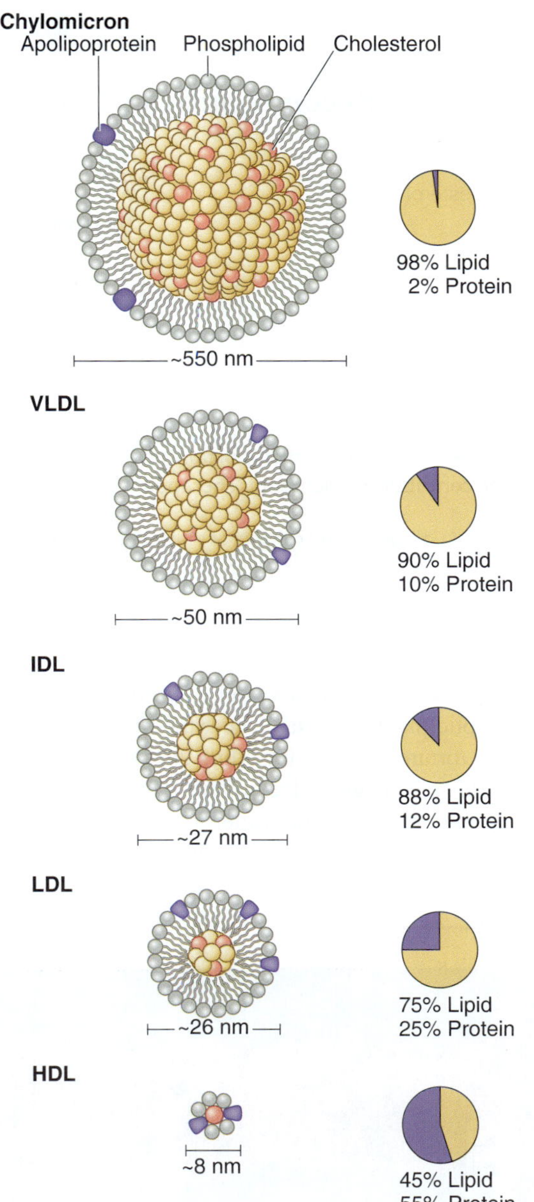

Figure 23.4

Representation of chylomicron and the various types of lipoproteins

The pie charts represent the ratio of lipid to protein across the various types of lipoproteins.

HDL = high-density lipoprotein; IDL = intermediate-density lipoprotein; LDL = low-density lipoprotein; nm = nanometre; VLDL = very-low-density lipoprotein.

The development of an atherosclerotic plaque

A number of theories have been proposed to explain the development of atherosclerotic plaques, all of which have unifying themes. First, it is important to note that an atherosclerotic plaque will not only damage the wall of the blood vessel and reduce blood flow, as noted above, it will also change

CLINICAL BOX 23.1

Recommendations for serum cholesterol and triglyceride levels

	Male	Female
HDL cholesterol	0.9–2.0 mmol/L Therapeutic target > 1 mmol/L	1.0–2.2 mmol/L Therapeutic target > 1 mmol/L
LDL cholesterol	2.0–3.4 mmol/L Therapeutic target < 2.5 mmol/L	2.0–3.4 mmol/L Therapeutic target < 2.5 mmol/L

Lipid profiles form only a small portion of a person's cardiovascular risk, and therefore should be considered in the context of all the other contributory elements. Therapeutic targets for these values depend on the individual risk factors present in the person.

Source: Royal College of Pathologists of Australasia (2019).

the architecture of the blood vessel (see Figure 23.5). Once an atherosclerotic plaque is established, the blood vessel becomes twisted and tortured, further impeding the free flow of blood. So, how does this plaque get lodged in the wall of the vessel?

Formation of an atherosclerotic plaque requires an initiating event, for which two primary circumstances have been identified: *damage to the endothelial cells* that line the wall; and *retention of LDL and VLDL* in the blood vessel wall. Within every artery, cholesterol will move passively into the blood vessel wall, and micro-tears will form in the wall due to hypertension and the turbulence of blood flow. *Hypertension*, or high blood pressure, represents an increased pressure of the blood against the blood vessel wall that can cause damage to the endothelial cells. Likewise, an area of turbulence can occur when a *blood vessel curves or splits (bifurcates)*, which can also lead to endothelial cell damage. In at-risk individuals, these episodes, either singly or in combination, lead to the development of a focal zone for the establishment of an atherosclerotic plaque (see Figure 23.6). Immediately following any damage to the endothelial wall of the blood vessel, leukocytes are recruited and the *inflammatory process* is initiated.

An increased entry of circulating fat and cholesterol into the vessel wall is associated with the formation of *micro-aggregates*, which are difficult to dislodge. Under normal circumstances, a small proportion of the LDL is converted to an oxidised version of cholesterol, or *Ox-LDL*. This Ox-LDL attracts circulating monocytes (which become macrophages when in the tissue), local macrophages, T cells and smooth muscle cells to this focal zone. The macrophages increase the oxidation of LDL in order to attract more macrophages so as to remove the LDL and restore the vessel wall integrity.

As part of this inflammatory and healing process, *inflammatory mediators* such as cytokines, as well as *growth factors* such as endothelial-derived growth factor, are released. Smooth muscle cells from the muscular tunica media of the arterial wall are stimulated to grow and enter into the developing focal zone. The recruited macrophages and migrating smooth muscle cells consume the fat, cholesterol and oxidised cholesterol in order to remove them from the area of the growing lesion. Under the microscope, these cholesterol- and fat-laden cells appear to be full of bubbles, leading to their common name—*foam cells*.

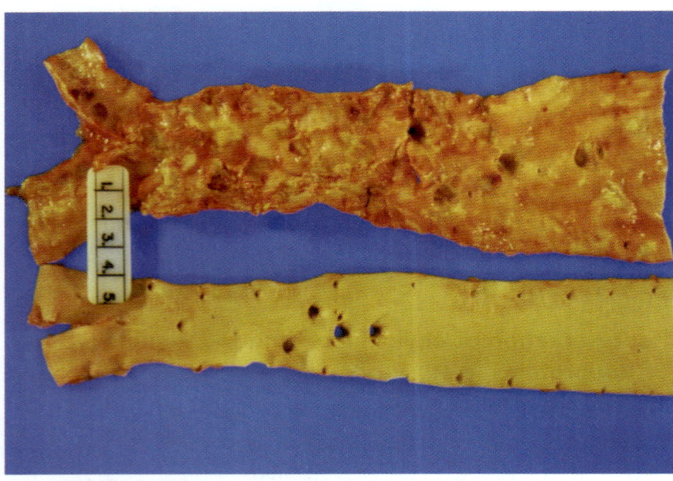

Figure 23.5

Comparison of healthy (bottom) and atherosclerotic (top) arteries

A longitudinal dissection of two blood vessels. The top image shows an atherosclerotic artery. Notice the fatty build-up and signs of old thrombi (red granular areas). It is important to note that in addition to the changes in the walls of the vessel, the entire architecture of the vessel has changed, with the margins uneven, tortured and twisted. The bottom image shows a healthy blood vessel.

Source: Dr E. Walker/Science Photo Library.

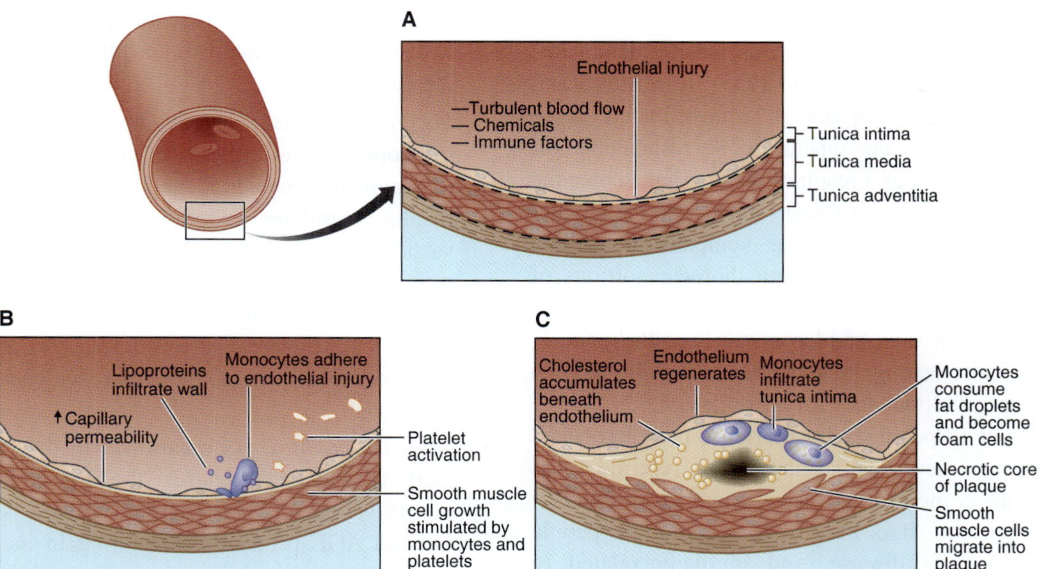

Figure 23.6

Overview of the development of an atherosclerotic plaque

(A) Endothelial injury promoting atherosclerotic plaque formation.

(B) Penetration of lipoproteins, such as LDL and VLDL, into the artery wall at the site of injury, and the subsequent oxidation of LDL, attracts monocytes to the focal zone.

(C) Smooth muscle cells and macrophages consume the lipoproteins and oxidised cholesterol (Ox-LDL), with the latter resulting in cell death and the deposition of dead cell debris, cholesterol crystals and cellular contents into a growing necrotic core. Fibrin infiltration, the generation of a fibrous cap and an attempt by endothelial cells to regenerate over the growing plaque complete the picture.

Unfortunately, Ox-LDL is cytotoxic at elevated levels, and individuals at risk of atherosclerosis generally have more active oxidation than other people. This leads to the death of the macrophages and smooth muscle cells, and the deposition of cellular contents (e.g. H^+, ATP, enzymes), membrane fragments and cholesterol crystals in the focal zone. A *necrotic core* now develops in the arterial wall, leading to fibrin infiltration and the establishment of a *fibrous cap*, which resembles the scab on a cut. This infiltration and cap formation contributes to the stiffening of the vessel wall and the characteristic 'hardening of the artery' classically associated with atherosclerosis. Calcium is deposited, which also contributes to this 'hardening' of the blood vessel wall. In many circumstances, endothelial cells will attempt to grow over the developing plaque, but as the plaque enlarges, this process becomes incomplete.

The growing plaque with its stiff cap is now prone to rupture due to the mechanical (shear) stress on fibrous cap, the increased matrix degradation and the decreased matrix synthesis related to chronic inflammation. As the immunological influence on atherosclerotic plaque stability increases, new therapeutic options are in development.

Once the atherosclerotic plaque ruptures, platelet activation and aggregation occurs as a result of exposure to the subendothelial collagen. As required in the initial steps of haemostasis, the release of pro-thrombotic factors contributes to platelet plug formation and support of the clotting cascade in order to achieve thrombus formation. Although the innate thrombolytic system exists to try to prevent pathogenic thrombus formation, the clot development exceeds clot lysis and therefore a thrombus is formed. Excessive thrombosis formation further reduces the diameter of the blood vessel lumen. Additionally, the availability of NO, the primary local vasodilator in the body, is reduced, hence *reducing the blood vessel diameter* because of unopposed vasoconstriction.

The relationship between atherosclerosis and coronary artery disease

The combination of an atherosclerotic plaque, unopposed vasoconstriction and the possibility of an associated thrombus leads to an imbalance between the supply of blood to the cells of the heart and the demand for that blood created by the normal functioning of the heart. This situation is exacerbated by feedback from a number of structures, such as baroreceptors and chemoreceptors, which leads to an increased demand on the heart as the cardiovascular centres of the pons and medulla increase sympathetic outflow to the heart in an effort to re-establish adequate cardiac output through an increase in heart rate and contraction force.

When the cells of the heart receive inadequate oxygen in the face of increased workload, they switch to *anaerobic metabolism*. Furthermore, insufficient levels of nutrients will compromise the generation of energy (ATP), which is required for a number of cellular events, not the least of which are the contraction and the relaxation of cardiac muscle. As a result of anaerobic metabolism, substances such as lactate, adenosine, bradykinins, serotonin, histamines and ROS are released and stimulate chemosensitive receptors of unmyelinated nerve fibres. Adenosine in particular appears to be responsible for much of the pain signalling as a result of myocardial ischaemia. Impulses from these *nociceptors* ('pain' fibres; see the chapter 'Nociception and pain') travel along sympathetic ganglia between the seventh cervical and fourth thoracic portions of the spinal cord. There are extensive connections in the somatic and visceral afferent pathways, and 'cross-talk' results in poorly localised pain signals, leading to the crushing, referred pain experienced by many individuals with heart disease.

Interestingly, not all people will experience pain associated with damage to their heart. This condition is referred to as *'silent' angina*, and is more likely in women than in men for as-yet-unknown reasons. It is also more common in people with peripheral vascular disease, and is likely related to nerve damage.

RISK FACTORS FOR ATHEROSCLEROSIS

LEARNING OBJECTIVE 4

Identify the risk factors associated with atherosclerosis.

There are numerous risk factors for atherosclerosis, which can be divided into major and non-modifiable risk factors. Many of these are similar to the modifiable lifestyle risk factors associated with hypertension discussed in the chapter 'Vascular disorders and circulatory shock' (see Figure 22.1).

Major modifiable risk factors

Major modifiable risk factors commonly associated with atherosclerosis include:

- *Hyperlipidaemia*: Elevated LDL levels promote atherosclerosis through the increased deposition of LDLs and triglycerides into the vessel wall. This contributes to endothelial dysfunction and induces endothelial inflammatory pathways. Low levels of HDLs result in reduced reverse cholesterol transport (from the vessel wall to the liver); the mechanism to reduce atherosclerotic growth is thereby diminished.
- *Hypertension*: As discussed in the chapter 'Vascular disorders and circulatory shock', hypertension is pro-atherogenic (promoting atherogenic activity) as it leads to increased vascular inflammation. Angiotensin II causes macrophages, smooth muscle cells and endothelial cells to produce pro-inflammatory cytokines, superoxide anions, and pro-thrombotic factors, which ultimately result in further endothelial damage. Hypertension also causes the up-regulation of *lectin-like oxidised LDL receptor-1 (LOX-1)*, which is associated with accelerated atherosclerotic lesion formation and increased inflammation.
- *Cigarette smoking*: Numerous toxic chemicals from cigarette smoke are inhaled and delivered to the bloodstream. Smoking not only promotes vasoconstriction and increases oxidative stress, it also increases platelet aggregation. It is also known to disrupt lipid metabolism, resulting in decreased HDLs and increased LDLs.
- *Insulin resistance*: Insulin resistance commonly occurs in people who are obese, as visceral adiposity contributes to significant metabolic and cardiovascular derangement. Insulin stimulates endothelial production of the critical vasodilator NO. NO is also important in limiting *vascular smooth muscle cell (VSMC)* growth and migration; therefore, when insulin signalling fails, vasoconstriction and increased VSMCs are encouraged to migrate into the intima, with a combined effect of a smaller vessel lumen and thicker, stiffer vessel wall.
- *Diabetes mellitus*: As mentioned in the chapter 'Diabetes mellitus', diabetes causes the formation of *advanced glycation end products (AGE)*. Diabetes is pro-atherogenic through AGE production, resulting in increased oxidative stress and reactive oxygen radicals, and the release of pro-inflammatory cytokines.
- *Lack of physical activity and obesity*: Obesity is associated with hypertension, dyslipidaemia and type 2 diabetes mellitus. Nevertheless, independently, obesity is considered pro-atherogenic because of its influence on endothelial dysfunction. A person with a body mass index (BMI) of more than 30 kg/m^2 has a more than four times greater likelihood of developing cardiovascular disease than an individual with a BMI of 25 kg/m^2 or less. *Visceral adiposity* (fat stored within the abdominal cavity) occurs when there is an imbalance of energy intake and energy expenditure. Increased fat mass causes white adipose tissue dysfunction, which in turn results in insulin resistance, activation of the sympathetic nervous system and the renin–angiotensin–aldosterone system, which subsequently leads to endothelial dysfunction. As with the ageing process, visceral adiposity causes a reduction of vasodilating substances and an increase in vasoconstricting substances. Finally, obesity contributes to the increase of pro-inflammatory mediators and oxidative stress.
- *Unhealthy diet*: Foods high in saturated fats (such as whole milk, high-fat cheese and ice cream) and foods high in trans-fat (such as fried foods, pizza, cake and biscuits) increase the *atheroma burden*. The avoidance of additional salt is also beneficial to reducing the risk of hypertension. The consumption of fruit and vegetables, whole grains, lean meats, seafood and low-fat or fat-free milk and dairy products is important to reduce the risk of atherosclerosis. Consistently consuming an unhealthy diet can also lead to obesity, diabetes mellitus and hypertension, further increasing atherosclerotic risk.
- *Obstructive sleep apnoea (OSA)*: Most people with obstructive apnoea are obese and have diabetes mellitus and hypertension; however, independently, OSA can contribute to an atherogenic risk. Individuals with untreated OSA experience intermittent cessation of breathing and resulting hypoxia, as a result of a mechanical obstruction from increased pharyngeal fat deposits or loss of upper airway

tone. This repeated hypoxia–reoxygenation cycle appears to lead to an overproduction of ROS and a subsequent increase in oxidative stress, and increasing pro-inflammatory signalling.

- *Alcohol intake*: Recently, a major UK study has concluded that there is a causal association between habitual alcohol consumption (at even modest intake) and an increased risk of hypertension and CAD, increasing exponentially with consumption rates. Although light consumption was associated with minimal risk, it dispels the claim the small alcohol intake can be cardioprotective. Excessive alcohol intake is associated with hypertension, not only because of the reduced NO, but also because of an increase in adrenergic activity resulting in increased vascular smooth-muscle tone and activation of the renin–angiotensin–aldosterone system.
- *Hyperhomocysteinaemia*: Homocysteine is a metabolic substance resulting from the consumption of methionine-containing food, such as meat, fish and dairy products. Methionine is transformed into *homocysteine* and then to *cysteine* (facilitated by vitamin B_6). Cysteine has many cellular functions, including an important role in protein structure and stability, and is necessary in the metabolism of several metals, such as zinc, iron and copper. Homocysteine may also be converted back to methionine (facilitated by vitamin B_{12} and folic acid). If homocysteine is unable to be converted to cysteine or is converted back to methionine, high levels of homocysteine can be found in the blood (known as *hyperhomocysteinaemia*). Hyperhomocysteinaemia is known to be atherogenic through various mechanisms, such as its ability to cause a reduction of NO, increase reactive oxygen species and lipid peroxidation, and also increase platelet aggregation.

Non-modifiable risk factors

Age, male gender and a positive family history of early heart disease are all risk factors for atherosclerosis that are not influenced by diet or lifestyle choices.

Figure 23.7 relates the risk factors for coronary artery disease to pathophysiology and to general management principles.

LEARNING OBJECTIVE 5

Discuss the influence of the immune system on cardiovascular disease.

Many of the risk factors mentioned above promote an increased inflammatory response. What might not be obvious is that the chronic inflammatory processes pre-date the observable clinical effects of atherosclerosis by several decades. Both innate and specific immune systems contribute to this chronic inflammatory process. The *non-specific (innate) immune system* initiates, exaggerates and sustains numerous cellular mechanisms, contributing to a state of atherogenesis. The *adaptive immune system* also contributes to the atherogenic process, with T cells that transmigrate to the intima and, in response to antigens, initiate the production of even more pro-inflammatory mediators. To a lesser extent, B cells have also been found in atherosclerotic lesions, as have antibodies; however, their exact role and influence remain controversial.

LEARNING OBJECTIVE 6

Describe the relationship between gut microbiota and cardiovascular disease.

It is well established that inflammation plays a large role in the development of cardiovascular disease. The gastrointestinal tract mucosa is one of the largest immunologically active organs in the body. Recently, data are suggesting that the composition of a person's intestinal microorganisms (*gut microbiota* or *microbiome*) can significantly influence their propensity to develop atherosclerosis. After birth, our gastrointestinal tracts are colonised with many and various types of microorganisms. The microbial community appears to be relatively stable across one's lifespan, although it can change rapidly in response to changes in diet and environment.

Although our current understanding of intestinal microbiota's influence is relatively primitive, early evidence suggests that some bacterial species are more likely to have a *systemic anti-inflammatory effect*, while other species appear to induce a *systemic pro-inflammatory effect* that can augment the development of atherosclerosis. A mechanism suggested to mediate this influence includes altered cholesterol metabolism from biologically active gut microbe-derived metabolites such as *trimethylamine*-N-*oxide (TMAO)*, which is produced in large quantities in omnivores, but not in vegetarians. High levels of TMAO decrease reverse cholesterol transport, alter bile acid synthesis and composition, and increase platelet aggregation.

Other avenues of research focus on dietary choices as a cause of *dysbiosis*—an imbalance or maladaptation of gut microbiota. For example, the consumption of a high-fat and/or high-sugar diet causes some microbiota species to release *lipopolysaccharides* (*LPS*—also known as *endotoxin*), which increases macrophage activity, increases lipid accumulation, increases foam cell formation and ultimately provokes a strong inflammatory response. Further research may elucidate not only clarity in the relationship between gut microbiota and atherosclerosis, but also potentially the development of new therapeutic targets.

LEARNING OBJECTIVE 7

Explain how metabolic syndrome relates to coronary artery disease.

Metabolic syndrome *Metabolic syndrome* is a cluster of disorders such as abdominal obesity, insulin resistance/diabetes mellitus, abnormal glucose tolerance, hypercholesterolaemia and hypertension (see the chapter 'Diabetes mellitus'). While there is no doubt that this constellation of symptoms is likely to be associated with the development of atherosclerosis and coronary artery disease, there is still debate as to the extent to which they synergise to increase a person's risk several-fold. Once the condition has been better studied and more individuals followed up for longer periods, the impact of this combination of symptoms should become clear.

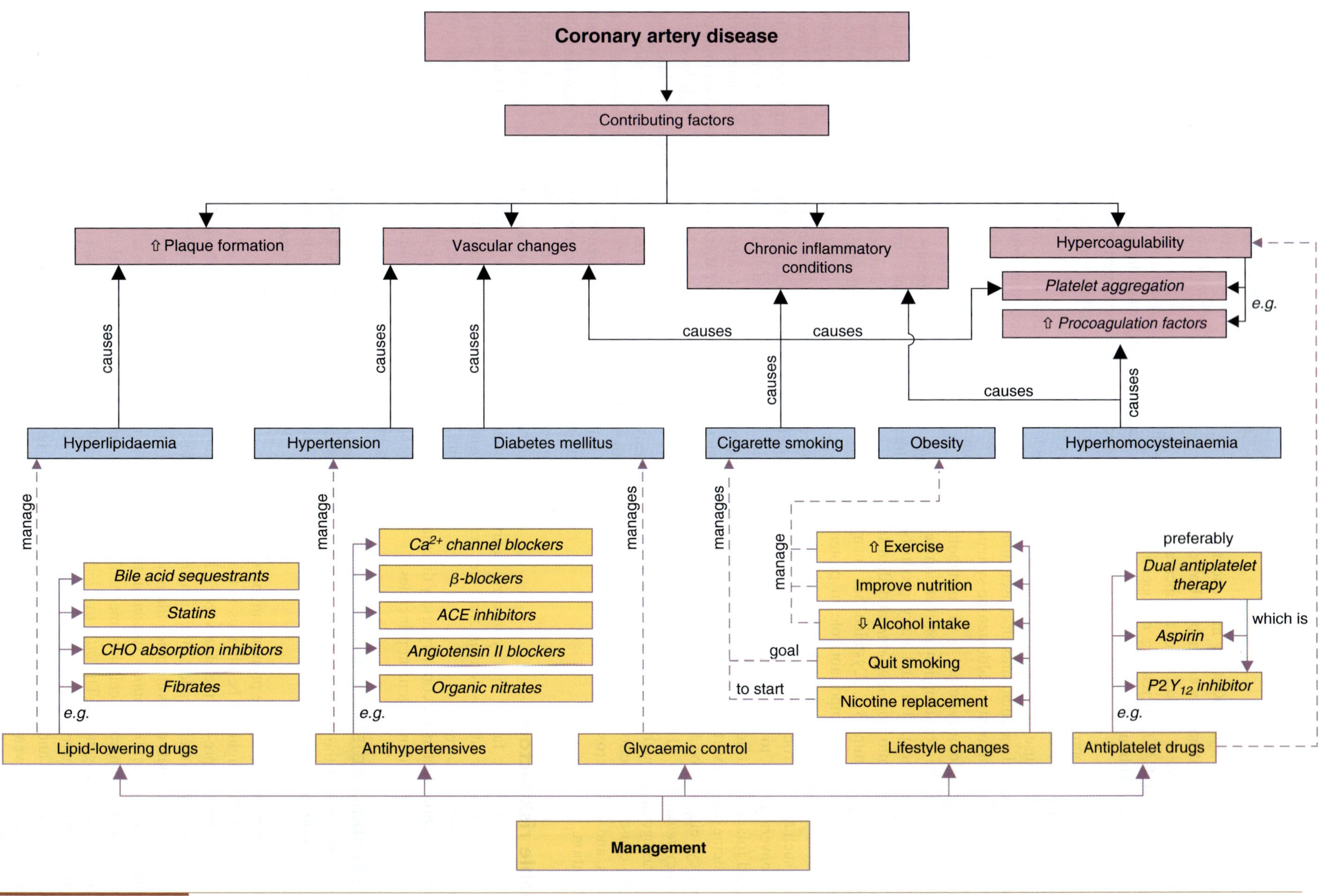

Figure 23.7

Clinical snapshot: Coronary artery disease

↓ = decrease in; ↑ = increase in; ACE inhibitors = angiotensin-converting enzyme inhibitors; β = beta; Ca^{2+} = calcium ion; CHO = carbohydrates; $P2Y_{12}$ inhibitor = an adenosine diphosphate (ADP) receptor inhibitor (antiplatelet medication).

Acute coronary syndrome

LEARNING OBJECTIVE 8

Define 'acute coronary syndrome', and describe its various presentations.

Acute coronary syndrome is a collective term for conditions that result in an *alteration to blood flow to a part of the myocardium*. This condition may be potentially reversible, such as with unstable angina pectoris (UAP), or result in irreversible cell death, such as in myocardial infarction (MI). Myocardial infarction can be further divided into:

- *non-ST elevation myocardial infarction* (*NSTEMI*, also known as *non-ST elevation acute coronary syndrome [NSTEACS]*), where a partial or transiently obstructive thrombus in the coronary artery results in ischaemia and necrosis; and
- *ST elevation myocardial infarction* (*STEMI*, also known as *ST elevation acute coronary syndrome [STEACS]*), where complete obstruction by a thrombus in the coronary artery results in ischaemia and necrosis.

ANGINA PECTORIS

Angina pectoris was first defined in 1744 as a disease marked by attacks of chest pain due to insufficient oxygenation of the heart. Although used as a generic term to refer to chest pain, it comprises a family of conditions marked by differences in the degree to which the coronary arteries are compromised. The three forms of angina are: stable, unstable and variant.

Stable angina

As can be seen in Figure 23.8, stable angina is the result of atherosclerotic plaque and inappropriate vasoconstriction within one or more blood vessels. The hallmark of stable angina is that blood flow is adequate at rest but compromised when the person exerts themselves, causing pain (for usually five minutes or less), which is relieved by rest. This form of angina may also be referred to as *exertional angina*.

Unstable angina

This condition is marked by an atherosclerotic plaque and an associated thrombus, which results in a greater degree of vascular obstruction than that seen with stable angina (see Figure 23.8). Clinically, the person has compromised blood flow at rest, leading most often to marked chest pain without exertion. The person may also experience nausea, shortness of breath, sweating and possibly vomiting.

Variant (Prinzmetal) angina

Originally described by Prinzmetal and his colleagues in 1959, this rare form of angina is marked by unexplained vasospasms rather than atherosclerotic plaque formation (see Figure 23.8). Prinzmetal angina occurs in conjunction with ST elevation on the electrocardiograph (ECG) trace. Individuals can experience angina pain at any time, even when sleeping, and there is no recognised trigger for their attacks. Furthermore, the person's capacity for exercise does not appear to be compromised and does not appear to trigger an attack.

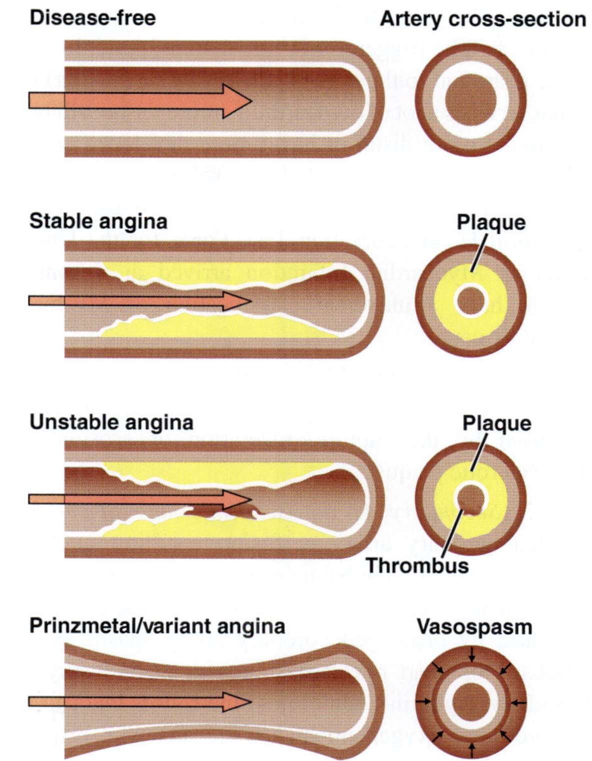

Figure 23.8

Changes to arteries associated with different types of angina

The difference in the physical symptoms of the types of angina can be linked back to the pathophysiological changes within the affected arteries. In stable angina, there is an atherosclerotic plaque and partial obstruction, but the flow is only insufficient when the person exerts themselves. The hallmark of unstable angina is an increase in the size and/or number of plaques, greater obstruction and the presence of an associated thrombus. In these individuals, blood flow is insufficient even at rest. Variant angina, also known as Prinzmetal angina, is the result of as-yet-unexplained vasospasm.

Source: © Sciencopia.

Some of the proposed reasons for the vasospasm include a marked reduction in the capacity of the endothelial cells to generate NO, an altered function of the calcium channels in the blood vessels, and changes in intracellular signalling cascades, but the exact mechanism remains unidentified. Interestingly, this condition is common in individuals of Japanese ancestry.

MYOCARDIAL INFARCTION

A myocardial infarction (MI; colloquially known as a heart attack), results in significantly *reduced blood flow such that myocardial cells die*. Depending on how much tissue is involved, the rest of the heart continues to function, and compensatory mechanisms will be triggered to try to restore blood flow to the rest of the heart and to the body. If the *lesion (occlusion)* is in a vessel that services a lot of myocardium, more tissue will be lost. If the lesion is more distal or has a more developed collateral circulation (as a result of chronic low-level tissue hypoxia from increasing vessel obstruction), less tissue will be lost.

The World Heart Federation Task Force for the Universal Definition of Myocardial Infarction arrived at a consensus decision to have a universal classification of MI by type categorised by cause:

- *Type 1: Spontaneous*—Most common type of MI; when impeded coronary artery perfusion resulting in necrosis is caused by the rupture, ulceration or erosion of an atherosclerotic plaque.
- *Type 2: Secondary to an ischaemic imbalance*—When impeded coronary artery perfusion resulting in necrosis occurs because of an imbalance between oxygen supply and oxygen demand (unrelated to a plaque). These events could be caused by prolonged coronary artery spasm, coronary embolism, or heart rate issues such or tachydysrhythmias or bradydysrhythmias. Other possible causes that can result in a profound oxygen imbalance are anaemia, respiratory failure, or blood pressure issues such as either hypotension or hypertension.
- *Type 3: Resulting in death when biomarker values are unavailable*—When there is impeded coronary artery perfusion resulting in cardiac death.
- *Type 4A: Related to percutaneous coronary intervention (PCI)*—When impeded coronary artery perfusion resulting in necrosis occurs from the iatrogenic effects of an angiogram, angioplasty or stent insertion.
- *Type 4B: Related to percutaneous stent thrombosis*—When impeded coronary artery perfusion resulting in necrosis occurs from the development of a clot on a previously inserted stent.
- *Type 5: Related to coronary artery bypass grafting*—When impeded coronary artery perfusion resulting in necrosis occurs as a result of coronary artery bypass grafting.

Clinically, these arbitrary classifications have been slow to make their way to the 'coal face'. Currently, MI classification is most often discussed in the context of the presence (or absence) of ST elevation.

To best understand the changes occurring at a cellular level, a discussion about an infarction's evolution, myocardial remodelling, and the risk and process of reperfusion injury following the infarction, is beneficial.

MI evolution and ventricular remodelling

Most myocardial infarctions occur in the presence of atherosclerosis. Once the fibrous cap of the atherosclerotic lesion ruptures, a cascade of events can cause significant tissue damage. The ruptured lesion exposes subendothelial collagen, which causes platelet aggregation and activation. The platelet plug is also entrapping red blood cells, and, once the coagulation cascade has converted the platelet plug into a thrombus by laying down fibrin (see the chapter 'Blood disorders'), the thrombus grows and propagates into and along the damaged vessel. As blood flow reduces, the ischaemia will cause a decrease in contractility, and the myocardium will become hypokinetic. Hypoxia may rapidly become *anoxia*.

In the absence of oxygen, cells switch to *anaerobic respiration*, resulting in the production of lactate and a shift to an increasingly acidic environment. This causes the sodium–hydrogen (Na^+/H^+) exchanger to work hard to remove the increased hydrogen by pumping it out in exchange for sodium. Subsequently a marked increase in intracellular sodium occurs. So then the sodium–calcium ($2Na^+/Ca^{2+}$) pump attempts to reduce the intracellular sodium by exchanging it with calcium, resulting in *too much intracellular calcium*. Exacerbating this whole sequence is the failure of the Na^+/K^+-ATPase pump (as a result of the ischaemia) adding to the *sodium overload*. The cells die and necrosis sets in. The cellular changes associated with hypoxia are further detailed in the chapter 'Pathophysiological terminology, cellular adaptation and injury'.

Subendocardial layers begin to become necrotic within a half an hour, and over the next three to six hours the *necrosis* grows outwards towards the epicardium. If blood flow is restored before this time, it can be called a *subendocardial MI*; if the necrosis spans the myocardial wall, it is called a *transmural MI*.

Over the next 4–12 hours, the tissue is broken down by a process of *coagulation necrosis* (see the chapter 'Pathophysiological terminology, cellular adaptation and injury'), which causes the cell to swell, the organelles to break down and the proteins to denature. Granulation tissue replaces the infarction zone after approximately three to four days, and for approximately two weeks the tissue is weak and capable of rupture. This is usually a catastrophic and fatal event, and contributes to approximately 10% of mortality related to MI. Within two to three months the infarct zone has healed into non-contractile, connective tissue, which is thinner and weaker than the unaffected myocardium.

Myocardial reperfusion injury

As we have previously discussed, prolonged and significant ischaemia affects cellular integrity and wreaks havoc with various intracellular ion concentrations. However, it is also important to acknowledge that, although necessary for tissue salvage, reperfusion interventions such as thrombolysis or PCI provide previously anoxic tissue with a sudden and immense flow of oxygen-rich blood. As the electron transport chain begins to work again, the mitochondria produce ROS and induce oxidative stress. With a dysfunctional sarcoplasmic reticulum adding to the intracellular calcium overload, the cell membrane is damaged by lipid peroxidation, and the oxidative effects damage the DNA. The cumulative effects of this cellular chaos can lead to more myocardial necrosis, and induce dysrhythmia, systolic dysfunction and heart failure. Reperfusion injury is estimated to contribute to up to 50% of the total myocardial damage. Consequently, the best way to reduce myocardial reperfusion injury is to attempt reperfusion as soon as possible.

COMPLICATIONS ASSOCIATED WITH CORONARY ARTERY DISEASE

Coronary artery disease, while potentially a life-threatening condition, increases a person's risk of many other disorders, such as heart failure and dysrhythmias, which in turn can also be life-threatening. Conversely, a history of heart failure and dysrhythmias puts a person at risk of angina and myocardial infarction (see the chapters 'Cardiac muscle and valve disorders' and 'Dysrhythmias').

CLINICAL MANIFESTATIONS

LEARNING OBJECTIVE 9

Discuss the clinical manifestations and management of acute coronary syndrome.

Common manifestations of acute coronary syndrome include an increase in the heart rate and the respiration rate, diaphoresis and sometimes nausea and vomiting. Chest pain may be felt, and a typical presentation may be reported as crushing central chest pain radiating into the person's jaw or arm. However, more than 50% of people who present to an emergency department have atypical symptoms, including syncope, fatigue, or epigastric, back or right-arm pain. Another characteristic that might make a presentation less typical is the description the person uses to report the pain. Typically, the pain is reported as crushing or as a feeling of heaviness; however, atypical presentations may include 'sharp' or 'burning' in quality. It is also important to note that older adults and people with neuropathic diseases or diabetes may not report pain at all. This is considered a *silent MI*.

CLINICAL DIAGNOSIS AND MANAGEMENT

Diagnosis

A definitive demonstration of the presence of atherosclerotic plaques requires imaging, such as an angiogram, although a presumptive diagnosis can be made if the person exhibits a combination of findings, such as elevated circulating lipid levels, pain on exertion or at rest, exercise intolerance and family history.

Diagnosis of a myocardial infarction relies primarily on the demonstration of cell death, by the measurement of cardiac markers. *Intracellular proteins* such as *cardiac troponin I (cTnI)* should not be found in the blood. Their presence signals myocardial cell damage. *Morphological changes* can also be seen on an *ECG*, which can identify not only the location of the events, but, often, also the difference between angina and an MI, as serial changes to the ECG trace, history and symptoms. *Angiograms* are beneficial to quantify the location and severity of the lesion, with the option of attempting to fix it at the same time with either an angioplasty or the insertion of a stent.

To determine a person's risk of acute coronary syndrome, Australian *cardiovascular risk calculators and charts* can be used, which take into consideration such factors as smoking status, gender and systolic blood pressure to assign a calculated five-year risk level for cardiovascular disease. More recently, a *non-invasive coronary artery calcium score* has been developed, which quantifies coronary artery calcification. Using a CT scan, measurements are taken and a risk value is reported on a 5-point scale, from zero risk to high risk, representing the likelihood of experiencing a cardiovascular event within five or 10 years (depending on how the provider reports). Both of these techniques can inform healthcare professionals how to assist the person to undertake risk reduction measures or direct prophylactic pharmacological intervention.

Management

Management of an individual presenting with an acute coronary syndrome needs to be divided into the immediate needs surrounding basic life support. As long as the person is breathing, is conscious and has a pulse, the other management options will centre on reducing pain, managing life-threatening complications such as hypotension and dysrhythmias, and ultimately attempting to undertake steps to achieve myocardial reperfusion as quickly as possible. A common saying in the emergency and cardiac environment is 'time is tissue', referring to the critical need to improve blood supply to the affected tissue as soon as possible.

Once the primary issues are resolved, the focus shifts to risk elimination, such as addressing dyslipidaemias, hypertension, glycaemic control and any other modifiable risk factors that exist. Lifestyle modifications and medications may form the structure of the management plan.

If a person demonstrates an increased clotting risk, consideration should be given to the administration of a dual antiplatelet medication (one that contains both aspirin and a $P2Y_{12}$ inhibitor) if possible. Figure 23.9 explores the common clinical manifestations and management of acute coronary syndrome.

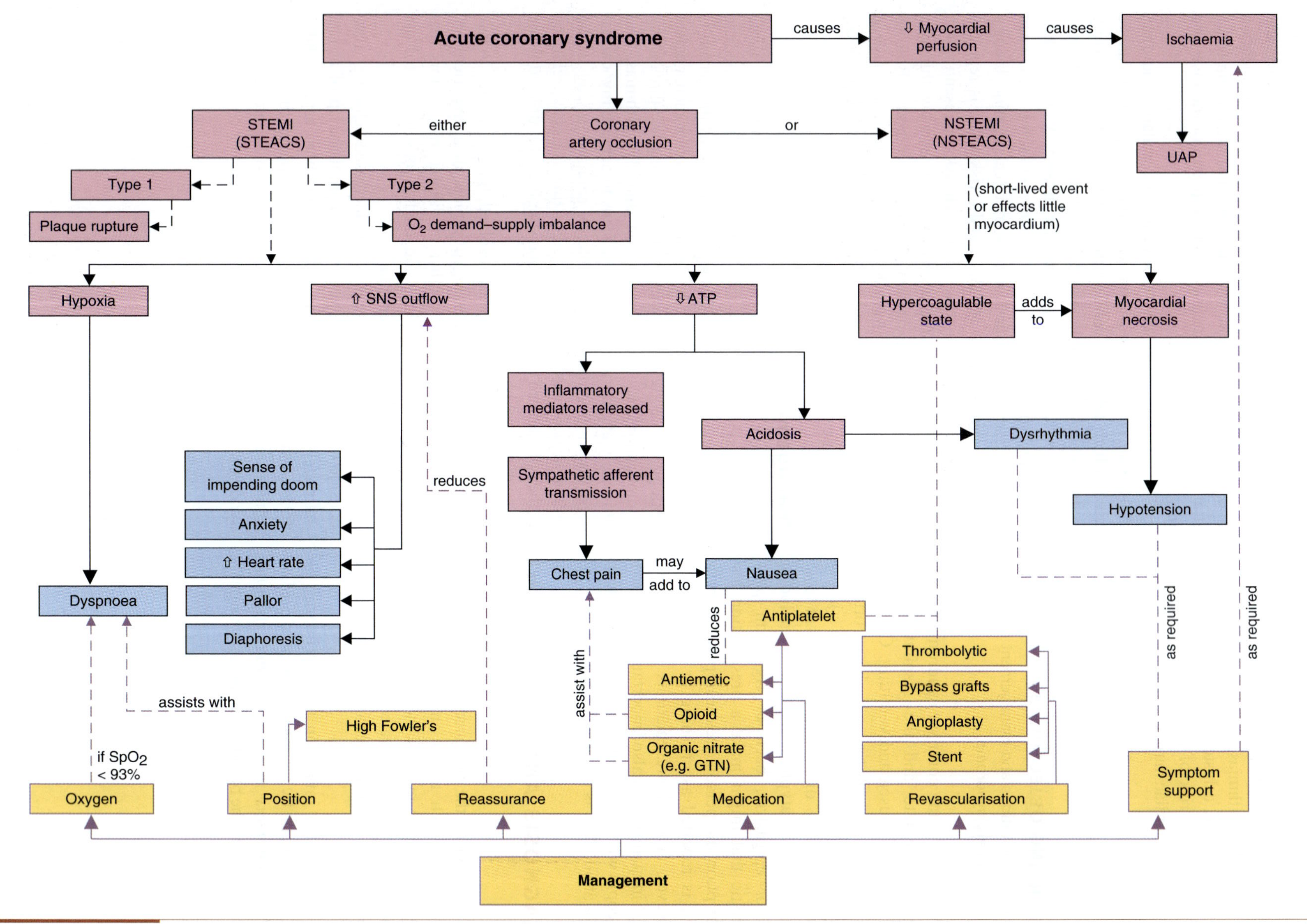

Figure 23.9

Clinical snapshot: Acute coronary syndrome

↓ = decrease in; ↑ = increase in; ATP = adenosine triphosphate; GTN = glyceryl trinitrate; NSTEACS = non-ST elevation acute coronary syndrome; NSTEMI = non-ST elevation myocardial infarction; O_2 = oxygen; SNS = sympathetic nervous system; SpO_2 = saturation of peripheral oxygen; STEACS = ST elevation acute coronary syndrome; STEMI = ST elevation myocardial infarction; UAP = unstable angina pectoris.

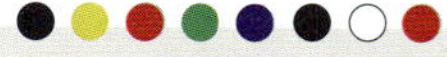

INDIGENOUS HEALTH FAST FACTS AND CULTURAL CONSIDERATIONS

FAST FACTS

- ***Aboriginal and Torres Strait Islander peoples are 2.1 times more likely to be diagnosed with, and 1.8 times more likely to die from, coronary artery disease. than non-Indigenous Australians.***
- ***Aboriginal and Torres Strait Islander peoples are less likely to receive coronary angiography (40% versus 46%) and revascularisation procedures (19%versus 24%) than non-Indigenous Australians.***
- ***Māori are 1.5 times more likely to be hospitalised and 2 times more likely s to die from ischaemic heart disease than European New Zealanders.***
- ***Pacific Islands people of New Zealand are 1.2 times more likely to develop heart disease and 4 times more likely to die from ischaemic heart disease than European New Zealanders.***

CULTURAL CONSIDERATIONS

- ***Participation in cardiac rehabilitation programs has been shown to reduce the risk of death from a cardiac event by up to 25%. Unfortunately, participation in cardiac rehabilitation is lower among Aboriginal and Torres Strait Islander peoples, some of which is related to the fact that up to 20% of Indigenous Australians reported feelings of being treated badly by healthcare professionals, and 30% had experienced racism in healthcare settings in the previous 12 months. There is a critical need for Aboriginal Health Workers, with Aboriginal Health Workers making up only 14% of the workforce within Aboriginal and Torres Strait Islander primary healthcare services. Funding, education and a focus on improving cultural competence may begin to assist with the significant health disparity experienced by Aboriginal and Torres Strait Islander peoples.***

Sources: Data from Australian Institute of Health and Welfare (2023); Heart Research Institute (2023); Winter-Smith et al. (2021).

CHILDREN AND ADOLESCENTS

- As obesity and other cardiovascular risk factors become more prevalent in children, the risk of atherosclerotic changes occurring within the coronary arteries of children increases. There is a direct correlation between the number of risk factors and the development of fatty streaks in the coronary arteries of children.
- Acquired heart disease (e.g. coronary artery disease) is uncommon in children; however, Kawasaki disease causes vasculitis and coronary artery lesions, resulting in myocardial infarction if untreated. Most affected children are under 5 years of age.

OLDER ADULTS

- In Australia in 2020, 85% of all deaths from coronary artery disease occurred in adults of 65 years of age or older.
- Coronary artery disease is the leading cause of death for men through all age groups after 45 years of age.
- Coronary artery disease is the second leading cause of death for women after 75 years of age.

KEY CLINICAL ISSUES

- Chest pain is experienced by almost everybody. It is important to be able to distinguish chest pain of cardiac origin from other causes.
- Hypertension, nicotine use and high glucose levels are also significant risk factors for cardiovascular disease. Cardiac assessment should include interventions to measure these risk factors.
- A person who is hypoxic is at an increased risk of experiencing myocardial ischaemia.
- Pain caused by myocardial ischaemia is relieved by vasodilators, such as the organic nitrate glyceryl trinitrate. Opioids can also be used as a second-line agent in the management of severe chest pain from myocardial ischaemia. Morphine or fentanyl will also reduce anxiety, decrease sympathetic nervous system outflow and reduce oxygen consumption. Morphine and fentanyl can also dilate coronary vasculature.
- Care must be taken when administering opioids to a person with myocardial dysfunction, as they can cause the blood pressure to drop (especially when used in conjunction with vasodilating agents). Morphine and fentanyl can also reduce respiratory rate, which may affect oxygenation.
- Cardiovascular disease is an increasing problem, and is the leading cause of death in Australia and New Zealand. A thorough history collection and a risk-factor assessment should be undertaken on all clients to ensure that further investigation and intervention can begin as soon as possible.
- The difference between stable and unstable angina is whether the pain occurs at rest. This factor is significant in the severity of vascular disease. Individuals with unstable angina are at more risk of coronary events.
- Care of a person experiencing chest pain should include putting them in a high Fowler's position, and the administration of supplemental oxygenation (only if their SpO_2 is $< 93\%$), a full set of observations, including blood pressure and ECG, and the administration of glyceryl trinitrate (as ordered) if the systolic blood pressure is over 100 mmHg (unless otherwise instructed).
- Myocardial infarction results in lost myocardium. The cells that have died will never be able to contribute to the pumping action of the heart again. Rapid intervention to gain reperfusion to the myocardium is critical, as 'time is tissue'.
- Weight loss in obese and overweight individuals can result in a significant reduction of risk factors. Exercise reduces insulin resistance and cholesterol levels. Cardiac rehabilitation is important to promote long-term health benefits.

CHAPTER REVIEW

- *Coronary artery disease* represents a family of conditions in which there is a reduced blood flow to the myocardium, leading to deficits in oxygen and nutrients, as well as a failure to remove metabolic waste from the tissue, which leads to the injury and, ultimately, death of heart cells.
- The primary underlying cause of coronary artery disease is the presence of *atherosclerotic plaques* in the coronary arteries.
- Atherosclerotic plaques form in the wall of the arteries, subsequent to an initial injury of the endothelial cells and penetration of circulating lipoproteins into the subendothelial layer.
- Of the numerous *risk factors* for atherosclerosis development, elevated circulating lipid levels, tobacco use, hypertension and diabetes mellitus are significant contributors.
- Other *modifiable risk factors* include decreased physical activity, obesity and elevated homocysteine.
- *Acute coronary syndrome* incorporates unstable angina pectoris and myocardial infarction.
- *Myocardial infarction* differs from angina in that cells of the heart have died, while the remainder of the heart attempts to maintain function around the dead zone.
- Angina and myocardial infarction predispose the person to a risk of heart failure and dysrhythmias; conversely, a history of heart failure or dysrhythmias predisposes the person to angina and myocardial infarction.

REVIEW QUESTIONS

1. Briefly outline the development of an atherosclerotic plaque.
2. List and differentiate between modifiable and non-modifiable risk factors for the development of atherosclerosis.
3. Discuss the significance of ischaemia and hypoxia in relation to cellular function.
4. Mrs Tonia Simpson is a 59-year-old woman with a history of hyperlipidaemia, diabetes and hypertension. She has just been diagnosed with a STEMI event. Discuss the mechanisms by which her previous medical history contributed to this event.
5. Mrs Simpson, from the previous question, is now recovering in the coronary care unit. A student asks you: 'What will happen to Mrs Simpson's myocardium over the next three weeks?' Discuss.

HEALTH PROFESSIONAL CONNECTIONS

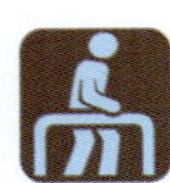

Physiotherapists Following cardiac surgery, physiotherapists are critical in pulmonary rehabilitation, especially if the use of a bypass machine and lung deflation occurred as part of the surgery. It is important to assist the person in deep breathing and coughing exercises. Early mobilisation is also pivotal, and physiotherapists must assist people in the early stages postoperatively to ensure maximum pulmonary rehabilitation. Early mobilisation is also critical to reduce the risk of thromboembolic events. When a median sternotomy approach is used, the person will often experience much upper-body and arm weakness. They may also experience sensory deficits in the fourth and fifth fingers of one or both hands. This may occur because of nerve compression or temporary injury from the chest retraction. When assisting people requiring cardiac rehabilitation, ensure that medical clearance has been obtained. Ensure that a medically appropriate, graduated increase in exercise is programmed.

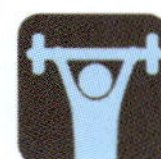

Exercise scientists Working with older individuals or athletes training for veteran events can pose unique challenges. Individuals should always seek medical advice before undertaking a radical change in exercise regimens. Exercise scientists should be aware of the risk factors associated with coronary artery disease, and advise people to seek medical attention or review if any concerns are identified. Sports requiring aerobic capacity or power events that increase intrathoracic pressures can be dangerous if precautions are not taken to ensure client safety.

When assisting people requiring cardiac rehabilitation, ensure that medical clearance has been obtained. Ensure that a medically appropriate, graduated increase in exercise is programmed. Exercise scientists can influence the success of compliance with medical management through well-developed professional–client relationships.

Nutritionists/Dieticians A significant contributing factor to the development of coronary artery disease is inappropriate diet or inadequate nutrition. People with CAD often have excess sodium, fat and sugar in their diet. They often make poor meal choices, and require much assistance to identify important nutrition information and food group characteristics. Individuals with CAD and metabolic syndrome tend to be obese and have a limited to non-existent exercise regimen. Interprofessional collaboration with medical and allied health professionals is required to effect the significant lifestyle changes that are required to have a positive effect on the disease progression.

All allied professionals Vigilance is required when working with individuals with CAD and diabetes mellitus. The neurological effects related to diabetes mellitus may prevent people from experiencing chest pain. Because of the neuropathy associated with the effects of glycosylation, pain signals may not be transmitted via the afferent nerve fibres for interpretation of a pain sensation in the brain. This situation can result in a 'silent myocardial infarction'. The lack of pain does not mean that no damage is occurring. Myocardial ischaemia and necrosis can still occur; however, the recognition of the damage is masked by neuropathy. This may result in worse outcomes, higher morbidity and mortality.

CASE STUDY

Mrs Betty Williams is a 62-year-old woman (UR number 947472) who has presented to the emergency department via an ambulance, experiencing an acute myocardial infarction. She has had pain for two hours. She has unstable angina pectoris, and was doing some light cleaning around the house prior to the onset of this pain. She had taken three glyceryl trinitrate tablets before calling the ambulance. These did little to relieve her pain. Mrs Williams has a history of hypertension and type 2 diabetes mellitus, and she smokes approximately one and a half to two packets of cigarettes a day. She has smoked for approximately 45 years. Her body mass index is 32. She has had no history of a cerebrovascular accident. She is to be assessed for suitability to thrombolyse. Her observations were as follows:

Temperature	Heart rate	Respiration rate	Blood pressure	SpO_2
37°C	92	28	92/58	91% (RA*)

*RA = room air.

Mrs Williams' skin was pale, and her peripheries were cool. Her admission pathology results have returned as follows:

HAEMATOLOGY

Patient location:	Ward 3	**UR:**	947472		
Consultant:	Smith	**NAME:**	Williams		
		Given name:	Betty	**Sex:**	F
		DOB:	01/04/XX	**Age:**	62

Time collected	15:30
Date collected	XX/XX
Year	XXXX
Lab #	75838294

FULL BLOOD COUNT		UNITS	REFERENCE RANGE
Haemoglobin	120	g/L	115–160
White cell count	8.2	$\times 10^9$/L	4.0–11.0

Platelets	320	$\times 10^9$/L	140–400
Haematocrit	0.39		0.33–0.47
Red cell count	4.02	$\times 10^{12}$/L	3.80–5.20
Reticulocyte count	0.6	%	0.2–2.0
MCV	92	fL	80–100
Neutrophils	7.81	$\times 10^9$/L	2.00–8.00
Lymphocytes	3.02	$\times 10^9$/L	1.00–4.00
Monocytes	0.38	$\times 10^9$/L	0.10–1.00
Eosinophils	0.35	$\times 10^9$/L	< 0.60
Basophils	0.12	$\times 10^9$/L	< 0.20
ESR	6	mm/h	< 12
COAGULATION PROFILE			
aPTT	32	secs	24–40
PT	14	secs	11–17
ABG			
pH	7.32		7.35–7.45
$PaCO_2$	48	mmHg	35–45
PaO_2	73	mmHg	> 80
HCO_3^-	21	mmHg	22–32
Oxygen saturations	92	%	> 95

BIOCHEMISTRY

Patient location:	Ward 3	**UR:**	947472		
Consultant:	Smith	**NAME:**	Williams		
		Given name:	Betty	**Sex:**	F
		DOB:	01/04/XX	**Age:**	62

Time collected	15:30
Date collected	XX/XX
Year	XXXX
Lab #	6658475

ELECTROLYTES		UNITS	REFERENCE RANGE
Sodium	138	mmol/L	135–145
Potassium	4.9	mmol/L	3.5–5.2
Chloride	97	mmol/L	95–110
Bicarbonate	21	mmol/L	22–32
Glucose	11.2	mmol/L	3.5–6.0
Iron	5.4	μmol/L	11–30
HbA_{1c}	7.9	%	3–6%
LIPID STUDIES			
Triglycerides	6.5	mmol/L	< 2.0
Total cholesterol	7.95	mmol/L	< 4.0 (at risk)
HDL cholesterol	2.1	mmol/L	> 1.0
LDL cholesterol	5.97	mmol/L	< 1.8 (at risk)

CRITICAL THINKING

1 Examine the pathology results for Mrs Williams. Identify the parameters that would inform your assessment of Mrs Williams' modifiable risk factors.

2 Identify Mrs Williams' signs and symptoms. Explain the physiological rationale for each of their occurrences. How would you manage Mrs Williams' care?

3 What is metabolic syndrome? Does Mrs Williams have metabolic syndrome? How could this influence an individual's cardiac history?

4 In relation to the interpretation of cardiac markers, why is it important to gain an understanding of when the myocardial insult may have occurred?

5 Identify all of Mrs Williams' modifiable risk factors. Develop a multifaceted plan to assist her to begin lifestyle changes. Identify and manage all of the factors that could contribute to the modifiable factors. Assisting an individual to participate in significant lifestyle changes is very difficult. Identify factors that will promote compliance, and factors that will impede compliance.

6 What are the contraindications for thrombolysis? Make a list, and explain the physiological reasons why each contraindication is necessary.

BIBLIOGRAPHY

Australian Bureau of Statistics (ABS) (2022a). *Causes of death, Australia, 2022.* Canberra: ABS. http://www.abs.gov.au/statistics/health/causes-death.

Australian Bureau of Statistics (ABS) (2022b). Death web report: Supplementary tables—2022. In *Deaths in Australia*. Canberra: ABS. https://www.aihw.gov.au/reports/life-expectancy-death/deaths-in-australia/data.

Australian Institute of Health and Welfare (AIHW) (2022a). *Australia's health 2022: data insights*. Australia's Health series No. 18. Cat. No. AUS 240. Canberra: AIHW. https://www.aihw.gov.au/reports/australias-health/australias-health-2022-data-insights/about.

Australian Institute of Health and Welfare (AIHW) (2022b). Data visualisation. Australia, 2020. *General Record of Incidence of Mortality (GRIM)* books. Canberra: AIHW. https://www.aihw.gov.au/reports/life-expectancy-death/grim-books/contents/general-record-of-incidence-of-mortality-grim-books.

Australian Institute of Health and Welfare (AIHW) (2022c). *Principal diagnosis data cubes: separation statistics by principal diagnosis (ICD-10-AM 11th edition), Australia, 2020–21.* Canberra: AIWH. https://www.aihw.gov.au/reports/hospitals/principal-diagnosis-data-cubes/contents/data-cubes.

Australian Institute of Health and Welfare (AIHW) (2023). *Aboriginal and Torres Strait Islander Health Performance Framework: summary report 2023.* Canberra: AIHW https://www.indigenoushpf.gov.au/Report-overview/Overview/Summary-Report.

Bauldoff, G., Gubrud-Howe, P.M., Carno, M.-A., Levett-Jones, T., Hales, M., Berry, K., … Stanley, D. (2020). *LeMone and Burke's medical–surgical nursing: critical thinking for person-centred care* (4th [Australian] edn). Sydney: Pearson Australia.

Best, O. & Fredericks, B. (2021). *Yatdjuligin: Aboriginal and Torres Strait Islander nursing and midwifery care.* (3rd edn). Port Melbourne, VIC: Cambridge University Press.

Biddinger, K.J., Emdin, C.A., Haas, M.E., Wang, M., Hindy, G., Ellinor, P.T., … Aragam, K.G. (2022). Association of habitual alcohol intake with risk of cardiovascular disease. *JAMA Network Open* 5(3):e223849. https://doi.org/10.1001/jamanetworkopen.2022.3849.

Bullock, S. & Manias, E. (2022). Fundamentals of pharmacology (9th edn). Sydney: Pearson Australia.

Burke, A.P. (2021). Pathology of myocardial infarction. *Emedicine*. https://emedicine.medscape.com/article/1960472-overview.

Chen, J., Lin, S. & Zeng, Y. (2021). An update on obstructive sleep apnea for atherosclerosis: mechanism, diagnosis, and treatment. *Frontiers in Cardiovascular Medicine* 8:647071. https://doi.org/10.3389/fcvm.2021.647071.

Coven, D.L. & Kalyanasundaram, A. (2020). Acute coronary syndrome. *Emedicine.* https://emedicine.medscape.com/article/1910735-overview.

Haber, M.D. & Brunell, T.A. (2021). Angina pectoris in emergency medicine. *Emedicine.* https://emedicine.medscape.com/article/761889-overview.

Jebari-Benslaiman, S., Galicia-García, U., Larrea-Sebal, A., Olaetxea, J.R., Alloza, I., Vandenbroeck, K., … Martin, C. (2022). Pathophysiology of atherosclerosis. *International Journal of Molecular Sciences* 23(6):3346. https://.doi.org/10.3390/ijms23063346.

Lilly, L.S. (2007). *Pathophysiology of heart disease* (3rd edn). Philadelphia, PA: Lippincott Williams and Wilkins.

Marieb, E.N. & Hoehn, K. (2016). *Human anatomy and physiology* (10th edn). San Francisco, CA: Pearson Benjamin Cummings.

National Heart Foundation of Australia (NHFA) (2019). *Cost-effective actions to tackle the biggest killer of men and women: heart disease.* Melbourne: National Heart Foundation of Australia. https://treasury.gov.au/sites/default/files/2019-03/C2016-052_National-Heart-Foundation-of-Australia.pdf.

Neri, M., Riezzo, I., Pascale, N., Pomara, C. & Turillazzi, E. (2017). Ischemia/reperfusion injury following acute myocardial infarction: a critical issue for clinicians and forensic pathologists. *Mediators of Inflammation* 17:7018393. https://doi.org/10.1155/2017/7018393.

Rahman, M., Islam, F., Or-Rashid, H., Al Mamun, A., Rahaman, S., Islam, M., Meem, A.F.K., … Cavalu, S. (2022). The gut microbiota (microbiome) in cardiovascular disease and its therapeutic regulation. *Frontiers in Cellular and Infection Microbiology* 12:903570. https://doi.org/10.3389/fcimb.2022.903570.

Sutton, N.R., Malhotra, R., St Hilaire, C., Aikawa, E., Blumenthal, R.S., Gackenbach, G., … Chen, Y. (2023). Molecular Mechanisms of Vascular Health: Insights From Vascular Aging and Calcification. *Arteriosclerosis, Thrombosis, and Vascular Biology* 43(1):15–29. https://doi.org/10.1161/ATVBAHA.122.317332.

24 Cardiac muscle and valve disorders

KEY TERMS

Afterloud
Atrial septal defect
Cardiomyopathy
Concentric hypertrophy
Congenital heart defects
Congestive heart failure
Eccentric hypertrophy
Heart failure
Inotropy
Patent ductus arteriosus
Preload
Rheumatic fever
Rheumatic heart disease
Tetralogy of Fallot
Valve regurgitation
Valve stenosis
Ventricular remodelling
Ventricular septal defect

LEARNING OBJECTIVES

After completing this chapter, you should be able to:

1 Outline the current heart failure classifications.
2 Describe the influence of compensatory responses on heart failure disease progression.
3 Identify the primary cellular changes associated with heart failure.
4 Describe the three main types of cardiomyopathies, and outline their relationship to heart failure.
5 Briefly describe the four types of congenital heart defects and their relationship to heart failure.
6 Differentiate between the various types of valve pathologies.
7 Explain how untreated rheumatic fever can lead to rheumatic heart disease and heart failure.
8 Identify the two primary sources of the organisms responsible for infective endocarditis, and briefly outline how they are thought to contribute to heart failure.
9 Describe the risk factors, clinical manifestations, complications, and diagnosis and management of heart failure.

WHAT YOU SHOULD KNOW BEFORE YOU START THIS CHAPTER

Can you identify the structures of the heart?
Can you outline the coronary circulation?
Can you identify the factors that determine cardiac output?
Can you describe the renin–angiotensin–aldosterone system?
Can you outline the organisation and responses of the autonomic nervous system associated with the heart?

Introduction

Valve integrity and muscle strength are critical to heart function. Both of these structures are important for the efficient forward flow of blood. If valve integrity is compromised, more stress is placed on the heart muscle through either increased volume from pooling blood, or increased pressure from inadequately open valves obstructing chamber outflow. Muscle function is reliant on structural integrity and a balanced supply and demand equation for oxygenation, nutrient delivery and the capacity to remove waste. When any of these components is compromised, the reduced capacity of the heart muscle to adequately contract or relax can challenge its ability to pump blood to the systemic, pulmonary and/or cardiac circuits. Therefore, both valve and muscle dysfunction often lead to heart failure. Heart failure can arise from various causes, such as myocardial infarction, hypertension, congenital heart defects, valve disease, rheumatic fever and varicose veins, and may be an acute or a chronic condition. The focus of this chapter is heart failure from conditions causing valve or myocardial dysfunction.

Heart failure

LEARNING OBJECTIVE 1

Outline the current heart failure classifications.

Heart failure occurs when *the heart is unable to supply sufficient oxygenated, nutrient-rich blood to meet the metabolic demands of the body*. This may result in a backflow of blood in the venous circuit, and lead to oedema.

Heart failure is most accurately described as a *syndrome*, in as much as it is really a collection of clinical manifestations rather than a single clinical disease. Recently, there has been an international attempt to improve the definition of heart failure. As a result, more terminology has been introduced to better capture the quality of the condition. The classification system relies on the measure of *ejection fraction (EF)*, which is the percentage of blood that is pumped out of the ventricles with each contraction. In health, a person's ejection fraction would be expected to be 55–70%. Classifying heart failure based on ejection fraction results in adding information as to whether compensatory changes to structure and function are presently sufficient to keep the ejection fraction at a reasonable percentage, or are failing to keep the ejection fraction above 55%. Although there have been many was to describe it, commonly the terms *systolic (contract)* and *diastolic (relax)* heart failure are used. Therefore, heart failure may be compromised because of an inability to either contract or relax adequately.

Heart failure can be staged using the American College of Cardiology/American Heart Association (ACC/AHA) Stages from A to D or the New York Heart Association (NYHA) Functional Classification system (see Table 24.1).

The main difference between these two systems is that the ACC/AHA Stages of heart failure focus on the severity of structural heart disease and the presence or absence of symptoms, whereas the NYHA Functional Classification focuses solely on the severity of symptoms.

The ACC/AHA Stages of heart failure are useful for determining the appropriate treatment and management strategies for people with heart failure, whereas the NYHA Functional Classification is useful for assessing the person's functional status and predicting prognosis.

In Australia, both the ACC/AHA Stages of heart failure and the NYHA Functional Classification are commonly used by healthcare professionals to evaluate and manage people with heart failure. The choice of system may depend on the individual's needs and the clinical context.

Further heart failure classification is achieved by describing left ventricular ejection fraction (LVEF), and, although this method of classification is still emerging at local levels in Australia, its use is important in refining clinical management internationally.

The recently updated classification system now includes four types. Table 24.2 describes the LVEF criteria necessary to categorise individuals into each type.

Table 24.1 American College of Cardiology/American Heart Association (ACC/AHA) Stages and New York Heart Association (NYHA) Classes of heart failure

ACC/AHA stage	NYHA class	Description of stage
Stage A At risk	Prefailure	At risk of heart failure because of comorbidities and risk factors, but as yet not displaying any structural heart disease, or cardiac biomarkers of stretch or injury.
Stage B Pre-HF	I	No signs or symptoms, but measurable structural heart disease, evidence of increased filling pressure, or have increased BNPs (or elevated cardiac troponin)—in the absence of competing diagnosis.
Stage C Symptomatic	II/III	Previous or current clinical manifestations with observable structures heart disease.
Stage D Advanced	IV	People with cardiac disease resulting in an inability to carry out any physical activity without discomfort. Symptoms of cardiac insufficiency or of the angina syndrome may be present even at rest. If any physical activity is undertaken, discomfort is increased.

BNP = B-type natriuretic peptide; HF = heart failure.

Source: Heidenreich et al. (2022).

Table 24.2 Classification of heart failure by left ventricular ejection fraction (LVEF)

Types	Acronym explained	Criteria
HFrEF	Heart Failure with reduced Ejection Fraction	LVEF $\leq$ 40
HFimpEF	Heart Failure with improved Ejection Fraction	Previous LVEF $\leq$ 40 LVEF > 40 following management
HFmrEF	Heart Failure with mid-range Ejection Fraction	LVEF 41–49%
HFpEF	Heart Failure with preserved Ejection Fraction	LVEF $\geq$ 50

HF = heart failure; LV = left ventricular; LVEF = left ventricular ejection fraction.

Sources: Heidenreich et al. (2022); Kalsi et al. (2022).

The phrase *Heart Failure with reduced Ejection Fraction (HFrEF)* is used when discussing systolic failure (EF $\leq$ 40%), and the phrase *Heart Failure with preserved Ejection Fraction (HFpEF)* is used when discussing diastolic failure (EF $\geq$ 50%). The newest term that has appeared in the European Society of Cardiology heart failure guidelines is called *Heart Failure with mid-range Ejection Fraction* (HFmrEF), and is used when discussing failure that lies somewhere between HFrEF and HFpEF (EF 41–49%). It is envisaged that more research will help clarify the characteristics of this classification, which attempts to bridge the gap for people who did not clearly fit in either one or the other previously identified categories. Figure 24.1 incorporates the newer descriptions of the various types of heart failure.

Currently, the ACC/AHA Stages of heart failure does not replace the New York Heart Association Functional Classification (both shown in Table 24.1), but it is said to complement current heart failure definition. The NYHA Functional Classification system is commonly used and helps to identify disease severity, and enables the person's condition to be quantified in relation to its effect on the activities of daily living. It can therefore be used to help guide management. There are currently moves by peak international bodies to adopt a Universal Definition and Classification of Heart Failure.

In the initial stages of the disease, the body attempts to compensate for the reduction in cardiac output by using an increase in sympathetic nervous system activity. This increases heart rate and contraction force, as well as vascular tone, and an increase in the activity of the renin–angiotensin–aldosterone system, which causes fluid retention to increase blood volume and increase blood pressure through vasoconstriction. In the short term, these measures do provide benefit to the person, but they are untenable as long-term compensations. In fact, the very systems that are attempting to improve cardiac function eventually contribute to the problem by aggravating the heart's deterioration. Due to the reduced ejection of blood, the person is at risk of angina and a myocardial infarction.

Remember that cardiac ischaemia is defined as an insufficient blood supply to meet the needs of the heart itself, so in heart failure if there is insufficient blood to meet the needs of the body, the heart, being part of the body, is also at risk (see the chapter 'Coronary heart disease'). The prevalence of heart failure in Australia is 1–2%, and increases with age (two-thirds of adults with heart failure are aged over 65). There is also a geographical and gender influence on heart failure prevalence, with remote and very remote areas experiencing heart failure rates 60% higher than those in major cities, and death rates from heart failure (as the underlying cause) 1.4 times higher in males than in females. Aboriginal and Torres Strait Islander peoples are more than twice as likely to die from heart failure than non-Indigenous Australians, but the risk is slightly higher in Indigenous women, at 2.2 times (and Indigenous men, 1.8 times) that of non-Indigenous Australians.

AETIOLOGY AND PATHOPHYSIOLOGY

LEARNING OBJECTIVE 2

Describe the influence of compensatory responses on heart failure disease progression.

The core problem in heart failure is the inability of the heart to eject a volume of oxygen- and nutrient-rich blood to meet the metabolic needs of the body. The initiating events that trigger the process resulting in heart failure are unique to each individual: for example, it might be myocyte damage from a myocardial infarction, an inherited condition such as cardiomyopathy, or acquired conditions such as hypertension or kidney disease. In many cases the initiating event may be unknown, thereby impeding our ability to understand the development of the disorder and provide appropriate interventions. Regardless of the identity of the trigger, what is clear is that heart function becomes compromised.

In the early stages, feedback from baroreceptors and chemoreceptors cause activation of the *sympathetic nervous system (SNS)* followed by the renin–angiotensin–aldosterone system in an attempt to correct the problem. Since *cardiac output (CO)* is the product of the *heart rate (HR)* and the *stroke volume (SV)* ejected due to adequate contraction force ($CO = HR \times SV$), an increased heart rate and calcium availability to the myocytes improves contractility and provides some short-term relief. Likewise, activation of the *renin–angiotensin–aldosterone system* will lead to increased blood volume, ventricular filling and stroke volume, in association with increased blood pressure from vasoconstriction. The

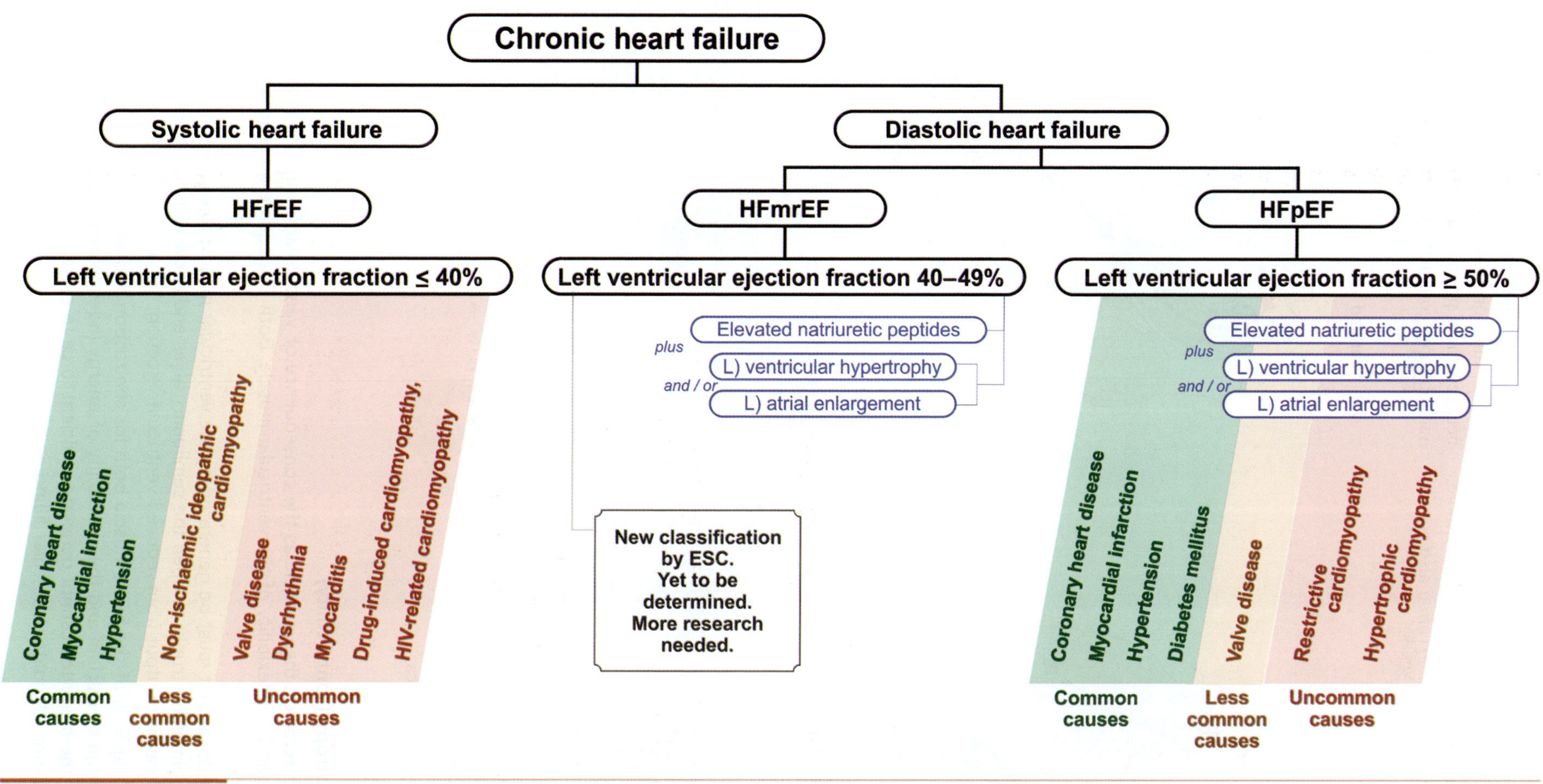

Figure 24.1

Types and causes of heart failure

ESC = European Society of Cardiology; HFmrEF = Heart Failure with mid-range Ejection Fraction; HFpEF = Heart Failure with preserved Ejection Fraction; HFrEF = Heart Failure with reduced Ejection Fraction; L) = Left.

continued myocyte workload results in hypertrophy. As the condition progresses, the basic function of the myocytes is fundamentally altered. SNS activity persists, yet there is *reduced responsiveness of cardiac tissue*, and furthermore, *reduced sensitivity to parasympathetic innervation* also occurs. Cumulatively, these chronic structural and functional changes are known as **ventricular remodelling**.

The functional integrity of the heart requires a balance between three primary cardiac parameters: preload, afterload and inotropy (contractility) (see Figure 24.2).

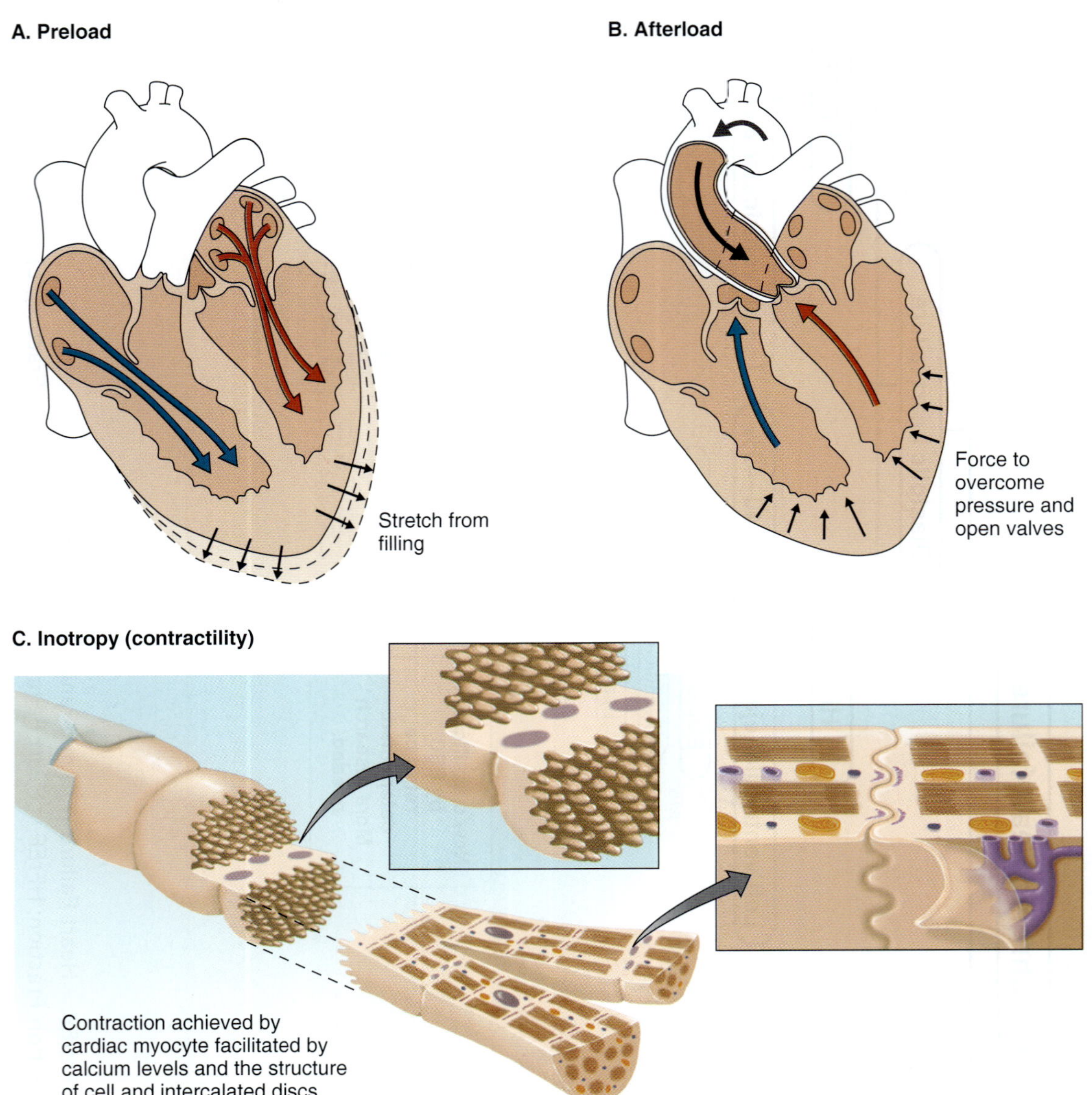

Figure 24.2

Preload, afterload and inotropy (contractility)

(A) Preload represents the stretch on the ventricle as the consequence of ventricular filling, and is an index both of the end-diastolic volume (EDV) and the flexibility of the ventricular muscle. Both inadequate and excess preload can be present in heart failure.

(B) Afterload represents the force that must be generated by the ventricular muscle to exceed the pressure in the outgoing vessel (aorta or pulmonary trunk) to open the semilunar valves and allow ventricular ejection. Excess afterload reduces stroke volume and cardiac output from reduced ventricular ejection.

(C) Inotropy represents the capacity of the heart muscle both for contraction and relaxation, both of which are dependent on the mobilisation of calcium and the availability of energy (adenosine triphosphate [ATP]). Cardiac function is compromised if the myocytes cannot generate sufficient force to eject blood, or if they cannot relax quickly or sufficiently enough to ensure adequate ventricular filling.

Source: Adapted from Marieb & Hoehn (2019), Figures 18.2 and 18.11.

Preload in heart failure

Preload represents the stretch on the ventricles as a consequence of *ventricular filling*. Preload problems can arise as the consequence of both inadequate and excess filling. One of the most likely causes of *insufficient preload* for the right ventricle is *varicose veins*. This will have a flow-on effect for the left ventricle, because insufficient stroke volume from the right ventricle into the pulmonary circuit will lead to inadequate filling of the left ventricle and, consequently, reduced cardiac output to the body. For the left side of the heart, additional causes of inadequate filling include *respiratory diseases* that prevent free movement of blood into and out of the lungs.

Excess preload presents a burden that is too great for the heart to manage efficiently. Excess blood volume may cause a burden exceeding the heart's capacity and it will struggle to efficiently eject a reasonable proportion of that blood. Although the Frank–Starling Law suggests that with increased ventricular wall stretch (because of increased incoming blood volume) there will be a concomitant increase in recoil from that stretch, leading to better ejection, there is a limit. The reason that the failing heart struggles with the *excess volume* and cannot take advantage of Frank–Starling forces is because the cells are no longer physiologically normal (see the 'Cellular changes in heart failure' section later in this chapter). However, reducing the volume even slightly can result in a larger ejected stroke volume and improved function. Although this might seem counterintuitive, it is a cornerstone of the pharmacological management of heart failure: a small reduction in the preload, the *end-diastolic volume (EDV)*, may actually result in an increase in stroke volume and therefore in cardiac output.

As the heart continues to fail, less blood is ejected and more is left in the ventricle after ejection. This is the *end-systolic volume (ESV)*. As the ESV increases, and returning blood also makes its way back to the heart, volume overload will continue. As the heart is forced to cope with this increased volume, excessive stretch on the myocytes can lead to a condition known as dilated cardiomyopathy (see later in this chapter). Alternatively, the stretch might trigger compensation in the form of hypertrophy of the myocytes. Initially, the hypertrophy might be beneficial, as larger myocytes can generate more contraction force, but in heart failure the hypertrophy quickly exacerbates the heart failure by making the muscle stiff and unable to either contract or relax efficiently, in large part because the hypertrophy is different from normal. This hypertrophy is discussed more in the 'Inotropy in heart failure' section.

Afterload in heart failure

Afterload is the pressure that the ventricle must overcome in order to *open the semilunar valves and eject the stroke volume*. The three primary sources of increased afterload are: atherosclerosis, hypertension and valve stenosis. *Narrowed and/or constricted vessels or valves* increase the force required by the ventricle to eject blood, and decrease the time available for ejection. Initially, the feedback from baroreceptors and chemoreceptors triggers a surge in sympathetic outflow from the brain, which, in this case, has the primary purpose of *increasing the calcium available* to the myocytes and, therefore, the force of contraction. This increased contractility allows the heart to reach the necessary ventricular pressure sooner in the cardiac cycle, providing an earlier, longer and hopefully more efficient ejection in cases of atherosclerosis and hypertension, but not necessarily with valve stenosis.

Unless the myocytes are compromised, this increased contraction will be associated with an improved relaxation and, therefore, filling. Sustained action of the SNS, as well as an increased availability of aldosterone, triggers hypertrophy of the myocytes, decreasing the dependence of the heart on increased sympathetic activity. However, as heart failure is a progressive condition, this compensation is useful only in the short term, as further deterioration necessitates repeated rounds of increased sympathetic intervention and further hypertrophy. Eventually, the ventricular chamber size is reduced due to the inward hypertrophy that arises because of the limited tolerance of the thoracic cavity to an increase in heart size. This hypertrophy creates a restructured heart that becomes muscle-bound and stiff (see Figure 24.3).

It is important to recognise that the hypertrophy associated with heart failure (*pathological hypertrophy*) is different from that associated with the normal adaptation of the heart to exercise (*physiological hypertrophy*). These maladaptive changes will often cause the person's condition to deteriorate.

Morphologically, physiological hypertrophy of the heart is balanced between lengthening the muscle fibres and an increased width. The hypertrophy associated with heart failure is either **eccentric hypertrophy** (due to volume overload), in which the *length* rather than the width is increased, or **concentric hypertrophy** (due to increased afterload), in which the *width* of the myocytes

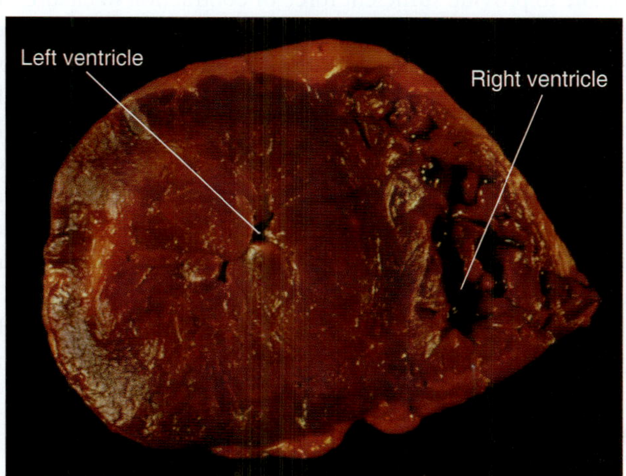

Figure 24.3

Left ventricular hypertrophy secondary to progressive hypertension

Severe left ventricular hypertrophy resulting in increased myocyte volume, causing an increased myocardial oxygen demand and reduced chamber size, causing decreased oxygen supply.

Source: Dr E. Walker/Science Photo Library.

increases, but not the length. In either case, the efficiency of the muscle is greatly reduced, leading to a reduction in cardiac output. Further complicating matters, regardless of the pressure that triggered it, this abnormal hypertrophy is aggravated and perpetuated by elevated circulating aldosterone levels. Therefore, the attempt to compensate for the loss of cardiac output by activating the renin–angiotensin–aldosterone system will actually worsen the reduced blood flow to the organs.

Acute heart failure is a sudden development of symptoms, often severe and as a result of a myocardial infarction or an ischaemic, inflammatory or toxic insult of some nature. Acute valve insufficiency or *pericardial tamponade* may also cause acute heart failure. It requires urgent evaluation and management, and may respond to treatment and improve rapidly. It may occur as a decompensation of chronic heart failure.

Conversely, *chronic heart failure* appears slowly over time, and gradually gets worse as heart function continues to deteriorate. It may continue as a result of an acute heart failure, or just as a long and slow deterioration in function because of continued challenges which exceed the cardiomyocytes' capacity. It requires frequent assessment and adjustment of the management regimen, and, although a person with chronic heart failure may have acute exacerbations from which they recover following the immediate life-threatening event, the person's heart function often continues on a slow and incessant decline despite intervention.

Inotropy in heart failure The word 'inotrope' comes from the Greek words *inos*, meaning 'fibre', and *tropos*, meaning 'behaviour', and refers to the ability of the muscle cells to function; namely, create a contraction and relax from it. In heart failure associated with reduced **inotropy**, the myocardium is unable to provide sufficient force of contraction to ensure that adequate stroke volume is ejected. A major cause of reduced inotropy is the loss of cells due to myocardial infarction. Additional triggers of inotropic failure include infiltration of the myocardium by iron, calcium, fibrin, amyloid or tumours. Like preload and afterload pressures, inotropic failure is associated with a *reduction in ejected stroke volume* and, consequently, an *increase in ESV*. Depending on the nature of the injury that set up the reduced inotropy, there will be either volume overload due to the combination of the incoming venous return and the ESV, or an increased wall pressure due to a limited capacity of the ventricular wall to relax, which leads to ventricular hypertrophy.

Cellular changes in heart failure

LEARNING OBJECTIVE 3

Identify the primary cellular changes associated with heart failure.

Unfortunately, it remains unclear whether heart failure causes the cellular changes that are seen in chronic disease, or whether these changes are the reason for heart failure developing. What is clear is the fact that the altered cellular integrity is integral to the self-perpetuating downward spiral that is the hallmark of chronic heart failure.

Altered myocyte integrity Myocytes affected by heart failure show a loss of α-myosin, with a concomitant increase in β-myosin, a reduction in myofilaments and altered excitation–contraction coupling, which will contribute to a decreased efficiency of contraction and, by extension, relaxation of the ventricular muscle. In addition, the abnormal hypertrophy is associated with the production of proteins that are normally only associated with fetal development, and it is proposed that these proteins also interfere with normal contractility.

As part of the altered excitation–contraction coupling, in heart failure, myocytes do not mobilise calcium quickly enough to ensure a robust contraction within the time allowed by the action potential. They also do not appear able to deal with the energy demands of contraction and relaxation, presumably through both reduced adenosine triphosphate (ATP) generation and increased ATP requirements for normal processes. These changes ensure that the heart failure will worsen rapidly in a self-perpetuating fashion.

Altered sympathetic–parasympathetic balance
A key feature of heart failure is a change in the sensitivity of the cardiovascular system to the two branches of the autonomic nervous system; namely, the sympathetic and parasympathetic nervous systems. As the disorder becomes chronic, the parasympathetic influence on heart rate is lost in the presence of tonic (persistent) activation of the SNS. This increased sympathetic activity is associated with both elevated nervous activity and an increased level of circulating noradrenaline, with the latter representing a good index of mortality rate. Interestingly, in the 1990s a specialised group of cells that act as neuroendocrine cells was identified in the heart; in other words, these cells resemble those in the adrenal medulla from which adrenaline is produced and released into the bloodstream. These cells, called *intrinsic adrenergic cells*, appear to be a key source of the increased circulating noradrenaline associated with heart failure. Despite this, however, there is a loss of β_1-adrenergic receptors on the cells of the heart. Paradoxically, when receptors are bombarded with constant signals (in this case, due to the increased nervous system and neuroendocrine activity), they *desensitise* (lose sensitivity) and can even *down-regulate* (reduce in number). Hence, you have a failing heart that is being pummelled with noradrenaline in order to try to maintain cardiac output, which only serves to make the heart less and less sensitive to noradrenaline, causing it to lose its ability to respond to the SNS.

Other causes of heart failure

In some cases of heart failure there is an underlying mechanical reason, and if this mechanical problem can be rectified, the heart failure may be reduced or even resolved. Some conditions can be divided into three different mechanisms, caused by cardiomyopathies, congenital heart defects or valve defects. An additional concern is infective endocarditis, which often arises secondary to valve defects and congenital heart defects. We provide a brief overview of each of these, and describe their contribution to heart failure.

CARDIOMYOPATHIES

LEARNING OBJECTIVE 4

Describe the three main types of cardiomyopathies, and outline their relationship to heart failure.

Cardiomyopathy refers to disorders of the heart muscle (*cardio* = 'heart', *myo* = 'muscle', *patho* = 'disease'), and can be grouped into dilated, hypertrophic and restrictive conditions (see Figure 24.4). *Dilated cardiomyopathies* are marked by a loss of elasticity of the myocardium and an overstretched, flaccid ventricular muscle mass. There are a variety of causes for dilated cardiomyopathy, including toxins such as chemotherapeutic drugs or alcohol, metabolic alterations such as those associated with pregnancy and hypothyroidism, and infections by bacteria, viruses or fungi.

Hypertrophic cardiomyopathies are associated with increased size of the ventricular muscle, and may be either an acquired or an inherited condition, with the latter more problematic as the increased size of the muscle is asymmetrical. Inherited hypertrophic cardiomyopathy is an autosomal dominant disorder marked by disorganised myocytes and weak connective tissue. Subvalvular hypertrophy often occurs, in which the muscle just beneath the valve is markedly enlarged, such that it contracts in front of the valve, blocking the ejection of blood, an event that is exacerbated by exercise. This type of cardiomyopathy is often referred to a *hypertrophic obstructive cardiomyopathy (HOCM)*.

Finally, *restrictive cardiomyopathies* involve infiltration of the myocardium by material that stiffens the muscle, inhibiting both contraction and relaxation. A key cause of restrictive cardiomyopathy is scar tissue formation post myocardial infarction, but other causes include infiltration by iron, amyloid or tumours.

Clinical manifestations

As cardiomyopathies can lead to pump failure, the signs and symptoms associated with cardiomyopathies include dyspnoea, fatigue and oedema. Other manifestations may include those typically associated with compensation, such as tachypnoea and tachycardia. Manifestations will vary, depending on whether there is left-sided or right-sided or biventricular involvement. See the section on the clinical manifestations of heart failure in this chapter.

Clinical diagnosis and management

Diagnosis Investigations to determine the presence of cardiomyopathy include: echocardiography; chest X-ray for chamber size, valve function and the presence of cardiomegaly;

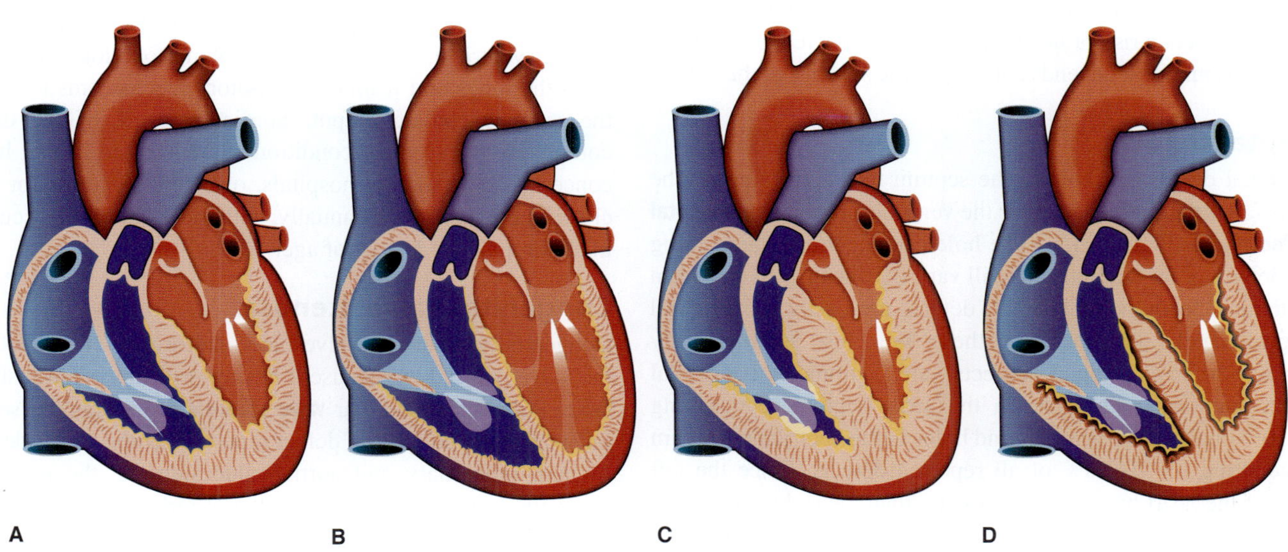

Figure 24.4

Dilated, hypertrophic and restrictive cardiomyopathies

These diagrams demonstrate the ways in which the heart muscle is altered in cardiomyopathies. (A) Normal heart. (B) Dilated cardiomyopathy: the chamber volume is increased, the ventricular walls are thin, and a systolic dysfunction develops. (C) Hypertrophic cardiomyopathy: the chamber volume is decreased, the ventricular walls are very thick, and a diastolic dysfunction develops. (D) Restrictive cardiomyopathy: the chamber volume may be normal; however, it may have infiltration of scar tissue, fibrin, amyloid, iron or tumours, making the wall very rigid, and both systolic and diastolic dysfunction develops.

Source: © Sciencopia.

and electrocardiography (ECG) in the exploration of possible dysrhythmia. Other investigations to rule out alternative causes of dyspnoea include iron studies and cardiac biomarkers, such as cardiac troponin I (cTnI), to determine the possibility of a myocardial infarction.

Management Management of cardiomyopathies is essentially the same as interventions for heart failure, such as control of blood pressure with medications to reduce or support, reduction of hypercoagulability with anticoagulants, and control of excess fluid with diuretics. For a deeper discussion regarding management, see the management of heart failure section in this chapter.

CONGENITAL HEART DEFECTS

LEARNING OBJECTIVE 5

Briefly describe the four types of congenital heart defects and their relationship to heart failure.

An estimated eight babies out of every 1,000 live births have a congenital heart defect, even though it might not be picked up until the child reaches adolescence or even adulthood. **Congenital heart defects** fall into two categories: *cyanotic* and *acyanotic*. Cyanosis is the blue colouration of lips, mucous membranes and even skin as the consequence of inadequate oxygenation. The hallmark of cyanosis is that the blood flow is adequate; however, perfusion is occurring with oxygen-poor haemoglobin resulting in tissue hypoxia. Both cyanotic and acyanotic defects present a risk of heart failure, and the degree to which the problems manifest depends entirely on the severity of the defect.

Septal defects

A septal defect is a hole in the septum that divides either the atria (an **atrial septal defect**) or the ventricles (a **ventricular septal defect**). (See Figure 24.5.) The hole can occur anywhere along the length of the septum, and will vary significantly in size from individual to individual. Small defects are easily missed, and approximately one-quarter of these will close spontaneously during infancy. Septal defects are common congenital malformations, with those in the atrial septum representing 5–10% of all malformations, and holes in the ventricular septum accounting for 20–30% of all reported defects. Since the left side of the heart has a higher pressure than the right side, blood is shunted from left to right through the hole, adding blood to the right side and presenting a growing volume overload problem for the right side, which can lead to hypertrophy.

Initially, increased ejection from the right side will increase venous return to the left side, which will also experience a greater volume that must be accommodated. Depending on the size of the hole, there might not be any appreciable loss of stroke volume and thus cardiac output. However, as the child grows, the hole can enlarge, and the heart's attempts to adapt can also enlarge the hole further. As the child ages, a greater and greater proportion of blood will be shunted to the right side, possibly leading to a compromise in cardiac output, and to signs of heart failure. Some people can reach middle age before any appreciable reduction in cardiac output is seen. Provided the shunt remains left to right, there will be no cyanosis. If the shunt becomes marked enough, however, it can actually reverse, as the right side, due to a combination of right-side compensation and volume-driven pulmonary hypertension, will become the high-pressure side and blood will be shunted from right to left, leading to cyanosis, because now a significant proportion of the blood ejected to the systemic circulation will be oxygen-poor. If picked up early, however, the hole can be surgically closed and the condition quickly resolves.

Patent ductus arteriosus

The ductus arteriosus is a blood vessel normally found only in utero; it connects the aorta and the pulmonary trunk (see Figure 24.6). Its role in the developing fetus is to shunt blood away from the lungs and into the systemic circulation, since the only blood needed in the lungs is that required for lung growth and development (approximately 5–10% of the flow from the left ventricle). (Remember that external fetal respiration occurs at the placenta.) The ductus arteriosus should close shortly after birth due to changes in both oxygen tension and prostaglandin levels.

In babies with **patent ductus arteriosus (PDA)**, the ductus fails to close, allowing blood from the aorta to be shunted into the pulmonary trunk. Shunting of blood from the aorta into the pulmonary trunk causes a reduction in the cardiac output delivered to the body, although what blood is delivered is fully oxygenated (so this is an *acyanotic defect*). Failure of the ductus to close will trigger hypertrophy of both the left atrium and the left ventricle, due, in part, to volume overload coming in from the lungs and from compensatory mechanisms to correct the reduced cardiac output. Surgical closure of the ductus completely resolves the condition and leaves no lasting health concerns. In Australian hospitals, over 650 surgeries for PDA closures are performed annually, with more than 74% occurring in children under 5 years of age.

Congenital valve stenosis

Congenitally stenosed valves are malformed either because the valve is fused or because it has fewer leaflets than it should have. Pulmonic semilunar **valve stenosis** represents the second most common congenital defect reported behind septal defects. In both pulmonary and aortic value stenosis, the respective ventricles experience an increase in afterload as they attempt to open the valve and eject blood. As ventricular ejection is impeded, cardiac output is reduced; however, arterial and venous blood is not mixing, and therefore it is not a cyanotic defect. Depending on the nature of the malformation, the valves can be either forced open using a balloon procedure or surgically replaced. Correction of the defect removes the pressure that led to signs of heart failure.

Tetralogy of Fallot

Tetralogy of Fallot is a cyanotic congenital condition that constitutes a set of four malformations: a *ventricular septal defect*, a *subvalvular pulmonic stenosis*, an *overarching aorta*

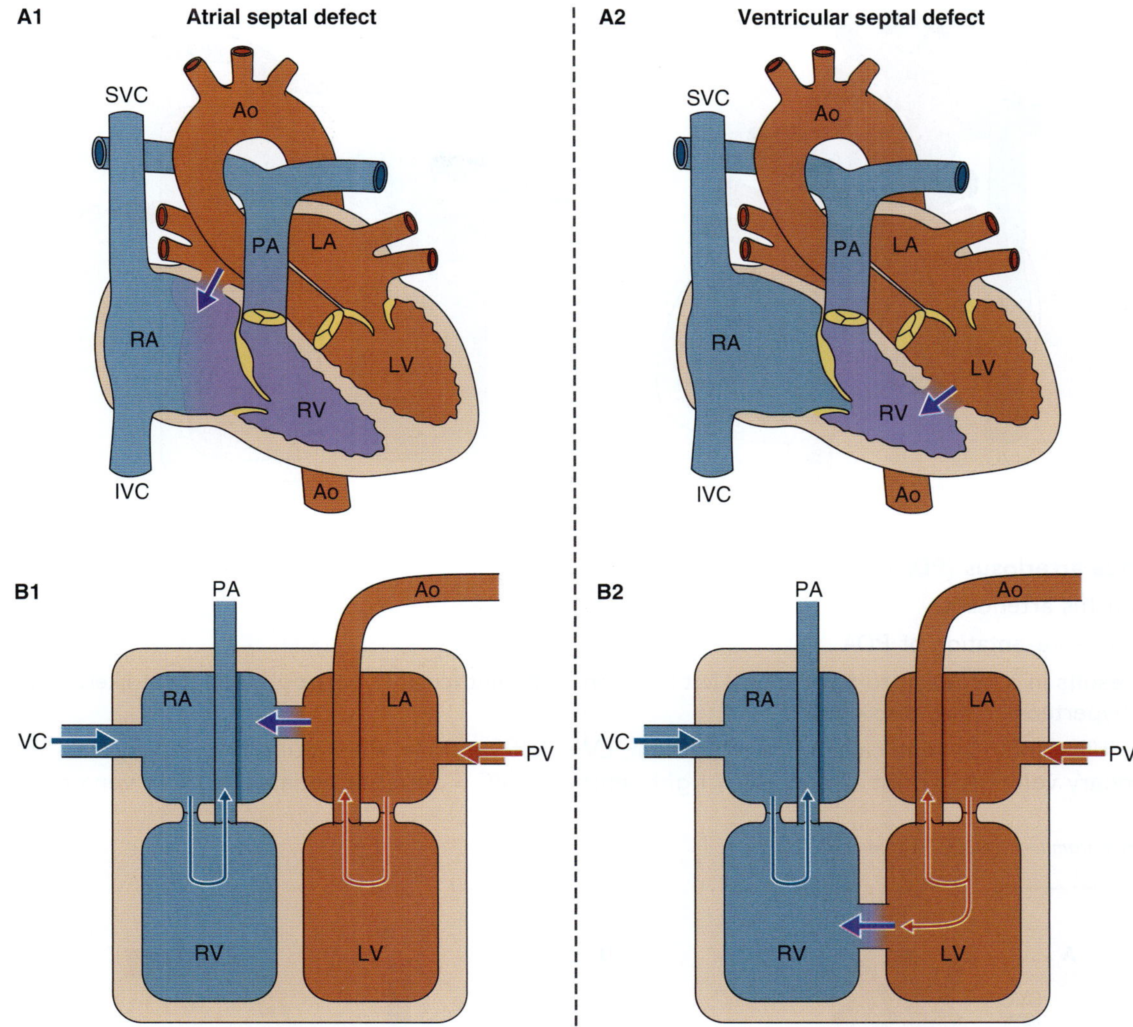

Figure 24.5

Atrial and ventricular septal defects

(A1) Atrial septal defect. (A2) Ventricular septal defect. (B1) Schematic representation of the blood flow associated with an atrial septal defect. (B2) Schematic representation of the blood flow associated with a ventricular septal defect. Septal defects can occur anywhere along the length of the septum. An atrial septal defect will trigger hypertrophy of the right atrium and ventricle due to the volume overload, whereas a ventricular septal defect can cause hypertrophy of the right ventricle, left atrium and left ventricle.

Ao = aorta; IVC = inferior vena cava; LA = left atrium; LV = left ventricle; PA = pulmonary artery; PV = pulmonary vein; RA = right atrium; RV = right ventricle; SVC = superior vena cava; *VC = vena cava.*

Sources: Adapted from Lily (2020); Morton et al. (2022).

and *right ventricular hypertrophy* (see Figure 24.7). Because of the subvalvular pulmonic stenosis, the blood is shunted from the right side into the left side through the ventricular septal defect and out through the aorta. Consequently, a mixing of oxygen-rich and oxygen-poor blood occurs, and the extent to which this happens determines the degree of cyanosis that the child experiences. The right ventricle hypertrophies in an attempt to compensate for the loss of blood to the left side, but this only aggravates the subvalvular stenosis, worsening the condition. It is well recognised that increased peripheral resistance eases the shunt, and children with this condition spontaneously adopt a crouched posture to allow the easing of the shunt. The condition creates a volume overload on the left ventricle, while compensatory hypertrophy of the right ventricle aggravates the right-to-left shunt. Surgical correction to replace the pulmonic valve and alleviate the subvalvular stenosis, as well as closure of the ventricular septal defect, allows those affected to live relatively normal lives.

Clinical manifestations

The clinical manifestations of someone with congenital heart disease are dependent on whether the condition is classed as *acyanotic* or *cyanotic*, and whether there has been any intervention. If there is arterial and venous blood mixing, the

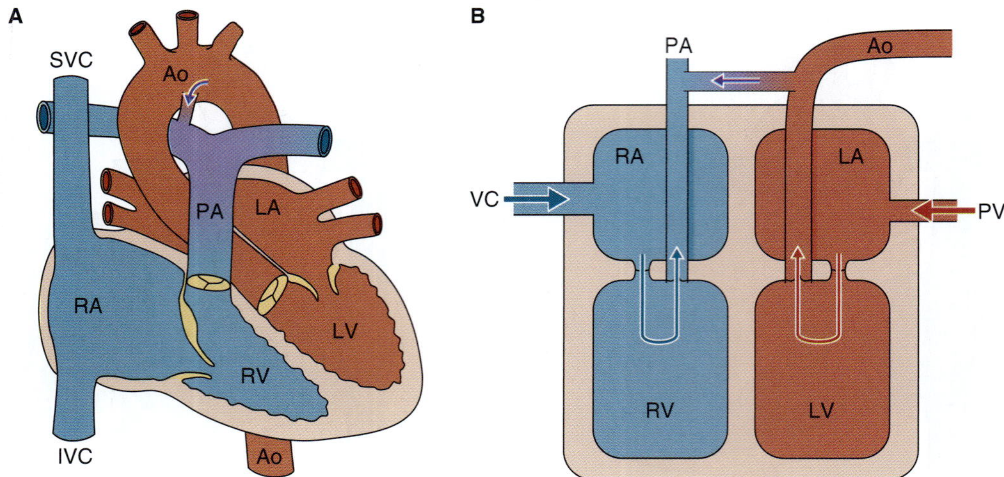

Figure 24.6

Patent ductus arteriosus (PDA)

(A) Patent ductus arteriosus.

(B) Schematic representation of PDA.

If the PDA results in a large left-to-right shunt, left atrial and left ventricular hypertrophy will most likely develop. Pulmonary hypertension may also occur.

Ao = aorta; IVC = inferior vena cava; LA = left atrium; LV = left ventricle; PA = pulmonary artery; PV = pulmonary vein; RA = right atrium; RV = right ventricle; SVC = superior vena cava; VC = vena cava.

Sources: Adapted from Lily (2020); Morton et al. (2022).

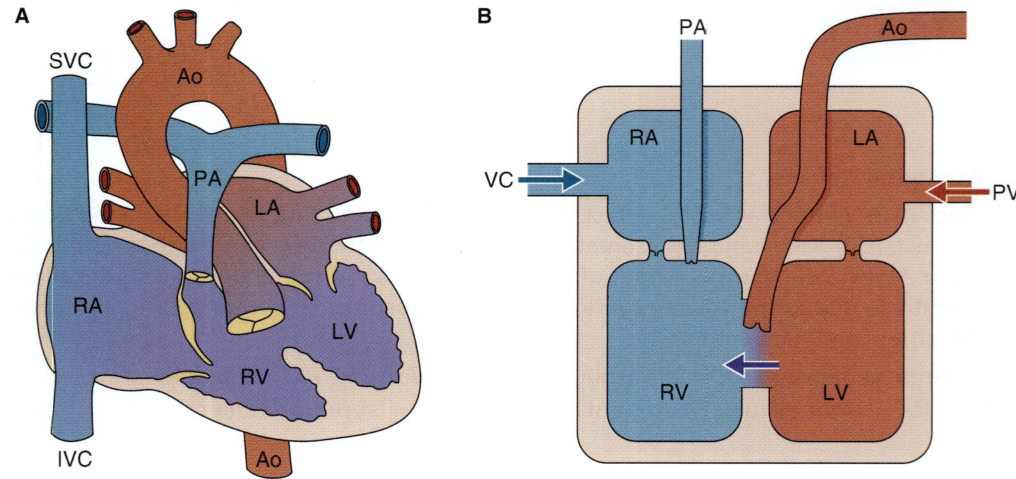

Figure 24.7

Tetralogy of Fallot

(A) Tetralogy of Fallot.

(B) Schematic representation of tetralogy of Fallot.

The combination of subvalvular stenosis (at the base of the PA), ventricular septal defect (dark blue arrow), overarching aorta and a hypertrophied right ventricle cause a right-to-left shunt of blood, leading to peripheral cyanosis and signs of heart failure.

Ao = aorta; IVC = inferior vena cava; LA = left atrium; LV = left ventricle; PA = pulmonary artery; PV = pulmonary vein; RA = right atrium; RV = right ventricle; SVC = superior vena cava; VC = vena cava.

Sources: Adapted from Lily (2020); Morton et al. (2022).

person will most probably have some degree of cyanosis and oxygen saturations that are normally around 80–85% (depending on the congenital lesion). Extra heart sounds and murmurs are likely, and typical heart-failure-like manifestations such as dyspnoea, fatigue and oedema may be obvious (see the section on the clinical manifestations of heart failure in this chapter).

Clinical diagnosis and management

Diagnosis Congenital heart defects, especially serious ones, may be detected at birth. A chest X-ray can be used to show the shape, size and position of the heart. On chest X-ray, the size of the heart should be less than 50% of the internal dimensions of the thorax. Other diagnostic techniques include cardiac catheterisation and ECGs. An echocardiogram can also be undertaken.

Management Surgical repair is usually required to close off abnormal openings and repair valves or damaged vessels. The timing of surgery depends on the ability of the person to withstand surgery and its impact on subsequent growth. Prophylactic antimicrobial therapy with amoxicillin may be required prior to surgery to prevent infective endocarditis.

VALVE DEFECTS

LEARNING OBJECTIVE 6

Differentiate between the various types of valve pathologies.

Valve defects can be *congenital* (as discussed above), or can be acquired as part of the ageing process through *calcification* of the valves, or through *rheumatic heart disease*.

Regardless of the underlying cause, valve defects fall into two categories: regurgitation and stenosis (see Figure 24.8). Irrespective of the category involved, the affected heart chamber will experience a volume overload either due to a failure to eject the appropriate volume (*stenosis*) or because the ejected volume returns to the chamber (*regurgitation*). Further, if stenosis is present, there is also increased wall tension, and both the volume overload and the wall tension will contribute to the inappropriate hypertrophy that contributes to the self-perpetuating nature of heart failure. Given the unique status of rheumatic heart disease, we will address this first before we address the generic issues associated with regurgitation and stenosis.

Clinical manifestations

As previously identified, valve conditions can cause heart failure, and therefore people may present with dyspnoea, oedema and maybe even chest pain, along with the typical manifestations seen in heart failure (see the section on the clinical manifestations of heart failure). People with valve defects may specifically present with presyncope (i.e. light-headedness and feeling faint), added heart sounds and dysrhythmias.

Clinical diagnosis and management

Diagnosis Apart from recording typical baseline observations—including heart rate, respirations, blood pressure and temperature—an echocardiogram would be valuable to measure the chamber size and detect the presence of valve incompetence. The degree of stenosis or regurgitation can be measured, as can the ejection fraction.

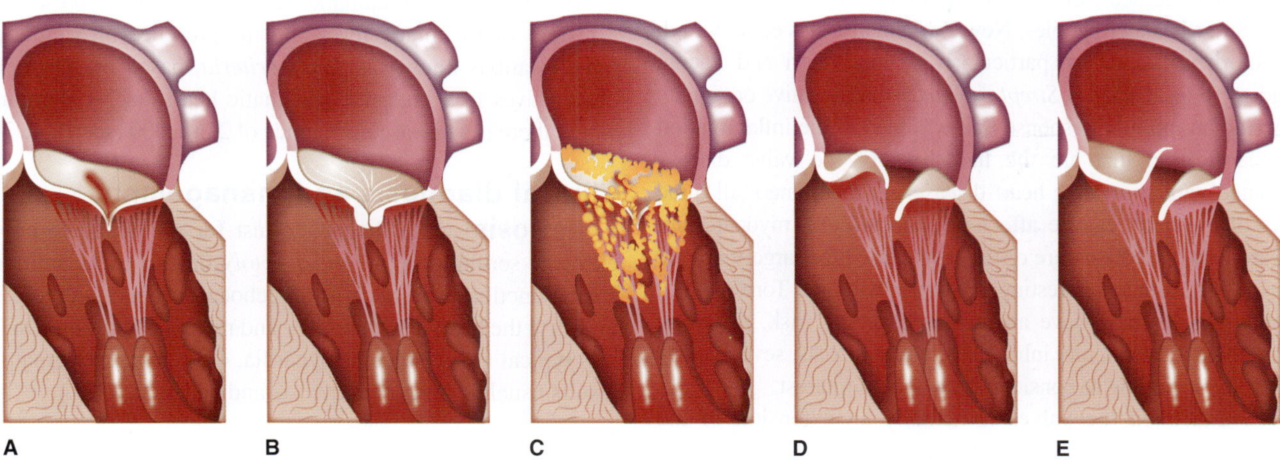

Figure 24.8

Common valvular pathologies

(A) Normal mitral valve. (B) Stenosis—occurs when the cusps are unable to open correctly, resulting in reduced ejection and increased pressure. (C) Infective vegetations—the colonisation of the valve by microorganisms and immune system cells, resulting in a thrombotic mass in and around the leaflets, annulus and chordae tendineae. (D) Regurgitation occurs when the cusps do not form an adequate seal and some previously ejected blood enters the chamber from which it has just come. (E) Valve prolapse from flail valve leaflet—occurs when the chordae tendineae or papillary muscle ruptures.

Source: © Sciencopia.

Management For many valve defects, surgical repair or replacement is the best option, and is commonly undertaken as an open procedure. An incision is made down the mediastinum and the person is placed on cardiopulmonary bypass so that the heart can be stopped while the surgery is performed. Alternatively, in some cases, for an aortic valve replacement a transcatheter aortic valve implantation (TAVI), or an transcatheter mitral valve replacement (TMVR) for the mitral valve, may be an option. In these procedures, there is no need for a sternotomy nor cardiopulmonary bypass, as the approach is a less invasive, 'off-pump' procedure.

Replacement valves can also be classed as tissue or mechanical. *Tissue valves* may be from animals such as pig (porcine), cow (bovine) and horse (equine). The value of tissue valves is in the limited need for continuous anticoagulation; however, they do not last as long and may need to be replaced in 10–20 years. *Mechanical valves* last longer; however, they require long-term anticoagulation, which poses an increased risk of bleeding. See the heart failure management options section in the chapter.

Rheumatic heart disease

LEARNING OBJECTIVE 7

Explain how untreated rheumatic fever can lead to rheumatic heart disease and heart failure.

Rheumatic heart disease is a consequence of prior, unmanaged **rheumatic fever**, and represents an autoimmune condition that attacks all three layers of the heart, as well as other organs. There is no clear understanding of why the manifestations of heart disease differ between people, but what is clear is that the valves of the heart are a common target of attack. In Australia, 92% of the incidence of all rheumatic heart disease is experienced by Aboriginal and Torres Strait Islander peoples. New Zealand also has equally high rates of rheumatic fever, particularly within Māori and Pacific Islander groups. Group A *Streptococcus* is the causative organism, triggering an immune response that will lead to the inflammation and scarification that are the hallmarks of the valve disease associated with rheumatic heart disease. As mentioned, all three layers of the heart can be affected (endocardium, myocardium, pericardium), and the nature of the damage will be largely unique to each individual. Interestingly, Aboriginal and Torres Strait Islander peoples may have an increased genetic risk. Although no single-gene Mendelian inheritance pattern exists, several early studies are beginning to consider a few loci of interest.

The attack on the valves is actually an extension of the damage to the myocardium, and is not thought to be a direct action on the valves themselves. What is critical, however, is the fact that the death of cells in the valves leads to a build-up of scar tissue, and this scar tissue can either cause the valves to stiffen or retract the valve leaflets, pulling the valves into a *permanently open* position.

Valve stenosis

Any of the valves can be affected, although those on the left side are more commonly damaged. Stenosis is often the consequence of *wear and tear on the valve with age*, and is generally accompanied by *calcification* (see Figure 24.8(B)). Vegetations develop on the valve, leading to a stiffening of the valve leaflets, and damage-induced scarification can fuse the leaflets (see Figure 24.8(C)). The chamber leading to the valve will have *difficulty opening* the valve, which will trigger hypertrophy of the myocytes of that chamber in response. This hypertrophy is particularly pronounced when a semilunar valve is affected. Stenosis of the valve presents an afterload pressure on the chamber facing the valve, and, if the valve is an atrioventricular valve, there will be insufficient preload (filling) for the ventricle, contributing a preload pressure to the developing heart failure.

Valve regurgitation

Any of the valves can be affected in **valve regurgitation**, with those on the left side more commonly damaged. In this case, the primary problem is a *volume overload* (excess preload) in the chamber leading to the damaged valve (see Figure 24.8(D) and (E)). Failure to eject an adequate stroke volume, and hence cardiac output, will trigger ventricular hypertrophy, which will be maladaptive, worsening the regurgitation.

Valve regurgitation can occur when the cusps do not form a seal, as a result of congenital conditions, disease or injury (such as chordae tendineae rupture).

Clinical manifestations

Rheumatic fever can present with many and various symptoms, including a sore throat, polyarthritis (usually in large joints and symmetrically), carditis, Sydenham chorea (irregular, rapid, involuntary movements of the arms and legs, trunk and facial muscles), and an eruption of non-pruritic, painless, erythematous skin lesions on the trunk. Other manifestations may include fever, abdominal pain and malaise.

A person with rheumatic heart disease may present with a history of rheumatic fever and the presence of a number of manifestations known as *Jones criteria*, based on whether the person lives in a high-risk rheumatic heart disease community where there is a disease prevalence of 2 in 1,000 (see Table 24.3).

Clinical diagnosis and management

Diagnosis The diagnostic test for rheumatic fever is an elevated serum titre of *antistreptolysin O (ASO)* antibodies. Heart function tests, such as an echocardiogram, are helpful to visualise the heart's morphology and measure function. On ECG it is typical to see sinus tachycardia, even at rest. Haematology results usually show leukocytosis and anaemia.

Management Continuous prophylaxis of antimicrobial therapy is usually required for those with a well-documented history of rheumatic fever. Common antimicrobial agents administered include benzathine penicillin intramuscularly or oral phenoxymethylpenicillin. Oral erythromycin is recommended if the person is allergic to penicillin. Treatment is often needed for five to 10 years in those with mild carditis or residual valve disease. On the other hand, life-long therapy is needed for people who have severe carditis or severe valve disease. If valvular disease develops as a complication of rheumatic fever, valve replacement surgery may be required.

Table 24.3 Manifestations of rheumatic heart disease in high-risk versus all other groups

Manifestation	Key points
Major manifestations	
Arthritis	Most common and usually extremely painful Usually asymmetrical, often affecting large joints especially knees and ankles
Sydenham chorea	Up to 25% of people experience jerky, uncoordinated movement, especially in the hands, feet, face and tongue
Carditis	Often presents with apical pansystolic murmur; however, a subclinical rheumatic valvulitis might be visible on echocardiography
Subcutaneous nodules	Small, round, painless nodules in numerous locations, including elbows, wrists, knees, ankles, occiput, and vertebral processes. Highly specific for carditis in Aboriginal and Torres Strait Islander peoples
Erythema marginatum	Circular, bright pink macules or papules on the trunk and proximal extremities. Difficult to detect in Aboriginal and Torres Strait Islander peoples
Minor manifestations	
Arthralgia	Most common and usually extremely painful Usually asymmetrical, often affecting large joints especially knees and ankles
Fever	Often low-grade and transient fever. Consider $> 38°C$ in high-risk groups and $< 38.5°C$ in low-risk groups
Elevated CRP and/or ESR	CRP ≥ 30 mg/L or ESR ≥ 30 mg/L in high-risk or ≥ 60 mg/L in low-risk groups
ECG changes	May demonstrate a prolonged PR interval (or other conduction abnormality). It is recommended to repeat the ECG in weeks to months to determine if resolved

CRP = C-reactive protein; ECG = electrocardiogram; ESR = erythrocyte sedimentation rate.

Source: Adapted from Rheumatic Heart Disease Australia (2022), Table 6.6.

INFECTIVE ENDOCARDITIS

LEARNING OBJECTIVE 8

Identify the two primary sources of the organisms responsible for infective endocarditis, and briefly outline how they are thought to contribute to heart failure.

Infective endocarditis is a common risk associated with valve and congenital defects, and people with these conditions require prophylactic antimicrobials prior to any surgical or dental intervention. Untreated, infective endocarditis is generally fatal; it has a mortality rate of approximately 14.5% in people who are treated. The two most common routes of access of the infective organism are intravenous needle use, particularly shared needles, and poor oral hygiene (see Figure 24.9). A number of organisms have been associated with infective endocarditis, particularly *Streptococcus* species and *Staphylococcus* species.

Clinical manifestations

Often, clinical manifestations of infective endocarditis are vague. Some people may complain of fever, anorexia, malaise and weight loss. They may also identify myalgias and arthralgias; however, when a person presents with dyspnoea, chest pain, overt symptoms of heart failure or even cerebrovascular accident, further investigations are necessary. A history of intravenous drug use may direct focus to tricuspid valve endocarditis.

Clinical diagnosis and management

Diagnosis There is a worldwide consensus that diagnosis for infective endocarditis is based on the modified *Duke diagnostic criteria*. The criteria relate to evidence obtained from microbiology, histology and clinical manifestations, and are designated as major and minor criteria. To be diagnosed with infective endocarditis, the person needs to have a combination of criteria. An example of a major criterion involves positive results obtained from blood cultures of typical organisms such as *Streptococcus bovis* or *Staphylococcus aureus*. Usually, two separate blood cultures need to be collected within two hours of presentation. However, *Coxiella burnetii*, a causative microorganism of infective endocarditis, is not readily detected in blood cultures. In this instance, a single positive blood culture result or a high immunoglobulin G (IgG) antibody titre for *Coxiella burnetii* will suffice.

Other major criteria include a positive echocardiogram result and evidence of new valvular regurgitation. A worsening or changing nature of a pre-existing murmur is not sufficient. Minor criteria include: a predisposition to infective endocarditis, including a prosthetic heart valve or a previous diagnosis of infective endocarditis; the presence of a fever of greater than

A
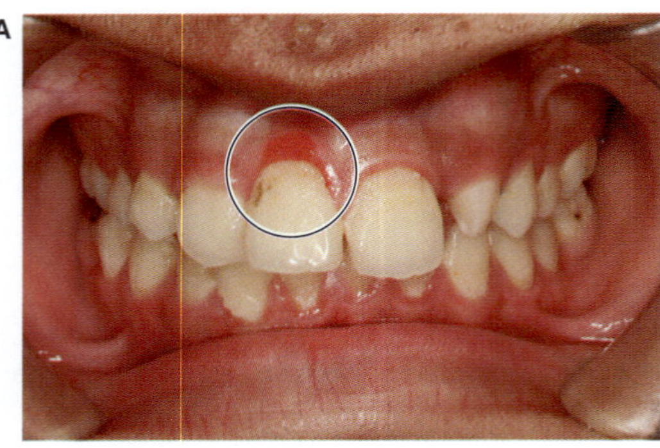
B
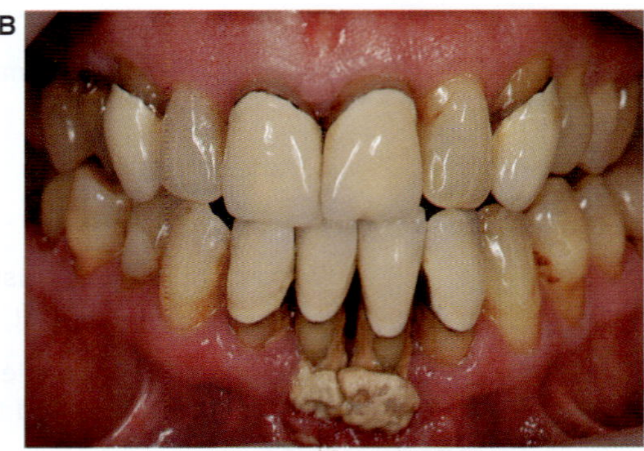

Figure 24.9

Gum disease as a source of infective endocarditis

Poor oral hygiene represents one of the two primary routes of access of the infective organisms responsible for infective endocarditis.

(A) Advanced gum disease (marked by the circle) is often missed, despite the fact that the gum appears swollen and angry.

(B) Aggressive gum disease is a serious condition and a recognised cause of infective endocarditis. Patients in hospital should be monitored, and a dental hygienist or dentist should be requested for people with signs of poor oral hygiene, as this is a preventable risk.

Sources: (A) watanyou/Getty Images; (B) thitinonjong/Shutterstock.

38°C; the presence of vascular phenomena, such as arterial emboli or pulmonary infarcts; the presence of immunological phenomena, such as glomerulonephritis and rheumatoid factor; and positive blood cultures that do not relate to major criteria.

Management Empirical treatment can be commenced before a definitive diagnosis of the causative organism is made. This treatment usually comprises benzylpenicillin, flucloxacillin and gentamicin. Benzyl-penicillin is a narrow-spectrum penicillin that is used for Gram-positive organisms. It is inactivated by β-lactamase, an enzyme produced by bacteria. Flucloxacillin is an anti-staphylococcal penicillin that is resistant to β-lactamase, so it can be used to cover β-lactamase-producing organisms, such as *Staphylococcus* spp. and *Streptococcus pyogenes*. Gentamicin is used to treat any Gram-negative organisms that may have caused the endocarditis. Targeted treatment is given once the causative organism has been determined.

Heart failure: risk factors, clinical manifestations, complications and diagnosis and management

LEARNING OBJECTIVE 9

Describe the risk factors, clinical manifestations, complications, and diagnosis and management of heart failure.

RISK FACTORS

The main risk factors for the development of heart failure are ischaemic heart disease, hypertension, venous insufficiency (e.g. varicose veins), valve disorders, cardiomyopathies and congenital heart defects. Consequently, it is not unusual for heart failure to represent a common secondary condition, and is rarely the identified cause of death. Acute heart failure is also often found in people post myocardial infarction, particularly those who have suffered an ST-elevation myocardial infarction (STEMI; see the chapter 'Coronary artery disease').

CLINICAL MANIFESTATIONS

As mentioned, the primary symptoms of heart failure are chronic tiredness, a decreased capacity for physical activity and shortness of breath, unless **congestive heart failure** has developed, in which case the location of the oedema is indicative of whether the heart failure is right-sided or left-sided (see Figure 24.10).

The loss of cardiac output causes muscle fatigue, urinary retention and signs of reduced central nervous system function (e.g. restlessness, confusion, anxiety, irritability and possibly personality changes), and these effects are the same regardless of whether it is the right side or the left side that is failing. If the heart failure has become congestive, then right versus left failure can be distinguished on the basis of the location of the oedema, with the right side causing an increased hydrostatic pressure in the periphery, while failure of the left side is associated with fluid in the lungs. This is easily remembered as *L* = *L*eft side = *L*ungs and *R* = *R*ight side = *R*est of the body.

Figure 24.11 explores the common clinical manifestations and management of left-sided heart failure and Figure 24.12 explores the common clinical manifestations and management of right-sided heart failure (*cor pulmonale*).

COMPLICATIONS

Several common complications are associated with heart failure; namely, atrial fibrillation, ventricular tachycardia or fibrillation,

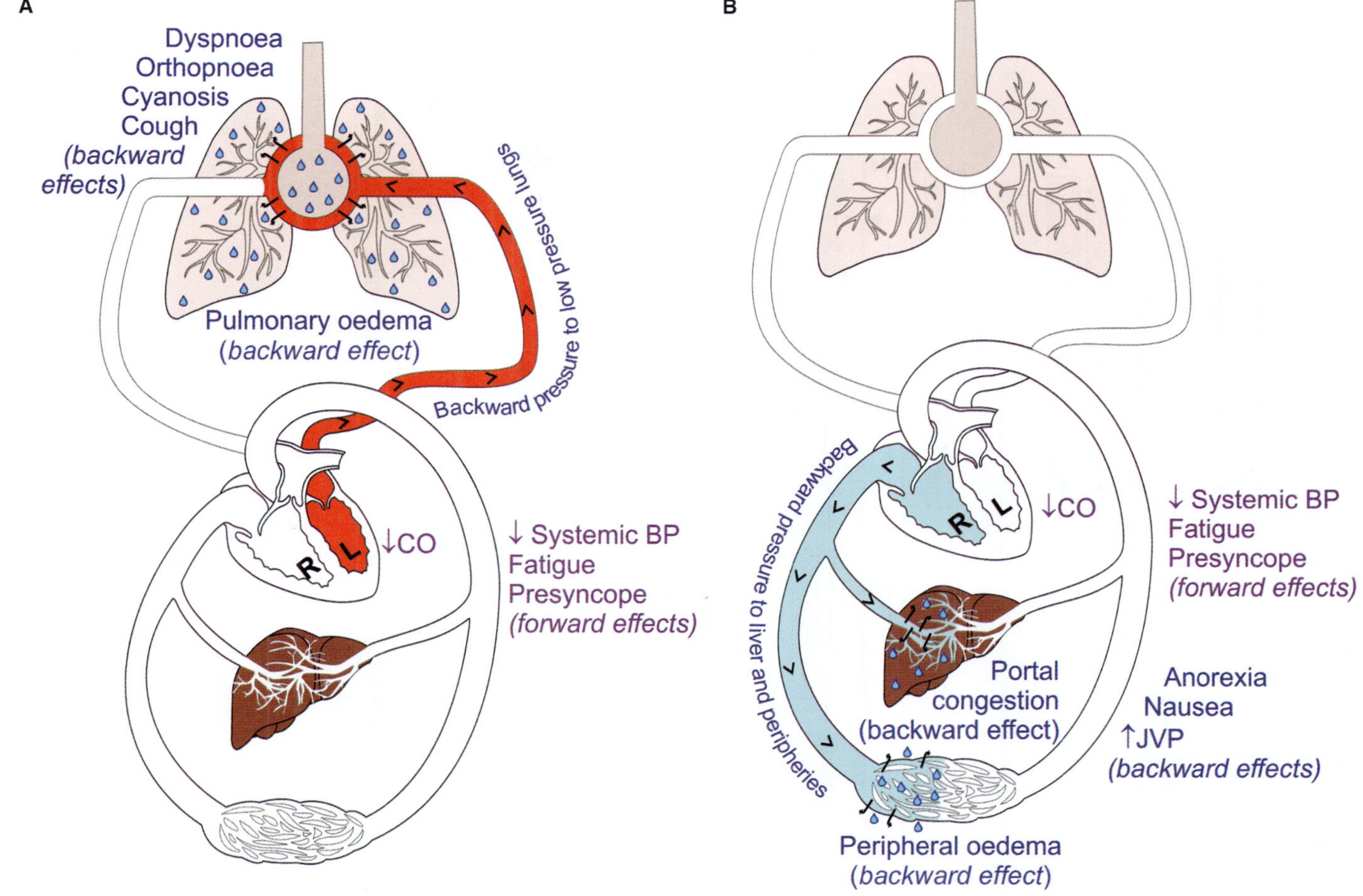

Figure 24.10

Signs of left-sided and right-sided heart failure

The forward effects of both (A) left-sided and (B) right-sided congestive heart failure are the same because they are directly related to the loss of cardiac output. The backward effects are the defining signs because they reflect the backlog of blood in the incoming venous circuit.

↓ = decrease in; ↑ = increase in; BP = blood pressure; CO = carbon monoxide; JVP = jugular venous pressure; L = left; R = right.

Source: Adapted from Bauldoff et al. (2020), Figures 30.1 and 30.2, p. 1045.

acute kidney failure, heart valve deterioration, myocardial infarction, stasis dermatitis and leg ulcers, and thromboembolism formation (and, therefore, stroke and myocardial infarction). *Atrial fibrillation* is generally the consequence of the remodelling of the myocardium, leading to instability of the resting membrane potential and episodic disruptions to atrial rhythm. Generally, these arise in the right atrium, and activity can be restricted to that chamber. *Ventricular tachycardias* and fibrillations also arise as a consequence of myocyte remodelling, with ventricular fibrillation the most dangerous rhythm disturbance, since in this case there is no cardiac output for the duration of the disrupted rhythm.

Acute kidney injury (see the chapter 'Acute kidney injury and chronic kidney disease') arises as a consequence of inadequate perfusion of the kidneys due to the generally reduced cardiac output. This can be aggravated by the prolonged use of non-steroidal anti-inflammatory drugs (NSAIDs), particularly aspirin, which can reduce renal blood flow in low cardiac output states. *Stasis dermatitis* is a condition in which the skin of the leg becomes thickened, shiny and scaly, and *ulcers* arise due to impaired venous return and increased hydrostatic pressure resulting in oedema and subsequently poor perfusion.

Myocardial infarction is the direct result of the ischaemic state of the heart due to the inadequate cardiac output (see the chapter 'Coronary artery disease'). Volume overload in the heart will strain the heart valves, as will remodelling changes to the myocardium, which will destabilise the integrity of the valves, further aggravating the heart failure.

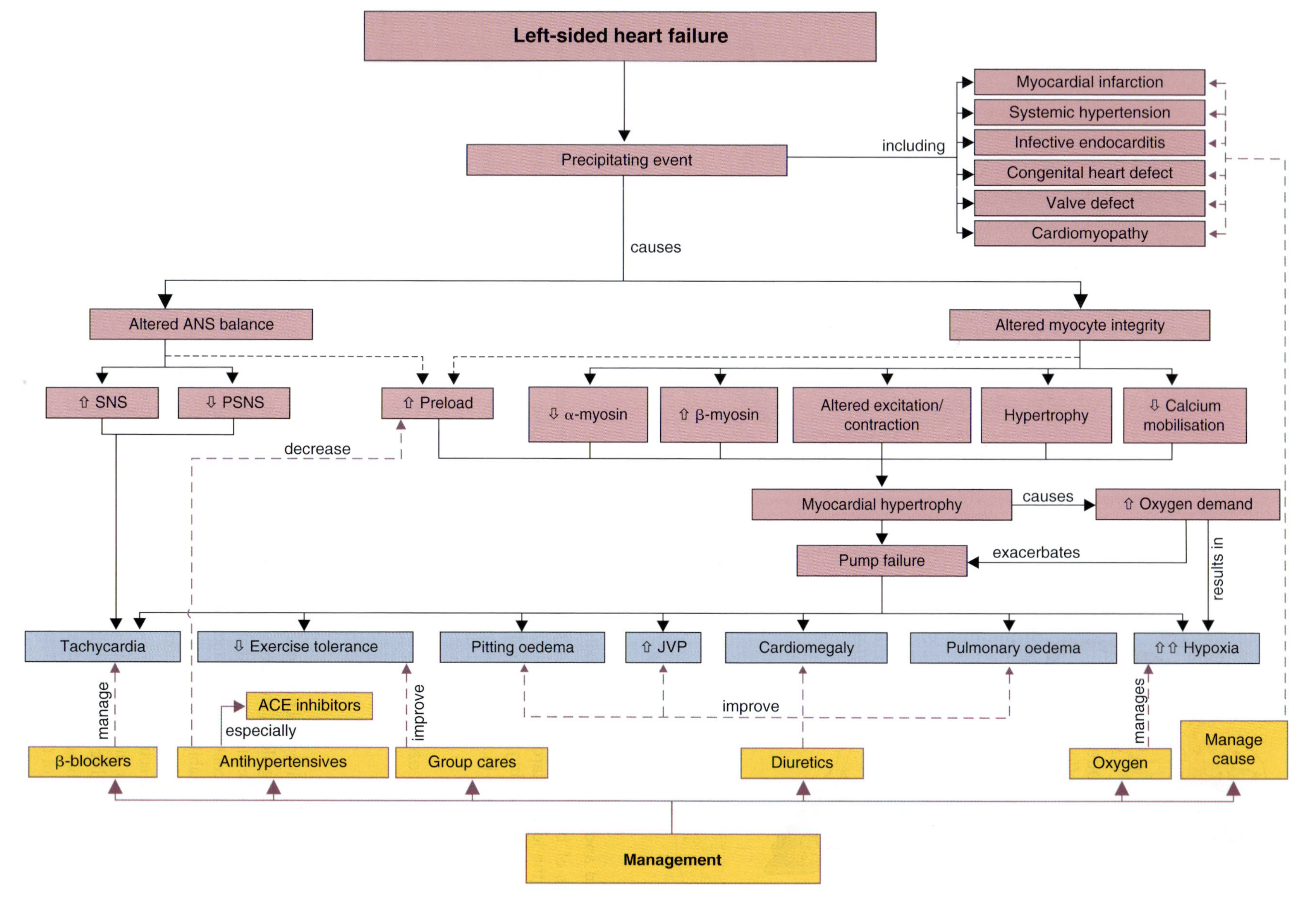

Figure 24.11

Clinical snapshot: Left-sided heart failure

↓ = decrease in; ↑ = increase in; α = alpha; β = beta; ACE = angiotensin-converting enzyme; ANS = autonomic nervous system; JVP = jugular venous pressure; PSNS = parasympathetic nervous system; SNS = sympathetic nervous system.

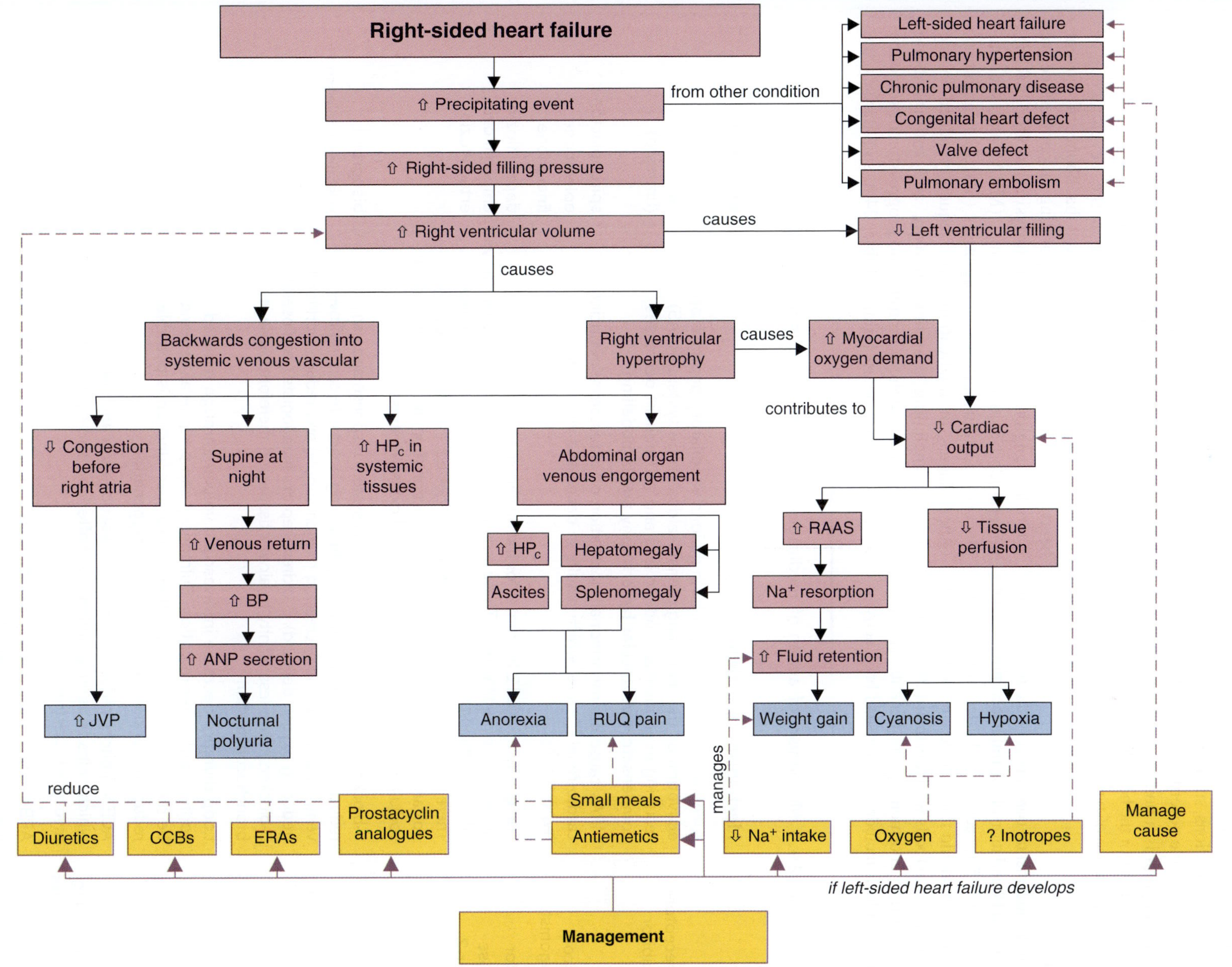

Figure 24.12

Clinical snapshot: Right-sided heart failure

↓ = decrease in; ↑ = increase in; ? = possibly; ANP = atrial natriuretic peptide; BP = blood pressure; CCBs = calcium channel blockers; ERAs = endothelin receptor antagonists; HP_c = capillary hydrostatic pressure; JVP = jugular venous pressure; Na^+ = sodium ion; RAAS = renin–angiogensin–aldosterone system; RUQ = right upper quadrant.

CLINICAL DIAGNOSIS AND MANAGEMENT

Diagnosis

The underlying cause of congestive heart failure can usually be identified from clinical assessment, electrocardiography (ECG) and chest X-ray. Other investigations, such as an echocardiogram, may be needed to determine the severity of the illness and the prognosis. An echocardiogram is a non-invasive procedure that evaluates the internal structures of the heart, valvular functioning, heart movement and the presence of pericardial fluid.

Management

Lifestyle changes are a fundamental component of the management of heart failure. The Heart Foundation of Australia recommends that fluid intake is limited to 1–1.5 L each day, adjusted as necessary. It is recommended that salt should not be added to food, and that salt intake should be limited to foods with less than 120 mg/100 g. Physical activity can lead to enormous health benefits, and it is recommended that individuals include 30 minutes of brisk activity for most days of the week. Alcohol intake should be restricted to two standard drinks a day (one standard drink = 10 g alcohol). Smoking is strongly discouraged. Individuals are advised to lose weight and to adopt good eating habits, including a balanced diet high in a range of fresh vegetables.

The underlying causes of heart failure, such as acute myocardial infarction, dysrhythmia and infections, should be treated promptly. As the prolonged use of NSAIDs can lead to heart failure, their use should be balanced between effectiveness and risk.

Recent advances have resulted in the development of a number of drugs which form the backbone of current heart failure management incorporating a cardioselective ß-blocker, angiotensin receptor–neprilysin inhibitor (ARNi), mineralocorticoid receptor antagonist (MRA) and sodium-glucose co-transporter-2 antagonist (SGLT2 inhibitor). Other classes of medications are frequently added to the regimen, including diuretics, digoxin, and antithrombotic therapy to manage the symptoms and progression of someone with congestive heart failure. Table 24.4 summarises the

Table 24.4 Mechanism of action of medications commonly used in heart failure

Class	Mechanism of action	Examples
ARNi Angiotensin receptor–neprilysin inhibitor	A combination drug which both inhibits vaodilatory peptides and activation of the renin–angiotensin–aldosterone system (RAAS) resulting in an increase sodium loss and subsequent decreases compensatory ventricular hypertrophy and remodelling	sacubitril/valsartan (Entresto)
MRA Mineralocorticoid receptor antagonist	MRAs cause neurohormonal modulation of aldosterone-reducing cardio-renal fibrosis, which results in decreased ventricular hypertrophy	spironolactone, eplerenone, finerenone
SGLT2 inhibitor Sodium-glucose co-transporter-2 antagonist	The effects of SGLT2 inhibitors for the management of heart failure appear to be multifactorial. These include the diuretic and antihypertensive effects (in the presence of hyperglycaemia—but not in euglycaemia). There are potential novel mechanisms suggested, including reduction of epicardial fat, improved ventricular contraction (from reduced intracellular sodium-calcium exchange), and reduced oxidative stress	dapagliflozin, empagliflozin, ertugliflozin
Cardioselective β-blocker	β-blockers reduce sympathetic nervous system response and can reduce heart rate and contractility. Reducing heart rate can improve ventricular filling time (increasing oxygen supply) and reduce workload (reducing oxygen demand). β_1-adrenoceptors antagonists (cardioselective β-blockers) have less affinity to airway tissue and therefore cause less bronchoconstriction	bisoprolol, sustained-release metoprolol, carvedilol
Diuretics	Loop diuretics decrease intravascular volume through reduced sodium and water retention. Pulmonary and peripheral oedema can be reduced, and an improvement in cardiac function is possible by reducing workload and increasing oxygenation	furosemide
ACEi Angiotensin-converting enzyme (ACE) inhibitors	ACE inhibitors reduce workload by vasodilation and sodium excretion which helps to reduce preload and afterload and subsequently cardiac myocyte hypertrophy.	enalapril perindopril
ARB Angiotensin receptor blockers	ARBs reduce workload, by vasodilation and sodium excretion working lower down on the RAAS than the ACEis. ARBs reduce preload and afterload and subsequently cardiac myocyte hypertrophy	candesartan irbesartan losartan valsartan

Sources: Data from Heidenreich et al. (2022); Kalsi et al. (2022); Kristjánsdóttir et al. (2020).

mechanism of action of medications commonly used in heart failure.

The use of *antithrombotic therapy* in heart failure is important to reduce the risk of thrombosis-related complications, such as stroke or myocardial infarction, in the presence of atrial fibrillation. The debate regarding the use of antithrombotic therapy for those with heart failure without atrial fibrillation is still ongoing, although early indications suggest that it may reduce the incidence of further adverse cardiovascular events.

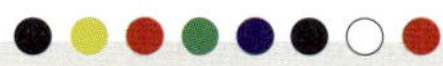

INDIGENOUS HEALTH FAST FACTS AND CULTURAL CONSIDERATIONS

FAST FACTS

- ***Aboriginal and Torres Strait Islander peoples accounted for 92% of all acute rheumatic fever in the five years preceding 2021.***
- ***Aboriginal and Torres Strait Islander peoples are 2.3 times more likely than non-Indigenous Australians to experience heart failure.***
- ***Aboriginal and Torres Strait Islander peoples are more than two times more likely than non-Indigenous Australians to die from heart failure.***
- ***Heart failure hospitalisation and mortality rates in Māori are 4 times higher than those for non-Māori New Zealanders.***
- ***Heart failure hospitalisation and mortality rates in New Zealand Pacific Islands people are more than 2 times higher than those for non-Māori New Zealanders.***
- ***Māori are 5.4 times more likely than European New Zealanders to die from rheumatic heart disease.***

CULTURAL CONSIDERATIONS

- ***A pivotal factor in reducing heart failure mortality is the commencement, maintenance and adjustment of the person's medication regimen. Aboriginal and Torres Strait Islander peoples may develop a distrust of healthcare services if they do not have a culturally appropriate, community-centred approach. Healthcare facilities are finding improved success when utilising Indigenous hospital liaison officers and cultural practice teams. Given that—irrespective of culture—heart failure mortality statistics within five years of diagnosis are already very high, any interventions that facilitate acceptance of treatment regimens by Aboriginal and Torres Strait Islander peoples would be beneficial.***

Sources: Data from Australian Commission on Safety and Quality in Health Care (2021); Australian Institute of Health and Welfare (2022b); Best Practice Advocacy Centre New Zealand (2022).

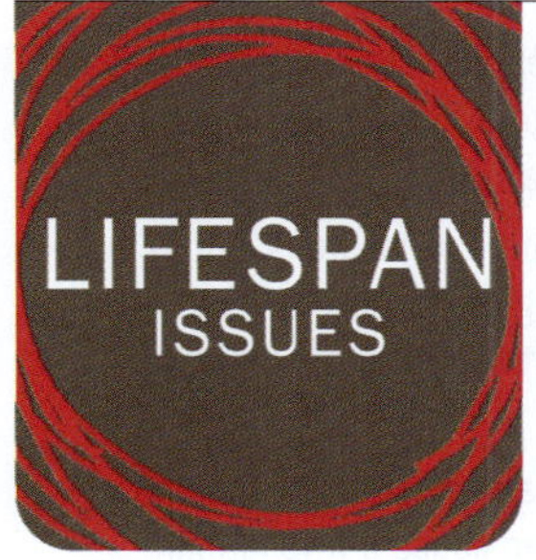

CHILDREN AND ADOLESCENTS

- Heart failure in children is significantly less common than in adults. Most heart failure deaths in children are as a result of congenital malformations of the circulatory system.
- Heart failure as a result of rheumatic heart disease may be more common in Australian and New Zealand children than in many other developed countries, as rheumatic heart disease is more common. However, statistics to support this hypothesis are difficult to locate.

OLDER ADULTS

- Heart failure is more common in older adults as a result of age-related decline in myocardial function and the increased incidence of coronary artery disease.
- Management of heart failure becomes more complex in the older adult as a result of differences in drug metabolism, increasing incidence of comorbidities, and the potential for adverse drug reactions from polypharmacy.

KEY CLINICAL ISSUES

- Community confusion exists between the terminology 'heart failure' and 'heart attack'. Be sure to educate those affected and those who care for them, where necessary.
- Heart failure can result in reduced blood pressure. In other conditions, hypotension is often treated with fluid support via a bolus of crystalloid or colloid solution. In heart failure, a fluid bolus is generally not indicated, and may actually exacerbate the hypotension. Counterintuitively, intravenous diuretics may actually be necessary to reduce myocardial load, improve contractility and increase blood pressure.
- Critical management interventions to reduce myocardial oxygen demand and increase myocardial oxygen supply can improve the clinical outcomes.
- Common risk factors for heart failure include hypertension, valve disorders, congenital heart defects and rheumatic fever. Ensure that cardiac assessment includes assessments and investigations to identify potential risk factors.
- People diagnosed with heart failure have a very complex and difficult life ahead of them. Many people do not live past five years after diagnosis. Mortality statistics are improving with better management of ischaemic heart disease; however, rigorous and complex management plans must be instituted to reduce mortality and morbidity risks.
- A key feature of heart failure is the *remodelling of the ventricular myocytes*, which results in cells that are less responsive to the sympathetic nervous system and markedly hypertrophied but energetically less efficient. This leads to a self-perpetuating loop that drives disease progress but makes the condition notoriously difficult to manage pharmacologically.
- Although many cases of heart failure have no recognised underlying trigger, *functional disruption* of the integrity of the heart, through congenital heart defects, cardiomyopathies or valve disorders, represents a common treatable cause.

CHAPTER REVIEW

- *Heart failure* occurs when the heart is unable to pump sufficient oxygenated, nutrient-rich blood to meet the demands of the tissues of the body.
- Heart failure may be described as either a *systolic* condition or a *diastolic* condition.
- Problems with *preload* are related to both insufficient venous return, often due to conditions such as paralysis and varicose veins, and excess venous return, providing too high a burden on the heart and compromising ejection efficiency.
- An excess *afterload* is most commonly associated with atherosclerosis and hypertension, and represents the force that the ventricle must overcome in order to eject the stroke volume.
- *Inotropic failure* is a loss of contractility of the heart muscle, most commonly due to previous myocardial infarction. A loss of ventricular muscle means that the heart is unable to generate sufficient force to eject blood, and may also have compromised relaxation, leading to inadequate ventricular filling.
- The compensatory mechanisms—namely activation of the *sympathetic nervous* system and *renin–angiotensin–aldosterone system*—can rectify some of the symptoms in the early stages of the development of heart failure, but will eventually exacerbate the condition, hastening its progression.

REVIEW QUESTIONS

1. What is heart failure, and to what does the word 'congestive' refer when a person is diagnosed as having congestive heart failure?
2. How does the hypertrophy seen in people with heart failure differ from that seen in athletes?
3. What are the two types of hypertrophy seen in heart failure, and what is the proposed cause of each?
4. Both insufficient and excessive preload can lead to heart failure. How is this possible?
5. What are the common sources of excess afterload in heart failure? How can heart failure symptoms arise as the result of this elevated afterload?
6. How does an undiagnosed ventricular septal defect cause heart failure?
7. How do both valve stenosis and valve regurgitation lead to a volume overload that can precipitate symptoms of heart failure?
8. Mrs Bonato is a 62-year-old woman who comes to see her general practitioner complaining of fatigue, poor appetite, and marked swelling in her hands and feet. She says that her family has been complaining that she's always moody and has a tendency to 'bite their heads off' if they disagree with her on anything. She has a history of mild asthma, has never been athletic, is markedly overweight, and isn't particularly attentive to her diet. The doctor diagnoses her with congestive heart failure and prescribes a diuretic and digoxin to manage her condition. The following questions refer to Mrs Bonato.
   a. Mrs Bonato doesn't understand what heart failure is, and is worried that whatever it is means that she's going to have a 'heart attack'. Explain the difference between 'heart failure' and a 'heart attack' to Mrs Bonato.
   b. Mrs Bonato's concern about having a myocardial infarction is justified. Explain how heart failure can cause a myocardial infarction.
   c. Mrs Bonato doesn't understand how she could have developed heart failure. Describe the three pressures on the heart that lead to heart failure, and how they can cause heart failure.
   d. Given Mrs Bonato's symptoms, is her heart failure right-sided or left-sided? Justify your answer.

HEALTH PROFESSIONAL CONNECTIONS

Midwives Congenital heart malformations can lead to acute heart failure in neonates. In an adult, a common method of determining heart malformations is listening to heart sounds. In neonates, auscultation can be difficult because the shunts required in utero are still in the process of closing. Because a neonate can only manipulate heart rate to increase cardiac output (a neonate's blood pressure is critically rate-dependent, as their myocardium is too immature to increase contractility), they can deteriorate very quickly. Other signs of heart function should be monitored closely, and changes in observations should be reported and acted on quickly.

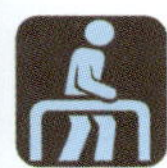

Physiotherapists Designing a rehabilitation program for people with heart failure is a common task for physiotherapists, but this task may be shared with cardiac rehabilitation exercise scientists. However, the role of a physiotherapist is critical in the rehabilitation and care of people with heart failure in intensive care units. Pulmonary physiotherapy is important for improving ventilation, reducing respiratory infections and increasing oxygenation. Range-of-movement exercises, strengthening, and assessment and assistance with mobilisation are also central to the care of critically ill people with heart failure.

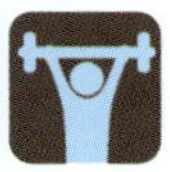

Exercise scientists Marked improvement in ventricular function and exercise tolerance can be achieved through appropriate exercise prescription and close monitoring in people with heart failure. An increase in stroke volume and, ultimately, cardiac output can be accompanied by a decrease in peripheral vascular resistance and better blood pressure control. Reduced levels of depression have also been reported when people with heart failure participate in individually tailored cardiac rehabilitation programs. Exercise scientists need to understand the balance between myocardial oxygen demand and supply, and the myocyte changes that occur in heart failure, to be able to design and prescribe appropriate programs. Communication with other members of the healthcare team is also imperative to ensure that a united approach can be achieved.

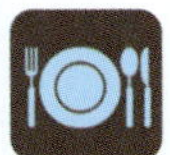

Nutritionists/Dieticians As with all individuals with cardiovascular system pathology, specific dietary programs are required. People with heart failure should be encouraged to decrease their sodium and fat intake, increase their fibre and potassium intake, and manage their fluid intake. Working with people experiencing heart failure can be difficult, as they are often obese as a result of many years of poor nutritional choices. Hypoxia and exercise intolerance can interfere with their daily activities; however, a hypermetabolic state to compensate for the inadequate tissue oxygenation can complicate calculation of caloric requirements. Individual planning and significant support and follow-up is often required to effect changes to a client's dietary choices.

CASE STUDY

Mr Fritz Matthews is a 75-year-old man (UR number 798455) who presented with paroxysmal nocturnal dyspnoea (PND) and orthopnoea from an episode of acute heart failure. He has a history of uncontrolled hypertension refractory to many different hypertensive agents trialled, although there is some concern about his ability to remember to take them. His observations were as follows:

Temperature	Heart rate	Respiration rate	Blood pressure	SpO_2
36.8°C	88	18	172/74	92% O_2 via NP * @4 L/min

*NP = nasal prongs.

Mr Matthews is newly widowed and lives alone. His diet consists of frozen meals. He weighs 117 kg and is 178 cm tall. His pathology results are as follows:

HAEMATOLOGY

Patient location:	Ward 3	**UR:**	798455		
Consultant:	Smith	**NAME:**	Matthews		
		Given name:	Fritz	**Sex:**	M
		DOB:	13/02/XX	**Age:**	75

Time collected	15:30
Date collected	XX/XX
Year	XXXX
Lab #	26783642

FULL BLOOD COUNT		UNITS	REFERENCE RANGE
Haemoglobin	120	g/L	115–160
White cell count	5.3	$\times 10^9$/L	4.0–11.0
Platelets	429	$\times 10^9$/L	140–400
Haematocrit	0.37		0.33–0.47
Red cell count	4.71	$\times 10^{12}$/L	3.80–5.20
Reticulocyte count	0.9	%	0.2–2.0
MCV	87	fL	80–100
Neutrophils	3.99	$\times 10^9$/L	2.00–8.00
Lymphocytes	2.18	$\times 10^9$/L	1.00–4.00
Monocytes	0.39	$\times 10^9$/L	0.10–1.00
Eosinophils	0.26	$\times 10^9$/L	<0.60
Basophils	0.12	$\times 10^9$/L	<0.20
ESR	7	mm/h	<12
COAGULATION PROFILE			
aPTT	22	secs	24–40
PT	13	secs	11–17
ABG			
pH	7.32		7.35–7.45
$PaCO_2$	49	mmHg	35–45
PaO_2	84	mmHg	>80
HCO_3^-	27	mmHg	22-26
Oxygen saturations	89	%	>95

BIOCHEMISTRY

Patient location:	Ward 3	**UR:**	798455		
Consultant:	Smith	**NAME:**	Matthews		
		Given name:	Fritz	**Sex:**	M
		DOB:	13/02/XX	**Age:**	75

Time collected	15:30
Date collected	XX/XX
Year	XXXX
Lab #	29874267

ELECTROLYTES		UNITS	REFERENCE RANGE
Sodium	138	mmol/L	135–145
Potassium	3.2	mmol/L	3.5–5.2
Chloride	105	mmol/L	95–110
Bicarbonate	27	mmol/L	22–32
Glucose	8.3	mmol/L	3.5–5.4
Iron	10	μmol/L	11–30

CRITICAL THINKING

1. Given Mr Matthews' history, explain the mechanisms that have contributed to the development of his acute heart failure.
2. What are PND and orthopnoea? Why have they developed in Mr Matthews' case?
3. Mr Matthews is hypoxic. Examine his haematology results and determine whether these are contributing to his hypoxia. Explain.
4. What interventions (pharmacological and non-pharmacological) should be undertaken to assist Mr Matthews with his respiratory compromise?
5. Mr Matthews has received intravenous diuretics. Observe his biochemistry results and determine which parameter is becoming problematic. Explain the mechanism of this change. What other observations should be undertaken? What interventions should be undertaken to assist with this situation?
6. What is Mr Matthews' body mass index (BMI) reading? Is this acceptable? Does this contribute to his acute heart failure? Note his glucose result. What is the relationship between his BMI, glucose and cardiovascular status?

BIBLIOGRAPHY

Adamo, M., Gardner, R.S., McDonagh, T.A. & Metra, M. (2022). The 'Ten Commandments' of the 2021 ESC Guidelines for the diagnosis and treatment of acute and chronic heart failure. *European Heart Journal* 43(6):440–41. https://doi.org/10.1093/eurheartj/ehab853.

American Heart Association (2017). *Heart failure in children and adolescents*. Dallas: American Heart Association. https://www.heart.org/en/health-topics/heart-failure/what-is-heart-failure/heart-failure-in-children-and-adolescents.

Australian Bureau of Statistics (ABS) (2016). *Causes of death, Australia, 2015.* Canberra: ABS. https://www.abs.gov.au/statistics/health/causes-death/causes-death-australia/.

Australian Commission on Safety and Quality in Healthcare (ACSQHC) (2021). 2.2 Heart failure. *The fourth Australian atlas of healthcare variation.* Sydney: ACSQHC. https://www.safetyandquality.gov.au/publications-and-resources/resource-library/fourth-atlas-2021-22-heart-failure.

Australian Health Ministers' Advisory Council's National and Aboriginal and Torres Strait Islander Health Standing Committee (2017). *Cultural respect framework 2016–2026: for Aboriginal and Torres Strait Islander health—a national approach to building a culturally respectful health system.* Canberra: Australian Government Department of Health. https://nacchocommunique.files.wordpress.com/2016/12/cultural_respect_framework_1december2016_1.pdf.

Australian Institute of Health and Welfare (AIHW) (2017). *Aboriginal and Torres Strait Islander Health Performance Framework: 2017 report*. Cat. No. 181. Canberra: AIHW. https://www.aihw.gov.au/reports/indigenous-australians/health-performance-framework-2017-sa/contents/table-of-contents.

Australian Institute of Health and Welfare (AIHW) (2019). *Principal diagnosis data cubes: separation statistics by principal diagnosis (ICD-10-AM, Australia,) 2018–19. National Hospital Morbidity Database.* Canberra: AIHW. https://www.aihw.gov.au/reports/hospitals/principal-diagnosis-data-cubes/contents/data-cubes.

Australian Institute of Health and Welfare (AIHW) (2021). *Heart, stroke and vascular disease—Australian facts: Congenital heart disease.* Canberra: AIHW. Retrieved from https://www.aihw.gov.au/reports/heart-stroke-vascular-diseases/hsvd-facts/contents/summary-of-coronary-heart-disease-and-stroke/coronary-heart-disease.

Australian Institute of Health and Welfare (AIHW) (2022a). *Acute rheumatic fever and rheumatic heart disease in Australia 2016–2022*. Cat. No. CVD 95. Canberra: AIHW. Retrieved from https://www.aihw.gov.au/reports/indigenous-australians/rheumatic-heart-disease-in-australia-2016-2020/summary.

Australian Institute of Health and Welfare (AIHW) (2022b). *Australia's health, 2022.* Australia's Health series No. 18. Cat. No. AUS 241. Canberra: AIHW. https://www.aihw.gov.au/reports/australias-health/australias-health-2022-in-brief/summary.

Bauldoff, G., Gubrud-Howe, P.M., Carno, M.-A., Levett-Jones, T., Hales, M., Berry, K., … Stanley, D. (2020). *LeMone and Burke's medical–surgical nursing : critical thinking for person-centred care* (4th [Australian] edn). Sydney: Pearson Australia.

Best, O. & Fredericks, B. (2021). *Yatdjuligin: Aboriginal and Torres Strait Islander nursing and midwifery care*. (3rd edn). Port Melbourne, VIC: Cambridge University Press.

Best Practice Advocacy Centre New Zealand (BPAC NZ) (2022). *Addressing heart failure in primary care: Part 1—Identifying and diagnosing heart failure.* Dunedin: BPAC NZ. https://bpac.org.nz/2022/heart-failure-part-1.aspx.

Brusch, J.L. (2022). Infective endocarditis. *Emedicine.* https://emedicine.medscape.com/article/216650-overview.

Bullock, S. & Manias, E. (2022). *Fundamentals of pharmacology* (9th edn). Sydney: Pearson Australia.

Dumitru, I. (2022). Heart failure. *Emedicine*. https://emedicine.medscape.com/article/163062-overview.

Guggilla, R.K., Sowa, P.M., Jamiolkowski, J., Sinnadurai, S., Amin, A. & Kaminski, K.A. (2020). Effects of neurohormonal antagonists on blood pressure in patients with heart failure with reduced ejection fraction (HFrEF): a systematic review protocol. *Systematic Reviews* 9(1):194. https://doi.org/10.1186/s13643-020-01452-0.

Heidenreich, P.A., Bozkurt, B., Aguilar, D., Allen, L.A., Byun, J.J., Colvin, M.M., … Yancy, C. W. (2022). 2022 AHA/ACC/HFSA Guideline for the Management of Heart Failure: a report of the American College of Cardiology/American Heart Association Joint Committee on clinical practice guidelines. *Journal of the American College of Cardiology* 79(17):e263–e421. https://doi.org/10.1016/j.jacc.2021.12.012.

Kalsi, M.S., Dayawansa, N., Winderlich, J. & Vaddadi, G. (2022). The evolving face of heart failure management. *Australian Journal of General Practice* 51(9):653–658. https://doi.org/10.31128/AJGP-03-22-6350.

Kristjánsdóttir, I., Thorvaldsen, T. & Lund, L.H. (2020). Congestion and diuretic resistance in acute or worsening heart failure. *Cardiac Failure Review* 6:e25–e25. https://doi.org/10.15420/cfr.2019.18.

Lameire, N. (2023). Renal mechanisms of diuretic resistance in congestive heart failure. *Kidney and Dialysis 3*(1):56–72. https://doi.org/10.3390/kidneydial3010005.

Lily, L.S. (ed.) (2020). *Pathophysiology of heart disease* (6th edn). Baltimore, MD: Lippincott Williams & Wilkins.

Marieb, E.N. & Hoehn, K. (2019). *Human anatomy and physiology* (11th edn). San Francisco, CA: Pearson Benjamin Cummings.

McDonagh, T.A., Metra, M., Adamo, M., Gardner, R.S., Baumbach, A., Böhm, M., … ESC Scientific Document Group. (2021). 2021 ESC guidelines for the diagnosis and treatment of acute and chronic heart failure. *European Heart Journal* 42(36):3599–3726. https://doi.org/10.1093/eurheartj/ehab368.

Morton, S.U., Quiat, D., Seidman, J.G. & Seidman, C.E. (2022). Genomic frontiers in congenital heart disease. *Nature Reviews Cardiology* 19(1):26–42. https://doi.org/10.1038/s41569-021-00587-4.

Muhamed, B., Parks, T. & Sliwa, K. (2020). Genetics of rheumatic fever and rheumatic heart disease. *Nature Reviews Cardiology* 17(3):145–54. https://doi.org/10.1038/s41569-019-0258-2.

National Heart Foundation of Australia (2016). *Guideline for the diagnosis and management of hypertension in adults*. Melbourne: National Heart Foundation of Australia. https://www.heartfoundation.org.au/getmedia/c83511ab-835a-4fcf-96f5-88d770582ddc/PRO-167_Hypertension-guideline-2016_WEB.pdf.

New Zealand Ministry of Health (2015). *Tatau kahukura: Māori health chart book 2015* (3rd edn). Wellington: Ministry of Health. https://www.health.govt.nz/publication/tatau-kahukura-maori-health-chart-book-2015-3rd-edition.

New Zealand Ministry of Health (2017). *Annual update of key results 2015/16: New Zealand health survey—interactive*. Wellington: Ministry of Health. https://www.health.govt.nz/publication/annual-update-key-results-2015-16-new-zealand-health-survey.

Rheumatic Hear Disease (RHD) Australia (ARF/RHD writing group). (2022). *The 2020 Australian guideline for prevention, diagnosis and management of acute rheumatic fever and rheumatic heart disease. (3.2 edn).* Casuarina, NT: National Heart Foundation of Australia & the Cardiac Society of Australia and New Zealand. https://www.rhdaustralia.org.au/system/files/fileuploads/arf_rhd_guidelines_3.2_edition_march_2022.pdf.

Satou, G.M. & Halnon, N.J. (2019). Pediatric congestive heart failure. *Emedicine.* https://emedicine.medscape.com/article/2069746-overview.

Savarese, G., Becher, P.M., Lund, L.H., Seferovic, P., Rosano, G.M.C. & Coats, A.J.S. (2023). Global burden of heart failure: a comprehensive and updated review of epidemiology. *Cardiovascular Research* 118(17):3272–3287. https://doi.org/10.1093/cvr/cvac013.

Sindone, A.P., De Pasquale, C., Amerena, J., Burdeniuk, C., Chan, A., Coats, A., … Atherton, J.J. (2022). Consensus statement on the current pharmacological prevention and management of heart failure. *Medical Journal of Australia* 217(4):212–17. https://doi.org/10.5694/mja2.51656.

Dysrhythmias

25

LEARNING OBJECTIVES

After completing this chapter, you should be able to:

1. Differentiate between tachycardia and bradycardia.
2. Explain how early after-depolarisation alters the rhythm of the heart.
3. Explain the relationship between potassium and digoxin in the context of dysrhythmia.
4. Differentiate between various conduction blocks.
5. Explain the difference between supraventricular tachycardia and ventricular tachycardia.

WHAT YOU SHOULD KNOW BEFORE YOU START THIS CHAPTER

Can you identify structures of the heart, and describe their functions?

Can you identify the major parts of the cardiac conduction system, and the contribution each part makes?

Can you identify the various waveforms on an electrocardiogram (ECG), and outline the cardiac event each represents?

KEY TERMS

Atrial fibrillation
Atrial flutter
Atrial tachycardia (AT)
Bradycardia
Conduction block
Delayed after-depolarisation (DAD)
Dysrhythmias
Early after-depolarisation (EAD)
Escape rhythm
Fibrillation
Premature ventricular complex
Re-entry
Supraventricular tachycardia (SVT)
Tachycardia
Ventricular fibrillation
Ventricular tachycardia (VT)

Introduction

LEARNING OBJECTIVE 1

Differentiate between tachycardia and bradycardia.

Disturbances of the rhythm of the heart are referred to as **dysrhythmias**. Clinically, and in some texts, these abnormalities are called *arrhythmias*. Although commonly used, the term 'arrhythmia' may be incorrect, as it literally means an 'absence of rhythm', when the condition is actually characterised by an *altered rhythm*. Dysrhythmias reflect an alteration of the electrical activity of the heart, either at the level of the conduction network of the heart or because of an altered electrical stability of the myocytes. Dysrhythmias are quite common, with *atrial fibrillation (AF)* by far the most common of all serious rhythm disturbances. Of the almost 115,000 people admitted with dysrhythmia as the principal diagnosis across Australian hospitals between 2020 and 2021, 66% were admitted with AF. The prevalence of AF is estimated at 2.2% of Australians, but 5.4% of people over 55 years of age. AF poses significant mortality and morbidity risks, including a two-fold increase in mortality and a five-fold increase in stroke. Dysrhythmias may be grouped into two broad categories: tachycardias and bradycardias.

By definition, a **tachycardia** is an adult heart rate greater than 100 beats per minute (bpm), while **bradycardia** is a rate less than 60 bpm in an adult. To be classed as *'sinus' dysrhythmia*, such as a sinus tachycardia, the *sinoatrial (SA) node* must control the rhythm, as evidenced by the presence of all three primary landmarks on the electrocardiogram (ECG), namely the P, R and T waves, such that each P wave is followed by a QRS complex and a T wave. The PR interval and QRS complex should be the ideal speed (between 120–200 ms/s and 80–120 ms/s, respectively) (see Figure 25.1).

Tachycardias can be restricted to either the upper chambers *(atria)* or the lower chambers *(ventricles)*, can be generalisable *(sinus tachycardia)* or can originate in the atria and spread to the ventricles *(supraventricular tachycardia)*. Despite the many variations, the root cause of a tachycardia comes down to one of three basic mechanisms: *re-entry*, which accounts for approximately 75% of all tachycardias. *early after-depolarisation* and *delayed after-depolarisation* (explained later in this chapter).

By contrast, a **fibrillation**, whether it occurs in the atria or the ventricles, represents a type of *electrical storm in the heart* (likened to epilepsy in brain tissue). As a result, individual myocytes contract independently instead of as a coordinated whole (a functional syncytium). While a person with a relatively healthy left ventricle can more readily tolerate an **atrial fibrillation**, a **ventricular fibrillation** constitutes a medical emergency, as the failure of the myocytes to contract in a coordinated fashion means that there is no stroke volume ejected from the heart and subsequently no cardiac output. Unless reversed quickly, ventricular fibrillation will result in death.

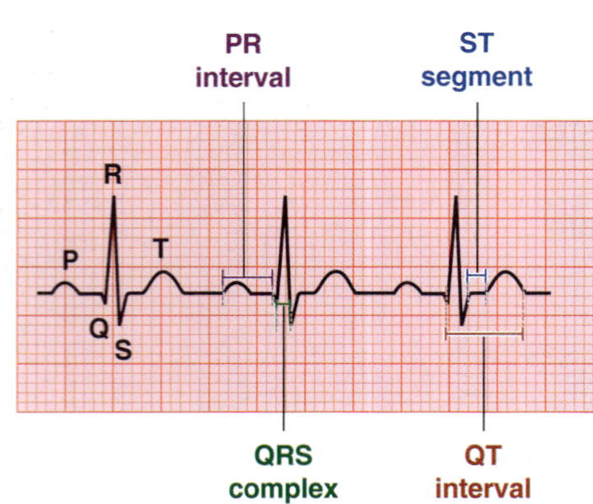

Figure 25.1

Landmarks on the electrocardiogram (ECG)

The first waveform demonstrates labelling of the P, Q, R, S and T components. The second waveform demonstrates the PR interval and QRS complex. The third waveform demonstrates the ST segment and QT interval.

Bradycardias comprise a small set of disturbances; namely, true bradycardias, escape rhythms and conduction blocks. The most common cause of a *true bradycardia* (also known as a *sinus bradycardia*) is treatment with beta-blockers. A person who experiences ventricular slowing is more likely to have an escape rhythm or a conduction block. A true **escape rhythm** occurs when the SA node has been destroyed, most commonly due to a myocardial infarction, causing control of the cardiac rhythm to default to the next most powerful pacemaker, namely the atrioventricular (AV) node. The intrinsic rate of the AV node is approximately 50–60 bpm, so this constitutes a bradycardia. In this case there is no atrial contraction, since SA node function is lost; hence, cardiac output will be reduced, as the final 20–30% of ventricular filling is due to the atrial contraction (otherwise known as 'atrial kick').

A **conduction block** occurs when the AV node or the bundles of His are damaged, again most often due to a myocardial infarction, leading to intermittent or interrupted conduction of the electrical signal between the atria and ventricles. The four basic types of AV conduction block range from the benign *first-degree block* to a complete block (*third-degree block*). In a complete block, the AV node or bundles of His have been destroyed and there is no communication between the atria and the ventricles. In this latter case, the ventricles experience a functional escape rhythm, as their pace will be set by the section of the conduction network with the fastest intrinsic rate located after the destroyed region.

Aetiology and pathophysiology

Despite the appearance of the various dysrhythmias on the ECG trace, a small set of underlying mechanisms are believed to be responsible. Interestingly, research into the genetic basis of some rhythm disturbances demonstrates that ion channel mutations contribute to these same mechanisms. In order to examine the pathophysiology of altered cardiac rhythm, dysrhythmias will be addressed in their two common groups: tachycardias/fibrillations and bradycardias/conduction blocks.

TACHYCARDIA AND FIBRILLATION

The mechanism most responsible for either a tachycardia or a fibrillation in any part of the heart is re-entry. The other two mechanisms are *early after-depolarisations* (*EADs*; also known as *early after-polarisations, EAPs*) and *delayed after-depolarisations* (*DADs*; or *delayed after-polarisations, DAPs*).

Re-entry

Re-entry mechanisms can occur in any part of the heart, be it a component of the conduction network or within the myocardium. The principal feature of **re-entry** is that an electrical signal is given an opportunity to re-excite the cells of the heart more than once. Normally, the electrical signal travels in a fixed path for a fixed period of time, and is extinguished once all of the cells are involved in the action potential (see Figure 25.2). In re-entry, a signal re-enters a patch of cells that it has already excited, often because the initial signal has followed an alternate pathway through the tissue or because the timing of the signal has been altered. Although any component of the heart can experience re-entry, we will focus on one example of a re-entry mechanism in the myocardium.

When an electrical signal is sent out from the SA node, it travels through the rapidly conducting fibres of the conduction network (see Figure 25.2). These cells then feed sodium and potassium ions into the surrounding myocytes through the gap junctions down the electrical gradient between the two cells. Once one myocyte gains positive ions in this way, the inside of its cell has a higher concentration than its neighbours, which drives these ions into the neighbouring cell. As each cell gains enough positive ions to hit the membrane threshold potential, the action potential takes hold and an enormous rush of positive ions now enters the cell, further driving the movement of ions between cells.

The direction of this wave of electrical activity (i.e. ion movement) is dictated by the position of the conduction network fibres and the presence of non-conducting features of the heart, such as the fibrous cytoskeleton, small blood vessels and capillaries, or possibly scar tissue. The electrical signal will need to bypass these structures, which is facilitated by the organisation of the myocytes. In a re-entry situation, however, the direction of the wave is disrupted, usually as a consequence of a *transient block* somewhere within the myocardium (see Figure 25.3).

The source of this transient block can be a small ischaemic episode that temporarily damages a set of cells, making them incapable of participating in the development of an action potential (which is why people with angina or post-myocardial infarction are at risk of dysrhythmia). Another cause might be a local electrolyte disturbance that lowers the resting membrane potential to a more negative value, which means that the cells are too far from threshold to participate in the action potential and subsequent contraction. Regardless of the underlying reason, the conduction of the signal is temporarily blocked, forcing the electrical wave to alter its normal pathway. This transient block is considered to be the first condition that must be met in order to set up a re-entry circuit.

In the example shown in Figure 25.3, this transient block is on one side of an electrically inert structure, in this case a small blood vessel or capillary. However, ions are still being conducted between the cells on the opposite side of this blood vessel. Normally, the two signals would meet at the bottom of the inert region as their transit time would be identical, but in a re-entry situation the signal from the 'normal' side does not encounter the signal from the other side. Since ions will freely move along their gradient and the gap junctions allow the movement of ions in both directions, the signal will now enter the side of the blood vessel on which the

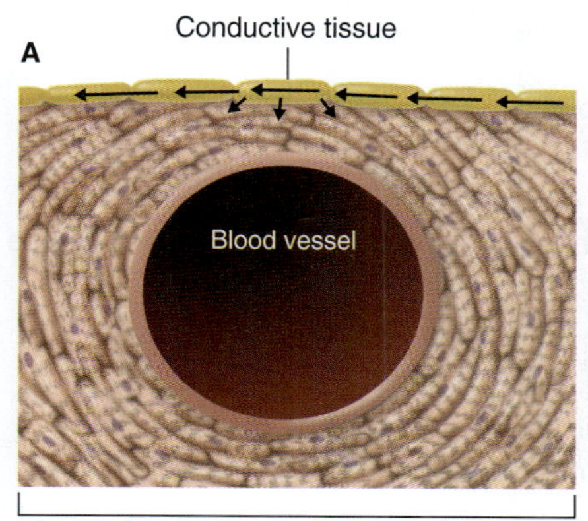

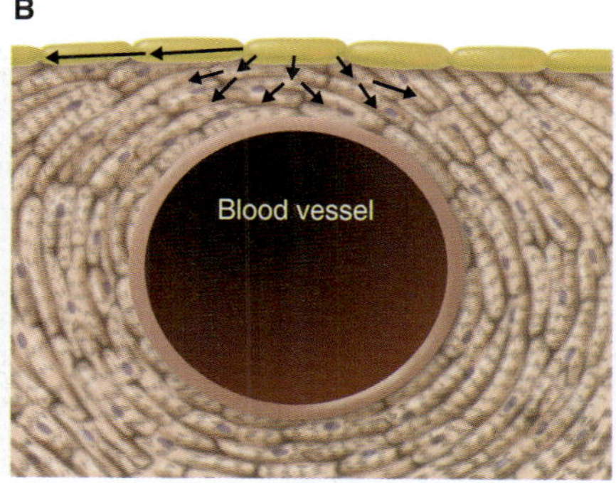

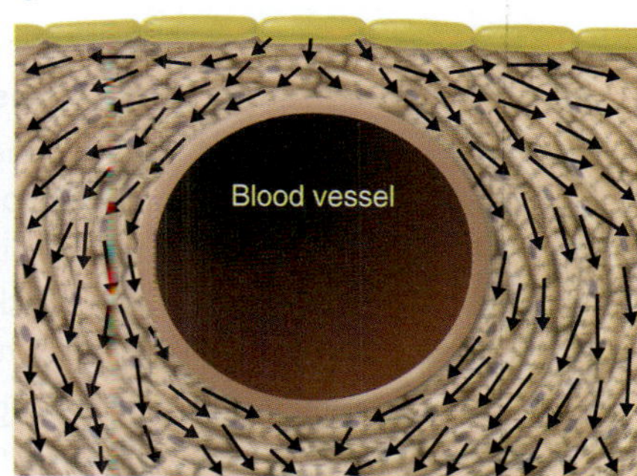

Figure 25.2

Normal pathway of conduction through the myocardium

(A) An electrical signal sent out from the sinoatrial node diffuses into the surrounding myocardium by the movement of positively charged ions into the myocytes.

(B) As the intracellular concentration of positive ions increases, a gradient is created between these cells and their neighbours. This gradient drives positive ions into the neighbouring myocytes through the gap junctions.

(C) As the myocytes are organised around non-conducting obstacles, such as a blood vessel, the electrical signal bypasses the obstacle, creating two avenues through which the signal traverses. As conduction speed is uniform throughout the normal myocardium, the cellular ion concentrations at the bottom of the obstacle are of equal value, cancelling out the gradient. All cells will now achieve threshold and begin the action potential that leads to a myocardial contraction.

Source: Anna-Marie Babey.

A

Blood vessel

The transient block is gone, and these cells start to receive the incoming signal

B

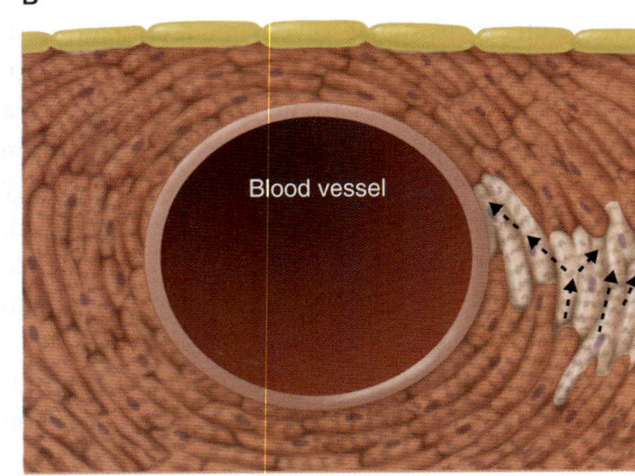

C

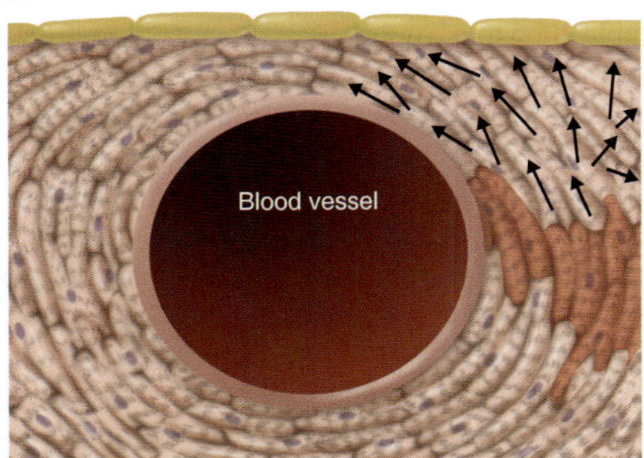

D

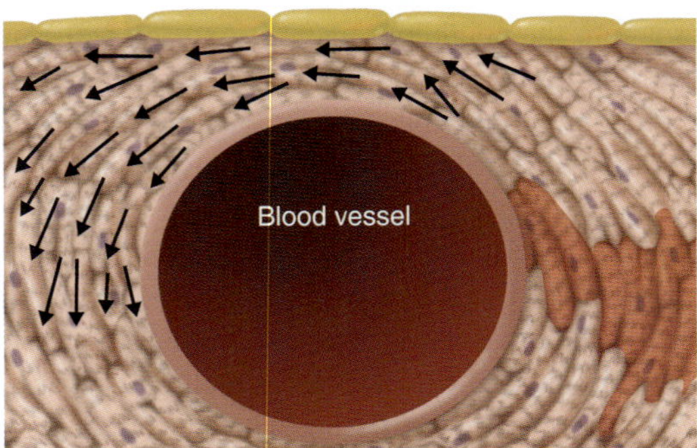

Figure 25.3

Altered electrical conduction as a consequence of re-entry

(A) Re-entry can be initiated by a number of factors, but a transient block is most common, resulting in a group of cells that either do not receive an inflow of positive ions or receive a reduced flow. Once the transient block has passed, these cells begin to receive an inflow of positive ions.

(B) Conduction through previously blocked cells is slowed, because these cells are not responding at a normal rate. During this delay, all of the other cells have entered into their action potential and begin to contract.

(C) If the delay is sufficiently long enough, the other cells will have completed their action potential by the time the signal finishes its transit through the previously blocked cells, which allows the signal to re-enter the unaffected cells.

(D) The previously blocked cells will experience a contraction. The re-entry signal now spreads throughout the myocardium, creating a second beat of the heart. As long as the previously blocked cells have delayed conduction, this signal can continue to repeat through the tissue and generate additional beats of the heart. If sufficient numbers are generated, the person can experience tachycardia.

Source: Anna-Marie Babey.

transient block was located, and start to move up that side in a direction backwards to the normal movement of the electrical wave.

By this time, whatever caused the transient block has passed, but has left the cells that were part of that block injured or otherwise experiencing a reduced function. Causes of this might include free radical damage to proteins, such as ion channels or those that create the gap junction pore, local changes to membrane potential or altered membrane stability. In any case, the key feature of this proposed injury is that these cells are unable to facilitate the free movement of ions between themselves. This is referred to as *delayed conduction*, and is considered the second condition that needs to be met to set up this particular type of re-entry.

As the ions move into the previously blocked cells, the conduction between these cells is slowed, taking more time than usual to move through this region of affected cells. Meanwhile the other cells have achieved threshold and an action potential has been generated, causing contraction of the heart. The longer it takes the ions to move between the previously blocked cells, the greater the probability that the action potential has passed through the 'normal' cells. If the delay of conduction is sufficient, then the last cells of this affected region will be ready to pass ions to the 'normal' cells, which have returned to the resting membrane potential. If this is the case, then a new action potential will be initiated and spread throughout the myocardium. For as long as the previously blocked cells have delayed conduction, the signal will repeat and repeat through the tissue, adding additional beats to the heart rate.

To summarise, the first condition that must be met to set up re-entry is a transient block that changes the direction of the electrical wave through the myocardium. As the wave travels backwards through the previously blocked region, the second condition that must be met is a delayed conduction through these cells, which allows the remaining cells to complete their initial action potential. The ions can now be transferred from the previously blocked cells into the 'normal' cells without interference, as if it were a new signal from the conduction network. The previously blocked cells now constitute an *ectopic focus*, which allows the generation of additional beats. The word 'ectopic' means 'outside the normal place' (e.g. an ectopic pregnancy). Normally, the source of the action potential is the SA node and the conduction network, but in this example the source of the extra beats is actually the myocardium itself.

It should be noted that there are alternatives to the two conditions discussed above. In some circumstances it is not delayed conduction but rather *more rapid conduction* through the 'normal' cells that sets up a re-entry circuit. Likewise, there might be an *anatomical reason* to set up re-entry, such as in people with Wolff–Parkinson–White syndrome, who have a second AV node and rudimentary bundle of His. In these people, a re-entry signal can be created because the two AV nodes bounce the electrical signals back and forth between each other, feeding those extra signals into the myocardium to become extra beats.

Early after-depolarisation

LEARNING OBJECTIVE 2

Explain how early after-depolarisation alters the rhythm of the heart.

This mechanism causes triggered activity independent of a previous action potential. An **early after-depolarisation (EAD)** (or early after-polarisation, EAP) occurs before the previous action potential is complete. It is also often caused by therapeutic drugs—a good example is the use of the K^+ channel blocker amiodarone. Other triggers include the gastrointestinal motility inhibitor cisapride, and the macrolide antimicrobial erythromycin. It can also be caused by bradycardia, hypoxia, acidosis and hypokalaemia.

The purpose of a K^+ channel blocker like amiodarone is to prolong the repolarisation phase of the action potential in order to prevent re-entry tachycardias. In normal cells, the action potential duration is coordinated with the absolute refractory period, which is defined by the return to rest of the voltage-gated Na^+ channels. Regardless of the reason, if the membrane potential of the cell is above threshold when these channels return to rest, an action potential is automatically triggered; therefore, it is important for the repolarisation to be near-complete and for the cell to be below threshold when these channels are ready to be reactivated (see Figure 25.4A). However, if the dose used is too high or if the person is particularly sensitive, then the delay in repolarisation

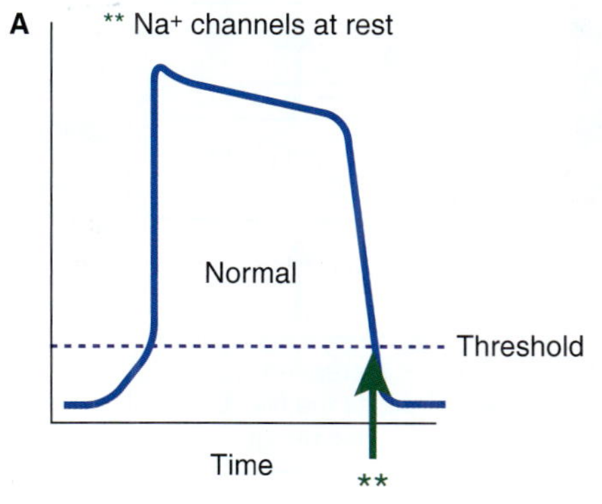

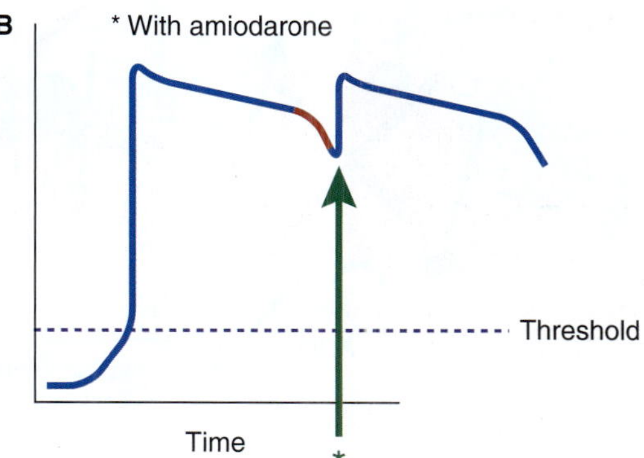

Figure 25.4

Early after-depolarisation triggered by a potassium channel blocker

(A) During a normal action potential, the duration of the action potential is coordinated with the return to rest of the voltage-gated Na^+ channels such that they return to a resting state when the cell's membrane potential is below threshold.

(B) Activation of the Na^+ channels through the use of K^+ channel blockers leads to a second action potential that piggybacks off the first. Each piggybacked action potential leads to an additional beat of the heart.

Source: Anna-Marie Babey.

is too long. In this case, the membrane potential of the cell will still be above threshold when the voltage-gated Na^+ channels return to rest and will automatically be activated. This causes the initiation of a second action potential before the first action potential is complete, giving them a 'piggyback' appearance (see Figure 24.5B). As long as the repolarisation is delayed to this extent, additional action potentials will emerge off the back of the previous action potential, adding additional beats to the heart.

Delayed after-depolarisation

Delayed after-depolarisation (DAD) (or delayed after-polarisation, DAP) is commonly caused by digoxin; however, it can also be caused by ischaemia, hypercalcaemia or as a consequence of mutations of ion channels, sarcoplasmic reticulum or transporters. In DAD, a set of cells generates an electrical signal through some action of the cell itself, and not through repetition of a previous signal (such as in re-entry). The key determinant of DADs is an *elevation in free intracellular calcium (Ca^{2+}) levels*, which raise the cell's membrane potential to threshold, and therefore triggers an extra action potential. Consequently, this also represents an ectopic focus in the heart, because once one cell is driven to threshold, it can affect its neighbours and the propagated signal becomes an extra beat.

LEARNING OBJECTIVE 3

Explain the relationship between potassium and digoxin in the context of dysrhythmia.

An excellent example of how a DAD can occur involves the action of the drug digoxin on cardiomyocytes. Digoxin can be given to people with heart failure in order to make more calcium available so that a stronger contraction can be generated. This fluctuation in calcium levels can trigger a DAD. It is important to remember that digoxin has two basic mechanisms of action, and it is the mechanism at work in heart failure, involving an inhibition of the Na^+/K^+-ATPase pump, that is of concern here (see Figure 25.5). The first thing to note about this pump is that its activity is controlled by a *phosphorylation event*. If the pump is phosphorylated (i.e. has a phosphate group attached to it), then it has a high affinity for digoxin. If the pump is dephosphorylated, then it has a low affinity for digoxin. This means that the dose of digoxin can remain exactly the same, but that the dose will have a different effect on the cell depending on whether or not the pump has been phosphorylated. As dephosphorylation is controlled by potassium availability, a person who is hypokalaemic can experience an overdose of digoxin, even if their treatment dose is within the therapeutic range, because of the changed state of the pump.

If the dose of digoxin is high or the person has hypokalaemia, more of these pumps will be blocked. This means that Na^+ efflux is delayed, resulting in a local accumulation of Na^+ near the cell membrane. This creates a change in the Na^+ gradient across the membrane, which will decrease the activity of the passive Na^+/Ca^{2+} exchanger, as this protein is dependent on a low intracellular Na^+ concentration to function. Reduced Na^+/Ca^{2+} exchanger activity will cause a delay in Ca^{2+} efflux from the cell. At standard doses of digoxin, or when K^+ levels are normal, the accumulated Ca^{2+} level is small and is easily moved to the sarcoplasmic reticulum. However, with digoxin

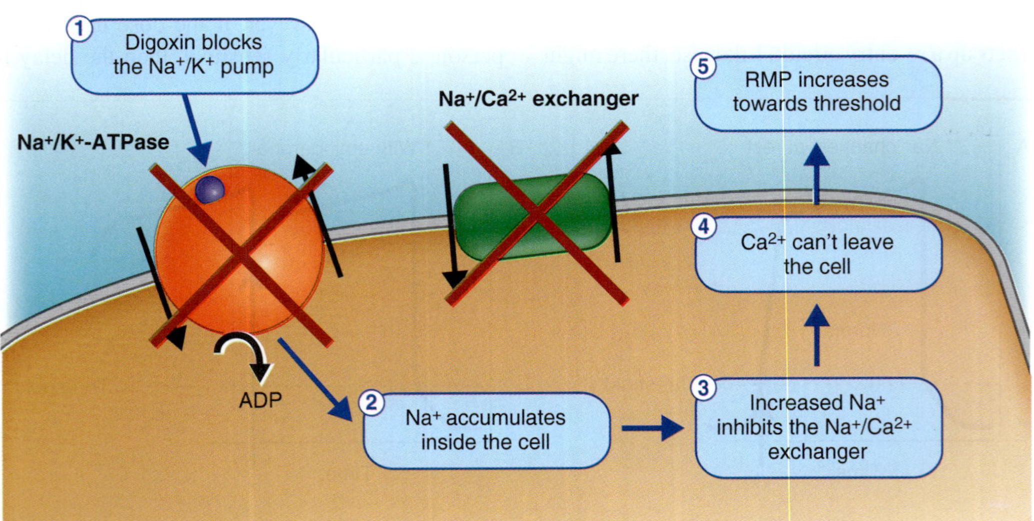

Figure 25.5

Delayed after-depolarisation triggered by digoxin

Digoxin blocks the Na^+/K^+-ATPase pump, which is responsible for resetting the concentrations of Na^+ and K^+ ions inside the cell.

ADP = adenosine diphosphate; ATPase = adenosine triphosphatase; Ca^{2+} = calcium ion; K^+ = potassium ion; Na^+ = sodium ion; RMP = resting membrane potential.

Source: Adapted from an image by Anna-Marie Babey.

levels high or K^+ levels low, there is too much intracellular Ca^{2+} to be stored by the sarcoplasmic reticulum, so Na^+ and Ca^{2+} are retained in the cytoplasm. If the delay in the removal of these positive ions is sufficient, the membrane potential of the cell will be above threshold when the voltage-gated Na^+ channels return to rest, triggering an action potential.

In a person who either receives too much digoxin or whose potassium levels are low (often occurring as a result of taking concomitant potassium-wasting diuretics such as loop or thiazide diuretics), blockage of the Na^+/K^+-ATPase pump by digoxin will be increased, posing a risk of a tachycardia due to DAD.

If DADs are due to elevated calcium levels, what does this have to do with the Na^+/K^+-ATPase pump? The role of the Na^+/K^+-ATPase pump is to remove the sodium ions (Na^+) that came into the cell during depolarisation, and retrieve the potassium ions (K^+) lost during repolarisation. Since the movement of both sodium and potassium is against the concentration gradients, energy is required, hence the ATPase function of the pump. Therefore, when digoxin blocks the pump, it delays the removal of Na^+ from inside the cell, allowing it to accumulate near the cell membrane. This results in an increase in the intracellular concentration of Na^+, which stops the activity of the passive Na^+/Ca^{2+} exchanger. This protein relies on the Na^+ gradient across the membrane to bring a small quantity of Na^+ into the cell in order to remove calcium (Ca^{2+}) from the cell. Remember that during the plateau phase of the action potential, a small amount of Ca^{2+} comes into the cell, triggering the release of the Ca^{2+} from the sarcoplasmic reticulum. At the end of the action potential, the majority of the Ca^{2+} returns to the sarcoplasmic reticulum, but the remainder must be excreted from the cell. So, if the passive Na^+/Ca^{2+} exchanger stops working, then free Ca^{2+} is allowed to accumulate inside the cell.

As long as the cell remains in its refractory period, the retention of positive ions (Na^+, Ca^{2+}) inside the cell creates no problems. However, once the cell has returned to a resting state, it is ready for another action potential, and if the membrane potential, which is defined by the number of positive ions inside the cell, is at threshold, then the cell will automatically initiate another action potential. So, in the presence of either too high a dose of digoxin or when digoxin is used in a person with hypokalaemia, the intracellular concentrations of Na^+ and Ca^{2+} will be potentially too high, due to the failure of the pump and the exchanger. If these concentrations are sufficient to reach threshold, the cell will fire, and so will its neighbours, resulting in an additional heart beat.

BRADYCARDIA AND CONDUCTION BLOCKS

LEARNING OBJECTIVE 4

Differentiate between various conduction blocks.

As mentioned, true bradycardias are commonly caused by drugs such as beta-blockers. These agents tip the balance between the parasympathetic and sympathetic nervous systems in the control of the intrinsic heart rate to favour a reduced heart rate. Modification of the drug dose normally rectifies the situation.

Escape rhythms and conduction blocks are generally the result of damage to the conduction network, namely the SA node and AV node/bundles of His, respectively. A common source of this damage is a myocardial infarction. Quite often the focus of attention after a myocardial infarction is the myocardium, as the loss of these muscle cells compromises the heart as a pump. However, the conduction network is equally vulnerable.

Atrial tachycardia (AT) is relatively rare in adults, representing less than 10% of supraventricular dysrhythmias. By contrast, AT is more common in children, representing 14–23% of cases. Interestingly, AT has even been observed in utero. Cases of re-entry in the AV node arising from an accessory pathway often present early in childhood (approximately one-third of cases), and may persist into adulthood, where it is seen as an episodic ventricular tachycardia.

When considering the risk factors that contribute to disrupted cardiac rhythm, it is necessary to recognise that the primary healthcare burden is from tachycardias and fibrillations. The main cause of conduction blocks is myocardial infarction, and therefore management of ischaemic heart disease is important. However, angina and myocardial infarction are also risks for re-entry tachycardias. In fact, post-myocardial-infarction tachycardias and fibrillations are quite common. Other risk factors associated with tachycardias and fibrillations include valve disease, congenital heart defects, heart failure, cardiomyopathy, hypertension and structural changes in the heart due to ageing.

Unfortunately, control of the primary condition does not necessarily decrease the dysrhythmia risk. *Sinus tachycardia* can be triggered by a host of conditions, such as hyperthyroidism, anaemia, infection, dehydration, orthostatic hypotension, diabetic autonomic dysregulation, phaeochromocytoma and treatment with certain drugs. In this case, the sinus tachycardia is generally managed by controlling the primary condition. *Supraventricular tachycardias* are more common during pregnancy, particularly when there is a pre-existing structural heart defect (e.g. congenital heart defects, valve disease, cardiomyopathy).

Clinical manifestations

LEARNING OBJECTIVE 5

Explain the difference between supraventricular tachycardia and ventricular tachycardia.

Most of the basic dysrhythmias are associated with recognisable changes to the ECG trace. **Atrial flutter** and atrial fibrillation show characteristic changes to the P wave (see Figure 25.6).

Supraventricular tachycardia (SVT) is often difficult to distinguish from ventricular tachycardias, as these closely resemble each other on the ECG trace. It is generally necessary to use further investigations, such as the administration of adenosine, which slows the rate and enables SVT and ventricular tachycardia to be more readily differentiated. Figure 25.7 explores the clinical manifestations and management of common atrial dysrhythmias.

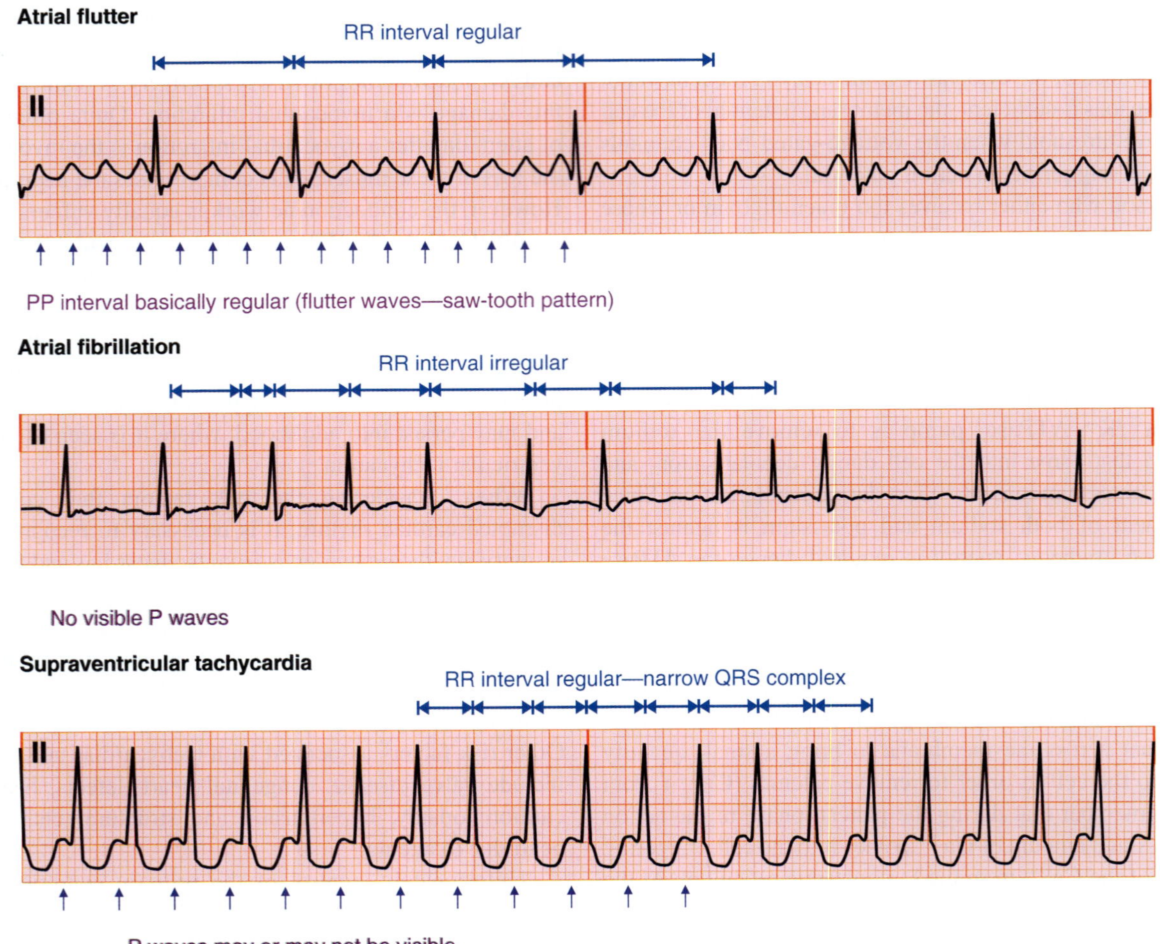

Figure 25.6

Characteristic ECG traces of common dysrhythmias

Ventricular tachycardia (VT), defined as *three or more ventricular ectopic beats in a succession*, has a characteristic sharp R wave with 'shoulders' that may be P or T waves (see Figure 25.8B). The polymorphic ventricular tachycardia known as *torsades de pointes* is marked by rhythmic tall and short undefined waves (see Figure 25.8C). Torsades de pointes is a variation of ventricular tachycardia, and can be caused by long QT syndrome. *Ventricular fibrillation* (see Figure 25.8D) is marked by a complete absence of any recognisable wave complexes.

Figure 25.9 shows the clinical manifestations and management of common ventricular dysrhythmias.

It is important to remember that episodic dysrhythmias may present on the ECG trace as *single atypical beats* (e.g. **premature ventricular complexes**); also known as premature ventricular contractions (see Figure 25.10) or *short runs of inappropriate activity*. The electrical activity may also fluctuate between fast and slow signals, such as seen in sick sinus syndrome. *Sick sinus syndrome* is a condition where degeneration of the conduction system from either scar tissue or non-specific causes results in a failure of the sinus node to adequately maintain control of a normal rhythm. Initially, this condition may result in alternating tachycardic and bradycardic rhythms, but, as the dysfunction of the sinus node continues, prolonged profound bradycardia may develop. Individuals with sick sinus syndrome will often require an implanted pacemaker to promote a more regular, reliable rhythm.

A *true bradycardia* (see Figure 25.11A) is marked by a prolonged TP segment and an adult heart rate of less than 60 bpm, while an *escape rhythm* (see Figure 25.11B) has no P wave due to dysfunction of the SA node. The rate of the escape rhythm will depend on which component of the conduction network is now controlling the rate; if it is the AV node, it will be approximately 50–60 bpm. Conduction blocks may go completely unnoticed because they do not affect cardiac output (see Figure 25.12A), or will be monitored and, if necessary, a pacemaker may be inserted to control the heart rate (see Figure 25.12B–D).

Figure 25.13 explores the clinical manifestations and management of common atrioventricular dysrhythmias.

The clinical presentation will depend entirely on the nature of the dysrhythmia. In tachycardias, patients might experience fatigue, shortness of breath, dizziness or fainting. For episodic dysrhythmias, the patient might experience a 'grabbing' sensation

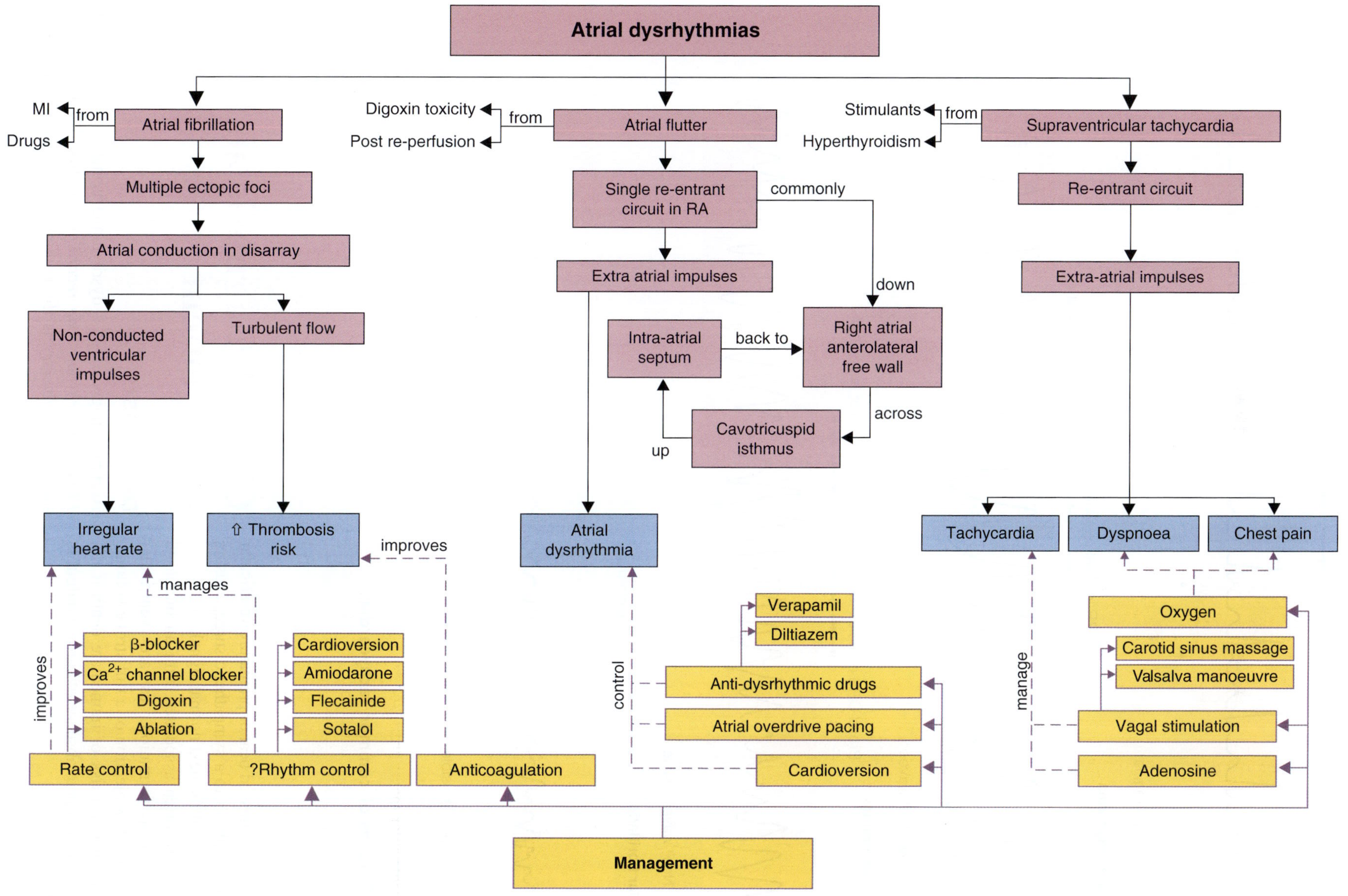

Figure 25.7

Clinical snapshot: Some common atrial dysrhythmias

↑ = increased; ? = possibly; β = beta; Ca^{2+} = calcium ion; MI = myocardial infarction; RA = right atrium.

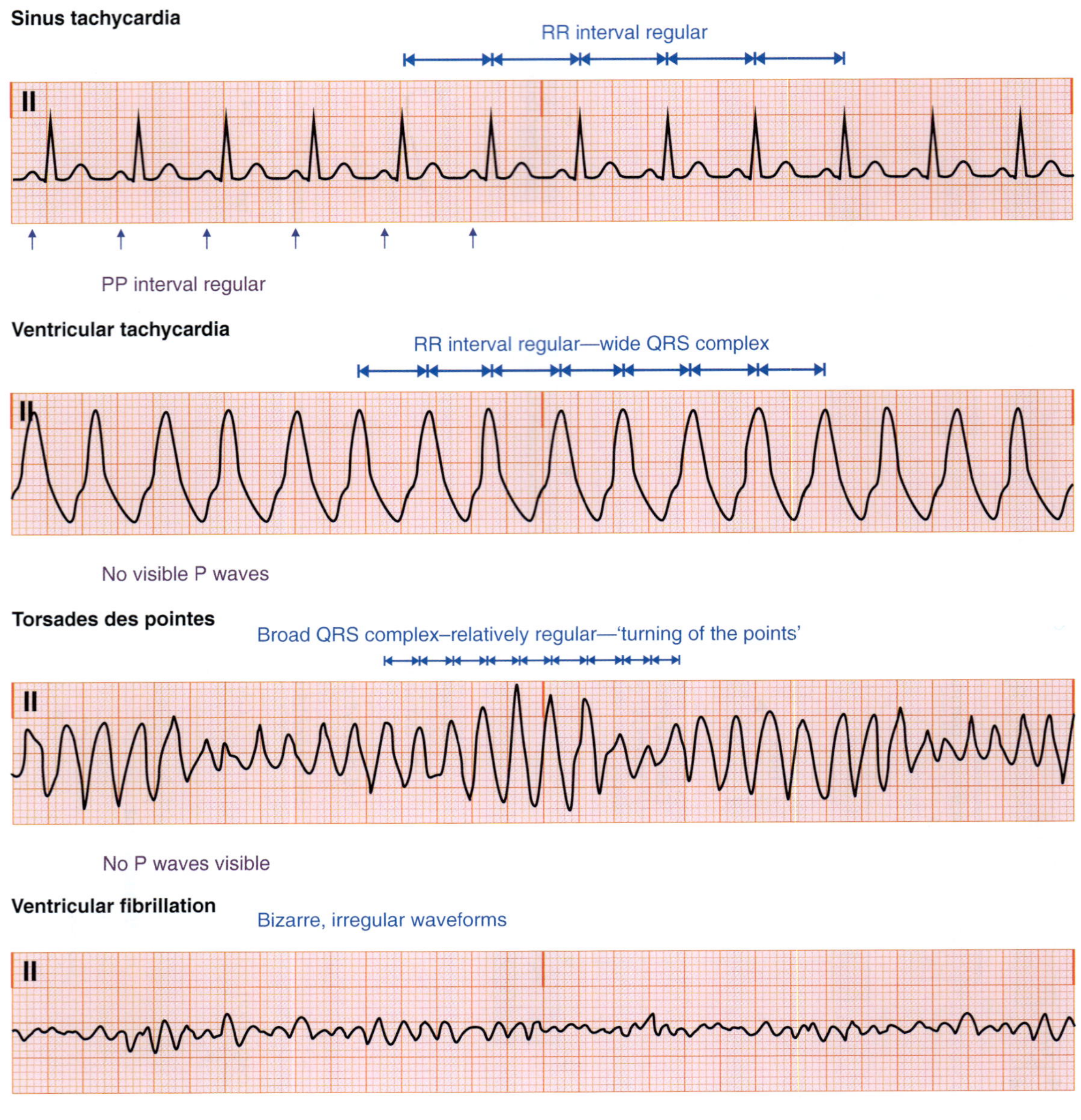

Figure 25.8
Characteristic ECG traces of common tachycardias

from the beat that follows a missed beat or premature ventricular complex as the heart is subject to a sympathetic surge, causing increased contraction force of the next normal signal.

Atrial fibrillations are often associated with an increased risk of thromboembolism formation, as are ventricular tachycardias that do not allow ejection of a full stroke volume. Ventricular fibrillation poses a risk of immediate death if not reversed, due to the near-complete absence of cardiac output in these individuals.

Clinical diagnosis and management

DIAGNOSIS

Accurate diagnosis of a dysrhythmia is made with a *12-lead ECG*. *Long rhythm strip recordings* are also used to make a diagnosis. *Telemetry* is the continuous recording of electrical

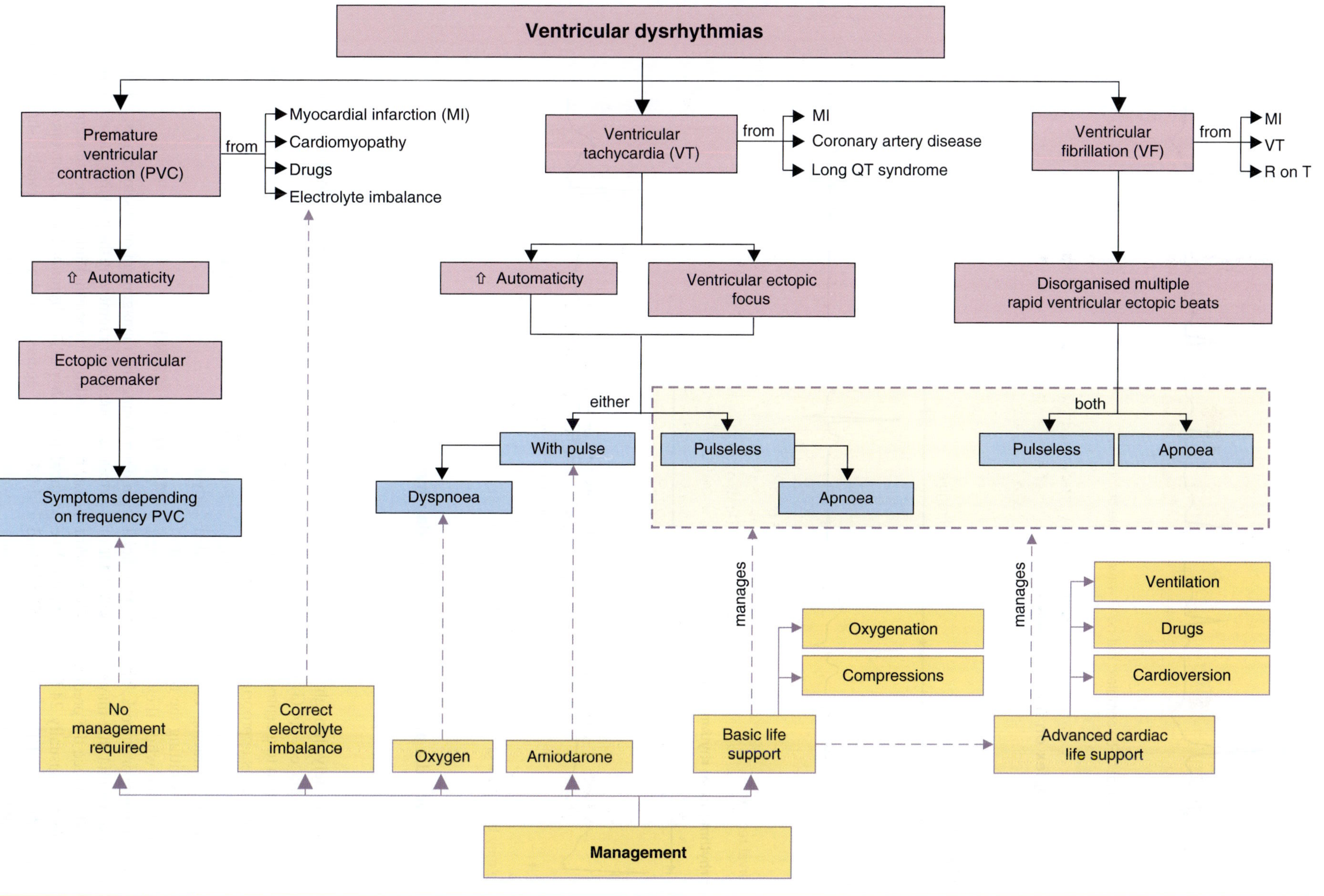

Figure 25.9

Clinical snapshot: Common ventricular dysrhythmias

↑ = increased; MI = myocardial infarction; PVC = premature ventricular contraction; VT = ventricular tachycardia.

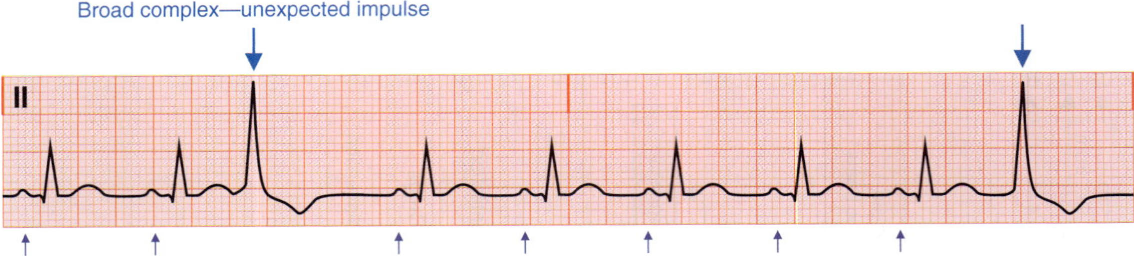

Figure 25.10

Premature ventricular complex on an ECG trace

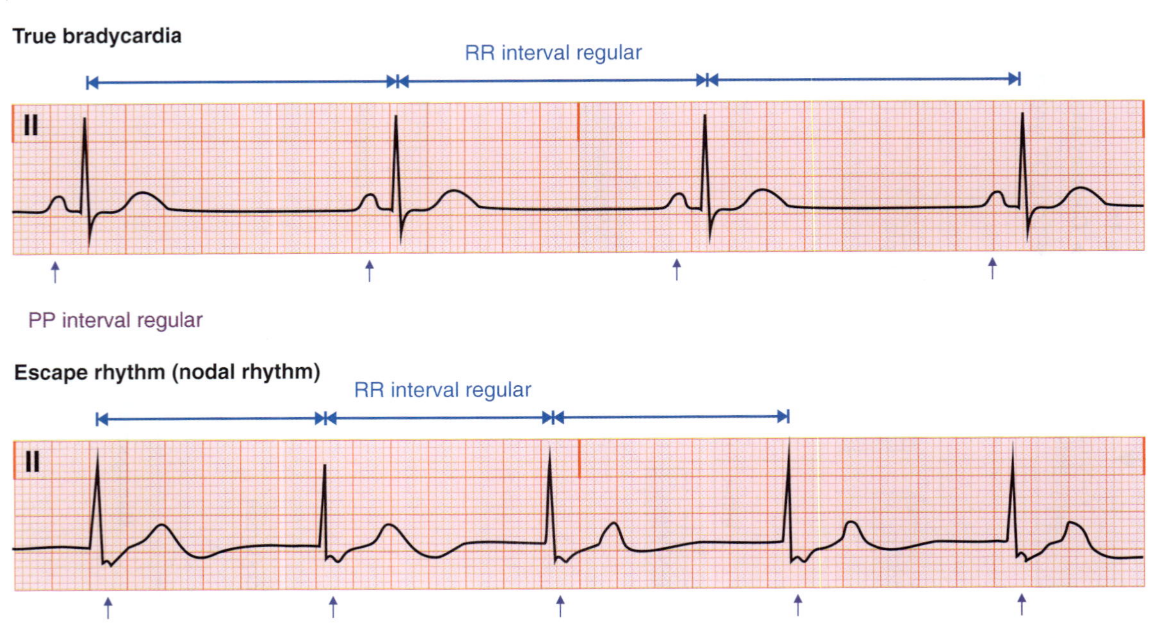

Figure 25.11

ECG traces of true bradycardia and escape rhythm (nodal rhythm)

rhythms, often achieved remotely through the use of a device attached to appropriately placed ECG dots. This device transmits the individual's rhythm to a central monitoring desk in the nurses' station or wherever is appropriate for the particular environment. Telemetry is more common in healthcare settings. *Holter monitoring* is an ECG tracing continuously recorded onto a device; instead of transmitting the rhythm to a monitor, the individual wears the device while they carry on with their activities of daily living at home or at work. This test is beneficial to detect intermittent dysrhythmia that may occur as a result of a certain stimulus or activity. Once the predetermined period of Holter monitoring is complete (usually 24 hours, but it may be repeated several times), the stored ECG data is retrieved and interpreted. The Holter monitoring device is more commonly applied and removed in healthcare settings, but the individual returns to their normal activities outside the healthcare setting while it is in situ.

Electrolyte blood levels are also taken, because electrolyte imbalances are a common cause of cardiac dysrhythmia. Potassium, magnesium and calcium imbalances may cause dysrhythmias.

MANAGEMENT

In determining the management of dysrhythmias, it is important to consider treating or removing the possible cause. *Dysrhythmias* can be caused by myocardial infarction, ischaemia, electrolyte imbalances, hypoxia, thyroid disease, pneumonia and pro-dysrhythmic agents. Health professionals should consider whether to commence administering anti-dysrhythmic agents at all, since several have pro-dysrhythmic activity. This means

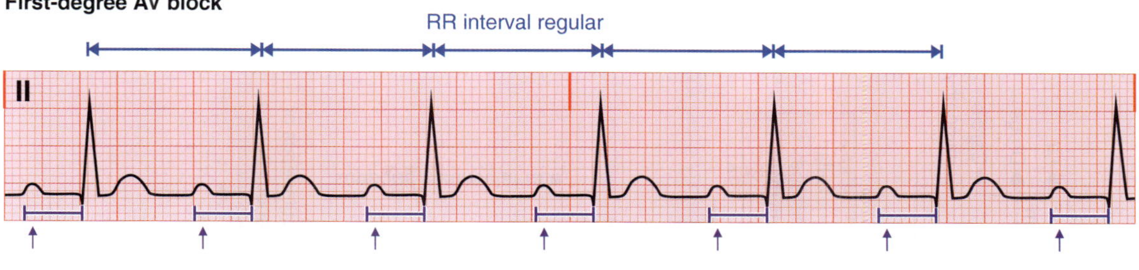

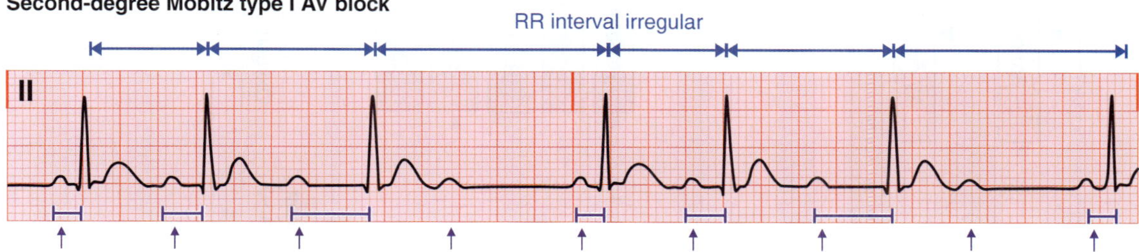

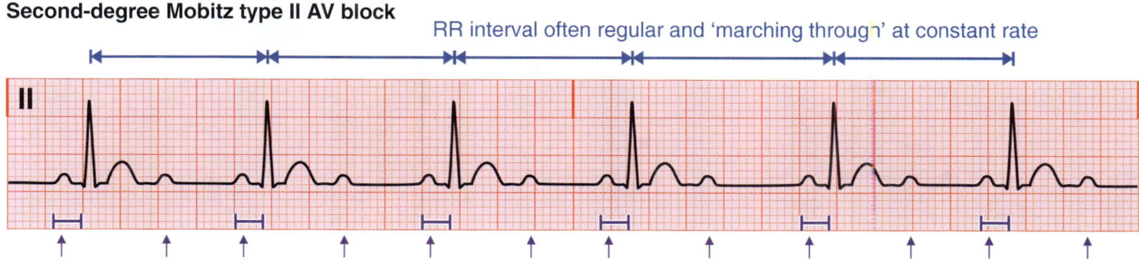

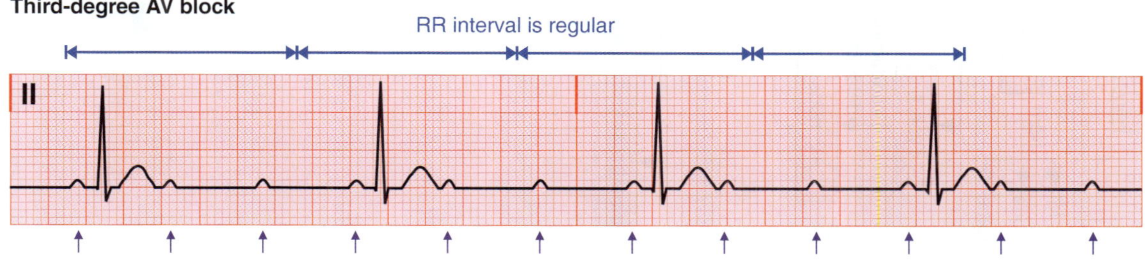

Figure 25.12

ECG traces of atrioventricular (AV) conduction blocks

that these agents can actually make the symptoms worse or even cause death.

Bradycardias are treated with anti-dysrhythmic agents only if individuals show symptoms of a slow heart rate. Atropine, a muscarinic antagonist, or isoprenaline, a sympathomimetic agent, are effective in increasing the heart rate. A pacemaker may be inserted for persistent bradycardia.

The aim of treating *atrial fibrillation* is to achieve a ventricular rate of less than 90 bpm at rest and less than 180 bpm during exercise. Preferred agents include beta-blockers or the calcium channel antagonists verapamil or diltiazem. Cardioversion—the application of electricity or administration of drugs to convert a dysrhythmia back into an acceptable rhythm—may be required for persistent atrial fibrillation in order to restore sinus rhythm. Cardioversion may be required for persistent atrial fibrillation to restore sinus rhythm, which can be undertaken electrically or chemically. For chemical cardioversion, flecainide, disopyramide, sotalol and amiodarone can be used.

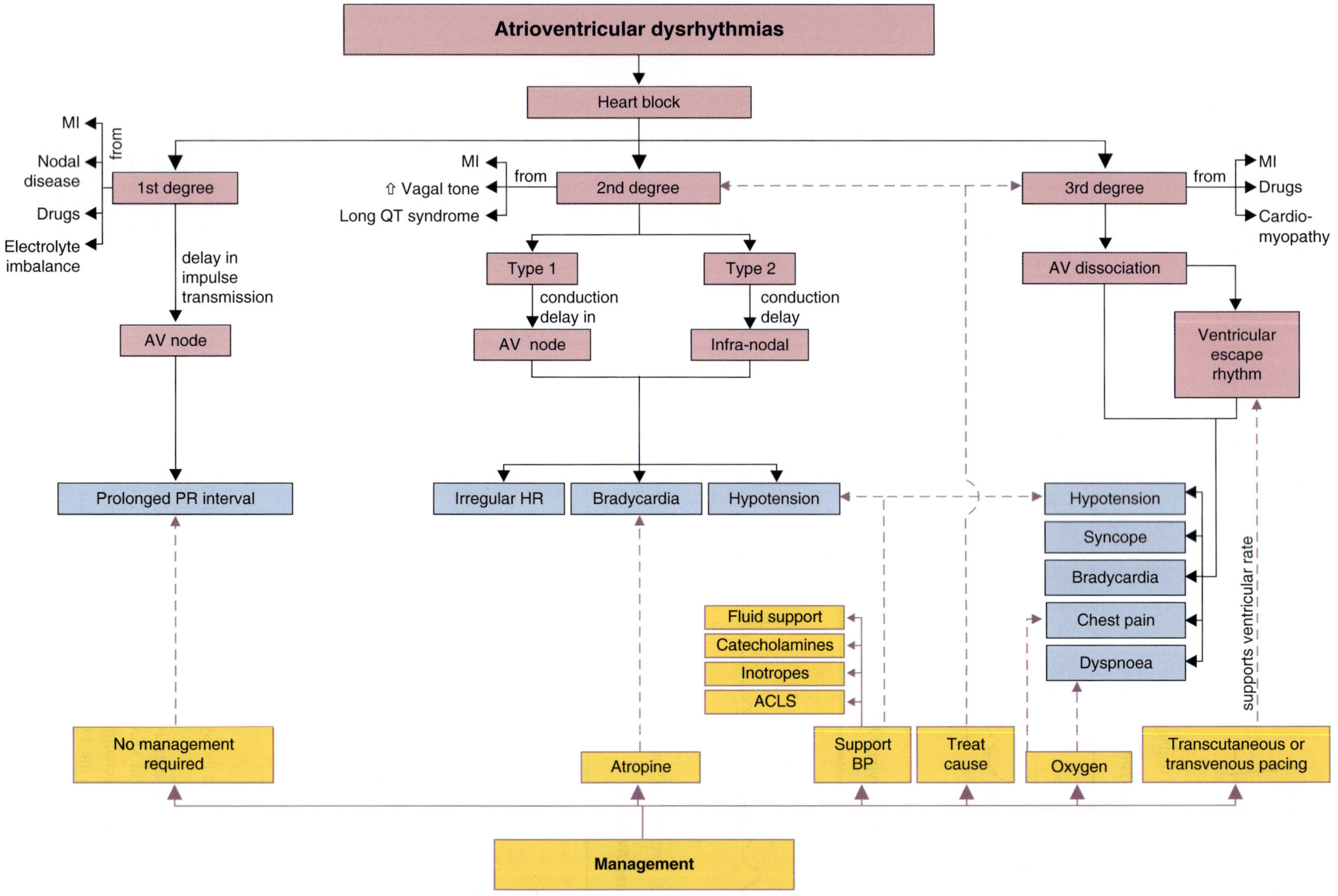

Figure 25.13

Clinical snapshot: Some common atrioventricular dysrhythmias

↑ = increased; ACLS = advanced cardiac life support; AV = atrioventricular; BP = blood pressure; HR = heart rate; MI = myocardial infarction.

Individuals who have had atrial fibrillation are at risk of developing thromboembolism. Although aspirin is still commonly used, current evidence is mounting to suggest that it has little benefit in reducing thromboembolic events in atrial fibrillation. The use of the oral vitamin K antagonist warfarin has been used for many years as an effective therapy in this condition. However, it presents a significant risk of bleeding and numerous drug–drug and drug–food interactions. Recently, *non-vitamin K antagonist oral anticoagulants (NOACs)* have transformed the anticoagulation options in the prevention of thromboembolic events in AF. NOACs provide exciting advantages when compared to warfarin, with fewer drug interactions and fixed dosing schedules that do not require regular monitoring of anticoagulation levels. Although NOACs have similar risks of major bleeding, and slightly more risk of gastrointestinal bleeding when compared to warfarin, they provide significant risk reductions in intracranial haemorrhage, stroke and mortality.

Atrial flutter responds well to cardioversion using electronic rather than chemical means. If cardioversion is not successful, then treatment is directed towards control of the ventricular rate using agents such as digoxin, a beta-blocker, or the calcium channel antagonist verapamil.

Supraventricular tachycardia is usually treated with vagal stimulation, using techniques such as the Valsalva manoeuvre or swallowing ice-cold water. Carotid sinus massage, which is sometimes used, should be avoided in older people because of the possible risk of arterial emboli. If the dysrhythmia persists, verapamil or adenosine are usually effective.

In the case of *unsustained ventricular tachycardia*, medication is given only if an individual experiences haemodynamic compromise, such as a drop in blood pressure. If haemodynamic compromise occurs with unsustained ventricular tachycardia, lignocaine is given initially, followed by amiodarone or sotalol. If a person experiences a sustained ventricular tachycardia, direct current cardioversion is usually the preferred option.

Both the Australian Resuscitation Council and the New Zealand Resuscitation Council have an agreed set of guidelines for basic life support and advanced life support that include the management of life-threatening dysrhythmias in infants, children and adults.

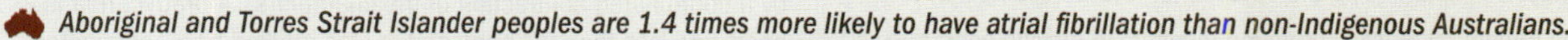

INDIGENOUS HEALTH FAST FACTS AND CULTURAL CONSIDERATIONS

FAST FACTS

- *Aboriginal and Torres Strait Islander peoples are 1.4 times more likely to have atrial fibrillation than non-Indigenous Australians.*
- *Māori and Pacific Islands people experience higher rates of atrial fibrillation and are diagnosed with it, on average, 10 years before non-Māori/non-Pacific Islands New Zealanders.*

CULTURAL CONSIDERATIONS

- *Cardiac rehabilitation can be important to reduce the morbidity and mortality associated with cardiac conditions. Many Aboriginal and Torres Strait Islander peoples prefer to receive services within their community, rather than going to a larger facility further away from home. Although it is not always possible, providing outreach cardiac rehabilitation services to local Aboriginal community-controlled health services can maximise therapeutic outcomes for individuals affected by cardiac dysrhythmia.*

Sources: Data from Australian Institute of Health and Welfare (2020); Miner-Williams (2017); Selak et al. (2020).

CHILDREN AND ADOLESCENTS

- Young children, especially neonates, can be considered 'rate-dependent'. This means that, because they have not developed sufficient physiological cardiac muscle hypertrophy to manipulate cardiac output by increasing contractility, the only way they may influence cardiac output is through heart rate. Bradycardias can severely affect the blood pressure of young children and neonates.
- It is very uncommon for a child to experience ventricular dysrhythmias, such as ventricular tachycardia and ventricular fibrillation. Cardiac arrest in children will generally result from a bradycardia or asystole.
- Supraventricular tachycardias are the most common sustained dysrhythmias in children. Use of adenosine or vagal stimulation methods, such as the application of ice or the Valsalva manoeuvre, may assist in terminating the supraventricular tachycardia.

OLDER ADULTS

- Age-related changes to the autonomic nervous system and cardiac conduction system generally result in decreased resting heart rates. The number of sinoatrial nodal cells decreases significantly with age, and parasympathetic control dominates.
- Baroreceptor reflex sensitivity decreases with age, and sinus node depression may result in an increased risk of syncope in the older adult.
- Atrial fibrillation is common in older adults. Some individuals do not even realise that there is a problem with their rhythm. Atrial fibrillation is clinically significant because of the increased risk of thrombosis and emboli caused by the turbulence, resulting in increased platelet aggregation and blood viscosity.
- The observation and reporting of atrial fibrillation in previously undiagnosed older adults should be undertaken so that further investigation of the cause and implementation of a management plan may ensue.

KEY CLINICAL ISSUES

- Any episode of a loss of consciousness can be as a result of a dysrhythmia. After neurological and circulatory causes have been ruled out, investigations into the individual's conduction system function may be beneficial. Electrocardiograms (ECG), telemetry and Holter monitors may demonstrate dysrhythmia. Unfortunately, with many dysrhythmias, the person must be experiencing the episode for it to be seen on ECG.
- Do not rely on peripheral oxygen saturation monitors to provide heart rate observations. Direct observation by palpation should be used to observe pulse rate and regularity. The oxygen saturation monitor does not identify the rate or rhythm accurately in an individual experiencing a dysrhythmia.
- Atrial dysrhythmias are generally tolerated better than ventricular dysrhythmias. However, this is specifically reliant on the capacity of the ventricular myocardium. The 'atrial kick' (atrial contraction) generates approximately 30% of cardiac output. If an individual has sufficiently good cardiac output, a drop of 30% may not necessarily result in clinically appreciable issues. However, if an individual has very low cardiac output, a further 30% drop may have a devastating effect on blood pressure and circulation.
- Ventricular tachycardia can present in two ways: pulseless and with a pulse. Individuals with stable ventricular tachycardia may present feeling unwell, dizzy or nauseous. However, when attached to a monitor they may display ventricular tachycardia. Although the level of urgency is less than that of a cardiac arrest from pulseless ventricular tachycardia, it is still important to have the individual revert to sinus rhythm. The myocardium cannot sustain ventricular tachycardia for extended periods of time, and ventricular tachycardia can progress to ventricular fibrillation quickly. On the monitor, ventricular tachycardia appears the same whether the person is pulseless or not. The distinguishing feature between these two types of ventricular tachycardia is whether there is sufficient cardiac output achieved by the ventricles to support myocardial and cerebral blood flow. In pulseless ventricular tachycardia, there is no cardiac output, and therefore the person is unconscious and in 'cardiac arrest'. In ventricular tachycardia, where the person has a pulse, they are most often conscious and a pulse is palpable.
- The Australian and New Zealand Resuscitation Councils have recently reviewed the basic and advanced life support protocols. Ensure that you frequently achieve competency in life support protocols to guarantee that the best practice techniques, skills and sequences are put in place when an individual requires resuscitation.

CHAPTER REVIEW

- A *tachycardia* is a heart rate greater than 100 bpm, and is marked by a coordinated contraction of the chamber(s). A *bradycardia* is a heart rate less than 60 bpm, and is also marked by a coordinated contraction of the chambers. By contrast, a *fibrillation* is marked by disconnection of the myocytes such that each myocyte contracts independently. *Ventricular fibrillation* constitutes a medical emergency as there is no cardiac output.
- *Excess atrial activity* (atrial tachycardia, atrial flutter, atrial fibrillation) is generally better tolerated than excess ventricular activity, as there is a smaller degree of compromised ejection.
- *Re-entry* accounts for approximately 75% of all tachycardias, and fibrillations and can occur in any part of the heart.
- *Early and delayed after-depolarisations* are commonly the result of medications. These mechanisms provide a source of triggered activity in the heart, and the problem hinges on the timing of the return of the voltage-gated sodium channels to rest and the membrane potential of the cell at that point.
- A common cause of *escape rhythms* and *conduction blocks* is myocardial infarction.

REVIEW QUESTIONS

1. What is the difference between ventricular tachycardia and ventricular fibrillation? Why is ventricular fibrillation a medical emergency?
2. A person taking digoxin and a potassium-wasting diuretic (i.e. a loop or thiazide diuretic) for heart failure is at risk of tachycardia. What could possibly cause this tachycardia? Outline the mechanism.
3. What are the two conditions that must be met for re-entry to occur?
4. What is the difference between the two types of second-degree heart block?
5. How does tachycardia contribute to angina?

HEALTH PROFESSIONAL CONNECTIONS

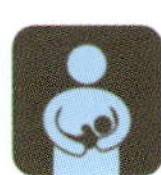

Midwives Congenital cardiac malformations can contribute to dysrhythmias, especially cardiac defects involving the atrial or ventricular septum. A thorough cardiac assessment will assist in identifying potential dysrhythmias. Cardiac monitoring should be undertaken when there is concern about irregular heart rates or aberrant cardiac assessments. Referral to medical officers and further investigation are critical when there is concern regarding the cardiac conduction system.

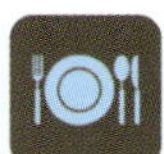

Nutritionists/Dieticians Electrolyte imbalances are a common cause of dysrhythmias. Dietary deficiencies in potassium, magnesium and calcium can all contribute to problems with the conduction system. Analysis of a person's diet is important to reduce the risk of dysrhythmia from electrolyte imbalances. If inadequate dietary intake is temporarily unavoidable, supplementation should be initiated to ensure appropriate electrolyte balance. Excessive stimulants and caffeine can also cause extra-systoles and other cardiac conduction issues. People should be dissuaded from an excessive intake of energy drinks containing stimulants such as caffeine and guarana.

All allied professionals When working with people who experience pre-syncope, syncope (transient loss of consciousness due to fall in blood pressure) or balance issues, referral to a medical officer for further investigation is warranted. Dysrhythmia can cause dizziness and, occasionally, loss of consciousness. When observation (or conversation) about experiences suggests a problem, dysrhythmia should be ruled out. All healthcare professionals have a responsibility to keep their first aid and resuscitation knowledge current. Annual cardiopulmonary resuscitation competency testing should be undertaken to ensure that any healthcare professional is prepared to assist an individual experiencing a life-threatening dysrhythmia. Automatic external defibrillators (AEDs) should be available in all treatment areas. Annual training and competency regarding their placement and use should be undertaken for AEDs as well. It is well established that competent compressions and early defibrillation significantly increase an individual's chance of survival if experiencing a witnessed cardiac arrest.

CASE STUDY

Ms Tanya Cooper is a 21-year-old woman (UR number 846117) with a three-year history of anorexia nervosa and laxative abuse. She presented with dehydration and fatigue. She is allergic to sulfur and penicillin. Her observations were as follows:

Temperature	Heart rate	Respiration rate	Blood pressure	SpO_2
36.1°C	56	26	90/56	96% (RA*)

*RA = room air.

Ms Cooper weighs 39 kg and is 169 cm tall. Her pathology results are as follows.

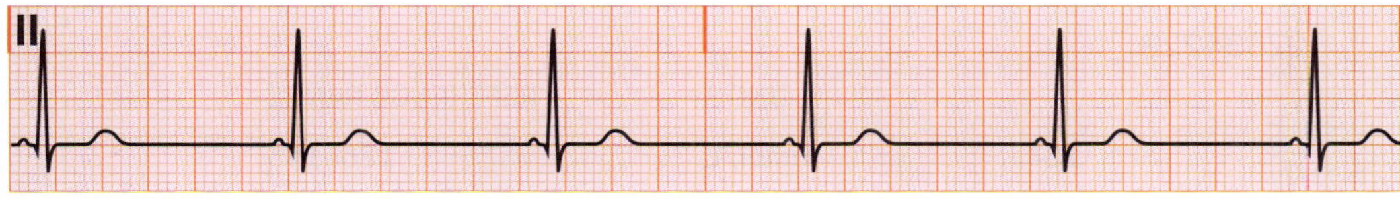

Ms Tanya Cooper's 6-second rhythm strip

Rate can be estimated by counting the number of R waves in 6 seconds and multiplying by 10.

HAEMATOLOGY

Patient location:	Ward 3	**UR:**	846117		
Consultant:	Smith	**NAME:**	Cooper		
		Given name:	Tanya	**Sex:**	F
		DOB:	06/04/XX	**Age:**	21
Time collected	11:05				
Date collected	XX/XX				
Year	XXXX				
Lab #	23234234				

FULL BLOOD COUNT		UNITS	REFERENCE RANGE
Haemoglobin	110	g/L	115–160
White cell count	3.8	$\times 10^9$/L	4.0–11.0
Platelets	135	$\times 10^9$/L	140–400
Haematocrit	0.32		0.33–0.47
Red cell count	3.79	$\times 10^{12}$/L	3.80–5.20
Reticulocyte count	0.9	%	0.2–2.0%
MCV	82	fL	80–100
Neutrophils	1.49	$\times 10^9$/L	2.00–8.00
Lymphocytes	1.21	$\times 10^9$/L	1.00–4.00
Monocytes	0.11	$\times 10^9$/L	0.10–1.00
Eosinophils	0.16	$\times 10^9$/L	$<$0.60
Basophils	0.11	$\times 10^9$/L	$<$0.20
ESR	7	mm/h	$<$12
COAGULATION PROFILE			
aPTT	25	secs	24–40
PT	11	secs	11–17

BIOCHEMISTRY

Patient location:	Ward 3	**UR:**	846117		
Consultant:	Smith	**NAME:**	Cooper		
		Given name:	Tanya	**Sex:**	F
		DOB:	06/04/XX	**Age:**	21

Time collected	11:05
Date collected	XX/XX
Year	XXXX
Lab #	12334222

ELECTROLYTES		UNITS	REFERENCE RANGE
Sodium	134	mmol/L	135–145
Potassium	2.9	mmol/L	3.5–5.2
Chloride	96	mmol/L	95–110
Bicarbonate	27	mmol/L	22–32
Glucose (random)	3.9	mmol/L	3.5–7.7
Iron	11	μmol/L	11–30

CRITICAL THINKING

1. Ms Cooper has many haematology and biochemistry parameters outside the reference range. Identify which aberrant results may contribute to cardiac conduction issues. Explain the relationship of the parameters that you have identified to cardiac conduction.
2. Observe Ms Cooper's rhythm strip. Calculate the rate, identify the rhythm, and determine the PR interval, the QRS width and the QT interval. Are the parameters within acceptable reference ranges? If not, explain.
3. How did Ms Cooper's anorexia contribute to her cardiac conduction issues? Explain.
4. Examine Ms Cooper's observations and the other details provided. Explain the pathophysiology that contributed to this outcome. (Begin with behaviours and diet.)
5. How could Ms Cooper's conduction issues be improved? What interventions could be initiated to improve her ECG and, ultimately, her cardiac conduction?

BIBLIOGRAPHY

Australian Bureau of Statistics (ABS) (2022). *Causes of death, Australia, 2021*. Canberra: ABS. https://www.abs.gov.au/statistics/health/causes-death/causes-death-australia/latest-release.

Australian Health Ministers' Advisory Council's National and Aboriginal and Torres Strait Islander Health Standing Committee (2017). *Cultural respect framework 2016–2026: for Aboriginal and Torres Strait Islander health—a national approach to building a culturally respectful health system.* Canberra: Australian Government Department of Health. https://nacchocommunique.files.wordpress.com/2016/12/cultural_respect_framework_1december2016_1.pdf.

Australian Institute of Health and Welfare (AIHW) (2020). *Aboriginal and Torres Strait Islander Health Performance Framework—summary report 2020.* Cat. No. IHPF 2. Canberra: AIHW. file:///C:/Users/User/Downloads/2020-summary-ihpf-2.pdf.

Australian Institute of Health and Welfare (AIHW) (2020). *Atrial fibrillation in Australia*. Web report. Canberra: AIHW. https://www.aihw.gov.au/reports/heart-stroke-vascular-diseases/atrial-fibrillation-in-australia/contents/what-is-atrial-fibrillation.

Australian Institute of Health and Welfare (AIHW) (2022). *Principal diagnosis data cubes: separation statistics by principal diagnosis (ICD-10-AM 11th edition), Australia, 2020–21.* Canberra: AIHW. https://www.aihw.gov.au/reports/hospitals/principal-diagnosis-data-cubes/contents/data-cubes.

Bauldoff, G., Gubrud-Howe, P.M., Carno, M.-A., Levett-Jones, T., Hales, M., Berry, K., … LeMone, P. (2020). *LeMone and Burke's medical-surgical nursing: Critical thinking for person-centred care* (4th [Australian] edn). Sydney: Pearson Australia.

Best, O. & Fredericks, B. (2021). *Yatdjuligin: Aboriginal and Torres Strait Islander nursing and midwifery care* (3rd edn). Port Melbourne, VIC: Cambridge University Press.

Bullock, S. & Manias, E. (2022). *Fundamentals of pharmacology* (9th edn). Sydney: Pearson Australia.

Chao, T.-F., Joung, B., Takahashi, Y., Lim, T.W., Choi, E.-K., Chan, Y.-H., … Lip, G.Y.H. (2022). 2021 focused update consensus guidelines of the Asia Pacific Heart Rhythm Society on stroke prevention in atrial fibrillation: executive summary. *Thrombosis and Haemostasis* 122(1):020–047. https://doi.org/10.1055/s-0041-1739411.

Gallagher, C., Hendriks, J.M., Giles, L., Karnon, J., Pham, C., Elliott, A.D., … Wong, C. X. (2019). Increasing trends in hospitalisations due to atrial fibrillation in Australia from 1993 to 2013. *Heart* 105(17):1358–63. https://doi.org/10.1136/heartjnl-2018-314471.

Kantharia, B.T., Sharma, M. & Shah, A.N. (2019). Atrial tachycardia. *Emedicine*. https://emedicine.medscape.com/article/151456-overview.

Marieb, E.N. & Hoehn, K. (2019). *Human anatomy and physiology* (11th edn). San Francisco, CA: Pearson Benjamin Cummings.

Miner-Williams, W. (2017). Racial inequities in cardiovascular disease in New Zealand. *Diversity and Equality in Health and Care* 14(1):23–33. https://diversityhealthcare.imedpub.com/racial-inequities-in-cardiovascular-disease-in-newzealand.pdf.

New Zealand Heart Foundation (2022). *Atrial fibrillation.* https://www.heartfoundation.org.nz/your-heart/heart-conditions/atrial-fibrillation/.

Rosenthal, L., McManus, D.D. & Sardana, M. (2019). Atrial fibrillation. *Emedicine*. https://emedicine.medscape.com/article/151066-overview.

Selak, V., Poppe, K., Grey, C. Mehta, S. Winter-Smith, J., … Harwood, M. (2020). Ethnic differences in cardiovascular risk profiles among 475,241 adults in primary care in Aotearoa, New Zealand. *New Zealand Medical Journal* 133(1521):14–27. https://journal.nzma.org.nz/journal-articles/ethnic-differences-in-cardiovascular-risk-profiles-among-475-241-adults-in-primary-care-in-aotearoa-new-zealand.

Yan, G.-X., Kowey, P.R. & Antzelevitch, C. (2020). *Management of cardiac arrhythmias* (3rd edn). Geneva: Springer International Publishing. https://doi.org/10.1007/978-3-030-41967-7.

PART

6

Pulmonary pathophysiology

26 Pulmonary dysfunction

KEY TERMS

Apnoea
Biot's breathing
Bradypnoea
Cheyne–Stokes breathing
Cyanosis
Digital clubbing
Dyspnoea
Eupnoea
Haemoptysis
Hypercapnia
Hyperoxia
Hypocapnia
Hypoxaemia
Orthopnoea
Respiratory compensation
Spirometry
Tachypnoea
Ventilatory failure
Wheeze

LEARNING OBJECTIVES

After completing this chapter, you should be able to:

1 Discuss the effects of illness on respiratory rate and depth.

2 Define the relationship between blood carbon dioxide levels and pH.

3 Distinguish between the various patterns of respiration associated with Kussmaul, Cheyne–Stokes, Biot's and apneustic breathing.

4 Review the significance of alterations in oxygen and carbon dioxide levels.

5 Explain the common clinical manifestations of pulmonary dysfunction, including dyspnoea, cough, haemoptysis, cyanosis and digital clubbing.

6 Describe the different types of respiratory assessments and investigations.

7 Examine the pathophysiology, clinical manifestations and management of respiratory failure.

WHAT YOU SHOULD YOU KNOW BEFORE YOU START THIS CHAPTER

Can you identify the structure and function of the respiratory membrane, and the factors that influence its function?

Can you define and apply important gas and pressure laws associated with the mechanics of breathing and gas exchange (such as Boyle's and Pascal's laws)?

Can you explain the principles of gas exchange in relation to oxygen and carbon dioxide?

Can you state the acceptable reference ranges for oxygen, carbon dioxide, sodium bicarbonate and pH in blood?

Can you describe the location of the apneustic and pneumotaxic centres, and explain the influence they have on respiration?

Can you identify acceptable rates for respiration across the lifespan?

Can you describe what factors affect respiratory rate and oxygenation?

Introduction

At some stage in their life, most people will experience an episode of shortness of breath, or suffer a coughing fit from either a poor attempt at swallowing or from an upper respiratory tract infection. As a healthcare professional, it is important to understand the various clinical manifestations of pulmonary dysfunction and the investigations that can be undertaken to determine the cause.

This chapter will explore the important concepts related to oxygenation and ventilation. Common clinical manifestations and causes of altered lung function will be considered. Alterations in gas exchange, symptoms of **dyspnoea** (difficulty in breathing) and signs of cough, **haemoptysis**, digital clubbing and cyanosis will be addressed. Common respiratory investigations will be explained. The causes, clinical manifestations and management of respiratory failure will also be examined.

Respiratory rate, rhythm and depth

LEARNING OBJECTIVE 1

Discuss the effects of illness on respiratory rate and depth.

When a person presents with a respiratory illness, the most important assessments are the rate, rhythm and depth of their respiratory effort. Various conditions can influence the nature and frequency of respirations. Disease processes interfering with oxygenation will generally result in a faster respiratory rate. Neurological and endocrine conditions can also influence respiratory rate, rhythm and depth. The common terminology used to describe respiratory observations is given in Table 26.1.

RATE

Assessment of respiration rate is important. As a child ages, the respiratory muscles mature (get stronger), allowing for increased tidal volume; therefore, the rate of breathing required for adequate oxygenation decreases (see Table 26.2).

Eupnoea is a normal respiratory rate (see Figure 26.1). **Tachypnoea** is a critical risk factor for significant clinical decline (see Figure 26.2). **Bradypnoea** can also be a sign of impending crisis, especially in the context of narcotic overdose or traumatic brain injury (see Figure 26.3).

Control of respiratory rate

LEARNING OBJECTIVE 2

Define the relationship between blood carbon dioxide levels and pH.

As *central and peripheral chemoreceptors* monitor carbon dioxide and oxygen partial pressures, changes in respiratory rate are mediated by the pneumotaxic and apneustic centres in the brainstem. Central receptors are stimulated by increased blood levels of carbon dioxide or decreased blood pH (i.e. *acidaemia*). Unbound carbon dioxide in the blood can be converted into carbonic acid in a reversible reaction. As a result, alterations in blood carbon dioxide levels can greatly influence blood pH (the higher the levels of carbon dioxide, the lower the blood pH—therefore the blood is more acidic). This relationship is described in detail in the 'Arterial blood gas analysis' section.

Peripheral chemoreceptors are stimulated by high carbon dioxide levels (hypercapnia), low oxygen levels (hypoxia) or decreased pH in the blood. In people with normally functioning respiratory systems, hypercapnia triggers an increase in the respiratory rate in order to 'breathe off' the excess carbon dioxide levels to correct acidaemia (*hypercapnic drive*).

Table 26.1 Terminology used to describe respiratory observations

Term	Definition	Usually can be associated with
Eupnoea	Respiratory rate and depth within acceptable limits	Good health
Tachypnoea	Respiratory rate faster than acceptable limits for age	Pain and most respiratory illnesses
Bradypnoea	Respiratory rate slower than acceptable limits for age	Excessive narcotic consumption
Dyspnoea	Difficulty breathing; shortness of breath	Any respiratory illness
Orthopnoea	Difficulty breathing when lying flat	Cardiac failure, pulmonary oedema and many respiratory illnesses
Paroxysmal nocturnal dyspnoea	Difficulty breathing at night—most often associated with reclined positioning, and rouses individual from sleep in respiratory distress	Cardiac failure
Hypoventilation	Generic term for not breathing enough to expel sufficient carbon dioxide; may relate to rate or depth or both	Narcotic overdose
Hyperventilation	Generic term for breathing too much and expelling too much carbon dioxide; may relate to rate or depth or both	Anxiety
Apnoea	Absence of breath	Respiratory arrest

Table 26.2 Reference ranges for respiratory observations across the lifespan

Age	Reference range (breaths/min)*	Important considerations
Premature	40–70	If born before 28 weeks, surfactant production is affected and the newborn will develop infant respiratory distress syndrome
0–3 months	35–55	Obligate nose breathers
3–6 months	30–45	If nasopharyngeal secretions become excessive, respiratory compromise can develop quickly. An abdominal breathing pattern occurs within this age group
6–12 months	25–45	Abdominal breathing pattern occurs within this age group. Significant changes to the size and shape of conducting airways occur during this time
1–2 years	20–45	
2–5 years	16–34	The narrowest section of the airway remains cricoid cartilage at this age
5–11 years	16–29	Abdominal breathing begins to cease by 7 years of age, when a costal breathing pattern becomes dominant
12 years–adulthood	12–20	
Older adult (> 65 years of age)	12–20	Age-associated changes to the pulmonary system may result in faster respiratory rates, especially in people with a history of cigarette smoking

For other differences in respiratory function between adults and children, see Table 26.7.

** = Commonly acceptable observations as deemed by various children's early warning tools/paediatric early warning scores.*

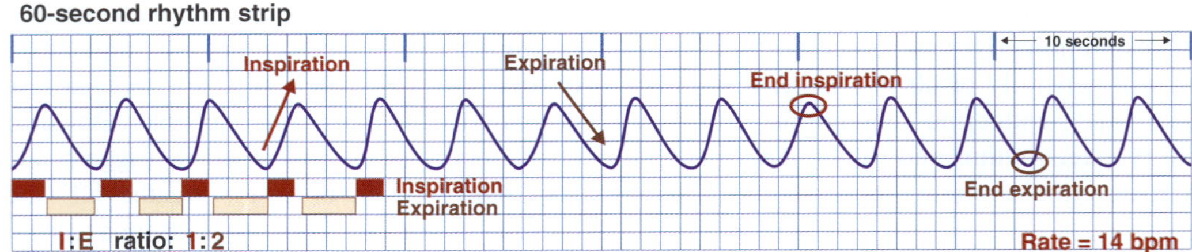

Figure 26.1

Normal respirations: eupnoea

The peaks represent inspiration, and the troughs represent expiration. Note that the depth and the frequency are consistent. The rate of the respiratory pattern shown is 14 breaths per minute. This can be calculated by counting the peaks. As the example represents 60 seconds, the number of peaks over 60 seconds signifies the respiratory rate.

bpm = breaths per minute; I:E ratio = inspiratory:expiratory ratio.

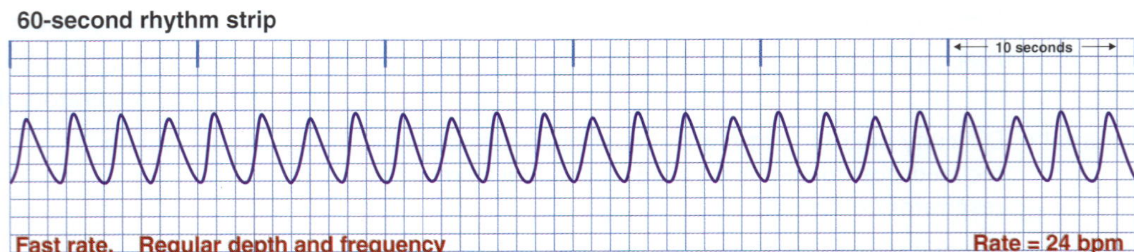

Figure 26.2

Tachypnoea

The respiratory rate in this example is 24 breaths per minute. This is considered tachypnoeic for an adult. Note that the frequency and the depth are regular, albeit more rapid than normal. Tachypnoea in someone at rest is a critical risk factor for significant clinical decline.

bpm = breaths per minute.

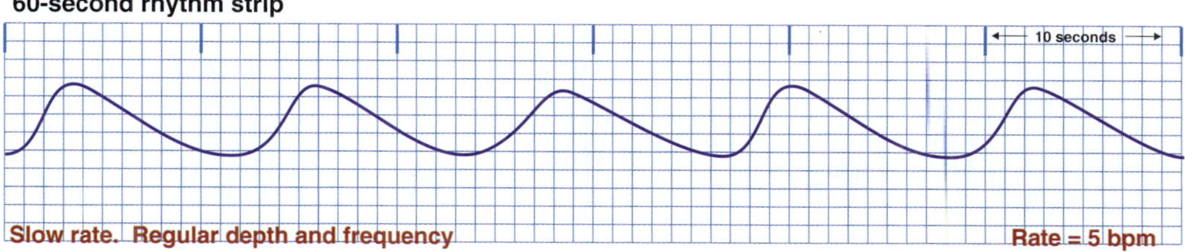

Figure 26.3

Bradypnoea

The respiratory rate in this example is five breaths per minute. This is considered bradypnoeic in adults and profound in children. Note that even though the rate is slow, the frequency and the depth are regular. Bradypnoea can be a sign of impending crisis, especially in the context of narcotic overdose or traumatic brain injury.

bpm = breaths per minute.

Hypoxia can also trigger an increase in the respiratory rate in an attempt to improve alveolar ventilation. An issue that may alter an individual's response to hypercapnia occurs in chronic airway disease. When a person is exposed to chronic carbon dioxide levels and acidosis, the chemoreceptor function becomes somewhat blunted and low levels of oxygen become the trigger for an increase in the respiratory rate (*hypoxic drive*). Many people with chronic obstructive pulmonary disease (COPD) have developed a hypoxic drive instead of a hypercapnic drive (see the chapter 'Obstructive pulmonary disorders').

Assessment of respiratory rate

Many factors can influence respiratory rate; therefore, rate is a powerful tool in the assessment of numerous conditions, and is a critical factor to guide clinical decision-making (see Table 26.3). As with any parameter, respiratory rate should not be considered in isolation, but rather in association with other assessments, such as oxygen saturation, the colour of the extremities, heart rate, and the other components of respiratory assessment, such as depth and rhythm.

Table 26.3 Some factors influencing respiratory rate

Factors decreasing respiratory rate	Factors increasing respiratory rate
• Increased intracranial pressure	• Anxiety
• Alcohol	• Caffeine
• Opioids	• Pain
• Rest/sleeping	• Exertion
• Hypocapnia	• Hypercapnia
• Hypothermia	• Fever
	• Haemorrhage
	• Acidosis
	• Lung disease
	• Cardiac disease
	• Young age

In considering respiratory rate, it is also important to understand that, just because a person is breathing quickly, it does not necessarily mean that they are breathing deeply or that the alveolar ventilation or gas exchange is effective. In health, an increase in respiratory rate and depth will cause an increase in alveolar ventilation and, to a point, an increase in oxygen saturation and decreased carbon dioxide levels within the blood. However, if any component of the respiratory system is compromised, the increased rate will not necessarily produce an improved arterial oxygenation, tissue oxygenation or reduced carbon dioxide level.

RHYTHM

LEARNING OBJECTIVE 3

Distinguish between the various patterns of respiration associated with Kussmaul, Cheyne–Stokes, Biot's and apneustic breathing.

Normal respirations

Normal respirations have a regular rhythm and an *inspiratory phase (I)* that is slightly shorter than the *expiratory phase (E)*. The *I:E ratio* is generally about 1:1.5 or 1:2 (see Figure 26.1) Several *structures* influence the control of respiratory rhythm, including the respiratory centres in the medulla oblongata and the pons. *Chemical factors* can also influence rhythm; however, respiratory rate and depth are more influenced by chemical stimuli than rhythm.

Some classic alterations in respiratory rhythm include patterns such as Kussmaul, Cheyne–Stokes, Biot's, cluster and apneustic breathing.

Kussmaul breathing

Kussmaul breathing can be described as *hyperventilation*. This breathing pattern is deep, laboured and rapid, and is commonly associated with conditions such as diabetic ketoacidosis and increased intracranial pressure (see Figure 26.4). Kussmaul breathing occurs as a respiratory compensation for severe metabolic acidosis (see 'Arterial blood gas analysis') through the expiration of carbon dioxide; as a result, arterial blood gas analysis will demonstrate hypocapnia in normally functioning lungs.

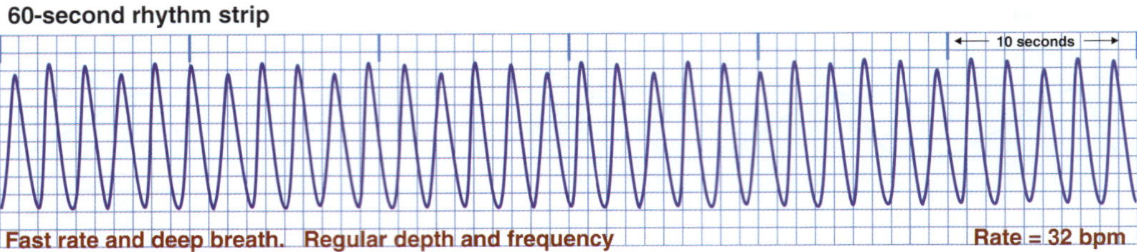

Figure 26.4

Kussmaul breathing

Note that the depth is consistent (although deeper than normal tachypnoea), and the frequency is rapid but still regular. This is commonly associated with metabolic acidosis, especially diabetic ketoacidosis. The respiratory rate in this example is 32 breaths per minute.

bpm = breaths per minute.

Cheyne–Stokes breathing

Cheyne-Stokes breathing has a cyclic pattern in a *crescendo–decrescendo* manner of deep, laboured breathing, which becomes shallower and slower until an episode of **apnoea** occurs. This is then followed by a pattern of shallow respirations becoming deeper and faster until they once again begin to slow (see Figure 26.5). The period of apnoea may be as short as 10 seconds or as long as 30–40 seconds. Although the rate is variable, the overall respiratory rate is generally recorded as quite slow because the apnoea reduces the frequency of breaths over the minute.

Cheyne–Stokes breathing is often associated with end-of-life situations, and is commonly seen in people receiving palliative care. Cheyne–Stokes breathing can also be associated with congestive heart failure when sleeping, and increases the risk of adverse cardiac events in this group of people.

The mechanism of Cheyne–Stokes breathing is not well understood. The pattern may develop as a result of altered brainstem function, poor cerebral circulation, alterations in the respiratory control centre or even cortical dysfunction. In individuals with cardiac failure, Cheyne–Stokes breathing may result in worsening diastolic dysfunction and dysrhythmia. This exacerbation results from excessive sympathetic nervous system stimulation in response to the apnoea, causing hypoxaemia.

Biot's breathing (aka ataxic breathing)

Biot's breathing, or pattern of respiration, has an *irregular period of rapid breathing followed by variable periods of apnoea*. The depth of breath is also inconsistent (see Figure 26.6). The critical difference between Cheyne–Stokes and Biot's breathing is the lack of crescendo–decrescendo cycle in Biot's breathing. Biot's breathing is commonly associated with neurological damage,

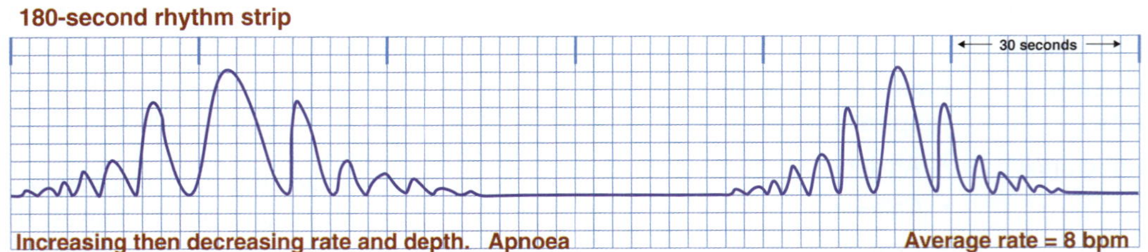

Figure 26.5

Cheyne–Stokes breathing

Note that the depth and the frequency increase, then decrease to a period of apnoea, then begin again with rapid, shallow breathing, once again reducing to deeper, slower breathing, and the cycle continues. This is common in end-of-life and palliative care situations. The respiratory rate in this example is an average of approximately 8 breaths per minute, but consists of periods of tachypnoea and apnoea.

bpm = breaths per minute.

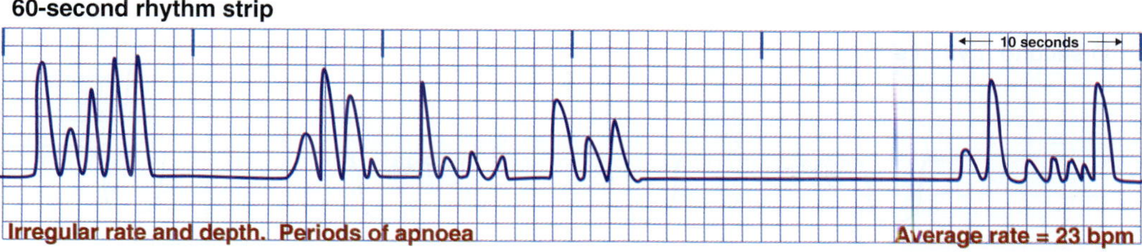

Figure 26.6

Biot's breathing

Note that the depth is inconsistent, the frequency is irregular and the periods of apnoea are variable. Biot's breathing is more irregular in rate, depth and rhythm than cluster breathing. The respiratory rate in this example is an average of approximately 23 breaths per minute, and consists of periods of tachypnoea and apnoea.

bpm = breaths per minute.

meningitis and sometimes increased intracranial pressure. This pattern can also be confused with cluster breathing; however, Biot's breathing is more irregular than cluster breathing.

Cluster breathing

Cluster breathing is characterised by *periods of tachypnoea separated by periods of apnoea*. The number of breaths per tachypnoeic set is variable, and the duration of apnoea is also irregular (see Figure 26.7). Cluster breathing is commonly associated with damage high in the medulla oblongata or low in the pons. This pattern can be confused with a Biot's breathing pattern, but, even though it is irregular, too, cluster breathing could be described as *more regular* than Biot's breathing.

Apneustic breathing (aka apneusis)

Apneustic breathing is characterised by *a slow, regular rhythm of gasping inspiration with a period of apnoea at end-inspiration* (see Figure 26.8). Apneustic breathing is associated with a basilar arterial occlusion resulting in damage to the pons. The pneumotaxic centre is affected. Apneustic breathing can be seen in people with severe stroke or head trauma. This respiratory pattern is comparatively uncommon.

Central neurogenic hyperventilation

Central neurogenic hyperventilation is a *tachypnoeic pattern of respiration with sustained respiratory rates* (in an adult) of approximately 40–60 breaths per minute (see Figure 26.9). Central neurogenic hyperventilation is commonly associated with neurological damage and increased intracranial pressure, causing compression of the pulmonary receptors within the brainstem and demonstrating pontine dysfunction. This pattern signifies advancing brainstem dysfunction, and results in severe hypocapnia and alkalosis if sedation, paralysis and mechanical ventilation are not initiated.

Apnoea

Apnoea is the total absence of any effective respiration for a period of greater than 20 seconds (see Figure 26.10). There are three types of apnoea. *Central apnoea* is caused by dysfunctional respiratory control mechanisms within the medulla oblongata. There is no attempt to breathe and no obvious chest wall movement. *Obstructive apnoea* is caused by an occlusion within the airway, interfering with airway patency. Obstructive apnoea may occur because of poor tone within

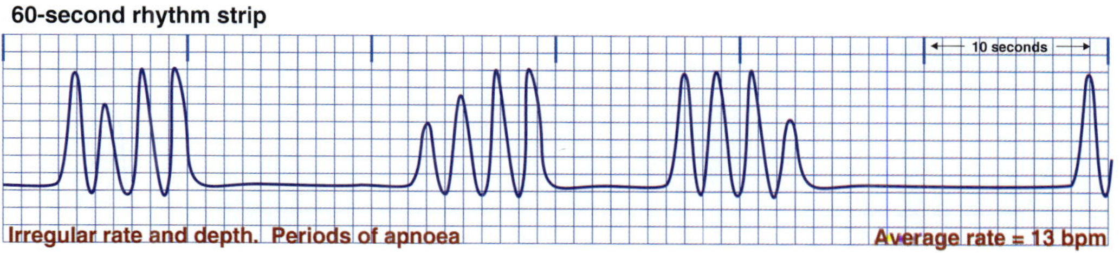

Figure 26.7

Cluster breathing

Note that the depth is inconsistent, the frequency is tachypnoeic, and it is interrupted by periods of apnoea. The periods of apnoea can be of different durations. However, the clusters are more regular than in Biot's breathing. The respiratory rate in this example is 13 breaths per minute, and consists of periods of tachypnoea and apnoea.

bpm = breaths per minute.

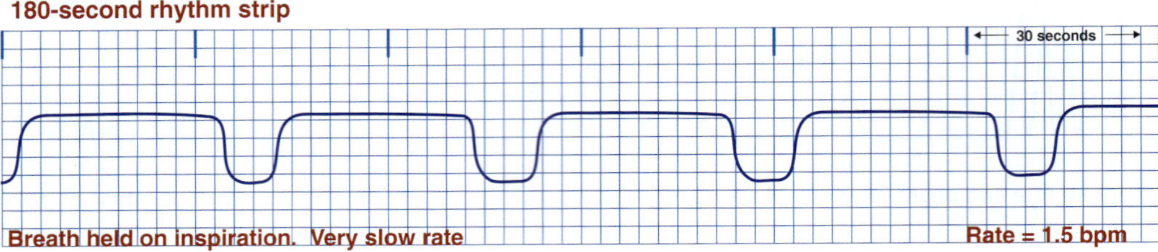

Figure 26.8

Apneustic breathing

This abnormal pattern of breathing is characterised by a deep, gasping inhalation with a pause at end-inspiration, where the breath is held for a period of time. This is followed by a brief exhalation and immediate inhalation, again continuing the cycle. This pattern can be seen in people with severe head trauma or stroke involving damage to the pons or the upper part of the medulla oblongata. The pneumotaxic centre is affected. The respiratory rate in this example is 1.5 breaths per minute.

bpm = breaths per minute.

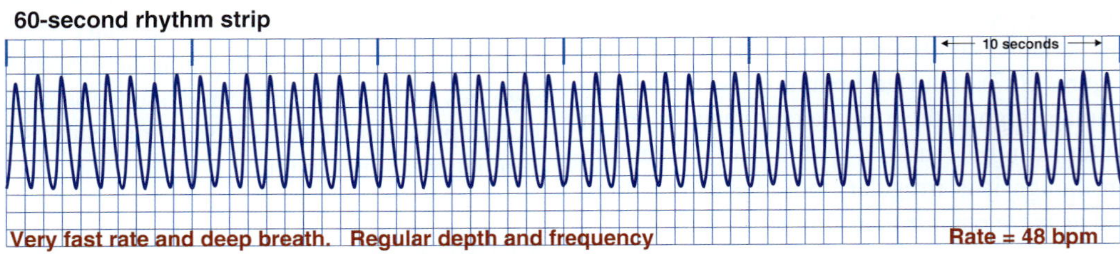

Figure 26.9

Central neurogenic hyperventilation

Note the sustained, rapid respiratory rate. The respiratory rate in this example is 48 breaths per minute.

bpm = breaths per minute.

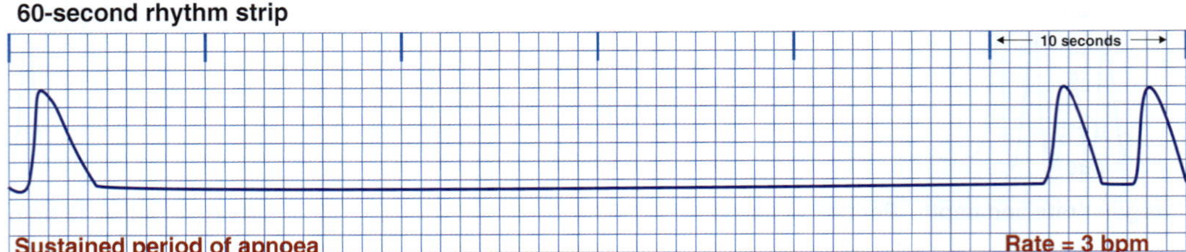

Figure 26.10

Apnoea

Apnoea is a total absence of any effective respiratory rate for greater than 20 seconds. The cause may be central or obstructive, or a mixture of both. The respiratory rate in this example is 3 breaths per minute; however, a sustained apnoea of almost 50 seconds occurred.

bpm = breaths per minute.

Table 26.4 Features of diaphragmatic and costal breathing

	Diaphragmatic breathing	Costal breathing
Specifics	Movement of the diaphragm to facilitate breathing. Contributes to a significant percentage of tidal volume (i.e. the volume of air moving in and out of the lungs with each normal breath).	Movement of the rib cage to assist with breathing. Contributes to a smaller percentage of tidal volume than diaphragmatic breathing.
Inhalation	Contraction of the diaphragm results in the downward movement of the diaphragm towards the abdominopelvic cavity. As a result of this movement and Boyle's law, a significant volume of air is *sucked* into the lungs. *Consider Boyle's law*	An upward movement of the rib cage by contracting intercostal muscles contributes to an increase in the transverse diameter of the thoracic cavity. A forward movement of the rib cage and sternum by contraction of the thoracic muscles results in an increase in the anterior–posterior diameter of the thoracic cavity. As a result of a combination of these two movements, some air is *sucked* into the lungs. *Consider Boyle's law*
Exhalation: Passive	Passive relaxation of the diaphragm results in an upward movement of the abdominopelvic cavity and the 'stored energy' within the muscles, and as it rebounds the diaphragm *pushes* air from the lungs. *Consider Pascal's law*	With intercostal relaxation, the cartilage is allowed to spring back, reducing the transverse diameter of the thorax. The elasticity of the thoracic cavity with intercostal muscle relaxation also assists in reducing the anterior–posterior diameter and subsequent movement of air *out* of the lungs. *Consider Pascal's law*
Forced	The thoracic diaphragm relaxes and the abdominal muscles contract, resulting in a more rapid and forceful movement that *pushes* air from the lungs. *Consider Pascal's law*	Some costal muscles contract, which results in a more rapid lowering of the rib cage. This helps *push* air from the lungs. *Consider Pascal's law*

the pharynx, obesity, foreign body aspiration, or some other factor resulting in airway obstruction. Often inspiratory effort is visible but ineffective. The third type of apnoea is caused by a combination of both central and obstructive apnoea, and is called *mixed apnoea*.

DEPTH

The depth of breathing is controlled by both *neurological and mechanical influences*, and is detected by *mechanoreceptors in the thorax*. When the pulmonary stretch receptors are stimulated, inspiratory time is shortened and expiratory time is lengthened. Other external factors can increase depth of breathing, too, as indicated by the following:

- *Pain* from rib fractures, infection or inflammatory conditions of the pleura can cause a person to take shallow breaths because deep breathing exacerbates the pain.
- *Metabolic disorders*, such as diabetic ketoacidosis, can cause deep, rapid breathing in an attempt to eliminate carbon dioxide in compensation of acidosis (see Kussmaul breathing).
- A person who is *exercising* will have a deeper, faster respiration rate in response to the metabolic demands of the activity.
- A person who is in *slow-wave sleep* will generally have a deeper and slower quality of respiration than someone who is awake. When the person cycles to *rapid eye movement (REM) sleep*, every 60–90 minutes, the respiratory depth (and rate) becomes more erratic in nature.

The two types of breathing are *diaphragmatic* and *costal*. Table 26.4 outlines the differences. The types of muscles engaged in breathing can influence respiratory depth.

Alterations in oxygen and carbon dioxide levels

LEARNING OBJECTIVE 4

Review the significance of alterations in oxygen and carbon dioxide levels.

Oxygen is mainly transported in red blood cells *bound to haemoglobin* (see Figure 26.11). Although hypoxia is the most common alteration, an excessive oxygen level is also dangerous. Several factors can influence the levels of oxygen within the blood; namely, body temperature, pH and the level of 2,3-diphosphoglycerate (2,3-DPG), an organic phosphate in erythrocytes that influences movement of oxygen to the tissues.

Carbon dioxide can be carried in three ways (see Figure 26.11). Approximately 7% is *dissolved in plasma*, 23% is

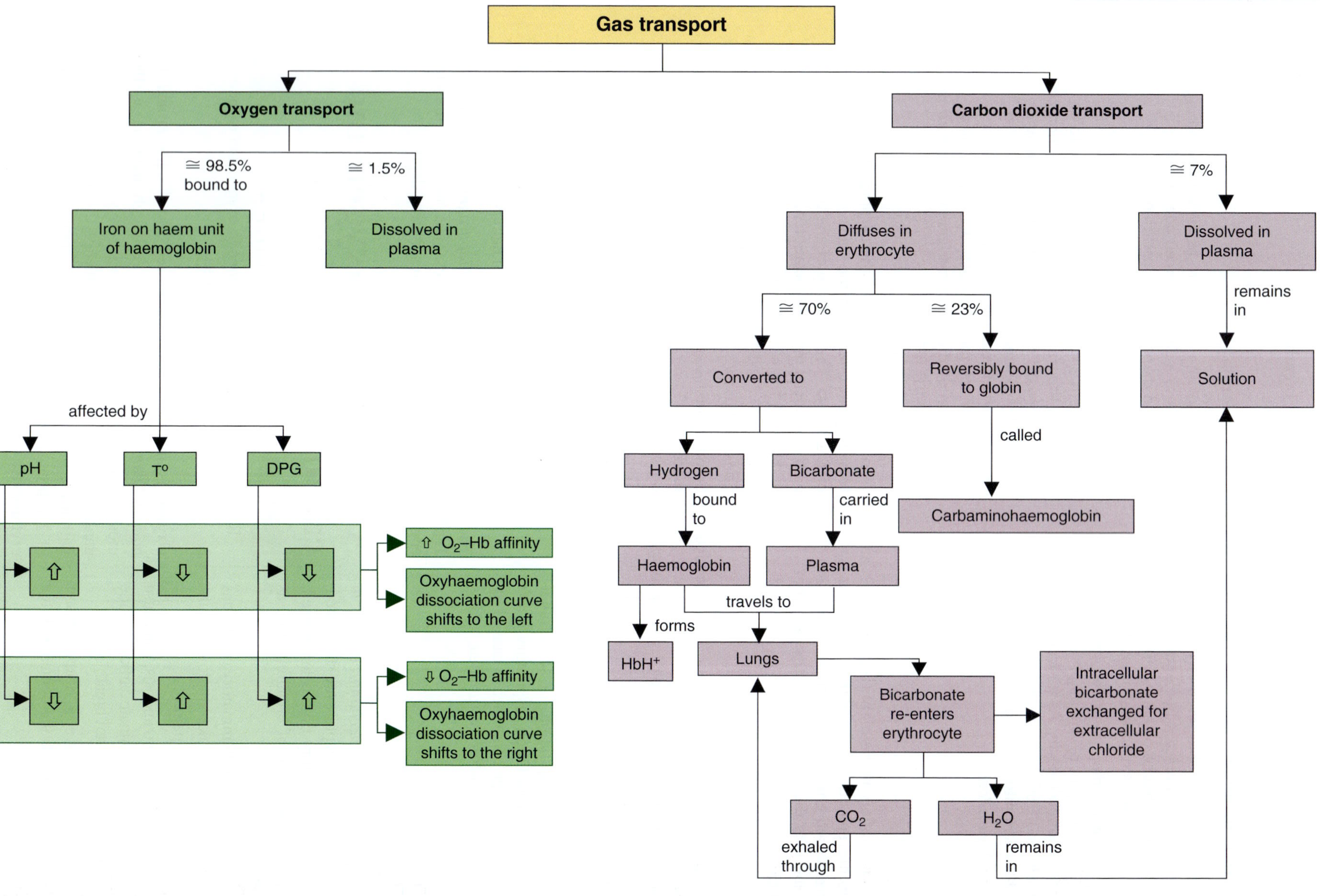

Figure 26.11

Gas transport

Oxygen is carried in two ways, and oxygen transport is affected by the acidity of the blood, changes in body temperature, and the presence of 2,3-diphosphoglycerate (2,3-DPG). Carbon dioxide can be carried in three ways. Elimination of the majority of carbon dioxide occurs through the lungs by exhalation. ↓ = decreased; ↑ = increased; CO_2 = carbon dioxide; DPG = diphosphoglycerate; HbH^+ = hydrogen–haemoglobin; H_2O = water; O_2–Hb = oxygen–haemoglobin; pH = potential of hydrogen; T° = temperature.

bound to the haemoglobin and the remaining 70% is *converted to bicarbonate*, which is carried in the plasma, and *hydrogen*, which is buffered by the haemoglobin. Once entering the lung vasculature, the bicarbonate re-enters the erythrocyte, in exchange for chloride, then is converted back to carbon dioxide, which is exhaled. Several factors can influence carbon dioxide levels.

ALTERATIONS IN OXYGEN LEVELS

Aetiology and pathophysiology

Arterial partial pressures of oxygen (PaO_2) should be maintained at approximately 80–100 mmHg. A low arterial oxygen level is called *hypoxaemia*, and an excessively high oxygen level is called *hyperoxia*. Oxygen transport is affected by the affinity of the haemoglobin. *Affinity* is the readiness to which the oxygen will bind to the haemoglobin. High affinity results in more binding, and this occurs at the alveolar–capillary interface within the lungs because the partial pressure of oxygen is high. Low affinity results in less binding, and this occurs at tissue level because the partial pressure of oxygen is low. The relationship between the partial pressure of oxygen and oxygen saturation can be demonstrated by the *oxyhaemoglobin dissociation curve*. As demonstrated by Figure 26.12A, the curve has a sigmoidal shape (S-shape). The plateau section of the curve shows that once the partial pressure of oxygen rises above 80 mmHg, the changes to oxygen saturation are minimal. However, in the steep section of the curve, minor changes to oxygen partial pressures will result in a significant change to oxygen saturations. An oxygen saturation of 50% equates to an oxygen partial pressure of approximately 27 mmHg.

Various factors can cause the curve to shift to the left or to the right. If the *curve shifts to the left, oxygen affinity increases*, and hence the ability to release oxygen to the tissues is reduced (see Figure 26.12B). The factors that cause the oxyhaemoglobin dissociation curve to shift to the left include:

- an increase in pH
- a decrease in temperature
- a decrease in 2,3-DPG
- an increase in circulating methaemoglobinaemia (MetHb)
- the presence of fetal haemoglobin (HbF)
- the presence of carbon monoxide (CO).

If the *curve shifts to the right, oxygen affinity reduces* and the ability to release oxygen at the tissues is improved (see Figure 26.12C). The factors that cause the oxydissociation curve to shift to the right include:

- a decrease in pH
- an increase in temperature
- an increase in 2,3-DPG.

The clinical significance of the oxyhaemoglobin dissociation curve relates to an understanding of what factors influence a left or right shift so that interventions can be initiated to counteract these factors. The concept of oxygen affinity is critical in developing ways of manipulating oxygen transport. Recognising the effect of changes in the partial pressures of oxygen and the relationship to oxygen saturations at various points on the curve will assist a healthcare professional when administering supplemental oxygen to individuals with hypoxaemia. Finally, administering more supplemental oxygen than is required to achieve adequate oxygen saturations will provide no clinical benefit and may, in fact, cause tissue and organ damage.

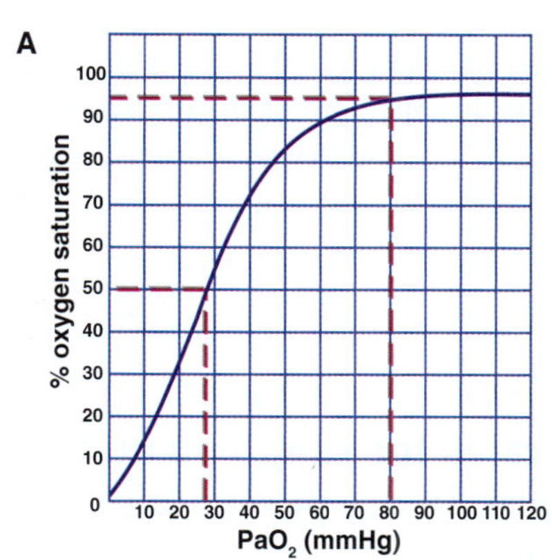

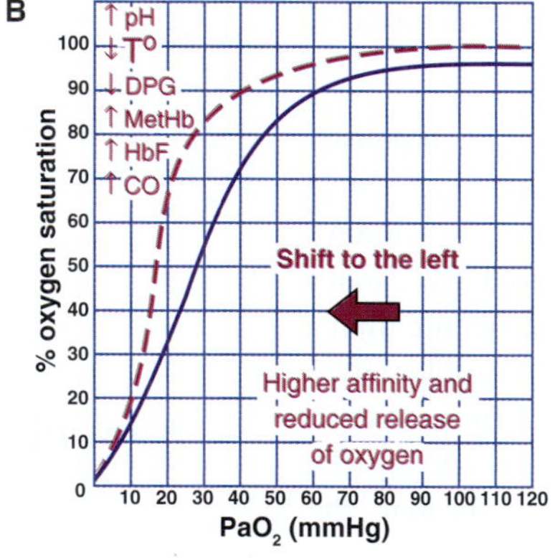

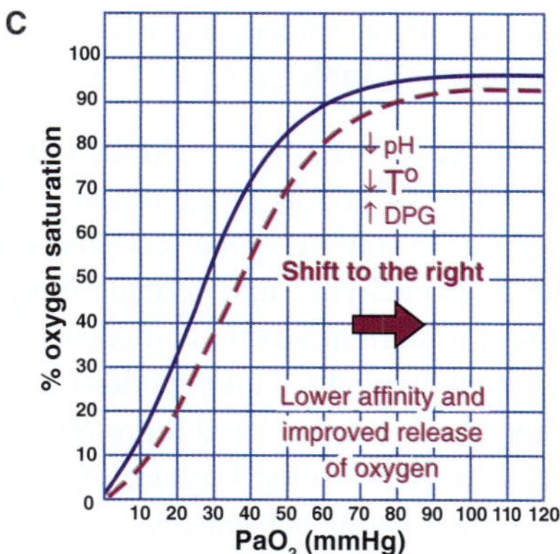

Figure 26.12

Oxyhaemoglobin dissociation curve

(A) The oxyhaemoglobin dissociation curve demonstrates the relationship between the partial pressure of oxygen and oxygen saturation. A higher PaO_2 increases oxygen saturation of the blood.

(B) A shift to the left results in higher affinity and reduced oxygen release.

(C) A shift to the right results in lower affinity and improved oxygen release.

CO = carbon monoxide; DPG = diphosphoglycerate; HbF = fetal haemoglobin; MetHb = methaemoglobinaemia; mmHg = millimetre of mercury; PaO_2 = arterial partial pressures of oxygen; pH = potential of hydrogen; T° = temperature.

Table 26.5 Factors affecting oxygenation

Factor	Cause
Decreased oxygen-carrying capacity	Hypovolaemia
	Anaemia
	Thalassaemia
	Carbon monoxide poisoning
Decreased inspired oxygen concentrations	Conditions affecting ventilation
	Conditions affecting the respiratory membrane
	Low atmospheric oxygen conditions—high altitude
Circulatory failure	
Increased metabolic rate	

Oxygen deficiency The terms 'hypoxia' and 'hypoxaemia' are commonly used interchangeably; however, they are technically different. *Hypoxaemia* is a *deficiency of oxygen in arterial blood*. This may be caused by either reduced partial pressure of oxygen, insufficient haemoglobin levels or a combination of both. *Hypoxia*, which is *reduced oxygen at the tissues*, can be caused by a reduction of blood flow to an area or decreased oxygen within the blood. Both hypoxia and hypoxaemia are *symptoms*, not a diagnosis.

Hypoxaemia can be defined as a partial pressure of arterial oxygen less than 60 mmHg (PaO_2 60 mmHg) or an oxygen saturation of less than 90%. The factors influencing oxygenation include any condition that affects cardiopulmonary functioning, as shown in Table 26.5.

Oxygen toxicity At the other end of the scale, **hyperoxia** is the state of *too much oxygen*. Oxygen toxicity can cause central nervous system effects and can damage tissue, including lung parenchyma and retinal tissue. Oxygen toxicity cannot occur in normal health, and occurs only as an iatrogenic injury (caused by medical intervention). If high levels of supplemental oxygen are administered for a prolonged period of time, oxygen toxicity can develop because of the production of oxygen free radicals. These substances cause cellular injury through the disruption of cell membranes and impaired energy production. Other effects include impaired neurotransmitter function and inhibition of protein synthesis.

Some important effects of oxygen toxicity are outlined below.

- *Pulmonary system*: Lung injury, including alveolar and interstitial oedema, alveolar haemorrhage and when inflammatory changes occur. Fibrotic changes occur with prolonged exposure to excess oxygen.
- *Retinas*: When excessive supplemental oxygen is administered to premature infants, oxygen-induced retinopathy can develop (known as *retinopathy of prematurity*). It is thought that, initially, retinal vasoconstriction occurs, resulting in endothelial destruction and ischaemia. As a result, neovascularisation (a proliferation of new capillaries) occurs; however, these vessels are immature, fragile and dysfunctional.
- *Central nervous system effects*: Oxygen toxicity has been associated with seizure activity from cerebral artery vasoconstriction, vasodilation, inflammatory processes and, ultimately, cellular damage. Neurotransmitters are also affected, especially in the context of hyperbaric oxygen administration.

Clinical manifestations

Some clinical manifestations commonly associated with hypoxaemia include tachycardia, tachypnoea and, in severe cases, hypoxaemia cyanosis.

Clinical manifestations commonly associated with oxygen toxicity include respiratory failure, loss of visual acuity or blindness, seizure, altered level of consciousness, and numerous other central nervous system signs and symptoms.

Management

Apart from managing the cause of the hypoxaemia, administration of supplemental oxygen will be beneficial. Interventions to improve cardiopulmonary function may be necessary, and, in the context of alterations in haemoglobin function, blood transfusion may assist to improve oxygenation.

When administering supplemental oxygen, it is important to understand the approximate percentage that the set flow rate will deliver (see Clinical Box 26.1). Atmospheric oxygen is approximately 21% of air.

Oxygen toxicity can be prevented by administering the least possible supplemental oxygen to maintain adequate oxygenation. Attempting to keep the *fraction of inspired oxygen (FiO_2)* to less than 0.6 (60%) may be beneficial; however, oxygen toxicity has developed at lower FiO_2. The use of positive end-expiratory pressure can be beneficial to facilitate improved oxygenation without the need to increase oxygen administration too high for too long.

CLINICAL BOX 26.1

Administration rates for supplemental oxygen and approximate percentage oxygen

HUDSON MASKS (OR EQUIVALENT)		NASAL PRONGS		VENTURI MASKS (OR EQUIVALENT)	
L/MIN	%	L/MIN	%	L/MIN	%
4	35	1	24	As per the required L/min settings described on the mask	24
6	45	2	28		28
8	50	3	32		35
10	65	4	35		40
					50

ALTERATIONS IN CARBON DIOXIDE LEVELS

Aetiology and pathophysiology

Arterial partial pressures of carbon dioxide ($PaCO_2$) need to be maintained at 35–45 mmHg. When a person's carbon dioxide level is lower than 35 mmHg, they are considered to have hypocapnia, and when a person's carbon dioxide level is higher than 45 mmHg they have hypercapnia. Carbon dioxide levels are controlled largely by the respiratory system manipulating the fine balance between carbon dioxide production and elimination. Generally speaking, an increase in respiratory rate and/or depth will result in a decrease in arterial carbon dioxide, and, conversely, a decrease in rate and/or depth will result in an increase in arterial carbon dioxide levels.

Hypocapnia The main cause of **hypocapnia** (also known as *hypocarbia*) is hyperventilation. Mild hypocapnia ($PaCO_2$ 30–35 mmHg) is not associated with serious effects; however, as hypocapnia increases, the blood pH becomes alkaline. Moderate hypocapnia is regarded as a $PaCO_2$ of 25–29 mmHg, and severe hypocapnia is a $PaCO_2$ below 25 mmHg. Cerebral vascular perfusion is reduced because of decreased nitric oxide production, which results in vasoconstriction and ultimately cerebral hypoxia. Hypocapnia is a risk factor for cerebral palsy, auditory defects, poor neurodevelopmental outcomes and periventricular leukomalacia (PVL). PVL is a common brain injury caused by ischaemia in the white matter adjacent to the lateral ventricles. PVL causes cerebral palsy, vision deficits and intellectual impairment. Hypocapnia can also affect the respiratory system, with reports of hypocapnic alkalosis aggravating acute lung injury following episodes of ischaemia and re-perfusion.

Hypercapnia The main cause of **hypercapnia** (also known as *hypercarbia*) is hypoventilation. Mild hypercapnia ($PaCO_2$ 45–50 mmHg) is not associated with serious effects; however, as hypercapnia increases, the blood pH becomes acidic. Moderate hypercapnia is regarded as a $PaCO_2$ of 51–60 mmHg, and severe hypercapnia is a $PaCO_2$ above 60 mmHg. Other causes of hypercapnia include increased carbon dioxide production and increased dead-space ventilation.

Neurological effects of worsening hypercapnia include increased cerebral blood flow and increased intracranial pressure. The pulmonary effects of hypercapnia include an increase in pulmonary vascular resistance, and, with increasing pulmonary hypertension, alterations in ventilation/perfusion ratios can occur. A decrease in tidal volume may also occur. The cardiovascular effects of hypercapnia may initially include reduced myocardial contractility. However, because of sympathetic nervous system stimulation, an increase in heart rate and a subsequent increase in contractility can increase cardiac output. Counterintuitively, hypercapnia may result in increased oxygen delivery through the increased cardiac output, the development of an intrapulmonary shunt and the movement of the oxyhaemoglobin dissociation curve to the right, which ultimately improves tissue oxygenation through decreased affinity.

Clinical manifestations

Hypocapnia results in alkalosis and, as the hypocapnia worsens, neurological issues such as dizziness, anxiety and syncope can occur. Other clinical manifestations can occur, including peripheral paraesthesia (pins and needles in the hands and feet) and muscle cramps. Hyperventilation causes hypocapnia; therefore, an increased respiratory rate and/or depth can be observed. Individuals may complain of dyspnoea. Other biochemical changes include hypokalaemia, hypocalcaemia, hyponatraemia and hypochloraemia. Acute hypocapnia will result in low bicarbonate levels, and chronic hypocapnia will further stimulate renal compensation and cause a more significant reduction in bicarbonate levels until a limit of approximately 12–15 mmol/L.

Hypercapnia results in acidosis and, as the hypercapnia worsens, neurological issues, such as confusion, headache and mental obtundation, occur. Dyspnoea may be observed, and, as hypoventilation is a major cause of hypercapnia, bradypnoea may be seen. Conversely, if a respiratory disease process is causing hypercapnia, tachypnoea may be observed.

Management

One of the most effective methods of achieving change in a person's carbon dioxide level is through the respiratory system. In someone who is spontaneously breathing, encouragement to either increase or decrease their respiration rate and depth can influence their arterial carbon dioxide level. In an individual who is receiving mechanical ventilation, manipulation of their carbon dioxide level can be achieved more readily through altering the respiratory rate and tidal volume. Table 26.6 demonstrates interventions that can be undertaken to assist a person with alterations in their $PaCO_2$.

The act of tolerating higher arterial carbon dioxide levels in the ventilated individual is called *permissive hypercapnia* (when using an appropriate tidal volume per the weight of the ventilated person). Some clinicians advocate the benefits of permissive hypercapnia in people with acute respiratory distress syndrome (ARDS) to prevent barotrauma and avoid the consequences of alveolar overdistension. In permissive hypercapnia, smaller tidal volumes are set, and higher carbon dioxide levels and some degree of acidosis are tolerated, provided that oxygenation is maintained. Contraindications include neurological conditions, such as cerebrovascular disease, increased intracranial pressure and seizure disorders. Caution should also be observed in people with cardiovascular conditions, such as coronary artery disease and heart failure. Recent meta-analysis suggests that permissive hypercapnia in those who are ventilated results in lower mortality. However, interestingly, imposed hypercapnia (where there was an active plan to induce a degree of hypercapnia in the ventilated person) was found to cause higher mortality.

Pulmonary dysfunction

LEARNING OBJECTIVE 5

Explain the common clinical manifestations of pulmonary dysfunction, including dyspnoea, cough, haemoptysis, cyanosis and digital clubbing.

Some clinical manifestations are common to many conditions of pulmonary dysfunction. Dyspnoea is one of the most common symptoms reported by people with respiratory conditions. Cough

Table 26.6 Possible interventions for various clinical scenarios relating to arterial CO_2 levels

Intervention	Hypocapnia (↓ $PaCO_2$)	Hypercapnia (↑ $PaCO_2$)
Spontaneously breathing	Goal: ↓ respiration rate/depth to ↓ CO_2 retention • Encourage the person to slow breathing rate • Provide reassurance to ↓ anxiety • Provide pain relief (consider opioids)	Goal: ↑ respiration rate/depth and recruit more alveoli to ↓ CO_2 retention • Encourage incentive spirometry • Encourage deep breathing and coughing • Reduce opioid drug administration • Ensure sufficient flow through the oxygen mask to 'wash out' the CO_2 (i.e. Hudson masks require at least 4 L/min of oxygen to promote adequate CO_2 washout); if the person is receiving less than 4 L/min of oxygen, consider changing the oxygen delivery device to nasal prongs • Administer bronchodilators (as ordered)
Ventilated	Goal: ↓ respiration rate/depth to ↑ CO_2 retention • Interventions as above (plus) • Alter ventilator settings to encourage more synchrony as the person may be 'fighting the ventilator', resulting in tachypnoea from distress • Consider sedating and paralysing to obtain respiratory rate control and reduce distress • Decrease the respiratory rate (frequency) • Decrease the tidal volume	Goal: ↑ respiration rate/depth and recruit more alveoli to ↓ CO_2 retention • Interventions as above (plus) • Alter ventilator settings to encourage more synchrony as the person may be 'fighting the ventilator', resulting in poor ventilation • Consider sedating and paralysing to obtain respiratory rate control and reduce distress • Perform endotracheal suction (if indicated) • Increase the respiratory rate (frequency) • Increase the tidal volume • Administer bronchodilators (as ordered)

and haemoptysis may also occur. In severe episodes of low oxygenation, cyanosis may be detected, and in chronic respiratory conditions, digital clubbing may occasionally develop.

DYSPNOEA

Aetiology and pathophysiology

Dyspnoea can be referred to by many names. *'Shortness of breath'* and *'difficulty breathing'* are two common phrases used to describe this subjective symptom. Dyspnoea may be either *acute* or *chronic*. It is frequently associated with other signs of respiratory or cardiovascular compromise, and the mechanism of dyspnoea varies between conditions.

Some factors that may influence the sensation of dyspnoea include an increased work of breathing, hypercapnia or hypoxia. Stimulation of receptors may influence the sensation of dyspnoea, including upper airway mechanoreceptors or various lung receptors that sense stretch, an irritant or interstitial congestion. Finally, a disparity between the efferent motor signals to the muscles of respiration and the afferent information to the cortex may also result in dyspnoea.

Dyspnoea may be ascribed to a sensation of chest tightness, increased work of breathing, or air hunger. Chest tightness may occur as a result of bronchoconstriction and changes in lung compliance. An increased work of breathing may occur as a result of muscle fatigue, paralysis or increased lung volume, and air hunger may occur from chemoreceptor stimulation.

The ascending pathways and processing structures in the cortex involved in the sensation of dyspnoea are not entirely understood; however, the anterior and posterior cingulate cortex, the amygdala, the insula and the cerebellum are all considered to be involved.

Clinical manifestations

Although dyspnoea is a symptom itself, secondary manifestations associated with dyspnoea include tachycardia, tachypnoea and anxiety. These manifestations are related to sympathetic nervous system stimulation in response to respiratory compromise.

Some measures of dyspnoea severity can include how far the person can walk on flat surfaces, how many stairs they can climb, whether they are able to speak in sentences without difficulty or if they can manage only single words before needing to take another breath, and whether they are able to lie flat without getting breathless.

Other types of breathlessness may also be described, such as dyspnoea at night that wakes a person from sleep (*paroxysmal nocturnal dyspnoea*), and dyspnoea that occurs when a person lies flat (**orthopnoea**), lies on a particular side (*trepopnoea*) or sits upright (*platypnoea*).

COUGH

Aetiology and pathophysiology

A cough is the *sudden, explosive, audible exhalation of air from the lungs*. Coughing is a *respiratory defence mechanism* in an attempt to manually clear the airway of debris, pathogens or secretions. It happens more commonly when the mucociliary escalator is overwhelmed with excess secretions, or it can occur in response to irritant stimulation from environmental triggers. Although respiratory mucus has three critical roles—mucociliary clearance, humidification and antibacterial activity—excessive secretion is undesirable and can cause cough and airway obstruction.

A cough begins with a deep inhalation, which is followed by a closure of the glottis, resulting in the breath being trapped within the respiratory airways. The diaphragm contracts, the nasopharynx is occluded by the soft palate, and, as the pressure overcomes the strength of the glottis, the air suddenly escapes at speeds measured to approximately 160 km/h.

Clinical manifestations

Cough is commonly experienced in respiratory disorders. The frequency and characteristics are important to consider in the assessment of a person with a respiratory condition. A cough may be described as productive or non-productive. *Productive* refers to the presence of sputum. In productive coughs, the colour, consistency and odour of sputum can be of importance (see Clinical Box 26.2).

A *non-productive* cough does not produce any secretions. It may be persistent, and sometimes occurs in *paroxysms* (bouts of coughing). A non-productive cough may develop because of an irritant, allergy, viral infection or other respiratory disease. Cardiovascular conditions can also cause a dry cough, including congestive cardiac failure, mitral stenosis, bacterial endocarditis and congenital heart disease. Some medications, such as angiotensin-converting enzyme (ACE) inhibitors, may also cause a cough. The mechanism of cough induced by ACE inhibitors is thought to be due to an excess of tussive mediators bradykinin and substance P, which would normally be degraded by ACE.

A unique type of cough, caused by an infectious respiratory disease, is known as *pertussis (whooping cough)*. Whooping cough is associated with highly contagious bacteria that cause significant respiratory compromise, and a distinctive cough that comes in paroxysms and ends in a high-pitched 'whoop' on inspiration.

CLINICAL BOX 26.2

Various characteristics of sputum and their significance

- *Blood-stained sputum—haemoptysis*; suggests tissue damage or trauma to the respiratory airways; common causes of haemoptysis include trauma, pulmonary infections, lung cancer, pulmonary embolism and bleeding disorders
- *Rust-coloured sputum*—a sign of old blood, and can be associated with tuberculosis or lung cancer
- *Purulent sputum (green or yellow)*—common in lung infections and pneumonia
- *Black-flecked sputum*—commonly seen in smokers, and can be tar or smoke particulates
- *Frothy sputum (white or pink)*—highly suggestive of pulmonary oedema
- *Feculant (foul-smelling) sputum*—commonly found in anaerobic infections
- *Excessive volume* (> 50 mL/day) or *bronchorrhoea* (> 100 mL/day)—often occurs in respiratory conditions such as bronchiectasis, cystic fibrosis, tuberculosis, chronic bronchitis or lung abscess with bronchopleural fistula

HAEMOPTYSIS

Aetiology and pathophysiology

Haemoptysis is defined as coughing up blood from a source in the respiratory system below the level of the glottis. Haemoptysis can range in volume, with significant bleeding potentially resulting in airway obstruction or, occasionally, effects on haemodynamic stability. Various pathologies may cause haemoptysis, and the acronym TILDA can be beneficial in recalling them: *T*rachobronchial disorders (including aspiration and bronchogenic carcinoma), *I*atrogenic causes (including intubation and suctioning), *L*ocalised parenchymal diseases (including pneumonia, metastatic cancers and pulmonary embolism), *D*iffuse parenchymal diseases (including viral pneumonitis and systemic lupus erythematosus) and *A*nticoagulants or bleeding diathesis (including warfarin, thrombocytopenia or disseminated intravascular coagulation).

Clinical manifestations

By definition, haemoptysis is a sign; however, it may be associated with other clinical manifestations resulting from the condition causing the haemoptysis. These may include dyspnoea, tachypnoea, chest pain, fever, vomiting, melaena or even haematemesis (vomiting blood).

CYANOSIS

Aetiology and pathophysiology

Cyanosis is a bluish discolouration to the skin and mucous membranes from an increase in *deoxyhaemoglobin* (oxygen-poor haemoglobin). The three distinct forms of cyanosis are peripheral, central and acrocyanosis (a blue discolouration of the hands and feet). *Peripheral cyanosis* occurs in the fingers and toes, and is associated with decreased peripheral blood flow and increased oxygen extraction in the peripheral tissue (see Figure 26.13). It occurs when the blood contains greater than 5% deoxyhaemoglobin and in hypoxaemia. However, anaemia

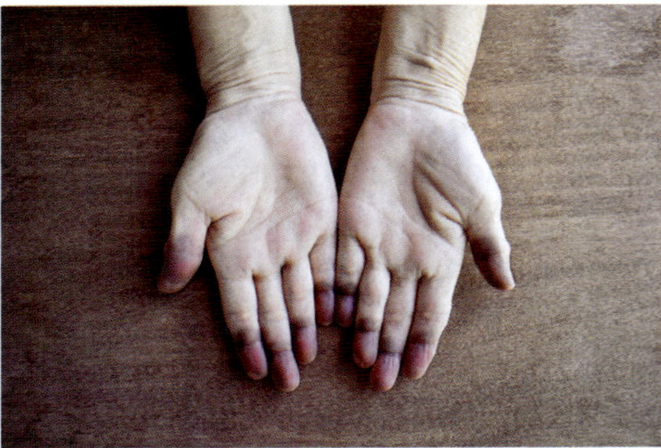

Figure 26.13

Peripheral cyanosis

Hand of a woman with peripheral cyanosis.

Source: Zay Nyi Nyi/Shutterstock.

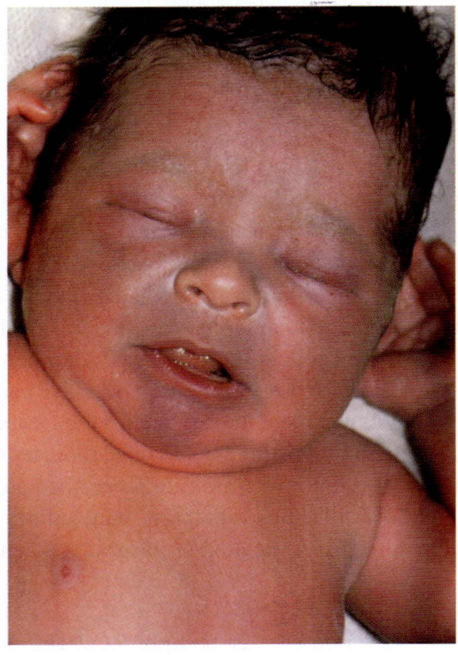

Figure 26.14

Central cyanosis

Baby with central cyanosis around the mouth and middle face.

Source: St Bartholomew's Hospital, London/Science Photo Library.

can mask this sign. The peripheries are often cool in peripheral cyanosis. All causes of central cyanosis will also cause peripheral cyanosis, but other causes of peripheral cyanosis include vasoconstriction from cool ambient temperatures, Raynaud's syndrome, low cardiac output states such as heart failure, and arterial or venous obstruction.

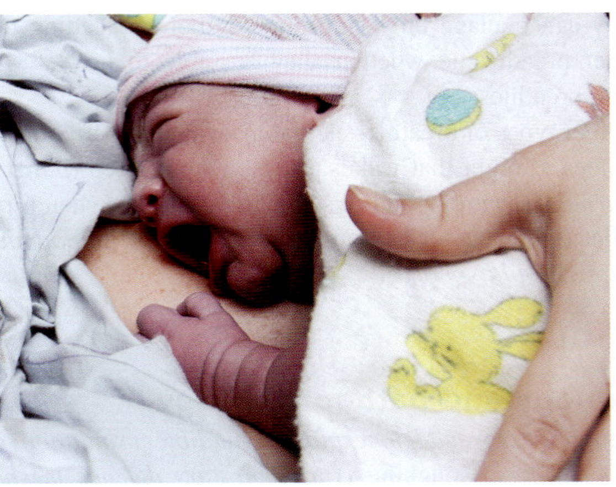

Figure 26.15

Acrocyanosis

Baby with acrocyanosis. Note the bluish discolouration of the hand. Compare this to the skin tone of the mother's hand.

Source: © Paul Hakimata Photography/Shutterstock.

Central cyanosis is a more serious sign, and occurs around the lips, tongue and mucous membranes when the oxygen saturation is less than 85%. It results from insufficient oxygen intake, decreased pulmonary blood flow, the mixing of arterial and venous blood, or from methaemoglobinaemia or polycythaemia (see Figure 26.14). The peripheries may be warm in central cyanosis.

Acrocyanosis (a painless condition also causing a bluish discoloration of the peripheral extremities) may sometimes involve the face as well. Acrocyanosis can be associated with sweating in the affected areas, too. Although the mechanism is not properly understood, it is thought to involve cutaneous arteriolar vasospasm, causing the cyanosis, and compensatory post-capillary venodilation, causing sweating because of the disparity in vessel tone, the volume of blood and, therefore, the retention of heat. Acrocyanosis is most commonly associated with newborns in the first 24 hours of life (see Figure 26.15).

Clinical manifestations

Peripheral cyanosis results in the bluish discolouration of the fingers and toes. Central cyanosis involves the fingers, toes and the mucous membranes, such as the lips and tongue. Acrocyanosis involves the hands and feet, and may also involve the perioral area, but is distinguished from central cyanosis by a pink tongue. None of these conditions is painful.

DIGITAL CLUBBING

Digital clubbing is a bulbous enlargement of the distal portion of the fingers and toes, and is most frequently associated with *chronic hypoxia* (secondary), although it can also be *idiopathic* (primary). Primary clubbing may have a genetic component. Secondary clubbing is generally associated with cardiac and respiratory conditions; however, it has also been described in endocrine, gastrointestinal and skin conditions.

A

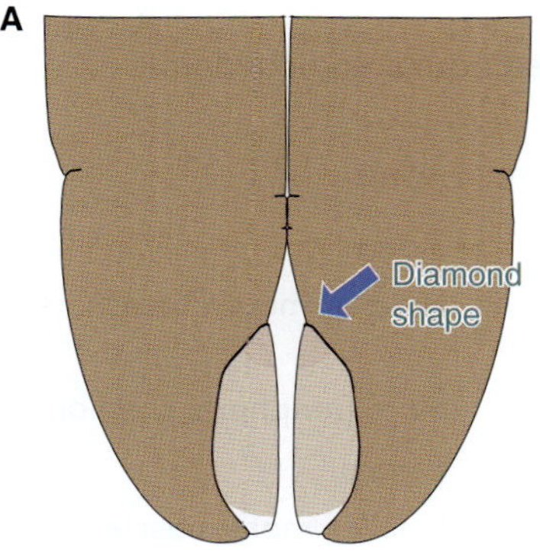

B

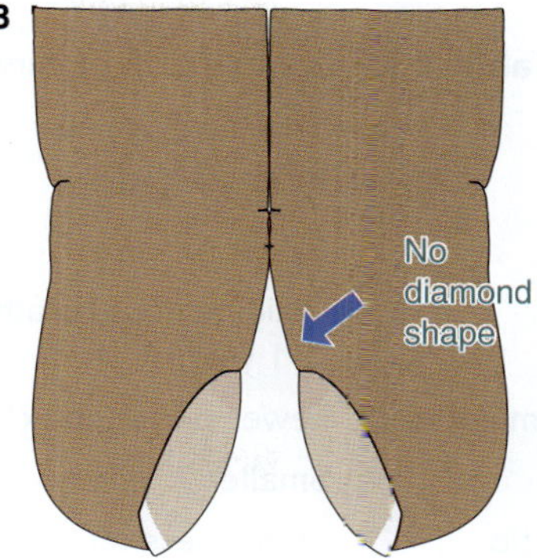

C

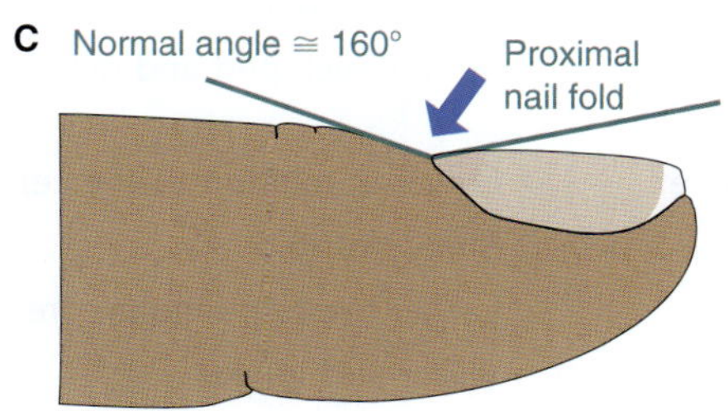

D

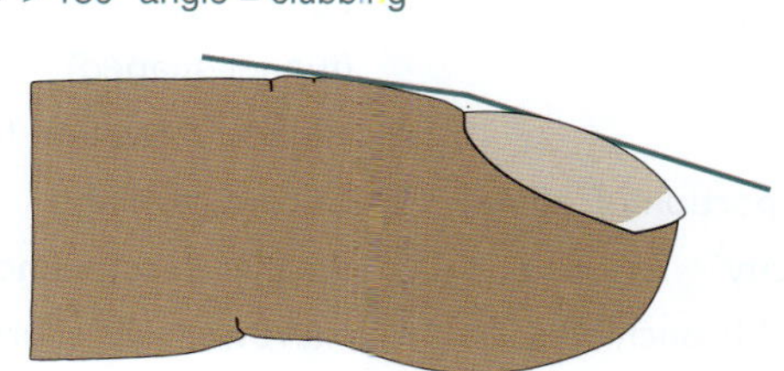

Figure 26.16

Digital clubbing

(A) Normal fingers create diamond shape when placed side by side.
(B) Clubbed fingers do not create a diamond shape in this position.
(C) Normal fingers have an angle of approximately 160° at the proximal nail fold.
(D) Clubbed fingers have an angle of > 180° at the proximal nail fold.

Aetiology and pathophysiology

Although the pathophysiology of digital clubbing is not well understood, it is thought to occur as a result of interstitial oedema, which progresses to produce changes in the vascular connective tissue. Focal vasodilation and increased blood flow occurs, which may be caused by local vasodilating agents or from neural mechanisms.

Clinical manifestations

Digital clubbing is most frequently observed in the fingers as a component of a respiratory assessment; however, toes can also be clubbed. The affected digits appear to have a bulbous enlargement distally (see Figure 26.16). This enlargement is painless and most often symmetrical.

Respiratory assessments and investigations

LEARNING OBJECTIVE 6

Describe the different types of respiratory assessments and investigations.

There are several ways to quantify a person's respiratory system function. This section will review the principles of physical assessment, auscultation, pulse oximetry, arterial blood gas analysis, spirometry and peak flow measurements. One important aspect to remember when undertaking respiratory assessment is that the structure and function of a child's respiratory system differs from that of an adult (see Table 26.7). These differences will influence not only the interpretation of the data gathered from the physical assessment, but also potentially management decisions.

PHYSICAL ASSESSMENT

Mental status

Respiratory conditions resulting in hypoxia can cause alterations in level of consciousness. An individual may present with altered levels of consciousness ranging from confusion, delirium, somnolence, obtundation, stupor or coma (see the chapters 'Brain and spinal cord dysfunction' and 'Neurotrauma'). A Glasgow coma scale assessment should be undertaken.

General physical appearance

An assessment of the person's general appearance will be beneficial in considering their respiratory function. As previously discussed, skin colour can suggest hypoxia when cyanosis is present. Their body position should be observed. It is rare for someone with respiratory compromise to tolerate lying down; they are commonly sitting upright, and may be leaning forward

Table 26.7 Comparison of airway differences between adults and children

Feature	Infant/child	Adult
Respiratory rate	Faster	Slower
Breathing	Obligate nose breathers (infants up to ≈ 1 year)	Nose or mouth breathers
Central nervous system control	Fewer peripheral chemoreceptors	More peripheral chemoreceptors
Nostrils	Smaller	Larger
Tongue:oropharynx ratio	Larger, less muscle tone	Smaller, more muscle tone
Epiglottis	Longer, less flexible and more horizontal	Shorter, more flexible and less horizontal
Trachea	Shorter, narrower and less rigid	Longer, wider and more rigid
Cricoid cartilage	Less developed and less rigid (funnel-shaped)	More developed and more rigid
Larynx	Higher in relation to the cervical spine	Lower in relation to the cervical spine
Narrowest portion of airway	Cricoid cartilage	Rima glottidis
Lung capacity	Smaller (less pulmonary reserve)	Larger (more pulmonary reserve)
Bronchi and bronchioles	Narrower and shorter	Wider and longer
Chest wall (bony structure)	Twice as compliant (prone to retractions)	Less compliant (less prone to retractions)
Rib orientation	Horizontal (less intercostal muscle leverage to lift the ribs)	45° angle (more intercostal muscle leverage to lift the ribs)
Diaphragm	Located higher in the thorax and horizontal; heavily reliant on the diaphragm	Located lower in the thorax and oblique; not as heavily reliant on the diaphragm
Intercostal muscles	Less developed (strength and coordination)	More developed (strength and coordination)
Alveolar tissue	Less elastin (less recoil and more loss of patency)	More elastin (more recoil and less loss of patency)

in a tripod position. In situations of profound dyspnoea or hypoxia, a person may not be able to sit still as their air hunger, anxiety and sense of impending doom is so overwhelming.

A person's physical condition can influence respiratory function. Someone who is obese or pregnant may have respiratory compromise from diaphragmatic malposition due to either abdominal distension or an enlarged uterus (more of an issue in the third trimester). The presence of chest trauma may affect a person's capacity to take a breath sufficient to maintain adequate gas exchange. This may be from either pain (pleuritic pain) or from loss of negative intrapleural pressures interfering with inspiration.

As previously discussed, the rate, rhythm and quality of respirations are important, and so is the ease with which the person can speak in sentences. Dyspnoea that results in a person taking a breath in between each word is serious, and urgent intervention is necessary to prevent rapid decompensation from fatigue.

A respiratory assessment includes the inspection, palpation and percussion of the person's thorax.

Inspection

When assessing the chest, the presence of deformities should be noted, because these may interfere with tidal volume. Kyphoscoliosis, rib fractures or penetrating injuries can have a profound influence on gas exchange. The anterior–posterior (AP) diameter of the chest should also be quantified, as large AP diameters suggest chronic obstructive conditions resulting in gas trapping (see the chapter 'Obstructive pulmonary disorders'). If the person has a productive cough, their sputum should also be inspected for volume and characteristics, because self-reporting of sputum quality is often not reliable.

Palpation

Palpating the thorax can give an impression of symmetry of movement during inspiration and expiration. Palpable vibrations of the chest wall over the lung fields felt while breathing are called *fremitus*. Increased tactile fremitus may be caused by consolidation, and decreased fremitus may result from pleural effusion, pneumothorax or bronchial obstruction.

Percussion

The use of a technique called percussion can elucidate whether the person's chest wall produces sounds that are normal, dull or hyperresonant in certain regions. Sounds travel easily through air, less well through fluid and poorly through solids. Therefore, listening to the quality and characteristics of sounds generated by this technique can give an impression of the state of the tissue beneath the area assessed. Hyperresonant sounds can be indicative of pneumothorax, dull sounds can suggest consolidation or collapse, and very dull sounds can suggest a pleural effusion.

AUSCULTATION

Respiratory assessments include auscultation of breath sounds with a stethoscope. Normal breath sounds are commonly loud and harsh over the trachea, and loud and high-pitched over the bronchi. Bronchovesicular sounds are softer than bronchial sounds and have a tubular quality. They are heard in the posterior chest between the scapulae, and also in the central anterior chest. Vesicular sounds are heard throughout the lung fields, are low-pitched and have a soft, breezy quality.

Adventitious sounds are abnormal sounds, and are frequently divided into wheezes, crackles and rubs. *Stridor* is also a lung sound that can often be heard without a stethoscope.

Wheezing

A **wheeze** is a high-pitched sound, often of a musical quality, caused by a narrowing of the tracheobronchial tree and small airways. Wheezes are most often heard in expiration. *Rhonchi* are lower-pitched sounds, and are more like a snore or a rumble. They represent secretions in the large airways.

Crackles

Crackles (formerly known as *rales*) are non-musical, brief sounds that are more commonly heard during inspiration. Crackles can be described as fine, medium and coarse. *Fine crackles* tend to be high-pitched, and are heard at end-inspiration, most commonly at the bases. They are caused by alveolar and a small airway opening. *Medium crackles* tend to be lower-pitched, and are heard at mid-inspiration. They represent the sounds of the opening of small bronchioles. *Coarse crackles* can be heard on both inspiration and expiration, and represent the movement of mucus within the larger airways. Coarse crackles frequently clear with endotracheal suctioning or following a cough.

Pleural friction rub

A pleural friction rub sounds like a creaking or grating sound, such as leather rubbing against itself. It is not cleared by coughing. Pleural friction rubs are due to the inflammation of the pleura, and occur with respiration. Pleural rubs are associated with severe pleuritic pain.

Stridor

Stridor can be heard without a stethoscope, and is a high-pitched, harsh sound heard during inspiration. It represents upper airway obstruction, and requires immediate attention as it is a sign of respiratory compromise.

PULSE OXIMETRY

Technique

The non-invasive measurement of peripheral oxygen saturation can be achieved by devices that gauge the absorption of two wavelengths of light emitted from a device in a process called *spectrophotometry*. Haemoglobin changes shape in response to the amount of oxygen bound to it. *Oxygen-rich haemoglobin* reflects wavelengths around 660 nm (red light), and *oxygen-poor haemoglobin* reflects wavelengths around 940 nm (infrared light). These differences can be used to quantify *oxygen saturation* by comparing how much red light is absorbed (or reflected) compared to how much infrared light is absorbed (or reflected). The pulse oximeter has photodetectors that detect light from pulsating arteries. This is important so that measurements are *calculated on peripheral arterial blood* instead of on venous blood or tissue.

Currently, there are two types of pulse oximetry devices. In *transmission pulse oximetry (TPO)*, the original type of oximetry, the detector is on the opposite side of the device to the light emitters (see Figure 26.17A). Recently, a technology called *reflectance pulse oximetry (RPO)* has gained popularity. In reflectance pulse oximetry, the detectors are placed beside the light emitters (see Figure 26.17B).

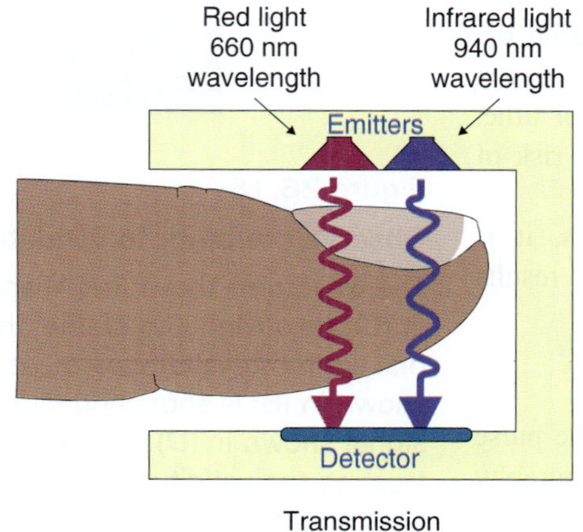

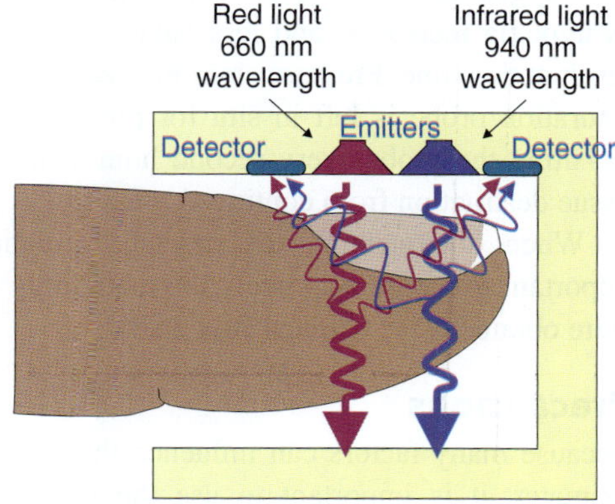

Figure 26.17

Oxygen saturation monitoring

(A) In transmission pulse oximetry, the photodetector is on the opposite side of the light emitters.

(B) In reflectance pulse oximetry, the photodetector is on the same side as the light emitters.

Light that is shone through tissue is both partly transmitted and partly absorbed. Transmission pulse oximetry works on the principle of detecting the amount of light that is absorbed. Reflectance pulse oximetry works on the principle of detecting the amount of light that is reflected back from within the tissue being monitored (not the light that is reflected back from the surface).

TPO measurements require an area of the body that can be circumscribed, and are frequently influenced by poor peripheral perfusion, because the required sites are generally digits or ears. With RPO, however, more central monitoring is becoming possible, because the device does not need to span a digit. Hence, it is less affected by poor peripheral perfusion, because the design can increase the number of sites available for monitoring; therefore, more central locations, such as the forehead or torso, can be used for monitoring. RPO may overcome the difficulties encountered with TPO in people who have poor peripheral perfusion either from vascular disease or circulatory volume issues.

Clinical interpretation

The ability to measure oxygen saturation provides valuable data that can be used to consider more about a person's respiratory function. Just like any other observation, oxygen saturation results should be interpreted in the context of the whole clinical picture and not relied upon in isolation. When used appropriately, pulse oximetry provides information about the peripheral oxygen saturation of an individual. Although understanding the oxygen status of a person is valuable, pulse oximeters do not measure carbon dioxide, and therefore only one of the two important respiratory gases is quantified. A person may demonstrate acceptable oxygen saturation levels; however, they may be profoundly hypercapnic or hypocapnic. Pulse oximetry also does not measure ventilation.

When combined with other data, such as heart rate, physical assessment and auscultation, pulse oximeters can demonstrate the need to investigate respiratory function further or provide more treatment, such as increasing supplemental oxygen or administering bronchodilating agents.

Oxygen saturation levels below 85% become less accurate as hypoxia increases, and less value should be placed on the result at this time. Pressure areas may also develop if an oxygen saturation probe is left in situ for prolonged periods of time. Re-siting the probe every second hour will reduce the risk of tissue destruction from continued pressure.

When documenting the oxygen saturation results, it is important to record accurately the method by which the results were obtained (see Clinical Box 26.3).

Precautions

Because many factors can influence the accuracy of the pulse oximeter, it is important to use the *pleth* (plethysmography waveform) to assist in determining the validity of the reading (see Table 26.8). The pleth may be shown as a waveform (see Figure 26.18A and B), or it may be shown as a set of bars (see Figure 26.18C and D). If the pleth suggests a poor signal, do not consider the reading as accurate.

Although second-generation machines are striving to overcome some of the common factors that influence oxygen saturation level accuracy, the capacity and limitations of the individual machine should be understood before placing any emphasis on readings.

CLINICAL BOX 26.3

Correct terminology when documenting oxygen saturation

SpO_2	Used when obtaining oxygen saturations from a pulse oximeter. This is the only way that oxygen saturation from an oximeter should be documented.
SaO_2	Used when obtaining an oxygen saturation result from an arterial blood sample.
SvO_2	Used when obtaining an oxygen saturation result from a venous blood sample.
SAO_2	Used more in research when referring to alveolar oxygen saturation.
PaO_2	Used when referring to the partial pressure of oxygen from an arterial blood sample.

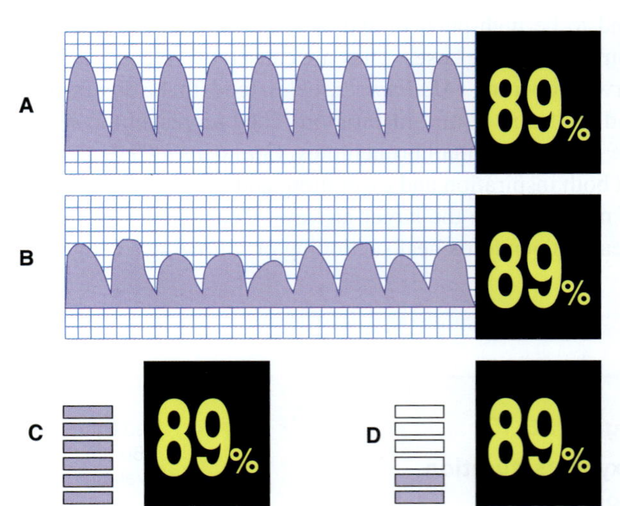

Figure 26.18

Observe the pleth to validate the reading

The waveform shown in (A) and the pleth signal shown in (C) are strong and stable; therefore, confidence can be placed in the validity of these readings. The waveform shown in (B) is short and variable in height, and the pleth signal shown in (D) is weak. Caution should be taken with trusting the validity of either of these two findings. In such situations, attempt to find another monitoring site, or rely more heavily on other data and the clinical picture as a sum of all the observations and assessments.

Table 26.8 Factors that can influence the validity of oxygen saturations measured via an oximeter

Influencing factor	Description	Resolution
Movement	Because many pulse oximeters are placed on the finger (or the foot with a neonate), the device may experience a lot of movement. Shivering can also affect the readings.	Movement of the probe alters the light absorption (or reflection) measurements and makes the reported value inaccurate. Attempt to place the probe in a location with limited movement (e.g. ear lobe). A different probe type may be required to resolve this issue.
Too much ambient light	Poorly fitting or inappropriately applied probes will enable ambient light from the room to interfere with the detector.	Ensure that the correct probe size is applied. Remove and re-site the probe to ensure a correct fit.
Poor peripheral perfusion	People with alterations to perfusion, either from peripheral vascular disease or a circulating blood volume issue, will cause the transcutaneous device to measure inaccurately because the signal will be too low.	Select a digit or location that is warm or is better perfused. Attempt to warm the location site to promote vasodilation. Choose another site. If using an RPO, select a location that is more central, and therefore better perfused (e.g. forehead).
Abnormal haemoglobin	Severe anaemia can affect the oxygen saturation reading. However, irrespective of the reported value, in a person with anaemia the volume of haemoglobin is reduced, and therefore the percentage of oxyhaemoglobin is high. A reported high oxygen saturation level does not truly represent the tissue hypoxia that occurs in anaemia.	Consider oxygen saturation reporting in the context of anaemia. A blood transfusion will improve anaemia, and therefore tissue hypoxia. A blood transfusion may be indicated for the management of hypoxia. Improving the accuracy of the oximetry measurement is only a benefit of treatment, not the goal.
	Polycythaemia causes the opposite situation to anaemia. If significantly more red blood cells exist in the circulation, it is more difficult to saturate the number of haemoglobin molecules with the available oxygen, and therefore oxygen saturations may be falsely reported as low.	Consider oxygen saturation reporting in the context of polycythaemia. Venesection will reduce the volume of excess red blood cells. A blood transfusion may or may not be indicated for the management of the clinical situation. Improving the accuracy of the oximetry measurement is only a benefit of treatment, not the goal.
	Methaemoglobin (metHb) and carbaminohaemoglobin (CoHb) are non-functional forms of haemoglobin produced in some forms of chemical exposure or certain disease. In health, these levels are low. In a person with higher levels of non-functional haemoglobin, the oximeter cannot differentiate between functional and non-functional haemoglobin, and reports artificially lower.	Consider the oxygen saturation reading in the context of methaemoglobinaemia and carboxyhaemoglobinaemia. Arterial blood gas analysis can identify these levels. A newer type of machine, the 'co-oximeter', can accurately differentiate between haemoglobin types and will report more reliable results; however, these machines are expensive, bulky and specialist equipment.
	Carbon monoxide (CO) binds preferentially to haemoglobin, displacing oxygen; therefore, it produces another situation of non-functional haemoglobin. The oximeter cannot distinguish between oxyhaemoglobin and carboxyhaemoglobin, and erroneously reports the oxygen saturation as high.	Do not consider oxygen saturations from oximeters in the context of carbon monoxide poisoning.
Nail polish	Coloured nail polish can interfere with the signal, which may result in an artificially low oxygen saturation.	Remove nail polish or select a site not affected by nail polish (e.g. ear lobe).

(continued)

Table 26.8 Factors that can influence the validity of oxygen saturations measured via an oximeter (*continued*)

Influencing factor	Description	Resolution
Intermittent inadequate blood flow	Placing an oxygen saturation probe on the same arm as a blood pressure cuff will result in intermittent loss of signal when blood pressure is being measured.	Place the pulse oximeter probe on the opposite arm to a sphygmomanometer.
Perinatal right-to-left shunts, such as patent ductus arteriosis	If mixing of arterial and venous blood is occurring because of a shunt, the oxygen saturations will differ between the right hand (preductal blood) and the other limbs (postductal blood). This may result in documentation of large oxygen saturation swings each time the oximetry probe is re-sited.	Alternate using the postductal sites (feet or left hand) and avoid the right hand. Sometimes, for assessment purposes, placing oxygen saturation probes on both preductal and postductal sites and noting if there is a greater than 15% difference is a way of determining whether a significant shunt exists.

Remote respiratory assessment and SARS-CoV-2 (COVID-19) infection

The recent worldwide COVID-19 pandemic spawned creativity to enable at-home monitoring of critical measures such as respiratory rate. Keeping COVID-infected individuals who do not require intensive medical support at home not only improves their comfort and reduces costs for the person and health service, but also reduces infection risks, and strain on an already overburdened system.

For the safety of the person receiving care, new technologies were developed to support alternative methods of care, and enable intermittent or continuous respiratory monitoring. The ability to determine improvement or deterioration in a person's condition is necessary to inform care decisions and determine the need to change medication regimens or facilitate urgent admission.

Oxygen saturation monitors were commonly provided in the Australian 'at-home' COVID response. However, although valuable, they only measure oxygen saturation (a late measure of hypoxia), and so new techniques were developed to monitor respiratory rates (which are an early measure of deterioration).

The various minimally-intrusive, contact-free technologies for measuring respiratory rate can be divided into three categories: camera-based, laser-based and radio-frequency based systems. It will be interesting to see the evolution of this technology and its acceptance in more telehealth programs, and potentially even into acute care monitoring systems.

ARTERIAL BLOOD GAS ANALYSIS

Test

An *arterial blood gas (ABG) analysis* measures several arterial blood parameters, including oxygen, carbon dioxide, pH and bicarbonate, and is generally sampled from the radial artery. Occasionally, the brachial artery is used, and in resuscitation situations an ABG may be sampled from the femoral artery. This test is particularly painful and, where possible, should be preceded by the administration of a local anaesthetic; however, clinically, this is often not done. A small-gauge needle connected to an ABG syringe (a specially designed syringe that contains heparin and will fill without pulling the plunger back) is inserted into the area that has been palpated for a strong pulse.

An *Allen's test* should be undertaken before sampling for an ABG analysis. This test determines the patency of the ulnar artery, so that if the radial artery is occluded, perfusion can be maintained to the hand. Most people have dual arterial supply to the hand, but damage to the artery in a person with only one functioning artery is serious, and occlusion can result in the total loss of perfusion to the hand.

Parameters

Some parameters are directly measured and some are calculated. Obviously, direct measurement is most accurate; however, as the technology advances and the quality of the machines improves, the disparity between the two values is becoming less clinically significant.

Each institution will generally have its own set of 'normal' values. These values are arbitrary but relatively consistent. A common set of arbitrary 'norms' has been provided in this text as the reference range in Clinical Box 26.4. The most important consideration is that any value obtained from any test is scrutinised against the clinical presentation of the person.

Clinical Box 26.4 also describes whether the ABG value is most likely directly measured or a calculated value. Consultation with the pathologist or a review of the ABG machine's specification literature should provide specific details.

Before attempting to analyse ABG results, it is important to understand the concepts of acidosis and alkalosis, and the two possible causes—either respiratory or metabolic.

In chemistry, a value of 7 represents neutral on the pH scale, and any value less than 7 is considered acidic, and any value greater than 7 is considered alkaline. In blood chemistry, the scale is shifted slightly (see Figure 26.19). Blood is considered

CLINICAL BOX 26.4

Some parameters measured or calculated in an ABG analysis

PARAMETER	ABBREVIATION	REFERENCE RANGE	UNIT OF MEASURE	MEASURED OR CALCULATED
Blood acidity	pH	7.35–7.45		Measured
Partial pressure of oxygen	PaO_2	80–100	mmHg	Measured
Partial pressure of carbon dioxide	$PaCO_2$	35–45	mmHg	Measured
Bicarbonate	HCO_3^-	22–26	mEq/L	Calculated
Saturation of arterial oxygen	SaO_2	>95	%	Calculated
Base excess	BE	-2 to $+2$	mEq/L	Calculated

to be more acidic when its pH is lower than 7.4, and more alkaline when its pH is higher than 7.4. However, when the pH, carbon dioxide level and bicarbonate level are within their respective reference ranges, it is not common to assign the words *acidosis* or *alkalosis* to the ABG value.

The most important chemical equation in understanding the regulation of blood pH describes the *carbonic acid–bicarbonate buffering system*:

$$\underset{\text{water}}{H_2O} + \underset{\text{carbon dioxide}}{CO_2} \leftrightarrow \underset{\text{carbonic acid}}{H_2CO_3} \leftrightarrow \underset{\text{bicarbonate ion}}{HCO_3^-} + \underset{\text{hydrogen ion}}{H^+}$$

This reversible reaction describes how water and carbon dioxide combine to form carbonic acid, and how a hydrogen ion is buffered by bicarbonate to form carbonic acid. This equation demonstrates how, depending on the needs of the body, blood pH can be altered by either buffering with bicarbonate to increase blood pH, or releasing hydrogen ions from bicarbonate to decrease blood pH. Carbonic acid can dissociate to form water and carbon dioxide, which can be exhaled from the respiratory system if the carbon dioxide levels are too high.

The two systems responsible for the regulation of blood pH are the *respiratory system* and the *renal system*. The respiratory

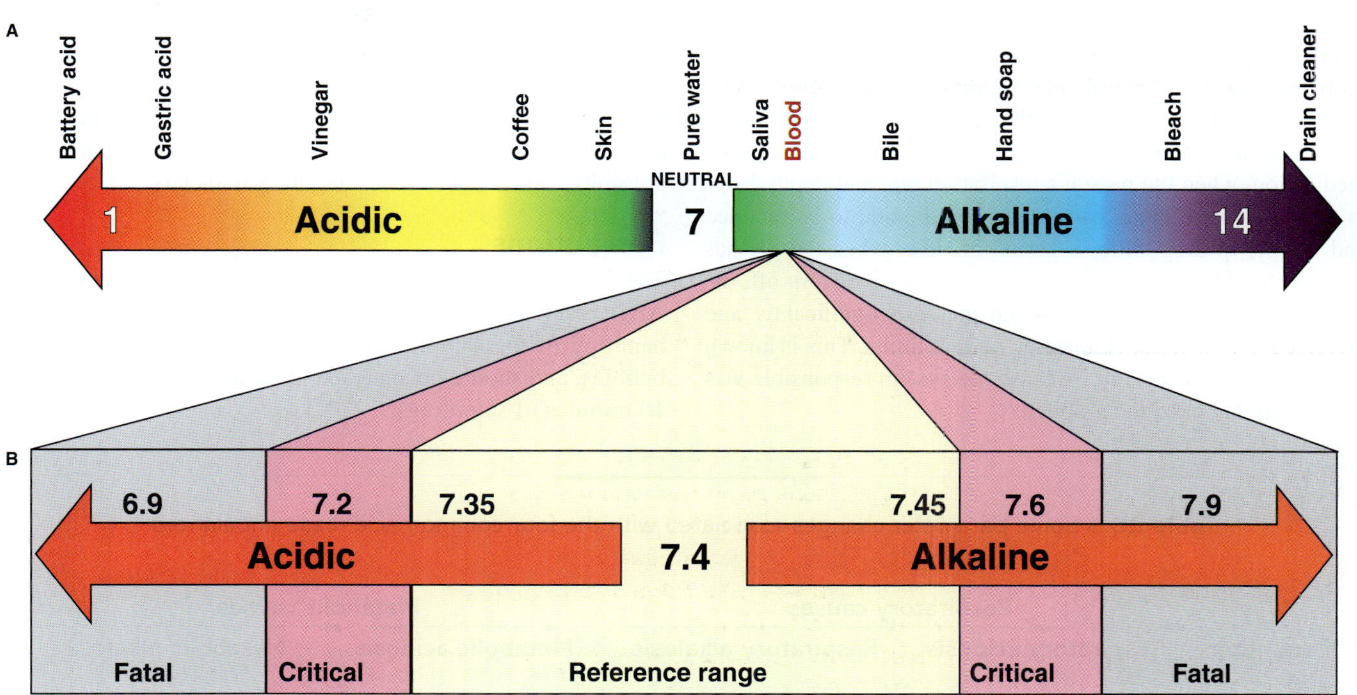

Figure 26.19

pH range of household products and blood

(A) The pH of various products found around the home and in the body.

(B) The pH of blood.

system regulates the volume of carbon dioxide through changes in breathing rate and depth (as explained in the section above). Carbon dioxide is 'blown off' with faster, deeper respirations, and 'retained' with slower, shallower or ineffective respiratory effort.

When excessive respirations result in low carbon dioxide levels, the blood pH rises (increases beyond 7.45—don't forget it is a negative logarithmic scale) and the person develops alkalosis. If the respiratory system is the only contributor to the high blood pH, this is described as *respiratory alkalosis*. Conversely, when ineffective respirations result in carbon dioxide retention, blood pH falls (decreases below 7.35) and the person develops acidosis. If the respiratory system is the only contributor to the low blood pH, this is described as *respiratory acidosis*. The respiratory system is considered a rapid manipulator of blood pH, and changes in respiration rate and depth will cause an increase or decrease in blood pH within minutes.

The kidneys have a slower response, so manipulation of blood pH will take hours to days. If a person's kidneys produce too much bicarbonate, this will buffer the hydrogen ions and the pH will rise, making the blood alkalotic. If the kidneys are the sole cause of higher blood pH, the problem is called *metabolic alkalosis*. Conversely, if the kidneys do not produce enough bicarbonate to buffer the free H^+, a low blood pH develops, this problem is called *metabolic acidosis*.

Although there are several more permutations, this description identifies some important concepts about the manipulation of blood pH by either the kidneys or the lungs. Two other important terms to understand are the words 'correction' and 'compensation'. Correction is 'fixing' the problem; however, this term can be used only when the system fixing the problem is the one that caused it. An example of this would be following the administration of too much opioid medication, when the person's respiration rate and depth drops to 6 breaths per minute, causing carbon dioxide to be retained and the pH to drop. After a period of time, when the pH has dropped too far and the effects of the opioid have worn off, the person's respiration rate and depth increase significantly and the blood pH comes back towards normal limits. This is known as respiratory 'correction', because the system responsible was the system that fixed the problem.

However, if a person has an kidney injury resulting in metabolic acidosis, because there is insufficient bicarbonate to buffer the excess hydrogen, and their respiratory rate is fast enough to breathe off sufficient carbon dioxide to correct the acidosis, this is an example of **respiratory 'compensation'**. The system that caused the problem (the kidneys) was incapable of fixing the problem, so the 'other system' (the lungs) fixed the problem. Compensation can be identified on one ABG analysis; however, correction can be seen only on a subsequent or serial ABG analysis.

Base excess is also calculated and reported in many ABG analyses. This is a way of looking at the metabolic component of an ABG analysis. When it is reported as a positive number, it is called a *base excess* and represents *metabolic alkalosis*; when it is reported as a negative number, it is called a *base deficit* and represents *metabolic acidosis*. If it is true metabolic acidosis, it can be used to calculate the dose of bicarbonate that needs to be administered. Care must be taken when interpreting this value, however, as it is calculated and will be inaccurate if the carbon dioxide level is abnormal.

Many respiratory and endocrine diseases can result in alterations to blood pH. The respiratory system and the renal system are the two systems responsible for manipulating the blood pH in order to regain homeostasis. Consultation of other resources will be required to gain a step-by-step understanding of methods to analyse ABG results; however, Table 26.9 represents parameter changes based on the four common acid–base imbalances.

Step-by-step analysis working through each of the parameters will elucidate the most accurate ABG analysis, especially when performed in the context of the clinical picture; however, some rapid interpretation tools may provide a quick and easy overview of the numbers (see Figure 26.20). It must be acknowledged that tools like this are limited in their application, as they treat the analysis as more of a mathematical calculation exercise, rather than considering the clinical circumstances and physiological changes influencing the parameters.

Precautions

The majority of factors that influence the accuracy of an ABG result are pre-analytical, such as the collection and handling of the sample. The sample should not contain air bubbles, and should be analysed immediately (at least within 10 minutes of sampling).

Table 26.9 Some parameter changes associated with the four common acid–base imbalances

	Respiratory causes		Metabolic causes	
Parameter	**Respiratory acidosis**	**Respiratory alkalosis**	**Metabolic acidosis**	**Metabolic alkalosis**
pH	↓	↑	↓	↑
$PaCO_2$	↑	↓	↓ Compensated ≈ Uncompensated	↑ Compensated ≈ Uncompensated
HCO_3	↑ Compensated ≈ Uncompensated	↓ Compensated ≈ Uncompensated	↓	↑

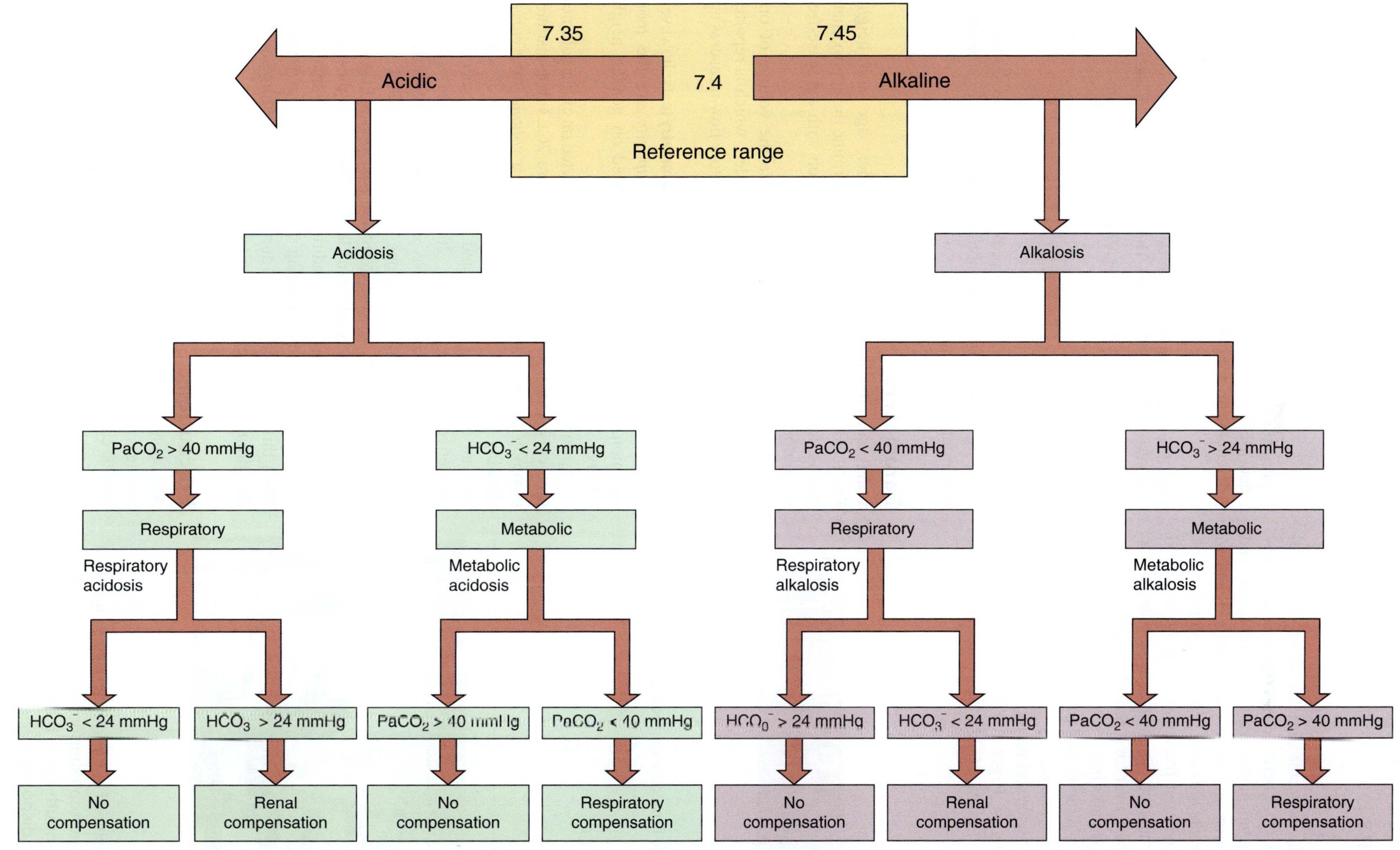

Figure 26.20

Guide to rapid ABG interpretation

This type of tool may provide quick and easy answers to the parameters obtained from an ABG analysis; however, its application is limited, and the information derived is incomplete and without regard for the clinical picture. A step-by-step analysis considering each parameter and the clinical picture is more beneficial and reliable.

HCO_3^- = bicarbonate ion; mmHg = millimetres of mercury; $PaCO_2$ = partial pressure of carbon dioxide from an arterial blood sample.

PEAK FLOW MEASUREMENTS AND SPIROMETRY

Tests

A *peak flow meter* is a device to measure the speed of forceful expiration (see Figure 26.21). There are two types of peak flow meters. Low peak flow meters have a scale of 0–300 L/min, and are used for young children and some older adults. Standard peak flow meters have a scale of 0–800 L/min. Monitoring peak flow prior to treatment and after treatment can provide a good insight into the effectiveness of the management plan. Home measurement documentation over long periods of time can also provide insights into seasonal changes to lung function, and identify whether further respiratory assessment or adjustment of the management plan is necessary.

A *spirometer* is a device primarily used by healthcare professionals; spirometers are larger and more expensive than peak flow devices (see Figure 26.22). Spirometers provide much more information than peak flow meters, and are used to assist in the diagnosis, or to monitor progress and treatment, of respiratory conditions.

CLINICAL BOX 26.5

Calculating predicted values for peak expiratory flow

Calculation of an individual's predicted *peak expiratory flow (PEF)* is based on height. An equation can be used to determine an approximate predicted value:

$$\text{PEF (L/min)} = [\text{Height (cm)} - 80] \times 5$$

So, if an individual is 170 cm tall, their predicted peak expiratory flow is 450 L/min. The calculation looks like this:

$$(170 - 80) \times 5 = 90 \times 5 = 450 \text{ L/min}$$

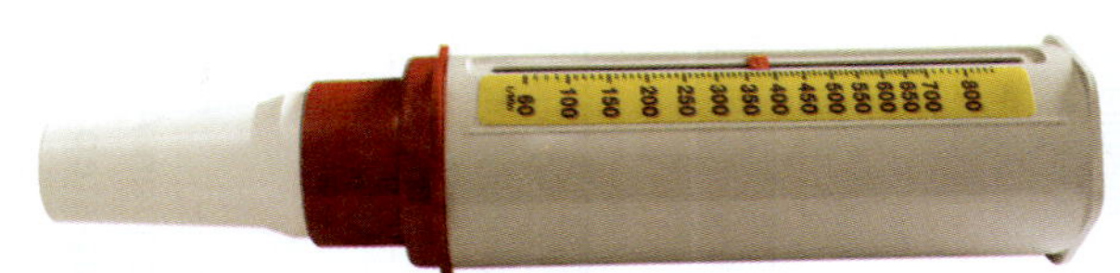

Figure 26.21

Peak flow device

A standard adult's peak flow device recording flow from 0 L/min to 800 L/min.

Source: MarkUK97/Shutterstock

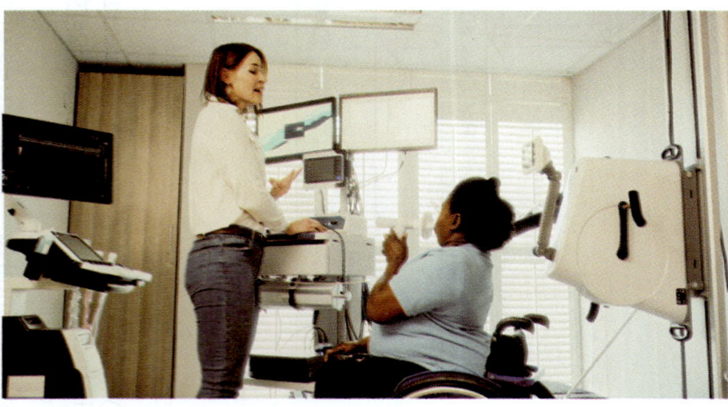

Figure 26.22

Spirometer

Newer spirometers consist of a hand-held device with a cable connected to a laptop computer with specialist software installed. The mouth piece that sits on the hand-held device is generally disposable.

Source: Kobus Louw/Getty Images.

Parameters

Lung capacity is influenced by gender, age and height. Predicted values can be calculated to determine the approximate results that should be obtained in a person with a disease-free respiratory system.

Peak expiratory flow meters measure the volume of one breath of air quickly and forcefully exhaled, which is reported in litres per minute. Predicted peak expiratory flow measures are based on height (see Clinical Box 26.5).

There are many different types of **spirometry** tests; however, *forced expiratory volume* and *vital capacity* are the most common. Predicted values are calculated on gender, height and age.

Spirometry results are most often reported on either volume–time curves or flow–volume loops. Figure 26.23 demonstrates common spirometry results collected as a *volume–time curve*, showing a normal spirogram result, one typical of a person with an obstructive disease, and one typical of someone with restrictive disease. Figure 26.24 demonstrates common spirometry results collected as a *flow–volume loop*, showing a normal spirogram result, one typical of a person with an obstructive disease, and one typical of someone with restrictive disease. Spirometry results can clearly demonstrate the type and severity of the respiratory condition experienced. Valuable data can also be obtained regarding the effectiveness of treatment when this test is performed a number of times before and after the administration of bronchodilating agents.

Precautions

Although valuable, it is important to ensure that the result of testing is accurate and reproducible. Some common unacceptable results can be obtained if the person coughs during the test, starts or finishes incorrectly, or there is a leak in the circuit (less common with newer devices). Figure 26.25 demonstrates some common influences on the spirometry loop or curve related to the type of problem experienced. The spirometry needs to be repeated to enable accurate results.

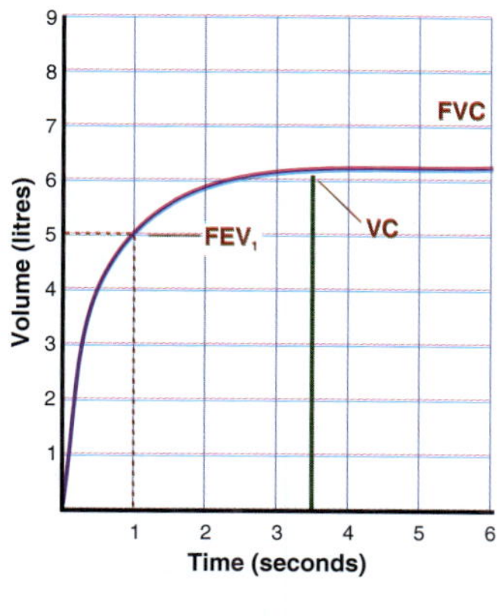

A. Normal spirogram

FEV_1 = Normal (near predicted)
FVC = Normal
VC = Normal (≅FVC)
FEV_1/FVC ratio = Normal

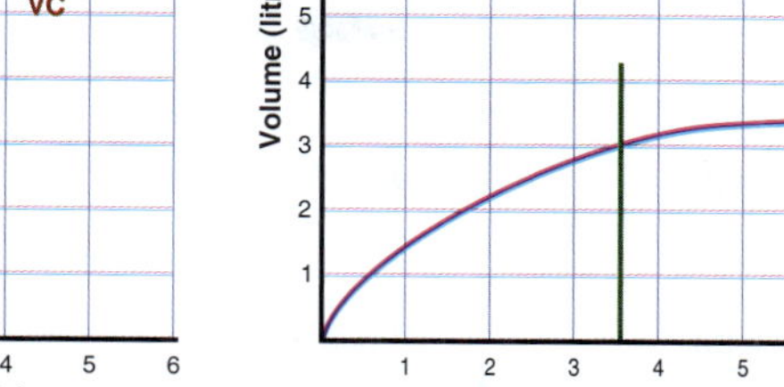

B. Typical obstructive pattern

FEV_1 = Reduced (below predicted)
FVC = Reduced (or normal)
VC = Increased (above FVC)
FEV_1/FVC ratio = Reduced

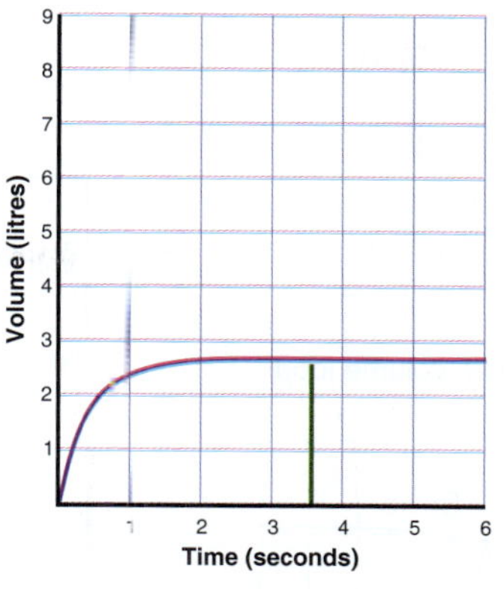

C. Typical restrictive pattern

FEV_1 = Reduced (below predicted)
FVC = Reduced (or normal)
VC = Reduced (≅FVC)
FEV_1/FVC ratio = Reduced

Figure 26.23

Spirometry: volume–time curve showing various results

FEV_1 = forced expiratory volume at 1 second; FVC = forced vital capacity; FEV_1/FVC ratio = ratio between forced expiratory volume at 1 second and forced vital capacity; VC = vital capacity.

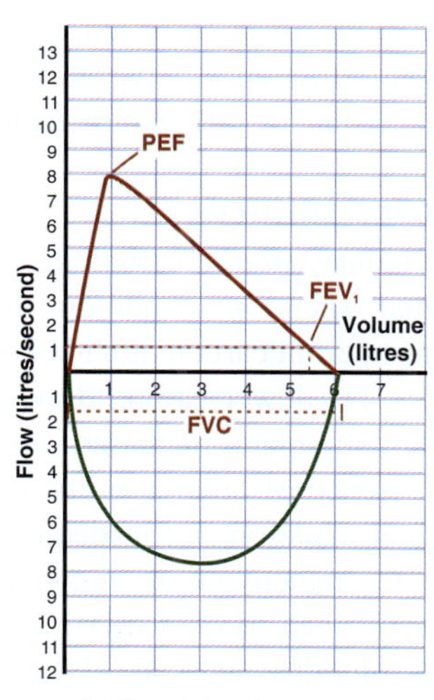

A. Normal spirogram

Expiration in red.
Inspiration in green.

PEF = Peak expiratory flow
FEV_1 = Forced expiratory volume (@1 second)
FVC = Forced expiratory volume

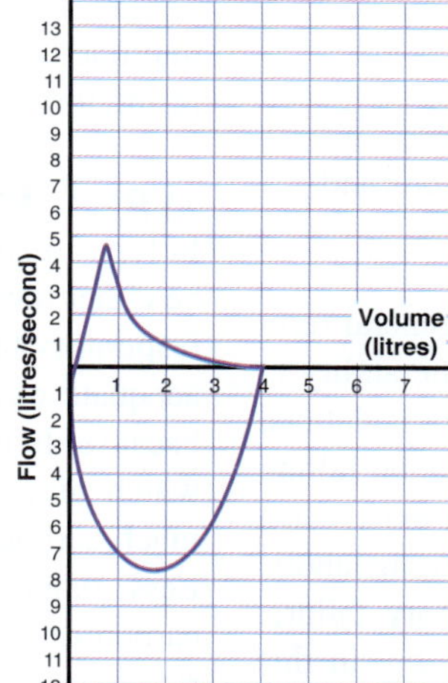

B. Typical obstructive pattern

Collapse of airways in early expiration.

Inspiration is not affected because of support from intraluminal pressure during inspiration.

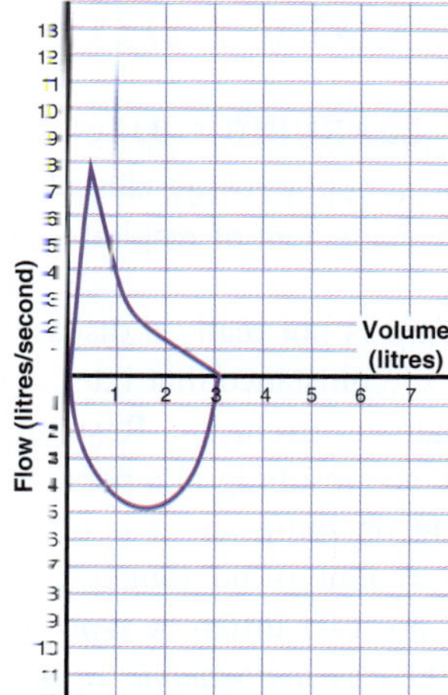

C. Typical restrictive pattern

Reduced volume expired. High flow in expiration from abnormally increased recoil.

Inspiratory volume and flow are reduced from lung or chest cavity restriction.

Figure 26.24

Spirometry: flow–volume loop showing various results

On the normal spirogram, the inspiratory phase of the loop is shown in green and the expiratory phase of the loop is shown in red.

FEV_1 = forced expiratory volume at 1 second; FVC = forced vital capacity; PEF = peak expiratory flow.

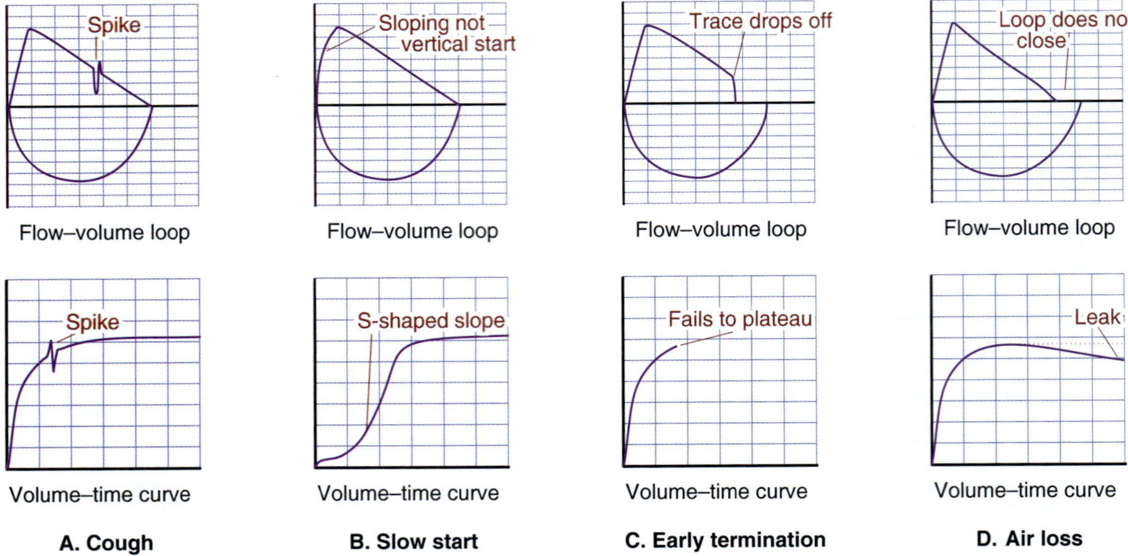

Figure 26.25

Spirometry: some common unacceptable results requiring retest

Early termination-finishing before breath is complete.

Respiratory failure

LEARNING OBJECTIVE 7

Examine the pathophysiology, clinical manifestations and management of respiratory failure.

Respiratory failure is not really a disease; it is a general term to describe any circumstance that interferes with the ability to maintain adequate gas exchange. Respiratory failure is defined as any circumstance resulting in a person's oxygenation falling below 60 mmHg on room air; it is considered to exist when the respiratory system is no longer able to meet metabolic demand. There are two different types of respiratory failure. *Type I* is classified as *hypoxaemic respiratory failure*. In this type, oxygenation is compromised; however, carbon dioxide levels may be either low or normal. *Type II* respiratory failure is also known as **ventilatory failure**, in which both oxygenation and carbon dioxide elimination are compromised. Figure 26.26 explores the common clinical manifestations and management of respiratory failure.

AETIOLOGY AND PATHOPHYSIOLOGY

The collection of statistics for respiratory failure is difficult as it is not a disease *per se*, and any condition that results in serious oxygen compromise can be categorised as respiratory failure. Data collection is inconsistent for both mortality and morbidity. Nonetheless, there is an ICD-10 code for 'Respiratory Failure, not classified elsewhere', for which over 6,500 people were admitted to Australian hospitals in 2020–21, and of which 69 people died.

The pathophysiology of respiratory failure is complex and multifactorial. The main difference between type I and type II respiratory failure is the state of carbon dioxide levels.

Type I respiratory failure

In type I respiratory failure, arterial carbon dioxide levels may be either low or normal. Therefore, conditions that cause type I respiratory failure must permit carbon dioxide exchange but not adequate oxygenation. The lower carbon dioxide level occurs because hypoxia can stimulate increased respiration rates, which may (in the absence of other conditions) result in too much carbon dioxide elimination, yet inadequate oxygenation. Less functional lung parenchyma is required to facilitate carbon dioxide transport than oxygen transport. The diffusion rate is influenced by solubility and mass. Even though carbon dioxide is larger than oxygen, it is 22 times more soluble, and therefore is more readily able to diffuse.

Factors contributing to poor arterial oxygenation include decreased alveolar oxygenation, ventilation/perfusion mismatch and decreased oxyhaemoglobin saturation.

Decreased alveolar oxygenation Alveolar ventilation is influenced by many factors, including conditions modifying environmental oxygen tension (i.e. affected by altitude, fire and oxygen supplementation). At altitude, the partial pressure of oxygen decreases and the *fraction of inspired oxygen* (FiO_2) reduces to less than 0.21 (21% of atmospheric air at sea level). Fires consume the environmental oxygen in the process of combustion. People exposed to an environment with a large fire will experience a period of low oxygen tension, resulting in a transient decrease in alveolar oxygenation.

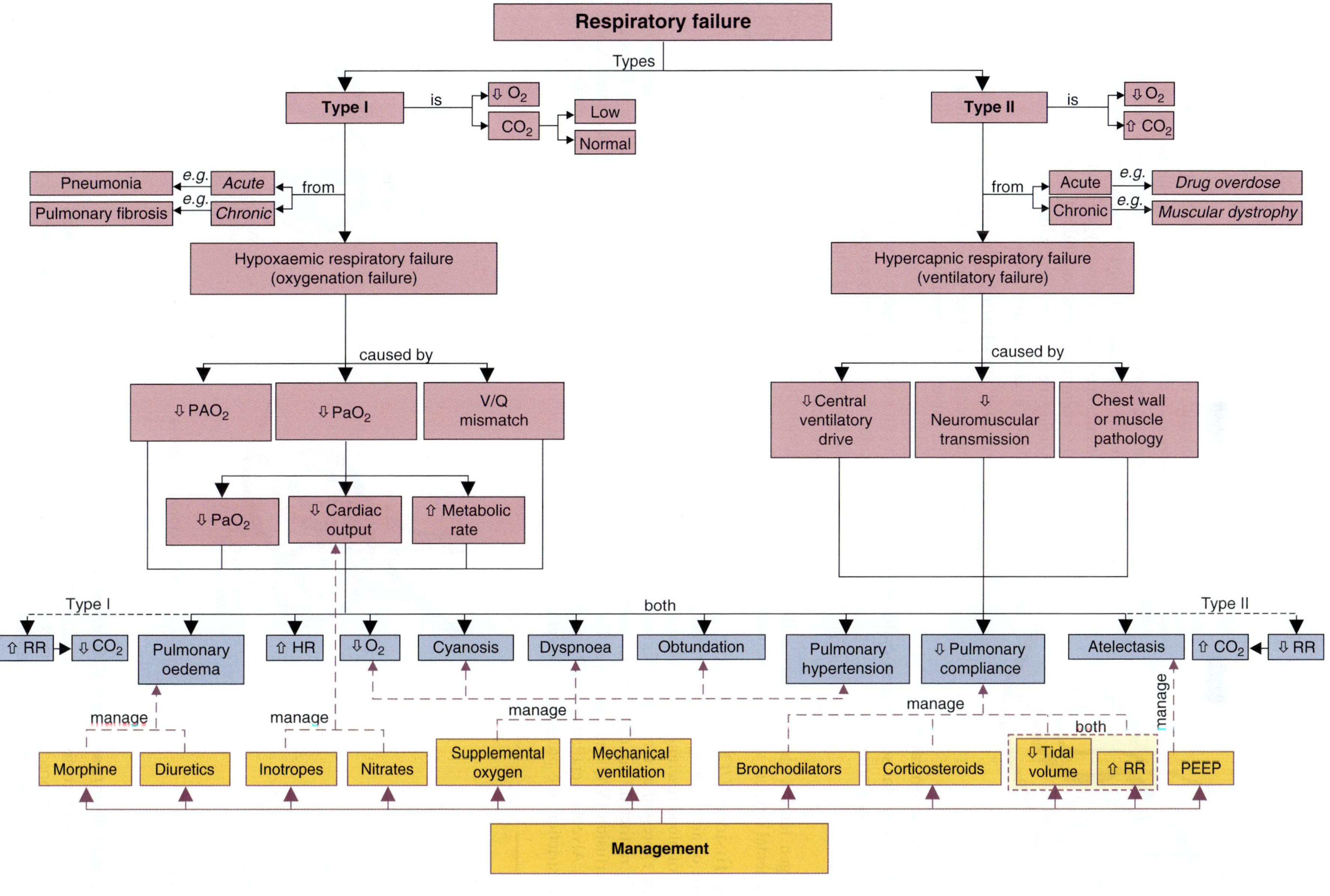

Figure 26.26

Clinical snapshot: Respiratory failure

↓ = decreased; ↑ = increased; CO_2 = carbon dioxide; HR = heart rate; O_2 = oxygen; PAO_2 = partial pressure of alveolar oxygen; PaO_2 = partial pressure of arterial oxygen; PEEP = positive end-expiratory pressure; RR = respiratory rate; V/Q = ventilation/perfusion.

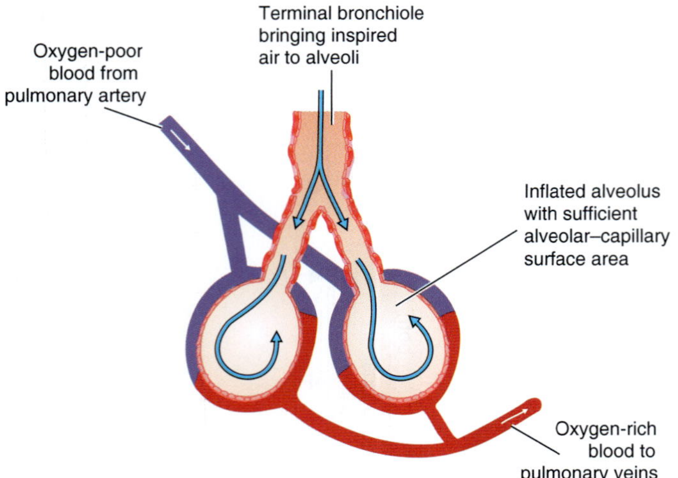

Figure 26.27

Normal ventilation/perfusion ratio

The relative volume of alveolar surface area matches the function of the alveolar capillaries.

An increase in oxygen tension can be achieved through the initiation of supplemental oxygen, which will increase FiO_2.

Ventilation/perfusion (V/Q) mismatch *Ventilation* refers to the volume of air reaching the alveoli, and *perfusion* refers to the volume of blood reaching the vessels supplying the alveoli. This can be expressed as a ratio (see Figure 26.27). If either component is restricted, gas exchange is compromised and a ventilation perfusion (V/Q) mismatch results. This can occur in many ways. Alveolar ventilation is affected by factors such as bronchoconstriction, the presence of secretions in the airway and the surface area of the alveoli. Atelectasis (alveolar collapse) decreases surface area, and so does emphysema and fluid within the alveoli (see Figure 26.28). Perfusion is affected by any condition causing reduced blood flow to the pulmonary capillaries. Pulmonary artery vasospasm and pulmonary embolism can cause reduced perfusion (see Figure 26.29).

Unlike any other organ system which experiences vasodilation in response to hypoxia, hypoxia in the lungs leads to hypoxic pulmonary *vasoconstriction*, thus preventing a V/Q mismatch, because the vasculature supplying the poorly ventilated alveoli will constrict in response to low oxygen levels (see Figure 26.30). Hypoxic pulmonary vasoconstriction fails to occur when inflammatory mediators interfere with this mechanism and cause vasodilation in areas of dysfunctional alveoli.

Decreased oxyhaemoglobin saturation Apart from the factors impeding gas exchange, other influences can affect the amount of oxygen binding to haemoglobin. Increased carbon monoxide levels from exposure to fire or automotive exhaust can severely impede oxygen transport, because carbon monoxide has a significantly greater affinity to haemoglobin; it not only has greater binding capacity, but it will also displace already bound oxygen. An increased metabolic rate may result from disease or from the increased work of breathing. Increased oxygen demand generates the need for increased supply. Deformed haemoglobin or reduced levels of haemoglobin will also affect oxygenation.

Type II respiratory failure

In type II respiratory failure, *oxygen levels are low* and *carbon dioxide levels are high*. Type II respiratory failure is known as *ventilatory failure,* and occurs as a result of decreased central ventilatory drive, decreased neuromuscular transmission, or chest wall or muscle pathology.

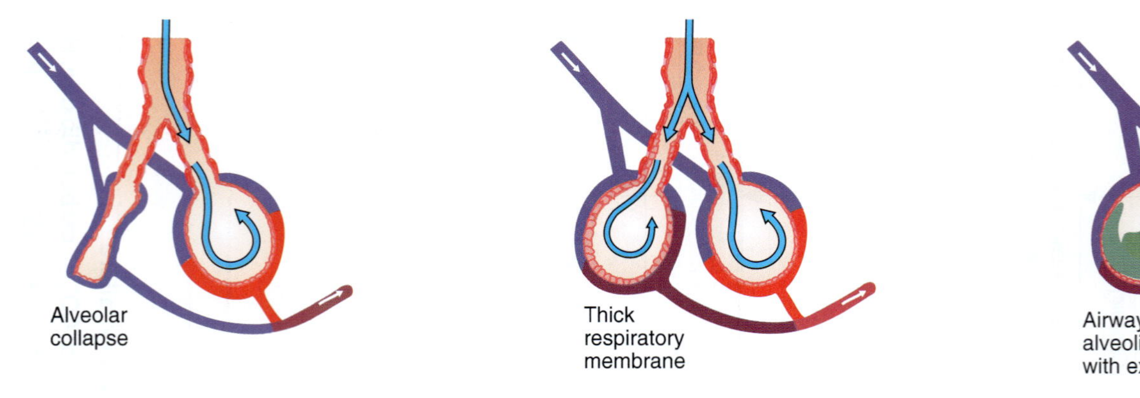

Figure 26.28

Factors affecting ventilation/perfusion (V/Q) ratio: ventilation

(A) V/Q mismatch from atelectasis. In this example, the alveoli collapse, yet the perfusion remains unchanged.
(B) V/Q mismatch from pulmonary oedema. In this example, the cells that form the alveolar wall and the interstitial space swell from oedema, the respiratory membrane becomes thick and causes poor gas exchange.
(C) V/Q mismatch from pneumonia. In this example, airways and alveoli become filled with exudate, which results in poor gas exchange.

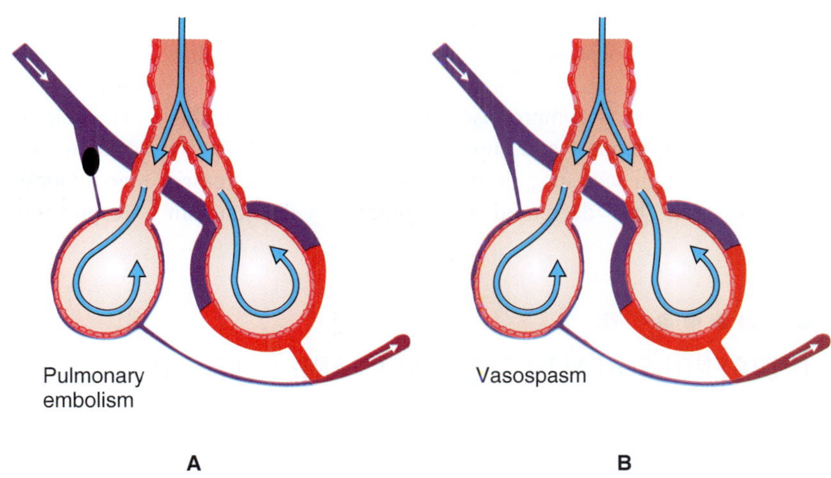

Figure 26.29

Factors affecting ventilation/perfusion (V/Q) ratio: perfusion

(A) V/Q mismatch from pulmonary embolism. In this example, if a clot forms anywhere in the pulmonary vasculature, the affected alveoli can still be ventilated; however, gas exchange is compromised because there is no flow past the ventilated alveoli.

(B) V/Q mismatch from vasospasm. In this example, if the pulmonary vasculature constricts gas exchange, it is still compromised because the ventilated alveoli receives little to no blood flow.

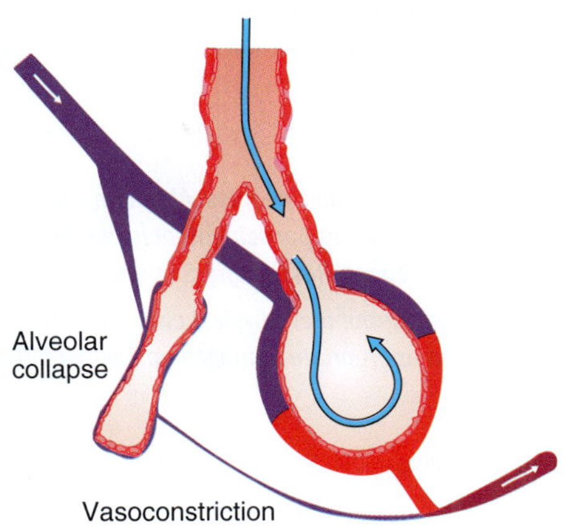

Figure 26.30

Hypoxic pulmonary vasoconstriction

In the lungs, hypoxia normally stimulates vasoconstriction, unlike in other body tissues, where hypoxia stimulates vasodilation.

Decreased central ventilatory drive Conditions that alter the respiratory drive include brainstem compression from haemorrhage or tumour, metabolic encephalopathy, and overdose of depressant drugs, such as anaesthetic agents, opioids or benzodiazepines. The respiratory rate decreases, oxygenation falls and carbon dioxide levels increase.

Decreased neuromuscular transmission Conditions affecting the neuromuscular units supplying the respiratory muscles include spinal cord injury, multiple sclerosis, myasthenia gravis and Gullain–Barré syndrome. Drugs with neuromuscular junction antagonistic effects can also cause ventilatory failure.

Chest wall or muscle pathology Conditions that affect respiratory muscles include fatigue, disuse atrophy, polymyositis and muscular dystrophy. A flail chest, kyphoscoliosis, morbid obesity and pneumothorax can also cause respiratory failure because of their effect on the chest wall.

CLINICAL MANIFESTATIONS

Respiratory failure can be either acute or chronic depending on the cause. Apart from hypoxia and the difference in carbon dioxide levels, there are many causes, including dyspnoea, potentially cyanosis, and obtundation from hypoxaemia. Tachycardia will develop, and the person may be either hypotensive from pulmonary embolus or sepsis, or hypertensive from sympathetic nervous system compensation and maybe even cardiogenic pulmonary oedema.

Pulmonary oedema may develop because of either increased hydrostatic pressure or increased permeability. Airway pressures may be high, and pulmonary compliance may be low. Jugular venous pressure may be elevated, and pulmonary hypertension may develop with right ventricular dysfunction.

DIAGNOSIS AND MANAGEMENT

Diagnosis

Investigations for both types of respiratory failure are the same. Arterial blood can be sampled for analysis of blood gases to quantify oxygen and carbon dioxide levels. A measurement of pH and bicarbonate values will also be valuable. Other biochemical parameters—such as sodium, potassium, lactate and carbaminohaemoglobin values—may also be available, depending on the machine and the kits used. Venous blood may demonstrate anaemia or polycythaemia to assist in understanding the cause. Leukocytosis can suggest infection, and thrombocytopenia may suggest sepsis. Other investigations may include a chest X-ray or computed tomography (CT) scan, or a ventilation/perfusion scan to identify other potential causes.

Management

One major difference between type I and type II respiratory failure is that, generally, type I is refractory to supplemental oxygen, whereas the hypoxaemia of type II will often correct with supplemental oxygen.

The principles of managing respiratory failure revolve around treating the underlying condition. Interventions to manage the cause may include antimicrobial agents for infection, bronchodilators for obstruction or inotropes to improve cardiac function.

As oxygenation is compromised, the person will probably need ventilatory support and supplemental oxygen. If airway pressures are high and lung compliance is low, an increased respiratory rate but decreased tidal volume will maintain minute volume but reduce the risk of barotrauma. However, if airway pressures are acceptable, the application of positive end-expiratory pressure (PEEP) and a prolonged inspiratory phase can help with lung recruitment of atelectatic alveoli. The person may require sedation and paralysis to cope with the mechanical ventilation early in their management. In people with chronic respiratory failure, non-invasive ventilation may be beneficial.

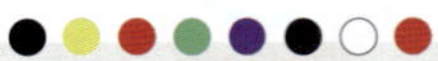

INDIGENOUS HEALTH FAST FACTS AND CULTURAL CONSIDERATIONS

FAST FACTS

- *There are no statistics regarding respiratory failure in Aboriginal and Torres Strait Islander peoples. However, given that the burden of respiratory disease in Aboriginal and Torres Strait Islander Australians is 2.7 higher than in non-Indigenous Australians, it stands to reason that respiratory failure would be more common. (Note that the latest statistics up until 2019—prior to the COVID-19 pandemic).*
- *There are no statistics regarding respiratory failure in Māori or Pacific Islands New Zealanders. However, given that Māori and Pacific Islands New Zealanders are 3.2 times more likely than European New Zealanders to be hospitalised for respiratory conditions, it stands to reason that respiratory failure would be more common.*

CULTURAL CONSIDERATIONS

- *There are currently no evidence-based spirometry reference values for Aboriginal and Torres Strait Islander peoples. Although some studies have attempted to develop reference values, the study designs were less than ideal, and none adhered to participant inclusion and exclusion criteria as outlined by the two peak bodies—the American Thoracic Society and the European Respiratory Society.*
- *Use of ethnicity-based predicted values—spirometry reference ranges developed using racial background or physical characteristics—is important for the accurate diagnosis of lung conditions. Accurate diagnosis leads to timely and appropriate management, which ultimately reduces morbidity and mortality.*

Source: Data from Australian Bureau of Statistics (2022); Australian Institute of Health and Welfare (2023); Barnard & Zhang (2021).

CHILDREN AND ADOLESCENTS

- Neonates often have an irregular respiratory rate and depth. This is especially common in premature infants because of an underdeveloped respiratory control centre.
- The respiratory system of a child is vastly different from that of an adult, and does not anatomically begin to resemble a small version of an adult's airway until after approximately 8 years of age.

OLDER ADULTS

- The respiration rate of an older adult is slightly higher, and the depth is more shallow, because of the reduced vital capacity.
- Age-related changes to the respiratory system include decreased lung elasticity and decreasing strength in the muscles of respiration. These two changes result in hypoventilation and increased carbon dioxide retention.

KEY CLINICAL ISSUES

- Respiratory rate, rhythm and depth should always be observed when assessing the respiratory system.
- Familiarity with common respiratory terminology is important, especially in the context of descriptions related to alterations in breathing, such as tachypnoea, bradypnoea, dyspnoea, orthopnoea and apnoea.
- Hyperventilation may occur as a result of excessive respiratory rate or depth, or a combination of both. In people with healthy lungs, it is more common to develop hypocapnia from hyperventilation.
- A child's respiratory system is not just a miniature version of an adult's system. Several significant differences in anatomy and physiology exist until approximately 7 years of age.
- Many factors influence respiratory rate. These should be considered when undertaking a respiratory assessment that does not conform to predicted observations.
- Although oxygen is considered a drug and should be administered with an order, in urgent and emergent circumstances relating to hypoxia, appropriately qualified healthcare professionals may initiate oxygen if expected parameters are breached. They should subsequently seek medical assistance urgently (Medical assistance is required within 30 minutes from initiation).
- Oximetry results from a peripheral oxygen saturation oximeter should be considered with caution, as many factors can influence the validity of a reading.
- Various observations can inform a health professional about the respiratory function of a person in their care.
- A person with a chronic lung condition can have acute periods of severe dyspnoea.
- When assessing spirometry or peak flow measurements, it is important to compare people with their own predicted measurements, not with those of other people.
- Any condition interfering with ventilation and oxygenation can cause respiratory failure.
- *Oxygen toxicity* may develop in a person receiving extremely high-flow oxygen ($FiO_2 > 0.6$ [60%]). Neonates are particularly at risk of damage to retinas and lung parenchyma.
- Cough can be a sign of respiratory dysfunction, and normally develops when other respiratory defence mechanisms are dysfunctional.
- The characteristics and quantity of sputum can reveal important information about the function of the respiratory system.
- *Central cyanosis* is a very critical clinical manifestation of respiratory dysfunction, and will only appear in cases of extreme hypoxia. Cyanosis develops as a result of decreasing oxygen saturation of haemoglobin. Severe anaemia can delay the appearance of cyanosis, as fewer erythrocytes are present; therefore, the amount of deoxyhaemoglobin may be low. However, tissue hypoxia still exists.
- *Digital clubbing* is a sign of chronic hypoxia.
- Data collected from *respiratory assessment* should be considered in the context of all information; an isolated value is meaningless without a context informed by other information.

CHAPTER REVIEW

- Both *tachypnoea* and *bradypnoea* can be indicators of impending respiratory crisis.
- As a neonate grows and matures, *respiratory muscle hypertrophy* is the primary mechanism that results in the reduction of respiratory rate across the lifespan.
- *Hypoventilation* can result in *hypercapnia*, which causes *acidaemia*. In a person with an intact hypercapnic drive, increasing levels of carbon dioxide or acidaemia should initiate an increase in respiratory rate. An increase in respiratory rate may cause *hypocapnia* or develop as a result of hypercapnia.
- A person with chronic hypoxia may develop a *hypoxic drive*, which is where low levels of oxygen become the stimulus to breathe instead of high levels of carbon dioxide. People with a hypoxic drive should not receive high-flow oxygen for a prolonged period of time.

REVIEW QUESTIONS

1. What conditions can interfere with respiratory rate and depth?
2. How do respiratory rate and depth influence carbon dioxide levels?
3. What are the distinguishing features of the following types of breathing patterns?
   a. Kussmaul
   b. Cheyne-Stokes
   c. Biot's breathing
   d. apneustic breathing
4. How do alterations in oxygen and carbon dioxide levels affect body systems?
5. Define the following terms:
   a. dyspnoea
   b. haemoptysis
   c. orthopnoea
   d. paroxysmal nocturnal dyspnoea
   e. cyanosis
   f. digital clubbing
6. What are some common components of a respiratory assessment?
7. What are adventitious lung sounds? Identify and explain three types.
8. What parameters are measured in arterial blood gas analysis?
9. What is the difference between peak flow and spirometry?
10. What considerations should one make when determining the validity of pulse oximetry?
11. What is respiratory failure?
12. What differentiates the two types of respiratory failure?
13. What are the common clinical manifestations associated with respiratory failure?
14. How are the most common clinical manifestations of respiratory failure managed?

HEALTH PROFESSIONAL CONNECTIONS

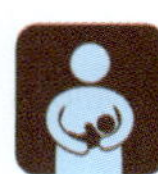

Midwives Care must be taken with administering oxygen therapy to a neonate, as excessive or fluctuating concentrations of oxygen can cause 'retinopathy of prematurity'. Hyperoxia should be avoided through administering as little oxygen as required to maintain adequate oxygenation. Oxygen saturations should be monitored, and weaning off supplemental oxygen should be undertaken as soon as possible.

Other considerations include the respiratory system of women, which may be compromised by the pregnancy in the third trimester, especially in the presence of an existing respiratory condition. Hormonal changes may result in respiratory tract mucosal oedema, resulting in nasal congestion or upper respiratory tract infection. Although compensatory lung changes can increase lung volume from increased anterior–posterior and transverse diameters, upward lung displacement of several centimetres can result from diaphragmatic elevation by a gravid uterus. Careful positioning to reduce the upward pressure of the uterus on the diaphragm can reduce significant loss of volume in women in their second and third trimester.

During labour, oxygen demands may increase by almost 60% due to increased cardiac and respiratory workload. Also, a left shift of the oxyhaemoglobin dissociation curve can result from excessive hyperventilation, causing hypocapnia and alkalosis for both mother and fetus. Increased affinity results in reduced oxygen release. Furthermore, in this state, hypoxia is exacerbated by uteroplacental and cerebral vasoconstriction.

Physiotherapists Chest physiotherapy can improve ventilation and oxygenation in people with respiratory conditions. Active cycle breathing and positive expiratory pressure (PEP) therapy techniques can be taught to assist with airway clearance and improve ventilation. Flutter valves are devices that increase the expiratory resistance; they therefore increase the positive expiratory pressure, preventing early airway collapse. The oscillation produced by the flutter of the ball approximates the cilia 'beat' at a frequency of approximately 12 Hz, which promotes the mobilisation of mucus.

Autogenic drainage techniques attempt to achieve the highest possible airflow in different generations of bronchi, the use of controlled tidal breathing and the prevention of early airway closure. Historically, it was standard practice that most ventilated individuals would receive prophylactic chest physiotherapy with manual techniques such as percussion and vibration to improve impaired mucociliary clearance and reduced lung volume. These techniques are no longer recognised as best practice, as the evidence suggests that they are limited in value. Coughing and huffing and postural drainage techniques are also less preferred to new and more easily self-administered techniques.

Exercise scientists Exercise intensity will directly affect oxygen consumption. An oxygen imbalance may develop if oxygen demand exceeds oxygen supply. Alveolar ventilation can increase by almost 20 times from the resting state; however, if respiratory membrane function or oxygen transport is deficient, increased alveolar ventilation will be of little use. Lung function should be considered when working with individuals. Measurement of lung function via spirometry or a peak flow meter may be beneficial to assist in the appropriate and safe design of exercise programs in both athletes and those undertaking rehabilitation programs.

CASE STUDY

Mr James Mohr (UR number 615947) is a 25-year-old man who was involved in a motor vehicle accident three days ago, in which he sustained head, neck and chest injuries. Because of a high demand for bed availability in the intensive care unit, he was transferred to the ward six hours ago. He still requires significant nursing care and close observation. A CT scan has ruled out spinal cord injury; however, there are some changes to his head CT. Mr Mohr's Glasgow coma scale (GCS) score is 12 (E = 4; V = 4; M = 4). He has a tracheostomy in situ, is receiving oxygen at 4 L/min via a tracheostomy mask, and is requiring at least second-hourly suctioning. He has a flail section involving the fourth to sixth ribs on his right chest. Initially, on transfer to the ward, no paradoxical movement of the flail section was observed. Mr Mohr did not receive any other orthopaedic injuries. Some venous and arterial blood was drawn for testing before he was transferred to the ward.

His observations are as follows:

Temperature	Heart rate	Respiration rate	Blood pressure	SpO_2
37.3°C	84	22 (shallow)	120/60	94% (4 L/min—tracheostomy mask)

On assessment it appears as though Mr Mohr's pain control is an issue. Although he has an altered level of consciousness, he still grimaces during pressure area cares and when he coughs. He has morphine and some simple analgesia ordered; however, only the paracetamol has been given. No opioid analgesia has been administered.

As the shift progresses, Mr Mohr's respiration rate increases to 38 bpm, shallow and irregular. Accessory muscles of respiration are engaged, and it appears as though there is a paradoxical movement in the flail section of his thorax. His GCS score remains at 12. His other observations are as follows. An urgent medical review is requested.

Temperature	Heart rate	Respiration rate	Blood pressure	SpO_2
37.5°C	112	38 (shallow and irregular)	138/84	86% (4 L/min—tracheostomy mask)

HAEMATOLOGY

Patient location:	Ward 3	**UR:**	615947		
Consultant:	Smith	**NAME:**	Mohr		
		Given name:	James	**Sex:**	M
		DOB:	31/12/XX	**Age:**	25

Time collected	07:30
Date collected	XX/XX
Year	XXXX
Lab #	3456544

FULL BLOOD COUNT		UNITS	REFERENCE RANGE
Haemoglobin	111	g/L	115–160
White cell count	4.9	$\times 10^9$/L	4.0–11.0
Platelets	138	$\times 10^9$/L	140–400
Haematocrit	0.34		0.33–0.47
Red cell count	3.78	$\times 10^{12}$/L	3.80–5.20
Reticulocyte count	2.9	%	0.2–2.0
MCV	98	fL	80–100
COAGULATION PROFILE			
aPTT	26	secs	24–40
PT	15	secs	11–17

BIOCHEMISTRY

Patient location:	Ward 3	**UR:**	615947		
Consultant:	Smith	**NAME:**	Mohr		
		Given name:	James	**Sex:**	M
		DOB:	31/12/XX	**Age:**	25

Time collected	07:30	19:30
Date collected	XX/XX	XX/XX
Year	XXXX	XXXX
Lab #	3456544	1654321

ELECTROLYTES			UNITS	REFERENCE RANGE
Sodium	139		mmol/L	135–145
Potassium	3.9		mmol/L	3.5–5.2
Chloride	105		mmol/L	95–110
Glucose (random)	5.2		mmol/L	3.5–7.7
RENAL FUNCTION				
Urea	6.2		mmol/L	2.5–7.5
Creatinine	68		μmol/L	60–110
ARTERIAL BLOOD GAS				
pH	7.39	7.49		7.35–7.45
PaO_2	82	58	mmHg	80–100
$PaCO_2$	41	49	mmHg	35–45
Bicarbonate	24	24	mEq/L	22–26

He is transferred back to the intensive care unit and placed on a ventilator. An arterial line is re-inserted and a blood gas analysis is obtained (see the biochemistry results).

CRITICAL THINKING

1. What risk factors does Mr Mohr have for the development of respiratory failure? (*Hint:* Consider all of the components of the case study, including his head injury, other injuries and some management interventions, too.)
2. How can a flail segment of chest interfere with Mr Mohr's ventilation and oxygenation? What is a paradoxical movement?
3. Identify all of the components of a respiratory assessment, and predict what types of results might be observed for Mr Mohr. Explain your answers. You notice that Mr Mohr's oxygenation is not ideal. What is the best position for him to promote adequate gas exchange? What other interventions could you undertake to promote his oxygenation and ventilation?
4. No opioid analgesia has been administered. Why might there be concern regarding this agent? What are the risks and benefits of administering an opioid analgesic agent to a person with thoracic (and/or head) injuries?
5. When Mr Mohr was taken back to the intensive care unit, an arterial blood gas was sampled. Explain the results of this blood gas analysis. Considering the factors that manipulate gas exchange, and taking into account Mr Mohr's respiratory rate, explain what different result may have been predicted for his carbon dioxide level. Why might his carbon dioxide level be so high? (*Hint:* Consider the *two* factors that can influence minute volume.) Given these results, what type of respiratory failure is Mr Mohr experiencing?
6. Mr Mohr is placed back on the ventilator. The paradoxical movement in the flail portion of his thorax ceases immediately. Why was the positive pressure mechanical ventilator so effective at controlling the paradoxical movement in Mr Mohr's chest? (*Hint:* When not ventilated, how do we normally breathe?)

BIBLIOGRAPHY

Australian Bureau of Statistics (ABS) (2022). *Causes of death, Australia, 2021.* Canberra: ABS. . https://www.abs.gov.au/statistics/health/causes-death/causes-death-australia/latest-release.

Australian Health Ministers' Advisory Council's National and Aboriginal and Torres Strait Islander Health Standing Committee (2017). *Cultural respect framework 2016–2026: for Aboriginal and Torres Strait Islander health—a national approach to building a culturally respectful health system.* Canberra: Australian Government Department of Health. https://nacchocommunique.files.wordpress.com/2016/12/cultural_respect_framework_1december2016_1.pdf.

Australian Institute of Health and Welfare (2020). *Aboriginal and Torres Strait Islander Health Performance Framework—summary report 2020.* Canberra: AIHW. https://www.indigenoushpf.gov.au/publications/hpf-summary-2020.

Australian Institute of Health and Welfare (AIHW) (2022a). *Australia's health, 2022: data insights.* Australia's Health series No. 18. Cat. No. AUS 240. Canberra: AIHW. https://www.aihw.gov.au/reports/australias-health/australias-health-2022-data-insights/about.

Australian Institute of Health and Welfare (AIHW) (2022b). *Principal diagnosis data cubes: separation statistics by principal diagnosis (ICD-10-AM 11th edition), Australia, 2020–21.* Canberra: AIHW. https://www.aihw.gov.au/reports/hospitals/principal-diagnosis-data-cubes/contents/data-cubes.

Australian Institute of Health and Welfare (AIHW) (2023). *Aboriginal and Torres Strait Islander Health Performance Framework—summary report 2023.* Canberra: AIHW. https://www.indigenoushpf.gov.au/Report-overview/Overview/Summary-Report.

Barnard, L.T. & Zhang, J. (2021). *The impact of respiratory disease in New Zealand: 2020 update.* Wellington: Asthma and Respiratory Foundation NZ. https://www.asthmafoundation.org.nz/assets/documents/Respiratory-Impact-report-final-2021Aug11.pdf.

Bauldoff, G., Gubrud-Howe, P.M., Carno, M.-A., Levett-Jones, T., Hales, M., Berry, K., … Stanley, D. (2020). *LeMone and Burke's medical–surgical nursing: critical thinking for person-centred care* (4th [Australian] edn). Sydney: Pearson Australia.

Best, O. & Fredericks, B. (2021). *Yatdjuligin: Aboriginal and Torres Strait Islander nursing and midwifery care* (3rd edn). Port Melbourne, VIC: Cambridge University Press.

Bullock, S. & Manias, E. (2022). *Fundamentals of pharmacology* (9th edn). Sydney: Pearson Australia.

Gendreau, S., Geri, G., Pham, T., Vieillard-Baron, A. & Mekontso Dessap, A. (2022). The role of acute hypercapnia on mortality and short-term physiology in patients mechanically ventilated for ARDS: a systematic review and meta-analysis. *Intensive Care Medicine* 48(5):517–34. https://doi.org/10.1007/s00134-022-06640-1.

Kaynar, A.M. & Sharma, S. (2020). Respiratory failure. *Emedicine*. https://emedicine.medscape.com/article/167981-overview.

Lone, N.A. & Abid, H. (2019). Pulmonary examination technique. *Emedicine.* https://emedicine.medscape.com/article/1909159-technique.

McCarthy, K., & Dweik, R.A. (2020). Pulmonary function testing. *Emedicine.* https://emedicine.medscape.com/article/303239-overview.

Scanlon, P.D. & Hyatt, R.E. (2019). *Hyatt's interpretation of pulmonary function tests: a practical guide* (5th edn). Philadelphia: Wolters Kluwer Health.

Springer, S.C., Priestley, M.A. & Huh, J.W. (2022). Pediatric respiratory failure. *Emedicine*. https://emedicine.medscape.com/article/908172-overview.

Stahlheber, C.L., Oba, Y., Patel, S. & Peralta, A.R. (2022). Breath sound assessment. *Emedicine.* https://emedicine.medscape.com/article/1894146-overview.

Tortora, G.J., Derrickson, B., Burkett, B., Peoples, G., Dye, D., Cooke, J., … Green, H. (2022). *Principles of anatomy and physiology* (3rd Asia-Pacific edn). Milton, QLD: John Wiley and Sons.

Obstructive pulmonary disorders

27

LEARNING OBJECTIVES

After completing this chapter, you should be able to:

1 Describe the pathophysiology, clinical manifestations and management of asthma.

2 Differentiate between acute bronchitis and chronic bronchitis.

3 Describe the pathophysiology, clinical manifestations and management of emphysema.

4 Examine the causes and the effects of the different types of gas trapping.

5 Discuss the pathophysiology, clinical manifestations and management of cystic fibrosis.

6 Describe the pathophysiology, clinical manifestations and management of bronchiectasis.

WHAT YOU SHOULD KNOW BEFORE YOU START THIS CHAPTER

Can you differentiate between the structure and function of the conducting and the respiratory airways?

Can you identify the structure and the role of the respiratory membrane?

Can you discuss the factors that influence the function of the respiratory membrane?

Can you recognise the main defences within the respiratory system?

Can you identify the structures that constitute lung parenchyma?

Can you explain the relationship between ventilation and perfusion?

Can you explain the influence that the diameter of the conducting airways has on gas exchange?

Can you discuss the structure and the function of the mucous and sweat glands?

KEY TERMS

Airway hyperresponsiveness

α_1-antitrypsin

Asthma

Asthma–COPD overlap

Atelectasis

Atopy

Ball-valving

Bronchiectasis

Bronchitis

Chronic obstructive pulmonary disorders (COPD)

Cor pulmonale

Cystic fibrosis (CF)

Emphysema

Hyperinflation

Status asthmaticus

Introduction

Breathing is a body function that we generally take for granted. It occurs spontaneously with little conscious input. So the inability to breathe can be acutely distressing. Respiratory illnesses that greatly compromise our breathing ability are considered serious and potentially life-threatening conditions.

Obstructive disorders are one of the most common groups of respiratory illness experienced, and can affect people of all ages. These conditions may occur as acute or chronic presentations, and they may be intermittent or persistent in nature. The mortality and morbidity rates associated with many obstructive disorders are so serious that significant resources are allocated by governments, healthcare providers and community organisations to address the physical and financial burdens.

This chapter will examine some of the most common obstructive disorders, such as asthma, bronchitis and emphysema. Other less common, but equally debilitating, respiratory disorders—cystic fibrosis and bronchiectasis—will also be discussed.

Chronic obstructive pulmonary disorders (COPD) are a group of lung disorders that result in difficulty breathing. The two main conditions associated with COPD are chronic bronchitis and emphysema. One of the significant characteristics of a COPD is airflow limitation that is not fully reversible. Although asthma and COPD have similar characteristics, asthma is not classed as a COPD. With treatment, individuals with asthma have near normal lung function when free from exacerbation. Cystic fibrosis causes chronic airflow limitation that is not fully reversible; however, it is not classified as a COPD because these disorders must also be preventable and treatable. Cystic fibrosis is an inheritable genetic disorder that results in early mortality.

Asthma

AETIOLOGY AND PATHOPHYSIOLOGY

LEARNING OBJECTIVE 1

Describe the pathophysiology, clinical manifestations and management of asthma.

In 2022, the Global Initiative for Asthma (GINA) defined **asthma** as '… a heterogeneous disease, usually characterized by chronic airway inflammation. It is defined by the history of respiratory symptoms such as wheeze, shortness of breath, chest tightness and cough that vary over time and in intensity, together with variable expiratory airflow limitation'. The comprehensive definition was formed to distinguish asthma from other types of respiratory conditions. The focus of this section will largely be on allergic asthma, as this is the most common type; however, there are actually several types of asthma, some of which will be discussed.

In asthma, a complex cascade of events occurs, which begins with exposure to a trigger and ends in expiratory airway obstruction. Release of inflammatory mediators results in **airway hyperresponsiveness**, causing bronchoconstriction and subsequent airflow limitation.

A method of classification differentiates asthma in relation to its trigger, and uses the terms 'extrinsic' and 'intrinsic'. *Extrinsic asthma* is also known as *allergic asthma* (the focus of this section), whereas *intrinsic asthma* can be triggered by numerous factors including exercise, stress, obesity, or drugs such as aspirin, or as an exacerbation of a respiratory infection.

Airway oedema and mucus hypersecretion cause further obstruction. Figure 27.1 explores the common clinical manifestations and management of allergic asthma.

Allergic asthma

Two distinct phases can be identified in allergic (extrinsic/allergen-induced) asthma: early-phase reaction and late-phase reaction. The *inflammatory response* occurs as a result of immunoglobulin-E (IgE)-dependent release of inflammatory mediators from mast cells. The *degranulation* results in the release of preformed mediators, and therefore happens rapidly (beginning immediately and lasting up to two hours), and so represents the *early-phase reaction*. When mast cells degranulate, they release histamine, leukotrienes and cytokines. This results in bronchoconstriction, vasodilation of the airway vasculature, hyperaemia and subsequent vascular congestion. Increased capillary permeability also occurs, which ultimately results in airway oedema.

The *late-phase reaction* occurs approximately four hours later, and can last up to 24 hours. T cells induce the production of mediators that cause the production of subpopulations of cytokines. Interleukin-5 (IL-5) then causes the differentiation of eosinophils in the bone marrow, which are then released into the circulation, where they migrate to the airway. Eosinophils release more leukotrienes and granule proteins, which continue to exaggerate the inflammatory response in the airways. This process is delayed because of the complexity and remoteness of the events that need to occur. The granule proteins released from the eosinophils are toxic products, and can result in epithelial damage, even more bronchoconstriction and impaired mucociliary function.

The presence of *inflammatory mediators* within the airway and the failure of normal neuroregulation cause *airway hyperresponsiveness*. Muscle bands surrounding the outside of the bronchioles contract, and this results in *bronchoconstriction*, which further causes airflow limitation. Not only are the airways inflamed, oedematous and constricted, but also *mucus hypersecretion* further exacerbates intraluminal obstruction (see Figure 27.2). In severe and persistent asthma, the chronic inflammatory state causes *airway remodelling*, such as changes to the basement membrane, goblet cell hyperplasia and smooth muscle hypertrophy. Clinical Box 27.1 identifies evolving classifications which help explain and direct management of people with severe asthma.

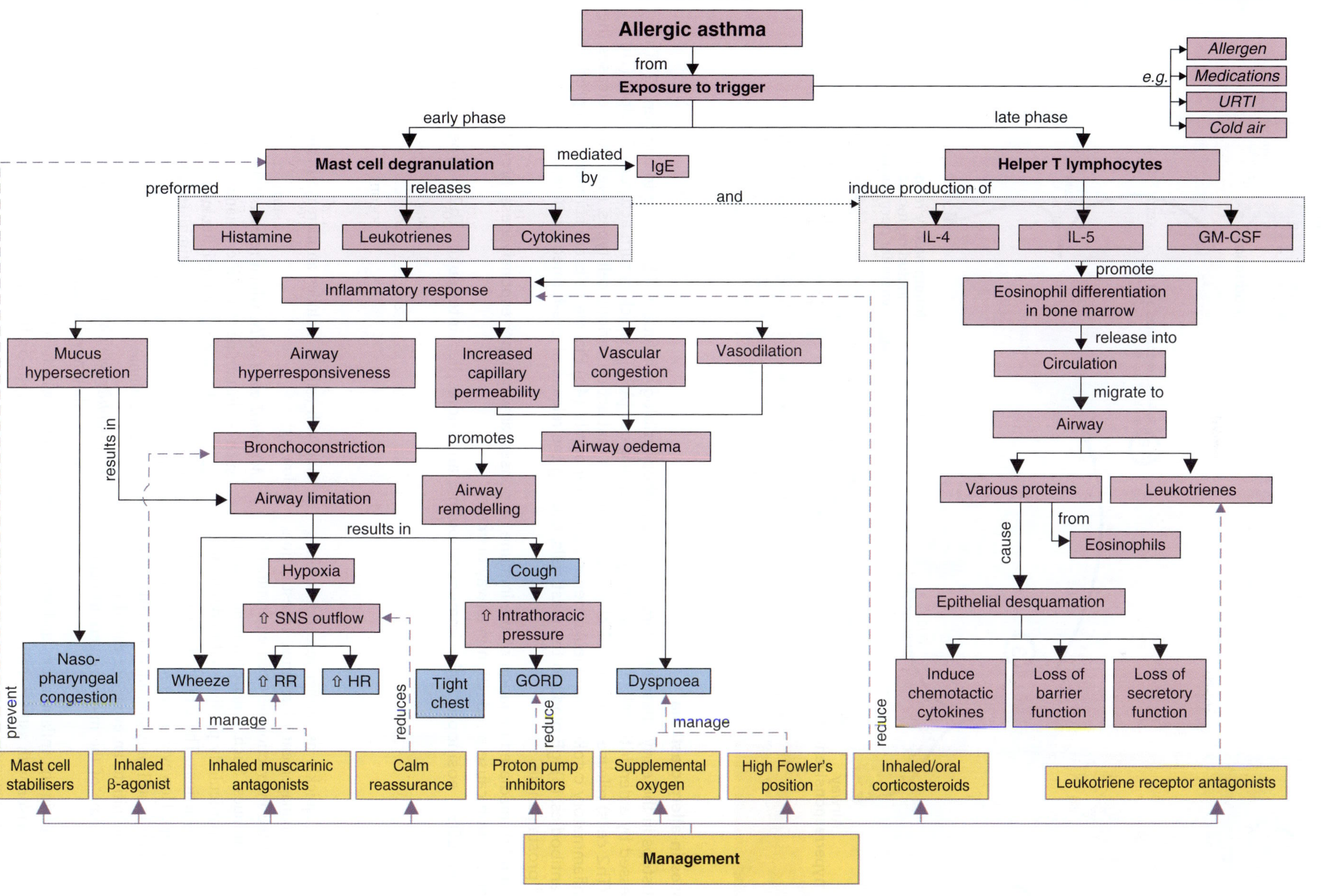

Figure 27.1

Clinical snapshot: Allergic asthma

↑ = increased; β = beta; GM-CSF = granulocyte-macrophage colony-stimulating factor; GORD = gastro-oesophageal reflux disease; *HR* = *heart rate*; IgE = immunoglobulin E; IL = interleukin; RR = respiratory rate; SNS = sympathetic nervous system; URTI = upper respiratory tract infection.

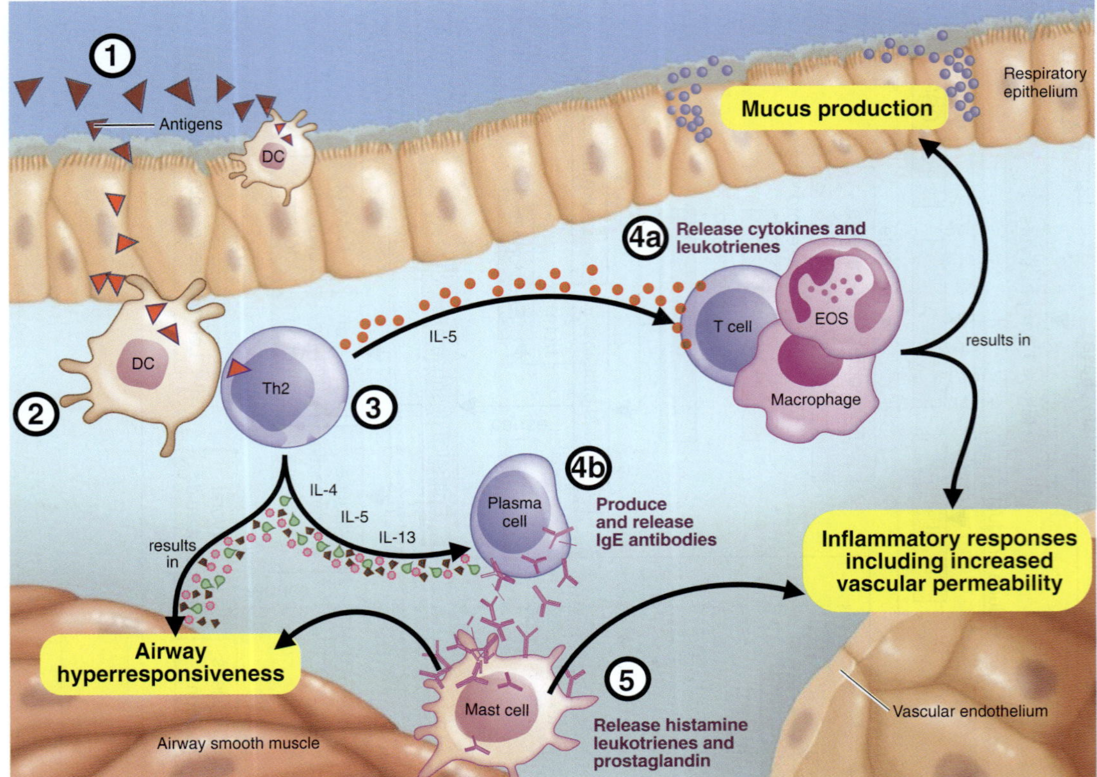

Figure 27.2

Cellular responses in allergic asthma

Some important steps in the early phase of allergic asthma pathophysiology include: (1) Exposure to allergen. (2) The allergen is processed by a dendritic cell (aka—an antigen-presenting cell [APC]), which in turn activates T helper (Th) cells. (3) T cells (Th2 cells) release a number of chemical mediators that act on various cell types. (4a) This increases the release of pro-inflammatory cytokines and leukotrienes from eosinophils. (4b) Plasma cells are stimulated to produce and release IgE antibodies. (5) IgE binds to the mast cells, causing the release of pre-formed granules of histamines, leukotrienes and prostaglandin.

Therefore, following IgE-mediated initiation of the immune responses, airway hyperresponsiveness, bronchoconstriction and mucus hypersecretion cause a reduction in airway diameter.

DC = dendritic cell; EOS = eosinophil; IgE = immunoglobulin-E antibodies; IL = interleukin; Th2 = type 2 helper T cell.

This field is evolving quickly as further research informs the understanding and management of asthma. Investigation into the importance of the interaction between environmental and genetic factors continues. Such *genetic influence* can be seen in people who are particularly predisposed to developing allergic hypersensitivity reactions. These individuals are known as *atopic* (i.e. have **atopy**). However, *environmental influences* must also exist, as atopy is still only considered a risk factor, not a cause. Factors that initiate an event are called *triggers*. Clinical Box 27.2 lists some of the many triggers associated with asthma.

Various changes occur in the inflammatory and structural cells in the airway of a person with asthma, and these are well described by the GINA's management and prevention document. A summary of the inflammatory cell changes in the airway of a person with asthma includes an increase in the number of the following:

- ***Mucosal mast cells***, which release inflammatory mediators such as histamine, leukotrienes and prostaglandin D_2, are activated by several stimuli, including immunoglobulin-E (IgE)-mediated responses stimulated by allergens and also by changes in osmotic stimuli (see the section on exercise-induced asthma).
- ***Eosinophils***, which release leukotrienes, growth factors and proteins that may damage epithelial cells in the airway.
- ***T cells***, which release cytokines, including interleukins (IL) IL-4, IL-5, IL-9 and IL-13, which are responsible for facilitating eosinophil-mediated inflammation, and an increase in the production of IgE by B cells.

CLINICAL BOX 27.1

Inflammatory phenotype classification T2-High and T2-Low

For individuals with severe asthma, a new method of classifying extrinsic asthma characterises the condition relating to the nature and process of inflammation induced. Subsequently, the terms T2-high and T2-low are becoming more common to help define the mechanism by which a person's asthma develops, and this knowledge then guides the best method for symptom control (see the figure below). 'T2' stands for a subtype of T cells known as type 2 helper T cells (Th2 cells), which have long been considered a significant driver of asthma.

The T2-high asthma phenotype is considered to have high eosinophilic values as two interleukins (IL-4 and IL-13) activate B cells which produce IgE and subsequently cause mast cells to be sensitised. This process then causes IL-5 to promote eosinophil recruitment to the lungs. This phenotype is often associated with severe, persistent asthma, with frequent exacerbations and poor quality of life. Biological drugs (such as monoclonal antibodies— '-mAbs') have been developed to target this process. In Australia, there are currently four monoclonal antibodies—dupilumab, omalizumab, mepolizumab and benralizumab—used in the management of severe asthma (where asthma control is not reached despite the use of high-dose inhaled corticosteroids).

The T2-low (non-T2 pathways) asthma phenotype is considered to be non-eosinophilic, which is often further categorised into endotypes as neutrophilic (with high neutrophil counts) or paucigranulocytic (with low inflammatory cell counts of any type).

The neutrophilic T2-low endotype is associated with IL-8 and IL-17 promotion of neutrophil recruitment to the lungs. This endotype is considered to be adult-onset and can also be associated with severe persistent and frequent exacerbations and a fixed airway obstruction. Neutrophilic T2-low asthma is commonly associated with co-morbidities which complicate symptom management, such as nasal polyps, obesity, obstructive sleep apnoea, and gastro-oesophageal reflux disease.

The paucigranulocytic T2-low endotype is most commonly associated with stable asthma; however, a subgroup of people with paucigranulocytic asthma can experience severe and persistent asthma which is unresponsive to corticosteroids.

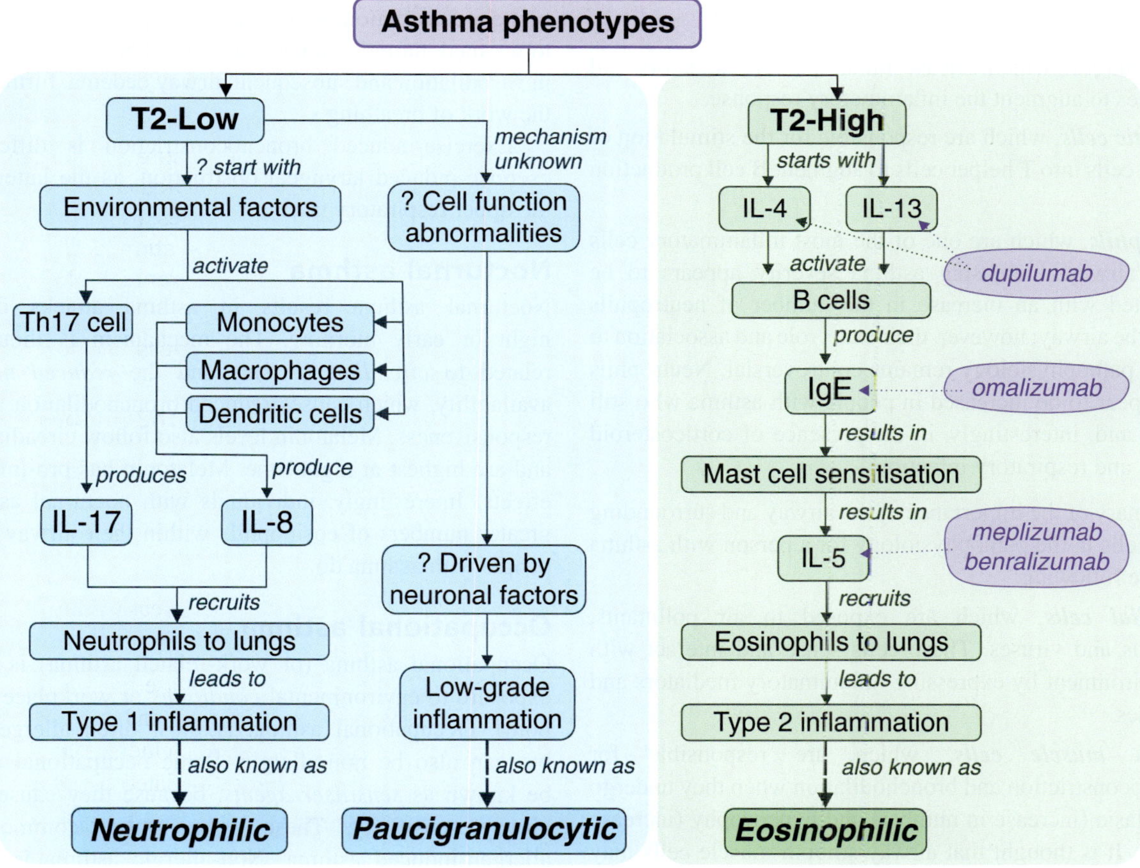

Asthma phenotypes and emerging therapies important for management of symptoms in people with severe asthma

Sources: Data from Bullock & Manias (2022); Hinks et al. (2021); Kardas et al. (2022); Papaioannou et al. (2022); Ricciardolo (2022); Syabbalo (2020).

CLINICAL BOX 27.2

Triggers associated with asthma

- Exposure to an allergen:
  - dust mites
  - pet dander
  - air pollutants
  - pollens
  - moulds
- Exercise
- Cold air
- Cigarette or wood smoke
- Medications:
  - non-steroidal anti-inflammatory drugs (NSAIDs), especially aspirin
  - beta-antagonist medications
- Upper respiratory tract infections
- Stress
- Strong odours or fumes
- Gastro-oesophageal reflux disease (GORD)

- ***Macrophages***, which release inflammatory mediators and cytokines to augment the inflammatory response.
- ***Dendritic cells***, which are responsible for the stimulation of naïve T cells into T helper cells to augment B cell production of IgE.
- ***Neutrophils***, which are one of the most inflammatory cells in the airway. Increasing asthma severity appears to be associated with an increase in the number of neutrophils within the airway; however, their exact role and association to asthma pathophysiology remains controversial. Neutrophils also appear to be increased in people with asthma who still smoke, and, interestingly, in the presence of corticosteroid therapy and respiratory infection.

A summary of the importance of the airway and surrounding structural cells in the pathophysiology for a person with asthma includes the following:

- ***Epithelial cells***, which are exposed to air pollutants, allergens and viruses. These cells sense and interact with the environment by expressing inflammatory mediators and cytokines.
- ***Smooth muscle cells***, which are responsible for bronchoconstriction and bronchodilation when they undergo hyperplasia (increase in number) and hypertrophy (increase in size). It is thought that airway smooth muscle cells may also express inflammatory proteins.
- ***Endothelial cells***, which are important for the recruitment of inflammatory cells from the circulation, and which then migrate into the airway.
- ***Fibroblasts and myofibroblasts***, which are responsible for airway remodelling through their ability to produce collagens and proteoglycans.
- ***Airway nerves***, which may become sensitised and undergo more reflexive activation as a result of triggers. Cholinergic nerve activation results in bronchoconstriction and mucus secretion.

Exercise-induced asthma

Exercise-induced asthma (also known as *exercise-induced bronchoconstriction*) occurs within 5–20 minutes of exercise beginning. In this type of asthma, the trigger is physical exertion. As the person's respiratory rate and velocity increases, a change from nasopharyngeal breathing to oropharyngeal breathing results in a greater quantity of unhumidified air being inspired, and a greater loss of heat and water from the respiratory tract. The resulting higher osmolarity causes intracellular shrinkage, and transudate enters the airway. Mast cells, eosinophils and neutrophils subsequently release inflammatory mediators, whereby an increase in airway hyperresponsiveness causes bronchoconstriction and increases the work of breathing. Initially, the colder air causes vasoconstriction, and may also activate the parasympathetic nervous system, resulting in further bronchoconstriction. As the person stops exercising, they return to warmed, humidified nasopharyngeal breathing, which results in vasodilation and subsequent airway oedema, further affecting the work of breathing.

Exercise-induced bronchoconstriction is different from exercise-induced laryngeal obstruction, as the latter occurs in the upper respiratory tract.

Nocturnal asthma

Nocturnal asthma results in asthma attacks during the night or early morning. The mechanism is thought to be related to *circadian rhythms* and the *reduced nitric oxide* availability, which causes reduced bronchodilation and airway responsiveness. Melatonin levels also follow circadian rhythms and are highest at night time. Melatonin has pro-inflammatory effects. Interestingly, individuals with nocturnal asthma have greater numbers of eosinophils within their airway than other people with asthma do.

Occupational asthma

Occupational asthma (or work-related asthma) is caused by exposure to environmental *conditions* or workplace *agents* (or both). Occupational asthma is most often allergen-induced, but can also be non-allergic. Some occupational agents can be known as *sensitiser agents*, because they cause increased airway sensitivity. These agents more commonly cause allergen-induced asthma. Non-allergic asthma is caused by *respiratory irritants*, such as smoke, fumes or gas. Irritant-induced asthma can arise from a large single 'dose' or from multiple exposures to an irritant. Occupational asthma may develop over a prolonged period of time, or it may occur with a sudden onset appearing within hours of the exposure. An *inflammatory response* is most probably the cause of irritant-induced occupational asthma.

Asthma and GORD

The association of asthma and *gastro-oesophageal reflux disease (GORD)* (see the chapter 'Gastro-oesophageal reflux disease and peptic ulcer disease') is interesting. The exact relationship is unknown; however, a significant number of adults with asthma also experience GORD. People with asthma are twice as likely as those without asthma to develop GORD. Individuals over 60 years of age are 13 times more likely than those under 20 years of age to experience asthma and GORD. Two theories on the coexistence of GORD and asthma suggest that either the refluxed and aspirated gastric acid damages the pulmonary tree (*reflux theory*), or the vagal nerve stimulation from nerve endings in the oesophagus causes bronchoconstriction induced by the parasympathetic nervous system (*reflex theory*). An exacerbation of GORD is probably induced from increased intrathoracic pressures as a result of coughing, which causes increased pressure gradients across the lower oesophageal sphincter, leading to further reflux. Early evidence suggests that the initiation of an anti-reflux medication, such as a proton-pump inhibitor or H_2-receptor antagonist (see the chapter 'Gastro-oesophageal reflux disease and peptic ulcer disease') in people with asthma who also have GORD, enables a reduction in asthma treatment.

EPIDEMIOLOGY

The World Health Organization estimates that more than 262 million people have asthma worldwide, and there are approximately 455,000 asthma deaths per year. Although urbanisation has been associated with an increase in asthma, the highest mortality is experienced in low- to lower-middle-income countries.

Australia has a relatively high prevalence of asthma, with 10.7% of Australians (or 2.7 million people) experiencing asthma. In children, prevalence is higher in boys (9.5:7.9); However, in adults it is higher in women (12:9.4). In 2021, 345 people died of asthma in Australia.

In New Zealand, national prevalence is 12.5%. In children, in 2021, asthma prevalence had reduced to 6%.

CLINICAL MANIFESTATIONS

People with asthma can present with various signs and symptoms. However, the common clinical manifestations include a high-pitched, end-expiratory wheeze, dyspnoea, non-productive cough, tight chest and hypoxia. Nasal congestion may also be reported. In response to hypoxia, sympathetic nervous system (SNS) activation can induce tachycardia and tachypnoea.

In severe asthma attacks, the individual may experience excessive bronchoconstriction and respiratory muscle fatigue associated with the increased work of breathing. If this occurs, then they may develop 'silent asthma' (or *silent chest*), an ominous sign as it represents significant deterioration. Wheezing ceases because there is very little airflow occurring (see the section on status asthmaticus, later in the chapter). Aggressive management to improve oxygenation is required. Intubation and mechanical ventilation may be necessary at this stage. Other signs that may be observed in a severe asthma attack include peripheral or central cyanosis. Also, because of the fight-or-flight response, the SNS response causes a further surge of catecholamines in an attempt to promote bronchodilation. This results in the individual developing significant anxiety and potentially a sense of 'impending doom'. A person with severe dyspnoea will most often be exceedingly restless in an attempt to try to catch their breath.

CLINICAL DIAGNOSIS AND MANAGEMENT

Diagnosis

Collection of a thorough history is necessary, including factors known to be triggers, such as atopy history, cohabitation with pets, the cleaning routine for the home or the presence of mould. A physical examination, including observation of chest diameter (anterior–posterior) and chest auscultation, should be undertaken. Pulse oximetry should be commenced immediately, and continued for the duration of the acute episode. Imaging investigations, such as chest X-ray, may be beneficial to eliminate other respiratory conditions, but should not delay treatment in an acute attack. Arterial blood gas (ABG) analysis is beneficial to quantify hypoxia, hypercapnia and acidaemia, and to direct further management.

During an acute asthma attack, a peak flow or spirometry measurement is beneficial (see the chapter 'Pulmonary dysfunction'), but depending on the acuity of the asthma attack, this may not be possible. A comparison of spirometry results pre- and post treatment is useful. Allergy testing may be beneficial to assist in the identification of triggers. A bacterial upper respiratory tract infection may have caused the exacerbation of asthma. A collection of sputum for microscopy, culture and sensitivity is valuable if the cough is productive.

The term **asthma-COPD overlap** has been recommended to accommodate the fact that some individuals have components of both conditions, which concomitantly results in worse morbidity and mortality outcomes.

The guidelines from the National Asthma Council Australia provide useful criteria in the diagnosis of asthma:

- An individual presents with variable symptoms, including dyspnoea, wheeze, cough and chest tightness, and demonstrates a significant, reversible airflow limitation on spirometry.
- A positive diagnosis of asthma can be considered if the individual demonstrates at least one spirometry with a reduced

FEV_1/FVC ratio (normally > 0.8 for adults and > 0.9 for children). (A FEV_1/FVC ratio is the ratio between forced expiratory volume at 1 second and forced vital capacity.) Peak flow measurements are less relied upon as a diagnostic device, and are retained more as a monitoring device.

- The diagnosis is supported if the person demonstrates an improvement in peak flow by at least 20% in response to asthma treatment.

Management

Asthma is a chronic condition with intermittent acute exacerbations. GINA recommendations suggest a five-step approach; however, at the time of publication the National Asthma Council Australia has not yet updated its resources with the latest management recommendations. See Figure 27.3 for the GINA stepwise approach to control symptoms and reduce future exacerbation risk. However, it is critical to note that one of the single most important considerations with significant evidence is ensuring that the person uses their inhaler devices correctly. Improper technique and use of inhaled medications results in significantly worse symptom control issues and morbidity outcomes.

The National Asthma Council Australia's four-step asthma first-aid plan for the community is an easy-to-follow procedure for appropriate and consistent management of individuals experiencing an acute asthma attack (see Table 27.1).

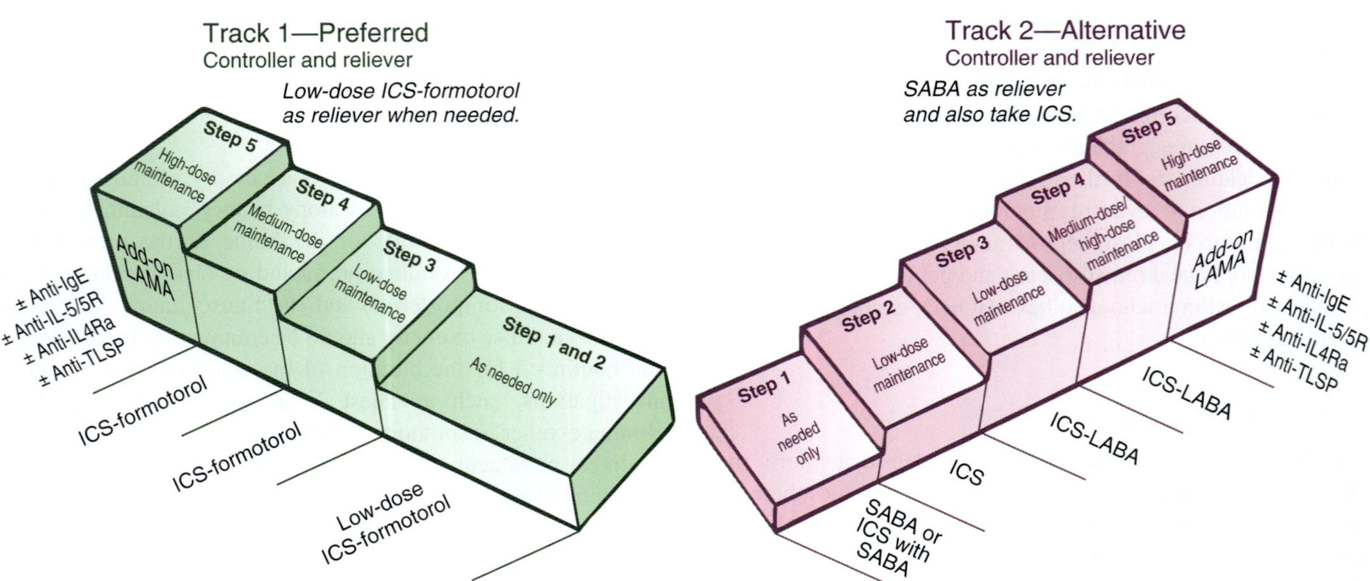

Figure 27.3

A representation of the GINA stepwise approach for asthma management in people 12 years and older

After diagnosis, the provision of—and education regarding the use of—a reliever medication (short-acting β_2-agonist) should be commenced. From there, the stepwise plan should be followed and escalated as required. A process of assessment, adjusting treatment, and reviewing response is necessary before escalating.

- Not for children younger than 12 years old.
- For children 6–11 years old, the preferred step 3 treatment is medium-dose ICS.
- Low-dose ICS-formoterol or low-dose beclomethasone/formoterol maintenance and reliever therapy.
- Tiotropium (antimuscarinic agent) by mist inhaler is an add-on treatment for those with a history of exacerbations; it is not indicated in children younger than 12 years of age.

anti-IgE = anti-immunoglobulin E; anti-IL4aR = interleukin-4a receptor antagonist; anti-IL5/5R = IL-5/IL-5 receptor antagonist; anti-TSLP = anti-thymic stromal lymphopoietin; ICS = inhaled corticosteroids; LABA = long-acting β_2-agonist; LAMA = long-acting muscarinic agonist; SABA = short-acting β_2-agonist.

Source: Adapted from Global Initiative for Asthma (2022). Global strategy for asthma management, and prevention. Gobal Initiative for Asthma, Box 3-5a, p. 61.

Table 27.1 National Asthma Council Australia's four-step asthma first-aid plan

Step	Plan
1	Sit the person upright, be calm and reassuring. Do not leave the person alone.
2	Give 4 separate puffs of a blue/grey reliever (Ventolin, Asmol or Airomir). Use a spacer, if available. That is, 1 puff, then 4 breaths after each puff. Use the person's own inhaler if possible. If not, use the first-aid kit inhaler, or borrow one.
3	Wait 4 minutes. If the person still cannot breathe normally, give 4 more puffs.
4	If the person still cannot breathe normally, CALL AN AMBULANCE IMMEDIATELY (DIAL 000) Say someone is having an asthma attack. Keep giving 4 puffs every 4 minutes until the ambulance arrives. Children: 4 puffs each time is a safe dose. Adults: For a severe attack, you can give up to 6–8 puffs every 4 minutes.

Source: New South Wales Health SHPN and Asthma Australia. Licensed under a CC BY International 4.0 licence, https://creativecommons.org/licenses/by/4.0/.

When caring for an individual experiencing an asthma attack, three priority interventions should be undertaken:

1 high-flow oxygen should be applied
2 where possible, the person should be positioned upright in a high Fowler's or semi-Fowler's position
3 a short-acting β_2-agonist should be administered, preferably via nebulisation.

It is also important to provide calm reassurance to reduce the excessive SNS outflow.

As understanding of the pathophysiology of asthma evolves, new medications to manage the clinical manifestations of this condition will be added to the current treatment options (Figure 27.3). Medication options are extending from the current 'Relievers (rescue)', 'Controllers' and 'Add-on therapies' to more targeted biological interventions such as monoclonal antibodies directed at asthma-specific causing properties. Generically, *relievers* are *short-acting β_2-agonists (SABAs)*, and achieve a rapid alleviation of dyspnoea and wheeze through SNS-mediated bronchodilation. β_2-agonists also stabilise mast cell membranes to prevent degranulation. Their effects are apparent within minutes, and may continue for up to four hours. The muscarinic antagonist ipratropium is used as an adjunct in more severe episodes. Relievers are administered through inhalation, either from a *metered-dose inhaler (MDI)* or nebulised.

Controllers are often *corticosteroids,* and can either be inhaled or be taken as oral medications. In severe episodes, parenteral formulations may also be used. Corticosteroids reduce the inflammatory response and bronchial hyperresponsiveness. *Antileukotrienes* (leukotriene receptor antagonists) are non-steroidal preventers that reduce the synthesis, release and action of leukotrienes, which cause inflammation, bronchoconstriction and increased intraluminal mucus and oedema. Another group of controllers are the *mast cell stabilisers* cromoglycate and nedocromil, which are considered inhaled prophylactic agents in maintenance therapy.

Symptom controllers are *long-acting β_2-agonists (LABAs)*, and cause extended smooth muscle relaxation (lasting up to 12 hours), resulting in bronchodilation. Symptom controllers are generally taken twice a day, and are used when people are still experiencing asthma symptoms even when taking regular corticosteroids.

Other important interventions include education regarding the control of environmental exposures to known triggers, such as animal dander, dust mites and pollen. Activity levels should be monitored. It is common for individuals with asthma to avoid exercise due to fear of exacerbating their disease. People with allergen-induced asthma or exercise-induced asthma may benefit from undertaking indoor physical activity to reduce exposure to environmental triggers and the degree of or change in humidity or temperature within their airways. People with asthma should be strongly encouraged not to smoke cigarettes, and to avoid exertion during periods of high pollution. Avoidance of some drugs, including aspirin and other non-steroidal anti-inflammatory drugs (NSAIDs), should be encouraged, as these may result in the exacerbation of symptoms.

Status asthmaticus

Status asthmaticus is a severe exacerbation of asthma that is refractory to the usual appropriate therapy. It constitutes a medical emergency.

AETIOLOGY AND PATHOPHYSIOLOGY

In status asthmaticus, there is an exacerbation of the asthma pathophysiological process that is so severe that the bronchospasm, mucosal oedema and mucus plugging are more extreme. Premature airway closure (obstruction of the small airways before the expiratory phase of the breath is complete) on expiration causes gas trapping, alveolar **hyperinflation** and hypercapnia, which can become so extreme that individuals may need intubation and mechanical ventilation.

CLINICAL MANIFESTATIONS

In status asthmaticus, the individual will generally have tachycardia, tachypnoea and hypertension. The use of the accessory muscles of respiration may be observed, and the ability to speak in sentences will decline. As the episode progresses in severity, the individual will progressively develop hypoxaemia, hypercapnia and acidaemia, which can result in seizures and coma.

Auscultation may initially reveal bilateral expiratory wheeze, but this may progress to pan respiratory wheeze (wheeze during both the inspiratory and the expiratory phases), and crackles may also develop. As the individual deteriorates further, they may develop a 'silent chest' as a result of very limited airflow. This ominous sign may indicate imminent respiratory collapse.

Clinical diagnosis and management

As status asthmaticus is a severe form of asthma, all of the diagnostic interventions used to assess asthma will be beneficial. The management of status asthmaticus only differs in the degree of urgency with which the asthma symptoms must be controlled (see Figure 27.3).

Bronchitis

LEARNING OBJECTIVE 2

Differentiate between acute bronchitis and chronic bronchitis.

Bronchitis is an *inflammation of the bronchi*. It is commonly classified as either acute or chronic. Bronchitis causes shortness of breath, cough and an increased production of mucus. Although the incidence is high, mortality associated with bronchitis is very low. Risk factors for bronchitis include cigarette smoking and being overweight. People who have smoked cigarettes at any time are 1.6 times more likely to have bronchitis, and those who smoke and are overweight are 2.8 times more likely to have bronchitis than non-smoking people of an acceptable weight. Other risk factors include exposure to second-hand cigarette smoke, pollution or chemical irritants. People with other chronic respiratory conditions are also at increased risk of bronchitis.

The air quality index is a measure reporting the volume of pollution within the air. The Australian Bureau of Meteorology and the New Zealand National Institute of Water and Atmospheric Research (NIWAR) frequently publish results of air quality on their websites. Health alerts are released through the media when levels become high. People with respiratory conditions exacerbated by pollution can benefit from this knowledge regarding their local area, and modify their outdoor activities accordingly. *Acute bronchitis* is most often caused by a viral illness and lasts longer than three weeks. *Chronic bronchitis* is defined as the presence of bronchitis symptoms for at least three months a year over a period of two consecutive years. Figure 27.4 explores the common clinical manifestations and management of bronchitis.

ACUTE BRONCHITIS

Aetiology and pathophysiology

Acute bronchitis results in the inflammation of and irritation to the bronchial mucosa following an upper respiratory tract infection. Viral infections are the most common cause of acute bronchitis. Bacterial infections can cause bronchitis, albeit less frequently. People with chronic lung conditions, such as emphysema, develop bacterial infections causing acute bronchitis more frequently than those who are otherwise normally healthy.

Following infection, an inflammatory response initiates increased mucus production, resulting in increased secretions to assist the mucociliary escalator function. However, the excess mucus production actually exceeds requirements and impedes function. Leukocytes are attracted to the area, and once they infiltrate the bronchial walls and lumen they contribute to destruction of the ciliated epithelium. As a result of the failure of the overwhelmed mucociliary escalator, coughing bouts occur in an attempt to expel the excess secretions. Inflammatory mediators can cause bronchospasm and further obstruct the bronchial lumen.

Clinical manifestations

As the common cause of acute bronchitis is most often a viral infection, prodromal symptoms such as headache, fever, myalgia and malaise are generally experienced. Upper respiratory tract symptoms such as sore throat and rhinorrhoea will occur. The development of lower respiratory tract symptoms, such as dyspnoea, wheezing and a cough that may be either productive or non-productive, marks the development of bronchitis. The individual will often experience chest discomfort or pleuritic chest pain, which may occur because of the coughing.

Clinical diagnosis and management

Diagnosis Diagnosis can be complex, as acute bronchitis from a viral cause may resemble asthma, and from a bacterial cause may resemble bacterial pneumonia. Acute bronchitis is generally considered a diagnosis of exclusion. Following collection of a thorough history and a physical assessment, the individual may be subjected to pulse oximetry to determine their oxygen saturation. Blood may be drawn for a full blood count and blood cultures if the person is febrile; however, this is not diagnostic, just informative. A sputum culture may be taken for microscopy, culture and sensitivity in those with a purulent, productive cough, as this may inform the choice of antimicrobials if a bacterial infection is considered to be the cause.

A chest X-ray may be indicated if more serious symptoms exist, and is especially useful in eliminating bacterial pneumonia as the cause. Spirometry can be informative, and may also assist in the exclusion of asthma as the cause of the symptoms.

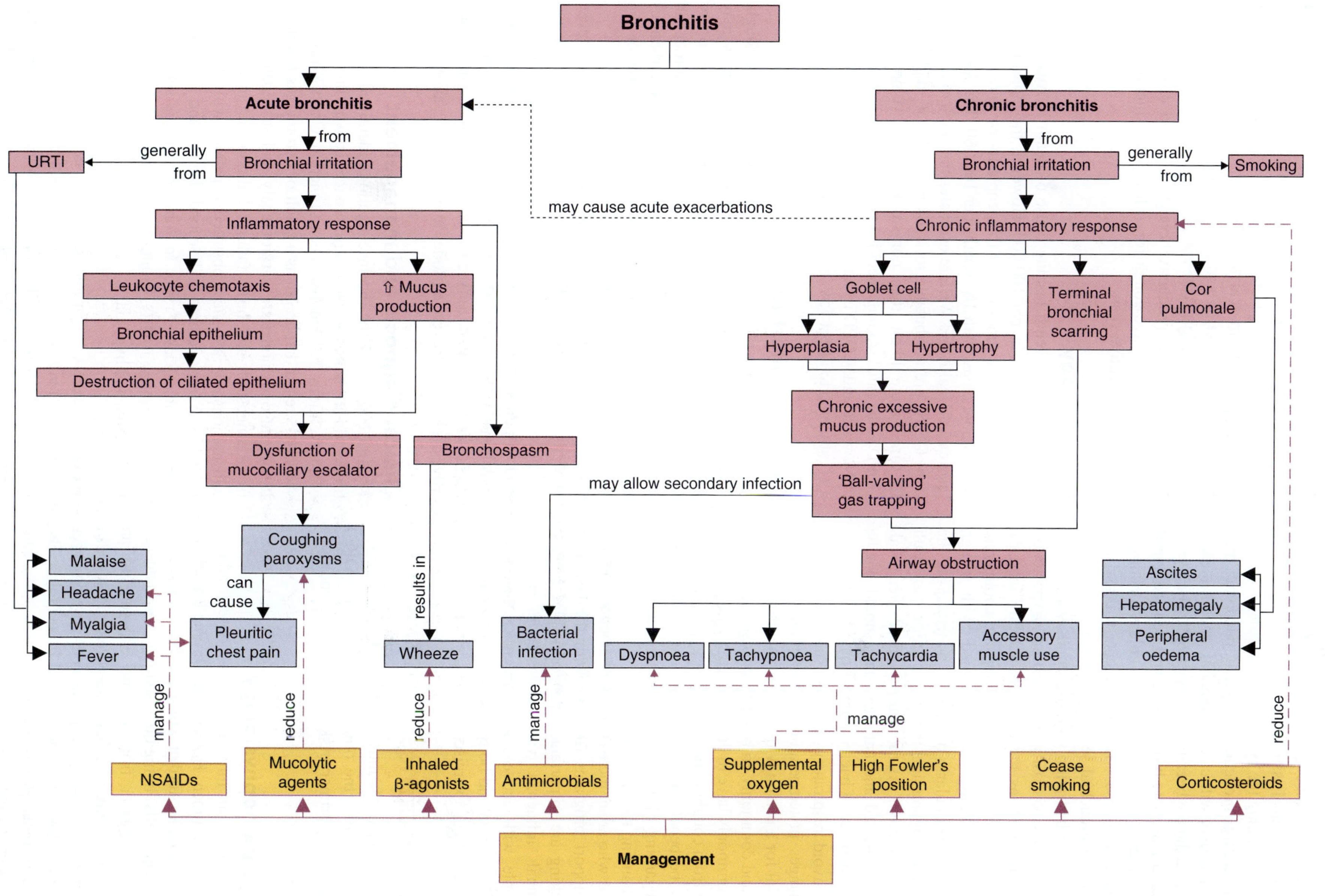

Figure 27.4

Clinical snapshot: Bronchitis

↑ = increased; β = beta; NSAIDs = non-steroidal anti-inflammatory drugs; URTI = upper respiratory tract infection.

Management Acute bronchitis is generally self-limiting and can be managed without medical assistance. Admission is not frequently required. If medical assistance is sought, management plans are aimed at alleviating the symptoms. As acute bronchitis is an obstructive condition, bronchodilators and mucolytics may be beneficial. β_2-agonists will cause bronchial smooth muscle relaxation, and will reduce wheezing and dyspnoea. The use of bronchodilator therapy in acute bronchitis is still debated, but if symptom relief is achieved, then it is warranted unless concurrent disorders contraindicate its use. Mucolytic agents will assist to reduce the viscosity of bronchial secretions; however, it should be said that maintaining hydration with oral fluids will also be beneficial in reducing the viscosity of secretions. Expectorant agents should not be used, as these agents actually increase the volume of mucus secretion by stimulating the cholinergic pathways. When expectorants are combined with cough suppressants, they are particularly dangerous, as increasing the mucus secretions and suppressing the cough reflex can result in further airway obstruction. As the cause is most often viral, supportive care is indicated and antimicrobials should not be administered in the absence of bacterial infection.

Education to avoid respiratory irritants, such as cigarette smoke, rapid changes in temperature and extreme pollution, would be beneficial for a person with acute bronchitis. Bed rest is recommended and commonly embraced, because the affected individuals will commonly have malaise from the viral infection and often fatigue from coughing paroxysms.

NSAIDs may be beneficial for relief of chest discomfort, and education regarding chest splinting when coughing may assist further in reducing the discomfort.

For individuals who are at increased risk of acute bronchitis, education and support programs to assist with the cessation of cigarette smoking are important. Other principles include maintaining annual influenza vaccinations and reducing exposure to people with active respiratory tract infections. Maintaining good nutrition and body weight is important, as is achieving adequate rest and exercise.

CHRONIC BRONCHITIS

Chronic bronchitis is one of the most common COPDs. Chronic bronchitis and emphysema (the other most common COPD) often coexist, because the primary risk factor for both conditions is cigarette smoking.

Aetiology and pathophysiology

As with acute bronchitis, an inflammatory response results in damage to the bronchial lumen. However, in chronic bronchitis, chronic irritation results in further consequences. The goblet cells (mucus-producing cells) lining the respiratory tract undergo hypertrophy and hyperplasia from chronic exposure to an irritating substance. Consequently, there is a chronic increase in the production of mucus. Furthermore, goblet cells develop lower in the respiratory tract down near the terminal bronchioles. The ciliated cells of the respiratory tract also reduce in number and, combined with the overproduction of mucus, the capacity of the mucociliary escalator is exceeded, further obstructing the lumen.

As respiratory defences become chronically reduced, repeated infections occur, resulting in a defective cycle of inflammation. As the alveolar epithelium is damaged, it initiates more inflammation, causing more destruction. Permanent changes develop from scarring in the distal airway, and this contributes to obstruction and gas trapping. As one of the only respiratory defences left is the cough reflex, the person generally develops a chronic, productive cough. Chronic bronchitis is defined as a productive cough for at least three months a year over two consecutive years.

Epidemiology

COPD was the seventh leading cause of death in Australia in 2021, with 31 deaths per 100,000. However, the mortality rate is more than three times higher for people living in remote and very remote areas, with 103 deaths per 100,000. The Australian Institute of Health and Welfare estimates that 71% of all deaths from COPD are attributable to smoking, and that smokers are 13 times more likely than non-smokers to develop COPD. COPD is the third leading specific cause of total disease burden. In New Zealand, COPD is the fourth leading cause of death, and it is estimated to affect 15% of people over 44 years of age.

Clinical manifestations

The most common clinical manifestation is a productive cough. All of the clinical manifestations from acute bronchitis may also develop, such as dyspnoea and wheeze. Signs of upper respiratory tract infection, including rhinorrhoea, sore throat and pleuritic chest pain, may also be present. Acute exacerbations may also cause tachypnoea, tachycardia and the use of the accessory muscles of respiration.

Other signs of more chronic respiratory compromise may also be present, and include hepatomegaly, ascites and peripheral oedema from heart failure. Chronic bronchitis can lead to pulmonary hypertension (see the chapter 'Respiratory infections, cancers and vascular conditions') and cor pulmonale (right-sided heart failure) (see the chapter 'Cardiac muscle and valve disorders'). Severe episodes may result in cyanosis.

Clinical diagnosis and management

Diagnosis All of the investigations identified for acute bronchitis are indicated in chronic bronchitis, with the addition of interventions that can assess heart function. Chest X-ray may show a flattened diaphragm as a result of chronic gas trapping. It may also demonstrate cardiomegaly and/or hepatomegaly from congestion and heart failure. Pulmonary function tests will demonstrate a typical obstructive pattern with decreased forced expiratory volume at 1 second (FEV_1) and FEV_1/FVC (forced vital capacity) ratio. In someone who is seriously ill and deteriorating, ABG results will demonstrate acidaemia, hypercapnia and hypoxia.

Management Chronic bronchitis is incurable, so the management plan focuses on symptom control and the prevention of acute exacerbations. All of the interventions identified in the management of acute bronchitis may be indicated in chronic bronchitis. Other interventions may include the administration of supplemental oxygen for acute exacerbations associated with hypoxia. Cessation of cigarette smoking is critical to the management of chronic bronchitis, and therefore significant effort and support should be focused on Quit programs.

The addition of inhaled muscarinic antagonists, such as ipratropium, may be beneficial when added to an inhaled β_2-agonist regimen for bronchodilation. Oral or inhaled corticosteroids may also be useful in dampening down the inflammatory response. Secondary bacterial infections can be treated with antimicrobials.

Emphysema

LEARNING OBJECTIVE 3

Describe the pathophysiology, clinical manifestations and management of emphysema.

Emphysema is another COPD, and is an incurable airway disease that is most commonly associated with smoking. Emphysema results in the enlargement of the terminal bronchioles, and a loss of elasticity and the destruction of the alveoli. Figure 27.5 explores the common clinical manifestations and management of emphysema.

AETIOLOGY AND PATHOPHYSIOLOGY

Emphysema is characterised by *the destruction of elastin and collagen by a protease–antiprotease imbalance*. The resulting parenchymal destruction causes a reduction in elastic recoil, reduced intra-alveolar pressure and airflow limitation. Permanent enlargement of the alveolar spaces occurs. The damage is initiated or exacerbated by cigarette smoking, and the inflammatory process results in chemotaxis of macrophages, neutrophils and T cells. The neutrophils play a significant role in the degradation of elastin and collagen fibre. The neutrophils appear to be recruited by the macrophages and tissue necrosis factor-alpha (TNF-α). The T cells (usually $CD8^+$ cells) contribute to the destruction of the alveolar walls, potentially through the release of TNF-α and perforins. T cell-mediated apoptosis also contributes to the destruction of lung parenchyma.

There are several types of emphysema. The four main types, distinguished by the diseased regions involved, are explained in Table 27.2. The risk factors for emphysema are outlined in Clinical Box 27.3.

α_1-antitrypsin deficiency

A condition associated with emphysema in younger individuals (under 40 years of age) is called α_1-antitrypsin deficiency. **α_1-antitrypsin** is a protease inhibitor that reduces the function of the enzymes responsible for the destruction of elastin and collagen. An inherited deficiency of α_1-antitrypsin prevents the release of α_1-antitrypsin from hepatocytes. Excess accumulation of α_1-antitrypsin within hepatocytes causes liver disease, and reduced circulating α_1-antitrypsin results in an increased destruction of the elastic and structural proteins around the terminal bronchioles and the outside of the alveolus, causing emphysema.

CLINICAL BOX 27.3

Risk factors for emphysema

Risk factors associated with the development of emphysema include:

- exposure to particles, particularly:
  - tobacco smoke
  - occupational dusts
  - pollution
- sex–male
- age–> 50 years of age
- frequent respiratory infections
- socioeconomic status–poor
- poor nutrition
- respiratory comorbidities.

EPIDEMIOLOGY

It is difficult to find statistics solely reporting the incidence or prevalence of emphysema, as it is commonly reported as COPD and includes chronic bronchitis as well. In Australia, men are almost twice as likely as women to die from emphysema, and approximately 2.7 people in 1,000 die from emphysema each year. In New Zealand, 1 in 15 people over 45 years of age have COPD (either bronchitis or emphysema). Over 80% of emphysema deaths are attributable to smoking. In fact, current smokers are almost four times more likely than non-smokers to have emphysema. People who have ever smoked are 6.3 times more likely than non-smokers to have emphysema. Comorbid respiratory conditions are common in COPD. People with asthma are 5.4 times more likely than those without asthma to have emphysema or chronic bronchitis.

CLINICAL MANIFESTATIONS

As emphysema is a chronic disease occurring over the course of many years, the progression of the disease is less noticeable to the individual, and the degree of respiratory compromise may be significant before serious assistance is sought. Affected people often experience several years of respiratory symptoms and infective exacerbations before a full respiratory assessment is undertaken. Commonly, these people reduce their activities of daily living and exertion over time to adjust for their worsening respiratory function. They normally present in their fifth decade of life; younger people presenting with symptoms of emphysema should be tested for α_1-antitrypsin deficiency.

People presenting with frequent upper respiratory tract infections, dyspnoea, wheezing and tachypnoea should be investigated further. A history of smoking is almost universally present, as are frequent productive coughing episodes. Initially, exertional dyspnoea is experienced. However, as the disease progresses, dyspnoea will occur with minimal effort. As the volume of gas trapping increases, the chronic force of the trapped air begins to influence the structure of the ribs and a widening of the anterior–posterior diameter occurs. This change results

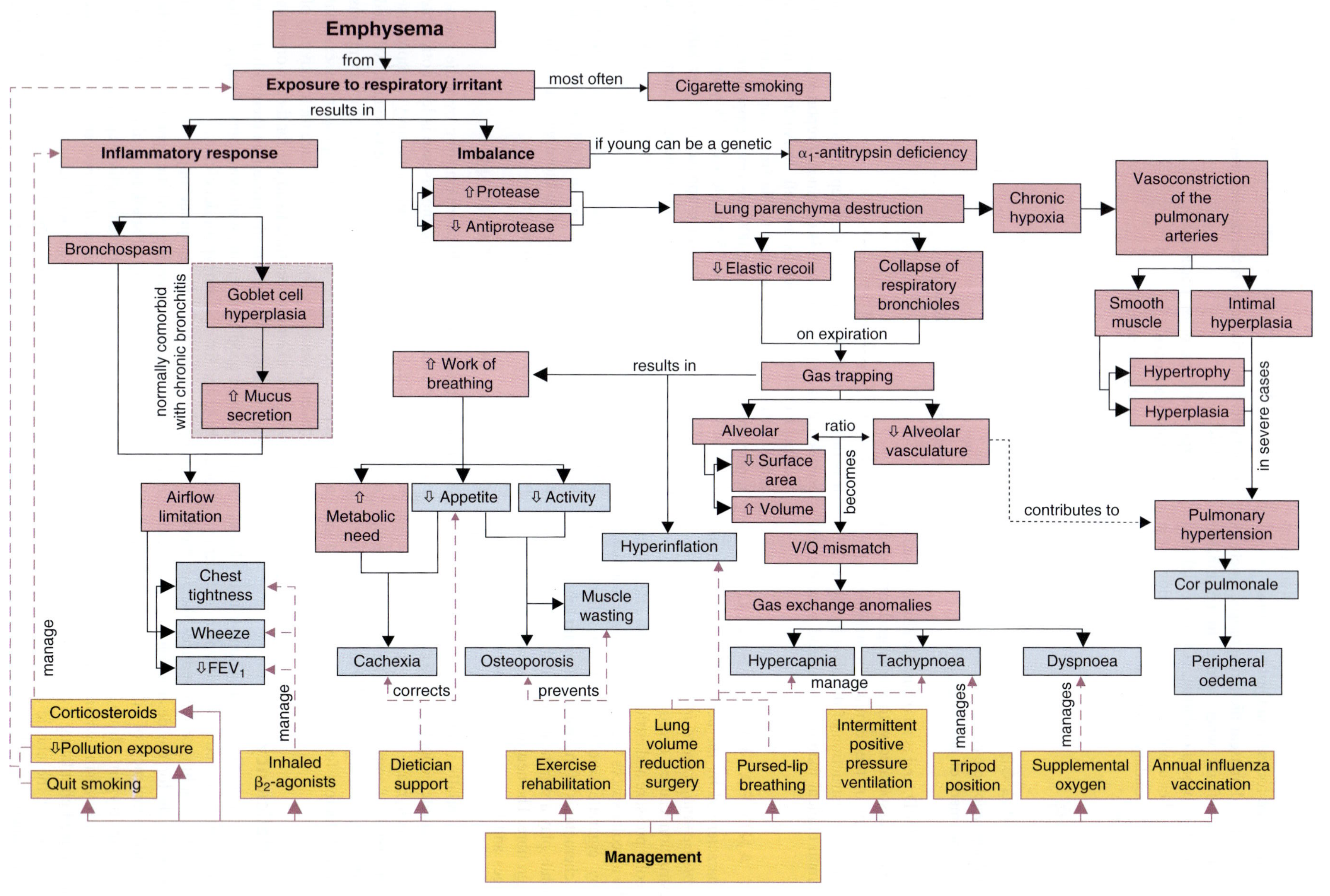

Figure 27.5

Clinical snapshot: Emphysema

↓ = decreased; ↑ = increased; α = alpha; β = beta; FEV_1 = forced expiratory volume at 1 second; V/Q = ventilation/perfusion.

Table 27.2 Four main types of emphysema

Type	Characteristics
Centriacinar emphysema	Centriacinar (aka centrilobar) emphysema involves focal destruction, beginning in the respiratory bronchioles and extending to the central portions of the acinus. The destroyed respiratory bronchioles coalesce and form emphysematous spaces, but are separated from the distal acinar by normally sized alveolar ducts and sacs (see Figure 27.6B and compare with Figure 27.6A). Centriacinar emphysema is typical in smokers, and lesions are commonly found in the upper lobes of the lung, particularly towards the posterior, apically. As the disease progresses, the destruction continues distally towards the periphery, making it difficult to differentiate between centriacinar and panacinar emphysema.
Panacinar emphysema	Panacinar (aka panlobar) emphysema involves the destruction of all portions of the acinus, and is typical in individuals with α_1-antitrypsin deficiency (see Figure 27.6C and compare with Figure 27.6A). Panacinar and centriacinar emphysema commonly occur in the same individuals, and are most commonly observed in smokers. Panacinar emphysema is most often worse in the lower lobes. As the disease progresses, differentiation between alveoli and alveolar ducts becomes less clear as the units enlarge and lose their shape.
Paraseptal emphysema	Paraseptal emphysema involves the destruction of the distal structures, such as the alveolar ducts, sacs and the lung periphery. Paraseptal emphysema is often most severe in the lung apices, where subpleural bullae occur. Individuals with this type of emphysema are at higher risk of developing a spontaneous pneumothorax (see the chapter 'Respiratory infections, cancers and vascular conditions').
Paracicatricial emphysema	Paracicatricial (aka 'cicatricial' or 'irregular') emphysema is seen adjacent to localised parenchymal scarring in individuals with inflammatory conditions, such as pneumoconiosis with progressive massive fibrosis, sarcoidosis, radiation injury and tuberculosis. Paracicatrial emphysema can develop anywhere, and can be diffuse or focal.

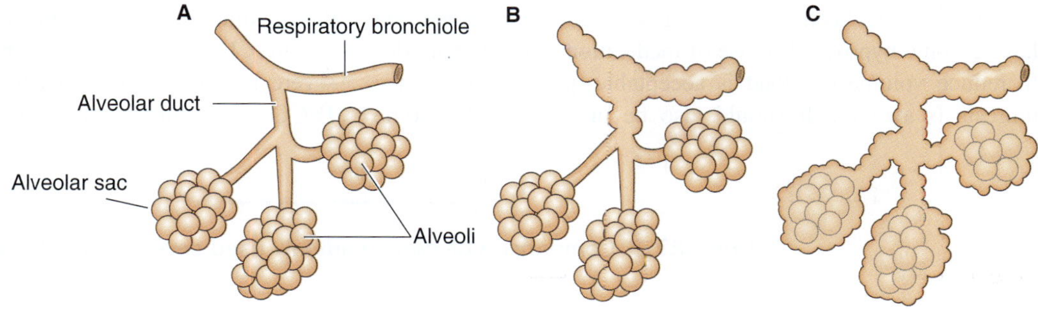

Figure 27.6

Two common types of emphysema: panacinar and centriacinar emphysema

(A) Normal acinar.

(B) Centriacinar emphysema.

(C) Panacinar emphysema.

in the distinctive barrel chest common in people with advanced emphysema. As chronic dyspnoea interferes with appetite and the work of breathing increases, individuals lose weight and become easily fatigued.

Seasonal or intermittent exacerbations often occur and result in significantly reduced respiratory function, which resolves over time with treatment. Depression is common in people with emphysema, and has been associated with many factors, including social isolation from reduced activity capacity and mobility. An assessment to identify depression in individuals with chronic respiratory disease is important so that holistic approaches can be implemented to improve the success of all interventions.

CLINICAL DIAGNOSIS AND MANAGEMENT

Diagnosis

Following a thorough collection of history and a physical assessment, blood may be collected for ABG analysis and a full blood count. Individuals with emphysema may develop polycythaemia (see the chapter 'Blood disorders') as compensation for chronic hypoxia. ABG analysis will demonstrate respiratory acidosis that may progress to compensatory metabolic alkalosis. Individuals will also demonstrate hypoxaemia and hypercapnia.

Imaging investigations, such as X-ray, are important to quantify the degree of lung damage. Common changes associated with chronic emphysema include long lung fields and a flattened diaphragm from gas trapping (see Figure 27.7). The anterior–posterior diameter of the individual's chest cavity increases as the gas trapping worsens over time. Comparison of a current lateral chest X-ray with a previous chest X-ray of several years earlier demonstrates the development of a barrel chest.

In an acute, infective exacerbation of emphysema, a sputum sample can be collected for microscopy, culture and sensitivity. Respiratory function tests can confirm the diagnosis of emphysema, and should be done to quantify respiratory function. Respiratory function tests can be done when the person is well, as a baseline, and also when ill to determine the degree of respiratory compromise. In those with emphysema, the FEV_1 exhibits a typical reduced obstructive pattern. Staging of the disease progression can be achieved by comparing FEV_1 and the FEV_1/FVC ratio to the Global initiative for chronic Obstruction Lung Disease (GOLD) classifications (see Table 27.3).

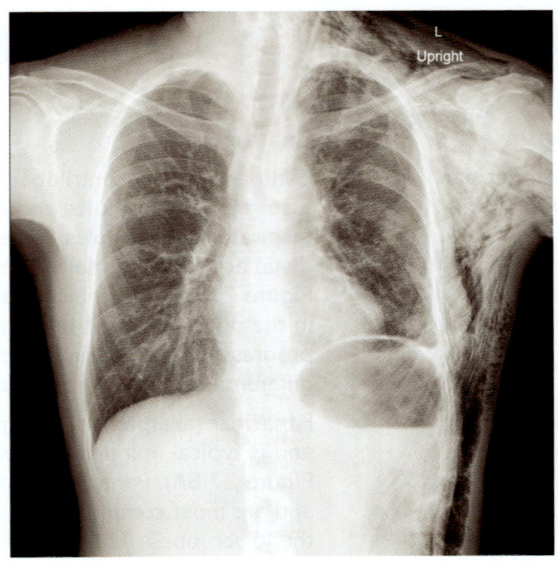

Figure 27.7

X-ray of an individual with emphysema

Notice the long lung fields, relatively flat diaphragm and the elongated cardiac silhouette.

Source: Pom_Wongsathorn/Shutterstock.

Management

The management of people with emphysema needs to focus on the general principles of reducing disease progression and preventing exacerbation. A primary intervention is the assistance to quit cigarette smoking through Quit programs, counselling and, if appropriate, nicotine replacement products. Some chemicals in cigarettes increase the amount of elastase destruction, contributing significantly to the development of the disease. Other considerations include encouraging the individual to have an annual influenza vaccination, and exploring ways to reduce exposure to pollution and passive smoking.

To optimise lung function, management of exacerbating conditions should be a priority. Oxygen therapy for more than 15 hours a day has been found to improve morbidity in people who have chronic hypoxia. The use of medications such as diuretics to reduce volume overload is acceptable, provided excessive diuresis is avoided. It should also be understood that some diuretics may cause a metabolic alkalosis, which may suppress ventilatory drive. Lung volume reduction surgery has not yet been proven as a sufficiently safe and effective intervention at this time. Nor is there evidence to support opioid use for the treatment of severe breathlessness (including nebulised opioids). Lung transplant may be an option for individuals with severe hypoxia ($PaO_2 < 60$ mmHg) and/or a hypercapnia of $PaCO_2 > 50$ mmHg plus numerous other inclusion criteria;

Table 27.3 Comparison of two commonly used severity classifications

Classification	**Mild**	**Moderate**	**Severe**
Typical symptoms	Few symptoms	Breathless walking on level ground	Breathless on minimal exertion
	Breathlessness on moderate exertion	Increasing limitation of daily activities	Daily activities severely curtailed
	Cough and sputum production	Recurrent chest infections	Exacerbations of increasing frequency and severity
	Little or no effect on daily activities	Exacerbations requiring oral corticosteroids and/or antimicrobials	
Lung function	$FEV_1 \approx 60–80\%$ predicted	$FEV_1 \approx 40–59\%$ predicted	$FEV_1 < 40\%$ predicted

FEV_1 = forced expiratory volume in 1 second.

Source: Yang et al. (2022a), Box 4, p. 32.

however, there are a significant number of exclusion criteria, including any type of substance dependence in the previous six months and prior treatment compliance issues.

Although individuals often begin to discover it themselves, teaching people with emphysema to perform pursed-lip breathing by exhaling through mostly closed lips (imagine the position the lips are in when drinking through a straw) will assist with dyspnoea and reduce gas trapping. Pursed-lip breathing works by slowing the expiratory flow and increasing positive end-expiratory pressure, which assists to reduce small airway collapse. Alveolar ventilation is improved, carbon dioxide levels decrease and hyperventilation reduces.

Inhaled β_2-agonists and muscarinic antagonists become central in the treatment regimen in order to reduce bronchoconstriction and maximise airflow. However, the Lung Foundation of Australia and the Thoracic Society of Australia and New Zealand want it well known that there is strong evidence that incorrect inhaler technique is common and is associated with worse outcomes. Therefore, education about how to use inhaler devices is critical in the process to stop exacerbations. Infective exacerbations will require treatment with appropriate antimicrobials.

In very severe emphysema or in acute exacerbations, application of intermittent positive pressure ventilation may be valuable to reduce carbon dioxide retention and improve dyspnoea. The decision to use this modality is entirely personal, as some individuals have difficulty tolerating the device, because the mask may cause an overwhelming feeling of claustrophobia. Initially, supplemental oxygen may only be necessary in times of acute exacerbation. However, as the person's lung function declines, continuous home oxygen may become necessary. Oxygen concentration units are available through government programs to people whose physiological condition meets specific parameters (see Figure 27.8). The Thoracic Society of Australia and New Zealand has developed guidelines suggesting that long-term home oxygen should be prescribed when an individual's PaO_2 falls beneath 60 mmHg or their oxygen saturations are consistently less than 90%. Flow rates should be set to between 0.5 and 2 L/min, and titrated to administer the lowest possible rate to maintain a resting PaO_2 of 60 mmHg. It is suggested that the flow rate is increased by 1 L/min during exercise. Supplemental oxygen therapy should be reviewed between one and two months after initiation, when a decision should be made as to whether or not the therapy should continue.

Other education programs should include appropriate positioning to maximise gas exchange. A high Fowler's position will reduce the effect of the upward pressure of the abdominal contents, further reducing lung expansion, and the tripod position (leaning slightly forward by supporting hands on knees) may optimise the recruitment of accessory muscles of respiration. Although there are limited studies supporting the use of breathing positions, it is common for individuals to use positioning in order to provide relief from dyspnoea.

As the disease process directly affects exercise capacity and appetite, significant muscle wasting and cachexia may develop. Inactivity can also lead to osteoporosis, which is exacerbated by inhaled or systemic corticosteroids. Education and advice from a physiotherapist to assist with exercise rehabilitation plans, and assistance from dieticians with nutrition and food selection, are important to manage loss of strength and condition.

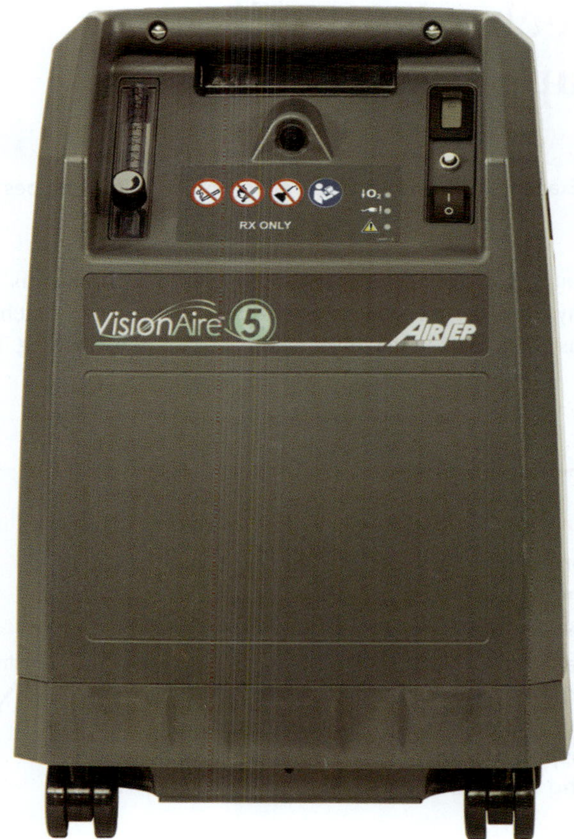

Figure 27.8

Oxygen concentrator

This device processes ambient air by removing the nitrogen and providing a pulsed flow of increased oxygen that can be 'dialled up' to the prescribed rate.

Source: © 2023 CAIRE Inc. All rights reserved.

Management of **cor pulmonale** (a form of right-sided heart failure) induced by pulmonary hypertension is multifaceted and complex. Administration of oxygen, bronchodilators and inotropes may assist. Oxygen and bronchodilators are administered to reduce the pulmonary vasculature vasoconstriction induced by hypoxia. The use of vasodilators to assist has been identified as ineffective, and may actually exacerbate hypoxia as a result of systemic hypotension. Inotropes increase cardiac contractility and may be beneficial to increase stroke volume, but are most valuable in the context of left-sided heart failure. In people who have developed polycythaemia in response to chronic hypoxia, venesection (the removal of excess red blood cells and the replacement of the lost volume with crystalloid solution) may be used to cause haemodilution, reducing blood viscosity and improving pulmonary haemodynamics. Peripheral oedema may be managed with diuretics, but care is required so as not to cause significant dehydration, resulting in worsening blood viscosity and increasing cardiac workload.

Mechanisms of gas trapping

LEARNING OBJECTIVE 4

Examine the causes and the effects of the different types of gas trapping.

Although gas trapping occurs in both chronic bronchitis and emphysema, the mechanism is different. In chronic bronchitis, mucus collections in the lower airways result in **ball-valving**. This is a phenomenon where, on inspiration, the air is able to enter the alveoli past the mucus secretion; however, on expiration, the mucus is influenced by the air pressure and can move into position to obstruct the outflow of air. Conversely, in emphysema, loss of elastin around the outside of the airways results in the loss of structural integrity and the collapse of the airway on expiration (see Figures 27.9 and 27.10). As this chronic gas trapping continues, further structural changes will occur within the lung, including the elongation of the lung fields, a flattening of the diaphragm and an increase in the anterior–posterior chest diameter (see Figure 27.11).

Figure 27.9

Different mechanisms of gas trapping: ball-valving

The mechanism of gas trapping in bronchitis and asthma occurs through the obstruction of expired air from a mucus plug acting as a valve, permitting air to enter the alveoli on inspiration, but preventing the air from leaving the alveoli on expiration.

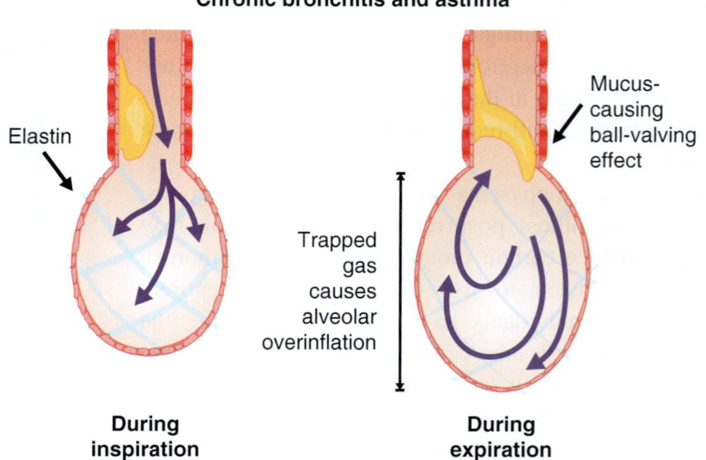

Figure 27.10

Different mechanisms of gas trapping: collapse

The mechanism of gas trapping in emphysema occurs through the collapse of the distal respiratory airway from loss of elastin. The walls are held open by the pressure of the airflow on inspiration, but on expiration the loss of structural integrity causes the walls to obstruct the airflow.

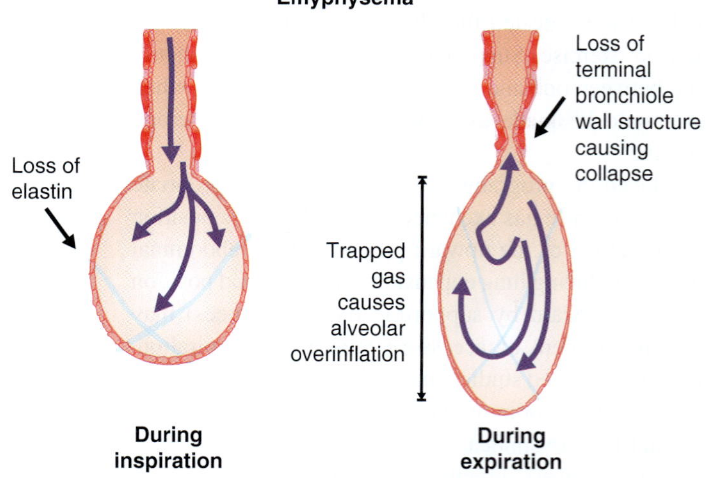

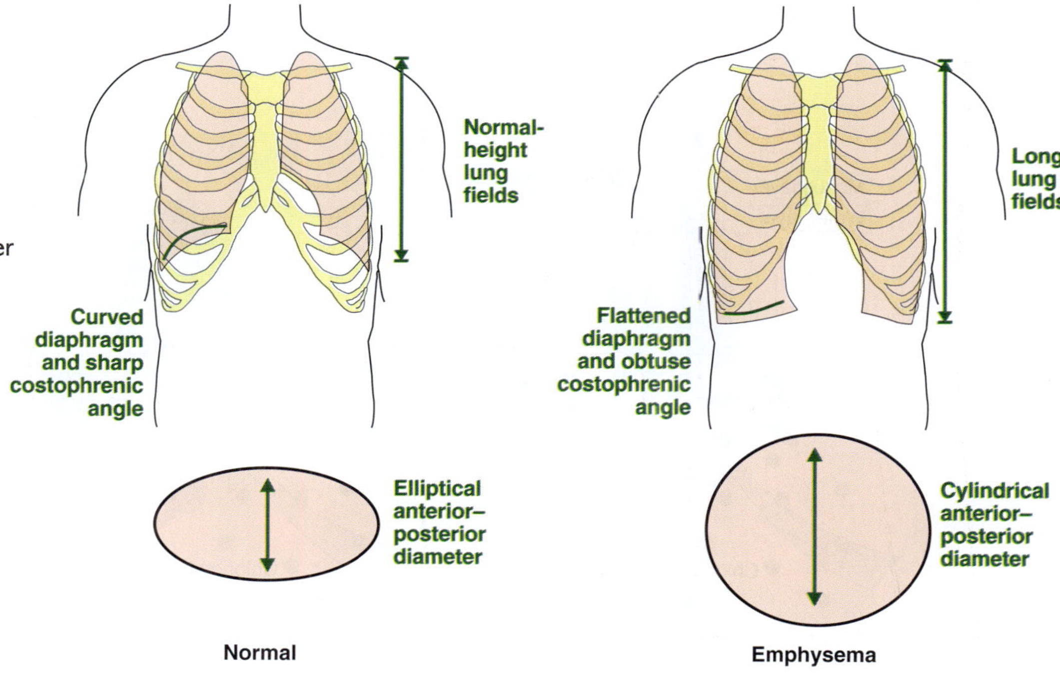

Figure 27.11

Gross anatomical changes associated with emphysema

Not only are the lung fields elongated and the diaphragm flattened, the anterior–posterior diameter of the chest is also larger in chronic emphysema.

Cystic fibrosis

LEARNING OBJECTIVE 5

Discuss the pathophysiology, clinical manifestations and management of cystic fibrosis.

Cystic fibrosis (CF) is an inherited disease affecting many body systems. However, end-stage lung disease is the most common cause of death in symptomatic individuals.

AETIOLOGY AND PATHOPHYSIOLOGY

CF has an autosomal recessive pattern of inheritance. A faulty recessive gene on the long arm of chromosome 7 coding for the protein *cystic fibrosis transmembrane conductance regulator (CFTR)* is pivotal to the development of this disease. CFTR is a salt transport protein, and defects in this gene result in chloride transport abnormalities, causing a decreased secretion of chloride and an increased resorption of sodium and water affecting the mucosal surfaces of epithelial cells (see Figure 27.12).

Although there are more than 1,600 possible defects to the CFTR gene, over two-thirds of people with CF have the same *delta-F508 mutation*, which causes a deletion of three nucleotides, resulting in the loss of phenylalanine (F) at position 508. Consistent with an autosomal recessive pattern of inheritance, the presence of one defective gene results in the individual being a CF carrier. The presence of two defective genes results in the individual having CF. If both parents are carriers, there is a 25% chance of having a baby who is not a carrier or a baby who is affected, and a 50% chance of having a baby who is a carrier (see Figure 27.13). If one person in the couple is a carrier, there is a 50% chance of having a baby who is a carrier and a 50% chance of having a baby who is not a carrier (see Figure 27.14).

The genotype–phenotype correlation is poor in many CFTR mutations. This means that the severity of the signs and symptoms (the phenotype) in people with the same mutation (the genotype) is not necessarily predictable.

Although over 1,000 CFTR defects exist, classification into six different classes based on the processing or the effect on the protein has been achievable. Figure 27.15 demonstrates the six classes of CFTR mutation.

EPIDEMIOLOGY

CF is most often found in people of northern European descent, and is rare in Asians and Polynesians. In both Australia and New Zealand, all babies are screened for CF shortly after birth. In Australia, according to the Australian Cystic Fibrosis Data Registry, approximately 80–90 babies a year are born with CF, which is about 1 in 2,800 births, and 1 in 25 people carry the CF gene. There are approximately 3,000 people with CF in Australia. In New Zealand, 1 in 3,000–3,500 children are born with CF, and approximately 1 in 25 people carry the CF gene.

CLINICAL MANIFESTATIONS

CFTR protein dysfunction causes multisystem effects involving the lungs, pancreas, intestines and liver. Other body systems can also be affected, with varying effects.

Respiratory effects

The most common cause of death in individuals with CF is bronchiectasis and end-stage lung disease. Babies are normally diagnosed within the first year, either by screening programs or from the development of symptoms. Common respiratory clinical manifestations include dyspnoea, tachypnoea, paroxysmal cough, wheezing, mucoid or purulent rhinorrhoea or sputum, and nasal

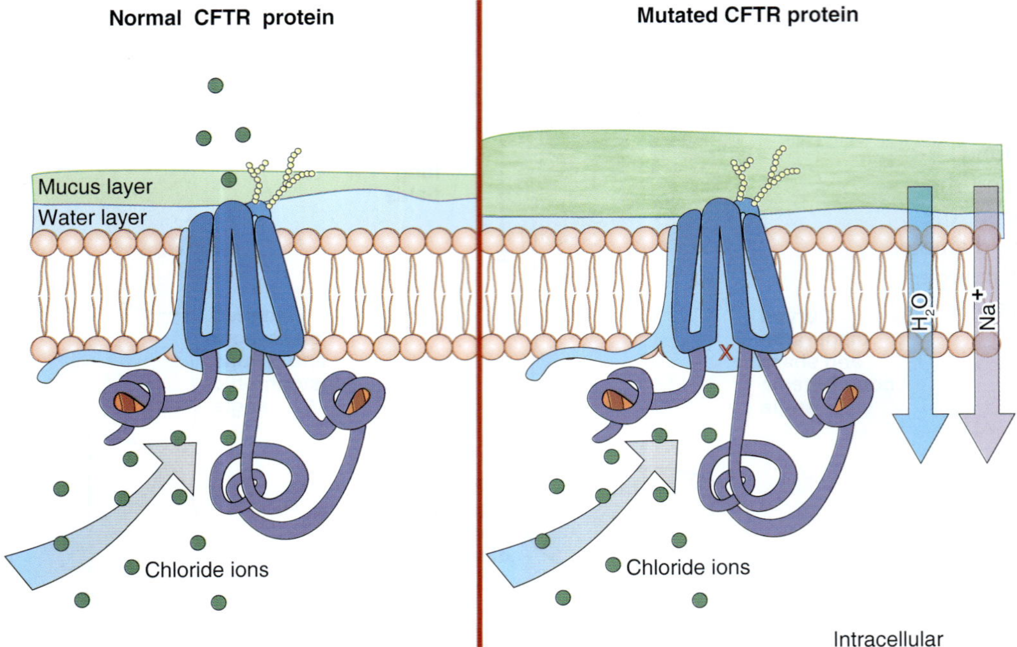

Figure 27.12

Effects of CFTR gene mutation

The CFTR protein defect results in chloride transport abnormalities, causing a decreased secretion of chloride ions and an increased reabsorption of sodium and water, affecting the mucosal surfaces of epithelial cells.

CFTR = cystic fibrosis transmembrane conductance regulator; H_2O = water; Na^+ = sodium ion.

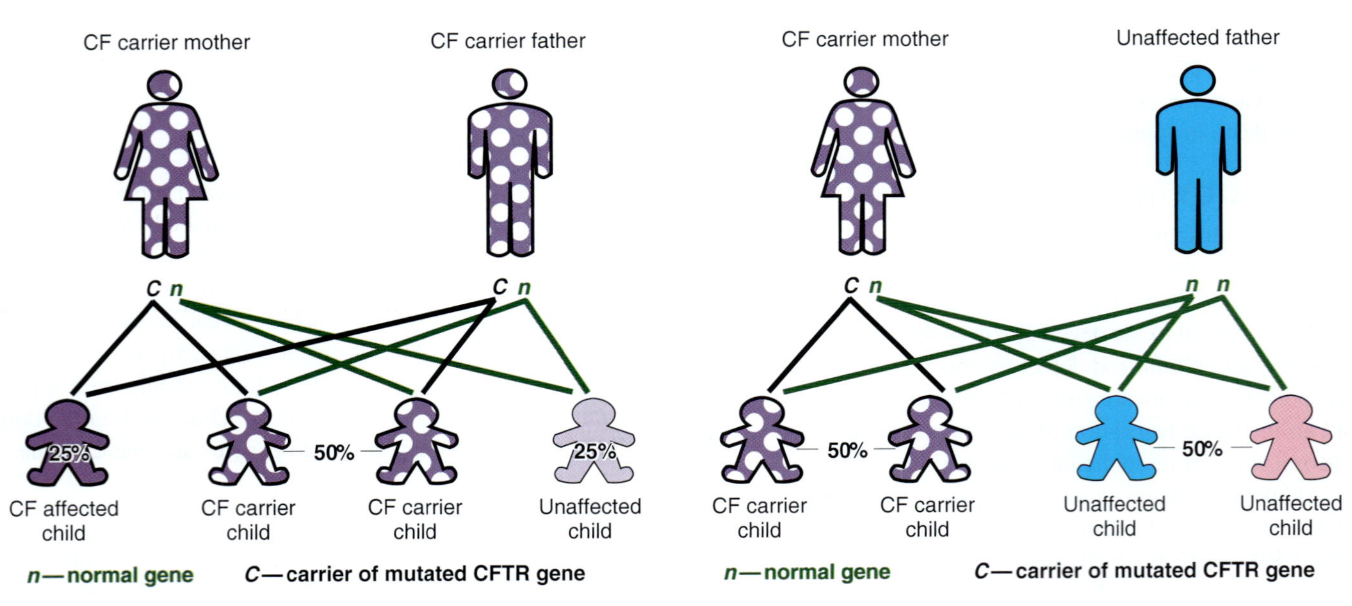

Figure 27.13

Autosomal recessive inheritance: both parents are carriers

When both parents are carriers, there is a 25% chance of having an unaffected child, a 25% chance of having a child with cystic fibrosis, and a 50% chance of having a child who is a carrier.

Figure 27.14

Autosomal recessive inheritance: one parent is a carrier

When one parent is a carrier, there is a 50% chance of having a child unaffected by cystic fibrosis, and a 50% chance of having a child who is a carrier.

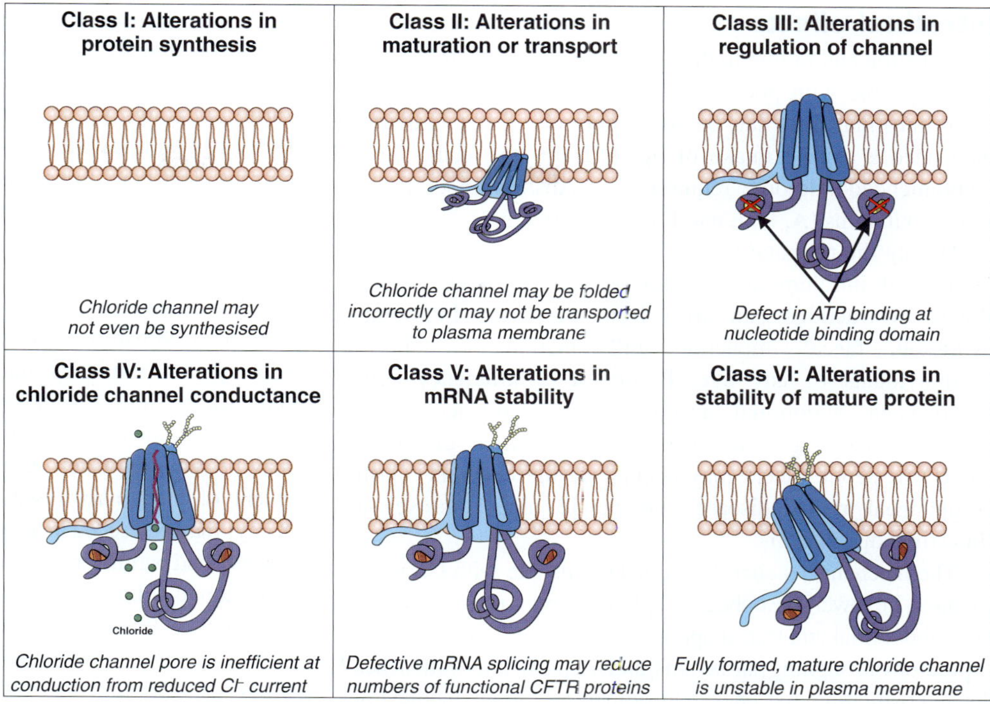

Figure 27.15

Classes of CFTR gene mutation

Of the six classes of CFTR gene mutation, class II is the most common, as the delta-F508 mutation is grouped in this class. Over two-thirds of people with CF have this type of mutation. Classes I–III are known as 'classic' or 'typical' CF, and classes IV–VI are known as 'atypical' CF.

ATP = adenosine triphosphate; CF = cystic fibrosis; CFTR = cystic fibrosis transmembrane conductance regulator; Cl^- = chloride ion; mRNA = messenger RNA.

obstruction. Trauma from coughing paroxysms may cause haemoptysis, pneumothorax or pleuritic chest pains. As the disease progresses, signs of chronic hypoxia become visible in the form of finger clubbing (see the chapter 'Pulmonary dysfunction').

Initially, a newborn's lungs are unaffected; however, the chloride transport defects begin to affect goblet cell function. Sodium ion and water are reabsorbed and cause viscous mucus production. Additionally, mucociliary dysfunction encourages bacterial colonisation, infection and initiation of the inflammatory process. Endobronchial and peribronchial spaces (spaces in and around the bronchi) are affected by an intense neutrophilic response, and a cycle of inflammation and infection that continues throughout life. Antiprotease chemicals are released by the neutrophils (elastase) and structural damage to the parenchyma occurs as elastin degrades. Chondrolysis also results in the airways becoming dilated. Bronchiectasis (the irreversible dilation of the airways) and **atelectasis** (alveolar collapse) follow as the chronic disease progresses. The pathophysiological characteristics, epidemiology, clinical manifestations, diagnosis and management of bronchiectasis are covered in detail in the next section of this chapter.

In Australasia, the most common pathogens cultured in individuals with CF are *Pseudomonas aeruginosa* and *Staphylococcus aureus*. Both of these organisms have multidrug-resistant strains: multidrug-resistant *P. aeruginosa* (MDR-PA) and multi-resistant methicillin-resistant *S. aureus* (mrMRSA). Other important organisms include *Burkholderia cepacia* and *Haemophilus influenzae*. *S. aureus* and *H. influenzae* are most common in children under 1 year of age. In CF, *P. aeruginosa* is the most clinically significant organism, because it leads to lung damage more quickly and contributes more to mortality than the other organisms. Strict infection control protocols are necessary to prevent cross-infection to *P. aeruginosa*-naïve individuals.

Pancreatic effects

Pancreatic dysfunction in CF causes malabsorption and results in failure to thrive or weight loss. This aspect of CF is further discussed in the chapter 'Disorders of the liver, the gall bladder and the pancreas'. Various mechanisms cause the reduced secretion of pancreatic enzymes, including the plugging of the pancreatic ductules and acini from viscous secretions that are deficient of water. Also, reduced pancreatic bicarbonate levels result in an unfavourable pH, further interfering with pancreatic enzyme function.

As the disease progresses, individuals can develop pancreatitis from autodigestion. As the pancreatic cells are slowly replaced by fat and fibrosis, some individuals may develop *cystic-fibrosis-related diabetes (CFRD)*. Individuals with CFRD experience more respiratory exacerbations and more severe pulmonary disease. The management of nutritional requirements becomes even more critical, and can negatively affect clinical outcomes. If poorly managed, microvascular, macrovascular and neuropathic effects of long-term, poorly controlled hyperglycaemia may develop.

Hepatic effects

Cholestatic jaundice may develop, especially in the neonatal period. Bile synthesis is significantly compromised from the effects of chloride deficiency. Bile becomes viscous, and biliary ductules can become obstructed.

Hepatomegaly and splenomegaly can develop from portal hypertension and fatty liver. If liver disease progresses, obstructive biliary cirrhosis develops, and can result in oesophageal varices and gastrointestinal bleeding. Liver disease is the second most common cause of mortality, behind respiratory complications. Other common hepatic-related clinical manifestations include nausea and vomiting, abdominal pain, jaundice and pruritus.

Intestinal effects

Malnutrition and failure to thrive are common prior to diagnosis and in people with poorly managed CF. Absorption from the gastrointestinal tract can be so compromised that individuals may need a caloric intake of up to 200% above the normal recommended kilojoule requirements. Absorption of the fat-soluble vitamins (A, D, E and K) is also affected.

During the neonatal period, a meconium ileus may develop because of intraluminal dehydration and increased viscosity. Bowel obstructions can arise from decreased intraluminal hydration, faecal impaction, inflammation or adhesions in individuals of any age. Pancreatic insufficiency causes steatorrhoea, abdominal distension and flatulence. As the affected person ages, issues such as intestinal obstruction, GORD or peptic ulcers may occur (see the chapters 'Gastro-oesophageal reflux disease and peptic ulcer disease' and 'Intestinal disorders').

The mechanisms cited for GORD in people with CF include changes in lower oesophageal sphincter pressures, changes in intra-abdominal and transdiaphragmatic pressure from the forced expiration of coughing paroxysms, and frequent, intermittent head-down positioning for chest physiotherapy. Some medications, including drugs in the muscarinic antagonist, β-agonist, tricyclic antidepressant and benzodiazapine classes, reduce lower oesophageal sphincter tone, as does glyceryl trinitrate.

Other effects

Reproductive effects, such as infertility or sterility, are common in males with CF. Although most men with CF are able to produce sperm, many have a congenital bilateral absence of the vas deferens, and therefore have no spermatozoa present in the semen. Women may have reduced fertility because of cervical mucus abnormalities, making fertilisation more difficult. Poor nutrition may also influence endocrine function and reduce fertility further; however, carrying a healthy child to term is possible when closely supervised and managed well.

Individuals with CF can develop osteoporosis because of long-term steroid use, inadequate calcium or vitamin D intake or absorption, and, sometimes, reduced physical activity.

Chronic sinus infections are common in individuals with CF, due to deceased mucociliary function and often colonisation with *P. aeruginosa.*

CLINICAL DIAGNOSIS AND MANAGEMENT

Diagnosis

The effectiveness of neonatal screening for CF is approximately 95%, but some individuals are not diagnosed until they present with symptoms. A Guthrie test measuring *immunoreactive trypsinogen* is sampled by a heel prick about three days after birth. A positive test indicates the need for DNA testing. DNA testing explores approximately 12 CFTR mutations, which covers almost 80% of the common mutations in Australasia. Most children are diagnosed before they are 2 years old. However, a few individuals with milder clinical manifestations are not diagnosed until adulthood.

Sweat testing (*pilocarpine iontopheresis testing*) is a definitive diagnostic investigation for CF, and is generally undertaken after 6 weeks of age. Sweat tests can be attempted earlier, although sweat volumes may not be sufficient. Sweat testing is non-invasive and is undertaken by placing low-current electrodes impregnated with pilocarpine onto the skin to stimulate sweat. Once the current is removed, the sweat is collected on a filter paper and sent for chemical testing. A high chloride level is considered a positive result.

Respiratory function tests will be undertaken frequently after approximately 5 years of age to monitor lung function. Alternative techniques may be attempted to measure lung function in children younger than 5 years of age.

In individuals with clinical deterioration, *periodic imaging* may be required. Chest X-ray may be necessary to measure the extent of pulmonary disease and cardiac changes. Abdominal X-rays may be needed to assess for intestinal obstruction or hepatic disease, and barium enemas may also be used to assess obstruction. Occasionally, bronchoalveolar lavage may be necessary, and sputum is collected for microscopy, culture and sensitivity.

Assessment of liver function may be necessary as the disease progresses. *Monitoring of blood glucose levels and glycosylated haemoglobin* (HbA_{1c}) should be undertaken in individuals when beta cell function declines. Observation for the signs and symptoms of chronic hyperglycaemia, such as microvascular and macrovascular complications, should be undertaken. Renal function should be monitored frequently, and eye tests should be done annually.

Assessment of bone density using *dual energy X-ray absorptiometry (DEXA)* will be necessary to ensure that osteoporosis is not developing (see the chapter 'Bone and joint disorders').

Management

As with any chronic disease, management of those with CF involves promoting optimum health and reducing the frequency of exacerbations. CF management plans need to focus on respiratory health, infection control and nutrition; and now, as people with CF are living well into adulthood, issues relating to fertility and other life choices become important.

Daily regimens for maintaining respiratory function may include:

- inhaled β_2-agonists and muscarinic antagonists to promote bronchodilation
- inhaled mucolytic agents, maintenance of adequate hydration and chest physiotherapy to promote airway clearance—chest physiotherapy may include percussion and vibration and the use of flutter devices, and, ideally, should be done in combination with bronchodilator therapy
- occasionally, prolonged use of inhaled or oral antimicrobials for the control and elimination of bacterial or fungal infections (especially *P. aeruginosa* and *Aspergillus fumigatus*)
- anti-inflammatory drugs to reduce airway inflammation.

Respiratory exacerbations may be caused by bacterial, viral or fungal infections. If respiratory function becomes too compromised, hospital admission may be necessary to facilitate the systemic administration of antimicrobials. Indications of exacerbation include increasing rhinorrhoea, coughing or dyspnoea. An elevated temperature and fatigue or malaise may develop. Changes in weight or the presence of anorexia may also be demonstrated in an individual with an infective respiratory exacerbation.

A critical component of caring for individuals with CF is the prevention of infection through comprehensive infection control policies and procedures. Common infections in the CF community include *P. aeruginosa, S. aureus, B. cepacia* complex, nontuberculous mycobacteria (NTM), influenza and *A. fumigatus*. If more than one person with cystic fibrosis is within the same environment, it is strongly recommended that they should remain at least 4 metres apart so as to reduce the risk of pathogen transmission. When caring for people with CF in an acute care, inpatient facility, healthcare professionals should ensure individuals known to be infected (or colonised) with nontuberculous mycobacterium *Mycobacteriodes abcessus* and *B. cepacia* should be provided with their own negative pressure room with en suite. Transmission-based precautions are critical to reduce person-to-person and environment-to-person transmission to reduce the spread of multi-resistant organisms.

Education regarding methods of transmission and general hygiene measures is paramount to reducing infection within and outside the CF community. Some important factors include not sharing toys, respiratory equipment or eating utensils. During infection with the common pathogens, consideration must be given regarding exposure to others in the CF community (including outpatient clinics, hospital schools and camps). During any hospital admission, room-sharing arrangements will be influenced by the presence or absence or these organisms. Ideally, individuals with CF should have a single room, with their own en suite where possible. Individuals with *B. cepacia* infection will often be nursed with contact and/or droplet precautions, depending on institution policy. A mask should be worn when within 1 m of the infected individual. The psychosocial implications of isolation for infection control measures can be challenging, and support during this time is important.

Interventions to promote good nutrition, and hepatic and endocrine function, include the following:

- As it may be difficult to achieve an adequate caloric intake, oral or parenteral supplementation (via percutaneous gastrostomy tube) may be used to maintain a kilojoule intake of 110–200% above normal recommended requirements.
- Enteric-coated purified pancreatic enzymes may be taken to support pancreatic insufficiency.
- Supplemental fat-soluble vitamins may be necessary to offset the effects of their poor absorption.
- If pancreatitis develops and beta cell function deteriorates in the context of CF-related diabetes, monitoring of blood glucose and the administration of exogenous insulin may be required.

Osteoporosis can be managed with bisphosphonates by reducing bone density loss through preventing calcium resorption (see the chapter 'Bone and joint disorders'). Treatment may be complicated by reduced gastrointestinal absorption. Although systemic preparations are available, administering bisphosphonates by this route has been known to cause bone pain and flu-like symptoms. Further research is needed to resolve some complex issues in this area.

Although reduced fertility is experienced by both males and females, the life expectancy of people with CF is now well into adulthood. Studies have shown that parenthood can have positive effects on individuals with CF. Some research suggests that the presence of children greatly influenced a person's desire to adhere to treatment regimens. Although children can be physically demanding and reduce the time for self-care, the psychological and emotional benefits of having children can contribute to long-term clinical outcomes, provided sufficient support and time-management planning is instituted.

Bronchiectasis

LEARNING OBJECTIVE 6

Describe the pathophysiology, clinical manifestations and management of bronchiectasis.

Bronchiectasis is a permanent and abnormal dilation of the bronchial airway, and is generally associated with chronic lung infection and impaired airway defences. Bronchiectasis is common in CF, and can also be associated with chronic bronchitis, asthma and emphysema.

AETIOLOGY AND PATHOPHYSIOLOGY

Bronchiectasis shares some similarities with asthma and emphysema. Bronchial dilation is related to *airway musculature changes* and the *destruction of elastin* from neutrophilic proteases and inflammatory mediators. *Transmural inflammation* and *oedema* develop and further compromise gas exchange. The impaired clearance of organisms and impaired body defence result in chronic changes to lung parenchyma. Bronchiectasis can be focal or diffuse in presentation. *Focal lesions* affect a lobe or a segment, whereas *diffuse lesions* affect most of both lungs.

Bronchiectasis is classified as cystic/saccular, cylindrical/tubular or varicose:

- *Cystic/saccular bronchiectasis* is the most severe form, and results in dilated, thick, cyst-like bronchiolar walls.
- *Cylindrical/tubular bronchiectasis* results in dilated airways with smooth wall thickening and uniform luminal dilation.
- *Varicose bronchiectasis* results in irregular and distorted bronchioles, appearing almost as a string of pearls.

EPIDEMIOLOGY

In Australia, the prevalence of bronchiectasis is unknown; however, in recent studies, an estimation of bronchiectasis rates in central Australian Aboriginal children is thought to be at least 1,470 per 100,000 children. Interestingly, approximately 70% of these children have chronic suppurative otitis media.

New Zealand reports an incidence of 99 per 100,000; however, Maori and Pacific Island people are overrepresented with rates of 128 and 228 per 100,000, respectively.

CLINICAL MANIFESTATIONS

People with bronchiectasis may present with typical COPD symptoms, including cough, tachypnoea, wheezing and dyspnoea. They may also produce excessive mucopurulent sputum. Haemoptysis and pleuritic chest pain may occur during an infective exacerbation, and this is often accompanied by a typical pneumonia-like presentation, such as fever, malaise, adventitious sounds on auscultation and hypoxia. Anorexia and weight loss may occur in severe bronchiectasis. Another indication of severe bronchiectasis is the presence of cor pulmonale.

CLINICAL DIAGNOSIS AND MANAGEMENT

Diagnosis

The collection of a thorough history and a comprehensive physical examination are important in the initial stage of investigations. Peripheral oximetry will demonstrate low oxygen saturations. An ABG analysis will indicate the degree of pulmonary dysfunction by the severity of hypoxia and hypercapnia. Although not diagnostic of bronchiectasis, it is important for informing the development of a management plan.

Imaging investigations, such a chest X-ray, will demonstrate either focal or diffuse irregularities with dilated and thickened airways. Computed tomography (CT) scans will show a bronchial wall thickening, and a greater diameter of the internal bronchi when compared to the adjacent pulmonary artery.

Elimination of other causes of respiratory dysfunction may include testing for tuberculosis, asthma and other chronic obstructive diseases. The presence of another COPD does not eliminate the diagnosis of bronchiectasis, however. Anaphylaxis, pneumothorax and pulmonary embolism should also be ruled out as a cause of respiratory distress.

Management

Management principles for bronchiectasis include limitation of the acute exacerbation, confirmation of the respiratory disease and comorbidities, stabilisation and prevention of further complications.

Acute exacerbations are managed with supplemental oxygen, macrolide antibacterials (sometimes long-term), bronchodilators and mucolytic agents. Chest physiotherapy may also be necessary to assist in clearing secretions and improving gas exchange. Use of bubble-positive expiratory pressure devices increases the effectiveness of physiotherapy. Inhaled anti-inflammatory agents and oral or systemic corticosteroids may assist with controlling the transluminal oedema and inflammation. Dietary support is important, and supplemental nutrition may be necessary to manage anorexia and weight loss. As exacerbation recedes, improving exercise tolerance with pulmonary rehabilitation and individually tailored exercise programs will benefit clinical outcomes.

The identification and management of comorbidities, especially chronic respiratory disease, is important in the development of an appropriate long-term plan. Maintenance programs are similar to the treatments identified for exacerbation; however, antimicrobial therapy may not be necessary. Active management of comorbid respiratory conditions can assist in delaying the progression of the disease or contributing to acute exacerbations.

Prevention of further complications includes encouraging annual and periodic vaccinations (as required), education regarding avoidance of smoke (including cigarette or pollution), and avoidance of people with active upper respiratory tract infections. A focus on mechanisms to prevent respiratory infections is particularly important in the current context of the COVID-19 pandemic. Clinical Box 27.4 explores how an infection with SARS-CoV-2 in individuals with asthma can be particularly serious.

CLINICAL BOX 27.4

COVID-19 infection in people with chronic respiratory compromise

The risk of serious illness from exposure to infection with severe acute respiratory syndrome coronavirus 2 (SARS-CoV-2) is dependent on many factors, including personal immune system maturity and resilience, virus variant, comorbidities and a number of other elements. Fortunately, although the infectivity of the SARS-CoV-2 appeared to increase, the pathogenicity has decreased across time. Also, targeted vaccine development has meant that one's immune system preparedness can be increased without/before exposure to the virus.

Unfortunately, SARS-CoV-2 infection in people with comorbid respiratory illnesses such as chronic obstructive pulmonary disease are at greater risk of severe illness or even death. Many factors to consider include:

- pre-existing airway obstruction
- pre-existing heightened levels of inflammation reducing the threshold for inducing inflammatory storm
- possible co-infection, with other pre-existing pathogens exacerbating inflammatory responses
- pre-existing innate immune system dysregulation interfering with capacity to mount adequate immune response
- immunomodifying medications (such as corticosteroids) further compromising the person's innate immune system and promoting viral replication and survival
- potential behaviours such as cigarette smoking which reduce respiratory immunity and promote chronic inflammation
- precocious differentiation of naïve T cells, resulting in greater tissue damage and increased inflammatory mediators.

As further research into the influence of COVID-19 and respiratory conditions such as COPD continues, hopefully new or novel methods to improve clinical outcomes for people with respiratory conditions will emerge.

INDIGENOUS HEALTH FAST FACTS AND CULTURAL CONSIDERATIONS

FAST FACTS

- ***Aboriginal and Torres Strait Islander peoples are 1.6 times more likely to be diagnosed with asthma, and more than 2.2 times more likely to die from asthma, than non-Indigenous Australians.***
- ***Aboriginal and Torres Strait Islander peoples are nearly twice as likely as non-Indigenous Australians to develop bronchitis, and 2.3 times more likely to be diagnosed with COPD.***
- ***It is estimated that Aboriginal and Torres Strait Islander children under 5 years of age are 3 times more likely than non-Indigenous Australian children to develop bronchiectasis.***
- ***Māori are 3 times more likely than European New Zealanders to be hospitalised and 3 times more likely to die from asthma.***
- ***Pacific Islands people are 3.2 times more likely than European New Zealanders to be hospitalised and 2.7 times more likely to die from asthma.***
- ***Māori are 3.7 times more likely than European New Zealanders to be hospitalised and 2.3 times more likely to die from COPD.***
- ***Pacific Islands people are 2.6 times more likely than European New Zealanders to be hospitalised and 1.5 times more likely to die from COPD.***
- ***Māori are over 3.5 times more likely, and Pacific Islands people over 5.5 times more likely, than European New Zealanders to develop bronchiectasis.***

CULTURAL CONSIDERATIONS

- ***There has been some excellent progress in relation to reducing smoking rates in Aboriginal and Torres Strait Islander peoples. This will in years to come have a dramatic effect on the number of people with obstructive lung conditions.***
- ***The National Asthma Council Australia has identified some important cultural considerations, which include the need to always ensure to ask about the presence of a cough when collecting a history, as the person may not offer that information unprompted. In the presence of a cough, consider coexisting lung conditions, and investigate to rule out their existence. If bronchiectasis cannot be ruled out, a computed tomography and the offer of a referral to a specialist are highly recommended.***

Sources: Data from Asthma and Respiratory Foundation NZ (2022); Barnard & Zhang (2021); National Asthma Council Australia (2022a).

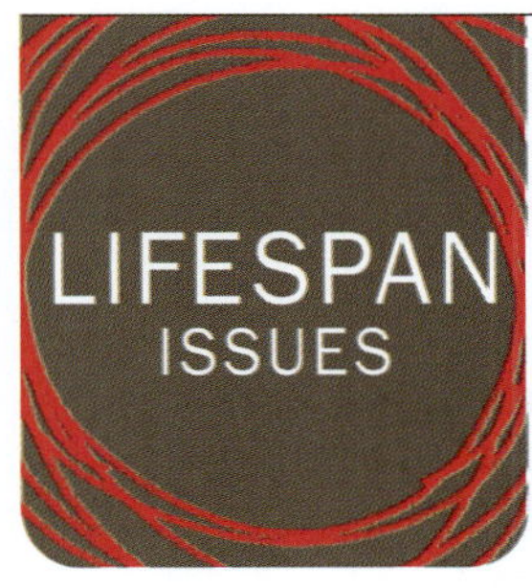

CHILDREN AND ADOLESCENTS

- Breastfed infants have a lower risk of developing asthma during their infancy.
- Infants with asthma or wheezing are more common with mothers who have asthma or who smoked during the pregnancy.
- Children who live with people who smoke are more likely to develop asthma and chronic bronchitis.
- The bronchodilator effects of β_2-agonist drugs in children under 2 years of age are unpredictable.

OLDER ADULTS

- More than 80% of Australians who die of bronchiectasis are over 70 years of age.
- Spirometry interpretation in older adults is complicated, as ageing-associated changes to the respiratory system result in spirometry flow patterns resembling airflow obstruction.
- Chronic obstructive pulmonary disease becomes apparent in individuals over 60 years of age.
- Older adults have altered perception and are less sensitive than younger adults to dyspnoea and significant bronchoconstriction.

KEY CLINICAL ISSUES

- Identifying asthma triggers can assist in reducing disease exacerbation, as plans can be developed to reduce or eliminate trigger exposure.
- Some people with chronic obstructive pulmonary disease still smoke cigarettes. In such instances, it is important to educate people on home oxygen about the dangers associated with oxygen supporting combustion, and the implications for the smoking habit.
- People with asthma may also have gastro-oesophageal reflux disease (GORD), which can contribute to poorer disease control. Identification and management of GORD is therefore important for asthma stabilisation.
- Discharge planning should include education about the asthma four-step first-aid plan and an individualised asthma management plan.
- Early detection and aggressive management of a person in status asthmaticus is important to reduce the risk of asthma-related death.
- Cigarette smoking is the principal contributing factor for chronic bronchitis and emphysema. Assistance and support with Quit programs is a critical component in the management plan assisting those with chronic respiratory disease.
- Acute bronchitis is generally self-limiting; however, chronic bronchitis can cause significant changes to lung parenchyma and reduce quality of life. Prevention of exacerbation is important to reduce the amount of lung damage.
- Pursed-lip breathing can assist in reducing gas trapping, by slowing the expiratory phase of the breath, increasing peak end-expiratory pressure and maintaining airway patency.
- Respiratory comorbidities are common, and people with asthma are more likely to have either emphysema or chronic bronchitis as well.
- Gas trapping results in changes to the thoracic cavity by increasing the anterior–posterior diameter of the chest. Finger clubbing and increased anterior–posterior chest diameter are signs of chronic hypoxia and gas trapping.
- As people with cystic fibrosis (CF) now have a longer life expectancy, issues related to fertility and adulthood become more important considerations.
- Reducing cross-infection in people with CF by adhering to best practice through infection control policies reduces the risk of lung damage within the CF community.
- Significant and various extrapulmonary effects occur in CF. Although respiratory failure is the most common cause of death, extrapulmonary complications can contribute to respiratory exacerbations.
- Although rare in isolation, bronchiectasis is a common comorbidity in people with other respiratory diseases. It is underdiagnosed, complicates the management of other respiratory illnesses, and is a significant cause of death in individuals over 65 years of age with other respiratory disease.

CHAPTER REVIEW

- The key pathological manifestations of *asthma* are airway *hyperresponsiveness, bronchoconstriction* and *airflow limitation*, resulting in airway oedema, mucus hypersecretion and respiratory compromise.
- The IgE-mediated response in asthma results in a *two-phase reaction* whereby initially preformed inflammatory mediators (e.g. histamine, leukotrienes and cytokines) are released from mast cells, causing initial bronchoconstriction, vascular congestion and airway oedema. In the late-phase reaction, other inflammatory mediators from eosinophils are released that have just been produced in response to the initial stimulus. Subsequently, epithelial damage, further bronchodilation and impaired mucociliary function occur.
- *Chronic bronchitis* results in the loss of the mucociliary escalator function from an overwhelming production of purulent secretions, which initiate an inflammatory process and promote a cycle causing chronic airway disease.
- Although asthma and emphysema are both obstructive airway diseases, asthma results in *bronchoconstriction* from IgE-mediated inflammatory responses, and emphysema results in *destruction* of elastin from cigarette smoking–related reduction of α_1-antitrypsin deficiency.
- The mechanism of *gas trapping* between emphysema and chronic bronchitis is different, but the result is the same: reduced gas exchange occurs from ventilation/perfusion mismatch as the ratio between alveolar surface area and vasculature skews.
- *Cystic fibrosis* occurs as a result of a faulty chromosome on the long arm of chromosome 7. This region codes for a protein called *cystic fibrosis transmembrane conductance regulator*, and is responsible for the movement of chloride out of the cell. Failure of this process results in viscous body secretions in all affected exocrine cells, causing multisystem effects. Individuals with cystic fibrosis have an average life expectancy of approximately 56 years.
- *Bronchiectasis* is a permanent abnormal dilation of the bronchial airway, which is associated with other respiratory diseases, and results in significantly worse clinical outcomes, especially for older adults.

REVIEW QUESTIONS

1. Define the following terms, and explain their relationship with obstructive respiratory disorders:
   a. digital clubbing
   b. cyanosis (peripheral and central)
   c. expiratory wheeze
   d. mucociliary escalator
   e. V/Q mismatch
   f. accessory muscles of respiration
2. What are common asthma triggers? Make a list, and beside each trigger identify at least one method of reducing exposure to that trigger.
3. Explain atopy and its significance in asthma.
4. Explain the changes that may occur in respiration rate and heart rate in response to dyspnoea, and to the administration of bronchodilators. Make sure that your explanation explores the physiological and pharmacological effects of these interactions.
5. Compare and contrast the major characteristics of acute and chronic bronchitis. Make sure that you address the predominant contributing factors, age of onset, pathophysiological changes and management options.
6. If a 4-year-old child was just diagnosed with asthma after a two-week episode of wheezing and dyspnoea that was associated with an upper respiratory tract infection and was relieved with short-acting bronchodilators, would you expect to see digital clubbing and changes in the anterior–posterior diameter of their chest wall? Explain your answer.

7 Identify the mechanism of action, precautions and adverse reactions for common respiratory drugs, and for each class below give some example of Australasian trade and generic names:
   a short-acting bronchodilators
   b long-acting bronchodilators
   c inhaled muscarinic antagonists
   d inhaled corticosteroids
   e mucolytic agents
   f leukotriene receptor antagonists
   g mast cells stabilisers

8 A person with emphysema is on oxygen via nasal prongs at 4 L/min and wants to have a cigarette. What education is needed?

9 Chronic respiratory diseases can cause cor pulmonale. Fully describe cor pulmonale, and identify its most common effects and management.

10 Spirometry testing is an important component of respiratory assessment in obstructive diseases. What is it, and how does it inform treatment?

11 What is the difference between spirometry and peak expiratory flow measurement?

12 What other methods are used to assess lung function or disease?

13 Explain the mechanism that results in elongated lung fields and changes in anterior–posterior chest diameter.

14 In caring for a person with respiratory issues, the common, general interventions include:
   a positioning in a semi- or high Fowler's position (as possible)
   b administration of oxygen
   c administration of bronchodilator (as ordered).

   For each of these interventions, explain the mechanism by which they assist the situation.

HEALTH PROFESSIONAL CONNECTIONS

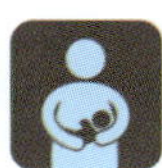

Midwives Women with cystic fibrosis (CF) can conceive and carry a baby to term. However, they are considered high risk and require significant multidisciplinary team support. If the pregnancy is planned, striving for optimum nutritional status, target weight and maximal lung function are critical. Preconception weight can be a predictor of pregnancy outcomes, and respiratory function will be further compromised by pregnancy. Genetic counselling is beneficial to ensure that both partners understand the risks associated with having a child who is either a carrier or has CF. Prenatal diagnosis from chorionic villi sampling can provide options for parents if they so choose. Following delivery, respiratory function generally improves within weeks; however, if self-cares are not maintained because of fatigue or lack of support, respiratory function can also decline. Further nutritional assessment and supplementation is required if the woman chooses to breastfeed. All medications should be reviewed in the context of their pregnancy category, and antimicrobials should be avoided if possible.

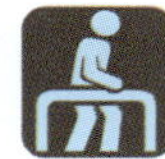

Physiotherapists Physiotherapy is critical in the management of CF. Both pulmonary and extrapulmonary issues are managed by physiotherapists from diagnosis to end-stage disease. Common treatment techniques for pulmonary issues include positive expiratory pressure (PEP) therapy, oscillating PEP and autogenic draining. Individuals and families need to be taught how to perform these techniques. The use of bronchodilators and mucolytics can be more beneficial when associated with chest physiotherapy. Extrapulmonary support, including exercise prescription and assistance with musculoskeletal pain, are also important functions of a physiotherapist when caring for an individual with CF.

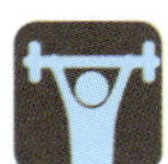

Exercise scientists Exercise scientists can be of great assistance to people with chronic respiratory conditions. Exercise prescription and pulmonary rehabilitation can reduce exacerbations, reduce disease progression and improve clinical outcomes. Once measures of current lung capacity, aerobic fitness, strength and flexibility have been undertaken, a program can be designed encapsulating the person's goals. The program should include exercises to improve upper limb strength, lower extremity strength, and aerobic training with a VO_2 peak of approximately 60–70%. Critical components of the program include psychosocial support and education regarding the disease process, rehabilitation and training program.

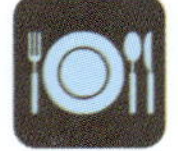

Nutritionists/Dieticians Nutrition professionals play a pivotal role in the management of individuals with CF. Although individual dietary needs will vary, common principles include a significant increase in caloric requirements, sometimes to as much as 200% of the normal recommended daily intake. Pancreatic enzyme replacement therapy (PERT) will be necessary, and, among other differences, unrestricted fat intake, often more than 100 g/day, is common. Protein requirements are increased to approximately 0.75–1 g/day, depending on age. Carbohydrate needs will vary, especially if CF-related diabetes develops, in which case carbohydrate intake will need to be spread throughout the day and insulin administration titrated appropriately. Fibre requirements are suggested at 10–30 g/day, which can be beneficial in controlling unwanted gastrointestinal symptoms. Fat-soluble vitamin and iron deficiencies are common, and supplementation should be guided by biochemical values.

CASE STUDY

Ms Amy Campbell (UR number 560623) is a 30-year-old woman with a long history of severe asthma. Ms Campbell has had three previous intensive care admissions for acute asthma exacerbation. She states that she has been unwell the past week with a minor upper respiratory tract infection, and also that she had run out of her medications—salmeterol and ipratropium.

This morning, Ms Campbell was brought to the emergency department by paramedics. Suffering a severe asthma attack, she had followed the four-step asthma first-aid plan and experienced little improvement, so a friend called the ambulance. She was experiencing dyspnoea, tachypnoea and coughing paroxysms, and her oxygen saturation was 92% on room air. En route she was given continuous nebulised salbutamol, and a cannula was inserted. On arrival at the emergency department, she had an inspiratory and expiratory wheeze, although her dyspnoea and coughing paroxysms had settled.

On spirometry, her FEV_1 was 65% of the predicted value. Following several more doses of nebulised salbutamol and some intravenous methylprednisolone, she settled and was transferred to the ward. Ms Campbell is not using any accessory muscles of respiration. An end-expiratory wheeze is still audible on auscultation, and she still has an occasional cough. She has been on the ward for three hours now, and her observations are as follows:

Temperature	Heart rate	Respiration rate	Blood pressure	SpO_2
37.2°C	64	26	124/84	94% (4 L/min via NP*)

*NP = nasal prongs.

In the emergency department some blood was taken. Her pathology results are as follows:

HAEMATOLOGY

Patient location:	Ward 3	**UR:**	560623		
Consultant:	Smith	**NAME:**	Campbell		
		Given name:	Amy	**Sex:**	F
		DOB:	13/03/XX	**Age:**	30

Time collected	12:35
Date collected	XX/XX
Year	XXXX
Lab #	2423345

FULL BLOOD COUNT		UNITS	REFERENCE RANGE
Haemoglobin	120	g/L	115–160
White cell count	5.4	$\times 10^9$/L	4.0–11.0
Platelets	250	$\times 10^9$/L	140–400
Haematocrit	0.39		0.33–0.47
Red cell count	4.35	$\times 10^{12}$/L	3.80–5.20
Reticulocyte count	1.2	%	0.2–2.0
MCV	91	fL	80–100
Neutrophils	3.42	$\times 10^9$/L	2.00–8.00
Lymphocytes	2.34	$\times 10^9$/L	1.00–4.00
Monocytes	0.37	$\times 10^9$/L	0.10–1.00
Eosinophils	0.28	$\times 10^9$/L	<0.60
Basophils	0.09	$\times 10^9$/L	<0.20
ESR	8	mm/h	<12
ABG ANALYSIS			
pH	7.33	mmHg	7.35–7.45
$PaCO_2$	49	mmHg	35–45
PaO_2	78	mmHg	> 80
HCO_3^-	23	%	22–32
Oxygen saturations	92		> 95

BIOCHEMISTRY

Patient location:	Ward 3	**UR:**	560623		
Consultant:	Smith	**NAME:**	Campbell		
		Given name:	Amy	**Sex:**	F
		DOB:	13/03/XX	**Age:**	30

Time collected	12:35
Date collected	XX/XX
Year	XXXX
Lab #	34534533

ELECTROLYTES		UNITS	REFERENCE RANGE
Sodium	142	mmol/L	135–145
Potassium	3.9	mmol/L	3.5–5.2
Chloride	106	mmol/L	95–110
Glucose (random)	7.5	mmol/L	3.5–8.0
Iron	16	μmol/L	11–30

Ms Campbell is currently ordered q2h salbutamol, q6h ipratropium, bd salmeterol and fluticasone, and montelukast nocte. She is currently resting in bed in the semi-Fowler's position. She denies any pain, discomfort or dyspnoea. She is to have hourly observations for the next four hours. If her oxygen saturation drops below 90%, she is to have continuous salbutamol and an immediate medical review. Otherwise, continue with regular medications and report concerns.

The air quality index was 165 today, as a large bushfire has been burning locally for the past two days. Ms Campbell states she had been vacuuming this morning, and that she had been outside raking the dry leaves from the back of the yard. There had been a high bushfire warning, and she wanted to make sure that her house was safe.

CRITICAL THINKING

1. Given the history provided by Ms Campbell, what factors may have precipitated this exacerbation?
2. Analyse Ms Campbell's observations. What is interesting about her heart rate, given that she has been having a β_2-agonist bronchodilator? Would you expect a different heart rate for an individual with dyspnoea or who has had a bronchodilator? If her last dose of salbutamol was an hour and a half ago, would this make any difference to your assessment of her heart rate? (*Hint:* What is the mechanism of action and duration of action of salbutamol?)
3. Ms Campbell is ordered many drugs. Create a table with five columns. Title the columns 'Drug name', 'Drug class', 'Mechanism of action', 'Precautions' and 'Adverse reactions'. Write each drug on a separate row and complete the table.
4. What is important about the following information?
   a. Ms Campbell has been admitted to an intensive care unit for asthma exacerbation previously.
   b. Her FEV_1 was 65% of the predicted value.
   c. She has recently had an upper respiratory tract infection.
   d. She let some of her medications run out.
5. What discharge education will Ms Campbell require? Consider all of the aspects mentioned in the case study, and develop a comprehensive education plan. Ensure that some focus is also placed on factors that may have contributed to Ms Campbell's exacerbation.

BIBLIOGRAPHY

Asthma Australia (2021). *Asthma first aid.* Chatswood, NSW: Asthma Australia. https://asthma.org.au/treatment-diagnosis/asthma-first-aid/.

Asthma and Respiratory Foundation (2022). *Te Hā ora annual report 2022.* Wellington: Asthma and Respiratory Foundation. https://www.asthmafoundation.org.nz/assets/documents/Te-Ha%CC%84-Ora-Annual-Report-2022-web_compressed.pdf.

Asthma and Respiratory Foundation (2023). *Key statistic: respiratory disease in New Zealand.* Wellington: Asthma and Respiratory Foundation NZ. https://www.asthmafoundation.org.nz/research/key-statistics.

Australian Bureau of Statistics (ABS) (2021). *Causes of death, Australia, 2022.* Canberra: ABS. https://www.abs.gov.au/statistics/health/causes-death/causes-death-australia/2021.

Australian Bureau of Statistics. (2022). *National Health Measures Survey.* Canberra: ABS. https://www.abs.gov.au/participate-survey/household-survey/national-health-measures-survey.

Australian Institute of Health and Welfare (2020). *Aboriginal and Torres Strait Islander Health Performance Framework 2020—summary report.* Cat. No. IHPF 2. Canberra: Australian Government Department of Health. https://www.indigenoushpf.gov.au/publications/hpf-summary-2020.

Australian Institute of Health and Welfare (AIHW) (2022a). Data insights. *Australia's health 2022.* Australia's Health series no. 18. Cat. No. AUS 240. Canberra: AIHW. https://www.aihw.gov.au/reports/australias-health/australias-health-2022-data-insights/summary.

Australian Institute of Health and Welfare (AIHW) (2022b). *Principal diagnosis data cubes: separation statistics by principal diagnosis (ICD-10-AM 11th edition), Australia, 2020–21.* Canberra: AIHW. https://www.aihw.gov.au/reports/hospitals/principal-diagnosis-data-cubes/contents/data-cubes.

Australian Institute of Health and Welfare (AIHW) (2023). *Aboriginal and Torres Strait Islander Health Performance Framework: summary report 2023.* Canberra: AIHW. https://www.indigenoushpf.gov.au/Report-overview/Overview/Summary-Report.

Barnard, L.T. & Zhang, J. (2021). *The impact of respiratory disease in New Zealand: 2020 update.* Dunedin: Asthma and Respiratory Foundation NZ. https://www.asthmafoundation.org.nz/assets/documents/Respiratory-Impact-report-final-2021Aug11.pdf.

Bauldoff, G., Gubrud-Howe, P.M., Carno, M.-A., Levett-Jones, T., Hales, M., Berry, K., … LeMone, P. (2020). *LeMone and Burke's medical–surgical nursing: critical thinking for person-centred care* (4th [Australian] edition.). Sydney: Pearson Australia.

Best, O. & Fredericks, B. (2021). *Yatdjuligin: Aboriginal and Torres Strait Islander nursing and midwifery care* (3rd edn). Port Melbourne, VIC: Cambridge University Press.

Boka, K. & Ouellette, D.R.(2019). Emphysema. *Emedicine.* https://emedicine.medscape.com/article/298283-overview.

Brusselle, G.G. & Koppelman, G.H. (2022). Biologic therapies for severe asthma. *New England Journal of Medicine* 386(2):157–171. https://doi.org/10.1056/NEJMra2032506.

Bullock, S. & Manias, E. (2022). *Fundamentals of pharmacology* (9th edn). Sydney: Pearson Australia.

Caggiano, S., Cutrera, R., Di Marco, A. & Turchetta, A. (2017). Exercise-induced bronchospasm and allergy. *Frontiers in Pediatrics* 5(131):1–8. https://doi.org/10.3389/fped.2017.00131.

Carolan, P.L. (2019). Pediatric bronchitis. *Emedicine*. https://emedicine.medscape.com/article/1001332-overview.

Centre for Genetics Education (2021). Cystic fibrosis: Fact sheet 41. *The Australasian Genetics Resource Book*. St Leonards, NSW: Centre for Genetics Education. https://www.genetics.edu.au/PDF/Cystic_fibrosis_fact_sheet-CGE.pdf.

Cystic Fibrosis Australia (2020). *Reducing the risk of infections in everyday life: information for people with cystic fibrosis and their carers in Australia.* North Ryde, NSW: Cystic Fibrosis Australia. https://www.cysticfibrosis.org.au/getmedia/3107361a-2a73-47c9-b9c0-59dc32fbdfa1/Infection-Control-Document-Oct-2020.pdf.aspx.

Cystic Fibrosis Australia (2022). *Australian Cystic Fibrosis Data Registry annual report 2021.* Melbourne, VIC: Cystic Fibrosis Australia. https://www. https://www.cysticfibrosis.org.au/dataregistry.

Emmerson, K.M. & Keywood, M.D. (2021). *Australia state of the environment 2021: air quality*: Indepe3ndent report to the Australian Government Minister for the Environment, Commonwealth of Australia. Canberra: Australian Government Department of the Environment and Energy. https://soe.dcceew.gov.au/sites/default/files/2022-07/soe2021-air-quality.pdf

Fanta, C.H. & Barrett, N.A. (2023). An overview of asthma management. *UpToDate*. https://www.uptodate.com/contents/an-overview-of-asthma-management.

Fayyaz, J., Olade, R.B. & Lessnau, K.-D. (2021). Bronchitis. *Emedicine.* https://emedicine.medscape.com/article/297108-overview.

Global Initiative for Asthma (2022). *Global strategy for asthma management and prevention*. Fontana, WI: Global Initiative for Asthma. http://ginasthma.org/gina-reports/.

Global Initiative for Chronic Obstructive Lung Disease (GOLD) (2023). *Global strategy for the diagnosis, management, and prevention of chronic obstructive pulmonary disease: 2023 report.* Global Initiative for Chronic Obstructive Lung Disease. https://goldcopd.org/2023-gold-report-2/.

Grandes, X.A., Talanki Manjunatha, R., Habib, S., Sangaraju, S.L. & Yepez, D. (2022). Gastroesophageal reflux disease and asthma: a narrative review. *Cureus* 14(5):e24917. https://doi.org/10.7759/cureus.24917.

Hayes, T. & Charlesworth, M. (2022). Lung volume reduction surgery—a narrative review of clinical evidence, patient selection and peri-operative care. *Shanghai Chest* 6(3):1–7. https://shc.amegroups.com/article/view/7679/html.

Hinks, T.S.C., Levine, S.J. & Brusselle, G.G. (2021). Treatment options in type-2 low asthma. *European Respiratory Journal* 57(1):2000528. https://doi.org/10.1183/13993003.00528-2020.

Howarth, T., Heraganahally, S.S. & Heraganahally, S.S. (2023). Bronchiectasis among adult First Nations indigenous people: a scoping review. *Current Respiratory Medicine Reviews* 19(1):36–51. https://doi.org/10.2174/1573398X19666221212164215.

Kardas, G., Panek, M., Kuna, P., Damiański, P. & Kupczyk., M. (2022). Monoclonal antibodies in the management of asthma: dead ends, current status and future perspectives. *Frontiers in Immunology* 13:983852. https://doi.org/10.3389/fimmu.2022.983852.

Khosa, J.K., Louie, S., Lobo Moreno, P., Abramov, D., Rogstad, D.K., Alismail, A.,… Tan, L.D. (2023). Asthma care in the elderly: practical guidance and challenges for clinical management—a framework of 5 'Ps'. *Journal of Asthma and Allergy* 16:33–43. https://doi.org/10.2147/JAA.S293081.

Klain, A., Indolfi, C., Dinardo, G., Contieri, M., Decimo, F. & Del Giudice, M.M. (2022). Exercise-induced bronchoconstriction in children. *Frontiers in Medicine* 8:814976. https://doi.org/10.3389/fmed.2021.814976.

National Asthma Council Australia (NACA) (2022a). *Australian asthma management handbook 2016.* South Melbourne: NACA. http://www.asthmahandbook.org.au.

National Asthma Council Australia (NACA) (2022b). *Diagnosing and assessing asthma in Aboriginal and Torres Strait Islander people:* South Melbourne: NACA. https://www.asthmahandbook.org.au/populations/indigenous-people/diagnosis.

National Asthma Council Australia (NACA) (2022c). *First aid for asthma chart ages 12+.* South Melbourne: NACA. https://www.nationalasthma.org.au/living-with-asthma/resources/patients-carers/charts/first-aid-for-asthma-chart.

New South Wales Ministry of Health (2022). *Air quality factsheets.* North Sydney: New South Wales Department of Health. https://www.health.nsw.gov.au/environment/air/Pages/air-factsheets.aspx.

Papaioannou, A.I., Fouka, E., Ntontsi, P., Stratakos, G. & Papiris, S. (2022). Paucigranulocytic asthma: potential pathogenetic mechanisms, clinical features and therapeutic management. *Journal of Personalized Medicine* 12(5):850. https://doi.org/10.3390/jpm12050850.

Pilewski J.M. (2022). Update on lung transplantation for cystic fibrosis. *Clinics in Chest Medicine* 43(4):821–40. https://doi.org/10.1016/j.ccm.2022.07.002.

Rafeeq, M.M. & Murad, H.A.S. (2017). Cystic fibrosis: current therapeutic targets and future approaches. *Journal of Translational Medicine* 15(1):84. https//:doi.org/10.1186/s12967-017-1193-9.

Ricciardolo, F., Carriero, V. & Bertolini, F. (2022). Which therapy for non-type(T)2/T2-low asthma. *Journal of Personalized Medicine* 12(1):10. https://doi.org/10.3390/jpm12010010.

Rogers, L. (2016). Role of sleep apnea and gastroesophageal reflux in severe asthma. *Immunology and Allergy Clinics of North America* 36(3):461–71. https://doi.org/10.1016/j.iac.2016.03.008.

Saadeh, C.K. (2020). Status asthmaticus. *Emedicine.* https://emedicine.medscape.com/article/2129484-overview.

Saxby, N., Painter, C., Kench, A., King, S., Crowder, T., van der Haak, N. & the Australian and New Zealand Cystic Fibrosis Nutrition Guideline Authorship Group(2017). *Nutrition guidelines for cystic fibrosis in Australia and New Zealand*. Sydney: Thoracic Society of Australia and New Zealand. https://www.cysticfibrosis.org.au/CysticFibrosis/media/CFA/Policies/NHMRC-NutritionGuidelines-CF-ANZ-final-web.pdf.

Sharma, G.D. (2022). Cystic fibrosis. *Emedicine*. Retrieved from https://emedicine.medscape.com/article/1001602-overview.

Sharma, G.D. & Gupta, P. (2021). Pediatric asthma. *Emedicine.* https://emedicine.medscape.com/article/1000997-overview.

Singh, D., Mathioudakis, A.G. & Higham, A. (2022). Chronic obstructive pulmonary disease and COVID-19: interrelationships. *Current Opinion in Pulmonary Medicine* 28(2):76–83. https://doi.org/10.1097/MCP.0000000000000834RI.

Subhas, E. & Rees, M. (2022). Bronchiectasis. *Australian Journal of General Practice* 51(12), 945–49. https://doi.org/10.311128/AJGP-08-22-6520.

Syabbalo, N. (2020). Clinical features and management of paucigranulocytic asthma. *Annals of Clinical Medicine and Research* 1(3):1011. https://www.remedypublications.com/.

Tortora. G.J., Derrickson, B., Burkett, B., Peoples, G., Dye, D., Cooke, J.,… Green, H. (2022). *Principles of anatomy and physiology* (3rd Asia-Pacific edn). Milton, QLD: John Wiley and Sons.

World Health Organization (WHO) (2022). *Asthma*. Geneva: WHO. https://www.who.int/news-room/fact-sheets/detail/asthma.

Yan, X., Song, Y., Shen, C., Xu, W., Chen, L., Zhang, J.,… Bai, C. (2017). Mucoactive and antioxidant medicines for COPD: consensus of a group of Chinese pulmonary physicians. *International Journal of Chronic Obstructive Pulmonary Disease* 12:803–12. http://doi.org/10.2147/COPD.S114423.

Yang, I.A., George, J., McDonald, C.F., McDonald, V., O'Brien, M., Craig, S.,… Dabscheck, E. (2022). *The COPD-X Plan: Australian and New Zealand Guidelines for the management of chronic obstructive pulmonary disease 2025.* (Version 2.66, April 2022). https:// https://copdx.org.au/copd-x-plan/.

Yang, Y., Wei, L., Wang, S., Ke, L., Zhao, H., Mao, J.,… Mao, Z. (2022). The effects of pursed lip breathing combined with diaphragmatic breathing on pulmonary function and exercise capacity in patients with COPD: a systematic review and meta-analysis. *Physiotherapy Theory and Practice* 38(7), 847–57. https://doi.org/10.1080/09593985.2020.1805834.

28 Restrictive respiratory disorders

KEY TERMS

Asbestosis
Effusions
Extraparenchymal lung disorders
Hypersensitivity pneumonitis
Infant respiratory distress syndrome (IRDS)
Neuromuscular junction
Parenchymal lung disorders
Pleura
Pleurodesis
Pneumoconiosis
Pneumothorax
Surfactant
Transudate

LEARNING OBJECTIVES

After completing this chapter, you should be able to:

1. Differentiate between the causes, clinical manifestations and management of infant respiratory distress syndrome and acute (adult) respiratory distress syndrome.
2. Explain the effects of environmental and occupational exposures to substances that damage lung parenchyma.
3. Identify several drugs responsible for causing interstitial lung disease.
4. Recognise several connective tissue diseases that cause interstitial lung disease.
5. Discuss the effects of common neuromuscular conditions on respiratory function.
6. Discuss common extraparenchymal, non-neuromuscular conditions affecting respiratory function.

WHAT YOU SHOULD KNOW BEFORE YOU START THIS CHAPTER

Can you identify the structure and function of pneumocytes? Can you differentiate between type I and type II pneumocytes?

Can you explain the function of surfactant? Can you identify when surfactant is first produced in a developing fetus?

Can you describe the structure and function of lung parenchyma?

Can you explain the process of inflammation? Can you identify what effect chronic inflammation has on tissue?

Can you describe the processes that facilitate expansion in the thorax (i.e. what tissue allows rib movement and where is it located)?

Can you identify the components that constitute a neuromuscular junction? Can you explain how a neuromuscular junction functions?

Can you describe the structure, function and location of connective tissue?

Introduction

Conditions which impede the expansion of lung parenchyma or the thorax are called *restrictive lung disorders*. Restrictive lung disorders reduce tidal volume and interfere with oxygenation, and can be classified as either **parenchymal lung disorders** or **extraparenchymal lung disorders**. There are hundreds of restrictive pulmonary disorders, each with their own mechanism affecting respiratory function. Figure 28.1 organises restrictive conditions in broad categories. Only a selection of conditions will be discussed in this chapter: the respiratory distress syndromes (RDS), occupational and environmental diseases, drug-induced inflammatory conditions and connective tissue disorders. The general concepts of how some extraparenchymal lung disorders affect lung function will also be discussed.

Lower respiratory tract infections, such as pneumonia or tuberculosis, are also regarded as interstitial lung diseases; however, these are covered in the chapter 'Respiratory infections, cancers and vascular conditions' along with other respiratory infections.

Parenchymal lung disorders

LEARNING OBJECTIVE 1

Differentiate between the causes, clinical manifestations and management of infant respiratory distress syndrome and acute (adult) respiratory distress syndrome.

INFANT RESPIRATORY DISTRESS SYNDROME

Aetiology and pathophysiology

Infant respiratory distress syndrome (IRDS) was formerly known as *hyaline membrane disease (HMD)*, because of the proteinaceous, fibrous matrix that forms in the distal airways. IRDS is an interstitial lung disease that develops in premature neonates as a result of immature lungs. It is more common in neonates with a gestational age of less than 37 weeks, and occurs because of a deficiency in pulmonary surfactant. Although type II alveolar cells begin producing surfactant at approximately 28 weeks' gestational age, the lungs take many more weeks to develop fully. The risk of developing IRDS is inversely proportional to the degree of prematurity.

Insufficient pulmonary **surfactant** increases surface tension, causing alveolar collapse (*atelectasis*). The resulting ventilation/perfusion (V/Q) mismatch and decrease in lung compliance leads to parenchymal dysfunction, causing hypoxia and hypercapnia. Hypoxia causes pulmonary vasoconstriction and pulmonary hypertension. An inflammatory response results in increased capillary permeability, leading to pulmonary oedema, and the deposition of proteinaceous exudates, developing from necrotic debris and eosinophilic materials.

Other risk factors for the development of IRDS include multiple births, possibly as they often have a reduced gestational age. Children of mothers with diabetes have an increased risk of IRDS, as fetal hyperinsulinaemia interferes with the glucocorticoid-facilitated surfactant synthesis. Caucasian children, especially males, are also at an increased risk. Risk factors for IRDS are reduced with pre-eclampsia and prolonged ruptured membranes. Maternal corticosteroid administration can assist with lung maturation and surfactant production, reducing the risk of IRDS.

Clinical manifestations

Common clinical manifestations of IRDS include tachypnoea, suprasternal and substernal retractions, and nasal flaring, as a direct result of the increased work of breathing from atelectic lungs. An expiratory grunt can develop, and is an attempt at increasing positive end-expiratory pressure to reduce alveolar collapse. A significant respiratory effort is required to overcome closed alveoli. Accessory muscles of respiration are engaged, and the scalene and sternocleidomastoid muscles are engaged to assist with ventilation. However, the neck extensor muscles are not sufficiently developed to stabilise the baby's head, resulting in head bob. An excessive workload and increased metabolic demand follows, where the baby can fatigue and rapidly deteriorate. A respiratory acidosis can develop from the hypercapnia, and, if profound, can cause a hypercapnic encephalopathy. Severe neurological complications of IRDS can cause intraventricular haemorrhage and injury to the periventricular white matter from hypoxia, hypercapnia and altered cerebral perfusion. Other complications can include tension pneumothorax and bronchopulmonary dysplasia. Figure 28.2 explores the common clinical manifestations and management of IRDS.

Figure 28.1

Restrictive pulmonary conditions organised by category

ILD = interstitial lung disease; RDS = respiratory distress syndrome.

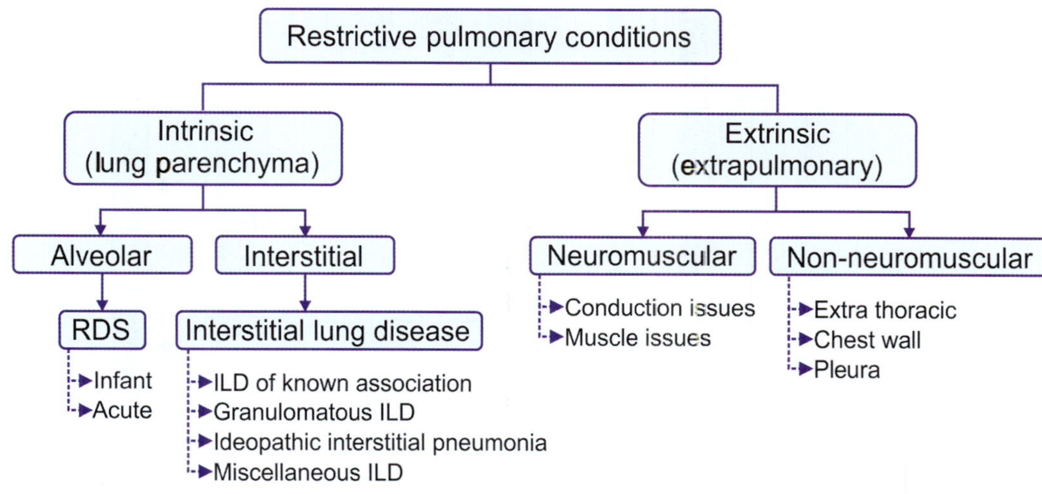

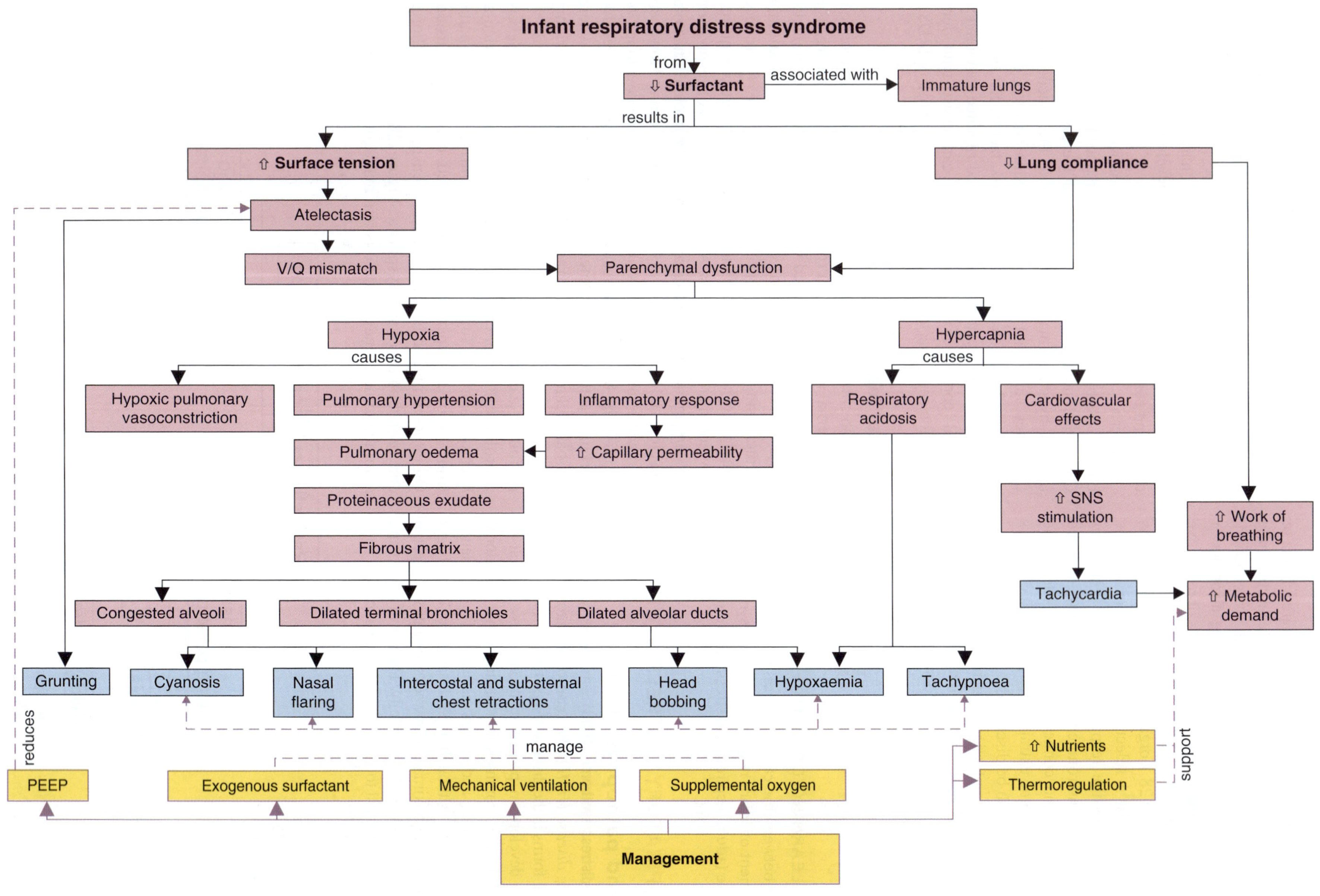

Figure 28.2

Clinical snapshot: Infant respiratory distress syndrome

↓ = decreased; ↑ = increased; PEEP = positive end-expiratory pressure; SNS = sympathetic nervous system; V/Q = ventilation/perfusion.

Clinical diagnosis and management

Diagnosis Physical assessment will demonstrate a neonate with an obvious state of compromised respiratory function. Venous blood may be drawn for a full blood count and biochemistry to rule out anaemia and assess for a possible infection. Blood cultures will also be beneficial to rule out sepsis. Arterial blood can be drawn to quantify the extent of hypoxia and hypercapnia. Assessment of the pH, and lactate and bicarbonate levels will also be beneficial. A chest X-ray may show a typical 'ground-glass' appearance, with diffuse atelectasis and visible air bronchograms. Air bronchograms are areas on an X-ray with clearly defined air-filled bronchi that contrast with the opacified surrounding tissue (from oedema or collapse) (see Figure 28.3).

Management Infants with severe surfactant deficiency will need to be intubated and mechanically ventilated. Exogenous surfactant can be administered through the endotracheal tube. Supplemental oxygen will need to be titrated to ensure a balance of the least oxygen flow necessary to maintain adequate oxygenation but not cause further pulmonary damage or retinopathy. Nutritional support needs to be frequently assessed and adjusted as required, because the metabolic demands from the compensatory sympathetic nervous system stimulation can increase the fluid and caloric needs of the infant. Thermoregulation is important to reduce the risk of hypothermia or further increased metabolic demands from heat stress. Electrolytes should be administered as required to maintain the appropriate normal levels. Psychosocial support for the mother and her partner should also be provided in the context of holistic care.

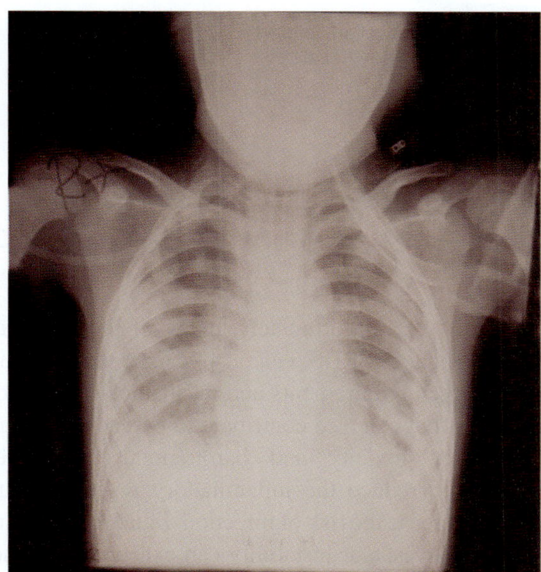

Figure 28.3

X-ray of a child with infant respiratory distress syndrome

Note the diffuse, bilateral and symmetrical ground-glass appearance of the lungs and a number of air bronchograms.

Source: Santibhavank P/Shutterstock.

ACUTE RESPIRATORY DISTRESS SYNDROME

Aetiology and pathophysiology

Acute respiratory distress syndrome (ARDS), formerly known as *adult respiratory distress syndrome*, has similar parenchymal characteristics to IRDS, but a different cause. ARDS is an acute interstitial lung disease resulting in respiratory failure from either pulmonary or extrapulmonary causes. *Pulmonary causes* of ARDS include lung contusion, pneumonia, toxic gas or smoke inhalation, gastric contents aspiration, oxygen toxicity and pulmonary embolism. *Extrapulmonary causes* of ARDS include any state that can initiate a profound inflammatory response, such as sepsis, systemic inflammatory response syndrome, SARS CoV-2 infection, acute pancreatitis, massive transfusion and disseminated intravascular coagulation. *Iatrogenic extrapulmonary causes* of ARDS include cardiopulmonary bypass, and medications such as opioids, salicylates and tocolytics (drugs that inhibit labour).

Pulmonary causes of ARDS result in damage to the alveolar membrane, which then initiates an inflammatory response. Extrapulmonary causes result in a profound systemic inflammatory response, which first results in changes to the pulmonary vascular endothelium followed by an increased capillary permeability. Ultimately, despite the cause, the result is still respiratory failure.

The three stages of ARDS are: exudative, proliferative and fibrotic. The *exudative stage* occurs within the first week. The inflammatory response triggers increased capillary membrane permeability, which results in interstitial oedema and microvascular thrombi (see Figure 28.4). Pulmonary emboli also cause proteinaceous deposits in the alveoli. Surfactant production is affected, alveolar cell destruction occurs and the inflammatory response is further fuelled. Atelectasis results in decreased lung compliance and ventilation/perfusion mismatch.

The *proliferative stage* occurs within the next two weeks, with fibroblast activation and fibrinolysis resulting in collagen deposition. Cellular regeneration also begins in this stage. Those with issues may begin to experience a resolution of symptoms or progress to the third stage, known as the *fibrotic stage*, where a coagulation–fibrinolysis imbalance develops from increased fibrinolysis, causing capillary microthrombi and more alveolar proteinaceous debris. Interstitial fibrin is deposited and results in chronic fibrosis and decreased compliance.

Clinical manifestations

The primary clinical manifestations are hypoxaemia, hypercapnia, dyspnoea and cyanosis. Sympathetic nervous system responses to hypoxia will cause tachycardia and tachypnoea. Generally, the use of accessory muscles of respiration occurs. Pulmonary hypertension and pulmonary oedema develop, interfering further with oxygenation, ventilation and lung compliance.

Extrapulmonary causes of ARDS will also result in typical manifestations specific to the cause. Signs of cardiovascular compromise often develop, and cardiac output falls. An increased risk of infection can lead to sepsis, or sepsis may cause ARDS.

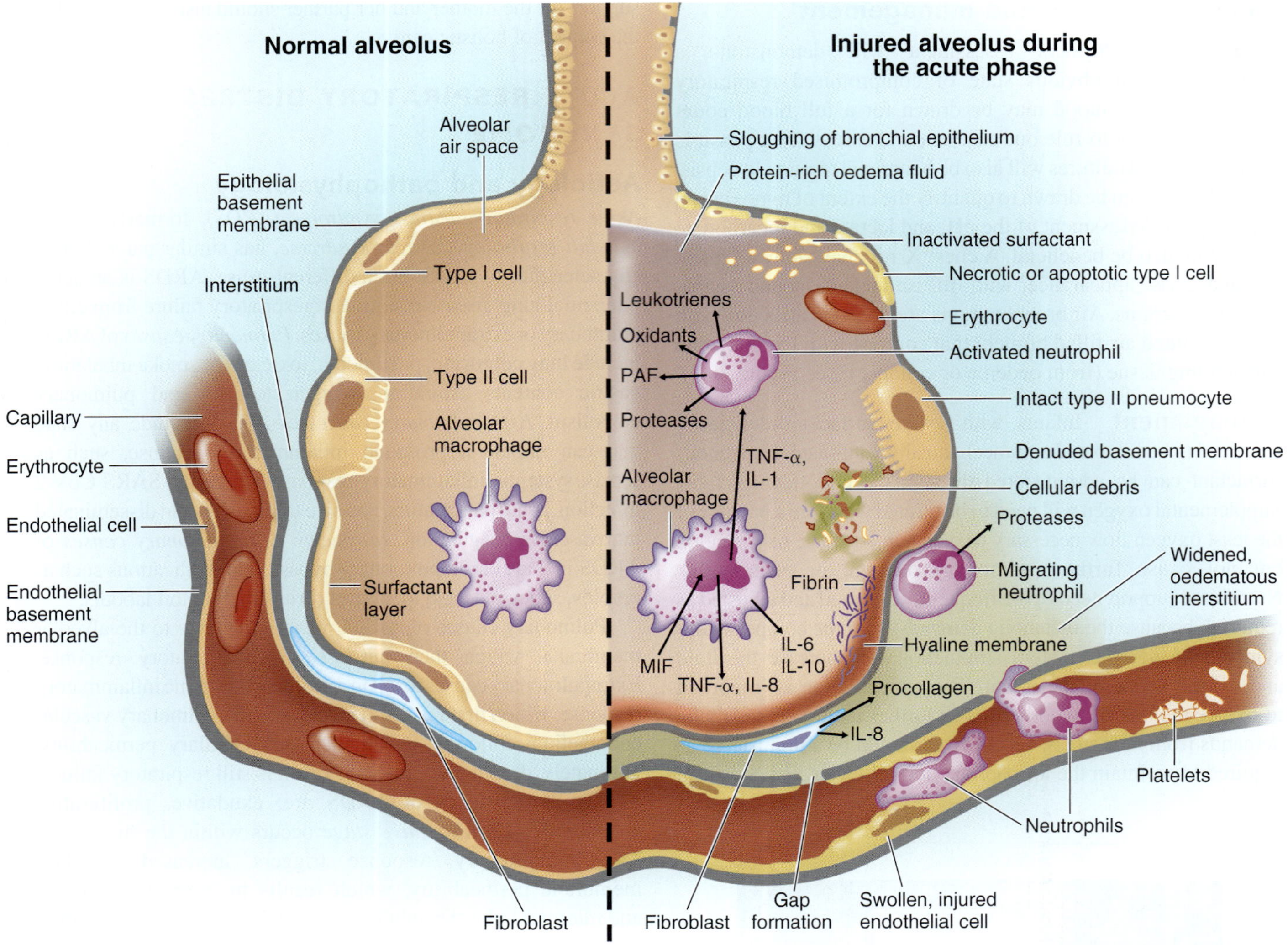

Figure 28.4

Alveolar changes associated with the exudative phase of ARDS

IL = interleukin; MIF = migration inhibitory factor; PAF = platelet-activating factor; TNF-α = tumour necrosis factor-alpha.

Those with ARDS may develop multisystem organ failure. Figure 28.5 explores the common clinical manifestations and management of ARDS.

Clinical diagnosis and management

Diagnosis Physical assessment will reveal someone who is critically ill, with worsening respiratory failure. Auscultation may demonstrate quiet lung fields, and bilateral crackles are also common. Venous blood can be drawn for a full blood count and biochemistry to identify causes or to help manage the haematological or electrolyte derangement. An arterial line will be placed so that arterial blood gases (ABGs) can be sampled frequently. ABGs will show hypoxaemia, hypercapnia, and respiratory and/or mixed acidosis, depending on the cause. Diagnostic imaging, such as X-ray or computed tomography (CT), will reveal the typical ground-glass appearance of the parenchyma. Air bronchograms are also commonly identified.

Management Unfortunately, many of the interventions required to manage ARDS can also cause further damage. Escalating oxygen requirements and mechanical ventilation are both necessary, but can also contribute to parenchymal damage through oxygen toxicity and barotrauma. Corticosteroids are beneficial to reduce the inflammatory response, but also significantly increase the risk of infection. Fluid resuscitation for increasing cardiovascular instability can exacerbate pulmonary oedema. Positive end-expiratory pressures can assist in the recruitment of more alveoli and reduce atelectasis; however, they can also contribute to barotrauma.

The primary goals of care are supportive, and include inotropic therapy to improve cardiac output and antimicrobials to prevent or treat infection. Sedation and paralysis can improve tolerance of the ventilator, reduce the risk of self-extubation and provide much-needed rest to reduce metabolic demands.

Multisystem organ failure may develop, reducing the chances of recovery.

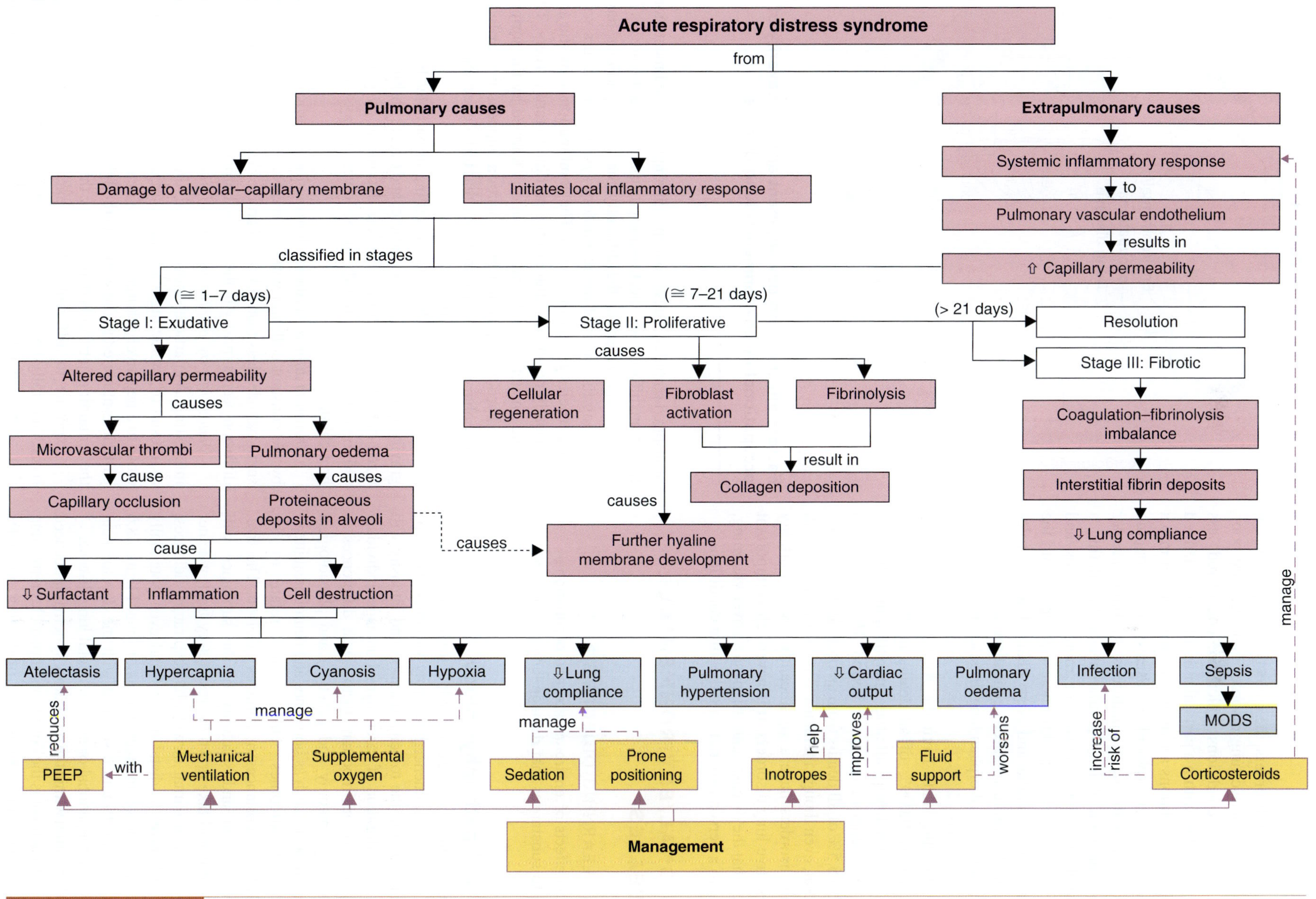

Figure 28.5

Clinical snapshot: Acute respiratory distress syndrome

↓ = decreased; ↑ = increased; MODS = multiple organ dysfunction syndrome; PEEP = positive end-expiratory pressure.

EPIDEMIOLOGY OF RESTRICTIVE LUNG DISEASES

Unlike obstructive lung disorders, the collection and publication of data on current restrictive lung disorder incidence are poor. There are many lung conditions which are considered less common and may not fit within a particular traditionally-defined lung disease. These conditions are often grouped together into a composite category called 'orphan lung disease'. This grouping enables individuals with these conditions to build greater numbers of people with at least similar needs, facilitating a voice to advocate for the provision of more resources and support. There are now even special-interest groups within the Thoracic Society of Australia and New Zealand whose roles are to foster collaboration, research, education, advocacy and professional engagement of orphan lung diseases, most of which are restrictive conditions.

Australian mortality data from the Australian Bureau of Statistics report only 0.009% of all deaths in 2019–20 were related to ARDS. Mortality for all other interstitial lung diseases was 2.7% of all deaths in the same period. However, when compared with 16.5% of all deaths from an obstructive disorder, it can be seen that, even though incidence is not formally tracked, restrictive lung disorders have a significantly lower mortality rate than obstructive lung disorders. It is nevertheless important to acknowledge that the diseases can still pose an overwhelming, chronic burden to a person experiencing the lung condition.

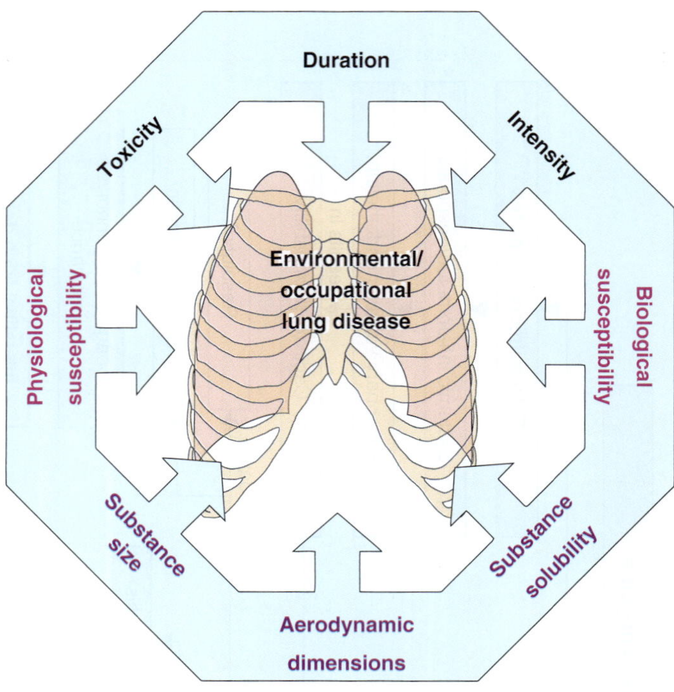

Figure 28.6

Factors affecting the development and the severity of occupational or environmental lung disease

OCCUPATIONAL/ENVIRONMENTAL LUNG DISEASES

LEARNING OBJECTIVE 2

Explain the effects of environmental and occupational exposures to substances that damage lung parenchyma.

Aetiology and pathophysiology

The development of lung disease as a result of toxins or substances from the environment is influenced by many variables. The type of exposure in relation to the toxicity, duration and intensity will affect the speed and duration of parenchymal damage. Individual susceptibility can play an important factor, with differences in biological (e.g. lung anatomy and genetics) and physiological (e.g. biochemical aspects, such as hormones and neurotransmitters) elements affecting outcomes. Other issues relate to the characteristics of the substances or particles involved. The size, aerodynamic dimension and solubility of the substance will influence the path it will take down the respiratory tract, whether it will be stopped in proximal airways by respiratory defences, or whether it will travel to distal airways and even potentially migrate to other previously unaffected areas of lung. Figure 28.6 demonstrates the many factors associated with the development and the severity of occupational or environmental lung disease.

Particulate deposition within the respiratory system is influenced by many factors. An aerosol is the collection of particles remaining air-borne for a period of time. Knowledge of the four principles of aerosol deposition is important to predict the path and distribution of inspired particles. These concepts are impaction, sedimentation, Brownian diffusion and electrostatic precipitation (see Figure 28.7).

Impaction refers to the difficulty the larger particles have navigating the turns of the respiratory system, and occurs with large particles greater than 5 μm. The combination of inertia and size usually results in failure of the particle to turn corners. The particle impacts with the mucosa and is trapped by the surface mucus. Particle deposition by impaction happens primarily in the nasopharynx and other areas of great turbulence, such as the bifurcation of large airways.

Sedimentation is the gradual settling of particles because of gravity and the weight of the particle, and occurs within medium-sized particles of 2–5 μm. Particle deposition by gravitational sedimentation occurs mostly in the lower airways and terminal bronchioles.

Brownian diffusion is the random motion of particles influenced by the constant collision with gas molecules; this occurs within small particles less than 0.1 μm. Particle deposition by Brownian diffusion occurs mostly in the terminal bronchioles and alveoli.

Deposition by electrostatic precipitation is negligible, but interesting. As particles move around, they can become charged as a result of interacting with other particles. If a particle comes close to a negatively charged particle near an airway surface, the particle is attracted to the wall. It is thought that less than 10% of the remaining aerosol is deposited by this mechanism.

Exposure to different environments will result in varying risks. Generally speaking, blue-collar workers are more at risk than white-collar workers. The location and type of industry will present different exposures.

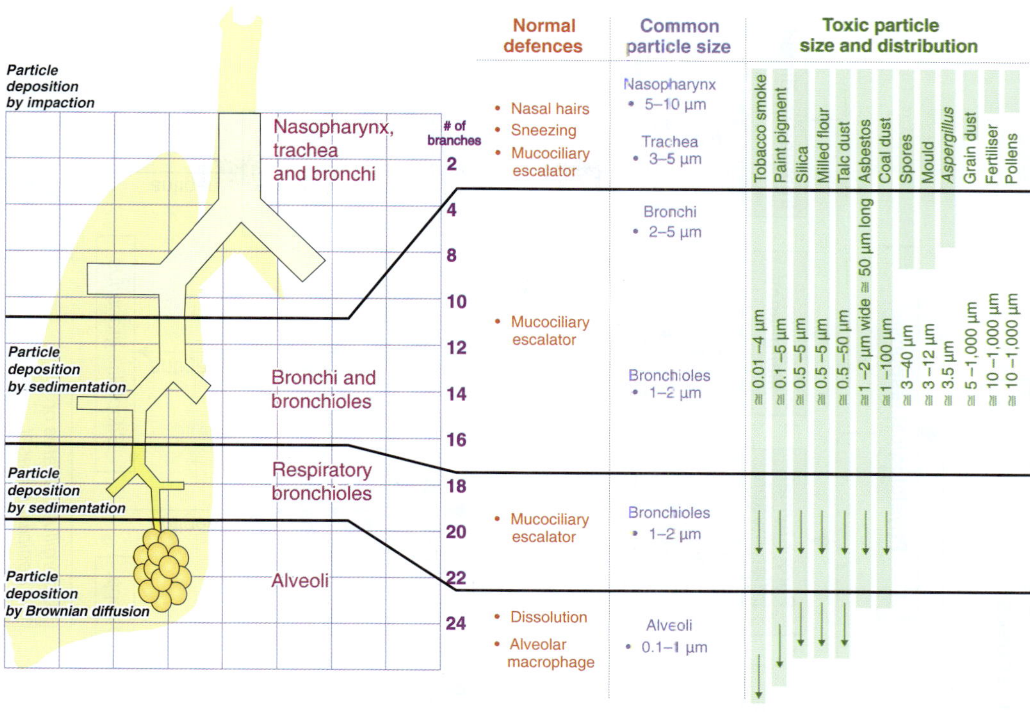

Figure 28.7
Inhaled particle sizes: principles of deposition

The difference between occupational and environmental lung disease is purely that if exposure occurs while undertaking employment, it is classed as an 'occupational' cause. Any other exposure would be classed as 'non-occupational' or 'environmental'.

Occupational lung diseases may be organised in many ways. Classification by anatomical effects, physiological effects or by the substance inhaled may be valuable (see Figure 28.8). A common method of classifying occupational lung diseases is by dividing the diseases into those causing hypersensitivity pneumonitis and those resulting in pneumoconiosis.

Hypersensitivity pneumonitis

Hypersensitivity pneumonitis is caused by exposure of lung parenchyma to an antigen that results in a cell-mediated immune reaction. On the second exposure to the antigen, an immune response results in an increase in neutrophils, lymphocytes and plasma cells. Inflammatory mediators and proteolytic enzymes are released. Inflammation will develop around the bronchi or the bronchioles, but alveolitis can also develop. The hypersensitivity reaction causes the development of non-caseating granulomas (see the chapters 'Inflammation and healing' and 'Immune disorders').

Pneumoconiosis

Pneumoconiosis is the accumulation of inhaled inorganic dust in the respiratory system, causing tissue reaction and parenchymal lung disease. The type of inorganic particles can determine a different outcome. Coal dust can cause the release of a greater volume of inflammatory mediators because of the presence of more free radicals from the mining process. Silica deposited in alveoli is consumed by macrophages, which are then destroyed by cytolysis from the toxicity of the substance, initiating an inflammatory process reaction **Asbestosis** can cause parenchymal degradation through inflammation and the release of oxygen free radicals by the macrophages. Asbestos fibres are small in diameter, but they are long and are not able to be phagocytosed. As a result, they remain in the lungs and generate chronic inflammation. Asbestos fibres are also able to migrate to other parenchyma because fibres less than 3 mm are able to penetrate the alveolar wall. There are many other types of pneumoconiosis not covered in this text.

Depending on the cause, the clinical progression may vary. For example, early stages of asbestos-related lung disease will cause a benign pleural issue with few symptoms. However, after 10 years of prolonged exposure, asbestosis may develop, followed by lung cancer or mesothelioma.

Clinical manifestations

Initially, someone with an occupational or environmental lung disease may be asymptomatic. As exposure continues, a productive cough may develop. More serious manifestations can develop over many years. As lung function declines, dyspnoea and hypoxia increases. Cor pulmonale may develop.

Clinical diagnosis and management

Diagnosis

Blood may be drawn to rule out other causes of dyspnoea, such as anaemia. The presence of infection may also be identified or ruled out. Biochemical imbalances may be identified and corrected. Imaging techniques such as X-ray and CT are most beneficial in the diagnosis of occupational lung diseases. A bronchoalveolar lavage may be undertaken to sample respiratory secretions, or a sputum sample may be collected and analysed for microscopy, culture and sensitivity. Respiratory function tests can also assist with diagnosis by demonstrating a typical restrictive pattern (see Figure 28.9).

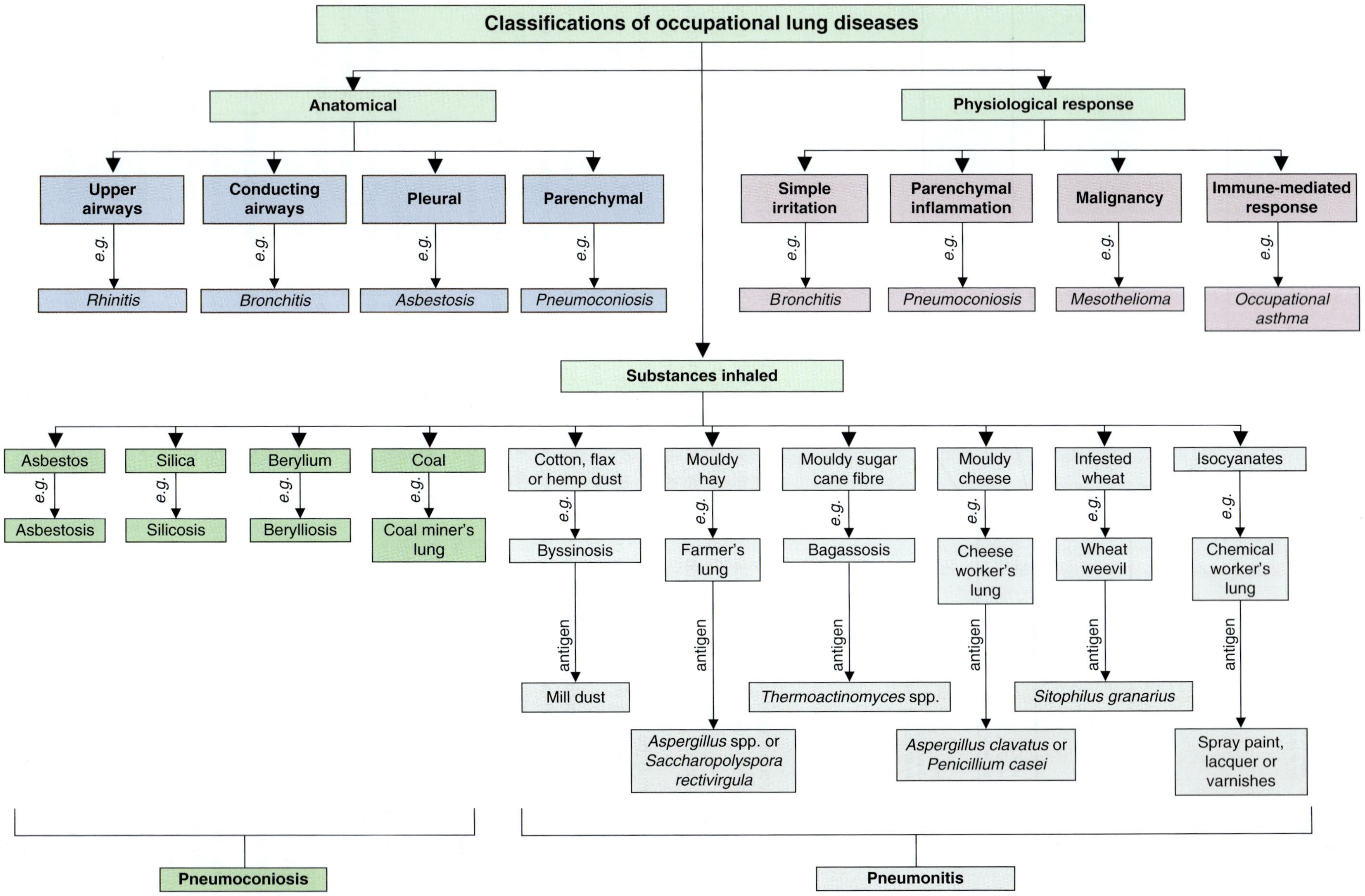

Figure 28.8

Various classifications of occupational lung diseases

Occupational lung diseases may be classified in various ways: anatomically, by the physiological response that occurs in response to the exposure, or by the substance inhaled.

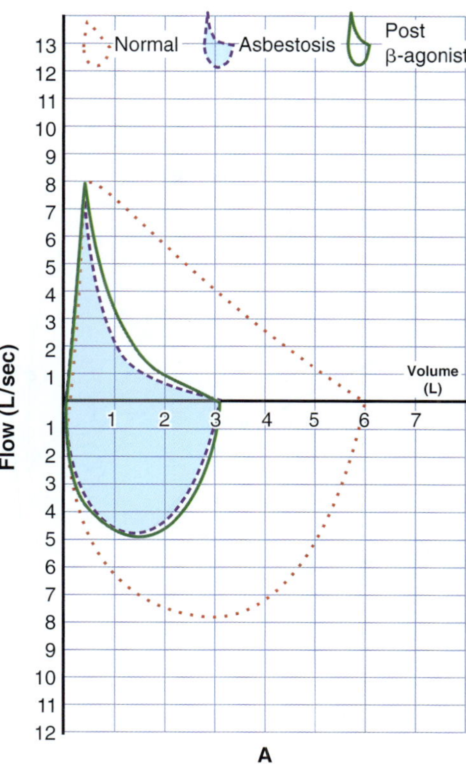

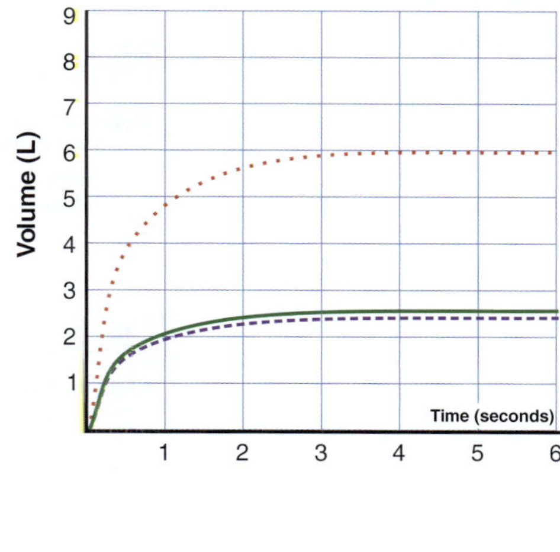

Figure 28.9

Typical restrictive pattern on spirometry

(A) Flow–volume loop.

(B) Volume–time spirogram. The typical restrictive pattern demonstrated on spirometry demonstrates a reduced inspired and expired volume from the chest cavity or lung restriction, and a high flow as a result of abnormally increased recoil.

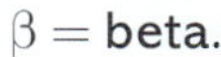
β = beta.

Management Improvements in workplace health and safety laws have assisted in the prevention of occupational lung diseases in recent history. However, some people will still develop either hypersensitivity pneumonitis or pneumoconiosis. If exposure continues, symptoms will increase. Failing prevention, the primary intervention is removing the cause. This may result in the need to find a different career. Cigarette smoking exacerbates lung conditions; therefore, if an exposed person smokes, assistance should be provided to help them quit.

Treatment of occupational and environmental lung disease is aimed at managing the clinical manifestations. Supplemental oxygen and bronchodilators form the mainstay of the management plan. Other interventions may include promoting annual vaccinations, and reducing exposure to people with active upper respiratory tract infections.

DRUG-INDUCED LUNG DISEASE

LEARNING OBJECTIVE 3

Identify several drugs responsible for causing interstitial lung disease.

Aetiology and pathophysiology

Lung disease of a restrictive nature can result from iatrogenic damage to lung parenchyma. Although different medications can induce injury to different components of the respiratory system, chemicals causing restrictive conditions affect parenchymal tissues and result in diffuse lung disease, hypersensitivity-type disease, alveolar haemorrhage, pleural disease or pulmonary oedema. Figure 28.10 outlines examples of various medications which may cause damage to the respiratory system.

Pulmonary toxicity may develop from any number of mechanisms. Some medications can accelerate the generation of oxygen free radicals, *stimulating inflammatory and fibrotic reactions* that cause diffuse lung injury. Examples include the antidysrhythmic amiodarone, the immune suppressant cyclophosphamide and the antimicrobial agent nitrofurantoin. Illicit drugs such as cocaine 'cut' with talc can result in *granulomatosis* and *fibrosis* due to a diffuse reaction from the talc particles. The reaction can result in the development of changes similar to pneumoconiosis.

Some medications may alter the vascular permeability or hydrostatic pressure, or interfere with coagulation, causing *pulmonary vascular damage*. Examples include amiodarone, cocaine or the oral anticoagulants. Other medicines may have a *direct cytotoxic effect* on the parenchymal cells through a toxic reaction to the drug, its metabolites or from idiosyncratic reactions. Examples include amiodarone and methotrexate.

Parenchymal damage can result in decreased total lung capacity and forced vital capacity from fibrosing alveolitis or any number of other mechanisms.

Clinical manifestations

People may present with a non-specific, insidious progression of respiratory manifestations, including cough, dyspnoea, bronchospasm, wheeze and/or crackles. Depending on the type of pathophysiological reaction, decreased breath sounds

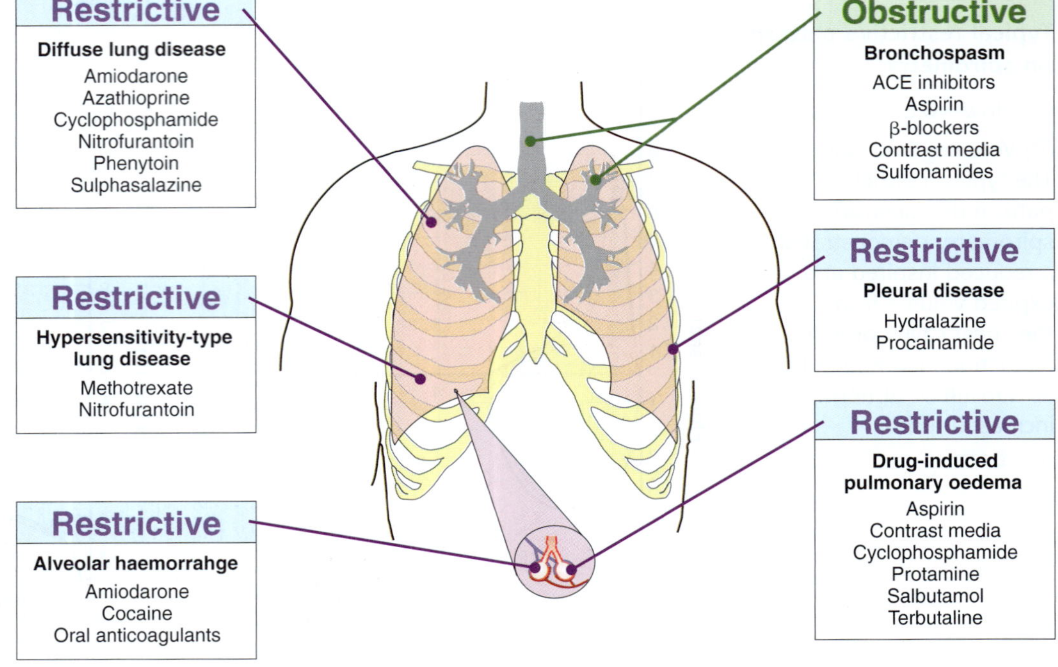

Figure 28.10

Drug-induced lung disease

Some examples of drugs that cause drug-induced lung disease.
ACE = angiotensin-converting enzyme;
β = beta.

may develop. Increasing severity may result in hypoxia and pulmonary oedema. In chronic drug-induced lung disease, right-sided heart failure and digital clubbing may develop.

Clinical diagnosis and management

Diagnosis The diagnosis of drug-induced lung disease is based on exclusion. When other causes of respiratory compromise, such as infection, are ruled out, attention may turn to the medication history.

A physical examination, a full respiratory assessment and a collection of a history involving all of the drugs the person has recently taken are pivotal to identifying the agent that may have caused the respiratory compromise. Blood may be drawn to assist with excluding other causes. Imaging studies, such as chest X-ray and CT scan, are beneficial in determining the degree of damage present. These studies will also assist in ruling out other respiratory conditions that may cause a similar presentation. Bronchoalveolar lavage may be undertaken, and, although specific findings cannot confirm drug-induced lung disease, it may exclude infective or metastatic causes.

Management Apart from removing exposure to the causative agent, management plans focus on symptom control. Administration of corticosteroids may assist to reduce the inflammatory reaction, and antimicrobials may assist in the control of any concomitant respiratory tract infections. Supplemental oxygen may be needed, depending on the nature and severity of the reaction. Reducing exposure to other agents that may affect lung function is recommended. Management of pulmonary oedema may require the use of loop diuretics.

CONNECTIVE-TISSUE–ASSOCIATED LUNG DISEASE

LEARNING OBJECTIVE 4

Recognise several connective tissue diseases that cause interstitial lung disease.

Aetiology and pathophysiology

People with connective tissue disorders as a result of autoimmune, collagen-related, vascular or rheumatological mechanisms often develop interstitial lung disease. While the mechanism is still unclear, people with systemic lupus erythematosus, polymyositis or even rheumatoid arthritis can develop pulmonary fibrosis.

Clinical manifestations

As with most respiratory conditions, people may present with shortness of breath. Other manifestations may include cough, and maybe even adventitious (added) lung sounds, such as crackles. Fatigue is common; however, it is difficult to determine whether it is associated with hypoxia or the pre-existing connective tissue disorder.

Clinical diagnosis and management

Diagnosis Blood may be drawn in order to exclude other conditions, such as infection or anaemia. Various antibody tests may assist with diagnosis. Pulmonary function tests can demonstrate a restrictive pattern, and imaging studies may determine the severity of the condition.

Management Symptom relief is the mainstay of treatment. Corticosteroids can be used to reduce the inflammatory processes.

Immunomodulating drugs, such as azathioprine, tacrolimus or mycophenolate, can be used to provide immunosuppression as a means of controlling the connective tissue disorder.

Extraparenchymal lung disorders

A variety of conditions can affect lung expansion. Extraparenchymal restrictive lung diseases are divided into neuromuscular and non-neuromuscular conditions. *Neuromuscular conditions* may result from neurological, neuromuscular or myopathic causes. *Non-neuromuscular conditions* may result from diaphragmatic compression, chest wall deformity, disease of the **pleura**, or as an iatrogenic effect from the surgical removal of lung tissue, such as a lobectomy or pneumonectomy, to manage diseased lung. Figure 28.11 explores the common clinical manifestations and management of extraparenchymal restrictive lung diseases.

NEUROMUSCULAR CONDITIONS

LEARNING OBJECTIVE 5

Discuss the effects of common neuromuscular conditions on respiratory function.

Aetiology and pathophysiology

Neuromuscular conditions occur as a result of an underlying pathology of either the nerves or the muscles involved in respiration. Neurological causes of restrictive lung disease can be classed as central or peripheral. *Central* causes are conditions affecting the cerebral cortex, brainstem, basal ganglia or spinal cord. These conditions can result in alterations in the control of breathing—either voluntary or involuntary. A stroke, head injury or tumour may cause damage to any of these structures. Neurological conditions resulting in dysfunction of *peripheral* nerves can also result in decreased lung volume. Two examples of this are motor neurone disease (see the chapter 'Neurodegenerative disorders') and Guillain–Barré syndrome (see the chapter 'Brain and spinal cord dysfunction').

Peripheral neuromuscular conditions resulting in restrictive lung disease also arise from a failure at the **neuromuscular junction**. Muscle contraction is inhibited by drugs that alter the release of acetylcholine, or its binding to nicotinic cholinergic receptors on the surface of the skeletal muscle, or receptor responsiveness. Otherwise known as *neuromuscular blockers*, these muscle relaxants, or paralysing agents, are used to facilitate endotracheal intubation or maintain paralysis in a person undergoing surgery or on a mechanical ventilator. Toxins such as botulism (from the bacteria *Clostridium botulinum*) or neurotoxins from many snake venoms can result in either presynaptic or postsynaptic neuromuscular junction failure. Damage to the phrenic nerve from either surgery or disease can result in a paralysed diaphragm (usually hemi-diaphragm). Other conditions causing chest wall muscle weakness and subsequent reduced lung volume include myasthenia gravis. Myasthenia gravis is an autoimmune disorder that results in damage to skeletal muscles from the complement-mediated destruction of the acetylcholine receptor at the postsynaptic neuromuscular junction (see the chapter 'Musculoskeletal trauma and muscle disorders').

Myopathy can also cause neuromuscular restrictive lung disease. Muscular dystrophy (see the chapter 'Musculoskeletal trauma and muscle disorders') is an example of an inherited condition causing the progressive degeneration and destruction of muscle fibres, ultimately resulting in respiratory failure. Any condition causing myotonia involving the muscles of respiration can cause extraparenchymal restrictive lung diseases.

Clinical manifestations

Depending on the condition, the common clinical manifestations will include dyspnoea, hypoxia and possibly respiratory failure. The signs and symptoms may develop rapidly, as in a stroke, head injury or spinal cord injury, or they may progress slowly, as in disorders such as myasthenia gravis, motor neurone disease or muscular dystrophy.

Clinical diagnosis and management

Diagnosis The standard investigations, such as respiratory assessment, chest X-ray, CT scan, respiratory function tests and blood tests, may be employed to investigate the cause.

Management Management is directed at the cause of the condition and symptom relief. Unfortunately, there is no definitive treatment for many restrictive disorders. As respiratory failure ensues, mechanical ventilation may need to be instigated. If the condition is chronic, the person may choose not to receive mechanical ventilation. In this circumstance, they are provided with palliative care until their respiratory system fails to provide sufficient oxygen and ventilation to sustain life.

NON-NEUROMUSCULAR CONDITIONS

LEARNING OBJECTIVE 6

Discuss common extraparenchymal, non-neuromuscular conditions affecting respiratory function.

Any extraparenchymal condition that does not involve the nerve, muscle or neuromuscular junction but still causes a restrictive respiratory condition is considered a *non-neuromuscular cause*. There are many conditions in this category.

Aetiology and pathophysiology

Causes of non-neuromuscular restrictive lung disease can be organised into conditions causing diaphragmatic compression, chest wall deformity, pleural disease or even surgical removal of lung tissue.

Pulmonary tumours (see the chapter 'Respiratory infections, cancers and vascular conditions'), ascites (see the chapter 'Disorders of the liver, the gall bladder and the pancreas') and effusions can all affect the ability of the lung tissue to expand, and cause a type of restrictive lung disease.

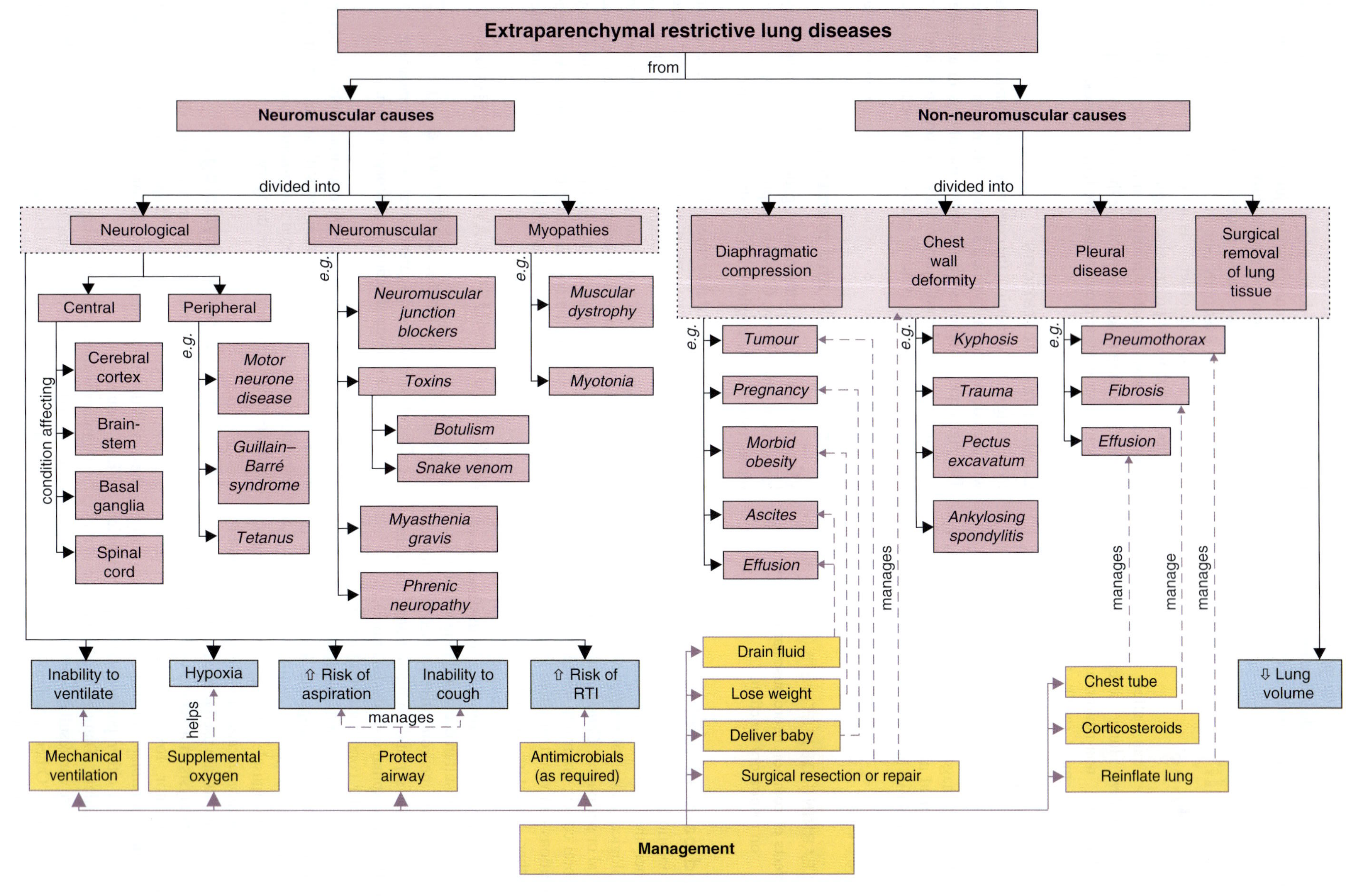

Figure 28.11

Clinical snapshot: Extraparenchymal restrictive lung diseases

↓ = decreased; ↑ = increased; RTI = respiratory tract infection.

Table 28.1 Types of pulmonary effusions

Effusion	Contents of collection	Source
Haemothorax	Blood	Trauma or (less commonly) rupture of major blood vessel
Empyema	Pus	Complication of infection
Chylothorax	Milky fluid high in triglycerides	Complication of damaged thoracic duct or superior vena cava obstruction
Cholesterol (pseudochylous ascites)	Milky fluid high in cholesterol (but low in triglycerides)	Chronic release of cholesterol from lysed erythrocytes and neutrophils
Iatrogenic	Nasogastric feed or intravenous solution	From migration or malinsertion of tubes into the pleural space; from a nasogastric tube into the trachea or from central venous catheter perforating the superior vena cava

Effusion A *pleural effusion* is the accumulation of fluid in the pleural space (between the visceral and the parietal pleura). Pleural **effusions** develop either as a result of excessive fluid production or from decreased absorption. They are commonly classified by the type of fluid contained within this space. Pleural effusions can be either transudative or exudative.

Transudative pleural effusions occur as a consequence of either increased hydrostatic pressure or decreased plasma oncotic pressure in the context of an intact endothelial–capillary barrier (i.e. not affected by inflammation). A **transudate** develops most commonly in congestive cardiac failure, end-stage liver disease, hypoalbuminaemia, nephrotic syndrome and glomerulonephritis.

Exudative pleural effusions occur as a consequence of either increased capillary permeability or decreased drainage through the lymphatic system. An *exudate* develops from an inflammatory process of the pleura as a result of infection, malignancy, renal failure, ascites, or breast or lung cancer.

Effusions are known by many names based on the type of fluid collected. Table 28.1 describes the different types of effusions.

Effusions cause dyspnoea and often pleuritic chest pain (where the pain is worse, often sharp, with inspiration). Effusions can be seen on X-ray. As fluid is affected by gravity, the first signs of an effusion are blunted costophrenic angles (see Figure 28.12). A blunted costophrenic angle suggests at least 75 mL of fluid within the pleural space (in an average-sized adult). Free-flowing fluid will take a level and a straight line will be visible on an upright X-ray. The image may change between X-rays, depending on the position of the individual. A thoracentesis is generally done to sample the pleural fluid to determine the type of effusion and whether an infective component is involved (see Figure 28.13). Depending on the size, type and cause of the collection, an effusion may be left to reduce itself or an intercostal catheter may be inserted to assist in draining the effusion. Provision of non-steroidal

Figure 28.12

Costophrenic angles

Costophrenic angles are the triangle at the base of both lungs. In health, costophrenic angles are sharp. In pleural effusions, blunt costophrenic angles can suggest a collection of approximately 75 mL of fluid (in an average adult chest X-ray).

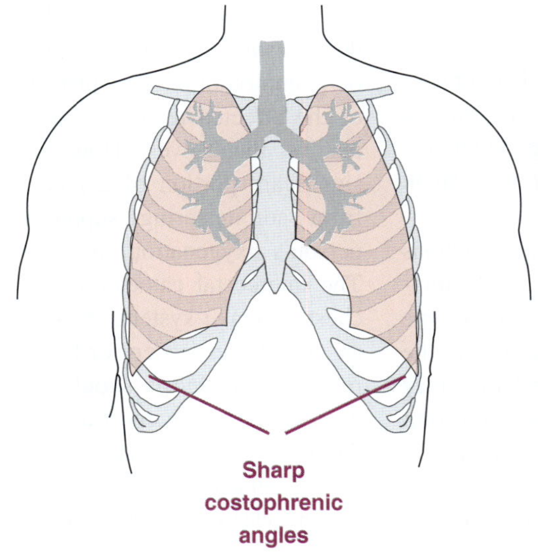

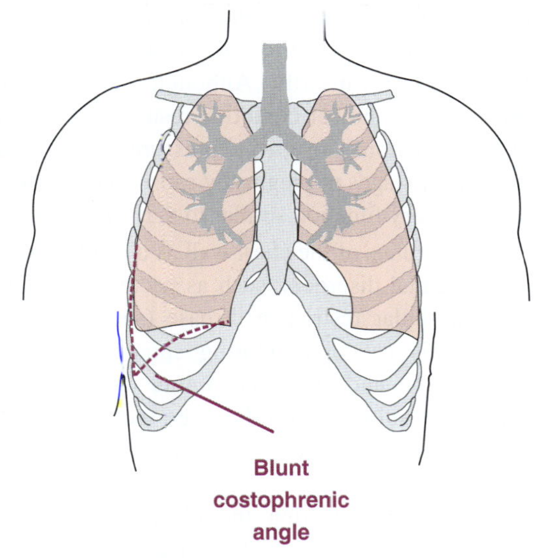

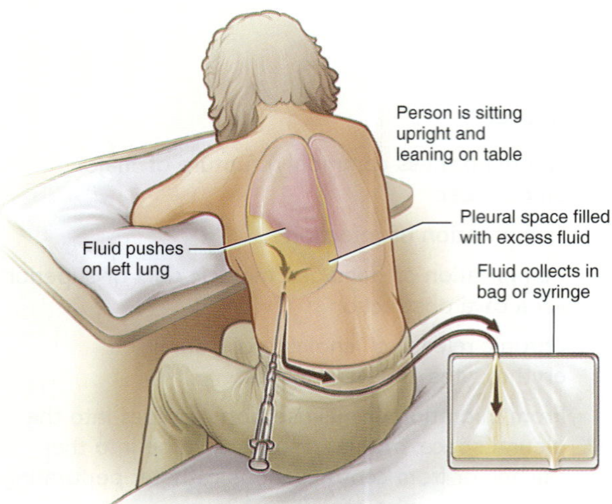

Figure 28.13

Thoracentesis

A needle is inserted into the pleural space, and fluid is sampled from the collection.

Source: Skimage/Alamy Stock Photo.

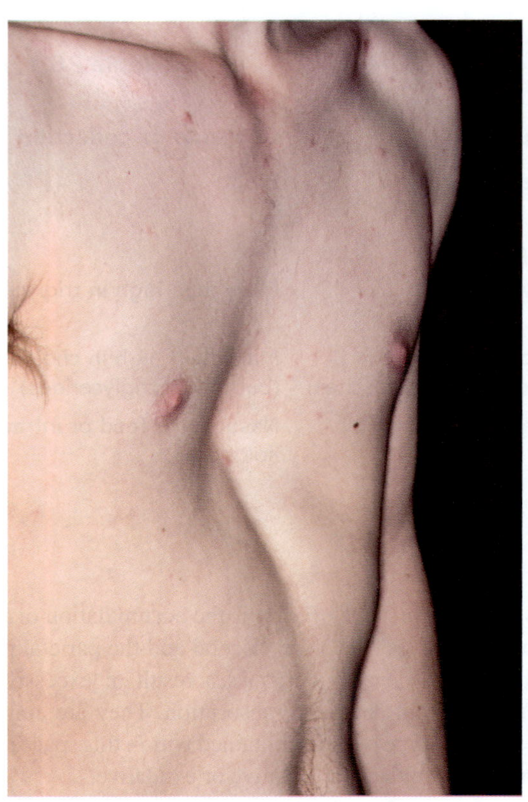

Figure 28.14

Pectus excavatum

Severe pectus excavatum can cause non-neuromuscular restrictive lung disease.

Source: Dr P. Marazzi/Science Photo Library.

anti-inflammatory drugs can reduce the inflammation and have beneficial effects on the intensity of the pleuritic pain. If the pain is excessive, narcotic analgesics may be necessary.

Diaphragmatic compression and chest wall deformity There are many other non-neuromuscular causes of extraparenchymal lung disorders of varying degrees of severity. Even in the absence of a respiratory disease, the vital capacity and total lung capacity of a morbidly obese person is compromised because of decreased chest wall compliance and impaired respiratory muscle function. The increased load on the chest wall and abdomen contribute to this reduction in respiratory function. Alveolar recruitment in the lung bases is often compromised from the contents of the abdominal cavity applying upward pressure, affecting the thoracic cavity's capacity to expand downwards. Although generally well tolerated, pregnancy is another condition resulting in a restrictive pattern of lung function. The upward pressure exerted by a gravid uterus in the later stages of pregnancy causes a mechanical impairment to respiratory function similar to that with obesity.

Deformities of the chest wall as a result of trauma, kyphosis or congenital disorders, such as pectus excavatum, cause non-neuromuscular restrictive disease (see Figure 28.14). A type of arthritis called ankylosing spondylitis can result in the lower spine and sacroiliac joints undergoing inflammatory changes, resulting in rigidity (see the chapter 'Bone and joint disorders'). These changes can cause a significant reduction in chest expansion.

Conditions affecting the pleura can result in restrictive physiology. A collapsed lobe or lung (pneumothorax) interferes with the capacity of the lung parenchyma to expand.

Pneumothorax A **pneumothorax** is the collection of air between the visceral and the parietal pleura (pleural space) due to a breach of either the visceral or the parietal pleura. A pneumothorax may develop spontaneously or secondary to another condition. Table 28.2 outlines the pathophysiology and clinical manifestations of various types of pneumothoraces.

Although the cause will influence management to some degree, some management principles are common to each type of pneumothorax. The primary goal is to achieve reinflation of the affected region. Small pneumothoraces may be left to resolve themselves. However, pneumothoraces involving a significant portion of a lobe will require intervention. Apart from administering supplemental oxygen to support the person's oxygenation, an intercostal catheter will be inserted. The intercostal catheter (chest tube) is attached to a closed-chest drainage system, which achieves negative pressure with an underwater system or by attaching it to a low-flow suction regulator. Analgesia should be provided regularly, and hourly observation of the chest drain should be undertaken to monitor the progress and safety.

If a person experiences frequent spontaneous pneumothoraces, a pleurodesis may be undertaken to reduce the chances of pneumothorax occurring again in that region of the lung. A **pleurodesis** is a surgical intervention whereby a granular substance

Table 28.2 Three types of pneumothorax

Type	Pathophysiology	Manifestations
(A) Spontaneous 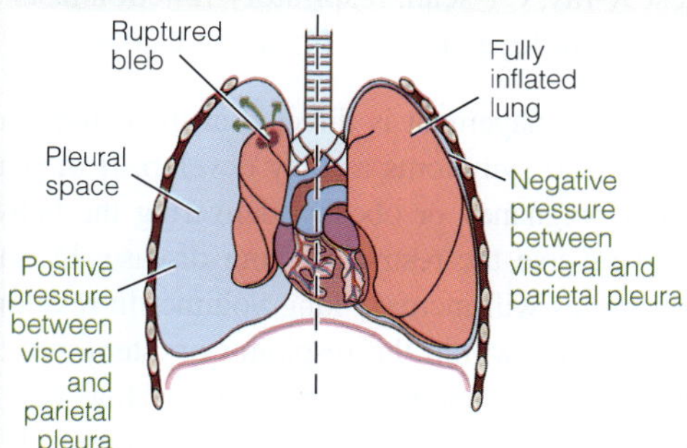 	Rupture of a bleb on the lung surface allows air to enter the pleural space from the airways. • *Primary pneumothorax* affects previously healthy people. • *Secondary pneumothorax* affects people with pre-existing lung disease (e.g. COPD).	• Abrupt onset • Pleuritic chest pain • Dyspnoea, shortness of breath • Tachypnoea, tachycardia • Unequal lung excursion • Decreased breath sounds and hyperresonant percussion tone on the affected side
(B) Traumatic 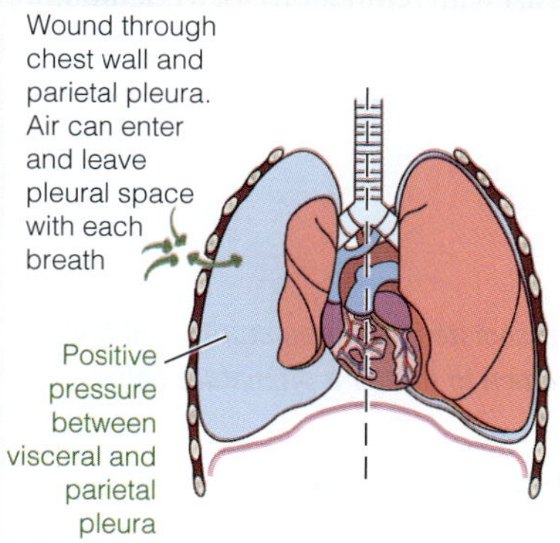 	Trauma to the chest wall or pleura disrupts the pleural membrane. • *Open* occurs with penetrating chest trauma that allows air from the environment to enter the pleural space. • *Closed* occurs with blunt trauma that allows air from the lung to enter the pleural space. • *Iatrogenic* involves laceration of visceral pleura during a procedure such as thoracentesis or central-line insertion.	• Pain • Dyspnoea • Tachypnoea, tachycardia • Decreased respiratory excursion • Absent breath sounds in the affected area • Air movement through an open wound
(C) Tension 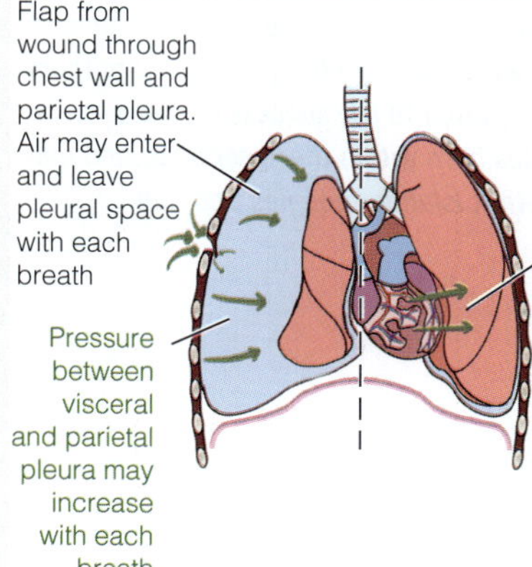 	Air enters the pleural space through the chest wall or from airways but is unable to escape, resulting in rapid accumulation. The lung on the affected side collapses. As intrapleural pressure increases, the heart, great vessels, trachea and oesophagus shift towards the unaffected side.	• Hypotension, shock • Distended neck veins • Severe dyspnoea • Tachypnoea, tachycardia • Decreased respiratory excursion • Absent breath sounds on the affected side • Tracheal deviation towards unaffected side

COPD = chronic obstructive pulmonary disease.

Source: Illustrations S. Elliott © Sciencopia.

(talc or synthetic equivalent) or physical abrasion (with a gauze on the parietal pleura) causes an inflammatory process that uses the endogenous response to trauma to cause inflammation and adhesion, effectively 'gluing' the visceral and the parietal pleura together around the region of the trauma.

A pneumothorax is a restrictive condition during lung collapse, which resolves when the collapse inflates. However, a pleurodesis actually causes another type of restrictive condition known as a 'trapped lung'. In this instance, although iatrogenic, the trapped lung is preventing another pneumothorax in that region, and reducing the risk of significant danger from tension pneumothorax at a later time.

Other conditions associated with restrictive lung disease *Pleural fibrosis* will also restrict lung function through the development of pleural thickening and sometimes calcifications. Conditions that require the removal of pathological lung tissue (e.g. lung cancer) cause an *iatrogenic restrictive lung disease*. Those affected may require surgery to have a lobe removed (*lobectomy*) or a whole lung removed (*pneumonectomy*), ultimately decreasing lung volume by virtue of removing some lung tissue.

Clinical diagnosis and management

Diagnosis The standard investigations, such as respiratory assessment, chest X-ray, CT scan, respiratory function tests and blood tests, may be employed to investigate the cause.

Management Management is directed at the cause and at supporting the signs and symptoms as they develop. If the cause of the restriction is pregnancy or obesity, delivering the baby or losing weight will reverse the restrictive lung disease. Drainage of an effusion or ascites will increase lung volume. In relation to management of a tumour within the respiratory system, removal may be required to prevent spread of the cancer. However, any removal of lung tissue also constitutes a restrictive cause. If the condition is caused by a chest wall deformity, surgical correction may be able to resolve the issue in some instances. If the origin of the condition involves the pleura, an intercostal catheter can remove fluid (for an effusion) or assist with reinflation (for a pneumothorax).

INDIGENOUS HEALTH FAST FACTS AND CULTURAL CONSIDERATIONS

FAST FACTS

- *No formal incidence of infant respiratory distress syndrome (IRDS) is recorded. Given that IRDS is associated with prematurity, and that Aboriginal and Torres Strait Islander women are 1.7 times as likely as non-Indigenous Australian women to deliver a premature baby, it stands to reason that the incidence of IRDS may be higher in Indigenous neonates.*
- *IRDS is associated with prematurity. Māori women are 1.7 times more likely to deliver a baby before 37 weeks gestation and Pacific Islander women are 1.2 times more likely to deliver prematurely than European New Zealand women.*

CULTURAL CONSIDERATIONS

- *Programs and activities to reduce preterm birth in Aboriginal and Torres Strait Islander women will reduce rates of IRDS. The establishment of an Aboriginal Maternal and Infant Health Service in New South Wales, and Moort Boodjari Mia in Western Australia—focusing on culturally sensitive, women-centred, quality services using primary healthcare principles—have managed to reduce preterm birth to almost half of the previously recorded rates for the areas in which these services operate. Techniques such as employing Aboriginal grandmothers and Aboriginal and Torres Strait Islander Health Workers to provide support and education have contributed to the success of these programs. These measures will have an extraordinary impact on the respiratory health of the neonates born within these services, and may begin to contribute to reducing the immense healthcare disparities between Aboriginal and Torres Strait Islander peoples and non-Indigenous Australians.*

Sources: Data from AIHW (2022a, 2022b); New Zealand Ministry of Health (2022).

CHILDREN AND ADOLESCENTS

- Restrictive lung diseases are less common in children. However, interstitial lung disease can still develop from pneumonitis or pulmonary fibrosis. Non-neuromuscular restrictive lung disease in an adult can technically develop in a child.

OLDER ADULTS

- Age-associated changes to the respiratory system result in restrictive-type patterns from a reduction in chest expansion related to reduced tissue elasticity, impaired chest expansion and thoracic spinal deformities.
- Senescence can cause decreased respiratory muscle strength.

KEY CLINICAL ISSUES

- Low birth weight and premature delivery are associated with infant respiratory distress syndrome (IRDS). There is an inverse relationship between the prematurity of a neonate and the severity of IRDS. Therefore, extra attention must be paid to a newborn of less than 32 weeks' gestation.
- Respiratory distress can develop quickly in a neonate. Grunting, head bobbing and nasal flaring are all signs of increased work of breathing that need to be managed urgently.
- Endotracheal surfactant administration is the treatment for IRDS.
- Care must be taken to avoid oxygen toxicity, especially in a premature baby. Administration of the lowest amount of oxygen to maintain adequate oxygenation is the goal.
- Hypoxaemia and hypercapnia will generally occur as a result of acute respiratory distress syndrome (ARDS). Severe ARDS can progress to multisystem organ failure.
- A balance must be determined between the administration of corticosteroids to reduce the overactive inflammatory response and the increased risk of infection, especially in the context of an intubated person where several respiratory defences are bypassed.
- Iatrogenic lung disease may develop from the administration of a number of different drugs. Agents that pose an increased risk of causing damage to a person's respiratory system should be considered carefully before administration, especially where the person has existing lung disease.
- A significant number of conditions can cause restrictive lung disease. Adequate observations skills, and a knowledge of the respiratory system's anatomy and physiology, as well as of the use of drugs in restrictive lung disorders, are critical for healthcare professionals.

CHAPTER REVIEW

- Restrictive lung diseases can be divided into parenchymal and extraparenchymal causes.
- *Parenchymal causes* of restrictive lung disease include infant respiratory distress syndrome (IRDS), acute respiratory distress syndrome (ARDS), occupational lung diseases, drug-induced lung disease and connective-tissue–associated lung disease.
- *IRDS* differs from *ARDS* in that the principal cause of IRDS is a surfactant deficiency, whereas there are many causes of ARDS.
- *Occupational lung diseases* can result from exposure to many different types of toxins or substances. The substance or toxin, duration of exposure and intensity of exposure will influence the severity of disease.
- *Respiratory particle deposition* is influenced by four important principles of particle deposition: impaction, sedimentation, Brownian diffusion and, less importantly, electrostatic precipitation.
- Occupational lung diseases may be acute or chronic, and the primary management is prevention. Failing this, removal from the causative agent is critical to reduce the inflammatory process contributing to chronic interstitial lung damage.
- Agents causing *drug-induced lung disease* are thought to cause destruction of lung tissue through the increased generation of oxygen free radicals that stimulate inflammatory and fibrotic reactions. Other agents may manipulate hydrostatic pressure, interfere with oral anticoagulants or direct cytotoxicity.
- Although the mechanism is not entirely understood, systemic lupus erythematosus, polymyositis and rheumatoid arthritis increase a person's risk of developing pulmonary fibrosis.
- *Extraparenchymal lung diseases* can be classified as neuromuscular or non-neuromuscular.
- *Neuromuscular extraparenchymal restrictive lung conditions* include any condition that affects the nerves, muscles or neuromuscular junction involved in respiration.
- *Non-neuromuscular extraparenchymal restrictive lung conditions* include any condition affecting diaphragmatic function, chest wall structure, the pleura or reduced volume of lung tissue (e.g. lung resection or pneumonectomy).

REVIEW QUESTIONS

1. Explain how a deficiency in surfactant can result in increased work of breathing and atelectasis.
2. Why does grunting occur in a neonate with infant respiratory distress syndrome (IRDS)? What physiological benefit is gained by exhaling against a partially closed glottis?
3. How does IRDS affect the metabolic demands of a neonate?
4. What are the general concepts involved in interstitial lung injury (i.e. what is the overall mechanism of parenchymal damage)?
5. How do the conditions covered in this chapter cause a restrictive disorder? Make a list of all the conditions covered, and identify the specific reasons that cause each condition to be included in the classification of restrictive respiratory disorders.
6. What causes acute respiratory distress syndrome (ARDS)? How does lung contusion, pneumonia, exposure to toxic gases or aspiration of gastric contents cause ARDS?
7. What are air bronchograms? Why do they occur?
8. What are the four principles of aerosol particle deposition? How do they influence the placement of substances within the lung parenchyma?
9. How are occupational lung diseases classified? What differentiates one class from the other?
10. What mechanisms are considered to cause drug-induced lung disease?
11. Differentiate between the causes of extraparenchymal neuromuscular restrictive disorders.
12. What are four common classifications of extraparenchymal non-neuromuscular restrictive disorders? How can each type of non-neuromuscular restrictive disorder be managed?

HEALTH PROFESSIONAL CONNECTIONS

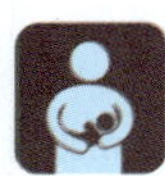

Midwives Preterm delivery is defined as occurring at a gestational age of less than 37 weeks. Very premature is defined as a gestational age of less than 32 weeks. The majority of neonatal deaths occur in preterm infants. Increasing prematurity increases the neonatal risk of developing infant respiratory distress syndrome. Full assessment and collection of a comprehensive history may assist to identify factors that increase the risk of preterm delivery. Prediction of preterm delivery is imprecise. However, some characteristics are common to premature births, including a history of premature births, extremes of maternal age (older than 35 years of age and younger than 17 years of age), light pre-pregnancy weight, and stressful environments or events, including domestic violence or the death of a close family member. Tocolytic agents (drugs that inhibit labour) may be administered. However, judgment regarding the viability of the fetus becomes an issue. Neonates of less than 23 weeks' gestational age have little chance of surviving, and maternal risks may complicate the decision to administer aggressive tocolysis. Maternal administration of corticosteroids prior to delivery can improve respiratory outcomes by encouraging lung maturation. In the first 48 hours following delivery, preterm neonates should be closely monitored for signs of increased work of breathing and respiratory distress. Deterioration can occur quickly, as neonates have no respiratory reserve upon which to rely. Early assessment and management of the deteriorating infant may provide an opportunity for planned intervention rather than rapid induction and emergency intubation in response to a critical respiratory or circulatory collapse.

Physiotherapists Physiotherapy techniques to assist people with restrictive lung disease should be tailored to the needs of the individual, and may include: techniques to promote effective coughing for clearance of airway secretions; respiratory muscle training and breathing exercises to prevent or delay deconditioning; functional electrical stimulation of the abdominal muscles to promote increased lung volumes; appropriate positioning to maximise vital capacity and improve pulmonary function; administration of non-invasive ventilation as neuromuscular disease progresses; and, potentially, even instruction on glossopharyngeal breathing to promote lung expansion and improve cough strength.

CASE STUDY

Miss Seraphina Walker (UR number 942480) is 12 hours old. She was born by caesarean section because of abruptio placentae. Mrs Walker (Seraphina's mother) was given corticosteroids pre-caesarean section. Seraphina's mum also has type 1 diabetes mellitus. Seraphina is 33 weeks' gestational age and weighs 2521 g. Her head circumference is 32.4 cm and her length is 42 cm. Initially her APGAR scores were 9/9; however, she quickly deteriorated and was brought to the neonatal intensive care unit in respiratory distress. She had moderate intercostal and subcostal retractions, nasal flaring, head bobbing and grunting. Her air entry was equal but globally quiet, and her chest movement was symmetrical.

Temperature	Heart rate	Respiration rate	Blood pressure	SpO_2
36.3°C	158	82	62/32	95% (2 L/min via NP*)

* NP = nasal prongs.

She was peripherally tepid, and had capillary refill of less than three seconds. Her abdomen was soft, she had normal bowel sounds and no organomegaly. Her reflexes were normal, but she was mildly hypotonic. Over the next few hours she deteriorated further, was intubated and placed on positive pressure ventilation. A nasogastric tube was inserted, and an umbilical intravenous cannula placed for drugs and fluid support. An arterial line was also inserted. Some blood was drawn for haematology and biochemistry. Her pathology results are as follows:

HAEMATOLOGY

Patient location:	Ward NICU	UR:	942480		
Consultant:	Jones	NAME:	Walker		
		Given name:	Seraphina	Sex:	F
		DOB:	6/10/XX	Age:	1d

Time collected	17:15
Date collected	XX/XX
Year	XXXX
Lab #	654315

FULL BLOOD COUNT		UNITS	REFERENCE RANGE
Haemoglobin	111	g/L	115–160
White cell count	6.9	$\times 10^9$/L	4.0–11.0
Platelets	250	$\times 10^9$/L	140–400
Haematocrit	0.55		0.33–0.47
Red cell count	3.41	$\times 10^{12}$/L	3.80–5.20
Reticulocyte count	1.6	%	0.2–2.0
MCV	87	fL	80–100
COAGULATION PROFILE			
aPTT	29	secs	24–40
PT	14	secs	11–17

BIOCHEMISTRY

Patient location:	Ward NICU	UR:	942480		
Consultant:	Jones	NAME:	Walker		
		Given name:	Seraphina	Sex:	F
		DOB:	6/10/XX	Age:	1d

Time collected	17:15
Date collected	XX/XX
Year	XXXX
Lab #	654213

ELECTROLYTES		UNITS	REFERENCE RANGE
Sodium	139	mmol/L	135–145
Potassium	3.9	mmol/L	3.5–5.2
Chloride	105	mmol/L	95–110
Glucose (random)	3.2	mmol/L	3.5–6.0
RENAL FUNCTION			
Urea	4.5	mmol/L	(2.5–7.5)
Creatinine	48	μmol/L	(45–90)
ARTERIAL BLOOD GAS			
pH	7.48		7.35–7.45
PaO_2	62	mmHg	80–100
$PaCO_2$	55	mmHg	35–45
Bicarbonate	24	mEq/L	22–26

Seraphina had a chest X-ray, which demonstrated diffuse symmetrical reticulogranular lung fields (ground-glass appearance), air bronchograms and decreased lung inflation. She was commenced on exogenous surfactant replacement therapy through the endotracheal tube. Seraphina was also receiving supplemental oxygen at an FiO_2 of 0.55 (55%) to maintain a PaO_2 greater than 60 mmHg.

Seraphina is receiving 10% glucose intravenously, and nasogastric feeds of expressed breast milk have been commenced. She is being nursed in an intensive care cot with overhead radiant and mattress heating. She has also been commenced on intravenous antimicrobials.

CRITICAL THINKING

1. What risk factors does Seraphina have for the development of infant respiratory distress syndrome (IRDS)? Make a list of each risk factor, and explain the mechanism for each of the risks. Draw a line under the list and add all of the other risk factors (that Seraphina didn't have) associated with IRDS. (Include the mechanism associated with each of these risk factors, too.)
2. Make a list of all the respiratory clinical manifestations that suggested Seraphina was having difficulty breathing. Note all the other observations listed. Are these within the reference range for a neonate?
3. Observe Seraphina's arterial blood gas results. What are the oxygen and carbon dioxide results? Explain why these results have developed.
4. Seraphina was intubated, placed on a mechanical ventilator and administered exogenous surfactant. How does each of these interventions assist Seraphina? Why doesn't she have enough endogenous surfactant? What does surfactant do? The case study specifically mentioned temperature control and adequate nutrition. Why might these two things be important to manage Seraphina's care and her IRDS?
5. When Seraphina is better and discharged from the intensive care unit, what expectations are there for her lung function in years to come? Explain your answer.

BIBLIOGRAPHY

Ajibowo, A.O., Kolawole, O.A., Sadia, H., Amedu, O.S., Chaudhry, H.A., Hussaini, H., … Khan, A. (2022). A comprehensive review of the management of acute respiratory distress syndrome. *Curēus*:14(10):e30669. https://doi.org/10.7759/cureus.30669.

Australian Bureau of Statistics (ABS) (2022). *Causes of death, Australia, 2021.* Canberra: ABS. https://www.abs.gov.au/statistics/health/causes-death/causes-death-australia/2021.

Australian Health Ministers' Advisory Council's National and Aboriginal and Torres Strait Islander Health Standing Committee (2017). *Cultural respect framework 2016–2026: for Aboriginal and Torres Strait Islander health—a national approach to building a culturally respectful health system.* Canberra: Australian Government Department of Health. https://nacchocommunique.files.wordpress.com.

Australian Health Ministers' Advisory Council (2023). *Aboriginal and Torres Strait Islander Health Performance Framework 2023 report.* Canberra: Australian Government Department of Health. https://www.indigenoushpf.gov.au/.

Australian Institute of Health and Welfare (AIHW) (2022a). *Australia's children: web report—data.* Canberra: AIHW. https://www.aihw.gov.au/reports/children-youth/australias-children/data.

Australian Institute of Health and Welfare (AIHW) (2022b). *Australia's health, 2022*: Data insights. Australia's Health series No. 18, Cat. No. AUS 240. Canberra: AIHW. https://www.aihw.gov.au/getmedia/c91a05ef-307f-4c18-8ed3-dfe33d0c603d/aihw-aus-240.pdf.aspx?inline=true.

Bauldoff, G., Gubrud-Howe, P.M., Carno, M.-A., Levett-Jones, T., Hales, M., Berry, K., … LeMone, P. (2020). *LeMone and Burke's medical-surgical nursing: critical thinking for person-centred care* (4th [Australian] edn). Sydney: Pearson Australia.

Best, O. & Fredericks, B. (2021). *Yatdjuligin: Aboriginal and Torres Strait Islander nursing and midwifery care* (3rd edn). Port Melbourne, VIC: Cambridge University Press.

Bos, L.D.J. & Ware, L.B. (2022). Acute respiratory distress syndrome: causes, pathophysiology, and phenotypes. *The Lancet*, 400(10358):1145–1156. https://doi.org/10.1016/S0140-6736(22)01485-4.

Bullock, S. & Manias, E. (2022). *Fundamentals of pharmacology* (9th edn). Sydney: Pearson Australia.

Department of Health and Aged Care (2020) *Clinical Practice Guidelines: Pregnancy care.* Canberra: Australian Government Department of Health. https://www.health.gov.au/resources/pregnancy-care-guidelines.

Harman, E.M. & Riley, L.E. (2022). Acute respiratory distress syndrome (ARDS). *Emedicine.* https://emedicine.medscape.com/article/165139-overview.

Hsieh, C. & Kamangar, N. (2020). Hypersensitivity pneumonitis. *Emedicine.* https://emedicine.medscape.com/article/299174-overview.

Jackson, C.D. & Muthiah, M.P. (2020). Asbestosis. *Emedicine.* https://emedicine.medscape.com/article/295966-overview.

Lessnau, K-D., & Lazo, K.G.G. (2019). Drug-induced pulmonary toxicity. *Emedicine.* https://emedicine.medscape.com/article/1343451-overview.

Mendes, R.G., Castello-Simões, V., Trimer, R., Garcia-Araújo, A.S., Gonçalves Da Silva, A.L., Dixit, S., … & Borghi-Silva. A. (2021). Exercise-based pulmonary rehabilitation for interstitial lung diseases: a review of components, prescription, efficacy, and safety. *Frontiers in Rehabilitation Sciences*, 2. https://doi.org/10.3389/fresc.2021.744102.

New South Wales Government (2023). *Aboriginal Maternal Infant Health Services (AMIHS).* https://mnclhd.health.nsw.gov.au/child-youth-and-family-services/aboriginal-maternal-infant-health-service-amihs/.

New Zealand Ministry of Health (2022). *New Zealand Maternity Clinical Indicators: background document.* Wellington: Te Whatu Ora. https://www.tewhatuora.govt.nz/assets/Our-health-system/Data-and-statistics/nz-maternity-clinical-indicators-background-document-feb23.pdf.

Pramanik, A.K. (2020). Respiratory distress syndrome. *Emedicine.* https://emedicine.medscape.com/article/976034-overview.

Wong, F.J., Dudney, T.N. & McCormack, M.T. (2019). Coal worker's pneumoconiosis (black lung disease). *Emedicine.* https://emedicine.medscape.com/article/297887-overview.

Yenduri, N.J.S., Guillerman, R.P. & Farber, H.J. (2022). Pediatric hypersensitivity hneumonitis. *Emedicine.* https://emedicine.medscape.com/article/1005107-overview.

Respiratory infections, cancers and vascular conditions

29

LEARNING OBJECTIVES

After completing this chapter, you should be able to:

1 Differentiate between several different types of respiratory infections.

2 Discuss the various types of pneumonia, the clinical implications of their diagnosis and their management.

3 Examine the effects and management of tuberculosis.

4 Differentiate between the different types of lung cancer.

5 Identify the complications commonly associated with lung cancer.

6 Discuss the mechanisms by which a pulmonary embolism may develop.

7 Explore the pathophysiology, diagnosis and management of pulmonary oedema.

8 Examine the causes and consequences of pulmonary hypertension.

WHAT YOU SHOULD KNOW BEFORE YOU START THIS CHAPTER

Can you distinguish between the conducting and the respiratory structures of the respiratory system?

Can you make a list of all the respiratory defences in the nasopharynx, trachea, bronchus, terminal airways and alveoli?

Can you differentiate between various pathogens and their management?

Can you describe the causes and processes of cellular changes leading to neoplasia?

Can you identify factors that contribute to hypercoagulability?

Can you explain what happens to tissue that fails to receive any blood flow?

Can you identify the structure and function of the respiratory membrane, and the factors that can alter its function?

Can you explain the mechanisms controlling blood pressure within the pulmonary vasculature system?

Can you describe the principles associated with capillary dynamics, including colloid osmotic pressure and hydrostatic pressure?

KEY TERMS

Bronchiolitis

Coagulopathy

Lower respiratory tract infection (LRTI)

Lung cancer

Pneumonia

Pulmonary embolism (PE)

Pulmonary hypertension (PH)

Pulmonary oedema

Respiratory syncytial virus (RSV)

Tuberculosis (TB)

Upper respiratory tract infection (URTI)

Ventilation/perfusion (V/Q) mismatch

Virchow's triad

Introduction

The principles of cancer and infection have been described in the chapters 'Neoplasia' and 'Infection'. In this chapter, the specific effects and complications associated with respiratory infections and lung cancers are explored. Furthermore, alterations in pulmonary vascular function can also profoundly affect the processes of oxygenation and tissue perfusion. The effects of pulmonary embolism, oedema and hypertension are described.

Respiratory infections

LEARNING OBJECTIVE 1

Differentiate between several different types of respiratory infections.

Respiratory infections are divided into upper and lower at the level of the *vocal cords (vocal folds)*, a landmark that represents the dividing line between the *extrapulmonary* and *intrapulmonary* parts of the respiratory tract (see Figure 29.1). However, sometimes upper and lower respiratory tract infections can be difficult to distinguish clinically because an infection may begin as an **upper respiratory tract infection (URTI)**, but can quickly spread to become a **lower respiratory tract infection (LRTI)**. *Rhinovirus* is considered to be the most common cause of URTIs, and **respiratory syncytial virus (RSV)** is considered to be the most common cause of LRTIs. However, many pathogens can cause both upper and lower respiratory tract manifestations. See the 'Infection' chapter for more detail on SARS-CoV-2 infection.

Upper respiratory tract infections

AETIOLOGY AND PATHOPHYSIOLOGY

URTIs occur after direct inoculation and invasion by viral, bacterial or fungal pathogens. Common URTIs and the pathogens involved are listed in Table 29.1. The methods of transmission of organisms that cause URTIs include directly via hand-to-hand contact with infected secretions, via droplet infection or by aerosol. For successful infection to occur, the invading pathogen must overcome the various upper respiratory tract defences in order to become established within the mucosal tissues. Incubation times vary between pathogens, and can be as short as one to three days in the case of parainfluenza virus, or as long as 40 days for infection with Epstein–Barr virus.

Following incubation, the organism proliferates and an inflammatory reaction begins as a direct result of the immune response to invasion or the toxins that are produced by the pathogen, or a combination of both. Inflammation is characterised by vascular and cellular responses. *Vascular responses* involve hyperaemia, increased capillary permeability and tissue swelling,

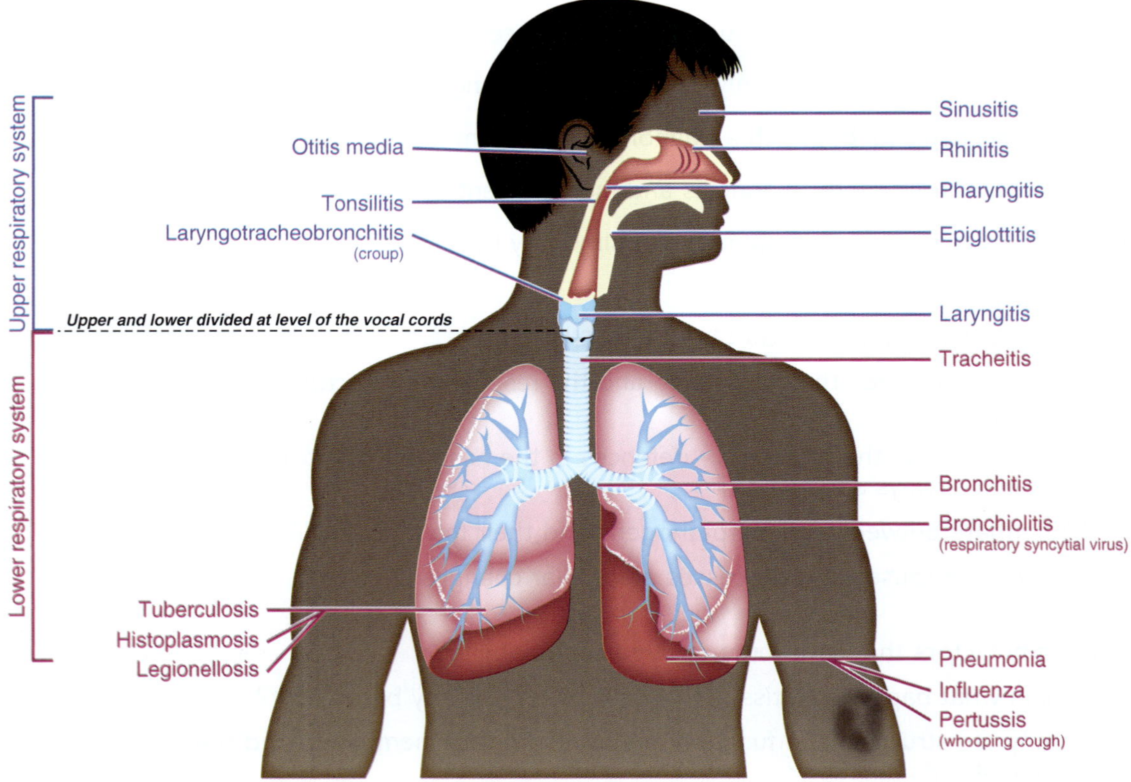

Figure 29.1

Classification of respiratory infections by the anatomical region affected

Upper respiratory tract infections are those above the level of the vocal cords (folds), and lower respiratory tract infections are those below the level of the vocal cords.

Table 29.1 Common upper respiratory tract infections

Infection	Anatomy involved	Pathogen	Comments
Sinusitis	Inflammation of the paranasal sinuses	Can be bacterial, viral or fungal. Most commonly *Haemophilus influenzae* and *Streptococcus pneumoniae*	Mostly occurs with concurrent rhinitis
Rhinitis	Inflammation of the nasal membranes	Can be bacterial, viral or fungal. Most commonly *H. influenzae* and *S. pneumoniae*	Mostly occurs with concurrent sinusitis
Pharyngitis	Inflammation of the pharynx and/or tonsils	Usually bacterial or viral. Most commonly β-haemolytic streptococci, adenovirus, rhinovirus, influenza A or B, coronavirus	Rheumatic heart disease can be a consequence of β-haemolytic streptococcal pharyngitis
Otitis media	Inflammation of the eustachian tube	Most commonly bacterial or viral: *Staphylococcus*, *Streptococcus* and *Pseudomonas* species, respiratory syncytial virus (RSV), influenza A and adenovirus	See 'Disorders of the special senses' chapter
Tonsillitis	Inflammation of the tonsils	Can be bacterial or viral: *Streptococcus pyogenes*, *H. influenzae* and *Staphylococcus aureus*	Can occasionally develop into rheumatic fever or acute glomerulonephritis
Epiglottitis	Inflammation of the epiglottis, vocal folds, arytenoids and sometimes uvula	Most commonly *H. influenzae* type B (Hib)	Can cause airway obstruction in a child if severe. Far less common now with Hib vaccine
Croup	Inflammation of the larynx, trachea and bronchi	Most commonly parainfluenza virus and RSV	Also known as laryngotracheobronchitis. Most commonly affects children. Involves copious subglottic mucus secretion
Laryngitis	Inflammation of the larynx and vocal folds	Can be bacterial, viral or fungal: most commonly parainfluenza virus and RSV	Persistent vocal hoarseness beyond 3 weeks is commonly fungal in origin; occurs more in those who are immunodeficient
Tracheitis	Inflammation of the trachea and subglottic area	Most commonly parainfluenza virus and RSV, *S. aureus* or Hib	Children often present with croup-like symptoms. Bacterial tracheitis is commonly a complication of preceding viral upper respiratory tract infection

while the *cellular response* is mediated by neutrophils and macrophages. Mucosal membranes are damaged as a result of the interaction between the host's immune response and the pathogen. An exudate develops, which may be either serous or mucopurulent.

CLINICAL MANIFESTATIONS

The clinical manifestations of URTIs depend on the severity, causative organism and anatomical region involved. Common signs and symptoms include a sore throat, rhinorrhoea, wheezing, dysphonia or hoarseness, sneezing, fever, headache, malaise and myalgia. Specific infections can cause distinctive symptoms, such as a seal-like barking cough in laryngotracheobronchitis or a classic whooping-sounding cough associated with pertussis infection (pertussis is an LRTI, but can present as a URTI).

DIAGNOSIS AND MANAGEMENT

Diagnosis

Most URTIs are managed in a community setting by the general practitioner. Presentation and admission to a hospital usually only occur when symptoms become severe, such as airway compromise, high temperatures, dehydration or altered consciousness.

Initially, physical assessment and obtaining a history are a primary focus. The investigation of the person's oxygenation status by peripheral oxygen saturation monitoring, temperature and hydration are also important. In some cases, care should be taken to avoid the use of instrumentation (e.g. tongue depressors) as pharyngeal stimulation may provoke airway spasm and further compromise oxygenation. A chest X-ray may be obtained for those with serious or complex presentations. Throat swabs or nasopharyngeal aspirates may be taken to assist with determining the causative organism. In more complex presentations, a blood sample may be collected for serology testing, and a full blood count may be collected to determine the presence of leukocytosis.

Management

URTIs are generally self-limiting in duration. However, in situations where admission is indicated, symptom management is undertaken. For obvious or confirmed bacterial infections, the use of appropriate antimicrobial agents will assist in controlling the infection.

Airway compromise may be managed with supplemental oxygen and/or adrenaline (administered as an aerosol) if mucosal oedema becomes clinically significant. Humidified oxygen will be better tolerated and reduce the risk of exacerbating inflammation or throat discomfort. Airway management, including intubation and mechanical ventilation, may be necessary if respiratory deterioration or fatigue develop. In extreme circumstances, if complete airway obstruction and respiratory arrest occur so that nasopharyngeal or endotracheal intubation is impossible, cricothyroidotomy may be necessary.

High temperatures may be managed with antipyretic agents, such as paracetamol, to prevent febrile seizures in very young children. However, it must be noted that fever is a non-specific defence mechanism and is beneficial to reduce viral replication. Difficulty arises when the metabolic consequences of fever negatively affect clinical outcomes through promoting dehydration and increasing oxygen demand. Temperatures over 39°C may result in the need for antipyretic administration.

Dehydration can occur as a result of insensible loss from diaphoresis or from dysphagia. If oral fluids are not well tolerated or are too painful, the administration of intravenous fluids can improve vital signs, increase comfort and reduce the risk of electrolyte imbalance.

In a child showing an altered level of consciousness, such as obtundation, then severe airway compromise and/or systemic infection should be suspected. Airway management and continuous vital sign monitoring are important. Management in a critical care environment is necessary to promote safety and decrease the risk of morbidity or mortality. Determination of the cause should be a priority following airway management and the initiation of cardiovascular support.

Lower respiratory tract infections

Table 29.2 lists the common LRTIs, the region affected and the pathogens often implicated. It should be noted that the causative organism in these infections may be difficult to identify. Most LRTIs are presumed to be caused by a virus, and in children the most common pathogen is respiratory syncytial virus (RSV).

Clinically important LRTIs, such as bronchiolitis, pneumonia and tuberculosis, are covered in detail below.

BRONCHIOLITIS

Aetiology and pathophysiology

Bronchiolitis is a common LRTI, especially in children under 2 years of age. It can present as both a URTI and an LRTI infection. Bronchiolitis is most often caused by RSV, is very contagious and is transmitted by droplet infection.

An inflammatory response results in mucus hypersecretion, submucosal oedema and the destruction of ciliated epithelial cells. Widespread obstruction of the small airways is caused by peribronchiolar infiltrate and oedema. Expiration further narrows the bronchioles, causing gas trapping, increasing the work of breathing and exacerbating hypoxia and **ventilation/perfusion (V/Q) mismatch**. This is especially true in infants, because the respiratory system is still developing and lung compliance is low.

Factors that increase the risk of a child developing bronchiolitis include premature birth, a history of chronic respiratory conditions, immunodeficiency, congenital cardiac disease and some neurological conditions.

Clinical manifestations

Bronchiolitis commonly presents with both upper and lower clinical manifestations. Upper respiratory tract signs include rhinitis, tachypnoea, nasal flaring and coughing. Lower respiratory tract signs include wheezing, crackles, the use of accessory muscles and hypoxia. Other clinical manifestations can include apnoea, poor feeding and a low-grade fever.

Diagnosis and management

Diagnosis The collection of a thorough history and physical assessment data is a critical primary step. In infants, their feeding history, as well as any evidence of irritability and malaise, should be noted. The infant's measurement of oxygen saturation on room air, both at rest and during feeding, is warranted to obtain an impression about oxygenation. On auscultation, a wheeze or expiratory crackles may be heard. The work associated with breathing should be observed, and the presence of nasal flaring, tracheal tug, head bobbing (see the chapter 'Restrictive respiratory disorders') and chest wall retraction will indicate more severe airway limitation. Oxygen saturations lower than 90% and periods of apnoea are significant observations, and, if present, should prompt management in a critical care environment. Endotracheal intubation and oxygen support with mechanical ventilation are the appropriate interventions in such cases.

If the airway compromise and oxygenation are of significant concern, and the clinical picture appears more complex than typical bronchiolitis, further investigations, such as nasopharyngeal aspiration and chest X-ray, may be beneficial; however, routine chest X-ray and viral testing are not recommended. If the child is receiving intravenous fluid support, blood may be drawn for the assessment of electrolyte levels. Arterial blood gas determinations will be necessary to appropriately manage mechanical ventilation in critically ill infants, and an arterial line should be put in place.

Table 29.2 Common lower respiratory tract infections

Infection	Anatomy involved	Pathogen	Comments
Bronchitis	Inflammation of the bronchus	Most commonly caused by respiratory syncytial virus (RSV) and parainfluenza virus, but can also be bacterial (e.g. *Streptococcus pneumoniae, Haemophilus influenzae* or *Moraxella catarrhalis*)	See 'Obstructive pulmonary disorders' chapter
Bronchiolitis	Inflammation of the bronchioles	Most commonly caused by RSV, but can also be caused by influenza, parainfluenza, adenovirus or metapneumovirus	Can affect up to 30% of children under 12 months of age
Pneumonia	Lung parenchyma	Most commonly caused by RSV and SARS-CoV-2 virus, but can also be bacterial from *S. pneumoniae*. Other important causes include *Mycoplasma pneumoniae, Chlamydophila pneumoniae* and *Legionella* spp.	There are distinct differences in the types of pathogens that cause pneumonia when comparing community-acquired to hospital-acquired forms
Influenza	Bronchial epithelium and lung parenchyma	Influenza virus	Often associated with upper and lower respiratory tract infections.
Pertussis	Structures of both the upper and lower respiratory tracts	*Bordetella pertussis*	Also known as whooping cough. Epidemics of pertussis occur every 3–4 years
Tuberculosis	Tubercle development in the lung parenchyma	*Mycobacterium tuberculosis*	Can remain latent and reactivate at any time, especially when immunocompromised
Histoplasmosis	Lung parenchyma	*Histoplasma capsulatum*	Organism, which is inhaled, is a soil-based fungus found within the top 20 cm of soil
Legionellosis	Lung parenchyma	*Legionella pneumophila* or *Legionella longbeachae*	*L. pneumophila* is transmitted from aerosolised contaminated water, and *L. longbeachae* from potting mix

Management A mild episode of bronchiolitis can be managed at home, as long as the parents and caregivers are guided about positioning, feeding and when to seek medical attention. Supportive therapy is indicated, as no treatment will shorten the course of the condition, nor hasten the resolution of the symptoms. A child with an oxygen saturation of 90–93%, who shows the use of accessory muscles, tachypnoea and/or brief apnoeas should be admitted for observation, oxygen supplementation and intravenous fluid support. Corticosteroids, bronchodilator therapy and noradrenaline are recommended. An infant with severe bronchiolitis will require continuous cardiorespiratory monitoring in a critical care unit in order to address the need for ventilation support from either non-invasive continuous positive airway pressure or fully invasive mechanical ventilation.

VACCINE-PREVENTABLE DISEASES

A number of respiratory diseases are preventable by vaccination. These diseases are notifiable, and their incidence is monitored by federal government communicable diseases intelligence units. In both Australia and New Zealand, notifiable respiratory diseases include tuberculosis, *Haemophilus influenzae* type b (Hib) meningitis, influenza, pertussis, legionellosis and diphtheria. The efficacy of vaccination programs relies on *herd immunity (community immunity)*, whereby the maximum numbers of people are vaccinated and immune to an infectious disease to protect those who are not immune. Healthcare professionals need to encourage vaccinations aligned with the national vaccination program to reduce communicable respiratory disease.

Influenza rates are under-reported as most people ill with the flu will not necessarily present to the doctor, or, if they do, will not necessarily have virology tests collected. Countries are starting to report values by multiple surveillance sources, and are describing rates as influenza-like illness to represent a more realistic situation.

The coronavirus disease (COVID-19) caused by the SARS-CoV-2 virus had an immense influence on influenza incidence. In 2019 (pre-pandemic), Australia experienced the worst ever influenza outbreak, recording more than 313,000 (laboratory-confirmed) notified cases. Then with the infection control measures instituted for COVID-19, the following two years reduced to fewer than 21,000 in 2020 and fewer than 800 in 2022. Unfortunately however, as the COVID-19 measures lifted and Australia emerged from the pandemic, the influenza incidence increased once again to over 233,000 in 2022.

Healthcare workers are also at significant risk of developing respiratory tract infections in the course of their work through exposure to people with the infection. Healthcare workers should therefore ensure that their own immunisation status is current, and practise good-quality, appropriate infection control measures with everyone they are in contact with, irrespective of whether they are known to be infected or not.

PNEUMONIA

LEARNING OBJECTIVE 2

Discuss the various types of pneumonia, the clinical implications of their diagnosis and their management.

Aetiology and pathophysiology

Pneumonia is an inflammation of lung parenchyma resulting in altered gas exchange. Pneumonia may be caused by bacteria, viruses, fungi or other pathogens. Pneumonia can also have a non-infectious cause, such as inhalation of volatile or irritating substances, or aspiration of gastric contents. A number of factors can contribute to the development of pneumonia (see Clinical Box 29.1).

If the pneumonia is associated with an infection, pathogens can access the respiratory system via a variety of routes of entry:

- *Aspiration* of normal anaerobic flora or aerobic Gram-negative bacilli that have colonised the oropharynx. Aspiration pneumonia may also occur as a result of aspiration of refluxed bacterial-laden gastric contents.
- *Inhalation* of infected aerosols, which can deposit into the lower respiratory tract.
- *Haematogenous spread* of pathogens deposited into the lung via the vascular system as a result of bacterial translocation from infected cannulas or catheters, or from the gastrointestinal tract.
- *Direct inoculation* of pathogens, such as from an infected endotracheal tube biofilm or secretions on the outside or inside of the airway equipment. Direct inoculation may also occur during surgery from infected equipment (e.g. bronchoscopy scopes) or from direct extension from a breached, infected area contiguous to the lung.
- *Reactivation* of latent infection can occur with some pathogens (*Mycobacterium tuberculosis*, *Pneumocystis jiroveci* or cytomegalovirus), especially in someone who is immunodeficient.

Once the pathogen has gained entry to the respiratory system, it multiplies and releases toxic substances onto the lung parenchyma. An inflammatory response begins. As the inflammatory mediators are released, the person's core temperature may increase and they may develop pleuritic chest pain. Alveolar oedema and vascular congestion occur. Depending on the pathogen, the epithelial cells may be damaged, thereby exacerbating the situation. Cellular debris and exudate accumulate in the alveoli, causing consolidation and reducing lung compliance. Changes in sputum colour and consistency may occur, depending on the cause. Green sputum most often indicates infection with *Pseudomonas* species. Rusty/red-coloured sputum indicates a large amount of erythrocytes, and may suggest *Streptococcus pneumoniae*. Foul-smelling sputum may indicate anaerobic bacteria, and gelatinous sputum may suggest *Klebsiella pneumoniae*.

When pneumonia arises from non-infectious causes, an inflammatory reaction to the trauma occurs. The inflammatory processes cause parenchymal damage and produce similar clinical manifestations to pneumonia caused by an infectious agent. It is not uncommon for this condition to be complicated by a secondary bacterial infection.

CLINICAL BOX 29.1

Factors that increase the risk of pneumonia

- Altered level of consciousness
  - Anaesthesia
  - Head injury
  - Cerebrovascular accident
  - Seizure disorder
  - Drug overdose
  - Alcohol intoxication
- Neuromuscular dysfunction resulting in dysphagia
  - Parkinson's disease
  - Multiple sclerosis
  - Muscular dystrophy
  - Cerebral palsy
  - Myasthenia gravis
- Oesophageal obstruction
  - Oesophageal stricture
  - Cancer (e.g. thyroid, lung, pharynx, oesophagus)
- Use of invasive instrumentation
  - Nasogastric tube
  - Endotracheal/tracheostomy tube
  - Investigation scopes (e.g. bronchoscopy, upper gastrointestinal endoscopy)
  - Dental procedures
- Gastro-oesophageal reflux disease
- Tracheo-oesophageal fistula
- Supine positioning
- Advanced age

Types of pneumonia

Pattern of lung involvement Pneumonia can be classified according to the patterns of lung involvement. Two common examples of this type are lobar pneumonia and bronchopneumonia (see Figure 29.2). *Lobar pneumonia* is a form of exudative inflammation affecting a whole lobe or a large portion of a lobe, while *bronchopneumonia* is a suppurative inflammation distributed in a multifocal or patchy manner involving one or more lobes.

Another common pattern is *interstitial pneumonia*, which is a patchy or diffuse inflammation primarily involving the alveolar walls and bronchial tree connective tissue (interstitium). A less common type is *miliary pneumonia*, which occurs as a result of haematogenous spread and presents as numerous small, diffuse lesions throughout both lungs.

Setting in which pneumonia is acquired Pneumonia can also be classified by the setting associated with its development. The three major categories are hospital-acquired pneumonia, healthcare-associated pneumonia and community-acquired pneumonia. *Hospital-acquired pneumonia* develops as a result of exposure to a pathogen within a hospital (also known as *nosocomial pneumonia*). *Healthcare-associated pneumonia* develops as a result of exposure to a pathogen from an aged-care facility, outpatient clinic or dialysis unit. *Community-acquired pneumonia* develops as a result of exposure to a pathogen outside the hospital or healthcare-associated facilities.

In the literature, consensus has not been reached as to these definitions. Some authors define pneumonia developed in an aged-care facility as a type of community-acquired pneumonia. Others consider healthcare-associated pneumonia as a subcategory of hospital-acquired pneumonia. Clarification of the nomenclature surrounding this topic is still required.

Causative organism Identifying the microbe causing the pneumonia is imperative to ensure that an appropriate management plan can be developed. Microscopy, culture and sensitivity testing of respiratory secretions can inform antimicrobial selection and prevent the misuse of antimicrobials if circumstances do not warrant antimicrobial treatment. The setting in which pneumonia develops can significantly influence the type of pathogen exposure (see Table 29.3).

Figure 29.2

Comparison of (A) bronchopneumonia and (B) lobar pneumonia

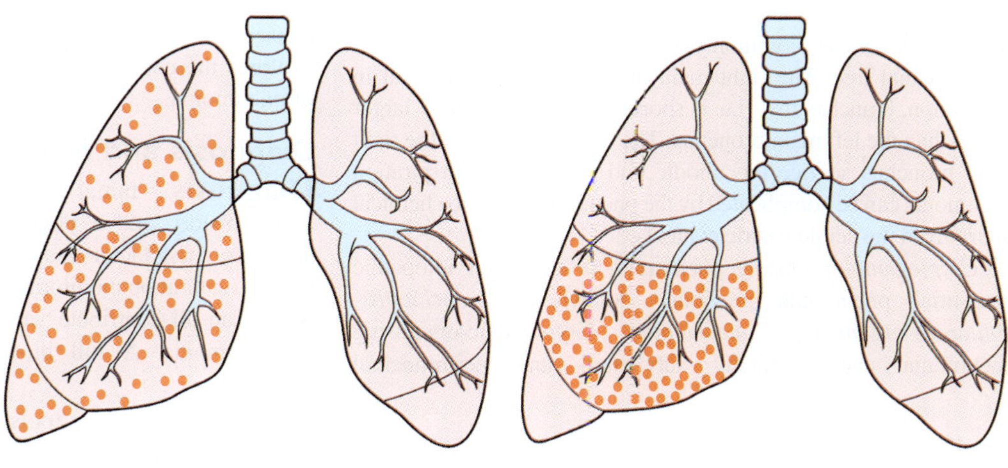

Table 29.3 Common organisms associated with pneumonia in adults

Hospital-acquired pneumonia	Healthcare-associated pneumonia	Community-acquired pneumonia	Opportunistic pneumonia
• *Staphylococcus aureus*	• *Streptococcus pneumoniae*	• *Streptococcus pneumoniae*	• *Pneumocystis jiroveci*
• *Pseudomonas aeruginosa*	• *Staphylococcus aureus*	• *Mycoplasma pneumoniae*	• *Mycobacterium tuberculosis*
• *Klebsiella pneumoniae*	• *Haemophilus influenzae*	• *Haemophilus influenzae*	• Cytomegalovirus
• *Legionella* spp.	• Influenza virus	• *Chlamydia pneumoniae*	• Atypical mycobacteria
• *Escherichia coli*	• *Enterobacter* spp.	• *Legionella* spp.	• Fungi
		• *Pneumophila* spp.	
		• Influenza virus	

Opportunistic pneumonia *Opportunistic pneumonia* is another type of inflammatory lung disease caused by microorganisms that are generally harmless to those who are immunocompetent. However, they can induce pneumonia in people with inadequate immune system responses. Factors that increase the risk of opportunistic pneumonia are shown in Table 29.4.

Other types of pneumonia Other types of pneumonia can develop, such as ventilator-associated pneumonia, aspiration pneumonia and cryptogenic-organising pneumonia.

Ventilator-associated pneumonia is common in the intensive care setting where someone who is critically ill is receiving assisted ventilation. Invasive ventilation (ventilation requiring the placement of an endotracheal or tracheostomy tube) bypasses all of the upper airway respiratory defences, exposes the person to potentially pathogen-inoculated respiratory equipment, and occurs in those who are most likely immunocompromised as a result of their condition.

Aspiration pneumonia is common in aged-care settings and in people who have dysphagia or altered levels of consciousness. When gastric secretions colonised with pathogenic bacteria are refluxed into the oropharynx and the cough and gag reflexes are diminished, the secretions can be inhaled into the larynx and lower respiratory tract. The lobes on the right side (particularly the middle and lower lobes) are commonly affected, because of the shape of the bronchial tree. The right main bronchus is more vertical in orientation, branches first (i.e. is shorter), and has a slightly larger lumen than the left main bronchus. The early branches of the right main bronchus service the middle and lower lobes. Aspiration pneumonia can be complicated by the pneumonitis due to chemical injury from the acidic gastric contents.

Cryptogenic-organising pneumonia is a type of idiopathic interstitial pneumonia previously known as *bronchiolitis-obliterans-organising pneumonia*. Cryptogenic-organising pneumonia causes patchy subpleural and peribronchial consolidation, and intraluminal polyps. The pathogenesis of cryptogenic-organising pneumonia remains unknown, but it is commonly associated with chronic alveolar inflammation.

Table 29.4 Factors that increase the risk of opportunistic pneumonia

- Medication-induced immunosuppresants, such as corticosteroids
- Cancer
- Acquired immunodeficiency syndrome (AIDS)
- Leukocyte defects
- Lymphocyte defects
- Immunoglobulin defects
- Pregnancy
- Chemotherapy agents
- Conditions causing hyperglycaemia
- Asplenia
- Autoimmune diseases

Epidemiology

In Westernised countries such as Australia and New Zealand, pneumonia has a relatively low annual mortality rate (about 1.7%). However, worldwide, some countries report mortality rates due to pneumonia of up to 33% in children under 5 years of age. The World Health Organization (WHO) reports a median childhood mortality rate from pneumonia of 13%.

In Australia, approximately 2,000 people die of pneumonia each year. Women have predominantly experienced greater mortality than men, and at a level higher than the total population. New Zealand mortality statistics do not separate influenza and pneumonia. Over 700 New Zealanders die from influenza and pneumonia each year, and the propensity for women to experience higher mortality rates persists.

Clinical manifestations

As with most respiratory conditions, the common clinical manifestations of pneumonia may include dyspnoea, tachypnoea, cough and tachycardia. Increased sputum production, fever and chest pain are also common issues. Malaise and fatigue may also develop. Severe hypoxia can result in an altered level of consciousness, such as confusion or agitation. Figure 29.3 explores the common clinical manifestations and management of pneumonia.

Diagnosis and management

Diagnosis Initial assessments include the collection of a full history and a physical examination, paying particular attention to risk factors that increase the likelihood of pneumonia. Oxygen saturation monitoring, assessment of vital signs and chest X-ray can all contribute valuable information in the diagnosis of pneumonia. A full blood examination may demonstrate leukocytosis.

Various assessment tools have been developed to quantify the severity of an individual's presentation. There are numerous pneumonia severity scoring tools commonly used in Australia and New Zealand.

- *Pneumonia Severity Index*—The Pneumonia Severity Index is a two-part assessment to quantify a risk of morbidity and mortality for individuals presenting with pneumonia. The risk stratification results in the tallying of a score within five risk classes, and as the score increases so does the risk of mortality within 30 days.
- *CORB*—CORB is a quick assessment that quantifies an individual's condition into severe or not severe. This can enable prediction of the need to provide mechanical ventilation or inotropic support measures. Each letter of the acronym identifies a parameter that contributes 1 point to a score value (C = confusion; O = oxygenation of $\leq 90\%$; R = respiratory rate of ≥ 30 breaths per minute; B = blood pressure of < 90 mmHg [systolic] or < 60 mmHg [diastolic]). Severe pneumonia is defined as a score of 2 or more.

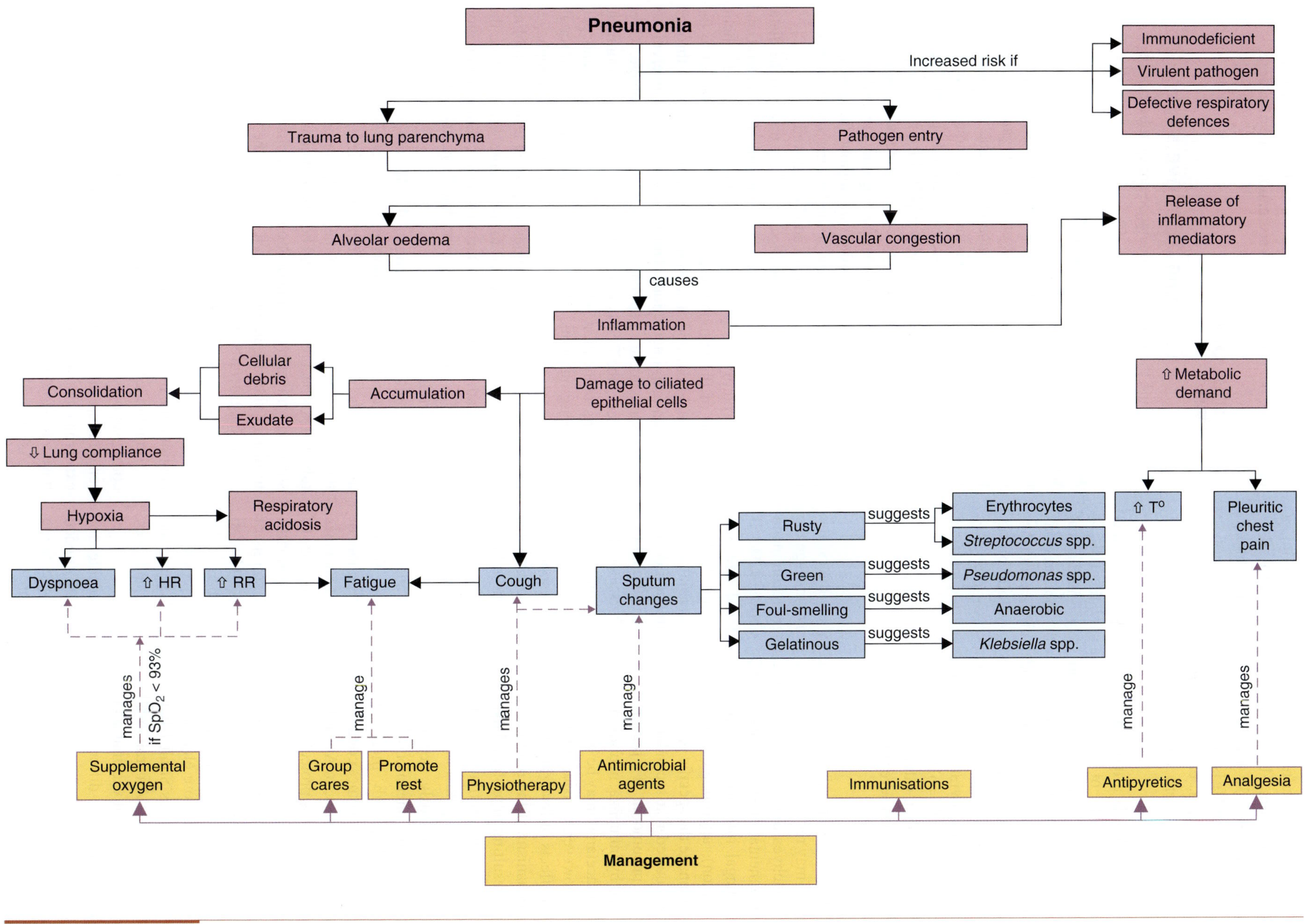

Figure 29.3

Clinical snapshot: Pneumonia

↓ = decreased; ↑ = increased; HR = heart rate; RR = respiratory rate; SpO_2 = saturation of peripheral oxygen; T° = temperature.

- *CURB-65*—This is a variation on CORB utilising a couple of different criteria to assist with quantifying a value (C = confusion; U = urea of >7 mmol/L; R = respiratory rate of ≥ 30 breaths per minute; B = blood pressure of < 90 mmHg [systolic] or < 60 mmHg [diastolic]; 65 = age ≥ 65). Again, each value outside the parameter is worth 1, and a severe value is defined as a score of 2 or more.
- *SMART-COP*—This is a moderately quick assessment that quantifies the severity of the pneumonia and the risk of requiring intensive respiratory support (e.g. mechanical ventilation) or inotropic support. As with the previous assessments, each letter of the acronym identifies a parameter that contributes to the score value (S = systolic blood pressure; M = multilobar lesions on chest X – ray; A = albumin R = respiratory rate; T = tachycardia; C = confusion; O = oxygenation; P = pH). When values fall outside prescribed limits, that value obtains a score of 1 and any score of ≥ 5 indicates severe pneumonia.

Management Depending on the severity of illness, the affected person may require supplemental oxygen to manage the dyspnoea and tachycardia. Recent guideline changes recommend oxygen supplementation to maintain SpO_2 above 92%. If bacterial or fungal infection is suspected (bacterial infection is more common), appropriate antimicrobial therapy will be necessary to manage the specific pathogen. Antimicrobial agents may also be required if a secondary bacterial infection occurs following viral pneumonia. If a person's condition is thought to be complicated by influenza, neuraminidase inhibitors should be considered. Paracetamol may be beneficial to control pain and to reduce fever; however, consideration should be made regarding the beneficial effects of fever and the inflammatory response as a defence mechanism. If the individual's condition deteriorates due to sepsis, resulting in profound hypoxaemia and poor blood pressure, mechanical ventilation and inotropic drug support (e.g. the dopaminergic agonist dobutamine) will be necessary.

Prevention is obviously better than cure. Immunisation can be obtained for pneumococcal pneumonia caused by *S. pneumoniae*. Although there are almost 100 strains of *S. pneumoniae*, the vaccines contain only a limited number of clinically important strains. In Australia, two different vaccines are available. One vaccine protects against 13 different types of *S. pneumoniae* and is given free to children at 2, 4 and 6 months of age. Another vaccine protects against 23 different strains of *S. pneumoniae* and is given to older children and adults. Certain groups are more at risk of pneumonia than other members of the community, and are therefore eligible to receive vaccines at no cost. Aboriginal and Torres Strait Islander people 50 years and over, and non-Indigenous Australian adults 65 years and over, can receive pneumococcal vaccination free of charge.

In New Zealand, three different vaccines are available: for 10 strains, 13 strains and 23 strains. The nationally funded vaccination program is limited to specific groups of people. Some children under 5 years of age are at very high risk of invasive pneumococcal disease, and any New Zealander with asplenia is eligible for free vaccinations. Māori and Pacific Islands children under 15 years of age have a high rate of pneumococcal pneumonia, but do not receive vaccinations free of charge.

TUBERCULOSIS

LEARNING OBJECTIVE 3

Examine the effects and management of tuberculosis.

Aetiology and pathophysiology

Tuberculosis (TB) is a contagious, air-borne, bacterial infection that commonly affects the lungs. It is characterised by a productive cough, weight loss and night sweats. Two organisms can cause tuberculosis: *Mycobacterium tuberculosis* and *Mycobacterium bovis*, although *M. tuberculosis* is the more common agent. Droplet nuclei containing the rod-shaped, wax-coated, aerobic, acid-fast bacteria that have been forcefully expelled from the respiratory system of an infected person by a cough can remain suspended in the air for several hours. Someone passing may inhale the infected droplets, which will be deposited throughout the unsuspecting person's airways. The majority of the bacteria will be subject to the various defence mechanisms and be removed.

If the *M. tuberculosis* bacilli successfully travel to the distal airways, alveolar macrophages will consume the bacteria and release proteolytic enzymes and cytokines to degrade them. As a part of the immune response, T cells are attracted to the site of infection, and macrophages signal these cells through surface antigen interactions. During this time, the tuberculosis microorganisms are replicating inside the macrophage. Over several weeks the T cells and macrophages create an environment that limits replication by reducing the oxygen levels and pH, and limiting nutrients. The lesion becomes walled-off through the processes of fibrosis and calcification. The macrophages die, and the affected area becomes a necrosed lesion resembling cottage cheese; this is referred to as *caseous necrosis* (see the chapter 'Pathophysiological terminology, cellular adaptation and injury'). At this stage, some bacilli remain alive, albeit trapped, within this lesion.

In immunocompetent people, the *M. tuberculosis* bacilli will remain contained and dormant in a state of latency. If at any stage the person becomes immunodeficient, the integrity of the containment wall encasing the bacilli can be breached. The tuberculosis bacteria escape and begin to spread to other alveoli; some can travel by haematogenous or lymphatic mechanisms to distant sites in the body, such as bone, the central nervous system or structures within the abdomen, in an infection referred to as *extrapulmonary TB*. Other bacilli can remain in the lungs to be picked up by droplets and forcefully exhaled again, to continue the transmission of infection to other people.

Immunodeficiency is exacerbated by the use of long-term corticosteroids, smoking, chemotherapy, malnutrition, diabetes, renal failure and sepsis. Co-infection with another pathogen can exacerbate the situation. Many of those with HIV/AIDS and TB have a ten-fold risk of disease progression.

As the pathogen has developed resistance to antitubercular drugs, newer strains have become particularly concerning in their capacity to withstand the effects of a number of the drugs that make up the standard TB treatment regimen. The acronym *MDR-TB* is used to describe *multiple-drug–resistant tuberculosis* (resistant to at least isoniazid and rifampicin—two first-line antitubercular drugs), and *XDR-TB* is used to describe *extensively drug-resistant tuberculosis* (resistant to at least four first-line antitubercular drugs).

Epidemiology

The WHO estimates that TB kills approximately 1.4 million people every year worldwide. In 2021, seven countries contributed to more than 61% of the total number of new cases of tuberculosis diagnosed in the world (India, Indonesia, China, the Philippines, Pakistan, Nigeria and Bangladesh).

TB rates in Australian and New Zealand are quite low, at an estimated 7 cases per 100,000 people However, many countries have incidence of more than 200 cases per 100,000, and some are as high as 650 cases per 100,000 people (the Philippines).

Clinical manifestations

Clinical manifestations depend on the stage at which the person seeks medical assistance and on their degree of immunocompetence (see Figure 29.4), but can include fever, weight loss, productive cough, haemoptysis, dyspnoea, night sweats and sometimes chest pain.

Diagnosis and management

Diagnosis The primary investigation in the assessment of TB is the collection of three quality, early morning sputum samples over three different days. It is important that sputum (not saliva) is collected, so instructions to promote respiratory secretion collection may be necessary. An example of this is beforehand taking a hot, steamy shower, which can loosen secretions. Sample collection should also occur first thing in the morning before eating, drinking, brushing teeth or rinsing the mouth.

A sputum smear to detect the presence of acid-fast bacilli can take approximately 24 hours. A sputum culture to identify *M. tuberculosis* can take approximately three weeks due to the slow growth of the microbe. The *polymerase chain reaction* can be used to detect mycobacteria exposure within 48 hours.

Collection of a thorough history and a physical assessment are also necessary. This should include discussions exploring the risk of exposure and time spent in locations where TB is prevalent. Any history of coughing, weight loss and night sweats is also important to note. Chest X-ray and tuberculin skin testing are also important in the diagnosis of TB.

Chest X-ray can be used to determine the presence of infiltrates with cavitation (small gas-filled cavities or hollows that are the centre of nodules or areas of consolidations within the lung). Tuberculin skin testing (the Mantoux test) is an intradermal injection of a purified protein derivative of tuberculin with the intention of measuring the hypersensitivity reaction (see Figure 29.5). If the transverse diameter of the induration measures less than 5 mm, the reading is considered negative. However, it is important to understand and account for any factors that may influence the reaction, such as the presence of immunosuppression from corticosteroid therapy or disease, poor nutrition or viral infection. Immunisation against TB is achieved using a suspension of live attenuated *M. bovis* organisms, called the *bacille Calmette–Guérin (BCG) vaccine*. Those who have had a previous BCG immunisation will demonstrate a quicker response.

Investigations for co-infection with human immunodeficiency virus (HIV) or other conditions causing immunodeficiency should be undertaken. Microscopy, culture and sensitivity testing should be performed to determine the most appropriate antimicrobial drug regimen, and to determine the presence of multidrug-resistant tuberculosis. An assessment for symptoms of extrapulmonary TB should be initiated, focusing on evidence of altered mental status, bone pain, paralysis or organomegaly.

Management The management of TB includes the administration of antimicrobial agents to the affected person, as well as contact screening and infection control measures to protect others. Those with suspected or confirmed active TB should be cared for in a negative-pressure room, with staff and visitors putting on appropriate transmission-based personal protective equipment (e.g. high-efficiency particulate filtering masks) before entering the room. Visitor numbers should be kept to a minimum. Immunocompromised relatives, children and other at-risk individuals should be discouraged from visiting. When leaving the room for investigations, the person should wear an appropriate mask. Isolation should continue until three consecutive negative sputum smears are obtained.

A regimen of four antimicrobial drugs (i.e. ethambutol, isoniazid, rifampicin and pyrazinamide) is the standard treatment for TB. An assessment of drug resistance should be undertaken, and regimens should be adjusted as necessary. The management of co-infection with HIV may be necessary for some people. In these people, concomitant treatment can complicate the management plan, as a paradoxical strong immune response to the TB can cause exacerbation of pulmonary infiltrates, worsening fever and lymphadenopathy.

Nutritional support is important, as people with TB can develop cachexia. The relationship between infection and weight loss can be accounted for by energy regulation imbalances, altered gastrointestinal absorption, anorexia from shortness of breath and malaise, and the influences of infection on leptin (an important mediator between nutrition and immunity). Excessive diaphoresis and anorexia may also lead to dehydration. Healthcare professionals should encourage the patient to increase their fluid intake.

Critically ill people with TB who require mechanical ventilation should be cared for in a negative-pressure room. A closed endotracheal suction system should be used, and bacterial filters should be placed on the expiratory circuit to reduce infected aerosolised droplets. Masks, gloggles, and gowns should be worn by staff and visitors entering the room.

Psychological support and counselling are important in the management of people with TB. Those with chronic disease are at a high risk of depression. Good communication with them and their carers is important to ensure adherence to the drug regimen, as treatment for up to a year may be necessary to ensure the

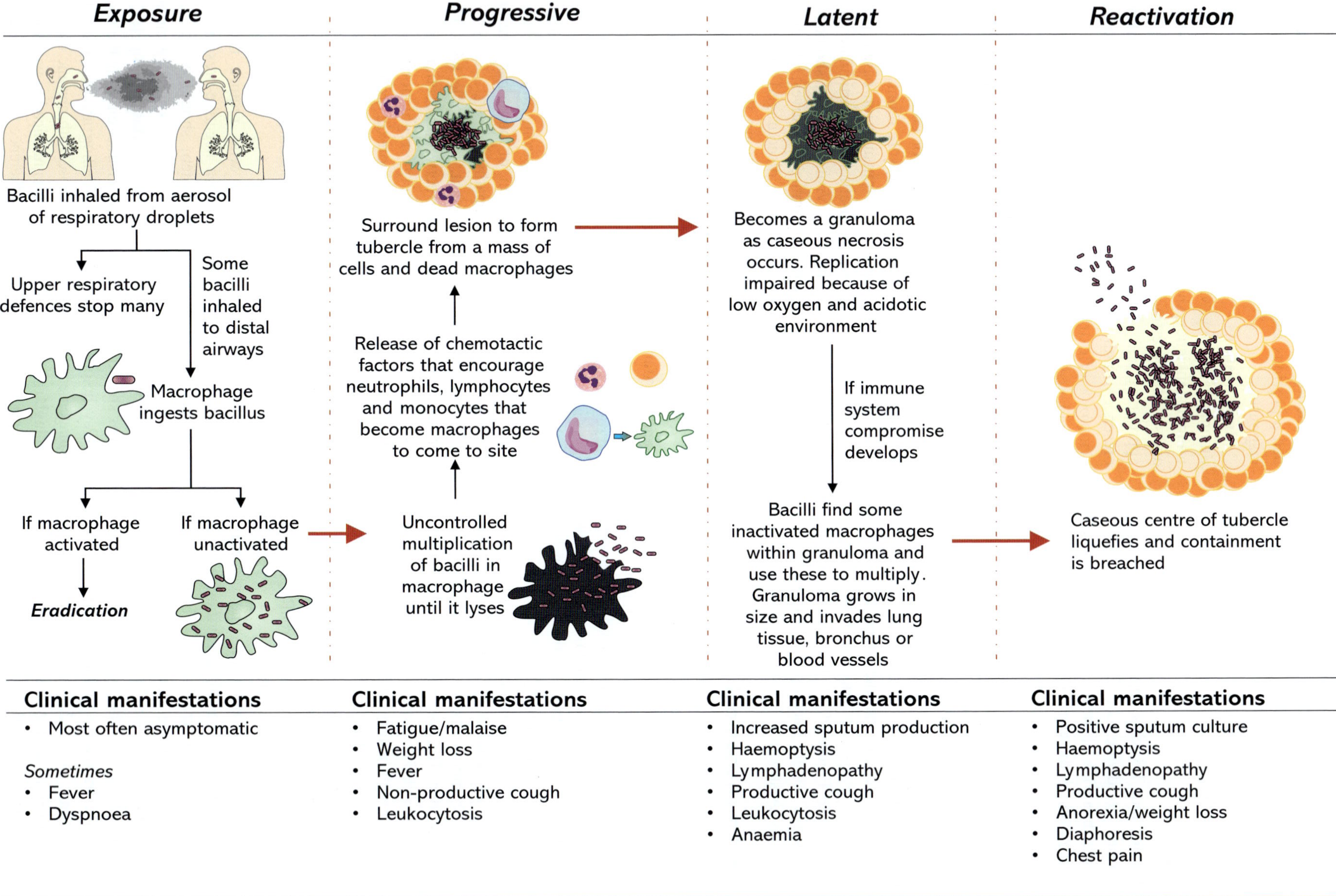

Figure 29.4
Stages of tuberculosis and commonly associated clinical manifestations

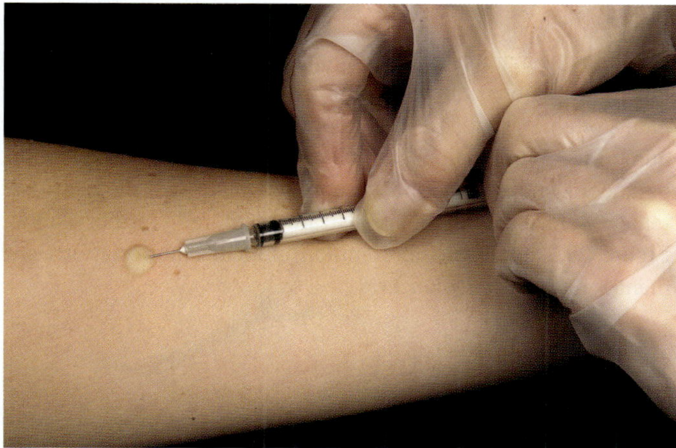

Figure 29.5

The Mantoux test

The Mantoux test involves an intradermal injection of purified protein derivative of tuberculin. Hypersensitivity reaction will be measured 48–72 hours later.

Source: CDC/Gabrielle Benenson.

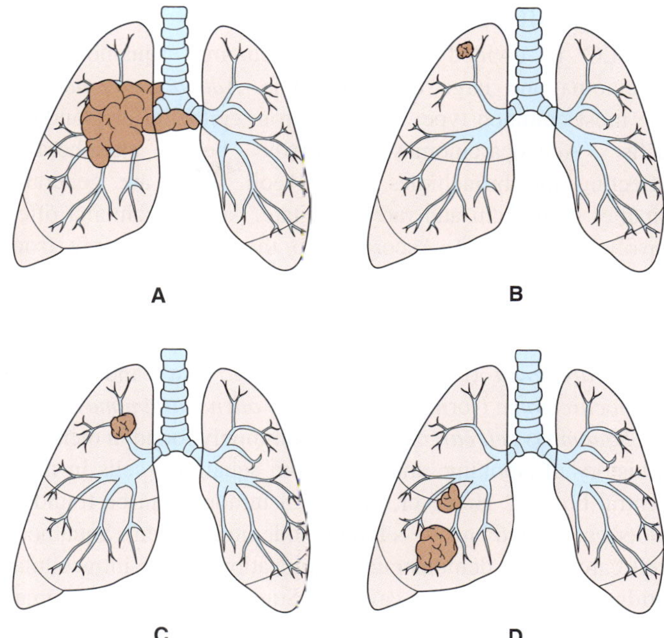

Figure 29.6

Comparison of lung cancer cell types

(A) Small cell lung cancer.
(B) Adenocarcinoma.
(C) Squamous cell carcinoma.
(D) Large cell carcinoma.

Source: Adapted from Bauldoff et al. (2020), Table 35.7, p. 1291.

successful elimination of TB and to reduce the risk of promoting further drug resistance or bacterial dormancy and reactivation.

Lung cancer

LEARNING OBJECTIVE 4

Differentiate between the different types of lung cancer.

Lung cancer is a term to describe a number of malignancies that can occur anywhere within the respiratory system. Lung cancer is initially classified into two types based on histological characteristics: *small cell lung cancer* and *non-small cell lung cancer (NSCLC)*. NSCLC can then be further subdivided into adenocarcinoma, squamous cell carcinoma and large cell carcinoma (see Figure 29.6). NSCLC is the most common type of lung cancer, and is responsible for approximately 80% of all lung cancers. It most often begins in the bronchi and the smaller airways. Small cell lung cancer is responsible for the remaining 20% of all lung cancers, and generally begins in the more central locations of the lung.

Lung cancer can also be classified into primary and secondary forms. *Primary lung cancer* originates in the lung, while *secondary lung cancer* is a neoplastic lesion that has been deposited in the lung from a distant location via either the lymphatic system or the vascular system. The principal focus of this section is primary lung cancer. However, secondary lung cancer is explained briefly.

AETIOLOGY AND PATHOPHYSIOLOGY

The general principles of cancer, terminology and tumorigenesis are covered in the chapter 'Neoplasia'. Carcinomas of the lung occur as a result of disordered cell growth and a failure of the normal immune surveillance systems, permitting growth of abnormal cells in the bronchi, bronchioles and/or alveoli to mutate and proliferate. The proto-oncogenes—genes that, when mutated, have the potential of becoming an oncogene and contributing to cancer development—thought to be involved in lung cancer development include *K-ras* and *c-Myc*. *K-ras* is important for the promotion of cell growth and proliferation, while *c-Myc* is important for DNA synthesis, cell cycle regulation, proliferation and the induction apoptosis. Tumour suppressor genes, such as *p53*, control neoplastic cell formation and manage cell senescence. Epidermal growth factor receptors influence proliferation, differentiation and apoptosis. Vascular endothelial growth factors influence tumour angiogenesis. Mutations in any or all of these genes, receptors and factors may contribute to tumour growth.

Small cell lung cancer

Although there are different types of small cell carcinoma, the most common are called *oat cell carcinoma*. Other types include *mixed small/large cell carcinoma* and *combined small cell carcinoma*. While small cell lung cancer is less common than NSCLC, it grows more rapidly and metastasises faster. Histologically, small cell lung cancer shows sparse cytoplasm and discreet nucleoli, and it is commonly associated with paraneoplastic syndromes (see the 'Neoplasia' chapter).

Non-small cell lung cancer

NSCLC is divided into adenocarcinoma, squamous cell carcinoma and large cell carcinoma. *Adenocarcinomas* are the most common type, and arise from epithelial or glandular cells. Adenocarcinomas primarily begin peripherally, affecting the bronchioles and alveoli. They are generally smaller than 5 cm and rarely cavitate. Adenocarcinoma often involves the pleura. According to the new taxonomy from the International Association for the Study of Lung Cancer, adenocarcinoma can be further divided into *adenocarcinoma in situ* (formerly *bronchoalveolar carcinoma*), *minimally invasive adenocarcinoma* (tissue invasion of ≤ 5 mm) and *invasive adenocarcinoma* (formerly *mixed-type adenocarcinoma*).

Squamous cell carcinomas are commonly found in men with a history of smoking, and arise from squamous cells in more central bronchi. However, peripheral tumours can be found in older people and have less lymph node involvement. Squamous cell carcinomas demonstrate keritinisation and/or intracellular bridges and frequently cavitate. Squamous cell carcinomas are renowned for their association with the paraneoplastic syndrome, resulting in hypercalcaemia.

Large cell carcinomas are less common than the other types of lung cancer. They are moderately large polygonal cells with ample cytoplasm and prominent nucleoli. Large cell carcinoma is most often found in lung periphery, and is frequently diagnosed by exclusion of the other types because they lack squamous, glandular or small cell features.

EPIDEMIOLOGY

Smoking is a major cause of lung cancer. Other factors that increase the risk of lung cancer include a genetic predisposition and exposure to carcinogenic substances, such as asbestos. A dose relationship exists between the exposure to inhaled carcinogens and the development of lung cancer. A person's risk of developing lung cancer is significantly increased by an earlier age of starting to smoke cigarettes, the more frequently cigarettes are smoked in a week, and the number of years of smoking cigarettes. Smokers can have a risk of developing lung cancer of up to 25 times that of a non-smoker. Women appear to have an increased risk compared to men, and require less exposure to develop lung cancer. Fortunately, over the past 20 years smoking rates in Australia have been declining. In 2001, more than 28% of the Australian population were daily smokers; however, by 2021–22, only 10.1% of the population were daily smokers.

In Australia, lung cancer is the second most common cause of death in males, and the fourth most common in females. Overall, lung cancer is the leading cause of cancer death and the fourth most common cancer diagnosed (excluding skin cancer). In New Zealand, lung cancer is the second most common cause of death in males, and the fourth most common in females. Overall, lung cancer is the most common cause of cancer death in men and women. Despite advances in knowledge and treatment, mortality statistics for lung cancer are very poor, with few people surviving beyond five years from the time of their diagnosis.

CLINICAL MANIFESTATIONS

The clinical manifestations of lung cancer can be divided into local and regional effects. Common *local effects* include chest pain, cough, dyspnoea and haemoptysis. *Regional effects* include numerous complications, which can be divided into metabolic, paraneoplastic, endocrine, haematological, neurological and renal. Selected complications are explored further below. Figure 29.7 explores the common clinical manifestations and management of lung cancer.

DIAGNOSIS AND MANAGEMENT

Diagnosis

Various diagnostic modalities may be employed when investigating someone presenting with a suspected lung cancer. The collection of a thorough history is important, especially in the context of determining past cigarette smoking behaviours and exposure to second-hand smoke or other carcinogenic chemicals from occupational or environmental encounters.

Imaging studies, such as chest X-ray or computed tomography (CT), may be used initially to determine the presence and possible lesion location. More conclusive investigations, such as fine-needle aspiration biopsy, bronchoscopy, sputum cytology or video-assisted thoroscopy, may be used to determine the type of cancer. It is important that the presence of metastasis be identified. Bone scans and positron emission tomography (PET) may be used to quantify the presence and extent of secondary growths.

The most important undertaking in preparation for the development of a management plan is cancer staging. Lung cancer staging is performed using the internationally accepted *tumour–node–metastases (TNM) staging system* given in Table 29.5.

Table 29.5 TNM lung cancer staging

T = tumour: a code of T0–T4 can be assigned to quantify the size of the tumour; T0 means no tumour and a higher code signifies a larger tumour.

N = node: a code of N0–N3 may be assigned to quantify the presence of metastasis to regional lymph nodes; N0 means no lymph node involvement and a higher number signifies more prolific lymph node involvement.

M = metastasis: a code of either M0 or M1 can be assigned; M0 means that there are no metastases, M1a means that there are local thoracic metastases, and M1b identifies extrathoracic metastases.

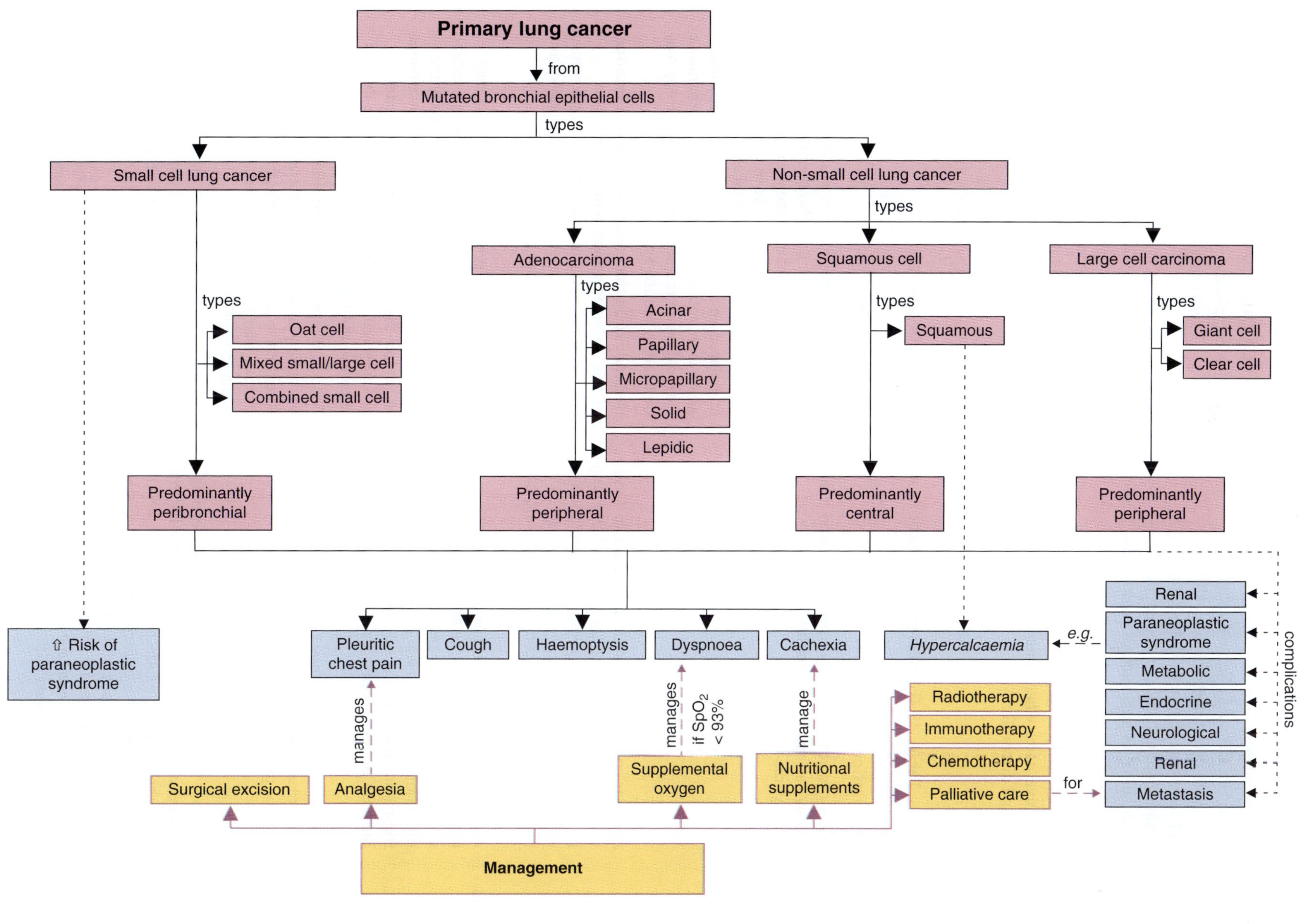

Figure 29.7

Clinical snapshot: Lung cancer

↑ = increased; SpO_2 = saturation of peripheral oxygen.

Management

The TNM system equates to a lung cancer staging from stage 0 to stage IV. A higher number signifies a more serious disease and a worse prognosis. Treatment plans are developed, and are primarily informed by the lung cancer stage. Some management options may include surgery to remove the lesion, although this is not possible for all lung cancer types. Radiotherapy or chemotherapy may be administered to reduce or control the size of the cancer. Immunomodulating agents, such as interferons, interleukins or colony-stimulating factors, may be administered in order to stimulate endogenous defence or replenish cells types lost in the treatment process. In stage IV, the person may be offered supportive palliative care, where interventions are offered only to reduce pain and discomfort.

SELECTED COMPLICATIONS COMMONLY ASSOCIATED WITH LUNG CANCER

LEARNING OBJECTIVE 5

Identify the complications commonly associated with lung cancer.

Although lung cancer alone is a significant disease causing substantial morbidity and mortality, it can also be associated with a considerable number of complications that occur secondary to lung cancer and complicate management or hasten deterioration. Table 29.6 identifies selected complications, their mechanisms of development and possible management considerations.

Table 29.6 Selected complications associated with lung cancer

Complication	Description/Mechanism	Management
Airway obstruction	Local growth of a tumour near or around a large airway can result in respiratory compromise and hypoxia.	Depending on the location, acuity and severity of the obstruction, bronchoplasty (airway dilation), placement of a stent or microdebriding via bronchoscopy may improve outcomes. Electrocautery or LASER (light amplification by stimulated emission of radiation) therapy may assist with debulking the tumour. Cryotherapy or external beam radiation and brachytherapy may be used to reduce airway obstruction.
Atelectasis	Alveolar collapse can occur as a result of lung cancer, either through compression of the lung parenchyma by tumour or fluid accumulation within the pleural cavity, or as a result of respiratory infection secondary to the lung cancer.	Depending on the cause, severity and location of the atelectasis, lung function may be improved by postural drainage, management of respiratory infections, incentive spirometry and management of the primary tumour where possible.
Bronchopleural fistula	A potentially life-threatening communication between the bronchial tree and the pleural space may develop as a result of lung cancer. A bronchopleural fistula will cause displacement of the mediastinum to the opposite side of the fistula because of the trapped air.	Management of a bronchopleural fistula may include a bronchoscopy to determine the location and severity of the fistula, and potentially the application of sealing compounds in an attempt to control the leak. A chest tube connected to an underwater sealed drain may be required to decrease the trapped air or empyema.
Dysphagia/ oesophageal obstruction	Difficulty swallowing may occur as a result of compression of the oesophagus from tumour growth.	Balloon dilation or the placement of an oesophageal stent may assist with dysphagia. Attempts to control the growth of the primary tumour also play an important part in the management plan.
Empyema/lung abscess	Cavitary lesions from lung cancer may become seeded with a pathogen and cause an inflammatory response. Purulent exudate is produced, which can result in either a collection that is loculated (abscess) or frank pus and infected pleural fluid within the pleural cavity. Empyema may also cause a bronchopleural fistula. Empyema is also commonly associated with bacterial pneumonia.	Antimicrobials are the most important treatment. A microscopy, culture and sensitivity test should be undertaken on the exudate to ensure the appropriateness of the antimicrobials selection. Depending on the size and severity of the empyema or abscess, video-assisted thoracoscopic surgery may be considered for mechanical removal or debridement of purulent material.

Table 29.6 Selected complications associated with lung cancer (*continued*)

Complication	Description/Mechanism	Management
Haemoptysis	Coughing up blood from the respiratory tract may occur as a result of the invasion of the tumour into superficial mucosa or the erosion of blood vessels. Lung cancer may also cause respiratory tract infections, which may result in haemoptysis.	There are really no management options for haemoptysis other than managing the cause, such as antimicrobials for bacterial respiratory infection or reducing the bronchogenic tumour size.
Horner's syndrome	A constellation of symptoms from sympathetic nerve damage to any of the nerve fibres that innervate the eye. The nerve fibres exit the spinal cord at T1 and T2. Lung cancer tumour growth in this region may cause compression, affecting any of the nerve pathways. The classic symptoms include partial ptosis, miosis and anhidrosis on the affected side.	Other than primary tumour control, there are no management options available.
Paraneoplastic syndromes	A collection of symptoms that occur remote from the primary tumour but are a direct result of the tumour itself. The chapter 'Neoplasia' explores paraneoplastic syndromes further. A variety of symptoms may develop, depending on the tissue involved. The clinical manifestations may occur as endocrine, haematological, cardiovascular, cutaneous, renal or musculoskeletal symptoms.	Management of the paraneoplastic syndrome depends on the location and presenting clinical manifestations. Ultimately, management of the primary tumour is important.
Pericardial effusion	A collection of extra fluid within the pericardial sac may develop as a result of the lung cancer or the treatment itself. Clinical manifestations can include chest pain, dyspnoea, tachycardia, tachypnoea, orthopnoea, cough, hypoxia and cardiac tamponade. Pericardial effusion is more common in late-stage disease.	Management of pericardial effusion may include pericardiocentesis, pericardotomy or pericardectomy.
Pleural effusion	A collection of extra fluid within the pleural space can develop secondary to lymphatic obstruction, pneumonia or congestive cardiac failure from the effects of lung cancer.	Depending on the severity of the effusion, the acuity of the affected person and the stage of disease, interventions may include placement of a thoracotomy tube, chemotherapy or talc pleurodesis (a procedure to obliterate the pleural space).
Pneumonia	Lung infections, such as viral and bacterial pneumonia, are closely associated with lung cancer and the treatment of lung cancer, such as chemotherapy. Mechanisms contributing to the development of pneumonia in the context of lung cancer may be related to immunocompromise, altered respiratory defences or some unknown cause. Some people with lung cancer may experience frequent and recurrent episodes of pneumonia.	Bacterial pneumonia may be treated with appropriate antimicrobials. Antiviral agents may be used in an attempt to manage viral pneumonia. If someone with viral pneumonia develops a secondary bacterial infection, appropriate antimicrobials will also be beneficial. Supportive care may be necessary, including supplemental oxygen, fluid support and rest promotion. Incentive spirometry and methods to improve pulmonary hygiene, such as physiotherapy, may also be necessary in the management of pneumonia.
Pneumonitis	An inflammation of the lung tissue is common in people with lung cancer who receive radiotherapy. Pneumonitis often develops between 1 and 6 months after the treatments have finished. Concomitant chemotherapy treatment can exacerbate the effects. Clinical manifestations of pneumonitis include chest pain, dyspnoea, fever and a cough.	The main treatment for inflammation is the administration of corticosteroids; however, pulmonary fibrosis will often develop and lead to a chronic reduction in lung function.

(*continued*)

Table 29.6 Selected complications associated with lung cancer (*continued*)

Complication	Description/Mechanism	Management
Pneumothorax	A collapsed portion of lung can develop as a result of lung cancer. The mechanisms contributing to this collapse may include the development of a bronchial obstruction, resulting in the formation of interstitial air, the rupture of a subpleural bleb or the development of necrotic parenchymal tissue.	The development of a pneumothorax can be an ominous sign and suggest late-stage disease. Management will depend on the clinical presentation, and may include thoracocentesis, placement of a chest tube connected to an underwater seal drain or Heimlich valve, or pleurodesis. Supportive care, such as supplemental oxygen, pain relief and methods to promote oxygenation, such as appropriate positioning, may also be necessary.
Pulmonary embolism (PE)/venous thromboembolism (VTE)	A potentially fatal blood clot in the pulmonary vasculature (PE) or a blood clot in another location that embolises (VTE) may develop as a result of lung cancer. Although the exact mechanism is unknown, people with lung cancer appear to be at greater risk of developing a PE or VTE if they have surgery, receive chemotherapy, have an adenocarcinoma-type lung cancer, high haemoglobin levels or are in late-stage disease.	Management options depend on the type of embolism (PE or VTE), the acuity of the affected person and their prognosis. A large PE may be immediately fatal. Otherwise embolectomy, anticoagulation and, potentially, thrombolysis may be attempted. PE or VTE may develop in a person with lung cancer despite the institution of prophylactic measures. Regardless of this, VTE and PE prophylaxis should be instituted in those with lung cancer.
Superior vena cava (SVC) syndrome	A potentially fatal obstruction of the superior vena cava by tumour invasion or compression will result in reduced venous return. A person with SVC syndrome will generally present with dyspnoea, cough, and oedema in the face or arm. Other symptoms may include chest pain, syncope, headache, dysphagia or altered level of consciousness.	Apart from primary tumour control, the most important management concern is surgical revascularisation of the superior vena cava.

SECONDARY LUNG CANCER

Secondary lung cancer forms as a neoplastic lesion in another body region that spreads to the lungs via the lymphatic or vascular systems. Some secondary lung cancers may develop by direct invasion from tissue neighbouring the lung, such as the chest wall, thyroid, oesophagus or thymus. The lungs are a common site of metastasis in breast, prostate, bladder, colon and some nervous tissue cancers. Metastatic cancer is distinguished from primary cancer by histological characteristics, genetic sequencing or immunohistochemical markers. In some cases, the site of the primary cancer is not discernible. This is known as *carcinoma of unknown primary*.

The clinical manifestations and diagnosis of secondary lung cancer are the same as for primary lung cancer. Unfortunately, the prognosis for secondary lung cancer is quite poor.

Pulmonary vascular conditions

Conditions associated with the pulmonary vasculature can be acute or chronic. They result in hypoxia and can be life-threatening. Three important conditions are pulmonary embolism, pulmonary oedema and pulmonary hypertension.

PULMONARY EMBOLISM

LEARNING OBJECTIVE 6

Discuss the mechanisms by which a pulmonary embolism may develop.

Aetiology and pathophysiology

A **pulmonary embolism (PE)** is an occlusion of a pulmonary artery, which prevents blood flow to lung parenchyma, and results in hypoxia, tissue damage and, in severe cases, death. A PE can be caused by either a thrombotic or a non-thrombotic event. The most common cause is related to thrombosis, often from a *deep vein thrombosis (DVT)*, also known as *venous thromboembolism (VTE)*.

Pulmonary embolism from a thrombotic cause VTE generally precedes PE (see the chapter 'Vascular disorders and circulatory shock'). In **Virchow's triad**, increased venous stasis, hypercoagulability and vessel injury increase the risks of thrombus formation. The same risk factors are associated with PE as those that contribute to VTE. Any condition that increases venous stasis, such as prolonged bed rest or sitting for long hours (e.g. long-haul flights or long-distance travel), will increase the risk of PE. Along with that, vessel wall injury (e.g. due to fracture or surgery), and increased coagulation (e.g. due to dehydration, **coagulopathy**, oral contraceptives, pregnancy or cancer) will increase the risk of VTE, and therefore PE.

When a thrombus has formed, it may dislodge and embolise. Once dislodged, an embolus will flow through the venous system to the right atrium, through the right ventricle and then into the pulmonary artery. The size of the thrombus dictates the point at which the occlusion will occur. Some clots may be large enough to occlude the main pulmonary artery. This is a life-threatening situation and can cause death within minutes. However, smaller thrombi lodge in the arterial vasculature more distally. In this situation, the person may experience pleuritic chest pain and some shortness of breath. Sometimes, people with PE might remain asymptomatic and never be diagnosed.

The effects of occlusion on the pulmonary arterial vasculature will vary depending on several factors. *Bronchospasm* may result from the local release of histamine, and *vasospasm* can arise from the local release of serotonin. *Hypoxaemia* can develop as a result of V/Q mismatch, as some areas may be well perfused but have poor ventilation as a result of atelectasis (as surfactant production is affected), and other areas may be adequately ventilated but have no perfusion (due to thrombus or vasospasm). Carbon dioxide levels may rise, as obstruction associated with the pulmonary vasculature increases dead space and can reduce end tidal carbon dioxide. In more serious cases of PE, cardiac output can be affected because hypoxaemia results in an increased cardiac workload due to increased pulmonary artery and right ventricular pressures. A sympathetic nervous system response to hypoxia will cause tachycardia and further exacerbate myocardial workload. As myocardial perfusion decreases, right ventricular and then left ventricular function diminishes. Hypotension will develop, and systemic perfusion is further decreased. Mortality from pulmonary embolism occurs as a result of circulatory failure.

Pulmonary embolism from a non-thrombotic cause Pulmonary arteries can also be occluded by the introduction of non-thrombotic emboli, such as fat particles, septic growths, tumour fragments, foreign bodies, amniotic fluid or even air bubbles.

Fat embolism Occasionally, when long bones fracture, bone marrow particles may enter the circulation and become lodged in the pulmonary vasculature. The pathophysiology of how a fat embolus causes a PE is not entirely understood. Direct mechanical obstruction may contribute to the condition. It has been proposed that free fatty acids (converted from triglycerides) cause a toxic reaction in the endothelium. This reaction results in the accumulation of inflammatory cells, and further contributes to the occlusion of the pulmonary artery. Neurological effects are very common in fat embolism, and may even be the first indication of a problem.

Septic growths Intravenous drug users are at risk of developing PE for a number of reasons. Bacterial endocarditis can develop in the right side of the heart (especially on the tricuspid valve) when pathogens from the skin are introduced into the circulatory system due to unhygienic techniques or reused needles. As the vegetations on the valve grow larger, the risk of them breaking off and travelling through the venous system to the right ventricle and then the pulmonary artery is increased. Often with endocarditis, multiple small emboli develop and cause numerous pulmonary insults and bacteraemia.

Septic thrombophlebitis may develop as a result of an infected skin injury that permits bacteria to enter the bloodstream. Interestingly, other causes of thrombophlebitis may result from contaminated vena caval filters used to prevent stroke in those with a high risk of thrombosis.

Tumour fragments Tumour cells may embolise and travel through the circulatory system. Adenocarcinomas from a number of different body sites are associated with tumour emboli. Once in the venous system, they can travel to the right side of the heart and then to the pulmonary artery. Tumour pulmonary emboli are often less acute medical situations, as the person may develop symptoms over days to weeks.

Foreign bodies As previously mentioned, intravenous drug users have an increased risk of PE. Apart from the risks associated with endocarditis, substances used to 'cut' the illicit drugs may also cause PE. Magnesium trisilicate (talc) is commonly used in street drugs as a filler to increase the drug volume. When injected intravenously, talc can travel to the pulmonary vasculature and cause parenchymal damage. Multiple small PE may cause pulmonary hypertension and chronic lung disease. Cotton fibres from swabs are also associated with intravenous drug use. Iatrogenic causes (caused by medical intervention) of foreign body emboli include pacemaker wires or pieces of a central venous catheter.

Amniotic fluid Fortunately, amniotic fluid emboli are not common. Occasionally, amniotic fluid debris (e.g. fetal cells, lanugo or meconium) may enter the maternal circulatory system and can result in maternal and/or fetal death. Although the mechanism of amniotic fluid emboli is not well understood, the effects are thought to be associated with an inflammatory, complement or anaphylactic response, as opposed to a purely mechanical obstruction.

Air bubbles Air may enter an individual's circulatory system as a result of chest trauma, during a diving accident or from iatrogenic causes. Chest trauma can cause injury to the great vessels, resulting in an air embolus, which can travel to the pulmonary artery. Diving accidents may result in barotrauma-induced tears to pulmonary parenchyma, which enables air to escape and travel to the pulmonary vasculature. Once there, air emboli may travel to the pulmonary artery and obstruct blood flow. Iatrogenic causes of air embolism include the accidental rapid injection of air during the intravenous administration of radiocontrast agents, during haemodialysis, or from any intravenous device. Other iatrogenic causes of air embolism include during surgery, fine-needle aspiration biopsy or through the use of positive pressure ventilation.

Epidemiology

Approximately 12,000 people are admitted with PE to Australian hospitals per year. In 2021, 371 people lost their lives to this condition, which accounts for 0.22% of all deaths. The mortality rate among males (52%) was slightly higher than that for females (48%). Notably, there has been a significant 4% shift in the gender distribution of PE cases over the past six years. Surprisingly, more males are now experiencing fatal outcomes from PE. Once diagnosed, and with treatment, chances of recovery are good.

Clinical manifestations

The clinical manifestations of PE can be divided into respiratory consequences and non-respiratory consequences. *Respiratory consequences* include dyspnoea and tachypnoea as a result of the hypoxia and V/Q defect. Pleuritic chest pain (i.e. sharp chest pain that increases with inspiration) is also commonly reported. Sometimes, individuals will experience haemoptysis as a result of pulmonary parenchymal trauma or necrosis.

The *non-respiratory consequences* of PE are often associated with more serious emboli. A sympathetic nervous system response to hypoxia will result in an increased heart rate, diaphoresis and anxiety. Worsening myocardial perfusion can cause syncope and ultimately disrupt blood pressure. Many people will experience low-grade fever; however, those with septic causes may develop significant temperatures. Figure 29.8 explores the common clinical manifestations and management of PE.

Diagnosis and management

Diagnosis

Collecting a full and comprehensive history can assist in identifying the risk factors associated with VTE and, ultimately, PE. Although several tools have been developed to assist with this assessment, recent evidence-based analysis suggests that they may be less reliably predictive than one would hope. Increased predictive efficacy may be achieved through the use of a combination of tools such as the *Wells Score* followed by the *Pulmonary Embolism Rule out Criteria (PERC)*. With the Wells Score, the addition of points for various criteria suggests a two-tier likelihood of pulmonary embolism (i.e. likely or unlikely). In the scenario of a person with typical symptoms but a low likelihood of PE, the PERC should be assessed. This assessment contains a number of criteria: age, heart rate, oxygen saturations, the presence of leg swelling, haemoptysis, a history of thrombosis or recent trauma/surgery, and consumption of exogenous oestrogen. Negative responses for all of the criteria suggest that the person does not have a pulmonary embolism, and therefore does not require any further investigation. A positive response for any of the criteria suggests the need for further testing, such as D-dimer. Although D-dimer does not diagnose PE, it is a marker of inflammation, and so a negative D-dimer result can exclude the likelihood of the presenting manifestations being caused by a PE. If the D-dimer result is positive, V/Q scans may be indicated. V/Q scans can clearly identify V/Q defects and confirm the diagnosis of PE. Some facilities may choose other imaging techniques, such as CT scans.

Management

The primary objectives for managing the care of someone with PE include reducing the risk of further clot formation. This can be achieved through the administration of anticoagulant agents, such as low molecular weight heparin or unfractionated heparin initially, and either the novel oral anticoagulants (NOACs) or the vitamin K antagonist, warfarin.

Other priorities include the support of oxygenation and blood pressure. Someone experiencing a PE may require supplemental oxygenation to manage the hypoxia, and circulatory system support is provided through the administration of intravenous fluids and vasopressor agents. Antipyretics may be given for fever, but are generally reserved for excessive fever (> 39°C). Simple analgesia may be used for the pleuritic chest pain; however, stronger agents may be required. In considering the latter option, it is important to recognise the risks of administering an opioid agent to a person with respiratory compromise. All care must be taken to prevent exacerbating the hypoxia associated with respiratory depression. Calm reassurance should be used to reduce the sympathetic nervous system effects of stress, which, if unaddressed, will ultimately aggravate the clinical situation.

If anticoagulation is contraindicated, the placement of an inferior or superior vena cava filter may be considered to reduce the risk of future PE. Depending on the capacity of the facility, if a clot is large, a decision may be made to remove it (embolectomy). Because mortality risks can be higher than 15%, a massive pulmonary embolism event with haemodynamic instability may require systemic intravenous thrombolysis (if no contraindication for thrombolysis exists).

PULMONARY OEDEMA

LEARNING OBJECTIVE 7

Explore the pathophysiology, diagnosis and management of pulmonary oedema.

Aetiology and pathophysiology

Pulmonary oedema is the accumulation of fluid within pulmonary interstitial spaces, and ultimately within the alveoli. This excess fluid occurs as a result of either an alteration to pressure within the pulmonary vessels, or changes in vascular permeability (see the chapter 'Fluid imbalances').

Two broad categories of pulmonary oedema exist: cardiogenic and non-cardiogenic. *Cardiogenic pulmonary oedema* is associated with left ventricular dysfunction from cardiovascular diseases, such as ischaemic heart disease, hypertension, dysrhythmia, myocardial infarction or valve disease. Cardiogenic pulmonary oedema results in left ventricular dysfunction, which causes increased atrial pressures. This pressure results in a pulmonary capillary pressure that exceeds the plasma oncotic pressure and forces fluid into the alveoli, interfering with gas exchange.

Common causes of *non-cardiogenic pulmonary oedema* include cardiopulmonary bypass surgery, prolonged exposure to high altitudes, eclampsia, brain trauma, drugs, PE and blocked lymphatic drainage.

Cardiopulmonary bypass surgery

Any surgery requiring the use of a cardiopulmonary bypass pump and the deflation of the lungs can induce pulmonary oedema. The trauma associated with reinflation, the effect of the surgery

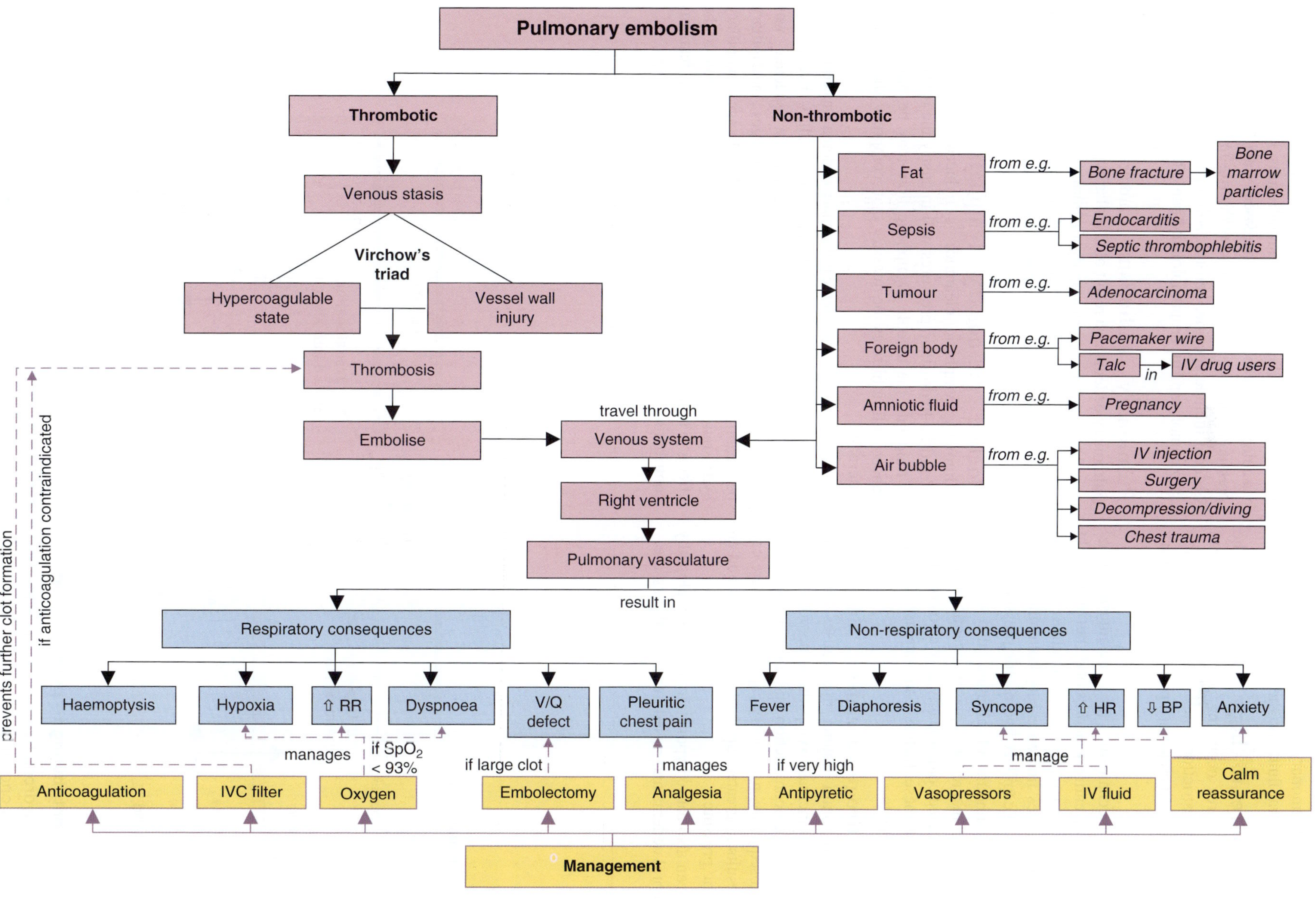

Figure 29.8

Clinical snapshot: Pulmonary embolism

↓ = decreased; ↑ = increased; BP = blood pressure; HR = heart rate; IV = intravenous; IVC = inferior vena cava; RR = respiration rate; SpO_2 = saturation of peripheral oxygen; V/Q = ventilation/perfusion.

on surfactant production, and periods of hypotension all contribute to increased pulmonary capillary permeability and the translocation of interstitial fluid into the alveoli.

Prolonged exposure to high altitudes The altered atmospheric pressures occurring at high altitude can result in pulmonary vasoconstriction, causing trauma, increasing hydrostatic pressure and increasing pulmonary capillary permeability.

Eclampsia The mechanism of eclampsia-related pulmonary oedema is not entirely understood, but is thought to involve a profound increase in sympathetic nervous system discharge that causes immense catecholamine release, hypertension and increased capillary hydrostatic pressure.

A reduction in the amount of albumin also occurs in eclampsia. This can result in a reduced plasma oncotic pressure. The presence of disseminated coagulopathy may also contribute to the condition. All of these factors can increase vascular permeability within the lungs.

Brain trauma (neurogenic cause) Although not completely understood, brain trauma that causes increased intracranial pressure can increase sympathetic nervous system discharge, resulting in vasoconstriction and an increase in left atrial pressure. Subsequently, pulmonary capillary pressure can increase, which results in greater capillary permeability and an elevated hydrostatic pressure.

Brain trauma can also cause hyponatraemic encephalopathy as a result of cerebral oedema and raised intracranial pressure.

Drugs Drug-induced pulmonary oedema is generally associated with cytotoxic damage to the endothelial cells of the pulmonary capillaries. This trauma results in both increased vascular permeability and increased capillary hydrostatic pressure. Some drugs associated with drug-induced pulmonary oedema include cocaine, heroin, radio-opaque contrast agents, salbutamol, aspirin, propranolol and penicillin.

Pulmonary embolism Chronic PE can induce pulmonary oedema as a result of alveolar hypoxia, which causes vasodilation, left ventricular dysfunction, increased left atrial pressures and right ventricular dilation. These changes increase both capillary permeability and hydrostatic pressures.

Blocked pulmonary lymphatic vessels If pulmonary lymphatic clearance is reduced, an increase in interstitial hydrostatic pressures will intensify the translocation of fluid into the alveoli. Lymphatic flow may be blocked by cancer cell infiltrates or masses that compress the vessels externally.

Traditionally, cardiogenic pulmonary oedema was considered to be primarily related to changes in capillary hydrostatic pressure, while non-cardiogenic pulmonary oedema was considered to be primarily related to changes in capillary permeability. More recently, it is believed that changes in capillary hydrostatic pressure and capillary permeability contribute to the effects in both forms. Figure 29.9 shows the various mechanisms contributing to pulmonary oedema.

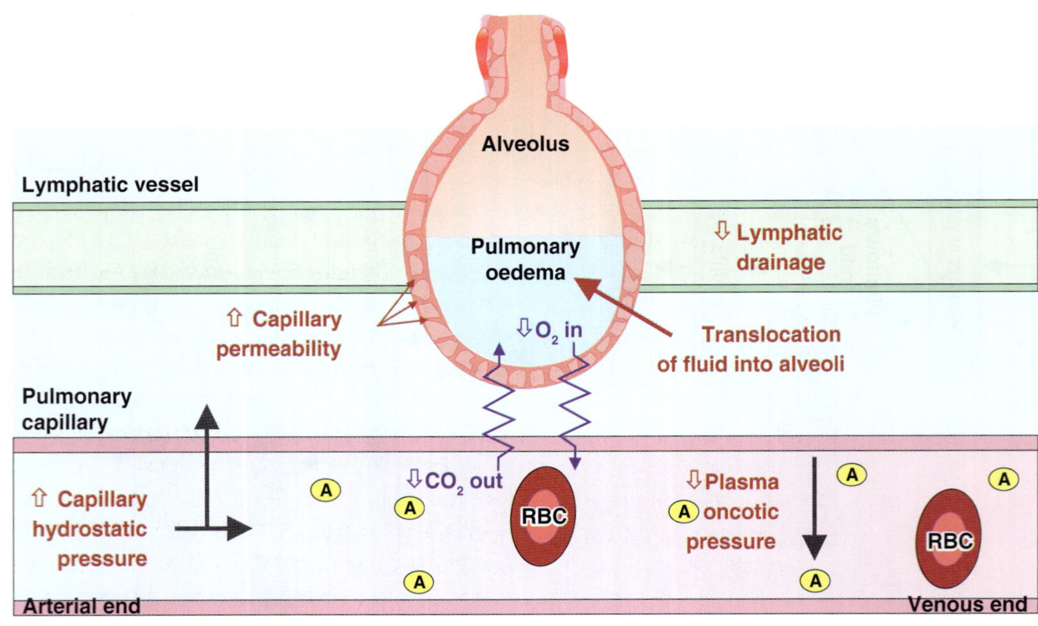

Figure 29.9

Various mechanisms contributing to pulmonary oedema

An increase in capillary hydrostatic pressure, an alteration in capillary permeability, a decrease in lymphatic drainage and a decrease in plasma oncotic pressure can, independently or in any combination, increase the amount of fluid within the alveoli, resulting in pulmonary oedema and altered gas exchange.

↓ = decreased; ↑ = increased; A = albumin; CO_2 = carbon dioxide; O_2 = oxygen; RBC = red blood cell.

Epidemiology

Approximately 570 people are admitted to Australian hospitals with pulmonary oedema each year, and, according to the Australian Bureau of Statistics, approximately 60 people die. Of all known causes, pulmonary oedema is most commonly associated with heart failure (see the chapter 'Cardiac muscle and valve disorders'). In Australia and New Zealand, the prevalence of heart failure is reported as occurring in 1–2% of the total population (although it is > 13% in the eighth decade of life), and it is estimated that most people with heart failure will experience at least one episode of pulmonary oedema. The risk is even greater in older population groups.

Clinical manifestations

The signs and symptoms associated with hypoxia will manifest in pulmonary oedema. This condition is life-threatening, and a significant number of people with heart failure will die as a result of pulmonary oedema. Extreme dyspnoea, tachycardia and tachypnoea will develop. Because of the immense sympathetic nervous system response to the hypoxia, a sense of impending doom may also be experienced by a person with pulmonary oedema. Often it is difficult to keep a person with pulmonary oedema sitting in one place, as they are so overwhelmed with the extreme dyspnoea that they become very agitated in an attempt to relieve it. If the degree of hypoxia increases, cyanosis may develop and the person may develop an altered level of consciousness. Other clinical manifestations include crackles on auscultation and the presence of pink, frothy sputum. Figure 29.10 explores the common clinical manifestations and management of pulmonary oedema.

Diagnosis and management

Diagnosis An assessment of pulmonary oedema should be undertaken quickly, as delays in treatment will increase mortality risk. An assessment of full blood count, electrolyte, urea and creatinine levels may be useful in confirming the presence of anaemia, electrolyte imbalance or organ failure, which are known to contribute to the development of signs and symptoms. If febrile, a blood culture may demonstrate the presence of sepsis. Arterial blood gases may be sampled and analysed to determine oxygenation, carbon dioxide and blood pH. A chest X-ray may be beneficial as well. However, it should be done without delay in the emergency department, as transport to the X-ray department could result in earlier fatigue and respiratory collapse. Respiratory auscultation will be beneficial in determining the presence of crepitation or wheezes. The collection of an appropriate medical and social history, and a current list of medications, may assist in the discovery of the cause.

Management The primary goal in the management of pulmonary oedema is improving oxygenation. The administration of supplemental oxygen may be required, and in severe cases intubation and mechanical ventilation may be indicated. A focus on reducing pulmonary capillary pressures and systemic vascular resistance can be achieved through the administration of vasodilators, such as the organic nitrate glyceryl trinitrate to reduce ventricular afterload, diuretics (e.g. the loop diuretic, furosemide) and morphine. Careful monitoring and titration of these agents is required so as not to cause profound hypotension. The use of inotropic agents (e.g. dopamine or dobutamine) may be required to increase myocardial contractility and support blood pressure. As the sympathetic nervous system response to hypoxia results in catecholamine release, an adrenaline surge can cause a sense of impending doom. Calm reassurance and the administration of morphine may assist in reducing anxiety.

In severe heart failure, critical interventions must be administered immediately, including sedation, chemical paralysis, emergency intubation and mechanical ventilation. It is preferable to undertake intubation and mechanical ventilation at an earlier stage in a more controlled environment; however, occasionally, a person may fatigue quickly, and profound respiratory compromise may develop abruptly. Ultimately, identification and management of the primary cause (e.g. coronary artery disease, hypertension, valve disease or cardiomyopathy) is critical to successful outcomes.

PULMONARY HYPERTENSION

LEARNING OBJECTIVE 8

Examine the causes and consequences of pulmonary hypertension.

Aetiology and pathophysiology

Pulmonary arterial hypertension (PAH) is defined as an increased blood pressure within the pulmonary arteries. For the sake of brevity, in clinical environments it is most commonly called **pulmonary hypertension (PH)**. Normal systolic pulmonary artery pressure is about 15–30 mmHg (mean pulmonary artery pressure, 6–16 mmHg). PH is defined as a systolic pulmonary artery pressure > 30 mmHg (or mean pulmonary artery pressure > 20 mmHg). Paradoxically, although the pulmonary vasculature receives higher flows than the systemic system, pulmonary resistance is lower because of the greater distensibility of the vessels and the potential for the recruitment of previously unused blood vessels. Figure 29.11 compares the pressures between the systemic and pulmonary systems.

Causes of PH can be divided into primary or secondary forms. *Primary pulmonary hypertension*, which is sometimes called *idiopathic PH*, has no known aetiology and is relatively uncommon. *Secondary PH* is a complication of another condition, and is common in many pulmonary and cardiac diseases. At the 5th World Symposium on Pulmonary Hypertension, the five-grouping system was modified to ensure clarity within the subgroups. Table 29.7 shows the current PH classification.

Although the mechanisms by which PH occurs differ depending on the original cause, the common pathophysiological mechanisms include endothelial dysfunction leading to constriction, hypertrophy and vascular wall remodelling of the pulmonary arteries. It is now accepted that, irrespective of the cause, a degree of inflammation and thrombosis always occurs. These changes result in increased pulmonary vascular resistance and, therefore, increased pressure.

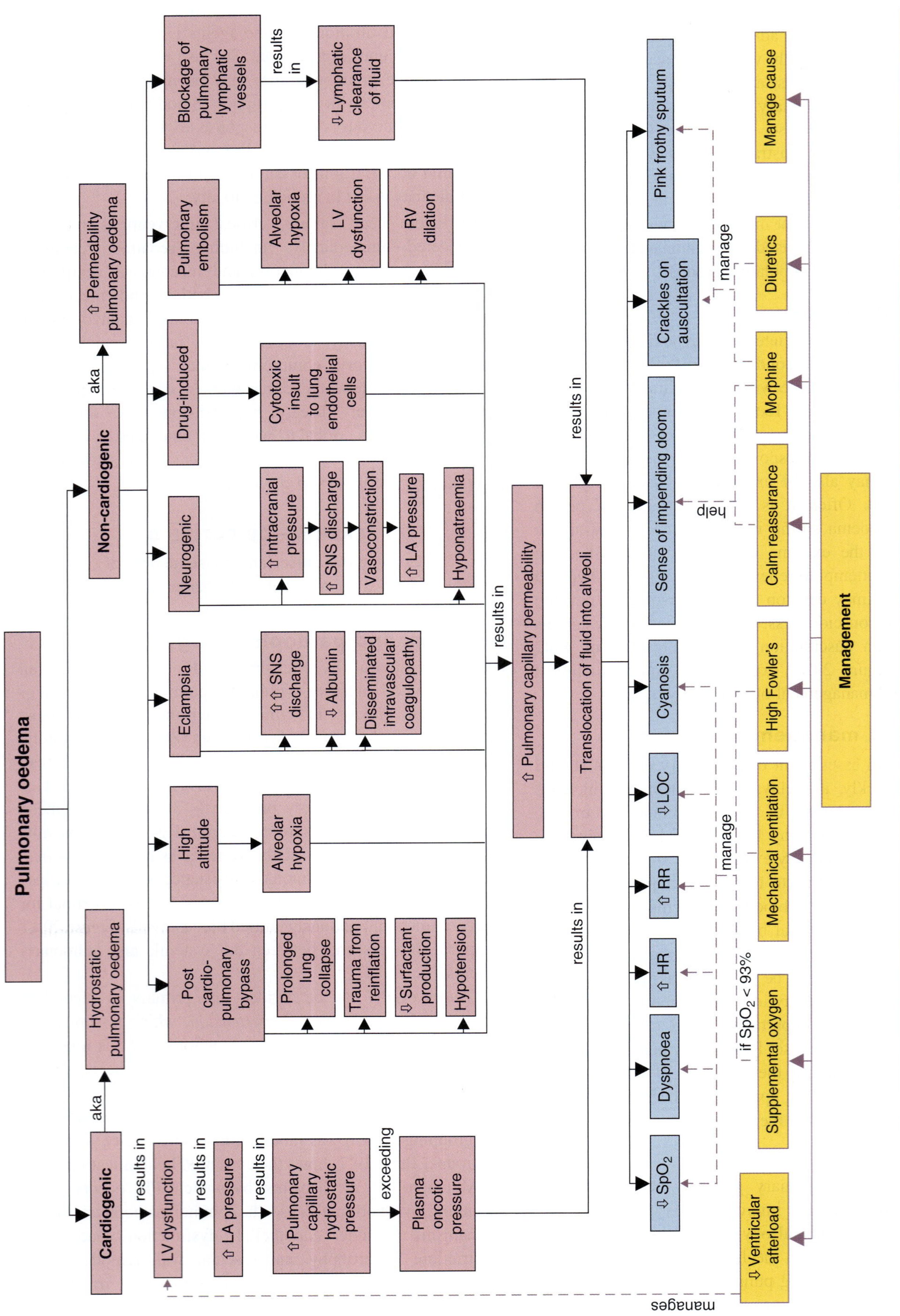

Figure 29.10

Clinical snapshot: Pulmonary oedema

↓ = decreased; ↑ = increased; aka = also known as; HR = heart rate; LA = left atrial; LOC = level of consciousness; LV = left ventricular; RR = respiration rate; RV = right ventricular; SNS = sympathetic nervous system; SpO_2 = saturation of peripheral oxygen.

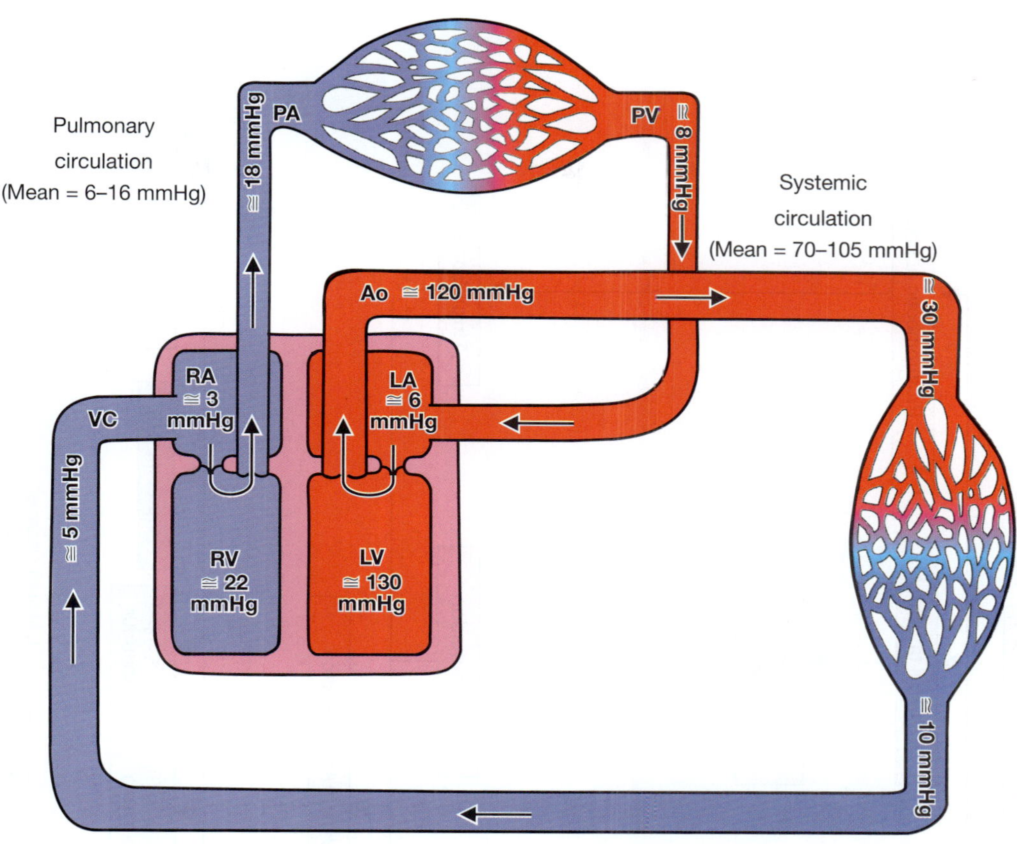

Figure 29.11

Comparison of pressures between systemic and pulmonary systems

The mean pulmonary arterial pressure range is 6–16 mmHg, whereas the mean systemic arterial blood pressure range is 70–105 mmHg.

Ao = aortic;
LA = left atrial;
LV = left ventricular;
PA = pulmonary artery;
PV = pulmonary vein;
RA = right atrial;
RV = right ventricular;
VC = vena cava.

Table 29.7 Classification of pulmonary hypertension (PH)

Group	Type
1	Pulmonary arterial hypertension (PAH)
2	Pulmonary hypertension associated with left heart disease
3	Pulmonary hypertension associated with lung disease and/or hypoxia
4	Pulmonary hypertension associated with pulmonary artery obstructions
5	Pulmonary hypertension with unclear and/or multifactorial mechanisms

Source: Data from Humbert et al. (2022), Table 6, p. 3638.

In *PH caused by left heart disease*, the excessive pressure is transmitted back towards the right side of the heart, resulting in a vasoconstrictive reflex, which ultimately causes endothelial dysfunction and vessel wall changes.

In *PH caused by lung disease*, hypoxic vasoconstriction is a major contributing factor to the vascular changes. Other influencing elements include mechanical stress from hyperinflated lungs, and possible inflammatory and cytotoxic effects from cigarette smoke.

In *PH caused by thromboembolism*, the obstruction of the pulmonary arteries influences the pressure and promotes a procoagulant environment. This condition may be further exacerbated by platelet anomalies, resulting in the increased pulmonary vascular resistance and subsequent PH.

Clinical manifestations

PH is more common in children than in adults. The most common clinical manifestation of PH is dyspnoea. In the early stages of disease, dyspnoea is exertional. However, as the individual's condition deteriorates, end-stage PH will cause shortness of breath even at rest. Other signs and symptoms include an increased heart rate and respiratory rate as a compensatory response to hypoxia. Some people may report pre-syncope and chest pain. A deconditioning towards physical activity and exercise develops, which can exacerbate the symptoms. As the individual's condition deteriorates, signs of right-sided heart failure and then left-sided heart failure will develop (see the chapter 'Cardiac muscle and valve disorders').

Any condition that interferes with the ability to breathe can affect mental health and result in anxiety and depression. Other issues include peripheral oedema, hepatomegaly and an elevated jugular venous pressure. The pressure-induced changes to the right side of the heart can heighten a tricuspid murmur and S3 heart sound. People with PH must have their condition actively managed, as those who do not receive treatment are unlikely to survive more than a few years. Figure 29.12 explores the common clinical manifestations and management of PH.

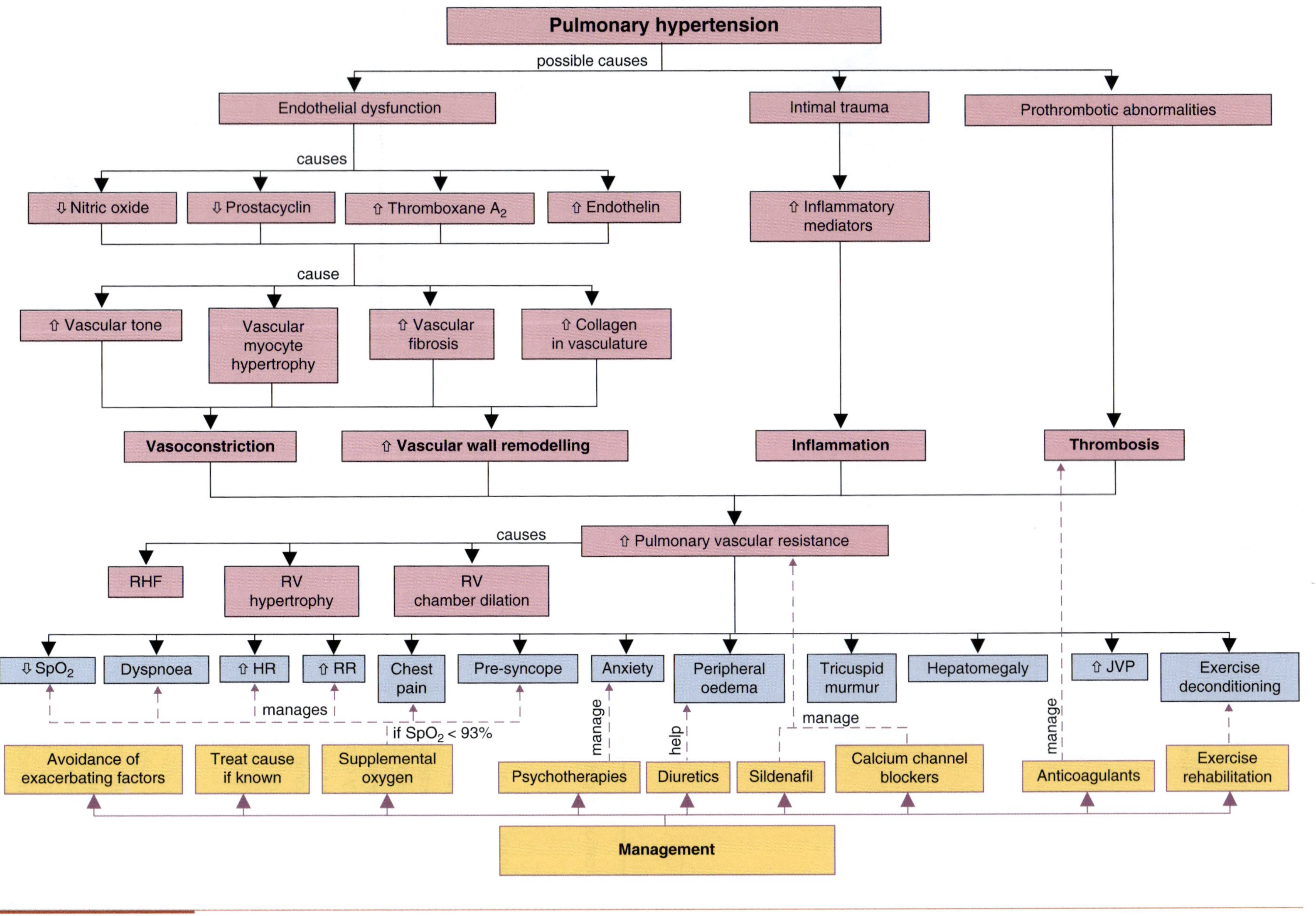

Figure 29.12

Clinical snapshot: Pulmonary hypertension

↓ = decreased; ↑ = increased; HR = heart rate; JVP = jugular venous pressure; RHF = right-sided heart failure; RR = respiration rate; RV = right ventricular; SpO_2 = saturation of peripheral oxygen.

Diagnosis and management

Diagnosis A systematic assessment to determine the presence and the possible cause of PH begins with a consideration of the history, a physical assessment and clinical manifestations observed. If the initial assessment is suggestive of PH, further investigation is warranted to determine whether the cause is cardiac or respiratory in origin. An electrocardiogram (ECG), chest X-ray, transthoracic echocardiography or respiratory function tests may be used to establish the cause. If a thromboembolic component is considered, a V/Q scan is indicated. Other investigations that may be beneficial include a full blood count, electrolyte levels, liver function test and coagulation profile to determine the presence of anaemia, chronic haemolysis, liver pathology or coagulopathy. An investigation for human immunodeficiency virus (HIV) and an antibody test for schistosomiasis may be valuable, as either of these infections can contribute to PH. An abdominal ultrasound may also help to exclude or reveal cirrhosis and portal hypertension as contributing factors.

Management Although PH is relatively uncommon, and there is little current treatment available to manage it, the consequences of PH exacerbation can be death. New drugs are being developed and released, so perhaps future interventions may offer more successful management.

As hypoxia is the most likely cause of tachycardia, tachypnoea, chest pain and pre-syncope, the administration of oxygen may assist in the management of these manifestations. Calm reassurance and assistance with organising mental health support are very important in the management of someone with PH. Education about avoiding exacerbating factors, such as cigarette smoking and consumption of vasoconstricting agents (e.g. caffeine, some anti-migraine agents and catecholamines), is essential.

Diuretics (e.g. the loop diuretic furosemide) can be used to treat peripheral oedema, hepatomegaly, increased jugular venous pressure and tricuspid murmur. Anticoagulants and antiplatelet agents are necessary to reduce the hypercoagulable state. Vasodilators, such as the calcium channel blockers and sildenafil, can be used to manage the increased peripheral resistance. Exercise deconditioning can be managed using the development of an individually tailored exercise rehabilitation program from an appropriately qualified exercise health professional, such as a physiotherapist or an exercise scientist.

INDIGENOUS HEALTH FAST FACTS AND CULTURAL CONSIDERATIONS

FAST FACTS

- *Aboriginal and Torres Strait Islander peoples are 3.1 times more likely than non-Indigenous Australians to be hospitalised for pneumonia.*
- *Aboriginal and Torres Strait Islander peoples are 2.7 times more likely than non-Indigenous Australians to smoke cigarettes on a daily basis.*
- *Aboriginal and Torres Strait Islander peoples are 2–3 times more likely than non-Indigenous Australians be hospitalised with lung cancer, and 1.7 times more likely to die from it.*
- *Aboriginal and Torres Strait Islander peoples are 11.3 times more likely than non-Indigenous Australians to develop tuberculosis.*
- *Māori children are 3.3 times more likely, and Pacific Islands children 4.8 times more likely, than European New Zealander children to die from pneumonia.*
- *Māori women are 3.8 times more likely and men 3 times more likely than European New Zealander women to develop lung cancer.*
- *Pacific Islands men are more likely than European New Zealander men, but less likely than Māori men, to die of lung cancer.*
- *Pacific Islands women are more likely than non-Pacific Islands women to die of lung cancer.*

CULTURAL CONSIDERATIONS

- *Smoking is strongly linked to lung cancer risk, with a smoker over 20 times more likely than a non-smoker to develop lung cancer. Many studies have reviewed attitudes and beliefs about smoking in Aboriginal and Torres Strait Islander communities, and have found that there are strong influences in smoking behaviours, such as stress relief, the importance of reinforcing relationships by sharing tobacco, and the effect of maintaining social cohesion and strengthening kinships through the communal act. Other reasons suggested for smoking include habit, relief of boredom or as an aid for weight loss. A strong influence in relation to young people adopting the behaviour is associated with the desire to look older or 'tough'. These factors can complicate the process of assisting people to change their behaviours and attributes to smoking cigarettes, and must be considered when designing culturally appropriate primary health programmes.*

Sources: Data from Australian Health Ministers' Advisory Council (2017); Australian Indigenous HealthInfoNet (2017); Greenhalgh et al. (2022); New Zealand Ministry of Health (2017b).

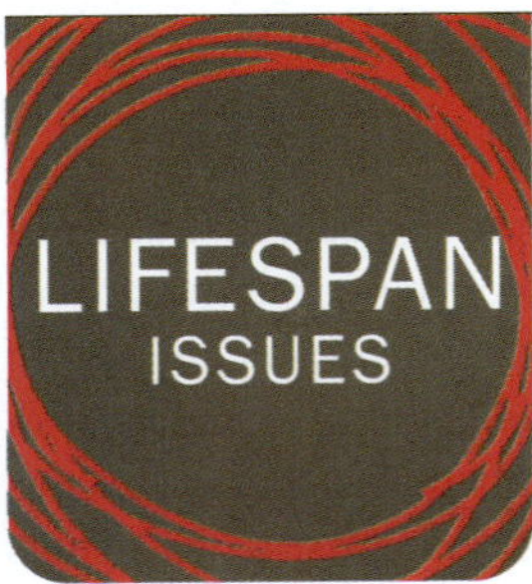

CHILDREN AND ADOLESCENTS

- In developing countries, childhood mortality statistics for pneumonia can be as high as 33%, because of malnutrition and the lack of access to immunisation programs and clean running water, as well as exposure to indoor pollution from the burning of solid fuels, such as wood and charcoal for cooking.
- Although pulmonary hypertension is rare, it is more common in children than in adults.
- Children living at high altitudes may develop pulmonary oedema as a result of the high altitude, especially if they also have chronic cardiopulmonary abnormalities, such as pulmonary hypertension.
- Primary lung cancer in children is less common than in adults, with the most common forms being carcinoid tumours and pleuropulmonary blastomas. Secondary lung cancer in children is more common than primary lung cancer.

OLDER ADULTS

- Almost two-thirds of people diagnosed with lung cancer are over 65 years of age.
- Older adults are more likely to develop secondary pulmonary hypertension than primary idiopathic pulmonary hypertension.
- Age-related changes of the cardiopulmonary system and cardiac failure significantly increase the risk of pulmonary oedema in adults older than 65 years of age.
- Residents living in an aged-care facility are 10 times more likely to develop pneumonia and 30 times more likely to be admitted to hospital than an older person living in their own home.
- Pneumonia-related mortality accounts for one-third to almost one-half of all deaths in residents of aged-care facilities in Australia.

KEY CLINICAL ISSUES

- Most respiratory conditions require similar management in order to improve oxygenation. Management strategies include appropriate positioning, administration of supplemental oxygen and bronchodilators (where appropriate).
- Healthcare workers are at significant risk of becoming infected through droplet or contact transmission with respiratory pathogens. Frequent hand-washing, appropriate infection control mechanisms and keeping vaccinations up to date will decrease the risk of succumbing to infection.
- In children, respiratory infections can increase the risk of airway obstruction.
- Neonates and children with respiratory compromise can fatigue quickly. Frequent observations for work of breathing and oxygenation can reduce the risk of rapid deterioration to respiratory arrest.
- Encouraging parents to maintain up-to-date vaccinations and documentation will not only protect the child, but will also ease the burden associated with proving vaccination status to qualify for support, government incentives and admission into educational facilities.
- The prevention of aspiration pneumonia is critical to reduce mortality in older people.
- Pneumonia severity scales enable a quantification of the risk of mortality associated with this condition.
- Care of a person with tuberculosis requires the appropriate environmental controls, such as negative-pressure rooms, and the provision of equipment, such as highly efficient filtering masks.
- Antimicrobial medication adherence is critical in order to prevent further development of multidrug-resistant strains of tuberculosis.
- Mortality rates for lung cancer are very poor, despite advances in knowledge regarding cancer development and immunotherapy. Adequate pain control should be provided, and the need for palliative care should be identified and instituted quickly. Assistance with psychosocial needs is imperative for those receiving end-of-life care.
- Pulmonary oedema requires urgent attention. A knowledge of the mechanism of its development, clinical manifestations and treatment can significantly reduce the risk of death.

CHAPTER REVIEW

- Respiratory infections are classified as upper and lower according to the anatomical relationship to the vocal folds. An *upper respiratory tract infection* can quickly spread to involve the lower respiratory tract. The most common pathogens associated with these infections are viruses and bacteria.
- *Bronchiolitis* is a common *lower respiratory tract infection*, particularly in young children. The common causative agent is the respiratory syncytial virus. The condition is highly contagious.
- A number of respiratory infections are *preventable by vaccination*, including tuberculosis, *Haemophilus influenzae* type b meningitis, influenza, pertussis, legionellosis and diphtheria. They are *notifiable conditions* that require reporting to the federal government.

- *Pneumonia* is a clinically important respiratory condition. It may be caused by an infectious agent, such as bacteria, viruses or fungi, but can also be induced by non-infectious means (e.g. aspiration of an irritating substance, such as gastric juice).
- *Pneumonia*, as an infection, can be classified by the pattern of lung involvement, the setting in which it was acquired and the causative microorganism involved. An effective assessment of the severity of the condition can result in better management.
- *Tuberculosis* is a clinically important infection commonly associated with *Mycobacterium tuberculosis*. Transmission is via the respiratory system. The infection can remain dormant in affected people, becoming active if the person becomes immunocompromised. Immunodeficiency is associated with the long-term use of corticosteroids, smoking, chemotherapy, malnutrition, diabetes mellitus, renal failure, HIV/AIDS and sepsis.
- *Lung cancer* is a common cause of death in men and women. Cigarette smoking is considered a major cause of the condition. Lung cancer is initially classified into two types based on histological characteristics: *small cell lung cancer* and *non-small cell lung cancer*.
- The complications associated with lung cancer can include metabolic, paraneoplastic, endocrine, haematological, neurological and renal effects. The lungs are a common site of metastasis in breast, prostate, bladder, colon and some nervous tissue cancer.
- A *pulmonary embolism* is an occlusion of a pulmonary artery preventing blood flow to lung parenchyma, resulting in hypoxia, tissue damage and, in severe cases, death. The condition can be caused by either a thrombotic or a non-thrombotic event. The most common cause is related to *thromboembolism*, often from a deep vein thrombosis. *Non-thrombotic emboli* have a variety of causes, including fat particles, septic growths, tumour fragments, foreign bodies, amniotic fluid or even air bubbles.
- *Pulmonary oedema* is the accumulation of fluid within pulmonary interstitial spaces, and ultimately within the alveoli. This excess fluid occurs as a result of either alteration to pressure within the pulmonary vessels or from changes in vascular permeability. Pulmonary oedema is categorised as either cardiogenic or non-cardiogenic. *Cardiogenic pulmonary oedema* is associated with left ventricular dysfunction from cardiovascular diseases. *Non-cardiogenic pulmonary oedema* can be associated with a variety of causes, such as cardiopulmonary bypass surgery, prolonged exposure to high altitudes, eclampsia, brain trauma, drugs, pulmonary embolism and blocked lymphatic drainage.
- *Pulmonary hypertension* is defined as an increased blood pressure within the pulmonary arteries. Pulmonary hypertension can be divided into primary or secondary forms. *Primary pulmonary hypertension*, sometimes called *idiopathic pulmonary hypertension*, has no known aetiology and is relatively uncommon. *Secondary pulmonary hypertension* is a complication of another condition and is common in many pulmonary and cardiac diseases. The most common clinical manifestation of pulmonary hypertension is *dyspnoea*.

REVIEW QUESTIONS

1. Compare and contrast the characteristics of upper and lower respiratory tract infections.
2. Describe how the failure of respiratory defences contributes to the development of pneumonia. List six factors that increase the risk of pneumonia.
3. Distinguish between the following types of pneumonia:
   a. lobar pneumonia and bronchopneumonia
   b. community-acquired and hospital-acquired pneumonia
   c. opportunistic and aspiration pneumonia
4. Briefly describe the pathophysiology of tuberculosis.
5. Within our community, who is at particular risk of developing tuberculosis, and why?
6. Compare and contrast the characteristics of the two types of lung cancer.
7. Describe three complications associated with lung cancer.
8. Which cancers commonly induce secondary lung cancer?
9. Describe the mechanisms by which a pulmonary thromboembolism develops.
10. List two types of non-thrombotic pulmonary embolism, and briefly describe the mechanism of development.
11. Briefly describe the pathophysiology of pulmonary oedema. From a clinical point of view, what is the main goal of management?
12. Outline the management of pulmonary hypertension.

HEALTH PROFESSIONAL CONNECTIONS

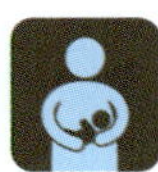

Midwives Pregnancy increases the risk of venous thromboembolism by up to 35 times that of a non-pregnant woman. Pulmonary embolism is one of the largest threats to a pregnant woman. All three elements of Virchow's triad are altered as a result of pregnancy. Venous stasis is exacerbated by hormone-associated venodilation, and, as the fetus gets larger, by compression of the pelvic vessels and the left iliac vein. Vessel damage occurs as a result of venous compression from the gravid uterus and from the trauma of delivery. Hypercoagulability is influenced by procoagulant changes occurring in pregnancy, such as reduced protein S, increased protein C and thrombin. Midwives should understand the significance, risk factors, mechanism, diagnostic challenges and management options available to a pregnant woman with suspected pulmonary embolism. Prevention of this potentially fatal complication of pregnancy can be achieved through thorough risk assessment, observation, consultation and appropriate management of a pregnant woman.

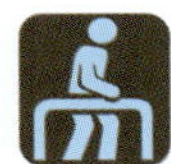

Physiotherapists Physiotherapists play an integral role in the promotion of improved oxygenation, optimising pulmonary mechanics, movement of respiratory secretion and airway clearance for people with lower respiratory tract infections. Important techniques that may be employed to assist with symptoms of lower respiratory tract infection may include use of oscillatory positive expiratory pressure devices and autogenic drainage. Encouraging increased hydration, cough assist and deep breathing exercises can also improve sputum clearance and pulmonary hygiene. Infection control practices and awareness of the dangers of droplet transmission of respiratory tract pathogens should be foremost in a physiotherapist's mind so that maximal protection is taken against contracting the infection oneself or transmitting the infection to other people.

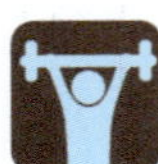

Exercise scientists Upper respiratory tract infections are common in athletes with heavy training programs because of the immune-modifying effects of exercise. Although moderate exercise has been associated with stimulation of the immune system, heavy exercise increases oxidative stress, inflammation and post-exercise immune system inhibition. Exercise professionals also need to consider the effect that age and gender can have on the immune system function of those they are working with. Respiratory tract infections can compromise oxygenation, induce fever states, increase metabolic demand, and cause fatigue and malaise. Appropriate exercise training programs, education and guidance for athletes to promote health and reduce illness are critical in ensuring that respiratory tract infections do not impair exercise goals or sporting achievements.

Nutritionists/Dieticians Challenges to promote appropriate and adequate nutrition in those with respiratory compromise can complicate a nutrition professional's role. Age-specific needs should be considered, especially regarding the influence of infection and hypoxia on the metabolic needs of neonates and infants. Although breastfeeding provides the best immune system support, the energy demands required for suckling may be more than an infant with respiratory compromise can sustain. Preterm babies are also at risk because of the difficulties in coordinating the need to suck, breath and swallow. Enteral feeding of expressed breast milk may be necessary. Increased work of breathing will significantly increase caloric requirements, and glucose infusions or supplemental nutrition may be required to reduce the risk of hypoglycaemia and failure to thrive. Insensible water loss from increased respiratory rates may also affect hydration status. A neonate's maturation, weight, age, activity, thermal environment and nature of feeding should be considered in determining appropriate caloric needs. Ill babies may require up to 90–125 calories/kg/day, depending on the presence of stress from infection. Extra proteins, vitamins and trace elements may be necessary to provide support in babies with respiratory tract infections.

CASE STUDY

Miss Jacqui Dignan (UR number 848426) is 32 days old. She is 'twin two' and weighs 2.2 kg. She and her sister were born at 37 weeks' gestation. After their birth, Jacqui and her sister were discharged on day 9, and have been home for almost three weeks. Mrs Dignan brought Jacqui into the children's emergency department with episodes of cyanosis and apnoea. Although the other twin is unwell, too, Jacqui's apnoeic and cyanotic episodes scared her parents. Jacqui's father was at home with twin one and their 4-year-old sister. After assessing Jacqui and suspecting respiratory syncytial virus (RSV) bronchiolitis, the medical team asked Mrs Dignan to call her husband to bring the other twin in for assessment. Jacqui's observations are as follows:

Temperature	Heart rate	Respiration rate	Blood pressure	SpO_2
34.3°C	171	64	89/67	94% (RA*)

*RA = room air.

Jacqui's respiratory function was extremely compromised on arrival to the emergency department. She had tachypnoea, head bobbing and evidence of the use of accessory muscles of respiration. She also had rhinorrhoea and bilateral crackles. Her chest X-ray showed increased perihilar lung markings. Her blood glucose level was 6.3 mmol/L. During the assessment she had an episode of apnoea, and was intubated and mechanically ventilated on a respiratory rate of 25 breaths per minute, a tidal volume of 14 mL and oxygen of 45%. Her peak inspiratory pressures were approximately 17 cm H_2O. She was transferred to the intensive care unit. An intravenous (IV) line and an intra-arterial line (IAL) were inserted, and blood was taken for pathology testing.

HAEMATOLOGY

Patient location:	PICU	**UR:**	848426		
Consultant:	Johns	**NAME:**	Dignan		
		Given name:	Jacqui	**Sex:**	F
		DOB:	35/XX/XX	**Age:**	32 d
Time collected	07:30				
Date collected	XX/XX				
Year	XXXX				
Lab #	3456544				

FULL BLOOD COUNT		UNITS	REFERENCE RANGE
Haemoglobin	101	g/L	115–160
White cell count	7.8	$\times 10^9$/L	4.0–11.0
Platelets	515	$\times 10^9$/L	140–400
Haematocrit	0.28		0.33–0.47
Red cell count	3.08	$\times 10^{12}$/L	3.80–5.20
Reticulocyte count	1.5	%	0.2–2.0
MCV	93	fL	80–100

BIOCHEMISTRY

Patient location:	PICU	**UR:**	848426		
Consultant:	Johns	**NAME:**	Dignan		
		Given name:	Jacqui	**Sex:**	F
		DOB:	16/XX/XX	**Age:**	32 d
Time collected	07:30	07:35			
Date collected	XX/XX	XX/XX			
Year	XXXX	XXXX			
Lab #	3456546	3456558			

ELECTROLYTES		UNITS	REFERENCE RANGE
Sodium	135	mmol/L	135–145
Potassium	4.1	mmol/L	3.5–5.2
Chloride	107	mmol/L	95–110
Calcium (total)	2.5	mmol/L	2.1–2.6
Magnesium	0.9	mmol/L	0.7–1.0
Glucose (random)	6.4	mmol/L	3.5–7.7
RENAL FUNCTION			
Urea	2.9	mmol/L	3.0–8.5
Creatinine	31	μmol/L	60–110
ARTERIAL BLOOD GAS			
pH	7.28		7.35–7.45
PaO_2	64	mmHg	80–100
$PaCO_2$	51	mmHg	35–45
Bicarbonate	24	mEq/L	22–32

Jacqui had a nasopharyngeal aspirate sent to pathology for microscopy, culture and sensitivity testing. She was also administered the cephalosporin antimicrobial cefotaxime, in case there was a bacterial component to her respiratory compromise or the provisional diagnosis was incorrect.

A nasogastric tube was inserted and feeds were commenced. She also had a 10% glucose infusion running. Thermoregulation was achieved by an overhead heater and a temperature-controlled mattress. A diagnosis of respiratory syncytial virus (RSV) was later confirmed.

CRITICAL THINKING

1. What risk factors does Jacqui have for the development of bronchiolitis from an RSV infection? List them all, and explain how each factor contributes to an increased risk.
2. Analyse Jacqui's observations. Are these physical assessments within the acceptable ranges for a child of her age? Explain.
3. Jacqui had many signs of respiratory compromise. List these, and explain the mechanism contributing to each sign.
4. Make a list of all of Jacqui's signs and symptoms. In a second column, list the interventions and treatments identified in the case study. Attempt to associate the intervention or treatment with the sign or symptom.
5. Jacqui had a nasopharyngeal aspirate. What is this, and why was it sent for microscopy, culture and sensitivity testing? Would this identify the pathogen causing a viral infection?
6. Jacqui was commenced on the cephalosporin antimicrobial cefotaxime. Would this manage the RSV? Explain.

BIBLIOGRAPHY

Asthma and Respiratory Foundation NZ (2023). *Key statistic: respiratory disease in New Zealand.* Wellington: Asthma and Respiratory Foundation NZ. https://www.asthmafoundation.org.nz/research/key-statistics.

Australian Bureau of Statistics (ABS) (2022a). *Causes of death, Australia, 2021.* Canberra: ABS. https://www.abs.gov.au/statistics/health/causes-death/causes-death-australia/latest-release#data-downloads.

Australian Bureau of Statistics (ABS) (2022b). *Insights into Australian smokers, 2021–22. Snapshot of smoking in Australia.* Canberra: ABS. https://www.abs.gov.au/articles/insights-australian-smokers-2021-22.

Australian Health Ministers' Advisory Council (2023). *Aboriginal and Torres Strait Islander Health Performance Framework 2023 report*. Canberra: Australian Government Department of Health. https://www.indigenoushpf.gov.au/.

Australian Health Ministers' Advisory Council's National and Aboriginal and Torres Strait Islander Health Standing Committee (2017). *Cultural respect framework 2016–2026: for Aboriginal and Torres Strait Islander health—a national approach to building a culturally respectful health system*. Canberra: Australian Government Department of Health. https://nacchocommunique.files.wordpress.com/2016/12/cultural_respect_framework_1december2016_1.pdf.

Australian Institute of Health and Welfare (AIHW) (2022a). *Australia's health, 2022. Data insights.* Australia's Health series No. 18. Cat. No. AUS 240. Canberra: AIHW. https://www.aihw.gov.au/getmedia/c91a05ef-307f-4c18-8ed3-dfe33d0c603d/aihw-aus-240.pdf.aspx?inline=true.

Australian Institute of Health and Welfare (AIHW) (2022b). *Cancer in Australia, 2021*. Cancer series No. 133. Cat. No. CAN 122. Canberra: AIHW. https://www.aihw.gov.au/reports/cancer/cancer-in-australia-2021/summary.

Australian Institute of Health and Welfare (AIHW) (2022c). *Principal diagnosis data cubes: separation statistics by principal diagnosis (ICD-10-AM 11th edition), Australia, 2020–21.* Canberra: AIHW. https://www.aihw.gov.au/reports/hospitals/principal-diagnosis-data-cubes/contents/data-cubes.

Bauldoff, G., Gubrud-Howe, P.M., Carno, M.-A., Levett-Jones, T., Hales, M., Berry, K.,... LeMone, P. (2020). *LeMone and Burke's medical–surgical nursing: critical thinking for person-centred care* (4th [Australian] edn). Sydney: Pearson Australia.

Best, O. & Fredericks, B. (2022). *Yatdjuligin: Aboriginal and Torres Strait Islander nursing and midwifery care* (3rd edn). Port Melbourne, VIC: Cambridge University Press.

Bullock, S. & Manias, E. (2022). *Fundamentals of pharmacology* (9th edn). Sydney: Pearson Australia.

Department of Health and Aged Care (2022). *Tuberculosis (TB)*. Canberra: Department of Health. https://www.health.gov.au/diseases/tuberculosis-tb.

Department of Health and Aged Care (2023). *Influenza*. National Notifiable Disease Surveillance System. Canberra: Department of Health. https://www.health.gov.au/diseases/influenza-flu.

Geran, A.R. (2023). Pathophysiology of cardiogenic pulmonary edema. *UpToDate*. https://www.medilib.ir/uptodate/show/3487.

Greenhalgh, E., Scollo, M. & Winstanley, M. (2022). Prevalence of tobacco use among Aboriginal peoples and Torres Strait Islanders. https://www.tobaccoinaustralia.org.au/chapter-1-prevalence/1-9-prevalence-of-tobacco-use-among-aboriginal-peo.

Humbert, M., Kovacs, G., Hoeper, M.M., Badagliacca, R., Berger, R.M.F., Brida, M.,... ESC/ERS Scientific Document Group (2022). 2022 ESC/ERS Guidelines for the diagnosis and treatment of pulmonary hypertension. *European Heart Journal* 43(38), 3618–3731. https://doi.org/10.1093/eurheartj/ehac237.

International Association for the Study of Lung Cancer (IASLC) (2016). *Staging manual in thoracic oncology* (2nd edn). North Fort Myers, FL: Editorial Rx Press. https://www.iaslc.org/research-education/publications-resources-guidelines/staging-manual-thoracic-oncology-2nd-edition.

Maraqa, N.F. (2021). Bronchiolitis. *Emedicine*. https://emedicine.medscape.com/article/961963-overview.

Meneghetti, A. (2020). Upper respiratory tract infection clinical presentation. *Emedicine*. https://emedicine.medscape.com/article/302460-clinical.

Naik, T.K. & Soo Hoo, G.W. (2020). Neurogenic pulmonary edema. *Emedicine*. https://emedicine.medscape.com/article/300813-overview.

New Zealand Ministry of Health (2022). *Births and deaths: year ended September 2022.* Wellington: Ministry of Health. https://www.stats.govt.nz/information-releases/births-and-deaths-year-ended-september-2022/.

New Zealand Ministry of Health (2023). *New Zealand immunisation schedule.* Wellington: Ministry of Health. https://www.health.govt.nz/our-work/preventative-health-wellness/immunisation/new-zealand-immunisation-schedule.

Pulmonary Hypertension Association of Australia (PHAA) (2017). *Classification of pulmonary hypertension*. PHAA. https://www.phaaustralia.com/page/74/p-class.

Schwab, K.E. & Kamangar, N. (2023). Pulmonary arterial hypertension. *Emedicine*. https://emedicine.medscape.com/article/303098-overview.

Sovari, A.A., Kocheril, A.G. & Baas, A.S. (2020). Cardiogenic pulmonary edema. *Emedicine*. https://emedicine.medscape.com/article/157452-overview.

Tortora. G.J., Derrickson, B., Burkett, B., Peoples, G., Dye, D., Cooke, J.,… Green, H. (2022). *Principles of anatomy and physiology* (3rd Asia-Pacific edn). Milton, QLD: John Wiley and Sons.

World Health Organization (WHO) (2022a). *Global tuberculosis report 2022*. Geneva: WHO. https://www.who.int/teams/global-tuberculosis-programme/tb-reports/global-tuberculosis-report-2022.

World Health Organization (WHO) (2022b). *Tuberculosis*. Geneva: WHO. https://www.who.int/health-topics/tuberculosis#tab=tab_1.

PART

7

Fluid, electrolyte and renal pathophysiology

30 Fluid imbalances

KEY TERMS

Dehydration
Euvolaemia
Fluid balance
Fluid deficit
Fluid excess
Hydrostatic pressure
Hypertonic solution
Hypotonic solution
Hypovolaemia
Isotonic solution
Oedema
Osmolality
Osmosis
Osmotic pressure
Tonicity

LEARNING OBJECTIVES

After completing this chapter, you should be able to:

1. State the normal distribution of water across the body compartments.
2. Identify the major determinants of body fluid balance.
3. Define 'osmosis', and differentiate it from osmolality.
4. Describe the net movement of water between the intracellular and extracellular compartments when solute concentrations change.
5. Identify the common causes and clinical manifestations of fluid-deficient states.
6. Outline the changes in the capillary and tissue environment that can lead to oedema.
7. State the common clinical manifestations of oedema.

WHAT YOU SHOULD KNOW BEFORE YOU START THIS CHAPTER

Can you define the terms 'diffusion' and 'osmosis', and differentiate between the two?

Can you describe the properties of solutes and solvents?

Can you define 'tonicity'?

Can you describe capillary dynamics?

Can you explain the function of antidiuretic hormone (ADH)?

Introduction

Water is essential to human life. Cells contain water, tissues are bathed in it, and it is the primary constituent of blood. Therefore, water acts as the major medium to connect all parts of the body. As the principal body solvent, substances (solutes) such as nutrients, electrolytes and chemical messengers are dissolved into water and transported around the body to serve the needs of all body cells.

As you will see, significant alterations in body fluid levels can have deleterious effects on homeostasis.

Distribution of body water and fluid balance

LEARNING OBJECTIVE 1

State the normal distribution of water across the body compartments.

LEARNING OBJECTIVE 2

Identify the major determinants of body fluid balance.

Water represents about 60% of adult body weight. It is not distributed uniformly throughout the body. Most body fluid—approximately two-thirds of the total body water—is located inside cells (intracellular), while the remainder is outside cells (extracellular). The fluid in the *extracellular* compartment can be subdivided into *blood volume (intravascular volume)* and *tissue volume (interstitial fluid)*. Intravascular fluid represents 80% of the extracellular compartment (see Figure 30.1).

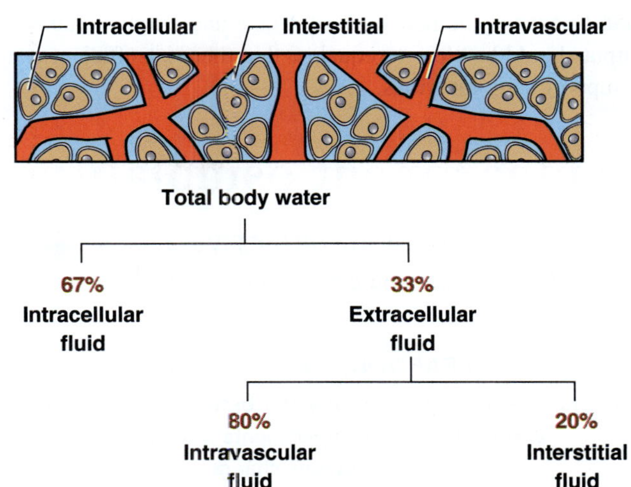

Figure 30.1

Water distribution across body compartments

Normal body water level, **euvolaemia**, is a balance between fluid intake and loss (see Figure 30.2). Normal water intake is via the gastrointestinal tract through the beverages we drink and the food we eat. Water is also a common product of metabolic reactions within the body. Humans normally excrete water as a part of urine formed in the kidney, within faeces eliminated via the gastrointestinal tract, in sweating, and in the insensible (or unregulated) loss of water through the skin and in the air expelled by our lungs. In critical clinical situations, fluid intake can be supplemented through a variety of routes, such as intravenously, rectally, via enteral feeding and via the peritoneum in dialysis.

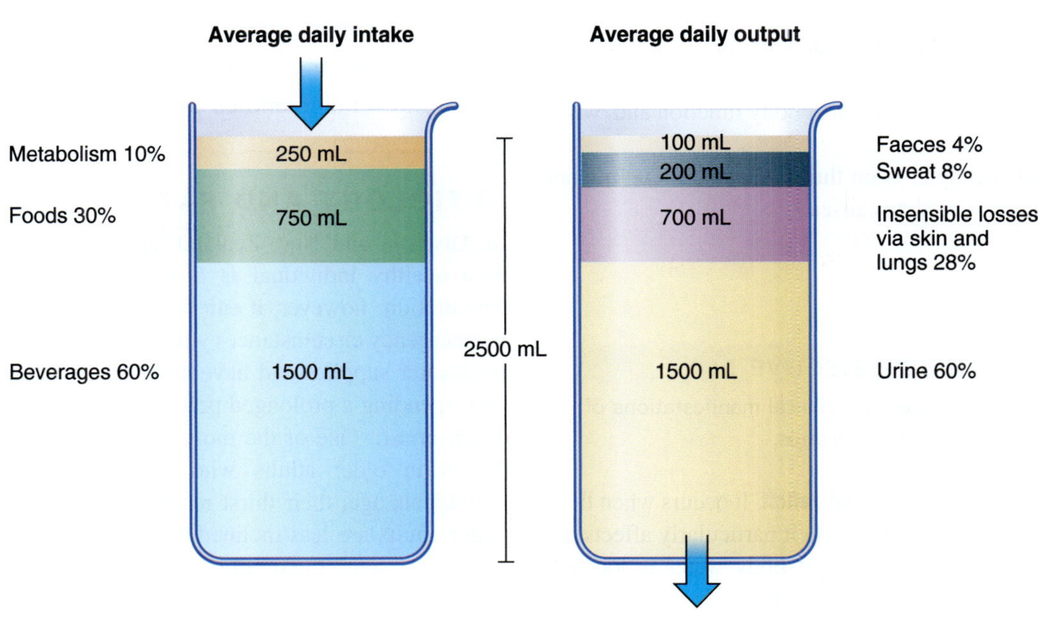

Figure 30.2

Body fluid balance

Source: Based on Marieb & Hoehn (2019), Figure 26.4, p 1048.

Fluid balance is the net result of intake and output. Intake and output should be close to equal so that there is sufficient water to support body functions.

Compartment osmolality

LEARNING OBJECTIVE 3

Define 'osmosis', and differentiate it from osmolality.

LEARNING OBJECTIVE 4

Describe the net movement of water between the intracellular and extracellular compartments when solute concentrations change.

Osmosis is the passive diffusion of water between body compartments. Like diffusion of any solute that is allowed to pass through a semipermeable membrane, water moves from an area of high concentration (which has the most dilute solute concentration) to one that is lower (the most concentrated solute solution) until equilibrium is reached. The relative solute concentrations in the extracellular and intracellular compartments create an **osmotic pressure**, which determines osmosis.

The solute concentration within a compartment is referred to by the term *osmolarity*. However, the accepted term is **osmolality**, which is the solute concentration per kilogram of water (in units of mOsm/kg). The normal value for compartment osmolality is 280 mOsm/kg. The concept of compartment osmolality and osmosis is represented in Figure 30.3.

A

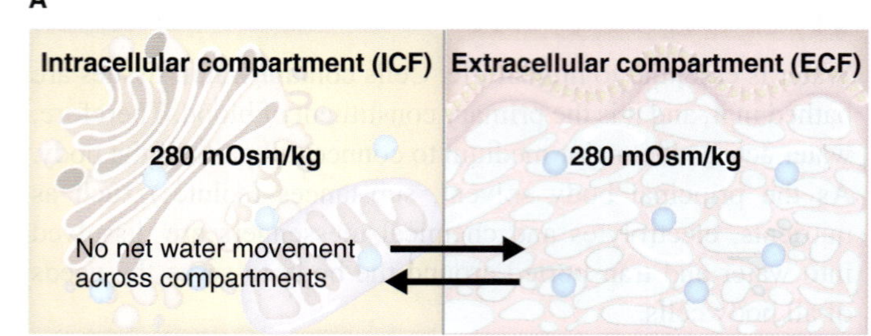

B

Intracellular compartment (ICF)
Extracellular compartment (ECF)
280 mOsm/kg
320 mOsm/kg
Net water movement from ICF to ECF until equilibrium (both compartments at 320 mOsm/kg). This leads to a contracted ICF and an expanded ECF.

C

Intracellular compartment (ICF)
Extracellular compartment (ECF)
280 mOsm/kg
265 mOsm/kg
Net water movement from ECF to ICF until equilibrium (both compartments at 265 mOsm/kg). This leads to an expanded ICF and a contracted ECF.

Figure 30.3

Compartment osmolality and osmosis

(A) Normal state.

(B) Hyperosmolar extracellular environment.

(C) Hypo-osmolar extracellular environment.

mOsm/kg = milliosmoles per kilogram.

Alterations in body fluid levels

Fluid imbalances arise as either deficits or excesses. The standard terms for these alterations are *dehydration* and *oedema*, respectively. These states greatly affect body function and, when severe, can lead to death.

The focus of this chapter is on fluid imbalances that are not due to haemorrhagic or cardiac causes.

Fluid deficits

LEARNING OBJECTIVE 5

Identify the common causes and clinical manifestations of fluid-deficient states.

Dehydration is a standard form of **fluid deficit**. It occurs when fluid intake falls well below output. The deficit particularly affects the intracellular compartment, where most body water is located. To some extent, water can be shunted from the extracellular compartment to compensate for the imbalance, but this is limited.

Severe dehydration can lead to **hypovolaemia**. Prolonged hypovolaemia can decrease tissue perfusion and organ failure, leading to an increased risk of mortality.

AETIOLOGY AND PATHOPHYSIOLOGY

In Australia and New Zealand, an inadequate intake of fluid in a healthy individual is a relatively uncommon cause of dehydration; however, it can occur in comatose individuals or in emergency circumstances where people do not have sufficient freshwater supplies and have no access to them in the vicinity (e.g. spending a prolonged period lost at sea or in remote bush/desert areas). One of the most common causes of dehydration occurs in older adults who are dependent on carers. As individuals age, their thirst response (thirst reflex) diminishes. Older adults are less inclined to sense thirst. People reliant on carers may sense thirst but may not be able to communicate the need, or they may be neglected as carers focus on other tasks.

The more common cause is a disproportionate loss through excessive diuresis. Examples of this include diabetic hyperglycaemia (see the chapter 'Diabetes mellitus'), excessive use of diuretic medications, or the inadequate secretion of (or responsiveness to) antidiuretic hormone (ADH) in diabetes insipidus, resulting in poor water reabsorption in the renal distal tubules. Insensible water loss through excessive sweating and expiration can, in some circumstances, also contribute to dehydration. Other causes of dehydration from fluid loss result from burns, diarrhoea or vomiting.

EPIDEMIOLOGY AND RISK FACTORS

The prevalence of dehydration in our community is not really known. Experts believe that it is most likely to be underestimated. In 2016 it was reported that most of the Australian population did not meet adequate intake (AI) levels for total water and total fluid intake, with the elderly at greatest risk. Indeed, across Westernised nations dehydration is considered a common chronic health issue in the elderly.

A person may be at risk of dehydration if they overexercise, are an older adult or a very young child, live at high altitudes, or work in hot, humid weather conditions. People with chronic illnesses, such as diabetes mellitus, diabetes insipidus, kidney disease or alcoholism, can also be prone to dehydration. The use of diuretic medication can also increase the risk of dehydration.

CLINICAL MANIFESTATIONS

The state of dehydration particularly affects body cell appearance and function (especially the cells of the brain, skin and mucous membranes), intravascular volume (inducing hypovolaemia) and the character of formed urine. The classic signs and symptoms include dry skin and mucous membranes, increased thirst, increased body temperature, weight loss (not surprising given the proportion of body weight accounted for by water), and the formation of a concentrated urine (except when the cause of dehydration is associated with hyperglycaemia or diabetes insipidus). In more severe cases, an affected person may show dark, sunken eyes, impaired consciousness and poor tissue turgor (turgor is measured by the elasticity of skin when pinched up, and is related to the water content of the skin cells).

Figure 30.4 explores the common clinical manifestations and management of dehydration.

CLINICAL DIAGNOSIS AND MANAGEMENT

Diagnosis

Dehydration is diagnosed by a combination of history taking, a physical examination and laboratory testing. During a physical examination, a health professional will look for changes in the appearance of the eyes, frequency of urination, blood pressure, pulse rate, tissue turgor, state of consciousness and body temperature. Decreases in body weight can also be used to indicate a fluid deficit.

Blood and urine tests can indicate the degree of dehydration and the likely cause, by providing information on parameters such as electrolyte levels (especially sodium, potassium and bicarbonate), blood glucose, blood urea nitrogen, creatinine and osmolality.

In those who are critically ill with hypovolaemia, ultrasonography in combination with physical examination is useful in determining the extent of the fluid deficit, its effects on vital organs and the optimal management.

Management

When fluid deficit occurs, the individual will require fluid volume replacement. If they are able to drink, encouraging the imbibing of oral fluids is the least invasive method. If the dehydration is too severe or the individual is unable to drink, parenteral fluid replacement is required. In acute care settings, intravenous fluid resuscitation is common practice, but this method requires a level of skill to perform intravenous cannulation. In aged-care, palliative care and other facilities, this skill is not available and subcutaneous fluid replacement is undertaken. Much smaller volumes can be infused with subcutaneous infusions when compared to the intravenous route. The placement of a subcutaneous cannula is less complex and can be achieved quickly.

The type of fluid chosen depends on the clinical situation. The fluid **tonicity** will determine the type of solution used. An **isotonic solution** has the same tonicity as plasma. This type of fluid distributes equally between intravascular, interstitial and intracellular spaces. A **hypotonic solution** has a lower tonicity than plasma, and encourages fluid from intravascular spaces to shift into interstitial and intracellular spaces. A **hypertonic solution** has a higher tonicity than plasma, and causes fluid to shift from interstitial and intracellular spaces into intravascular spaces (see Tables 30.1 and 30.2).

It is very important in emergency situations that fluid resuscitation is administered in a controlled rather than an aggressive way. If it is too aggressive, there is a risk of tipping the imbalance towards fluid overload. One complication of the latter approach is *intra-abdominal hypertension (IAH)* and *abdominal compartment syndrome (ACS)*. Like the skull, the abdominal cavity is considered a closed compartment. Rapid fluid resuscitation can readily increase abdominal pressure, leading to IAH and ACS. In this state, hypoperfusion and ischaemia of the abdominal viscera can develop, leading to the release of pro-inflammatory cytokines and tissue damage, increasing the risk of mortality.

Fluid excesses

LEARNING OBJECTIVE 6

Outline the changes in the capillary and tissue environment that can lead to oedema.

Fluid excesses develop when one or more body compartments become inundated with fluid. The focus of the discussion in this section is on the formation of oedema and excessive fluid intake.

AETIOLOGY AND PATHOPHYSIOLOGY

The development of oedema is related to alterations in filtration pressure, osmotic pressures and permeability at the level of the capillary. The capillary wall is selectively permeable to extracellular fluid solutes. A number of opposing pressures, both hydrostatic and osmotic, determine the net movement of fluid between the intravascular and interstitial compartments.

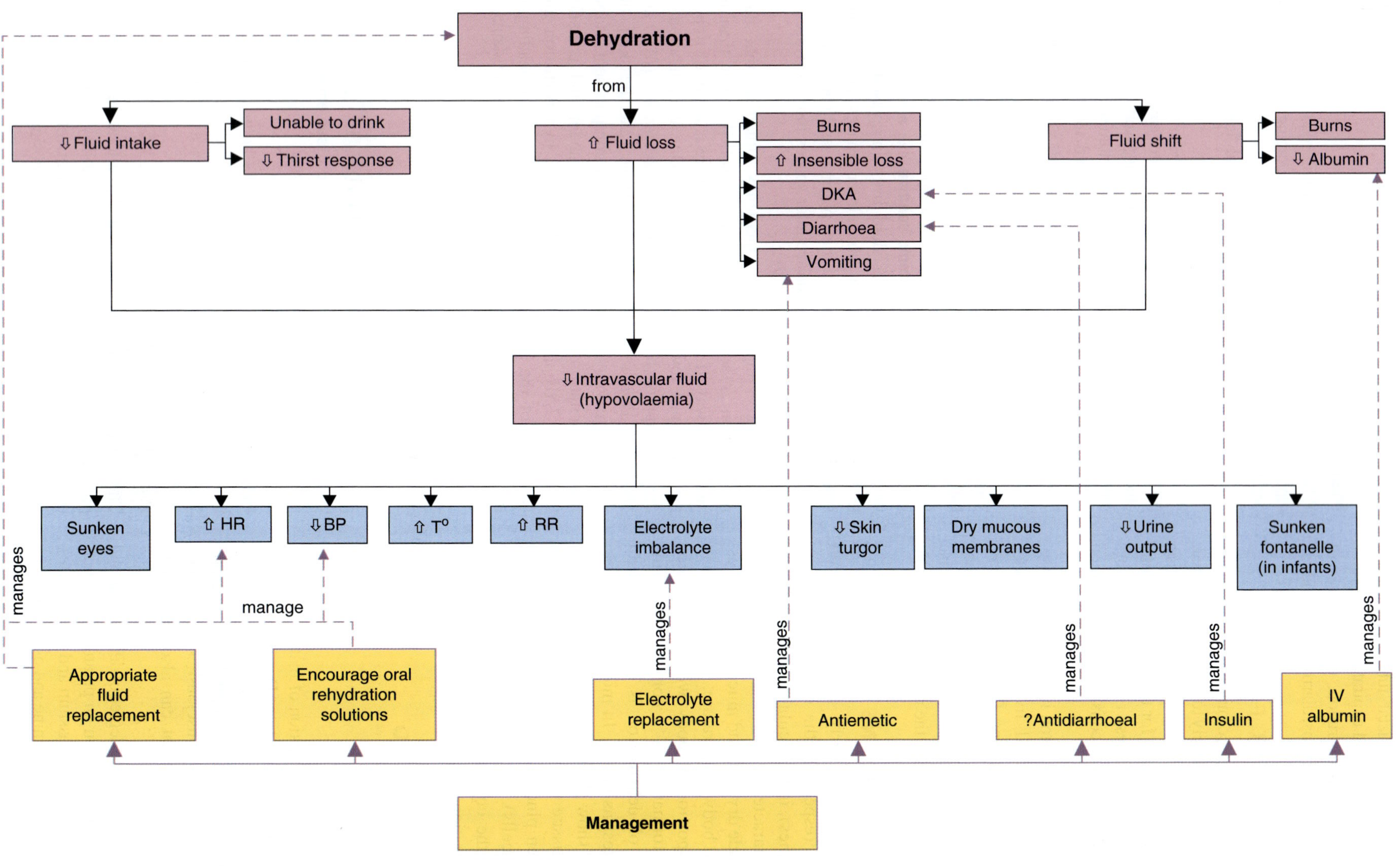

Figure 30.4

Clinical snapshot: Dehydration

Antidiarrhoeal agents may be considered, but they are not recommended in gastrointestinal infection as they can exacerbate the intestinal bacterial load. ↓ = decreased; ↑ = increased; ? = possible; BP = blood pressure; DKA = diabetic ketoacidosis; HR = heart rate; IV = intravenous; RR = respiration rate; T° = temperature.

Table 30.1 Types of crystalloid fluid and their effects on fluid movement

Fluid	Examples	Influence	Use
Isotonic (crystalloid)	0.9% sodium chloride Ringer's lactate solution 5% dextrose in water Hartmann's solution	**Isotonic solution** 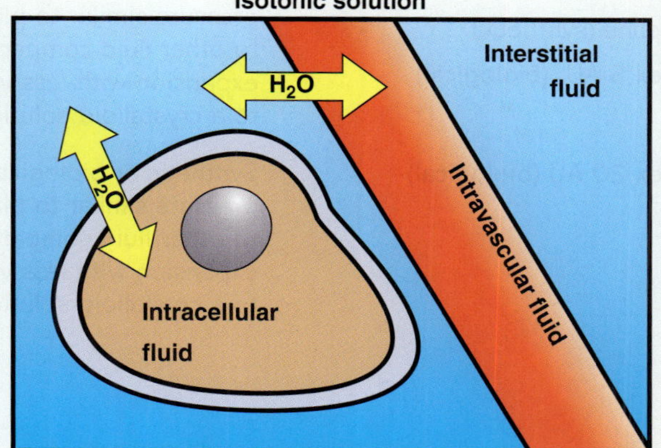 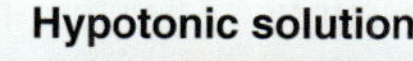	Rehydration. Depending on solution, may replace some electrolytes.
Hypotonic (crystalloid)	0.45% sodium chloride	**Hypotonic solution** 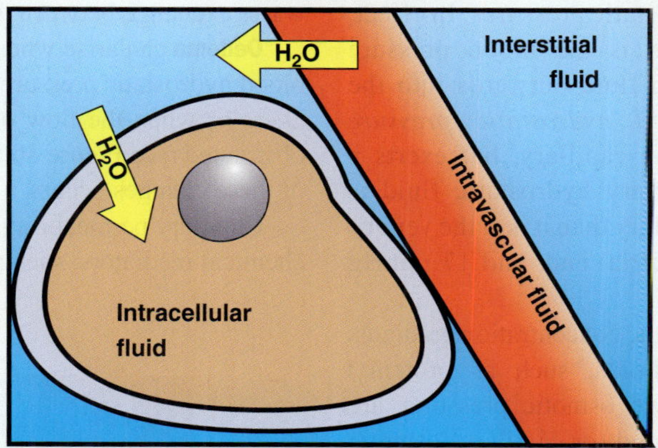 **Net osmosis into cell**	Depending on the solution, replaces sodium, chloride and free water. Can be used in the management of hyperosmolar diabetes and metabolic alkalosis states.
Hypertonic (crystalloid)	10% dextrose in water 20% dextrose in water 50% dextrose in water (mannitol)	**Hypertonic solution** 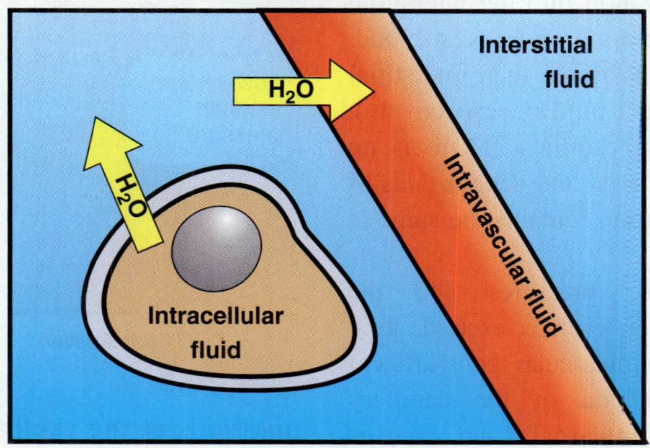 **Net osmosis out of cell**	Used more for glucose replacement than as an influence on fluid volume. Can be used to promote diuresis in some circumstances (mannitol).

Table 30.2 Types of colloidal fluids and their effects on fluid movement

Fluid	Examples	Use
Gelatin (colloid)	Gelofusine (synthetic) Polygeline (synthetic) Alburex 5 AU (biological)	Synthetic or biological proteins with an oncotic pressure similar to plasma to reduce redistribution to other fluid compartments, enabling volume expansion with less volume required when compared to a crystalloid solution.
Human albumin (colloid)	Alburex 20 AU (biological)	Synthetic or biological proteins with an oncotic pressure similar to plasma to reduce redistribution to other fluid compartments, enabling volume expansion with less volume required when compared to a crystalloid solution.

Hydrostatic pressure refers to fluid pressures acting on the wall of the capillary. There are two hydrostatic pressures: capillary and interstitial fluid hydrostatic pressures. In effect, the *capillary hydrostatic pressure* is the blood pressure within the capillary acting to push fluid outwards into the interstitium. The *interstitial fluid hydrostatic pressure* attempts to push the fluid into the capillary, but exerts a negligible force (0 mmHg). Capillary hydrostatic fluid is higher at the arterial end of the capillary than it is at the venous end (normally 35 mmHg at the arterial end, and 17 mmHg at the venous end).

Osmotic pressures are created by the concentration gradients of non-diffusible solutes (e.g. colloids, such as proteins) between the two compartments. Two osmotic pressures are at work at the capillary level: the blood (or capillary) osmotic pressure and the interstitial fluid osmotic pressure. The *blood osmotic pressure* pulls fluid from the interstitial space back into the bloodstream, while the opposing *interstitial fluid osmotic pressure* exerts a weak force pulling fluid into the interstitial space. Due to the concentration of plasma proteins in blood, blood osmotic pressure is significantly higher than interstitial osmotic pressure fluid (26 mmHg and 1 mmHg, respectively), and should draw fluid back into the capillary. There is no difference in these pressures at the arterial and venous ends of the capillary, as the colloid concentration remains the same at either end.

Taking into account the four pressures and the direction across the capillary wall that each is exerted, fluid normally tends to move from the intravascular compartment to the interstitium at the arterial end of the capillary [(35 − 0) − (26 − 1) = 10 mmHg outwards] and moves from the interstitial space back into the capillary at the venous end [(17 − 0) − (26 − 1) = 8 mmHg inwards]. Excess fluid remaining in the tissue (2 mmHg) is removed by lymphatic system transport. This system allows for efficient nutrient and waste exchange between the capillary blood and tissues.

Oedema can arise when capillary permeability increases, the blood hydrostatic pressure increases, the blood osmotic pressure alters or when the flow of lymphatic fluid out of the tissue is obstructed (see Figure 30.5). In some conditions, a combination of these changes occurs.

Capillary permeability increases in response to the release of chemical mediators, such as prostaglandins and histamine, from

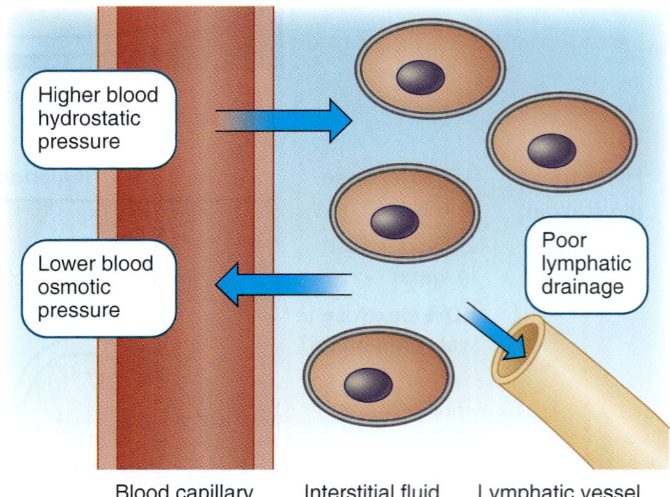

Figure 30.5
Conditions at the capillary–tissue interface that lead to oedema

cells that are damaged or are activated when injured. Gaps open up between the endothelial cells that form the capillary wall, allowing for the movement of intravascular fluid and plasma proteins into the interstitial space. This can occur in severe burns, as well as in immune or inflammatory reactions (see the chapters 'Inflammation and healing' and 'Immune disorders'). The passage of plasma proteins from the intravascular compartment decreases blood osmotic pressure and promotes the movement of water into the tissues. A plasma protein deficit also decreases blood osmotic pressure, and can arise in liver disease through the inadequate production of plasma proteins, or where there is an excessive loss, such as in severe malnutrition, where plasma proteins are used for energy production when food protein is unavailable, or as a result of serous exudate drainage from an open wound (see the chapter 'Inflammation and healing').

Conditions that increase blood hydrostatic pressure include hypertensive states, venous obstruction, excessive fluid intake or diseases characterised by fluid and sodium retention. A common cause of venous obstruction is the formation of a venous thrombosis or embolism. Blood hydrostatic pressure increases because blood flow past the obstruction is restricted. Excessive fluid intake can result from inappropriate intravenous fluid therapy, where the infusion rate is too quick or the dose is miscalculated. Fluid overload can occur when a person ingests an excessive amount of fluid; this is known as *water intoxication*, and is usually associated with psychiatric illness. Water intoxication has also been reported in people using recreational drugs, such as ecstasy, at dance parties, who have been fearful of developing severe dehydration. Fluid and sodium retention is usually associated with kidney disease (see the chapters 'Common inflammatory disorders of the kidneys and urinary tract', 'Renal neoplasms and obstructions' and 'Acute kidney injury and chronic kidney disease'), congestive cardiac failure (see the chapter 'Cardiac muscle and valve disorders') and endocrine imbalances (e.g. hyperaldosteronism, Cushing's disease and syndrome of inappropriate ADH secretion [SIADH]; see the chapters 'Hypothalamic–pituitary disorders' and 'Adrenal gland disorders'). In each case, the pressure favouring the movement of fluid into tissues from the blood outweighs the combination of the pressure moving fluid back and lymphatic drainage.

The lymphatic system is responsible for the removal of a small but significant amount of tissue fluid, as well as the transport of proteins and other large molecules from the tissues. Lymphatic obstruction can occur in the presence of a tissue infection, inflammation or a tumour, and can lead to a form of oedema called *lymphoedema*. Lymphoedema may also result from the surgical removal of neighbouring lymph nodes when a tumour within a tissue is excised, impairing lymphatic flow out of the surrounding tissues. A common example of this is associated with radical mastectomy as a part of the treatment of breast carcinoma.

As oedema develops, the expansion of the tissue space leads to an increased distance between tissue blood vessels and cells. As a result, the distance that nutrients and wastes need to traverse within the tissue space increases. While healthy tissues may be able to compensate adequately under these conditions, injured or healing tissues may be compromised, leading to slowed healing processes, and an increased risk of infection and ulceration. Another complication is that in severe oedema the accumulated tissue fluid may not be easily returned to the intravascular compartment, becoming sequestered out of the circulation. This situation may induce a state of dehydration.

EPIDEMIOLOGY AND RISK FACTORS

The incidence of oedema in our community due to all causes is not known. Risk factors for oedematous states include pregnancy, congestive cardiac failure, kidney disease, obstructive liver diseases such as cirrhosis, lymphatic obstructions, deep venous thrombosis and chronic venous insufficiency. Medications such as vasodilators and non-steroidal anti-inflammatory drugs can also increase the risk of oedema.

CLINICAL MANIFESTATIONS

LEARNING OBJECTIVE 7

State the common clinical manifestations of oedema.

Oedema can occur as a result of a pathophysiological process or naturally in a healthy person of any age (e.g. localised oedema can occur in the hands and feet in warm weather or in the feet during prolonged standing). Oedema can be localised to one region of the body, such as the foot, fingers or within an organ (e.g. pulmonary oedema), or be systemic. It can be referred to as *dependent oedema* due to the effects of gravity associated with prolonged periods in one position, such as standing (where it pools in the feet) or being bed-ridden (where it pools around the buttocks and sacrum). Dependent oedema may also be known as *pitting oedema* (where lightly poking a finger into the oedematous tissue leaves an indentation after the finger is withdrawn). When indentation does not occur, it is known as *non-pitting oedema*.

Common manifestations of oedema include weight gain, puffiness and swelling. In some cases, the degree of swelling can induce pain. Other indicators include tight-fitting shoes or jewellery (e.g. rings may be hard to remove or put on).

Depending on the tissues affected by the oedema, the function of an organ may be significantly impaired. Indeed, if the lungs, heart or brain are affected, the consequences could be life-threatening. Under these circumstances, symptoms might include hypoxaemia, hypercapnia, alterations in blood pressure and tissue perfusion, headache, convulsions and loss of consciousness. Figure 30.6 explores the common clinical manifestations and management of oedema.

CLINICAL DIAGNOSIS AND MANAGEMENT

Diagnosis

A diagnosis of oedema is made after taking a medical history, conducting a physical examination and considering the results of other investigations. It is important to identify the specific cause of the fluid excess so that the correct management can be instigated.

Depending on the probable cause/s, the investigations may involve chest X-ray, electrocardiogram (ECG), ultrasound imaging, full blood examination and urinalysis. These tests will provide important information about current heart, liver and kidney functioning, and imaging can reveal possible obstructions.

Management

The clinical management of oedema depends on its location. Oedema in limbs can be reduced by the use of gravity. Ensuring that legs do not remain dependent when sitting (by elevating the legs) and the use of compression stockings are two important interventions that should be undertaken for limb oedema. *Ascites* is oedema in the abdomen. Management of ascites is addressed in the chapter 'Disorders of the liver, gallbladder and pancreas'. Oedema in brain tissue is critical, and is exacerbated by the fact that the brain is trapped within the cranial vault, which does not allow for much expansion. Management of brain oedema is addressed in the chapter 'Neurotrauma'. Oedema in the lungs is called pulmonary oedema and is addressed in the chapter 'Pulmonary dysfunction'.

General principles of management should focus on the cause of the oedema. Oedema may be multifactorial; however, there are ultimately some common principles. Generally speaking, either an increase in the capillary hydrostatic pressure or the tissue osmotic pressure occurs, or there is a decrease in the capillary osmotic pressure.

An increase in the capillary hydrostatic pressure can result from an increase in blood pressure at the venous end of the capillary. Elevating the legs will somewhat reduce tissue hydrostatic pressure, thereby reducing oedema. Applying compression stockings will increase tissue hydrostatic pressure, forcing more fluid back into the vessel (or into lymph vessels) and, ultimately, reducing oedema.

A reduction in albumin production (a plasma protein produced by the liver and largely responsible for blood osmotic pressure) contributes to oedema. If an individual has liver failure and is not producing sufficient albumin, it can be administered intravenously to increase blood osmotic pressure, and thereby reduce oedema.

Excessive fluid can be 'dragged' from the tissue and encouraged back into the intravascular space, which will ultimately be processed by the kidneys and excreted. This process can be accelerated through the use of diuretics. A class of drugs that exerts significant 'pull' is the osmotic diuretics. This class of drugs increases the volume of solutes within the intravascular space, which exerts an osmotic pull, encouraging interstitial and intracellular fluid to shift into the intravascular space. This fluid then continues in the circulation, and at some stage will be processed by the kidneys and turned into urine, which is then voided, reducing oedema. Care must be taken so as not to give too much diuretic (especially osmotic diuretics) as they can cause dehydration.

INDIGENOUS HEALTH FAST FACTS AND CULTURAL CONSIDERATIONS

FAST FACTS

- ***Access to safe, clean water, sanitation and hygiene are considered by the United Nations to be basic human rights. A Western Australian Office of the Auditor General report in 2021 found that water sampling across 37 remote communities still tested positive for chemical and biological contaminants that exposed community members to a risk of illness.***
- ***In 2020–21, the prevalence rate for children to be given solid foods before 4 months of age is 6.7%. This behaviour increases the risk of dehydration. Māori children are 2.05 times as likely as European New Zealander children to be given solid foods before 4 months of age. Pacific Islands children are 1.77 times as likely as non-Pacific Islands children to be given solid foods before 4 months of age.***

CULTURAL CONSIDERATIONS

- ***For many Aboriginal and Torres Strait Islander communities, water plays significant cultural, social and economic roles. It is important that healthcare professionals and public health officials understand the complexities of balancing the traditional and cultural needs of the Indigenous community with the critical and potentially divergent needs of natural resource management and sewage treatment.***

Sources: Data from New Zealand Ministry of Health (2021); United Nations Sustainable Development Goals Report (2022); Western Australian Office of the Auditor General (2021).

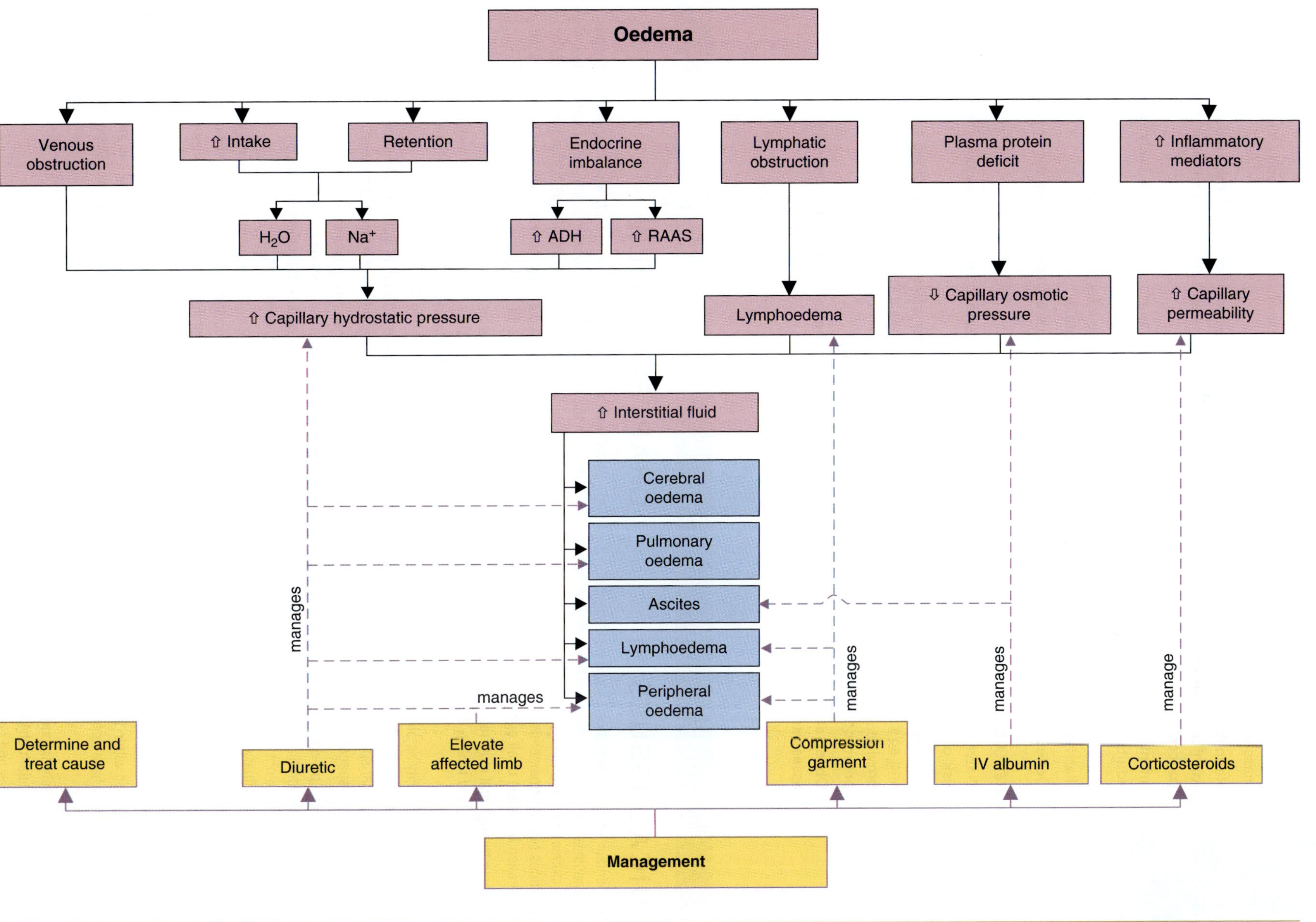

Figure 30.6

Clinical snapshot: Oedema

↓ = decreased; ↑ = increased; ADH = antidiuretic hormone; H_2O = water; IV = intravenous; Na^+ = sodium ion; RAAS = renin-angiotensin-aldosterone system.

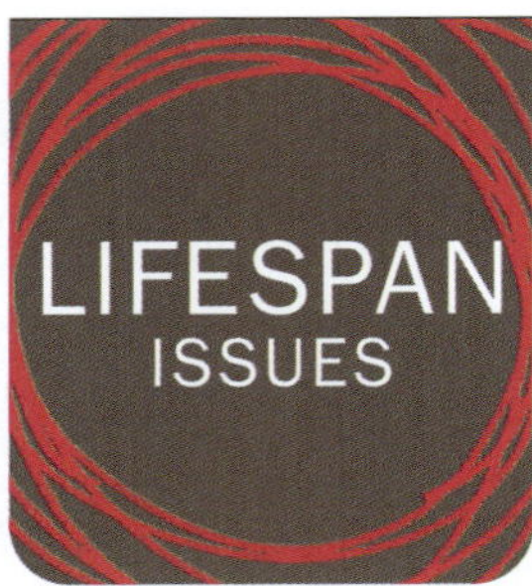

CHILDREN AND ADOLESCENTS

- Infants and children can become dehydrated quickly, because of an increased body surface area to mass index ratio and a faster metabolic rate than adults.
- Neonates have an increased risk of dehydration or fluid overload because of their reduced ability to influence intravascular fluid volume status. This risk occurs as a result of their poor renal concentration capabilities.
- Infants have approximately 70% body water, children have approximately 65% body water and adults have approximately 60% body water.
- The most common causes of dehydration in children include infections that result in vomiting and diarrhoea (especially gastroenteritis) and inadequate oral intake.
- Oedema is less common in children, and can represent issues with cardiac, hepatic or renal function.

OLDER ADULTS

- Water homeostasis becomes complex in an older adult as cardiac and renal function decreases. The risk of dehydration and oedema increases.
- Osmoreceptor and chemoreceptor function blunts, and older adults are less inclined to sense thirst, and so can become dehydrated very quickly. Also, in individuals who are reliant on other people to provide support with nutrition (i.e. feeding), dehydration can occur from infrequent or insufficient provision of fluid.
- Observations for dry oral mucosa and turgor testing have been found to be more reliable than assessment for orthostatic hypotension and thirst.

KEY CLINICAL ISSUES

- Interventions to maintain adequate hydration should be instigated to ensure fluid homeostasis. Provision of frequent and sufficient oral fluids, appropriate clothing for the environment, control of fever and prevention of infections (e.g. gastroenteritis) will assist in reducing the incidence of dehydration in people of all ages.
- Rehydration can occur through oral rehydration therapies or intravenous therapy using various types of fluid tonicity (depending on the causes of the dehydration).
- Isotonic fluids have the same tonicity as plasma, and will distribute equally between the various spaces. Hypotonic fluid will encourage fluid into interstitial and intracellular spaces. Hypertonic fluids will encourage fluid into intravascular spaces.
- Weighing individuals regularly can provide an insight into fluid status, and may suggest oedema or dehydration (serial weights, not a single value). Rapid changes in weight do not occur as a result of fat, but are most likely to occur as a result of fluid changes.
- Oedema can occur from cardiac, renal or hepatic issues, or as a result of failure of the lymphatic system to cope with the volume of interstitial fluid.
- Oedema can be localised or systemic. Oedema may be described as pitting (dependent) or non-pitting.
- Ascites is oedema that is contained within the abdominal region. Someone with severe ascites may have approximately 20 L of fluid interstitially around the abdomen.
- A person can have oedema and dehydration at the same time. They may have hypotension or even cellular dehydration as a result of excess fluid in the interstitial spaces and not in the intravascular or intracellular spaces.

CHAPTER REVIEW

- Water represents about *60% of adult body weight*. Approximately two-thirds of the total body water is located inside cells (*intracellular*), while the remainder is outside cells (*extracellular*). Within the extracellular compartment, *intravascular fluid* represents 80% and the *interstitial* compartment 20% of total fluid.
- Normal body water level is a *balance between fluid intake and loss*. The major forms of water are as beverages, food and metabolism. Water is excreted as urine, within faeces, in sweat, and in the insensible loss of water through the skin and lungs.
- *Osmosis* is the passive diffusion of water between body compartments from the highest concentration of water to the lowest.
- *Dehydration* occurs when fluid intake falls well below output. The classic signs and symptoms include dry skin and mucous membranes, increased thirst, increased body temperature, weight loss and the formation of a concentrated urine.
- *Oedema*—a build-up of fluid in the interstitial space—can arise when capillary permeability increases, the blood hydrostatic pressure increases, the blood osmotic pressure alters or when lymphatic fluid flow out of the tissue is obstructed.
- Common manifestations of oedema include weight gain, puffiness and swelling. In some cases, the degree of swelling can induce pain. Other indicators include tight-fitting shoes or jewellery. Depending on the tissues affected by the oedema, the function of organs, such as the lungs or brain, may be significantly impaired.

REVIEW QUESTIONS

1 What percentage of body water is located in each of the following compartments?
   a intracellular compartment
   b intravascular compartment

2 If an adult weighs 70 kg, what weight of water would be expected to be present inside that person's body cells?

3 In which direction would the net water movement be expected in each the following conditions?
   a a hyperosmolar intracellular compartment
   b a hyperosmolar extracellular compartment

4 How would the conditions within the capillary and tissue environment be expected to change in each of the following cases in order for oedema to develop?
   a blood osmotic pressure
   b lymphatic drainage
   c blood hydrostatic pressure

HEALTH PROFESSIONAL CONNECTIONS

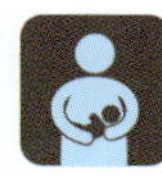

Midwives Neonates can become dehydrated very quickly. Assessment for a depressed fontanelle, poor skin turgor, dry mucous membranes and sunken eye sockets will assist the midwife in determining whether the neonate is dehydrated. Excess fluid support as an iatrogenic error is also a risk to neonates. Bulging fontanelle and periorbital oedema can be observed in a neonate with fluid overload.

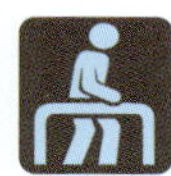

Physiotherapists Assisting people with range-of-movement exercises can be beneficial to reduce oedema. This process can enable excess fluid to be removed by nearby lymph vessels if localised vessels are not functioning well. Dehydration can impede chest physiotherapy by causing thick, tenacious mucus that is difficult to move. Ensuring adequate hydration will assist with pulmonary hygiene.

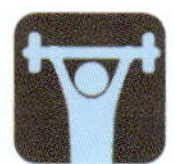

Exercise scientists Oedema is common after a soft tissue injury. This results from increased tissue oncotic pressure, which will delay wound healing. The general principles of rest, ice, compression and elevation (RICE) will assist with the reduction of swelling, and an earlier return to training through manipulation of oncotic pressures and hydrostatic pressures in the tissue and the capillary. Fluid loss with endurance athletes can be 1–2 L an hour. It is imperative that appropriate fluid replacement be provided to athletes training or competing in endurance events. Monitoring fluid loss in non-endurance athletes is also important. To ensure that your client is safe and well hydrated, observe for physical signs of dehydration.

Nutritionists/Dieticians Individuals with oedema may benefit from decreased sodium and increased protein in their diet. A high sodium intake or a loss of protein from kidney disease are two factors that commonly contribute to oedema. Individuals with diabetes can become dehydrated when their glucose levels begin to rise as a result of the increase in capillary osmotic pressure, causing the intravascular volume to increase, which is then filtered by the kidney and excreted as urine. The higher a person's glucose level rises, the more the risk of dehydration. Individuals with eating disorders (particularly anorexia nervosa) are commonly dehydrated. People with liver disease can become oedematous easily. An individual's provisional diagnosis will greatly influence the diet education that they will receive.

CASE STUDY

Ms Rachel Chelan is a 23-year-old woman (UR number 547614) presenting with dehydration after falling asleep in the sun when she was sunbathing at the beach. She has sustained partial thickness burns to 5% of her total body surface. Her observations were as follows:

Temperature	Heart rate	Respiration rate	Blood pressure	SpO_2
39°C	94	26	116/76	99% (RA*)

* RA = room air.

Ms Chelan was commenced on 1 L of 0.9% sodium chloride to be infused over eight hours. She has had some blood taken for testing urea and electrolyte levels, and a full blood count. She is to have the antibacterial agent silver sulfadiazine (SSD) cream applied to all affected areas. She has been given some non-steroidal anti-inflammatory drugs with effect. Ms Chelan has also had the antiemetic metoclopramide with effect two hours ago. Her pathology results were as follows:

HAEMATOLOGY

Patient location:	Ward 3	**UR:**	547614		
Consultant:	Smith	**NAME:**	Chelan		
		Given name:	Rachel	**Sex:**	F
		DOB:	12/06/XX	**Age:**	23

Time collected	14:20
Date collected	XX/XX
Year	XXXX
Lab #	34524325

FULL BLOOD COUNT		UNITS	REFERENCE RANGE
Haemoglobin	163	g/L	115–160
White cell count	6.5	$\times 10^9$/L	4.0–11.0
Platelets	290	$\times 10^9$/L	140–400
Haematocrit	0.50		0.33–0.47
Red cell count	5.1	$\times 10^{12}$/L	3.80–5.20
Reticulocyte count	0.8		0.2–2.0%
MCV	94	fL	80–100
Neutrophils	3.2	$\times 10^9$/L	2.00–8.00
Lymphocytes	2.41	$\times 10^9$/L	1.00–4.00
Monocytes	0.37	$\times 10^9$/L	0.10–1.00
Eosinophils	0.36	$\times 10^9$/L	$<$ 0.60
Basophils	0.11	$\times 10^9$/L	$<$ 0.20
ESR	2.6	mm/h	$<$ 12

BIOCHEMISTRY

Patient location:	Ward 3	**UR:**	547614		
Consultant:	Smith	**NAME:**	Chelan		
		Given name:	Rachel	**Sex:**	F
		DOB:	12/06/XX	**Age:**	23

Time collected	14:20
Date collected	XX/XX
Year	XXXX
Lab #	554334532

ELECTROLYTES		UNITS	REFERENCE RANGE
Sodium	134	mmol/L	135–145
Potassium	3.4	mmol/L	3.5–5.2
Chloride	95	mmol/L	95–110
Bicarbonate	20	mmol/L	22–32
Glucose (random)	6.2	mmol/L	3.5–8.0
Iron	21	μmol/L	11–30

CRITICAL THINKING

1 Consider Ms Chelan's clinical picture. Identify her observations, and determine which parameters are consistent with dehydration. Explain.

2 What other physical signs (including skin and mucous membranes) would assist with the conclusion that Ms Chelan is dehydrated? How would these be assessed?

3 What factors would have contributed to Ms Chelan's dehydration? Explain the mechanism of dehydration as a result of prolonged sun exposure.

4 Observe Ms Chelan's pathology results. What parameters suggest dehydration? Explain.

5 Apart from fluid support, what other interventions/education should be initiated to assist Ms Chelan with the current situation and also to prevent any recurrence in the future?

BIBLIOGRAPHY

Australian Indigenous Health*Info*Net (2022). *Overview of Aboriginal and Torres Strait Islander health status, 2021.* Perth, WA: Australian Indigenous Health*Info*Net. http://www.healthinfonet.ecu.edu.au.

Australian Institute of Health and Welfare (AIHW) (2016). *Australia's health, 2016*. Australia's Health series No. 15. Cat. No. AUS 199. Canberra: AIHW. https://www.aihw.gov.au/reports/australias-health/australias-health-2016/contents/summary.

Australian Institute of Health and Welfare (AIHW) (2022). *Australia's health, 2022: data insights.* Australia's Health series No. 18. Cat. No. AUS 241. Canberra: AIHW. https://www.aihw.gov.au/reports/australias-health/australias-health-2022-data-insights/about.

Bauldoff, G., Gubrud-Howe, P.M., Carno, M.-A., Levett-Jones, T., Hales, M., Berry, K., … Stanley, D. (2020). *LeMone and Burke's medical–surgical nursing: critical thinking for person-centred care* (4th [Australian] edn). Sydney: Pearson Australia.

Beck, A.M., Seemer, J., Knudsen, A.W. & Munk, T. (2021) Narrative review of low-intake dehydration in older adults. *Nutrients* 13(9):3142. https://doi.org/10.3390/nu13093142.

Best, O. & Fredericks, B. (2021). *Yatdjuligin: Aboriginal and Torres Strait Islander nursing and midwifery care* (3rd edn). Port Melbourne, VIC: Cambridge University Press.

Bullock, S. & Manias, E. (2022). *Fundamentals of pharmacology* (9th edn). Sydney: Pearson Australia.

Huang, L.H., Anchala, K.R., Ellsbury, D.L. & George, C.S. (2018). Dehydration treatment and management. *Emedicine*. http://emedicine.medscape.com/article/906999.

Marieb, E.N. & Hoehn, K. (2019). *Human anatomy and physiology* (11th edn). San Francisco, CA: Pearson Benjamin Cummings.

Milano, R. (2017). Fluid resuscitation of the adult trauma patient: where have we been and where are we going? *Nursing Clinics of North America* 52:237–47. https://doi.org/10.1016/j.cnur.2017.01.001.

New Zealand Ministry of Health (2021). *New Zealand Health Survey, 2020–2021.* Wellington: Ministry of Health. https://www.health.govt.nz/publication/annual-update-key-results-2020-21-new-zealand-health-survey.

Schwartz, R.A. & Kapila, R. (2021). Lymphedema. *Emedicine*. https://emedicine.medscape.com/article/1087313-overview.

Sterns, R.H. (2022). Etiology, clinical manifestations, and diagnosis of volume depletion in adults. *UpToDate*. https://www.medilib.ir/uptodate/show/2298.

Sui, Z., Zheng, M., Zhang, M. & Rangan, A. (2016) Water and beverage consumption: analysis of the Australian 2011–2012 National Nutrition and Physical Activity Survey. *Nutrients* 8(11): 678. https://doi.org/10.3390/nu8110678.

United Nations (2022). *United Nations Sustainable Development Goals Report 2022.* Geneva: United Nations. https://unstats.un.org/sdgs/report/2022/.

Western Australian Office of the Auditor General (2021). *Delivering essential services to remote Aboriginal communities: follow-up*. Report 25:2020–21. Perth: Office of the Auditor General. https://audit.wa.gov.au/reports-and-publications/reports/delivering-essential-services-to-remote-aboriginal-communities-follow-up/.

31 Electrolyte imbalances

KEY TERMS

Calcium
Electrolytes
Hypercalcaemia
Hyperkalaemia
Hypermagnesaemia
Hypernatraemia
Hyperphosphataemia
Hypocalcaemia
Hypokalaemia
Hypomagnesaemia
Hyponatraemia
Hypophosphataemia
Magnesium
Phosphate
Potassium
Sodium

LEARNING OBJECTIVES

After completing this chapter, you should be able to:

1 Identify the main functions of the electrolytes sodium, potassium, calcium, phosphate and magnesium, and state their normal serum levels.

2 State the common causes of imbalances in the blood levels of these electrolytes.

3 Describe the consequences of imbalances in the levels of these electrolytes.

4 State the clinical manifestations associated with each of these imbalances.

WHAT YOU SHOULD KNOW BEFORE YOU START THIS CHAPTER

Can you define the resting membrane state?

Can you describe the process of action potential generation in excitable cells?

Can you describe the roles and distribution of important electrolytes in the body?

Can you differentiate between symport and antiport membrane transport mechanisms?

Can you state the principles of osmosis and tonicity?

Can you outline the influence of 2,3-diphosphoglycerate on the oxygen–haemoglobin dissociation curve?

Introduction

LEARNING OBJECTIVE 1

Identify the main functions of the electrolytes sodium, potassium, calcium, phosphate and magnesium, and state their normal serum levels.

A key group of solutes found in water are known as **electrolytes**. These are charged particles or ions. Common electrolytes include the mineral ions of sodium, potassium, calcium and chloride, and organic molecules such as sulfates or phosphates. Electrolytes perform essential functions in the body (see Table 31.1). It should come as no surprise that as electrolytes are dissolved particles in water, their concentrations are strongly influenced by body water levels.

Table 31.1 The functional roles of key electrolytes in the body

Electrolyte	Normal serum levels (mmol/L)	Functions
Sodium	135–145	Most abundant extracellular ion; body fluid balance; action potential generation and conduction in muscle and nervous tissue.
Potassium	3.5–5.2	Most abundant intracellular ion; action potential generation and conduction in muscle and nervous tissue; intracellular protein synthesis; body fluid and acid–base balance.
Calcium	2.1–2.6	Strong bones and teeth; plays a role in coagulation; neurotransmitter release; muscle contraction; endocytosis and exocytosis, excitability of muscle and nervous tissue.
Phosphate	0.75–1.5	Component of key blood buffer system; contributes to the structure of bones and teeth; forms part of cell membranes; participates in cellular energy storage and release; DNA and RNA nucleotide structure.
Magnesium	0.70–1.10	Part of bone structure; cofactor in some enzyme reactions; neuromuscular function; nerve impulse generation; required normal myocardial function.

Distribution of electrolytes

Like water, the distribution of electrolytes is not uniform across the body compartments. The concentration of particular electrolytes is usually relatively higher in one of the compartments, either intracellularly or extracellularly. Indeed, while the electrolyte concentrations within the intravascular and interstitial compartments are similar, they are not identical. Overall, in order to maintain osmotic balance, the total number of particles inside and outside the cell should be equal.

The unequal distribution of particular electrolytes across compartments depends on aspects such as the nature of the cell membrane transport mechanisms (e.g. the presence of antiport and symport transporters or ion channels), as well as the type and magnitude of the charge of the ions involved. The distribution of key electrolytes across the body compartments is summarised in Figure 31.1.

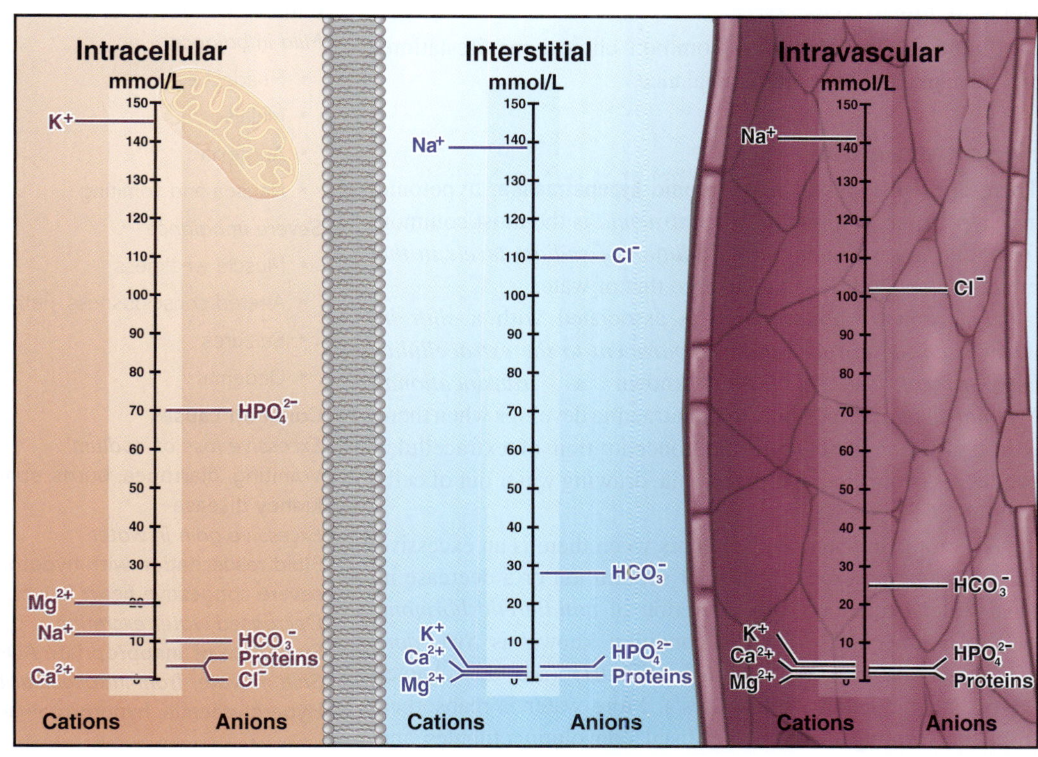

Figure 31.1

Distribution of electrolytes in blood, interstitial fluid and intracellular fluid

Ca^{2+} = calcium ion;
Cl^{-} = chloride ion;
HCO_3^{-} = bicarbonate;
HPO_4^{2-} = hydrogen phosphate;
K^{+} = potassium ion;
Mg^{2+} = magnesium ion;
Na^{+} = sodium ion.

Electrolyte imbalances

LEARNING OBJECTIVE 2

State the common causes of imbalances in the blood levels of these electrolytes.

LEARNING OBJECTIVE 3

Describe the consequences of imbalances in the levels of these electrolytes.

LEARNING OBJECTIVE 4

State the clinical manifestations associated with each of these imbalances.

Alterations in the normal body levels of certain key electrolytes, such as sodium, potassium, calcium, phosphate and magnesium, can have important clinical consequences, and are the focus of this section.

ALTERATIONS IN SODIUM BALANCE

The sodium ion is the most abundant electrolyte in extracellular fluid. The normal range for plasma sodium concentration is 135–145 mmol/L. The main roles of **sodium** are to determine the osmolality of the extracellular compartment and to contribute to the membrane potential of excitable cells. The discussion here will focus on the non-isotonic forms of sodium ion imbalance in the blood: hyponatraemia and hypernatraemia. These terms are derived from the Latin name for sodium, *natrium*, from which the symbol for sodium, *Na*, originates. An understanding of sodium imbalances is important clinically, as dysnatraemia in critical care settings is an important predictor of poor prognosis and mortality.

Figure 31.2 explores the common clinical manifestations and management of sodium imbalance.

Hyponatraemia

There are two types of non-isotonic **hyponatraemia**: hypotonic and hypertonic. *Hypotonic hyponatraemia* is the most common form, and is associated with a *dilution of sodium levels in the extracellular fluid (ECF)* relative to that of water.

Hypertonic hyponatraemia is associated with a *shift in water from the intracellular compartment to the extracellular compartment*, and is also known as *translocational hyponatraemia*. Hypertonic hyponatraemia develops when there is a significant increase in the concentration of extracellular solutes, as occurs in hyperglycaemia, drawing water out of cells into the ECF.

Hypotonic hyponatraemia occurs when there is an excessive gain in water, an excessive loss of sodium ion or a decrease in renal water excretion. Hypersecretion of *antidiuretic hormone (ADH)* is associated with the condition known as *Syndrome of Inappropriate ADH secretion (SIADH)* (see the chapter 'Hypothalamic–pituitary disorders'). More water is reabsorbed from the forming urine in the distal convoluting tubules and collecting ducts. The urine formed is quite concentrated. In a person so affected the sodium concentration in the ECF is diluted, but they remain euvolaemic. In this state of *dilutional hyponatraemia*, the relatively low sodium levels and elevated water content will inhibit the release of aldosterone, contributing to sodium loss.

In another situation, a person with a psychological disorder can compulsively drink water to a point where they induce a hyponatraemic state. This is known as *water intoxication*. An excessive loss of sodium can also develop during diuretic therapy or in kidney disease.

Hypovolaemic hyponatraemia can also occur in people who have a subarachnoid haemorrhage caused by a ruptured aneurysm. It is thought that this brain injury alters sympathetic nervous system activity and natriuretic peptide release, resulting in dysfunctional renal sodium transport. This condition has been termed *cerebral wasting syndrome*. It is important to differentiate between hypovolaemic and euvolaemic hyponatraemia, as the treatment required for each differs markedly.

Common examples of the causes of hyponatraemia are provided in Clinical Box 31.1.

The clinical manifestations reflect an alteration in cell function, particularly neurons. In mild to moderate hyponatraemia, headache, malaise, anorexia, nausea and vomiting occur. More severe manifestations involve muscle weakness, oedema, alterations in consciousness (lethargy progressing to coma) and

CLINICAL BOX 31.1

Characteristics of hyponatraemia

Serum sodium levels

$<$ 135 mmol/L

Clinical manifestations

Mild imbalance

- Headache
- Malaise
- Anorexia
- Nausea and vomiting

Severe imbalance

- Muscle weakness
- Altered consciousness (lethargy → coma)
- Seizures
- Oedema

Common causes

Excessive loss of sodium

Vomiting, diarrhoea, burns, some diuretic therapies, kidney disease

Excessive gain in water

Fluid resuscitation with hypotonic solutions, excessive thirst, severe congestive heart failure, water intoxication

Decreased water excretion

Syndrome of Inappropriate ADH secretion (SIADH)

Shift in water from intracellular to extracellular compartment

Hyperglycaemia, hyperproteinaemia

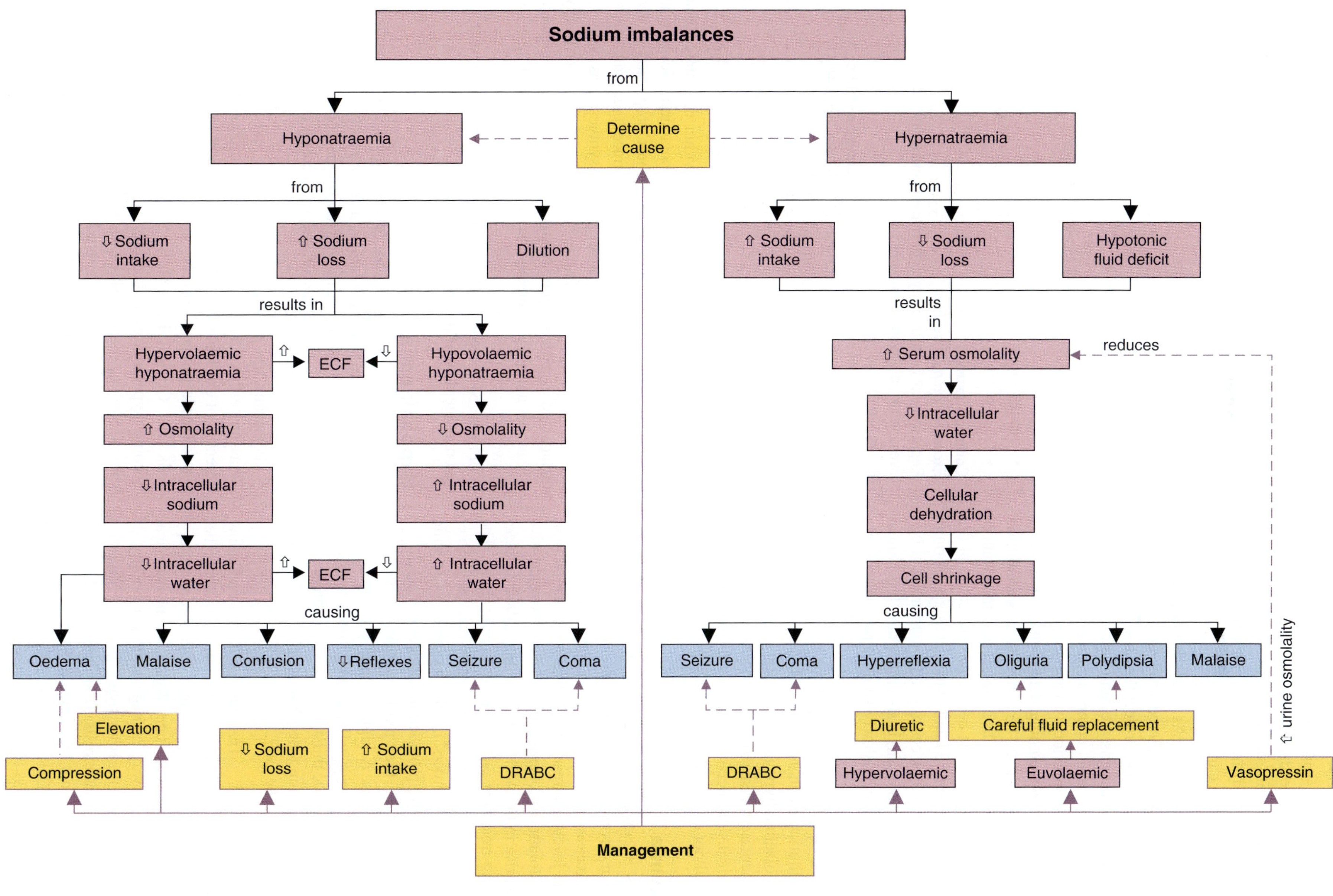

Figure 31.2

Clinical snapshot: Sodium imbalances

↓ = decreased; ↑ = increased; DRABC = danger, response, airway, breathing, circulation; ECF = extracellular fluid.

seizures (see Clinical Box 31.1). The latter symptoms develop as the imbalance in osmotic pressure between the intracellular and extracellular compartments leads to a fluid influx into neurons and cell swelling. The severity of symptoms changes with the degree of hyponatraemia and the rate at which it develops. A severe case of hyponatraemia can be fatal.

Clinical management As the consequences of hyponatraemia can result in an altered level of consciousness, initial interventions to assess and protect the airway are critical. However, these neurological signs are quite late in the clinical progression, so frequent and comprehensive neurological assessment is indicated in individuals with suspected sodium imbalances to prevent life-threatening deterioration. Generally speaking, sodium deficiency should be corrected, as should fluid depletion if present. In someone with an intact gag and swallow reflex, oral supplementation is most beneficial. The cause of the sodium deficit should be identified and managed as appropriate. Reducing sodium loss through ceasing any natriuretic drugs (such as furosemide or vasopressin) is also important. It is critical that hyponatraemia is corrected slowly so as to prevent osmotic demyelination syndrome.

Fluid restrictions may be necessary if the hyponatraemia is related to haemodilution, such as in SIADH. This would not be the case in hypovolaemic hyponatraemia. Hypertonic solutions may be used to increase the speed of hyponatraemia correction if severe neurological signs occur; however, this must be closely monitored and still not corrected too quickly.

Hypernatraemia

Hypernatraemia is an *excessive concentration of sodium ions in the ECF*. It can develop as a result of an excessive gain in sodium ions, an excessive loss of water, or a combination of both. Excessive sodium levels can result from fluid resuscitation with hypertonic saline solution or overuse of salt tablets. An excessive loss of fluid can arise in the ADH-deficient state called *diabetes insipidus* or during treatment with osmotic diuretic drugs. The former can occur as a result of pituitary surgery (see the chapter 'Hypothalamic–pituitary disorders'). Other examples of specific causes under this heading are provided in Clinical Box 31.2.

As in hyponatraemia, the most vulnerable cells to hypernatraemia are neurones. A high osmotic pressure within the ECF draws fluid out of nerve cells, leading to cell shrinkage. Clinical manifestations include thirst and confusion, progressing to lethargy, seizures and coma (see Clinical Box 31.2). When severe, hypernatraemia can be fatal.

Clinical management Treatment will vary depending on how hypernatraemic an individual becomes, and whether the person is hypervolaemic or euvolaemic. The aim of therapy is to restore a normal osmotic state. Again, as neurological complications are a risk, airway management is a priority. If an individual has a hypernatraemic hypervolaemia, diuretics are indicated to encourage natriuresis. If an individual becomes hypernatraemic in a euvolaemic state, hypotonic fluids are often administered. Vasopressin (ADH) is occasionally administered to decrease the ratio of sodium to free water. Symptom relief from nausea and vomiting can be achieved with antiemetic agents.

CLINICAL BOX 31.2

Characteristics of hypernatraemia

Serum sodium levels

>145 mmol/L

Clinical manifestations

- Thirst
- Nausea and vomiting
- Confusion
- Altered consciousness (lethargy → coma)
- Seizures
- Hypotension
- Oliguria

Common causes

Excessive gain of sodium

Replacement fluid therapy with hypertonic saline solutions, overuse of salt tablets, impaired thirst

Excessive loss of water

Inadequate ADH secretion (diabetes insipidus), osmotic diuretic therapy, fever, insufficient water intake, profuse sweating, respiratory infection

ALTERATIONS IN POTASSIUM BALANCE

Potassium ions are highly concentrated within the intracellular compartment. Therefore, the blood potassium levels, at 3.5–5.2 mmol/L, do not reflect the highest proportion of the ion in the body. **Potassium** is involved in intracellular ion balance, acid–base balance, intracellular protein synthesis, as well as muscle and neuronal function. Potassium intake is primarily dietary, and excretion is predominantly via the kidneys, although it can be normally excreted via the gastrointestinal tract or in sweat.

Figure 31.3 explores the common clinical manifestations and management of potassium imbalance.

Hypokalaemia

Lower than normal potassium levels can be due to multiple causes: *decreased dietary intake*, a *large translocational shift* out of the ECF into cells, *increased excretion* or a combination of all of these. Examples of specific causes are provided in Clinical Box 31.3.

Potassium has a major role in muscle and nerve function. Potassium efflux across the membrane determines the membrane potential of excitable cells. Therefore, clinical manifestations of **hypokalaemia** primarily involve all types of muscles and nerve cells (see Clinical Box 31.3). Skeletal and smooth muscle become hyperpolarised, making them more unresponsive to stimuli. Skeletal muscles show weakness and flaccidity. Smooth muscle of the gut becomes distended, bowel sounds are reduced and paralytic ileus may develop. Vascular smooth muscle may relax, leading to hypotension. The effects on cardiac muscle are more complex. Conduction through the atrioventricular node is slowed, and cardiac action potentials are prolonged. This leads

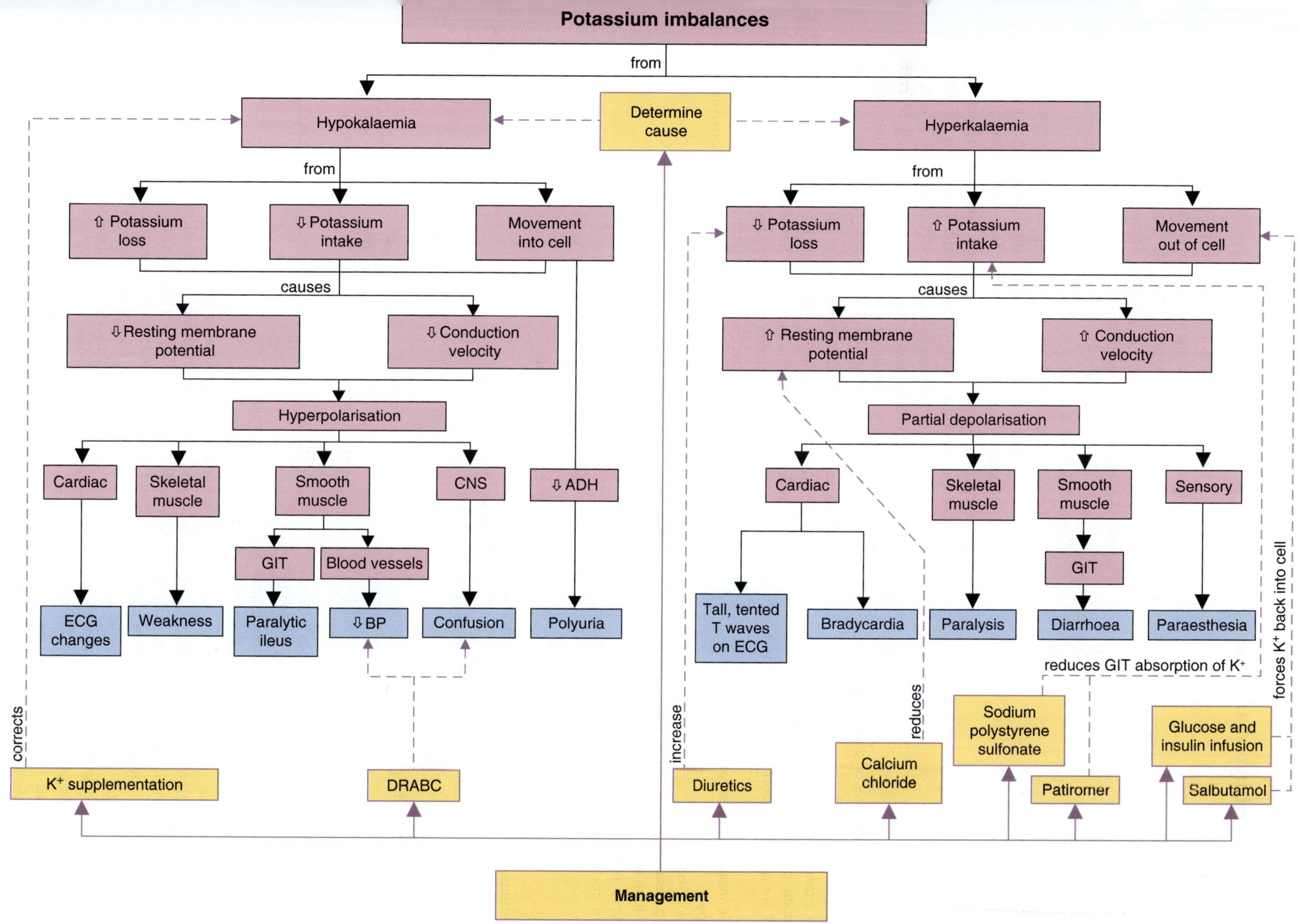

Potassium imbalances
from
Hypokalaemia
Determine cause
Hyperkalaemia
from
⇧ Potassium loss
⇩ Potassium intake
Movement into cell
causes
⇩ Resting membrane potential
⇩ Conduction velocity
Hyperpolarisation
Cardiac
Skeletal muscle
Smooth muscle
CNS
⇩ ADH
GIT
Blood vessels
ECG changes
Weakness
Paralytic ileus
⇩ BP
Confusion
Polyuria
from
⇩ Potassium loss
⇧ Potassium intake
Movement out of cell
causes
⇧ Resting membrane potential
⇧ Conduction velocity
Partial depolarisation
Cardiac
Skeletal muscle
Smooth muscle
Sensory
GIT
Tall, tented T waves on ECG
Bradycardia
Paralysis
Diarrhoea
Paraesthesia
reduces GIT absorption of K^+
forces K^+ back into cell
corrects
increase
reduces
K^+ supplementation
DRABC
Diuretics
Calcium chloride
Sodium polystyrene sulfonate
Patiromer
Glucose and insulin infusion
Salbutamol
Management

Figure 31.3

Clinical snapshot: Potassium imbalances

↓ = decreased; ↑ = increased; ADH = antidiuretic hormone; BP = blood pressure; CNS = central nervous system; DRABC = danger, response, airway, breathing, circulation; ECG = electrocardiogram; GIT = gastrointestinal system; K^+ = potassium ion.

CLINICAL BOX 31.3

Characteristics of hypokalaemia

Serum potassium levels
< 3.5 mmol/L

Clinical manifestations

- Skeletal muscle weakness and flaccidity
- Fatigue
- Respiratory muscle paralysis
- Reduced bowel sounds
- Paralytic ileus
- Cardiac dysrhythmias
- Mental confusion
- Hypotension
- Polyuria
- Vomiting
- Increased sensitivity to the action of digoxin

Common causes

Decreased dietary intake
Malnutrition, anorexia, poor-quality diets
Translocation shift out of the extracellular to the intracellular compartment
Alkalosis, excessive insulin administration, excessive β_2-agonist therapy
Increased potassium losses
Diarrhoea, vomiting, laxative misuse, some forms of diuretic therapy (especially loop or thiazide diuretics), gastrointestinal suctioning procedures, profuse sweating, primary hyperaldosteronism, corticosteroid therapy, Cushing's disease

to cardiac dysrhythmias. Within the brain, nerve cells become easier to excite, leading to mental confusion.

Hypokalaemia also disrupts ADH action on the nephron, leading to higher urine volumes and polyuria.

Clinical management Hypokalaemia is generally managed with either oral or intravenous potassium supplementation. If hypokalaemia is mild, potassium-sparing medication and oral potassium supplements will generally be sufficient. As a low serum potassium level can often cause frequent premature ventricular contractions and other electrocardiographic (ECG) changes, cardiac monitoring should be undertaken either continuously, or with serial ECGs while the hypokalaemia is being affected.

If intravenous potassium supplementation is required, the dose should be administered via a volume control pump instead of using a gravity-feed giving set. The use of an infusion pump reduces the risk of life-threatening potassium overdose as a result of accidental failure of the gravity-feed system, causing the rapid infusion of a large dose of potassium. However, many cardiac arrests have also occurred from potassium overdose caused by health care professionals erroneously programming infusion rates into an infusion pump, so additional care and attention should be undertaken if an intravenous potassium infusion is to be administered.

Hyperkalaemia

A rise in blood potassium levels above 5.2 mmol/L is referred to as **hyperkalaemia**. Common causes of hyperkalaemia include an *excessive and/or rapid intake* of potassium, *excessive cell injury* resulting in a shift of intracellular potassium into the extracellular compartment, or *poor renal excretion* of potassium. Examples of specific causes are provided in Clinical Box 31.4.

Hyperkalaemia has significant implications for normal muscle function. Due to the ion's positive charge, higher than normal potassium levels shift the resting membrane potential to a partially depolarised state. Skeletal and smooth muscle can become more easily excited. Depending on how quickly the hyperkalaemic state develops and how severe it becomes, the resting membrane potential can match or rise above that of the threshold potential, leading to membrane unresponsiveness and profound dysfunction of skeletal, smooth and cardiac muscle. There are also changes in cardiac conduction and the duration of cardiac action potentials.

In mild hyperkalaemia, the common clinical manifestations are intestinal cramps, diarrhoea and restlessness (see Clinical Box 31.4). In more severe cases, skeletal muscle weakness and loss of tone occurs. Intestinal smooth muscle unresponsiveness

CLINICAL BOX 31.4

Characteristics of hyperkalaemia

Serum potassium levels
> 5.2 mmol/L

Clinical manifestations

- Mild imbalance
  - Restlessness
  - Diarrhoea
  - Intestinal cramping
- Severe imbalances
  - Skeletal muscle weakness
  - Nausea
  - Cardiac depression (bradycardia, dysrhythmias, cardiac arrest)
  - Paraesthesias

Common causes

Excessive/rapid potassium intake
Excessive/rapid intravenous potassium infusion, excessive doses of drugs containing potassium salts
Shift out of the intracellular to the extracellular compartment
Acidosis, crush injuries, excessive β-receptor antagonism, massive cell death, erythrocyte haemolysis, digoxin toxicity
Decreased potassium losses
Potassium-sparing diuretic therapy, chronic kidney disease, treatment with angiotensin-converting enzyme (ACE) inhibitors or angiotensin II antagonists, hypoaldosteronism

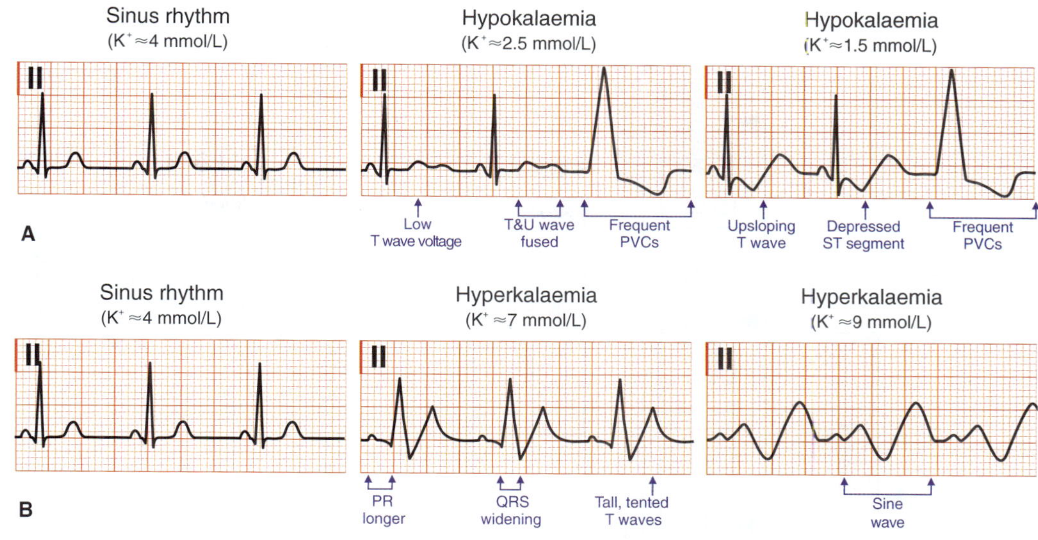

Figure 31.4

ECG changes to serum potassium concentrations

(A) Hypokalaemia. (B) Hyperkalaemia. K^+ = potassium ion.

leads to decreased bowel sounds, and can result in paralytic ileus. In the heart, bradycardia occurs. Severe hyperkalaemia will induce cardiac arrest. Figure 31.4 demonstrates the changes that may be seen on ECG with different serum potassium levels. However, it is important to understand that ECG changes should not be relied on to suggest potassium level. If ECG changes consistent with potassium level imbalances are identified, investigation of serum potassium should occur.

Clinical management Hyperkalaemia can be lethal. The higher the serum potassium level, the more risk of cardiac arrest. The two major approaches to treatment are to increase either potassium excretion or potassium uptake into cells. Mild hyperkalaemia can be treated with oral sodium polystyrene sulfonate (Resonium A) or patiromer. These substances bind to the potassium in the gastrointestinal system and promote excretion. Non-potassium-sparing diuretics (e.g. loop or thiazide diuretics) may also be used to increase potassium excretion. If concern is held for the individual's cardiac rhythm, intravenous calcium chloride can be administered to reduce the membrane potential, decreasing the risk of dysrhythmia. For dangerously high hyperkalaemia, a glucose and insulin infusion will reduce the serum potassium level rapidly. The insulin encourages the extracellular potassium to shift into cells, and the glucose prevents hypoglycaemia. Nebulised salbutamol may also be beneficial. Finally, in critical individuals and those with chronic kidney disease, dialysis will readily decrease serum potassium levels.

ALTERATIONS IN CALCIUM BALANCE

Calcium plays significant roles in blood coagulation, neurotransmission, muscle contraction, excitable membrane potential, cardiac conduction, cell division, cell motility, endocytosis and exocytosis, and in forming the structure of bones and teeth. Calcium is present in the blood in three forms: *bound to plasma proteins, bound to small organic molecules* and as *free ions*. About 40% of the blood calcium level is unbound. The bound forms are physiologically inert, leaving only the free ionised form to exert a physiological action. The range in total blood calcium levels is 2.1–2.6 mmol/L. If necessary, the serum concentration of ionised calcium can also be measured clinically so as to more accurately reflect physiological activity. Figure 31.5 explores the common clinical manifestations and management of calcium imbalance.

Hypocalcaemia

Hypocalcaemia occurs when the serum level of calcium drops below 2.1 mmol/L. It is a straight-forward situation when the total serum calcium levels drop. However, functional hypocalcaemia can develop even when total serum calcium levels are normal. This occurs when the proportion of bound blood calcium increases.

Common causes of hypocalcaemia include *inadequate dietary absorption, increased calcium excretion* and *poor availability of ionised calcium*. Poor dietary absorption can be due to either an inadequate level of calcium in the diet, or the calcium is present but not enough is absorbed. In the latter case, calcium is bound to other molecules in the gut, or the level of activated vitamin D is deficient. Examples of specific causes are provided in Clinical Box 31.5.

Hypocalcaemia is characterised by increased muscle and nerve excitability. The threshold potential of these cells is decreased closer to the resting membrane state. As a consequence, it is easier to induce action potentials (see Figure 31.6). Common clinical manifestations include muscle twitches and spasms, hyperreflexia, paraesthesias, seizures, laryngospasm and cardiac dysrhythmias (see Clinical Box 31.5). As calcium ion influx plays an important role in the plateau phase of the action potential, and in particular in atrioventricular conduction, ventricular conduction and myocardial contractility become impaired.

Two important diagnostic tests are helpful in the evaluation of increased neuromuscular excitability: the Chvostek and

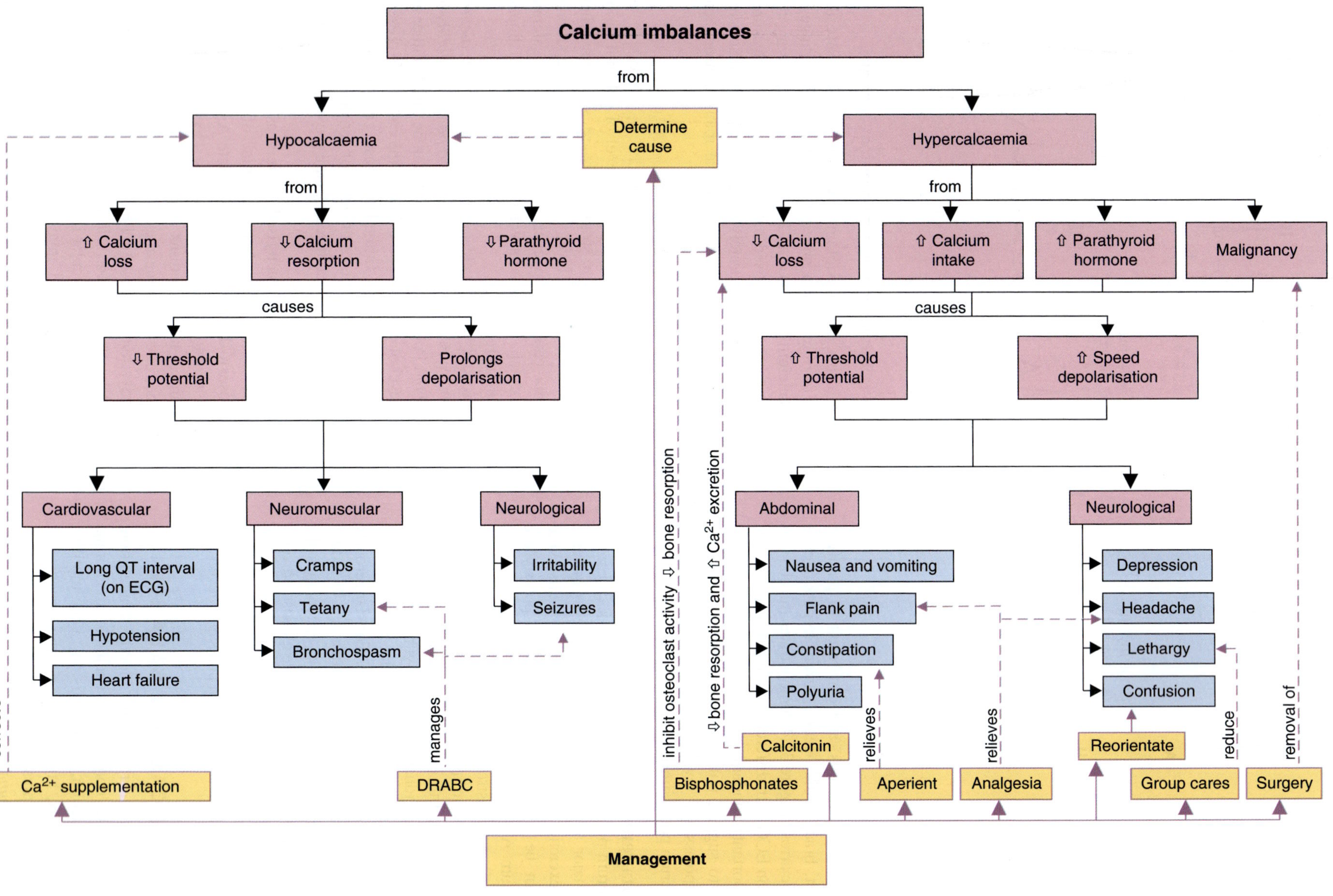

Figure 31.5

Clinical snapshot: Calcium imbalances

↓ = decreased; ↑ = increased; Ca^{2+} = calcium ion; DRABC = danger, response, airway, breathing, circulation; ECG = electrocardiogram.

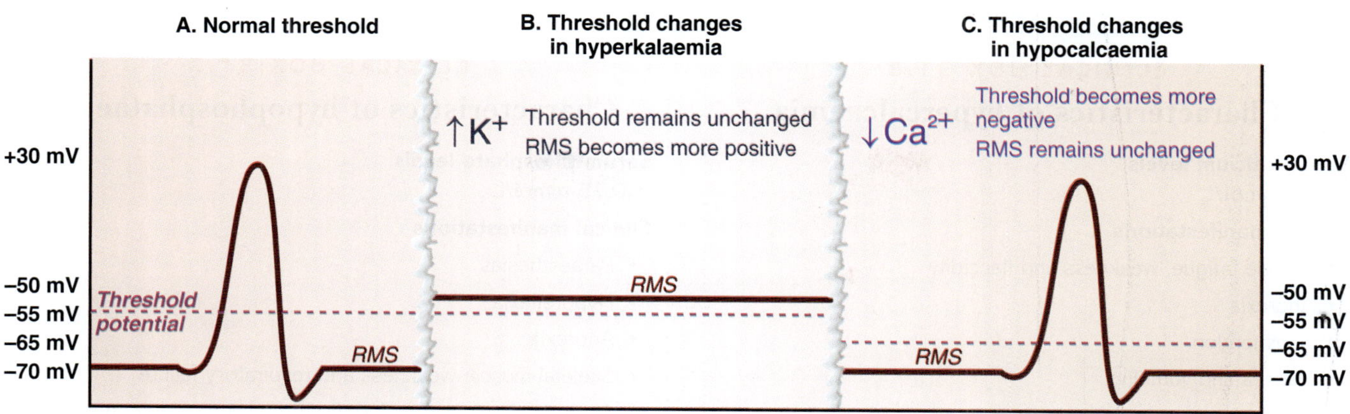

Figure 31.6

Changes in membrane threshold potential in electrolyte imbalances

(A) Normally, the resting membrane state is well below that of the threshold potential. When a stimulus is strong enough to depolarise the membrane to the point of the threshold potential, the membrane will generate an action potential.

(B) In hyperkalaemia, the resting membrane state is equal to or above that of the threshold potential at which the membrane will generate an action potential. The membrane becomes unresponsive and no action potential occurs.

(C) In hypocalcaemia, the threshold membrane potential is lowered closer to the resting membrane state. It is easier for weaker stimuli to generate an action potential in this situation, leading to increased membrane excitability.

↓ = decreased; ↑ = increased; Ca^{2+} = calcium ion; K^+ = potassium ion; mV = millivolts; RMS = resting membrane state.

CLINICAL BOX 31.5

Characteristics of hypocalcaemia

Serum calcium levels

< 2.1 mmol/L

Clinical manifestations

- Muscle twitches and spasms
- Intestinal cramps
- Positive Chvostek sign
- Positive Trousseau sign
- Hyperreflexia
- Paraesthesias
- Seizures
- Laryngospasm
- Cardiac dysrhythmia
- Dry skin and hair, brittle nails

Common causes

Inadequate absorption of calcium

Poor diet in calcium and vitamin D, excessive levels of small organic molecules that bind calcium ions in the gastrointestinal tract (e.g. phytates), high dietary levels of phosphate, malabsorption, alcoholism, chronic diarrhoea, laxative misuse

Poor availability of ionised calcium

Hypoparathyroidism, alkalosis, hypomagnesaemia, elevated plasma free fatty acids, citrated blood transfusions, acute pancreatitis

Excessive excretion of calcium

Loop diuretic therapy

Trousseau signs. A positive *Chvostek sign* is associated with a spasm of the facial muscles. In a state of heightened neuromuscular excitability, tapping the facial cranial nerve in front of the ear triggers a unilateral spasm of the cheek and mouth muscles. A positive *Trousseau sign* develops when a sphygmomanometer applied to the upper arm is partially inflated for a few minutes, leading to decreased blood flow to the hand. This triggers a clearly identifiable carpal spasm.

Clinical management The general principle in the management of hypocalcaemia is supplementation. Calcium can be administered orally via tablets or a powder. Alternatively, intravenous calcium may be used to manage more severe episodes of hypocalcaemia. Assessment and management of the airway are critical in periods of tetany, bronchospasm and seizure. Investigation and management of the cause is also imperative to the appropriate management of an individual with hypocalcaemia.

Hypercalcaemia

Hypercalcaemia occurs when the serum calcium levels rise above 2.6 mmol/L. The typical causes of this condition are *increased gastrointestinal calcium absorption, decreased excretion* and a *shift of calcium* from stores in the bone to the blood. Examples of specific causes are provided in Clinical Box 31.6.

The primary consequence of hypercalcaemia is decreased excitability of the nerve and muscle membranes due to an increase in threshold potential. This is due to the greater intracellular levels of calcium that develop in this state, opposing depolarisation. Common clinical manifestations include constipation, muscle fatigue and weakness, hyporeflexia, headache, confusion and

CLINICAL BOX 31.6

Characteristics of hypercalcaemia

Serum calcium levels
$>$ 2.6 mmol/L

Clinical manifestations

- Muscle fatigue, weakness and flaccidity
- Anorexia
- Constipation
- Nausea and vomiting
- Headache
- Hyporeflexia
- Altered consciousness (confusion → lethargy → stupor → coma)
- Cardiac dysrhythmias
- Polyuria
- Risk of pathological fractures
- Kidney stones

Common causes

Increased absorption of calcium
Excess vitamin D
Shift of calcium from bone to blood
Hyperparathyroidism, Paget's disease of the bone, bone or haematological cancers, prolonged period of immobility
Decreased excretion of calcium
Thiazide diuretic therapy, chronic kidney disease

CLINICAL BOX 31.7

Characteristics of hypophosphataemia

Serum phosphate levels
$<$ 0.75 mmol/L

Clinical manifestations

- Paraesthesias
- Hyporeflexia
- Anorexia
- Skeletal muscle weakness and respiratory failure
- Altered consciousness (confusion → stupor → coma)
- Seizures
- Decreased cardiac output and cardiomyopathies
- Bone pain and pathological fractures

Common causes

Inadequate absorption of phosphate
Chronic diarrhoea, vomiting, malabsorption, misuse of phosphate-binding antacids, chronic alcoholism, vitamin D deficiency
Shift of phosphate from blood into cells (increased cell metabolism)
Total parenteral nutrition, respiratory alkalosis, insulin administration, adrenaline administration
Excessive excretion of phosphate
Increased diuresis, hyperparathyroidism

lethargy. Anorexia, nausea and vomiting, and polyuria also occur (see Clinical Box 31.6). Cardiac dysrhythmias are associated with a shortened plateau phase and delayed atrioventricular conduction. If there is an excessive loss of calcium from the bone, then the affected person is at great risk of kidney stones and pathological fractures.

Clinical management A number of agents can reduce osteoclast activity. Calcitonin can be administered to inhibit bone resorption and increase calcium excretion. Bisphosphonates also affect osteoclast function and inhibit bone resorption actions through binding to the hydroxyapatite in the bone matrix. Depending on the cause, diuretics may also be used to encourage calcium excretion and prevent fluid overload from increased intravenous fluid therapy. Other electrolytes must be monitored during diuretic therapy, as this may result in losses of sodium and potassium as well. If the cause of the hypercalcaemia is related to malignancy or parathyroid hormone imbalance, surgery or radiotherapy may be necessary.

ALTERATIONS IN PHOSPHATE BALANCE

Phosphate plays a key role in intracellular signalling, nucleotide formation and neuromuscular function. It is an essential constituent of the key energy storage molecules, adenosine triphosphate (ATP) and creatine phosphate, and some enzymes, and is an important blood buffer system. The levels of calcium and phosphate in the blood are tightly regulated, so when the levels of one goes up, the other falls. The normal blood concentration of phosphate is 0.75–1.5 mmol/L. Figure 31.7 explores the common clinical manifestations and management of phosphate imbalance.

Hypophosphataemia

Hypophosphataemia occurs when the blood phosphate levels drop below 0.75 mmol/L. Hypophosphataemia can develop when there is a *decreased gastrointestinal absorption* of phosphate, a *shift from the blood into cells* or when the *excretion of phosphate is excessive*. A decrease in phosphate absorption can be associated with either poor dietary intake or excessive loss from the gastrointestinal tract prior to it being absorbed. A shift from the ECF to the intracellular compartment is usually associated with a stimulus that leads to increased cellular metabolism. Examples of specific causes are provided in Clinical Box 31.7.

A key consequence of hypophosphataemia is a lack of readily available ATP for cellular processes. This results in tissue hypoxia. Oxygen transport to cells can be further compromised because of impaired 2,3-diphosphoglycerate (2,3-DPG) formation. 2,3-DPG plays an important role in oxygen–haemoglobin dissociation. Common manifestations include anorexia, paraesthesias, hyporeflexia, muscle weakness that can result in respiratory failure, confusion, stupor, seizures, coma and cardiomyopathies due to impaired cardiac output (see Clinical Box 31.7). Compensatory bone resorption in order to raise blood phosphate levels may lead to bone pain and pathological fractures.

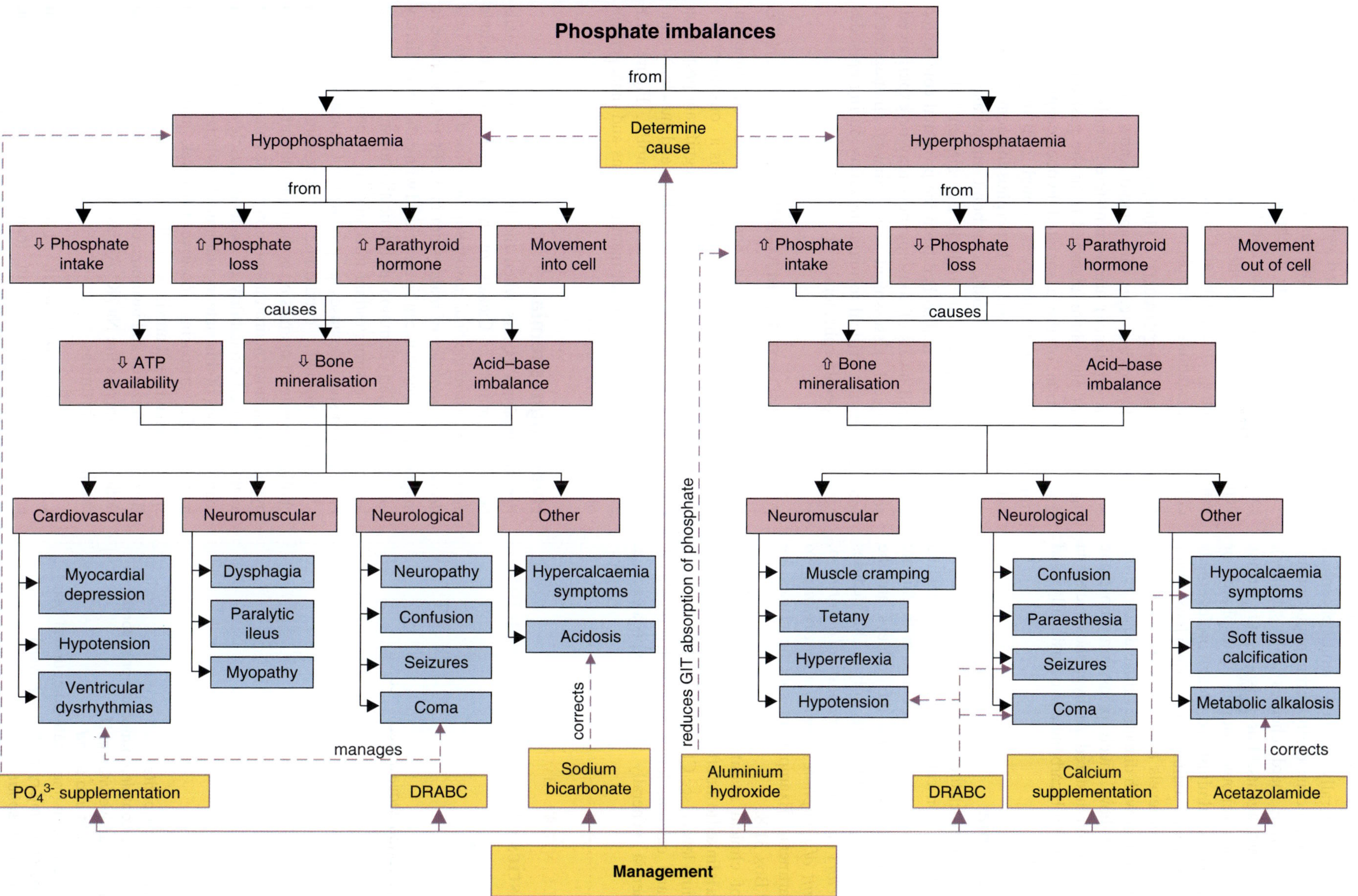

Figure 31.7

Clinical snapshot: Phosphate imbalances

↓ = decreased; ↑ = increased; ATP = adenosine triphosphate; DRABC = danger, response, airway, breathing, circulation; GIT = gastrointestinal tract; PO_4^{3-} = phosphate ion.

Clinical management Irrespective of the cause, hypophosphataemia is generally treated with phosphate supplementation. This may occur orally through phosphate-rich foods (including liver, hard cheeses and sardines), or phosphate replacement agents. For episodes of serious hypophosphataemia, intravenous sodium phosphate or potassium phosphate may be administered. Health professionals should take care to quantify the sodium or potassium levels prior to administration. Potassium levels may be low in individuals with chronic alcohol abuse or with diabetic ketoacidosis. Serum potassium may influence how much potassium phosphate supplementation may be administered. As hypophosphataemia can result in acidosis, sodium bicarbonate is occasionally used to buffer the excess acids.

Hyperphosphataemia

Hyperphosphataemia occurs when the serum phosphate levels rise above 1.5 mmol/L. A common cause of hyperphosphataemia is *decreased excretion* of phosphates associated with chronic kidney disease. This develops because the kidneys are the major normal route of excretion of this electrolyte. Other causes include *increased dietary intake and gastrointestinal absorption*, and a significant *shift of phosphates from the intracellular to extracellular* compartments. Examples of specific causes are provided in Clinical Box 31.8.

The main set of clinical manifestations associated with hyperphosphataemia is linked to the effects of changing phosphate levels on blood calcium levels (see Clinical Box 31.8). As stated earlier, phosphate and calcium levels are tightly regulated, so hyperphosphataemia generally induces hypocalcaemia.

CLINICAL BOX 31.8

Characteristics of hyperphosphataemia

Serum phosphate levels

$>$1.5 mmol/L

Clinical manifestations

- Associated with hypocalcaemia
  - Muscle twitches and spasms
  - Paraesthesias
  - Seizures
- Calcification of soft tissues
  - Itching skin
  - Aching, stiff joints
  - Impaired lung function
- Cardiac dysrhythmias

Common causes

Increased absorption of phosphate

Chronic use of phosphate-containing medications (some laxatives or enemas), excessive vitamin D

Shift of phosphate from cells into blood

High levels of cell destruction (metastatic tumour cell lysis during chemotherapy, crush injury, rhabdomyolysis)

Inadequate excretion of phosphate

Chronic kidney disease, hypoparathyroidism

As indicated earlier in this chapter, hypocalcaemia increases neuromuscular excitability and will result in muscle twitches and spasms, as well as paraesthesias and seizures.

Hyperphosphataemia due to chronic kidney disease leads to calcification of soft tissues due to calcium phosphate salt deposition in tissues such as the skin, lungs and joints. Itching skin and aching, stiff joints and impaired lung function are clinical manifestations of this phenomenon.

Clinical management Phosphate binders such as aluminium hydroxide (e.g. the antacid known as Mylanta contains this substance) are administered orally to reduce the amount of phosphate absorbed from the gastrointestinal tract. Correction of the associated hypocalcaemia is also important. This can be achieved through oral or parenteral calcium supplementation. As hyperphosphataemia can also result in metabolic alkalosis, a carbonic anhydrase inhibitor may be administered to reduce the amount of sodium bicarbonate that is reabsorbed from the proximal convoluted tubule. Altered levels of consciousness may be experienced, so neurological assessment and airway management interventions are critical to maintain safety during episodes of severe hyperphosphataemia.

ALTERATIONS IN MAGNESIUM BALANCE

Magnesium plays a role in nerve and muscle function, neurotransmission and bone structure, and is a constituent of a number of important enzyme systems. A significant proportion (about 50%) of magnesium is stored in bone and muscle. Normal blood levels are between 0.7 and 1.1 mmol/L. Figure 31.8 explores the common clinical manifestations and management of magnesium imbalance.

Hypomagnesaemia

Hypomagnesaemia occurs when the blood concentration falls below 0.7 mmol/L. Causes of hypomagnesaemia include *decreased gastrointestinal absorption, increased excretion* or a *decreased availability* of magnesium in the ECF. A decrease in magnesium absorption can be associated with either poor dietary intake (particularly common in chronic alcoholism) or excessive loss from the gastrointestinal tract prior to it being absorbed. Examples of specific causes are provided in Clinical Box 31.9.

Under normal conditions, magnesium suppresses cholinergic neurotransmission at the neuromuscular junction. In hypomagnesaemia, neurotransmission here is enhanced, leading to the increased excitability of skeletal muscles. The clinical manifestations of this state include muscle twitches and cramps, hyperreflexia, grimacing, positive Chvostek and Trousseau signs, dysphagia and ataxia, as well as nystagmus (see Clinical Box 31.9). Seizures and insomnia can also occur. A magnesium deficiency impairs the Na^+/K^+-ATPase enzymes, which leads to cardiac dysrhythmias.

Clinical management Low levels of magnesium are generally managed with magnesium supplementation, either orally or parenterally. For mild magnesium deficiency, an increased consumption of magnesium-rich foods may

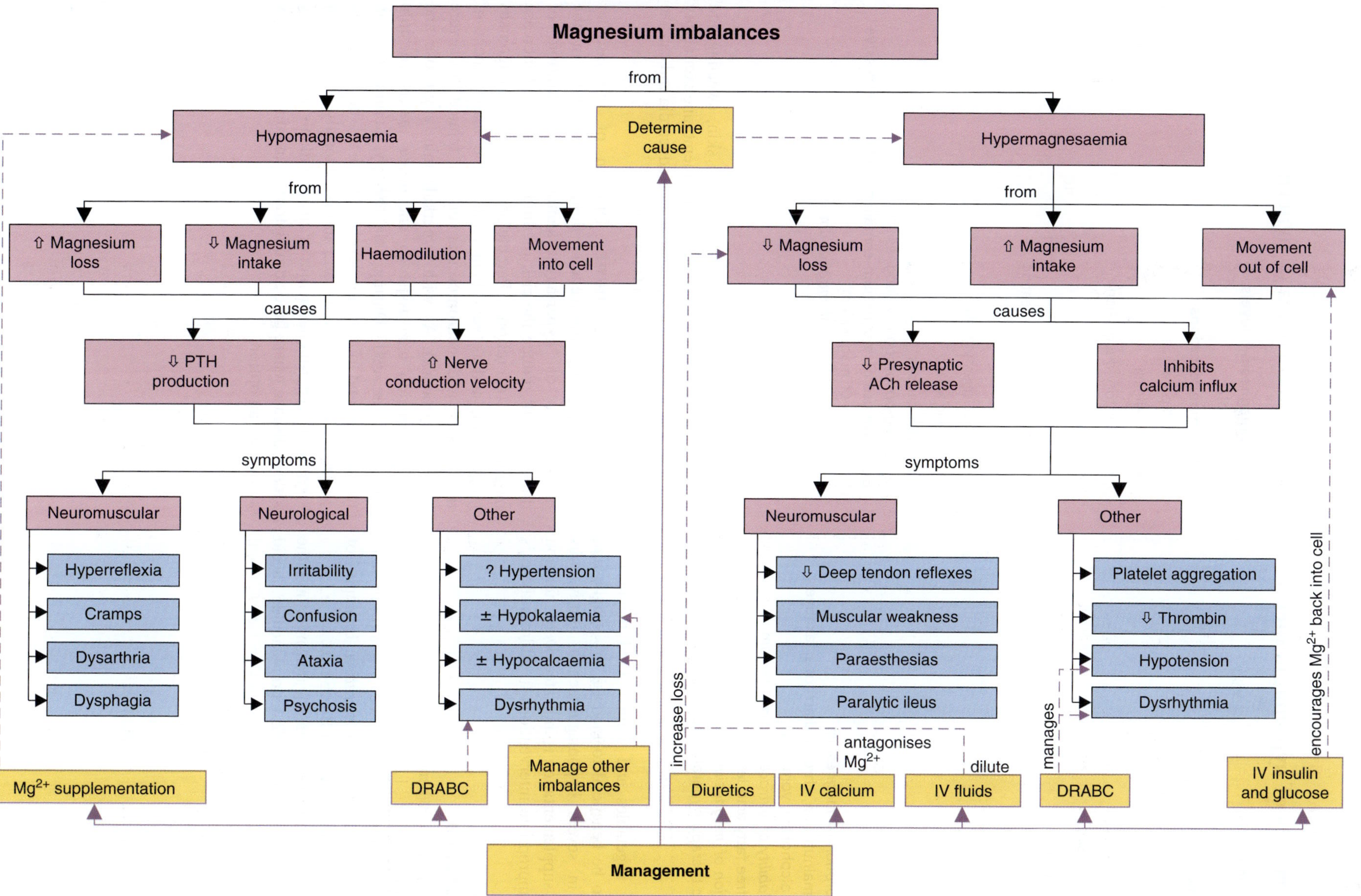

Figure 31.8

Clinical snapshot: Magnesium imbalances

↓ = decreased; ↑ = increased; ? = possible; ± = with or without; ACh = acetylcholine; DRABC = danger, response, airway, breathing, circulation; IV = intravenous; Mg^{2+} = magnesium ion; PTH = parathyroid hormone.

CLINICAL BOX 31.9

Characteristics of hypomagnesaemia

Serum magnesium levels

$<$ 0.70 mmol/L

Clinical manifestations

- Muscle twitches and cramps
- Grimacing
- Hyperreflexia
- Positive Chvostek sign
- Positive Trousseau sign
- Dysphagia
- Ataxia
- Nystagmus
- Seizures
- Insomnia
- Cardiac dysrhythmias

Common causes

Inadequate absorption of magnesium

Malabsorption, malnutrition, chronic diarrhoea, laxative misuse, chronic alcoholism, vomiting

Decreased availability of extracellular magnesium

Elevated blood free fatty acid levels

Excessive excretion of magnesium

Thiazide diuretic therapy, hyperaldosteronism

be beneficial (e.g. vegetables and grains). Oral magnesium gluconate may also be beneficial to increase low magnesium levels. However, in severe hypomagnesaemia, intravenous magnesium sulfate supplementation is indicated. Determination of the cause and appropriate interventions to address these is also critical.

Hypermagnesaemia

Hypermagnesaemia occurs when the blood concentration of magnesium rises above 1.1 mmol/L. The causes of hypermagnesaemia include increased *gastrointestinal magnesium absorption* and *decreased excretion*. Examples of specific causes are provided in Clinical Box 31.10.

Hypermagnesaemia depresses cholinergic transmission at the neuromuscular junction. Clinical manifestations include flaccid paralysis, hyporeflexia and respiratory depression (see Clinical Box 31.10). Lethargy, drowsiness, flushed skin, sweating and hypotension can also be observed. Cardiac membrane excitability is depressed in this condition, leading to bradycardia and cardiac dysrhythmias, possibly even cardiac arrest.

CLINICAL BOX 31.10

Characteristics of hypermagnesaemia

Serum magnesium levels

$>$ 1.1 mmol/L

Clinical manifestations

- Flaccid paralysis
- Hyporeflexia
- Respiratory depression
- Drowsiness
- Lethargy
- Flushed skin and sweating
- Hypotension
- Cardiac dysrhythmias
- Cardiac arrest

Common causes

Increased absorption of magnesium

Excessive use of magnesium-containing antacids, excessive IV infusion of magnesium

Decreased excretion of magnesium

Chronic kidney disease

Clinical management Dilution of intravascular magnesium using intravenous fluid is important in the management of hypermagnesaemia. Administration of diuretics will reduce the risk of fluid overload and increase magnesium excretion. Parenteral calcium antagonises magnesium, and is very beneficial in the management of the cardiac and neuromuscular effects related to severe hypermagnesaemia. As with hyperkalaemia, a glucose and insulin infusion can assist to encourage the magnesium back into the cell. During this therapy, serum glucose, magnesium and potassium levels should all be monitored closely. A glucose–insulin infusion is generally reserved for significant hypermagnesaemia or in individuals with chronic kidney disease where fluid administration and diuretic therapy are less of an option.

INDIGENOUS HEALTH FAST FACTS AND CULTURAL CONSIDERATIONS

FAST FACTS

- ***Based on 2016–17 data, the hospitalisation rates for acute gastroenteritis in Aboriginal and Torres Strait Islander infants in major cities and inner regional areas are around twice those of non-Indigenous children. Hospitalisation rates are nearly 50 times higher in the most socially disadvantaged areas compared to in the least disadvataged areas. Severe diarrhoea from the gastroenteritis can result in electrolyte imbalances, such as hypokalaemia and hyponatraemia.***

CULTURAL CONSIDERATIONS

- ***Aboriginal and Torres Strait Islander peoples' traditional diets included seasonal fruit, roots, vegetables, fish and wild meats, which were low in energy density and rich in nutrients; ideal to ensure an intake of appropriate amounts of important electrolytes such as potassium, calcium and sodium. However, post-European settlement, as more non-traditional foods became available, and fewer Indigenous bush foods were consumed, Western diets high in salt and lower in potassium and calcium came to dominate Indigenous Australians' diets.***
- ***Aboriginal and Torres Strait Islander peoples aged 2 and over living in remote areas are more likely to eat bush foods, such as non-commercially caught fish, crustacea and molluscs, wild harvested meat and reptiles.***

Source: Data from Australian Indigenous HealthInfoNet (2022); Centre for Epidemiology and Evidence (2018); Lee & Ride (2018).

CHILDREN AND ADOLESCENTS

- Maternal electrolyte status may influence a neonate's electrolyte analysis within the first 12–24 hours. Administration of hypotonic intravenous fluids can cause neonatal hyponatraemia, as can excessive oxytocin use.
- Children with diarrhoea or vomiting can rapidly develop sodium, potassium and chloride deficiencies. Oral rehydration therapies (ORT) can support sodium, potassium and chloride levels. ORT also contains glucose.
- The use of antidiarrhoeal agents is not recommended for infants and children, as they may mask a child's decline, resulting in treatment delay.

OLDER ADULTS

- Age-related decreases in glomerular filtration rate occur as a result of reducing renal blood flow, and from renal cortical cell loss. Even in health, these changes can result in hyponatraemia. Hyponatraemia is very common in older people, and can result in cognitive impairment and increased falls.
- Hypokalaemia is common in older adults treated with diuretics. Potassium supplementation or use of potassium-sparing diuretics may be necessary to prevent the development of hypokalaemia.
- Hypernatraemia occurring in the older person is commonly associated with a decreased thirst sensation (causing decreased water intake) and the inability to concentrate urine (causing increased water loss without loss of sodium).

KEY CLINICAL ISSUES

- Assessment of an ind vidual's electrolyte status is important, as fluid and electrolyte homeostasis is imperative for cellular function. Alterations in level of consciousness, electrocardiography changes, abdominal pain and excessive fluid losses should all trigger investigation with a view to the urgent management of electrolyte imbalances.
- The choice of intravenous therapy, fluids and additives will directly influence an individual's fluid and electrolyte status. Frequent reassessment should be undertaken to ensure that supplementation for electrolyte deficiencies does not result in dangerous electrolyte excess.
- Sodium deficiencies should be corrected slowly, as rapid correction can result in dangerous neurological events.
- Potassium supplementation administered intravenously should always be undertaken using a pump or syringe driver to ensure that a bolus potassium dose is not inadvertently administered. Having a colleague double-check the program on a potassium infusion is also good practice, and can reduce the risk of potassium overdose, resulting in cardiac arrest and death.

- Hyperkalaemia can be managed in a number of ways, depending on the severity of the excess. Mildly elevated potassium can be managed with agents that reduce potassium absorption from the gastrointestinal tract. Higher levels may require a more aggressive use of loop diuretics, and excessively high potassium levels may need to be managed with insulin-glucose infusion, or even dialysis.
- Calcium imbalances are less common than sodium and potassium issues; however, they can still be dangerous. Observations for neurological deficits can assist in the clinical assessment of calcium imbalance.
- Phosphate imbalances can be common in individuals with kidney disease. The use of phosphate binders can reduce hyperphosphataemia, and phosphate supplementation can assist with hypophosphataemia. Phosphate imbalances will directly influence calcium levels.
- Magnesium and potassium imbalances may result in dysrhythmias, such as frequent ventricular ectopic beats. Assessment of an individual's biochemistry blood test may be clinically indicated if cardiac signs are noticed.

CHAPTER REVIEW

- *Electrolytes* are important solutes found in body fluids, where they exist as charged particles that contribute to body functioning.
- The distribution of electrolytes is not uniform across the body compartments.
- *Hyponatraemia* occurs when blood sodium levels drop below 135 mmol/L. It can develop due to an inadequate intake, an excessive gain in water, or as a result of a shift in water from the intracellular to the extracellular compartment. Clinical manifestations include anorexia, nausea and vomiting, altered consciousness and seizures.
- *Hypernatraemia* occurs when blood sodium levels rise above 145 mmol/L. It can develop due to an excessive sodium gain or an excessive loss of water. Clinical manifestations include thirst, confusion, altered consciousness and seizures.
- *Hypokalaemia* occurs when blood potassium levels drop below 3.5 mmol/L. It can develop due to an inadequate intake, an excessive loss or as a result of a shift from the extracellular to the intracellular compartment. Clinical manifestations include skeletal muscle weakness, paralytic ileus, hypotension, cardiac dysrhythmias and polyuria.
- *Hyperkalaemia* occurs when blood potassium levels rise above 5.2 mmol/L. It can develop due to an excessive or rapid intake, decreased losses or as a result of a shift from the intracellular to the extracellular compartment. Clinical manifestations include diarrhoea, intestinal cramps, muscle weakness, paralytic ileus, bradycardia and cardiac arrest.
- *Hypocalcaemia* occurs when blood calcium levels drop below 2.1 mmol/L. It can develop due to inadequate calcium absorption, an excessive loss or poor availability of the physiologically active ionised form. Clinical manifestations include muscle twitches and spasms, hyperreflexia, paraesthesias, seizures, cardiac dysrhythmias and positive Chvostek and Trousseau signs.
- *Hypercalcaemia* occurs when blood calcium levels rise above 2.6 mmol/L. It can develop due to increased calcium absorption, decreased losses or a shift from bone to blood. Clinical manifestations include muscle fatigue and weakness, constipation, altered consciousness, anorexia, nausea and vomiting, cardiac dysrhythmias, pathological fractures and kidney stones.
- *Hypophosphataemia* occurs when blood phosphate levels drop below 0.75 mmol/L. It can develop due to inadequate phosphate absorption, an excessive loss or a shift from blood into cells. Clinical manifestations include paraesthesias, hyporeflexia, muscle weakness, altered consciousness, seizures, cardiomyopathies and pathological fractures.
- *Hyperphosphataemia* occurs when blood phosphate levels rise above 1.5 mmol/L. It can develop due to increased phosphate absorption, decreased losses or a shift from cells into blood. Clinical manifestations include paraesthesias, muscle twitches, seizures and calcification of soft tissues.
- *Hypomagnesaemia* occurs when blood magnesium levels drop below 0.7 mmol/L. It can develop due to inadequate magnesium absorption, an excessive loss or a decreased availability of extracellular magnesium. Clinical manifestations include muscle twitches and cramps, hyperreflexia, dysphagia, ataxia, seizures and cardiac dysrhythmias.
- *Hypermagnesaemia* occurs when blood magnesium levels rise above 1.1 mmol/L. It can develop due to increased magnesium absorption or decreased excretion. Clinical manifestations include flaccid paralysis, hyporeflexia, respiratory depression, altered consciousness, hypotension, cardiac dysrhythmias and cardiac arrest.

REVIEW QUESTIONS

1 Define the term 'electrolyte'.

2 a What is the most abundant intracellular electrolyte?
  b What is the most abundant electrolyte in the blood?

3 State two normal functions of each of the following electrolytes:
  a potassium
  b calcium
  c sodium
  d magnesium

4 State the serum electrolyte level that characterises each of the following imbalances:
  a hypophosphataemia
  b hyperkalaemia
  c hypocalcaemia

5 How does muscle function change in each of the following electrolyte imbalances?
  a hyperkalaemia
  b hypocalcaemia
  c hypermagnesaemia

6 State two clinical manifestations associated with each of the following electrolyte imbalances:
  a hypokalaemia
  b hypomagnesaemia
  c hyperphosphataemia
  d hyponatraemia

7 Mr George Stein is a 60-year-old man who has been diagnosed with hyperaldosteronism. He is showing uncharacteristic weakness in his arms, cardiac dysrhythmia, some confused thoughts and is voiding urine more frequently. Which electrolyte imbalance does Mr Stein appear to be experiencing?

8 Mrs Fran Peters is a 72-year-old woman who is living alone after her husband died a year ago. Her son stays in touch with her regularly by telephone, but he hasn't seen her for a couple of weeks. The son suspects that his mother is not eating well, and asks her to go and have a medical check-up. She goes to her doctor, who while taking her blood pressure notices that her wrist muscles spasm when the cuff on her right arm is partially inflated. The doctor checks her reflexes and notes that they are more reactive. He taps her cheek bone just in front of her right ear and notes twitching of the corner of her mouth.

a Identify each of the muscle responses described in this case.

b What are the likely electrolyte imbalances that manifest these responses?

c Following on from your answer to question b, how could you determine which imbalance is present?

HEALTH PROFESSIONAL CONNECTIONS

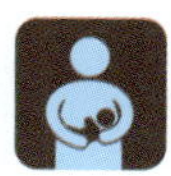

Midwives Hyperemesis can result in fluid and electrolyte imbalances in a pregnant woman. Good communication, interview and physical assessment skills are important to prevent fluid and electrolyte imbalance in a woman, or to detect such an imbalance and assist her if it has already occurred. The newborn's kidney is immature and unable to concentrate urine well. Large sodium losses can occur, and other electrolyte imbalances may result, too. Generally speaking, well babies will cope; however, concerns regarding a neonate's fluid or electrolyte balance should be investigated and managed quickly. Consultation with other health care professionals is important to ensure the safety and early intervention of ill babies.

Physiotherapists Fluid and electrolyte levels can cause muscle cramping. If during a treatment a muscle cramp occurs, massage and stretching of the affected area are indicated. Client education regarding diet and fluid replacement is important, especially when you notice a person experiencing several cramp episodes. Many people in intensive care units experience electrolyte imbalances, and many electrolyte imbalances can cause dysrhythmia. When working with critically ill individuals, good communication skills are important between staff to ensure that all of the necessary information is available to the physiotherapist, so that the team may plan the most appropriate times and interventions to best assist the client.

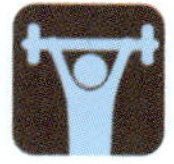

Exercise scientists Electrolyte imbalances are common following aerobic events. Significant electrolyte imbalances can have major effects on cardiac and skeletal muscle and nerve function. Measured preparation prior to such an event and appropriate replacements after an event can have a positive effect on outcomes.

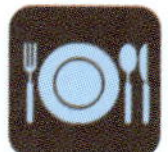

Nutritionists/Dieticians Diet can have a significant influence on fluid and electrolyte balance. Both enteral and parenteral nutrition can manipulate fluid and ionic shifts between fluid compartments. Working with clients to maintain this balance can be complicated by disease, food preferences and commitment. Client education is a major step in encouraging adherence to appropriate meal plans. Knowledge of how fluid and electrolytes can affect health outcomes may be the factor that promotes success.

CASE STUDY

Mrs Myrtle Fox is an 85-year-old woman (UR number 184927) transferred from the intensive care unit this morning following an unconscious collapse in her home three days ago. Mrs Fox is widowed and lives alone in a two-storey house. She has no family, but a close friend visits a couple of times a week. The police broke into her house when her friend raised the alarm. Mrs Fox was found unconscious on the floor near the telephone. She was lying semi-prone in what appeared to be a large amount of urine. It was surmised that she fell and was not able to get back up. There were no apparent skeletal injuries. The paramedics were unable to determine how long ago this had occurred, but feel that it had been a few days. Some soft tissue injuries on her right knee and right elbow were obvious. Her mucous membranes were dry, and she had decreased skin turgor. An oropharyngeal airway was placed and supplemental oxygen was applied. Following transfer by ambulance, on admission her observations were as follows:

Temperature	Heart rate	Respiration rate	Blood pressure	SpO_2
35.6°C	124	10	72/34	94% (6L/min via mask)

On arrival, Mrs Fox was unconscious, and her Glasgow coma scale (GCS) score was 6 (E = 1, V = 1, M = 4); her deep tendon reflexes were diminished. She was intubated and ventilated, and blood was taken for a full blood count and electrolyte levels. Her pathology results were as follows:

HAEMATOLOGY

Patient location:	Ward 3	**UR:**	184927		
Consultant:	Smith	**NAME:**	Fox		
		Given name:	Myrtle	**Sex:**	F
		DOB:	03/02/XX	**Age:**	85

Time collected 11:22
Date collected XX/XX
Year XXXX
Lab # 53244534

FULL BLOOD COUNT		UNITS	REFERENCE RANGE
Haemoglobin	115	g/L	115–160
White cell count	9.3	$\times 10^9$/L	4.0–11.0
Platelets	150	$\times 10^9$/L	140–400
Haematocrit	0.34		0.33–0.47
Red cell count	3.89	$\times 10^{12}$/L	3.80–5.20
Reticulocyte count	1.8	%	0.2–2.0
MCV	82	fL	80–100
Neutrophils	3.2	$\times 10^9$/L	2.00–8.00
Lymphocytes	2.23	$\times 10^9$/L	1.00–4.00
Monocytes	0.35	$\times 10^9$/L	0.10–1.00
Eosinophils	0.32	$\times 10^9$/L	< 0.60
Basophils	0.15	$\times 10^9$/L	< 0.20
ESR	11	mm/h	< 12

BIOCHEMISTRY

Patient location:	Ward 3	**UR:**	184927		
Consultant:	Smith	**NAME:**	Fox		
		Given name:	Myrtle	**Sex:**	F
		DOB:	03/02/XX	**Age:**	85

Time collected 11:22
Date collected XX/XX
Year XXXX
Lab # 64646745

ELECTROLYTES		UNITS	REFERENCE RANGE
Sodium	119	mmol/L	135-145
Potassium	3.5	mmol/L	3.5-5.2
Chloride	95	mmol/L	95-110
Bicarbonate	18	mmol/L	22-32
Glucose (random)	2.9	mmol/L	3.5-5.4
Iron	15	μmol/L	11-30

Although limited history was available, a bottle of thiazide diuretics was found (with her name on it) on the kitchen table.

Following stabilisation, fluid support and management of her hyponatraemia and hypoglycaemia, she was extubated on day 2 and has been transferred to the ward this morning. Her GCS score is 13 (E = 3, V = 4, M = 6), and she is intermittently confused. Her observations were as follows:

*NP = nasal prongs.

Temperature	Heart rate	Respiration rate	Blood pressure	SpO_2
36°C	78	18	140/86	96% (4L/min via NP*)

CRITICAL THINKING

1. Consider Mrs Fox's history. What factors contributed to the development of her hyponatraemia? Explain the mechanism of each factor that you identify.
2. Observe her first set of observations (and history). What can be deduced from this information regarding Mrs Fox's initial fluid status? Identify each of the factors used to make this judgment, and explain what is occurring in the intravascular and intracellular fluid compartments.
3. Explain the significance of correcting the hyponatraemia slowly. Why is this important? What may occur if the sodium level rises too rapidly? Explain the mechanism.
4. What assessments and interventions are appropriate in caring for Mrs Fox? Ensure that consideration is made regarding the neurological effects of sodium imbalance.
5. Given the mechanism of her developing the hyponatraemia and her current social situation, what interventions should be considered prior to discharge?

BIBLIOGRAPHY

Agraharkar, M., Dellinger, O.D. & Gangakhedkar, A.K. (2021). Hypercalcemia. *Emedicine*. https://emedicine.medscape.com/article/240681-overview.

Australian Indigenous Health*Info*Net (2022). *Overview of Aboriginal and Torres Strait Islander health status, 2021.* Perth, WA: Australian Indigenous Health*Info*Net. https://healthinfonet.ecu.edu.au/learn/health-facts/overview-aboriginal-torres-strait-islander-health-status.

Bauldoff, G., Gubrud-Howe, P.M., Carno, M.-A., Levett-Jones, T., Hales, M., Berry, K., … Stanley, D. (2020). *LeMone and Burke's medical–surgical nursing: critical thinking for person-centred care* (4th [Australian] edn). Sydney: Pearson Australia.

Best, O. & Fredericks, B. (2021). *Yatdjuligin: Aboriginal and Torres Strait Islander nursing and midwifery care* (3rd edn). Port Melbourne, VIC: Cambridge University Press.

Bullock, S. & Manias, E. (2022). *Fundamentals of pharmacology* (9th edn). Sydney: Pearson Australia.

Centre for Epidemiology and Evidence (2018). *Aboriginal kids—a healthy start to life: Report of the Chief Health Officer 2018*. Sydney: NSW Ministry of Health. https://www.health.nsw.gov.au/hsnsw/Publications/chief-health-officers-report-2018.pdf.

Hamrahian, S.M., Maarouf, O.H., Teran, F.J. & Simon, E.E. (2022). Hyponatremia. *Emedicine*. https://emedicine.medscape.com/article/242166-overview.

Lederer, E., Alsauskas, Z.C., Mackelaite, L. & Nayak, V. (2021a). Hyperkalemia. *Emedicine*. https://emedicine.medscape.com/article/240903-overview.

Lederer, E., Alsauskas, Z.C., Mackelaite, L. & Nayak, V. (2021b). Hypokalemia. *Emedicine*. https://emedicine.medscape.com/article/242008-overview.

Lee, A. & Ride, K. (2018). Review of nutrition among Aboriginal and Torres Strait Islander people. *Australian Indigenous Health*Bulletin 18(1). https://healthbulletin.org.au/wp-content/uploads/2018/02/Nutrition-Review-Bulletin-2018_Final.pdf.

Lukitsch, I. (2023). Hypernatremia. *Emedicine*. https://emedicine.medscape.com/article/241094-overview.

Marieb, E.N. & Hoehn, K. (2019). *Human anatomy and physiology* (11th edn). San Francisco, CA: Pearson Benjamin Cummings.

32 Common inflammatory disorders of the kidneys and urinary tract

KEY TERMS

Acute tubular necrosis (ATN)
Cystitis
Diabetic nephropathy
Dysuria
Haematogenous urinary tract infection
Haematuria
Nephritic syndrome
Nephrotic syndrome
Nitrite
Nosocomial infection
Pyelonephritis
Pyuria
Tubulointerstitial nephritis
Urethritis
Urinary incontinence
Urinary stasis

LEARNING OBJECTIVES

After completing this chapter, you should be able to:

1 Describe the effects of infection within the kidneys and urinary tract.

2 Describe how nephron functions may be compromised in pyelonephritis and glomerulonephritis.

3 Explore the mechanism of nephropathy secondary to diabetes.

4 Compare and contrast tubulointerstitial nephritis and acute tubular necrosis.

5 Describe urinary incontinence and its various causes.

WHAT YOU SHOULD KNOW BEFORE YOU START THIS CHAPTER

Can you identify the structure of the urinary tract, and describe its functions?

Can you identify the major structures of the kidney, and describe their functions?

Can you identify the structure of the nephron, and describe its functions?

Can you describe the phases of acute inflammation?

Can you describe the stages of the healing process?

Can you differentiate between acute and chronic inflammation?

Introduction

The kidneys (adj. *renal*), working together with various hormones, the autonomic nervous system and the body's thirst-sensing mechanism, maintain the volume and composition of the body's extracellular fluids. The focus of this chapter is on the common infections and inflammatory conditions that affect the kidneys and the urinary tract. By way of introduction, a brief overview of the organisation of the kidneys and urinary tract is given below.

The normal kidneys

Each kidney is covered by a connective tissue capsule and enclosed in a protective layer of fat. The anterior surface is covered in peritoneum. The kidneys are supplied with blood through the renal arteries, which are derived from branches of the abdominal aorta, and drain through renal veins into the inferior vena cava.

Within the kidney, three zones can be identified macroscopically (see Figure 32.1):

1. the *cortex* (outer zone)
2. the *medulla*, consisting of cone-shaped renal pyramids—the apex of each pyramid is a *renal papilla* that delivers urine to the renal pelvis
3. the *renal sinus*, the central part of the kidney, that contains the branches of the *renal artery*, the tributaries of the *renal vein* and the *renal pelvis*.

The renal pelvis is a funnel-shaped tube that is continuous at one end with the ureter, and branches at the other end to form the *major calyces*. Each major calyx, in turn, subdivides into *minor calyces* that receive urine from the papillae.

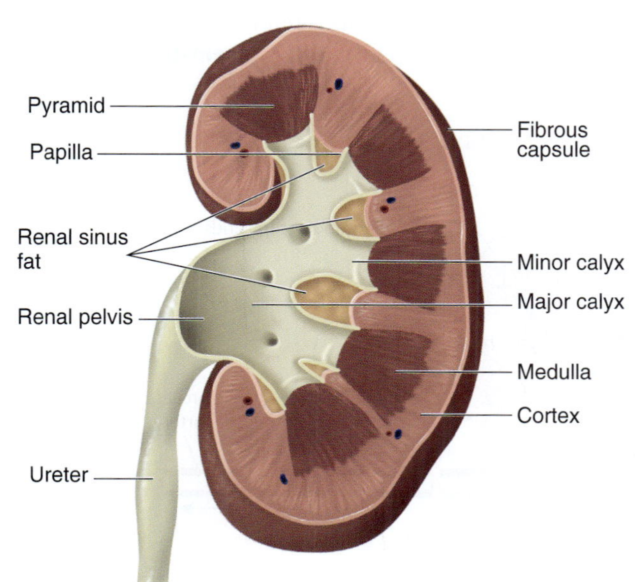

Figure 32.1
Zones of the kidney

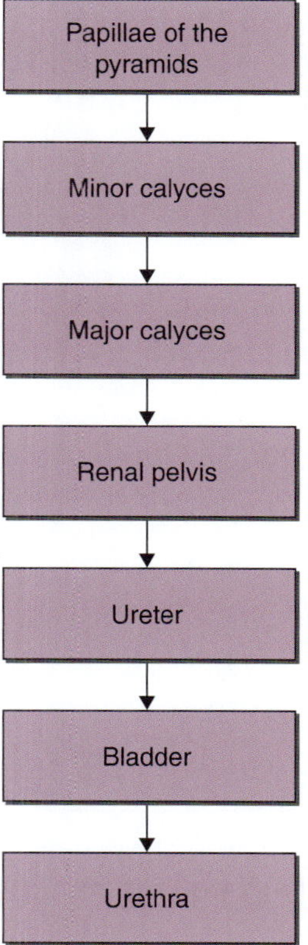

Figure 32.2
Path of urine flow from the kidneys to the urethra

The urine drains from the papillae of the pyramids down to the bladder and out of the body along the path indicated in Figure 32.2. The urinary system of each sex is represented in Figure 32.3.

The walls of the calyces, pelvis and ureters contain smooth muscle. Coordinated contractions of the smooth muscle enable these structures to actively propel urine towards the bladder. A *vesicoureteral valve* at the junction of each ureter with the bladder ensures that this movement occurs in one direction only.

The *nephron* is the microscopic functional unit of the kidney. Each kidney contains roughly 1.5 million nephrons. The nephron filters the blood and, through a variety of mechanisms, subsequently adjusts the levels within it both of wastes and useful substances, such as water and electrolytes. Each nephron (see Figure 32.4) is subdivided into:

- a *glomerulus*, also known as a *renal corpuscle*—a tight cluster of capillaries (*glomerular capillaries*) surrounded by an epithelial glomerular capsule (*Bowman's capsule*)
- a *renal tubule*—a long thin tube surrounded by a second network of capillaries (*peritubular capillaries*).

The urine, as it forms, empties from the renal tubule into a collecting tubule, then into a collecting duct, with each duct receiving urine from many nephrons. The collecting ducts run through the medullary pyramids and combine to form papillary ducts, which deliver urine via the papillae to the minor calyces. Glomeruli are located in the kidney cortex, while tubules and collecting ducts extend from the cortex into the medulla.

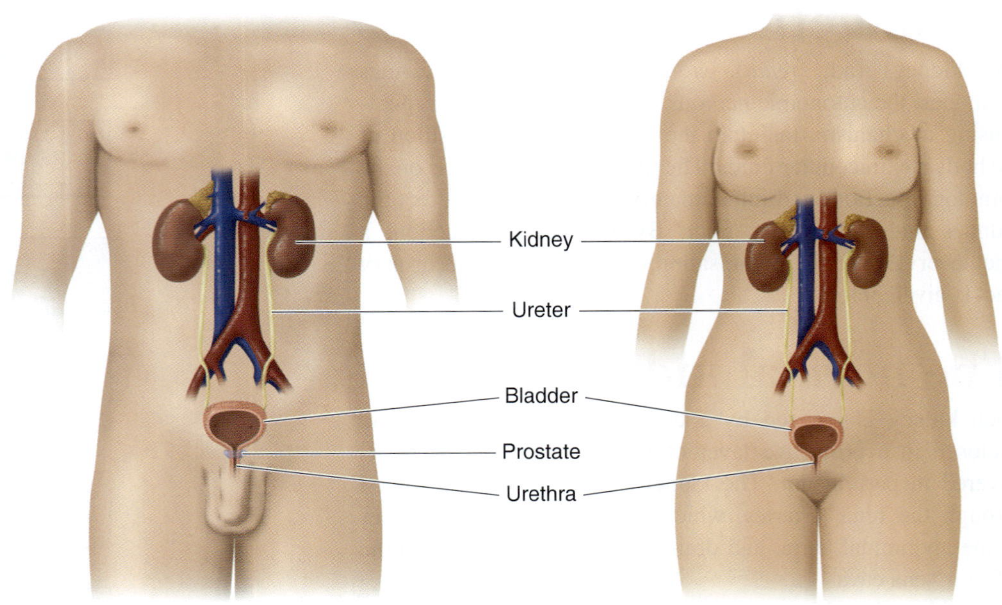

Figure 32.3

Urinary systems of male (left) and female (right)

Bacterial urinary tract infections

AETIOLOGY AND PATHOPHYSIOLOGY

LEARNING OBJECTIVE 1

Describe the effects of infection within the kidneys and urinary tract.

The kidneys, ureters, bladder and proximal urethra are normally sterile. Sterility is maintained by the frequent flushing action of urine. Moreover, specific immune protection is afforded to the lining of the bladder by *secretory antibody (IgA)*. It is only in the distal urethra near the external opening that a resident microbial community exists. This consists mainly of Gram-positive skin bacteria (e.g. *Staphylococcus epidermidis*) and Gram-negative enteric bacteria (e.g. *Escherichia coli*, otherwise called *E. coli*). Thus, while urine is normally sterile in the bladder, it becomes contaminated with microbes during its passage through the urethra. When the mechanical, chemical and immune defences of the urinary tract are compromised, the risk of infection is increased.

Most *urinary tract infections (UTIs)* arise from the person's own bowel flora. Bacteria from faeces can enter the urinary tract at the urethral opening (see Figure 32.5) and ascend to the bladder, sometimes progressing higher up to the kidneys (called an *ascending UTI*). Less often, the pathogen may be carried by the bloodstream from a distant focus of infection to the kidney. This is referred to as *haematogenous spread* (see Figure 32.6) or a **haematogenous urinary tract infection**.

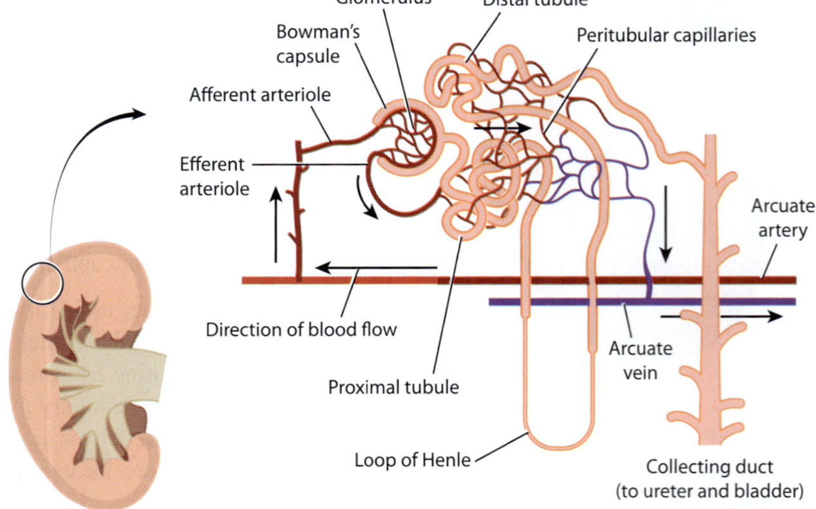

Figure 32.4

The nephron, Bowman's capsule and glomerular capillaries

Source: Blamb/Shutterstock.

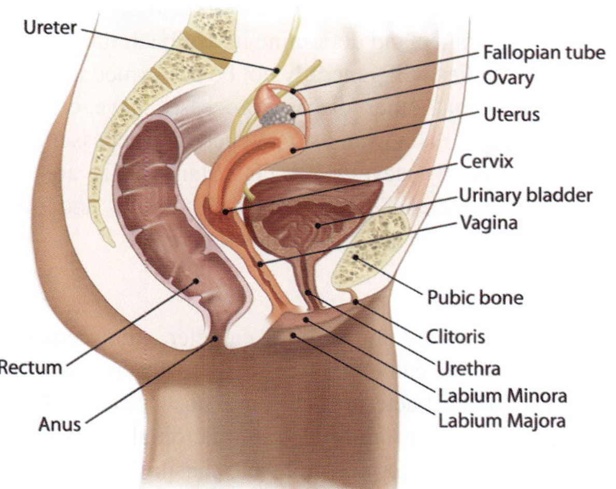

Figure 32.5

The urethral opening in women

Bacteria from the gastrointestinal tract can enter the urethra. Wiping incorrectly from the rectum towards the urethra may permit translocation of enteric bacteria into the urethra.

Source: kocakayaali/Shutterstock.

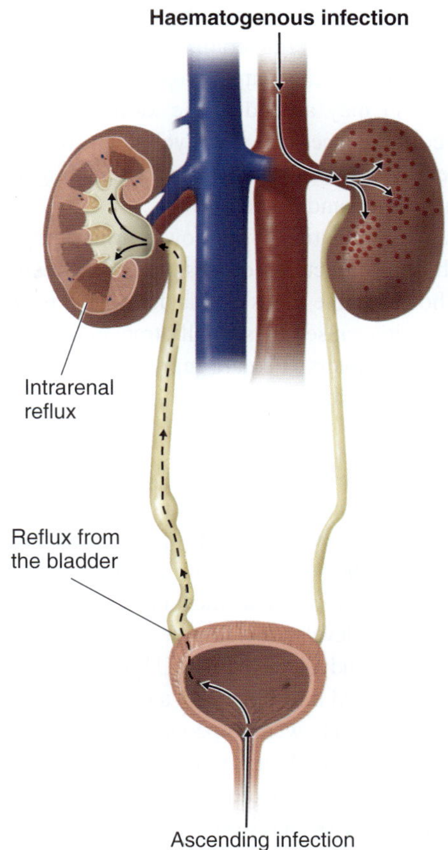

Figure 32.6

Ascending urinary tract infections versus haematogenous spread

In hospitals, UTIs occur mainly as a result of urological instrumentation, especially catheterisation. Bacteria from the person's endogenous flora, from instruments or even from carers' hands, may be carried by the instruments into the urinary tract. They may also ascend in the layer of exudate that forms between an indwelling catheter and the urethral wall. Bacteria can proliferate in the drainage reservoir of a catheter and, if drainage is not properly arranged, may ascend the column of urine to enter the bladder.

The major cause of both community-acquired and hospital-acquired (**nosocomial infection**) UTIs is *E. coli*. In nosocomial UTIs, other causative organisms are *Proteus, Klebsiella* and *Pseudomonas* (Gram-negative rods) and *Enterococcus faecalis*. The risk of infection increases with the length of time that the indwelling catheter is in place, and can occur within 14 days. In short-term catheterisation, infection is often associated with endogenous organisms. Long-term catheterisation is more often associated with exogenous organisms derived from instruments and equipment, or from the hands of carers.

Other risk factors for UTIs are:

- *gender*—females are 30 times more likely to develop UTIs than are males due to the shortness of the female urethra and the small distance between the urethral opening and the anus; sexual activity further increases the risk in women
- *age*—higher rates of UTIs are associated with increased age; this is believed to be due to age-related bladder dysfunction, urinary and faecal incontinence, as well as changes in oestrogen levels in women
- *obstruction*—kidney stones, congenital malformations of the vesicoureteral valves in children and prostate enlargement in ageing men may obstruct the flow of urine, and also cause urinary reflux from the bladder to the ureters (this is known as *vesicoureteral reflux*)
- *incomplete voiding of urine*—the flow of urine along the urinary tract and emptying of the bladder has an important role in cleansing the tract of bacteria; without the flushing action of urine, bacteria in the tract can proliferate to cause infection
- *metabolic factors*—diabetes mellitus significantly increases the risk of UTIs and many other infections; the increased risk is associated with elevated urine glucose levels and decreased immune function in diabetes.

When a pathogenic microbe, such as *E. coli,* enters the urinary tract, it attaches to the urethral epithelial cells and damages the lining of the urethra, precipitating an inflammatory state called **urethritis**. *E. coli* can continue to ascend the urinary tract, entering the urinary bladder, where it attaches to bladder epithelial cells. Damage to the epithelial lining of the bladder in the form of cell apoptosis and exfoliation elicits inflammation, which in this location is called **cystitis**. *E. coli* can be incorporated into the epithelial cell cytoplasm, where it forms a quiescent intracellular bacterial pool that can be released back into the bladder lumen to infect other bladder cells. This is one of the ways in which a recurrent UTI develops. Recurrent infection may also occur after reinfection with the microbe, or infection caused by a different bacterial strain.

Urethritis and cystitis are classified as *lower UTIs*. Ultimately, a UTI may ascend to the kidney with potentially very serious consequences (see the 'Pyelonephritis' section later in this chapter). A UTI can become chronic, leading to a state of chronic inflammation and tissue necrosis.

Of course, inflammation of the lower urinary tract can also be induced by non-infectious causes, such as chemical agents and trauma; however, the focus of this discussion is on bacterial infection. Urethritis caused by sexually transmitted infections is discussed in the chapters 'Female reproductive disorders' and 'Male reproductive disorders'.

EPIDEMIOLOGY

Bacterial UTIs are among the most common community-acquired infections that arise in previously healthy people. Due to anatomical differences between the sexes in the urinary system, UTIs are far more common among women than men: in Australia, 1 in 4 women and 1 in 20 men will develop a UTI over their lifetime. In 2019, a multisite Australian study revealed that UTIs were among the top three hospital-associated infections with a prevalence rate of 2.4%; 50% of the reported UTIs were in people with catheters inserted. In general, nosocomial UTIs are more serious than community-acquired infections, as many of the causative bacteria in the former have developed antimicrobial resistance.

CLINICAL MANIFESTATIONS

The symptoms of urethritis or cystitis caused by bacterial infection are **dysuria** (pain on urination) and increased frequency and urgency of urination. Figure 32.7 explores the common clinical manifestations and management of urinary tract infections.

CLINICAL DIAGNOSIS AND MANAGEMENT

Diagnosis

Investigation may begin on the ward. The urine often has an offensive smell, its colour may be abnormal (see Figures 32.8 and 32.9) and it may be cloudy (turbid). A test with a urinary dipstick may yield positive results for blood and nitrite. Such findings on the ward warrant further investigation.

A *midstream urine (MSU)* sample should be collected. When there is bacterial infection, laboratory findings from the MSU will reveal:

- *neutrophils*—in other words, 'pus cells' (i.e. **pyuria**; see Figure 32.10)
- a high concentration of bacteria (i.e. *bacteriuria*; see Figure 32.10)—note that a finding of a low concentration of bacteria in urine does not in itself, in the absence of clinical findings, lead to a diagnosis of urinary tract disease
- **nitrite** (NO_2^-), a characteristic product of bacterial metabolism
- *blood* (in some cases).

A culture of the urine sample should also be carried out to identify the pathogen and determine its antibacterial sensitivity.

Imaging studies will generally not be performed unless there is a suspicion that other disease processes have contributed to the infection. Such studies may become necessary where a person repeatedly develops UTIs. Many UTIs are caused by ineffective hygiene practices, so aggressive and invasive diagnostic procedures are not usually warranted.

Management

If someone has an indwelling catheter, the removal or replacement of the catheter often leads to the resolution of a UTI. Many of the bacteria that cause nosocomial UTIs have acquired resistance to multiple antimicrobial agents. While awaiting results of bacterial culture and sensitivity testing, initial antimicrobial therapy will, therefore, utilise a broad-spectrum agent. Common antibacterial drugs used to manage a UTI include co-trimoxazole, nitrofurantoin and the fluoroquinolones (which tend to be reserved for more serious infections).

Other management considerations include encouraging fluid intake in order to help flush bacteria through the urinary tract. Urinary alkalisers may assist in reducing the dysuria, as may having a warm bath several times a day. The use of cranberry derivatives to reduce the adhesion of bacteria to the epithelial lining of the urinary tract is commonplace, and may be beneficial as a supplement to the other interventions.

Kidney disorders

Inflammatory conditions of the nephron and associated structures can greatly affect renal function. In this section, we will focus on pyelonephritis, glomerulonephritis, diabetic nephropathy, tubulointerstitial nephritis and acute tubular necrosis. These conditions may be acute or chronic, and may range in severity from mild to life-threatening, as they may end in end-stage kidney disease (see the chapter 'Acute kidney injury and chronic kidney disease').

LEARNING OBJECTIVE 2

Describe how nephron functions may be compromised in pyelonephritis and glomerulonephritis.

PYELONEPHRITIS

Aetiology and pathophysiology

Pyelonephritis is infection and inflammation of the kidney (see Figure 32.11). Infection of the urinary system usually begins downstream of the kidney in the urethra and bladder (see the previous section on bacterial UTIs). It can ascend from the bladder to reach the renal pelvis and spread to the calyces and medullary tissues, including the tubules of the nephrons. Infection and inflammation may eventually extend to the cortex and involve the glomeruli. The microbes responsible for this condition are usually bacteria, most often *E. coli*.

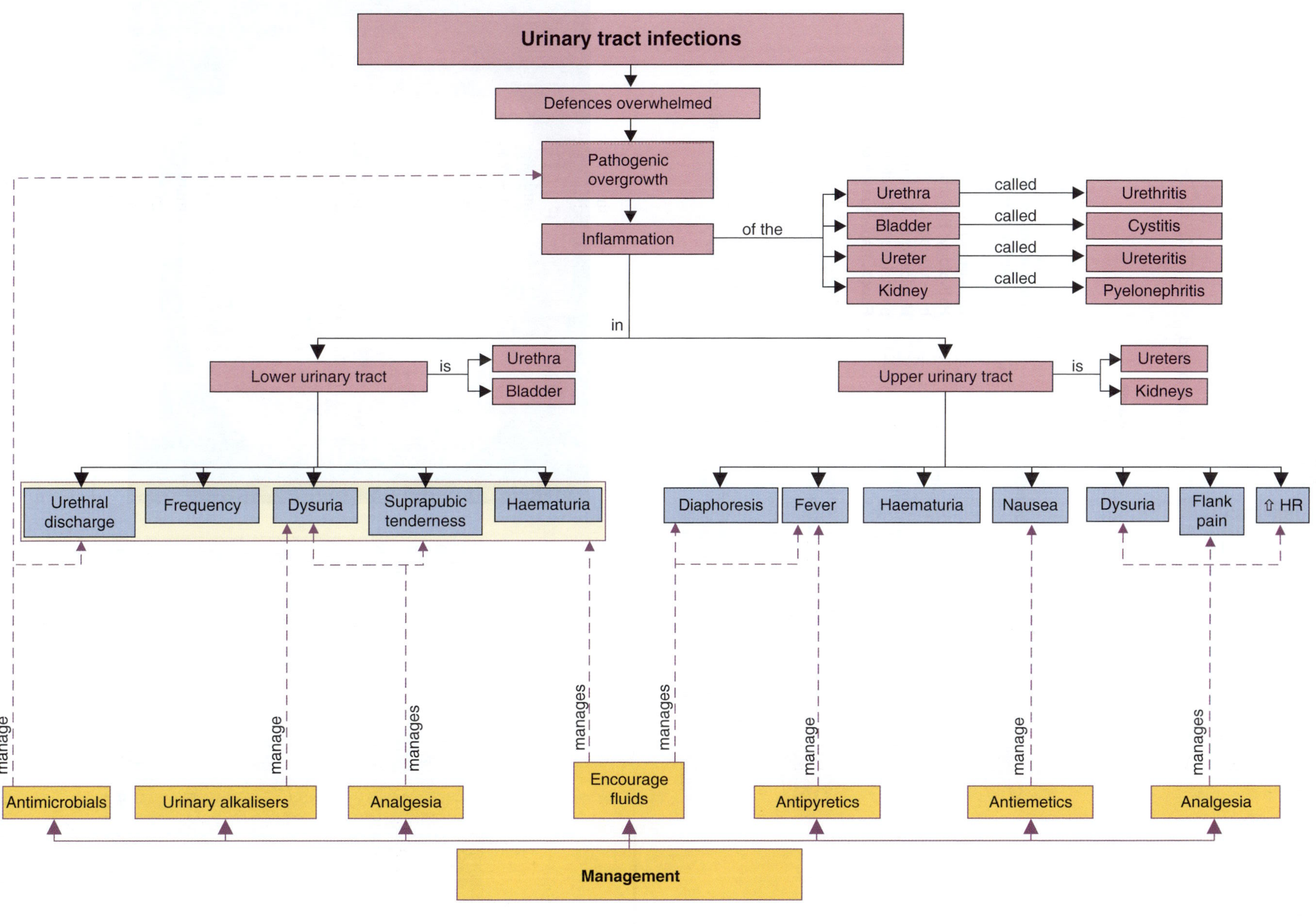

Figure 32.7

Clinical snapshot: Urinary tract infections

↑ = increased; HR = heart rate.

Figure 32.8

Common colour changes of urine related to hydration status

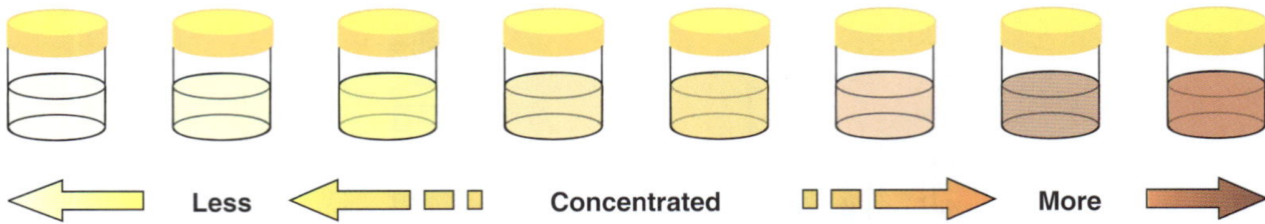

Figure 32.9

Common colour changes of urine requiring further investigation

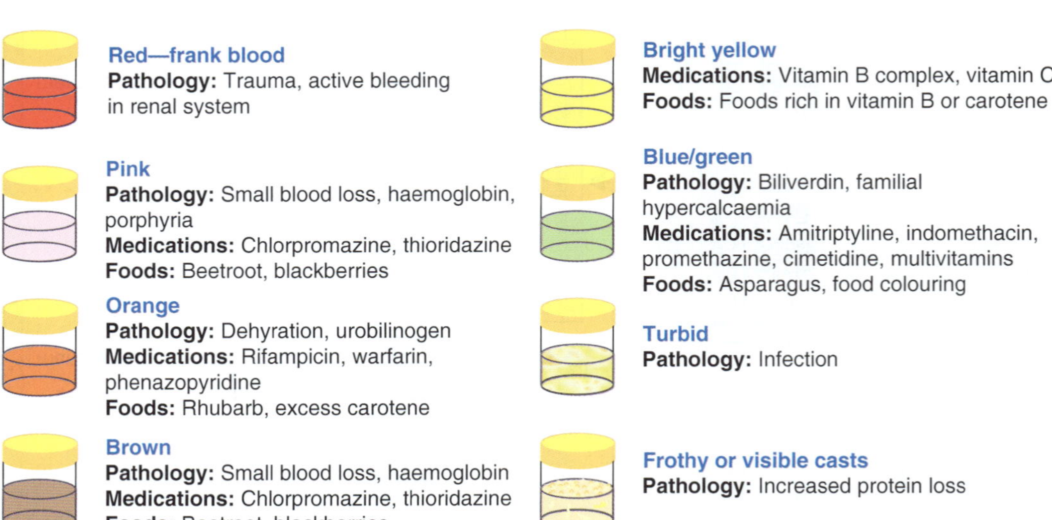

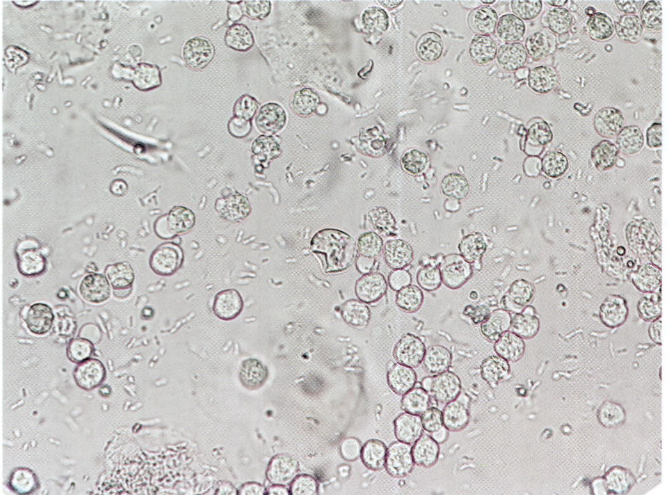

Figure 32.10

Neutrophils and bacteria in the urine

Source: Chamaiporn Naprom/Shutterstock.

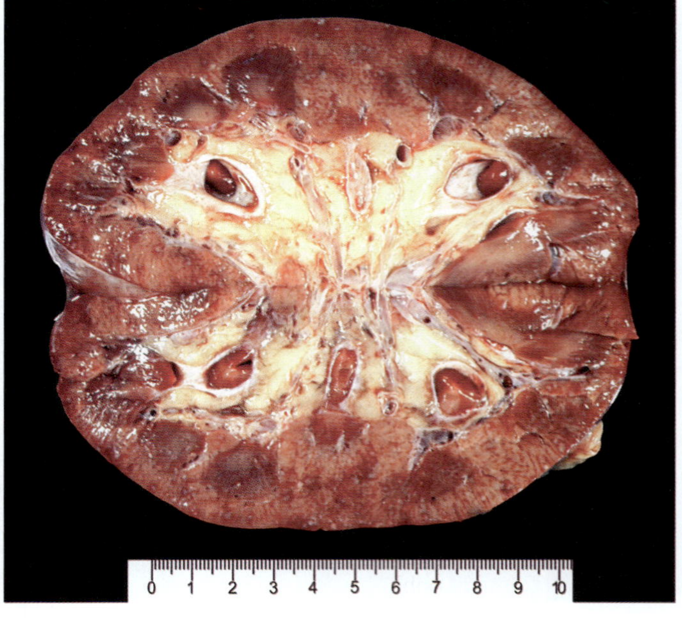

Figure 32.11

Pyelonephritis

Acute pyelonephritis showing pale abcesses.

Source: Jose Calvo/Science Photo Library.

Acute pyelonephritis In the acute inflammatory processes, phagocytes and inflammatory exudate move from the blood into the affected area, impeding tubule function. There may also be suppuration (production of pus) and bleeding. In people with diabetes mellitus who suffer acute pyelonephritis, the papillae of the medullary pyramids may become necrotic.

Ultimately, infection of the kidney may spread to the bloodstream, causing sepsis.

Chronic pyelonephritis Chronic pyelonephritis is a condition in which persistent or repeated infection causes gradual damage and loss of functional kidney tissue, which is replaced by scar tissue. It is often asymptomatic until considerable irreversible tissue loss has occurred and progression to chronic kidney disease (see the chapter 'Acute kidney injury and chronic kidney disease') is inevitable.

Urinary obstruction with **urinary stasis**, characterised by incomplete bladder emptying, or even urinary reflux from the bladder to the ureters (see Figure 32.12) may occur in people with kidney stones, children with congenital malformations of the vesicoureteral valves, and ageing men with prostate enlargement. In such circumstances, the likelihood of infection becoming established in the urinary system and causing the progressive damage of chronic pyelonephritis is greatly increased.

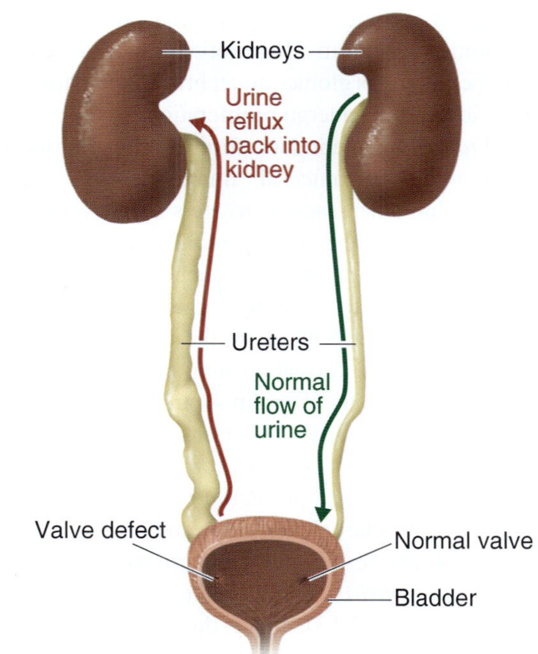

Figure 32.12
Urinary reflux

Clinical manifestations

In addition to dysuria and increased frequency and urgency of urination, which are characteristic of all UTIs, pyelonephritis is characterised by flank pain, high fever and tachycardia. Where the condition is chronic, flank pain may be more diffuse and the other overt symptoms of a UTI may not be present.

If the person develops sepsis, they will develop hypotension and more tachycardia. If they progress to septic shock (see the chapter 'Vascular disorders and circulatory shock'), they will develop profound hypotension, yet they may remain peripherally warm. Peripheral vasoconstriction will be counteracted by the very inflammatory mediators that were responsible for the systemic inflammatory response in the first place, and this will exacerbate the state of distributive shock.

Clinical diagnosis and management

Diagnosis As for lower UTIs, urine is tested on the ward with a dipstick, and an MSU sample is obtained for microscopic examination and bacterial culture. Results will be similar to those for lower UTIs.

In addition, blood may be drawn for laboratory investigation, especially if the individual is febrile and may be heading towards sepsis (see the chapter 'Infectious disease'). There may be an increase in white blood cells (leukocytosis), with elevation specifically of neutrophils (neutrophilia). Blood culture may also be attempted, but negative results will not rule out infection, especially if antibiotic treatment has already commenced.

Although imaging tests will not be necessary in most cases, some people may require an intravenous pyelogram, ultrasound or computed tomography (CT) scan (often using contrast) to rule out other causes of disease.

A careful history and physical assessment will assist with the diagnosis.

Management Administration of antimicrobial agents is crucial to the management of pyelonephritis. Oral antimicrobials may be sufficient, depending on the severity of infection. Analgesia and control of fever will be required to relieve symptoms. Individuals should be encouraged to increase their fluid intake. However, if they are dehydrated or unable to tolerate fluids by mouth, they may require hospital admission for intravenous hydration and antibiotics.

If an individual develops sepsis, they may require adrenergic agents or other inotropic support, as well as fluid volume support to compensate for the distributive shock. At this stage, intravenous antimicrobials will be required. Transfer to a critical care unit will be necessary, as continuous haemodynamic monitoring and the administration of vasoactive drugs are not generally managed on a ward.

GLOMERULONEPHRITIS

Aetiology and pathophysiology

Glomerulonephritis is a group of conditions characterised by damage to the glomeruli. A common classification of glomerulonephritis is to divide the presentations into nephritic and nephrotic syndromes. **Nephrotic syndrome** is characterised by aetiologies which result in an excessive loss of protein (i.e. *proteinuria*), whereas **nephritic syndrome** is associated with an excessive loss of blood (i.e. *haematuria*). Conditions that are nephritic in character include IgA nephropathy (Berger's disease), rapidly progressive glomerulonephritis and post-infectious glomerulonephritis. Nephrotic forms include minimal change and membranous glomerulonephritis. In nephritic forms, cells of the glomerulus undergo proliferation.

IgA nephropathy is a common form of glomerulonephritis. IgA is important in mucosal immunity. In susceptible individuals, an immune reaction triggers the release of large amounts of structurally altered IgA into the blood, which other natural plasma immunoglobulins (such as IgG) recognise as antigenic and bind to, forming large immune complexes that are not readily metabolised by the liver. The magnitude of the immune complex formation may be heightened during infection by certain strains of group A streptococci (which has been a historically important cause) or other pathogens, such as the hepatitis B virus or *Staphylococcus aureus*, leading to higher levels of reactive IgG present in the blood. The immune complexes lodge in the glomerulus, and activate an acute inflammatory process, resulting in glomerulonephritis.

In *glomerulonephritis*, the glomerulus becomes acutely inflamed (see Figure 32.13). Since the inflamed glomerulus is less efficient in allowing the formation of a filtrate, the glomerular filtration rate will fall. This will cause the volume of urine to fall, while the blood will retain water and nitrogenous wastes.

In addition, inflammation causes the filtration membrane to become excessively leaky to blood cells, and somewhat leaky to large proteins as well. This allows their movement into the filtrate, and, since they cannot be reabsorbed in the tubule, they will appear in the urine. Eventually, the concentration of proteins in plasma will fall, reducing its osmotic pressure. This will cause oedema.

In some cases, the glomerulus may recover from the inflammation and normal nephron function will be restored. However, if the inflammatory process intensifies or persists, the glomerulus may die. Since all of the blood supply of the nephron downstream of the glomerulus (i.e. the tubules) is derived from the glomerular capillaries (see Figure 32.4), this means that the entire nephron will die. If this happens to a large proportion of nephrons, the kidney will fail.

Clinical manifestations

Common clinical manifestations of glomerulonephritis are hypertension and oedema, together with degrees of haematuria and proteinuria (depending on whether the aetiology is nephritic or nephrotic), as well as the presence of erythrocyte and leukocyte casts in the urine. A person may complain of headache secondary to hypertension, and display symptoms of oedema, including obvious peripheral oedema and shortness of breath secondary to pulmonary oedema. Anaemia may develop as fluid retention leads to haemodilution. People often complain of flank pain and skin rashes, and may also suffer from nausea, vomiting and anorexia. As the damage continues, they may develop oliguria.

Figure 32.14 explores the common clinical manifestations and management of glomerulonephritis.

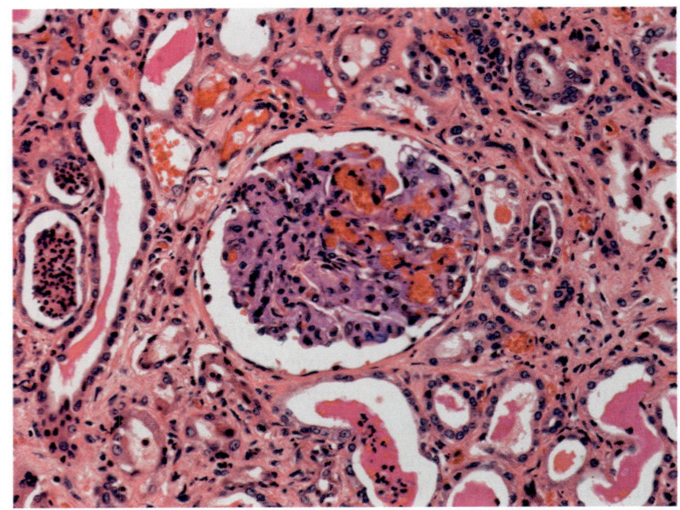

Figure 32.13

Inflamed glomerulus

Light micrograph of a section of kidney tissue with acute nephritis. Areas of the glomerulus are necrotic. Inflammatory cells have infiltrated glomerular tissue. Haematoxylin and eosin stain.

Source: Steve Gschmeissner/Science Photo Library.

Clinical diagnosis and management

Diagnosis Urine and blood is collected for assessment. Urinalysis will generally demonstrate haematuria, cell casts and marked proteinuria. A full blood examination may demonstrate leukocytosis if the glomerulonephritis is related to infection (e.g. in post-streptococcal glomerulonephritis). If the person is febrile, blood cultures should be carried out. The erythrocyte sedimentation rate (ESR) and C-reactive protein levels are generally elevated as non-specific markers of inflammation. Kidney impairment consequent on the reduction in glomerular filtration rate will allow increases in blood urea, creatinine and electrolytes, such as potassium. Autoantibodies may be found if the disease has originated in an autoimmune process.

Imaging techniques, such as ultrasonography, can be used to measure kidney size for the assessment of inflammation. Chest and abdominal X-rays and CT scans may be useful in detecting or excluding the presence of other pathology, such as tumours and abscesses.

Management In the case of post-streptococcal glomerulonephritis, antibacterials are appropriate, but care must be taken not to further compromise kidney function with drugs that are nephrotoxic. Oedema should be managed by fluid restriction and, depending on the clinical picture, loop diuretics. Profound hypertension can exacerbate kidney damage, and

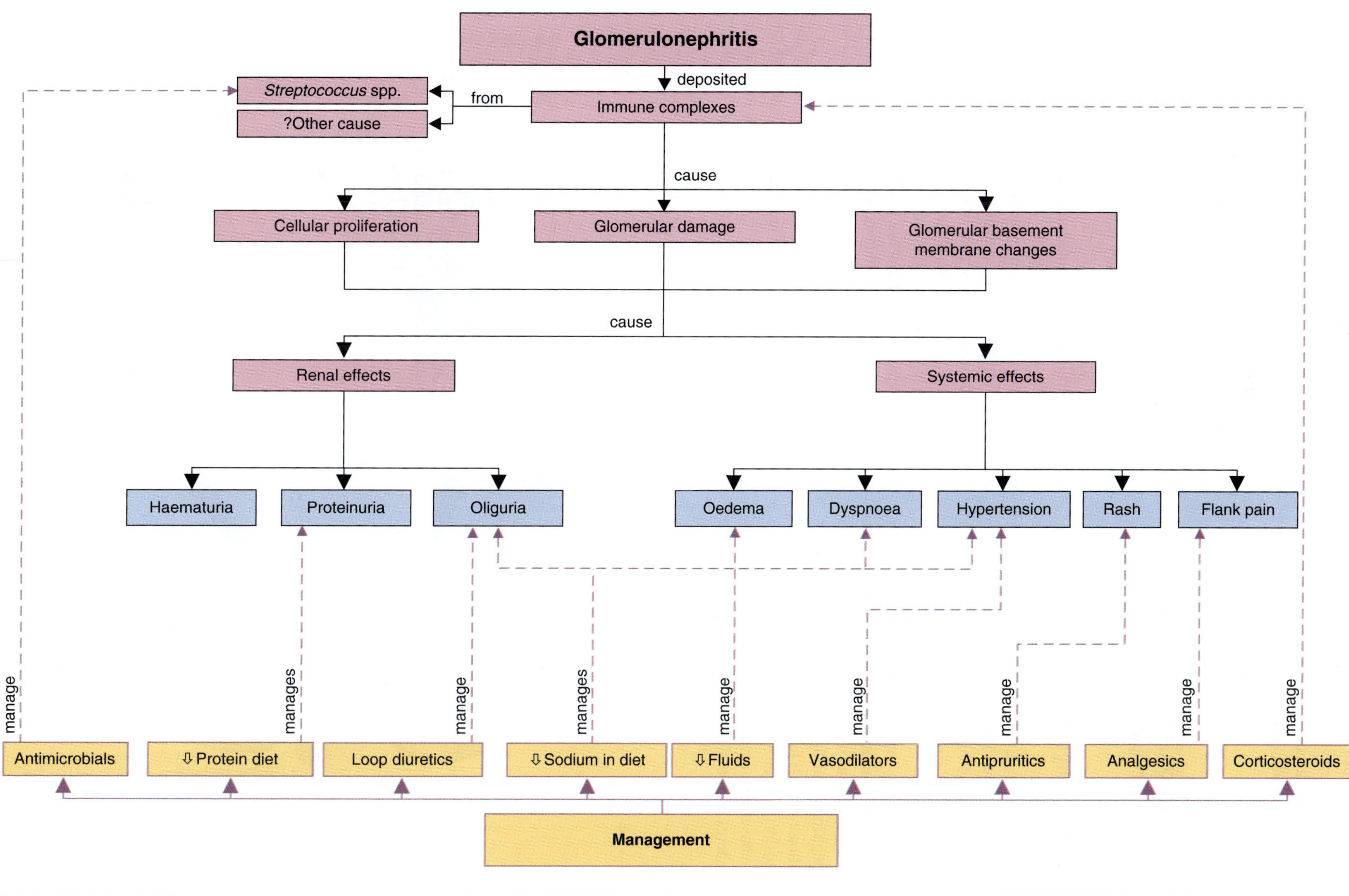

Figure 32.14

Clinical snapshot: Glomerulonephritis

↑ = decreased; ? = possible.

should be controlled with diuretics and antihypertensive agents. In the event of oliguria or anuria, dialysis may be required. Control of overactive or self-directed immune responses may be attempted with corticosteroid medications.

DIABETIC NEPHROPATHY

LEARNING OBJECTIVE 3

Explore the mechanism of nephropathy secondary to diabetes.

Aetiology and pathophysiology

Diabetic nephropathy, or *diabetic kidney disease*, is a major complication of diabetes mellitus. Around 40% of people with this condition progress to chronic kidney disease and end-stage kidney disease. Good control of blood glucose levels has been shown to be important in decreasing the rate of development of diabetic nephropathy.

Diabetic nephropathy may be preceded by many years of deterioration of kidney function. Initially, the glomerular filtration rate of healthy nephrons may increase (*hyperfiltration*) to compensate for nephrons that have been lost, but eventually the glomerular filtration rate will fall.

Diabetic nephropathy is a microvascular disease characterised by a thickening of the basement membrane of small blood vessels (see the chapter 'Diabetes mellitus'). Prolonged hyperglycaemia causes the glycosylation of cell proteins and lipids, and alters cellular signalling. This leads to the release of cytokines, chemokines, growth factors and transcription factors, as well as oxidative stress. Under these conditions in the kidneys, the intraglomerular mesangial cells—which support the glomerulus and regulate its blood flow—expand, and the glomerular basement membrane becomes thicker, with the glomerulus becoming far more permeable to proteins (see Figure 32.15). Diffuse scarring of the glomerular capillaries develops, which is known as *glomerulosclerosis*. Glomerulosclerosis impedes glomerular filtration and causes ischaemic damage to the cortex and medulla.

In glomerulosclerosis, large amounts of plasma protein are lost in the urine (*proteinuria*), and the level in the blood falls (*hypoalbuminaemia*) more rapidly and to a much greater extent than in glomerulonephritis. The pathophysiology of hypoalbuminaemia is represented in Figure 32.16.

The clinical manifestations that arise from glomerulosclerosis are collectively associated with nephrotic syndrome. The key feature is extensive loss of plasma proteins in urine. In the long term, this will itself contribute to nephron damage, but the more immediate consequence will be hypoalbuminaemia leading to oedema.

Additional consequences of the extensive loss of plasma proteins in nephrotic syndrome are increased susceptibility to infection, as antibodies and complement proteins are lost in the urine, and a high blood level of lipid (*hyperlipidaemia*), as

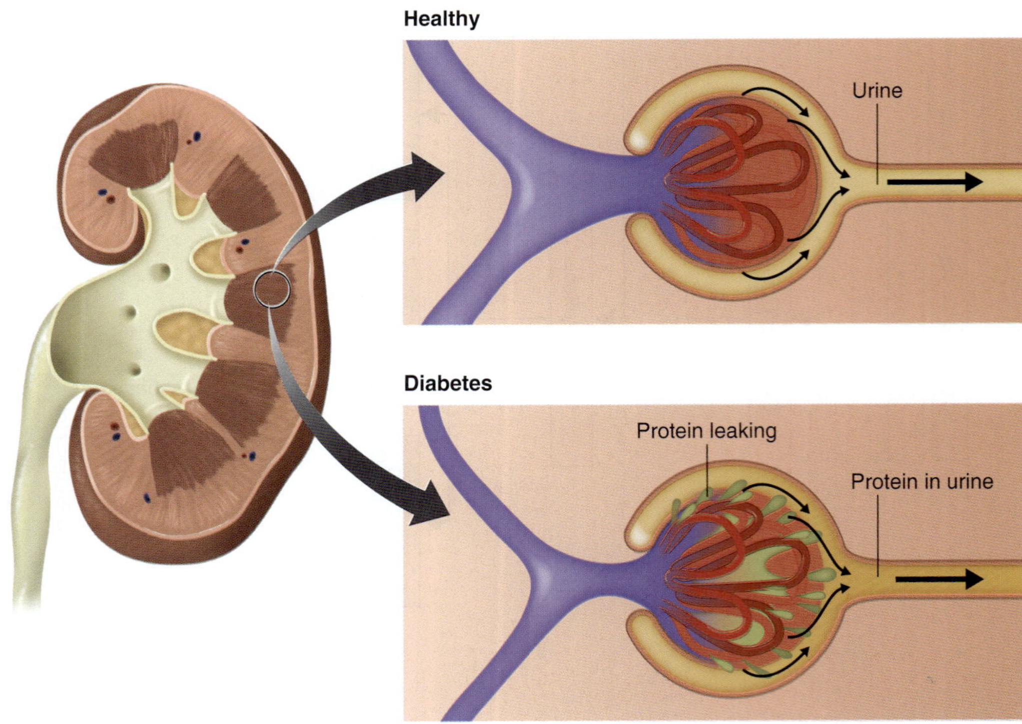

Figure 32.15

Thickening of the glomerular capillary wall injured by diabetes

Results in loss of protein (albumin) leading to hypoalbuminaemia.

Figure 32.16

Pathophysiology of hypoalbuminaemia

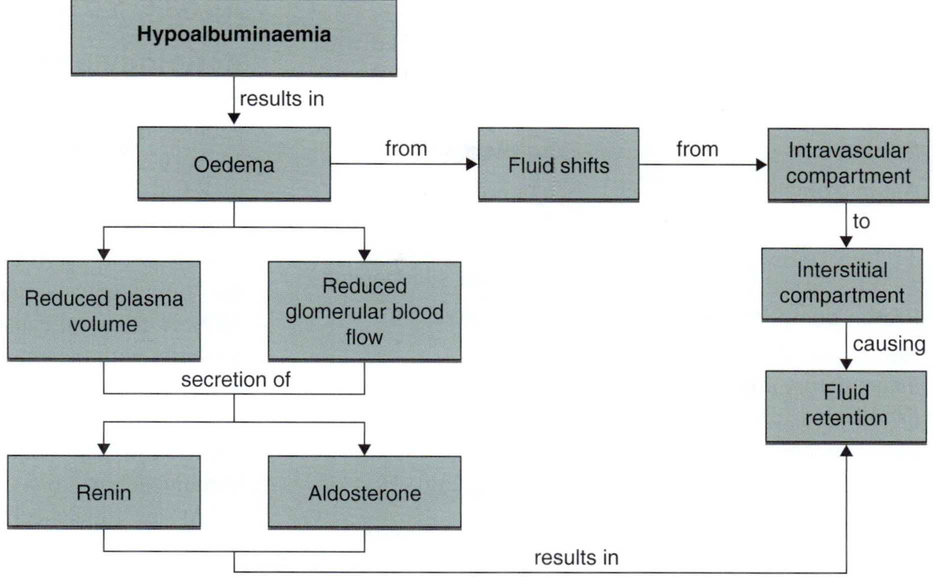

the liver exports large amounts of lipoproteins to the blood in an attempt to compensate for the lost plasma protein.

LEARNING OBJECTIVE 4

Compare and contrast tubulointerstitial nephritis and acute tubular necrosis.

TUBULOINTERSTITIAL NEPHRITIS

Aetiology and pathophysiology

Because of the large amount of blood that flows through the kidneys, nephrons may be exposed to high levels of certain blood-borne substances that can damage them by triggering hypersensitivity reactions within the kidney. Among these substances are some therapeutic drugs. Such damage occurs mainly in the tubules and associated structures of the medulla, and is known as **tubulointerstitial nephritis**. It can be either acute or chronic.

Acute process In the acute inflammatory processes associated with hypersensitivity, phagocytes and inflammatory exudate move from the blood into the affected area, impeding tubule function (see Figure 32.17). Eosinophils—leukocytes central to many allergic processes—play key roles in these hypersensitivity reactions.

In very severe cases, necrosis of medullary tissues may occur. The most serious outcome of acute tubulointerstitial nephritis is acute kidney injury (see the chapter 'Acute kidney injury and chronic kidney disease').

Substances known to cause hypersensitivity reactions or toxicity in the kidney medulla are listed in Table 32.1. In some cases, withdrawing exposure to the substance allows the renal tubules an opportunity to regenerate.

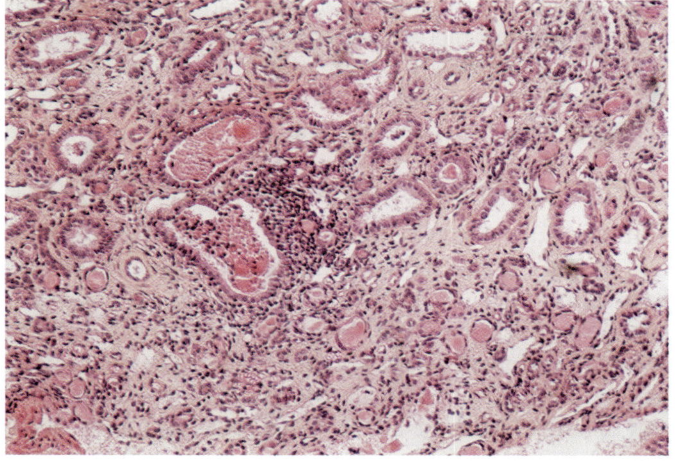

Figure 32.17

Eosinophils and neutrophils within inflamed tissue

An inflamed interstitium with fibrosis, tubular atrophy (trichrome stain).

Source: CNRI/Science Photo Library.

Chronic process The chronic process consists of the gradual replacement of functional structures with fibrous (scar) tissue following repeated episodes of acute inflammation.

Clinical manifestations

Early in the disease process, blood and some protein may be detected in the urine. If the disease progresses to acute kidney injury, urine output will fall steeply, with the person developing oliguria and then perhaps anuria, and manifesting the consequences of fluid overload and uraemia. Fluid overload

Table 32.1 Examples of substances associated with kidney toxicity or hypersensitivity reactions

Substances	Examples
Antimicrobials	Rifampicin, β-lactams (e.g. penicillins), aminoglycosides (e.g. gentamicin), sulfonamides
Proton pump inhibitors	Esomeprazole
Non-steroidal anti-inflammatory agents (NSAIDs)	Aspirin
Immunosuppressive agents	Ciclosporin
Psychotropic agents	Lithium carbonate
Organic solvents	Carbon tetrachloride

will cause hypertension and oedema. If the lungs become oedematous, pulmonary gas exchange will be compromised. Depending on the degree of uraemia, neurological symptoms may also develop: this can be averted by the use of continuous venovenous haemodialysis. Occasionally, the individual may develop a rash; depending on the extent of the medullary damage, symptoms of anaemia may also appear.

Clinical diagnosis and management

Diagnosis Samples of urine and blood may be obtained for testing. Urinalysis may demonstrate proteinuria and **haematuria**. Chemical pathology tests may show uraemia if damage to the nephrons is severe and protracted. Red blood cell and haematocrit values will fall if anaemia develops. If the disease process has arisen from hypersensitivity, eosinophils may appear in the urine and be found at elevated levels in the blood.

Depending on the suspected cause of the disease, imaging studies, such as ultrasound, CT or intravenous pyelogram, may be used to confirm or rule out other sources of kidney damage, such as stones or tumours. None of these studies is definitively diagnostic for tubulointerstitial nephritis.

Management Where a causative substance is identified, it must be removed immediately. However, depending on the degree of damage, this may not necessarily result in a rapid recovery. In the interim, supportive management of kidney impairment, hypertension and perhaps anaemia will be necessary. If nephron function is reduced so far that the person becomes uraemic, dialysis will be required. Antihypertensive agents and a low-sodium diet may assist with blood pressure control. If anaemia develops, the administration of oxygen or even a red blood cell transfusion may be appropriate. Unfortunately, transfusions can lead to increased haemolysis and increased blood potassium levels, and so may increase the workload of the kidneys.

ACUTE TUBULAR NECROSIS

Aetiology and pathophysiology

When the epithelial cells that make up the tubules of the nephron die, **acute tubular necrosis (ATN)** can result. These cells are very sensitive to hypoxia, and may therefore die when their blood supply fails. *Renal hypoperfusion* can develop in cases of significant blood loss, severe hypotension, circulatory shock or sepsis. Exposure to nephrotoxic chemicals, particularly in the clinical environment, can also kill tubule cells, resulting in ATN. A common cause is toxicity from radiographic contrast medium, with the characteristic chemical pathology becoming evident within two to three days after the radiological investigation. Treatment with anticancer drugs or antimicrobial agents can also lead to ATN. ATN can also result from immune attack.

As the tubule cells are responsible for reabsorption and secretion subsequent to glomerular filtration, the death of a significant number without replacement leads to kidney impairment. ATN is a common cause of acute kidney injury (see the chapter 'Acute kidney injury and chronic kidney disease').

While there are similarities between ATN and tubulointerstitial nephritis with regard to aetiology, the latter develops more insidiously. ATN develops as a result of direct renal epithelial injury, and a rapid deterioration in renal function is observed. The characteristics of both ATN and tubulointerstitial nephritis are compared in Figure 32.18.

Clinical manifestations

The cause of the acute tubular necrosis will influence an individual's presentation. If kidney ischaemia is due to hypovolaemic shock (see the chapter 'Vascular disorders and circulatory shock'), the person will have hypotension, tachycardia and oliguria. If it is due to distributive shock, such as in sepsis, arising in the course of anaphylaxis or a systemic inflammatory response, the person may also have a fever or rash. If disseminated intravascular coagulopathy is present in a systemic inflammatory response, the person may display petechiae and suffer the effects both of microthrombi and increased blood clotting time. However, acute tubular necrosis may, in some cases, be identified solely from laboratory results if the individual has not developed clinical manifestations apart from reduced urine output.

Clinical diagnosis and management

Diagnosis Physical examination, urinalysis, full blood examination and appropriate chemical pathology will be required. Centrifugation of the urine sample may reveal brown, granular cell casts. These represent dead tubular epithelial cells that have been shed into the lumen of the tubule. Blood levels of urea and creatinine will be elevated, and electrolytes may be disordered. Imaging studies, such as ultrasound, CT and magnetic resonance imaging, may be undertaken to rule out other causes.

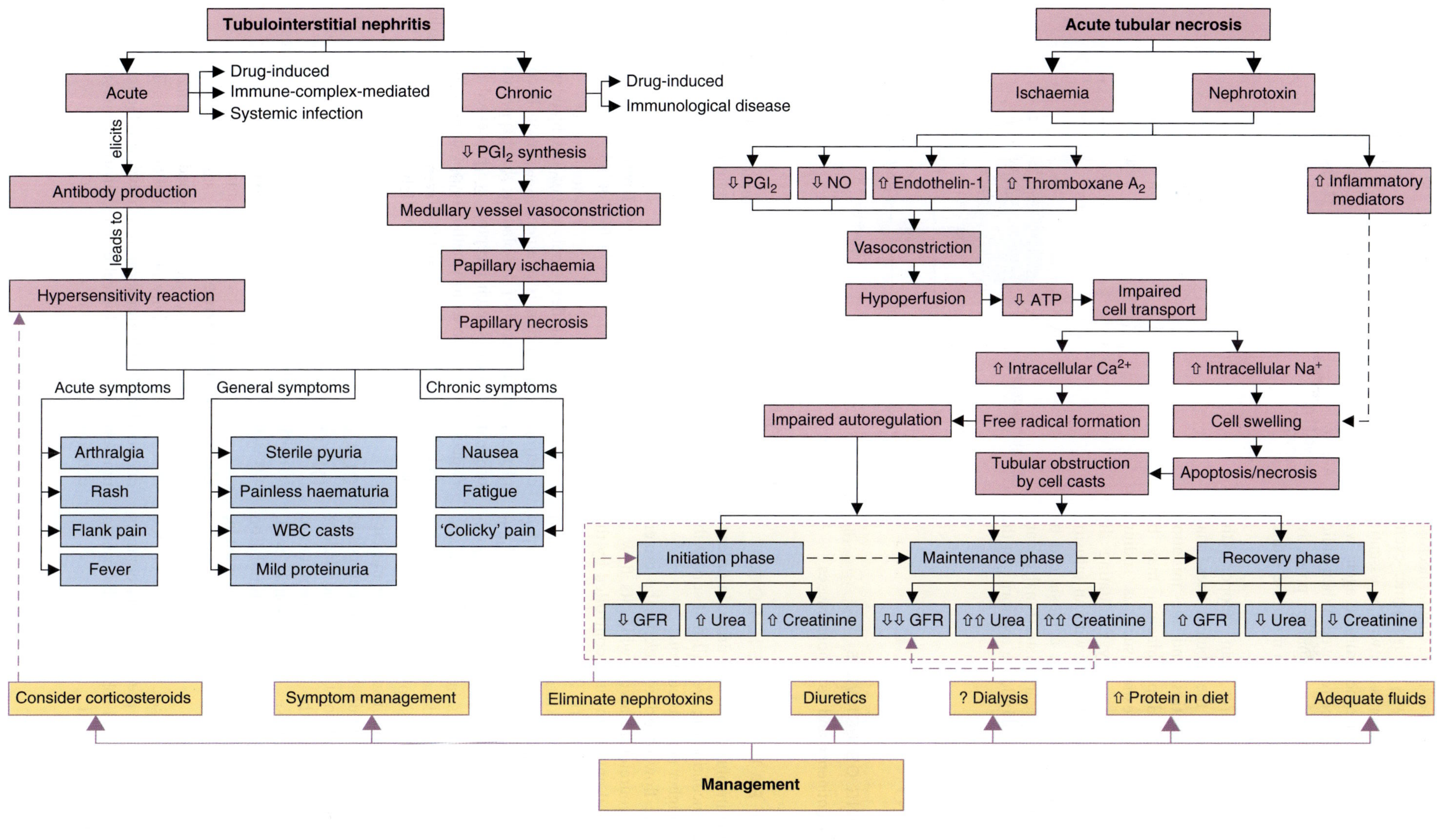

Figure 32.18

Clinical snapshot: Tubulointerstitial nephritis and acute tubular necrosis

↓ = decreased; ↑ = increased; ? = possible; ATP = adenosine triphosphate; Ca^{2+} = calcium ion; GFR = glomerular filtration rate; Na^+ = sodium ion; NO = nitric oxide; PGI_2 = prostacyclin; WBC = white blood cell.

Management The management of acute tubular necrosis is based on the cause. If the cause was an ischaemic event, support of blood volume and blood pressure will be essential to ensure recovery of the tubules. If a nephrotoxic agent was responsible for the damage, it should be removed. When radio-opaque contrast medium is required for investigations, protective drugs such as *N*-acetylcysteine can be used to minimise kidney damage.

Additional management measures can support the resorptive and secretory functions of the tubules. These may include the administration of diuretics, and the initiation of haemodialysis when required. Hyperkalaemia may be corrected with potassium-binding resins, such as sodium polystyrene sulfonate (Resonium A), or by facilitating the movement of potassium back inside the cell with an infusion containing insulin and glucose. Developing acidosis can be corrected with intravenous sodium bicarbonate. Finally, care regarding nephrotoxic medications should be a priority in the ordering and administration of drugs.

Urinary incontinence

LEARNING OBJECTIVE 5

Describe urinary incontinence and its various causes.

AETIOLOGY AND PATHOPHYSIOLOGY

Urinary incontinence is the involuntary loss of urine. In order to understand the nature of incontinence, we will first survey the micturition reflex and its higher nervous control.

From the bladder, the flow of urine back to the ureters is prevented by the vesicoureteral valves, while its flow to the urethra and the external environment is controlled by the internal and external urethral sphincters. The internal sphincter consists of smooth muscle, while the external sphincter, located within the pelvic floor, is composed of skeletal muscle. The internal sphincter receives sympathetic innervation, which causes contraction of its smooth muscle and, thus, closure of the sphincter; the external sphincter is innervated by somatic motor neurons that travel in the pudendal nerve and cause muscle contraction and closure of this sphincter.

The muscular wall of the bladder itself (detrusor muscle) consists of smooth muscle fibres, contains stretch receptors and is innervated by parasympathetic motor fibres. As the bladder becomes full and its wall stretches, the stretch receptors are stimulated and send afferent impulses to the spinal cord. Through spinal reflex pathways, these induce both stimulation of parasympathetic motor pathways to the detrusor muscle, and inhibition of the sympathetic pathways to the internal sphincter.

Parasympathetic stimulation causes contraction of the detrusor muscle, which increases the pressure of its contents and also tends to pull open the internal sphincter; such opening is now unopposed by sympathetic input.

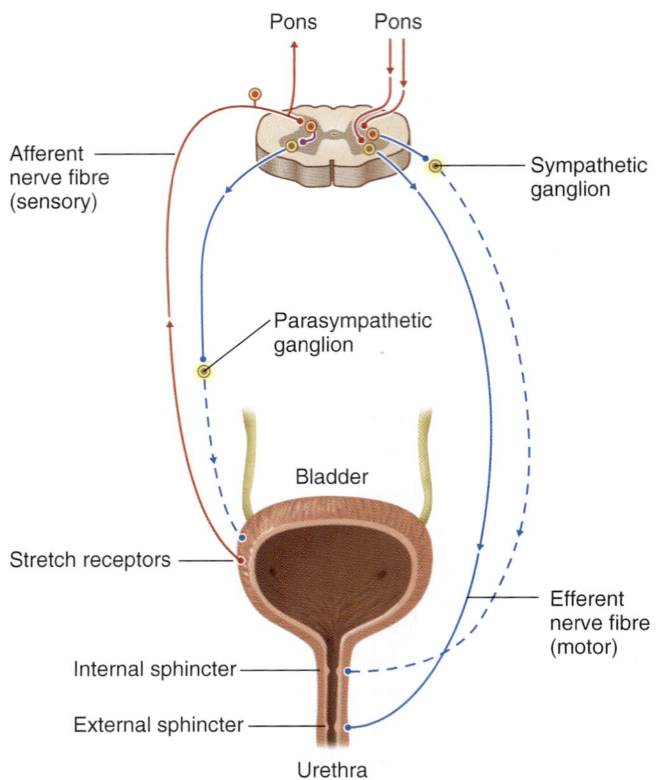

Figure 32.19

Urinary bladder control

Micturition is controlled by an interaction between afferent inputs from the bladder wall and efferent outputs from the autonomic and somatic nervous systems.

In a person who is not yet toilet-trained, or who has suffered a spinal cord injury, urine is now emptied from the bladder (see Figure 32.19).

In contrast to reflex emptying of the bladder, conscious control of micturition is attained as a person becomes aware of the state of stretch of the bladder; this happens as impulses originating in the stretch receptors are processed in the brain. A decision is made as to whether or not urine will be passed, and the tone of the external urethral sphincter is accordingly adjusted through somatic motor pathways.

CLASSIFICATION OF URINARY INCONTINENCE

Urinary incontinence can be classified into four categories: urge, stress, overflow and functional incontinence.

Urge incontinence

Urge incontinence, also known as *overactive bladder syndrome*, arises from hyperactivity of the detrusor muscle. This may be due to bladder inflammation as a result of infection, stones or tumours, or to neurological damage arising from stroke, spinal cord injury or Parkinson's disease.

Urge incontinence is characterised by urgency and frequency of urination, usually with an inability to maintain bladder control once fullness is consciously perceived.

Stress incontinence

This type of incontinence is caused by *weakness of the external urethral sphincter or of the pelvic floor muscles* around it, even though the relevant neural pathways are intact. Typically, small volumes of urine are lost when intra-abdominal pressure—and thus the pressure of the bladder—is sharply increased during activities such as coughing, sneezing or laughing.

Damage to the external urethral sphincter may be caused by surgery; more often, stress incontinence is caused by pelvic floor weakness that develops with childbearing and with ageing.

Overflow incontinence

Overflow incontinence may occur when the bladder cannot empty sufficiently during urination and subsequently fills excessively. This may happen as a result of *obstruction* to the flow of urine (e.g. when the prostate is enlarged) or where the detrusor muscle may *not be able to contract* with sufficient strength. Such weakness may be caused by neurological defects, such as spinal cord injury or diabetic neuropathy. Overflow incontinence is manifested as frequent leakage of small volumes of urine.

Functional incontinence

This is defined as incontinence that occurs when you have a healthy bladder but, for some unrelated reason, cannot get to the toilet on time.

CLINICAL MANIFESTATIONS

The clinical manifestations will reflect the cause of the urinary incontinence. If an individual is experiencing urge incontinence, they will be overwhelmed by a sudden desire to pass urine frequently, and possibly also at night. If stress incontinence is the problem, an individual will report accidental urination associated with situations of increased abdominal pressure: this may happen because of sneezing, laughing or coughing. In overflow incontinence, individuals will experience frequent, small-volume urine leakage as a result of incomplete emptying. Figure 32.20 explores the common clinical manifestations and management of incontinence.

CLINICAL DIAGNOSIS AND MANAGEMENT

Diagnosis

Urinalysis should be performed to confirm or exclude UTI as the primary cause of the incontinence. A blood glucose test to detect diabetes mellitus is important when polyuria and polydipsia, symptoms of this disease, are also reported. The lining of the urethra and the bladder may be examined by cystourethroscopy. The degree of incontinence can be quantified by urodynamic tests, which include uroflowmetry and cystometry. A post-void residual test may be useful, especially for the diagnosis of overflow incontinence. Pelvic floor muscle strength can be assessed using electromyography.

A blood glucose test is important when polyuria and polydipsia are also reported. Other blood tests may not be of much benefit, but may identify other issues that need to be managed. Imaging studies are of little benefit in the diagnosis of incontinence, but may be necessary to confirm or exclude underlying problems, such as tumours, stones or inflammation.

Management

The type of incontinence dictates the management plan.

- *Urge incontinence* is often treated with antimuscarinic agents to inhibit detrusor contractions and increase effective bladder capacity. Tricyclic antidepressants may be used to modify neurotransmission in the central nervous system. Their effect is to increase somatic motor output to the external urethral sphincter, and thus enhance its tone.
- *Stress incontinence* may be treated with α-adrenergic agonists to improve tone in the internal urethral sphincter. Tricyclic antidepressants may also be used for urge incontinence. Surgical interventions to stabilise the bladder neck are available, but these techniques are aggressive and yield variable results.
- *Overflow incontinence* is generally caused by an anatomical obstruction; thus, removal of the obstruction may improve the symptoms. However, the procedure itself may exacerbate the symptoms. In men, a transurethral resection of the prostate can remove the excess tissue of benign prostatic hypertrophy or prostate cancer. Pharmacological methods include the use of α-adrenergic antagonists to relax the smooth muscle of the internal urethral sphincter to improve flow.

More general approaches include strengthening of the pelvic floor with the use of Kegel exercises. For women, weighted vaginal cones can be inserted twice a day to help perform the Kegel exercises effectively. Biofeedback devices for males and females are also available. Weight loss should be undertaken where necessary, as obesity increases incontinence. Occasionally, in postmenopausal women hypersensitive bladders may respond to oestrogen therapy. When most interventions fail, some types of incontinence may benefit from intermittent self-catheterisation.

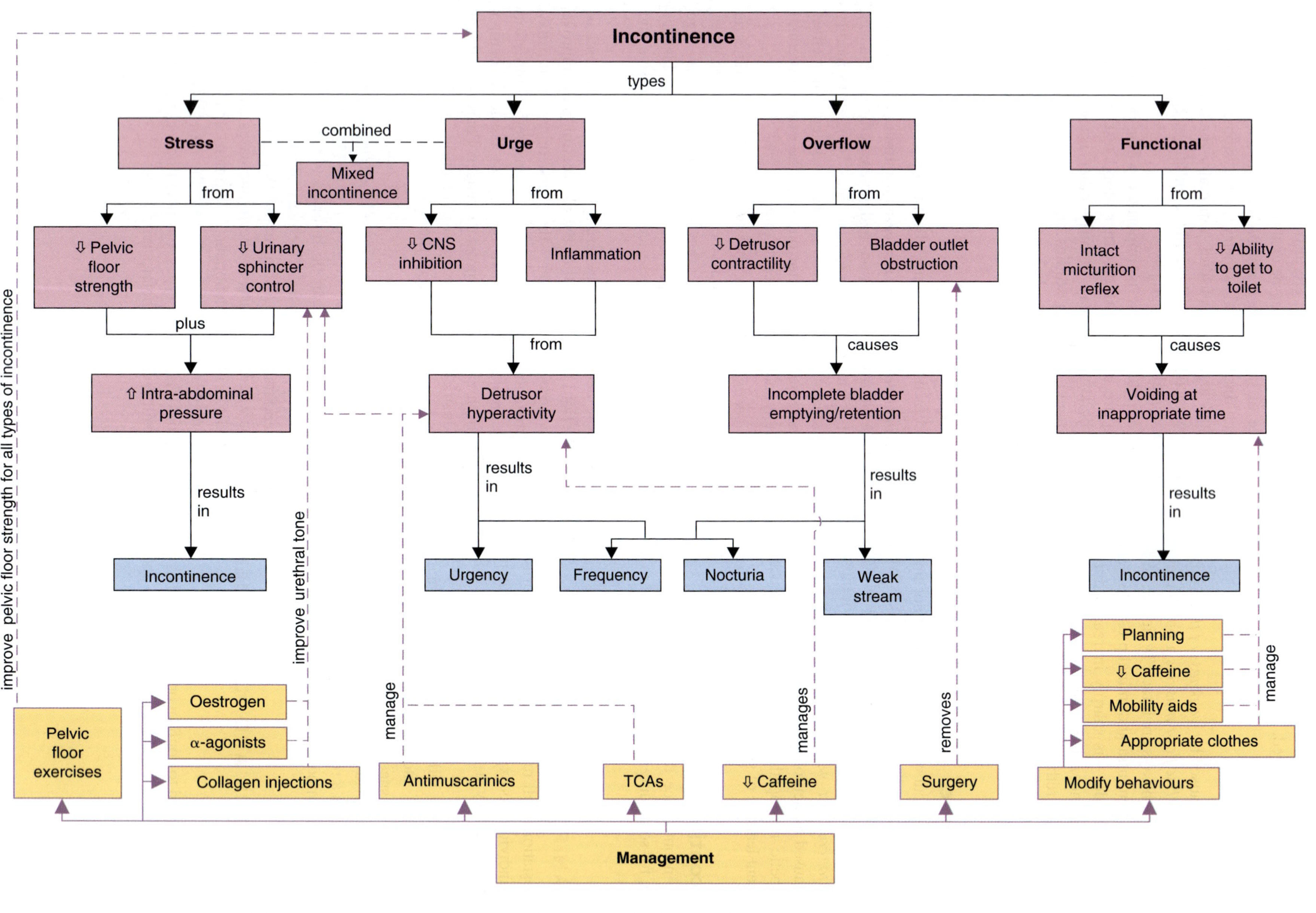

Figure 32.20

Clinical snapshot: Incontinence

↓ = decreased; ↑ = increased; α = alpha; CNS = central nervous system; TCAs = tricyclic antidepressants.

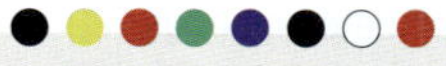

INDIGENOUS HEALTH FAST FACTS AND CULTURAL CONSIDERATIONS

FAST FACTS

- *Rates of urinary tract infections (UTIs) are 2.2 times higher in Aboriginal and Torres Strait Islander peoples than in non-Indigenous Australians.*
- *Urinary tract infection is among the top five causes of preventable hospitalisations in Aboriginal and Torres Strait Islander peoples. Around 50% of these preventable hospitalisations were for people aged 65 years and over.*
- *Māori children are 6 times and Pacific Islands children are 17.5 times more at risk than European New Zealander children of developing post-streptococcal glomerulonephritis.*
- *Māori women experience urinary incontinence almost 3.6 times more than European New Zealand women.*

CULTURAL CONSIDERATIONS

- *People who live in hot conditions have an increased risk of dehydration and UTI. Coupled with the increased risk for people who live in regional areas and the significant incidence of type 2 diabetes in Aboriginal and Torres Strait Islander peoples, there is clearly more threat to Indigenous Australians. However, these biological considerations are not the only factors contributing to the disparity in statistics. Cultural factors such as low levels of trust in healthcare professionals, low health literacy, and the lack of provision and availability of culturally appropriate services contribute to the risks experienced by Aboriginal and Torres Strait Islander peoples.*

Source: Data from Australian Institute of Health and Welfare (2020); Wong et al. (2013).

CHILDREN AND ADOLESCENTS

- Urinary tract infections (UTIs) are common in children, and *E. coli* is the most common organism isolated.
- After 2 years of age, girls have a significantly higher incidence than boys of UTIs.
- Glomerulonephritis occurs most commonly in children aged 5–15 years, with the post-infectious form the most common cause of acute glomerulonephritis in children. Generally, the prognosis and recovery from the post-infectious form is excellent.
- A child has generally developed the capacity to control bladder function by 2 years of age.
- A child of 2–3 years of age generally develops the capacity to voluntarily postpone voiding.
- Paediatric nocturnal enuresis is twice as common in boys as in girls.
- After the age of 5 years, incontinence is defined as repeated loss of control, resulting in voiding into bed or clothes at least twice a week for at least three months.

OLDER ADULTS

- Incontinence rates increase with age. Numerous causes of incontinence include cognitive, physical, structural or pharmacological reasons. Incontinence in the older adult may be a result of numerous causes, making management plans more complex.
- Age-related changes to the renal system do not cause incontinence, but may contribute to reducing continence. Age-related changes include reducing sphincter strength, impaired detrusor contractility, changes in vasopressin and atrial natriuretic hormone secretion, prostate size, and functional changes, such as arthritis, interfering with the ability to remove clothing in time, or the ability to make it to the toilet in time.

KEY CLINICAL ISSUES

- Nosocomial (or hospital-associated) urinary tract infections (UTIs) tend to be more dangerous than community-acquired infections, as they are often more resistant to antimicrobials. Therefore, clinicians should follow all infection control procedures and principles to reduce the risk of causing a UTI.
- Children and individuals who develop frequent UTIs should be taught how to reduce them through improved personal hygiene behaviours.
- Assisting an individual to obtain a midstream urine sample should include education on the appropriate technique to ensure that the sample is not contaminated.
- When an individual presents with pyelonephritis, they may have severe flank pain, fever and dysuria. Administration of analgesia, antibacterials and fluids will be important in the management plan.
- Many chemicals are nephrotoxic. Clinicians should be aware of nephrotoxic substances and institute methods to reduce the potential negative effects by increasing the volume of fluid and the time over which the agent is administered, as well as using other substances that may reduce the risk of kidney damage. Knowledge of a person's renal function is important when administering potentially nephrotoxic agents.

CHAPTER REVIEW

- When pathogenic microbes enter the urinary tract and damage the lining of the urethra, they precipitate an inflammatory state called *urethritis*. The microbes can continue to ascend the urinary tract, entering the urinary bladder. Damage to the lining of the bladder elicits inflammation, which is called *cystitis* in this location. Urethritis and cystitis are classified as lower *urinary tract infections (UTIs)*. Ultimately, a UTI may ascend to the kidney with potentially very serious consequences. Inflammation of the lower urinary tract can also be induced by non-infectious causes, such as chemical agents and trauma.
- UTIs are usually caused by bacteria. They are among the most common community-acquired infections, which arise in previously healthy people. Most UTIs arise endogenously from the person's *bowel flora*. Less often, the pathogen may be carried to the kidney in the bloodstream. This is known as *haematogenous spread*. Risk factors for the development of UTIs include gender, catheterisation, urinary tract obstructions, and metabolic disorders, such as diabetes mellitus.
- *Pyelonephritis* is infection and inflammation of the kidney. Infection usually begins downstream of the kidney in the urethra and bladder. It ascends from the bladder to reach the kidney pelvis, and spreads through the kidney tissue. There are acute and chronic forms of this condition.
- *Glomerulonephritis* is inflammation of the glomerulus. The inflamed glomerulus is less efficient in the formation of a filtrate, leading to a fall in the glomerular filtration rate. Inflammation also causes the filtration membrane to become excessively leaky to blood cells and large proteins. The ensuing loss of protein from blood reduces its osmotic pressure and results in *oedema*.
- *Nephropathy* is a serious complication of diabetes mellitus. It may be preceded by many years of deterioration of kidney function. Initially, hyperfiltration occurs to compensate for the nephrons that have been lost, but eventually the glomerular filtration rate will fall. *Diabetic nephropathy* is a microvascular disease characterised by a thickening of the glomerular basement membrane, and the development of glomerulosclerosis. *Proteinuria* and *hypoalbuminaemia* are important clinical manifestations of the condition. These alterations develop more rapidly and to a greater extent compared to glomerulonephritis.
- *Tubulointerstitial nephritis* is associated with hypersensitivity reactions within the kidney. Such damage, with the inflammatory responses that it evokes, occurs mainly in the tubules and associated structures of the renal medulla.
- *Acute tubular necrosis* is a condition characterised by the death of nephron tubule epithelial cells. It occurs as a result of renal ischaemia, nephrotoxic chemical damage or immune attack. It is a common cause of acute kidney injury.
- *Urinary incontinence* may be caused by overactivity of the smooth muscle of the bladder, weakness of the voluntary muscles at the outlet of the bladder, the inability of the bladder to empty sufficiently during urination, or a timing problem in an otherwise healthy bladder.

REVIEW QUESTIONS

1. Explain the risk factors for urinary tract infection in:
   a. a sexually active young female
   b. an elderly man with benign prostatic enlargement
   c. a person in hospital with a urinary catheter
2. What component/s of the nephron would you suspect to be damaged in a person whose urine contained a significant amount of protein? Explain your answer.
3. What are the major symptoms of each of the following?
   a. cystitis
   b. pyelonephritis
   c. glomerulonephritis
4. Explain why oliguria is a major feature of inflammatory disorders of the kidney.
5. What is the significance of a finding of eosinophils in the urine of a person with inflammatory kidney disease?
6. How might an infection with group A streptococcus or hepatitis B virus that does not reach the kidneys nevertheless cause inflammation of glomeruli?
7. What are the major causes of acute tubular necrosis?
8. Outline the autonomic pathways that govern the functions of the urinary bladder.
9. What are the major differences between urge, stress and overflow incontinence?

HEALTH PROFESSIONAL CONNECTIONS

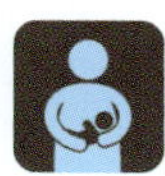

Midwives The risk of urinary tract infections (UTIs) increases with advancing pregnancy due to anatomical and hormonal changes. As the fetus grows, the urinary bladder is displaced, and smooth muscle tone decreases due to high progesterone levels. These changes can result in increased urinary storage and urinary stasis. Vesicoureteral reflux may also develop (see the chapter 'Renal neoplasms and obstructions'). Post-voiding hygiene practices become difficult as the size of the abdomen increases. Glucosuria may also develop, making local conditions favourable for the growth of pathogens. Prevention of UTIs through appropriate hygiene practices still remains the most beneficial intervention. However, if a UTI does occur, antimicrobials may be necessary. Care must be taken to ensure the administration of antimicrobials with appropriate pregnancy categories to protect the health of the developing fetus.

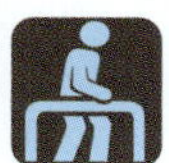

Physiotherapists Assessment of a person's pelvic floor muscle (PFM) function, and education and development of therapeutic modalities to assist with strengthening, are central to a physiotherapist's role in assisting a person with incontinence issues. Facilitating PFM awareness and exercises for strength, use of anticipatory PFM contraction, and biofeedback may all be elements of a beneficial program. It is also important to note that when assessing a person who reports back pain, referral to a medical officer may be required if investigation suggests a UTI. Dysuria, frequency, haematuria and offensive urine are all indications of a UTI. Assess clients for these signs and symptoms, especially if they are experiencing back pain with no associated history of injury.

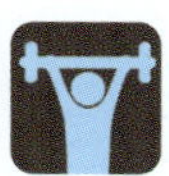

Exercise scientists Appropriate exercise prescription and follow-up can assist an individual with incontinence problems. Exercises that can help include pelvic floor conditioning and core work. As they develop a stronger core, they are less likely to experience UTIs and incontinence.

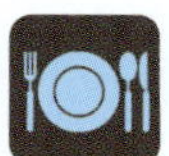

Nutritionists/Dieticians Increased fluid intake and appropriate nutrition can reduce the risk or frequency of UTI. Where appropriate, increased fluid intake results in increased urine output, ultimately reducing urinary stasis. After consultation with the medical team, urinary alkalisers may be advised, along with the reduced consumption of foods which increase urinary acidity. People should be encouraged to avoid coffee and spicy foods during an active UTI, as they may aggravate the symptoms. Cranberry juice may reduce the capacity of the bacteria to attach to the bladder wall.

CASE STUDY

Mrs Agnes Gibson is an 84-year-old woman (UR number 886132) presenting for investigation of incontinence, confusion and suspected urinary tract infection (UTI). She was admitted two hours ago via ambulance from a local nursing home. Her observations were as follows:

Temperature	Heart rate	Respiration rate	Blood pressure	SpO_2
36.1°C	88	20	140/90	97% (RA*)

*RA = room air.

On collection of a ward urine test, her urine was found to be turbid with an offensive odour. It was positive for protein, blood and nitrite. The pH was 6.0, and the specific gravity was 1.020. Although Mrs Gibson is difficult to assess because of her confusion, it appeared that voiding caused her pain. She appears to be dehydrated, her skin turgor is poor, and her mucous membranes are dry and cracked. She also has an excoriated perianal area. She commenced antibacterial therapy with co-trimoxazole (trimethoprim and sulfamethoxazole), and had a urine sample collected for microscopy, culture and sensitivity (MCS). A blood sample was also taken.

Her pathology results were as follows.

HAEMATOLOGY

Patient location:	Ward 3	**UR:**	886132		
Consultant:	Smith	**NAME:**	Gibson		
		Given name:	Agnes	**Sex:**	F
		DOB:	01/01/XX	**Age:**	84

Time collected	14:20
Date collected	XX/XX
Year	XXXX
Lab #	34524325

FULL BLOOD COUNT		UNITS	REFERENCE RANGE
Haemoglobin	121	g/L	115–160
White cell count	12.2	$\times 10^9/L$	4.0–11.0
Platelets	178	$\times 10^9/L$	140–400
Haematocrit	0.35		0.33–0.47
Red cell count	4.0	$\times 10^{12}/L$	3.80–5.20
Reticulocyte count	0.6	%	0.2–2.0
MCV	94	fL	80–100
Neutrophils	9.2	$\times 10^9/L$	2.00–8.00
Lymphocytes	3.41	$\times 10^9/L$	1.00–4.00
Monocytes	0.52	$\times 10^9/L$	0.10–1.00
Eosinophils	0.36	$\times 10^9/L$	< 0.60
Basophils	0.12	$\times 10^9/L$	< 0.20
ESR	14	mm/h	< 12

BIOCHEMISTRY

Patient location:	Ward 3	**UR:**	886132		
Consultant:	Smith	**NAME:**	Gibson		
		Given name:	Agnes	**Sex:**	F
		DOB:	01/01/XX	**Age:**	84

Time collected	14:20
Date collected	XX/XX
Year	XXXX
Lab #	554334532

ELECTROLYTES		UNITS	REFERENCE RANGE
Sodium	134	mmol/L	135–145
Potassium	3.3	mmol/L	3.5–5.2
Chloride	94	mmol/L	95–110
Bicarbonate	19	mmol/L	22–32
Glucose (random)	3.4	mmol/L	3.5–7.7
Iron	9	μmol/L	11–30

Mrs Gibson has been commenced on intravenous fluid–sodium chloride 0.9% q8h. The current plan until further review is to encourage oral fluid intake. She has been commenced on a fluid balance chart for intake, and she is to be observed for signs of fluid overload. Her output may be difficult to track and record. Incontinence pads have been provided to her and she is to have all episodes of incontinence recorded, but it is not required that the pads be weighed at this stage. Her temperature should be monitored: she was given two paracetamol before transfer as her temperature was 38.1°C. Frequent observation of her intravenous cannula will be required, as Mrs Gibson is quite confused and may accidentally remove it.

CRITICAL THINKING

1 Consider Mrs Gibson's presentation. What is the clinical significance of her age, confusion, incontinence and urinary tract infection? Explain.
2 A ward urine test shows protein, blood and nitrite. Should these substances be found in the urine of a healthy individual? Explain.
3 Mrs Gibson was commenced on antibacterial agents even though the results of the urine MCS were unknown. What data supported the possibility that she had a UTI? Why shouldn't the medical officer have waited until the urine MCS had come back?
4 Observe Mrs Gibson's pathology results. What values suggest that an inflammatory process is occurring? Explain.
5 Identify all of the interventions necessary to manage Mrs Gibson's UTI (including, but not limited to, the ones mentioned in this case study). Explain the rationale of each intervention.

BIBLIOGRAPHY

Australian Institute of Health and Welfare (AIHW) (2020). *Disparities in potentially preventable hospitalisations across Australia 2012–13 to 2017–18.* Cat. No. HPF 50. Canberra: AIHW. https://www.aihw.gov.au/reports/primary-health-care/disparities-in-potentially-preventable-hospitalisations-australia.

Australian Institute of Health and Welfare (AIHW) (2022). *Australia's health, 2022.* Australia's Health series No. 18. Canberra: AIHW. https://www.aihw.gov.au/reports-data/australias-health.

Batuman, V., Schmidt, R.J., Soman, A.S. & Soman, S.S. (2021). Diabetic nephropathy. *Emedicine*. Retrieved from https://emedicine.medscape.com/article/238946-overview.

Bauldoff, G., Gubrud-Howe, P.M., Carno, M.-A., Levett-Jones, T., Hales, M., Berry, K.,… Stanley, D. (2020). *LeMone and Burke's medical–surgical nursing: critical thinking for person-centred care* (4th [Australian] edn). Sydney: Pearson Australia.

Best, O. & Fredericks, B. (2021). *Yatdjuligin: Aboriginal and Torres Strait Islander nursing and midwifery care* (3rd edn). Port Melbourne, VIC: Cambridge University Press.

Brusch, J.L., Bavaro, M.F. & Tessier, J.M. (2023). Urinary tract infection (UTI) and cystitis (bladder infection) in females. *Emedicine*. https://emedicine.medscape.com/article/233101-treatment.

Bullock, S. & Manias, E. (2022). *Fundamentals of pharmacology* (9th edn). Sydney: Pearson Australia.

Herness, J., Buttolph, A. & Hammer, N.C. (2020). Acute pyelonephritis in adults: rapid evidence review. *American Family Physician* 102(3):173–80. https://www.aafp.org/pubs/afp/issues/2020/0801/p173.html.

Hughes, T., Juliebø-Jones, P., Saada, L., Saeed, K. & Somani, B.K. (2021). Recurrent urinary tract infections in adults: a practical guide. *British Journal of Hospital Medicine* 82(12). https://doi.org/10.12968/hmed.2021.0337.

Lam, A. (2021). Advancing your practice: urinary incontinence. *Australian Journal of Pharmacy* 102(1202):62–66. https://doi.org/10.3316/informit.671681366542046.

Marieb, E.N. & Hoehn, K. (2019). *Human anatomy and physiology* (11th edn). San Francisco, CA: Pearson Benjamin Cummings.

Mohammad, D. & Baracco, R. (2020). Postinfectious glomerulonephritis. *Pediatric Annals* 49(6):e273–e277. doi:10.3928/19382359-20200519-01.

Mutnuri, S., Agraharker, M. & Lerma, E.V. (2021). Acute tubular necrosis. *Emedicine*. https://emedicine.medscape.com/article/238064-overview.

Russo, P.L., Stewardson, A.J., Cheng, A.C., Bucknall, T. & Mitchell, B.G. (2019). The prevalence of healthcare associated infections among adult inpatients at nineteen large Australian acute-care public hospitals: a point prevalence survey. *Antimicrobial Resistance and Infection Control* 8:article 114. https://doi.org/10.1186/s13756-019-0570-y.

Vasavada, S.P., Barat, O. & Leone, G. (2021). Urinary incontinence. *Emedicine*. https://emedicine.medscape.com/article/452289-overview.

Wong, W., Lennon, D.R., Crone, S., Neutze, J.M. & Reed, P.W. (2013). Prospective population-based study on the burden of disease from post-streptococcal glomerulonephritis of hospitalised children in New Zealand: epidemiology, clinical features and complications. *Journal of Paediatrics and Child Health* 49(10):850–55. https://doi.org/10.1111/jpc.12295.

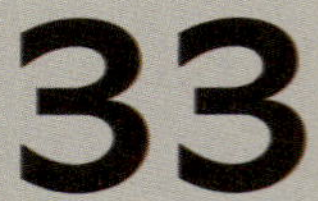

33 Renal neoplasms and obstructions

KEY TERMS

Extracorporeal shock wave lithotripsy (ESWL)
Hydronephrosis
Intravenous pyelogram (IVP)
Nephrolithiasis
Nephrotoxicity
Oxalate
Polycystic kidney disease
Struvite
Uric acid
Urothelium
Vesicoureteral reflux (VUR)

LEARNING OBJECTIVES

After completing this chapter, you should be able to:

1. Identify the types of neoplasms that can influence renal system function.
2. Describe the characteristics and management of polycystic kidney disease.
3. Differentiate between the different types of cancer that can occur within the renal system.
4. Characterise the effects of renal flow obstruction and hydronephrosis.
5. Compare and contrast the different substances that cause kidney stone formation.
6. Describe the characteristics of vesicoureteral reflux and hydronephrosis.

WHAT YOU SHOULD KNOW BEFORE STARTING THIS CHAPTER

Can you identify the major parts of the renal system, and outline their functions?

Can you identify the structures of the kidney?

Can you identify the parts of the nephron, and describe their functions?

Can you describe the phases of inflammation?

Can you differentiate between acute and chronic inflammation?

Can you outline the stages of the healing process?

Can you describe the major concepts associated with neoplasia?

Introduction

LEARNING OBJECTIVE 1

Identify the types of neoplasms that can influence renal system function.

The focus of this chapter is to describe conditions that obstruct the formation or passage of urine through the renal system, and the consequences of such obstruction. Neoplastic disorders affecting the kidneys and the bladder are covered in this chapter. As discussed in the chapter 'Neoplasia', neoplasms grow in a relatively accelerated and uncontrolled fashion. As they develop, neoplasms compress and obstruct the normal tissues, leading to a significant disruption of normal function. Some types of renal neoplasm may metastasise to distant areas of the body.

Other conditions primarily characterised by the obstruction of normal urine flow, such as kidney stones and vesicoureteral reflux, are also described in this chapter. Benign prostate hypertrophy and prostate cancer can obstruct urine flow in males. These conditions are covered in the chapter 'Male reproductive disorders'.

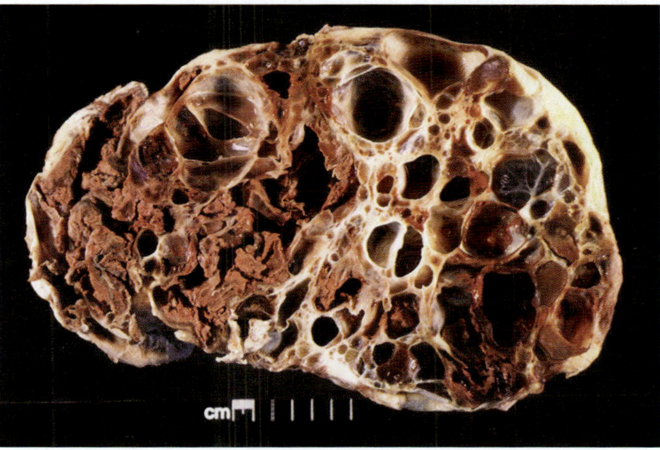

Figure 33.1

A kidney from a person affected by adult polycystic disease

A cross-section of a kidney from a person affected by polycystic kidney disease shows multiple cysts throughout the damaged organ.

Source: Ed Uthman.

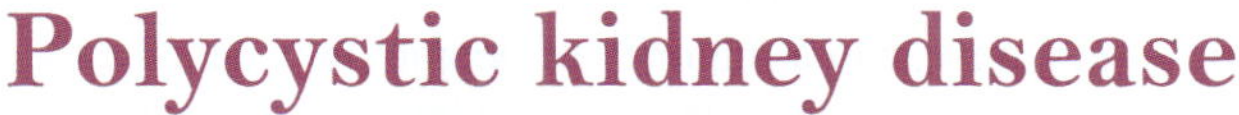

Polycystic kidney disease

LEARNING OBJECTIVE 2

Describe the characteristics and management of polycystic kidney disease.

Aetiology and pathophysiology

Polycystic kidney disease is genetically determined. The most common form, *autosomal dominant polycystic disease,* or *adult polycystic kidney disease*, affects 1 in 1,000 people (see Figure 33.1). In this condition, hundreds of cysts develop from the nephrons. Mutations in the *PKD-1* and *PKD-2* genes affect the formation of the proteins polycystin-1 and polycystin-2. The abnormal proteins induce a proliferation of the tubular epithelium and increased fluid secretion, which leads to the formation of the cysts. As the cysts grow, they block the renal vasculature, causing ischaemia and activation of the renin–angiotensin system.

The process usually begins in the teenage years. By early middle age, the kidneys will be greatly distended (see Figure 33.2), and the signs and symptoms of kidney impairment will appear. In time, the kidneys may fail, and affected people will require either a kidney transplant or life-long dialysis.

This condition may also be associated with systemic disorders. Cysts form in the liver, pancreas and other organs, but may remain asymptomatic. Affected people may also develop cerebral and aortic aneurysms, heart valve disorders and diverticular disease.

Another rarer type of polycystic kidney disease, which is associated with an autosomal recessive inheritance pattern, manifests in infancy. It may be referred to as *infantile polycystic kidney disease*. Most of those affected die in childhood. Cysts develop in both the kidneys and the liver, leading to significant fibrosis in both organs. Asymptomatic infants and children have

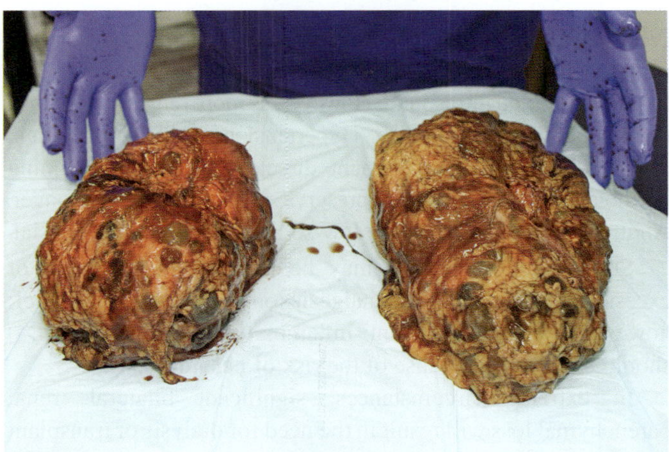

Figure 33.2

Distended and grossly disfigured kidneys

Explanted kidneys from a bilateral nephrectomy for a person with a 14-year history of polycystic kidney disease in preparation for a renal transplant at a later date. The combined weight of kidneys was 21.9 kg, which represented 21.6% of the person's total body weight. A transplant from a living related donor three months later was successful, with normal renal function noted at the two-year post-transplant review.

Source: Life in view/Science Photo Library.

been identified. Increased survival rates have been observed when associated with early intervention and improved screening of at-risk children.

Clinical manifestations

The clinical manifestations of someone with polycystic kidney disease include hypertension, enlarged painful abdomen, urinary tract infections and haematuria. Flank pain is one of the most common presenting complaints. If an individual presents late in the disease process when chronic renal disease has begun, dry skin, oedema and uraemia may also be observed.

Clinical diagnosis and management

Diagnosis Diagnosis is based on family history, age, physical examination and the number of cysts. Genetic testing for *PKD-1* and *PKD-2* is valuable and accurate. Urea and creatinine levels will give an indication of renal function, and an increased haematocrit indicates an increase in erythropoietin secretion from some of the cysts. Urinalysis should be performed to determine the presence of a urinary tract infection.

Imaging studies are beneficial to determine renal anatomy. An ultrasound is non-invasive, relatively inexpensive and accurate to detect cysts and measure kidney size. Computed tomography (CT) and magnetic resonance imaging (MRI) can also assist with diagnosis.

A full blood count and blood biochemistry may be beneficial to identify other issues requiring management; however, they are not diagnostic of polycystic kidney disease.

Management Depending on the progression of the disease, management plans may be as simple as annual renal function tests and ultrasound. However, as more renal tissue is lost, renal function will diminish. Hypertension exacerbates chronic kidney disease, so management directed towards maintaining normotensive pressures will preserve renal function for longer. Antihypertensive agents and a low-sodium diet will be beneficial.

Surgery to drain cysts may be required in the event of excessive pain. Narcotic analgesics may offer some relief; however, non-steroidal anti-inflammatory drugs (NSAIDs) should be avoided because of the risk of **nephrotoxicity**.

In extreme circumstances, significant bilateral, renal parenchymal loss will result in the need for dialysis or transplant if chronic kidney failure develops or nephrectomy is required for intractable pain.

Renal system cancers

In this section, common renal system cancers are described, such as kidney cancer, Wilms' tumour and urinary bladder cancer. Figure 33.3 explores the common clinical manifestations and management of renal system cancers.

LEARNING OBJECTIVE 3

Differentiate between the different types of cancer that can occur within the renal system.

KIDNEY CANCER

Aetiology and pathophysiology

Renal cell carcinoma (see Figure 33.4) originates from epithelial cells of the tubule. It is relatively uncommon, accounting for 2% of all cancers. However, it is the most common renal malignancy, and is considered to be aggressive, with a poor prognosis. About 1 in 10 renal cell cancers will have metastasised by the time they are diagnosed, with the most common sites being nearby lymph nodes, bones and lungs.

Epidemiology

The causes and risk factors for this disease are not well defined. Cigarette smoking, obesity, exposure to asbestos and heavy metals, a defect on chromosome 3, hypertension and other kidney diseases have been cited as risk factors. The incidence of renal cell carcinoma is about twice as high in men as in women. According to data from the Australian Institute of Health and Welfare, in 2022 the estimated age-standardised incidence rates are 20.6 cases per 100,000 persons in men, and 9.1 cases per 100,000 persons in women.

Clinical manifestations

The classic signs and symptoms of renal cell carcinoma are haematuria, the presence of a palpable mass, and flank pain, although these appear in a minority of people only. Many cases are discovered incidentally when the abdomen is investigated for other reasons. Hypertension is common, as is weight loss and fever.

If metastases develop in bones, severe bone pain is observed. Hypercalcaemia and pathological fractures may also occur.

Clinical diagnosis and management

Diagnosis Diagnosis of renal cell cancer is definitive by cell collection guided by CT or ultrasound. Histological examination of cells reveals classification and grading. Other imaging studies, such as MRI, positron emission tomography (PET) scans and bone scans, are important to quantify the extent of the tumour invasion and to detect metastatic lesions.

A full blood count and electrolyte levels will be beneficial to determine other issues that need management. They may also identify the presence of hypercalcaemia. Renal and liver function tests are also valuable, although not diagnostic.

Management Surgery is the central treatment for early renal cell carcinoma, with chemotherapy and radiotherapy of very limited use for this tumour. A person with a stage I tumour, in which the cancer is confined to one kidney and is not more than 7 cm in diameter, has a five-year survival of 90% following surgery. Bisphosphonate therapy can prevent the bone pain, hypercalcaemia and pathological fractures associated with bone metastases.

Immunomodulators, such as interferon-α, may be used to reduce tumour growth and improve outcomes. The tyrosine kinase inhibitor sunitinib is useful in the management of advanced renal cell carcinoma.

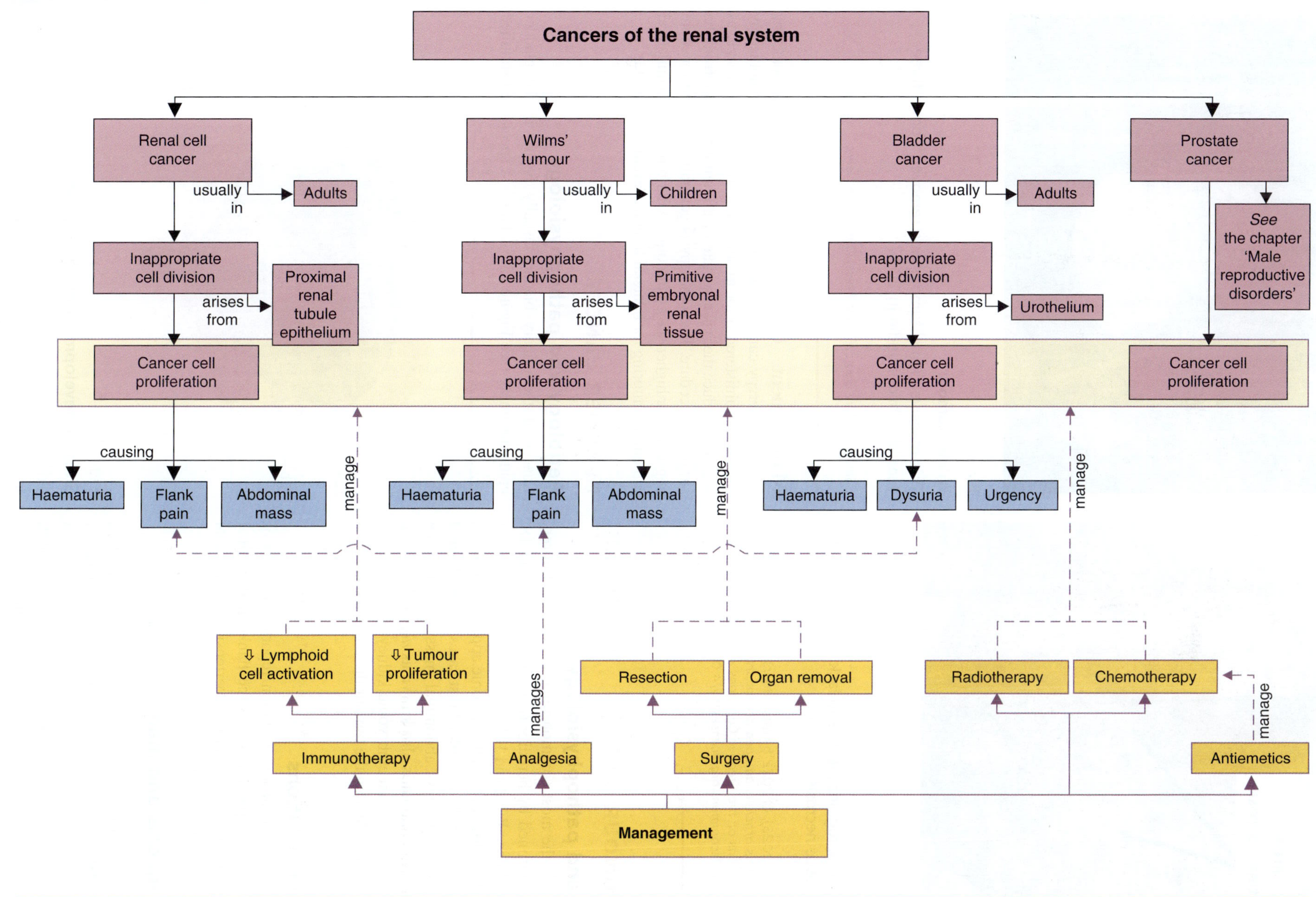

Figure 33.3

Clinical snapshot: Renal system cancers

↓ = decreased.

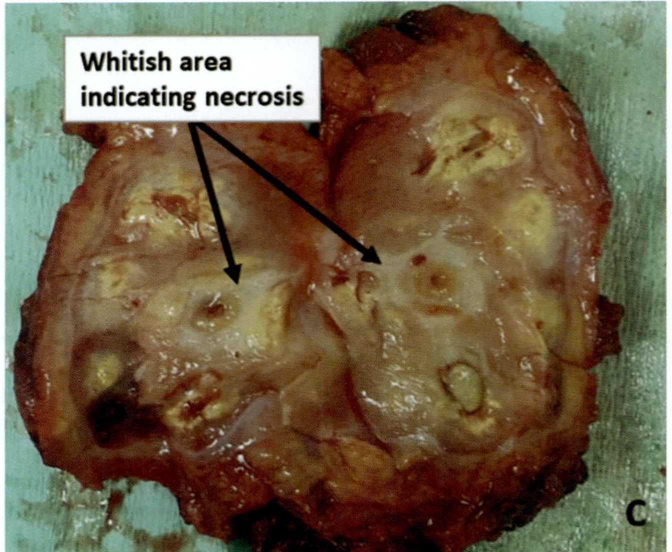

Figure 33.4

Renal carcinoma

The indicated white regions are due to lack of blood supply, which causes tissue necrosis.

Source: Gaudji et al. (2023);

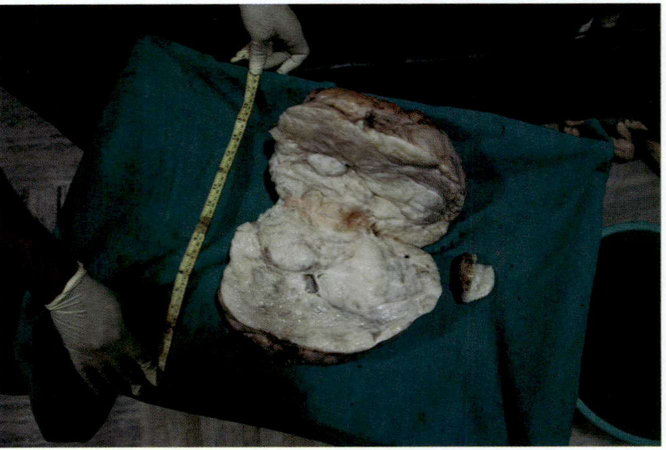

Figure 33.5

Wilms' tumour

This massive Wilms' tumour was removed from a three-year-old child in India in 2017.

Source: Akshay Gupta/Pacific Press/Alamy Live News.

WILMS' TUMOUR

Aetiology and pathophysiology

Wilms' tumour is the most common renal tumour in children. It is largely determined by heredity (e.g. trisomies 13 and 18, mutations in the genes *WT-2* and *WT-1*), and is probably present at birth, although it does not usually become apparent for years. Peak incidence age is 3–4 years old. Most cases are discovered accidentally when a painless abdominal mass is found (see Figure 33.5). Wilms' tumour is also known as *nephroblastoma*, as it is believed to arise from embryonic kidney cells that have persisted beyond birth. Within the tumour there may be necrosis and cyst development.

Clinical manifestations

The most common clinical manifestation reported in cases of Wilms' tumour is a palpable mass in the flank or abdominal area. Other manifestations include hypertension, abdominal pain and microscopic haematuria.

Clinical diagnosis and management

Diagnosis Imaging studies include the use of ultrasound, CT scans and MRI to determine the extent of the disease. A bone scan is also necessary with advanced disease, as is a chest X-ray to quantify metastatic spread. A full blood count, electrolyte levels, liver and renal function tests, although not diagnostic, are beneficial to determine whether there are other issues that require management.

Management Current treatment with surgery, chemotherapy and radiotherapy can cure at least 85% of cases. Chemotherapy may be administered prior to surgery to reduce tumour size, as well as to reduce the risk associated with tumour spillage from the surgical procedure. Radiotherapy is generally reserved for more aggressive or higher-staged tumours. After removal of a unilateral tumour, monitoring for bilateral tumour development occurs.

BLADDER CANCER

Aetiology and pathophysiology

Cancer of the urinary bladder usually begins in the bladder epithelial lining (see Figure 33.6). This is a specialised stratified

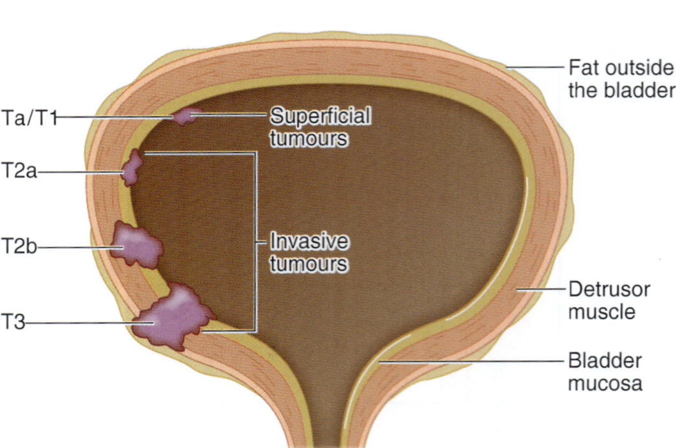

Figure 33.6

Sites of development of urinary bladder cancers

Urinary bladder cancers can grow superficially within the mucosa, or can infiltrate into deeper layers of the bladder wall. The Tn staging refers to the size/extent of the primary tumour. T3 is more extensive than T1.

epithelium known as *transitional epithelium* or **urothelium**. In this tissue, cells of the basal layer are cuboidal but gradually become flatter as they mature and reach the luminal surface. Bladder cancer begins when the urothelium is irritated; these cells proliferate (i.e. become hyperplastic) and proto-oncogenes (see the chapter 'Neoplasia') are activated. Inflammation can induce the release of pro-tumour chemical factors that promote cancer cell survival.

Bladder cancers are urothelial cell carcinomas. They may be superficial or invasive. *Superficial transitional cell carcinomas* are the most common types. They tend not to be invasive, and form flat or papillary (projecting) growths while remaining confined to the urothelium. *Invasive transitional cell carcinomas* are much less common. Such cancers invade deeper layers of the bladder, such as the smooth muscle, and metastasise to the lymph nodes, bones, lungs and the liver.

In some parts of the world where parasitic infections of the bladder, such as schistosomiasis (see Figure 33.7), are common, cancer may arise as a consequence of chronic bladder inflammation. The rate of mitosis of surviving urothelial cells will increase in an attempt to replace those lost by infection and inflammation; this provides opportunities to arise for spontaneous mutations, including those that create oncogenes.

Epidemiology

Bladder cancers tend to be diagnosed earlier than renal cell carcinomas, as they give rise to characteristic early symptoms of haematuria and urinary irritation. Cancers of the bladder are uncommon in people under 60 years of age. According to statistics from the Australian Institute of Health and Welfare, in 2022 the estimated risk of developing bladder cancer by the age of 85 years for an Australian is 1%. Age-related changes that may contribute to the increased risk in older adults include alteration of the *p53* tumour suppressor gene, smoking, increased cellular mutation and unchecked replication.

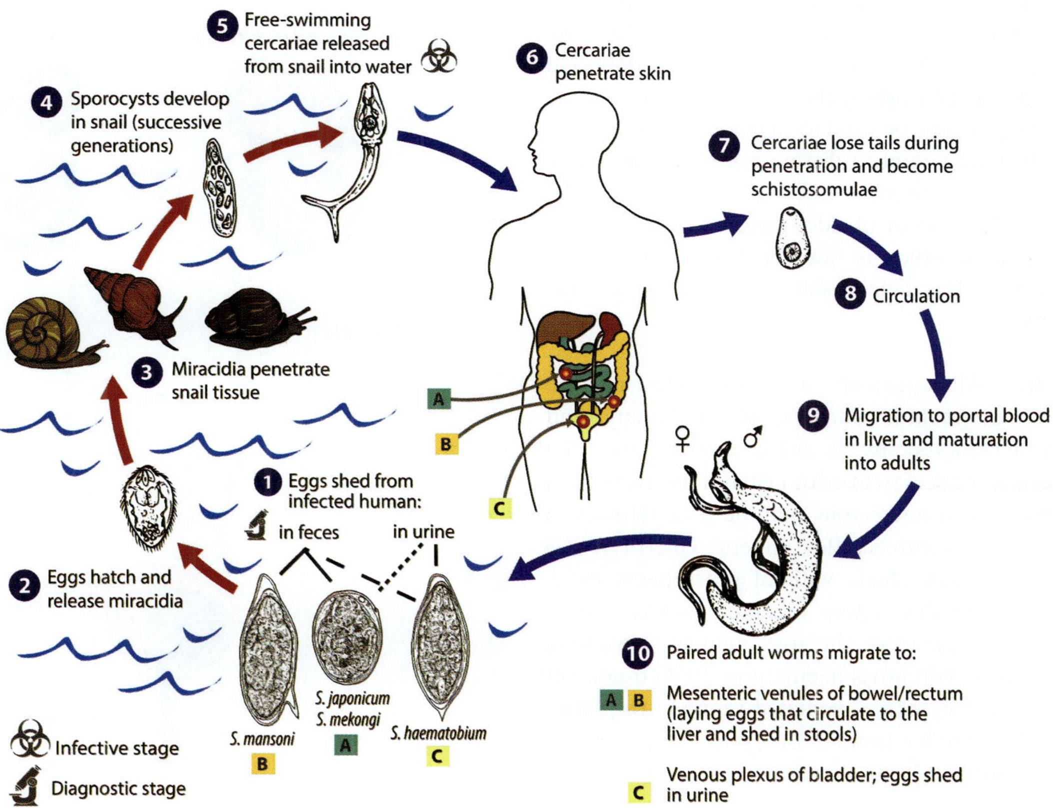

Figure 33.7

Schistosomiasis: parasitic infection of the bladder

The risk of bladder cancer is increased following exposure to parasitic infections as the inflammatory process causes cellular changes that may result in the spontaneous mutations leading to bladder cancer.

Source: Centers for Disease Control and Prevention, USA.

Like kidney cancer, there is a marked sex difference in incidence: the age-standardised incidence rate in 2022 is estimated at 16 in 100,000 persons for men and 4 in 100,000 persons in women.

The major factors that are thought to contribute to bladder cancer are:

- age—the greatest risk is between 85 and 89 years old
- cigarette smoking—many carcinogens from cigarette smoke, and their metabolites formed within the body, end up in the bladder and may spend considerable time there before being voided
- exposure to certain industrial dyes, such as anilines
- use of cyclophosphamide, a drug used to treat certain cancers and autoimmune disorders.

Clinical manifestations

Haematuria is an important initial clinical manifestation in bladder cancer. The haematuria is commonly gross and painless. Occasionally, individuals may present with dysuria, as well as increased frequency and urgency of micturition.

Clinical diagnosis and management

Diagnosis Urinalysis should be performed to quantify the presence or extent of a urinary tract infection. Imaging studies may include an X-ray of the kidneys, ureters and bladder (KUB), **intravenous pyelogram (IVP)** and ultrasound. A cystoscopy and biopsy may be used to diagnose and grade the bladder cancer. It is important to distinguish between *muscle invasive* and *non-muscle invasive disease* as this directs the management plan. The use of bladder cancer markers is still debatable, and their accuracy is not yet proven. Blood and urine sampling may be beneficial to determine other issues that require management.

Management Management of non-muscle invasive bladder cancer can include surgery, chemotherapy and immunotherapy. Chemotherapy is often inserted into the bladder (intravesical) or it may be administered intravenously. Immunomodulation with interferons may be used. However, intravesicular treatments with bacille Calmette–Guérin (BCG) may be beneficial in individuals without gross haematuria. An individual's risk of developing tuberculosis-like illness from haematogenous spread of the live attenuated bacteria increases significantly with gross haematuria. BCG treatment is thought to initiate a cytokine-mediated immune response. A resection of the bladder tumour or cystectomy may be required if immunotherapy and chemotherapy fail to control the cancer.

Management of muscle invasive bladder cancer may also include surgery and chemotherapy. The mortality rates for muscle invasive cancer with metastasis are very high. Radical surgical procedures are required to increase the chance of survival.

Renal obstructions

LEARNING OBJECTIVE 4

Characterise the effects of renal flow obstruction and hydronephrosis.

LEARNING OBJECTIVE 5

Compare and contrast the different substances that cause kidney stone formation.

LEARNING OBJECTIVE 6

Describe the characteristics of vesicoureteral reflux and hydronephrosis.

Obstruction of the urinary tract (see Figure 33.8) can occur at any point from the renal tubules to the external urethral opening. It may be caused by pregnancy, kidney stones, tumours, blood clots, infection and inflammation, enlargement of the prostate gland (see the chapter 'Male reproductive disorders'), and

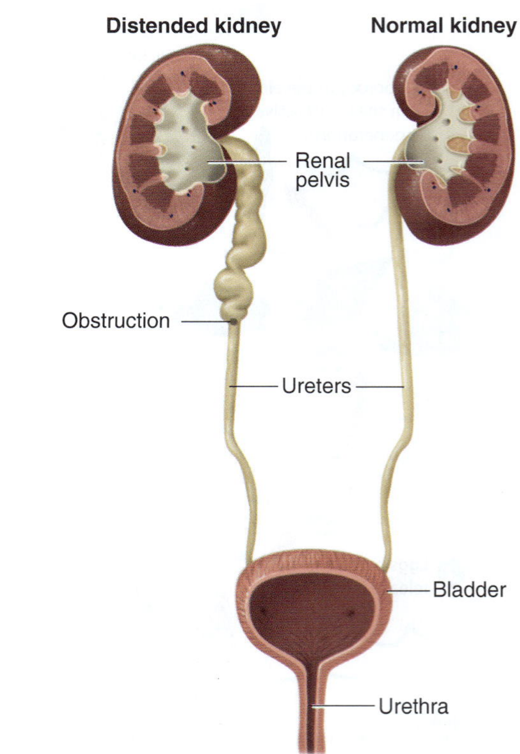

Figure 33.8

Consequences of an obstruction of the urinary tract

An obstruction in a ureter can lead to a back pressure that causes distension of the proximal end of the ureter and the renal pelvis.

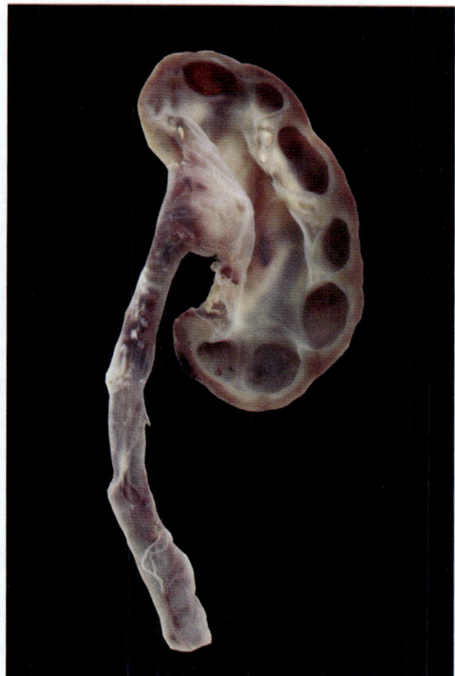

Figure 33.9

Hydronephrosis

The image shows a markedly enlarged kidney. The ureter is obstructed, and the corresponding renal pelvis and calyx are distended.

Source: Copied with permission from ACT Pathology.

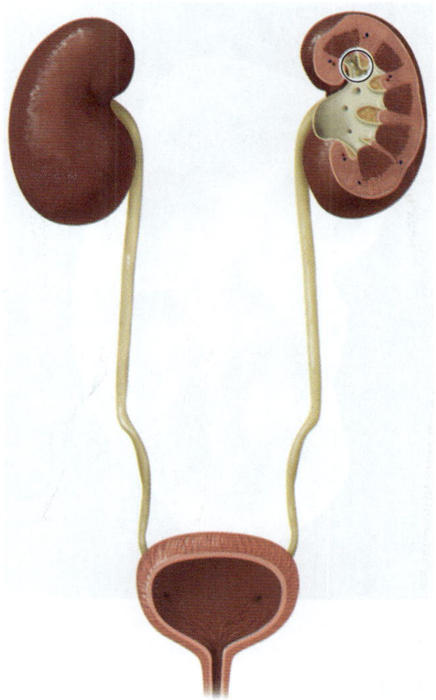

Figure 33.10

Formation of urinary calculus in the renal pelvis

A calculus is shown to have developed in the upper region of the renal pelvis of the left kidney.

blockages in a catheter. When a ureter deforms and becomes tortuous, it is known as *hydroureter*.

When a blockage occurs, urine will accumulate upstream of the blockage. This is called *urinary stasis*. While filtration continues at the glomeruli, urine will accumulate in the kidney pelvis and calyces and distend them as its hydrostatic pressure rises. This is called **hydronephrosis** (see Figure 33.9). Eventually, the nephrons, together with their blood supply, will be squeezed. If the obstruction is not relieved, permanent kidney damage will occur as the nephrons die; the tubules will die first because their blood supply is choked off.

Obstruction is also a risk factor for the development of urinary tract infections (see the chapter 'Common inflammatory disorders of the kidneys and urinary tract'). The sterility of the healthy urinary tract is maintained largely by the flushing action of urine. When the flow of urine is impeded, there is a greatly increased risk that infection will ascend from the distal end of the tract.

KIDNEY STONES

Aetiology and pathophysiology

Insoluble stones or urinary calculi may form in the urinary tract, usually in the renal pelvis, as ions precipitate from solution in the urine (see Figure 33.10). This process is termed **nephrolithiasis** or *urolithiasis*.

The major component involved in the formation of kidney stones is *calcium ions* (Ca^{2+}), which forms precipitates with **oxalate**, phosphate or urate ions to form calcium oxalate, calcium phosphate or calcium urate. The substance of the stone may also consist of **uric acid** crystals, cystine (two cysteine residues joined by a disulfide bond) and **struvite** (a crystalline compound made up of ammonium magnesium phosphate). Kidney stones tend to form when the concentration of Ca^{2+} is high in urine (i.e. *hypercalciuria*). This may be due to a reduced water content of urine (e.g. in dehydration) or it can occur during treatment with loop diuretics.

Some kidney stones are compounds of magnesium. This type of kidney stone tends to form in urinary tract infections involving bacteria that produce the enzyme urease. This enzyme releases ammonia from urea, rendering the urine alkaline and promoting precipitation of the magnesium compounds.

Small stones may be asymptomatic, whether they remain in the urinary tract or are passed through it. Larger stones can cause urinary tract obstruction and damage to structures of the urinary tract. The entry of a large stone into the urinary tract causes intense pain that originates at the ureter and often radiates considerable distances. Chills and fever often occur, and, as the stone damages tissue in its descent, blood appears in the urine.

Some stones may remain in the renal pelvis and grow there, extending into the calyces. Their shape is moulded by these structures, and they are named, accordingly, 'staghorn calculi' (see Figure 33.11).

Epidemiology

Four to eight per cent of Australians develop symptomatic kidney stones over their lifetime, with men at greater risk than women: about 1 in 10 men will suffer from kidney stones, compared to 1 in 35 women.

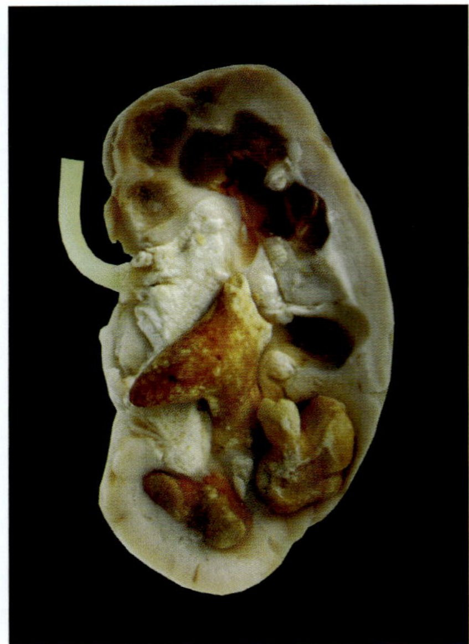

Figure 33.11

Staghorn calculi

Calculi have grown and moulded into the renal pelvis and calyces to resemble the antlers of a stag.

Source: Copied with permission from ACT Pathology.

Clinical manifestations

The main clinical manifestation associated with kidney stones is pain. Generally, the pain is associated with the presence of a stone within the ureter, which distends the ureteral wall. The onset of pain is usually abrupt and can be severe. This is called *ureteral colic*. The pain increases in intensity as the urine flow is obstructed and the ureteral wall is further distended by the build-up of urine behind the stone. The pain is rhythmic and ipsilateral. The pain begins in the flank area and, as the stone moves towards the bladder, it radiates down to the groin area. Nausea and vomiting are often experienced, but fever is generally only present in nephrolithiasis complicated by infection. In males, the testicles may be painful.

Clinical diagnosis and management

Diagnosis Imaging studies include the use of KUB X-rays, CT and ultrasound. An IVP can be beneficial. However, since other imaging methods have become more widely available, clinicians may rely more on CT studies, as significantly more information can be determined.

A full blood count, electrolyte levels and renal function tests (urea and creatinine) will be beneficial to determine whether there are adverse effects on renal function, but they are not diagnostic. Individuals with calcium phosphate stones may demonstrate hypokalaemia and low bicarbonate levels. The renal function test can also influence the decision as to whether radio-opaque contrast is used, or prophylactic renal preservation measures (against contrast-induced nephrotoxicity), such as the administration of *N*-acetylcysteine, are used before contrast is administered.

Urinalysis should be undertaken, and will generally demonstrate haematuria and, depending on whether the nephrolithiasis is complicated by infection, there may also be a degree of pyuria. Individuals with struvite stones may demonstrate nitrites and a urinary pH greater than 7. All urine should be strained for stone collection.

Management One of the priorities in the management of renal calculi is pain control. Depending on the severity of pain, NSAIDs (e.g. ketorolac or naproxen) may be used, as they reduce the formation of prostaglandin E_2. However, NSAIDs can have nephrotoxic effects, so care must be taken. Opioids (e.g. morphine) are very useful in severe pain. Although antiemetics are generally administered prophylactically when opioids are given, they are almost always required to manage the nausea and vomiting associated with renal calculi. As such, intravenous fluids are generally required as a result of dehydration. Some debate exists about the value of fluid support in non-dehydrated individuals from concern that the increased volume may exacerbate the pain from stone movement.

Thiazide diuretics, unlike the loop diuretics, tend to oppose hypercalciuria, and as such are useful in the prevention of recurrent kidney stones.

Extracorporeal shock wave lithotripsy (ESWL) uses focused ultrasound shock waves to break the stones into smaller pieces. Medications such as α-adrenergic antagonists and (less commonly) calcium channel blockers can also be beneficial by increasing ureteral peristalsis. This combined approach increases the likelihood of passing the stone without the need for surgical intervention.

Depending on the size and type of stone, and the facilities available, ESWL may not be an option. In this instance, surgical removal will be necessary. Surgical intervention is particularly important in individuals with significant renal compromise, intractable pain, or those with only one functioning kidney.

VESICOURETERAL REFLUX

Aetiology and pathophysiology

At the junction of each ureter with the urinary bladder, the vesicoureteral valve ensures that urine flows in one direction only—distally into the bladder. In **vesicoureteral reflux (VUR)**, coordinated peristaltic muscle contractions that propel the urine bolus distally are disrupted either by functional or structural causes. The flow of urine is reversed and it re-enters the ureters.

VUR can be classified as primary or secondary. In the *primary form*, an affected person is born with the condition, which is due to an impairment in the development of the valve. As a result, the valve does not close completely. It is possible that, as the child grows, the growth of the ureters may enable more complete closure. In children, 30–40% of urinary tract infection diagnoses are associated with primary VUR. In the *secondary form*, an obstruction in the urinary tract may lead to distended or swollen ureters in the valvular region, so that the valve mechanism cannot achieve a proper seal. A neurogenic bladder can also lead to VUR, when the smooth muscle of the bladder does not relax or contract at the time of bladder emptying.

Clinical manifestations

The most common presentation of an individual with VUR is related to that of a urinary tract infection. Dysuria, haematuria and urinary frequency are common. A fever may develop, and, depending on the extent of the infection and reflux, flank pain and renal compromise may develop.

Clinical diagnosis and management

Diagnosis Occasionally, VUR may be discovered accidentally on investigations for other conditions. Urinalysis is important, and may demonstrate nitrites, haematuria and proteinuria. A full blood count and electrolyte levels may identify other issues that require management, but are not diagnostic for this condition. Renal function tests, including urea and creatinine, are used to determine the degree of compromise occurring.

Imaging studies may include an ultrasound and a nuclear renal scan using technetium-99m DMSA (dimercaptosuccinic acid). This is administered intravenously, and measures renal function and the development of pyelonephritis as a result of the reflux. A voiding cystourethrogram is valuable to demonstrate the degree of voiding dysfunction, and direct visualisation of the bladder may be undertaken with cystoscopy, but as the issue is generally higher, a risk–benefit analysis may not support its value.

Management Depending on the severity and the clinical presentation resulting in the diagnosis of VUR, the management options may range from observation and annual review through to a more aggressive approach with surgical intervention necessary. Prophylactic antimicrobial administration may be used to reduce potential damage from pyelonephritis. The use of α-receptor antagonists or antimuscarinic agents may decrease smooth muscle contraction and reduce spasm. Finally, severe VUR may require surgical intervention in which the ureters are repaired or reimplanted. An endoscopic technique may be beneficial, whereby a bulking compound is injected into the ureteral orifice to increase obstruction of the ureter when the bladder contracts.

INDIGENOUS HEALTH FAST FACTS AND CULTURAL CONSIDERATIONS

FAST FACTS

- *Aboriginal and Torres Strait Islander children living in remote tropical and desert areas of Australia are over two times more likely than non-Indigenous children to experience urolithiasis.*
- *Aboriginal and Torres Strait Islander peoples are less likely than non-Indigenous Australians to be diagnosed with kidney cancer (0.8:1), but 1.1 times more likely to die. A similar trend was observed for Māori compared to European New Zealanders.*
- *Māori are less likely than European New Zealanders to develop urolithiasis.*

CULTURAL CONSIDERATIONS

- *High rates of urolithiasis in Aboriginal and Torres Strait Islander children are thought to be associated with socioeconomic risk factors, such as poor water quality, widespread endemic diarrhoea and recurrent infectious disease. Coupled with the more common risk factors of dry, hot environmental conditions, children living in remote areas are at extreme risk. This is reinforced by the fact that urolithiasis is rare in Aboriginal and Torres Strait Islander children living in urban areas. Therefore, culturally appropriate, community-centred programs focusing on public health factors, such as improving poor living conditions with a particular focus on upgraded water supply and waste disposal systems, could hopefully help close the disease burden gap for at least this parameter.*

Sources: Data from ANZDATA Registry (2021); Australian Institute of Health and Welfare (2018); Stumpers & Thomson (2013).

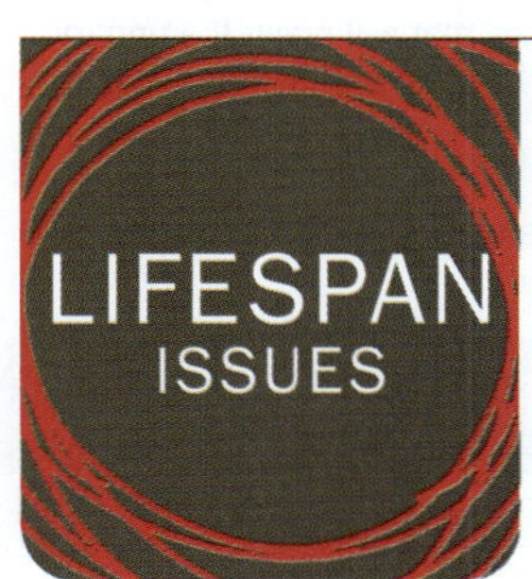

CHILDREN AND ADOLESCENTS

- Children are less likely than adults to develop polycystic kidney disease.
- Children are less likely than adults to develop urolithiasis. The aetiology of stone formation in children is often different from that of adults, and children with a diagnosis of urolithiasis should undergo metabolic evaluations.
- Wilms' tumour is most commonly found in children (average age at diagnosis is 3.5 years) and rarely found in individuals older than 16 years of age.
- Bladder cancer is extremely rare in children.

OLDER ADULTS

- The risk of developing bladder cancer in the older adult increases, and the chance of favourable outcomes decreases.
- An increased incidence of urolithiasis in the older adult can often be attributed to dehydration, aggressive management of hypertension (with diuretics) and declining renal function.
- Extracorporeal shockwave lithotripsy for the management of urolithiasis in the older adult is safe, and can be associated with low complication rates when appropriate planning and management of comorbidities is instituted.

KEY CLINICAL ISSUES

- Individuals with alterations to renal function require close monitoring of fluid balance and other assessment data that may suggest fluid homeostasis issues, such as electrolyte levels, skin turgor, urine output, blood pressure, lung sounds and oedema.
- Many antimicrobial and analgesic agents are nephrotoxic. Care should be taken when an individual is recovering from renal surgery so as not to exacerbate kidney impairment from chemical damage.
- Although survival rates are improving, mortality statistics for urological cancers are of concern to newly diagnosed individuals. Ensure that the management plan, treatment options and prognosis are clearly explained to the client and significant others. Ensure the lines of communication are open, and that appropriate time is given to answer questions and support all involved.
- Individuals should be encouraged and supported to modify lifestyle choices, such as ceasing smoking and making healthy eating choices, which have been demonstrated to assist with weight loss for issues such as urological cancer and renal obstructions. These two factors can assist with the disease process and recovery.

CHAPTER REVIEW

- *Polycystic kidney diseases* are genetically determined. The most common is *autosomal dominant polycystic disease* or *adult polycystic disease*. In this condition, hundreds of cysts develop from nephrons. As the cysts expand into the tissue, they compromise the viability of normal renal tissue and its vasculature. In time, the kidneys may fail, and the person will require either a kidney transplant or life-long dialysis.
- *Renal cell carcinoma* originates from epithelial cells of the tubule. It is relatively uncommon, but it is an aggressive malignancy. About 1 in 10 renal cell cancers will have metastasised by the time they are diagnosed, with the most common sites being nearby lymph nodes and the bones and lungs. The incidence is twice as high in men as in women.
- *Wilms' tumour* is the most common renal tumour in children. It is largely determined by heredity. Most cases are discovered accidentally when an abdominal mass is found. Wilms' tumour is also known as *nephroblastoma*, as it is believed to arise from embryonic kidney cells that have persisted beyond birth.
- *Cancer of the urinary bladder* usually begins in its epithelial lining, known as the urothelium. Bladder cancers tend to be diagnosed earlier than renal cell carcinomas, as they give rise to characteristic early symptoms of haematuria and urinary irritation. Cancers of the bladder are uncommon in people under 60 years of age. The major factors that are thought to contribute to bladder cancer are cigarette smoking, exposure to certain industrial dyes, such as anilines, and cyclophosphamide, a drug used to treat certain cancers and autoimmune disorders. In some parts of the world where parasitic infections of the bladder are common, cancer may arise as a consequence of chronic bladder inflammation.
- *Obstruction of the urinary tract* can occur at any point from the renal tubules to the external urethral opening. It may be caused by pregnancy, kidney stones, tumours, blood clots, infection and inflammation, enlargement of the prostate gland and blockages in a catheter. When this happens, urinary stasis develops and hydrostatic pressure rises. Eventually, nephrons together with their blood supply will be squeezed. If the obstruction is not relieved, permanent kidney damage will occur as nephrons die.
- *Insoluble stones or urinary calculi* may form in the urinary tract, usually in the renal pelvis, as ions precipitate from solution in the urine. This process is termed *nephrolithiasis* or *urolithiasis*. The major component involved in the formation of kidney stones is calcium ions (Ca^{2+}), which forms precipitates with oxalate, phosphate or urate ions to form calcium oxalate, calcium phosphate or calcium urate. *Kidney stones* tend to form when the concentration of Ca^{2+} is high in urine (i.e. hypercalciuria). Small stones may be asymptomatic, whether they remain in the urinary tract or are passed through it. Larger stones can cause urinary tract obstruction and damage to structures of the urinary tract. The entry of a large stone into the urinary tract causes intense pain that originates at the ureter, and often radiates considerable distances.
- When a vesicoureteral valve controlling urine flow into the bladder does not close properly, *vesicoureteral reflux* can occur. This is where the flow of urine is reversed, so that it re-enters the ureters. This condition may be due to a congenital disorder or develop as a result of urinary tract obstruction.

REVIEW QUESTIONS

1. What types of cells or tissues give rise to the following?
   a. the cysts of polycystic disease
   b. renal cell carcinoma
   c. Wilms' tumour
   d. the most common type of bladder cancer
2. What are the major causes of urinary obstruction?
3. Outline the series of pathological processes that will occur if a urinary obstruction develops and is not resolved.
4. What factors may increase the likelihood that kidney stones develop?
5. What are the major causes and consequences of vesicoureteral reflux?

HEALTH PROFESSIONAL CONNECTIONS

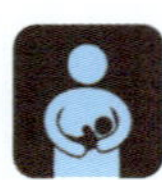

Midwives During pregnancy, changes in urinary calcium excretion may increase the risk of nephrolithiasis. Calcium intake is often increased during pregnancy, and absorption from the gastrointestinal tract increases. These factors may result in the development of calcium oxalate stones that may complicate a pregnancy. Other renal difficulties in pregnancy include exacerbation of polycystic disease symptoms in women with autosomal dominant polycystic kidney disease and hypertension. Polycystic kidney disease increases the risk of fetal and maternal complications in women who are also hypertensive. Adequate data collection when taking a history should elucidate these potential complications.

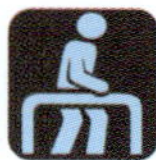

Physiotherapists Rehabilitation of clients following procedures for renal pathology is important. Early mobilisation reduces the risks of thrombosis and embolus formation, and also reduces respiratory complications. People who have had large renal surgical procedures often have significant wounds involving much underlying muscle in the abdominal and/or flank regions. Although the surgical procedures and the size of the surgical site access have changed radically in the past few decades, individuals may still experience pain that dissuades them from moving much postoperatively. A physiotherapist should work with the healthcare team to ensure that the postoperative recovery routine includes appropriate rehabilitation exercises.

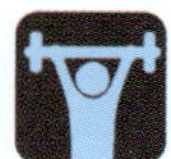

Exercise scientists Strenuous exercise resulting in dehydration can increase the risk of nephrolithiasis formation. It is critical that fluid replacement is a primary focus prior, during and after exercise, especially if the training duration is extended. Knowledge of the causes and manifestations associated with nephrolithiasis can help an exercise physiologist to identify the potential development of kidney stones in those in their care.

Nutritionists/Dieticians Promoting adequate hydration and changes to a person's diet can reduce the risk of kidney stone formation. Different food consumption can result in different types of stone development. Individuals who have a high intake of animal protein may develop oxalate stones, especially when this diet is coupled with poor fluid intake and obesity. Reducing animal proteins can reduce the risks through decreasing the urinary excretion of oxalate, calcium and uric acid. Individuals who consume vegetarian diets excrete lower volumes of oxalate, calcium and uric acid. Consumption of whole grains may also be associated with a significant risk reduction in the formation of kidney stones. Although hydration is an important factor, the type of drink consumed may increase or decrease the risk of stone formation. Tea, coffee and cola drinks increase calcium and oxalate excretion, yet consuming wine may decrease the risk provided that other fluids are also consumed to prevent dehydration from developing. Calcium intake is very important, especially in certain groups of people, such as pregnant women and older individuals. Early studies suggest that calcium consumption within a meal time does not increase the risk of kidney stone formation as much as it does in between meals. Education and guidance to change dietary behaviours will not only improve an individual's overall health, but also decrease the risk of nephrolithiasis.

CASE STUDY

Mr Robert Rant is a 65-year-old man (UR number 545451) presenting with severe right flank pain, nausea and vomiting, and suspected renal calculi. He has a history of hyperparathyroidism. His observations were as follows:

Temperature	Heart rate	Respiration rate	Blood pressure	SpO_2
36.3°C	100	24	168/94	98% (RA*)

*RA = room air.

In the emergency department, he has had an intravenous cannula inserted and has received several doses of morphine over the past two hours with limited effect. He has had blood taken for a full blood count and electrolyte levels. He is to have a KUB X-ray today. He is also booked for an IVP and a CT scan. His pathology results were as follows:

HAEMATOLOGY

Patient location:	Ward 3	**UR:**	545451		
Consultant:	Smith	**NAME:**	Rant		
		Given name:	Robert	**Sex:**	M
		DOB:	13/10/XX	**Age:**	65

Time collected 11:29
Date collected XX/XX
Year XXXX
Lab # 5479837

FULL BLOOD COUNT		UNITS	REFERENCE RANGE
Haemoglobin	132	g/L	115–160
White cell count	8.2	$\times 10^9$/L	4.0–11.0
Platelets	290	$\times 10^9$/L	140–400
Haematocrit	0.42		0.33–0.47
Red cell count	4.9	$\times 10^{12}$/L	3.80–5.20
Reticulocyte count	1.1	%	0.2–2.0
MCV	92	fL	80–100
Neutrophils	5.3	$\times 10^9$/L	2.00–8.00
Lymphocytes	2.5	$\times 10^9$/L	1.00–4.00
Monocytes	0.55	$\times 10^9$/L	0.10–1.00
Eosinophils	0.42	$\times 10^9$/L	< 0.60
Basophils	0.08	$\times 10^9$/L	< 0.20
ESR	16	mm/h	< 12

BIOCHEMISTRY

Patient location:	Ward 3	**UR:**	545451		
Consultant:	Smith	**NAME:**	Rant		
		Given name:	Robert	**Sex:**	M
		DOB:	13/10/XX	**Age:**	65

Time collected 11:29
Date collected XX/XX
Year XXXX
Lab # 5543534564

ELECTROLYTES		UNITS	REFERENCE RANGE
Sodium	139	mmol/L	135–145
Potassium	3.4	mmol/L	3.5–5.2
Chloride	101	mmol/L	95–110
Calcium	2.9	mmol/L	2.1–2.6
Phosphate	0.6	mmol/L	0.75–1.5
Bicarbonate	19	mmol/L	22–32
Glucose (random)	4.2	mmol/L	3.5–5.4
Iron	11	μmol/L	11–30
Urea	3.4	mmol/L	2.1–8.5
Creatinine	68	μmol/L	40–120

Mr Rant had a midstream urine sample collected, and his ward urine test demonstrated large amounts of blood and protein. His urine is haematuric.

CRITICAL THINKING

1 Consider Mr Rant's presentation and observations. Why is he requiring so many doses of the opioid morphine? Explain.

2 Observe Mr Rant's history and pathology reports. Of the four types of kidney stone, what is the most likely type of stone that Mr Rant is experiencing? What data did you use to determine this? Explain.

3 Mr Rant is ordered an IVP. Intravenous contrast is injected while the X-rays are being taken. This contrast can be nephrotoxic. What parameters on the pathology report give an indication of appropriate renal function? Are these within the limits to risk an IVP? What other interventions could be instituted to reduce the risk of nephrotoxicity from the contrast?

4 What treatment options are available to Mr Rant? Compare and contrast all of the different management approaches that may be taken for renal calculi. Which method may be the best choice for Mr Rant?

5 What other cares are required for the management of Mr Rant's condition? (*Hint:* Think of interventions beyond that of dealing with the stone.)

BIBLIOGRAPHY

Australia and New Zealand Dialysis and Transplant Registry (ANZDATA Registry) (2021). Chapter 10: End stage kidney disease in Aboriginal and Torres Strait Islander Australians. *ANZDATA annual report.* Adelaide: ANZDATA Registry. https://www.anzdata.org.au/wp-content/uploads/2021/09/c10_indigenous_2020_ar_2021_v1.0_20220224_Final.pdf.

Australian Institute of Health and Welfare (AIHW) (2018). *Cancer in Aboriginal and Torres Strait Islander people of Australia*. Cat. No. CAN 109. Canberra: AIHW. https://www.aihw.gov.au/reports/cancer/cancer-in-indigenous-australians/contents/cancer-type/kidney-cancer-c64.

Australian Institute of Health and Welfare (AIHW) (2022a). Tier 1—Health status and outcomes. 1.10 Kidney disease. *Aboriginal and Torres Strait Islander High performance framework.* https://www.indigenoushpf.gov.au/measures/1-10-kidney-disease.

Australian Institute of Health and Welfare (AIHW) (2022b). *Cancer data in Australia.* https://www.aihw.gov.au/reports/cancer/cancer-data-in-australia/contents/cancer-summary-data-visualisation.

Bauldoff, G., Gubrud-Howe, P.M., Carno, M.-A., Levett-Jones, T., Hales, M., Berry, K., ... Stanley, D. (2020). *LeMone and Burke's medical–surgical nursing: critical thinking for person-centred care* (4th [Australian] edn). Sydney: Pearson Australia.

Best, O. & Fredericks, B. (2021). *Yatdjuligin: Aboriginal and Torres Strait Islander nursing and midwifery care* (3rd edn). Port Melbourne, VIC: Cambridge University Press.

Bullock, S. & Manias, E. (2022). *Fundamentals of pharmacology* (9th edn). Sydney: Pearson Australia.

Dave, C.N., Mehta, S., Meier, K. & Shetty. (2021). Nephrolithiasis. *Emedicine*. https://emedicine.medscape.com/article/437096-overview.

Dobruch, J. & Oszczudłowski, M. (2021). Bladder cancer: current challenges and future directions. *Medicina* 57(8):749. https://doi.org/10.3390/medicina57080749.

Gaudji, G.R., Bida, M., Conradie, M., Damane, B.P. & Bester, M.J. (2023). Renal papillary necrosis (RPN) in an African population: disease patterns, relevant pathways, and management. *Biomedicines* 11(1):93. https://doi.org/10.3390/biomedicines11010093.

Goldfarb, D.S. (2019). Empiric therapy for kidney stones. *Urolithiasis* 47:107–13. https://doi.org/10.1007/s00240-018-1090-6.

Likartsis, C., Printza, N. & Notopoulos, A. (2020). Radionuclide techniques for the detection of vesicoureteral reflux and their clinical significance. *Hellenic Journal of Nuclear Medicine* 23(2):180–87. https://pubmed.ncbi.nlm.nih.gov/32716409/.

Marieb, E.N. & Hoehn, K. (2019). *Human anatomy and physiology* (11th edn). San Francisco, CA: Pearson Benjamin Cummings.

Policastro, M.A., Sinert, R.H. & Guerrero, P. (2021). Urinary obstruction management in the ED. *Emedicine*. https://emedicine.medscape.com/article/778456-overview.

Polycystic kidney disease (2018). *Nature Review Disease Primers* 4:51. https://doi.org/10.1038/s41572-018-0053-0.

Sachdeva, K., Jana, B.R.P. & Curti, B. (2021). Renal cell carcinoma. *Emedicine*. http://emedicine.medscape.com/article/281340-overview.

Stumpers, S. & Thomson, N. (2013). *Review of kidney disease and urologic disorders among Indigenous people.* Australian Indigenous Health Reviews No. 11. Perth, WA: Australian Indigenous Health*Info*Net. http://www.healthinfonet.ecu.edu.au/chronic-conditions/kidney/reviews/kidney_review.

Thompson, D.B., Siref, L.E., Feloney, M.P., Hauke, R.J. & Agrawal, D.K. (2015). Immunological basis in the pathogenesis and treatment of bladder cancer. *Expert Reviews in Clinical Immunology* 11(2):265–79.

34 Acute kidney injury and chronic kidney disease

KEY TERMS

Acute kidney injury (AKI)
Anuria
Arteriovenous (AV) fistula
Azotaemia
Blood urea nitrogen (BUN)
Bruit
Chronic kidney disease (CKD)
Creatinine
End-stage kidney disease (ESKD)
Glomerular filtration rate (GFR)
Haemodialysis
Oliguria
Peritoneal dialysis
Pruritus
Uraemia
Urea

LEARNING OBJECTIVES

After completing this chapter, you should be able to:

1 Explain how altered nephron function leads to the clinical manifestations of kidney impairment.

2 Differentiate between the three types of acute kidney injury.

3 Associate appropriate management plans related to the specific cause of each type of acute kidney injury.

4 Contrast the clinical progression of acute kidney injury to that of chronic kidney disease.

5 Explain the important principles for managing someone with end-stage kidney disease.

WHAT YOU SHOULD KNOW BEFORE YOU START THIS CHAPTER

Can you identify the major parts of the renal system, and outline their functions?

Can you identify the structures of the kidney?

Can you identify the parts of the nephron, and describe their functions?

Can you describe the phases of inflammation?

Can you differentiate between acute and chronic inflammation?

Can you outline the stages of the healing process?

Can you describe the major concepts associated with neoplasia?

Can you identify the key electrolytes in body fluids?

Can you describe the effects associated with imbalances in the levels of these key electrolytes?

Introduction

LEARNING OBJECTIVE 1

Explain how altered nephron function leads to the clinical manifestations of kidney impairment.

The normal structure of the kidneys is outlined in the chapter 'Common inflammatory disorders of the kidneys and urinary tract'. The kidneys are very important in maintaining homeostasis of the blood. In filtering the blood, the kidneys keep fluid and electrolytes, particularly potassium ions (K^+) and hydrogen ions (H^+), as well as other solutes within their normal range. They also work to excrete nitrogenous wastes, such as **urea**, measured in the laboratory as **blood urea nitrogen (BUN)**, and **creatinine**, and eliminate potentially harmful chemicals and drugs. The kidneys play a key role in maintaining normal acid-base balance, and converting vitamin D into its active form, as well as regulating blood pressure and red blood cell production.

An important measure of kidney function is the **glomerular filtration rate (GFR)**, which represents the amount of blood filtered into the kidneys per minute. Although there are direct measures of GFR available clinically, the most common estimate (eGFR) is the monitoring of creatinine clearance.

When the kidneys are injured, the consequences can be clinically significant. The kidney has 'excess capacity', and a considerable proportion of nephrons (80–90%) may be lost before the overall ability of the kidney to process blood is in a clinical sense significantly reduced. However, if this stage is reached, kidney function will be greatly compromised. If a nephron does not regenerate, it will be replaced by fibrous (scar) tissue.

When the kidney function is impaired, the volume of urine will fall, and blood will retain water, electrolytes and nitrogenous wastes. Severe impairments can develop suddenly and rapidly in the course of an acute insult to the kidneys. This is called **acute kidney injury (AKI)**. Acute kidney injury can be sustained when events occur either internal or external to the kidney, but ultimately directly affect renal structure and function.

Long-term, progressive and permanent damage to the kidneys can result from renal and systemic disorders. This is known as **chronic kidney disease (CKD)**.

Acute kidney injury

AETIOLOGY AND PATHOPHYSIOLOGY

LEARNING OBJECTIVE 2

Differentiate between the three types of acute kidney injury.

LEARNING OBJECTIVE 3

Associate appropriate management plans related to the specific cause of each type of acute kidney injury.

Acute kidney injury (AKI) is classified as prerenal, intrarenal and postrenal (see Figure 34.1). *Prerenal* AKI develops upstream of the kidneys, and is usually due to disruptions in renal blood supply. *Intrarenal* AKI develops when the insult occurs within the kidney tissue. *Postrenal* AKI is due to obstructions of urine flow distal of the kidneys.

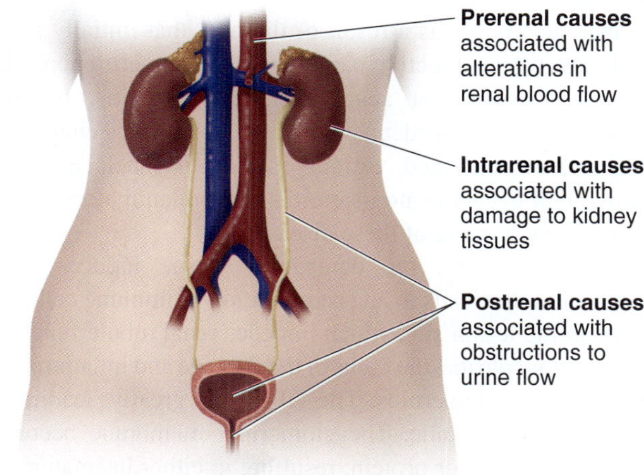

Figure 34.1

Types of causes of acute kidney injury

AKI is commonly associated with hospitalisation. Statistical data provided by the Australian Institute of Health and Welfare (AIHW) indicates that for the period 2017–18 the average crude rate of AKI hospitalisation for Australia was 911.6 cases per 100,000 people, with hospitalisation rates above the average for the Northern Territory (1,147 cases per 100,000 people), Queensland (1,043 per 100,000) and South Australia (949 per 100,000). The rates were much higher in males and for people aged 75 years and older.

Prerenal AKI

This type of AKI is most often caused by *renal ischaemia*, which leads to an abrupt decrease in the GFR. Blood flow to the kidneys can be reduced when there has been blood loss due to trauma or major surgery, loss of water from blood due to dehydration or burns, heart disease with reduced cardiac output (e.g. in myocardial infarction or congestive cardiac failure), hypotension in liver disease, notably with portal hypertension and ascites, severe hypotension in sepsis (i.e. septic shock) or in anaphylaxis, stenosis of renal arteries, or due to an occlusion of small blood vessels within the kidney. In the case of an occlusion of the small renal blood vessels, arterioles may be occluded as a result of atherosclerosis, and capillaries may become blocked by microemboli due to disseminated intravascular coagulation or by products of haemolysis due to haemolytic diseases or 'muscle meltdown' (referred to as *rhabdomyolysis*).

The most significant result of ischaemic damage to the kidney is *tubular necrosis*. Tubule cells are very sensitive to hypoxia, and may therefore die when their blood supply fails. Nevertheless, the tubule has a considerable ability to regenerate. This depends on the glomerulus, since all of the blood that supplies a nephron reaches it through the afferent arteriole of the glomerulus before travelling through its two sets of capillaries (glomerular and peritubular capillaries). Thus, the entire nephron may be restored if, and only if, the glomerulus has survived. So if the cause of ischaemia is rectified, and the person is supported by dialysis during the period of kidney injury, it can usually be expected that kidney function will return over several weeks.

Intrarenal AKI

AKI may also occur as a result of diseases that initially affect the kidney tissue directly; namely, acute glomerulonephritis, acute pyelonephritis or acute interstitial nephritis. Immune hypersensitivity disorders, infections, toxic chemicals, endogenous toxins and certain medicines (such as some antimicrobial agents or non-steroidal anti-inflammatory drugs) can cause one or more of these diseases.

In *pyelonephritis*, the damage to tissue induces acute inflammation that leads to an accumulation of immune cells and exudate in the lesion site, which impedes renal tubule function. In *glomerulonephritis*, the focus of the damage and inflammatory response is the glomerulus. The GFR falls greatly, leading to decreased urine volume. The glomerular membrane becomes permeable to blood or protein, resulting in either haematuria or proteinuria, respectively. These conditions are covered in more detail in the chapter 'Common inflammatory disorders of the kidneys and urinary tract'.

COVID-19 infection has been linked with the development of AKI. While the focus of COVID-19 pathophysiology is within the respiratory system, haematuria and proteinuria have been noted in those with COVID-19 within three weeks of the onset of the infection. It has been suggested that this may be due to a combination of both direct and indirect effects. The SARS-CoV-2 virus competes with the vasoconstrictor angiotensin II at the angiotensin-converting enzyme-2 (ACE-2) receptor to enter cells, leading to direct viral damage within the tubular interstitium. This leads to a down-regulation of expressed ACE-2 receptors, decreasing the protective anti-inflammatory effects mediated at this receptor while increasing the vasoconstrictor action. Indirect effects may involve altered immune responses, including cytokine storms and enhanced complement activity, as well as hypercoagulation and hypoxia.

Postrenal AKI

This type of AKI may be caused by *obstruction of the flow of urine* from both kidneys, at the level of the ureters, urinary bladder or urethra. Examples of obstructive conditions include kidney stones, prostate hypertrophy, cancerous tumours, blocked or improperly inserted urinary catheters (see the chapter 'Renal neoplasms and obstructions').

Formed urine accumulates proximal to the obstruction, leading to *urinary stasis*. As urine formation continues unabated, an increase in hydrostatic pressure develops within the renal pelvis and calyces, distending them. If this situation is allowed to persist, the compression of renal tissue will compromise vascular supply, leading to a permanent loss of nephrons.

CLINICAL MANIFESTATIONS

In AKI, renal function impairment is measured by a reduction in GFR and elevations in serum creatinine levels and BUN. The affected person can experience a sudden drop in urine volume (**oliguria**) that lasts for hours, in some cases even a complete cessation of urine production (**anuria**). Oliguria is defined clinically as a urine output of less than 0.5 mL/kg/hr.

In prerenal AKI, hypotension and possibly tachycardia may be observed. In the intrarenal or postrenal forms, hypertension may be demonstrated. Flank pain is a common clinical manifestation of kidney injury. Impairment of kidney function can lead to the retention of potassium. Oedema is associated with significant reductions in GFR. In glomerulonephritis, oedema can develop in response to the altered blood osmotic pressure associated with proteinuria.

CLINICAL DIAGNOSIS AND MANAGEMENT

Diagnosis

AKI is strongly associated with a sudden drop in GFR. Blood testing for full blood count, electrolyte levels and renal function, as well as urinalysis, are important in the clinical diagnosis of AKI. Such investigations may assist to distinguish between acute and chronic kidney disease, especially when previous results are available for comparison.

A useful and widely accepted classification system reflecting the degree of impairment in AKI is termed KDIGO (Kidney Disease Improving Global Outcomes). The parameters that are used to measure renal function are serum creatinine levels and urine output. (See Table 34.1 for more detail.)

An increase in blood cell casts may be observed in urinalysis, especially if the AKI is intrarenal. The presence of white blood cells or nitrites will suggest an infective component.

Imaging studies, such as ultrasound and computed tomography (CT), may be valuable to determine the type of

Table 34.1 The KDIGO classification system

Stage	Serum creatinine levels	Urine output
1	1.5–1.9 × baseline OR 26.5 μmol/L increase	< 0.5 mL/kg/hr for 6–12 hours
2	2–2.9 × baseline	0.5 mL/kg/hr for at least 12 hours
3	> 3 × baseline OR increase in serum creatinine > 353.6 μmol/L OR initiation of renal replacement therapy OR in patients < 18 years old decrease in eGFR to < 35 mL/min/1.73m^2	0.3 mL/kg/hr for at least 24 hours OR anuria for at least 12 hours

Source: Langham et al. (2014).

AKI; however, the use of contrast media should be used with caution, as it can significantly exacerbate the injury owing to its nephrotoxic effects. If a renovascular cause is considered, aortorenal angiography may be beneficial to assist with diagnosis.

Management

The focus of a management plan must be directed at the type of AKI. It is imperative that determination of the cause is accomplished as a priority. As the cause of the injury is removed and the repair processes can proceed, renal function recovers. Normal kidney function may take several months to be restored, and in some cases full recovery may not be possible.

It is important to note that the administration of treatment for one type of AKI may result in serious exacerbation if the cause is erroneously thought to be another type. For example, the administration of diuretics is appropriate for treating an intrarenal AKI, but if the type of injury was actually prerenal AKI, serious complications may occur, such as an exacerbation of profound circulating blood volume deficit. This kind of error may result in death.

Prerenal AKI Correction of fluid volume deficits or improvement of heart failure using inotropic agents is necessary. Care must be taken in prerenal AKI to isolate the exact cause, as it is imperative that hypovolaemia is corrected before inotropes are administered. However, volume should not be administered if there is heart failure caused by fluid overload. Reducing postoperative hypotension is a major step in preventing prerenal AKI.

Intrarenal AKI In acute pyelonephritis, acute glomerulonephritis or acute interstitial nephritis, manage the cause of the kidney damage, be it infection, chemical or immune in origin (see the chapter, 'Common inflammatory disorders of the kidneys and urinary tract'). Many therapeutic agents can cause intrarenal AKI. An evaluation of a person's medication regimen is important, and elimination of all possible nephrotoxic agents is crucial.

Postrenal AKI Managing the cause of the obstruction will assist with recovery. However, depending on the duration and severity of the renal damage, recovery may take a significant time after the obstruction has been removed.

Figure 34.2 explores the common clinical manifestations and management of AKI.

Chronic kidney disease

AETIOLOGY AND PATHOPHYSIOLOGY

LEARNING OBJECTIVE 4

Contrast the clinical progression of acute kidney injury to that of chronic kidney disease.

Chronic kidney disease (CKD) develops in long-standing diseases that affect the kidney, such as *chronic glomerular disease* and *chronic pyelonephritis* (see the chapter 'Common inflammatory disorders of the kidneys and urinary tract'). It is also associated with *diabetes mellitus* and *hypertension*, as well as *polycystic kidney disease* (see the chapter 'Neoplasms and obstructions'). CKD is considered an important risk factor for cardiovascular disease. Furthermore, CKD is considered a higher risk for more severe COVID-19 infection and increased mortality due to the relationship between ACE-2 receptors and the SARS-CoV-2 virus.

CKD is classified as kidney impairment persisting for more than three months, and is characterised by a progressive loss in nephron function, which is most readily measured in reductions of the GFR (see Table 34.2). The cause of the kidney impairment and the degree of albuminuria also contribute to the final classification.

The affected person's kidneys have a significant capacity to adapt to the loss of nephrons. Clinical manifestations of renal impairment—such as changes in nitrogenous wastes, fluid, sodium and potassium—are not apparent until renal function is reduced by 70–75% of normal. Progressive structural and functional changes in the glomerulus (i.e. *glomerular hypertension, hyperfiltration* and *glomerosclerosis*), *tubulointerstitial inflammation* and *renal fibrosis* are the hallmarks of the pathophysiological process.

Proteinuria is an important clinical sign in CKD. The proportion of the blood protein albumin in total protein is usually increased in proteinuria, and its measurement is considered an important laboratory test in CKD. It is usually measured as *albumin/creatinine ratio*, and normal excretion is higher in women (3.5 mg/mmol versus 2.5 mg/mmol for men). *Microalbuminuria* is defined as 3.5–35 mg/mmol for women and 2.5–25 mg/mmol for men, while *macroalbuminuria* is classified as values above the upper limit for microalbuminuria.

Statistical data from the AIHW indicates that 11% of people—equivalent to 1.7 million Australians aged 18 years or older—have biomedical signs of CKD in blood and urine tests. The prevalence of CKD increases with age, with around 44% of people aged 75 years and older being affected. In 2018 the AIHW reported that the contribution of CKD to the overall burden of disease in Australia is 1%. Burden of disease increases with age.

End-stage kidney disease (ESKD) is the end-point of CKD, and occurs when the GFR falls below 60 mL/min/1.73m^2 and

Table 34.2 Classification of chronic kidney disease

Stage	Description	GFR (mL/min/1.73m^2)
1	Kidney damage with normal or increased GFR	> 89
2	Kidney damage with mild reduced GFR	60–89
3A	Moderately reduced GFR	40–59
3B	Moderately reduced GFR	30–44
4	Severely reduced GFR	15–29
5	Kidney failure	< 15 or on dialysis

GFR = glomerular filtration rate.

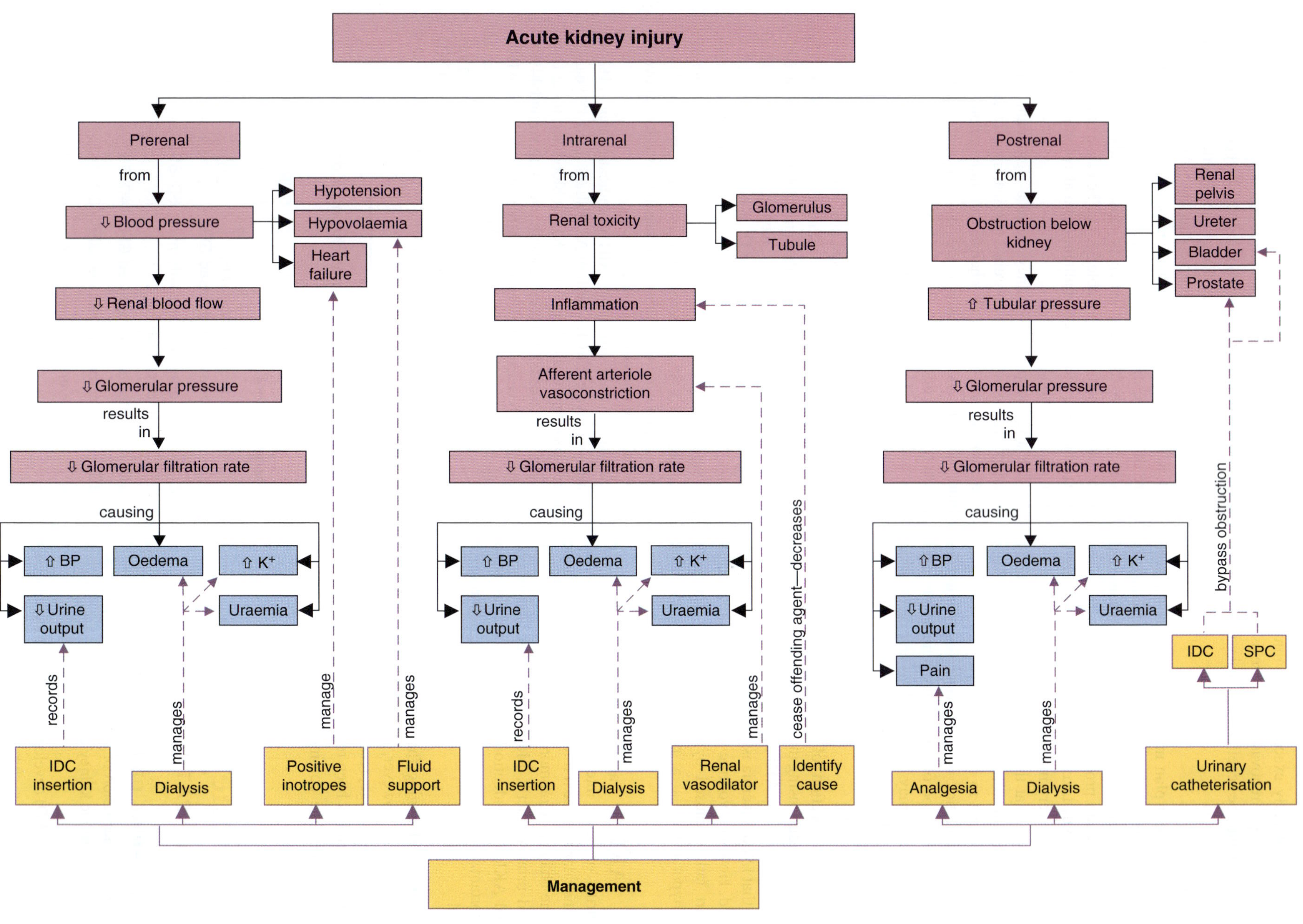

Figure 34.2

Clinical snapshot: Acute kidney injury

↓ = decreased; ↑ = increased; BP = blood pressure; IDC = indwelling catheter; K^+ = potassium ion; SPC = suprapubic catheter.

persists for greater than three months. It manifests clinically when more than 90% of nephron function is lost. Unlike the outlook in AKI, there is no possibility of recovery of nephron function. People with end-stage kidney disease require regular dialysis for the rest of their lives, or a kidney transplant.

The consequences of severe, sustained impairments of nephron function for the whole body are shown in Table 34.3.

In Australia, ESKD is an increasingly common cause of death, particularly in Indigenous communities (see 'Indigenous health fast facts and cultural connections') and in lower socioeconomic groups, where the incidence of diabetes and hypertension is high.

CLINICAL MANIFESTATIONS

In CKD, nitrogenous wastes accumulate in the blood, resulting in **azotaemia**. The affected person progresses to experience **uraemia** (i.e. the components of urine in the blood). Once adaptation to the loss of nephrons fails, early clinical manifestations associated with azotaemia and uraemia can include hypertension, nocturia, restless legs, haematuria, dyspnoea, lethargy, malaise, fatigue, anorexia and weight loss. As uraemia increases, the individual may experience **pruritus**, dry skin and an increased risk of infection from scratching the skin.

Those presenting with ESKD generally have multisystem effects. *Fluid and electrolyte imbalances* include elevated potassium levels (which can induce life-threatening cardiac dysrhythmias), sodium and water retention, leading to oedema, and the development of metabolic acidosis. *Cardiovascular dysfunction* includes hypertension, hyperlipidaemia (leading to atherosclerosis) and heart failure. *Haematological alterations* include anaemia and platelet dysfunction. *Gastrointestinal/endocrine problems* include nausea, vomiting, anorexia, diarrhoea, malnutrition and insulin resistance. *Skeletal problems* include vitamin D deficiency, hypocalcaemia, hyperphosphataemia, osteopathologies and an increased risk of fractures. *Neurological dysfunction* includes peripheral neuropathy and encephalopathy. *Other problems* include immune suppression, reduced blood sex hormone levels, decreased libido and infertility. *Renal system manifestations* include oliguria or anuria.

CLINICAL DIAGNOSIS AND MANAGEMENT

Diagnosis

Blood testing for full blood count, electrolyte levels, renal function and liver function is necessary to determine the progression of the disease, especially when previous results are available for comparison. Urinalysis will generally demonstrate

Table 34.3 The systemic consequences of severe sustained kidney impairment

Nephron function	Consequences for blood or other body fluids	Consequences for whole body
Removal of water from the blood	Blood will retain water. The volume of urine will fall: this is termed *anuria* if no urine is produced, or *oliguria* if it is produced in only small volumes.	High blood volume and high blood pressure may lead to congestive heart failure. Oedema may occur, as blood that is diluted by an excessive content of water will have low osmotic pressure. Both pulmonary and systemic oedema may develop.
Removal of nitrogenous wastes: urea, creatinine, uric acid	The blood concentrations of urea and creatinine increase: this is termed *azotaemia*.	Urea and creatinine at high concentrations are toxic to the nervous system, causing confusion, seizures and coma (encephalopathy). Effects on the digestive system: loss of appetite, nausea, vomiting; mucosal bleeding. Effects on the skin: high concentrations of nitrogenous wastes cause itching, and urea may crystallise from sweat as 'uraemic frost' on the skin. Characteristic smells appear on the breath and in sweat.
Removal of potassium	High blood potassium (*hyperkalaemia*).	The membrane potentials of excitable tissues, such as cardiac muscle and nerves, are disrupted. This may cause dysrhythmias or cardiac arrest.
Removal of hydrogen ions and production of bicarbonate ions	Metabolic acidosis.	Contributes to disruption of excitable tissue.
Kidney endocrine functions: erythropoietin secretion, activation of vitamin D	Low blood calcium (*hypocalcaemia*) from failure to activate vitamin D.	Anaemia from lack of erythropoietin. Hypocalcaemia leads to bone disease and contributes to the disruption of excitable tissue.
Complex mechanisms, not fully understood		Blood clotting disorders; may exacerbate mucosal bleeding in the digestive tract. Increased susceptibility to infection. Pericarditis.

haematuria, and maybe even white blood cells if there is an active infection. Proteinuria is also generally observed.

Imaging studies are not generally indicated unless they are to be used to determine other issues requiring management, or the development of new signs and symptoms, or the exacerbation of old ones. Ultrasound may assist with determining the size and morphology of the kidneys. Imaging studies requiring contrast should be avoided because of the nephrotoxic effects. Magnetic resonance imaging (MRI) may be beneficial to determine the various causes, including vascular conditions.

LEARNING OBJECTIVE 5

Explain the important principles for managing someone with end-stage kidney disease.

Management

End-stage kidney disease cannot be cured. Management plans focus on reducing the progression of the disease or, if possible, stopping the disease process altogether. In order to be systematic in representing all of the diverse effects associated with the management plan required for those with CKD, they have been organised below according to the interventions with which they are associated.

- *Systemic effects*: Control of hypertension is crucial. The higher the blood pressure, the more renal damage occurs. Antihypertensive agents are generally required. Anaemia may be managed with erythropoietin injections.
- *Electrolyte effects*: Hyperkalaemia can be managed with decreasing potassium within the diet. Hypocalcaemia and hyperphosphataemia (see the chapter 'Electrolyte imbalances') can be controlled with phosphate binders, such as aluminium hydroxide, magnesium hydroxide and simethicone (Mylanta).
- *Urine effects*: A low-protein diet may assist with reducing proteinuria. Multidisciplinary consultations should be undertaken, as a dietician can ensure that a low-protein diet contains sufficient protein to ensure that excessive catabolism does not occur, especially in someone who has previously been malnourished.
- *Metabolic effects*: Uraemia can be managed with dialysis, as can acidosis. Sodium bicarbonate may also assist with acidosis.
- *Gastrointestinal effects*: A person with anorexia, nausea and vomiting will quickly become malnourished. Management of uraemia is important. Antiemetic agents may also assist in the control of nausea and vomiting.
- *Other effects*: Pruritus is difficult to manage; however, EMLA cream and ultraviolet-B therapy may be of some value. 'Restless' legs are sometimes a by-product of the calcium and phosphate levels, and therefore phosphate binders may be of some benefit.

The mainstay of management for those with ESKD is dialysis. There are two types of dialysis: haemodialysis and peritoneal dialysis. **Haemodialysis** removes the blood, and filters it in a haemodialysis machine to remove waste products and excess fluid. It is required approximately three times a week, and each session will normally last between five and six hours. When long-term haemodialysis is required, an **arteriovenous (AV) fistula** is often surgically created by joining a vein and an artery (see Figure 34.3). This procedure results in vein engorgement and distension. Haemodialysis requires two venous access sites. An AV fistula makes the frequent, multiple cannulation easier, and provides a larger surface area of vein in which to obtain venous access. Assessment of the AV fistula is important to ensure that it remains patent. When auscultated, a patent AV fistula will make a 'whooshing' sound called a **bruit**, and will feel like a thrill (or vibration). The bruit and thrill are caused by the turbulence of the blood flow.

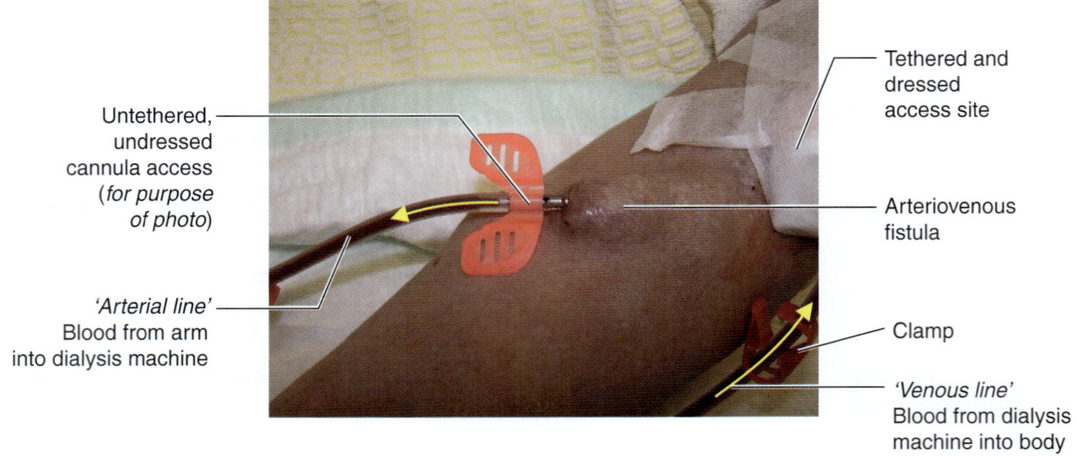

Figure 34.3

Arteriovenous (AV) fistula

A surgically created connection between a vein and an artery, resulting in vessel enlargement and an increased surface area, making it easier to cannulate for haemodialysis.

Source: Image adapted from Terrapanthera/Shutterstock.

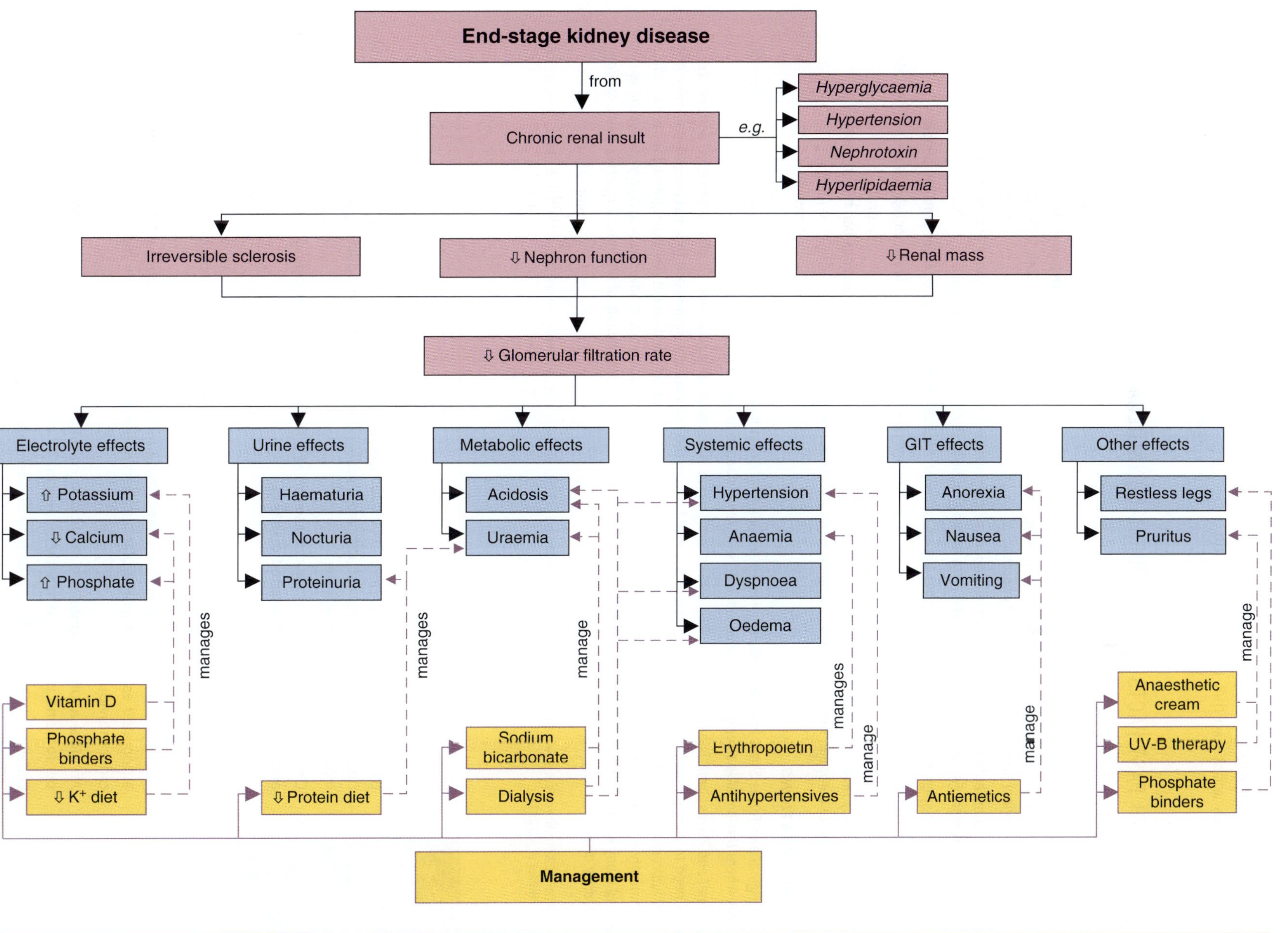

Figure 34.4

Clinical snapshot: End-stage kidney disease

↓ = decreased; ↑ = increased; GIT = gastrointestinal tract; K^+ = potassium ion; UV-B = ultraviolet B.

A significant proportion of people with ESKD choose haemodialysis; however, some opt for peritoneal dialysis. **Peritoneal dialysis** uses the body's own peritoneal membrane as the filter, following the insertion of a special catheter that remains in situ and provides access, so that the dialysate fluid can be introduced and removed. It requires less training and equipment, and is performed at home.

Figure 34.4 shows the common clinical manifestations and management of end-stage kidney disease.

INDIGENOUS HEALTH FAST FACTS AND CULTURAL CONSIDERATIONS

FAST FACTS

- *Chronic kidney disease (CKD) is 2.1 times more prevalent among Indigenous Australians compared with non-Indigenous Australians. The burden of disease accounted for by CKD is 7.8 times higher than for non-Indigenous Australians, and is the 10th leading cause of total disease burden for Aboriginal and Torres Strait Islander peoples.*
- *The burden of disease contributed by CKD is greater in Indigenous women, where it is the 8th leading cause of total burden at 3.1% of the total burden for women. For Indigenous men, it is the 13th leading cause at 2.3% of the total burden.*
- *Notification rates for end-stage kidney disease (ESKD), after age-adjustment, from 2016 to 2020 was 616 per 1 million people.*
- *In 2018 the incidence of ESKD was reported at 19% in European New Zealanders, 67% in Maori, 64% in Pacific Islands people, and 55% in Asian New Zealanders.*
- *Renal replacement therapy rates are much higher in Maori and Pacific Islands people (494 and 244 persons per million people, respectively) compared to European New Zealanders (72 persons per million people).*

CULTURAL CONSIDERATIONS

- *In many Aboriginal and Torres Strait Islander cultures, there is a traditional belief that the kidneys hold the spirit. By extension, people in communities where this belief is strong will consider a person with renal disease to have a sick spirit.*
- *Also, Aboriginal and Torres Strait Islander peoples often feel uncomfortable and displaced in hospitals. Those living in rural and remote areas would need to relocate and attend a dialysis clinic or hospital far from their community. In the past, this had a significant influence on achieving appropriate care, with dialysis schedules being up to 12–15 hours a week. In more recent times, programs that are locally run and community-controlled take dialysis and renal support services to remote communities, and have become highly successful in not only offsetting many of the effects of the people's chronic kidney disease, but also improving quality of life, reducing stress and enabling those with kidney disease to stay 'close to country'.*

Sources: Data from AIHW (2022a); Australia and New Zealand Dialysis and Transplant Registry (2019); Australian Indigenous Governance Institute (2016); Australian Indigenous HealthInfoNet (2022); Walker et al. (2019).

CHILDREN AND ADOLESCENTS

- Children with chronic kidney disease tend to experience growth failure as a product of poor metabolic waste management, increased phosphorus (antagonising calcium deposition in bones), reduced oxygen-carrying capacity from reduced erythropoietin production, and a potentially negative influence on growth hormone.
- Children with chronic kidney disease are at a higher risk of developing hypertension, atherosclerosis and cardiovascular-associated diseases.

OLDER ADULTS

- Thirty per cent of adults over 65 years of age have moderate, severe or end-stage kidney disease (stages 3–5).
- The serum creatinine level can overestimate renal function in an older adult. Therefore, the use of an automated estimated glomerular filtration rate may provide a better indication of renal function in older individuals.
- An older adult's prognosis in relation to chronic kidney disease is poorer than that of a younger person, and is also significantly influenced by cognitive, psychosocial and functional capacity.
- Older adults with end-stage kidney disease tend to be placed on peritoneal dialysis (instead of haemodialysis) more frequently than younger adults, even though there appears to be evidence that they would prefer haemodialysis when given the choice.

KEY CLINICAL ISSUES

- Acute kidney injury (AKI) has numerous causes. A knowledge of prerenal, intrarenal and postrenal causes and their specific management is important. Inappropriate management of AKI can be fatal. The management plan of prerenal failure can include interventions that are directly contraindicated for intrarenal or postrenal AKI.
- Many agents are nephrotoxic. A clinician should know the nephrotoxic risk of any agent they are administering, and implement methods to reduce toxicity, such as reducing the speed of administration or the concentration of the agent (where possible).
- End-stage kidney disease will occur when more than 90% of kidney function is lost. Therefore, close monitoring of fluid balance, skin turgor, urine output, blood pressure and oedema is critical to assist in the early identification of renal insufficiency.
- End-stage kidney disease affects almost every body system. Complex management plans are required to ensure that all of the issues caused are identified and addressed.

CHAPTER REVIEW

- When a significant proportion of *nephrons shut down*, the overall ability of the kidney to process blood is significantly reduced. If this stage is reached, end-stage kidney disease will occur. When the kidneys fail, the volume of urine will fall, and the blood will retain water, potassium, hydrogen and nitrogenous wastes, such as urea and creatinine.
- Renal impairment may develop rapidly in the course of acute disease within the kidney. This is called *acute kidney injury. Chronic kidney disease* may result from the long-term, progressive and permanent loss of nephrons.
- The types of acute kidney injury are classified according to three categories: prerenal, intrarenal and postrenal. *Prerenal acute kidney injury* occurs upstream of the kidneys, and is usually due to disruptions in renal blood supply. *Intrarenal acute kidney injury* develops within the kidney tissue. *Postrenal acute kidney injury* is due to obstructions of urine flow downstream of the kidneys.
- In chronic kidney disease, the person begins to experience the symptoms of *uraemia*, which become obvious when kidney function falls below 25–30% of normal. A sudden drop in urine volume (*oliguria*) also occurs, or even a complete cessation of urine production (*anuria*). Waste products accumulate in the body and cause a disruption in the major functions of all body systems.
- *End-stage kidney disease* is the result of long-term progressive and permanent loss of nephrons, and becomes evident when more than 90% of nephron function is lost. Unlike the outlook in acute kidney injury, there is no possibility of recovery of nephron function. People with end-stage kidney disease require regular *dialysis* for the rest of their lives, or a kidney *transplant*.

REVIEW QUESTIONS

1 Explain the major causes of:
   a acute kidney injury
   b chronic kidney disease
2 In each of the following conditions that induce acute kidney injury, indicate whether the cause is prerenal, renal or postrenal:
   a acute pyelonephritis
   b a blocked urinary catheter
   c severe haemorrhage
   d treatment with the aminoglycoside gentamicin
3 Outline the main aspects of the management of acute kidney injury.
4 What are the major indicators of chronic kidney disease?
5 What are the two most significant clinical manifestations of chronic kidney disease?
6 In end-stage kidney disease, explain:
   a the reason/s for fluid retention
   b the consequences of fluid retention
7 Explain how end-stage kidney disease affects the blood concentrations of electrolytes. What are the major pathological consequences of these disturbances of electrolyte concentrations?
8 Explain how end-stage kidney disease affects the blood concentrations of nitrogenous wastes. What are the major pathological consequences of these changes in blood concentrations of nitrogenous wastes?
9 What clinical manifestations are expected to develop in someone with poorly managed end-stage kidney disease?

HEALTH PROFESSIONAL CONNECTIONS

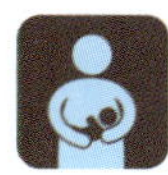

Midwives In rare certain circumstances, a pregnant woman may develop acute kidney injury. In the early stages of pregnancy, the cause is most commonly prerenal (from hyperemesis gravidarum) or intrarenal (from acute tubular necrosis). In late pregnancy, HELLP syndrome (haemolysis, elevated liver enzymes, low platelet count) or pre-eclampsia may cause acute kidney injury. Management of the cause is the primary focus, but early diagnosis is very important to ensure positive fetal outcomes. Fetal loss can be high in women who develop renal failure during the pregnancy. Although those with pre-existing kidney disease are considered a high-risk group, a prediction of clinical outcomes and the development of appropriate management plans may result in better outcomes. While women with chronic kidney disease experience a decrease in fertility, they may still become pregnant. Acceleration of the renal impairment may also occur during this time. Other complicating factors include the risk that the medications required for the management of the maternal disease affect the health and safety of the developing fetus. Healthcare team communication and planning are critical when caring for women with renal disease, whether they develop it during the pregnancy or it existed prior to the gravid state.

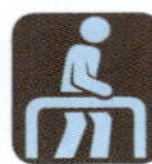

Physiotherapists Rehabilitation and physiotherapy for people with chronic kidney disease are becoming more common. Research has even found a benefit for those who exercise on bicycles during dialysis sessions. Early results demonstrate that the increased exercise improves overall health, and may even improve the benefits of the dialysis treatment. People with renal disease tend to be obese and have numerous comorbidities. Using exercise to modify waist:hip ratios can decrease insulin resistance and reduce the effects of type 2 diabetes. A reduction of diabetic nephropathy may be achieved through more work in this area.

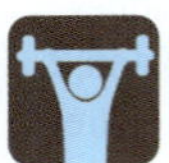

Exercise scientists When working with a person experiencing renal insufficiency, it is important for an exercise scientist to understand the impact of fluid and electrolyte management. Collaboration with other members of the healthcare team is imperative to ensure that exercise prescription and fluid and electrolyte management are not going to exacerbate the person's poor health. Exercise is important in reducing some effects of renal disease. However, individual consideration regarding the person's disease progression and their clinical health should always be a priority.

Nutritionists/Dieticians When working with someone experiencing chronic kidney disease, dietary modifications may depend on whether they are receiving haemodialysis (HD) or peritoneal dialysis (PD), and the frequency of their treatment. PD uses a carbohydrate-rich fluid to mediate the exchange; however, this causes a passive increase in calorie intake and may complicate weight loss and/or blood glucose control. Therefore, when undertaking PD, changes to the person's dietary carbohydrate intake may be necessary. Protein loss can occur in both HD and PD, and supplementation of high-quality dietary protein may be necessary to reduce the risk of catabolism. Sodium intake should be monitored and reduced as necessary, and is comparable for both types of dialysis. Phosphorus contained within food can be removed by both types of dialysis, but excess intake should be avoided. The addition of phosphate binders may be beneficial for hyperphosphataemia. The addition of vitamin D may be considered to improve calcium levels. Depending on the frequency of haemodialysis, potassium levels vary. Most frequently those on HD require potassium restriction, but, with PD, restriction is not generally necessary, as dialysis is occurring daily. Sometimes, potassium supplementation may be required.

CASE STUDY

Mr Stephen McEvoy is a 45-year-old man (UR number 623793) with end-stage kidney disease. He is anaemic, nauseous and complains of malaise. He has pitting oedema bilaterally on his lower extremities and his fingers and hands. He is complaining of pruritus and feels very depressed. He has a history of type 1 diabetes mellitus, hypertension and diabetic nephropathy. His urine is dark, frothy and scant. His observations were as follows:

Temperature	Heart rate	Respiration rate	Blood pressure	SpO_2
37.1°C	96	20	170/110	91% (on 4 L/min via NP*)

*NP = nasal prongs.

In the emergency department, Mr McEvoy has had blood taken for pathology testing. His ward urine test showed haematuria and a large amount of protein. His last glomerular filtration rate (GFR) was measured at 6.2 mL/min. Mr McEvoy is indicated for a strict fluid-balance chart and fluid restrictions. He requires daily weighing, as well as social worker and dietician consultation. He will also need to see the diabetic and renal educator during this admission. His pathology results were as follows:

HAEMATOLOGY

Patient location:	Ward 3	**UR:**	623793		
Consultant:	Smith	**NAME:**	McEvoy		
		Given name:	Stephen	**Sex:**	M
		DOB:	13/10/XX	**Age:**	45

Time collected 13:05
Date collected XX/XX
Year XXXX
Lab # 6776456

FULL BLOOD COUNT		UNITS	REFERENCE RANGE
Haemoglobin	92	g/L	115–160
White cell count	16.3	$\times 10^9$/L	4.0–11.0
Platelets	390	$\times 10^9$/L	140–400
Haematocrit	0.26		0.33–0.47
Red cell count	3.2	$\times 10^{12}$/L	3.80–5.20
Reticulocyte count	1.3	%	0.2–2.0%
MCV	79	fL	80–100
Neutrophils	13.1	$\times 10^9$/L	2.00–8.00
Lymphocytes	2.4	$\times 10^9$/L	1.00–4.00
Monocytes	0.46	$\times 10^9$/L	0.10–1.00
Eosinophils	0.38	$\times 10^9$/L	< 0.60
Basophils	0.09	$\times 10^9$/L	< 0.20
ESR	18	mm/h	< 12

BIOCHEMISTRY

Patient location:	Ward 3	**UR:**	623793		
Consultant:	Smith	**NAME:**	McEvoy		
		Given name:	Stephen	**Sex:**	M
		DOB:	13/10/XX	**Age:**	45

Time collected 13:05
Date collected XX/XX
Year XXXX
Lab # 75564566

ELECTROLYTES		UNITS	REFERENCE RANGE
Sodium	139	mmol/L	135–145
Potassium	5.6	mmol/L	3.5–5.2
Chloride	101	mmol/L	95–110
Calcium	1.87	mmol/L	2.1–2.6
Phosphate	2.1	mmol/L	0.75–1.5
Bicarbonate	16	mmol/L	22–32
Glucose (random)	17.4	mmol/L	3.5–7.7
Iron	6.2	μmol/L	11–30
Alkaline phosphatase (ALP)	412	u/L	30–120
Gamma-glutamyltranspeptidase (GGT)	8	u/L	10–45
Urea	32.6	mmol/L	2.1–8.5
Creatinine	832	μmol/L	40–120

CRITICAL THINKING

1. Explain the relationship between Mr McEvoy's observations (temperature, pulse, respirations and blood pressure) and the disease process affecting him.
2. What is the relationship between the haemoglobin, red cell count and his disease process? Would someone with acute (prerenal or postrenal) kidney injury experience this problem? Explain.
3. Consider Mr McEvoy's previous medical history. What contributed to his end-stage kidney disease? Explain the mechanism/s.
4. What type of management should be expected for Mr McEvoy? Create a table and list all of his signs and symptoms in the first column. In the second column, identify the management required to assist Mr McEvoy with each issue, and in the third column explain the mechanism of each intervention.
5. Mr McEvoy will require dialysis for the rest of his life unless he receives a kidney transplant. Compare and contrast the risks associated with both options (dialysis for life versus renal transplant).

BIBLIOGRAPHY

Ahmadian, E., Hosseiniyan Khatibi, S.M., Razi Soofiyani, S., Abediazar, S., Shoja, M.M., Ardalan, M. & Zununi Vahed, S. (2021). Covid-19 and kidney injury: pathophysiology and molecular mechanisms. *Reviews in Medical Virology* 31(3):e2176. https://doi.org/10.1002/rmv.2176.

Akchurin, O.M. (2019). Chronic kidney disease and dietary measures to improve outcomes. *Pediatric Clinics of North America* 66(1):247–67. https://doi.org/10.1016/j.pcl.2018.09.007.

Australia and New Zealand Dialysis and Transplant Registry (ANZDATA Registry) (2019). Chapter 9: End stage kidney disease in Aotearoa New Zealand. *42nd Report*. Adelaide, SA: ANZDATA Registry. http://www.anzdata.org.au.

Australia and New Zealand Dialysis and Transplant Registry (ANZDATA Registry) (2021). Chapter 10: Indigenous people and end stage kidney disease. *44th Report*. Adelaide, SA: ANZDATA Registry. https://www.anzdata.org.au/.

Australian Indigenous Governance Institute (AIGI) (2016). *Congratulations to the 2016 Indigenous Governance Awards winners*. Acton, ACT: AIGI. http://www.aigi.com.au.

Australian Indigenous Health*Info*Net (2022). *Overview of Aboriginal and Torres Strait Islander health status, 2021*. Perth, WA: Australian Indigenous Health*Info*Net. http://www.healthinfonet.ecu.edu.au.

Australian Institute of Health and Welfare (AIHW) (2021). *Geographical variation in disease: diabetes, cardiovascular disease and chronic kidney disease. Acute Kidney Injury Dashboard.* Canberra: AIHW. https://www.aihw.gov.au/reports/chronic-disease/geographical-variation-in-disease/contents/chronic-kidney-disease-dashboards/acute-kidney-injury-dashboards.

Australian Institute of Health and Welfare (AIHW) (2022a). *Australia's health, 2022: in brief*. Australia's Health series No. 18, Cat. No. AUS 241. Canberra: AIHW. https://www.aihw.gov.au/reports/australias-health/australias-health-2022-in-brief/summary..

Australian Institute of Health and Welfare (2022b). *Chronic kidney disease: Australian facts*. Canberra: AIHW. https://www.aihw.gov.au/reports/chronic-kidney-disease/chronic-kidney-disease/contents/summary.

Bauldoff, G., Gubrud-Howe, P.M., Carno, M.-A., Levett-Jones, T., Hales, M., Berry, K., … Stanley, D. (2020). *LeMone and Burke's medical–surgical nursing: critical thinking for person-centred care* (4th [Australian] edn). Sydney: Pearson Australia.

Beyerstedt, S., Casaro, E.B. & Rangel, É.B. (2021). COVID-19: angiotensin-converting enzyme 2 (ACE2) expression and tissue susceptibility to SARS-CoV-2 infection. *European Journal of Clinical Microbiology and Infectious Diseases* 40(5):905–19. https://doi.org/10.1007/s10096-020-04138-6.

Bullock, S. & Manias, E. (2022). *Fundamentals of pharmacology* (9th edn). Sydney: Pearson Australia.

Chen, T.K., Knicely, D.H. & Grams, M.E. (2019). Chronic kidney disease diagnosis and management: a review. *JAMA* 322(13):1294–304. https://doi.org/10.1001/jama.2019.14745.

Langham, R.G., Bellomo, R., D'Intini, V., Endre, Z., Hickey, B.B., McGuinness, S., … Gallagher, M.P. (2014). KHA-CARI guideline: KHA-CARI adaptation of the KDIGO Clinical Practice Guideline for Acute Kidney Injury. *Nephrology* 19(5):261–65. https://doi.org/10.1111/nep.12220.

Marieb, E.N. & Hoehn, K. (2019). *Human anatomy and physiology* (11th edn). San Francisco, CA: Pearson Benjamin Cummings.

Okusa, M. & Rosner, M. (2022). Overview of the management of acute kidney injury (AKI) in adults. *UpToDate*. https://www.uptodate.com/contents/overview-of-the-management-of-acute-kidney-injury-aki-in-adults.

Walker, R.J., Tafunai, M. & Krishnan, A. (2019). Chronic kidney disease in New Zealand Maori and Pacific people. *Seminars in Nephrology* 39(3):297–99. https://doi.org/10.1016/j.semnephrol.2019.03.001.

PART

8

Gastrointestinal pathophysiology

35 Gastro-oesophageal reflux disease and peptic ulcer disease

KEY TERMS

Barrett's oesophagus
Duodenal ulcers
Gastric (stomach) ulcers
Gastro-oesophageal reflux disease (GORD)
Helicobacter pylori infection
Non-steroidal anti-inflammatory drugs (NSAIDs)
Oesophagitis
Peptic ulcer disease (PUD)
Zollinger–Ellison syndrome

LEARNING OBJECTIVES

After completing this chapter, you should be able to:

1. Define the term 'gastro-oesophageal reflux disease (GORD)'.
2. Describe the pathophysiology and epidemiology of GORD.
3. Differentiate between GORD and non-erosive reflux disease (NERD).
4. Outline the complications of GORD.
5. Describe the clinical diagnosis and management of GORD.
6. Describe the pathophysiology and epidemiology of peptic ulcer disease (PUD).
7. Explain the role of *Helicobacter pylori* infection and chronic NSAID use in the development of PUD.
8. Outline the complications of PUD.
9. Describe the clinical diagnosis and management of PUD.

WHAT YOU SHOULD KNOW BEFORE YOU START THIS CHAPTER

Can you outline the processes involved in cellular adaptation and injury?

Can you describe the main stages of inflammation and healing?

What are the principles of the pathophysiology and management of infectious diseases?

Can you describe the normal stomach structures and functions?

Can you identify the cell types in the stomach, and outline their function?

Can you outline the structure and function of the duodenum and oesophagus?

Introduction

In this chapter, the focus of the discussion is on two conditions characterised by increased gastric juice production: *gastro-oesophageal reflux disease (GORD)* and *peptic ulcer disease (PUD)*. These are relatively common disorders in Western countries and can have serious complications.

Gastro-oesophageal reflux disease

LEARNING OBJECTIVE 1

Define the term 'gastro-oesophageal reflux disease (GORD)'.

LEARNING OBJECTIVE 2

Describe the pathophysiology and epidemiology of GORD.

LEARNING OBJECTIVE 3

Differentiate between GORD and non-erosive reflux disease (NERD).

LEARNING OBJECTIVE 4

Outline the complications of GORD.

The transient involuntary reflux of gastric juices into the oesophagus is considered a normal occurrence in healthy humans across the lifespan. However, if the symptoms of *reflux* (i.e. heartburn and regurgitation) impair the quality of life of a person or put them at risk of complications, it is regarded as a dysfunction and is termed **gastro-oesophageal reflux disease (GORD)**.

AETIOLOGY AND PATHOPHYSIOLOGY

A key factor in the development of GORD is believed to be *lower oesophageal sphincter (LOS) dysfunction*, such that there is a failure of tonic LOS contraction. The sphincter becomes incompetent, allowing the regurgitation of gastric contents into the oesophagus (see Figure 35.1). The exposure of the gastric contents to the oesophageal lining may lead to mucosal damage, but this is not always the case. GORD can occur in adults, children and young infants.

When reflux disease does not lead to mucosal damage, it is called *NERD (non-erosive reflux disease)*. NERD is the most common presentation of reflux disease. It is characterised as being endoscopy-negative with an abnormal oesophageal acid exposure time and positive symptomology.

The dysfunction of the LOS is due to altered neuromuscular control, which increases the potential for mucosal damage by prolonging the clearance of the contents from the oesophagus. Therefore, the *integrity of nervous system innervation* to this region of the gut and the *level of gastrointestinal motility* are also contributing factors in the development of this condition.

A number of other factors also play a role in GORD, including gastric and abdominal distension, delayed gastric emptying, increased secretion of pro-inflammatory mediators, increased intragastric and abdominal pressure, poor posture, obesity, reduced level of physical activity, and smoking. The increased rate of gastric reflux symptoms in relatives of those people with GORD suggests a genetic link. Associations with poor sleep quality and with alcohol consumption have been proposed, but on current evidence are not considered causal in GORD. Both nicotine and alcohol have been shown to relax the LOS.

Serious complications associated with GORD in adults include oesophagitis, Barrett's oesophagus, strictures, and oesophageal cancer. In **oesophagitis**, the oesophageal mucosa becomes inflamed. This can lead to discomfort and pain when

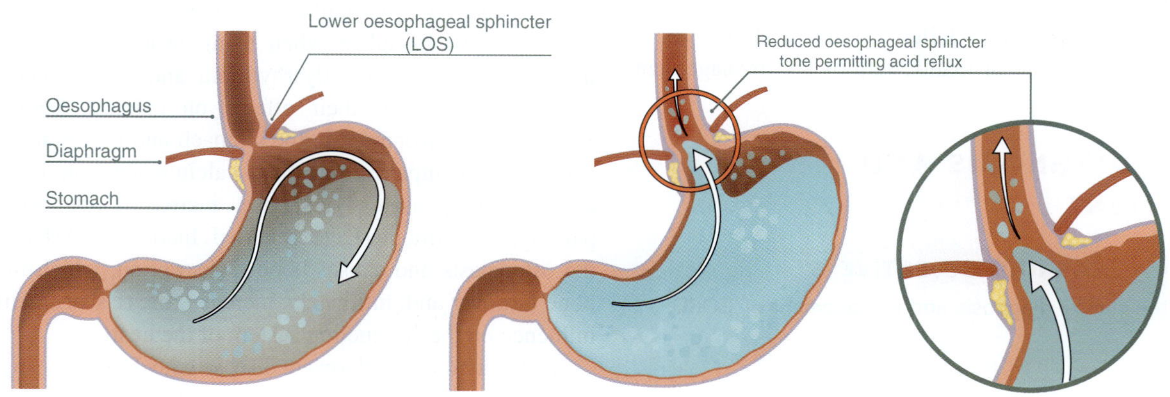

Figure 35.1

Oesophageal reflux

Competent lower oesophageal sphincter (LOS) prevents reflux, and a dysfunctional LOS contributes to gastro-oesophageal reflux disease (GORD).

Source: elenabsl/Shutterstock.

eating certain foods or drinking hot drinks. In severe cases, the oesophagus can become ulcerated and scarred. The region of scarred tissue can narrow the oesophageal lumen, referred to as *strictures*. Chronic episodes of oesophagitis may lead to the pre-cancerous state known as **Barrett's oesophagus**, which is characterised by metaplasia of the oesophageal lining. Barrett's oesophagus can lead to *oesophageal adenocarcinoma* developing. In infants, GORD can induce respiratory complications. These complications are not common, but gastric contents can be aspirated into the lungs, leading to pneumonia or interstitial lung disease.

EPIDEMIOLOGY

The prevalence of GORD in Western countries is estimated at 4–30% in adults, 3.5% in adolescents aged between 10 and 17 years, 1.8% in children aged 3–9 years, and 5–9% in infants. The prevalence of GORD symptoms in Australia is estimated in the 10–14.9% range, while in New Zealand it is slightly higher, in the 15–19.9% range. Australian and New Zealand data indicate a relatively high and increasing general prevalence rate of diagnosed GORD, at about 20%. More than 70,000 people are admitted to Australian hospitals each year with GORD as the principal diagnosis. Statistics from the Australian Institute of Health and Welfare indicate that the rate increases with age: 3.4% in people aged under 25 years, rising to 34.3% in those aged over 65 years. No differences were detected in the rates for males and females.

CLINICAL MANIFESTATIONS

The common clinical manifestations of GORD in adults include heartburn, regurgitation, epigastric or chest pain, nausea, flatulence, chronic cough, hoarseness and earache.

In infants, GORD can be difficult to distinguish from normal physiological gastro-oesophageal reflux characterised by regurgitation. Infants with GORD commonly show regurgitation, accompanied by occasional projectile vomiting, feeding aversion, anorexia, abdominal pain and failure to thrive. Figure 35.2 explores the common clinical manifestations and management of GORD.

CLINICAL DIAGNOSIS AND MANAGEMENT

LEARNING OBJECTIVE 5

Describe the clinical diagnosis and management of GORD.

Diagnosis

Gastroscopy (oesophagogastroduodenoscopy) will enable visualisation of the mucosa, quantify and monitor the severity of oesophagitis, and confirm or exclude the presence of other diseases. If gastroscopy is contraindicated or otherwise not desired, another method used is the 24-hour pH level measurement, permitting correlation of symptoms with reflux episodes. Histological examination and pH monitoring are important in differentiating GORD and NERD. The response to the administration of proton pump inhibitors can assist in the diagnosis of GORD.

Capsule endoscopy has revolutionised the previously invasive surgical diagnostic procedure, through the use of a special pill-shaped device that can be swallowed (see Figure 35.3). The capsule contains a camera and a light. Once it is swallowed, it transmits data to a recording device strapped to the waist of the person being investigated. Capsule endoscopy enables visualisation of the oesophagus, stomach, intestines and rectum as it passes through the gastrointestinal tract.

Oesophageal manometry, which involves the insertion of a tube to measure the function of the oesophagus and the lower oesophageal sphincter, may be beneficial to exclude other diseases.

Management

Lifestyle modifications are important in the management of GORD. As obesity is a risk factor for GORD, prevention through appropriate weight management is a most desirable approach. For those who have developed GORD, other lifestyle modifications include those that decrease the volume of gastric acid secretion. Some methods involve avoiding large meals and waiting several hours before lying down after a meal. Avoidance of acidic food may be beneficial, but current research is generating a review of this concept. Elevating the head of the bed (15–20 cm) or sleeping on a couple of pillows will also reduce the discomfort from GORD.

For mild intermittent symptoms, initial treatment with antacids may be beneficial. If adequate relief cannot be attained using antacids, then a drug group that reduces gastric acid secretion is recommended. Proton pump inhibitors (such as esomeprazole or pantoprazole) are efficacious drugs, and are the first choice in the control of GORD and oesophagitis. Histamine H_2-receptor antagonists (such as famotidine or nizatidine) can be effective, especially for those allergic to the proton pump inhibitors. H_2-receptor antagonists can bring about immediate relief of heartburn, particularly at night.

Care must be taken when using proton pump inhibitors in people with cardiac dysrhythmia and in postmenopausal women, because of their effects on calcium homeostasis. A less acid environment in the stomach and the small intestine can result in impaired intestinal calcium absorption, and can cause a compensatory response, increasing the amount of parathyroid hormone (PTH) released. Increased PTH stimulates the osteoclasts and causes bone reabsorption, which increases bone turnover and, ultimately, increases the risk of fracture and influence on the conduction system of the heart.

For individuals with severe disease who develop oesophageal strictures or Barrett's oesophagus, fundoplication surgery may be necessary. The goal of this surgical procedure is to increase the strength of the sphincter so as to reduce reflux. This can be achieved by wrapping a portion of the stomach around the base of the oesophagus and suturing it in place. When the stomach contracts, the wrapped section will also contract and this can assist sphincter strength, thereby reducing reflux.

The surgical approach is better than the proton pump inhibitors in inducing healing in this condition and in

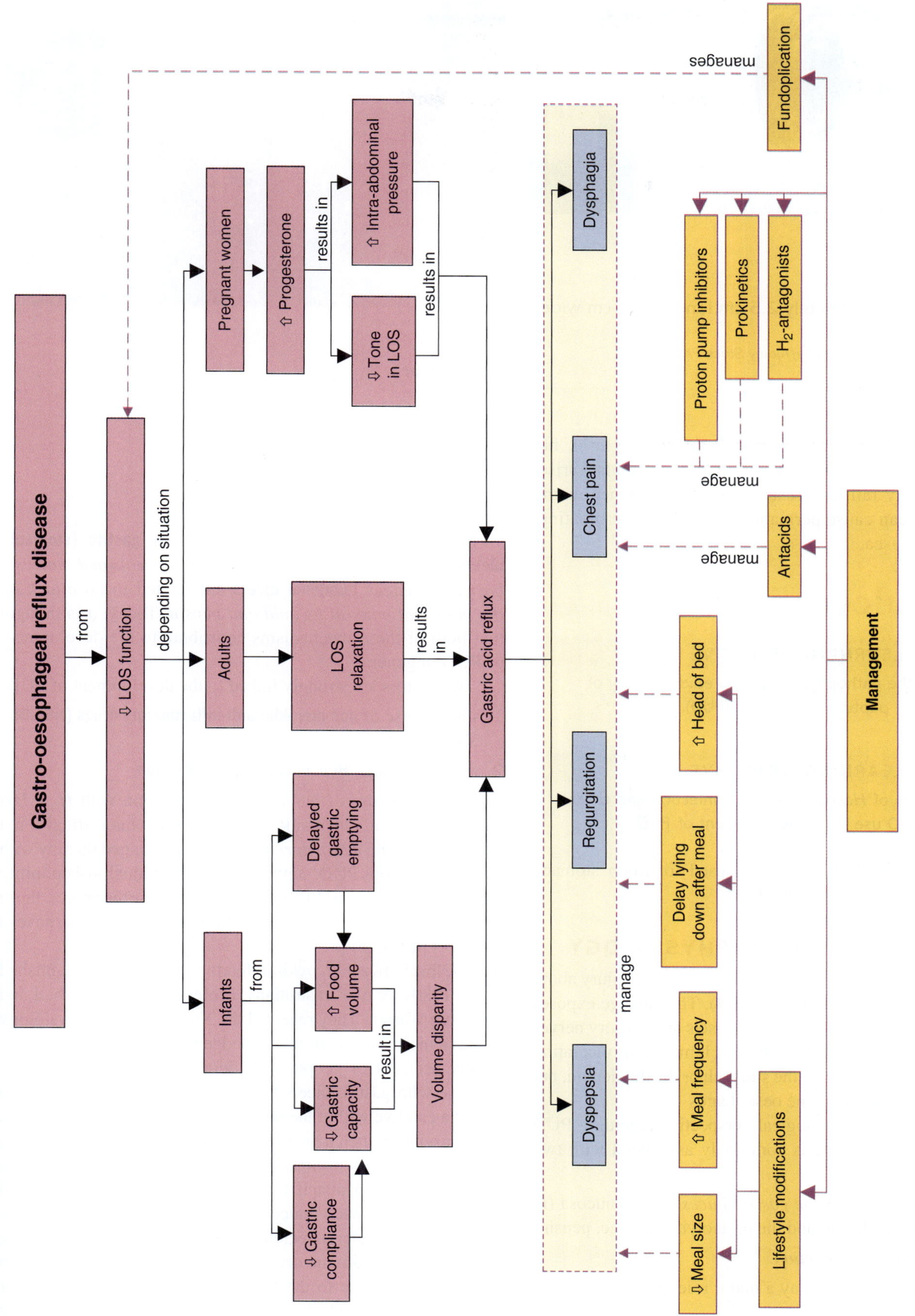

Figure 35.2

Clinical snapshot: Gastro-oesophageal reflux disease

↓ = decreased; ↑ = increased; H_2 = histamine-2 receptor; LOS = lower oesophageal sphincter.

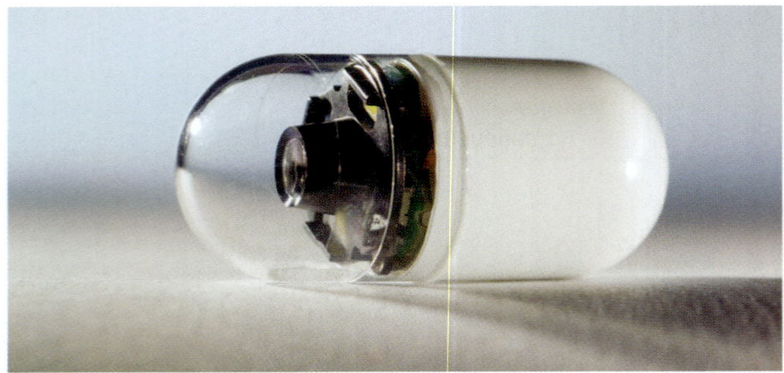

Figure 35.3

Capsule endoscopy

This capsule is approximately 2.5 cm long and 1 cm wide.

Source: David Bleeker Photography/Alamy Stock Photo.

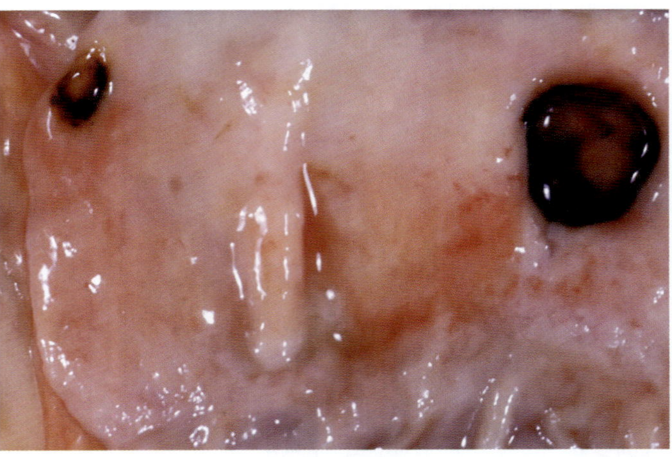

Figure 35.4

Peptic ulcer

Source: Jose Luis Calvo/Shutterstock.

reducing the number of relapses over the longer term, but is more costly. Post-surgical complications can also arise: the treatment may fail, can result in dysphagia when eating solid food, and can cause permanent side-effects in bloating, diarrhoea and nausea.

Peptic ulcer disease

LEARNING OBJECTIVE 6

Describe the pathophysiology and epidemiology of peptic ulcer disease (PUD).

LEARNING OBJECTIVE 7

Explain the role of *Helicobacter pylori* infection and chronic NSAID use in the development of PUD.

Peptic ulcer disease (PUD) is a term used to group stomach (gastric) and duodenal ulcers together.

AETIOLOGY AND PATHOPHYSIOLOGY

A *peptic ulcer* is characterised by a mucosal erosive injury about 5 mm or more in depth (see Figure 35.4). The damage exposes the underlying smooth muscle, blood vessels and sensory nerves to the gastrointestinal contents within the lumen. This ulceration tends to commonly develop in the stomach or the duodenum, but less commonly can occur in the oesophagus.

The current pathophysiological perspective regarding PUD is that the mucosal damage is commonly associated with two primary mechanisms:

1 an *aggressive action of the gastric juices* on the mucosa (in particular, stomach acid and the proteolytic enzyme, pepsin)
2 *weakened mucosal protection*.

Inflammatory processes play a major role in triggering both of these mechanisms.

Traditionally, the view has been that **gastric (stomach) ulcers** are primarily associated with a *weakened mucosal barrier*, whereas **duodenal ulcers** are related to an *attack on the intestinal mucosa by acid and pepsin*. Today, it is thought that both of these mechanisms contribute to the development of PUD in general.

Two factors are strongly linked to the development of PUD:

1 chronic use of **non-steroidal anti-inflammatory drugs (NSAIDs)**, such as aspirin
2 gastrointestinal ***Helicobacter pylori* infection**.

Indeed, the use of NSAIDs in combination with *H. pylori* infection have a synergistic effect in PUD. Interestingly, not every person with a *H. pylori* infection or prolonged therapy with NSAIDs develops PUD, suggesting that individual susceptibility also plays a part in PUD development. Furthermore, those people who have prolonged NSAID therapy tend to have a *H. pylori* infection.

The link between *H. pylori* infection and PUD was established in the 1980s by two Australians, Professor Barry Marshall and Dr Robin Warren. They received the Nobel Prize for Physiology or Medicine in 2005 as an acknowledgement of their achievement. Ninety per cent of people with duodenal ulcers and 70–90% of those with gastric ulcers have *H. pylori* infection. *H. pylori* bacteria can live within the hostile environment of the stomach. They survive in such a hostile environment by secreting *urease*, making the local environment more alkaline. They secrete factors to enable them to attach to the gastric epithelium. Infection damages the stomach mucosa by inducing an inflammatory response. The bacteria secrete a range of *cytokines*, including interleukins and tumour necrosis factor. Gastric acid secretion changes in response to the inflammatory mediators. Hypo- or hyperchlorhydria can develop. An increased release of the gastrointestinal hormone gastrin may occur. *H. pylori* infection also decreases the release of somatostatin, a potent inhibitor of gastric acid secretion. *H. pylori* breaks down mucosal defences by reducing the thickness of the mucosal protective layer and reducing mucosal blood flow. *H. pylori* infection is also linked to chronic gastritis, gastric adenocarcinoma and a type of lymphoma associated with stomach lymphoid tissue.

NSAIDs act to *reduce prostaglandin (PG) synthesis* from cell membrane phospholipids through the *inhibition of the enzyme cyclo-oxygenase (COX)*. Prostaglandins have a constitutive homeostatic role in the gastrointestinal tract (see Figure 35.5), considered to be more associated with the activity of the COX-1 isoenzyme. These prostaglandins, particularly PGE_2, are involved in the maintenance of the mucosal barrier, and also reduce gastric acid secretion. Regular doses of NSAIDs high enough to produce effective anti-inflammatory effects can significantly reduce gastrointestinal PG availability, predisposing the person receiving treatment to PUD. The risk of gastrointestinal toxicity is considered lowest for the habitual administration of the NSAIDs celecoxib and ibuprofen, and highest for piroxicam and ketorolac. The prevalence rate of PUD in chronic NSAID users is about 25%. The risk of PUD is even increased in those people taking regular low-dose aspirin therapy to reduce the chance of thrombotic episodes that underlie myocardial infarction or stroke. It is also more likely that the complications of PUD (see later in this section) will develop in people taking NSAIDs.

Around 20% of PUD is not associated with *H. pylori* infection or NSAID therapy, and is known as *idiopathic PUD*. Factors implicated in this type of PUD include chronic stress, cigarette smoking, age, oral bisphosphonates (used in osteoporosis therapy), glucocorticoid treatment and potassium chloride therapy. Conditions that increase gastric acid/pepsin secretion, such as **Zollinger-Ellison syndrome** (a gastrin-secreting tumour), cholinergic hypersensitivity or gastric cell hyperplasia, are cofactors in the development of idiopathic PUD. Idiopathic PUD is characterised by slower healing, higher recurrence rates and higher mortality compared to the more common aetiologies.

LEARNING OBJECTIVE 8

Outline the complications of PUD.

The most serious complications of PUD are *gastrointestinal bleeding perforation* and *gastric outlet obstruction*. Perforation is associated with continued erosion at the ulcer site until it creates a hole in the gastrointestinal tract wall. The gastrointestinal contents are then able to leak out into the peritoneal cavity, leading to peritonitis. A perforation usually manifests as sudden intense pain in the upper abdomen. Erosive injury damages the blood vessels of the gastrointestinal wall, leading to bleeding into the lumen. These complications can remain asymptomatic until they are well advanced. NSAID use *inhibits thromboxane* A_2, which is involved in platelet aggregation and coagulation. The risk of bleeding is therefore enhanced.

EPIDEMIOLOGY

The estimated lifetime prevalence of PUD is 5–10%, affecting around 4 million people globally. The prevalence of this condition has declined over the past 100 years. Identification and enhanced management of *H. pylori* infection and the use of potent drugs are believed to be the major contributors to this decline. Based on the available National Health Survey statistics, 2.7% of Australians self-reported as having PUD.

There are concerns that antibacterial drug resistance with respect to *H. pylori* eradication is a threat to the control of this condition. In 2017, the WHO listed *H. pylori* in the high-priority category of antimicrobial-resistant bacteria that pose the greatest risk to human health.

CLINICAL MANIFESTATIONS

Common manifestations of PUD include pain, nausea, vomiting, bloating, weight loss and loss of appetite. The pain is epigastric, usually described as burning, and occurs when the stomach is empty, particularly before meals and overnight.

There are some differences observed in the common clinical manifestations for duodenal ulcers and gastric ulcers. In duodenal ulcers an affected person can feel hungry and experience nocturnal abdominal pain, while in gastric ulcers a person tends to experience post-prandial abdominal pain, nausea, vomiting and weight loss.

The manifestation of gastrointestinal bleeding will vary according to the volume lost and the time interval. Anaemia

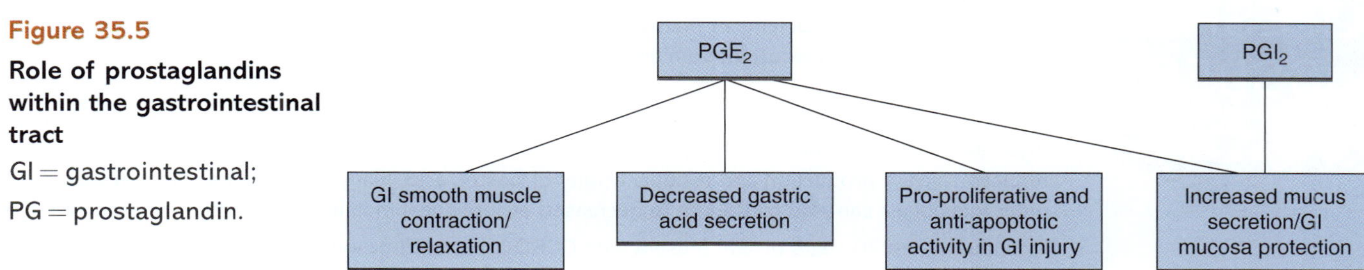

Figure 35.5

Role of prostaglandins within the gastrointestinal tract

GI = gastrointestinal; PG = prostaglandin.

may develop, with the affected person being pale, tired, feeling dizzy or fainting. If the bleeding involves a greater blood loss, the person may experience emesis, where the vomitus is blood-stained (haematemesis). Blood can also be present in the faeces, producing dark red or black tarry stools. Peritonitis will manifest as sudden and severe abdominal pain. Figure 35.6 explores the common clinical manifestations and management of peptic ulcer disease.

CLINICAL DIAGNOSIS AND MANAGEMENT

LEARNING OBJECTIVE 9

Describe the clinical diagnosis and management of PUD.

Diagnosis

Measurement of haematology and biochemistry values will not confirm a diagnosis of PUD. However, it will assist with determining whether there are any associated issues that need managing. Anaemia may be experienced if chronic or severe PUD has developed. Anaemia may also be one of the presenting symptoms in children.

A critical investigation in the diagnosis of PUD is detecting the presence of *H. pylori*. The gold standard diagnostic test is an endoscopy which is undertaken to visualise gastric mucosa, take biopsies, exclude malignancies and perform a rapid urease test to help with the detection of *H. pylori*. Breath, blood, stool tests and histological examination may be used to determine its presence.

Management

Cessation of NSAIDs and smoking is important in the management of PUD. The other important approach is aimed at eliminating the infection. This promotes healing, and prevents relapse and recurrent bleeding.

Drugs that reduce acid secretion (proton pump inhibitors and histamine H_2-receptor antagonists) are important in management; however, any signs of side-effects and drug interactions should be monitored closely. Drugs that coat or protect the ulcerated mucosal layer, such as sucralfate, bismuth or the prostaglandin E_2 analogue misoprostol, are useful. Misoprostol preserves the constitutive effects of this prostaglandin on the stomach where NSAID therapy is required.

In Australia, triple therapy of a proton pump inhibitor and two antimicrobials (generally clarithromycin plus either amoxicillin or metronidazole) are necessary to eliminate PUD caused by *H. pylori*. Some strains of *H. pylori* are becoming resistant to metronidazole, so monitoring and assessment of efficacy is needed.

INDIGENOUS HEALTH FAST FACTS AND CULTURAL CONNECTIONS

FAST FACTS

- *The prevalence of* Helicobacter pylori *has been shown to be higher in Indigenous populations compared to non-Indigenous ones. A Western Australian study found the prevalence in a remote Aboriginal community to be 76% compared to the pooled prevalence of 24.6%.*
- H. pylori *infection is more likely in Māori, Pacific Islands and Asian communities compared to European New Zealanders. The prevalence of* H. pylori *infection is 34.9% in Māori and 29.6% in Pacific Islands people, compared to 7.7% in European New Zealanders.*

CULTURAL CONSIDERATIONS

- *Aboriginal and Torres Strait Islander peoples have long used bush foods for medicinal purposes. For example, the Emu bush 'Yadhandah' (*Eremophila longifolia*), which is common in Western Australia, has been used to treat stomach ulcers. More recently, research has found other Australian flora to have gastroprotective or mucoprotective properties against* Helicobacter pylori. *A perennial creeping herb,* Bacopa monnieri, *and other flora such as* Solanum lyratum, *and even camomile oil, are being investigated for their effects on the bacteria that cause peptic ulcers.*

Sources: Data from Best Practice Advocacy Centre New Zealand (BPAC NZ) (2022); Congedi et al. (2022); Williams (2013); Wise et al. (2019).

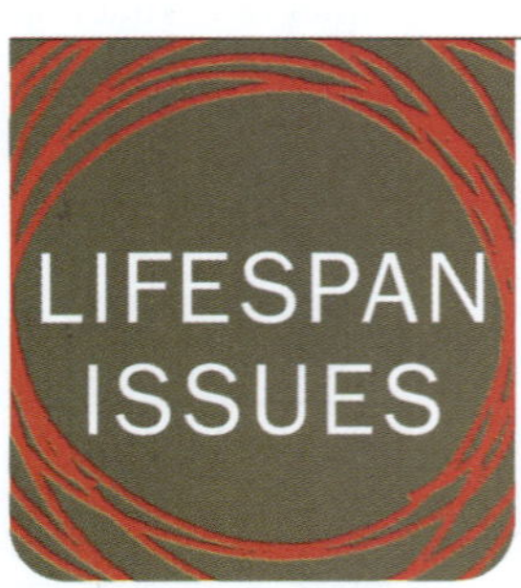

CHILDREN AND ADOLESCENTS

- Gastro-oesophageal reflux disease (GORD) in children may be caused by an immature lower oesophageal sphincter, increased abdominal pressure, dysfunctional motility, prematurity, neurodevelopmental problems or hiatus hernias. Children with a failure to thrive, abdominal pain, feeding difficulties and recurrent vomiting should be investigated for GORD.

OLDER ADULTS

- Age-related changes contributing to the development of GORD include reduced oesophageal motility, reduced salivary production and residual acidity of gastric acid. Many medications commonly used by older individuals can also contribute to decreased oesophageal motility and result in increased reflux.
- Individuals over 70 years of age present with GORD-associated oesophagitis three times more frequently than younger adults.

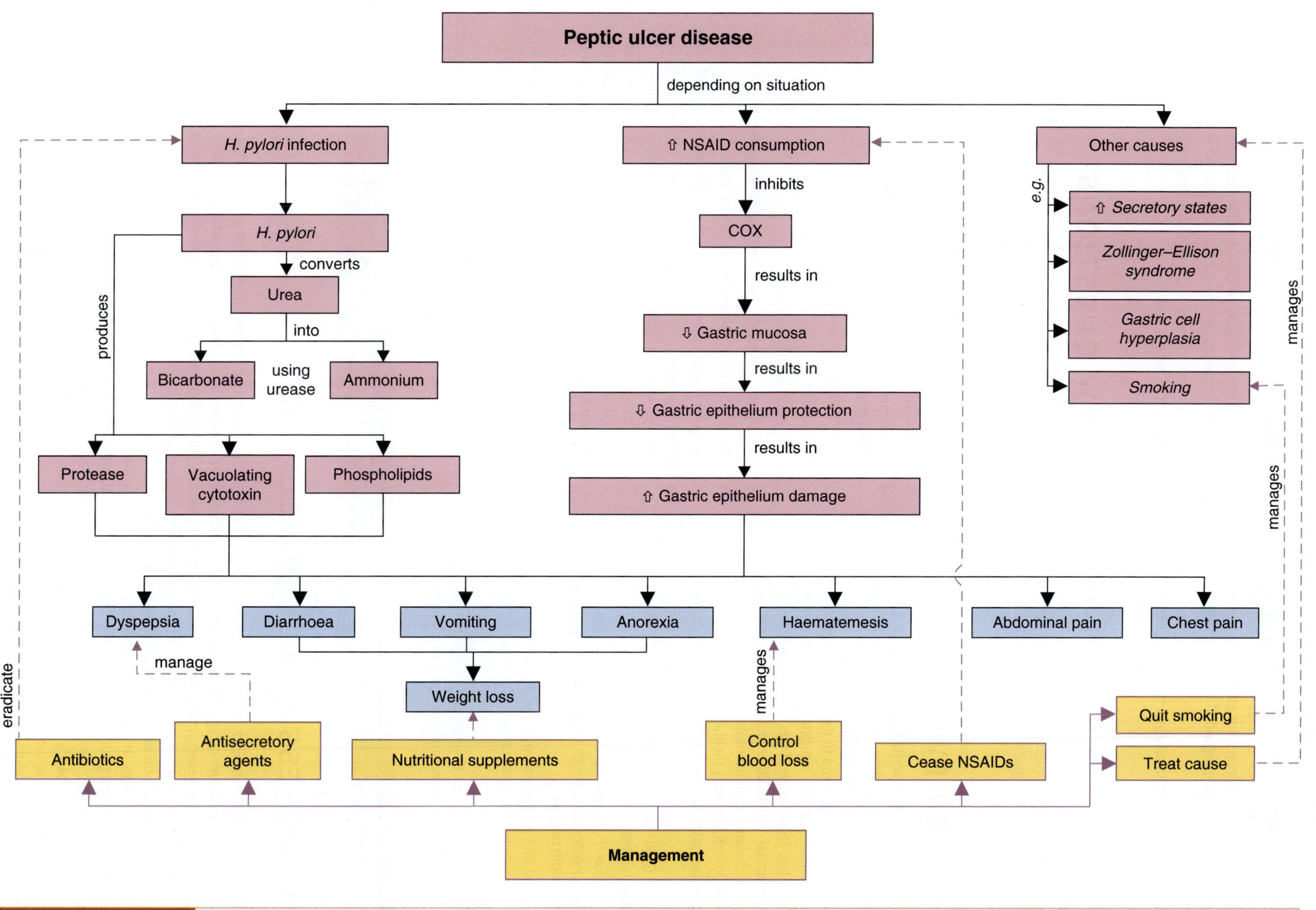

Figure 35.6

Clinical snapshot: Peptic ulcer disease

↓ = decreased; ↑ = increased; COX = cyclo-oxygenase; H. = Helicobacter; NSAIDs = non-steroidal anti-inflammatory drugs.

KEY CLINICAL ISSUES

- Management plans for individuals with GORD should include education regarding methods to reduce reflux, such as reducing meal size, remaining upright for at least half an hour after eating, avoiding particularly acidic food, and sleeping with the head of the bed slightly elevated.
- Overuse of non-steroidal anti-inflammatory drugs (NSAIDs) can result in peptic ulcer disease.
- Lifestyle modifications, such as smoking cessation and reducing chronic stress, may assist in reducing the incidence of peptic ulcer disease.
- Individuals presenting with haematemesis, gastrointestinal bleeding and/or anaemia should be investigated for peptic ulcer disease.

CHAPTER REVIEW

- *Gastro-oesophageal reflux disease (GORD)* occurs when the symptoms of reflex, heartburn and regurgitation impair quality of life and put the affected person at risk of complications.
- The development of GORD is linked to *dysfunction of the lower oesophageal sphincter*, allowing regurgitation of gastric contents into the oesophagus. Dysfunction of this sphincter is associated with altered neuromuscular control. Other factors playing a role in GORD include gastric and abdominal distension, delayed gastric emptying, the presence of pro-inflammatory mediators, increased intragastric and abdominal pressure, poor posture, obesity, low level of activity, smoking and genetics.
- Complications of GORD include *oesophagitis, Barrett's oesophagus* and *oesophageal cancer*.
- *Peptic ulcer disease (PUD)* represents the grouping of gastric and duodenal ulcers. Peptic ulcers are characterised by a *mucosal erosive injury of 5 mm depth* or more.
- PUD is associated with an *aggressive action of gastric juices* on the mucosa and a *weakened mucosal barrier*. Inflammation plays a major role in these processes.
- Two factors strongly linked to the development of PUD are the *chronic use of non-steroidal anti-inflammatory drugs* and gastrointestinal infection by the bacterium *Helicobacter pylori*. There is also *idiopathic PUD*, which accounts for 20% of cases. Factors contributing to idiopathic PUD include chronic stress, smoking, age and treatments with certain drugs. Conditions that increase gastric juice secretion—such as Zollinger-Ellison syndrome, cholinergic hypersensitivity or gastric cell hyperplasia—are considered cofactors in idiopathic PUD.
- *Serious complications* of PUD are gastrointestinal bleeding and perforation of the gut wall.

REVIEW QUESTIONS

1. Define the following acronyms:
   a. PUD
   b. NERD
   c. GORD
2. How does the prevalence of GORD vary across the lifespan?
3. Briefly describe the pathophysiology of GORD.
4. Outline how each of the following factors contributes to the development of GORD:
   a. increased intragastric pressure
   b. smoking
   c. delayed gastric emptying
5. Differentiate between Barrett's oesophagus and oesophageal cancer.
6. What are the two mechanisms associated with PUD?
7. How does *H. pylori* infection contribute to the development of PUD?
8. Mr Tom Yee is 56 years old. He has rheumatoid arthritis, which is being managed with an NSAID. He has been experiencing moderate epigastric pain over the past month. The pain tends to occur in bed overnight and before lunch. He has been feeling tired and lacking in energy, but has put it down to a busy period at work. Mr Yee went to see his doctor, who ordered blood tests and a gastroscopy.
   a. What do you think is the most likely condition affecting Mr Yee?
   b. What would you expect to be the findings from the investigations ordered by the doctor?
   c. What, if any, is the relationship between Mr Yee's condition and his drug treatment?

HEALTH PROFESSIONAL CONNECTIONS

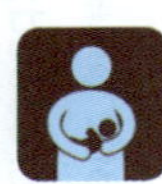

Midwives Gastro-oesophageal reflux disease (GORD) is common in pregnancy. The proposed mechanisms include a decrease in the lower oesophageal sphincter strength related to an increase in female sex hormones. Increased intra-abdominal pressure may also contribute to GORD development in a woman with a gravid uterus. A critical challenge in managing pregnant women with GORD is related to the potential teratogenicity of medications commonly used to treat GORD. Antacids are accepted as relatively safe in appropriate doses. However, they should be avoided in the last weeks of pregnancy, as they may have a tocolytic effect (i.e. stimulate uterine contractions). Proton pump inhibitors, H_2-receptor antagonists and pro-motility drugs all have pregnancy categories that cause concern in relation to administration in pregnant women. Many of these drugs are also not recommended for lactating women. Lifestyle modifications are important in pregnant women with GORD. As with all individuals, eating small meals frequently, and waiting for two to three hours after meals before lying down will have a positive effect on GORD symptoms. Other methods to reduce GORD discomfort include sleeping with the head of the bed raised and taking antacids in appropriate doses. Care should be taken with antacids containing aluminium, however, as they may be constipating and are dangerous in large doses. The antacids containing sodium bicarbonate are less beneficial, as they can increase sodium, resulting in water retention.

Nutritionists/Dieticians Nutrition professionals have a difficult task educating people on ways to manage GORD, as the volume of incorrect, non-medical information available on the internet is overwhelming. Some myths that need to be dispelled include drinking milk before bed. Although this may initially result in a decrease in acid reflux, it will ultimately increase gastric acid secretion. Sometimes quite inappropriate diets are proposed on the internet to reduce acid reflux. An important method in reducing symptoms is related to the volume of food eaten at one time. Eating smaller meals more frequently is proven to reduce GORD symptoms. Other dietary changes that should be promoted include increasing complex carbohydrates to ensure that the gastric acid secreted has food on which to work. Decreasing the fat content of meals will reduce the time that food stays in the stomach, ultimately reducing gastric acid secretion.

CASE STUDY

Mrs Jenny Waite (UR number 842111) is a 32-year-old woman who has been admitted for an upper gastrointestinal endoscopy and an *H. pylori* breath test to confirm peptic ulcer disease (PUD). She has a history of severe dysmenorrhoea for which she takes ibuprofen, naproxen and, occasionally, aspirin. Mrs Waite is a personal assistant to a busy executive officer in a construction business. She works long hours, and states that her diet is 'not good'. She has three children and a very supportive husband. Mrs Waite was referred by her local medical officer. Her observations were as follows:

Temperature	Heart rate	Respiration rate	Blood pressure	SpO_2
36.7°C	68	16	124/82	100% (RA*)

*RA = room air.

Mrs Waite has returned from theatre post-endoscopy and is resting comfortably. Peptic ulcer disease is confirmed, and she will begin a treatment regimen commencing today. The *H. pylori* breath test results have not yet been reported. She remains nil by mouth for the next hour. The pathology results taken on admission are as follows:

HAEMATOLOGY

Patient location:	Ward 3	**UR:**	842111		
Consultant:	Smith	**NAME:**	Waite		
		Given name:	Jenny	**Sex:**	F
		DOB:	24/04/XX	**Age:**	32
Time collected	09:30				
Date collected	XX/XX				
Year	XXXX				
Lab #	4353456				

FULL BLOOD COUNT		UNITS	REFERENCE RANGE
Haemoglobin	116	g/L	115–160
White cell count	6.2	$\times 10^9$/L	4.0–11.0
Platelets	270	$\times 10^9$/L	140–400
Haematocrit	0.33		0.33–0.47
Red cell count	3.81	$\times 10^{12}$/L	3.80–5.20
Reticulocyte count	0.8	%	0.2–2.0
MCV	82	fL	80–100

Neutrophils	4.56	$\times 10^9$/L	2.00–8.00
Lymphocytes	2.34	$\times 10^9$/L	1.00–4.00
Monocytes	0.35	$\times 10^9$/L	0.10–1.00
Eosinophils	0.26	$\times 10^9$/L	< 0.60
Basophils	0.11	$\times 10^9$/L	< 0.20
ESR	13	mm/h	< 12

BIOCHEMISTRY

Patient location:	Ward 3	**UR:**	842111		
Consultant:	Smith	**NAME:**	Waite		
		Given name:	Jenny	**Sex:**	F
		DOB:	24/04/XX	**Age:**	32

Time collected	09:30
Date collected	XX/XX
Year	XXXX
Lab #	2345454

ELECTROLYTES		UNITS	REFERENCE RANGE
Sodium	142	mmol/L	135–145
Potassium	3.8	mmol/L	3.5–5.2
Chloride	99	mmol/L	95–110
Bicarbonate	23	mmol/L	22–32
Glucose (random)	4.1	mmol/L	3.5–5.4
Iron	17	μmol/L	11–30

CRITICAL THINKING

1 Consider Mrs Waite's history. Outline the mechanism resulting in the development of peptic ulcer disease.

2 Consider Mrs Waite's pathology results. Are these results of any value in understanding Mrs Waite's condition? Explain.

3 Given Mrs Waite's history, the mechanism causing her PUD may already be established. What results may be revealed by the *H. pylori* breath test? Will this change the management plan?

4 In the light of this diagnosis and the mechanism of its development, what management options are possible for Mrs Waite?

5 What client education does Mrs Waite require?

BIBLIOGRAPHY

Abbasi-Kangevari, M., Ahmadi, N., Fattahi, N., Rezaei, N., Malekpour, M.-R., Ghamari, S.-H., … Farzadfar, F. (2022). Quality of care of peptic ulcer disease worldwide: a systematic analysis for the Global Burden of Disease Study, 1990–2019. *PLoS ONE* 17(8):e0271284. https://doi.org/10.1371/journal.pone.0271284.

Anand, B.S. (2021). Peptic ulcer disease. *Emedicine*. https://emedicine.medscape.com/article/181753-overview.

Australian Institute of Health and Welfare (AIHW) (2022). *Australia's health, 2022: in brief*. Australia's Health series No. 18. Cat. No. AUS 241. Canberra: AIHW. https://www.aihw.gov.au/reports/australias-health/australias-health-2022-in-brief/summary.

Bauldoff, G., Gubrud-Howe, P.M., Carno, M.-A., Levett-Jones, T., Hales, M., Berry, K., … Stanley, D. (2020). *LeMone and Burke's medical–surgical nursing: critical thinking for person-centred care* (4th [Australian] edn). Sydney: Pearson Australia.

Best, O. & Fredericks, B. (2021). *Yatdjuligin: Aboriginal and Torres Strait Islander nursing and midwifery care* (3rd edn). Port Melbourne, VIC: Cambridge University Press.

Best Practice Advocacy Centre New Zealand (BPAC NZ) (2022). H pylori: *who to test and how to treat*. Dunedin: BPAC NZ. https://bpac.org.nz/2022/h-pylori.aspx.

Bullock, S. & Manias, E. (2022). *Fundamentals of pharmacology* (9th edn). Sydney: Pearson Australia.

Congedi, J., Williams, C. & Baldock, K.L. (2022). Epidemiology of *Helicobacter pylori* in Australia: a scoping review. *PeerJ* 10:e13430. http://doi.org/10.7717/peerj.13430.

Fass, R., Boeckxstaens, G.E., El-Serag, H., Rosen, R., Sifrim, D. & Vaezi, M.F. (2021). Gastro-oesophageal reflux disease. *Nature Reviews. Disease Primers* 7(1):55. https://doi.org/10.1038/s41572-021-00287-w.

Marieb, E.N. & Hoehn, K. (2019). *Human anatomy and physiology* (11th edn). San Francisco, CA: Pearson Benjamin Cummings.

Nista, E.C., Pellegrino, A., Giuli, L., Candelli, M., Schepis, T., De Lucia, S.S., … Gasbarrini, A. (2022). Clinical implications of *Helicobacter pylori* antibiotic resistance in Italy: a review of the literature. *Antibiotics* 11(10):1452. https://doi.org/10.3390/antibiotics11101452.

Williams, C. (2013). *Medicinal plants in Australia. Volume 4—an antipodean apothecary*. Dural, NSW: Rosenberg Publishing.

Wise, M.J., Lamichhane, B. & Webberley, K.M. (2019). A longitudinal, population-level, big-data study of *Helicobacter pylori*-related disease across Western Australia. *Journal of Clinical Medicine* 8(11):1821. https://doi.org/10.3390/jcm8111821.

36 Malabsorption syndromes

KEY TERMS

Coeliac sprue/coeliac disease
Diarrhoea
Giardiasis
Gluten
Hypolactasia
Lactase deficiency
Lactose intolerance
Malabsorption
Maldigestion
Microvilli
Steatorrhoea
Tropical sprue
Whipple's disease

LEARNING OBJECTIVES

After completing this chapter, you should be able to:

1. Define the terms 'malabsorption' and 'malabsorption syndromes'.
2. Describe the common clinical manifestations of the malabsorption syndromes.
3. State the general way in which malabsorption syndromes are classified.
4. Describe how maldigestion can lead to malabsorption, and outline the pathophysiology of common conditions in this category.
5. Describe the pathophysiology of hypolactasia.
6. Describe how impaired mucosal function can lead to malabsorption, and outline the pathophysiology of common conditions in this category.
7. Outline the basis by which coeliac disease and tropical sprue can be differentiated.
8. Describe how alterations in microbial gut flora can lead to malabsorption, and outline the pathophysiology of common conditions in this category.

WHAT YOU SHOULD KNOW BEFORE YOU START THIS CHAPTER

Can you outline the types of cellular adaptation?

Can you describe the responses to both reversible and irreversible cellular injury?

Can you identify the major parts of the gastrointestinal system, and describe their functions?

Can you describe the process of normal gastrointestinal digestion and absorption?

Introduction

LEARNING OBJECTIVE 1

Define the terms 'malabsorption' and 'malabsorption syndromes'.

LEARNING OBJECTIVE 2

Describe the common clinical manifestations of the malabsorption syndromes.

The normal absorption of nutrients such as proteins, fats, carbohydrates, vitamins and minerals from the gastrointestinal tract requires effective digestion, an intact mucosa and nutrient transport mechanisms, as well as the presence of a normal intestinal flora. When these elements become disrupted, **maldigestion** and malabsorption can develop.

Malabsorption can lead to a variety of clinical manifestations, including **diarrhoea** and abdominal distension, **steatorrhoea** (increased fat content in stools), malnutrition, weight loss and anaemia. Collectively, these manifestations are referred to as *malabsorption syndromes*. The malabsorption syndromes are generally classified according to their primary aetiologies: maldigestion, impaired mucosal function and impaired microbial flora.

Maldigestion

LEARNING OBJECTIVE 3

State the general way in which malabsorption syndromes are classified.

LEARNING OBJECTIVE 4

Describe how maldigestion can lead to malabsorption, and outline the pathophysiology of common conditions in this category.

AETIOLOGY AND PATHOPHYSIOLOGY

Normal digestion is dependent on a combination of mechanical and chemical processes. These processes start in the mouth through chewing and the mixing of saliva. The bolus of food enters the stomach to be churned and mixed with gastric juices. The liquefied chyme is squirted into the duodenum in a regulated way to be mixed with pancreatic, biliary and intestinal secretions ready for absorption in the intestines.

Gastric surgery can result in a loss of control of gastric emptying into the intestines. This leads to partially digested food entering the intestines, with incomplete mixing of pancreatic secretions and bile with the bolus. This is known as *dumping syndrome*. The partially digested chyme exerts an elevated osmotic pressure, drawing fluid from the blood into the gastrointestinal tract lumen. An increase in intraluminal pressure stimulates gastrointestinal motility, triggers explosive diarrhoea and may lead to malabsorption. Rapid absorption of glucose with a rebound hypoglycaemia may also occur.

A number of conditions affect the pancreas and liver (see the chapter 'Disorders of the liver, gall bladder and pancreas') and the intestines (see the chapter 'Intestinal disorders'). These conditions alter the availability of digestive chemicals within the gastrointestinal tract, and can lead to malabsorption (see Figure 36.1). Gall bladder diseases, such as *cholelithiasis* (gallstones in the gall bladder) and *choledocholithiasis* (gallstones in the common bile duct), affect bile formation and transport, as do *biliary atresia* (a congenital obstruction of the common bile duct) and *hepatic inflammatory conditions. Autoimmune and chronic pancreatitis* can lead to a reduction in pancreatic acini (exocrine cells), which decreases the formation of pancreatic secretions. In *cystic fibrosis* (see the chapter 'Obstructive pulmonary disorders'), viscous mucus plugs block the outflow of pancreatic juices into the duodenum.

Surgical removal of too much bowel after traumatic abdominal injuries or resection for cancer will also induce an incurable malabsorption condition known as *short bowel*

Figure 36.1

Factors leading to malabsorption

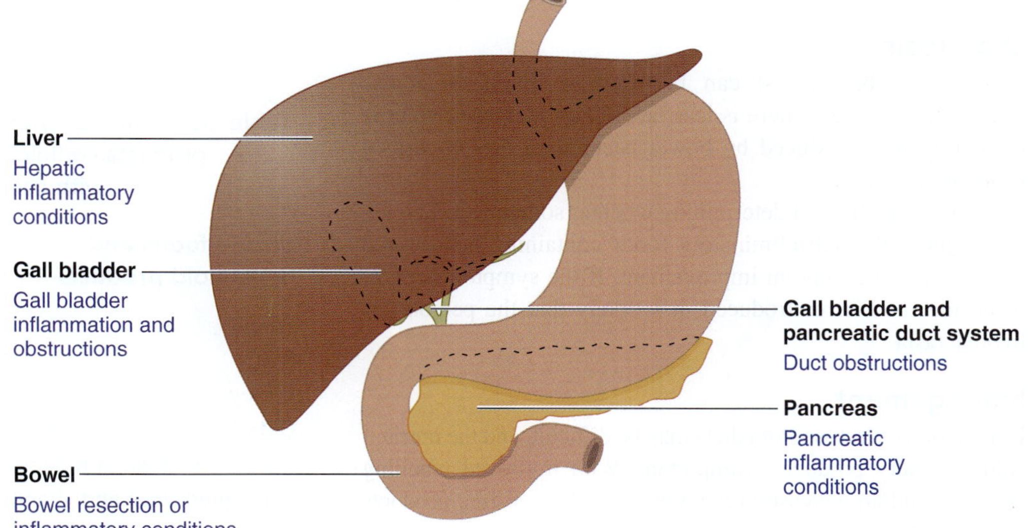

syndrome. This occurs purely because there is insufficient small bowel left to sustain the person's nutritional needs. In this event, the person will only be able to survive if they receive *total parenteral nutrition (TPN)*, which is a concentrated intravenous infusion of all the daily nutritional requirements for someone who is unable to absorb the nutrients necessary to sustain metabolic function, or a *bowel transplant*.

LEARNING OBJECTIVE 5

Describe the pathophysiology of hypolactasia.

The **microvilli** of the intestines also produce digestive enzymes, some of which are disaccharidases involved in carbohydrate metabolism. Deficiencies in the production of these enzymes can develop in what appears to be otherwise intact intestinal mucosa. **Lactase deficiency** or (**hypolactasia**), which disrupts the conversion of lactose into galactose and glucose, is the most common of these. This condition is widely known as **lactose intolerance** or *lactase deficiency*. It is important to note that this is a deficient state not an allergy, as there is no immune-mediated pathophysiology associated with the state. Lactase production normally decreases in early childhood, as the child is weaned. For some people the production of this enzyme may be low or even decrease to negligible levels. This represents a *primary lactase deficiency*. It is rare for a congenital lactase deficiency to occur.

In a person with lactase deficiency, lactose is fermented by the gut flora in the large bowel, leading to the accumulation of significant amounts of gas within the gut lumen. The gas distends the gut lumen and can result in abdominal discomfort. The undigested lactose can also increase gut osmotic pressure, stimulating motility and causing diarrhoea.

A less common *secondary lactase deficiency* can develop as a consequence of another gastrointestinal condition that injures the small intestinal mucosa, such as inflammation, infection or coeliac disease. A decrease or unavailability in lactase occurs without a true deficient state developing.

Figure 36.2 explores the common clinical manifestations and management of lactase deficiency.

CLINICAL DIAGNOSIS AND MANAGEMENT

Diagnosis

A hydrogen breath test can be used to diagnose lactose intolerance. Because there is less lactase, an increased volume of hydrogen is produced by bowel bacteria in the process of fermenting lactose.

Another method of determining whether someone is lactose-intolerant is through eliminating foods containing lactose and monitoring for symptom improvement. If the symptoms return when the food is reintroduced, it is likely that the person has hypolactasia.

Management

Elimination of lactose from diets may be difficult, and the nutrient value of dairy products is important. With improved labelling practices and an increase in the number of lactose-free products available, however, the task has become easier for those with hypolactasia. Lactose-free products are in fact manufactured by adding lactase to them to degrade the lactose. Lactose-free milks and other dairy products are now available, and the consumption of these can contribute to a significant reduction in abdominal discomfort. Calcium supplementation may be indicated, and should be considered on a case-by-case basis.

Some other dietary modifications to assist a person with lactose intolerance include substituting foods with soy alternatives. Other methods include eating dairy products that are more fermented, including mature cheeses and yoghurts, but they may still be problematic for some lactase-intolerant people. When choosing to drink milk, people with hypolactasia should be educated to drink full-fat milk and avoid low-fat or fat-free milk. The increased volume of fat within the gastrointestinal tract decreases the rate of motility, which increases the amount of time that the available lactase has to digest (hydrolyse) lactose.

Impaired mucosal function

LEARNING OBJECTIVE 6

Describe how impaired mucosal function can lead to malabsorption, and outline the pathophysiology of common conditions in this category.

This group of malabsorption syndromes is characterised by a loss of mucosal tissue, which decreases both the absorptive surface of the gut and the availability of intestinal enzymes. The group include coeliac sprue (coeliac disease) and tropical sprue.

LEARNING OBJECTIVE 7

Outline the basis by which coeliac disease and tropical sprue can be differentiated.

COELIAC DISEASE

Coeliac sprue/coeliac disease, or *gluten-sensitive enteropathy*, results from an improper immune response to the storage proteins known as **gluten**, which are found in a number of cereal grains (wheat, barley and rye), but not in rice, maize, millet or sorghum (Table 36.1).

Table 36.1 The safety of foods and other household products containing gluten for people with coeliac disease

Unsafe foods and household products	Safe foods
Wheat	Corn (maize)
Rye	Millet
Barley	Sorghum
Oats (for some affected people)	Rice
Stamp and envelope adhesives	Quinoa
Some medicines and vitamin preparations	

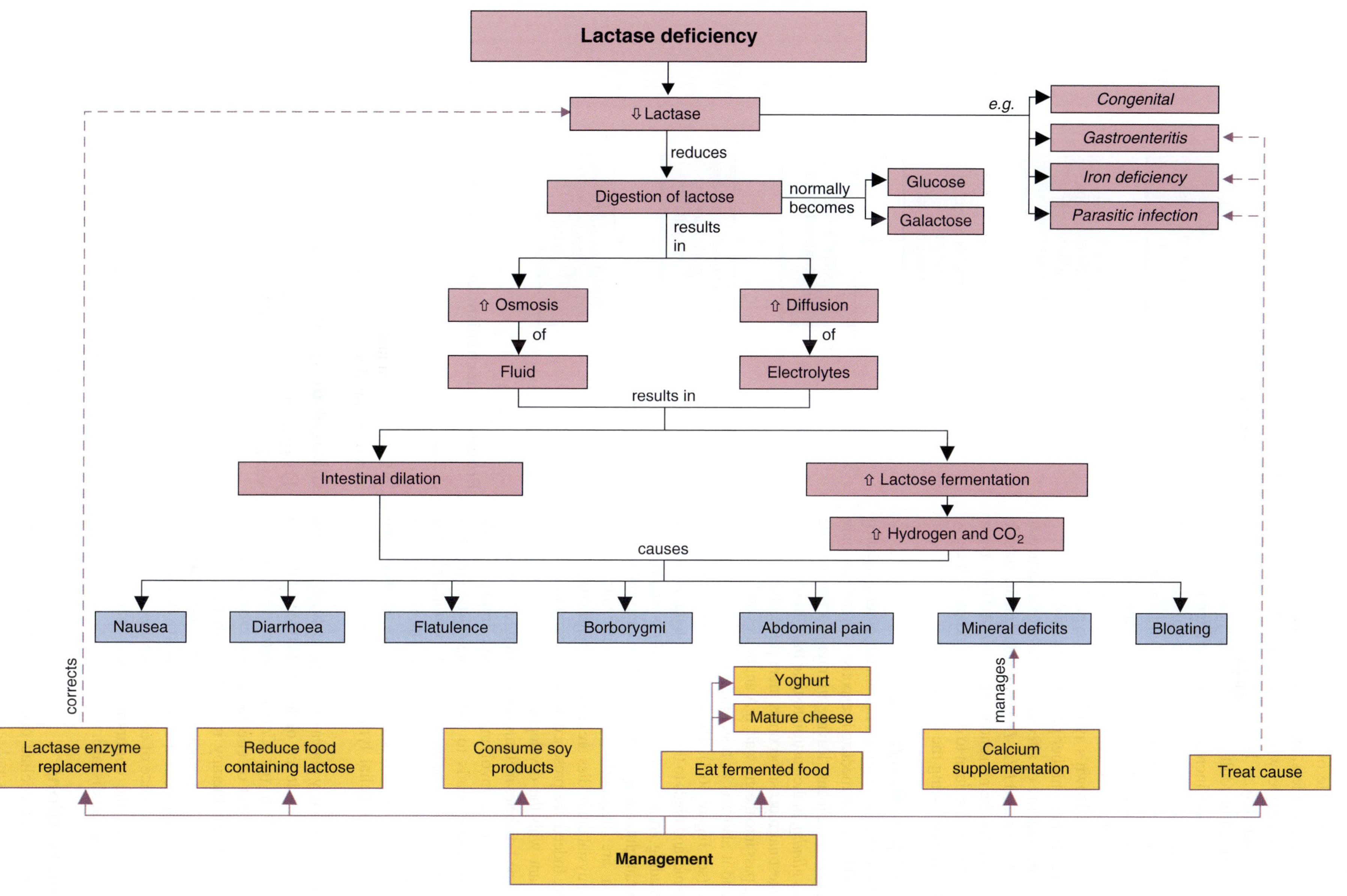

Figure 36.2

Clinical snapshot: Lactase deficiency

↓ = decreased; ↑ = increased; CO_2 = carbon dioxide.

Epidemiology

Coeliac disease affects people of European descent, including Australians and New Zealanders, and occurs in India. However, it is relatively rare in people with an African, Caribbean or East Asian background. It can be diagnosed at any age, but commonly it is identified in adults around 40–45 years old. The global prevalence rates are increasing. The Walter and Eliza Hall Institute estimates that prevalence rates in Australia are 1 case in 80 men and 1 case in 60 women, with a large proportion of the population undiagnosed. In New Zealand the Best Practice Advocacy Centre New Zealand estimates 1 affected in 100 adults. Children with Down's syndrome or type 1 diabetes mellitus are reported to have higher prevalence rates.

An overwhelming majority of affected people have a particular human leukocyte antigen called *HLA-DQ2* expressed on the surface of antigen-presenting cells; the remainder express *HLA-DQ8*. These genes are necessary for the condition to develop, but people can carry these genes without manifesting the disease.

Aetiology and pathophysiology

The condition is considered to be an autoimmune disorder associated with a reactive $CD4^+$ T-cell-mediated response. Gluten can only be partially digested in humans, leaving immunoreactive peptide fragments, such as *gliadin*, in the gastrointestinal tract. In susceptible individuals, the intestinal mucosa becomes more permeable to these peptides, and they pass into the gut wall. IgA antibodies are produced against gliadin, and it also acts as a substrate to the enzyme tissue *transglutaminase* (see Figure 36.3). The product of this reaction is particularly antigenic, and binds to the surfaces of antigen-presenting immune cells, leading to the formation of *antitransglutaminase antibodies*. Antitransglutaminases are related to antiendomysial antibodies, which are frequently associated with autoimmune disease. Antiendomysial antibodies are directed against components of smooth muscle. Indeed, the presence of this autoimmune disease may be concomitant with the development of other autoimmune diseases, such as type 1 diabetes mellitus and autoimmune thyroiditis.

The immune reaction, involving activated immune cells and mediator substances, leads to the characteristic mucosal damage. In coeliac disease, the *mucosal villi* become blunted or the *mucosa* may become totally flattened. The region most affected is the *proximal small intestines*. This is accompanied by an increase in intraepithelial lymphocytes and hyperplasia of the intestinal glands.

Environmental factors may play a role in the pathophysiology of the disease. There is evidence of a link between infection with rotavirus in children (or *Campylobacter* infection in adults) and the development of coeliac disease. Antimicrobial or proton pump inhibitor therapy may also increase the risk. The composition of the gut microbiome may influence the pathophysiological development in either a positive or a negative way, depending on the presence of certain microbes.

Figure 36.4 explores the common clinical manifestations and management of coeliac disease.

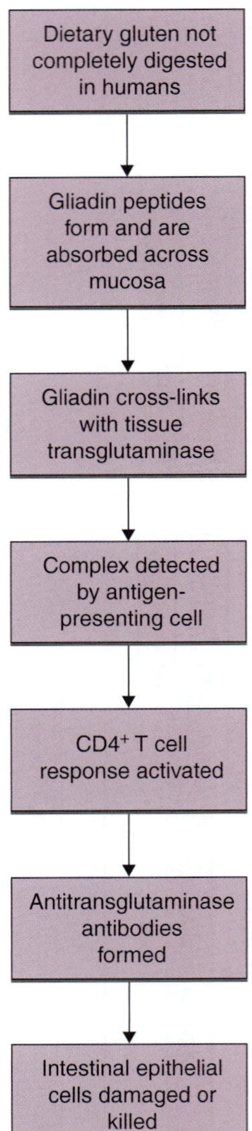

Figure 36.3

Proposed mechanism of gliadin pathogenicity

Clinical manifestations

The classic symptoms of coeliac disease in children include chronic diarrhoea, weight loss and failure to thrive; reflecting the clinical manifestations of malabsorption. Other symptoms seen in both children and adults include bloating, iron deficiency and anaemia, constipation, fatigue, abdominal pain and osteoporosis.

Clinical diagnosis and management

Diagnosis In adults, diagnosis is made by examination of serology (total IgA and IgA tissue transglutaminase levels) and tissue biopsy. The histological changes stated above are used diagnostically, and the degrees of severity can be categorised using the *Marsh classification system*. In Europe it has been recommended that children not undergo biopsy if there is a matching of symptoms and serology to the accepted criteria, but this has not been widely adopted in Australia. Human leukocyte antigen (HLA) testing is not routinely done for this condition.

Management The mainstay of treatment is to maintain a gluten-free diet. Assessment of micronutrient levels, such as vitamin B_{12}, D and folic acid, may require supplementation if deficient. Monitoring for osteoporosis is also recommended.

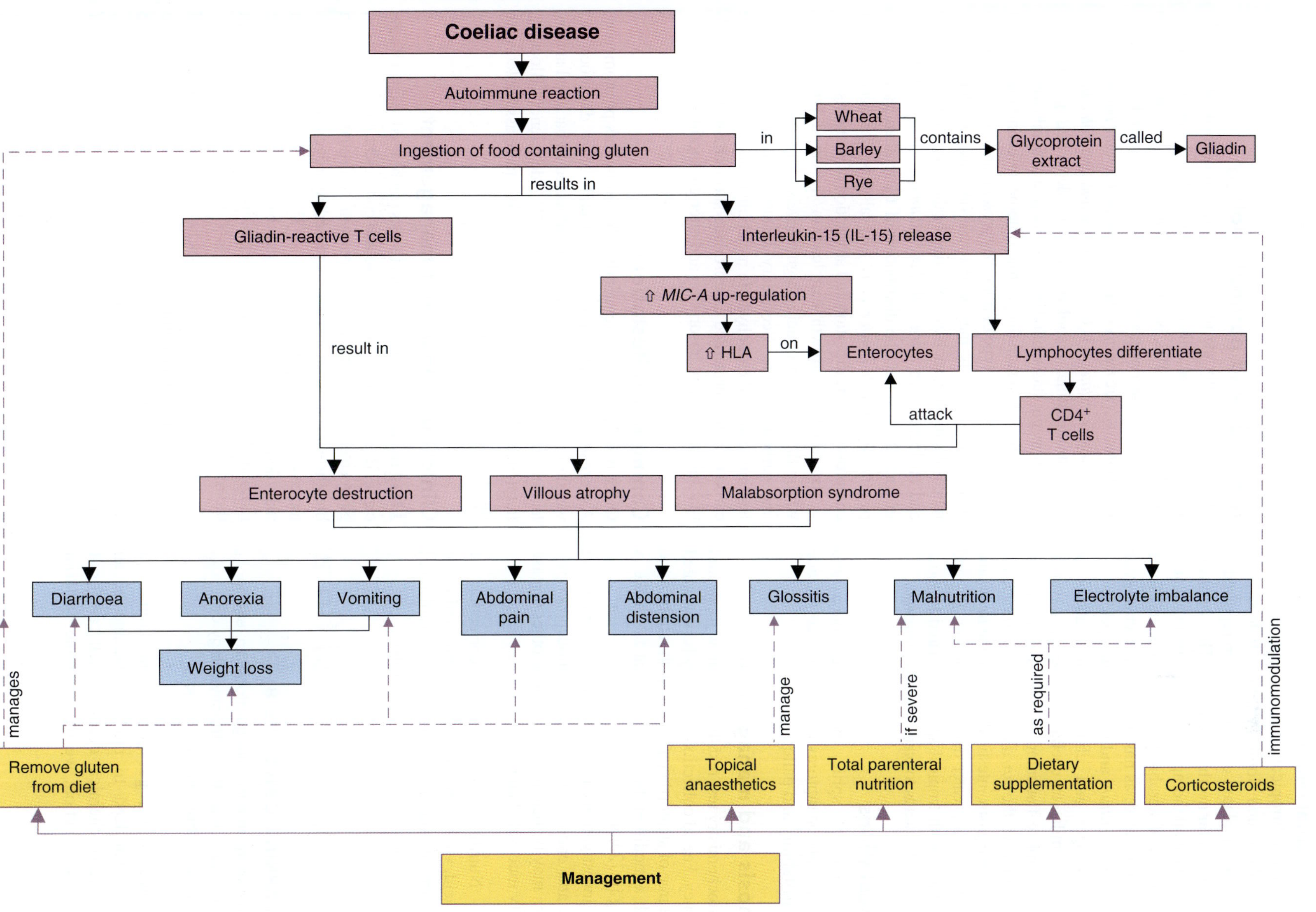

Figure 36.4

Clinical snapshot: Coeliac disease

↓ = decreased; ↑ = increased; $CD4^+$ = cluster of differentiation marker 4; HLA = human leukocyte antigen; IL = interleukin; MIC-A = MHC class I chain-related gene A.

TROPICAL SPRUE

Aetiology and pathophysiology

As the name suggests, **tropical sprue** is associated with living in, or visiting, tropical or subtropical areas, such as South-East Asia, India, the Caribbean and South America. Indeed, it is endemic in these regions. Isolated cases have been reported in Indigenous communities in far north Queensland. The condition responds well to antimicrobial therapy, suggesting that the cause is infectious. Overgrowth of aerobic gut organisms and toxin production has been implicated, as has parasitic infection with protozoa such as *Cryptosporidium* and *Cyclospora* species.

The histological changes and clinical manifestations of tropical sprue are very similar to coeliac disease. However, it is rare to observe a complete flattening of intestinal mucosa in tropical sprue. In addition to the *proximal small intestines*, the most affected regions of the gastrointestinal tract are the *ileum* and *proximal jejunum*. There is a greater degree of vitamin B_{12} and folate deficiency in those with tropical sprue compared to those with coeliac disease, and this leads to *megaloblastic anaemia*.

Clinical manifestations

Common manifestations of sprue include diarrhoea and steatorrhoea. The signs and symptoms of anaemia can include fatigue, weakness, irritability and pallor.

Clinical diagnosis and management

Diagnosis Biochemistry test results often show folate and vitamin B_{12} deficiency. Faecal collection tests may be warranted to determine the degree of steatorrhoea. This test should be done in conjunction with a modified diet to ensure that fat intake is not more than 100 g in 72 hours.

More invasive investigations may be indicated, including a barium swallow and endoscopy (oesophagoduodenoscopy). These investigations may be beneficial to exclude other disease processes or identify mucosal changes.

Management Nutritional support and correction of anaemia with folic acid, vitamin B_{12} or iron supplementation are the mainstays of treatment. Antimicrobials may be administered to eradicate pathogenic bacteria within the intestine.

Alterations in microbial flora

LEARNING OBJECTIVE 8

Describe how alterations in microbial gut flora can lead to malabsorption, and outline the pathophysiology of common conditions in this category.

An increase in growth of the gut flora or infection by a pathogenic organism can lead to mucosal damage or an alteration in the nature of chemical digestion that can result in malabsorption. In this section, we will examine bacterial overgrowth, Whipple's disease and a common parasitic infection called giardiasis.

BACTERIAL OVERGROWTH

Aetiology and pathophysiology

The gut is normally the most colonised compartment of the body, with more microbial cells in residence than the total number of cells in a human body. This is referred to as the *gut microbiome*. The majority of these organisms are bacteria. The microbiome in the *small intestines* are *mostly Gram-positive and aerobic bacteria*, while in the *large intestines* it is *Gram-negative and anaerobic bacteria*.

Gastrointestinal disorders—such as decreased gastric juice production, gut stasis, blind intestinal loops and fistula formation—can lead to a change in the gut microbiome, affecting the bacterial growth pattern, the type of microbes present, and their distribution within the gut. This may lead to accompanying alterations in mucosal structure, such as a blunting or flattening of the *microvilli* and an increase in *intraepithelial inflammatory cells*. However, in contrast to sprue, the distribution of these changes is usually patchy. The *brush border cells* may also be damaged, further compromising the digestion and absorption of nutrients.

Bacterial overgrowth can lead to increased fermentation within the lumen, producing higher levels of hydrogen, methane and carbon dioxide. Secondary lactase deficiency can arise, leading to altered carbohydrate metabolism and absorption. The carbohydrates fermented can produce short-chained fatty acids that inhibit nutrient absorption and alter gut motility.

Common manifestations

Older people are most frequently affected by this phenomenon. As a result of malabsorption, they usually show diarrhoea and weight loss. Bile salts may also be subjected to bacterial action, leading to steatorrhoea and vitamin B_{12} deficiency. Bloating, flatulence, abdominal distention and pain can be associated with increased gut fermentation.

Clinical diagnosis and management

Diagnosis A number of breath tests can be used to quantify the cause. Breath tests are non-invasive and convenient investigations in gastroenterology. In bacterial overgrowth syndrome, the hydrogen breath test may demonstrate increased hydrogen as a result of increased carbohydrate fermentation. The ^{14}C-Xylose breath test may detect increased Gram-negative bacteria through the use of radiolabelled xylose, which is metabolised by the bacteria with the release of radioactive carbon dioxide.

Blood should be drawn for biochemical and haematological testing. Anaemia is common, and, depending on the degree of malabsorption, various electrolyte imbalances can be demonstrated. As the individual will be experiencing diarrhoea, faecal analysis would be beneficial for deeper investigation of possible causes or to rule out other pathology.

Management The principal management includes the administration of antimicrobials to reduce the pathogenic bacteria and enable the enteric flora to increase. Probiotic therapy may be beneficial in restoring the gut microbiome, and may also suppress pro-inflammatory cytokine production. Other important considerations include management of malnutrition. Dietary support and vitamin and mineral supplementation should be considered, if necessary.

WHIPPLE'S DISEASE

Aetiology and pathophysiology

Whipple's disease is associated with an infection by a Gram-positive bacillus called *Tropheryma whipplei*. It is a systemic condition that affects the immune system, and is also associated with lymphadenopathy and endocarditis, in addition to pulmonary and central nervous system dysfunction. *T. whipplei* can be detected in the intestines, brain, heart, eyes, skin, monocytes, cerebrospinal fluid, saliva and faeces of affected people. Whipple's disease is relatively rare, and predominately affects middle-aged Caucasian men. A genetic predisposition to the condition has been suggested, associated with the *HLA-B27* gene.

The immune dysfunction is associated with alterations in *lymphocyte activity*, particularly a decrease in immunocompetent B cells. An examination of the affected intestinal mucosa shows that the intestinal folds become thickened and may contain yellow or white deposits. Lacteals within the villi are dilated and contain macrophages loaded with lipid and bacilli.

Clinical manifestations

This condition is usually characterised by diarrhoea, weight loss and abdominal pain, as well as fever and joint pain (arthralgia). Neurological symptoms can include dementia, personality changes and depression. It can also induce ocular disturbances.

Clinical diagnosis and management

Diagnosis Biopsy of lymph node or small intestine tissue and histological detection of the bacteria is the main diagnostic investigation. Investigations of malabsorption and anaemia, although important, are not specific for Whipple's disease. Other than DNA determination of *T. whippeli*, no tests are specific for this condition. Faecal fat studies may assist with determining the presence or degree of malabsorption.

Management Antimicrobial drug therapy is the primary method of management. Support for malabsorption and anaemia may be achieved through nutrient, vitamin and mineral supplementation. Recovery from severe neurological dysfunction is poor.

GIARDIASIS

Gastrointestinal infection by the parasite *Giardia lamblia*—also known *as Giardia intestinalis* or *Giardia duodenalis*—is highly prevalent globally. In developed countries such as Australia and New Zealand, its prevalence is 2–7%. In developing countries, its prevalence is much higher, at 2–30%. It is currently a notifiable infection in some Australian states and territories (ACT, Victoria, Tasmania and Western Australia) and in New Zealand. It is frequently associated with travelling in developing countries (one of the common causes of traveller's, or backpacker's, diarrhoea), and is a common parasitic infection acquired by those who are immunocompromised. Interestingly, recent evidence suggests that most cases in developed countries are acquired locally. It is most commonly seen in infants, small children and young adults.

Transmission is via the faecal–oral route or by sexual contact. Usually infective cysts are shed in faeces, and are present in contaminated water, food or fomites. Trophozoites hatch from these cysts and attach to the intestinal wall, where they cause inflammation, flattening of the intestinal villi and malabsorption. In the large intestines trophozoites form new cysts, which are expelled with faeces. It appears that the cysts may be more resistant to chlorine disinfectants than other microbes.

Clinical manifestations

The clinical manifestations of **giardiasis** include nausea, severe diarrhoea, steatorrhoea, bloating, flatulence, stomach cramps and abdominal distension. The condition may be associated with malabsorption and weight loss. However, in most people the condition will be asymptomatic. *Giardia* infection may also lead to secondary lactase deficiency.

Figure 36.5 explores the common clinical manifestations and management of giardiasis.

Clinical diagnosis and management

Diagnosis Faecal analysis identifying trophozoites or cysts is definitive. Faecal fat analysis may also be beneficial to demonstrate steatorrhoea. Eosinophilia may be demonstrated on haematology results. However, other blood tests are generally normal.

Management The primary management principle of giardiasis is antimicrobial therapy (with drugs such as metronidazole or albendazole) and fluid and electrolyte support. Education regarding dehydration and fluid and electrolyte imbalance is critical, especially in those who are very young or very old. Dietary modifications may assist with symptom relief. Limiting fat intake may reduce nausea, diarrhoea and steatorrhoea, and decreasing lactose intake may reduce abdominal pain. Probiotics may reduce trophozoite adhesion, and garlic is known for its antiparasitic properties, at least in vitro.

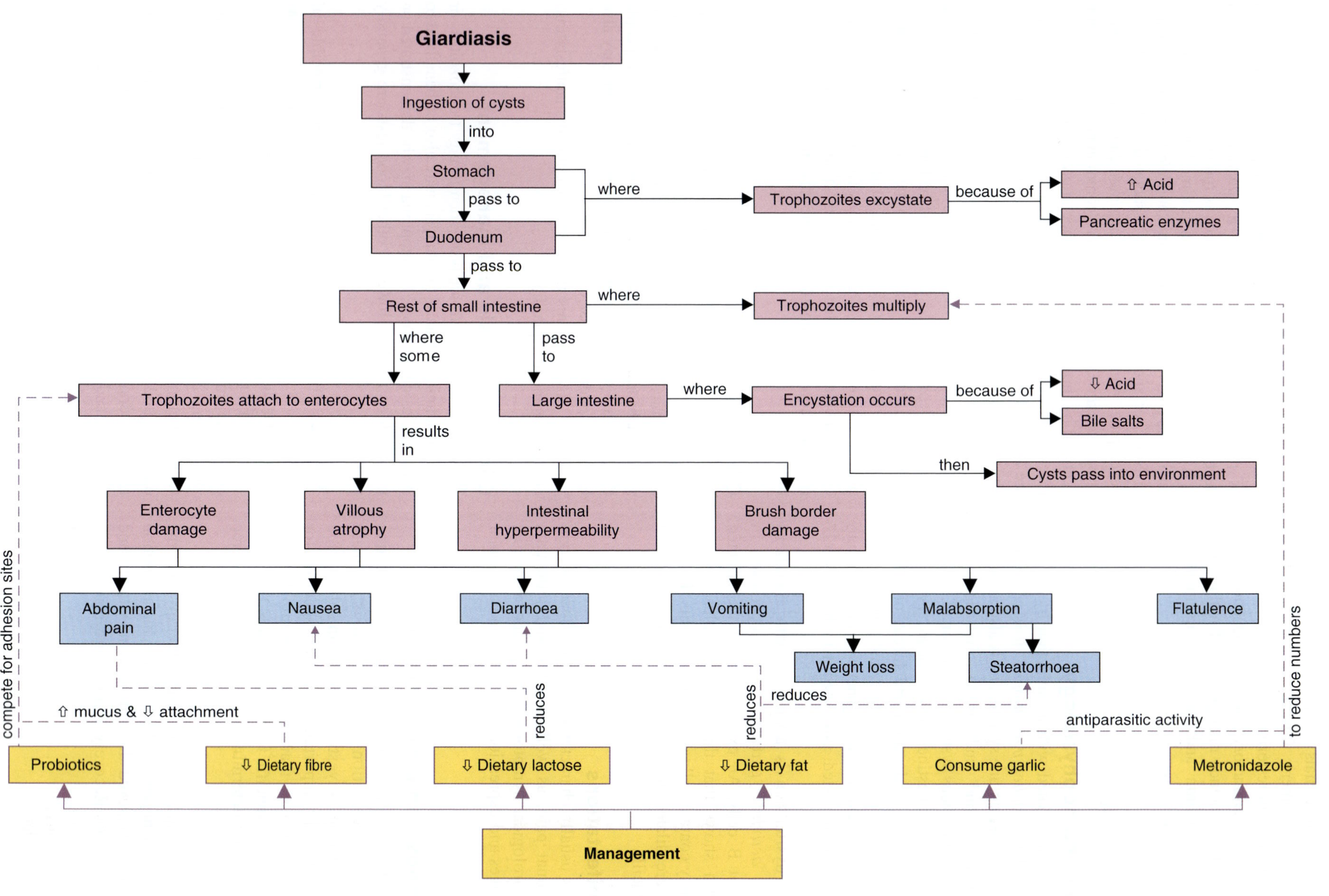

Figure 36.5

Clinical snapshot: Giardiasis

↓ = decreased; ↑ = increased.

INDIGENOUS HEALTH FAST FACTS AND CULTURAL CONSIDERATIONS

FAST FACTS

- *The burden of disease for giardiasis is greater in communities with poor access to water, sanitation and hygiene facilities. The Walter and Eliza Hall Institute has indicated that there are up to 600,000 cases reported in Australia per year. The condition is considered to be endemic in remote Indigenous Australians.*
- *Hospitalisation rates for gastroenteritis in Aboriginal and Torres Strait Islander children under 2 years of age are 11 times higher than in non-Indigenous children under 2 years of age.*
- *The incidence of gastroenteritis hospitalisations in Māori children under 2 years of age is slightly less (0.89:1) than in European New Zealanders.*
- *The incidence of gastroenteritis hospitalisations in Pacific Islands children under 2 years of age is approximately 1.5 times more than in European New Zealanders, and slightly higher than for Māori children.*

CULTURAL CONSIDERATIONS

- *In some rural and remote communities in Australia, access to good-quality drinking water with acceptably low levels of bacteria remains an ongoing concern. It is difficult to believe that in the 21st century, in Australia, there are still hundreds of Aboriginal and Torres Strait Islander communities nationwide that do not have reticulated water from the main town's water supply. Although the extent of drinking water quality differs across the nation, in Western Australia almost half of the remote Aboriginal communities have untreated drinking water without regular monthly testing. Little progress can be made to reduce the healthcare disparity crisis for Aboriginal and Torres Strait Islander peoples if even the most basic population health priority, such as provision of clean drinking water and sanitation, is not yet standard across all of our population.*

Sources: Data from Clifford et al. (2015); Simpson et al. (2017); Walter and Eliza Hall Institute (2022b); Zajaczkowski et al. (2019).

CHILDREN AND ADOLESCENTS

- Malabsorption in children can result in failure to thrive, and pubertal and psychomotor delay.
- Serology tests for coeliac disease (antiendomysial antibody, antireticulin antibody, antigliadin antibody) may not be reliable in children under 3 years of age, resulting in the need for histological diagnosis.

OLDER ADULTS

- Those over 80 years of age are at significant risk of malnutrition for reasons such as poor appetite, limited food options, and even issues relating to a decreasing ability to manipulate cutlery or food-preparing equipment.
- Vitamin D malabsorption increases with age, and older adults are at an increased risk of osteoporosis. Exposure to the sun and administration of calciferol may assist in reducing the risk of fracture.

KEY CLINICAL ISSUES

- The most important behaviours to reduce the spread of enteric pathogens include frequent hand-washing with good technique, and appropriate hygiene practices when dealing with food.
- People who have severe and prolonged malabsorption issues may require total parenteral nutrition (TPN). Care of people requiring TPN can be complex, and interprofessional teams—including nurses, dietitians and medical officers—must work together to improve the individual's condition.
- Lactase deficiency (lactose intolerance) tests can be performed quickly and easily with hydrogen breath tests. However, management plans for those with lactase deficiency can be complex and limiting, making compliance difficult.
- Children presenting with failure to thrive, chronic diarrhoea and anaemia may be investigated for coeliac disease, tropical sprue and/or problems such as chronic intestinal infections.

CHAPTER REVIEW

- *Malabsorption* is associated with a *disruption of normal nutrient absorption* from the gastrointestinal tract.
- Common clinical manifestations include diarrhoea, steatorrhoea, abdominal distension, malnutrition, weight loss and anaemia. Collectively, these symptoms are termed *malabsorption syndromes*.
- Conditions affecting the stomach, liver, pancreas and gall bladder can disrupt the normal digestive processes and lead to malabsorption.

- A deficiency in the disaccharidase *lactase (hypolactasia)* in an otherwise intact intestinal mucosa is relatively common. The condition is commonly known as *lactose intolerance*. The unmetabolised lactose is fermented by the gut flora, leading to an accumulation of gas in the gut lumen. This can cause abdominal discomfort and increase gut osmotic pressure, leading to diarrhoea.
- *Coeliac disease* is an immune disorder associated with an inappropriate response to the storage proteins called *gluten*. This leads to a $CD4^+$ T-cell-mediated inflammatory response. The peptides pass into the gut wall and trigger IgA *antitransglutaminase antibodies*. The intestinal mucosa undergoes a characteristic pattern of damage such that the microvilli become blunted, with an increase in intraepithelial lymphocytes and hyperplasia of intestinal glands. Sometimes the mucosal layer can be completely flattened in affected areas.
- *Tropical sprue* is thought to be associated with a *pathogenic infection or bacterial overgrowth*. The condition is endemic in tropical and subtropical regions. Tropical sprue manifests in a similar way to coeliac disease, differing in the regions of the intestines affected and the degree of vitamin deficiency. Complete flattening of the intestinal mucosa is rare in this condition.
- A change in the *distribution and type of microbes* present in the gut is associated with decreased gastric juice production, blind intestinal loops, fistulas, gut stasis and pathogenic infection, and can lead to malabsorption syndromes.

REVIEW QUESTIONS

1. Define the term 'malabsorption syndrome'.
2. List the common clinical manifestations of the malabsorption syndromes.
3. Explain how gall bladder disorders can lead to malabsorption.
4. Outline the pathophysiology of hypolactasia.
5. Mrs Gwen Thomas is a 70-year-old woman who has recently been diagnosed with diverticular disease. The diagnosis was made after a period in which she was experiencing diarrhoea, weight loss and anaemia. Discuss how this condition, characterised by gut stasis, could lead to malabsorption.
6. Dane Walker is a 15-year-old boy who has been experiencing significant gastrointestinal discomfort for some time. His doctor has traced the problem to his diet, determining that the gastrointestinal disturbance is worst when Dane eats food containing wheat and rye grains.
   a. Which condition do you think is affecting Dane?
   b. What is the usual epidemiology associated with this condition?
   c. Briefly describe the pathophysiology of this condition.
   d. What tests would be done to confirm the diagnosis?
   e. How would the appearance of the intestinal mucosa change in this condition?
   f. How is this condition usually managed?

HEALTH PROFESSIONAL CONNECTIONS

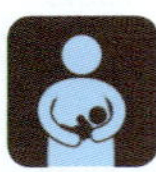

Midwives Congenital hypolactasia is an autosomal recessive form of lactase deficiency. It is rare; however, there is a trend suggesting that some babies weaned off breast milk and substituted with lactose-free substances are more prone. Failure to thrive and parental concern regarding dietary issues should be treated seriously, and appropriate investigation and parental education should be provided where necessary.

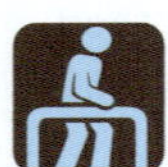

Physiotherapists Malabsorption can result in multiple and complex issues that may impede a physiotherapist's ability to assist the person in their care. Energy deficits may reduce a person's capacity to participate in the required rehabilitation. Mineral deficits may interfere with bone density, increasing the risk of injury during treatments. Physiotherapists play a critical role in the management of people with some malabsorption syndromes (e.g. cystic fibrosis). Clinicians must be familiar with the disease process, and how the clinical consequences will influence their management plan.

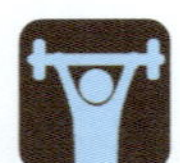

Exercise scientists People participating in competitive sports with weight categories can be at risk of dietary issues. Malnutrition and unhealthy eating habits may be experienced by athletes who are not properly monitored or educated regarding the importance of nutrition to their performance. In-depth discussion, planning and counselling should be undertaken to ensure that competition occurs in appropriate weight categories. Often, competing in a lower weight category may be appealing to the athlete who feels it may give them an advantage over lighter competitors. However, if inappropriate training or nutrition practices occur, the athlete should be encouraged to advance to the next weight category.

Nutritionists/Dieticians Management of people requiring total parenteral nutrition (TPN) is complex. Understanding the cause of malnutrition is important in the calculation of the formula required. Age, disease processes, medications and acuity will also influence the composition of the formula. Local issues and the cost and type of delivery systems will also influence TPN prescription. A multidisciplinary approach is necessary to ensure the best outcomes for those requiring TPN.

CASE STUDY

Mrs Grace Freeman (UR number 545819) is a 36-year-old woman who was involved in a motor vehicle accident five days ago. She sustained abdominal trauma and went straight to theatre for a laparotomy, partial colectomy small bowel resection and temporary colostomy. Postoperatively her observations were as follows:

Temperature	Heart rate	Respiration rate	Blood pressure	SpO^2
36.8°C	78	14	112/78	100% (4 L/min via NP*)

*NP = nasal prongs.

Over the past 24 hours her condition deteriorated. Her observations were as follows:

Temperature	Heart rate	Respiration rate	Blood pressure	SpO^2
39.3°C	112	28	86/44	86% (10 L/min via mask)

She was taken back to surgery for another laparotomy, and the surgeons discovered a large area of necrosis, resu ting in the need for a further significant small bowel resection. She now has short bowel syndrome. Mrs Freeman has been transferred to the intensive care unit. She is ventilated and on inotropic support and antimicrobials. She will need to commence total parenteral nutrition. The pathology results taken immediately prior to surgery have returned as follows:

HAEMATOLOGY

Patient location:	Ward 3	**UR:**	545819		
Consultant:	Smith	**NAME:**	Freeman		
		Given name:	Grace	**Sex:**	F
		DOB:	17/02/XX	**Age:**	36

Time collected	11:30
Date collected	XX/XX
Year	XXXX
Lab #	5738446

FULL BLOOD COUNT		UNITS	REFERENCE RANGE
Haemoglobin	92	g/L	115–160
White cell count	17.2	$\times 10^9/L$	4.0–11.0
Platelets	130	$\times 10^9/L$	140–400
Haematocrit	0.30		0.33–0.47
Red cell count	3.62	$\times 10^{12}/L$	3.80–5.20
Reticulocyte count	2.4	%	0.2–2.0
MCV	84	fL	80–100
Neutrophils	9.2	$\times 10^9/L$	2.00–8.00
Lymphocytes	3.83	$\times 10^9/L$	1.00–4.00
Monocytes	0.52	$\times 10^9/L$	0.10–1.00
Eosinophils	0.38	$\times 10^9/L$	< 0.60
Basophils	0.16	$\times 10^9/L$	< 0.20
ESR	19	mm/h	< 12

BIOCHEMISTRY

Patient location:	Ward 3	**UR:**	545819		
Consultant:	Smith	**NAME:**	Freeman		
		Given name:	Grace	**Sex:**	F
		DOB:	17/02/XX	**Age:**	36

Time collected	11:30
Date collected	XX/XX
Year	XXXX
Lab #	46384563

ELECTROLYTES		UNITS	REFERENCE RANGE
Sodium	137	mmol/L	135–145
Potassium	4.9	mmol/L	3.5–5.2
Chloride	98	mmol/L	95–110
Bicarbonate	18	mmol/L	22–32
Glucose (random)	9.2	mmol/L	3.5–7.7
Iron	9	μmol/L	11–30
pH	7.29		7.35–7.45
PaO_2	78	mmHg	> 80
$PaCO_2$	9	mmHg	35–45

CRITICAL THINKING

1 Consider Mrs Freeman's history. Outline the mechanism resulting in bowel necrosis following the first colectomy.

2 Contrast the first set of observations with the second set of observations. What has occurred to cause this change? Explain the mechanism resulting in the changes to each of her observations.

3 Consider Mrs Freeman's pathology results. Explore the parameters outside of the reference ranges. Why are each of these changes occurring?

4 How does the removal of too much bowel result in malabsorption? Explain.

5 Other than necrosis, what risks are associated with gastrointestinal surgery? How can these risks be reduced?

6 What are the risks, benefits and considerations associated with total parenteral nutrition? How can some of these risks be reduced?

BIBLIOGRAPHY

Australian Institute of Health and Welfare (AIHW) (2022). *Australia's health, 2022.* Australia's Health series No. 18. Cat. No. AUS 241. Canberra: AIHW. https://www.aihw.gov.au/reports/australias-health/australias-health-2022-in-brief/summary.

Bauldoff, G., Gubrud-Howe, P.M., Carno, M.-A., Levett-Jones, T., Hales, M., Berry, K., ... Stanley, D. (2020). *LeMone and Burke's medical-surgical nursing: critical thinking for person-centred care* (4th [Australian] edn). Sydney: Pearson Australia.

Best, O. & Fredericks, B. (2021). *Yatdjuligin: Aboriginal and Torres Strait Islander nursing and midwifery care* (3rd edn). Port Melbourne, VIC: Cambridge University Press.

Best Practice Advocacy Centre New Zealand (BPAC NZ) (2022). *Coeliac disease: investigations and management*. Dunedin: BPAC NZ. https://bpac.org.nz/2022/coeliac.aspx.

Bullock, S. & Manias, E. (2022). *Fundamentals of pharmacology* (9th edn). Sydney: Pearson Australia.

Catassi, C., Verdu, E.F., Bai, J.C. & Lionetti, E. (2022). Coeliac disease. *The Lancet* 399(10344):2413–26. https://doi.org/10.1016/S0140-6736(22)00794-2.

Clifford, H.D., Pearson, G., Franklin, P., Walker, R. & Zosky, G.R. (2015). Environmental health challenges in remote Aboriginal Australian communities: clean air, clean water and safe housing. *Australian Indigenous Health*Bulletin 15(2):1–14. http://healthbulletin.org.au/articles/environmental-health-challenges-in-remote-aboriginal-australian-communities-clean-air-clean-water-and-safe-housing.

Goebel, S.U. (2019). Celiac disease (sprue). *Emedicine*. https://emedicine.medscape.com/article/171805-overview.

Marieb, E.N. & Hoehn, K. (2019). *Human anatomy and physiology* (11h edn). San Francisco, CA: Pearson Benjamin Cumming.

Misselwitz, B., Butter, M., Verbeke, K. & Fox, M.R. (2019). Update on lactose malabsorption and intolerance: pathogenesis, diagnosis and clinical management. *Gut* 68(11):2080–2091. https://doi.org/10.1136/gutjnl-2019-318404.

Nazer, H. (2023). Giardiasis. *Emedicine*. https://emedicine.medscape.com/article/176718-overview.

Roy, P.K., Komanapalli, S.D., Shojamanesh, H. & Bashir, S. (2019). Lactose intolerance. *Emedicine*. https://emedicine.medscape.com/article/187249-overview.

Simpson, J., Duncanson, M., Oben, G., Adams, J., Wicken, A., Pierson, M., ... Gallagher, S. (2017). *Te ohonga ake: the health of Māori children and young people in New Zealand .Series Two.* Dunedin: New Zealand Child and Youth Epidemiology Service, University of Otago https://www.health.govt.nz/publication/te-ohonga-ake-health-status-maori-children-and-young-people-new-zealand-0.

Valkov, H., Kovacheva-Slavova, M., Lyutakov, I., Vladimirov, B. & Penchev, P. (2021). Whipple's disease. *British Journal of Hospital Medicine* 82(3):1–2. https://doi.org/10.12968/hmed.2020.0614.

Walter and Eliza Hall Institute (2022a). *Coeliac disease.* https://www.wehi.edu.au/research-diseases/immune-health-and-infection/coeliac-disease.

Walter and Eliza Hall Institute (2022b). Giardiasis. https://www.wehi.edu.au/research-diseases/immune-health-and-infection/giardiasis.

Zajaczkowski, P., Mazumdar, S., Conaty, S., Ellis, J.T. & Fletcher-Lartey, S.M. (2019). Epidemiology and associated risk factors of giardiasis in a peri-urban setting in New South Wales Australia. *Epidemiology and Infection* 147:e15, 1–9. https://doi.org/10.1017%2FS0950268818002637.

37 Intestinal disorders

KEY TERMS

Adenoma
Appendicitis
Colitis
Colon cancer
Crohn's disease
Diverticula
Diverticulitis
Familial adenomatous polyposis
Gastroenteritis
Haemolytic uraemic syndrome
Hernia
Ileus
Inflammatory bowel disease
Intussusception
Peritonitis
Rotavirus
Ulcerative colitis
Volvulus

LEARNING OBJECTIVES

After completing this chapter, you should be able to:

1. Outline the pathophysiological mechanisms of infectious diseases of the intestines.
2. Outline the disease processes associated with acute appendicitis and peritonitis.
3. Classify the major neoplasms of the intestines, and outline their characteristics.
4. Describe the pathophysiology of colon cancer.
5. Describe the pathophysiological processes in inflammatory bowel diseases.
6. Compare and contrast ulcerative colitis and Crohn's disease.
7. Outline the major causes of intestinal obstruction, and its pathophysiological consequences.

WHAT YOU SHOULD KNOW BEFORE YOU START THIS CHAPTER

Can you identify the parts of the gastrointestinal system, and outline their functions?

Can you identify the regions of the intestines, and the contribution each makes to digestive and absorptive processes?

Can you outline the principles associated with infections?

Can you describe the concepts associated with neoplasia?

Can you describe the stages of acute inflammation and healing?

Can you differentiate between acute and chronic inflammation?

Can you outline the major concepts associated with immune disorders?

Introduction

Diseases of the intestines kill and disable many millions of people around the world each year. In poorer parts of the world, diarrhoea caused by infection of the intestines is a major killer of the very young and the very old at all times. In the developed world, far fewer people die of intestinal infections, although many fall ill. Cancer of the large intestine is one of the most common causes of cancer deaths, becoming increasingly prevalent as the population ages.

In this chapter, we will address the major types of pathophysiological processes that affect the intestines and associated structures, such as infection, inflammation (both acute and chronic), cancer and obstruction.

Infectious conditions of the intestines

LEARNING OBJECTIVE 1

Outline the pathophysiological mechanisms of infectious diseases of the intestines.

AN INTRODUCTION TO INFECTIOUS DIARRHOEA

Infectious diseases of the intestines are among the most common causes of morbidity and mortality around the world. The term **gastroenteritis** is often used loosely to refer to acute infectious disease of the digestive tract, although infection of the stomach is not usually a major feature. Other usage that is more or less synonymous includes *enteritis* (strictly, inflammation of the small intestine, infectious or otherwise), **colitis** (inflammation of the large intestine) and *enterocolitis*.

The major symptom, and the major danger in such infections, is acute diarrhoea. Other clinical manifestations may include vomiting, nausea, fever and abdominal pain. Worldwide, the World Health Organization reports that there are around 1.7 billion cases of diarrhoeal disease in children, and that it kills 525,000 children under 5 years old each year. Among children diarrhoeal disease is second only to respiratory infection as a cause of death.

Diarrhoea is defined as a disruption in bowel habits, in which faeces become more fluid and are passed more frequently than usual. It is the result of increased secretion of water and electrolytes into the lumen of the intestine, or reduced fluid uptake from it.

The small intestine is the major site of absorption of water. When this process is disrupted by infection, faeces will be watery and voluminous. When the large intestine is affected, faeces tend to be smaller but very frequent. Diarrhoea also occurs in non-infectious conditions, such as malabsorption (see the chapter 'Malabsorption syndromes'), but such cases will not be reviewed in this chapter.

Most forms of infectious diarrhoea are acute, lasting a few days, and self-limiting. As affected people recover, the epithelium that may have been damaged regenerates rapidly. However, prolonged diarrhoea that persists for more than two or three days may cause extensive loss of fluid, which may be life-threatening, especially in small children. It will also contribute to malnutrition. *Dysentery* and *cholera* are examples of gastrointestinal infections that can be severe and result in death if not treated appropriately. Chronic diarrhoea that lasts more than a few weeks is usually not caused by infection, but may reflect a chronic condition, such as cancer or inflammatory bowel disease. People experiencing a form of immunosuppression, due to disease, drug treatment or older age, can be more susceptible to infectious diarrhoea.

The pathogens responsible for acute infectious diarrhoea include *bacteria*, *viruses* and *protozoa*. They are usually acquired by indirect *faecal–oral routes*, with transmission occurring via contaminated water, food or hands. Some viruses may be contracted through air-borne transmission.

In poor countries where sanitation and sewage disposal are inadequate, transmission is largely through contaminated water. When these services break down, in war or natural disasters, epidemics of cholera may occur. In developed countries, the pathogens are usually transmitted in food. Disease that is clearly associated with food is termed *food poisoning*.

The tissue damage that leads to diarrhoea is produced through a limited number of mechanisms, and in most cases the pathogens remain confined to the digestive tract, exerting local effects. The emphasis below will be on the pathophysiological processes of infectious diarrhoea rather than on the taxonomy of the pathogens or the epidemiology of infection.

Diarrhoea can be classified as secretory, osmotic or inflammatory. Various pathogens can cause different types of diarrhoea. *Secretory diarrhoea* results from increased ion transport processes from epithelial cells. Large volumes of water and a decreased sodium level occur in the small bowel as a result of reduced sodium reabsorption and increased crypt epithelial cell chloride secretion. *Osmotic diarrhoea* can occur as a result of consuming an increased volume of osmotically active substances. If the substances are isotonic, the water and solute are not absorbed; however, if the substances ingested are hypertonic, solutes and water are drawn into the lumen. Both mechanisms result in the typical abnormally high fluid content of the stool. *Inflammatory diarrhoea* results from disruption of the intestinal epithelium by cytotoxic substances. The function of the absorptive epithelial cells are disrupted, and therefore absorption of water is inefficient. Serum exudate and blood is also found in the lumen. Figure 37.1 explores the common clinical manifestations and management of infectious diarrhoea.

VIRAL DIARRHOEA

Aetiology and pathophysiology

Viruses that cause diarrhoea infect the *enterocytes (epithelial cells)* of the small intestine. Depending on the virus involved, the consequences can include the damage or death of the enterocytes, secretion of water and electrolytes into the lumen, a reduction in the absorptive capacity of the enterocytes for water and electrolytes, and a reduction in the capacity of the small intestine to digest and subsequently absorb carbohydrates. The latter can lead to an accumulation of osmotically active compounds in the lumen, which causes water to be retained in the lumen rather than be absorbed.

In most cases of viral infection, the diarrhoea is watery—this is termed *'non-inflammatory'*—in contrast to the diarrhoea caused by invasive bacterial infections (see the next section

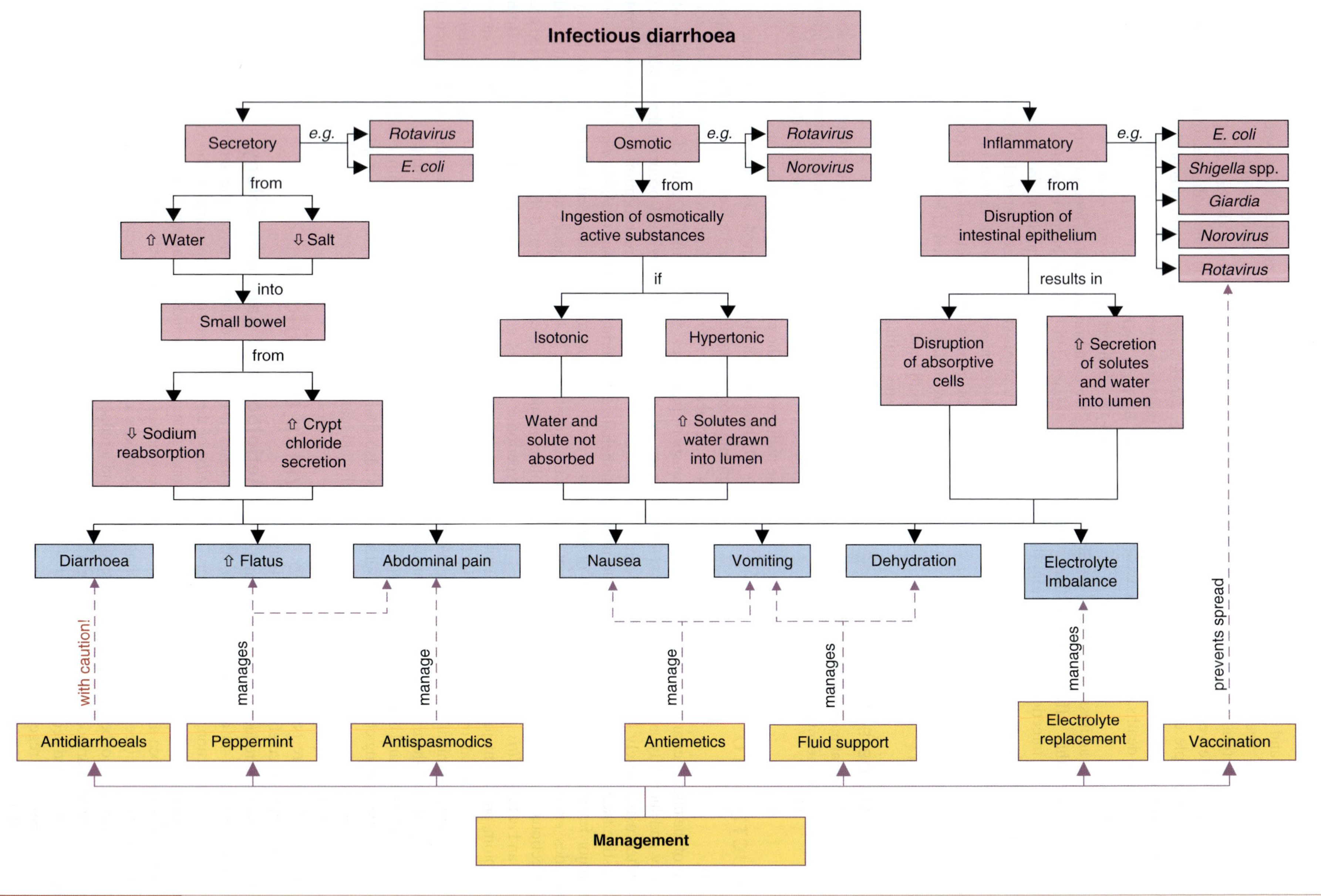

Figure 37.1

Clinical snapshot: Infectious diarrhoea

↓ = decreased; ↑ = increased; *E. coli* = *Escherichia coli; Shigella* spp. = *Shigella* species.

of this chapter). Vomiting, fever and abdominal pain may also accompany the diarrhoea.

Epidemiology

In Australia, New Zealand and other developed countries, most cases of infectious diarrhoea are caused by viruses, with **rotavirus** being the most common viral pathogen among children, and *norovirus (Norwalk virus)* the most common in adults.

It is estimated that in Australia, rotavirus infection is responsible for 7,000 hospitalisations each year in children under 5 years of age. In poorer countries, diarrhoea due to rotavirus infection causes over 2 million hospitalisations among children under 5 years old each year.

The pooled global prevalence for gastroenteritis in children and adults accounted for by norovirus infection is estimated at 16%.

BACTERIAL DIARRHOEA

Aetiology and pathophysiology

In poorer parts of the world, infectious diarrhoea caused by bacteria is a major cause of death. However, in developed countries, fewer cases of infectious diarrhoea are caused by bacteria than by viruses. The pathogens most often responsible are *Salmonella*, *Campylobacter*, *Shigella*, *Yersinia*, *Clostridium* and *Escherichia coli* (*E. coli*). In poorer countries and in disaster areas, *Vibrio cholerae* is the cause of epidemics of cholera.

The mechanisms by which bacteria may cause diarrhoea include invasion of the epithelium, attachment to the epithelial cell accompanied by production of exotoxins, and secretion of enterotoxins into the small intestinal lumen. Bacteria that invade the epithelium, usually of the large intestine, damage it and trigger an acute inflammatory response. This reduces the absorptive capacity of the epithelium, and stimulates secretion of water and mucus. *Salmonella*, *Campylobacter*, *Shigella* and some invasive strains of *E. coli* act in this way. The result is inflammatory diarrhoea: faeces will contain mucus or blood or both, together with neutrophils and protein from inflammatory exudate. Diarrhoea that is markedly bloody is sometimes termed *dysentery*, especially when the pathogen is identified as *Shigella* or as the protozoan *Entamoeba*.

In cases of infections with some of these pathogens, damage may extend beyond the intestine. *Salmonella* crosses the epithelial layer to enter the bloodstream or lymphatic system, and causes systemic infection. Infection by certain invasive toxigenic strains of *E. coli*, notably serotype O157:H7, may result in **haemolytic uraemic syndrome**. This occurs most often in children, and can be life-threatening. The syndrome is caused by a *shiga-like toxin* (also known as *verotoxin*) similar to that produced by *Shigella dysenteriae*. It is absorbed from the intestine into the bloodstream and targets vascular endothelium, especially that of the glomerular capillaries in the kidney. It kills endothelial cells by inhibiting protein synthesis within them, with damage to the endothelium triggering the blood clotting cascade. The consequences are: thrombosis of small blood vessels; damage to erythrocytes (i.e. haemolysis) as blood flows through damaged and partially blocked vessels; and thrombocytopenia as platelets aggregate at the sites of clotting. Acute kidney injury, which may be fatal, can ensue.

Bacteria such as *V. cholerae* and some non-invasive strains of *E. coli* attach to the epithelium of the small intestine without invading it, and there produce enterotoxins that cause the enterocytes to secrete water and electrolytes into the lumen. The resulting diarrhoea is profuse and watery (i.e. non-inflammatory). In cholera, the loss of water may be rapidly fatal.

Finally, bacteria may simply secrete enterotoxins into the lumen of the small intestine, or into food before it is eaten. The onset of symptoms (nausea, abdominal pain, vomiting and diarrhoea) is rapid, as it does not depend on microbial proliferation. Disease caused by the ingestion of preformed toxins may be classified as *intoxication* rather than infection.

When *Staphylococcus aureus*, *Bacillus cereus* or *Clostridium botulinum* grow on food (anaerobically in the case of *C. botulinum*), they can produce *heat-stable toxins* that are not inactivated by cooking. The toxins of *S. aureus* and *B. cereus* act in the small intestine to produce diarrhoea. The toxin from *C. botulinum*, botulinum toxin, is absorbed from the intestine, travels in the blood and blocks transmission at neuromuscular junctions, causing paralysis. Paralysis of the respiratory muscles is rapidly fatal if the person cannot be artificially ventilated.

PROTOZOAL DIARRHOEA

Aetiology

Protozoa are common causative agents of persistent diarrhoea in travellers associated with drinking contaminated water. The diarrhoea may occur during the trip or when the traveller returns home. Common protozoal species in this form of diarrhoea include *Giardia*, *Cryptosporidium* and *Entamoeba*.

CLINICAL MANIFESTATIONS

People with diarrhoea may present with increased flatus, abdominal pain and nausea. When protracted episodes of vomiting and diarrhoea have occurred, signs of dehydration may be exhibited, such as sunken eyes, dry mucous membranes and poor skin turgor. In neonates, a concerning sign of dehydration is a sunken anterior fontanelle. Electrolyte imbalances may also develop as the large volumes of potassium lost from the gastrointestinal tract result in hypokalaemia.

CLINICAL DIAGNOSIS AND MANAGEMENT

Diagnosis

Stools samples may be collected to isolate and identify the causative organism. Blood may be taken for analysis of electrolytes and observation of renal function. In chronic diarrhoea, intestinal biopsy may be considered in an attempt to determine the cause.

Management

Most cases of diarrhoea are self-limiting and may resolve over a short period of time (one or two days), which generally means that those affected do not seek medical assistance. When the quantity or duration of the diarrhoea exceeds the person's ability to self-manage, they will generally present with dehydration and electrolyte imbalances that require active intervention. Fluid and electrolyte replacement may be required intravenously. For a young child, breastfeeding should continue, as it is known to reduce the severity and duration of enteritis. In older children and adults, diet should be as tolerated, as an adequate caloric intake is necessary to assist with enterocyte repair. Food abstinence is not recommended. Easily digestible foods, such as bananas, apple sauce, toast and soups, will be tolerated more readily. Dairy foods should be avoided, because the amount of lactase necessary to process the dairy food may be inadequate as a result of the infection. Food and agents promoting gastric motility should also be avoided (e.g. caffeine, alcohol), as these will exacerbate the diarrhoea. Antimicrobial agents may be indicated for enteric bacterial and protozoan pathogens, and antiemetics may be indicated to help manage nausea and vomiting. Antispasmodic agents may assist with abdominal pain. Antidiarrhoeal agents based on opioid derivatives may be beneficial to reduce intestinal peristalsis; however, these agents should be avoided in the context of fever or bloody stools, as they may prolong the condition.

Rotavirus vaccination of infants has greatly reduced the rate of hospitalisation for this form of diarrhoeal infection in children aged under 5 years by 60–70%.

INFECTION ASSOCIATED WITH RESIDENT BACTERIA OF THE INTESTINES

Aetiology and pathophysiology

From the mouth to the anus, the normal healthy digestive tract harbours very large numbers of bacteria of great variety. These are known as *resident bacteria*, *commensal bacteria* or *normal flora*; those of the intestines are often termed *enteric bacteria*. Their concentration is very high in the mouth, low in the stomach and small intestine, and increases to a maximum in the large intestine. Here, there are hundreds of bacterial species, mainly anaerobes.

An ecological balance exists such that the overall numbers and species' distribution of microbes remain constant, as cells reproduce in the lumen of the digestive tract and are expelled in faeces.

The presence of a normal flora protects the host by excluding invading pathogens, and it may confer other benefits, such as the synthesis of vitamin K. However, some microbes of the normal flora may act as opportunistic pathogens in certain circumstances.

The ecological balance among resident microbes may be disturbed by antimicrobial treatment, which will affect some species but not others. The antimicrobial-resistant survivors may then undergo a population explosion and, in greatly increased numbers, cause disease.

Clostridium difficile is an anaerobic bacterium that is often present as a colonist in the intestine of people who are in hospital. While its numbers remain small, it is not pathogenic. However, when other components of the flora are disrupted by broad-spectrum antimicrobials, *C. difficile* may survive and proliferate to cause an infectious diarrhoea known as *pseudomembranous colitis* (also termed *antibiotic-associated colitis*). The 'pseudomembrane' in question consists of cell debris, and fibrin from the inflammatory exudate, which is formed in response to damage to epithelial cells caused by bacterial cytotoxins.

Bacterial overgrowth may also occur if the normal flow of intestinal contents is blocked. In abnormally large numbers, the otherwise harmless bacteria of the normal flora can cause rapid, extensive tissue destruction (i.e. gangrene), especially if necrotic tissue is already present as a result of ischaemia (see the 'Acute appendicitis' section).

Microbes of the normal flora can act as pathogens if they escape from the lumen of the digestive tract and enter sterile body compartments, such as the peritoneal cavity (see the 'Peritonitis' section). This may follow rupture of the tract from the inside as the end result of a sequence of obstruction and/or ischaemia, followed by bacterial overgrowth, tissue necrosis and gangrene (see the 'Acute appendicitis' section), or simply by erosion due to an ulcer or a tumour. The tract may also be perforated from the outside by trauma or surgical procedures.

Acute inflammatory conditions of the intestines

LEARNING OBJECTIVE 2

Outline the disease processes associated with acute appendicitis and peritonitis.

ACUTE APPENDICITIS

The appendix is a small, hollow, blind-ended projection of the caecum, the first part of the large intestine. Like other parts of the large intestine, it contains large numbers of resident bacteria in a steady state of replication and elimination.

Aetiology and pathophysiology

Acute **appendicitis** may arise if the lumen of the appendix becomes obstructed. As mucus continues to be secreted by the epithelium, pressure builds up within the appendix, while resident bacteria continue to replicate. The increasing pressure in the lumen damages the epithelial barrier, allowing the bacteria to infect the underlying tissue layers, provoking an acute inflammatory response. As pus forms, the luminal pressure is increased further, blood vessels of the appendix are compressed and its tissues suffer ischaemic damage. Necrotic tissue provides substrates for further bacterial growth with accelerating tissue destruction (i.e. *gangrene*). The process may move rapidly to the stage of rupture, with release of bacteria and pus from the appendix into the peritoneal cavity. This will cause peritonitis.

The cause of the initial obstruction of the appendix is often a faecalith, a hard mass of faeces. Obstruction may also be caused by a component of food that has not been digested, such as a pip, or it may be caused by increased activity and swelling of the subepithelial ('subepithelium') lymphoid tissue in response to an earlier infection.

In developed countries, acute appendicitis affects about 7% of the population. It can occur at any age, but is more common in older children and young adults, and is one of the major reasons for surgery in these age groups.

Clinical manifestations

People presenting with appendicitis generally complain of periumbilical or right lower quadrant pain. The pain may be relatively mild early in the disease process, but becomes intense when the inflamed appendix exerts pressure on the parietal peritoneum. Other manifestations in the early stage of development include low-grade fever, loss of appetite and nausea. Rebound tenderness is highly suggestive of appendicitis, and guarding and rigidity are common. Vomiting may follow as the severity of the pain increases. If vomiting precedes the pain, the possibility of intestinal obstruction should be considered. At a more advanced stage there is high fever, and the other symptoms persist longer.

Clinical diagnosis and management

Diagnosis A full blood examination and relevant chemical pathology testing should be performed. Leukocytosis (increased white blood cell count) with neutrophilia (increased neutrophil levels) is common. C-reactive protein levels (CRP) are also elevated. β-Human chorionic gonadotropin (β-hCG) measurements should also be performed in all women of childbearing age to exclude ectopic pregnancy as the cause of the abdominal pain.

Ultrasound, used either on its own or in conjunction with computed tomography (CT), can be used to inform decisions about surgery. An abdominal X-ray may have some role to play in the confirmation of appendicitis, but is more valuable when used to confirm or rule out other causes of abdominal pain.

Management The principles of managing people with acute appendicitis include pain control, fluid support for dehydration, and the administration of antimicrobials to prevent peritonitis. Antimicrobials are also used prophylactically when preparing for surgical intervention.

After appendectomy, antimicrobials may be continued, depending on the severity of presentation and on local policy. If the appendix has ruptured, they will be essential. Failure to manage the infection appropriately could result in the person developing peritonitis and sepsis.

PERITONITIS

The peritoneal cavity is normally sterile. **Peritonitis**, or inflammation of the peritoneum, will ensue when *bacteria* are introduced into the cavity, or if *chemical irritants*, such as bile, stomach acid or pancreatic juice, find their way into it.

Bacterial infection of the peritoneum may be 'spontaneous' in people with cirrhosis of the liver and ascites. In this condition, intestinal bacteria apparently move through the intestinal wall or through lymphatic vessels into the enlarged peritoneal cavity.

Aetiology and pathophysiology

Infection can originate internally or externally. It can develop internally following perforation of the digestive tract, or externally as a consequence of trauma or surgical procedures. It may also arise from infection of the female reproductive organs, especially the fallopian tubes, or from rupture of a ureter by disease or trauma. Such infections usually involve a mixture of bacterial species (i.e. they are *polymicrobial*).

The role of the peritoneum is to prevent the spread of infection by mounting an inflammatory response. The response is characterised by increased vascular perfusion, the attraction and accumulation of immune cells at the site of infection, the release of pro- and anti-inflammatory mediators and exudate formation. During the initial infection, fibrin in the inflammatory exudate may trap bacteria. At such sites, *abscesses* may form, which can cause persistent infection problems even after apparently successful treatment by surgery and antimicrobial therapy.

A further common complication of successfully treated peritonitis arises from *fibrosis* (i.e. the formation of scar tissue in the abdominopelvic cavity). This may cause adhesion between organs of the cavity, or between an organ and the cavity wall (see the 'Adhesions' section later in this chapter). Figure 37.2 explores the common clinical manifestations and management of peritonitis.

Clinical manifestations

The person presents with pain, originating mainly from the parietal layer of the peritoneum. Vomiting may also occur. They may present with a life-threatening systemic inflammatory process with fever, hypotension and tachycardia. The gastrointestinal tract may perforate if it has not already done so (see Figure 37.3).

Clinical diagnosis and management

Diagnosis A full blood examination and relevant chemical pathology testing should be performed. Leukocytosis with neutrophilia is common. β-hCG measurements should also be performed in all women of childbearing age to exclude ectopic pregnancy as the cause of the abdominal pain. If the person presents with fever, or if sepsis is developing, blood cultures will be required to identify the causative organisms.

A diagnostic peritoneal lavage (washout) may be useful if diagnosis is complicated. Ultrasound, computerised tomography (CT) and magnetic resonance imaging (MRI) scans can assist with diagnosis and assessment of the severity of the problem. However, when the diagnosis is conclusive, it is imperative that surgery is not delayed.

Management In severe cases of peritonitis, the essential interventions are laparotomy and thorough lavage of the peritoneum, control of bacteria, and identification of the cause and its location.

Medical management of peritonitis includes antimicrobial therapy to eliminate the causative organisms, as the problem is usually polymicrobial. Control of inflammatory processes and the continuing function of organs are also important, but may be complex and difficult if the peritonitis is severe. Nutritional support is important to ensure sufficient nutrients and energy to service the metabolic requirements of the hypermetabolic state, which arises in severe infection.

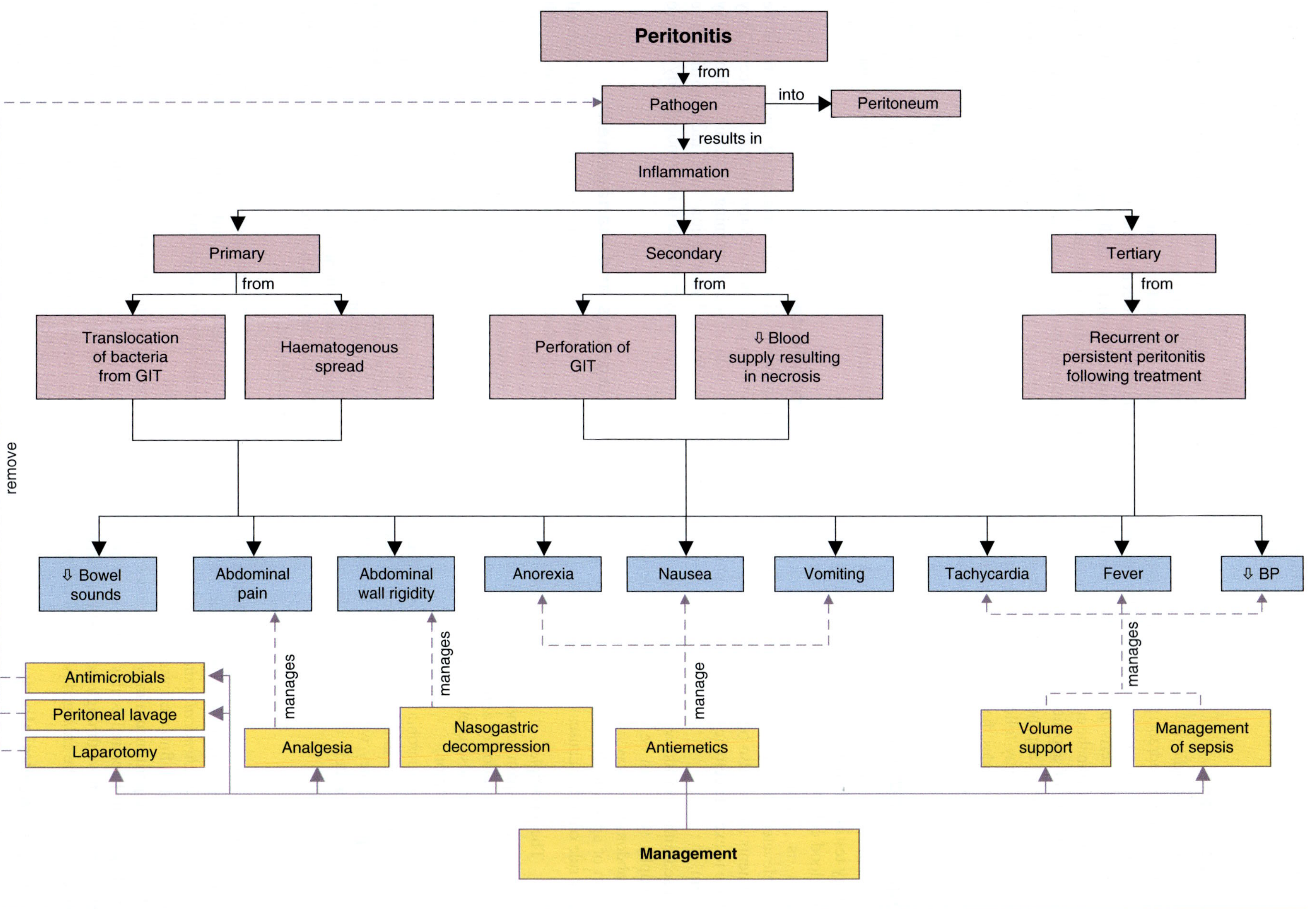

Figure 37.2

Clinical snapshot: Peritonitis

↓ = decreased; BP = blood pressure; GIT = gastrointestinal tract.

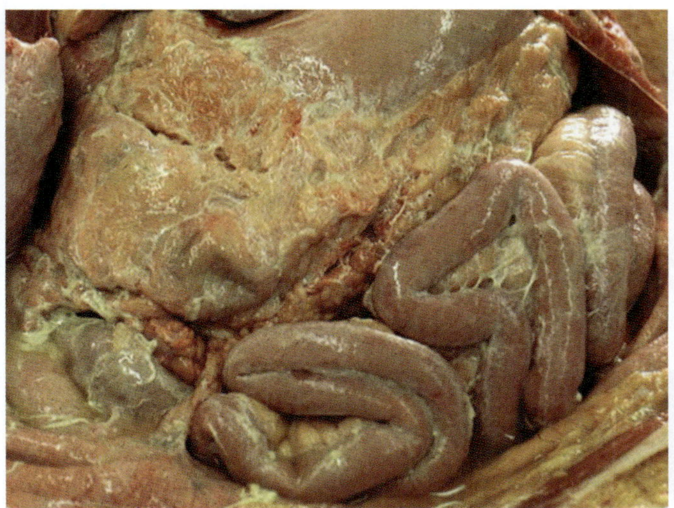

Figure 37.3

Acute peritonitis

Acute fibrinopurulent peritonitis in an open abdomen with evidence of inflammation and exudate (pus) following the rupture of a duodenal ulcer.

Source: © *PathoPic Pathorama.ch.*

Antimicrobial therapy is central to the control and elimination of the causative organisms, and is essential before and after surgery. Intra-abdominal antimicrobial lavages may also be carried out. Care must be taken with regard to the potential nephrotoxic and ototoxic effects of aggressive antimicrobial regimens, especially those that include aminoglycosides such as gentamicin.

If peritonitis occurred because of infection from a Tenckhoff catheter (used for peritoneal dialysis in people with renal failure), the catheter must be removed and dialysis via the peritoneum discontinued over the short or even long term. A switch to haemodialysis is generally required in these circumstances.

Intestinal neoplasms

LEARNING OBJECTIVE 3

Classify the major neoplasms of the intestines, and outline their characteristics.

LEARNING OBJECTIVE 4

Describe the pathophysiology of colon cancer.

Almost all tumours of the intestines occur in the large intestine (i.e. the colon). Tumours of the small intestine are very rare in humans and so will not be considered here. All of the common tumours of the large intestine begin as neoplastic growths of the cells of the epithelium.

In the developed world, cancer of the colon, also known as *colorectal cancer* or, simply, *'bowel cancer'*, is the most frequent malignancy of the digestive tract, and ranks among the four leading cancers, along with lung, breast and prostate cancers. According to recent Cancer Australia statistics, it is the second most common cause of cancer deaths. In Australia, 1 person in 19 (5.2%) risks being diagnosed with bowel cancer by 85 years of age, with a slightly higher risk for men (1 in 18) compared to women (1 in 21). The incidence and mortality rates are increased between the ages of 85–89 years old.

HYPERPLASTIC POLYPS

A *polyp* is a protrusion into the lumen of a hollow organ. Hyperplastic polyps are by far the most common type (90%) of polyp in the large intestine, and are found in most older people. These are almost always benign, composed of epithelial tissues, and less than 0.5 cm in diameter. Much larger hyperplastic polyps may have some potential to become malignant (see Figure 37.4).

ADENOMAS: PREMALIGNANT POLYPS

Most cancers (adenocarcinomas) of the colon develop from premalignant neoplasms known as **adenomas** (see Figure 37.5). Adenomas can occur anywhere in the colon, but are most commonly found in the rectum and sigmoid colon. Adenomas consist of epithelial cells that are dysplastic to some extent; that is, abnormal-looking under the microscope and presumably abnormal in various aspects of their behaviour, including a disturbance of growth control. The adenoma as a whole may be *pedunculated* (i.e. attached to the rest of the epithelium by a stalk) or *sessile* (flat).

Small adenomas are asymptomatic, whereas larger ones may cause bleeding. They all have malignant potential; that is, the cells of an adenoma have begun through successive mutations to accumulate oncogenes or to lose tumour suppressor genes (see the chapter 'Neoplasia'), setting them on the path to full-blown malignancy.

FAMILIAL ADENOMATOUS POLYPOSIS

Familial adenomatous polyposis is a rare condition, affecting about 1 in 10,000 people, and is inherited in an autosomal dominant fashion. It is caused by defects in the *adenomatous polyposis coli* (*APC*) gene, which in its normal form is a tumour suppressor gene. Those affected develop hundreds or thousands of adenomas of the colon in adolescence or early adulthood, some of which are bound to progress to cancer by middle age.

ADENOCARCINOMAS

The majority (70%) of **colon cancers** are located in the *rectum* and *sigmoid colon*. Almost all malignant tumours are *adenocarcinomas* that originate in the epithelium. Most develop from adenomas, while a minority arise from apparently normal areas of epithelium.

An accumulation of mutations is found in the progression from an adenoma to a fully malignant adenocarcinoma. A typical sequence involves:

- mutation of the *APC* tumour suppressor gene or inheritance of a defective *APC* allele
- mutation giving rise to a *K-ras* oncogene

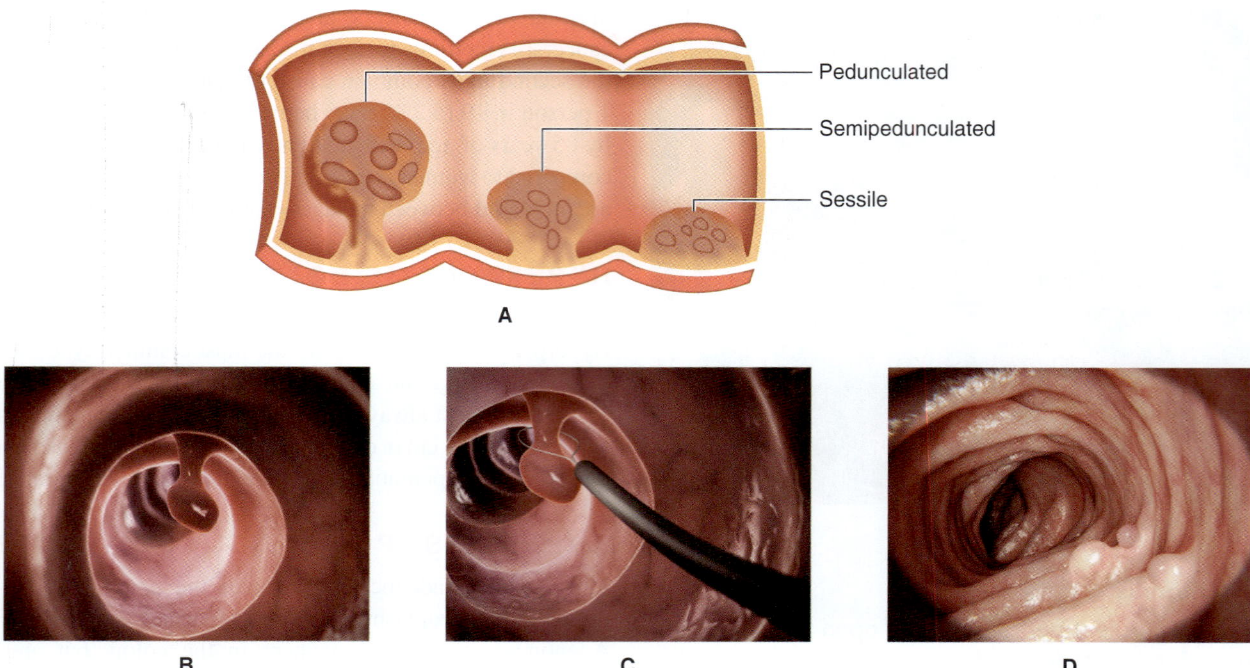

Figure 37.4

Hyperplastic polyps

(A) Common classification of polyps. (B) Endoscopic view of a pedunculated polyp. (C) Endoscopic loop removal of a peduculated polyp. (D) Endoscopic view of a sessile polyp.

Sources: (B) and (C) SciePro/Shutterstock; (D) Juan Gaertner/Shutterstock.

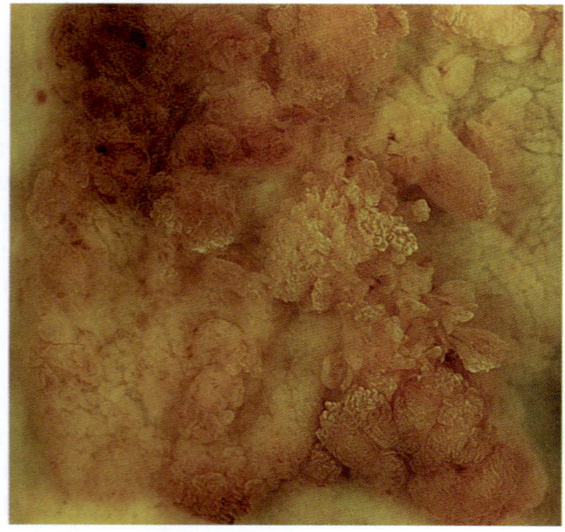

Figure 37.5

An adenoma of the colon

This adenoma can clearly be seen in an endoscopic image of the colon.

Source: Paul Fearn/Alamy Stock Photo.

- deletion of a 'deleted in colorectal cancer' (*DCC*) tumour suppressor gene
- deletion or inactivation of a *p53* tumour suppressor gene.

The known risk factors for colon cancer are: age, with a peak incidence at 68–72 years; gender, with a slightly higher risk for men; the presence of *large numbers of adenomas*, especially in familial adenomatous polyposis; and the presence of inherited *hereditary non-polyposis colon cancer (HNPCC) genes*. These are abnormal variants of genes for DNA 'proofreading' and repair. Their presence increases the likelihood that mutations will arise in many other genes, including proto-oncogenes and tumour suppressor genes, and predisposes the person to cancers of the colon, ovary, uterus and kidney.

The risk of colon cancer is also increased in people who have *ulcerative colitis* (see 'Chronic inflammatory bowel diseases' later in the chapter), in which chronic inflammation and tissue damage provoke a compensatory increase in the rate of mitosis among epithelial stem cells.

Specific mutagens have not been shown to contribute to colon cancer, despite a great deal of research on possible associations between diet and colon cancer. The constant regeneration of intestinal epithelial cells through mitosis in stem cells appears to provide ample opportunity for the emergence and accumulation of spontaneous mutations.

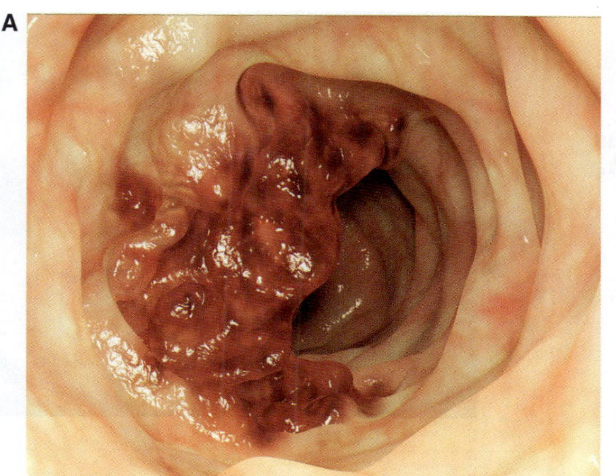

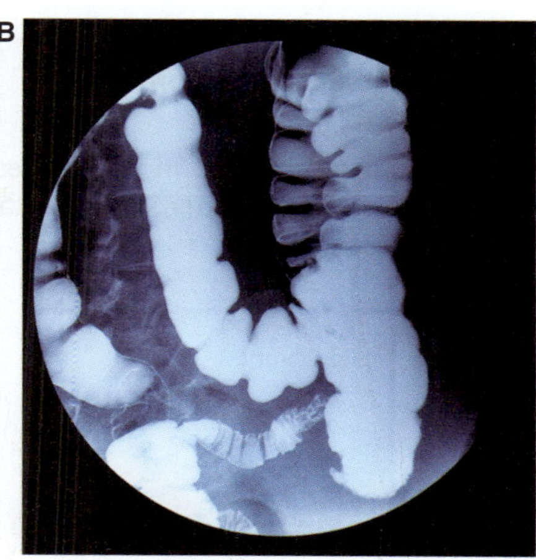

Figure 37.6

Transverse colon tumour

(A) Colonscopic view of an elevated tumour in the left side of the transverse colon.

(B) Fluoroscopic examination following barium enema demonstrating colon cancer. Note the reduced barium at the bottom of the image.

Sources: (A) Juan Gaertner/ Shutterstock; (B) Sutha Burawonk/Shutterstock.

AETIOLOGY AND PATHOPHYSIOLOGY

Chronic inflammation and immune dysfunction are strongly linked to neoplastic development. Significantly, tumour growth in the small intestines is relatively rare.

Tumours that arise in the proximal colon tend to grow by extending along one wall of the colon. Such tumours rarely cause obstruction, as the contents of the colon are liquid at this stage.

In contrast, a tumour arising in the distal colon tends to grow as a ring, causing constriction of the bowel with faecal obstruction (see Figure 37.6). The primary tumour will eventually invade the successive layers of the intestinal wall, possibly penetrating to the outer (serosal) surface (see Figure 37.7). It can spread to adjacent structures, and metastasise through lymph and blood to regional lymph nodes, the liver (see Figure 37.8), the lungs and bones, and many other sites, including the peritoneum.

Most colon cancers produce *carcinoembryonic antigen (CEA)*. This is a protein involved in cell adhesion that is produced in the fetus but is not usually found in adults. The production of CEA may simply reflect disorder in the internal regulation of tumour cells rather than an adaptation to their circumstances. The presence of CEA may be monitored in the blood of people who have been treated for colon cancer as a marker for its recurrence.

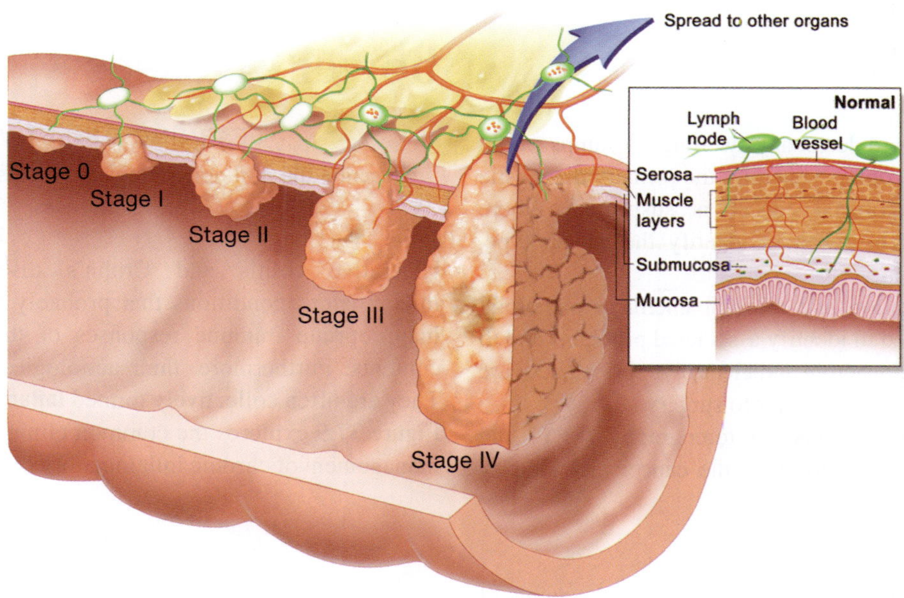

Figure 37.7

Stages of invasion through the intestinal wall

Stages of invasiveness of colon cancer from the lowest, stage 0, to the highest, stage IV.

Source: © 2005 Terese Winslow LLC, U.S. Govt. has certain rights.

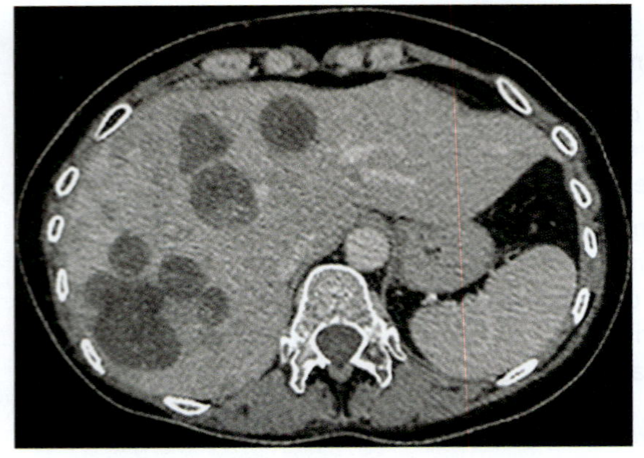

Figure 37.8

CT imaging showing colon cancer metastasis to the liver

The metastases show up in the images as shadows. There are numerous metastases in this person's liver.

Source: Centre Jean Perrin—ISM/Science Photo Library.

CLINICAL MANIFESTATIONS

Cancer of the colon is often asymptomatic in the early stages: the tumour may grow for years before diagnosis, by which time it may be incurable. Symptoms are usually caused by tumours that have reached an advanced stage. People may experience abdominal discomfort, change in bowel habits or pain. Advanced tumours are also responsible for fatigue, anorexia and weight loss. Less frequently, people will present with acute symptoms such as nausea, vomiting, pain and fever related to either obstruction or perforation, following which problems of infection by resident bacteria quickly develop.

When symptoms arise, they may be related to the location of the tumour. For example, a rectal cancer can cause blood to appear in the stool; however, bleeding in the ascending colon is not obvious and may only come to light because of the anaemia that results.

CLINICAL DIAGNOSIS AND MANAGEMENT

Diagnosis

A physical examination to detect any swellings or lumps would be conducted. Colonoscopy is generally the primary diagnostic intervention where colorectal cancer is suspected. Where possible, biopsies will be taken to identify the cancer type, differentiation and staging.

Full blood examination and relevant chemical pathology testing will be performed to identify associated problems and to measure CEA levels. If anaemia and electrolyte imbalances are found, they should be corrected prior to surgery.

CT scanning, positron emission tomography (PET) and MRI scanning may be used to stage the cancer and identify metastases.

Management

The stage of the cancer at diagnosis will determine the nature of management. If surgery is indicated, the extent of the cancer will dictate whether colectomy or colostomy is required. Surgery may be indicated even in palliative care situations to manage blood loss or assist with pain control.

Chemotherapy is a principal management intervention, and may be used in almost all stages of colon cancer, both before and after surgery. In addition to cytotoxic anticancer drugs, the use of immunomodifying agents is becoming more common in the treatment of colon cancer. These include angiogenesis inhibitors, which block the new blood vessel formation by the tumour, and monoclonal antibodies, such as cetuximab and bevacizumab. Radiotherapy may be used for rectal cancer, but it is not used as a matter of course in the management of colon cancer.

Other considerations in colon cancer include the evidence that diet influences the occurrence and recurrence of the cancer. Despite the absence of evidence for specific carcinogens from the diet that act on the intestine, a diet that is high in fresh fruit, vegetables and white meat may be preferable to one rich in red meat and highly processed foods. Reducing smoking and alcohol intake, and maintaining a healthy waist:hip ratio might also be beneficial.

Chronic inflammatory bowel diseases

LEARNING OBJECTIVE 5

Describe the pathophysiological processes in inflammatory bowel diseases.

Ulcerative colitis and Crohn's disease are long-term inflammatory conditions that probably have their origins in inappropriate immune responses of the intestines to their contents. Furthermore, their aetiologies are not understood. They are often collectively termed **inflammatory bowel disease**. Figure 37.9 explores the common clinical manifestations and management of chronic inflammatory diseases of the intestine.

LEARNING OBJECTIVE 6

Compare and contrast ulcerative colitis and Crohn's disease.

ULCERATIVE COLITIS

Aetiology and pathophysiology

In **ulcerative colitis**, it is thought that an abnormal activation of the immune processes leads to inflammation of the epithelium

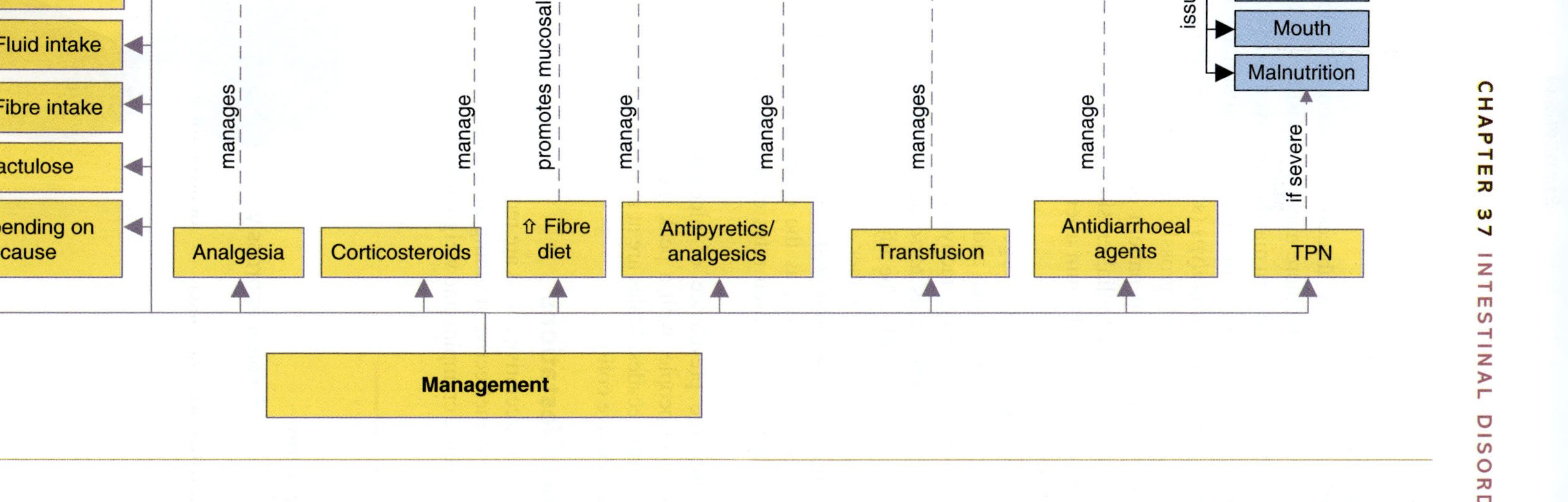

Figure 37.9

Clinical snapshot: Chronic inflammatory diseases of the intestines

↓ = decreased; ↑ = increased; GIT = gastrointestinal tract; TPN = total parenteral nutrition.

of the large intestine. This usually begins in the rectum and progresses proximally. Tissue layers other than the epithelium are not usually affected.

In the inflammatory process, abscesses, erosions and ulcers develop in the epithelium, and there may be a considerable loss of blood. Large areas of epithelium may be destroyed. Surviving patches that are left projecting from the damaged surface into the lumen are known as *pseudopolyps* (see Figure 37.10).

Ulcerative colitis is seen grossly in the colon at high magnification, with the typical pattern of pseudopolyps from severe inflammation and epithelial erosion. The pseudopolyps are remaining islands of epithelium after the bulk of the tissue has ulcerated away.

In the worst acute case, the large intestine may dilate and threaten to rupture, with signs and symptoms of systemic inflammatory response: fever, tachycardia, hypotension and leukocytosis. This is known as *toxic megacolon* and is life-threatening (see Figure 37.11). The adjective 'toxic' refers to the production of systemic effects rather than to any specific toxin.

In the long term, the likelihood that cancer will arise in the damaged area is increased, as the epithelium regenerates with a requirement for increased rates of mitosis in epithelial stem cells.

In Australia, the prevalence of ulcerative colitis is 334 cases per 100,000 people, with a peak incidence between the second and fourth decades. Males are at a slightly higher risk of developing ulcerative colitis.

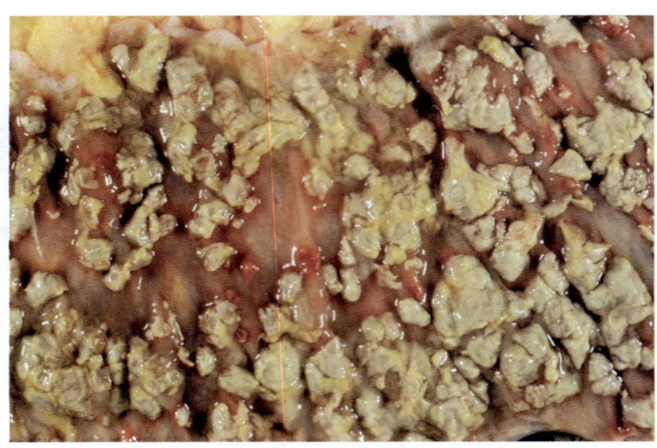

Figure 37.10

Pseudopolyps

Pseudopolyps visible in tissue following a colectomy for intractable chronic ulcerative colitis (CUC).

Source: CNRI/Science Photo Library.

Clinical manifestations

The symptoms of ulcerative colitis are rectal bleeding, diarrhoea and tenesmus (i.e. ineffective straining to defecate). The person may also experience cramping and weight loss. In severe disease, additional systemic symptoms may be experienced: there may be fever and, if the episode results in volume depletion, tachycardia and hypotension.

Clinical diagnosis and management

Diagnosis A full blood examination should be carried out and relevant chemical pathology tests investigated. These studies will often demonstrate anaemia and sometimes electrolyte imbalances. Together with blood studies, an investigation of stools

Figure 37.11

Toxic megacolon

In this condition, the colon is grossly distended.

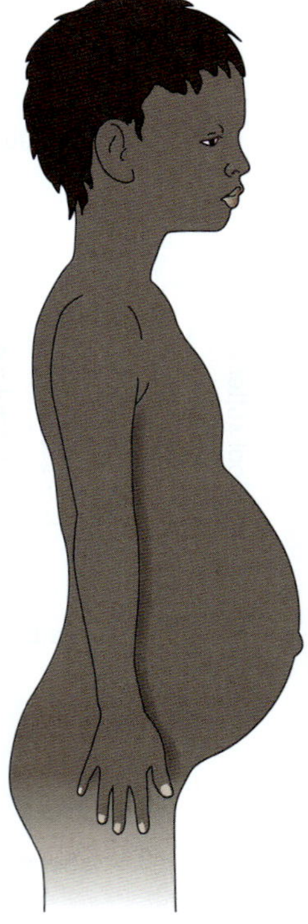

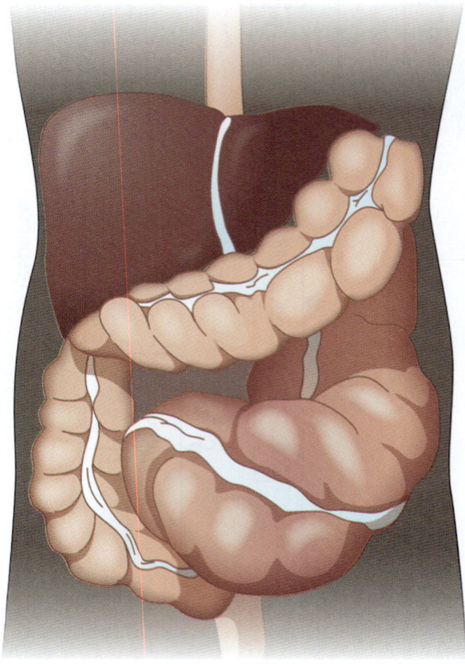

may be of use in confirming or ruling out other causes of the signs and symptoms.

Colonoscopy is the best imaging technique for diagnosing ulcerative colitis. Direct visualisation of the epithelium with biopsy of affected tissues will enable the severity of the disease to be assessed. X-rays may reveal megacolon or obstruction.

Management Treatment with the 5-aminosalicylates sulphasalazine, mesasalazine, balsalazide or olsalazine can be used in the treatment of this condition. The thiopurine immunosuppressants, mercaptopurine and azathioprine, are also useful in inducing remission. They are anti-inflammatory agents that act locally to inhibit the synthesis of prostaglandins. In acute episodes, corticosteroids may be used. Infliximab is a monoclonal antibody that blocks the cytokine tumour necrosis factor-α (TNF-α), which has a key role in autoimmune processes, or intravenous ciclosporin, can be effective. Collectively, these drugs can reduce bowel inflammation.

CROHN'S DISEASE

Crohn's disease may occur in any part of the digestive tract, from the mouth to the anus, but is most common in the ileum, the last part of the small intestine. Thus, it is also known as *regional ileitis* or *regional enteritis*.

Aetiology and pathophysiology

In Crohn's disease, inflammation occurs in all four layers of the intestinal wall (i.e. *transmural*). The *epithelium* develops ulcers that are initially very small, but soon extend as fissures to give a 'cobblestone' appearance to the luminal surface (see Figure 37.12).

The fissures may deepen to cause *perforations* of the intestinal wall, or form fistulas with nearby hollow organs or even with the skin. Abscesses may form around the anus (*perianal abscesses*).

The three other layers—*subepithelium*, *muscularis* and *serosa*—become *oedematous* as inflammation proceeds, then *fibrotic* (scarred) as the damaged tissues attempt to repair themselves. In the inflamed tissues, infiltrates of lymphocytes can be seen, and granulomas (see the chapter 'Immune disorders') are often present, indicating chronic cell-mediated immune processes. The affected region of the intestine becomes thickened, narrow and rigid. Affected regions tend to be separated by healthy areas; hence, there is a characteristic alternation of healthy tissue and *'skip lesions'*.

In Australia, the prevalence of Crohn's disease is 306 cases per 100,000 people, with women at a greater risk. Most are diagnosed before the age of 25 years. Crohn's disease carries an increased risk of colon cancer, but this is considerably lower than in ulcerative colitis.

Clinical manifestations

The symptoms of Crohn's disease are highly variable, and may include general malaise and lethargy, anorexia, abdominal pain, fever, malabsorption, nutritional deficiency, diarrhoea, bowel obstruction, abscesses and fistulas. There is a typical pattern of remission and relapse, but the disease will be present for a lifetime.

Clinical diagnosis and management

Diagnosis X-rays with barium contrast can help in assessment of the severity and the extent of disease. Colonoscopy allows biopsy and direct observations of the epithelium and lesions. Other imaging techniques, such as CT, MRI and ultrasonography, may also be useful.

Full blood examination and assessment of chemical pathology will often show anaemia and low levels of iron and folate. Leukocytes are usually elevated, as are markers of inflammation (erythrocyte sedimentation rate [ESR] and CRP). Measurement of the concentration of β-hCG should be performed in all women of childbearing age to exclude ectopic pregnancy as the cause of abdominal pain.

Management Immunomodifying agents, such as corticosteroids and the thiopurines (such as azathioprine), can control the inflammatory response. Adding allopurinol to the regimen can lower the dose requirement of thiopurine

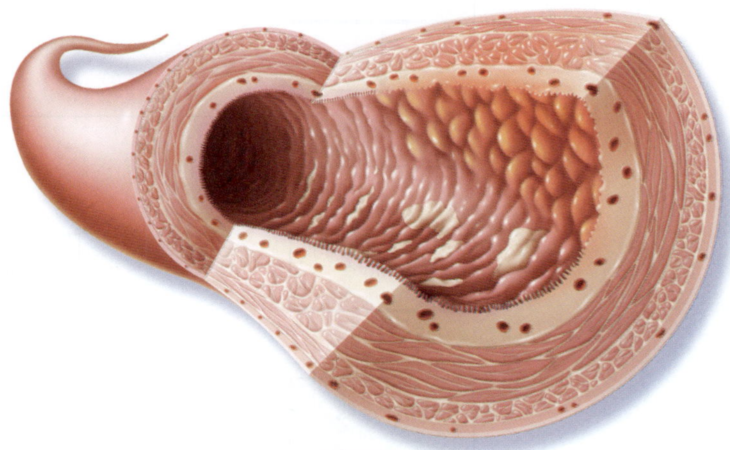

Figure 37.12

Cobblestone appearance of lumen wall in Crohn's disease

Source: JACOPIN/BSIP/Alamy Stock Photo.

therapy. Methotrexate is considered a useful alternative as an immunosuppressant. The use of agents that inhibit lymphocyte activation and control cytokine release—such as infliximab, adalimumab, ustekinumab or vedolizumab—may also be considered.

Symptom relief is important, and antidiarrhoeal agents can assist with diarrhoea, and antispasmodics may reduce the pain from abdominal cramping.

Intestinal obstruction

LEARNING OBJECTIVE 7

Outline the major causes of intestinal obstruction, and its pathophysiological consequences.

AETIOLOGY AND PATHOPHYSIOLOGY

Obstruction of the intestines is potentially life-threatening. There may be a *structural cause* of obstruction that is internal, such as a faecalith in the appendix, or external, as in the compression of a loop of intestine in an incarcerated hernia. Even a partial obstruction may be dangerous if it closes off a part of the intestinal lumen, as happens in appendicitis and diverticulitis. Obstruction may also arise from *'functional' disorders* in which the smooth muscle of the intestine fails to induce peristalsis.

In this section, we will address the major structural causes of obstruction in the small and large intestines, and then examine the causes of functional obstruction or *ileus*. The consequences of an intestinal obstruction have been described for acute appendicitis, and may be reviewed in Figure 37.13.

OBSTRUCTIONS AFFECTING THE SMALL INTESTINE

The most common structural disorders of the small intestine that lead to obstruction are *hernias* and *adhesions*, both of which cause compression from the outside. Much less often, the obstruction is caused by *intussusception* or *volvulus*. Figure 37.14 explores the common clinical manifestations and management of intestinal obstructions.

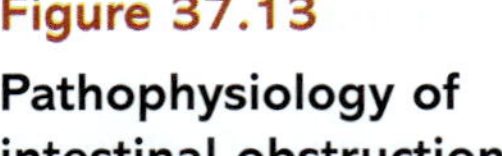

Figure 37.13

Pathophysiology of intestinal obstruction

Source: R. Arwas.

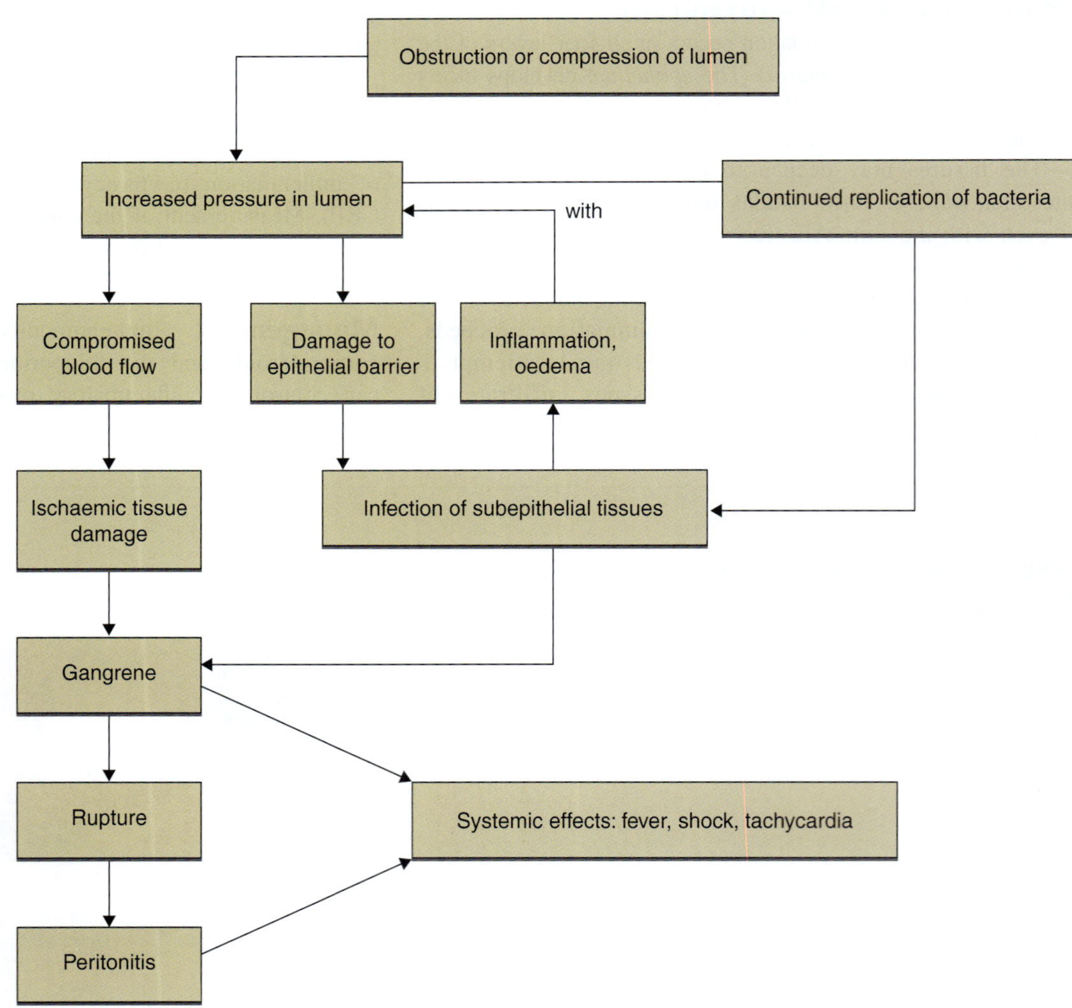

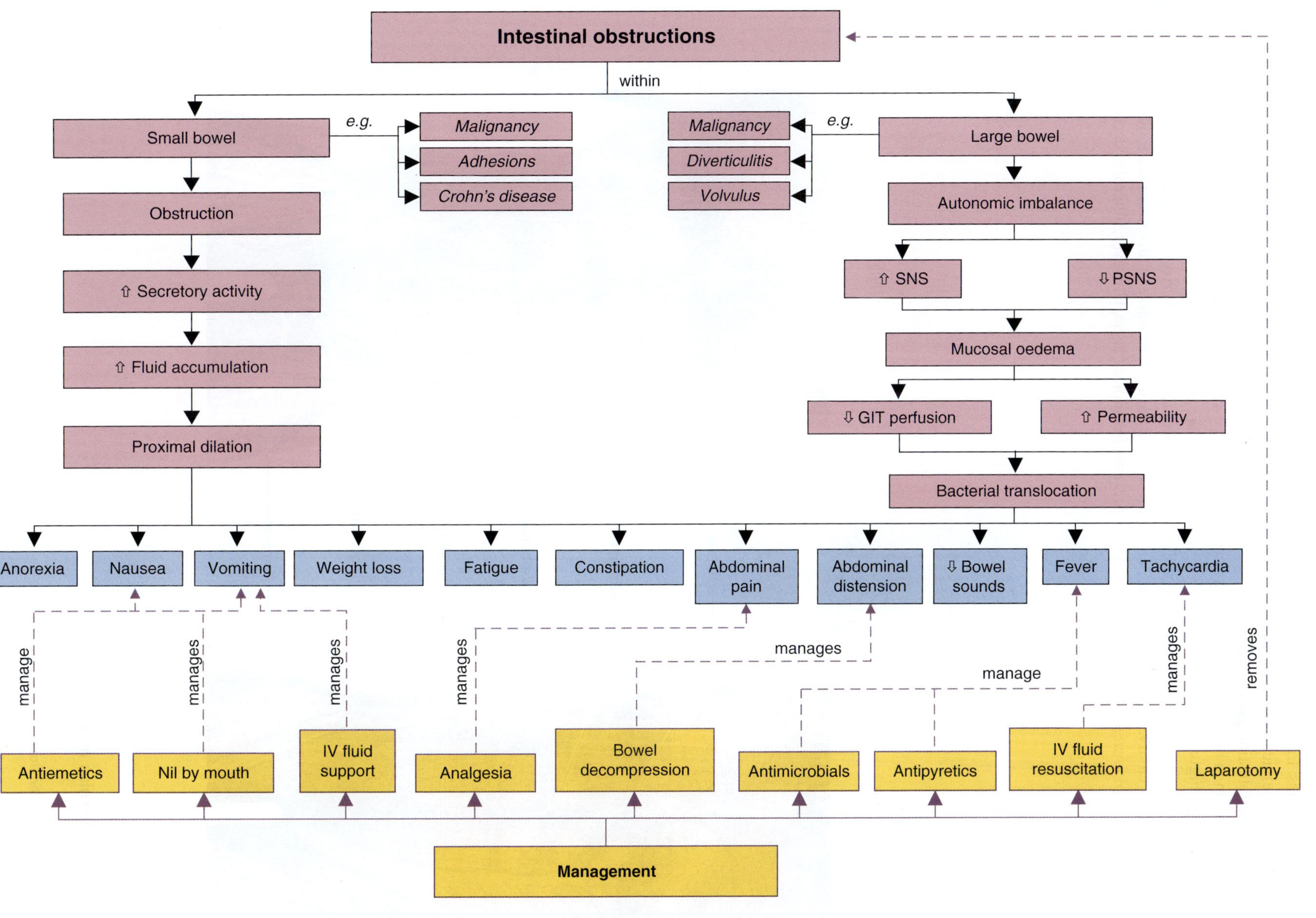

Figure 37.14

Clinical snapshot: Intestinal obstructions

↓ = decreased; ↑ = increased; GIT = gastrointestinal tract; IV = intravenous; PSNS = parasympathetic nervous system; SNS = sympathetic nervous system.

Hernias

Aetiology and pathophysiology A **hernia** occurs when a loop of intestine pushes through a weakness in the muscular wall of the abdominopelvic cavity. The most common site for a hernia of the small intestine is the inguinal ring of males, but they may also develop in other locations, such as the navel (an umbilical hernia) (see Figure 37.15).

In an *uncomplicated hernia*, the loop may spontaneously retract into the abdominopelvic cavity. If this cannot happen, the intestine is said to be *incarcerated* (see Figure 37.16A), and may be compressed by the encircling muscle wall, causing obstruction of its lumen. If the compression is sufficiently severe to squeeze veins and compromise blood flow, the hernia is said to be *strangulated* (see Figure 37.16B). In such cases, ischaemic damage and gangrene will progress rapidly.

Clinical manifestations Although pain and local deformity are common, symptoms of hernia differ, depending on the location, cause and severity. Asymptomatic hernias may be discovered during the course of an examination when the person presents for another issue. However, if hernias become painful or

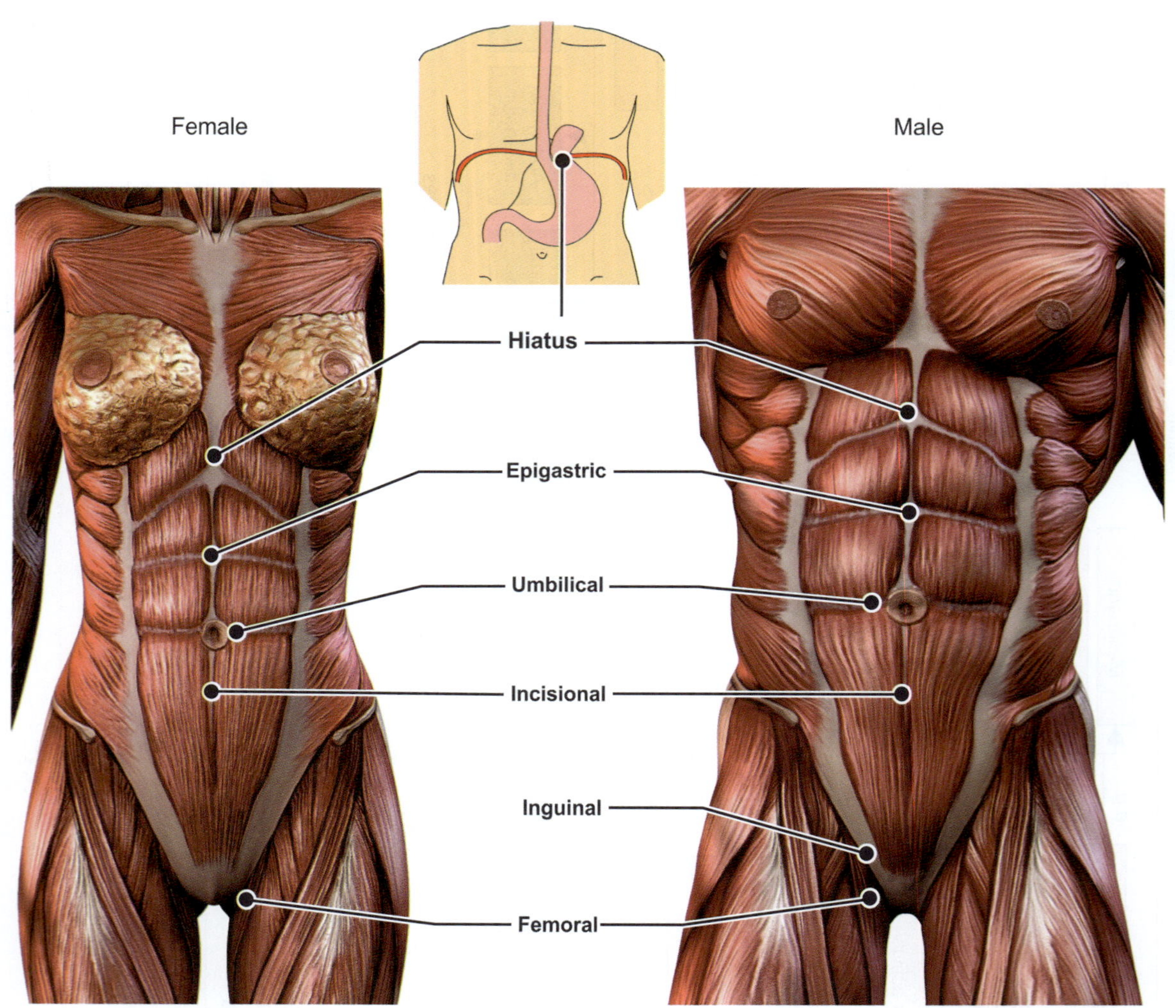

Figure 37.15

Hernia locations

Common locations where hernias may develop.

Source: Adapted from © SciePro/Shutterstock.

Figure 37.16

Types of hernia

(A) Non-reducible hernia.
(B) Strangulated hernia.

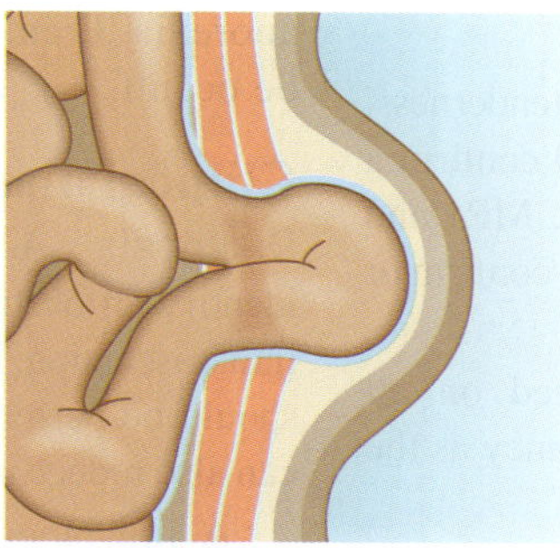

A. A **non-reducible hernia** results from the intestines becoming trapped within the abdominal wall, unable to be pushed back.

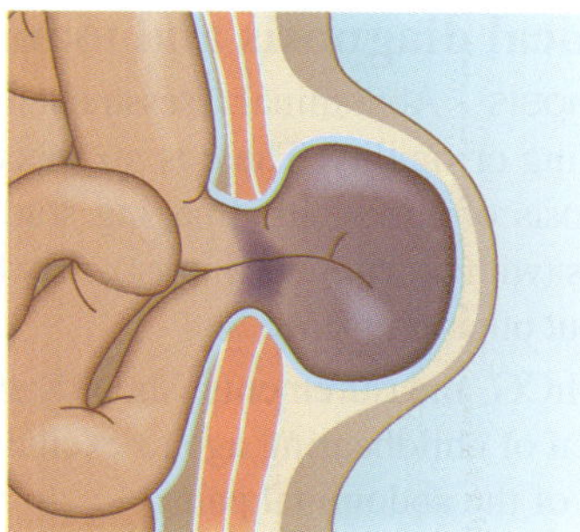

B. A **strangulated hernia** results from the intestines becoming trapped within the abdominal wall, compromising vascular supply to the trapped bowel tissue.

more serious, signs of incarceration (nausea, vomiting and pain) or strangulation (signs of sepsis, including tachycardia and fever) develop and intervention becomes critical.

Clinical diagnosis and management

Diagnosis Physical assessment is the primary method of detecting hernia. Full blood examination and chemical pathology tests are not diagnostic, but may be useful in confirming or ruling out other problems. X-ray, ultrasound, CT scans and endoscopy may be useful in diagnosis. In a serious episode of hernia, measurements of ESR and CRP suggest the presence of inflammation somewhere in the body.

Management Hernia reduction may be attempted manually with adequate sedation. Alternatively, surgery may be required to repair the hernia. Often, patches are surgically implanted to prevent the bowel from re-entering the muscular defect. If the hernia is strangulated, the hernia should not be manually reduced and surgery is indicated. If surgery is delayed, tissue loss will occur as a result of necrosis, which may ultimately cause peritonitis and complicate recovery.

Adhesions

Aetiology and pathophysiology *Scar tissue*, or *adhesions*, may form in the abdominopelvic cavity after abdominal surgery, after peritonitis or during the course of Crohn's disease. Such tissue growing between the organs of the cavity, or between the organs and the cavity walls, may cause obstruction by trapping loops of intestine, with consequences similar to those described for hernias, or by causing kinks in the intestine that obstruct the normal flow of intestinal contents (see Figure 37.17).

Clinical manifestations Adhesions are generally asymptomatic unless bowel obstruction occurs. A person may then present with abdominal pain, anorexia and vomiting.

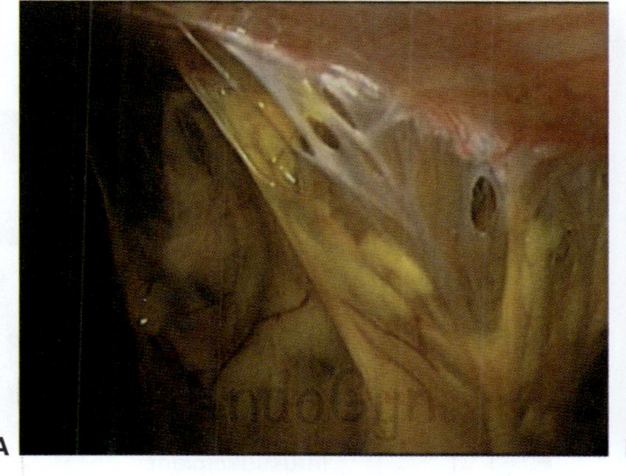

A

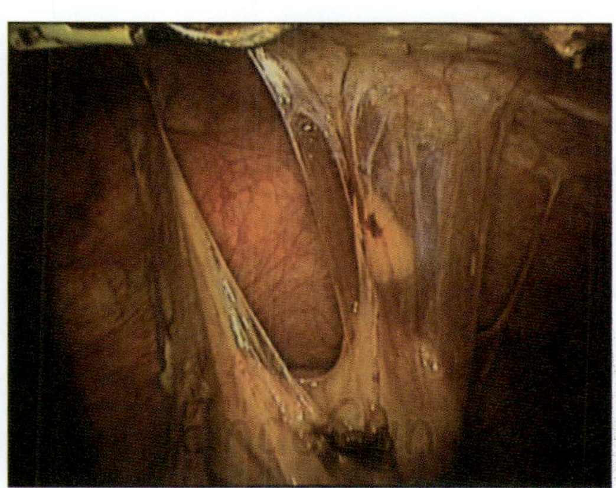

B

Figure 37.17

Kink in the intestines due to adhesions

Bowel adhesions in the right lower quadrant of a 25-year-old female with a previous history of ruptured appendix at 7 years of age.

(A) Bowel and omental adhesions. (B) Adhesions with fixation to the abdominal wall.

Source: © Dr Daniel Kruschinski/EndoGyn—Online Atlas on Adhesions.

Clinical diagnosis and management

Diagnosis Abdominal assessment may demonstrate tenderness, guarding or rigidity. There is no specific test that will confirm a diagnosis of adhesions. Imaging studies, such as CT, MRI and X-rays (with or without contrast), may be carried out to confirm or rule out other problems.

β-hCG measurements should also be performed on all women of childbearing age to exclude ectopic pregnancy as the cause of the abdominal pain.

Management Management of adhesions is complicated, because they can develop after surgery. Therefore, interventions to remove adhesions may themselves cause further problems. In the management of bowel obstructions, the person should have fasted, and then the stomach and small bowel should be decompressed through the insertion of a nasogastric tube. If the individual's condition deteriorates with a risk of perforation and peritonitis, surgery will be required.

Intussusception

Aetiology and pathophysiology In this rare disorder, the intestine folds in on itself like a telescope being closed (see Figure 37.18). The cause is probably a protrusion of some sort into the lumen, which snags on an adjacent part of the internal surface during a peristaltic contraction. Within the telescoped region, the lumen is narrowed and the blood vessels are squeezed.

Clinical manifestations If **intussusception** occurs, symptoms of obstruction will develop. A person may present with abdominal pain in paroxysms approximately 15 minutes apart. They may also complain of vomiting and anorexia. Frank blood may be visible in the stool, or it may be occult.

Clinical diagnosis and management

Diagnosis A plain abdominal X-ray may be undertaken, to identify an obstruction. Ultrasound is useful in the diagnosis of intussusception. If there are no signs of peritonitis, a barium enema should be performed. Although this is an imaging procedure, it can also reduce intussusceptions in a significant number of people.

A full blood examination and chemical pathology testing may help to identify other problems, but results will not be diagnostic for intussusception.

β-hCG measurements should also be performed in all women of childbearing age to exclude ectopic pregnancy as the cause of the abdominal pain.

Management If a barium enema fails to reduce the intussusception or perforation occurs, surgery will be required to reduce the risks of necrosis and peritonitis.

Volvulus

Volvulus is the *twisting of a loop* of intestine through 360 degrees. This occludes its lumen and collapses its blood vessels, with consequences as described for a strangulated hernia (see Figure 37.19).

OBSTRUCTIONS AFFECTING THE LARGE INTESTINE

Diverticular disease

In the large intestine, the major cause of obstruction is cancer (see 'Intestinal neoplasms' later in the chapter). Problems of obstruction may also occur in **diverticula**, which are projections

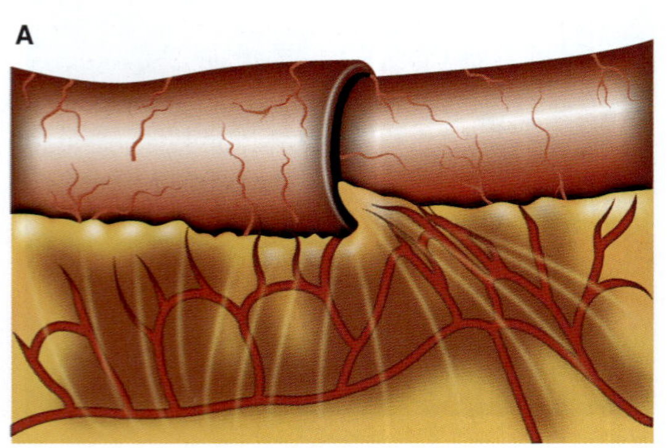

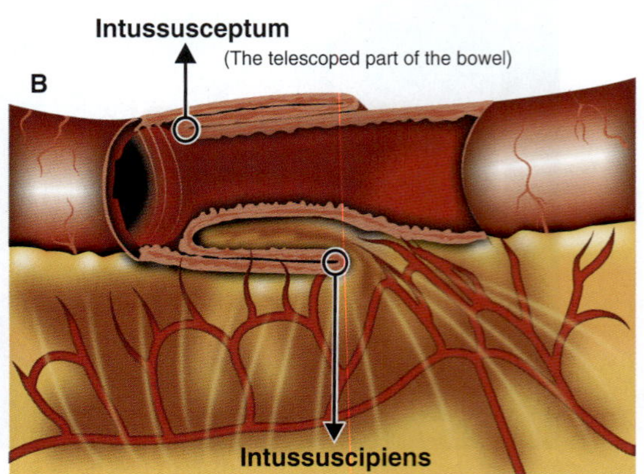

Figure 37.18

Intussusception

(A) Telescoping of the intestine into itself results in a narrowing of the lumen and potential compromising of blood flow.

(B) A cross-section of an intussusception showing the intussuscipiens, which is the region of intestine affected in intussusception, and the intussusceptum, which is the portion of telescoped intestine.

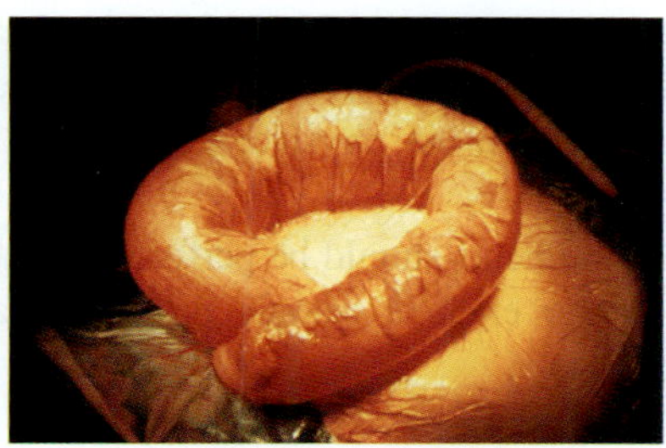

Figure 37.19
Volvulus
The intestinal area has become severely twisted, obstructing the lumen and blood vessels.

Source: DELALANDE/BSIP SA/Alamy Stock Photo.

of the large intestinal wall and lumen (see Figure 37.20). The disease process in one such structure, the appendix, has already been described.

Aetiology and pathophysiology Diverticula may form in the intestines of people who eat a low-fibre diet, form small, hard faeces and so have to generate high pressures in the intestine to move them along. Such high pressures induce a structural change in the colon wall, causing a ballooning out of the mucosa/submucosa through a defect in the muscle wall: this tends to happen in areas where the muscle wall is weakened by the passage of blood vessels through it. It is also more likely to happen in the distal parts of the large intestine, as faeces there are harder and more pressure is required to move them. The resultant structural change appears as a pocket in the colon wall.

Factors believed to contribute to the development of diverticula include *diet*, *changes to the microbiome*, *genetic susceptibility* and *poor colon motility*. There is evidence of a microscopic *inflammatory response* at the site associated with lymphocytic infiltration and the release of pro-inflammatory cytokines.

Diverticula of this nature are present in many older people who consume a low-fibre diet. The condition is termed *diverticulosis*, and is usually asymptomatic. However, as in appendicitis, infection by resident bacteria may occur if the lumen of the diverticulum becomes blocked, perhaps by a faecalith. This is **diverticulitis**. It is sometimes known as 'left-sided appendicitis', as diverticula are more common in the distal (i.e. left side) of the large intestine.

Diverticulitis usually resolves spontaneously, but may, in the worst cases, cause problems like those of acute appendicitis. Because diverticulosis is usually asymptomatic, and diverticulitis may develop and resolve spontaneously in people with diverticula, the conditions may collectively be termed *diverticular disease*.

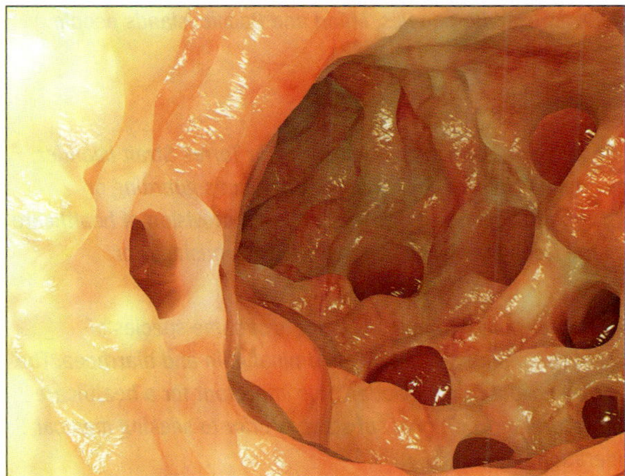

Figure 37.20
Diverticula
Colon with diverticula.

Source: Juan Gaertner/Shutterstock.

Clinical manifestations Someone experiencing diverticulitis may present with left lower quadrant pain. However, symptoms vary, depending on the location and severity of the disease. The person may also complain of nausea and vomiting, changes in bowel habits, diarrhoea and bloating. An abdominal mass may be palpable; however, this is unusual. In severe cases where perforation occurs, the person may present with peritonitis and sepsis.

Clinical diagnosis and management

Diagnosis Imaging techniques such as CT may be useful in confirming a diagnosis, especially when contrast medium is used. A full blood examination and chemical pathology testing to identify other problems may be performed, but results will not be diagnostic for diverticular disease.

β-hCG measurements should also be performed in all women of childbearing age to exclude ectopic pregnancy as the cause of the abdominal pain.

Management Conservative management is undertaken in most cases of uncomplicated diverticulitis. It is usually managed using a combination of increasing the fibre content of the diet, antimicrobials, spasmolytics, the anti-inflammatory agent mesasalazine and probiotics.

A regimen of antimicrobials and a clear fluid diet is effective in mild acute episodes, with normal diet slowly reintroduced as tolerated. If there are findings of peritonitis, persistent pain or marked leukocytosis, the person should be admitted to hospital. Analgesia and antimicrobials are important in the management of complicated diverticulitis, but, in the event of peritonitis, surgery will be required to eliminate intraperitoneal foci of infection and reduce the potential for sepsis.

FUNCTIONAL INTESTINAL OBSTRUCTION

Aetiology and pathophysiology

Intestinal motility may be reduced and the contents of the intestines may fail to move along even though there is no physical obstruction. This is known as **ileus**. (The terms *paralytic ileus*, *adynamic ileus* and *pseudo-obstruction* are all synonymous with 'ileus', although, confusingly, the term 'mechanical ileus' is sometimes used to refer to a physical obstruction.) Ileus is the consequence of a failure of the peristaltic contractions of the smooth muscle of the intestinal wall. Fluid and gas accumulate in the intestines, and the abdomen may become distended and tender.

The most common cause is abdominal surgery, after which ileus develops for a few days. In such cases, smooth muscle activity may be temporarily inhibited through neural reflexes. Less frequently, ileus may result from conditions such as systemic infection, hypokalaemia, kidney disease, peritonitis, spinal cord injury or ischaemia of the intestines. In the latter case, the grave problems of necrosis, gangrene and potential rupture may occur.

Clinical manifestations

As with all types of intestinal obstruction, a person may present with abdominal pain, vomiting and anorexia.

Clinical diagnosis and management

Diagnosis On physical examination, the abdomen may be distended and bowel sounds reduced or absent. An X-ray may demonstrate gas dilation in the small or large intestine. Other imaging studies, such as CT, MRI or ultrasound, may help to confirm or rule out physical obstruction as the cause of the problem.

β-hCG measurements should be performed in all women of childbearing age to exclude ectopic pregnancy as the cause of the abdominal pain.

Management The person should remain nil by mouth until the ileus has resolved. Gastrointestinal motility can be stimulated by encouraging mobilisation, and also by chewing gum.

Depending on the cause, an ileus may resolve with little or no intervention. In the meantime, symptom relief should be undertaken. It may be found that non-steroidal anti-inflammatory agents and the placement of a nasogastric tube may provide sufficient pain relief. Care should be taken to avoid medications that might exacerbate the ileus. For example, drugs such as opioids reduce motility. Note that surgery will not correct an ileus, but may cause it.

INDIGENOUS HEALTH FAST FACTS AND CULTURAL CONSIDERATIONS

FAST FACTS

- *Hospitalisation rates for gastroenteritis in Aboriginal and Torres Strait Islander children under 2 years of age are 11 times higher than in non-Indigenous children of the same age.*
- *The incidence of gastroenteritis hospitalisations in Māori children under 2 years of age is slightly less (0.89:1) than in European New Zealanders.*
- *The incidence of gastroenteritis hospitalisations in Pacific Islands children under 2 years of age is approximately 1.5 times more than in European New Zealanders, and slightly higher than for Māori children.*
- *Aboriginal and Torres Strait Islander infants and children were hospitalised with rotavirus gastroenteritis 3–5 times more commonly compared to non-Indigenous infants and children.*
- *Aboriginal and Torres Strait Islander peoples tend to have lower rates of stage I colorectal cancer, but higher rates of locally advanced or metastatic cancers compared to non-Indigenous Australians.*
- *The incidence of inflammatory bowel disease is lower in Aboriginal and Torres Strait Islander peoples, Māori and Pacific Islands people compared to Caucasian people.*

CULTURAL CONSIDERATIONS

- *The expression of abdominal pain may not be obvious to culturally naïve healthcare professionals. An Aboriginal or Torres Strait Islander person may choose not to discuss it, may become withdrawn and not exhibit common signs of abdominal pain, such as guarding or grimacing, or may even be embarrassed about the topic. To remove barriers in communication and assessment, the provision of healthcare providers of the same gender should always be attempted if at all possible, as the issue may be considered women's business or men's business.*
- *Traditionally, Aboriginal and Torres Strait Islander peoples have used pounded and/or boiled trunk core or roots of some species of pandanus trees (Pandanus spiralis—screw pine) for the treatment of a number of complaints, including abdominal pain and diarrhoea. The oil appears to possess analgesic and antispasmodic properties, and the roots may have a diuretic action. It is important for a healthcare professional to determine whether their client may have taken any prescribed, natural or traditional substances prior to seeking medical assistance for an acute abdominal pain, as drug interactions may be a consideration.*

Sources: Data from National Cancer Control Indicators (2018); Simpson et al. (2017); Wet Tropics Management Authority (WTMA) (2017).

CHILDREN AND ADOLESCENTS

- The largest number of hospitalisations in Australia and New Zealand for gastrointestinal infections occur in children aged 5 years and younger, with most of these in children aged under 2 years.
- Rotavirus is responsible for approximately 50% of gastroenteritis infections in children. Rotavirus vaccination programs have greatly reduced the hospitalisation rates for rotavirus infection.
- The incidence of Crohn's disease is increasing in the Australian paediatric community, but is rare in children under the age of 5 years.
- Intussusception is most common in infants and children of a couple of months to approximately 2 years of age.

OLDER ADULTS

- Colorectal cancer is common in older adults, with peak incidence rates in those of 68–72 years of age.
- The incidence of inflammatory bowel diseases in older adults is increasing.
- Age-related changes to the small and large intestine—such as muscle atrophy, reduced mucus secretion, decreased elasticity and reduced perception of distension of the rectal wall—can contribute to the diminishing gastrointestinal function seen in older adults. Some of these changes may predispose the person to gastrointestinal pathology.

KEY CLINICAL ISSUES

- Gastroenteritis is highly contagious, and requires appropriate and consistent infection control measures to prevent its spread. Families should also be educated about infection control procedures, as well as how to avoid contamination and spread through regular hand-washing techniques, and good personal hygiene and food preparation behaviours.
- Severe vomiting and diarrhoea can become dangerous in infants and older adults, as they may result in fluid and electrolyte imbalances. Undertake comprehensive physical assessments and hydration status regularly to ensure that dehydration or electrolyte imbalances do not develop. Aggressive management of fluid deficits may be required earlier in infants and older people compared to in other age groups.
- Colorectal screening is available from national government sources. Older people who match the criteria of the program should be encouraged to participate.
- People who present with blood in the stools, abdominal pain and changes in their bowel habits require clinical investigations.
- Inflammatory diseases of the bowel can cause significant discomfort, pain and embarrassment. Encourage anyone affected to seek assistance with the management of these diseases, as they can result in issues of malabsorption, and may even increase the risk of colorectal cancer in the long term.

CHAPTER REVIEW

- Infection by a range of *viral*, *bacterial* and *protozoal pathogens* may cause acute diarrhoea. The main danger associated with diarrhoeal disease is *dehydration*.
- *Resident bacteria* of the intestinal lumen may cause disease if their *ecological balance is upset*, if they *find their way into other parts of the body* or if the *intestines become obstructed*.
- *Tumours* in the small intestines are rare. Tumours of the large intestine originate in the epithelium. Benign, premalignant and malignant tumours are common, especially with increasing age. Detection of premalignant tumours is the key to prevention of malignant disease.
- *Chronic inflammatory diseases* of the intestines are believed to originate from inappropriate immune responses of the intestines to their contents. These diseases cannot be cured, but symptoms can be managed and the person monitored for the development of further disease, such as colon cancer.
- *Intestinal obstruction* may rapidly lead to ischaemic tissue damage and infection by resident bacteria, and is life-threatening. The cause is usually structural, as in the case of a strangulated hernia.

REVIEW QUESTIONS

1. Which major pathogens cause infectious diarrhoea in developed countries and in developing countries?
2. What are the modes of action of these pathogens?
3. Which measures are appropriate, and which are inappropriate, in the management of acute infectious diarrhoea?
4. In what ways may the normal bacterial flora of the digestive tract act as opportunistic pathogens?
5. What are the consequences of obstruction of the lumen of the appendix?
6. What is peritonitis, and how does it arise?

7 What are the similarities and the differences between hyperplastic polyps of the large intestine and adenomas?

8 What are the similarities and the differences between adenomas and adenocarcinomas of the large intestine?

9 How do the clinical manifestations of colon cancer arise from events at the cellular and tissue levels?

10 Which intestinal tissues are damaged in ulcerative colitis and in Crohn's disease?

11 What are the clinical manifestations of ulcerative colitis and Crohn's disease?

12 Explain how intestinal obstruction affects the flow of blood, and the activities of resident bacteria, in the affected region.

13 What are the consequences of intestinal obstruction for the body overall?

14 What are the major causes of intestinal obstruction?

15 What is diverticular disease?

HEALTH PROFESSIONAL CONNECTIONS

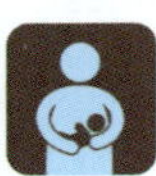

Midwives Severe vomiting and diarrhoea presents a significant risk to neonates. Irrespective of the cause, a thorough assessment should be undertaken to determine the degree of dehydration. Signs of dehydration in a neonate include a sunken fontanelle, crying without tears, decreased urine output, lethargy, and cool and dry skin. Although principles such as 'rooming-in' (where a neonate is kept in the same room as the mother) and improved hygiene practices have decreased the transmission of infectious agents compared with pathogenic spread in communal nurseries, infectious gastrointestinal diseases remain a problem in the community.

Common causes of diarrhoea include bacterial or viral infection, and the incorrect preparation of formula, leading to osmotic disturbance within the digestive tract. Other less common causes of diarrhoea include allergies and enzyme deficiencies. Parents should be taught the signs of dehydration in neonates, and be encouraged to seek help early when concerned about excess fluid loss. New parents also need to be educated about the characteristics of a newborn's stool. Frequently, neonates will pass soft (sometimes yellow) faeces several times a day. A change in a neonate's normal bowel habit should be considered, and investigation and intervention should occur if the baby has signs of failure to thrive. If a baby shows signs of dehydration, the mother should be encouraged to continue breastfeeding, and supplementation with oral rehydration solutions may be beneficial. However, urgent medical review is required if deterioration continues, and in extreme and prolonged situations, enteral or even parenteral nutrition may be required. It is imperative that parents do not attempt to medicate their neonate or child with antidiarrhoeal medications. These medications are not suitable for children under 12 years of age.

Nutritionists/Dieticians Diet and nutrition professionals are often consulted about digestive health. Although specific requirements will be determined following individualised consultations, some general principles can be followed. Diet can influence the production of gas, leading to abdominal bloating and flatulence, so the person may benefit from dietary modification. Nutrient malabsorption in intestinal diseases, such as Crohn's disease, ulcerative colitis or irritable bowel syndrome, may result in inadequate nutrition. Supplementation of specific vitamins and minerals may be appropriate in a wide range of circumstances; for example, zinc may promote wound healing after trauma or surgery.

CASE STUDY

Mr Paul Bruner (UR number 311468) is an 86-year-old man who presented with abdominal pain and a palpable mass. He has a history of weight loss, fatigue, anaemia and exertional dyspnoea. His stool was tested and was haemoccult. On examination he had an ill-defined right lower quadrant mass, which did not move with respiration. An ultrasound and CT (with contrast) scan confirmed the presence of a mass. Mr Bruner has begun to vomit, and his abdominal pain is increasing. His observations are as follows:

Temperature	Heart rate	Respiration rate	Blood pressure	SpO_2
38.4°C	88	26	150/86	96% (RA*)

*RA = room air.

Blood has been taken for full blood examination, chemical pathology tests and culture. In view of his current symptoms, Mr Bruner will have a laparotomy today. His pathology results are as follows:

HAEMATOLOGY

Patient location:	Ward 3	**UR:**	311468		
Consultant:	Smith	**NAME:**	Bruner		
		Given name:	Paul	**Sex:**	M
		DOB:	12/12/XX	**Age:**	86

Time collected	09:23
Date collected	XX/XX
Year	XXXX
Lab #	2465243

FULL BLOOD COUNT		UNITS	REFERENCE RANGE
Haemoglobin	94	g/L	115–160
White cell count	13.4	$\times 10^9$/L	4.0–11.0
Platelets	135	$\times 10^9$/L	140–400
Haematocrit	0.31		0.33–0.47
Red cell count	3.58	$\times 10^{12}$/L	3.80–5.20
Reticulocyte count	1.2	%	0.2–2.0
MCV	82	fL	80–100
Neutrophils	9.1	$\times 10^9$/L	2.00–8.00
Lymphocytes	3.45	$\times 10^9$/L	1.00–4.00
Monocytes	0.51	$\times 10^9$/L	0.10–1.00
Eosinophils	0.40	$\times 10^9$/L	< 0.60
Basophils	0.14	$\times 10^9$/L	< 0.20
ESR	17	mm/h	< 12

BIOCHEMISTRY

Patient location:	Ward 3	**UR:**	311468		
Consultant:	Smith	**NAME:**	Bruner		
		Given name:	Paul	**Sex:**	M
		DOB:	12/12/XX	**Age:**	86

Time collected	09:23
Date collected	XX/XX
Year	XXXX
Lab #	34576438

ELECTROLYTES		UNITS	REFERENCE RANGE
Sodium	136	mmol/L	135–145
Potassium	3.2	mmol/L	3.5–5.2
Chloride	97	mmol/L	95–110
Bicarbonate	23	mmol/L	22–32
Glucose (random)	3.5	mmol/L	3.5–7.7
Iron	5	µmol/L	11–30

CRITICAL THINKING

1 What genetic, environmental and lifestyle risks are associated with colon cancer? Use this information to generate questions that should be asked in assessing Mr Bruner's colon cancer risk.
2 The team made a decision not to perform a barium enema. What is the concern? What information supports this decision?
3 Consider Mr Bruner's history and presentation. What indicators suggest that he may have either an obstruction or a bowel perforation?
4 If a bowel resection is required and Mr Bruner has a right hemicolectomy, is there a risk that he could end up with short bowel syndrome or a malabsorption issue?
5 What other support is required for Mr Bruner following his right hemicolectomy? Identify all of the interventions required to care for him, considering all of the relevant biopsychosocial aspects of his case.
6 Australia has a bowel cancer screening program. Is Mr Bruner eligible to participate in this program? Explain.

BIBLIOGRAPHY

Australian Institute of Health and Welfare (AIHW) (2022). *Australia's health, 2022.* Australia's Health series No. 18. Canberra: AIHW. https://www.aihw.gov.au/reports-data/australias-health.

Bauldoff, G., Gubrud-Howe, P.M., Carno, M.-A., Levett-Jones, T., Hales, M., Berry, K.,... Stanley, D. (2020). *LeMone and Burke's medical-surgical nursing: critical thinking for person-centred care* (4th [Australian] edn). Sydney: Pearson Australia.

Bullock, S. & Manias, E. (2022). *Fundamentals of pharmacology* (9th edn). Sydney: Pearson Australia.

Busingye, D., Pollack, A. & Chidwick, K. (2021). Prevalence of inflammatory bowel disease in the Australian general practice population: a cross-sectional study. *PLoS ONE* 16(5):e0252458. https://doi.org/10.1371/journal.pone.0252458.

Cancer Australia (2018). Distribution of cancer stage. *National Cancer Control Indicators.* https://ncci.canceraustralia.gov.au/diagnosis/distribution-cancer-stage/distribution-cancer-stage.

Ghoulam, E.M., Clarrett, D.M. & Marsicano, E.V. (2019). Diverticulitis. *Emedicine*. https://emedicine.medscape.com/article/173388-overview.

Liao, Y., Hong, X., Wu, A., Jiang, Y., Liang, Y., Gao, J.,... Kou, X. (2021). Global prevalence of norovirus in cases of acute gastroenteritis from 1997 to 2021: an updated systematic review and meta-analysis. *Microbial Pathogenesis* 161(A):105259. https://doi.org/10.1016/j.micpath.2021.105259.

Marieb, E.N. & Hoehn, K. (2019). *Human anatomy and physiology* (11th edn). San Francisco, CA: Pearson Benjamin Cummings.

Mayo Clinic (2023). *Intussusception*. https://www.mayoclinic.org/diseases-conditions/intussusception/symptoms-causes/syc-20351452.

Rowe, W.A. & Lichtenstein, G.R. (2020). Inflammatory bowel disease. *Emedicine*. https://emedicine.medscape.com/article/179037-overview.

Simpson, J., Duncanson, M., Oben, G., Adams, J., Wicken, A., Pierson, M.,... Gallagher, S. (2017). *Te ohonga ake: the health of Māori children and young people in New Zealand. Series Two.* Dunedin: New Zealand Child and Youth Epidemiology Service, University of Otago. https://www.health.govt.nz/publication/te-ohonga-ake-health-status-maori-children-and-young-people-new-zealand-0.

Wet Tropics Management Authority (WTMA) (2017). *Australia's tropical rainforests world heritage fact sheet: bush medicine.* Cairns: WTMA. https://www.wettropics.gov.au/site/user-assets/docs/bushmedicine.pdf.

Disorders of the liver, the gall bladder and the pancreas

38

LEARNING OBJECTIVES

After completing this chapter, you should be able to:

1 List the major causes and consequences of damage to hepatocytes.

2 Describe the causes and consequences of fibrosis and scarring in the liver.

3 Explain the significance of bilirubin in the assessment of liver disease.

4 Describe the major disease processes in viral hepatitis.

5 Describe the pathophysiological processes in fatty liver disease, gallstone formation and hepatocellular carcinoma.

6 Describe the disease processes in pancreatitis and pancreatic cancer.

7 Describe the effects of cystic fibrosis on pancreatic structure and function.

WHAT YOU SHOULD KNOW BEFORE YOU START THIS CHAPTER

Can you identify the major structures of the liver, the pancreas and the gall bladder, and describe their functions?

Can you outline the nature of the blood supply and venous drainage of the liver and the pancreas?

Can you describe the processes of chemical digestion in the small intestine?

Can you describe the stages of acute inflammation and healing?

Can you differentiate between the characteristics of acute and chronic inflammation?

Can you describe the principles associated with immune dysfunction?

KEY TERMS

Ascites
Biliary calculi
Cholangitis
Cholecystitis
Cholelithiasis
Cirrhosis
Cystic fibrosis (CF)
Haemolysis
Hepatic encephalopathy
Jaundice
Kernicterus
Pancreatic ductal adenocarcinoma
Pancreatitis
Portal hypertension
Steatorrhoea
Varices

Introduction

Diseases that affect the liver, the gall bladder and the pancreas will cause widespread impairments in whole body function. The liver and the pancreas make important contributions to the digestive process, but their broader contributions to other body processes are significant, too. The liver carries out the storage of nutrients such as glycogen, the metabolism of many drugs including alcohol, the detoxification of ammonia and other noxious substances, and the excretion of wastes, such as bilirubin, as well as the synthesis of plasma proteins, notably albumin and the clotting proteins. The pancreas plays an important endocrine role in the control of blood glucose levels and the regulation of digestive processes. The contribution of the gall bladder is in the storage and release of the bile salts necessary in the digestion of fats.

An overview of the pathophysiology of hepatobiliary disease

AETIOLOGY AND PATHOPHYSIOLOGY

The common and serious hepatobiliary diseases are viral hepatitis, fatty liver disease, gallstones and cancer. These diseases have their own distinctive features, but some major functional alterations tend to occur in all of them. These are damage to or death of hepatocytes, reduced function of the liver, fibrosis and scarring, portal hypertension, impeded excretion of bile and pain. A brief discussion of each of these pathological processes is provided here.

Damage to or death of hepatocytes

LEARNING OBJECTIVE 1

List the major causes and consequences of damage to hepatocytes.

Common causes of damage to or death of hepatocytes are *alcohol intoxication* and *viral infection*, the latter triggering injurious immune and inflammatory responses. Other causes of hepatocyte damage are *cancer, chemical exposure* (such as medicines, carbon tetrachloride and chloroform), *haemochromatosis* (with iron accumulation in the hepatocytes) and other *rarer genetic disorders*.

In metabolic terms, the healthy liver has 'excess capacity'. Thus, a lot of hepatocyte damage can occur before the overall functions of the liver are significantly reduced.

Reduced function of the liver

A number of problems can arise as a consequence of impairment of liver function. The measurement of changes in liver function is outlined in Clinical Box 38.1. Impaired liver function can manifest in the following ways:

- *Failure of liver gluconeogenesis*—this can lead to hypoglycaemia.

CLINICAL BOX 38.1

The clinical importance of liver function testing

The extent of liver damage may be assessed by measuring the blood levels of enzymes that are normally contained within hepatocytes. These measures are an indirect assessment of liver function. More direct measures of liver function can be made by assessing the transport and conjugation of bilirubin, albumin and clotting factor synthesis, and the production of the platelet regulating hormone thrombopoietin.

The presence of liver enzymes at high concentrations in the bloodstream indicates that significant liver cell damage has occurred. The enzymes typically used for such assessments are those that are involved in amino acid metabolism in the hepatocytes; the most important of these are *alanine aminotransferase (ALT)* and *aspartate aminotransferase (AST)*. Impaired bile flow can be assessed by measurement of the biliary enzymes *gamma-glutamyl transferase (GGT)* and *alkaline phosphatase (ALP)*.

- *Reduced ability of the liver to convert ammonia to urea*—this leads to increased levels of ammonia in the blood. Ammonia is continually formed in the large intestine by the bacterial metabolism of amino acids. It is normally absorbed into portal blood and conveyed to the liver, where, like the ammonia that arises from the deamination of amino acids, it is converted to urea and returned to the blood to be excreted in urine. When failure of the liver allows the blood concentration of ammonia to rise, its toxicity is most markedly exerted in the brain, leading to a state called **hepatic encephalopathy**.
- *Reduced albumin production*—this leads to reduced osmotic pressure of the plasma. This gives rise to oedema, including oedema of the brain, and ascites (see the 'Portal hypertension' section).
- *Reduced production of clotting proteins*—this allows excessive bleeding.
- *Altered liver metabolism of sex hormones*—this leads to the development of gynaecomastia (abnormal breast development) in men.
- *Failure to produce and excrete components of bile*, such as bilirubin.
- *Systemic hypotension*—this possibly arises because of the failure of the liver to break down circulating vasodilators, such as nitric oxide. Kidney injury (hepatorenal syndrome) may ensue as perfusion of the kidneys fails.

Fibrosis and scarring

LEARNING OBJECTIVE 2

Describe the causes and consequences of fibrosis and scarring in the liver.

Hepatocytes are stable epithelial cells that retain the ability to divide when required throughout life. If individual hepatocytes are destroyed but the connective tissue scaffolding (*stroma*) of the lobules persists, the remaining hepatocytes will regenerate the normal liver structure.

However, in circumstances where the liver is exposed to a damaging stimulus, such as chronic alcohol misuse, for an extended period, a cycle of inflammation, necrosis, fibrosis and regeneration develops. Fibrosis and haphazard regeneration leads to a breakdown in the organised tissue framework, and extensive scarring results. This is known as **cirrhosis**. This causes major problems by impeding the flow of blood in sinusoids, and of bile in canaliculi.

A further complication is that any regeneration that occurs will produce only 'nodules' of hepatocytes that are incompletely perfused, so liver function overall will be reduced (see Figures 38.1 and 38.2).

It also should be remembered that in any tissue where rates of cell replication are chronically elevated—such as in a liver whose cells are constantly being damaged and killed by agents like alcohol or hepatitis viruses—the opportunity for oncogenes to arise is increased, resulting in an increased likelihood of malignancy (see the 'Liver cancer' section later in this chapter).

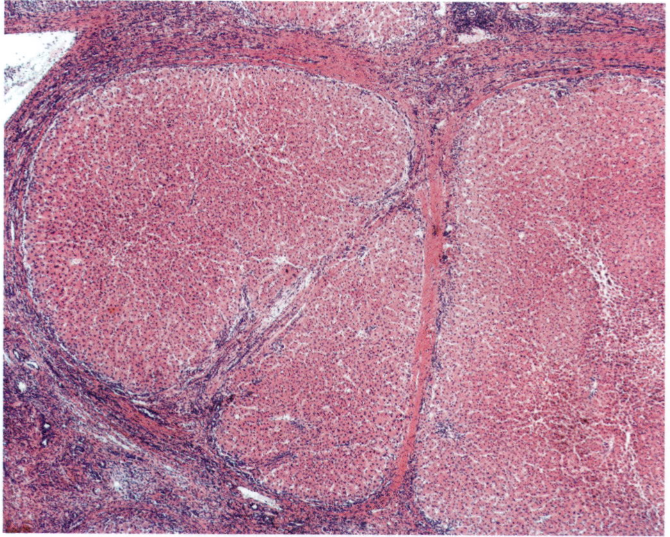

Figure 38.2

Histological changes in cirrhosis

This histological section of a cirrhotic liver shows fibrosis, regenerating nodules of hepatocytes and connecting tissue partitions.

Source: Jose Calvo/Science Photo Library.

Portal hypertension

When the *flow of blood from the portal vein through the sinusoids of the liver is impeded*, pressure rises in that vein. This most commonly occurs in cirrhosis, where normal liver organisation is disrupted by fibrous scar tissue. It may also occur when the portal vein is obstructed by a thrombus or tumour.

The changes that occur as **portal hypertension** arises are outlined below:

- Plasma and lymph leak under pressure from the liver into the peritoneal cavity, causing **ascites** (see Figure 38.3).
- Collateral systems of blood flow develop that bypass the portal vein; that is, tributaries of the portal vein form new connections, which allow them to drain directly into the general circulation.
- Hepatic encephalopathy develops. In portal hypertension, ammonia from the large intestine may bypass the detoxification mechanism in the liver (i.e. conversion to urea). Thus, it can move directly into the general circulation by means of collateral vessels and travel into the brain.

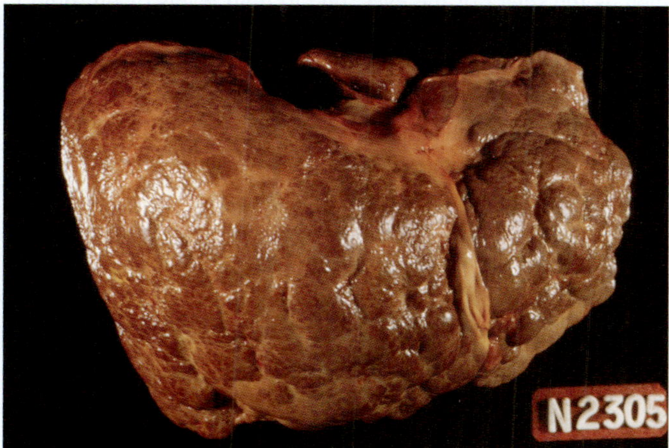

Figure 38.1

Large nodules in cirrhosis of the liver

The development of nodules and scarring in cirrhosis causes the organ to appear rough and lumpy.

Source: CNRI/Science Photo Library.

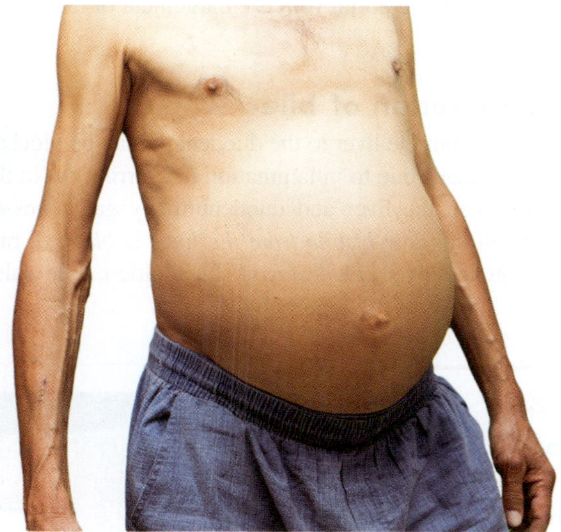

Figure 38.3

Ascites

The abdomen becomes distended in ascites due to the accumulation of fluid within the peritoneal cavity.

Source: donikz/Shutterstock.

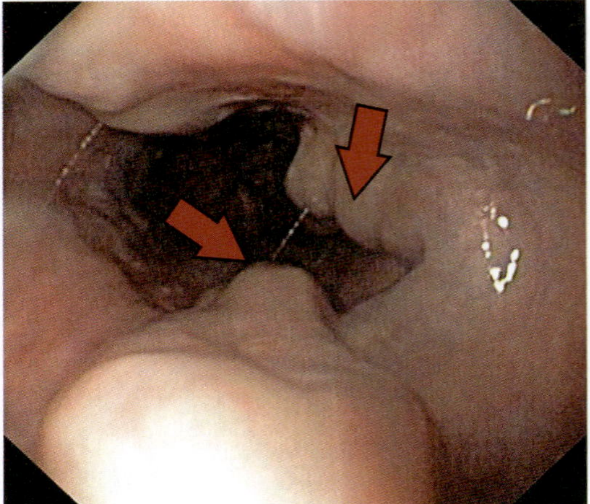

Figure 38.4

Endoscopic view of oesophageal varices

Endoscopy reveals large oesophageal varices (see red arrows). The red spots indicate a high risk of bleeding.

Source: Gastrolab/Science Photo Library.

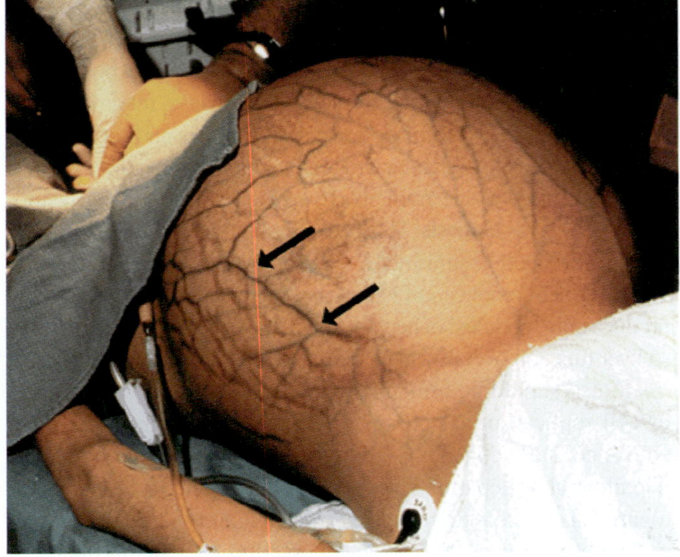

Figure 38.5

Caput medusae

The arrows indicate veins engorged with blood that are clearly visible through the skin surface.

Source: Henseler et al. (2001), Figure 10, pp. 691–704.

- Blood vessels that drain into the portal vein become congested, and thin-walled **varices** (as in varicose veins) may develop:
  - oesophageal varices (see Figure 38.4) are subject to rupture, with life-threatening haemorrhage
  - haemorrhoids may develop and bleed profusely
  - distended veins around the navel form a caput medusae (see Figure 38.5).

A less acute consequence of increased back pressure in the venous tributaries of the portal vein is enlargement of the spleen (splenomegaly).

Impeded excretion of bile

The flow of bile from the liver to the duodenum may be blocked within the liver itself (due to inflammation or scarring) or in the bile ducts between the liver and duodenum (by gallstones or tumours). When the *flow of bile from the liver is blocked*, bile accumulates in the liver (*cholestasis*). In addition, bile salts, conjugated bilirubin and other components of bile 'spill over' into the bloodstream in the liver and are carried into the general circulation. Since conjugated bilirubin is water-soluble, it will also appear in the urine, giving it a black tea appearance. The elevated blood level of bilirubin (*hyperbilirubinaemia*) manifests as *jaundice (icterus)*, while increased levels of *bile salts* in the blood may cause *itching (pruritus)*. Eventually, the accumulation of bile components in the liver will damage the hepatocytes. **Jaundice** is yellowing of the skin and certain other structures, such as the sclera of the eyes, due to high levels of bilirubin in the plasma and other extracellular fluids (see Figure 38.6).

When the flow of bile salts to the digestive tract is blocked, dietary fat will not be digested and will appear in the faeces (**steatorrhoea**). Faeces will also be pale due to the absence of bilirubin. Fat is not absorbed in the small intestine, so the fat-soluble vitamins (A, D, E and K) will not be absorbed at adequate levels.

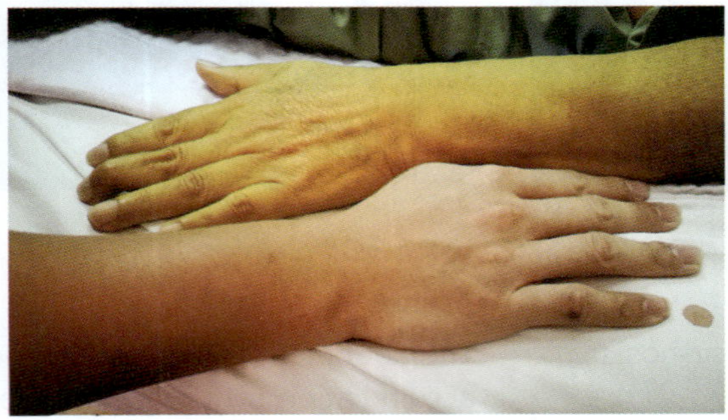

A

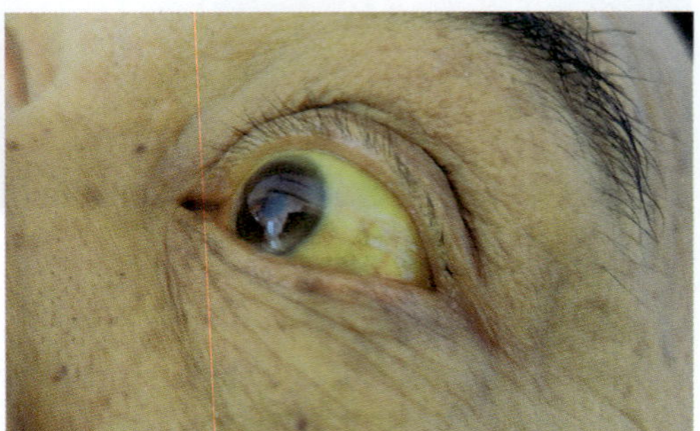

B

Figure 38.6

Jaundice

(A) Arm and hand of two individuals, one with jaundice, one without.
(B) Jaundice is often most visible in the sclera of a person's eye.

Source: Casa Nayafana/ Shutterstock.

LEARNING OBJECTIVE 3

Explain the significance of bilirubin in the assessment of liver disease.

Hyperbilirubinaemia may be caused by *biliary obstruction*. It may also occur when *liver metabolic functions fail*, with reduced uptake of *unconjugated (free) bilirubin* from blood and/or reduced conjugation and excretion of bilirubin. In such cases, both unconjugated bilirubin and conjugated bilirubin accumulate and rise to high levels in the blood. Even where liver function is normal, any process that causes the increased destruction of erythrocytes (**haemolysis**) may lead to hyperbilirubinaemia. In such diseases, destruction of the erythrocytes causes a rise in the blood levels of unconjugated bilirubin. Such levels may be higher than even a healthy liver can clear from the blood.

Hyperbilirubinaemia that is *physiological* rather than pathological may occur in the newborn, especially if the child is premature. In the first week or so after birth, the breakdown of fetal blood is extensive, and the metabolic capacities of the liver are not fully developed; thus, jaundice due to high blood levels of unconjugated bilirubin is common at this time. It is important that the level of unconjugated bilirubin in the blood of the newborn should not rise too high for too long. This substance, while insoluble in water, is highly soluble in fat, and can readily pass from the blood to the brain of the newborn. This may result in serious, irreversible damage to the child's brain (**kernicterus**). The simple treatment for this condition in babies is phototherapy. Exposure of the skin to bright light converts the unconjugated bilirubin in the blood, as it flows through the skin, into a metabolite that can be excreted in bile and urine.

Pain

The liver itself does not contain sensory receptors, but it is enclosed in a connective tissue capsule (*Glisson's capsule*) that contains nociceptors (see the chapter 'Nociception and pain'). In liver disease, pain is felt when the capsule is distended: this can occur when there are liver tumours or when the liver becomes enlarged as in acute hepatitis.

Pain is also experienced when the flow of bile is blocked in the bile ducts or cystic duct. In these circumstances, pain is exacerbated by spasm of the smooth muscle of the gall bladder. Figure 38.7 shows where pain from the abdominal region may be projected to the surface of the body.

SARS-CoV-2 and the liver

SARS-CoV-2 infection and its therapy have been reported to cause liver injury. Liver injury mainly manifests as abnormally high levels in the liver enzymes AST and ALT, and bilirubin, as well as low levels of albumin. The severity of COVID-19 infection correlates with these alterations in liver function.

The pathogenic mechanisms underlying the liver injury in COVID-19 infection are multifactorial. The SARS-CoV-2 virus enters cells by binding to angiotensin converting enzyme-2 (ACE-2) receptors, gaining access to liver cells where they can directly cause damage. Another mechanism is associated with immune response to the virus. It has been suggested that in severe COVID-19 infection a cytokine storm may damage liver cells. Other mechanisms of liver cell damage may be associated with ischaemia, hypoxia and thrombosis. It should also be noted that many of the antiviral agents used to treat COVID-19 infection are hepatotoxic, which may lead to liver injury.

Importantly in people with chronic liver disease, the pathogenic mechanisms associated with COVID-related liver injury will contribute to further compromising of liver function.

Figure 38.7

Referred pain common to abdominal pathologies

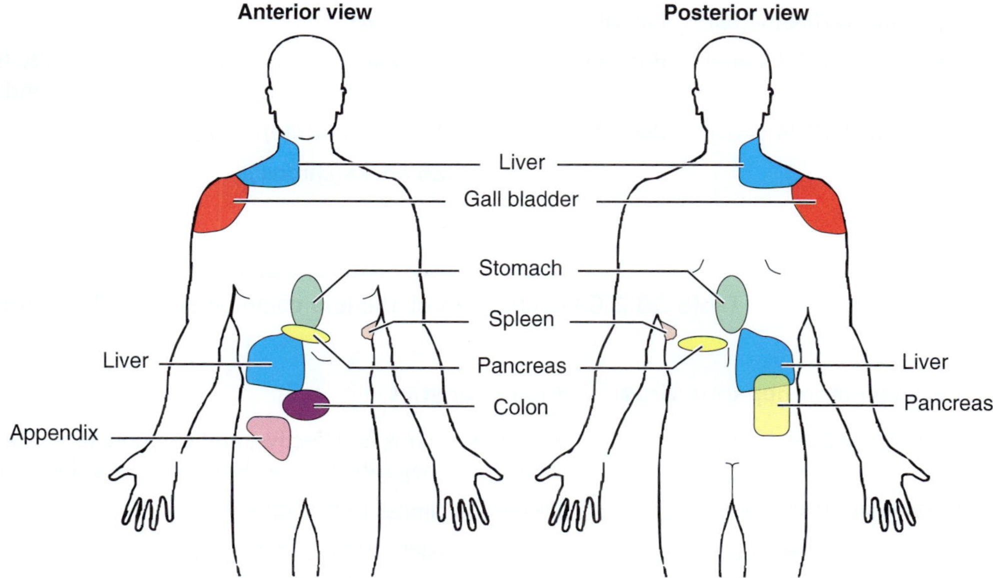

Major hepatobiliary diseases

VIRAL HEPATITIS

LEARNING OBJECTIVE 4

Describe the major disease processes in viral hepatitis.

Aetiology and pathophysiology

Hepatitis is liver inflammation associated with hepatocyte damage. It may arise from a number of causes; for example, *microbial pathogens* or *chemical toxicity*. The most important pathogens are the *hepatitis viruses*. Figure 38.8 explores the common clinical manifestations and management of viral hepatitis. Note that there is a great deal of variation in the clinical manifestations of viral hepatitis.

Viral hepatitis is a major health problem worldwide, causing millions of deaths each year. It often entails continuing problems, such as the existence of a chronic carrier state and an increased risk of further liver disease, notably cirrhosis and liver cancer.

A number of structurally unrelated viruses can infect the liver to cause hepatitis: currently these are hepatitis A, B, C, D, E and G. *Hepatitis A and E* are spread mainly by the *faecal–oral route*, while *hepatitis B, C, D and G* are spread by *blood* and, to a lesser extent, *other body fluids*. Table 38.1 shows the characteristics of the major hepatitis viruses. The characteristics of the less common hepatitis viruses are shown in Table 38.2.

Clinical manifestations

Inflammation of the liver may give rise to symptoms such as pain, fever, anorexia, nausea and vomiting, and jaundice. For any type of hepatitis, some or all of these symptoms may be absent. *Fulminant hepatitis* is a rapidly developing form of the disease that occurs in a small minority of infected people, and can cause total liver failure and death within weeks.

As all the hepatitis viruses can give rise to these symptoms, diagnosis of the specific pathogen cannot be made clinically, but must be based on detection of specific antibodies or identification of viral antigens in blood.

Hepatitis A

Aetiology and pathophysiology Hepatitis A virus (HAV) is a single-stranded RNA virus usually transmitted by the faecal–oral route as it is excreted in faeces. It is spread by contaminated food or water, or on hands. However, it may also be spread by intravenous drug use and/or by sexual activity (especially among men who have sex with men). After the virus is ingested, it spreads through the blood to the liver. Infective virus particles can be shed as *naked virions* in faeces or as *enveloped virions* from infected human cells. Infection only occurs in an acute form and is characteristically self-limiting, with an incubation period of 14–28 days.

Damage to the liver is believed to be due to the host's immune responses to infected hepatocytes.

Epidemiology There are an estimated 1.4 million cases of HAV per year globally. Prevalence is dependent on socioeconomic factors, and is higher in regions with poor sanitation and limited access to clean water. HAV is a notifiable infection in Australia. In 2022 the notification rate was 140 cases. The notification rate has decreased significantly since the 1990s, from more than 2,000 per year. In Australia and New Zealand, HAV infection is now regarded as relatively uncommon.

Table 38.1 Characteristics of the major hepatitis viruses

Major hepatitis virus	Transmission	Incubation period	Chronic infection	Vaccine
Hepatitis A (RNA virus)	Faecal–oral	14–28 days	No	Yes
Hepatitis B (DNA virus)	Body fluids	6–24 weeks	Yes (5–10% in adults; much higher in infants and children)	Yes
Hepatitis C (RNA virus)	Body fluids	6–10 weeks (acute) 2–25 weeks (chronic)	Yes (> 70%)	No

Table 38.2 Characteristics of the less common strains of hepatitis viruses

Less common hepatitis virus	Characteristics
Hepatitis D (RNA virus)	Hepatitis D virus is defective, and can only replicate in people who are also infected by hepatitis B virus. Hepatitis B vaccine protects against hepatitis D.
Hepatitis E (RNA virus)	Disease is similar to hepatitis A.
Hepatitis G (RNA virus)	Not as well described as other viral strains. There is some conjecture as to whether HGV induces clinically significant liver disease.

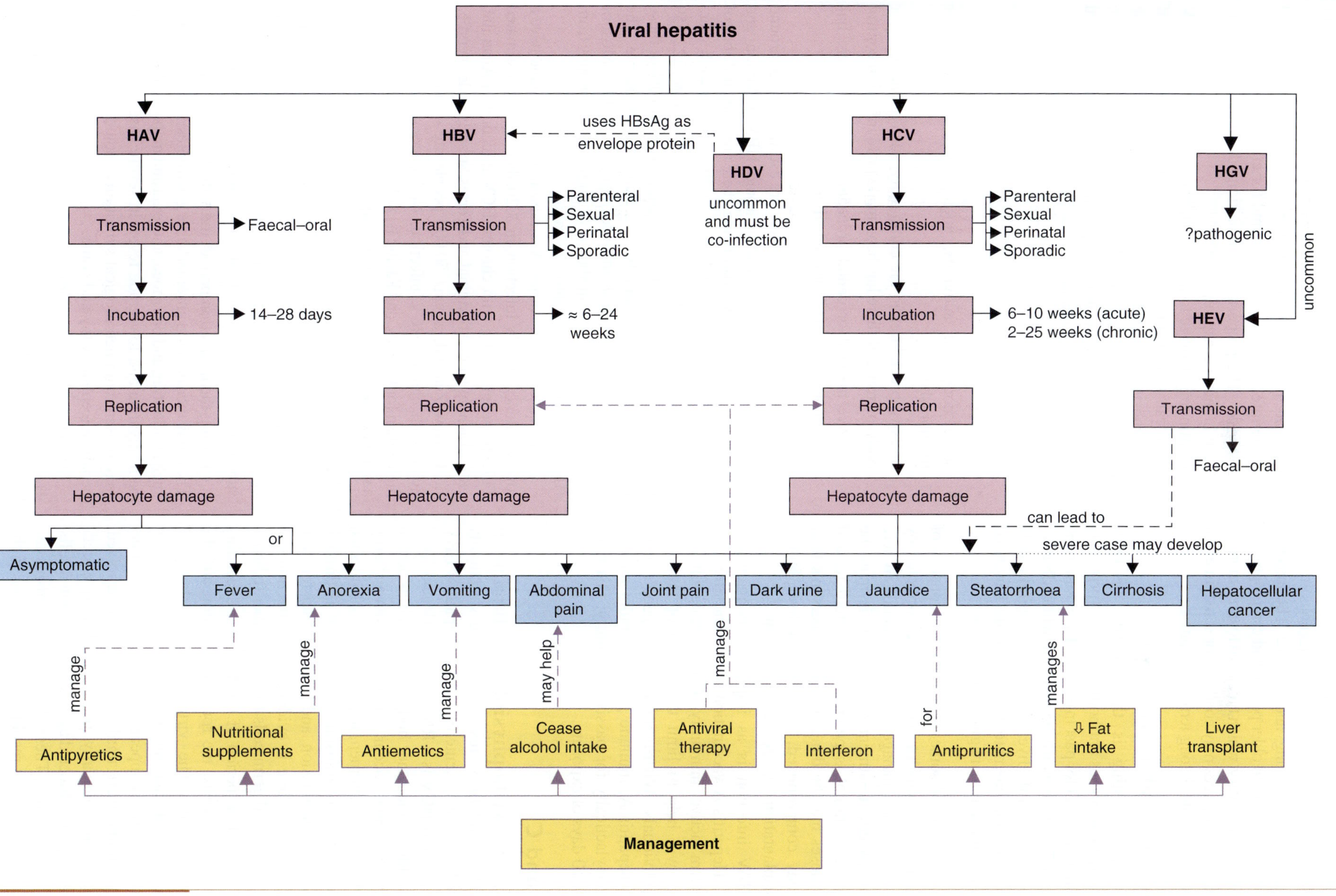

Figure 38.8

Clinical snapshot: Viral hepatitis

↓ = decreased; ? = possibly; HAV = hepatitis A virus; HBsAg = hepatitis B surface antigen; HBV = hepatitis B virus; HCV = hepatitis C virus; HDV = hepatitis D virus; HEV = hepatitis E virus; HGV = hepatitis G virus.

Clinical manifestations Symptoms vary from essentially none in young children (who are nonetheless infectious) to pain, fever, anorexia, nausea and vomiting, and jaundice. The infection tends to manifest more severely in older people and can progress to fulminant hepatitis. After recovery, which takes two to three months, the shedding of the virus in faeces may continue for some time, but there is no chronic carrier state or long-term liver damage.

Clinical diagnosis and management

Diagnosis Serological testing is the mainstay of HAV diagnosis: an infected person has antibodies to HAV (primarily IgM for current infection, IgG for past infection). Liver enzymes, such as AST and ALT, will generally be elevated, while albumin levels may decline if overall liver function is significantly reduced. Biochemistry and haematology results are beneficial to assist with identifying and managing other issues.

Management The care of someone with HAV consists of managing the symptoms. Dehydration should be corrected by volume support, and nausea managed with antiemetics. Where analgesic and antipyretic treatment is required, it must be remembered that paracetamol is potentially hepatotoxic, and even therapeutic doses may be dangerous if the person's liver function is already compromised. If fulminant liver failure occurs, liver transplantation may be the only option.

Preventing HAV infection is as important as managing active infections. Hepatitis A vaccination is safe and effective, providing long-term active immunity. Good sanitation and hygiene practices will help to limit the spread of the virus from infected individuals. Where unvaccinated people have been exposed to hepatitis A, immune gammaglobulin may be administered prophylactically for passive immunity; this must be done within 7–10 days of exposure.

Hepatitis B and C

Aetiology and pathophysiology Hepatitis B and C viruses (HBV and HCV, respectively) are structurally unrelated, but each can cause acute or chronic hepatitis. HBV is a DNA virus, whereas HCV is a RNA virus. HBV and HCV are transmitted in blood and other body fluids, such as sexual secretions. Most new cases occur among intravenous drug users, men who have sex with men, and the babies of infected mothers. The major mode of transmission of HCV is through infected blood. Sexual transmission, and 'vertical' transfer from mother to baby, are rare. There is evidence that infection can be transferred from infected germ cells from the father to baby.

HBV has an incubation period of 6–24 weeks, depending on the infecting dose of virus, the route of infection and the person's immune response. The virus replicates slowly in the liver without at first causing obvious liver damage or producing symptoms; viruses appear in the blood at this time, and continue to be found there until the infection is resolved. The liver damage that eventually occurs is due to a cell-mediated immune response directed against virus-infected cells, and consequent inflammation. These defence mechanisms are also responsible for the eventual resolution of the disease in the majority of cases, at least for HBV. The sequence of events in the course of HBV infection is shown in Figure 38.9.

In about 2–10% of HBV cases, usually after mild or unapparent initial disease, a chronic infection and thus a chronic carrier state may persist. In HCV cases, the incubation period for acute infection is 6–10 weeks, and for chronic infection it is 2–25 weeks. The proportion of infections that become chronic is much higher, perhaps up to 70%.

Continuing damage to the liver in chronic infection by HBV or HCV can lead to progressive liver damage in the forms of liver cirrhosis or cancer. Chronically infected people are the major sources of spread of HBV and HCV. HBV is viable in blood and other body fluids (e.g. saliva, semen and vaginal secretions). Transmission may occur during:

- sexual contact
- birth
- injecting drug use
- some household activities, such as sharing razors or toothbrushes
- invasive procedures in the community, such as tattooing or body-piercing, if there has been inadequate infection control
- invasive medical or dental procedures in which there has been inadequate infection control.

Epidemiology Globally, there are estimated to be around 360 million people living with chronic HBV infection and 200 million cases of HCV. Worldwide, there are many millions of carriers of HBV and HCV, and up to 1 million deaths each year.

In Australia in 2020 there were estimated to be 222,559 people living with chronic HBV infection. Around 10% of these cases are in Aboriginal and Torres Strait Islander people. The notification rate has been steadily declining since 2006. Most of the new HBV cases are attributed to migration of people from HBV-endemic countries into Australia.

Relative to other countries, Australia and New Zealand have a low prevalence of HCV infection. In 2020, there were an estimated 117,810 people living with chronic HCV infection in Australia, 18% of whom were Aboriginal and Torres Strait Islander people.

In New Zealand, around 50,000 people are estimated to be living with chronic HCV infection. Notifications for males are higher than for females, and Pacific Islander people and Māori have a significantly higher infection rate than European New Zealanders.

Clinical manifestations In both HBV and HCV infection, the clinical manifestations vary greatly, depending on whether the disease is acute or chronic. HCV causes acute symptoms similar to HBV, although they tend to be milder or subclinical. However, the rate of chronic infection is much higher.

During the incubation period, individuals are asymptomatic. They may then develop unremarkable gastrointestinal symptoms, such as vomiting and diarrhoea, anorexia and malaise, abdominal pain, myalgia and low-grade fever. In severe cases, individuals may present with neurological symptoms, including confusion, hepatic encephalopathy and coma.

In the chronic phase, individuals may also be asymptomatic. However, some people may complain of malaise and non-specific gastrointestinal symptoms, such as nausea and abdominal pain. Hepatomegaly, jaundice, ascites and fever may become apparent in severe cases that progress to liver failure.

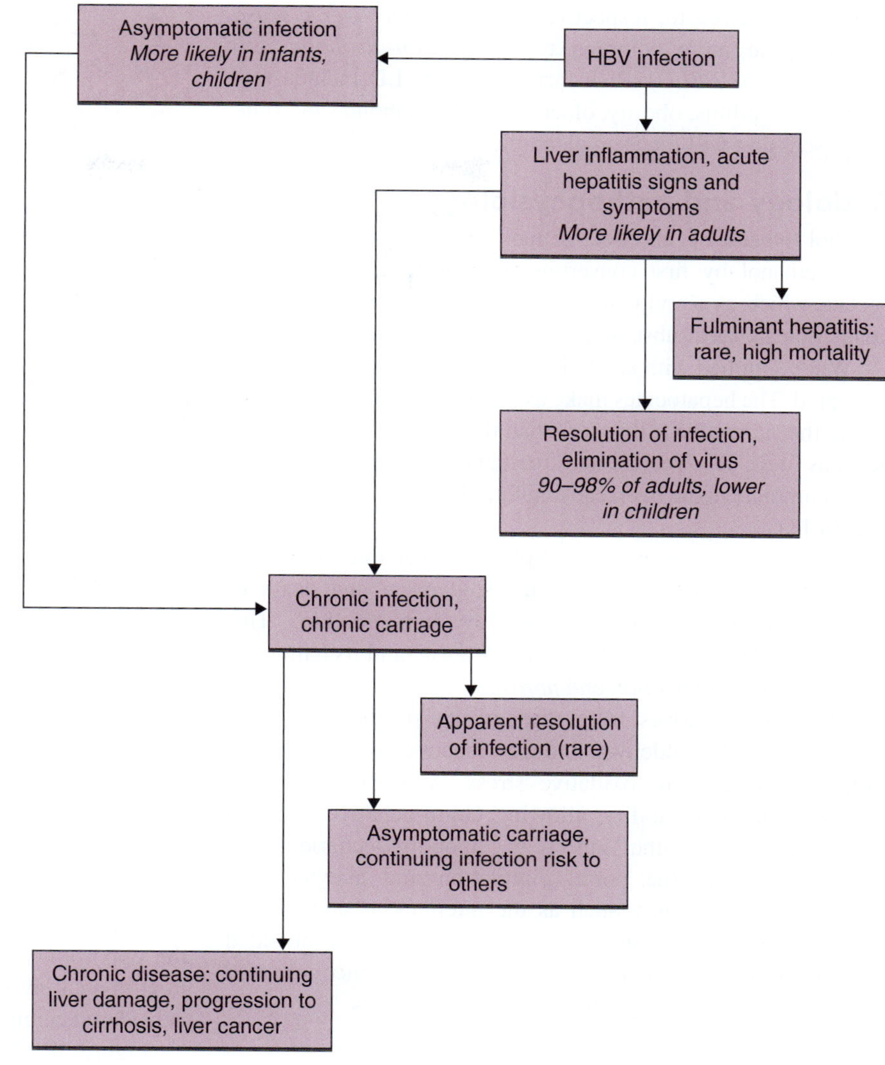

Figure 38.9
The course of hepatitis B virus (HBV) infection

Source: R. Arwas.

Clinical diagnosis and management

Diagnosis Diagnosis of HBV infection is by findings of HBV antigens or anti-HBV antibodies in the blood. Diagnosis of HCV infection is by finding anti-HCV antibodies and HCV RNA. Plasma concentrations of the liver enzymes ALT and AST will be elevated, as will levels of ALP, which is an indicator of biliary obstruction. Albumin is often low, and some degree of leukopenia may be present.

Management As for many viral diseases, there is no treatment for acute viral hepatitis other than hydration and the management of symptoms such as pain and nausea. Depending on the presentation and the clinical picture, antiviral medications, immunotherapy with peginterferon-α may be administered to reduce viral replication and thus reduce viral loads. An effective vaccine is available for HBV.

First-line antiviral medication used in HBV infection treatment comprise the DNA polymerase entecavir, and the nucleoside reverse transcriptase inhibitor tenofovir, in combination with peginterferon-α2a. Antiviral agents used in HCV therapy include NS3/4A protease inhibitors, RNA polymerase inhibitors and NS5A protein inhibitors in combination with peginterferon-α2a.

The prevention of spread of HBV depends on the identification of infectious cases and the safe management of carriers, the use of appropriate procedures to prevent the infection of health care workers (e.g. standard precautions), passive immunisation with immune gammaglobulin after accidental exposure, and vaccination. This can be done successfully even after exposure to the virus, because of the long incubation period for HBV.

At present, there is no vaccine for HCV. Like human immunodeficiency virus (HIV), HCV appears to be highly mutable, and so poses great challenges to vaccine development. Treatment of new HCV infections with peginterferon-α and ribavirin appears to be of benefit. Prevention strategies to reduce unsafe injection techniques, especially among high-risk groups, are important.

FATTY LIVER DISEASE

LEARNING OBJECTIVE 5

Describe the pathophysiological processes in fatty liver disease, gallstone formation and hepatocellular carcinoma.

Fatty liver disease is associated with either alcohol misuse or an excessive dietary intake of fats and monosaccharides. The two forms are referred to, respectively, as *alcoholic liver disease*, which is the more common type, and *non-alcoholic fatty liver disease (NAFLD)*. Risk factors for NAFLD include type 2 diabetes mellitus, obesity, older age and metabolic syndrome. The discussion will focus on alcoholic liver disease.

Aetiology and pathophysiology

Alcohol (ethanol) is an effective fuel for hepatocytes. The cells utilise ethanol by first converting it to acetaldehyde, then to acetate, which, as acetyl-CoA, can be used both for aerobic energy generation and as a substrate for the synthesis of fatty acids.

When supplied with alcohol as a major fuel, lipid turnover is disrupted. The hepatocytes make excess amounts of triglyceride, and at the same time utilise less than the usual amounts of fatty acids as fuels. Triglyceride and free fatty acids are not exported but accumulate in the liver, causing fatty liver (see Figures 38.10 and 38.11).

Fatty liver is, in itself, completely reversible. However, if excessive alcohol intake continues, damage and death of hepatocytes occurs, accompanied by inflammation. This condition is known as *alcoholic liver disease*, and its hallmarks are *steatosis, inflammation* and *fibrosis*.

The damage arises from the toxicity of the metabolite acetaldehyde. Acetaldehyde induces reactive oxygen species formation, leading to oxidative stress. Alcohol intake also increases gut permeability, allowing Gram-negative bacterial endotoxins within the gut (e.g. lipopolysaccharides) to be absorbed into the portal circulation and activate pro-inflammatory cytokines, such as the interleukins and tumour necrosis factor-α, enhancing the inflammation. Embedded macrophages within the liver called *Kupffer cells*, once activated in the inflammatory state, greatly stimulate fibrosis.

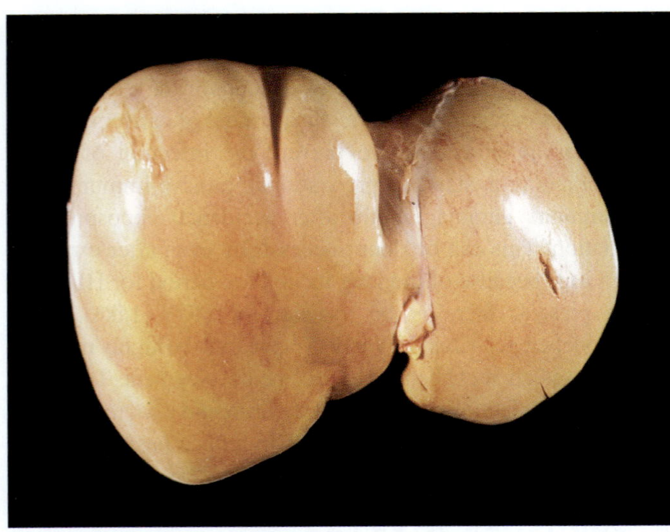

Figure 38.10

Fatty liver

This liver is slightly enlarged and has a pale yellow appearance. The uniform change is consistent with fatty metamorphosis (fatty change).

Source: CNRI/Science Photo Library.

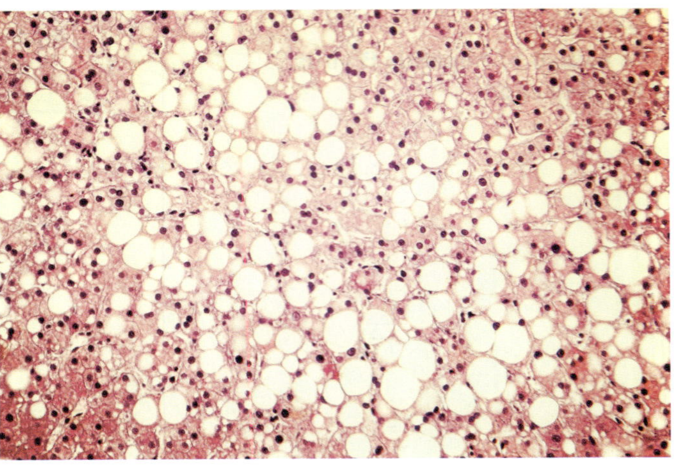

Figure 38.11

Histological section of a fatty liver

The histological appearance of hepatic fatty change shows lipid accumulation in the hepatocytes as vacuoles. The vacuoles have a clear appearance with this histological stain.

Source: Kateryna Kon/Shutterstock.

Where there is extensive damage to and death of hepatocytes, cirrhosis ensues and liver failure will develop. In addition, where cells are constantly being killed and then replaced through increased rates of cell replication among survivors, the opportunity for oncogenes to arise is increased, resulting in an increased likelihood of malignancy. Acetaldehyde is also considered carcinogenic.

Figure 38.12 explores the common clinical manifestations and management of alcoholic liver disease.

Clinical manifestations

As fatty liver disease involves inflammation, manifestations of this disease are generally similar to those of viral hepatitis. In the early stage, the affected person may be asymptomatic. When symptoms manifest, the person may present with gastrointestinal malaise and mild fever. However, more serious manifestations may include bleeding disorders, alcohol withdrawal symptoms, hepatomegaly, splenomegaly, ascites, malnutrition, muscle wasting, gynaecomastia (increased breast tissue) in men, spider angiomata (reddish-purple marks on the skin associated with dilated capillaries), palmar erythema and hepatic encephalopathy.

Clinical diagnosis and management

Diagnosis A comprehensive history with specific attention to alcohol intake is important. Liver function tests are crucial: these may reveal a reduction in serum albumin with elevations in ALT and AST (reflective of hepatocyte damage) and ALP (reflective of biliary obstruction). Hyperbilirubinaemia is common, and occasionally so is hyperkalaemia. Coagulopathy is frequently evident, and may be associated with anaemia. There may be signs of dehydration as a result of vomiting,

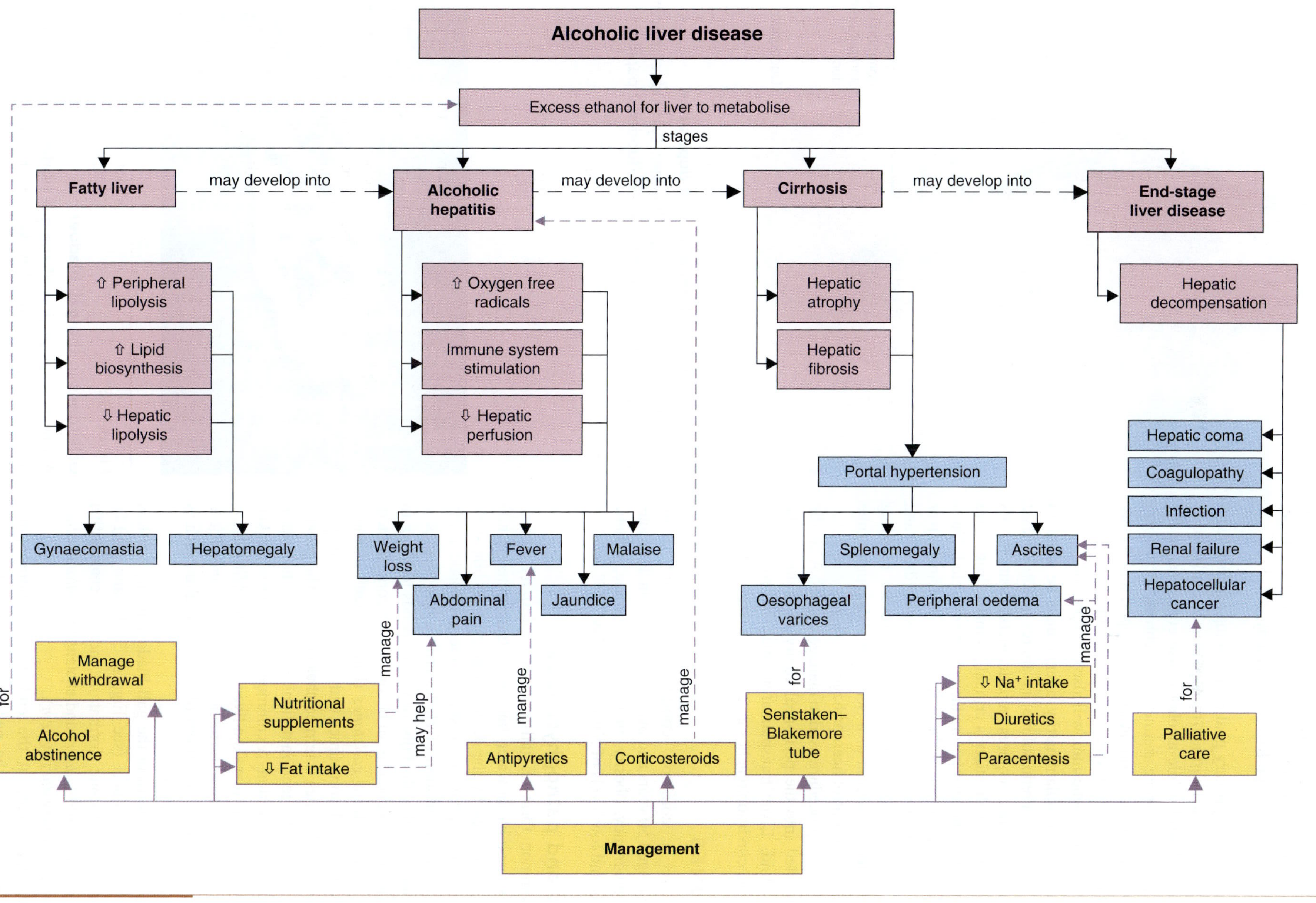

Figure 38.12
Clinical snapshot: Alcoholic liver disease
↓ = decreased; ↑ = increased; Na^+ = sodium ion.

and malnutrition may also be apparent. A liver biopsy may be considered, but this procedure entails a risk of haemorrhage, which increases with the degree of coagulopathy.

Management A primary goal of managing a person with alcoholic liver disease is to help them manage their alcohol misuse. No treatments will work while alcohol intake continues, so the focus of therapy is to promote abstinence. As chronic alcoholism generally results in malnutrition, nutritional support and dietary supplementation of micronutrients such as vitamins A, B, D and E, as well as zinc and magnesium, will also be important.

Corticosteroid anti-inflammatory agents may be used to reduce inflammation. Prednisolone is more effective than prednisone, as the latter requires hepatic metabolism for its activation. Care with medication is critical, as many drugs have to be metabolised by the liver before they can be excreted. Thus, in the medical management of those who have alcoholic liver disease, it is important to eliminate any unnecessary drugs and perhaps to modify the doses of others. For severe bleeding oesophageal varices, insertion of a Senstaken–Blakemore tube may be necessary to control haemorrhage.

Paracentesis is a procedure used to manage ascites. A needle or tube is inserted into the peritoneal cavity to drain off the accumulated fluid. Liver transplantation may be considered necessary as the condition reaches an advanced stage.

GALLSTONES

Gallstones are a common condition, affecting about 15% of people aged 50 years and over. Risk factors include age, female sex, pregnancy, obesity, metabolic syndrome, genetic predisposition and low levels of physical activity.

Aetiology and pathophysiology

The most common form of gallstones is *cholesterol stones*. Cholesterol is insoluble in water, but can be transported in bile because it is emulsified by the detergent activity of bile salts. Cholesterol may precipitate as crystals in the gall bladder and bile ducts if the concentration of cholesterol in bile increases, the concentration of bile salts falls, or if bile spends too long in the gall bladder and the cholesterol becomes over-concentrated. The crystals grow to form *gallstones* (**biliary calculi**) as more cholesterol is deposited, sometimes with bilirubin and calcium. The formation of gallstones is termed **cholelithiasis**. The genetic risk has been linked to gene mutations that affect cholesterol transport or bile composition. A common gene mutation linked to gallstone formation involves the liver transporter *ABCG8*.

Another type of gallstone formed is a *pigment stone*. These stones can develop under conditions of excess bilirubin, such as in anaemias or in liver cirrhosis.

Gallstones usually form in the gall bladder itself, and less commonly in the bile ducts (see Figures 38.13 and 38.14). Complications of gallstone formation include **cholecystitis** (*inflammation of the gallbladder*) and **cholangitis** (*inflammation or infection of the biliary duct system*).

Gallstones that lodge at the end of the common bile duct, where it joins with the pancreatic duct and empties its contents into the duodenum, may block both ducts. The

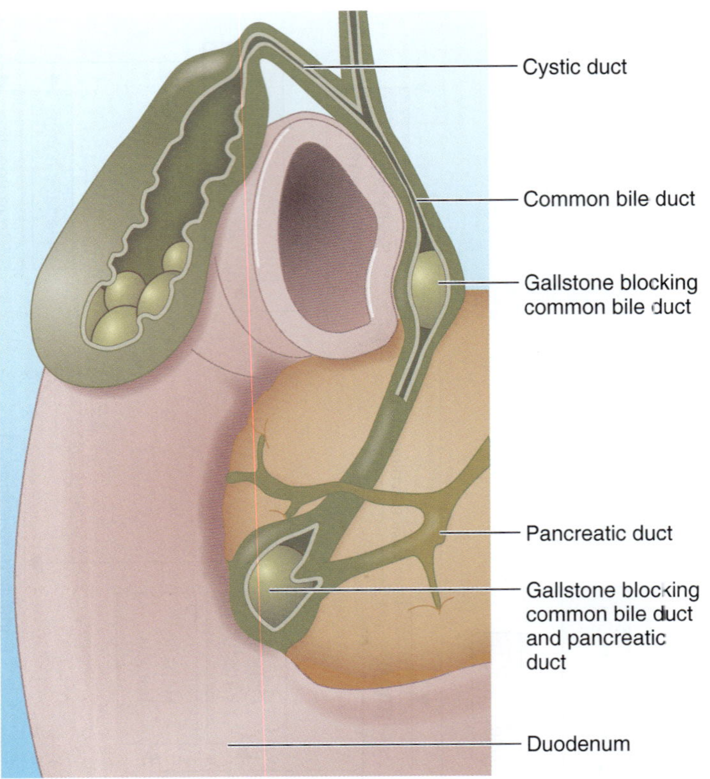

Figure 38.13

Sites of gallstone formation and deposition

Gallstones can form in the gall bladder, cystic duct, hepatic duct, common bile duct and greater duodenal papilla.

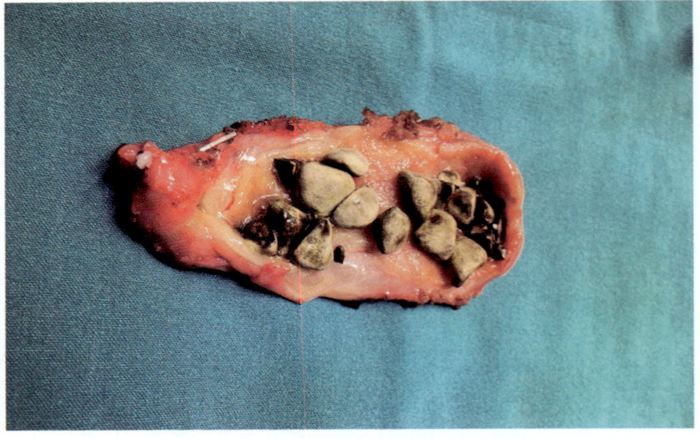

Figure 38.14

Gallstones in the gall bladder

A longitudinal section of the gall bladder shows a number of formed stones and a thickening of the bladder wall.

Source: Pthawatc/Shutterstock.

metabolic consequences of obstruction of the flow of bile have been described earlier, in the section on the pathophysiology of hepatobiliary disease. Blockage of the pancreatic duct will trap pancreatic digestive enzymes within the pancreas: the powerful enzymes then damage the pancreas, causing acute pancreatitis.

Clinical manifestations

Individuals may be asymptomatic; however, problems arise when the stones block ducts of the biliary system or, in some cases, the pancreatic duct as well. Blockage of the bile ducts causes pain in the upper abdomen. Blockage of the cystic duct, if prolonged, results in acute inflammation of the gall bladder (*cholecystitis*). This is often accompanied by secondary bacterial infection as bacteria ascend from the intestine.

When someone presents with an acute obstruction from cholelithiasis, they will complain of severe abdominal pain, which is poorly localised. This pain may be referred to the right shoulder. To moderate this, people put their hand behind their back with thumb pointing upwards. This is known as the Collins' sign. This is usually accompanied by nausea and vomiting. In most cases, sympathetic nervous system effects, such as tachycardia, hypertension and diaphoresis, may also occur. Less often, where vomiting has caused severe fluid depletion, the individual may be hypotensive despite the increase in sympathetic activity. Figure 38.15 explores the common clinical manifestations and management of cholelithiasis.

Clinical diagnosis and management

Diagnosis Ultrasound is often the imaging method of choice for the diagnosis of cholelithiasis, as it is quick and non-invasive. Computed tomography (CT) scans are useful in identifying the precise location/s of stones, and in assessing the extent of disease.

Although blood sampling for biochemistry and haematology tests may be beneficial to identify and manage other problems, pathology results are of little value in the diagnosis of cholelithiasis. Beta-human chorionic gonadotropin (β-hCG) measurements should also be performed in all women of childbearing age to exclude ectopic pregnancy as the cause of the abdominal pain.

Management Surgery, either open or laparoscopic cholecystectomy, is still considered the best treatment for symptomatic gallstones. Minimally invasive surgery to remove stones can be carried out with the use of an endoscope that is passed through the stomach into the duodenum and then up the common bile duct or the pancreatic duct. This is called *endoscopic retrograde cholangiopancreatography (ERCP)*.

Extracorporeal shock wave lithotripsy (ESWL) has been developed as a non-surgical approach in the management of cholelithiasis. This is used in combination with ultrasound, and supplemented by oral medications to help dissolve stone fragments. Recurrence is a risk of this approach, due mainly to an intact irritated gall bladder remaining in situ.

LIVER CANCER

Malignant tumours in the liver are classified as *primary* when originating in the liver itself, or *secondary* (i.e. of metastatic origin). Primary liver cancer may originate in the hepatocytes (*hepatocellular carcinoma* or *hepatocarcinoma*) or, less often, in the bile ducts (*cholangiocarcinoma*).

The major sites from which cancer spreads to the liver are the colon, breast, lung, stomach and pancreas. Cells from tumours in these organs utilise the rich, dual blood supply of the liver to reach and colonise it. Figure 38.16 explores the common clinical manifestations and management of liver cancer.

In Australia and other developed countries, secondary liver cancer is far more common than primary liver cancer. According to 1982–2018 data from the Australian Institute of Health and Welfare (AIHW), the age-standardised incidence for 2022 is estimated to be 8.8 cases per 100,000 people, and in 2022 the risk of dying from liver cancer by the age of 85 is 1 in 121 (0.83%). Men are at a greater risk than women.

Worldwide, hepatocellular carcinoma is the third most common cause of cancer death. It is associated with chronic infection by hepatitis viruses, and with alcoholic liver disease.

Hepatocellular carcinoma

The most common predisposing factor for hepatocellular carcinoma is cirrhosis (about 80% of cases), which develops in people with chronic infection with HBV or HCV, fatty liver disease or alcohol misuse. In these conditions, as dead cells are replaced by regenerating hepatocytes, the increased rate of mitosis of hepatocytes possibly provides scope for spontaneous mutations to appear, including those that create oncogenes.

Aetiology and pathophysiology Cirrhosis is present in most cases of hepatocellular carcinoma. This condition is characterised by cycles of inflammation, necrosis and regeneration that promotes the genetic mutations that underlie carcinogenesis (see the chapter 'Neoplasia').

A hepatocellular carcinoma may grow as a single mass (see Figure 38.17), as multiple nodules or as a diffuse infiltration. In many cases, the malignant cells produce a substance that is normally synthesised only in the liver of the fetus—α-fetoprotein—which may be used as a marker in the diagnosis and monitoring of the disease. Hepatocellular carcinomas may spread to adjacent organs in the abdominal cavity and metastasise to the lymph nodes.

Clinical manifestations In the early stages, hepatocellular carcinoma may not give rise to symptoms. The excess metabolic capacity of the liver means that it can continue to function normally even as healthy hepatocytes are lost, and the absence of sensory receptors within the liver means that the tumour can expand without causing pain.

In the later stages, the affected person may experience:

- pain in the upper right side quadrant of the abdomen, as the liver capsule is distended or the flow of bile is obstructed
- fever, which accompanies inflammatory responses to tissue destruction by the invasive tumour

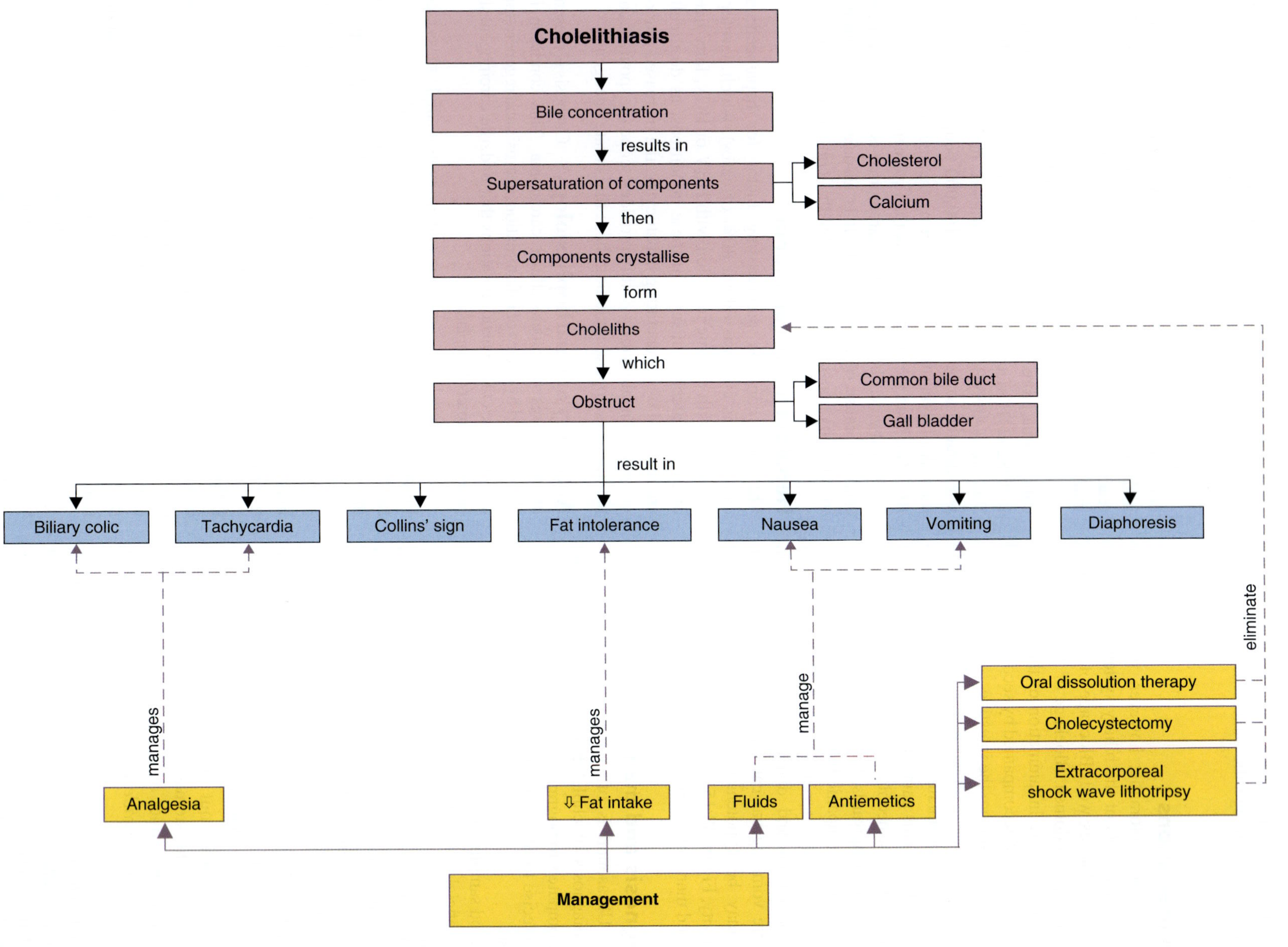

Figure 38.15
Clinical snapshot: Cholelithiasis
↓ = decreased.

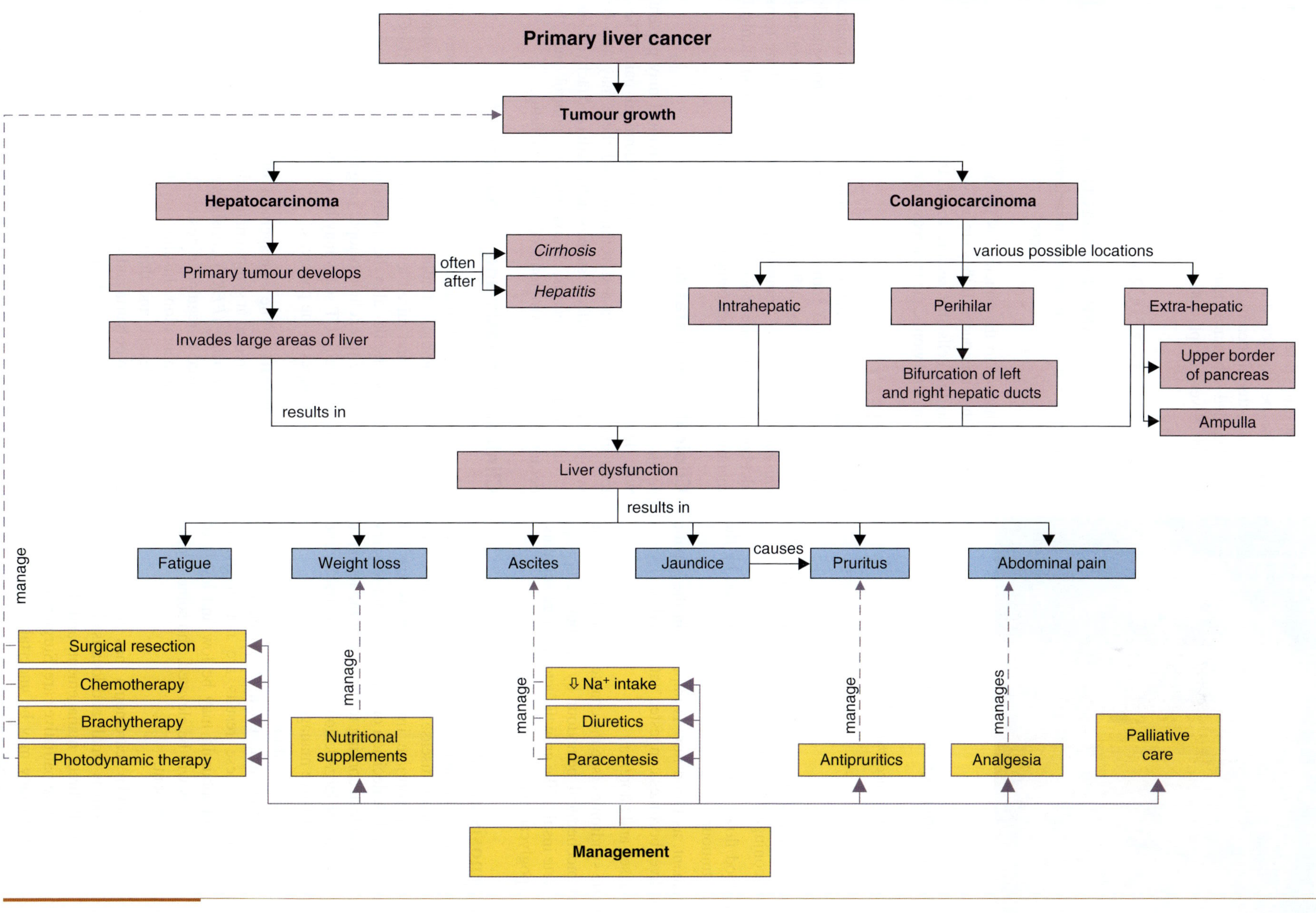

Figure 38.16

Clinical snapshot: Liver cancer

↓ = decreased; Na^+ = sodium ion.

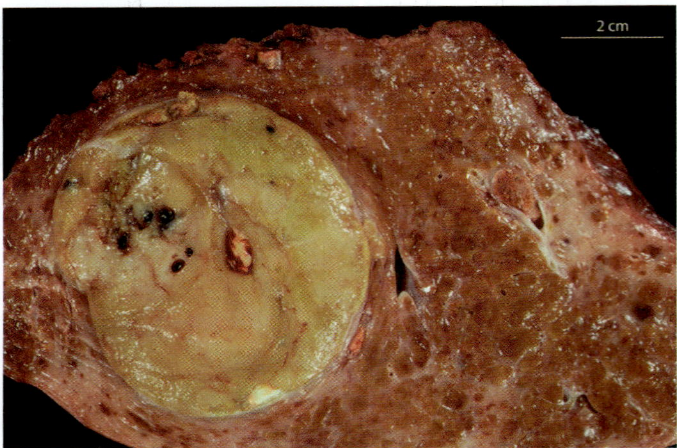

Figure 38.17

Hepatocellular carcinoma growing as a mass

Source: PR Benoit Terris, ISM/Science Photo Library.

- jaundice, as bile flow is obstructed and as the overall ability of the liver to conjugate bilirubin is reduced
- ascites, as blood flow in the portal vein is impeded by the growth of the tumour
- liver enlargement, as blood flow is impeded in the hepatic vein and the liver becomes congested with blood
- weakness, nausea and anorexia
- paraneoplastic syndromes (see the chapter 'Neoplasia'), due to abnormal biochemical behaviour by tumour cells (e.g. they may secrete insulin-like growth factor in large amounts, leading to hypoglycaemia).

Clinical diagnosis and management

Diagnosis Magnetic resonance imaging (MRI) allows assessment of the extent of disease, including the detection of metastases. Other appropriate imaging methods are CT scanning and ultrasound. A decision on whether or not to carry out a biopsy is often made according to the size of the lesion; it may not be appropriate for large lesions that are incurable, and which clearly require palliative management.

Haematology and chemical pathology tests may demonstrate anaemia, thrombocytopenia and, often, hyponatraemia and hypercalcaemia. However, these results are not diagnostic for the disease. Levels of albumin may be low and levels of bilirubin high, liver enzymes will be elevated, and some degree of coagulopathy may be present.

Management Hepatocellular carcinoma has a very poor prognosis unless the tumour is small and localised at the time of diagnosis. Staging will direct management, and those with advanced disease may receive palliative care. Surgical resection, chemotherapy and radiotherapy may be undertaken in various ways. As an alternative to surgical resection, cryosurgery may be used to destroy the cancer cells by freezing them. *Transcatheter arterial chemoembolisation (TACE)* may be used to deliver cytotoxic drugs directly into the tumour. For small lesions, alcohol may also be injected directly into the tumour. Radiotherapy using an external beam can be used to reduce tumour size, or radiolabelled substances that target the malignant cells may be injected. Liver transplantation may be a management option.

Major pancreatic diseases

LEARNING OBJECTIVE 6

Describe the disease processes in pancreatitis and pancreatic cancer.

A major hazard to the pancreas is the actions of the digestive enzymes that it produces. If they are activated prematurely, within or close to the cells that secrete them, they can cause severe damage. In other words, the pancreas undergoes *autodigestion*.

PANCREATITIS

Pancreatitis, an inflammation of the pancreas, is a consequence of such damage. Two forms of pancreatitis are recognised: *acute pancreatitis*, most often associated with gallstones, and *chronic pancreatitis*, commonly associated with long-term alcohol abuse. Figure 38.18 explores the common clinical manifestations and management of pancreatitis.

Clinical manifestations

In an acute episode of pancreatitis, an individual may present with fever and right upper quadrant abdominal pain. They may experience nausea and vomiting, and there may also be sympathetic nervous effects, such as tachycardia and tachypnoea.

In chronic pancreatitis, blood glucose control may be deranged, producing symptoms of diabetes mellitus.

Clinical diagnosis and management

Diagnosis Although blood tests are not diagnostic for pancreatitis, common findings may include leukocytosis, hyperglycaemia and raised levels of pancreatic lipase. β-hCG measurements should also be performed in all women of childbearing age to exclude ectopic pregnancy as the cause of the abdominal pain. CT scans may be useful in identifying any structural changes in the pancreas.

Management The management of someone who has pancreatitis is directed at symptomatic relief. *Pancreatic enzyme replacement therapy (PERT)* consisting of amylase, protease and lipase is used to regulate digestive function and fat-soluble vitamin supplementation. Insulin may be required to control blood glucose levels, and fluids may be necessary to correct dehydration from polyuria and vomiting. Pain relief is important and should be administered early, as pancreatitis can be intensely painful. Intractable pain may be managed using endoscopic surgery to relieve duct obstructions. Antiemetics may help with nausea and vomiting; if they are unsuccessful, a nasogastric tube may be placed to decompress the abdomen. Antimicrobials may be necessary to prevent or control secondary bacterial infection.

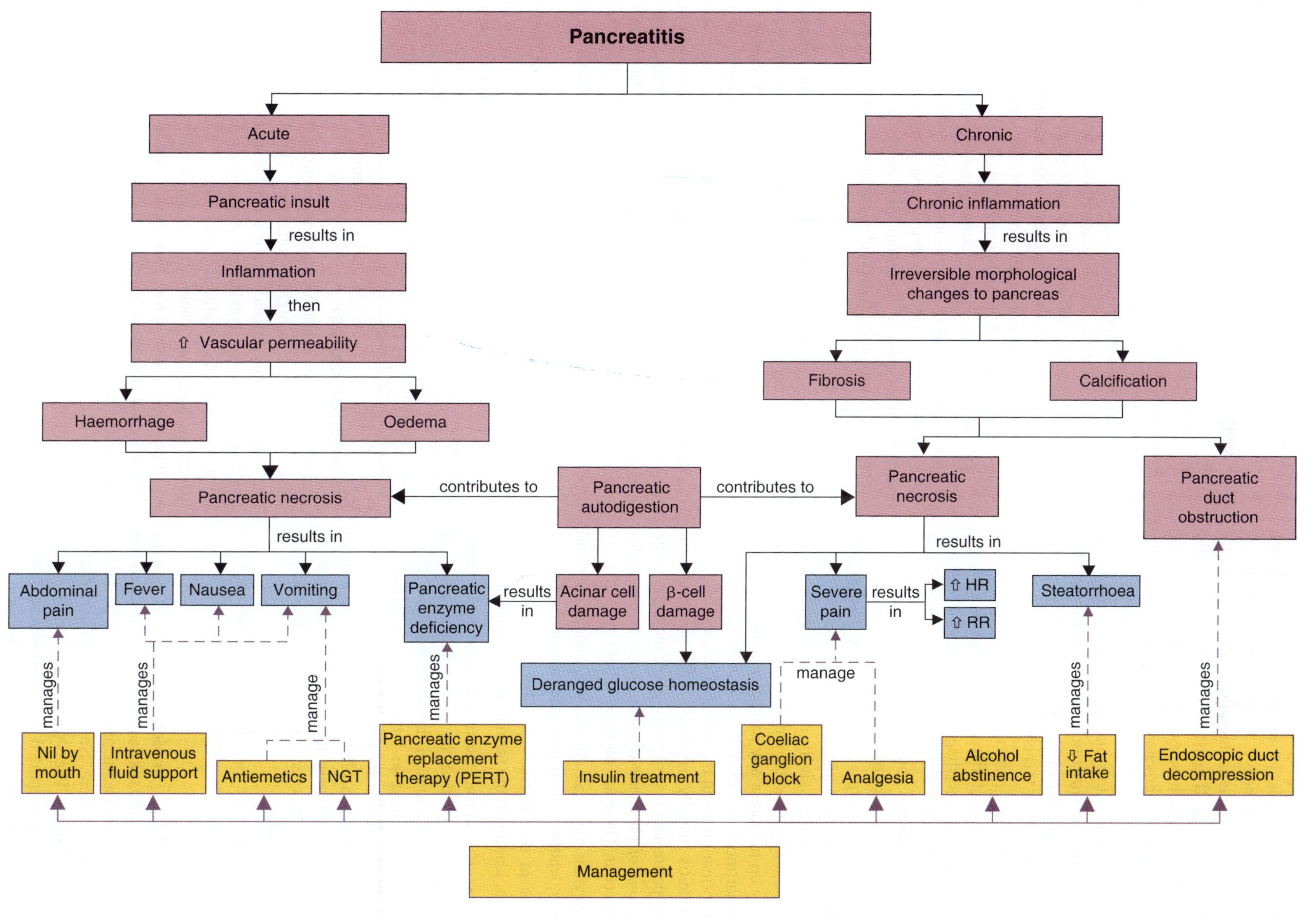

Figure 38.18

Clinical snapshot: Pancreatitis

↓ = decreased; ↑ = increased; β = beta; HR = heart rate; NGT = nasogastric tube; RR = respiration rate.

Acute pancreatitis

Aetiology and pathophysiology The role of alcohol in the disease process is not well understood. It cannot be straightforward, as most heavy drinkers do not develop pancreatitis. The role of gallstones in the pathophysiology of acute pancreatitis is, however, clear. If gallstones block the pancreatic duct, *digestive proenzymes* (such as trypsinogen) remain trapped within the pancreas, become activated and begin to destroy it. Damage to regional blood vessels by digestive enzymes leads to haemorrhage. Acute pancreatitis may also develop as a result of *viral, bacterial, fungal or parasitic infection*. It appears that viruses, particularly mumps, hepatitis or Coxsackie B infection, are the more common causes of this condition.

Tissue damage in the pancreas provokes an *acute inflammatory response* characterised by interstitial oedema, apoptosis, necrosis and haemorrhage. These responses may produce systemic effects, such as fever, circulatory shock (see the chapter 'Vascular disorders and circulatory shock'), kidney injury (see the chapter 'Acute kidney injury and chronic kidney disease') and respiratory distress syndrome (see the chapter 'Respiratory infections, cancers and vascular conditions').

As the pancreas is progressively damaged, enzymes such as pancreatic lipase and pancreatic amylase spill over into the bloodstream. They do not cause any pathophysiological effects in this fluid compartment, but their levels can be measured to yield valuable information about the extent of disease.

Acute pancreatitis usually resolves with no long-term symptoms and no permanent loss of function. However, in some cases, *complications of the acute disease*, some of them life-threatening, may occur. These are outlined below:

- Pancreatic enzymes may leak into the peritoneal cavity and cause irritation, leading to non-infectious peritonitis.
- Necrotic tissue in the pancreas may become infected by enteric bacteria, leading to the formation of abscesses.
- The destruction of exocrine tissue may lead to exocrine pancreatic insufficiency; that is, a reduced amount of pancreatic digestive enzymes in the small intestine. Thus, fat cannot be digested, and so fatty acids and fat-soluble vitamins (A, D, E and K) are not absorbed at adequate levels. The consequences of the insufficiency will be malnutrition with weakness and weight loss, steatorrhoea and deficiencies of fat-soluble vitamins. In severe cases, vitamin K deficiency will lead to coagulopathy.
- More rarely, the endocrine functions of the pancreas are affected, and diabetes mellitus develops.

Epidemiology Global incidence rates of acute pancreatitis are 3–138 per 100,000 and are increasing in most Western countries. Episodes of acute pancreatitis may be isolated or recurrent, and mild or severe. Severe acute pancreatitis is a life-threatening condition. The Australian mortality rates from pancreatitis have been reported by the AIHW at 0.08%. Males have a slightly higher rate compared with females. Acute pancreatitis is most often caused by gallstones (in women) or alcohol abuse (in men).

Chronic pancreatitis

Chronic pancreatitis is a complex group of conditions with different aetiologies. These aetiologies include *metabolic abnormalities* (such as hypercalcaemia, hyperlipidaemia and kidney disease), *autoimmune, obstructive* and *genetic causes*. There is also an atypical form that is not associated with tissue destruction but is characterised by *organ atrophy*.

Chronic pancreatitis is most often associated with alcohol abuse and cigarette smoking. It also develops in about 35% of people who have experienced at least one recurring episode of acute pancreatitis. In this condition, normal pancreatic tissues, both exocrine and endocrine, are replaced by scar tissue. The disease is progressive and irreversible, and predisposes to pancreatic cancer. However, the focus of this section is on the most common form of chronic pancreatitis.

The term 'chronic pancreatitis' may be misleading, as in this condition there is no long-term process of active inflammation. Rather, there is *destruction of normal tissue* and *gradual replacement of functional pancreatic cells by fibrous (scar) tissue*, probably the result of repeated episodes of acute inflammation.

Aetiology and pathophysiology In chronic pancreatitis, exocrine pancreatic insufficiency develops as functional tissue is lost. This results in reduced efficiency of digestive processes. The reduction in function is exacerbated by the stenosis (narrowing) of the pancreatic ducts by scar tissue; the stenosis may even extend to the duodenum. Nerves in the pancreas become trapped in scar tissue, which can cause upper abdominal pain, which may radiate to the back. The pain is sharp and often gets worse within half an hour of eating. Pain from pancreatitis may be somewhat relieved by sitting up or leaning forward.

In advanced cases, endocrine pancreatic insufficiency arises, leading to diabetes mellitus. People living with chronic pancreatitis are also at increased risk of developing pancreatic cancer. This is probably a consequence of increased rates of mitosis in regenerating glandular epithelial cells, as discussed earlier in this chapter in the context of alcoholic liver disease.

Pancreatic cancer

Pancreatic cancer is not common, accounting for 2% of cancer cases. However, it is highly aggressive. The AIHW estimated that the age-standardised incidence of pancreatic cancer in 2022 at 14 cases per 100,000 people, and a 1 in 85 (1.1%) risk of dying from the condition by the age of 85. Most cases of pancreatic cancer are pancreatic ductal adenocarcinomas.

The risk factors for pancreatic cancer are not well characterised. The most important risks appear to be advancing age—with the disease being very rare in people under 40 years of age—and a family history of pancreatic cancer. Other risk factors include cigarette smoking, male gender, diabetes mellitus, obesity, a high-fat diet, the presence of chronic pancreatitis and prior gastrectomy (surgical removal of the stomach).

The prognosis for pancreatic cancer is very poor. If the tumour is small and localised at the time of detection, surgery may be attempted, but most pancreatic cancers are well advanced and, hence, incurable at the time of diagnosis. Palliative treatment is directed at pain relief, and the removal of obstructions of the pancreatic, biliary or digestive tracts.

Aetiology and pathophysiology

A **pancreatic ductal adenocarcinoma** arises in the epithelium of the pancreatic duct system (see Figure 38.19). Like adenocarcinomas of the colon (see the chapter 'Intestinal disorders'), pancreatic ductal adenocarcinomas develop in several mutational steps over a number of years from normal pancreatic ductal epithelium, with 'benign' (or rather 'premalignant') neoplasms forming part of the progression. Typically, characteristic accumulations of oncogenes can be identified along the way. Researchers in this area are currently trying to find ways to identify earlier, less aggressive neoplasms before the emergence of full-blown malignancy.

Clinical manifestations

Most cancers of the pancreas originate in the head of the organ, and so may obstruct the pancreatic duct or bile duct. Such obstruction will give rise to abdominal pain, nausea and vomiting, jaundice, steatorrhoea, malnutrition and weight loss, as well as diabetes mellitus.

Tumours of the body and the tail of the pancreas cause pain as they invade the coeliac plexus. Like tumours of the pancreatic head, they cause nausea and weight loss, but are less likely, at least initially, to cause biliary obstruction and jaundice. Pancreatic cancers tend to invade locally to the duodenum or stomach (causing obstruction), liver or spleen (causing enlargement) and peritoneum (leading to ascites). Distant metastases also occur frequently.

Clinical diagnosis and management

Diagnosis Imaging studies are beneficial in identifying the disease severity. CT, MRI, ultrasound and positron emission tomography (PET) can all provide significant diagnostic information. Biopsy, using fine-needle aspiration that is guided by CT, will enable staging of the disease. Haematology and biochemistry measures may be beneficial in determining other issues that require management. However, no pathology measurements can be used to diagnose pancreatic cancer.

Management The staging of the cancer is used to guide management. Late-stage disease is associated with a very poor outcome, and palliation will often be the only option. Chemotherapy and radiotherapy may be used to reduce the size of a tumour, and surgical resection may be offered.

Pain relief and the management of discomfort caused by treatment are important, and in palliative care pain relief is paramount. If there is biliary obstruction, jaundice can cause pruritus. Pain, as well as the effects of biliary obstruction, may be managed by endoscopic decompression.

Cystic fibrosis

LEARNING OBJECTIVE 7

Describe the effects of cystic fibrosis on pancreatic structure and function.

Cystic fibrosis (CF) is one of the more common genetic diseases in Australia, affecting 1 in 2,500 births. In 2021 the Australian Cystic Fibrosis Data Registry reported 3,616 people with cystic fibrosis. People with the disease can have a greatly reduced life expectancy,

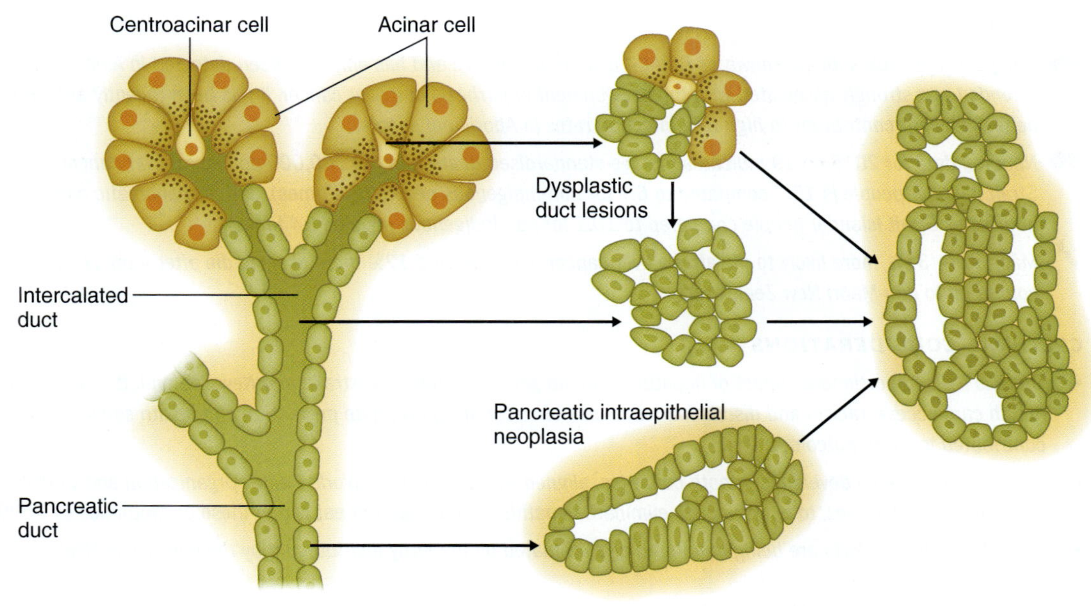

Figure 38.19
Pancreatic adenocarcinoma
Schematic presentation of the cytogenesis of pancreatic ductal adenocarcinomas induced in an animal model of the disease. Precursor lesions involve hyperplastic and dysplastic proliferation of the centroacinar cells, intercalated ducts and duct epithelium, but not of acinar cells.

tending to suffer from recurrent respiratory infections. The disorder is covered in detail in the chapter 'Obstructive pulmonary disorders', primarily as an obstructive pulmonary disorder. In addition to its effects on the respiratory system, the disease process may affect any mucus-secreting epithelium in the body, including that of the pancreatic ducts. The effects on the pancreas are clinically significant, and are the focus of this section.

AETIOLOGY AND PATHOPHYSIOLOGY

At the cellular level, the disease affects chloride transport across the cell membrane, with consequences for the movement of water across the membrane. In tissues that produce mucus secretions, the water content of the secretions is low, so the secretions are sticky and slow-moving. In the respiratory tract, this causes obstruction and predisposes the person to bacterial infections that eventually become life-threatening.

In the pancreas, the abnormally thick mucus secretion blocks the exocrine ducts, and blocks the ductal flow of secretions. The delivery of digestive enzymes to the duodenum is reduced, the digestion of dietary fat will be inadequate, and the person will suffer malabsoprtion unless digestive enzymes are therapeutically replaced. In severe disease, pancreatic enzyme production may be deficient. Furthermore, the loss of bicarbonate from the pancreas affects the neutralisation of gastric acid within the duodenum, and may result in tissue damage.

The trapping of digestive enzymes within the pancreas may induce inflammation that damages exocrine and endocrine tissue, as noted previously in the case of acute pancreatitis. This damage may be followed by fibrosis and scarring.

CLINICAL MANIFESTATIONS

CF affects the functions of many body systems. Gastrointestinal and nutritional problems related to CF arise from blockage of the pancreatic duct. When pancreatic lipase cannot flow to the small intestine, steatorrhoea will develop. The inability to chemically digest fat in the small intestine, and thus to absorb its products, will result in nutritional deficiencies, not only of energy but also of fat-soluble vitamins. Unless these deficiencies are corrected, an affected child will fail to thrive.

Long-term damage to the pancreas may involve endocrine as well as exocrine tissue, and thus can lead to diabetes mellitus. People with CF may also develop bowel obstructions from intussusceptions (see the chapter 'Intestinal disorders').

The clinical diagnosis and management of CF are covered in detail in the chapter 'Obstructive pulmonary disorders'. With respect to the pancreas, diagnosis will involve the assessment of fat absorption to the ingestion of a standardised dose, calculated from testing a faecal sample. Management will comprise PERT and fat-soluble vitamin supplementation.

INDIGENOUS HEALTH FAST FACTS AND CULTURAL CONSIDERATIONS

FAST FACTS

- *One particular HBV subtype known as HBV-C4 is quite aggressive and has only ever been detected in Australian Aboriginal populations. It tends to be strongly associated with the development of cirrhosis and liver cancer. It has been recently argued that this genotype may be a significant contributor to high HBV infection rates in Aboriginal people.*
- *National data for 2015–2019 indicates the age-standardised death rate per 100,000 people for liver cancer is Aboriginal and Torres Strait Islander people is 15.7 compared to 6.7 for non-Indigenous people (2.3 times), and for pancreatic cancer is 14.6 for Aboriginal and Torres Strait Islander people compared to 10.1 for non-Indigenous people (1.4 times).*
- *Māori were 31% more likely to die after a liver cancer diagnosis and 12% more likely to die after a pancreatic cancer diagnosis compared to non-Māori New Zealanders.*

CULTURAL CONSIDERATIONS

- *There is a disproportionate impact of hepatitis C on Indigenous people in Australia and New Zealand. It is acknowledged that inequalities in health care access, racism and discrimination, a lack of culturally appropriate prevention and health services, as well as other factors have contributed to these outcomes.*
- *Strategies have been developed in both countries, aligned with those of the World Health Organization and working with the respective Indigenous communities, to endeavour to eliminate hepatitis C as a health threat within these communities by 2030.*
- *In Australia these efforts are being monitored and evaluated by the Kirby Institute and by the Ministry of Health in New Zealand.*

Sources: Data from Australian Institute of Health and Welfare (2023); Gurney et al. (2020); Kirby Institute (2021); New Zealand Ministry of Health (2021); Plackett (2022).

LIFESPAN ISSUES

CHILDREN AND ADOLESCENTS

- It is not common for children with diagnosed and managed viral hepatitis to develop advanced liver disease from a hepatitis B or C infection. However, they should still be referred to specialist medical care so as to improve outcomes and reduce morbidity issues into adulthood.
- In Australia, approximately 7% of infants who are born to mothers with hepatitis C virus (HCV) infection will develop HCV.
- Chronic HCV infection in children may be asymptomatic, and, as such, there may be a risk for children to develop significant liver damage.
- Although uncommon, the incidence of idiopathic pancreatitis in children is increasing.
- Cholecystitis is rare in children.

OLDER ADULTS

- The incidence of liver cancer in those over 65 years of age is approximately 10 times that of those younger than 45 years, and half that of those aged 45–65 years.
- Older adults are more at risk than younger adults of developing cholelithiasis, because of the increased volume of cholesterol within the bile.
- Age-associated changes to the pancreas include pancreatic duct dilation and development of parenchymal calculi.
- Mortality rates of older adults from acute pancreatitis can be 2–2.5 times those of younger adults. The most common cause of pancreatitis in an older adult is cholelithiasis.

KEY CLINICAL ISSUES

- Most diseases and disorders in the abdominal cavity result in significant and complex clinical manifestations. Similar clinical manifestations occur irrespective of the cause. Comprehensive assessment and an analysis of history and various measurements will be required to assist in the differentiation of a cause.
- Those with pathology in the abdominal region can present with referred pain. Knowledge of where referred pain can occur and what it represents can assist a clinician in understanding a person's presentation.
- Transmission of viral hepatitis differs, depending on the type of virus involved. Knowledge of the different types, their transmission methods, incubation periods, clinical manifestations and whether a vaccine is available is critical for all health care professionals.
- Any pathology damaging hepatocytes can cause coagulopathy; therefore, the assessment of occult bleeding is important to prevent anaemia.
- The administration of medications to those with liver failure can be problematic. A knowledge of the role of the liver in the metabolism of drugs is essential to ensure that overdose or toxicity is prevented through dose adjustment and the early identification of adverse reactions.
- Assisting someone to manage an alcohol addiction requires the efforts of a multidisciplinary team, with significant emphasis on the skills provided by mental health professionals. Their families and their support people are also needed to increase the chances of success.
- Those with chronic pancreatitis often develop type 1 diabetes. Evaluation of a person's glucose status is important on admission and when the diagnosis of pancreatitis is made.

CHAPTER REVIEW

- Major functional alterations tend to occur in all of the common, serious hepatobiliary diseases. These are *damage to or death of hepatocytes, reduced metabolic activity of the liver*, *scarring*, the *impeded excretion of bile* and *pain*.
- *Hepatitis* is liver inflammation associated with hepatocyte damage. It may arise from a number of causes (e.g. *microbial pathogens* or *chemical toxicity*). The most important pathogens are the hepatitis viruses. A number of structurally unrelated viruses can infect the liver to cause hepatitis: these are *hepatitis A, B, C, D, E and G*. Hepatitis A and E are spread mainly by the faecal-oral route, whereas hepatitis B, C, D and G are spread by contact with blood and, to a lesser extent, other body fluids.
- *Serological testing* is the mainstay of viral hepatitis diagnosis: an infected person has antibodies to the virus, and in some cases viral antigens. There is no treatment for acute viral hepatitis other than hydration and the management of symptoms such as pain and nausea. Depending on the presentation and clinical picture, *antiviral and immunological medications* may be administered to decrease viral replication and thus reduce viral loads. *Preventative strategies* against infection are very important.
- *Fatty liver* is the first stage of fatty liver disease. It is completely reversible. In alcoholic liver disease, excessive alcohol intake leads to the *damage and death of hepatocytes*, accompanied by *inflammation*. If individual hepatocytes are destroyed but the connective tissue scaffolding of the lobules is not, the remaining hepatocytes will regenerate normal liver structure. However, where there is extensive damage and death of hepatocytes, extensive *scarring (cirrhosis)* will ensue and overall liver function will be reduced.

- *Gallstones (biliary calculi)* develop when cholesterol in the bile becomes over-concentrated and precipitates. They usually form in the gall bladder itself, and less commonly in the bile ducts. The formation of gallstones is termed *cholelithiasis*. Gallstones that lodge at the end of the common bile duct may block both that duct and the pancreatic duct. This can trap pancreatic digestive enzymes within the pancreas, damaging that organ.
- *Liver cancer* is one of the most common causes of cancer death worldwide. Primary liver cancer is associated with *chronic infection by hepatitis viruses* (especially hepatitis B virus) and with *alcoholic liver disease*. *Secondary cancers* often develop in the liver by metastasis from other organs, such as the lung, breast or colon.
- *Acute pancreatitis* may be isolated or recurrent, and mild or severe. Severe acute pancreatitis is a life-threatening condition. Acute pancreatitis is most often caused by gallstones (in women) or alcohol abuse (in men). Complications of the condition may include peritonitis, abscesses, exocrine pancreatic insufficiency and, more rarely, diabetes mellitus.
- *Chronic pancreatitis* is most often associated with alcohol abuse. In this condition, normal pancreatic cells, both exocrine and endocrine, are replaced by scar tissue. The disease is progressive and irreversible. In advanced cases endocrine pancreatic insufficiency arises, leading to diabetes mellitus. Those with chronic pancreatitis are also at increased risk of developing pancreatic cancer.
- *Pancreatic cancer* is not common. However, it is highly aggressive, with a correspondingly poor prognosis. The most common cancer of the pancreas arises in the epithelium of the pancreatic duct system, and is known as *pancreatic ductal adenocarcinoma*.
- *Cystic fibrosis (CF)* is one of the more common genetic diseases in Australia. At the cellular level, the disease affects chloride transport across the cell membrane. In tissues that produce mucus secretions, the water content of the secretions is low, and secretions are sticky and slow-moving. In the pancreas, the *abnormally thick mucus secretion blocks exocrine ducts*. The delivery of digestive enzymes to the duodenum is reduced, the digestion of dietary fat is inadequate, and the affected person will suffer malnutrition unless the enzymes are therapeutically replaced.

REVIEW QUESTIONS

1. In a cirrhotic liver, there are plenty of living hepatocytes, yet the liver does not function well. Explain.
2. Explain why the following might occur in severe liver disease:
   a. oedema
   b. excessive bleeding
   c. hepatic encephalopathy
   d. gynaecomastia in males
3. Explain why someone whose common bile duct is obstructed by a gallstone will display the following:
   a. jaundice with high blood levels of conjugated bilirubin
   b. itching
   c. dark urine
   d. pale, fatty faeces
4. Why does cirrhosis of the liver lead to portal hypertension?
5. Explain why the following might occur in portal hypertension:
   a. hepatic encephalopathy
   b. splenomegaly
   c. formation of oesophageal varices
6. Explain why gallstones may cause acute pancreatitis.
7. List the consequences of a pancreatic exocrine deficiency, and explain how they arise.
8. Explain why many people with cystic fibrosis develop diabetes mellitus.

HEALTH PROFESSIONAL CONNECTIONS

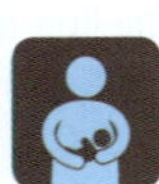

Midwives Pregnancy can increase the risk of cholelithiasis. The liver produces increased amounts of bile during pregnancy, and this may contain increased concentrations of cholesterol or reduced levels of some bile salts. Furthermore, high levels of progesterone in pregnancy will inhibit smooth muscle activity in the gall bladder. Early surgical intervention for gallstones carries a risk of fetal loss. Thus, where possible, medical management alone should be attempted during the first trimester, and surgery, preferably laparoscopic, should be delayed until the second trimester. Midwives should be mindful of the increased risk of gallstones in the pregnant woman. A multidisciplinary approach is required if cholelithiasis develops during pregnancy.

Physiotherapists Physiotherapists have a significant role in the care of those with cystic fibrosis (CF). Although most of the role is focused on caring for their respiratory health, a physiotherapist must understand the complex multi-organ effects of the disease. The gastrointestinal effects of CF may reduce a person's stamina or tolerance to rehabilitation. CF results in a condition of malabsorption, and poor management may result in caloric needs not being met. If not managed appropriately, this nutritional deficiency may interfere with the person's capacity to undertake the rigorous requirements of physiotherapy. All members of the health team caring for someone with CF should contribute to their assessment and management to ensure that appropriate and individualised care is provided.

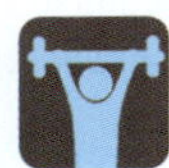

Exercise scientists Exercise is imperative to support and maintain many functions of the liver. Exercise professionals should educate those in their care about the importance of healthy diets and exercise to reduce the risk of developing a fatty liver. Fatty liver disease is associated with obesity and poor lifestyle choices. Those with liver disease from infection or excessive alcohol consumption can contribute to the decline of liver function through inactivity and weight gain.

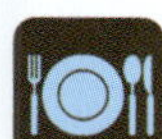

Nutritionists/Dieticians Nutrition professionals can influence the health of those with hepatic and pancreatic disease. Education and counselling surrounding good eating habits and the avoidance of fad and detox diets is important. The general principles of consuming low-fat, low-cholesterol diets and adequate amounts of fruit and vegetables can apply to all of the disease processes of the gastrointestinal accessory organs; however, specific conditions will benefit from a more individualised food plan. For those with liver disease, reducing or eliminating alcohol consumption is very beneficial. Protein needs should be monitored carefully, as excess protein will increase the risk of encephalopathy, but inadequate protein intake can increase liver damage. Vitamin supplementation should be monitored, as excess intake may worsen the disease. When assisting people with pancreatic issues, glucose control is important. Depending on the severity of disease, individuals with pancreatic disease may become diabetic. Other factors that may be beneficial include maintaining a low-fat diet, increasing fluid intake (but not coffee) and increasing the dietary intake of fruit and green vegetables. Reducing the amount of refined foods and red meats will help. Each diet plan should be individualised, and teamwork within the multidisciplinary team is imperative.

CASE STUDY

Ms Ruth Green (UR number 661243) is a 35-year-old woman who presented with right upper quadrant abdominal pain, a burning pain radiating to the left shoulder and nausea. This pain came on suddenly in the past 12 hours, and was not associated with any specific activity. Ms Green has been taking an oral contraceptive pill for many years, and is not currently in any steady relationship. She has lost approximately 20 kg in the past three months, and has recently experienced some emotional challenges in her life. Her body mass index (BMI) is 32. On assessment she appears in pain, dehydrated and pale, and is diaphoretic. After ultrasound and CT investigations, she was diagnosed with cholelithiasis. Her observations are as follows:

Temperature	Heart rate	Respiration rate	Blood pressure	SpO_2
37.2°C	90	24	140/84	96% (RA*)

*RA = room air.

Ms Green has been commenced on intravenous fluids; she has also been administered intravenous morphine and an antiemetic. Her preoperative documentation is completed; she only requires a blood glucose test and premedication on the call from the operating theatre. Ms Green is booked for a laparoscopic cholecystectomy, but, if the surgeon deems it necessary, she will have a laparotomy and open procedure instead. Her pathology results are as follows:

BIOCHEMISTRY

Patient location:	Ward 3	**UR:**	661243		
Consultant:	Smith	**NAME:**	Green		
		Given name:	Ruth	**Sex:**	F
		DOB:	11/04/XX	**Age:**	35

Time collected	14.23
Date collected	XX/XX
Year	XXXX
Lab #	5634543

ELECTROLYTES		UNITS	REFERENCE RANGE
Sodium	139	mmol/L	135–145
Potassium	3.6	mmol/L	3.5–5.2
Chloride	103	mmol/L	95–110
Bicarbonate	26	mmol/L	22–32
Glucose (random)	5.8	mmol/L	3.5–7.7
Iron	18	μmol/L	11–30
β-hCG	0	IU/L	> 25 IU/L pregnancy

HAEMATOLOGY

Patient location:	Ward 3	**UR:**	661243		
Consultant:	Smith	**NAME:**	Green		
		Given name:	Ruth	**Sex:**	F
		DOB:	11/04/XX	**Age:**	35

Time collected	14.23
Date collected	XX/XX
Year	XXXX
Lab #	3453455

FULL BLOOD COUNT		UNITS	REFERENCE RANGE
Haemoglobin	134	g/L	115–160
White cell count	9.4	$\times 10^9$/L	4.0–11.0
Platelets	265	$\times 10^9$/L	140–400
Haematocrit	0.39		0.33–0.47
Red cell count	4.52	$\times 10^{12}$/L	3.80–5.20
Reticulocyte count	1.3	%	0.2–2.0
MCV	88	fL	80–100
Neutrophils	3.61	$\times 10^9$/L	2.00–8.00
Lymphocytes	2.76	$\times 10^9$/L	1.00–4.00
Monocytes	0.57	$\times 10^9$/L	0.10–1.00
Eosinophils	0.30	$\times 10^9$/L	< 0.60
Basophils	0.12	$\times 10^9$/L	< 0.20
ESR	14	mm/h	< 12

CRITICAL THINKING

1. What risk factors does Ms Green have for the development of cholecystitis/cholelithiasis?
2. What useful information is provided in Ms Green's pathology results?
3. Ms Green complains of right upper quadrant pain and shoulder-tip pain. Explain how these symptoms arise.
4. There are many ways in which cholelithiasis may be managed. Draw up a table identifying all of the current management options, and the benefits and risks of each.
5. Following her cholecystectomy, what interventions and education does Ms Green require? (Don't forget dietary advice.) Draw up a table with each intervention or education principle, and in the next column explain each of these.

BIBLIOGRAPHY

Ahern, S., Salimi, F., Caruso, M., Ruseckaite, R., Wark, P., Schultz, A. & Armstrong, J. (2022). *The ACFDR Registry Annual Report, 2021*. Report No. 23. Melbourne: Department of Epidemiology and Preventive Medicine, Monash University. https://www.monash.edu/__data/assets/pdf_file/0004/3110269/2021-acfdr-annual-report-web.pdf.

Australian Institute of Health and Welfare (AIHW) (2018). *Hepatitis A in Australia: Fact Sheet.* Canberra: AIHW. Retrieved from https://www.aihw.gov.au/getmedia/6f006a38-4d3d-4926-b663-28f7b67e1d9f/aihw-phe-236_HepA.pdf.aspx.

Australian Institute of Health and Welfare (AIHW) & National Australian Indigenous Australians Agency (2023). Tier 1—Health status and outcomes. 1.08 Cancer. Data tables. *Aboriginal and Torres Strait Islander Health Performance Framework*. Canberra: AIHW. https://www.indigenoushpf.gov.au/measures/1-08-cancer.

Best, O. & Fredericks, B. (2021). *Yatdjuligin: Aboriginal and Torres Strait Islander nursing and midwifery care* (3rd edn). Port Melbourne, VIC: Cambridge University Press.

Bullock, S. & Manias, E. (2022). *Fundamentals of pharmacology* (9th edn). Sydney: Pearson Australia.

Cancer Australia (2022). *Liver cancer in Australia statistics.* Sydney: Cancer Australia. https://www.canceraustralia.gov.au/cancer-types/liver-cancer/statistics.

Cancer Australia (2022). *Pancreatic cancer in Australia statistics*. Sydney: Cancer Australia. https://www.canceraustralia.gov.au/cancer-types/pancreatic-cancer/statistics.

Department of Health and Aged Care (2023). National Communical Disease Surveillance Dashboard. *National Notifiable Disease Surveillance System.* https://nindss.health.gov.au/pbi-dashboard/.

González Grande, R., Santaella Leiva, I., López Ortega, S. & Jiménez Pérez, M. (2021). Present and future management of viral hepatitis. *World Journal of Gastroenterology* 27(47):8081–8102. https://doi.org/10.3748/wjg.v27.i47.8081.

Gurney, J., Stanley, J., McLeod, M., Koea, J., Jackson, C. & Sarfati, D. (2020). Disparities in cancer-specific survival between Māori and non-Māori New Zealanders, 2007–2016. *JCO Global Oncology* 6:766–74. https://doi.org/10.1200/GO.20.00028.

Howell, J., Pedrana, A., Cowie, B.C., Doyle, J., Getahun, A., Ward, J.,… Hellard, M.E. (2019). Aiming for the elimination of viral hepatitis in Australia, New Zealand, and the Pacific Islands and Territories: where are we now and barriers to meeting World Health Organization targets by 2030. *Journal of Gastroenterology and Hepatology* 34(1):40–48. https://doi.org/10.1111/jgh.14457.

Iannuzzi, J., Leung, J., Quan, J., Underwood, F., King, J.A., Windsor, J.W. & Kaplan, G.G. (2019). A256 global incidence of acute pancreatitis through time: a systematic review. *Journal of the Canadian Association of Gastroenterology* 2(2), 499–501. https://doi.org/10.1093/jcag/gwz006.255.

Kirby Institute (2021). *Progress towards hepatitis C elimination among Aboriginal and Torres Strait Islander people in Australia: monitoring and evaluation report, 2021.* Sydney: Kirby Institute, UNSW Sydney. https://kirby.unsw.edu.au/report/progress-towards-hepatitis-c-elimination-among-aboriginal-and-torres-strait-islander-people.

Marieb, E.N. & Hoehn, K. (2019). *Human anatomy and physiology* (11th edn). San Francisco, CA: Pearson Benjamin Cummings.

New Zealand Ministry of Health (2021). *National Hepatitis C Action Plan for Aotearoa New Zealand—Māhere Mahi mō te Ate Kakā C 2020–2030*. Wellington: Ministry of Health. https://www.globalhep.org/sites/default/files/content/resource/files/2022-12/hp7622_-_hep_c_action_plan_v11_web.pdf.

Odenwald, M.A. & Paul, S. (2022). Viral hepatitis: past, present, and future. *World Journal of Gastroenterology* 28(14):1405–29. https://doi.org/10.3748/wjg.v28.i14.1405.

Plackett, B. (2022). Hepatitis B: why hepatitis B hits Aboriginal Australians especially hard. *Nature Outlook* 603:562–63. https://www.nature.com/articles/d41586-022-00820-1.

Raftopulos, N.L., Torpy, D.J. & Rushworth, R.L. (2022). Epidemiology of acute pancreatitis in Australia from 2007–2019. *ANZ Journal of Surgery* 92(1–2):92–98. https://doi.org/10.1111/ans.17215.

Su, Y.-J., Chang, C.-W., Chen, M.-J. & Lai, Y.-C. (2021). Impact of COVID-19 on liver. *World Journal of Clinical Cases* 9(27):7998–8007. https://doi.org/10.12998/wjcc.v9.i27.7998.

Ueda, S., Fukamachi, K., Matsuoka, Y., Takasuka, N., Takeshita, F., Naito, A.,… Tsuda, H. (2006). Ductal origin of pancreatic adenocarcinomas induced by conditional activation of a human Ha-*ras* oncogene in rat pancreas. *Carcinogenesis* 27(12):2497–510. https://doi.org/10.1093/carcin/bgl090.

Wang, X., Lei, J., Li, Z. & Yan, L. (2021). Potential effects of coronaviruses on the liver: an update. *Frontiers of Medicine* 8:651658. https://doi.org/10.3389/fmed.2021.651658.

Zeng, D.-Y., Li, J.-M., Lin, S., Dong, X., You, J., Xing, Q.Q.,… Pan, J.-S. (2021). Global burden of acute viral hepatitis and its association with socioeconomic development status, 1990–2019. *Journal of Hepatology* 75(3):547–56. https://doi.org/10.1016/j.jhep.2021.04.035.

PART

9

Reproductive pathophysiology

39 Female reproductive disorders

KEY TERMS

Amenorrhoea
Anovulation
Benign breast diseases
Breast cancer
Cervical cancer
Cystocele
Dysmenorrhoea
Ectopic pregnancy
Endometriosis
Fibroadenoma
Fibrocystic disease
Infertility
Mastalgia
Mastitis
Menorrhagia
Metrorrhagia
Ovarian cancer
Ovarian cysts
Pelvic inflammatory disease (PID)
Polycystic ovary syndrome (PCOS)
Prolapse
Rectocele
Sexually transmitted infections (STIs)
Uterine (endometrial) cancer
Uterine fibroids/ leiomyomas
Vulvar cancer
Vulvovaginitis

LEARNING OBJECTIVES

After completing this chapter, you should be able to:

1. Describe the pathophysiology, diagnosis and clinical management of common menstrual disorders.
2. Differentiate between various types of genitourinary prolapse.
3. Describe the pathophysiology, diagnosis and clinical management of reproductive neoplasms.
4. Outline the pathophysiology, diagnosis and management of common inflammatory and infectious conditions affecting females.
5. Describe the causes and consequences of selected breast disorders such as mastitis and breast neoplasms.
6. Describe the pathophysiology, diagnosis and management of ectopic pregnancy.
7. Outline the current definitions of female infertility and some common conditions associated with decreased fertility.

WHAT YOU SHOULD KNOW BEFORE YOU START THIS CHAPTER

Can you describe normal endocrine system structures and functions?

Can you identify the normal female reproductive system structures, and describe their functions?

Can you describe the main stages of inflammation and healing?

Can you describe the principles of the pathophysiology and management of infection?

Can you outline the major concepts of neoplasia?

Introduction

In this chapter, the common disorders affecting the female reproductive system are discussed. These conditions can have profound effects on a woman's health, and unfortunately some conditions are still not yet fully understood. The content of this chapter includes menstrual disorders, reproductive complications of organ displacement, reproductive neoplasms, inflammatory and infectious conditions, breast disorders, ectopic pregnancies and important considerations regarding infertility.

Menstrual disorders

LEARNING OBJECTIVE 1

Describe the pathophysiology, diagnosis and clinical management of common menstrual disorders.

Common disruptions of menstrual cycle function are discussed in this section, including dysmenorrhoea, amenorrhoea and abnormal vaginal bleeding. These disruptions are common conditions that can greatly affect a woman's normal daily living pattern, and in some instances be quite debilitating. Figure 39.1 explores the common clinical manifestations and management of menstrual disorders.

DYSMENORRHOEA

Dysmenorrhoea is defined as painful monthly menstrual flow, and is characterised by cramping, lower abdominal pain. It is considered the most common gynaecological complaint. *Primary dysmenorrhoea* is associated with painful menses without evidence of microscopic pathology, whereas *secondary dysmenorrhoea* is linked to pelvic pathology.

Aetiology and pathophysiology

The pathophysiology of primary dysmenorrhoea is now considered to be strongly linked to an increased local secretion of the eicosanoids, especially the prostanoids, as well as other chemical mediators, such as vasopressin. These substances are known to be associated with increased myometrial contractility, cramping pain and changes in blood flow.

As the levels of progesterone decrease in the late post-ovulatory phase prior to menstruation, arachidonic acid from cell membranes is released, initiating the eicosanoid production cascade, and resulting in the production of prostaglandins, thromboxanes and leukotrienes. An inflammatory response ensues, accounting for the dysmenorrhagic symptoms. Prostaglandin $F2_{\alpha}$ is considered particularly important in this response, causing potent vasoconstriction, hypersensitisation of the nociceptive fibres and myometrial contraction, resulting in uterine ischaemia and pain. Prostaglandin E2 also has a key role to play in myometrial contraction. Both of these substances have been found to be present in higher than normal concentrations in the menstrual fluid of women with primary dysmenorrhoea. There is evidence that prostacyclin levels, which mediate vasodilation and uterine relaxation, appear to be reduced in this condition, enhancing the imbalance in uterine contraction and vascular responsiveness.

Epidemiology

Primary dysmenorrhoea is prevalent in adolescents and young women, decreasing in incidence with age. It can only occur in women with ovulatory cycles, so typically it does not begin with the first anovulatory menstrual cycles in adolescence. The condition is relatively uncommon during the first two to three years after menarche. The onset of secondary dysmenorrhoea is generally later in life, many years after menarche, but can occur in younger women who have endometriosis.

Risk factors for primary dysmenorrhoea include adolescence, excessive anxiety or stress, disrupted social networks, family history, menarche at a young age, cigarette smoking, nulliparity (i.e. yet to bear offspring) and being either underweight or obese.

Clinical manifestations

The symptoms of primary dysmenorrhoea occur around the start of menstrual flow, either prior to or shortly after its onset. The most common manifestation is cramping lower abdominal pain, but nausea, vomiting, bloating and headache may accompany this symptom. The symptoms typically last for the first 24–48 hours of menstruation. The pattern of symptoms in secondary dysmenorrhoea can vary considerably, manifesting as either cyclic or acyclic pain.

AMENORRHOEA

Amenorrhoea is the absence of menses. *Primary amenorrhoea* is associated with disruption to normal menstrual function. If normal sexual development is present, then it is defined as an absence of menses by age 15–16 years. If no secondary sexual characteristics have developed, then it is characterised as an absence of menses by age 13–14 years. *Secondary amenorrhoea* is considered to be an absence in menses for three months when regular menstruation had occurred previously, or for nine months in a woman who was formerly oligomenorrhoeic. Amenorrhoea is considered to be the normal physiological response prior to menarche, and in a woman who is pregnant or is postmenopausal.

Aetiology and pathophysiology

In *primary amenorrhoea*, an adolescent lacking secondary sexual characteristics and showing a delay in puberty may be demonstrating an impairment of the *hypothalamic–pituitary–gonadal axis*. This could occur at the level of the hypothalamus and pituitary where there is a failure to release the gonadotropins, or at the gonadal level when the ovaries fail to develop due to a congenital malformation, genetic disorders (e.g. Turner's syndrome) or exposure to radiation at an early age. *Chronic illnesses*, such as diabetes mellitus, thyroid disease, chronic renal insufficiency and immunodeficiency, can also delay normal growth and sexual development. Where normal sexual development has taken place, *impaired development* of the uterus or an alteration in vaginal anatomy (e.g. a transverse vaginal septum or an imperforate hymen) is usually suspected. Breast development with poor pubic hair growth may be associated with *androgen*

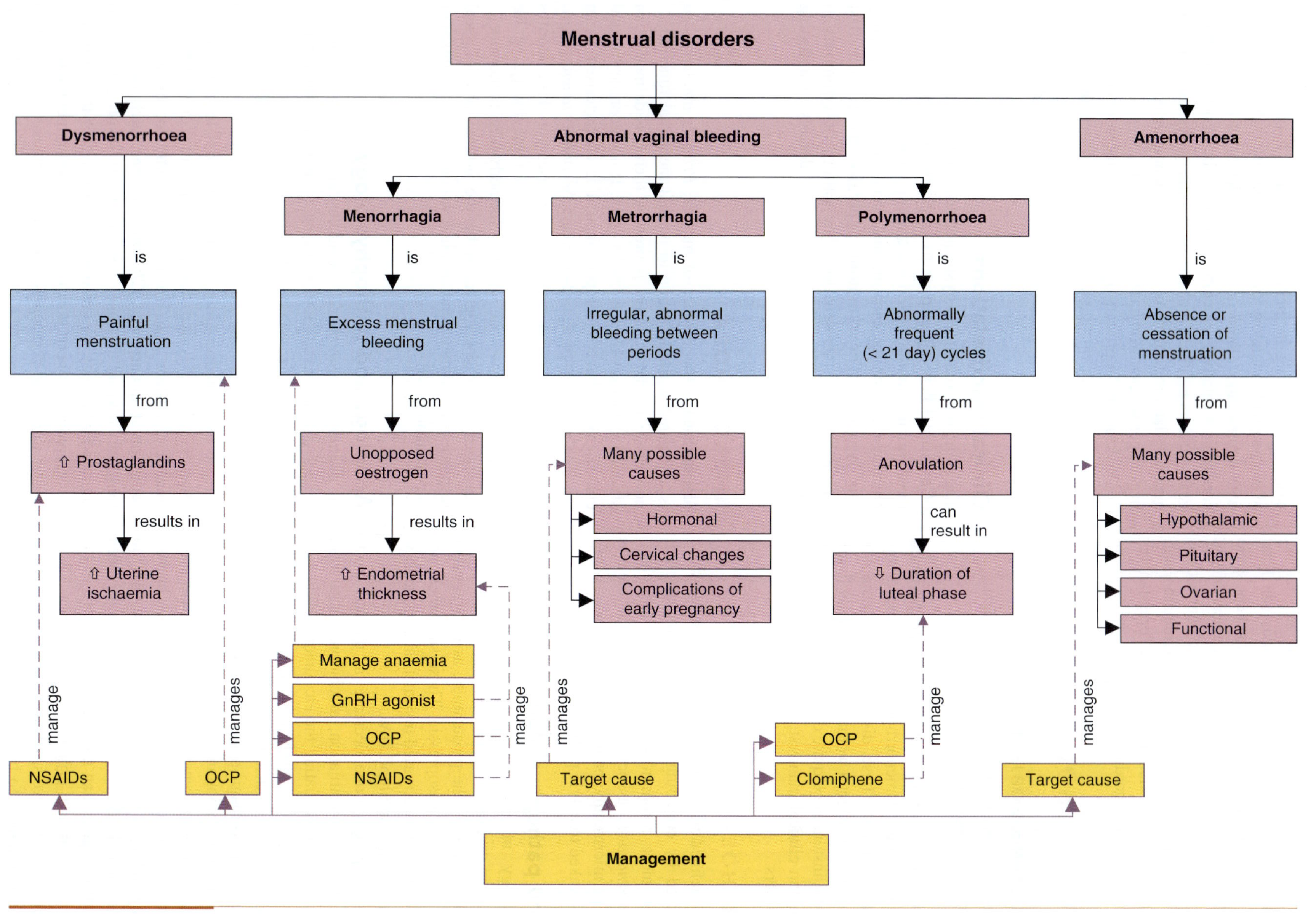

Figure 39.1

Clinical snapshot: Menstrual disorders

↓ = decreased; ↑ = increased; GnRH agonist = gonadotropin-releasing hormone agonist; NSAIDs = non-steroidal anti-inflammatory drugs; OCP = oral contraceptive pill.

insensitivity syndrome. In this case, the affected person is genotypically male, but phenotypically female because the reproductive tissues are incapable of responding to the androgen signal.

Secondary amenorrhoea can also occur following a disruption to the normal functioning of the hypothalamic–pituitary–gonadal axis. This can occur due to weight loss in *eating disorders* (e.g. anorexia nervosa or bulimia) or as a result of *excessive exercise* or *severe stress*. In the latter situations, women athletes may experience an episode of secondary amenorrhoea that may require clinical management. In these conditions, the normal secretion of gonadotropin-releasing hormone from the hypothalamus is impaired. A decrease in leptin levels, a protein hormone that regulates energy inputs and outputs, has also been implicated here.

Hyperprolactinaemia can disrupt anterior pituitary function, resulting in amenorrhoea. This condition can be caused by a pituitary tumour, may accompany thyroid disease or occur during treatment with certain medications, such as antipsychotic agents, tricyclic antidepressants, opioids, calcium channel antagonists or oestrogens. *Hypothyroidism* can also lead to secondary amenorrhoea. Normal menstruation is usually restored by drug treatment for this form of thyroid disease (see Part 4 for a fuller discussion of the endocrine disorders).

ABNORMAL VAGINAL BLEEDING

The term *abnormal (or dysfunctional) bleeding* covers a range of conditions associated with blood loss from the genital tract, including **menorrhagia** (heavy menstrual bleeding generally regarded to be in excess of 80 mL per cycle), **metrorrhagia** (prolonged irregular menstruation), *polymenorrhoea* (frequent menstruation), *oligomenorrhoea* (infrequent scanty menstruation), *postcoital bleeding* (bleeding following sexual intercourse), *intermenstrual bleeding* (bleeding not associated with menstruation or sexual intercourse, often known as 'spotting') and *postmenopausal bleeding. Amenorrhoea* may also be classified as abnormal vaginal bleeding.

Aetiology and pathophysiology

For some of these conditions, the site of the bleeding may not be the uterus, but could arise from anywhere along the genital tract or even the urinary tract. Furthermore, the possibility that intermenstrual bleeding in a woman of childbearing age is due to an undiagnosed pregnancy should not be excluded.

A common cause of menorrhagia is uterine fibroids (*leiomyomas*), benign smooth muscle tumours of the myometrium (discussed later in this chapter). Menorrhagia can occur in adolescence associated with *anovulatory cycles* as the immature hypothalamic–pituitary–gonadal axis develops. This state can persist for a couple of years after menarche. Menorrhagia is also associated with *liver or kidney disease, hypothyroidism, systemic lupus erythrematosus* and, not surprisingly, in *coagulation disorders* such as von Willebrand disease (where the risk of bleeding is increased).

Cervical lesions, such as polyps, neoplasias and cervicitis, are commonly associated with postcoital bleeding. Abnormal uterine bleeding is also associated with *endometrial cancer* and *endometrial hyperplasia*. The latter can manifest as postcoital or intermenstrual bleeding, or as menorrhagia. In endometrial cancer, postmenopausal bleeding may be a presenting sign, but it can also present as menorrhagia in a significant proportion of premenopausal women.

The use of a sex hormone preparation for contraception or to provide symptomatic relief for menopausal or postmenopausal women can cause intermittent bleeding or spotting.

CLINICAL DIAGNOSIS AND MANAGEMENT

Diagnosis

A clinical history that includes menstrual history should be collected, along with general health and lifestyle information, including weight changes and exercise levels. A physical examination, both general and pelvic, is also important.

Laboratory tests should include a Pap smear, blood tests, including β-human chorionic gonadotropin (β-hCG) to exclude pregnancy, a full blood count to exclude systemic causes, thyroid function tests (as thyroid imbalance may cause menstrual anomalies), gonadotropin levels (FSH and LH) to assess pituitary function, ovarian hormones (progesterone and oestradiol) to assess ovarian function, karyotyping for primary amenorrhoea to exclude genetic anomalies, such as Turner's syndrome, and cervical/vaginal cultures.

Diagnostic imaging procedures, including a transvaginal ultrasound and possibly also a saline infusion sonogram, should be done to detect neoplasms, including abnormalities in the uterus and the pelvic cavity. Such abnormalities include uterine fibroid tumours, ovarian cysts and polyps.

Hysteroscopy should be conducted to detect anomalies (e.g. fibroids and polyps) within the uterine cavity. An endometrial biopsy may also be taken at this time and sent for histopathological testing. Refer to Clinical Box 39.1 for more detailed information regarding this procedure. Diagnostic dilatation and curettage (D&C) of the uterine cavity can be done, with a tissue sample being sent for histopathological examination. Diagnostic laparoscopy will assist in detecting structural anomalies that may be associated with endometriosis, cysts or tumours.

Management

Management of menstrual disorders and abnormal uterine bleeding will depend on the clinical diagnosis, as well as the severity of the presenting condition, and may include medical, surgical and lifestyle approaches.

Medical approaches may include an oral contraceptive or the insertion of an intrauterine device to regulate menstruation. Analgesics, prostaglandin inhibitors (e.g. non-steroidal anti-inflammatory drugs [NSAIDs]) and hormone replacement medications (e.g. a progestin-like progesterone or medroxyprogesterone) can be used to regulate uterine bleeding. Iron supplements may be required to replace iron lost due to excessive uterine bleeding.

Surgical approaches may include a therapeutic dilation and curettage (D&C) to correct prolonged or excessive bleeding, endometrial ablation to permanently destroy the endometrial

CLINICAL BOX 39.1

Common procedures and investigations associated with female reproductive disorders, and the possible findings

Hysteroscopy
In hysteroscopy, a small fibreoptic scope is passed into the uterus via the cervical canal to enable visualisation of the uterine cavity.

Hysterosalpingogram (HSG)
In a hysterosalpingogram, a fine catheter is passed into the uterine cavity and contrast medium is instilled. Serial X-rays are used to monitor the passage of the radio-opaque medium through the uterus and fallopian tubes, to facilitate assessment of the uterine cavity and the patency of the fallopian tubes.

Hysterosalpingo-contrast sonography (HyCoSy)
In this procedure, an abdominal ultrasound or transvaginal ultrasound (TVUS) is used to monitor the passage of a small volume of fluid (saline or ExEm Foam) that is instilled into the uterine cavity via a fine catheter. This is used to assess the uterine cavity and the patency of the fallopian tubes. No anaesthetic is required, and it is performed as an outpatient procedure at a medical imaging practice.

Polymerase chain reaction (PCR)
PCR is generally performed on a first-catch urine sample. This test uses a technique that enables amplification of DNA present in the sample, indicating the presence of bacterial and/or parasite DNA (e.g. chlamydia, *Neisseria gonorrhoeae* or *Trichomonas*).

Intrauterine insemination (IUI)
This procedure is performed at or near the time of ovulation, and requires preparation of a sample of sperm (partner or donor) that is washed and concentrated. The male needs to have 'normal' semen analysis, and the female should have patent fallopian tubes to optimise the chance of 'normal' fertilisation occurring. The prepared sample is deposited into the uterine cavity via a small catheter inserted through the cervical canal.

In-vitro fertilisation (IVF)
This procedure involves ovarian stimulation using a combination of drugs that may include: gonadotropin-releasing hormone agonists (e.g. nafarelin acetate) or antagonists (e.g. ganirelix or cetrorelix), FSH and β-hCG. The procedure involves transvaginal oocyte retrieval, fertilisation of the oocytes in the laboratory, and embryo culture (for two to five days), followed by embryo transfer (this may be performed under ultrasound guidance) and cryopreservation of the suitable remaining embryos. The IVF procedures may require the use of donor gametes (i.e. eggs or sperm).

layer of the uterus in women who are not concerned about future fertility, and hysterectomy.

The management of menstrual disorders will vary depending on the presenting condition. Health professionals should ensure that the woman understands normal menstrual cycle physiology and self-care strategies. After assessment, care may include advice regarding treatment options, including promoting understanding of the proposed medical or surgical therapies, provision of information regarding the monitoring of basal body temperature to assess for the presence or absence of ovulation, assistance to prepare for operative procedures (including advice regarding postoperative care and the provision of emotional support), and the provision of postoperative care, including ongoing assessment (e.g. extent of bleeding) and pain management strategies. Lifestyle therapies may include regular physical exercise, a dietary review, and the use of local heat (low temperature heat packs/pad on the abdomen) to reduce pain.

Genitourinary prolapse

LEARNING OBJECTIVE 2

Differentiate between various types of genitourinary prolapse.

Prolapse, or descent, of pelvic organs into the vagina can occur when the supporting structures holding these organs in the normal anatomical position fail. The key supporting structures are the ligaments and muscles of the pelvic floor holding the pelvic organs in place (see Figure 39.2). Three common displacements of pelvic organs to be described in this section are uterine prolapse, cystocele and rectocele.

UTERINE PROLAPSE

Aetiology and pathophysiology

The uterus normally lies in an anteriorly flexed position over the urinary bladder. Holding it in place are the *broad, uterosacral, round and cardinal ligaments*. These structures allow some movement of the uterus, but usually prevent it from excessive descent into the vagina.

When this support system fails, intra-abdominal pressure will force the uterus downwards into the vagina. The prolapse may lead to the uterus appearing outside the vaginal opening. Under these circumstances, the exposed cervix may become damaged, leading to bleeding or ulceration (see Figure 39.3).

Risk factors for prolapse include family history, connective tissue disorders or congenital malformation, age, pregnancy, obesity, straining associated with constipation or chronic cough, and neuromuscular disorders.

CYSTOCELE

Aetiology and pathophysiology

A **cystocele** is when there is descent of a part of the urinary bladder into the vagina (see Figure 39.4B). It occurs when a weakness develops in the vaginal musculature. Common causes of vaginal weakness include trauma during childbirth or surgery, and advancing age.

RECTOCELE

Aetiology and pathophysiology

A **rectocele** is when there is a defect in the rectovaginal septum that results in part of the anterior wall of the rectum prolapsing into the posterior wall of the vagina (see Figure 39.4C). It occurs when the *perineal body* (the pyramidal fibromuscular central

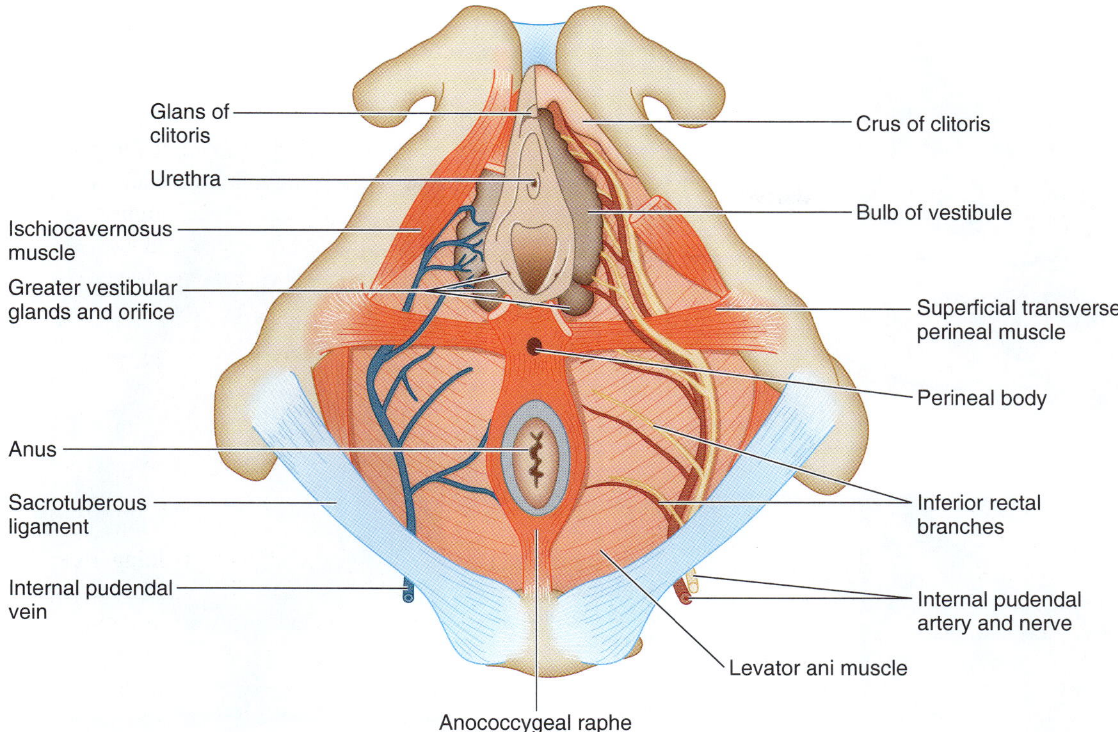

Figure 39.2

Cross-section showing the supporting structures of the pelvic floor

tendon of the perineum between the vaginal introitus and anus) detaches, resulting in perineal descent and ultimately, rectocele formation. Common causes include inherited or acquired weakness of the pelvic support structures, such as connective tissue disorders, vaginal childbirth, chronic increased intra-abdominal pressure (from constipation), obesity or surgery, and advancing age. If it is the small bowel that prolapses into the vagina, it is termed an *enterocele*.

CLINICAL MANIFESTATIONS

Clinical manifestations of pelvic floor prolapse can include vaginal discomfort, a sensation of pelvic pressure, back pain, urinary incontinence and/or dysuria. Dyspareunia (painful sexual intercourse) may also be reported. It may be possible to palpate or visualise some of the structure protruding through the vaginal opening (see Figure 39.3C).

CLINICAL DIAGNOSIS AND MANAGEMENT

Diagnosis

The person's past medical, surgical and reproductive history should be considered, and a physical/pelvic examination should be undertaken.

Management

The management is aimed at relieving/minimising symptoms, preventing infection and correcting or minimising the presenting condition. The treatment options may depend on the woman's age and the severity of the condition. Conservative, non-surgical management options are preferred, as they are associated with lower morbidity and mortality risks, and with relative success measured by satisfaction rates as reported by those in your care. Non-surgical interventions include pelvic floor exercises (Kegel exercises) and pessaries (vaginal pelvic support devices). Surgical options include repair of structural anomalies (also known as colporrhaphy), and in some cases a hysterectomy may be considered (commonly performed through the vagina, resulting in no external surgical scars).

The care will focus on identifying the woman's understanding of her condition (and the anatomy of a normal reproductive system) and of the proposed treatment options, with the provision of education as required. If surgical procedures are planned, then care will involve providing assistance with preoperative preparation (including an explanation of postoperative care and the provision of emotional support), postoperative care (including ongoing assessment, pain management strategies, monitoring fluid balance, the use of thromboembolic deterrent (TED) stockings and other devices as required). For non-surgical treatments, education focuses on the performance of pelvic floor exercises, the use of a pessary if required, and continence management strategies. Lifestyle factors are also an important consideration, regardless of the management approach, and these should include discussions regarding diet and weight loss, and also the reduction or elimination of caffeine consumption to reduce urinary symptoms such as frequency and urgency.

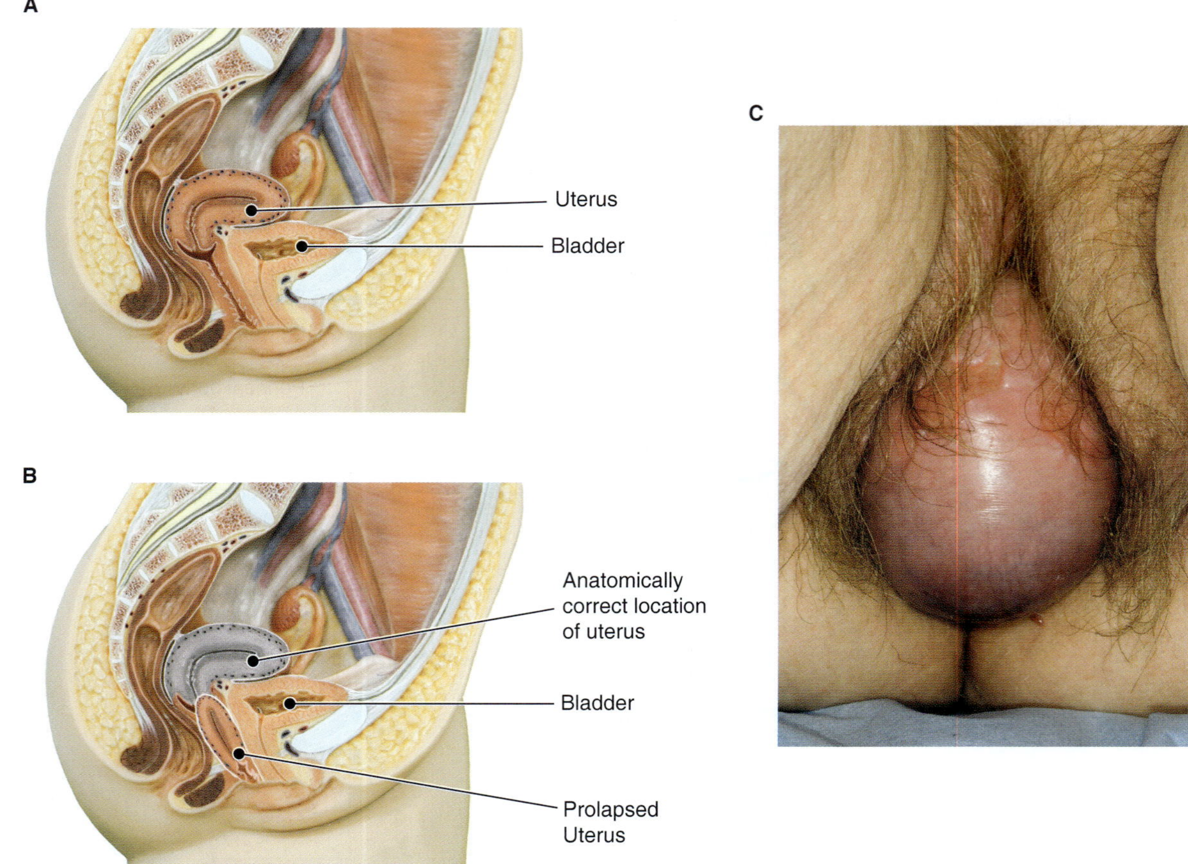

Figure 39.3

Uterine prolapse

(A) Normal uterine position. (B) Uterine prolapse where supporting tissue has failed and the uterus descends. (C) Third-degree prolapse of the uterus protruding beyond the vaginal canal.

Source: (A) and (B) modified from Puntasit Choksawatdikorn/123RF; (C) Dr P. Marazzi/Science Photo Library.

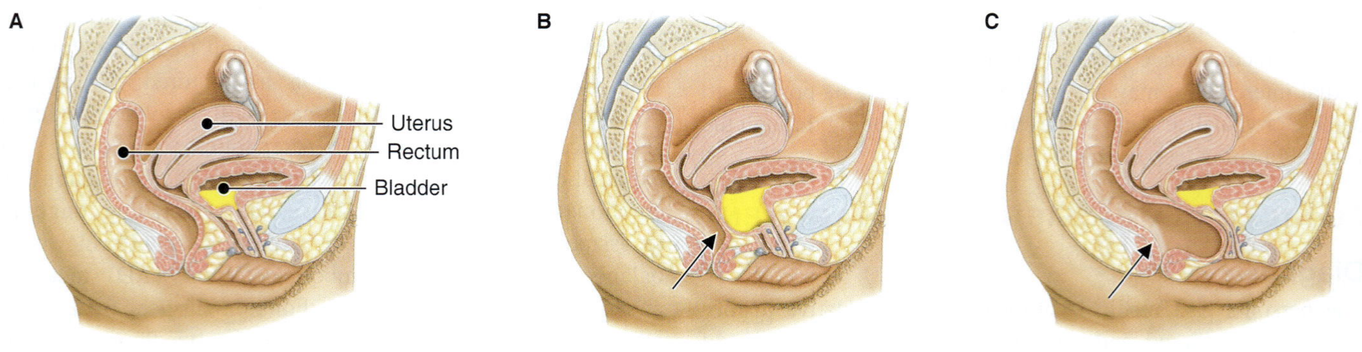

Figure 39.4

Pelvic organ prolapses: cystocele and rectocele

(A) Normal anatomy. (B) Cystocele: the pubocervical fascia can tear and permit prolapse or bulging of the urinary bladder into the vagina. (C) Rectocele: the front wall of the rectum can prolapse or herniate into the back wall of the vagina.

Reproductive neoplasms

LEARNING OBJECTIVE 3

Describe the pathophysiology, diagnosis and clinical management of reproductive neoplasms.

The principles of neoplastic disorders are well covered in the chapter 'Neoplasia'. A *neoplasm* can be defined as *abnormal proliferation of tissue* or the growth of an *abnormal mass of tissue that does not serve a physiological purpose*. Typically, we think of cancerous tumours when neoplasia is discussed, but equally the term can refer to a skin mole, a wart or a cyst.

Reproductive neoplasms, both benign and malignant, that arise in the abdominopelvic reproductive structures can affect the vulva, cervix, uterus and ovaries. Breast neoplasms and other forms of neoplasia (such as endometriosis, ovarian cysts and uterine fibroids) can also occur.

ENDOMETRIOSIS

Endometriosis is a common reproductive disorder affecting women of childbearing age. It affects about 5–10% of women in the general population.

Aetiology and pathophysiology

Endometriosis is characterised by the establishment of ectopic endometrial tissue, known as *endometrial implants*, outside the uterine cavity. The implants can grow on the ovaries, uterosacral and round ligaments, oviducts and the peritoneal surfaces, either within the pouch of Douglas or on the uterus (see Figure 39.5).

The widely accepted explanation of the pathophysiology of this condition was first proposed in the early 20th century. It is proposed that fragments of endometrial tissue enter the pelvic cavity through the open fallopian tubes via a process of *retrograde menstruation*. Individual susceptibility is the key to the progression of the condition, as the implants must firstly evade breakdown by the body's defence mechanisms, then adhere to the peritoneum and establish a self-sustaining system to continue to survive and grow in this environment. The ectopic endometrial implants are particularly sensitive to oestrogens for their proliferation. Recent studies have indicated that prostaglandin E2 plays a significant role in promoting the local expression of enzymes that result in increased oestrogen concentrations within the ectopic implants.

Individual susceptibility to endometriosis is believed to depend on a mix of *genetic and environmental factors*. Environmental agents with oestrogen-like endocrine disruptive properties, such as dioxin and diethylstilboestrol (DES), have been implicated in the pathogenesis of this condition.

Clinical manifestations

The clinical manifestations of endometriosis include chronic pelvic pain, painful sexual intercourse (dyspareunia), dysmenorrhoea and infertility. The complications of the condition include adhesions, as well as the compression and infiltration of the pelvic nerves.

Clinical diagnosis and management

Diagnosis A clinical history and a physical examination are undertaken, and diagnostic imaging procedures may include pelvic ultrasound and laparoscopy. If clinical evidence suggests bladder and bowel involvement, magnetic resonance imaging (MRI), intravenous pyelogram (IVP) and barium enema may be undertaken to assess the extent of the disease process. A full blood count may be performed to assess for anaemia and exclude infective processes.

Management The management of endometriosis will depend on the symptom severity, and the woman's age and fertility needs. Treatment may include medical and/or surgical approaches.

Medical treatment may involve the use of analgesic and prostaglandin synthesis inhibitors (e.g. the NSAIDs) to control pain, and hormone therapy (including oral contraceptives, progesterone or gonadotropin-releasing hormone [GnRH] agonist) to reduce systemic oestrogen levels, which, in turn, results in the shrinking/degeneration of the endometrial implants.

Surgical treatment involves laparoscopic (or in some cases laparotomy) ablation/excision of endometrial implants and endometriomas, as well as adhesiolysis (if indicated). Surgery may be followed by three to six months' treatment with GnRH agonist medication. A total hysterectomy may be performed in severe cases where fertility is not a concern.

The care will focus on identifying the woman's understanding of her condition and the provision of education as required, including the discussion of treatment options. Pre- and postoperative care will include ongoing assessment, pain management approaches and the provision of emotional support, as well as the identification and discussion of possible fertility concerns. Communication should also seek to include the woman's partner (if applicable). Lifestyle management approaches may include a discussion of the benefits of regular exercise, as well as weight management strategies.

OVARIAN CYSTS

Aetiology and pathophysiology

Ovarian cysts are *fluid-filled sacs on the ovary*, and can occur at any time from puberty to menopause. The cysts are *sex hormone sensitive*, and can alter their size in response to hormonal signalling at different stages of the menstrual cycle. The cysts can develop during the follicular stage if the ovum is not released, or later on when a corpus luteum fails to degenerate. Intact ovarian cysts can remain asymptomatic. If the cyst ruptures, there will be abdominal pain and haemorrhage, which may be severe enough to warrant surgery.

Polycystic ovary syndrome (PCOS) is a condition diagnosed when two of the three following criteria are present: irregular or no ovulation, hyperandrogenaemia and polycystic ovaries. Other causes of hyperandrogenaemia (e.g. Cushing's disease or an androgen-secreting tumour) should be excluded. The prevalence rate is estimated to be up to 8–13% of women of reproductive age. Symptoms of PCOS include hirsutism, acne, obesity, virilisation, amenorrhoea and infertility.

Figure 39.5

Common sites of endometriosis

Source: John Bavosi/Science Photo Library.

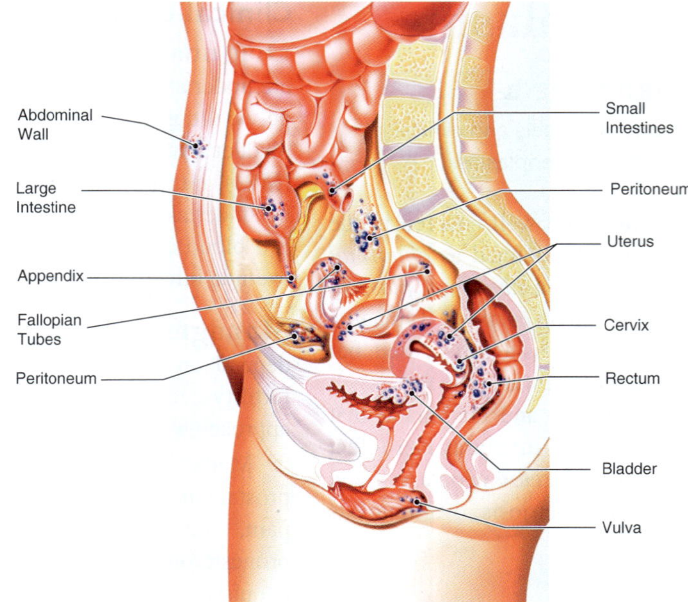

The main pathophysiological mechanisms underlying PCOS are alterations in the function of the hypothalamic–pituitary–ovary (HPO) and the hypothalamic–pituitary–adrenal (HPA) axes, as well as the onset of insulin resistance.

The *hyperandrogenaemia* seen in this condition is primarily associated with an increased production of ovarian androgens. This is due to an increased basal secretion of androgens from the ovaries, coupled with an altered pattern of luteinising hormone (LH) pulsatile secretion. The LH pulses are increased in amplitude, and become more irregular in response to an alteration in the secretion of gonadotropin-releasing hormone from the hypothalamus. Prior to diagnosis, women with PCOS show elevated circulating oestrogen levels due to the conversion of androgen at the level of peripheral tissues.

PCOS is also associated with *hyperactivity of the HPA axis*. However, processes within the adrenal gland also reduce synthesis of glucocorticoids and increase production of gonadocorticoids.

Insulin resistance is a characteristic of PCOS. In response to this state, the pancreatic β-cells secrete more insulin in order to meet metabolic demands. This leads to *hyperinsulinaemia*. It has also been proposed that hyperinsulinaemia may be due, at least in part, to impaired insulin clearance through the liver in PCOS. Hyperinsulinaemia also increases HPA axis activity, and decreases the production of the blood-borne binding protein for testosterone, sex hormone binding globulin, resulting in more free biologically active testosterone and further enhancing of the androgen hyperactivity.

A vicious cycle becomes established between insulin resistance and hyperandrogenaemia. Elevated testosterone levels secreted by the ovaries and adrenal glands can result in increased abdominal obesity, which further promotes insulin resistance. Abdominal obesity increases the levels of inflammatory mediators, such as chemokines, C-reactive protein and cytokines, and increases the activity of inflammatory cells. Increased secretion of these inflammatory mediators predicts metabolic syndrome, and increases the risk of diabetes mellitus (see the chapter 'Diabetes mellitus'). PCOS is recognised as having a strong association with diabetes.

PCOS is associated with an abnormal blood lipid profile—elevated cholesterol, triglyceride and low-density lipoprotein (LDL) levels, accompanied by lower high-density lipoprotein (HDL) levels. Women with PCOS are at a greater risk of hypertension and cardiovascular disease.

Clinical diagnosis and management

Diagnosis A clinical history and a physical examination are required. Diagnostic procedures may involve pelvic ultrasound and laparoscopy. Bloods tests may be performed to assess gonadotropin and ovarian hormone levels (including FSH, LH and testosterone). If PCOS is suspected, metabolic profiles may be assessed, including glucose tolerance, insulin resistance and lipid profiles.

Management The management of the condition may include medical, surgical and lifestyle approaches, and this will depend on the symptom severity, and the woman's age and fertility needs, with the aim being to normalise menstruation and resolve **anovulation** and subfertility.

Medical treatment options may include oral contraceptives, oral hypoglycaemic medications (e.g. metformin) and ovulation induction (using the partial oestrogen agonist clomiphene). Surgical approaches may include ultrasound-guided aspiration of functional cysts, and laparoscopic surgery for ovarian drilling for those with anovulatory PCOS, or ovarian cystectomy, depending on the type/size of ovarian cyst.

The care will focus on identifying the woman's understanding of her condition and the provision of education as required, including a discussion of treatment options. Pre- and postoperative care will include ongoing assessment, pain management approaches and the provision of emotional support. Lifestyle approaches are also an important adjunct to medical/surgical treatments, and will include weight loss (if obese), dietary review and the promotion of regular physical exercise.

UTERINE FIBROIDS

Uterine fibroids/leiomyomas are *benign tumours of the myometrium.* They are also known as *uterine myomas*.

Aetiology and pathophysiology

Uterine fibroids can develop within the uterine wall as intramural, submucosal, pedunculated or mixed growths (see Figure 39.6). *Intramural fibroids* are contained within the uterine wall, *submucosal fibroids* intrude into the uterine cavity and *pedunculated fibroids* are external to the uterine wall but remain tethered to the uterus. Submucosal fibroids appear to be more likely to be associated with menorrhagia. Fibroids are dependent on the presence of oestrogens and progesterone for proliferation. Initially, they are particularly sensitive to progesterone, but later become dependent on a mix of endogenous hormones.

In pregnancy, fibroids can lead to placental abruption (where the placenta separates from the uterine lining), pain and premature labour. Intramural fibroids can increase the risk of infertility.

Epidemiology

Uterine fibroids occur in 20–25% of women. Pathological examination of specimens taken during surgery suggests that the actual prevalence may be much higher, as high as 77%. Fibroids are not reported in prepubescent girls, occur occasionally in adolescents, and are most common in women in their 30s and 40s.

Risk factors for the development of fibroids include nulliparity, ethnicity, a family history of fibroids (the strongest association is when three first-degree relatives have had fibroids) and obesity. A link between the development of fibroids and the use of the oral contraceptive pill remains controversial, as studies have demonstrated mixed results; some show an increased risk, while others show a decreased risk or no association.

Clinical manifestations

The usual clinical manifestations of fibroids include excessively heavy menstrual bleeding, iron-deficiency anaemia, as well as pelvic pressure and pain. Pelvic pressure is due to uterine enlargement, which can be equivalent to the size of the pregnant uterus at 20 weeks. Typically, the presence of fibroids distorts the shape of the uterus. Fibroids located anteriorly tend to put pressure on the urinary bladder, causing urinary symptoms. Posteriorly located fibroids put pressure on the gastrointestinal tract, and can cause constipation.

Clinical diagnosis and management

Diagnosis A clinical history and a physical and pelvic examination are undertaken. Diagnostic procedures may involve a transvaginal or pelvic ultrasound, hysteroscopy, and possibly a laparoscopy and/or endometrial biopsy to exclude cancer.

Management The management of this condition will depend on the type/location of the fibroid/s, symptom severity, and the woman's age and her fertility needs. Medical treatments may include: analgesics and/or prostaglandin inhibitors (e.g. NSAIDs) for pain/cramps; oral contraceptives to control menorrhagia; GnRH agonist (e.g. nafarelin or leuprorelin) to reduce oestrogen levels and, in turn, reduce the tumour size; and iron supplementation for anaemia. Surgical and other treatments include: myomectomy (open or laparoscopic-assisted) to minimise the impact on reproductive ability; hysterectomy; or embolisation of the uterine arteries that provide the blood supply to the fibroid.

The care should focus on identifying the woman's understanding of her condition and the provision of education as required, including a discussion of treatment options. Pre- and postoperative care may include ongoing assessment,

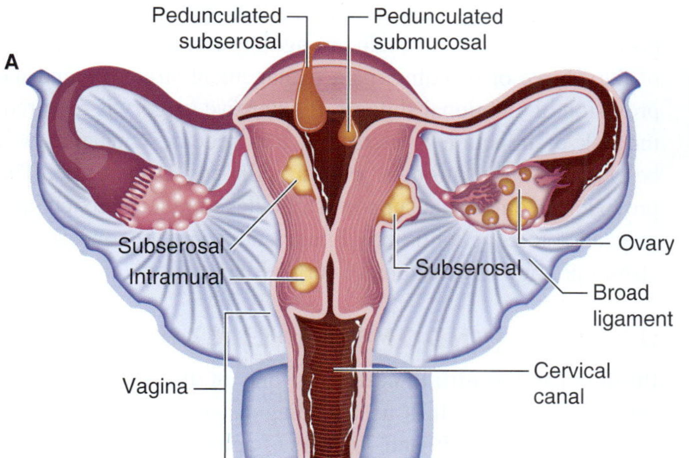

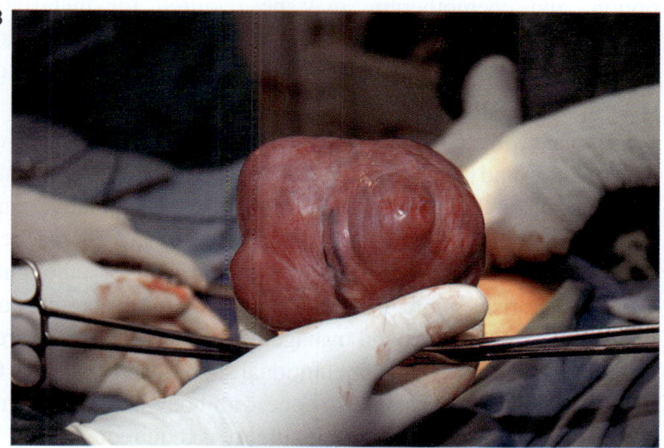

Figure 39.6

Uterine fibroids

(A) Types of uterine fibroids. (B) Surgical excision of a large uterine fibroid.

Sources: (A) Designua/Shutterstock; (B) Medicshots/Alamy Stock Photo.

pain management approaches and the provision of emotional support. Consideration should also be given to weight loss (if obese) and dietary review, including strategies to increase iron intake.

Female reproductive cancers

Figure 39.7 explores the common clinical manifestations and management of female reproductive system cancers.

VULVAR CANCER

Aetiology and pathophysiology

Vulvar cancer is considered the rarest of the gynaecological cancers. Usually it is diagnosed in postmenopausal women around the age of 65 years. The vast majority of vulvar cancers are squamous cell carcinomas. Risk factors for this form of cancer are advanced age, immunosuppression and being a current smoker.

A premalignant precursor lesion called *vulvar intraepithelial neoplasia (VIN)* occurs, which affects younger women. The peak incidence of this lesion is at 40 years of age. *Human papillomavirus infection (HPV)* is considered a strong correlation with VIN, with about 80% of women affected by the latter being seropositive for HPV.

Vulvar cancer may also develop as a result of a chronic inflammation in the genital area known as *lichen sclerosis*. The latter condition is characterised by a whitish plaque-like skin lesion, skin atrophy, tearing and bruising of tissue, and scarring.

Clinical diagnosis and management

Diagnosis Following a clinical history and a physical and pelvic examination, diagnosis is confirmed by biopsy of the lesion. If metastatic spread is suspected, then additional diagnostic procedures may include chest X-ray, computed tomography (CT)/MRI, cystoscopy/IVP and barium enema.

Management Surgical excision is the main treatment option, and chemotherapy may be required for metastatic disease. The extent of the surgery will depend on the stage of the cancer, and may range from local excision electrocautery or cryosurgery to simple or radical vulvectomy.

The care will focus on identifying the woman's understanding of her condition and the provision of education as required, including a discussion of treatment options. Pre- and postoperative care will include ongoing assessment, pain management approaches, urinary catheter management and the provision of emotional support. The risk of infection is high following vulvectomy, and thus advice regarding wound management and hygiene measures is important. The provision of emotional support and strategies to reduce anxiety and assistance to cope with body image concerns are also important when extensive surgery is required.

CERVICAL CANCER

Aetiology and pathophysiology

Cervical cancer is one of the leading causes of cancer death in the world, particularly in developing countries. In Western countries, cervical cancer screening programs have resulted in a significant decline in incidence and mortality. Most cervical cancers are squamous cell carcinomas, with the remainder arising from glandular tissue.

A causal relationship has been established between *HPV infection* (serotypes 16 and 18), the premalignant precursor lesion known as *cervical intraepithelial neoplasia (CIN)* and cervical cancer. *Other risk factors* include multiple sexual partners, sexually transmitted infection, age, cigarette smoking, immunosuppression and nutritional factors.

Clinical manifestations

Invasive cervical cancer may manifest as abnormal vaginal bleeding and chronic vaginal discharge, as well as dyspareunia and postcoital bleeding. This usually represents an advanced stage of cancer development, with earlier stages typically remaining asymptomatic.

Clinical diagnosis and management

Diagnosis A clinical history and a physical and pelvic examination are undertaken, and diagnosis may be confirmed by Pap smear, colposcopy and cervical biopsy. Pelvic CT or MRI may be required to assess the extent/spread of the tumour.

Management Management depends on the grading of the dysplastic changes. A loop electrosurgical excision procedure (LEEP) or loop electrosurgical excision of transformation zone (LEETZ) may be performed to simultaneously diagnose and treat lesions found on colposcopy. Surgical procedures may include cryosurgery, conisation and hysterectomy. If the cancer recurs and there is no lymphatic spread, then the pelvic contents may need to be surgically removed and replaced with an ileal conduit and/or colostomy. Radiation therapy (via external beam or intracavity implants) may be required to treat invasive cervical cancers. Preventative management should include HPV vaccination for girls aged 12–13 years, and early detection through biannual Pap smears.

The care will focus on identifying the affected woman's understanding of her condition and the provision of education as required, including a discussion of treatment options. Pre- and postoperative care will include ongoing assessment, including of the degree of bleeding, pain management strategies and the provision of emotional support. If extensive surgery is required, the risk of infection is increased, and specific education will be required in relation to wound, skin and stoma care. The provision of emotional support, strategies to reduce anxiety and assistance to cope with body image and sexuality concerns are also important when extensive surgery is required.

UTERINE (ENDOMETRIAL) CANCER

Uterine (endometrial) cancer is one of the most common cancers in women. It is usually diagnosed in postmenopausal women of between 50 and 70 years of age.

Aetiology and pathophysiology

The most common type of endometrial cancer arises from glandular tissue (*adenocarcinomas*). It tends to be diagnosed at an early stage of development and so has a good prognosis. *Mucinous carcinomas*, comprised of a large proportion of mucus, also have a good prognosis. Other forms of endometrial cancer

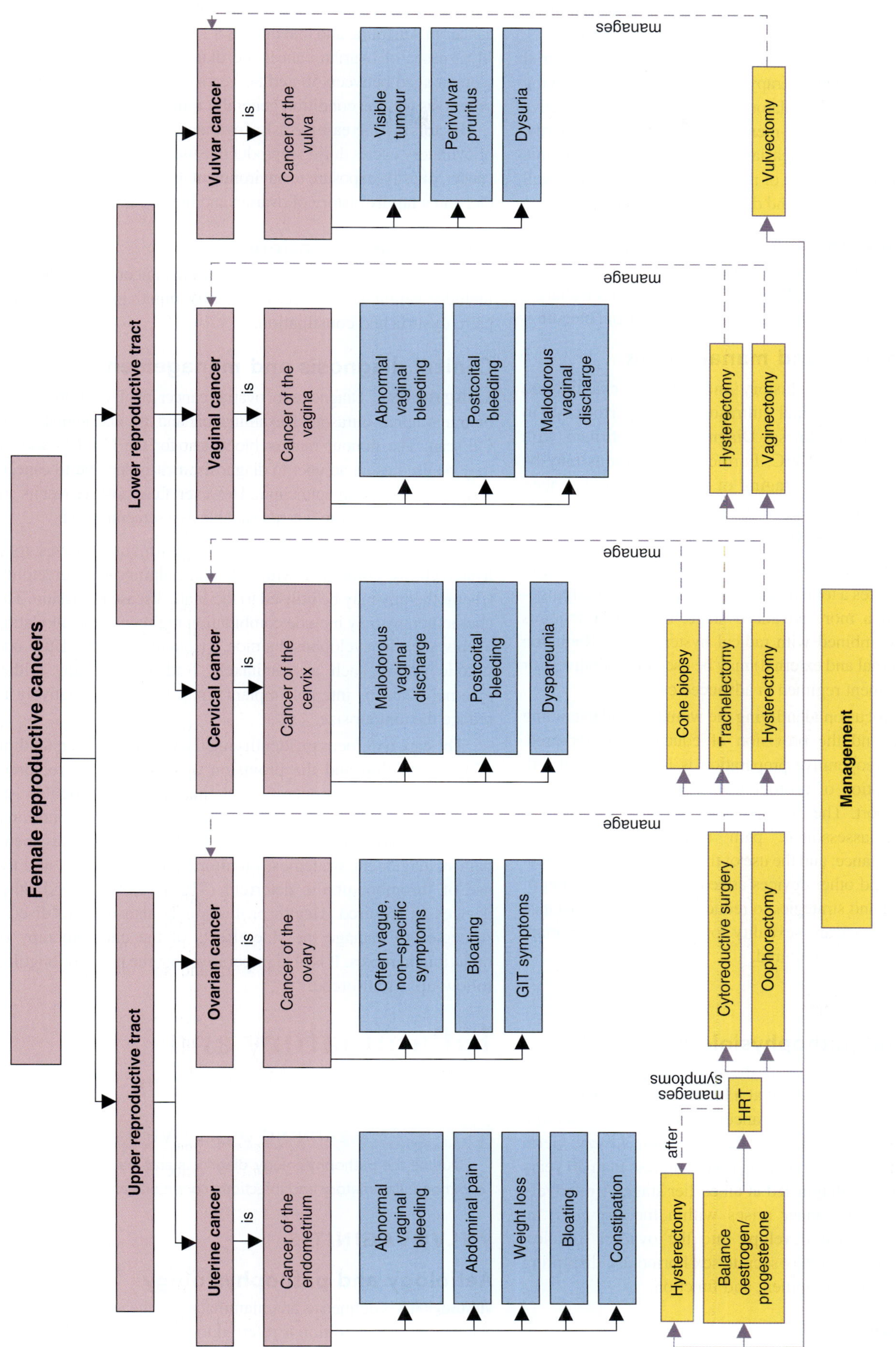

Figure 39.7

Clinical snapshot: Female reproductive system cancers

GIT = gastrointestinal tract; HRT = hormone replacement therapy.

arise from different types of epithelium (*serous and squamous epithelium*) and are more invasive, with a poorer prognosis.

Risk factors associated with the development of endometrial cancer include oestrogen therapy without an accompanying progestin, the number of ovulatory cycles during reproductive life (i.e. a long menarche-to-menopause interval), nulliparity, anovulation, advanced age, Caucasian genetics, high socioeconomic status, obesity and the presence of medical conditions such as gall bladder disease, hypertension and diabetes mellitus.

Clinical manifestations

Common symptoms of endometrial cancer include postmenopausal vaginal bleeding and chronic vaginal discharge. In premenopausal women, there may be intermenstrual bleeding.

Clinical diagnosis and management

Diagnosis A clinical history and a pelvic examination are performed. Transvaginal ultrasound is performed to measure endometrial thickness. Diagnosis is confirmed with an endometrial biopsy or D&C. Further investigations may be required, depending on the staging of the endometrial cancer, and these may include chest X-ray, MRI, bone scans, IVP, cystoscopy and a barium enema.

Management Surgery is the principal treatment. Cancer in its early stage requires a total hysterectomy and bilateral salpingo-oophorectomy. At a more advanced stage, the cancer requires node dissection combined with radical hysterectomy. Radiation therapy (both internal and external) may be used preoperatively or as part of the treatment regimen in advanced cases.

The care will focus on identifying the woman's understanding of her condition and the provision of education as required. Assistance with preoperative preparation is important, and will include an explanation of postoperative care and the provision of emotional support. The provision of postoperative care will include ongoing assessment, pain management strategies, monitoring fluid balance, and the use of thromboembolic deterrent (TED) stockings and other devices as required. The provision of emotional support and strategies to reduce anxiety and assistance to cope with body image and sexuality concerns are also important when extensive surgery is required.

OVARIAN CANCER

Aetiology and pathophysiology

Ovarian cancer mostly arises in the *epithelial surface* of the ovary, and tends to be diagnosed at a later, more advanced stage of development. Some ovarian cancers are *germ cell tumours*, which arise from one or more of the *embryonic layers*. Germ cell tumours tend to occur in younger women, less than 30 years old, and are generally diagnosed at an earlier stage. A relatively rarer form of ovarian cancer arises within the *sex cord*, an embryonic structure that develops into the ovarian follicles. Tumour cells of this form may secrete sex hormones, disrupting normal reproductive development and function.

Epidemiology

The death rate associated with ovarian cancer makes it one of the top gynaecological malignancies and a common cause of death in women. In 2022, it is estimated that 1,016 women died of ovarian cancer in Australia, and that there is a 1 in 84 risk of this diagnosis. Most cases of ovarian cancer are diagnosed in postmenopausal women aged between 50 and 80 years of age. Unfortunately, the prognosis for this condition generally remains poor.

Factors that increase the risk of ovarian cancer include the number of ovulatory cycles during reproductive life, nulliparity, prior breast cancer, obesity, exposure to environmental contaminants, a high-fat diet and a family history of ovarian and breast cancer.

Clinical manifestations

When symptoms associated with ovarian cancer occur, they can include weight loss, increases in abdominal girth, abdominal pain, dysuria and constipation.

Clinical diagnosis and management

Diagnosis Diagnosis for ovarian cancer involves an abdominal or transvaginal ultrasound examination and an abdominal/pelvic CT scan. The tumour marker blood test for the CA-125 antigen may be used as an adjunct to diagnosis, as it is specific to cancers arising in the ovarian epithelium. However, false positive results are common, and therefore it is not suitable as a screening test.

Management In most cases, treatment involves total hysterectomy combined with bilateral salpingo-oophorectomy. Chemotherapy may be utilised to facilitate disease remission. The chemotherapy may include combination regimens (e.g. alkylating agents such as cyclophosphamide, cisplatin or carboplatin, and mitotic poison such as paclitaxel). Radiation therapy (either external beam or internal implant) may be used palliatively to reduce the tumour size.

The care will focus on identifying the woman's understanding of her condition and the provision of education, as required. Assistance with preoperative preparation will include an explanation of postoperative care and the provision of emotional support. Postoperative care will include ongoing assessment, pain management strategies, monitoring fluid balance, and the use of thromboembolic deterrent (TED) stockings and other devices as required. Health professionals also need to discuss strategies to manage the side-effects of the chemotherapy or radiation therapies. It is also imperative that the need for ongoing follow-up is reinforced.

Inflammatory and infectious disorders

LEARNING OBJECTIVE 4

Outline the pathophysiology, diagnosis and management of common inflammatory and infectious conditions affecting females.

VULVOVAGINITIS

Aetiology and pathophysiology

Vulvovaginitis is defined as an inflammation of the vulva and vagina. Sometimes this condition is referred to simply as *vaginitis*. Given the anatomical proximity of the two structures, an inflammation of one of these structures can readily progress to involve the other.

The most common cause is an *infection*, but an inflammation could arise from *trauma*, a *reaction to chemicals* or to latex condoms, or *wetness from prolonged contact* with a sanitary pad or nappy. Most females will experience at least one episode of vulvovaginitis during their life.

The infectious organisms most commonly associated with vulvovaginitis are bacterial (*Haemophilus vaginalis, Chlamydia trachomatis* or *Neisseria gonorrhoeae*), fungal (*Candida albicans*), parasitic (*Trichomonas vaginalis*) or viral (human papillomavirus or herpes simplex virus type 2). With the exception of *C. albicans* infection, these infections are usually sexually transmitted. Conditions that predispose a female to vulvovaginal candidiasis are immunosuppression, antimicrobial therapy, pregnancy, diabetes mellitus and oestrogen therapy.

Clinical manifestations

Common manifestations of vulvovaginitis include vaginal or perineal itching, vaginal discharge, local irritation and burning sensations. In some cases, the infection may be asymptomatic.

Classically, *vulvovaginal candidiasis* (or *genital thrush*) manifests as a white 'cheesy' discharge from the vagina, irritation, redness and itching.

SEXUALLY TRANSMITTED INFECTIONS

The **sexually transmitted infections (STIs)** that are the focus of this section are chlamydia, *Trichomonas*, syphilis, gonorrhoea, genital warts and genital herpes.

Aetiology and pathophysiology

STIs can be acquired through vaginal, anal and/or oral sex with someone who has become infected. The STIs damage the local tissues and structures around the portal of entry and induce inflammation. If left untreated, the infections induce chronic inflammatory states that affect the organs and structures of the pelvic cavity (see 'Pelvic inflammatory disease'), and may spread to cause significant systemic lesions in major organs. Early treatment of these infections is, therefore, the most effective, although this is problematic, because the infection, especially in its early stages, may be asymptomatic. *C. trachomatis* is the bacterium that causes *chlamydia. Gonorrhoea* is caused by the bacterium *N. gonorrhoeae*. Co-infection is relatively common.

The pathological organism responsible for *syphilis, Treponema pallidum*, targets the endothelium from the earliest stages of infection. Initially, it triggers an inflammatory response, and smaller arteries and arterioles are damaged. Chronic inflammation of vascular tissue ensues, resulting in fibrosis and sclerosis. The three characteristic stages in syphilis are described below in the clinical manifestations section.

Genital herpes is caused by the *herpes simplex virus (HSV) type 2*, which is generally associated with genital, anal or perianal infection. HSV type 1 is more commonly related to cold sores on the lips and mouth. However, during oral sex, HSV type 2 can cause oral lesions.

Genital warts, also known as *condylomata acuminata*, are caused by a type of HPV. In effect, they are benign epithelial neoplasms. The warts are readily spread by sexual contact, and have the highest rate of incidence in adolescents and young adults.

Epidemiology

Recent notification data related to selected sexually transmitted diseases published by the Department of Health and Aged Care are shown in Table 39.1. As identified in the table, Northern Territory infection rates are significantly higher than the Australian average (which would be even lower if Northern Territory rates were removed from the averaging calculation).

Clinical manifestations

These infections may remain asymptomatic. When symptoms occur, they usually manifest 5–14 days post infection. These symptoms include cramping lower abdominal pain, dysuria, dysmenorrhoea accompanied by menorrhagia, intermenstrual bleeding, dyspareunia and abnormal vaginal discharge.

Occasionally, the infections can spread to involve systemic structures, particularly the joints. *Gonorrhoea* can involve the eye, while chlamydia may affect the liver. *Trichomonas* is associated with an infection triggered by the parasite *T. vaginalis*. When symptoms occur, they may include abnormal vaginal discharge, itchiness, lower abdominal pain, dyspareunia, dysuria and increased frequency of micturition. These organisms can also infect the Bartholin's glands, located either side of the vaginal opening, causing bartholinitis. This condition usually manifests by the development of an abscess, a Bartholin's cyst, which becomes tender and swollen.

In *syphilis*, the first stage involves the development of an ulcer, known as a chancre, in the anogenital area. It is usually painless and can develop on the vagina or, following anal sex, be hidden in the rectum. It can develop 1–12 weeks after

Table 39.1 Selected sexually transmissible infection notifications, 2021 (per 100,000)

Sexually transmitted infection	Notification rate—Australia (average)	Notification rate—Northern Territory	NT rates compared to Australian average
Chlamydia	417	1056	2.5 times higher
Gonorrhoea	159	669	4.2 times higher
Syphilis	34	110	3.1 times higher

Source: Data from Department of Health and Aged Care (2023). National Communicable Disease Surveillance Dashboard. National Notifiable Disease Surveillance System. https://nindss.health.gov.au.

infection, and usually heals within four weeks. In the second stage, the infection becomes systemic. A skin rash develops that may occur on the soles of the feet or the palms of the hands or cover the entire body, and is contagious to other people. Other accompanying manifestations include swollen lymph nodes, alopecia, genital lumps and flu-like symptoms. In the third stage of syphilitic infection, the infection can severely damage the brain and heart.

In symptomatic *genital herpes* infection, there is initially irritation and the appearance of blisters in the genital area after an incubation period of three to seven days. The blisters will rupture and leave shallow ulcers. The blistered area may or may not be painful; however, once the ulcers form, the affected region is quite painful. Some people will also experience the flu-like symptoms of fever and painful joints during this primary episode. Lymph nodes in the affected region may become swollen and tender. The initial lesions heal within three weeks, but the virus remains in the body and can be spread during sexual contact. The degree of blistering can vary greatly from person to person. For some people the initial infection can be asymptomatic. Once inside the body, herpes viruses tend to travel up nerve fibres, and can remain dormant within nerve cells until reactivated. A recurrent episode can be triggered by stress or during a period of immunosuppression.

Genital warts tend to have a long incubation period, usually about four months, but can develop anywhere between a month and up to a year after infection. Women tend to develop the warts on the vulva, but they can also form perianally. The appearance of the warts can vary in size (quite small to large) and in distribution (singularly or clumped together). They are generally painless, unsightly growths, but in some instances may be itchy. Figure 39.8 explores the common clinical manifestations and management of sexually transmitted infections.

Clinical diagnosis and management

Diagnosis Following assessment of a clinical history and a physical examination, tests will be undertaken to facilitate diagnosis of the STI. These tests will include swabs and urinary polymerase chain reaction (PCR) for chlamydia, gonorrhoea, herpes, *Mycoplasma* and *Trichomonas*, as well as syphilis serology blood tests and a Pap smear.

Management Treatment is based on the causative organism, and may include oral, topical and injectable medications. Appropriate antimicrobial therapy will generally provide effective resolution of bacterial STIs. Antiviral agents (e.g. aciclovir) will reduce the severity and degree of symptoms of genital herpes infection, but will not provide a permanent cure. Genital warts may be surgically excised or treated with cryotherapy, laser ablation or electrocautery.

The plan of care will vary depending on the diagnosis. It is important to ensure a non-judgmental approach during assessment, and to implement strategies to reduce anxiety and maintain privacy. Care approaches may include the provision of information and advice regarding treatment options (e.g. actions, risks, complications, treatment or failure to treat), the need to complete a full course of treatment, the need for sexual partner/s to be assessed and treated, as well as pre- and postoperative care if surgery is required. It is also imperative that strategies for the prevention of STIs are discussed and emphasised. This will include the use of barrier protection (male/female condoms and dental dams) and also the need for regular Pap smears.

PELVIC INFLAMMATORY DISEASE

Aetiology and pathophysiology

Infection by *N. gonorrhoeae* and/or *C. trachomatis* can ascend the genital tract, leading to *cervicitis*, an inflammation of the cervix. **Pelvic inflammatory disease (PID)** is also associated with infection of the reproductive tract by Gram-positive bacterial species such as staphylococci or streptococci, as well as Gram-negative bacteria such as *Pseudomonas* species and *Escherichia coli*. The infection can remain asymptomatic. When symptoms are present, the affected person may experience a mucopurulent cervical discharge, bleeding (intermenstrual or postcoital), dyspareunia and tenderness on movement of the cervix.

The infection can ascend further to involve other reproductive structures, including the *uterus (endometritis), oviducts (salpingitis)* and *ovaries (oophoritis)*. At this stage the condition is known as PID. PID can be an acute condition, but may persist as a subacute or chronic condition.

Clinical manifestations

The clinical manifestations usually consist of those associated with cervicitis accompanied by abdominal pain and fever. Complications of PID include scarring of the reproductive tract, pelvic adhesions, chronic pelvic pain and pelvic abscesses. The risk of subsequent ectopic pregnancy or infertility is significant.

Clinical diagnosis and management

Diagnosis Diagnostic procedures may include blood tests (full blood count and erythrocyte sedimentation rate [ESR]), cultures or PCR from cervical swabs, and, if severe, laparoscopy/laparotomy may be performed to facilitate assessment of the extent of pelvic involvement. Expected results may include elevated white blood cell counts and ESR levels. Laparoscopy may reveal evidence of inflammation, pelvic abscess and pelvic adhesions.

Management The management of PID is aimed at the relief of symptoms, the elimination of the infection and the minimisation of the risk of complications. Treatment will include analgesics, oral or intravenous antimicrobial therapy (depending on the severity of symptoms at the time of assessment) that typically involves two broad-spectrum antimicrobials (e.g. gentamicin or doxycycline plus cefoxitin or clindamycin) and in some cases intravenous fluids. Surgery may be required to drain pelvic abscesses.

The care plan will vary depending on the extent of the condition. Approaches may include the provision of information and advice regarding treatment options (including actions, risks and complications), the need to complete a full course of

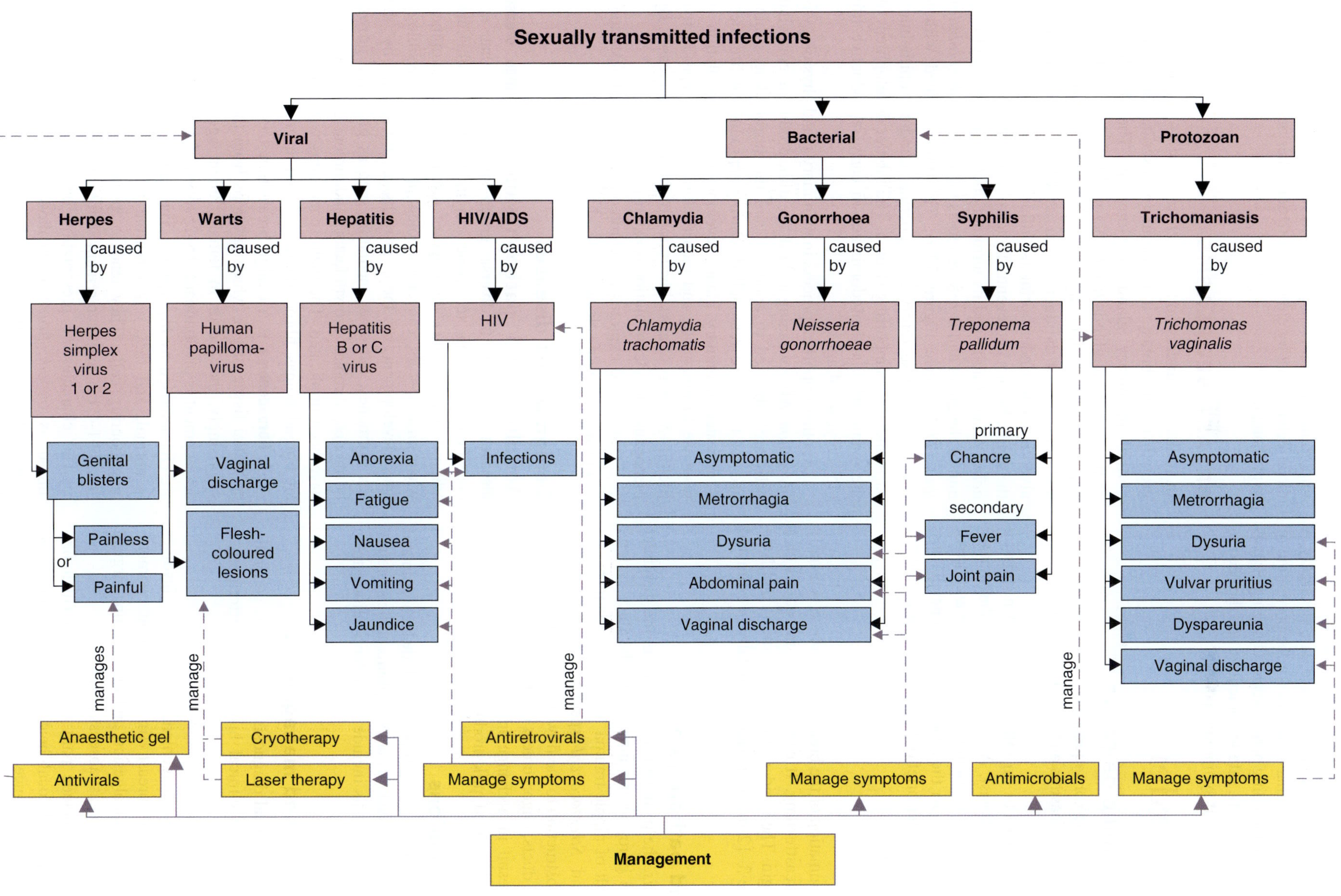

Figure 39.8

Clinical snapshot: Sexually transmitted infections

AIDS = acquired immunodeficiency syndrome; HIV = human immunodeficiency virus.

antimicrobials, the possible need for sexual partner/s to be assessed and treated, as well as pre- and postoperative care if surgery is required. It is also imperative that strategies for the prevention of infections are discussed, including perineal care, changing of pads or tampons at least four-hourly, safe sex practices, and the need to seek advice/treatment early if symptoms reoccur.

Breast disorders

LEARNING OBJECTIVE 5

Describe the causes and consequences of selected breast disorders such as mastitis and breast neoplasms.

In this section, we will focus on inflammatory and neoplastic conditions affecting the breast. Mastitis is the inflammatory condition affecting the breast. Benign breast disease and breast cancer will be examined under the heading of breast neoplasms, which will commence with a brief overview on the development of the mammary glands.

MASTITIS

Mastitis is an inflammation of the breast tissue, which is usually associated with breastfeeding. It can be of an infectious or a non-infectious origin. The incidence rate in Australia and New Zealand within the 3–12-month period postnatally is estimated to be 20–27%.

Aetiology and pathophysiology

In *infective mastitis*, the pathogen usually enters the glandular tissue through the pores in the nipple into the duct system, typically as a result of nipple trauma. Common organisms are *Staphylococcal* and *Streptococcal* species. In *non-infective mastitis*, there is obstruction to the flow of milk from the breast, such as in blocked ducts, engorgement or breast injury.

Mastitis can result in a change in the consistency of the breast milk and/or decreased milk production.

Clinical manifestations

The clinical manifestations of mastitis can include local pain and redness, as well as pyrexia and flu-like symptoms at the systemic level. Risk factors for mastitis include sleep deprivation, stress and excessive exercise.

Clinical diagnosis and management

Diagnosis

The clinical diagnosis of mastitis is generally determined after taking a clinical history and performing a physical examination.

Management

The management of mastitis involves regular emptying of the breast (in a lactating woman), antimicrobial therapy and analgesics, and may require surgical incision and drainage if a breast abscess develops.

Care strategies will include pain management (including the use of analgesics and local heat or cold therapy), and explanation about the importance of completing the full course of antimicrobial therapy. If surgery is required, then pre- and postoperative care and emotional support is required. For the lactating woman, specific advice will include a discussion of the importance of, and techniques to facilitate, regular emptying of the affected breast by either breastfeeding her baby or manually expressing milk.

BREAST NEOPLASMS

In order to understand the characteristics of neoplastic growth of the breast, it is useful to describe the nature of normal mammary gland development. The development of the mammary glands begins before birth. The duct system is present in a rudimentary form. At puberty, the proliferation and branching of the duct system, as well as the formation of alveoli, occurs under hormonal influence. Primary ducts from the nipple branch and eventually terminate in blind ends called *acini*. A set of acini and its terminal duct forms the functional unit of the gland and is referred to as the *terminal duct lobular unit (TDLU)* (see Figure 39.9). This unit is lined with a single layer of secretory and apocrine glandular epithelium, surrounded by supporting stroma. The lobular development of the mammary gland predominates in early reproductive life (15–25 years of age).

Another important process in mammary gland physiology is *involution*. After weaning a child, the milk-producing epithelial cells are subjected to apoptosis and the surrounding stroma and fat tissue are remodelled. During reproductive life there is repeated mammary gland development and involution in response to pregnancy and menstruation. In late reproductive life (35–55 years of age), involution of the lobules increases. By menopause, lobule involution is extensive.

Figure 39.10 explores the common clinical manifestations and management of selected breast disorders.

Benign breast diseases

Aetiology and pathophysiology

Benign breast diseases represent a diverse group of disorders that are classified according to tissue origin (stroma, epithelium, adipose and vascular), the stage of reproductive development when onset occurs, cancerous potential and pathophysiology. The development of these growths is influenced by the sex hormones, but other mediators such as prolactin, growth hormones, fibroblast growth factors and tumour growth factor-β have been implicated. The major conditions within this group are fibroadenomas, fibrocystic disease and severe mastalgia.

A **fibroadenoma** is a benign breast tumour of stromal and epithelial tissue origin, which develops from the lobules. Not surprisingly, they occur in females at an age when lobular development is predominant: 15–25 years of age. The tumours are characterised by *hyperplasia*. The morphology of the cells is normal, and they retain normal relationships with other neighbouring cells. They tend to grow to a particular size, usually 1–2 cm, and then remain at this constant size.

The characteristic presentation on palpation is that the tumour is *smooth, firm* and displays *high mobility*. In older women, they feel smooth and solid, with a similar density to the surrounding breast tissues. They may look like cysts, but on needle aspiration they are *not fluid-filled*.

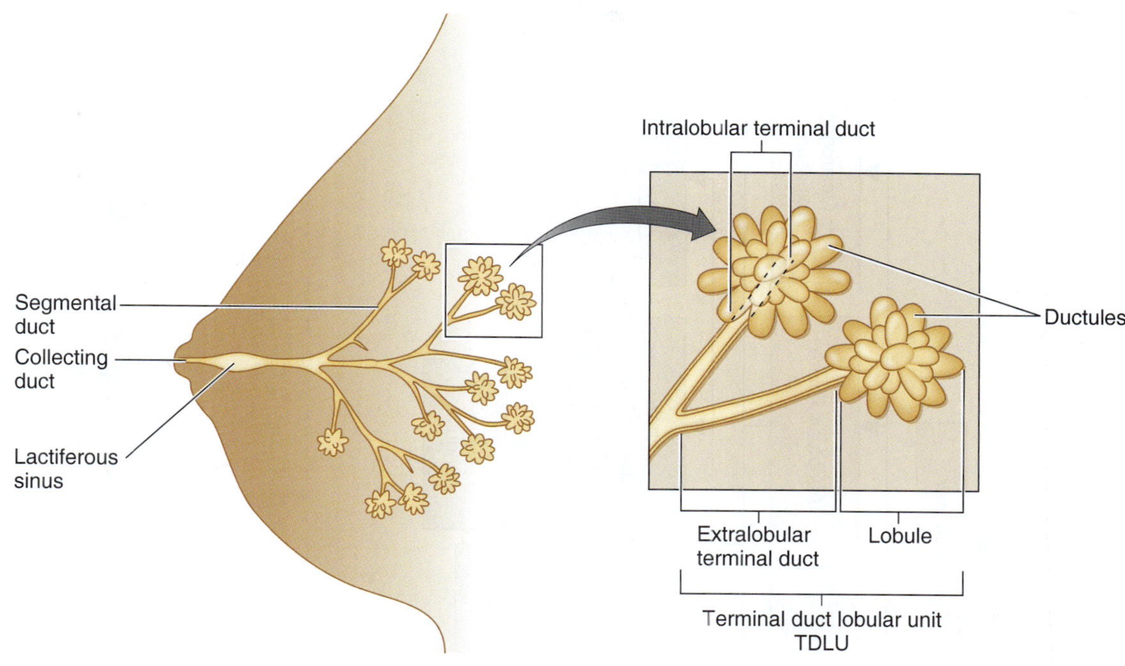

Figure 39.9
The terminal duct lobular unit

In **fibrocystic disease**, during the process of involution of lobules, acini may remain after the stroma is broken down. Cysts can form within the acini of the TDLU. Small cysts can become larger cysts. Cysts tend to occur in the later reproductive period, from 35 to 50 years of age. On presentation cysts are *smooth, firm* and *feel attached to breast tissue*. Cyst fluid can be aspirated with a needle.

Mastalgia is defined as *breast pain*. It can be categorised as cyclic or non-cyclic. *Cyclic mastalgia* is characterised as diffuse, bilateral tenderness with nodularity occurring postovulatory, and is usually seen in women in their 30s and 40s. The pain itself is described as an aching or soreness. The manifestations tend to ease as the cycle continues. *Non-cyclic mastalgia* is usually unilateral and described as sharp, localised and burning. The most common form of mastalgia is cyclic.

Clinical diagnosis and management

Diagnosis Clinical diagnosis in benign breast disease involves a comprehensive health history and a physical examination. Diagnostic imaging includes mammogram and possibly ultrasound examination. A biopsy may be taken (as either a fine-needle aspiration or open procedure) and histological/cytological examination performed.

Management Treatment will depend on the diagnosis, and may include mild analgesics and advice in relation to wearing a firm-fitting bra. Local application of cold or heat may also be effective to reduce breast pain. Cysts may be aspirated under local anaesthetic in cases where the cystic mass does not resolve spontaneously.

The care plan is similar to that identified above for mastitis.

Breast cancer

In 2022, more than 20,400 woman (and 200 men) were diagnosed with breast cancer. Approximately 6.4% of all cancer deaths in Australia are from breast cancer; however, fortunately, five-year survival rates are increasing, and are currently around 92% of those diagnosed.

Aetiology and pathophysiology

Breast cancer is the most common cancer in Western women. More rarely, breast cancer can occur in men. Risk factors for breast cancer include age, being female, the duration of reproductive life, a low number of children to which a woman gives birth, a later age for first pregnancy, the amount of saturated fat in the diet, obesity, alcohol intake, urban living, ethnicity, genetics, family history (a woman with a first-order relative who has had breast cancer is at a higher risk), radiation exposure and hormone therapy. In terms of genetics, specific gene mutations, such as *BRCA1* and *BRCA2*, have been shown to have strong associations with breast cancer risk.

The majority of breast cancers arise from the epithelium lining the TDLU—from the *milk ducts* and *lobules*. As such, they are referred to as *ductal* or *lobular carcinomas*. In ductal carcinoma in situ, the cancer growth remains within the boundaries of the duct or lobule lining. This form can progress to become invasive, infiltrating the surrounding breast tissue and eventually entering the lymphatic and blood vessels.

Breast cancers can *fungate*. This process occurs when a nodule develops that looks like a fungus. It may also have an ulcerated appearance. The *ulcer* may bleed and become infected and malodorous.

A number of different receptors are found on the surface of the cancerous breast cells, and these respond to the *growth factors* involved in promoting tumour proliferation. The sex hormones, *oestrogen* and *progesterone*, may be important growth factors in some forms of breast cancer. Other receptors, such as *human epithelial receptors-2 (HER-2)*, may be over-expressed on breast cancer cells. The presence of this receptor usually indicates a more aggressive form of the disease, with a

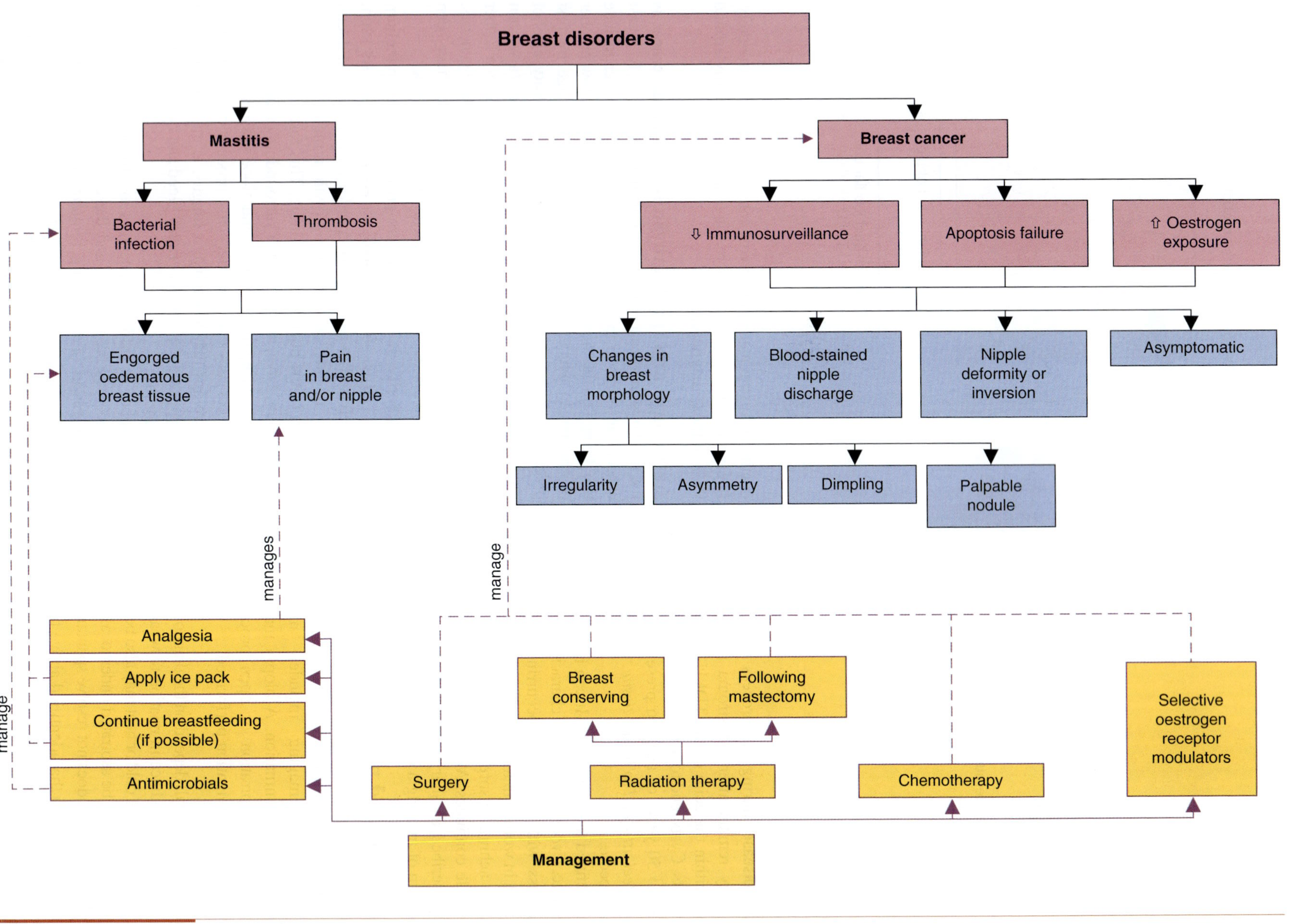

Figure 39.10
Clinical snapshot: Breast disorders
↓ = decreased; ↑ = increased.

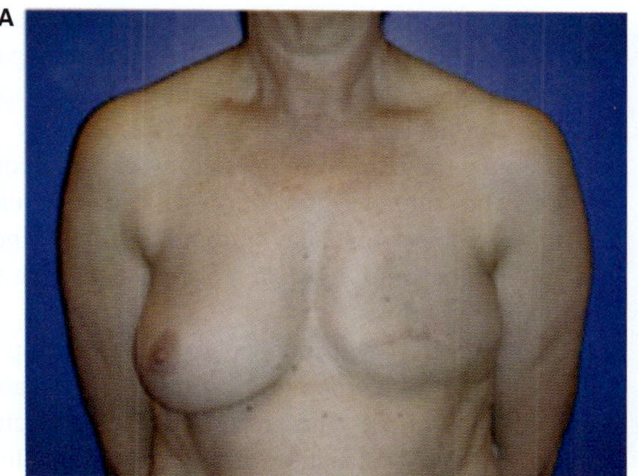

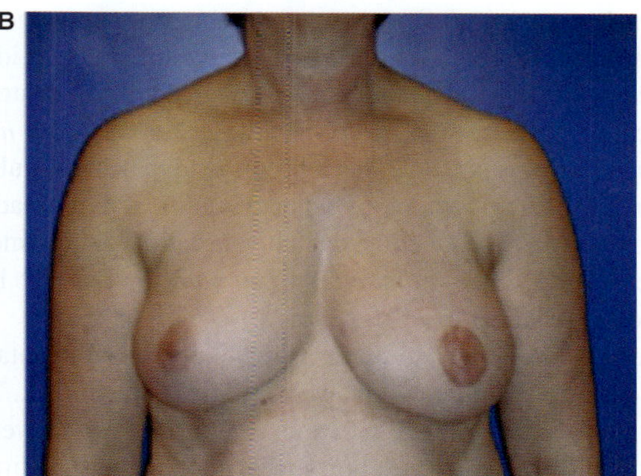

Figure 39.11

Breast Cancer

(A) Images from a 57-year-old woman two years after a left radical mastectomy and adjuvant radio-chemotherapy. (B) Four years after breast reconstruction following mastectomy.

poorer prognosis. Breast cancers that do not respond to the sex hormones oestrogen and progesterone, as well as HER-2, are referred to as *'triple-negative' breast cancer*.

Invasion of the skin, chest wall or lymph nodes by cancerous cells is called *local advanced breast disease*. Lymph nodes can become obstructed, leading to chronic swelling of the dependent limb (i.e. *lymphoedema*). *Metastatic breast cancer* involves the spread of cancerous cells to distant tissues via the bloodstream and lymphatics. Common sites for metastasis include bone, brain, liver and lungs. Metastases to bone tissue lead to significant destruction of the bony matrix; they can be quite painful, and the affected bones become more likely to fracture.

Clinical manifestations The common clinical manifestations of breast cancer include the presence of a breast lump (which can be painful), an altered position or orientation of the nipple, a change in the colour or the texture of the breast skin, and an abnormal discharge from the nipple (which may be clear or blood-stained).

Clinical diagnosis and management

Diagnosis Clinical diagnosis in suspected malignant breast disease involves a comprehensive health history and a physical examination. Diagnostic imaging includes mammogram and possibly ultrasound examination. A biopsy will be taken (either as a fine-needle aspiration or as an open procedure), and histological and cytological examination performed. Hormone receptor assays are also generally performed.

Management Breast cancer management will depend on the histology and staging of the tumour, as well as the woman's age and health history. Treatment may include surgery (lumpectomy or mastectomy, with or without axillary node dissection) and radiation therapy. Reconstruction surgery may be an option and occur immediately or some time after the original surgery (see Figure 39.11). Medications, including chemotherapeutic agents, hormone therapy (e.g. tamoxifen in oestrogen-sensitive tumours) and immunotherapy (e.g. trastuzumab, which binds to the HER-2 receptor to minimise proliferation of tumour cells) may be used. Ongoing psychological support and follow-up assessments are imperative.

The care strategies will vary depending on the proposed treatment plan, and may incorporate a discussion of treatment options, the provision of pre- and postoperative care (including specific education) and explanation of medications (including the duration of treatment and the potential risks and side-effects). Ongoing emotional support, incorporating strategies to reduce anxiety and assistance to cope with body image and sexuality concerns, are also important when extensive surgery is required. It is also imperative that the need for ongoing follow-up is reinforced.

Ectopic pregnancy

LEARNING OBJECTIVE 6

Describe the pathophysiology, diagnosis and management of ectopic pregnancy.

An **ectopic pregnancy** is a pregnancy that is implanted external to the uterine cavity. The vast majority of these pregnancies develop within the fallopian tube, but they can occur, rarely, within the abdominal cavity, cervix or on the ovaries.

AETIOLOGY AND PATHOPHYSIOLOGY

The current view is that two main factors determine ectopic pregnancy and the retention of the embryo within the fallopian tubes or other non-uterine sites: an impairment in the transport of the embryo along the fallopian tube; and an alteration in the local environment that allows early implantation to occur.

Impairment in tubal transport can be a consequence of decreased tubal smooth muscle contractility and a disruption to tubal ciliary activity. *Inflammatory processes* are implicated in these changes, as both *cyclo-oxygenase-2* and *inducible nitric oxide synthase levels (iNOS)* have been found to be up-regulated in animal models of ectopic pregnancy. iNOS activity leads to nitric oxide (NO) production, which relaxes the tubal smooth muscle. A *reduction of tubal ciliary cell numbers* has also been observed in tubal ectopic pregnancy.

The *altered local environment* of the ectopic implantation site is considered more conducive to embryo attachment. This is thought to be associated with a change in the responsiveness of the tubal tissues to the sex hormones, making the shedding of tissue less likely, and inducing the secretion of pro-inflammatory mediators and growth factors (e.g. vascular endothelial growth factor).

EPIDEMIOLOGY

In Western countries, the incidence rate of ectopic pregnancy is 1–2% of all pregnancies. In the developing world, the rate can be considerably higher. Australian public hospitals admitted over 6,100 women with an ectopic pregnancy in 2021. Ectopic pregnancy is a common cause of maternal death during the first trimester.

Key risk factors for ectopic pregnancy include chlamydia infection, cigarette smoking and in-vitro fertilisation (IVF) procedures. Chlamydia infection damages the reproductive tissue and induces inflammatory responses. There is evidence that smoking decreases both ciliary activity and tubal muscle contractility. The reasons why IVF may increase the risk of ectopic pregnancy are yet to be fully elucidated, but it has been proposed that embryo transfer procedures, the number of embryos implanted, changes to the local tissue environment caused by the ovarian hyperstimulation, and cell adhesive substances secreted by the transferred embryo may be implicated.

CLINICAL MANIFESTATIONS

Common clinical manifestations include lower abdominal cramping pain, which may also occur during micturition or defecation, tenderness and vaginal bleeding. In more severe cases, the pain may also spread to the lower back, pelvis and shoulder. The pain and tenderness may be felt unilaterally. Complications of ectopic pregnancy include severe bleeding associated with a rupture of tissue at the site of implantation, which can result in hypovolaemic shock and infertility.

CLINICAL DIAGNOSIS AND MANAGEMENT

Diagnosis

A clinical history and a pelvic examination are performed. The principal diagnostic procedures are transvaginal ultrasound and quantitative assessment of serum β-hCG.

Management

Management of an ectopic pregnancy depends on the stage of diagnosis, β-hCG level and the woman's condition, and may include medical or surgical approaches. Medical management involves injection/s of the chemotherapeutic drug methotrexate, which interferes with multiplication of the rapidly dividing cells. Surgical therapy is performed by laparoscopy predominantly. However, laparotomy may be required in some cases. The surgical procedure will involve either removal of the ectopic pregnancy through a small incision in the fallopian tube (*salpingostomy*) or removal of the fallopian tube (*salpingectomy*).

Care strategies will vary depending on the proposed treatment plan, and may incorporate a discussion of treatment options, the provision of pre- and postoperative care (including specific education) and explanation of medications (including duration of treatment and potential risks and side-effects). Ongoing emotional support and strategies to reduce anxiety and assistance to cope with concerns regarding future fertility are also important. It is also imperative to stress the need for ongoing follow-up with serial blood tests for β-hCG levels to monitor for reduction to the non-pregnant level ($<$ 2 IU/L).

Female infertility

AETIOLOGY AND PATHOPHYSIOLOGY

LEARNING OBJECTIVE 7

Outline the current definitions of female infertility and some common conditions associated with decreased fertility.

The definitions of infertility and subfertility are still subject to considerable discussion within the human reproduction literature. *Time-to-pregnancy (TTP)* is the fundamental measure used to determine the thresholds of degrees of infertility. The World Health Organization currently defines **infertility** as a couple where the woman is *under the age of 34 years and has not conceived within a 12-month period* of unprotected sexual intercourse (this decreases to a *six-month period* for a couple where the woman is *over the age of 35 years*).

Subfertility is generally regarded as reduced fertility in couples who are unsuccessful in trying to conceive. Clinical studies have shown that most pregnancies occur within the first six cycles of unprotected intercourse during the fertile phase. Possible subfertility is raised with couples when this criterion is not met.

Primary infertility refers to couples who have never conceived, while *secondary infertility* relates to couples who have conceived previously but are having difficulty in a subsequent attempt.

The key events in pregnancy involve the maturation and ovulation of a viable ovum, ovum transport along the fallopian tube to the uterine cavity, fertilisation of the ovum, the successful implantation and development of the conceptus within the endometrium, and the maintenance of a viable placenta (see Figure 39.12). This system also depends on the creation and maintenance of a suitable environment within the reproductive system by the endocrine system.

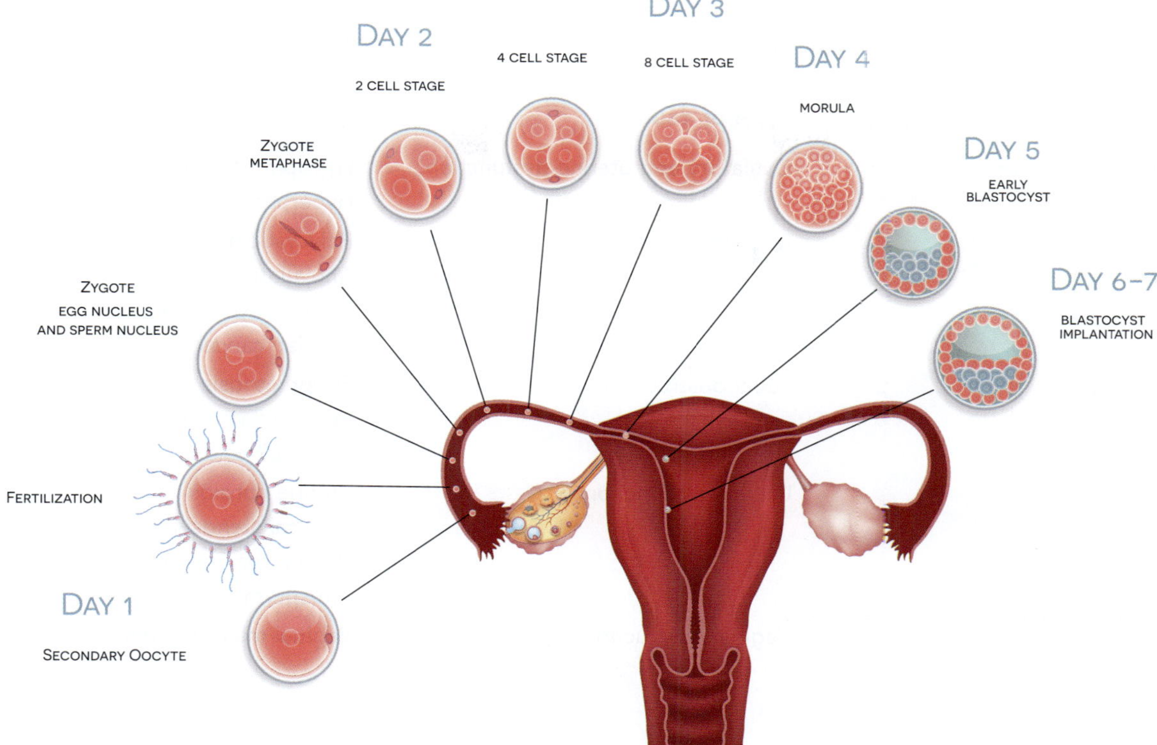

Figure 39.12

Key events in pregnancy

(A) An oocyte is released from the ovary.
(B) Haploid spermatozoa fertilises the haploid oocyte and becomes a diploid zygote.
(C) Cells divide.
(D) Continued mitosis results in a ball of cells called a morula.
(E) A fluid-filled space, called a blastocyst, forms by cell compaction. It hatches from the zona pellucida.
(F) The blastocyst implants into the uterine wall.

Source: guniita/123RF.

Common causes of female infertility include *ovulatory dysfunction, tubal obstruction, uterine dysfunction, vaginal obstruction* and *ageing*. The anatomical sites at which these problems originate can be the hypothalamus, pituitary, ovaries, fallopian tubes, uterus, cervix and vagina. Disruptions to the HPO axis are closely related to infertility. Examples of disorders and anatomical sites affected are provided in Table 39.2.

CLINICAL DIAGNOSIS AND MANAGEMENT

Diagnosis

Fertility assessment and diagnosis should incorporate both male and female assessments (refer to the chapter 'Male reproductive disorders' for specific male fertility diagnosis and management). Clinical diagnosis will include a comprehensive health history and a physical/pelvic examination. Diagnostic imaging will include a transvaginal ultrasound to assess the characteristics of the uterus, fallopian tubes and ovaries (including an antral follicle count). An assessment of tubal patency by *hysterosalpingogram (HSG)* or *hysterosalpingo-contrast sonography (HyCoSy)* will also be of assistance.

Laboratory tests may include gonadotropin hormone (timed on day 2 or 3 of the menstrual cycle) and ovarian hormone levels, anti-Mullerian hormone (a test of ovarian reserve) and thyroid function tests. Diagnostic laparoscopy and/or hysteroscopy may be performed.

Management

The management approach in infertility will depend on the clinical diagnosis, and the woman's age and individual needs. Treatment approaches may include expectant management with

Table 39.2 Anatomical sites and common conditions that may cause infertility

Anatomical site	Type of cause	Examples of condition
Hypothalamus–pituitary	Ovulatory and uterine dysfunction	Hypopituitarism Hyperprolactinaemia
Ovaries	Ovulatory dysfunction	Polycystic ovary syndrome Anovulation Turner's syndrome Ovarian cancer
Fallopian tubes	Tubal obstruction	Endometriosis Pelvic inflammatory disease (PID) Tubal adhesions
Uterus	Uterine dysfunction	Uterine fibroids Cervical stenosis Hostile cervical mucus Antisperm antibodies
Vagina	Vaginal obstruction	Vaginal malformations

a discussion of the timing of intercourse and self-management of lifestyle issues (including weight loss/gain and the cessation of smoking/alcohol/other drugs), and *assisted reproductive technologies (ART)*. ART may involve ovulation induction with either timed intercourse or intrauterine insemination (IUI), and IVF. (Refer to Clinical Box 39.1 for more details on ART procedures.) According to the National Perinatal Epidemiology and Statistics Unit, 87,206 ART super-ovulated treatment cycles that proceeded to oocyte retrieval were undertaken in Australia, and 8,493 treatment cycles in New Zealand, in 2020. As a result of these procedures, 16,439 live births were recorded in Australia and 2,023 in New Zealand.

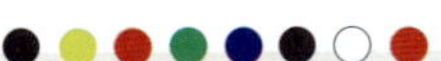

INDIGENOUS HEALTH FAST FACTS AND CULTURAL CONSIDERATIONS

FAST FACTS

- *Although the gap is closing, cervical cancer incidence rates in Aboriginal and Torres Strait Islander women are still 2.2 times higher than those in non-Indigenous Australian women, and mortality rates are 2.6 times higher than in non-Indigenous Australian women. It has been determined that the National Cervical Screening Program has not reduced incidence rates in Aboriginal and Torres Strait women due to under-screening from cultural, linguistic and access barriers.*
- *Breast cancer is the most common cancer in Aboriginal and Torres Strait Islander women. Aboriginal and Torres Strait Islander women are less likely to be diagnosed with breast cancer; however, they are 1.2 times more likely to die from breast cancer than non-Indigenous Australian women.*
- *The incidence of ovarian cancer in Aboriginal and Torres Strait Islander women is similar to that in non-Indigenous Australian women.*
- *Cervical cancer incidence in Māori women is 2 times more, and mortality is 2.5 times higher, than in European New Zealand women.*
- *Cervical cancer incidence in Pacific Islands women is 1.5 times more, and mortality is 5.2 times higher, than in European New Zealand women.*
- *Although better than two decades ago, Māori women are still 1.3 times more likely to be diagnosed with breast cancer than non-Māori women in New Zealand.*
- *Ten-year breast cancer survival rates for Māori women are 33% lower, and for Pacific Islands women 52% lower, than for non-Māori/non-Pacific Islands women in New Zealand.*
- *The incidence of ovarian cancer in Māori and Pacific Islands women is similar to that in European New Zealand women.*

CULTURAL CONSIDERATIONS

A focus on the basic logistical challenges to improve access to, and the timeliness and quality of, healthcare for women affected by reproductive health issues can form the basis of reducing the disparities observed within the various cultures of the Australian population. In addition, it is also critical to understand the importance of 'women's business' when considering the gender of the healthcare professional responsible for caring for Aboriginal and Torres Strait Islander women affected by reproductive health pathologies. However, just as important are the efforts to build collaborative cultural networks, especially in the context of reproductive cancers. Connecting women who have lived the experience to other women and to Aboriginal and Torres Strait Islander leaders is important in assisting a woman to feel more comfortable with the healthcare team and facility. Finally, the targeted, culturally appropriate use of social media to educate Aboriginal and Torres Strait Islander peoples and their communities appears to be an effective method of helping individuals and communities embrace the preventative health and screening resources available.

Sources: Data from Breast Cancer Foundation NZ (2022); Cancer Council Australia (2022); National Breast Cancer Foundation (2023); NHMRC Centre of Research Excellence in Cervical Cancer Control (2021);

CHILDREN AND ADOLESCENTS

- Children who begin pubertal development earlier than is considered normal are experiencing 'precocious puberty'. Generally speaking, this is considered to be girls younger than 8 years of age. Because of rapid bone maturation resulting in the early closure of the growth plates, children who experience precocious puberty will be shorter as adults.
- Premature thelarche is when breast development occurs in girls younger than 3 years of age, and when the breast development occurs without any other pubertal changes.
- Premature prebarche is when pubic hair develops in children younger than 7 years of age, and when the terminal hair occurs without other pubertal developments.

OLDER ADULTS

- Age-associated changes to a woman's reproductive system include reducing mucosal secretions and an increased incidence of vaginitis, which can be associated with decreasing libido. Labial atrophy and thinning vaginal walls with decreasing elasticity also occur.
- Decreasing muscle tone can result in prolapse of the vagina, uterus and/or bladder as a direct result of reproductive system senescence, and the significant reduction in oestrogen can result in osteoporosis.
- Mortality rates for ovarian cancer in women 85 years and older are more than 40 times those of women aged 40–44 years.
- Most women experience the onset of menopause around the age of 50 years.

KEY CLINICAL ISSUES

- Many women find it difficult to discuss issues related to reproductive health, and some cultures discourage discussion of 'women's business'. Therefore, health professionals must approach this topic with care and attention.
- It is suggested that a male healthcare professional should have a female healthcare professional in the room when performing an internal examination on a female.
- Reproductive health issues can be physically and psychologically challenging for women, especially when the risk of infertility is involved. Healthcare professionals may benefit from the assistance of mental health and counselling professionals to promote a woman's ability to cope with the diagnosis and the potential treatment outcomes.
- Menstrual disorders, such as dysmenorrhoea, can frequently disrupt a woman's life, result in significant sick leave and potentially cause issues with employers. Assisting a woman to reduce the effects of dysmenorrhoea is important to reduce the financial and physical burden for all involved.
- Evidence of reproductive cancers should be investigated thoroughly. Some gynaecological cancers can be treated quickly and with relative ease; however, other gynaecological cancers leave the team with limited treatment options and the woman with a poor prognosis. A multidisciplinary team is required to manage the total care of those with reproductive cancers.
- Sexually transmitted infections are common and increasing. More education for individuals and communities is needed to reduce their spread.

CHAPTER REVIEW

- *Dysmenorrhoea* is defined as painful monthly menstrual flow, and is characterised by cramping, lower abdominal pain. Primary dysmenorrhoea is associated with painful menses without evidence of pathology, while secondary dysmenorrhoea is linked to pelvic pathology.
- The pathophysiology of *primary dysmenorrhoea* is linked to increased local secretion of the eicosanoids and, possibly, other chemical mediators such as vasopressin. These substances are known to be associated with increased myometrial contractility, cramping pain and changes in blood flow.
- *Amenorrhoea* is the absence of menses. *Primary amenorrhoea* is associated with disruption to normal menstrual function. *Secondary amenorrhoea* is considered to be an absence of menses for three months when regular menstruation had occurred previously, or for nine months in a woman who was formerly oligomenorrhoeic. Amenorrhoea is considered to be the normal physiological response prior to menarche, in a woman who is pregnant, or postmenopausally.
- The term *abnormal bleeding* is associated with blood loss from the genital tract. Abnormal vaginal bleeding is classified as *menorrhagia* (heavy menstrual bleeding generally regarded to be in excess of 80 mL per cycle), *metrorrhagia* (prolonged irregular menstruation), *polymenorrhoea* (frequent menstruation), *oligomenorrhoea* (infrequent, scanty menstruation), *postcoital bleeding* (bleeding following sexual intercourse), *intermenstrual bleeding* (bleeding not associated with menstruation or sexual intercourse, often known as 'spotting') and *postmenopausal bleeding*.
- *Prolapse*, or descent, of pelvic organs into the vagina can occur when the supporting structures holding these organs in the normal anatomical position fail. When this support system fails, intra-abdominal pressure will force the uterus downwards into the vagina. A uterine prolapse may lead to the uterus appearing outside the vaginal opening. Under these circumstances, the exposed cervix may become damaged, leading to bleeding or ulceration.
- A *cystocoele* is when there is descent of a part of the urinary bladder into the vagina. It occurs when a weakness develops in the vaginal musculature. Common causes of vaginal weakness include trauma during childbirth or surgery, and advancing age.
- *Endometriosis* is a common reproductive disorder affecting women of childbearing age. It affects about 5–10% of women in the general population. Endometriosis is characterised by the establishment of ectopic endometrial tissue, known as *endometrial implants*, outside the uterine cavity. The accepted view is that fragments of endometrial tissue enter the pelvic cavity through the open fallopian tubes via a process of *retrograde menstruation*. Individual susceptibility is the key to the progression of the condition, as the implants must firstly evade breakdown by the body's defence mechanisms, then adhere to the peritoneum and establish a self-sustaining system to continue to survive and grow in this environment. Growth of the implants is particularly sensitive to oestrogen.
- *Ovarian cysts* are fluid-filled sacs on the ovary, and can occur any time from puberty to menopause. The cysts are *sex hormone sensitive* and can alter their size in response to hormonal signalling at different stages of the menstrual cycle.
- *Polycystic ovary syndrome (PCOS)* is a condition characterised by at least two of the three following criteria: irregular or no ovulation, hyperandrogenaemia and polycystic ovaries. The main pathophysiological mechanisms underlying PCOS are alterations in the function of the hypothalamic–pituitary–ovary (HPO) and the hypothalamic–pituitary–adrenal (HPA) axes, as well as the onset of insulin resistance and hyperinsulinaemia.
- *Uterine fibroids* are benign tumours of myometrium. They are also known as *uterine leiomyomas* or *myomas*. Uterine fibroids can develop within the uterine wall as intramural, submucosal, pedunculated or mixed growths. Fibroids are dependent on the presence of oestrogens and progesterone for proliferation. Initially, they are particularly sensitive to progesterone, but later become dependent on a mix of endogenous hormones.
- *Vulvar cancer* is considered to be the rarest of the gynaecological cancers. Usually it is diagnosed in postmenopausal women around the age of 65 years. The vast majority of vulvar cancers are squamous cell carcinomas. Risk factors for this form of cancer are advanced age, immunosuppression and being a current smoker. The development of vulvar cancer has been linked to infection by human papillomavirus (HPV) and chronic inflammation of the vulva.
- *Cervical cancer* is one of the leading causes of cancer death in the world, particularly within developing countries. Most cervical cancers are squamous cell carcinomas, with the remainder arising from glandular tissue. A causal relationship has been established between HPV infection (serotypes 16 and 18), the premalignant precursor lesion known as cervical intraepithelial neoplasia and cervical cancer.
- *Endometrial cancer* is one of the most common cancers in women. It is usually diagnosed in postmenopausal women between 50 and 70 years of age. The most common type of endometrial cancer arises from glandular tissue (adenocarcinomas). It tends to be diagnosed at an early stage of development, and so has a good prognosis.
- *Ovarian cancer* is considered one of the top gynaecological malignancies, and is a common cause of death in women. Most cases of ovarian cancer are diagnosed in postmenopausal women aged between 50 and 80 years of age. The prognosis for this condition generally remains poor. Most ovarian cancers arise in the epithelial surface of the ovary, and tend to be diagnosed at a later, more advanced stage of development.
- *Vulvovaginitis* is defined as an inflammation of the vulva and vagina. The most common cause is infectious, but an inflammation could arise from trauma, a reaction to chemicals or to latex condoms, or wetness from prolonged contact with a sanitary pad or nappy. Common manifestations of vulvovaginitis include vaginal or perineal itching, vaginal discharge, local irritation and burning sensations. In some cases, the infection may be asymptomatic.
- The infectious organisms most commonly associated with vulvovaginitis are bacterial (*Haemophilus vaginalis, Chlamydia trachomatis* or *Neisseria gonorrhoeae*), fungal (*Candida albicans*), parasitic (*Trichomonas vaginalis*) or viral (human papillomavirus or herpes simplex virus type 2). With the exception of *C. albicans* infection, these infections are usually sexually transmitted infections.
- Infection by *N. gonorrhoeae* and/or *C. trachomatis* can ascend the genital tract, leading to cervicitis, an inflammation of the cervix. The infection can ascend further to involve other reproductive structures, including the uterus (endometritis), oviducts (salpingitis) and ovaries (oophoritis). At this stage the condition is known as *pelvic inflammatory disease (PID)*.
- PID can be an *acute* condition, but may persist in a *subacute or chronic state*. The clinical manifestations usually consist of those associated with cervicitis accompanied by abdominal pain and fever. Complications of PID include scarring of the reproductive tract, pelvic adhesions, chronic pelvic pain and pelvic abscesses. The risk of subsequent ectopic pregnancy or infertility is significant.

- *Mastitis* is an inflammation of the breast tissue, which is usually associated with breastfeeding. It can be of an infectious or a non-infectious origin. The clinical manifestations of mastitis can include local pain and redness, as well as pyrexia and flu-like symptoms at the systemic level. Risk factors for mastitis include sleep deprivation, stress and excessive exercise.
- *Benign breast disorders* represent a diverse group of disorders that are classified according to tissue origin (stroma, epithelium, adipose and vascular), stage of reproductive development when onset occurs, cancerous potential and pathophysiology. The development of these growths is influenced by the sex hormones, but other mediators—such as prolactin, growth hormones, fibroblast growth factors and tumour growth factor-β—have been implicated. The major conditions within this group are *fibroadenomas, fibrocystic disease* and *severe mastalgia*.
- *Breast cancer* is the most common cancer in Western women. More rarely, breast cancer can occur in men. Risk factors for breast cancer include age, being female, the duration of reproductive life, a low number of children to which a woman gives birth, a later age for first pregnancy, the amount of saturated fat in the diet, obesity, alcohol intake, urban living, ethnicity, genetics, family history, radiation exposure and hormone therapy.
- The majority of breast cancers arise from the epithelium lining the milk ducts and lobules, and are referred to as *ductal or lobular carcinomas*. In ductal carcinoma in situ, the cancer growth remains within the boundaries of the duct or lobule lining. This form can progress to become invasive, infiltrating the surrounding breast tissue and eventually entering the lymphatic and blood vessels. Invasion by cancerous cells into the skin, chest wall or lymph nodes is called *local advanced breast disease. Metastatic breast cancer* involves the spread of cancerous cells to distant tissues via the bloodstream and lymphatics. Common sites for metastasis include bone, brain, liver and lungs.
- An *ectopic pregnancy* is one that is implanted external to the uterine cavity. The vast majority of these pregnancies develop within the fallopian tube, but they can occur, rarely, within the abdominal cavity, in the cervix or on the ovaries. The two main factors that are thought to determine ectopic pregnancy are an impairment in the transport of the embryo along the fallopian tube, and an *alteration in the local environment* that allows early implantation to occur. The *impairment in tubal transport* is a consequence of decreased tubal smooth muscle contractility and a disruption to tubal ciliary activity.
- The World Health Organization currently defines *infertility* as a couple where the woman is under the age of 34 years and has not conceived within a 12-month period of unprotected sexual intercourse (this decreases to a six-month period for a couple where the woman is over the age of 35 years). *Subfertility* is generally regarded as reduced fertility in couples who are unsuccessful in trying to conceive, usually within the first six cycles of unprotected intercourse during the fertile phase. Common causes of female infertility include ovulatory dysfunction, tubal obstruction, uterine dysfunction, vaginal obstruction and ageing.

REVIEW QUESTIONS

1. Differentiate between amenorrhoea and dysmenorrhoea.
2. Briefly outline the pathophysiology of primary dysmenorrhoea.
3. Differentiate between primary, secondary and physiological amenorrhoea.
4. Define the following forms of abnormal vaginal bleeding:
   a. spotting
   b. oligomenorrhoea
   c. menorrhagia
   d. metrorrhagia
5. Outline how a uterine prolapse may occur.
6. Briefly describe the pathophysiology of endometriosis.
7. Briefly describe the pathophysiology of polycystic ovary syndrome.
8. Differentiate between intramural, submucosal and pedunculated uterine fibroids.
9. Maggie Coles is 26 years old and is two months' pregnant. After a series of tests, uterine fibroids were detected. She asks you to tell her about the possible problems of having fibroids when pregnant. What do you tell her?
10. Compare and contrast the epidemiological and pathological characteristics of the following reproductive cancers: cervical, ovarian and vulvar.
11. Jess Marslee is 19 years old and comes to the clinic at which you are currently on placement. She allows you to sit in on the consultation. She is experiencing vaginal itching, burning sensations and a vaginal discharge. What is the likely diagnosis? She asks whether an infection is the only way to acquire this condition. What is your response?
12. Define 'pelvic inflammatory disease'. What are the common clinical manifestations on presentation, and what are the possible complications of this condition?
13. What are the ways in which you could differentiate between a breast cyst and a fibroadenoma?
14. Outline the pathophysiology of breast cancer development.
15. Identify and briefly describe the factors that determine an ectopic pregnancy.

HEALTH PROFESSIONAL CONNECTIONS

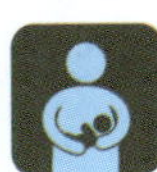

Midwives The incidence of sexually transmitted infections (STIs) is on the increase. Pregnancy is a consequence of unprotected vaginal sex and, therefore, the chance that a woman may have an STI when they are pregnant is becoming more common. The consequences of STI infection during pregnancy are a cause for concern not only to the mother, but also to the pregnancy and the fetus. Chlamydial infections can result in preterm delivery and low birth weights. Over half of the neonates exposed to chlamydia during pregnancy will develop a chlamydial infection, and can also develop infectious conjunctivitis and, potentially, nasopharyngeal infection. Neonates exposed to gonorrhoea can develop gonococcal ophthalmia neonatorum. Antenatal gonococcal infection may result in membrane rupture or sepsis. Almost half of the pregnancies where an untreated syphilis infection occurs will result in premature delivery or perinatal mortality. However, antenatal syphilis screening in Australia reduces this risk. Neonatal exposure to herpes simplex virus type 2 (HSV-2) during birth is high if the woman develops a primary infection in the third trimester. Vertical transmission is also very high for women with an acute hepatitis B infection in the third trimester. Human immunodeficiency virus (HIV) incidence in Australia is low; however, in HIV-positive women, vertical transmission rates are reduced to almost nothing as antiretroviral treatment and quality care is provided. Midwives should know the local incidence and prevalence rates of STIs, and understand the maternal and fetal risks.

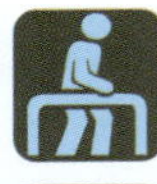

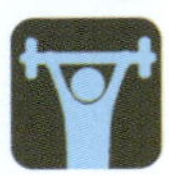

Physiotherapists/Exercise scientists Exercise professionals need to be aware of the risks associated with exercise-associated amenorrhoea. A female athlete who has not commenced menstruating before 16 years of age may have primary amenorrhoea. A female athlete who has previously menstruated but has missed three menstrual periods in the absence of pregnancy is considered to have secondary amenorrhoea. Intense exercise or abnormal eating behaviours may lead to malnutrition and excessively low body fat; therefore, a female athlete with amenorrhoea should be sent to a medical officer for investigation. Risks associated with amenorrhoea include decreased bone density, and could be a sign of overtraining, poor nutrition or an endocrine issue that needs to be investigated and managed. Exercise professionals should also understand that in sports where body weight influences selection into a particular division of the competition, a menstruating woman may be a few kilograms heavier (because of fluid retention). If a female athlete is attempting to qualify for a lower weight division, she needs to be aware of how the weigh-in date may coincide with her menstrual cycle. Extra body fat weight loss may be required to compensate for this situation; however, depending on an individual's body fat, this practice may not be safe, and the athlete should be counselled to compete in the heavier division.

CASE STUDY

Ms Tarina Morrissett (UR number 621892) is a 21-year-old woman who presented to the emergency department with acute abdominal pain, purulent vaginal discharge and fever. During her history interview, she disclosed that she has had multiple sexual partners in the past six months, and has frequently participated in unprotected sex. Ms Morrissett denied intravenous drug use, and there was no obvious evidence of such. On physical examination she demonstrated cervical pain and general abdominal discomfort and guarding. She reports that she has been experiencing dyspareunia in the past few days. Her most recent observations are:

Temperature	Heart rate	Respiration rate	Blood pressure	SpO_2
39.2°C	88	20	110/70	99% (RA*)

*RA = room air.

Ms Morrissett consented to an STI screen, and blood was collected for hepatitis B and HIV serology. A pharyngeal swab was taken for gonorrhoea (PCR), and she has also had first-catch urine collection for chlamydia and gonorrhoea (PCR). An endocervical swab was taken for microscopy, culture and sensitivity (MCS) of the discharge. Blood was also drawn for a full blood count and electrolyte and β-hCG levels. A urine ward test demonstrated leukocytes 3+ and blood 2+. A midstream urine sample was collected for urine MCS. In view of her temperature, blood was also drawn for cultures. Her available pathology results were as follows:

HAEMATOLOGY

Patient location:	Ward 3	**UR:**	621892		
Consultant:	Smith	**NAME:**	Morrissett		
		Given name:	Tarina	**Sex:**	F
		DOB:	01/11/XX	**Age:**	21

Time collected	15:30
Date collected	XX/XX
Year	XXXX
Lab #	5465633

FULL BLOOD COUNT		UNITS	REFERENCE RANGE
Haemoglobin	134	g/L	115–160
White cell count	12.2	$\times 10^9$/L	4.0–11.0
Platelets	283	$\times 10^9$/L	140–400
Haematocrit	0.44		0.33–0.47
Red cell count	4.42	$\times 10^{12}$/L	3.80–5.20
Reticulocyte count	0.6	%	0.2–2.0
MCV	86	fL	80–100
Neutrophils	8.31	$\times 10^9$/L	2.00–8.00
Lymphocytes	2.63	$\times 10^9$/L	1.00–4.00
Monocytes	0.42	$\times 10^9$/L	0.10–1.00
Eosinophils	0.32	$\times 10^9$/L	< 0.60
Basophils	0.11	$\times 10^9$/L	< 0.20
ESR	22	mm/h	< 12

BIOCHEMISTRY

Patient location:	Ward 3	**UR:**	621892		
Consultant:	Smith	**NAME:**	Morrissett		
		Given name:	Tarina	**Sex:**	F
		DOB:	01/11/XX	**Age:**	21

Time collected	15:30
Date collected	XX/XX
Year	XXXX
Lab #	54635564

ELECTROLYTES		UNITS	REFERENCE RANGE
Sodium	138	mmol/L	135–145
Potassium	4.1	mmol/L	3.5–5.2
Chloride	103	mmol/L	95–110
Bicarbonate	25	mmol/L	22–26
Glucose (random)	7.2	mmol/L	3.5–7.7
Iron	16	μmol/L	11–30
β-hCG	0	IU/L	> 25 IU/L pregnancy

Ms Morrissett was commenced on ceftriaxone and gentamicin intravenously. She has been given paracetamol, is self-caring and 'diet as tolerated'. Currently, she is resting in bed.

CRITICAL THINKING

1. From the history provided, what risk factors increase the possibility that Ms Morrissett has a sexually transmitted infection (STI)? Who is most at risk of STIs? Identify several different groups, and explain their risk profile.
2. Ms Morrissett had several samples taken for investigation. She also had a 'first-catch' urine and a 'midstream' urine sample collected. How do these two samples differ? How are they collected? For what purposes would they be used? What is PCR? How will it assist with the diagnosis? Will it inform the choice of treatment?
3. It is likely that Ms Morrissett has developed pelvic inflammatory disease (PID) from a *Chlamydia trachomatis* infection. Would the presence of an intrauterine device (IUD) increase or decrease the risk of PID? Explain. She tells you that she is worried about not being able to have babies in the future. Is this a realistic concern related to PID infection? What are the potential complications with PID? How can these be avoided?
4. Ms Morrissett states that she does not know what chlamydia is or how she got it. What is chlamydia, and how is it spread? What are her treatment options? What responsibilities does she have now to her previous sexual partners? Is a chlamydial infection always obvious? What should her previous sexual partners do?
5. The haematology and biochemistry results are the only results available. Are they of any benefit? What impression can be gained from these results? Why would a β-hCG test be performed? What might it show? Why is this test an important consideration? Why might the other results take more time? The microscopy, culture and sensitivity testing may cause the antimicrobial order to change. Why?
6. Ms Morrissett requires some client education. Develop a teaching plan to assist Ms Morrissett to avoid another episode of PID. What elements should this teaching plan include? Why? Will Ms Morrissett require follow-up after discharge from hospital? What community services would be beneficial for Ms Morrissett? How can she protect herself from other types of STIs?

BIBLIOGRAPHY

Australian Health Ministers' Advisory Council's National and Aboriginal and Torres Strait Islander Health Standing Committee (2017). *Cultural respect framework 2016–2026: for Aboriginal and Torres Strait Islander health—a national approach to building a culturally respectful health system*. Canberra: Australian Government Department of Health. https://nacchocommunique.files.wordpress.com.

Australian Institute of Health and Welfare (AIHW) (2022a). *Australia's health, 2022*. Data insights. Australia's Health series No. 18. Cat. AUS No. 240. Canberra: AIHW.

Australian Institute of Health and Welfare (AIHW) (2022b). *Principal diagnosis data cubes: separation statistics by principal diagnosis (ICD-10-AM 11th edition), Australia, 2020–21.* Canberra: AIHW. https://www.aihw.gov.au/reports/hospitals/principal-diagnosis-data-cubes/contents/data-cubes.

Australian Institute of Health and Welfare (2023). *Aboriginal and Torres Strait Islander Health Performance Framework: Summary report 2023.* Canberra: Australian Government Department of Health. htttps://www.indigenoushpf.gov.au/getattachment/d396ed0d-9347-4de6-8b41-ff56bf3dfa18/2023-ihpf-summary-report.pdf.

Australian Longitudinal Study on Women's Health (2020). *Evaluating the impact of the 2018 PCOS guideline.* https://alswh.org.au/projects/a1252-evaluating-the-impact-of-the-2018-pcos-guideline/.

Bauldoff, G., Gubrud-Howe, P. M., Carno, M.-A., Levett-Jones, T., Hales, M., Berry, K.,… LeMone, P. (2020). *LeMone and Burke's medical-surgical nursing: critical thinking for person-centred care* (4th [Australian] edn). Sydney: Pearson Australia.

Best, O. & Fredericks, B. (2021). *Yatdjuligin: Aboriginal and Torres Strait Islander nursing and midwifery care* (3rd edn). Port Melbourne, VIC: Cambridge University Press.

Boardman, C.H. & Matthews, K.J. (2022). Cervical cancer. *Emedicine.* https://emedicine.medscape.com/article/253513-overview.

Breast Cancer Foundation NZ (2022). 30,000 voices: Informing a better future for breast cancer in Aotearoa New Zealand. Auckland: Breast Cancer Foundation NZ. https://www.breastcancerfoundation.org.nz/what-we-do/advocacy/2022-register-report-launch.

Bullock, S. & Manias, E. (2022). *Fundamentals of pharmacology* (9th edn). Sydney: Pearson Australia.

Cancer Australia (2023a). *Breast cancer in Australia statistics*. Sydney: Cancer Australia. https://www.canceraustralia.gov.au/cancer-types/breast-cancer/statistics.

Cancer Australia (2023b). *Ovarian cancer statistics in Australia*. Sydney: Cancer Australia. https://www.canceraustralia.gov.au/cancer-types/ovarian-cancer/statistics.

Cancer Council Australia (2022). Clinical guidelines: cervical screening 12. HPV screening strategies for Aboriginal and Torres Strait Islander women. https://www.cancer.org.au/clinical-guidelines/cervical-cancer/cervical-cancer-screening/hpv-screening-in-aboriginal-and-torres-strait-islander-women.

Chiang, J. W. (2021). Uterine cancer. *Emedicine*. https://emedicine.medscape.com/article/258148-overview.

Davila, G.W., Kapoor, D., Alderman, E., Hiraoka, M.K.Y., Ghoniem, G.M. & Peskin, B.D. (2021). Endometriosis. *Emedicine*. https://emedicine.medscape.com/article/271899-overview.

Department of Health and Aged Care (2023a). *National cervical screening program—for healthcare providers*. Canberra: Department of Health and Aged Care. https://www.health.gov.au/our-work/national-cervical-screening-program.

Department of Health and Aged Care (2023b). National Communicable Disease Surveillance Dashboard. *National Notifiable Disease Surveillance System*. https://nindss.health.gov.au/pbi-dashboard/.

Horne, A.W. & Missmer, S.A. (2022). Pathophysiology, diagnosis, and management of endometriosis. *BMJ* 379, e070750. https://doi.org/10.1136/bmj-2022-070750.

Marieb, E.N. & Hoehn, K. (2019). *Human anatomy and physiology* (11th edn). San Francisco, CA: Pearson Benjamin Cummings.

National Breast Cancer Foundation (NBCF)(2023). *Breast cancer and Aboriginal And Torres Strait Islander peoples*. Sydney: NBCF. https://nbcf.org.au/about-breast-cancer/further-information-on-breast-cancer/breast-cancer-in-aboriginal-and-torres-strait-islander-peoples/.

Newman, J.E., Paul, R.C. & Chambers, G.M. (2022). *Assisted reproductive technology in Australia and New Zealand 2020.* Sydney: National Perinatal Epidemiology and Statistics Unit, the University of New South Wales, Sydney. https://npesu.unsw.edu.au/surveillance/assisted-reproductive-technology-australia-and-new-zealand-2020.

NHMRC Centre of Research Excellence in Cervical Cancer Control (2021). *Cervical cancer elimination progress report: Australia's progress towards the elimination of cervical cancer as a public health problem*. Melbourne: NHMRC Centre of Research Excellence in Cervical Cancer Control. https://www.cervicalcancercontrol.org.au/wp-content/uploads/2021/03/2021-C4-CRE-Elim-Report.pdf.

Sepilian, V.P. & Wood, E. (2022). Ectopic pregnancy. *Emedicine.* https://emedicine.medscape.com/article/2041923-overview.

Tortora. G.J., Derrickson, B., Burkett, B., Peoples, G., Dye, D., Cooke, J., … Green, H. (2022). *Principles of anatomy and physiology* (3rd Asia-Pacific edn). Milton, QLD: John Wiley and Sons.

40 Male reproductive disorders

KEY TERMS

Benign prostatic hyperplasia (BPH)
Chlamydia
Corpora cavernosa
Cryptorchidism
Epididymitis
Epispadias
Erectile dysfunction (ED)
Genital herpes
Genital warts
Gonorrhoea
Hydrocele
Hypospadias
Orchitis
Paraphimosis
Phimosis
Priapism
Prostate cancer
Prostatitis
Spermatocele
Syphilis
Testicular cancer
Varicocele

LEARNING OBJECTIVES

After completing this chapter, you should be able to:

1 Describe the pathophysiology, diagnosis and clinical management of common prostate disorders.

2 Describe the pathophysiology, diagnosis and clinical management of common penile and urethral disorders.

3 Describe the pathophysiology, diagnosis and clinical management of common scrotal and testicular disorders.

4 Identify the parameters used to measure male fertility, and outline some common conditions associated with decreased fertility.

5 Outline the pathophysiology, diagnosis and management of common sexually transmitted infections.

WHAT YOU SHOULD KNOW BEFORE YOU START THIS CHAPTER

Can you describe normal endocrine system structures and functions?

Can you identify the normal male reproductive system structures, and describe their functions?

Can you describe the main stages of inflammation and healing?

Can you describe the principles of the pathophysiology and management of infection?

Can you outline the major concepts of neoplasia?

Introduction

Disorders of the male reproductive system are either congenital or acquired conditions. These conditions can affect the structure and function of the urethra, penis, testes or accessory structures, such as the prostate or seminal vesicles. The effects of cancer and sexually transmitted infections (STIs) will also be explored in this chapter.

Prostate disorders

LEARNING OBJECTIVE 1

Describe the pathophysiology, diagnosis and clinical management of common prostate disorders.

In this section, the characteristics, diagnosis and management of common prostate conditions are described, including benign prostatic hyperplasia, prostatitis and prostate cancer.

The prostate is a doughnut-shaped structure located inferiorly to the urinary bladder and anterior to the rectum, surrounding the proximal end of the urethra. Its base is continuous with the neck of the bladder (see Figure 40.1). It consists of glandular, connective and smooth muscle tissue. The *connective tissue* is referred to as *stroma*, and the *glandular tissue* is embedded within this layer. The prostate secretes a milky, slightly acidic fluid contributing about 25% semen volume, which contains citrate for adenosine triphosphate (ATP) production, and several enzymes that will liquefy coagulated semen, such as prostate specific antigen (PSA), as well as zinc.

In the young adult male, the prostate can be divided into four layers (see Figure 40.2). The innermost layer is called the *transitional (or periurethral) zone*, and surrounds the urethra proximal to the entry of the ejaculatory ducts. It accounts for up to 10% of prostate mass. Positioned below the proximal urethral segment is the *central zone*. It represents about 20–25% of the organ's mass. Surrounding the central zone and occupying the prostate's apex is the *peripheral zone*. It accounts for 70–75% of the mass. The last third of the prostate mass is the *anterior fibromuscular stroma*, which is non-glandular tissue.

BENIGN PROSTATIC HYPERPLASIA

Aetiology and pathophysiology

Benign prostatic hyperplasia (BPH) is a common chronic disorder in men characterised by nodular prostatic tissue remodelling, primarily involving the stroma and, to a lesser extent, the epithelium. The *transitional zone* is usually where this process begins. The remodelling takes the form of *hyperplasia* (increased cell number) and, especially during the advanced phase, *hypertrophy* (increased cell size). (See the chapter 'Pathophysiological terminology, cellular adaptation and injury'.) The enlarged gland eventually constricts the proximal urethra, disrupting the flow of urine from the bladder. The bladder muscle contractions, particularly those of the detrusor system, become uncoordinated, triggering involuntary contractions during the filling phase of micturition—referred to as an *overactive bladder*—but allowing incomplete voiding. *Lower urinary tract symptoms (LUTS)* will ensue.

Alterations in the prostatic architecture can be seen in young men, even though the condition requires a long period of a man's life to fully develop. Studies of histological changes indicate a prevalence of 50% in men aged 50–60 years, increasing to 90% in men aged over 80 years.

These changes are dependent on *androgen levels*, particularly local concentrations of the testosterone metabolite, 5-α-dihydrotestosterone (5-α-DHT) and their *interaction with prostate androgen receptors*. This interaction triggers the secretion of a number of other growth factors by prostate cells that are believed to play crucial roles in the development of BPH, including fibroblast growth factors, transforming growth factor-β and insulin-like growth factors. Prostate cells also express oestrogen and progesterone receptors that may also have a role in BPH development. Chronic inflammatory reactions induced by the prostatic stromal cells have also been strongly implicated in the pathogenesis of this condition. The stromal cells are thought to activate $CD4^+$ T lymphocytes, and trigger the release of *pro-inflammatory cytokines*, such as interleukins, within the prostate microenvironment. These events lead to increased infiltration and proliferation of immune cells within the prostate.

Clinical manifestations

A man with BPH will remain asymptomatic until the enlarged gland obstructs the flow of urine from the bladder. The LUTS arising from this obstruction and the uncoordinated muscle

Figure 40.1

The prostate gland

The anatomical position of the prostate gland and its relationship with other reproductive structures.

Source: Human reproductive system/Alamy Stock Photo.

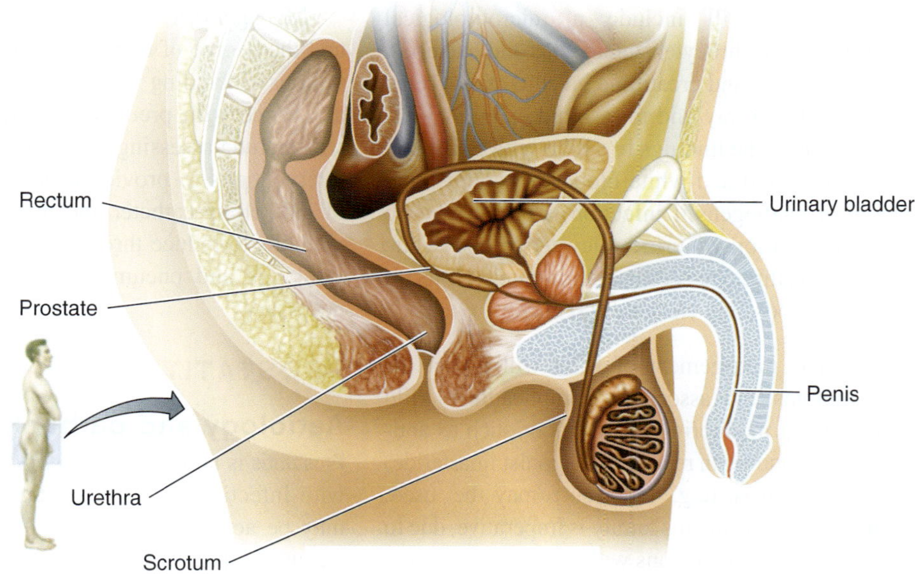

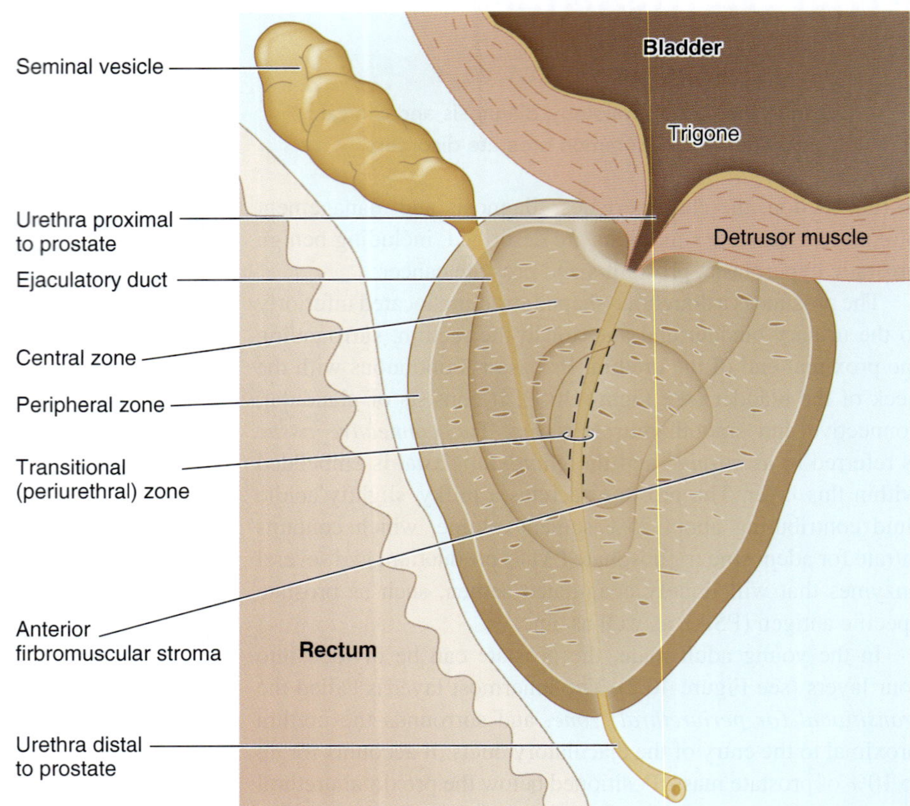

Figure 40.2

Layers of the prostate

The four layers of the prostate gland. The transitional zone accounts for up to 10% of prostate mass. The central zone represents about 20–25% of the organ's mass. The peripheral zone accounts for 70–75% of the mass. The anterior fibromuscular stroma is non-glandular tissue.

contractions include reduced urine flow, painful urination, urinary retention, urgency and urine reflux.

Figure 40.3 explores the common clinical manifestations and management of BPH and prostate cancer.

Clinical diagnosis and management

Diagnosis Diagnosis for BPH incorporates a health history, symptom scoring and an examination that includes a digital rectal examination (DRE) (refer to Clinical Box 40.1 for more information). The DRE can be used to identify the size, texture and degree of pain or tenderness of the prostate. Investigations performed will include a microbiological examination of urine (for erythrocytes, leukocytes and bacteria), blood tests (full blood count and creatinine level to assess renal function and PSA levels), X-ray and ultrasound examinations, as well as prostate biopsy. The findings in a man with BPH may include: elevated urinary red and white blood cell counts, and culture of bacterial uropathogens if infection is present due to the obstruction and retention of urine; elevated blood white blood cell counts and erythrocyte sedimentation rates (ESRs) if infection is present; and possibly elevated PSA levels.

Management The management of BPH will reflect the severity of the symptoms and associated complications. Mild cases will require ongoing monitoring. Medications such as anti-androgen agents (e.g. the androgen receptor antagonist finasteride) and α-adrenergic antagonists (e.g. terazocin) may be used. However, educating the person and his family is imperative, due to the potential side-effects and interactions with other medications.

Anti-androgen agents promote a reduction in the prostate size through the inhibition of the conversion of testosterone to 5-α-DHT, which mediates the growth of the prostate. α-Adrenergic antagonists may decrease the degree of smooth muscle contraction, decrease the degree of obstruction and increase urinary flow. Men experiencing retention of urine, recurrent urinary tract infection (UTI), bladder stones, haematuria or renal impairment generally benefit from surgical intervention, and this may be performed through minimally invasive, transurethral resection (TURP) (refer to Clinical Box 40.1 for more information), open or laser surgical approaches.

Management will include an assessment of the condition and the degree of urinary retention, advice regarding treatment options (including use, effects, risks and complications) and assistance with preoperative preparation. Post-procedure care will include assessing the degree of bleeding and fluid balance, interventions to provide adequate pain management, and care of indwelling catheter and bladder irrigations. Assistance with methods to reduce thrombosis, such as the use of anti-embolic stockings and pneumatic compression devices, may also be necessary.

PROSTATITIS

Aetiology and pathophysiology

Prostatitis is an *inflammation of the prostate*, frequently associated with infection by a urinary tract pathogen (a *uropathogen*). It may be accompanied by LUTS, such as pelvic pain, dysuria, frequency and urgency, as well as sexual dysfunction, or it

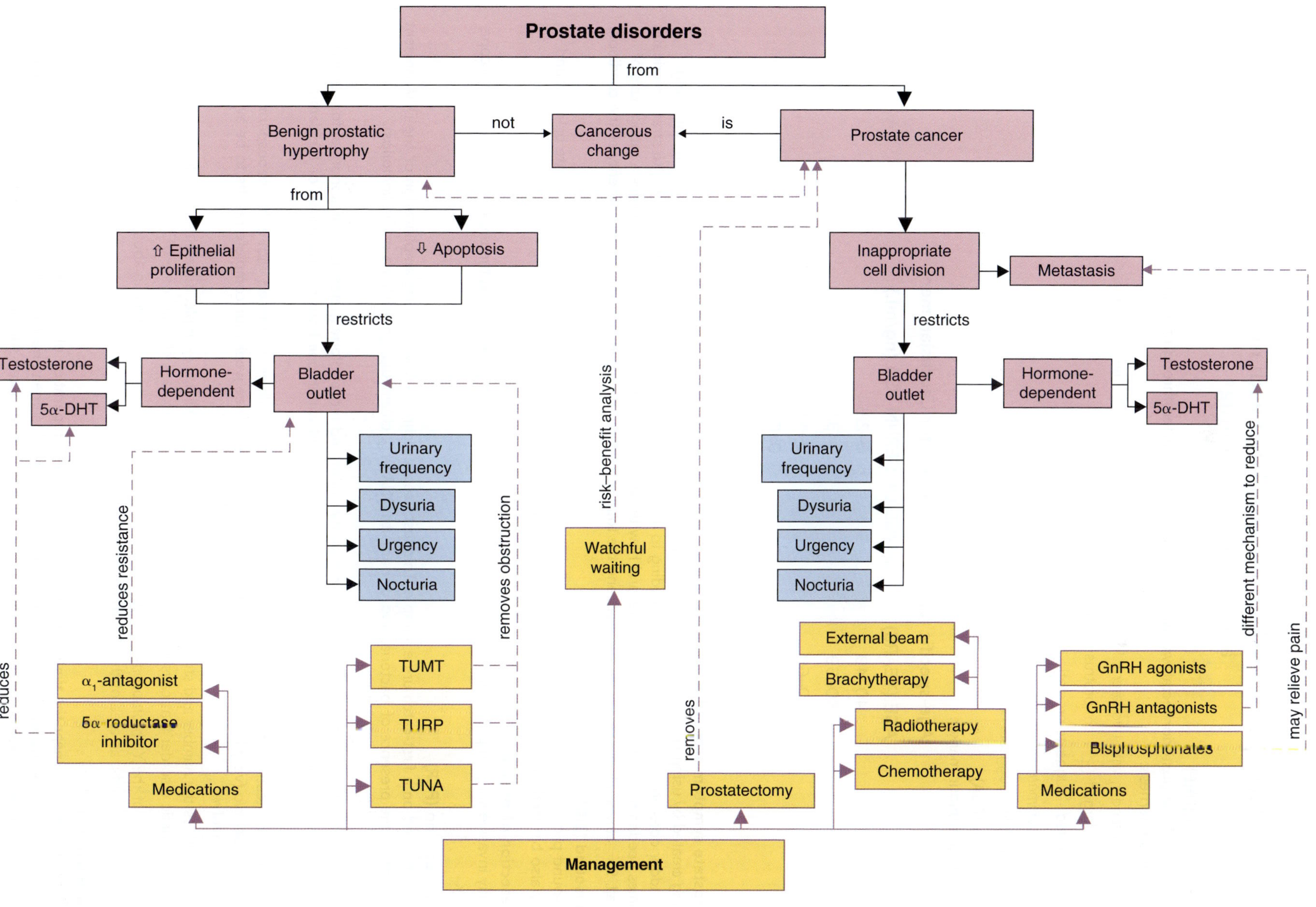

Figure 40.3

Clinical snapshot: Prostate disorders

↓ = decreased; ↑ = increased; α = alpha; 5α-DHT = 5-α-dihydrotestosterone; GnRH = gonadotropin-releasing hormone; TUMT = transurethral microwave therapy; TUNA = transurethral needle ablation; TURP = transurethral resection of the prostate.

CLINICAL BOX 40.1

Common procedures and investigations associated with male reproductive disorders and the possible findings

Digital rectal examination (DRE)

DRE involves palpation of the posterior rectal wall (with a gloved finger inserted through the anus) to assess prostate size, texture and degree of tenderness:

- *normal*—prostate non-tender, with two lateral lobes about 2 cm in length, smooth, median sulcus palpable
- *abnormal*—prostate enlarged ($\geq$ 1 cm protrusion into rectum)
- *median sulcus obliterated*—suggests prostatic hypertrophy
- *enlarged, tender and asymmetrical*—suggests prostatitis
- *hard with irregular nodule*—suggests carcinoma

Prostate specific antigen (PSA)

PSA is a prostate cancer tumour marker.

Age-specific range of PSA levels for Caucasian men

AGE (YEARS)	RANGE OF SERUM PSA (ng/mL)
40–49	0–2.5
50–59	0–3.5
60–69	0–4.5
70–79	0–6.5

Source: Brosman (2020).

International prostate symptom score (IPSS)

The IPSS is a rating created by using eight questions (seven symptom-based questions and one quality-of-life question), including: feeling that the bladder does not empty after urinating; needing to urinate within two hours after urination; needing to strain to urinate; the number of times needed to get up at night to urinate; and how the disorder makes the man feel. The IPSS uses a rating scale of 0–5 (0 = not at all; 5 = almost always) for each question, and the total score provides some indication of the severity of the condition.

Transrectal ultrasound (TRUS)

TRUS is an ultrasound procedure involving the insertion of a small probe into the rectum to visualise the prostate using sound waves. TRUS may also be used to guide a biopsy of the prostate for histological examination.

Transurethral resection of prostate (TURP)

TURP is a minimally invasive surgical procedure in which the enlarged prostate tissue is excised via the urethra using a resectoscope and electrocautery.

Polymerase chain reaction (PCR)

PCR is generally performed on a first-catch urine sample. This test uses a technique that enables amplification of the DNA present in the sample, indicating the presence of bacterial and/or parasite DNA (e.g. chlamydia, gonorrhoea or *Trichomonas*).

Semen analysis

Semen analysis is performed to assess: volume; pH; sperm motility, count and morphology (percentage of abnormal forms); white blood cell count; and antisperm antibody levels. Testing should be performed within one hour of production of the sample.

Genetic testing

These are specialised blood tests performed for males with severe infertility problems diagnosed with either *azoospermia* (no sperm) or *severe oligospermia* (very low sperm count). These tests take up to three weeks for complete results to be available. Common genetic tests involve:

- *karyotype*—this identifies the number and structure of chromosomes in each cell; for example, Klinefelter's syndrome is a relatively common genetic disorder that causes infertility—these men have an extra X chromosome (47XXY).
- *Y deletion testing*—parts of the Y chromosome are involved in the control of sperm production; in about 5% of males with zero or extremely low sperm counts, an area of the Y chromosome is missing.

Intrauterine insemination (IUI)

This procedure is performed at or near the time of ovulation, and requires preparation of a sample of sperm (from the partner or a donor) that is washed and concentrated. The male needs to have a 'normal' semen analysis and the female should have patent fallopian tubes to optimise the chance of 'normal' fertilisation occurring. The prepared sample is deposited into the uterine cavity via a small catheter inserted through the cervical canal.

In-vitro fertilisation (IVF)

This procedure involves ovarian stimulation using a combination of drugs that may include: gonadotropin-releasing hormone agonists (e.g. goserelin) or antagonists (e.g. ganirelix or cetrorelix), follicle-stimulating hormone and β-human chorionic gonadotropin. The procedure involves transvaginal oocyte retrieval, fertilisation of the oocytes in the laboratory, embryo culture (for two to five days) followed by embryo transfer (this may be performed under ultrasound guidance) and cryopreservation of suitable remaining embryos. IVF procedures may require the use of donor gametes (i.e. eggs or sperm).

Intracytoplasmic sperm injection (ICSI)

This is used in conjunction with an IVF procedure for severe male fertility issues. It involves the use of specialised microscopic and micro-injection equipment and techniques for the injection of a single sperm into each mature egg. The sperm may be selected from a prepared semen sample or recovered surgically from the epididymis or testis.

may be asymptomatic. It can occur in adult men of any age. It is considered the third most common urinary tract condition affecting men, after BPH and prostate cancer.

Due to the variability of the clinical presentation of this condition, the US National Institutes of Health has classified prostatitis into four main categories: acute bacterial prostatitis, chronic bacterial prostatitis, chronic prostatitis/chronic pelvic pain syndrome (CP/CPPS), and asymptomatic inflammatory prostatitis. Other less common forms of prostatitis outside of this classification system include *fungal and viral prostatitis*.

A man with *acute bacterial prostatitis (category I)* would present *acutely ill with symptoms of a UTI*. Bacteriuria, pelvic pain and pyuria would be expected. *Escherichia coli* is the most common uropathogen causing this form of the condition.

The prevalence of *chronic bacterial prostatitis (category II)* is low. The affected person presents with *recurrent bacterial UTI* caused by the same uropathogen. Common pathogens associated with this condition are those associated with urinary tract infections and sexually transmitted disease. As a part of this classification, the uropathogen should be isolated from the prostate in higher concentrations than those found in the urinary tract.

The prevalence of *chronic prostatitis/chronic pelvic pain syndrome (CP/CPPS) (category III)* is very high, representing the most common form of the condition. *Genitourinary pain* is the primary characteristic of this form. Implicit in this rather less specific definition is that other pelvic structures may be involved in the aetiology of this condition. The pain may be accompanied by LUTS and sexual dysfunction (e.g. painful ejaculation, premature ejaculation or erectile dysfunction). It may also be associated with infertility. This form of prostatitis can be very debilitating. This category differentiates between people experiencing current inflammation and those who are not, with the subdivisions based on white blood cells being present in expressed prostatic secretions and urine.

The presence of leukocytes is referred to as *category IIIA*, while their absence is referred to as *category IIIB*. The cause of this form of prostatitis is not considered to be primarily infectious. However, studies suggest that a bacterium that is difficult to culture may be present. It has been proposed that, in a situation analogous to the presence of *Helicobacter pylori* in peptic ulcer (see the chapter 'Gastro-oesophageal reflux disease and peptic ulcer disease'), this still unidentified bacterium may make a major contribution to the pathophysiological process. Other mechanisms that have been implicated are inflammation, autoimmunity and autonomic nervous system disorders.

A mechanism that may be involved in the development of chronic pelvic pain is where a dysfunction of the lower urinary tract transitional epithelium (bladder, urethral and prostatic) alters the balance between the protective and the injurious factors present in the lower urinary tract. Under these conditions, the permeability of the epithelium to potassium increases, allowing it to diffuse into the interstitium and depolarise sensory nerves and muscle. This sensitisation leads to urgency and pain.

Men diagnosed with *asymptomatic inflammatory prostatitis (category IV)* have no history of genitourinary pain or prostate infection. They present during evaluations of prostate cancer or infertility. They have an elevated PSA level, and white blood cells are present in prostatic secretions. This form is frequently associated with BPH.

Clinical diagnosis and management

Diagnosis Diagnosis for prostatitis incorporates a health history, symptom scoring and an examination that includes a DRE to identify the size, texture and degree of pain or tenderness of the prostate. Microbiological examination of urine, prostatic secretions and semen will include microscopic evaluation (for elevated levels of red and white blood cells), as well as bacterial cultures. If bacteria are identified, then antimicrobial sensitivity testing is performed to facilitate the appropriate antibacterial therapy, which will vary according to the causative organism.

Blood tests, including full blood count and PSA, as well as imaging of the prostate may also be undertaken. Findings in someone with prostatitis may include elevated urinary red and white blood cell counts and culture of bacterial uropathogens if infection is present, elevated blood white blood cell counts and ESR, and possibly elevated PSA levels.

Management Bacterial prostatitis requires long-term antimicrobial therapy. The antibacterial type will depend on the findings of the cultures and sensitivity testing. α-Antagonist therapy can alleviate the symptoms of urinary tract obstruction. Treatment for non-bacterial prostatitis may include non-steroidal anti-inflammatory drugs (NSAIDs), such as indomethacin or naproxen, and muscarinic receptor antagonist medications (e.g. oxybutynin hydrochloride or propantheline bromide). The NSAIDs reduce pain by inhibiting prostaglandin synthesis and producing anti-inflammatory and analgesic effects. The muscarinic receptor antagonist drugs reduce muscle spasms and decrease the frequency of urge to void.

Symptom management should be the major focus, and may include the use of analgesia, advice regarding the need to increase oral fluid intake, localised heat therapy (e.g. warm sitz baths), prevention of constipation that could exacerbate pain, advice on the importance of continuing antimicrobial therapy until the course is completed, and reassurance that prostatitis is not infectious and does not increase the risk of cancer.

PROSTATE CANCER

Aetiology and pathophysiology

The aetiology of **prostate cancer** is multifactorial. Genetic predisposition is important (research on women diagnosed with breast cancer before the age of 35 years indicated that their fathers and brothers had a five-fold increased risk of prostate cancer), as is ethnicity (in the United States, African American men have the highest prevalence, followed by Caucasians, with lower rates in men of Hispanic, Indigenous American and Asian/Pacific origin). Hormonal status, in terms of sex hormone levels, contributes to risk, as does dietary status (diets high in saturated fats may increase risk).

Most cases of prostate cancer arise in the glandular tissue of the organ (*adenocarcinomas*), while the remainder develop within the epithelial lining or from neuroendocrine stem cells present in the gland. In contrast to the pattern of development in BPH, the principal prostate layers affected are the *peripheral and central zones*.

In prostate cancer, 5-α-DHT and androgen receptor signalling is important. Studies reveal that men with a particular isoform of 5-α-reductase (*5-α-reductase type II*) had an increased risk of prostate cancer, whereas those that did not had a lower risk.

As the cancer advances, prostate cancer moves from being androgen-dependent to *androgen-independent or hormone refractory*. Other mediators, such as *growth factors and tyrosine kinase signalling*, may contribute to the progression of the condition at this stage.

Epidemiology

Cancer of the prostate is highly prevalent in our community, and in Australia is ranked second, after lung cancers, as a cause of cancer-related mortality in men. In New Zealand it is the third most common cancer in men. It was estimated to be the most commonly diagnosed cancer in Australia and New Zealand in 2022. The incidence rate of prostate cancer is highest for those men aged 75–79 years old. The age-standardised incidence rate in 2022 was estimated at 151 cases per 100,000 men.

Clinical diagnosis and management

Diagnosis Diagnosis for prostate cancer incorporates a health history, symptom scoring and an examination that includes a DRE to identify the size and texture of the prostate. Prostate biopsy via transrectal ultrasound (TRUS) (see Clinical Box 40.1) provides the only definitive diagnosis of prostate cancer. Other investigations performed may include urinalysis (for red and white blood cells and bacteria) and blood tests revealing PSA levels (this would generally be elevated). Bone scans, magnetic resonance imaging (MRI) or computed tomography (CT) examinations may be undertaken to identify metastasis.

Management Management is complex and dependent on the person's age, general health and preferences. Treatments include surgery, radiation therapy and hormonal manipulation. Surgery ranges from TURP (see Clinical Box 40.1) through to open/laparoscopic radical prostatectomy. Radiation may be used as a primary or palliative therapy via internal implants or an external beam.

Hormonal manipulation may range from orchidectomy to oral medications, and the effects vary from none to complete but temporary tumour reduction, as well as pain reduction. Oral hormonal therapies may include oestrogen compounds (diethylstilboestrol), luteinising-hormone-releasing hormone (LHRH, leuprolide), steroidal anti-androgens (megastrol acetate) or non-steroidal anti-androgens (flutamide), which may be combined with LHRH. Hormonal treatments may result in hot flushes, gynaecomastia, erectile dysfunction and loss of libido.

The management will include those aspects discussed in relation to BPH, as well as an additional focus on strategies for the management of urinary incontinence, pain and sexual dysfunction. Discussions should take place regarding the need for ongoing follow-up, the availability of support services and, if required, information regarding radiation therapy.

Urethral and penile disorders

LEARNING OBJECTIVE 2

Describe the pathophysiology, diagnosis and clinical management of common penile and urethral disorders.

The common urethral and penile conditions described within this section are urethral strictures, phimosis, paraphimosis, priapism, erectile dysfunction, hypospadias, epispadias and penile cancer. Figure 40.4 explores the clinical manifestations and management of common penile disorders.

URETHRAL STRICTURES

Aetiology and pathophysiology

Urethral strictures result from urethral fibrosis that narrows the urethra. The *fibrosis* may occur as a consequence of *infection or trauma*. Examples of trauma include straddle injuries (injury to the perineum or genitals following a fall where the person lands on an object in a straddled position) or invasive clinical procedures involving the insertion of a larger catheter or other instrument into the urethra.

Clinical manifestations

The narrowing of the urethra affects urine flow, causing a decreased urinary stream, urinary retention and bladder infection.

Clinical diagnosis and management

Diagnosis Diagnosis of urethral strictures incorporates a health history, a physical examination, diagnostic imaging

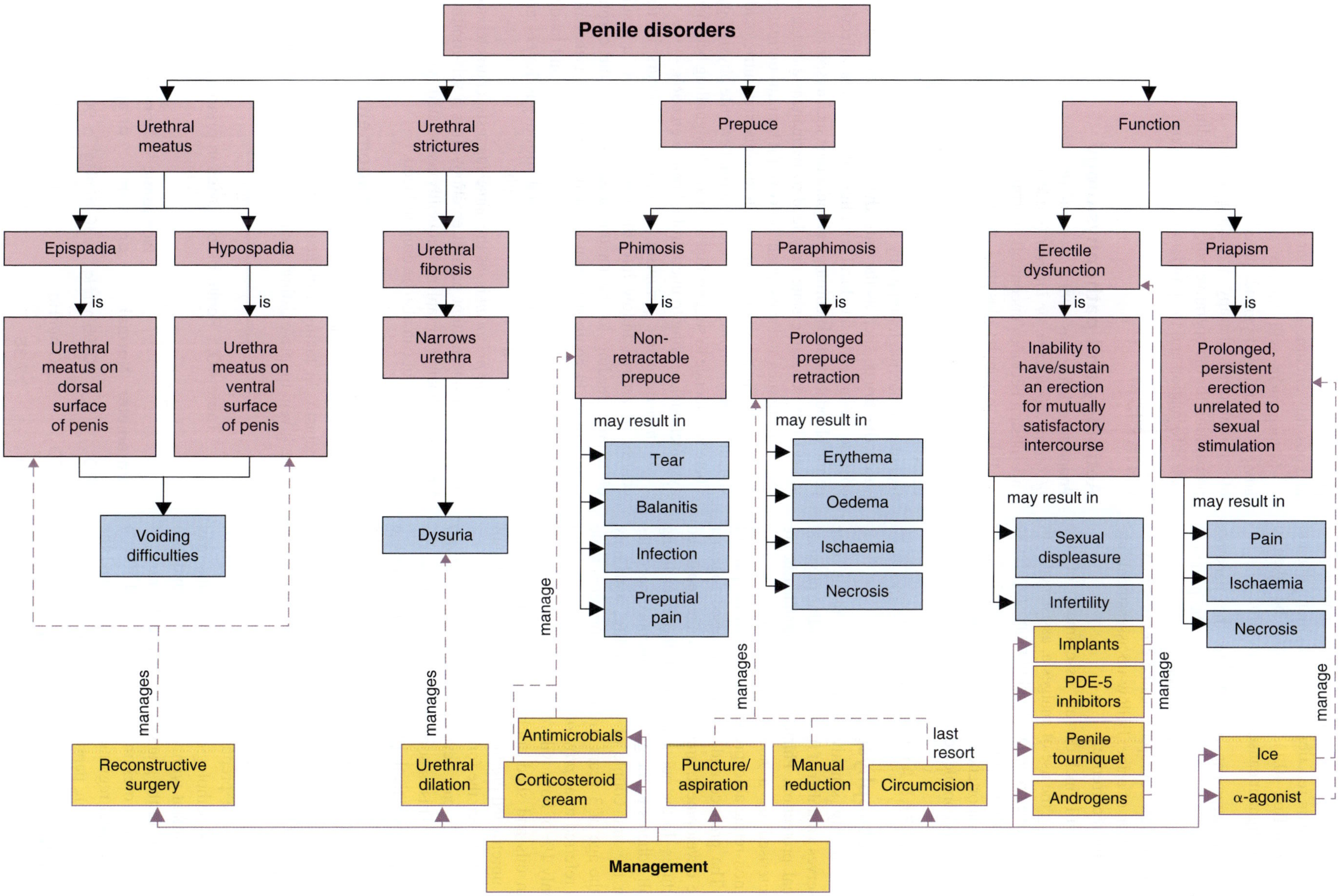

Figure 40.4

Clinical snapshot: Penile disorders

α = alpha; PDE-5 = phosphodiesterase type 5; SPC = superpubic catheterisation.

procedures to assess urinary flow (cystoscopy/urethroscopy and voiding cystourethrogram), urinalysis and microbiological cultures or polymerase chain reaction (PCR) for chlamydia and gonorrhoea (see Clinical Box 40.1). Biopsies may be taken to exclude or confirm a malignant cause for the stricture.

Management Management depends on the person's age and personal preference. However, surgery is the principal treatment, and may include dilation of the urethra, urethrotomy or open surgical procedures. Suprapubic catheterisation may be required for acute retention of urine. Follow-up assessments are important to monitor for recurrence.

The management will include an assessment of the condition, advice regarding the use of analgesia, assistance with preparation for the operative procedure (including postoperative care information and the provision of emotional support), as well as education on the importance of continuing antimicrobial therapy until the course is completed.

PHIMOSIS AND PARAPHIMOSIS

Aetiology and pathophysiology

The *prepuce* is a highly sensitive, retractable tissue (see Figure 40.5) that serves a number of functions, including physical and immunological protection. **Phimosis** and **paraphimosis** are conditions characterised by a *non-retractable prepuce* (see Figure 40.4). A non-retractable prepuce is a normal part of early childhood. The prepuce and glans were fused together during embryonic development, and at a later stage separated into distinct structures. In the neonatal period, the inner lining of the prepuce still adheres to the glans. The prepuce becomes retractable within the first couple of years of life, with only 10% of boys by the age of 3 years still having non-retractable foreskins. This is referred to as *physiological phimosis*, and by 16 years of age only 1% of boys will remain affected. *Smegma*, consisting of skin oils and shed epithelial cells, can become trapped under the unretracted prepuce, causing the formation of benign white lumps between the foreskin and glans.

Pathological phimosis can develop as a result of *distal scarring* of the prepuce. This is sometimes referred to as *true phimosis*, because physiological phimosis is usually just a developmental phenomenon. On examination, the pathological phimosis is observed as a white, fibrous ring around the preputial orifice, and the urethral opening may not be easily visualised. Another sign may be significant ballooning of the foreskin during urination, accompanied by a narrow urine stream. A recurrent episode of a severe inflammation of the glans penis (with or without involvement of the prepuce) is known as *balanitis*, and is the usual cause of pathological phimosis. Balanitis may also be observed in an infant with severe nappy rash, and as a consequence of infection of the glans by *Candida albicans*.

In paraphimosis, the foreskin remains retracted for a prolonged period, the distal regions of the glans penis and the foreskin may become swollen, painful and oedematous.

Clinical diagnosis and management

Diagnosis A health history and a physical examination are undertaken, and microbiological culture is performed if indicated.

Management Treatment may include changes in hygiene practices, manual reduction, antimicrobial therapy for infections, and possibly circumcision (after the infection has been treated).

Management will include assessment of the condition, advice regarding hygiene practices, advice about the use of antimicrobial therapy if required, and assistance with preparation for the operative procedure (including postoperative care information and the provision of emotional support).

PRIAPISM

Aetiology and pathophysiology

Priapism is defined as *persistent penile erection in the absence of sexual stimulation or interest* (see Figure 40.4). The corpus cavernosum becomes uncontrollably engorged with blood.

Priapism can be classified as ischaemic (low-flow), non-ischaemic (high-flow) or intermittent. *Ischaemic priapism* involves penile vascular stasis, where the venous outflow decreases. Conditions associated with ischaemic priapism include the haemoglobinopathy sickle cell anaemia, the use of vasoactive drugs, such as the antihypertensive agents, alcohol, cocaine or anaesthesia, local or metastatic cancers affecting penile blood flow, and neurological conditions such as spinal cord injury. The ischaemic state may lead to permanent damage of the penile tissues and subsequent fibrosis if it remains untreated. As described in the section on erectile dysfunction, nitric oxide signalling plays an important role in normal erectile physiology. There is evidence to suggest that nitric oxide signalling becomes dysfunctional, leading to uncontrolled penile erection.

In *non-ischaemic priapism*, a breakdown occurs in the control of arterial inflow into the penis, usually as a result of trauma, leading to the uncontrolled filling of the corpus cavernosum. In contrast to non-ischaemic priapism, ischaemic priapism is usually associated with a painful, rigid and tender penis. Aspirated blood is dark, and blood gas levels are abnormal (Table 40.1).

Intermittent priapism is, as the name suggests, characterised by recurrent intermittent painful erections. It is a self-limiting form of ischaemic priapism frequently associated with sickle cell anaemia, but can also be drug-induced.

Clinical diagnosis and management

Diagnosis Time is critical in the diagnosis and management of priapism. In taking a clinical history, consideration needs to be given to pre-existing medical conditions, recent drug

Table 40.1 Penile blood gases in priapism

Parameter	Normal	Ischaemic priapism	Non-ischaemic priapism
PO_2	90–95 mmHg	$<$ 30 mmHg	$>$ 90 mmHg
PCO_2	50 mmHg	$>$ 60 mmHg	$<$ 40 mmHg
pH	7.35	$<$ 7.25	7.40

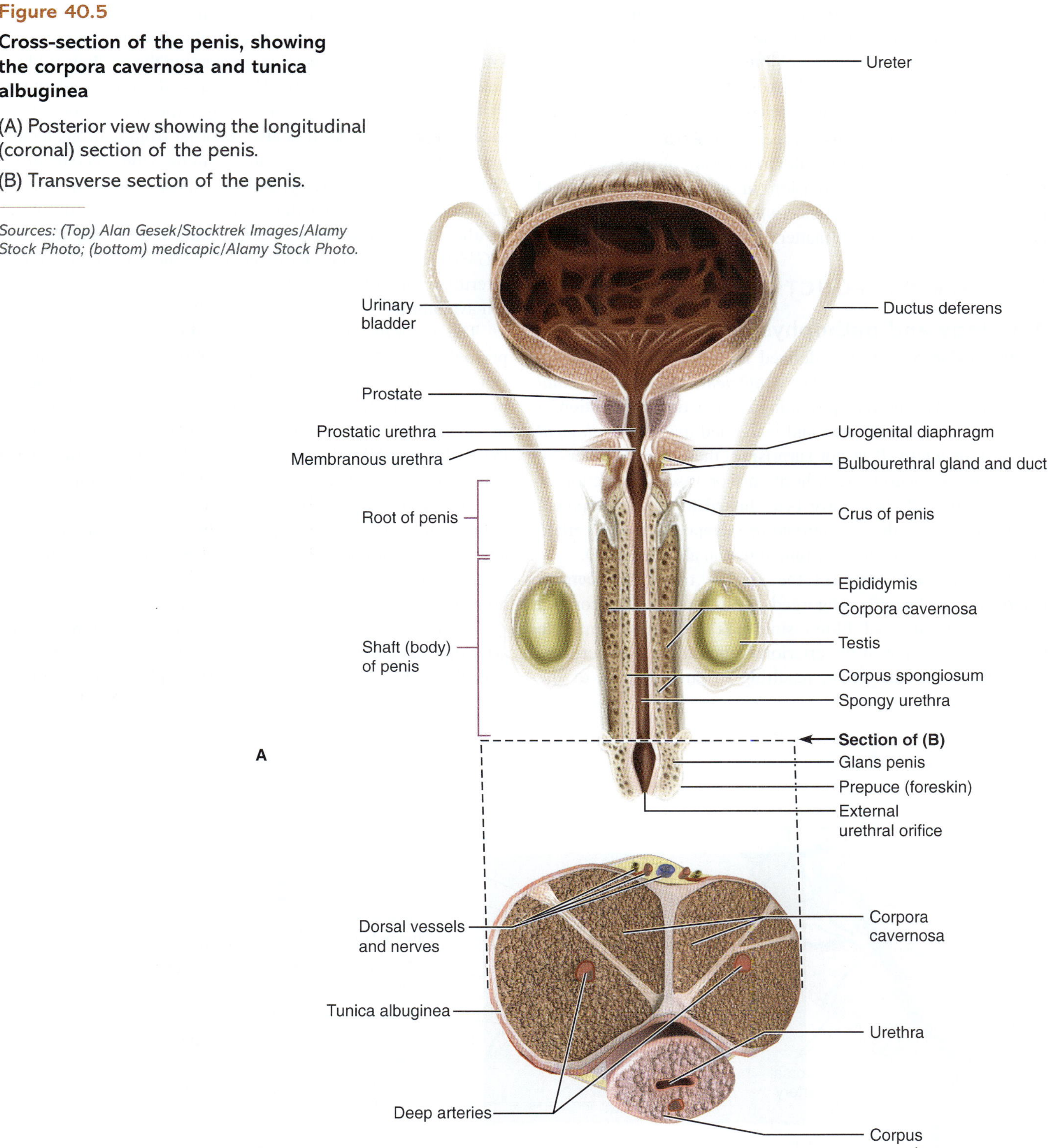

Figure 40.5

Cross-section of the penis, showing the corpora cavernosa and tunica albuginea

(A) Posterior view showing the longitudinal (coronal) section of the penis.

(B) Transverse section of the penis.

Sources: (Top) Alan Gesek/Stocktrek Images/Alamy Stock Photo; (bottom) medicapic/Alamy Stock Photo.

use (prescribed and illicit), any history of trauma, the extent of the pain, and a determination of the classification of the priapism (high-flow versus low-flow). Blood tests (full blood count, coagulation profile and blood gas analysis from the corpus cavernosum) may be performed. Diagnostic imaging using colour flow Doppler ultrasound may be used to facilitate classification of the priapism.

Management Treatment may include ice packs, external perineal compression, corporeal administration of adrenergic agonist medications to induce vasoconstriction of the arterioles and improved venous outflow (e.g. phenylephrine), aspiration of blood from the corpus cavernosum followed by urinary catheterisation and the application of pressure dressings, or creating a surgical shunt to drain deoxygenated blood from the corpus cavernosa. In intermittent priapism, hormonal treatment with oestrogens, antiandrogen, gonadotropin-releasing hormone analogues or 5-α-reductase inhibitors has been successful. In cases where priapism leads to damaged penile tissue, an inflatable penile prosthesis may be considered.

The care should focus on penile assessment (degree of erection, signs of ischaemia), the monitoring of urinary output, pain management, the provision of emotional support and reassurance, and also assistance with any procedures that may need to be undertaken as a matter of urgency.

ERECTILE DYSFUNCTION

Aetiology and pathophysiology

Erectile dysfunction (ED) is defined as an *inability to initiate and maintain penile erection sufficient to permit sexual intercourse*. The normal physiological reaction of erection is dependent on a coordinated and integrated *neuropsychological vascular response*. It is not surprising, then, that disorders in psychological, neurological, hormonal or vascular function or a combination of these have been linked to the development of ED. Moreover, the recreational or therapeutic use of certain drugs that affect any of these functions can also cause ED.

Penile erection requires the erectile tissue, the **corpora cavernosa**, to become engorged with blood. The corpora cavernosa consists of blood sinusoids and smooth muscle trabeculae. Dilation of the arteriolar smooth muscle increases blood flow into the penis, resulting in engorgement of the blood sinusoids. This response compresses the deep dorsal veins against the fibrous outer layer of the corpus cavernosum, known as the *tunica albuginea*, preventing the outflow of blood (see Figures 40.5 and 40.6). The endothelium plays a key role in the vasodilatory response through the production of the mediator, *nitric oxide*. It is also released from neurons locally under parasympathetic activation, along with *acetylcholine*. Nitric oxide and acetylcholine induce smooth muscle relaxation by activating the enzyme *guanylyl cyclase*, which results in an elevation of *cyclic guanosine monophosphate (cGMP)* levels intracellularly. cGMP induces the relaxation of arteriolar smooth muscle by decreasing intracellular calcium ion availability.

The *neuropsychological component* is associated with a person's libido. Thoughts and perceptions of particular stimuli can generate sexual arousal and erection. The *pudendal nerve*, part of the somatic nervous system, also has an important role in sexual arousal, as it transmits penile sensations back to the brain for processing, and is involved in the control of the extracorporeal striated muscle associated with the penis.

Androgens, especially testosterone, are important in the maintenance of libido, and play a role in nocturnal erections. Testosterone does not appear to be essential in the generation of an erection per se, but it is believed that a threshold level of these hormones may be necessary for an erection to occur.

Normally, penile *flaccidity* is restored by terminating the arteriolar vasodilatory response and *reinstating venous outflow*. cGMP is hydrolysed and inactivated by the phosphodiesterase-5

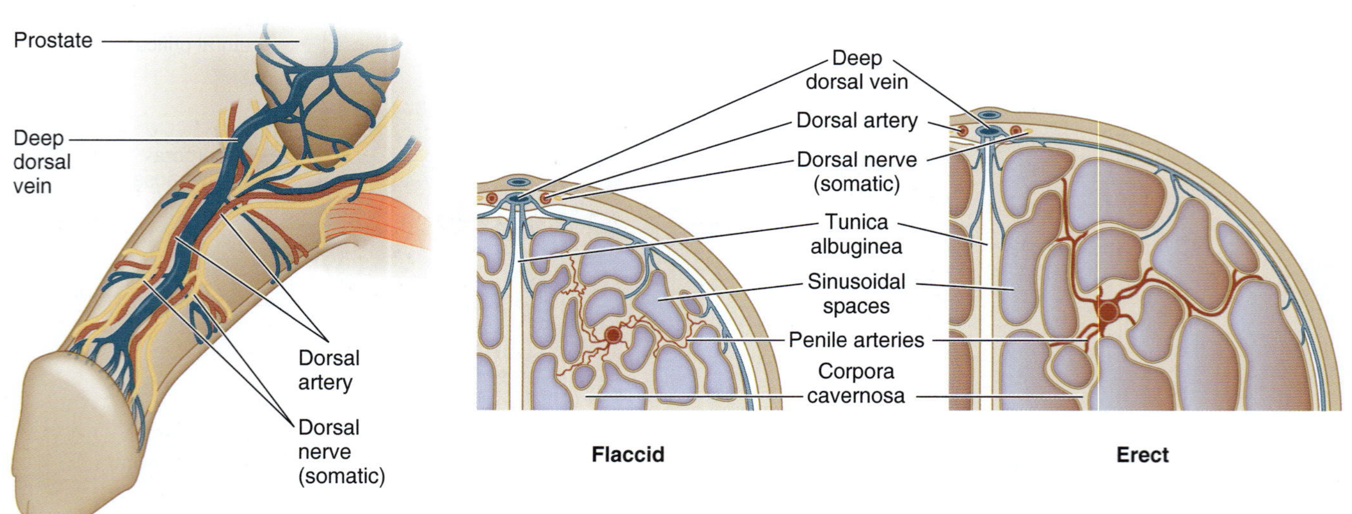

Figure 40.6

Dorsal external anatomy and corporal responses in erection

The mechanisms of erection and flaccidity are shown in the right and left images, respectively. During erection, relaxation of the trabecular smooth muscle and vasodilation of the arterioles result in a several-fold increase in blood flow, which expands the sinusoidal spaces to lengthen and enlarge the penis. The expansion of the sinusoids compresses the subtunical venular plexus against the tunica albuginea. In addition, stretching of the tunica compresses the emissary veins, thus reducing the outflow of blood to a minimum.

(PD5) enzyme. Smooth muscle contraction is also mediated by sympathetic nervous system activation, as well as the release of endothelins and prostaglandin $F_2\alpha$.

ED is broadly classified as either psychogenic or organic, although a combination of these two categories is very common.

Examples of *psychogenic ED* include performance anxiety, stress and a lack of sexual arousal. Men with psychiatric conditions, such as depression and schizophrenia, can also experience psychogenic ED. *Organic ED* can be of neurogenic, vascular, cavernosal or hormonal origin.

Neurogenic ED can develop in men with neurodegenerative diseases, such as Parkinson's disease or Alzheimer's disease. It can also occur in men who have had a stroke, brain trauma, spinal cord injury or radical pelvic surgery. There have also been reports in the literature of pudendal nerve entrapment in bicyclists and an increased incidence of ED.

Vascular conditions, such as hypertension, atherosclerosis, coronary disease, endothelial dysfunction, dyslipidaemias and diabetes mellitus, can be comorbidities with ED. Indeed, it is now believed that ED may be an early warning sign of impending cardiovascular disease. Medical practitioners are being asked to consider ED as a marker of people at risk of a premature cardiovascular event, and to manage accordingly.

Cavernosal dysfunction may occur as a result of traumatic injury, degenerative changes to the tunica albuginea or surgical procedures (e.g. to correct priapism). This tends to result in veno-occlusive dysfunction, where the veins do not completely close during the erectile response.

Endocrine disorders, such as hypogonadism, have been linked to ED. The link between hypogonadism and androgen levels is clear. Interestingly, hyperprolactinaemia inhibits the hypothalamic–pituitary–gonadal axis and causes hypogonadism through a disruption to dopaminergic transmission in the hypothalamus.

Drugs that are known to induce erectile dysfunction include centrally acting antihypertensives, antidepressants, anti-androgens and β-blockers. Cigarette smoking and chronic alcoholism lead to vascular and neuropathic changes, respectively, that result in penile dysfunction.

Epidemiology

There is epidemiological evidence that a degree of ED may be present in up to half of the male population between the ages of 40 and 70 years.

Clinical diagnosis and management

Diagnosis Diagnosis for ED incorporates an assessment of history (general and sexual health) and a physical examination (including a DRE). Lifestyle (diet, cigarette smoking, other recreational substance use, and alcohol ingestion) and the presence of cardiovascular disease, LUTS associated with BPH, or diabetes mellitus are known risk factors. Blood tests may be performed to assess for metabolic conditions (e.g. lipid and glucose levels, thyroid or kidney dysfunction) or altered levels of hormones (e.g. testosterone, luteinising hormone) and PSA. Penile monitoring may be undertaken at home or in a sleep laboratory to determine whether the origin of dysfunction is organic or psychological.

Management The management of this condition will vary depending on the reason for the dysfunction, as well as the preferences of the person and his partner. Strategies may include non-invasive therapy (oral medications; see below for more information on drug therapies), externally applied devices, such as vacuum pumps and penile rings, penile injections, hormone replacement therapy and surgery (e.g. vascular surgery or prosthetic implants). Changes in lifestyle can be quite effective, particularly in young men, and can include modifying diet, physical activity, medication and recreational substance use, as well as managing anxiety.

Drug therapies, either oral or injectable forms, include phosphodiesterase inhibitors, prostaglandin E_1 and the opioid papaverine. The *phosphodiesterase inhibitors*, such as sildenafil (Viagra), tadalafil (Cialis) and vardenafil (Levitra), are taken to inhibit PD5 in the corpus cavernosum, preventing the breakdown of cGMP. These drugs are contraindicated for people taking organic nitrate therapy, and there are increased risks of complications in those with cardiovascular disorders.

Alprostadil (Caverject) is *prostaglandin* E_1. It is administered via intracavernosal injection, and results in smooth muscle relaxation in the corpora cavernosa and corpus spongiosum, and dilation of the cavernosal arteries. The risk of priapism must be explained, and advice given about seeking urgent medical assistance if it persists for more than four hours.

Papaverine is an *opioid* that is administered via intracavernosal injection. It results in an erection through a relaxation of the penile arteriolar smooth muscle, which in turn increases blood flow and volume and compression of the venous channels. Again, the risk of priapism must be managed.

Management may also include referral to an endocrinologist, urologist or counsellor.

The care will incorporate assessment for risk factors, assessment of current sexual practices and dysfunction, discussion about coping strategies, and the provision of information regarding treatment options (including use, success rate, and risks and complications).

HYPOSPADIAS AND EPISPADIAS

Aetiology and pathophysiology

Hypospadias and epispadias are *congenital disorders affecting the positioning of the male urethral opening*, the *urethral meatus* (see Figure 40.7). The conditions arise during embryonic life, and affect the development of the male urinary tract. In **hypospadias**, the urethral meatus is located on the ventral undersurface of the penis. In **epispadias**, the meatus is found on the dorsal surface. Epispadias are less common than hypospadias. As these are conditions affecting normal development, *undescended testes* can also occur in hypospadias or epispadias.

There are varying degrees of severity. In the less severe form, the meatus is located distally, while in the more severe form, the meatus occurs proximally. In hypospadias, the meatus may even be located in the perineum. In more severe forms of this condition, the penis may also remain tethered downwards, leading to curvature of the shaft. This is known as *chordee*.

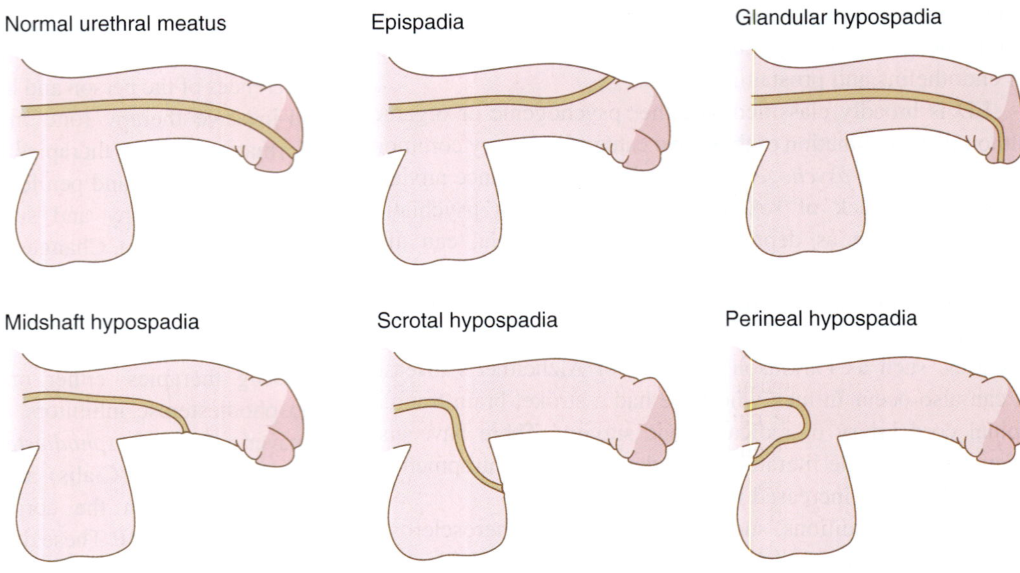

Figure 40.7
Hypospadias and epispadias

Epispadias is considered to be a mild form of *urinary bladder exstrophy*. Exstrophy is a condition where a hollow organ is turned inside out. In bladder exstrophy, the lower anterior abdominal wall and the anterior bladder wall do not form properly, allowing the posterior bladder wall and the penile mucosa to be exposed externally. If this condition arises more proximally, the urinary sphincter may also be involved, resulting in urinary incontinence.

Clinical diagnosis and management

Diagnosis Diagnosis involves a physical examination. Diagnostic imaging procedures may be used to exclude other associated congenital anomalies.

Management Treatment involves surgery to correct the defect, and normalise urinary control and cosmetic appearance. The timing and extent of surgery is dependent on the extent of the anomaly.

Management will include an assessment of the condition, advice regarding hygiene practices, and assistance with preparation for the operative procedure (including postoperative care information and the provision of emotional support). In the case of a young child, parental support and education about strategies for care are required.

PENILE CANCER

Aetiology and pathophysiology

Penile cancer is a relatively rare cancer that tends to occur predominantly in older men aged 60–70 years. Uncircumcised men, especially those with phimosis, are at particular risk of developing penile cancer. Poor penile hygiene, where smegma is retained, causing chronic irritation of the prepuce and glans, has been strongly implicated. Other risk factors include penile rashes and tears, urethral strictures, inflammatory conditions, cigarette smoking, phimosis (associated with chronic inflammation and balanitis), low socioeconomic status, the number of sexual partners and a history of STIs (especially infection with human papillomavirus [HPV]).

Most penile cancers are *squamous cell carcinomas* that arise from the glans and prepuce. Less than 5% of penile cancers arise on the shaft of the penis. Precursor cancerous lesions on the penis that are not associated with HPV are most commonly associated with a chronic inflammatory atrophic condition known as *lichen sclerosis*. This affects the prepuce and glans, causing pruritus, burning and soreness.

Epidemiology

The incidence rate of penile cancer in Western countries is about 0.5% of all malignancies, but appears to be increasing. However, the incidence is higher in the developing world, accounting for up to 1–2% of malignancies in men in some African, Asian and South American countries. In 2018, the age-standardised incidence rate globally was estimated at 0.08% per 100,000 person-years.

Clinical diagnosis and management

Diagnosis After taking a clinical history and performing a physical examination, a diagnosis of penile cancer is confirmed through biopsy of the lesion and any enlarged inguinal lymph nodes.

Management The treatment is dependent on the extent of the tumour and the degree of metastasis. It may include topical medication (e.g. the anticancer agent fluorouracil in a cream formulation), radiation, surgical excision, or partial or total amputation of the penis. Systemic forms of chemotherapy can be used, and may include bleomycin, cisplatin, fluorouracil and methotrexate.

The care will depend on the treatment undertaken, but may include advice regarding hygiene practices, the provision of information regarding pre- and postoperative care, strategies to facilitate urinary continence, and pain management. Provision of emotional support and strategies to reduce anxiety are also important.

Testicular and scrotal disorders

LEARNING OBJECTIVE 3

Describe the pathophysiology, diagnosis and clinical management of common scrotal and testicular disorders.

The *scrotum* is a sac of loose skin, superficial fascia and smooth muscle that contains the *testes*, the *epididymides* and the *spermatic cord* (consisting of the proximal part of the vas deferens, nerves, blood vessels and cremaster muscles). The testes are covered by a serous membrane called the *tunica vaginalis*, which is derived from the peritoneum (see Figure 40.8). The testes and accompanying structures are responsible for the production, maturation and transport of *spermatozoa*. The scrotum provides protection and helps to regulate the environment, particularly temperature, for maximum efficiency of sperm production.

Common scrotal and testicular disorders will be described here, including cryptorchidism, testicular torsion, epididymitis, orchitis, varicocele, hydrocele and spermatocele. Disorders of sperm production resulting in male infertility will also be discussed, as will testicular cancer. Figure 40.9 explores the clinical manifestations and management of common testicular and scrotal disorders.

CRYPTORCHIDISM

Aetiology and pathophysiology

Cryptorchidism occurs when one or both of the *testes fail to descend into the scrotum* along the inguinal canal from the abdominal cavity as a part of normal development. The term 'cryptorchidism' actually translates to *hidden testis*. A testicle that normally descends can also be regarded as cryptorchid if it retracts from the scrotum later in childhood. In the majority of cases the undescended testis is palpable, usually within the path of the inguinal canal, but an ectopic testis may also be palpated in front of the pubis, in the perineal region or in the upper thigh.

The causes of cryptorchidism are multiple, and are not completely understood. *Hormonal, environmental and genetic factors* have been implicated. The risk of cryptorchidism is increased in gestational diabetes, breech or caesarean delivery, when there is evidence of a family history of cryptorchidism, and in low-birth-weight infants. Cryptorchidism can also accompany hypospadias, inguinal hernia and hydrocele.

Complications of cryptorchidism include infertility and testicular cancer. The risk of these complications decreases the earlier surgical correction of the disorder occurs. In terms of fertility, studies indicate that men who had bilateral cryptorchidism as boys had lower sperm counts and paternity rates than those with a unilaterally undescended testis.

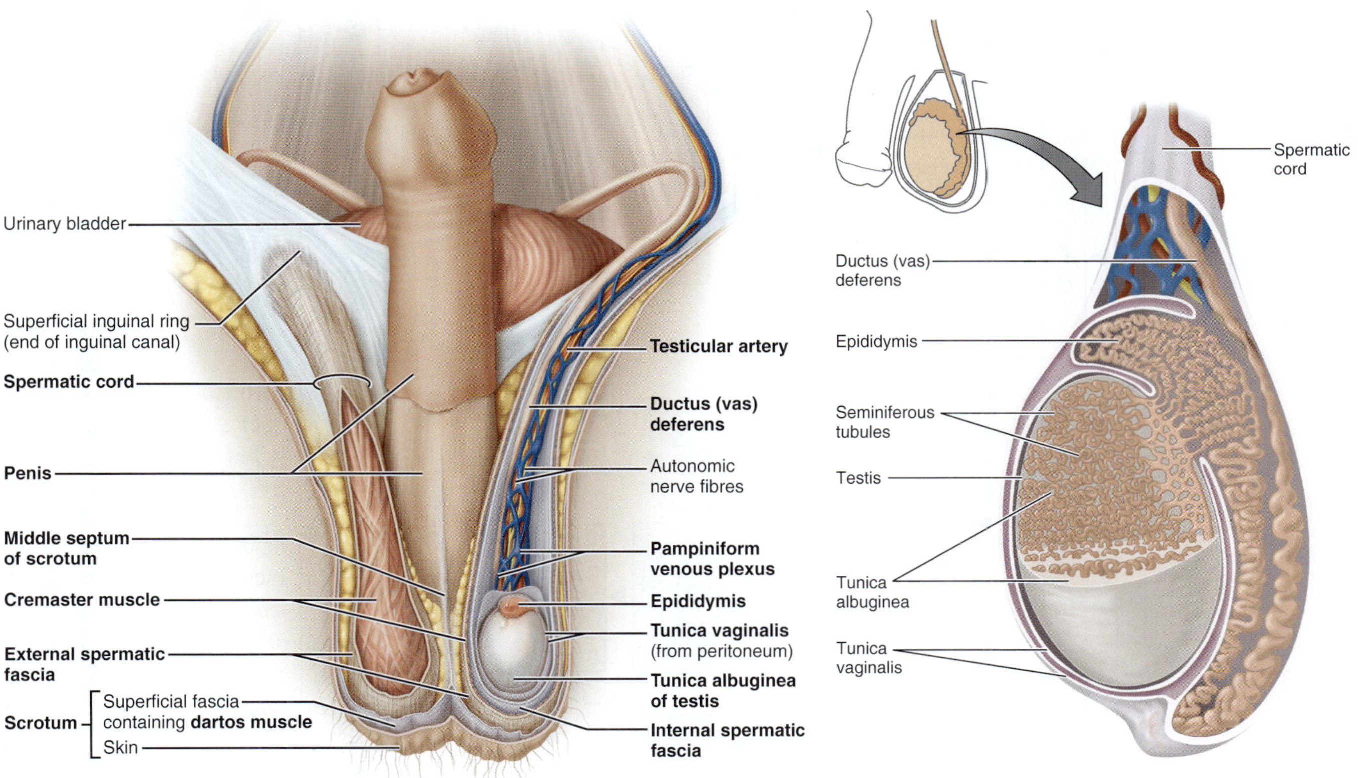

Figure 40.8

Scrotal and testicular structures

Sources: Adapted from (A) Marieb & Hoehn (2019), Figure 27.6; (B) Marieb & Hoehn (2019), Figure 27.7(a).

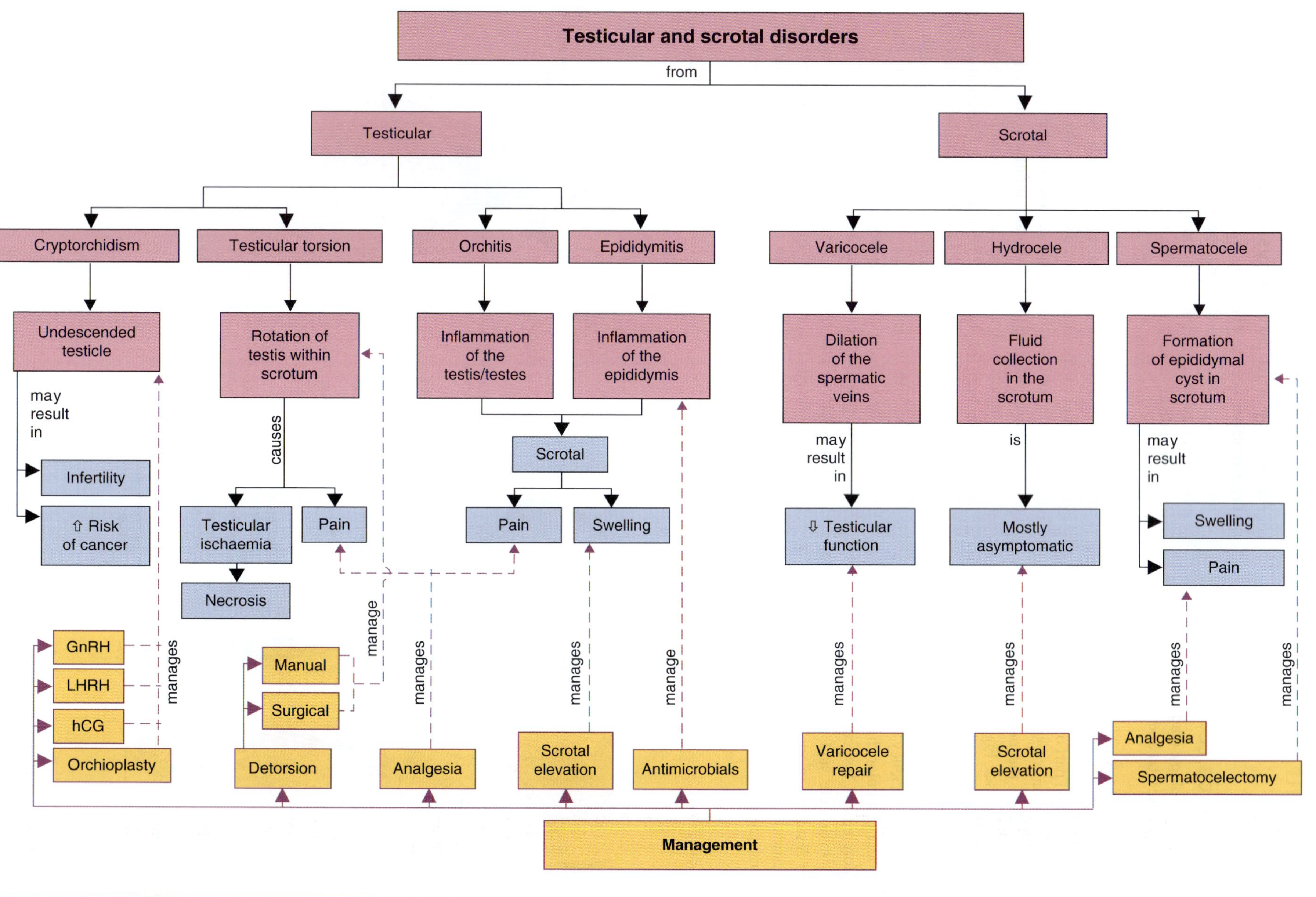

Figure 40.9

Clinical snapshot: Testicular and scrotal disorders

↓ = decreased; ↑ = increased; GnRH = gonadotropin-releasing hormone; hCG = human chorionic gonadotropin; LHRH = luteinising-hormone-releasing hormone.

Clinical diagnosis and management

Diagnosis Early identification of the condition results in the best outcomes. Physical examination is used to confirm that one or both testes has/ve not descended into the scrotum.

Management Surgery (*orchidopexy*) is required to move the undescended testicle down to the base of the scrotum. The surgery should be performed if the cryptorchidism persists after the child is 6 months of age, to minimise the risk of trauma, herniation, impaired self-image, impaired fertility and an increased risk of testicular cancer.

The care will focus on the provision of information regarding pre- and postoperative care, as well as strategies to reduce anxiety and pain before and after surgery. In the case of a young child, parental support and education regarding strategies for care are required.

Treatment with gonadotropin-releasing hormone analogues (also known as luteinising-hormone-releasing hormone [LHRH]) or human chorionic gonadotropin has been used in cases of bilateral cryptorchidism to improve testicular blood flow or increase fertility, but in most settings is currently discouraged.

TESTICULAR TORSION

Aetiology and pathophysiology

Testicular torsion is defined as a *twisting of a testis that compromises blood flow to the affected structure*. If prolonged ischaemia develops, the affected testicle may become necrotic and require surgical removal. The condition is characterised by sudden, acute pain, which can be very intense.

Trauma can lead to testicular torsion, but more commonly there is a *testicular or scrotal abnormality* that predisposes the affected person to testicular rotation. Examples of abnormalities include: the tunica vaginalis forming over the spermatic cord in such a way that it prevents the testicle from attaching to the posterior surface of the scrotum; cryptorchidism; a testicular cancer; or a testicle that tends to lie in a horizontal orientation rather than a vertical one.

Clinical diagnosis and management

Diagnosis A clinical history and a physical examination generally provide the information required for diagnosis of a testicular torsion. An ultrasound examination may be performed to identify testicular blood flow and exclude a tumour.

Management In some cases, urgent surgical management is indicated to relieve the torsion, fix the testis within the scrotum and restore blood flow. The testicular salvage rate is reported to be 90% if treatment occurs less than six hours after symptom onset, but can drop significantly if surgery is delayed. An orchidectomy may be required if the testis is necrotic or has sustained irreparable damage.

The care will focus on assessment, strategies to reduce anxiety, the provision of information regarding pre- and postoperative care, and pain management strategies, including the use of analgesics.

EPIDIDYMITIS AND ORCHITIS

Aetiology and pathophysiology

Epididymitis is an *inflammation of the epididymis*, the connecting tube between the testis and the vas deferens. **Orchitis** is an *inflammation of one or both of the testes*. These conditions are most commonly associated with infection. Both conditions can be caused by bacterial infections; orchitis can also be induced by viral infection. The most common *viral infection* associated with orchitis is mumps, when it occurs in males after puberty. The incidence of the orchitis related to mumps is in decline in Western countries due to mumps immunisation programs.

Bacterial infections leading to epididymitis/orchitis are most commonly observed in young adult men up to their mid-30s. It is usually associated with a bacterial infection of the urinary tract that spreads towards the testes. In this age group, orchitis is generally caused by the STIs **gonorrhoea** and **chlamydia**. In men older than 35 years, orchitis is often caused by translocation of *enteric bacteria*.

Risk factors for the development of these infections include sexual intercourse without the use of condoms, catheterisation and congenital abnormalities of the urogenital tract.

Clinical manifestations

Common manifestations include urethral discharge, dysuria, fever, groin/scrotal pain (which can be severe), testicular swelling, heaviness and tenderness, the presence of blood in the semen, pain during ejaculation and abdominal discomfort.

Clinical diagnosis and management

Diagnosis A clinical history and a physical examination are required, and should include the assessment of the degree of testicular pain, swelling and redness. It is imperative that testicular torsion as the cause of scrotal pain is eliminated Additional investigations may include a full blood count, which may show an elevated white blood cell count and raised ESR. In the case of suspected epididymitis, a swab and/or urine sample may be collected for PCR and culture for STIs. Commonly identified organisms include *Chlamydia trachomatis* and *Neisseria gonorrhoeae*, as well as *E. coli, Haemophilus influenzae* and *Cryptococcus* species in males who have practised unprotected anal intercourse.

Management Once epididymitis or orchitis has been determined, management strategies will include measures to manage pain and the infection, as well as to reduce anxiety. Administration of analgesia is a priority, and, as simple analgesia may not be sufficient to control pain, narcotic analgesia may be required. Ice packs and scrotal support can also assist with pain relief. Antiemetics may be required to manage the nausea and vomiting from the pain or from the emetic effects of narcotics. Antibacterial drugs will be required for the infection.

Information and advice regarding the possible need for long-term antimicrobial treatment, and the need for the sexual partner to be treated if diagnosed with an STI, are important aspects of communication. The possible longer-term effects on fertility should also be discussed. Strategies for the prevention of STIs should be discussed to prevent further recurrence of the infection.

VARICOCELES, HYDROCELES AND SPERMATOCELES

Aetiology and pathophysiology

Varicoceles, hydroceles and spermatoceles can be generally categorised as *fluid-filled masses* that are readily palpated within the scrotum (see Figures 40.9 and 40.10). They represent the most common of the scrotal abnormalities. However, each of these abnormalities has distinctly different anatomical origins and characteristics.

A **varicocele** is defined as a *dilation of the testicular vein*. Most varicoceles are *unilateral*, affecting the left testis. It has been suggested that this is due to the differing venodynamics normally apparent between each testicle. Varicoceles are considered the *main cause of male infertility*, being present in about 40% of infertile men. The accepted explanation for this is that poor venous drainage leads to scrotal overheating and impaired spermatogenesis. Altered sex hormones levels, oxidative stress and hypoxia within the testicular microcirculation triggered by the abnormality have also been proposed as explanations. Varicoceles usually develop in adolescence and are typically asymptomatic, although some males report a dull, throbbing pain brought on by physical exertion associated with this condition that improves when they lie down.

A **hydrocele** develops when *fluid accumulates between the layers of the tunica vaginalis*. This fluid may originate from the peritoneal space if the connection of the tunica vaginalis with the peritoneal membrane does not close properly, or if closure is delayed during infancy. If a hydrocele develops later in life, it is usually due to venous or lymphatic obstruction associated with trauma, infection, testicular torsion or surgery. Most hydroceles are asymptomatic, and are usually discovered by palpation during a physical examination.

Spermatoceles are *epididymal cysts* in the scrotum that are typically asymptomatic, and are usually discovered during a physical examination.

Clinical diagnosis and management

Diagnosis A clinical history and a physical examination (including transillumination of the scrotum) are undertaken. Ultrasound examination may also be performed to facilitate diagnosis.

Management The management of this condition may be conservative (e.g. scrotal support for small hydroceles) or require surgical intervention. Larger hydroceles may require aspiration and sclerosis of the tunica vaginalis to prevent recurrence. Surgical ligation to repair a varicocele, called a varicocelectomy, is indicated when fertility is of concern. Although there are few randomised controlled trials in this area, studies have revealed improvements in semen quality and pregnancy rates, as well as pain resolution in symptomatic cases associated with varicocelectomy.

In the treatment of spermatoceles, the care will focus on developing strategies to reduce anxiety, providing advice regarding scrotal support techniques, pre- and postoperative care information, as well as pain management strategies, including the use of analgesics, cool packs and supports.

SPERM PRODUCTION DISORDERS

LEARNING OBJECTIVE 4

Identify the parameters used to measure male fertility, and outline some common conditions associated with decreased fertility.

Aetiology and pathophysiology

It is estimated that about 1 in 20 men in Australia are infertile, and that for 30% of infertile couples the impairment lies with the male partner. A number of conditions can affect male fertility. An overview is provided here.

The main parameters of sperm concentration, percentage motility and percentage normal morphology within a sample of semen are generally used to discriminate between fertile and subfertile men (see Table 40.2 for reference values).

Infertility can be the result of a *failure in spermatogenesis* within the testes, *impaired sperm transport* along the genitourinary tract, or the *altered contribution to semen formation* from the accessory structures, such as the prostate or seminal vesicles. It is

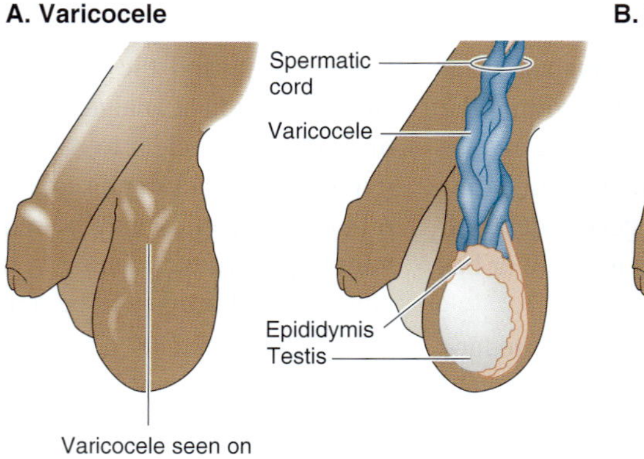

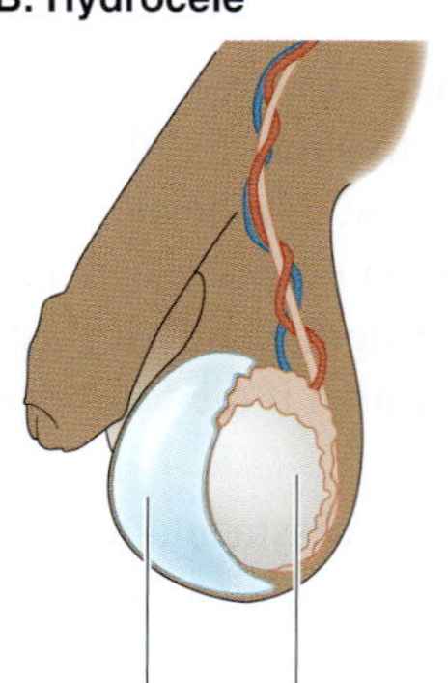

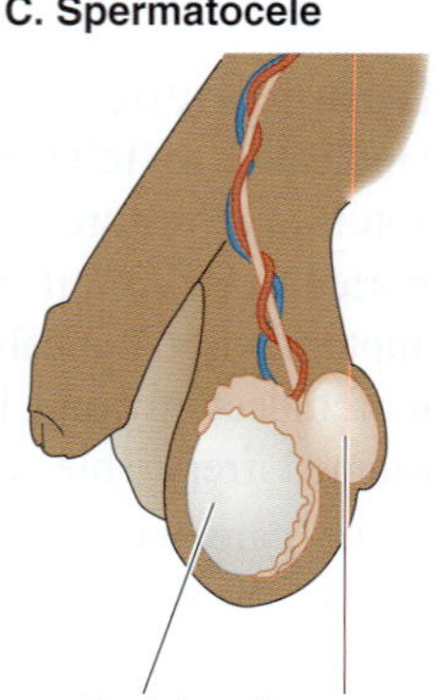

Figure 40.10

Varicoceles, hydroceles and spermatoceles

(A) A varicocele is a dilation of the testicular vein.

(B) A hydrocele develops when fluid accumulates between the layers of the tunica vaginalis.

(C) A spermatocele is an epididymal cyst.

Table 40.2 World Health Organization normal reference values for semen analysis*

Parameter	Normal value
Sperm volume	1.4 mL
Sperm concentration	39 million/mL
Sperm motility	42%
Sperm vitality	54%
Sperm morphology	4%

Other parameters, such as fructose levels and pH, may also be considered acceptable measures of fertility.

Source: World Health Organization (2021).

also possible for antibodies to form against spermatozoa. Under normal circumstances, immune cells are quarantined away from the process of sperm production and transport. If there is a breech in this system, *antisperm antibodies* can be formed. About 10% of infertile men will test positive for antisperm antibodies.

In *genetic disorders* such as Klinefelter's syndrome, polycystic kidney disease and cystic fibrosis, a consistent pattern shows a paucity of viable sperm in the ejaculate. Lower sperm counts, diminished motility and poorer morphology have also been noted in men with *diabetes mellitus*, or who have had an *STI*, are *obese* or who have a *varicocele*. In men with an STI, there is evidence of elevated titres of antisperm antibodies.

Prolonged exposure to *environmental toxins*, such as solvents, metals or pesticides, has also been shown to result in poor measures of sperm concentration, morphology and motility. This exposure may have occurred in an occupational or recreational context—the latter associated with a hobby such as restoring cars, houses or furniture, and painting or pottery.

A number of *medicines* can affect fertility, including calcium channel blockers, corticosteroids, antibacterials such as erythromycin or tetracycline, phenytoin and finasteride. *Recreational drugs*, such as tobacco, marijuana, cocaine and anabolic steroids, have all been shown to decrease sperm counts and alter sperm morphology.

Clinical diagnosis and management

Diagnosis A health history (including medications both prescribed and illicit, trauma, medical and surgical health problems) and a physical examination are undertaken. Diagnostic testing begins with semen analysis and an immunobead antibody test. Further testing will depend on the semen analysis results, but may include a repeat semen analysis, blood tests (levels of testosterone, LH, FSH), as well as genetic testing (including karyotype and Y deletion testing; see Clinical Box 40.1), urine testing for retrograde ejaculation and testicular biopsy.

Management Management will depend on the clinical diagnosis, and may include a change to or cessation of the causative medication to facilitate improvement in semen parameters, hormone replacement therapy and surgical treatment of varicocele.

Assisted reproductive technology (ART) treatments—including intrauterine insemination (IUI) or in-vitro fertilisation (IVF) with or without intracytoplasmic sperm injection (ICSI)—may be utilised for male factor fertility issues (see Clinical Box 40.1).

In some cases, sperm may also be recoverable directly from the testes through either fine-needle aspiration or open biopsy. In some genetic conditions, donor sperm treatment may be required to give the couple any chance of pregnancy. Infections are treated with appropriate antimicrobial therapy.

Management approaches will include both the male and his partner, discussions about treatment options, assessment of the health history, with a focus on lifestyle issues that may affect fertility (e.g. diet, exercise, body weight, smoking and caffeine, alcohol and other drug use), and the provision of information and advice regarding the planned treatments. If ART treatment is required, treatment-specific information and education as well as emotional support are key components for both the male and his partner.

TESTICULAR CANCER

Aetiology and pathophysiology

Germ cell testicular cancers account for over 90% of **testicular cancer**, with *stromal–spermatic cord tumours* accounting for the rest.

Clinical manifestations

Common symptoms include the presence of a testicular mass with accompanying testicular firmness and scrotal heaviness. Some men report testicular pain. Gynaecomastia (breast development) may occur in response to the secretion of β-hCG by the testicular tumour cells. Spread of the cancer may be identified by enlargement of the inguinal lymph nodes and by back pain, as well as abdominal or chest pain.

Epidemiology

The age-standardised incidence rate of testicular cancer in Australia in 2022 was estimated at 7.8 cases per 100,000 males. However, it is a leading cause of cancer among young males between 15 and 35 years of age (with a highest incidence at 30–34 years old).

Indeed, there is evidence that the annual incidence rate is increasing, with it nearly doubling over the past 40 years. Risk factors for testicular cancer include cryptorchidism, a family history of testicular cancer, previous testicular cancer, cigarette smoking, Caucasian genetics and infertility.

Clinical diagnosis and management

Diagnosis Diagnosis of testicular cancer involves a clinical history, a physical examination and ultrasound of the testes. Other tests may include blood tests for biochemical tumour markers, such as β-hCG, α-fetoprotein (AFP) and lactate dehydrogenase (LDH)—elevated levels provide strong support for a diagnosis of testicular cancer. Chest X-ray and CT scan can be used to exclude or confirm the spread of the cancer. Biopsy of the tumour is rarely performed, and diagnosis is confirmed after histological examination following orchidectomy.

Management Orchidectomy is the standard treatment of this condition. Chemotherapy and, in some cases, radiotherapy are used after surgery. Chemotherapy will vary, but the most common treatment regimens may include three or four cycles of combination therapy (cisplatin, bleomycin and etoposide or etoposide and cisplatin). Follow-up assessments should be undertaken for at least 10 years.

Management will incorporate those aspects discussed earlier in relation to orchidectomy. In addition, early discussions need to include fertility preservation strategies (freezing sperm prior to surgery or chemotherapy) and the provision of emotional support to help cope with possible concerns about future sexual function, fertility and body image. The male's partner, or in the case of younger males, families, also need to be involved. It is also imperative that the need for ongoing follow-up is reinforced.

Sexually transmitted infections

LEARNING OBJECTIVE 5

Describe the pathophysiology, diagnosis and clinical management of common sexually transmitted infections.

AETIOLOGY AND PATHOPHYSIOLOGY

The *sexually transmitted infections (STIs)* that are the focus of this section are chlamydia, gonorrhoea, syphilis, genital herpes and genital warts. HIV/AIDS and the various forms of hepatitis that can be sexually transmitted have been discussed in the chapters 'Immune disorders' and 'Female reproductive disorders'. Causative infectious organisms associated with STIs are *bacteria, viruses* or *parasites* (see Table 40.3).

STIs can be acquired through vaginal, anal and/or oral sex with someone who has become infected. STIs occur in men who engage in heterosexual sex and among men who have sex with men. The STIs damage the local tissues and structures around the portal of entry, and induce inflammation. STIs are associated with prostatitis, urethritis, epididymitis, orchitis and semen infection. Semen infection can transfer the infection to sexual partners, cause complications in pregnancy and induce fetal/neonate infection. If left untreated, the infections induce chronic inflammatory states that can decrease fertility, and can spread to cause significant systemic lesions in major organs. Early treatment of these infections is therefore the most effective management, although this is problematic because the infection, especially in its early stages, may be asymptomatic.

In 2017, the incidence of bacterial STIs in Australia was reported as 84,436 new cases. This included a chlamydial infection rate of approximately 395 per 100,000 people, and a gonorrhoeal rate of approximately 174 per 100,000 people. In New Zealand, the incidence reported was nearly 6000 cases. Adolescents, young adults and men who have sex with men show the highest rates of infection, and are the focus of major health education programs.

Usually, the infective organism is not definitively identified. Chlamydia, gonorrhoea or co-infection with both of these organisms is usually suspected. Genital ulcers can also be a presenting complaint in STIs, and usually indicate infection with either genital herpes or syphilis.

Gonorrhoea and chlamydia can also be spread through anal sex. Rectal pain and a discharge may develop, but the infection can be asymptomatic. Gonorrhoea transmitted by oral sex can cause a mild throat infection or remain asymptomatic. Men who are infected this way can pass on the STI via unprotected sex with a partner.

There are three stages of syphilitic infection (described in the 'Clinical manifestations' section below). The pathological organism responsible for **syphilis** targets the endothelium from the earliest stages of infection. Initially, it triggers an inflammatory response, and smaller arteries and arterioles are damaged. Chronic inflammation of vascular tissue ensues, resulting in fibrosis and sclerosis.

Genital herpes is caused by the *herpes simplex virus (HSV) type 2*, which is generally associated with genital, anal or perianal infection. HSV type 1 is more commonly related to cold sores on the lips and mouth. However, during oral sex HSV type 2 can cause oral lesions. Once inside the body, herpes viruses tend to travel up nerve fibres, and can remain dormant within nerve cells until reactivated. A recurrent episode can be triggered by stress or during a period of immunosuppression.

Genital warts, also known as *condylomata acuminata*, are caused by a type of *human papillomavirus (HPV)*. In effect, they are benign epithelial neoplasms. The warts are readily spread by sexual contact, and have the highest rate of incidence in adolescents and young adults. Genital warts tend to have a long incubation period, usually about four months, but can develop anywhere between a month up to a year after infection.

Table 40.3 Common causative organisms in sexually transmitted infections

Infection	Causative organism
Chlamydia	*Chlamydia trachomatis*
Genital herpes	Herpes simplex virus (HSV types 1 and 2)
Genital warts	Human papillomavirus (HPV)
Gonorrhoea	*Neisseria gonorrhoea*
Syphilis	*Treponema pallidum*
Urethritis	*Chlamydia trachomatis* *Mycoplasma genitalium* *Neisseria gonorrhoea* *Trichomonas vaginalis* (parasite)

CLINICAL MANIFESTATIONS

A man with an STI who is experiencing symptoms usually presents to his doctor with a patchy urethral inflammation (urethritis), as the tract epithelium is damaged. However, for some men the STI may remain asymptomatic. Urethritis is characterised by a mucopurulent discharge from the penis, dysuria and urethral itchiness or tingling. In chlamydial and gonorrhoeal infections, the organism may move beyond the urethra and cause injury and inflammation of the epididymis, testes or prostate (epididymitis, orchitis or prostatitis). The clinical manifestations of these conditions are covered elsewhere in this chapter.

The first stage of *syphilis* infection manifests as an ulcer, referred to as a *chancre*. It is usually painless and can develop on the penis, or following anal sex may be hidden in the rectum. It can develop between one to 12 weeks after infection, and usually heals within four weeks. In the second stage of infection, the infection becomes systemic. A skin rash develops, which may occur on the soles of the feet or the palms of the hands or cover the entire body, and is contagious to other people. Other accompanying manifestations include swollen lymph nodes, alopecia, genital lumps and flu-like symptoms. In the third stage of syphilitic infection, the infection can severely damage the brain and heart.

Initially, symptomatic *genital herpes* infection results in irritation and the appearance of blisters in the genital area after an incubation period of three to seven days. The blisters will rupture and leave shallow ulcers. The blistered area may or may not be painful; however, once the ulcers form, the affected region is quite painful. Some people will also experience the flu-like symptoms of fever and painful joints during this primary episode. Lymph nodes in the affected region may become swollen and tender. The initial lesions heal within three weeks, but the virus remains in the body and can be spread during sexual contact. The degree of blistering can vary greatly from person to person. For some people, the initial infection can be asymptomatic.

In men, *genital warts* tend to occur on the penis, but they can also form perianally. The appearance of the warts can vary in size (quite small to large) and in distribution (singularly or clumped together). They are generally painless, unsightly growths, but in some instances may be itchy.

CLINICAL DIAGNOSIS AND MANAGEMENT

Diagnosis

Following assessment of the clinical history and a physical examination, tests will be undertaken to facilitate diagnosis of the STI. These tests will include urinary PCR (see Clinical Box 40.1) for chlamydia, gonorrhoea, herpes and *Mycoplasma*, and blood tests for syphilis serology, hepatitis B and C, and HIV.

Management

Treatment is based on the causative organism, and may include oral, topical and injectable medications. Appropriate antimicrobial therapy will generally provide effective resolution of bacterial STIs. Antiviral agents (e.g. aciclovir) will reduce the severity and degree of symptoms of genital herpes infection, but will not provide a permanent cure. Genital warts may be surgically excised or treated with cryotherapy, laser ablation or electrocautery.

The plan of care will vary depending on the diagnosis. The main foci will include health and physical assessment, using a non-judgmental approach and ensuring privacy and confidentiality. Care strategies may include the provision of information and advice regarding treatment options (including actions, risks, complications of treatment or failure to treat), the need to complete the full course of medications, the need for sexual partner/s to be assessed and treated, and the provision of pre- and postoperative information if surgical treatment is required. It is also imperative that strategies for the prevention of STIs using barrier protection (including male/female condoms and dental dams) are discussed and emphasised.

INDIGENOUS HEALTH FAST FACTS AND CULTURAL CONSIDERATIONS

FAST FACTS

- *Aboriginal and Torres Strait Islander men have slightly less risk than non-Indigenous Australian men of developing prostate cancer (0.7 times).*
- *In 2021, mortality from malignant neoplasm of the prostate was 1.2 times higher in Aboriginal and Torres Strait Islander men when compared to non-Indigenous Australian men.*
- *Māori men have a lower risk of being diagnosed with prostate cancer compared to non-Māori men (0.8 times), but have a higher risk of dying from this form of cancer (1.5 times).*

Note: Lower rates of prostate cancer in Aboriginal, Torres Strait Islander, Māori and Pacific Islands men may be related to the under-recording of cancer incidence, and also to lower life expectancy, rather than an actual lower relative risk, and therefore these extraneous variables may be causing the data to skew.

CULTURAL CONSIDERATIONS

- *Aboriginal and Torres Strait Islander men are reticent to talk about health matters; furthermore, seeking assistance or counsel about sexual and reproductive health matters can be terribly challenging. Cultural understanding regarding the importance of 'men's business' should be considered when organising healthcare workers to assist an Indigenous Australian with gender-specific health matters. The culture of men supporting men is strong in Aboriginal and Torres Strait Islander communities, and the uncle–nephew relationship, which draws on the obligations of a related older male, may even at times be stronger than a father–son relationship. Understanding and utilising this bond may become a very powerful tool in ensuring culturally appropriate support and guidance of Aboriginal and Torres Strait Islander men affected by sexual and reproductive health conditions. Finally, cancer awareness in communities may best be serviced by educational resources through 'mates programs' and engagement with Elders and leaders in the community. Better knowledge, understanding and interaction with healthcare services and primary health programs could certainly assist in closing the healthcare gap in Australia.*

Sources: Data from Australian Bureau of Statistics (2022); Australian Indigenous HealthInfoNet (2020); Australian Institute of Health and Welfare (2018); Egan et al. (2020).

CHILDREN AND ADOLESCENTS

- A prepubescent boy's prostate weighs approximately 1.4 g. A 21-year-old male's prostate weighs approximately 18 g.
- At puberty, a boy's prostate increases to almost eight times the size of his prepubescent prostate.

OLDER ADULTS

- Lower testosterone levels occur in senescence, and contribute to a decreased libido and an increased risk of depression and osteoporosis.
- In an older man (over 70 years of age), the prostate increases to approximately double the size of the prostate in a 21-year-old male.
- Muscular tone decreases as a man ages, resulting in erections that are less firm and take longer to develop.

KEY CLINICAL ISSUES

- Many males, especially Indigenous men, are unwilling to discuss sexual or reproductive health concerns. This becomes even more difficult for many men when the healthcare professional is a woman. In the context of understanding cultural differences, a more reliable sexual or reproductive health history may best be collected by a male healthcare professional in some circumstances.
- The size of a man's prostate increases with age, and can begin to influence urinary stream. It is important to ensure that the man understands that issues influencing urinary function may not necessarily be cancer.
- A shift in clinical management for prostate issues may increase the number of men undergoing less aggressive treatment, having more frequent prostate specific antigen testing, and undergoing 'watchful waiting'.
- Congenital disorders affecting the location of a boy's urethral meatus may require surgical intervention to repair the defect.
- Erectile dysfunction can occur because of neurological, vascular, endocrine or psychological reasons, but can commonly be a complex combination of a few of these issues. Myriad treatment options are available to assist in regaining confidence and function.
- Some urological issues can be considered an emergency. Priapism and testicular torsion can be time-critical conditions that require rapid assessment and management to preserve function.
- Issues related to sperm production may be related to various causes, including diet, underwear, overall health, genetics or congenital issues. Options to assist subfertile or infertile men are increasing as medical research and technology grows. Management plans will vary depending on the cause, and may require assistive reproductive technologies.
- Sexually transmitted infections (STIs) are common in Australia and New Zealand. Education programs to reduce the transmission of STIs should include the use of condoms and dental dams, personal hygiene practices, and urogenital assessments to identify infection and commence treatment.

CHAPTER REVIEW

- *Benign prostatic hyperplasia (BPH)*, a common chronic disorder in men, is characterised by *nodular prostatic tissue remodelling*. The remodelling takes the form of hyperplasia and, especially during the advanced phase, hypertrophy. These changes are dependent on androgen levels. The enlarged gland eventually constricts the proximal urethra, *disrupting the flow of urine* from the bladder. This manifests clinically as reduced urine flow, painful urination, urinary retention, urgency and urine reflux.
- *Prostatitis* is an *inflammation of the prostate*, frequently associated with infection by a uropathogen. It may be accompanied by lower urinary tract symptoms, such as pelvic pain, dysuria, frequency and urgency, as well as sexual dysfunction, or it may be asymptomatic. It can occur in adult men of any age. It is classified according to whether it is *acute or chronic*, the *presence of a uropathogen* and *symptomology*.
- *Cancer of the prostate* is highly prevalent in our community. Generally, it tends to manifest in older men over 74 years of age. The aetiology of prostate cancer is *multifactorial*, and includes genetic predisposition, ethnicity, sex hormone status and dietary status. Most cases of prostate cancer are *adenocarcinomas*.
- *Hypospadias and epispadias* are congenital disorders affecting the *positioning of the urethral meatus*, the male urethral opening. In hypospadias, the urethral meatus is located on the ventral undersurface of the penis. In epispadias, the meatus is found on the dorsal surface. Epispadias is less common than hypospadias.
- *Urethral strictures* result from *urethral fibrosis* that narrows the urethra. The *narrowing of the urethra* affects urine flow, causing a decreased urinary stream, urinary retention and bladder infection.
- *Erectile dysfunction (ED)* occurs when a man shows an *inability to initiate and maintain penile erection sufficient to permit sexual intercourse*. Disorders in psychological, neurological, hormonal or vascular function, or a combination of these, have been linked to the development of ED. Moreover, the recreational or therapeutic use of certain drugs that affect any of these functions can also cause ED.
- *Priapism* is *persistent penile erection in the absence of sexual stimulation or interest*. Priapism can be classified as ischaemic (low-flow), non-ischaemic (high-flow) or intermittent.
- *Phimosis* is a condition characterised by a *non-retractable prepuce (foreskin)*. A *paraphimosis* develops when the foreskin remains retracted for a prolonged period. In this condition, the distal regions of the glans penis and the foreskin may become swollen, painful and oedematous.
- *Penile cancer* is a relatively rare cancer that tends to occur predominantly in older men aged 60–70 years. Uncircumcised men, especially those with phimosis, are at particular risk of developing penile cancer. Poor penile hygiene, penile rashes and tears, urethral strictures, inflammatory conditions, cigarette smoking, the number of sexual partners and a history of sexually transmitted infections (especially infection with human papillomavirus) have been identified as risk factors for this condition.

- *Cryptorchidism* occurs when one or both of the *testes fail to descend into the scrotum* along the inguinal canal from the abdominal cavity as a part of normal development, or the *testis retracts* from the scrotum later in childhood. The causes of cryptorchidism are multiple, and are not completely understood. Hormonal, environmental and genetic factors have been implicated. Complications of cryptorchidism include infertility and testicular cancer.
- Varicoceles, hydroceles and spermatoceles can be generally categorised as *fluid-filled masses* that are readily palpated within the scrotum. A *varicocele* is defined as a *dilation of the testicular vein*. Varicoceles are considered the main cause of male infertility, being present in about 40% of infertile men. A *hydrocele* develops when *fluid accumulates between the layers of the tunica vaginalis. Spermatoceles* are *epididymal cysts* that are typically asymptomatic, and are usually discovered during a physical examination.
- *Testicular torsion* is defined as a *twisting of a testis that compromises the blood flow to the affected structure*. If prolonged, ischaemia develops, and the affected testicle may become necrotic and require surgical removal.
- *Infertility* can be the result of a *failure in spermatogenesis* within the testes, *impaired sperm transport* along the genitourinary tract or *altered contribution to semen formation* from the accessory structures, such as the prostate or seminal vesicles. It is also possible for *antibodies* to form against spermatozoa. Genetic disorders, obesity, varicoceles, sexually transmitted infections (STIs), exposure to environmental toxins and drug use have been identified as risk factors for infertility.
- *Testicular cancer* is a relatively rare form of cancer, but is a leading cause of cancer among young males aged between 15 and 35 years. Risk factors for testicular cancer include cryptorchidism, a family history of testicular cancer, previous testicular cancer, cigarette smoking, Caucasian genetics and infertility.
- *STIs* can be acquired through vaginal, anal and/or oral sex with someone who has become infected. STIs occur in men who engage in heterosexual sex and among men who have sex with men. The STIs damage the local tissues and structures around the portal of entry, and induce *inflammation*. If left untreated, the infections induce *chronic inflammatory states* and can spread to cause significant *systemic lesions* in major organs. Common STIs affecting men include gonorrhoea, chlamydia, genital warts, genital herpes and syphilis.
- A man with an STI who is experiencing symptoms usually presents to their doctor with a patchy urethral inflammation (*urethritis*) as the tract epithelium is damaged. However, for some men, the STI may remain asymptomatic. Urethritis is characterised by a mucopurulent discharge from the penis, dysuria and urethral itchiness or tingling.

REVIEW QUESTIONS

1. Compare and contrast the pathophysiologies associated with benign prostatic hyperplasia and prostate cancer.
2. a Define category III prostatitis.
   b Why is this form considered very debilitating?
3. Differentiate between hypospadias and epispadias.
4. Briefly describe the physiology of penile erection, and indicate where dysfunction can occur, leading to erectile dysfunction.
5. Compare and contrast low- and high-flow priapism.
6. Differentiate between physiological and pathological phimosis.
7. Compare and contrast the characteristics of prostate, penile and testicular cancer in terms of tissue of origin, risk factors and the age group affected.
8. Differentiate between a varicocele, a spermatocele and a hydrocele.
9. Outline how male fertility is measured.
10. For the following sexually transmitted infections, briefly outline the pathogenesis and symptomatology:
    a genital herpes
    b gonorrhoea
    c syphilis

HEALTH PROFESSIONAL CONNECTIONS

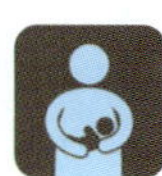

Midwives Urological dysfunction can be discovered during the first full physical assessment of the neonate. The least common occurrences include ambiguous genitalia. Problems associated with the position of the urethral meatus may result in hypospadia or epispadia. Examination of a male neonate's scrotum can indicate cryptorchidism. Urological consultations are necessary on discovery of such disorders, as urinary difficulties, self-perception and body image issues, or future fertility problems, may be reduced by early intervention.

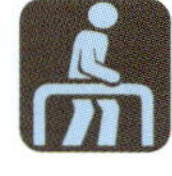

Physiotherapists Physiotherapists can assist males with incontinence and erectile dysfunction through exercise prescription and rehabilitation directed at the pelvic floor and abdominal muscles. Treatment options may also include the use of electromyography and electrical stimulation to improve outcomes. Physiotherapists may also have men with pelvic pain referred to them following the elimination of organic causes. Management plans for pelvic pain may include soft tissue mobilisation, proprioceptive neuromuscular facilitation and lymphatic drainage.

Exercise scientists Testicular torsion and injuries to the scrotum are possible during various sports. Blunt trauma to the scrotum may result in a haemocele (a collection of blood in the scrotum) or a hydrocele, and testicular torsion is a medical emergency as there is a risk of ischaemia to the testicle. Exercise professionals should encourage the use of athletic supports (jock straps) and protective cups (boxes) to prevent possible damage to the reproductive organs.

Nutritionists/Dieticians Although adequate nutrition through eating appropriate portions from the five food groups is important for health in general, men can benefit from ensuring that certain nutrients exist in their diets. Adequate zinc levels are important for reproductive health. Reduced testicular function, impotence and decreased libido have all been associated with low zinc levels. Vitamin C reduces sperm agglutination, improving fertility, and there are some suggestions that vitamin E improves sperm motility. Reducing excessive caffeine and alcohol consumption is important for sperm health. A well-balanced diet will include sufficient quantities of vitamins, minerals and all of the necessary nutrient values. However, if they have gastrointestinal or metabolic anomalies that interfere with the absorption or metabolism of vitamins and minerals, supplementation may be necessary.

CASE STUDY

Mr Joseph Citane (UR number 789872) is a 76-year-old man who is three days postoperation following a transurethral resection of the prostate (TURP) for benign prostate hypertrophy (BPH). His preoperative prostate serum antigen (PSA) level was measured at 9.1 ng/mL and he was experiencing dysuria, nocturia, frequency and occasionally urinary overflow incontinence. Mr Citane had taken prazosin for a few months; however, this was stopped because he experienced hypotension, pre-syncope, headaches and fatigue. As his symptoms increased, surgical management was recommended. His surgery went well, he experienced no immediate postoperative complications and the surgeon was satisfied with the result. This morning, he is for 'trial of void' following removal of his indwelling catheter (IDC) at 0600 hours. He has had some urinary incontinence and is complaining of penile discomfort, for which he has been given paracetamol 1 g at 0800 hours, but has not yet voided since IDC removal. His observations are as follows:

Temperature	Heart rate	Respiration rate	Blood pressure	SpO_2
37.0°C	82	16	158/82	98% (RA*)

*RA = room air.

Mr Citane needs encouragement to increase his oral fluid intake to 2–3 L/day. He has been asked to reduce his caffeine intake, and has been ordered stool softeners. He has intravenous antimicrobials ordered. His postoperative pathology results are as follows:

HAEMATOLOGY

Patient location:	Ward 3	**UR:**	789872		
Consultant:	Smith	**NAME:**	Citane		
		Given name:	Joseph	**Sex:**	M
		DOB:	03/03/XX	**Age:**	76

Time collected	08:34
Date collected	XX/XX
Year	XXXX
Lab #	5345345

FULL BLOOD COUNT		UNITS	REFERENCE RANGE
Haemoglobin	98	g/L	115–160
White cell count	6.3	$\times 10^9$/L	4.0–11.0
Platelets	160	$\times 10^9$/L	140–400
Haematocrit	0.31		0.33–0.47
Red cell count	3.79	$\times 10^{12}$/L	3.80–5.20
Reticulocyte count	2.6	%	0.2–2.0
MCV	88	fL	80–100
Neutrophils	3.61	$\times 10^9$/L	2.00–8.00
Lymphocytes	2.10	$\times 10^9$/L	1.00–4.00
Monocytes	0.52	$\times 10^9$/L	0.10–1.00
Eosinophils	0.43	$\times 10^9$/L	< 0.60
Basophils	0.08	$\times 10^9$/L	< 0.20
ESR	11	mm/h	< 12

BIOCHEMISTRY

Patient location:	Ward 3	**UR:**	789872		
Consultant:	Smith	**NAME:**	Citane		
		Given name:	Joseph	**Sex:**	M
		DOB:	03/03/XX	**Age:**	76

Time collected	08:34
Date collected	XX/XX
Year	XXXX
Lab #	34543234

ELECTROLYTES		UNITS	REFERENCE RANGE
Sodium	142	mmol/L	135–145
Potassium	4.4	mmol/L	3.5–5.2
Chloride	105	mmol/L	95–110
Bicarbonate	25	mmol/L	22–32
Glucose (random)	7.3	mmol/L	3.5–7.7
Iron	9	μmol/L	11–30

CRITICAL THINKING

1. What signs, symptoms and assessments were identified for Mr Citane that suggest possible BPH? Explain each of these in relation to their meaning and the mechanism resulting in their development. This may be best achieved using a table.
2. Preoperatively, Mr Citane experienced overflow incontinence. What is this, and why did it occur?
3. Initial medical management for Mr Citane included prazosin; however, he experienced some adverse reactions. What kind of drug is prazosin, and how does it work in the context of BPH? What adverse reactions did Mr Citane experience? Why?
4. Part of Mr Citane's postoperative management included an indwelling catheter, bladder irrigation, increased fluid intake and stool softeners. Why are these things necessary? Explain the rationale for each of these interventions.
5. Are any of Mr Citane's pathology results outside normal parameters? If so, what is the significance of these results? What further observations should be undertaken to inform the assessment? (*Hint:* Think of common postoperative complications.)
6. You overhear Mr Citane tell a family member that now that he has had his prostate removed, he doesn't have to worry about prostate cancer. What procedure did Mr Citane have? What response would be appropriate in this situation?

BIBLIOGRAPHY

Australian Bureau of Statistics (2022). Table 12.2: Underlying causes of death, leading causes by Aboriginal and Torres Strait Islander origin, Males, NSW, QLD, SA, WA and NT, 2021. *3303.0 Causes of death, Australia, 2021*. https://www.abs.gov.au/statistics/health/causes-death/causes-death-australia/latest-release#leading-causes-of-death-in-aboriginal-and-torres-strait-islander-people.

Australian Indigenous Health*Info*Net (2017). *Overview of Aboriginal and Torres Strait Islander health status, 2016.* Perth, WA: Australian Indigenous Health*Info*Net. http://www.healthinfonet.ecu.edu.au.

Australian Indigenous Health*Info*Net (2020). *Summary of cancer among Aboriginal and Torres Strait Islander people.* Perth, WA: Australian Indigenous Health*Info*Net. https://healthinfonet.ecu.edu.au/cancer.

Australian Indigenous Health*Info*Net (2022). *Overview of Aboriginal and Torres Strait Islander health status, 2021.* Perth, WA: Australian Indigenous Health*Info*Net. http://www.healthinfonet.ecu.edu.au.

Australian Institute of Health and Welfare (AIHW) (2018). *Cancer in Aboriginal and Torres Strait Islander peoples of Australia.* Cat. No. CAN 109. Canberra: AIHW. https://www.aihw.gov.au/reports/cancer/cancer-in-indigenous-australians/contents/about.

Australian Institute of Health and Welfare (AIHW) (2019). *The health of Australia's males.* Canberra: AIHW. https://www.aihw.gov.au/reports/men-women/male-health/contents/how-healthy/sexual-health.

Bauldoff, G., Gubrud-Howe, P.M., Carno, M.-A., Levett-Jones, T., Hales, M., Berry, K., … Stanley, D. (2020). *LeMone and Burke's medical–surgical nursing: critical thinking for person-centred care* (4th [Australian] edn). Sydney: Pearson Australia.

Best, O. & Fredericks, B. (2021). *Yatdjuligin: Aboriginal and Torres Strait Islander nursing and midwifery care* (3rd edn). Port Melbourne, VIC: Cambridge University Press.

Boitrelle, F., Shah, R., Saleh, R., Henkel, R., Kandil, H., Chung, E., … Agarwal, A. (2021). The sixth edition of the *WHO Manual for Human Semen Analysis*: a critical review and SWOT analysis. *Life* 11(12):1368. https://doi.org/10.3390/life11121368.

Brosman, S.A. (2020). Prostate-specific antigen testing. *Emedicine*. https://emedicine.medscape.com/article/457394-overview.

Bullock, S. & Manias, E. (2022). *Fundamentals of pharmacology* (9th edn). Sydney: Pearson Australia.

Cancer Australia (2022). *Prostate cancer in Australia statistics*. Sydney: Cancer Australia. https://www.canceraustralia.gov.au/cancer-types/prostate-cancer/statistics.

Cancer Australia (2022). *Testicular cancer in Australia statistics*. Sydney: Cancer Australia. https://www.canceraustralia.gov.au/cancer-types/testicular-cancer/statistics.

Deem, S.G., Rhee, J.R. & Costabile, R.A. (2022). Acute bacterial prostatitis. *Emedicine.* https://emedicine.medscape.com/article/2002872-overview.

Egan, R., Kidd, J., Lawrenson, R., Cassim, S., Black, S., Blundell, R., … Broughton, J. (2020). Inequalities between Māori and non-Māori men with prostate cancer in Aotearoa New Zealand. *New Zealand Medical Journal* 133(1521):69–76. https://journal.nzma.org.nz/journal-articles/inequalities-between-maori-and-non-maori-men-with-prostate-cancer-in-aotearoa-new-zealand.

Fu, L., Tian, T., Yao, K., Chen, X.-F., Luo, G., Gao, Y., … Zou, H. (2022). Global pattern and trends in penile cancer incidence: population-based study. *JMIR Public Health Surveillance* 8(7):e34874. https://doi.org/10.2196/34874.

Marieb, E.N. & Hoehn, K. (2019). *Human anatomy and physiology* (11th edn). San Francisco, CA: Pearson Benjamin Cummings.

McVary, K.T. (2021). Clinical manifestations and diagnostic evaluation of benign prostatic hyperplasia. *UpToDate.* https://www.uptodate.com/contents/clinical-manifestations-and-diagnostic-evaluation-of-benign-prostatic-hyperplasia.

Tracy, C.R., Brooks, N.A. & Said, M. (2023). Prostate cancer. *Emedicine*. https://emedicine.medscape.com/article/1967731-overview.

World Health Organization (WHO) (2021). *WHO laboratory manual for the examination and processing of human semen* (6th edn). Geneva: WHO.

Yafi, F.A., Jenkins, L., Albersen, M., Corona, G., Isidori, A.M., Goldfarb, S., … Hellstrom, W.J.G. (2017). Erectile dysfunction. *Nature Review Disease Primers* 2:16003. www.doi.org/10.1038/nrdp.2016.3.

PART

10

Musculoskeletal pathophysiology

41 Musculoskeletal trauma and muscle disorders

KEY TERMS

Allodynia
Avascular necrosis
Avulsion
Bursitis
Compartment syndrome
Cramps
Delayed onset muscle soreness (DOMS)
Delayed union
Denervation atrophy
Dislocation
Disuse atrophy
Dystrophin
Electromyography
Fasciotomy
Fibromyalgia
Fracture
Idiopathic inflammatory myositis
Infectious myositis
Malunion
Muscular dystrophy
Myalgia
Myalgic encephalomyelitis/ chronic fatigue syndrome (ME/CFS)
Myopathy
Myositis
NO HARM
Non-union
Pyomyositis
Rhabdomyolysis
RICER
Sprain
Strain
Subluxation
Tendinitis

LEARNING OBJECTIVES

After completing this chapter, you should be able to:

1 Describe the important principles of managing selected soft tissue injuries.

2 Differentiate between various fracture types, and explain the mechanism and their management.

3 Describe the common complications of fracture, including compartment syndrome, delayed union and non-union.

4 Examine the complexities of disorders resulting in muscle pain such as fibromyalgia and systemic exertion intolerance disease.

5 Explore various inflammatory myopathies, including idiopathic inflammatory myositis and infectious myositis.

6 Discuss the pathophysiology, clinical manifestations and management of muscular dystrophy.

7 Explore various muscle conditions, including atrophy, contractures, cramps and delayed-onset muscle soreness.

8 Identify the causes and management of rhabdomyolysis.

WHAT YOU SHOULD KNOW BEFORE YOU START THIS CHAPTER

Can you describe the process of bone growth and repair?

Can you identify the major nerves and blood vessels that support the extremities?

Can you outline the major concepts of pain perception?

Can you describe the main stages of inflammation and healing?

Can you describe the important anatomical components of a myocyte, and how they interact to promote movement?

Can you explain how the relationship between the nervous system and muscles contributes to neuromuscular events?

Introduction

Musculoskeletal trauma involves injuries to bones, cartilage, ligaments, tendons, muscles and fascia. These injuries are largely preventable. Although the body is robust and can withstand physical forces several times greater than its own weight, its component parts are still prone to injury. The first part of this chapter explores several different types of soft tissue injury, such as strains, dislocations and avulsions. Various types of factures and their potential complications are also discussed, as well as the various stages of bone healing.

This chapter also includes muscle diseases and disorders not directly related to a neurological cause. **Myopathy** (*muscle disease*) may present in many forms. Idiopathic inflammatory myopathy and infectious myopathy are introduced, and so are the pathophysiology and management of muscular dystrophy. The muscular complications of trauma, disease and illness are examined, including atrophy, contractures, cramp and rhabdomyolysis. Sometimes disorders can be difficult to classify as they affect multiple body systems; fibromyalgia and myalgic encephalomyelitis/chronic fatigue syndrome are good examples. These conditions have been included in this chapter, but they may also just as easily fit in other chapters.

Musculoskeletal trauma

SOFT TISSUE INJURIES

LEARNING OBJECTIVE 1

Describe the important principles of managing selected soft tissue injuries.

Sprains, strains, dislocations and avulsions

Aetiology and pathophysiology Soft tissue injuries include sprains, strains, dislocations, subluxations and avulsions. An understanding of the terminology is important in order to recognise the structures involved, and hence the clinical course and management options possible. Soft tissue injuries can be described by their *type* (e.g. sprain or strain). They can also be described by their *location* (e.g. ankle or knee) and by their *anatomical position* (e.g. medial—towards the midline; or lateral—away from the midline).

A **sprain** is an injury to a *ligament*. A ligament connects bone to bone or bone to cartilage. Ligaments also strengthen a joint. An injury to a ligament may occur as a result of a twisting or stretching action that continues beyond the normal range of movement for that joint. The joints that are most commonly sprained are the ankle, knee and wrist. Sprains can be graded as described in Table 41.1.

A **strain** is a stretching or tearing injury to a *muscle* or *tendon*. A tendon connects muscle to bone. Tendons facilitate movement by transmitting the force of a muscle contraction. An injury to a tendon or muscle generally occurs as a result of an action that continues beyond the normal range of movement for that joint. The joints that are most commonly strained are the ankle, knee and wrist. Strains can be graded as described in Table 41.2.

Approximately 4.1 million people seek assistance from their general practitioner for musculoskeletal injuries in Australia each

Table 41.1 Grading of sprains

Grading	Injury extent
1st degree	Overstretch or slight ligamentous tear Some oedema and pain on stretch No joint instability
2nd degree	Partial tear of ligament Oedema and pain
3rd degree	Complete rupture of the ligament Significant swelling and loss of function May be associated with joint dislocation and nerve or vascular compromise

Table 41.2 Grading of strains

Muscle injury		Tendon injury	
Grading	Injury extent	Grading	Injury extent
1st degree	Overstretch or slight muscle tear Some pain on stretch	Primary	Some inflammation—tendinitis
2nd degree	Partial tear Oedema and pain	Secondary	Partial tear Pain and oedema Some weakness
3rd degree	Complete tear of the muscle Significant swelling and loss of function	Tertiary	Complete tendon rupture Significant swelling and loss of function

year, of which approximately 1.6 million injuries were from sprains and strains. Over 10% of all soft tissue injuries in Australia occur when playing sport. Sprains and strains are two of the most frequent sports injuries experienced. Males are admitted to hospital significantly more frequently than females. Most sprains and strains are not serious. Some people may present to the emergency department, some to their GP, and many may not even seek medical assistance at all, as most of these injuries are self-limiting and can be easily managed at home. Therefore, when analysing hospital data representing all admissions for musculoskeletal injuries where the percentage for sprains, strains and dislocations is very small, it is important to consider that many injuries will not even be recorded (see Figure 41.1). In New Zealand, emergency department presentations for ankle injuries represent up to 10% of all injuries treated. Anecdotal evidence suggests that up to 20% of athletes have had a sprained ankle at some stage.

A **dislocation**, or *luxation*, is the displacement of one or more ends of articulating bones. A dislocation can occur when extreme forces damage a ligament, resulting in separation of the two bones. Extensive damage can occur to ligaments, blood vessels and nerves in the event of a dislocation. As a result of joint malposition, nerves and vessels can become trapped between two hard structures, resulting in compression damage. Any joint is at risk of dislocation; however, some joints are at more risk than others by the nature of their structure. The greater the range of motion a joint is able to provide, the less stable it is. The shoulder joint—which is a ball-and-socket joint that enables an extreme range of motion—is one of the most commonly dislocated joints. Other commonly dislocated joints are the fingers, ankles, knees and elbows.

A **subluxation** is the partial dislocation of one or more ends of articulating bones. In a subluxation, the ligaments anchoring the two bones may experience less damage than in a dislocation. Blood vessel and nerve entrapment is possible, but less likely. Sometimes, rotation may occur within the subluxation. As a result the bone is not only partially dislocated but is rotated as well. The joints that are the most likely to dislocate are also the most likely to experience subluxation.

An **avulsion** is the forcible detachment of a tendon, ligament, muscle or bone from its point of attachment. Technically, a third-degree sprain or strain (complete rupture) can be considered an avulsion. Bone can also be forcibly fractured off other bone, too. This is called an *avulsion fracture*, and is discussed further in the fracture section of this chapter.

A *tendon avulsion* occurs when the fibrous tissue that connects the muscle to the bone is overwhelmed by the force of the attachment. Tendons are very strong, and in some locations may withstand forces greater than five times the body weight of the person; however, certain factors can increase the risk of tendon avulsion (*rupture*). These factors include advancing age, a history of corticosteroid injections into the tendon, or some chronic diseases such as connective tissue disorders, including sarcoidosis, systemic lupus erythematosus, rheumatoid arthritis and gout. People with hyperparathyroidism also appear to have an increased risk of tendon rupture. Interestingly, people with type O blood are also over-represented in tendon rupture statistics. It is thought that this may be due to the reduced volume of *N*-acetylgalactosamine found in type O blood compared to other blood groups. *N*-acetylgalactosamine is an important component of connective tissue. Eccentric loading (when extra load is applied to an already contracting muscle) can also increase the risk of tendon rupture. Although complete tendon avulsion is uncommon, the four most frequent tendons ruptured are the quadriceps and Achilles tendons in the leg, the rotator cuff tendon in the shoulder, and the biceps tendon in the upper arm.

A *ligament avulsion* occurs when the connective tissue that attaches bone to bone is overwhelmed by the force on the attachment. Ligaments are non-contractile, collagenous tissue. Some ligaments are more elastic than others. The characteristic of the trauma appears to directly influence the location at which

Figure 41.1

Sprains, strains and dislocations as a percentage of all public hospital admissions for musculoskeletal injuries, per body region in Australia, 2020–21

The percentage is a portion of all of the admissions for sprains, strains and dislocations of that particular body part. The whole number is the total number of admissions recorded for musculoskeletal injuries of that body part.

Sources: Developed using data from Australian Institute of Health and Welfare (2022). Image modified from © Ralf Juergen Kraft/Shutterstock.

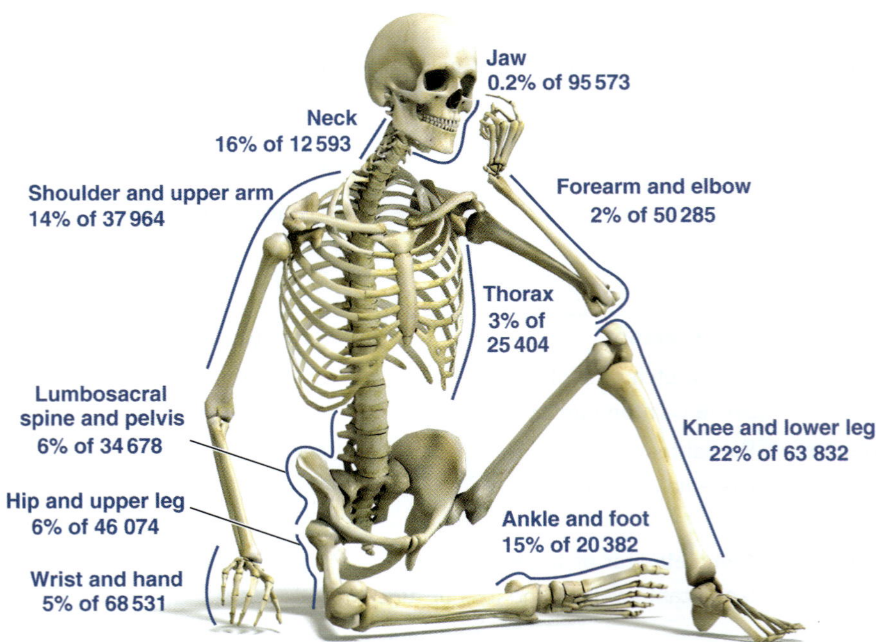

a ligament will fail. In third-degree strains, moderate force will generally cause failure at the ligament's insertion, causing it to avulse from the bone (often resulting in a fracture avulsion), whereas excessive force will generally cause failure within the ligament itself. Ligament strength is dependent on the quantity of the collagen fibres within its structure. States that reduce the strength of a ligament include advancing age, and chronic conditions such as osteoarthritis and fibromyalgia. Any condition influencing connective tissue health may also affect the quality and strength of a ligament. Pregnancy hormones are also known to influence ligament function and cause significant joint laxity. The most common ligaments injured are the cruciate ligaments in the knee, the lateral ankle ligaments, the acromioclavicular ligament of the shoulder, and various ligaments of the fingers and thumb.

Chronic or overuse injury to soft tissue, although less dramatic, can also be painful and interfere with activities of daily living. Bursitis and tendinitis are two examples of common chronic *soft tissue conditions*. **Bursitis** is a condition that results in inflammation and an accumulation of fluid in the subcutaneous bursae (the sac-like structures filled with fluid to reduce friction between two surfaces). The inflammation and volume added to the bursa causes the bursa to become painful and lose its friction-reducing properties. Bursitis often occurs as a result of excessive repetitive use and pressure to a joint. It is commonly found in the shoulder, knee or elbow, and can be eased by reducing the repetitive action causing the pain. **Tendinitis** is inflammation of a tendon, and can occur as a result of chronic overuse, which may be exacerbated by poor posture, obesity, poor or inappropriate technique, exercising with excessively heavy weights, bone spurs, and exercising in cold temperatures without warming up correctly. Tendinitis commonly affects the shoulder, wrist and heel tendons.

Clinical manifestations Most people with soft tissue injuries present with pain, a decreased range of motion and localised oedema. Some people may exhibit bleeding into the joint or adjacent structures, which manifests as localised bruising. If a complete rupture of a tendon has occurred, there may be an obvious tissue void or deformity in the affected area, and a lump or bulge in an area proximal to the injury from where the tendon has retracted back up the limb. Total loss of function will occur as a result of a third-degree sprain or strain, as an avulsion has occurred and there is no attachment to facilitate the specific action required at the joint (see Figure 41.2). In these types of injuries, the person may report hearing a 'pop' or a 'snap'. In the event of a dislocation, the joint can be remarkably deformed. If the blood supply is compromised distal to the injury, the skin will look pale and the area may also feel cool to touch. Peripheral pulses will be reduced or absent, and capillary refill will be delayed. Injuries that involve vascular compromise are limb-threatening injuries and require urgent attention. Failure to re-establish blood flow may result in the need for amputation. Figure 41.3 explores the common clinical manifestations and management of soft tissue injury.

Tendinitis and bursitis present as persistently swollen and painful joints, which may be associated with muscle weakness and a decreased range of movement. The affected site may also be warm to touch. As tendinitis or bursitis develops over time, no one instance of trauma or specific insult is required.

Clinical diagnosis and management

Diagnosis Following the primary survey and initial management of any impairments of airway, breathing and circulation, a secondary survey should include a neurovascular

A

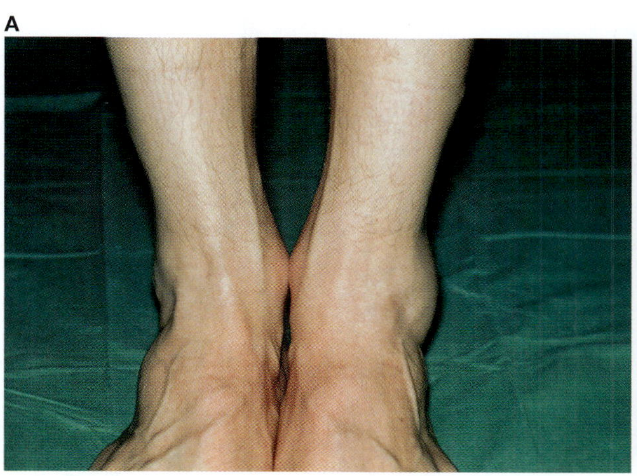

B

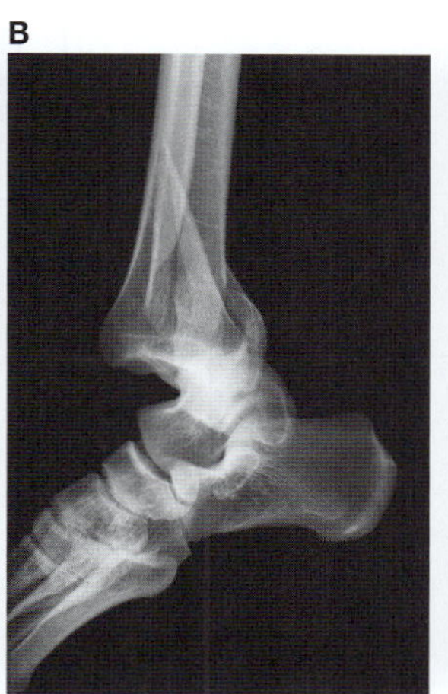

C

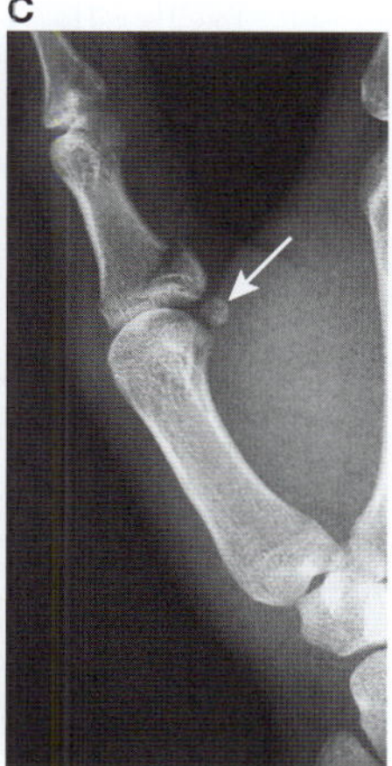

Figure 41.2

Various soft tissue injuries

(A) Sprained ankle. This photograph was taken 30 minutes after injury. Note the swelling around the left lateral malleolus.

(B) X-ray of a severely fractured and dislocated ankle joint. Serious soft tissue injuries are associated with this type of dislocation. If vascular compromise has occurred, this injury may be limb-threatening.

(C) Avulsion of the ulnar collateral ligament off the proximal phalanx (thumb). Although it is not possible to see soft tissue injury on X-ray, this ligamentous rupture is visible because it has caused an avulsion fracture.

Sources: (A) Dr P. Marazzi/Science Photo Library; (B) Puwadol Jaturawutthichai/Shutterstock; (C) Scott Camazine/Alamy Stock Photo.

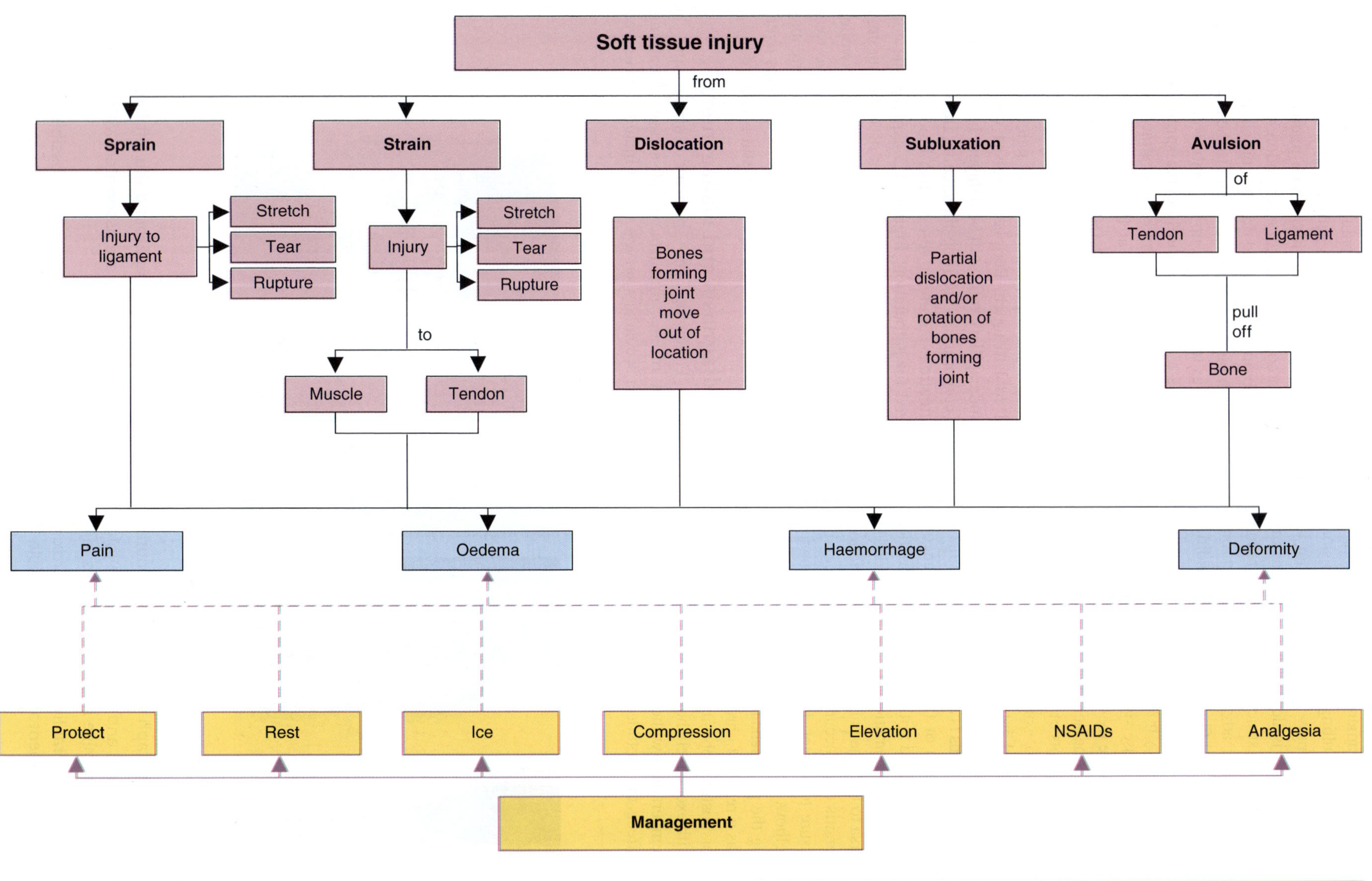

Figure 41.3

Clinical snapshot: Soft tissue injury

NSAIDs = non-steroidal anti-inflammatory drugs.

assessment. The affected limb should be assessed for colour, warmth, movement, sensation, capillary refill and peripheral pulses (see Table 41.3).

Irrespective of the sequence, a helpful method of assessing neurovascular observations can be done using the '*five Ps of neurovascular assessment*': pain, pallor, pulselessness, paraesthesia and poikilothermia (cool temperature). A medical history and an explanation of the mechanism of injury should be collected. A physical assessment should identify additional injuries or comorbidities that may complicate management.

A pain assessment should be undertaken and reassessed frequently. Depending on the details obtained from the history and the physical assessment, imaging tests may be indicated. If localised bone tenderness, suspicion of a foreign body or a tendon injury is present, then an X-ray should be taken of the affected area. If no bony tenderness is felt and a full range of motion is achievable, an X-ray is generally unnecessary. An ultrasound is indicated if there is suspicion of non-radio-opaque material, such as wood or glass, embedded in the injury.

Management For all soft tissue injuries the immediate first aid management is encompassed by the mnemonic **RICER** (rest, ice, compression, elevation, referral). Activity should be ceased and an ice pack should be applied to the area, ensuring that material (e.g. a towel) is placed between the skin and the ice pack to prevent damage to the skin and the underlying structures from an ice burn (frostbite). A compression bandage should be applied to reduce the swelling. This should be checked and reapplied regularly, so that it is not impeding blood flow. Regular neurovascular observations should be performed. If no neurovascular compromise is detected, the limb should be elevated. If neurovascular compromise is detected, the limb should not be elevated above the level of the heart, as this can further compromise blood flow.

Further assessment and intervention should be undertaken by an appropriately qualified health professional. Referral to a surgical team may be indicated in the presence of a dislocation or an avulsion. Unqualified people should not attempt to reduce a dislocation, as there is a significant risk of nerve or blood vessel entrapment, which will quickly result in a limb-threatening situation. Appropriate assessments, such as an X-ray, and administration of sufficient analgesia or sedation should be undertaken before any dislocation is reduced.

A dislocation may require a simple *closed reduction* (not requiring surgery) undertaken in the emergency department following appropriate assessment and pain relief. If the dislocation is severe and involves fractures, an *open reduction and internal fixation (ORIF)* may be required. Surgery for an avulsion is complex, and it can be difficult to locate and re-attach the tendon. Some ligamentous avulsions may heal without intervention over several months, whereas some may never heal without surgical intervention.

Following reduction of a dislocation, the joint will be immobilised with a splint or a cast to promote correct alignment and facilitate healing. Depending on the severity and location of the injury, mobility aids such as crutches or a wheelchair may be necessary during the initial stage of recovery. Physiotherapy should be started as soon as possible so as to reduce the risk of muscle atrophy or loss of joint function from prolonged splinting or disuse.

Table 41.3 Neurovascular assessment

Parameter	Desirable value	Observations of concern
Colour	Pink (or similar colour to other limb)	• White or pale (determine whether ice packs have been applied to the affected area) • Cyanotic (determine whether the person has Raynaud's syndrome or peripheral vascular disease) • Mottled
Warmth	Warm	• Cool or cold (determine whether ice packs have been applied to the affected area)
Movement	Full range of movement	• Severe pain on active or passive movement • No movement possible in a particular direction • No movement
Sensation	Touch distinguished in all areas of affected limb	• Touch not distinguished in all areas of affected limb • Complaints of 'pins and needles' • No sensation recognised (determine the presence of nerve block or epidural anaesthesia)
Capillary refill time	Blanching resolves in < 2 seconds	• Blanching does not resolve in < 2 seconds
Peripheral pulses	Intensity score of: 2—normal, or 3—bounding	Intensity score of: • 0—absent, or • 1—diminished

Education prior to discharge should cover all aspects of the **NO HARM** acronym—no heat, alcohol, running or massage. This acronym is important to ensure that the person knows that in the first 24 hours they should not apply *h*eat or drink *a*lcohol (as it can exacerbate swelling and reduce the pain threshold, meaning that further injury may occur). They should not *r*un or exercise in any form (so as not to increase blood flow to the area and further exacerbate the swelling). The area should not be *m*assaged for at least 72 hours, to reduce the risk of further internal bleeding. Other education should include the appropriate use of analgesic agents to promote maximal effect and reduce the risk of adverse effects.

The management of tendinitis and bursitis includes rest and re-evaluation of the activities that cause pain, as they are potentially the activities that contributed to the problem. Although these conditions usually improve without intervention, in some circumstances corticosteroid injections and weight loss may be indicated if the condition persists. If excessive exercise or training has contributed to the condition, technique and the training schedule should be reassessed to reduce the risk of further injury.

Fractures

LEARNING OBJECTIVE 2

Differentiate between various fracture types, and explain the mechanism and their management.

AETIOLOGY AND PATHOPHYSIOLOGY

The average fully formed human skeleton has 206 bones. The smallest bones are those in the ear, and the largest is the femur. A **fracture** is a break in a bone. Given the right circumstances, any bone is capable of breaking; however, it takes considerable force to break a healthy bone. Trauma and disease can cause fractures to occur all too frequently. Table 41.4 illustrates examples of the more common fracture-related terminology.

Table 41.4 Descriptions of various fracture types

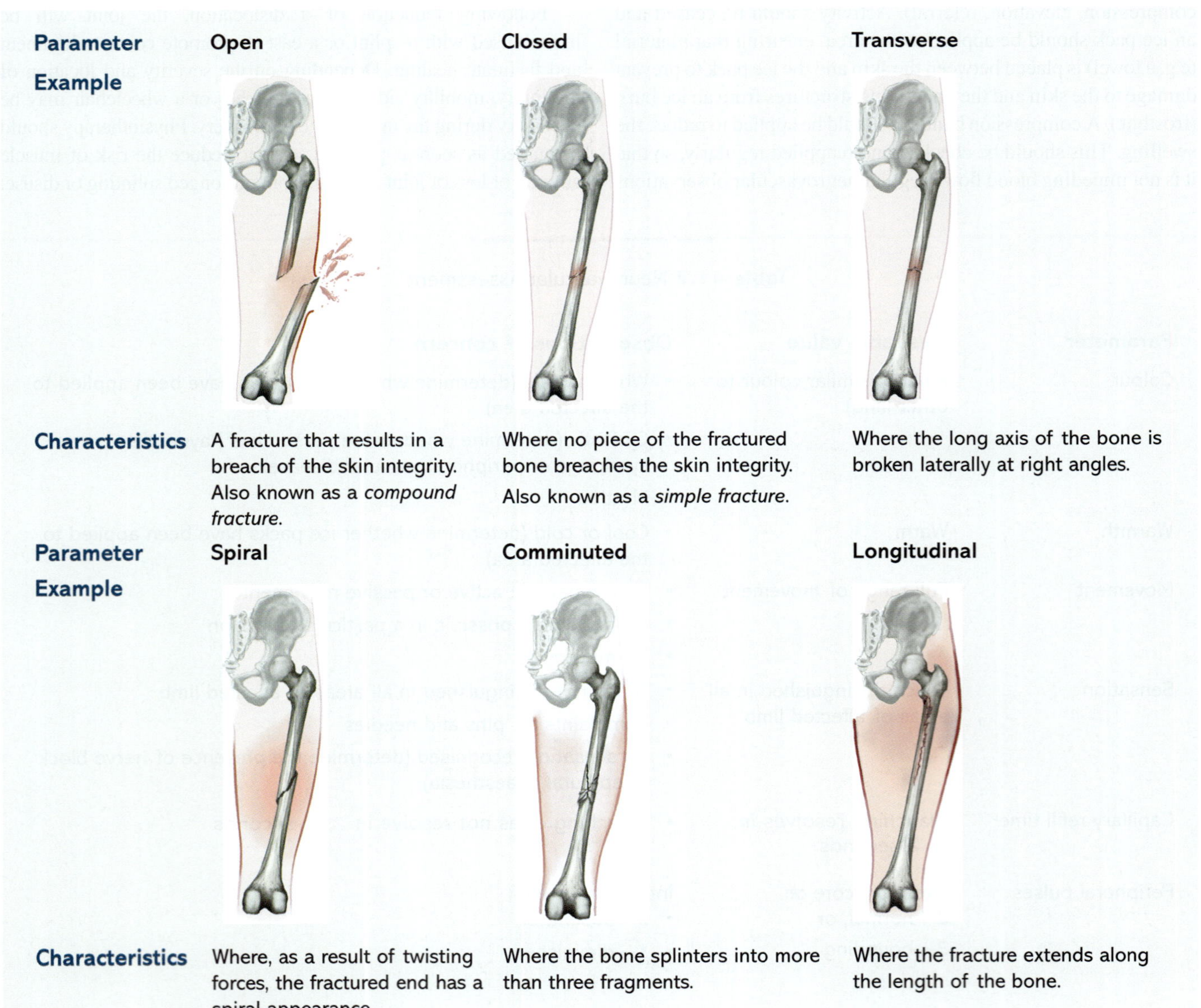

Parameter	Open	Closed	Transverse
Example			
Characteristics	A fracture that results in a breach of the skin integrity. Also known as a *compound fracture*.	Where no piece of the fractured bone breaches the skin integrity. Also known as a *simple fracture*.	Where the long axis of the bone is broken laterally at right angles.
Parameter	**Spiral**	**Comminuted**	**Longitudinal**
Example			
Characteristics	Where, as a result of twisting forces, the fractured end has a spiral appearance.	Where the bone splinters into more than three fragments.	Where the fracture extends along the length of the bone.

Table 41.4 Descriptions of various fracture types (*continued*)

Parameter	Segmental	Oblique	Greenstick
Example	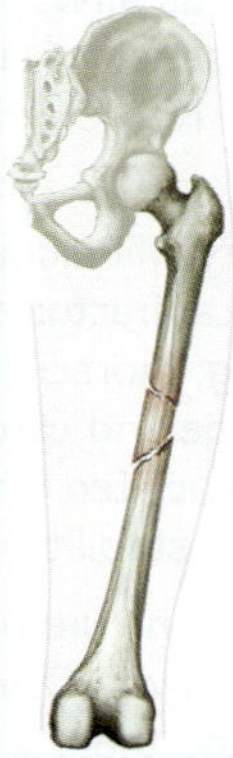	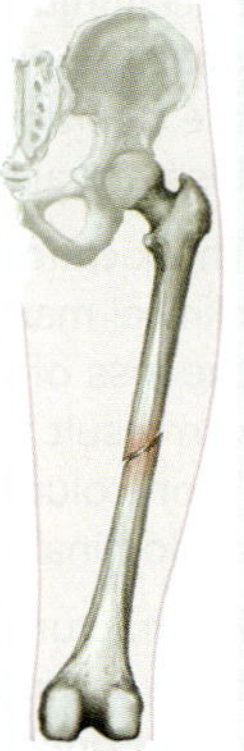	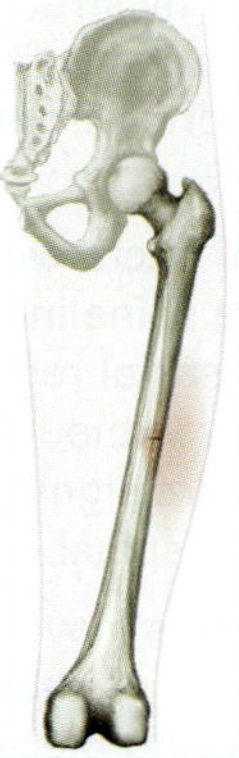
Characteristics	Where multiple complete fractures result in a free section of bone across the whole shaft.	Where a fracture extends down the shaft in a diagonal manner.	Where an immature bone (occurs in children) may bend and not break entirely. The cortex of the bone remains intact. Also known as a *interperiosteal fracture.*
Parameter	**Avulsion**	**Torus**	**Physeal**
Example	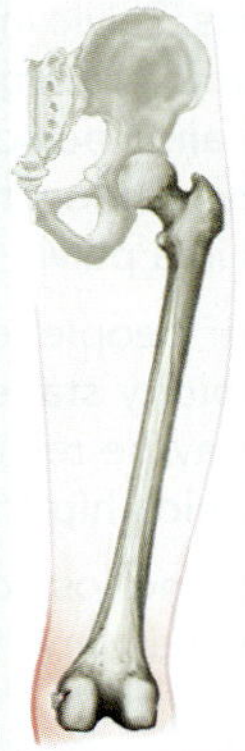	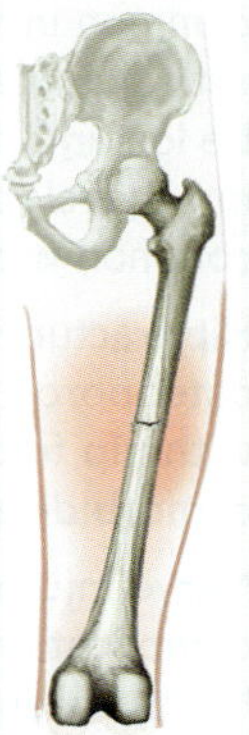	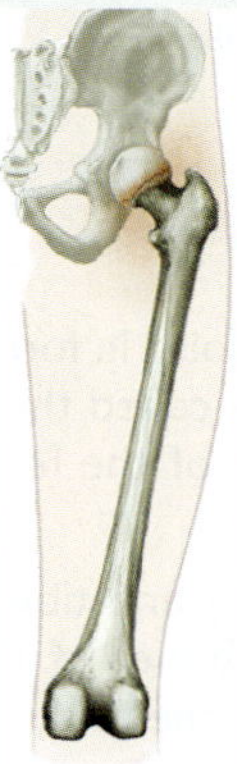
Characteristics	Where the section of bone at the site of a ligament or tendon is torn away with a fragment of bone attached.	Where bulging occurs from cortical compression after the trabeculae are crushed along a fracture line. Also known as a *buckle fracture.*	Where the fracture involves part of the growth plate (*epiphysis*).
Parameter	**Pathological**	**Compression**	**Depressed**
Example	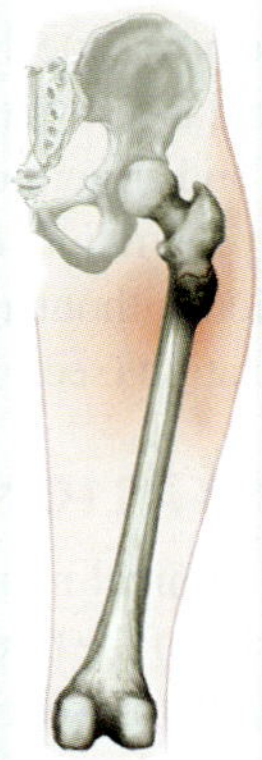	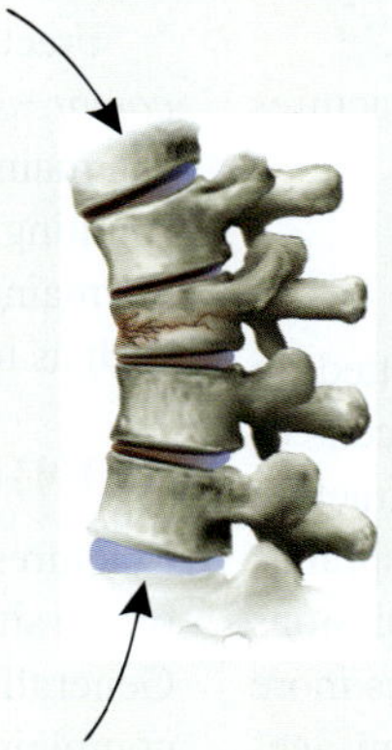	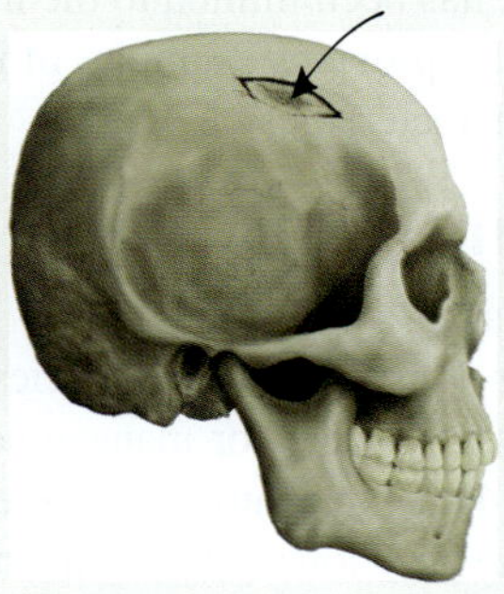
Characteristics	Where a fracture occurs as a result of severely diminished bone density or as a result of an innocuous movement.	Where a fracture occurs as a result of direct loading through the bone. Commonly seen in vertebrae.	Where a fractured section of a bone is pushed inwards. Generally in relation to a skull.

Source: Illustrations: Averil Bellert © Sciencopia.

Table 41.5 Specific fractures and their characteristics

Fracture	Description	Characteristics/considerations
Facial	Several bony structures form the face, including the maxilla and mandible, the zygoma, orbit, frontal bone and nose.	Facial injuries can be dangerous, as airway compromise is possible due to oedema, the presence of a foreign body or the position of a bone fragment. Neurological injury and vision loss are also a concern.
Vertebral	Vertebral fractures can occur anywhere along the spine in the cervical, thoracic or lumbosacral regions. Vertebral damage may occur without spinal injury; however, the risks are significant (see the chapter 'Brain and spinal cord dysfunction').	The location of the vertebral injury will dictate the range of clinical manifestations. High cervical fractures may result in the loss of spontaneous breathing; thoracic vertebral injuries can result in impaired gas exchange and cardiac dysfunction. Thoracolumbar injuries can be associated with concomitant abdominal trauma. Haemodynamic stability may be compromised.
Rib	Rib fractures may be single or multiple. If two parts of the same rib are broken, a free-moving piece, called a *flail section*, results.	Rib fractures may result in a lung puncture or occult blood loss from accumulation in the thoracic cavity. Oxygenation may be compromised with rib fractures, and there is an increased risk of chest infection as airway clearance may be suppressed because of pain. Brachial plexus injuries are also common with rib fractures.
Upper limb	Common upper limb fractures include the clavicle, proximal humerus, distal radius and the scaphoid.	Brachial plexus injuries and other nerve injuries may cause devastating loss of function; however, limb fractures are rarely life-threatening.
Pelvic	The pelvis is formed by the ilium, ischium and pubis.	It takes significant force to cause a pelvic injury, which are common in motor vehicle accidents. Pelvic injuries are associated with significant mortality and morbidity. Large blood volumes can be lost into the abdominal cavity, and haemodynamic compromise may develop quickly. Injury to other abdominal structures is also common with trauma that results in a pelvic fracture.
Hip	The hip joint is formed by a cup-like structure called the *acetabulum* into which the head of the femur sits.	Hip fractures are common in older people, especially those with osteoporosis. Mortality and morbidity statistics associated with hip fracture are high. This may be related to the age and comorbidities of the people in which hip fracture is common.
Lower limb	The femur and tibia are the major load-bearing bones of the leg. There are 26 bones in the foot.	Nerve injuries may cause devastating loss of function and complications with mobility; however, limb fractures are rarely life-threatening.

A number of bone disorders are associated with pathological fractures, including osteoporosis, osteogenesis imperfecta and osteomalacia (see the chapter 'Bone and joint disorders'). While range of other fracture types can also occur, the discussion in this chapter has been limited to the more common forms.

Table 41.5 provides examples of important specific fractures and their characteristics.

EPIDEMIOLOGY

In Australia in 2020–21, 615,537 people were admitted to hospital for musculoskeletal injuries. Forty-seven per cent of these admissions were for management of people with fracture (see Figure 41.4). In contrast, it is interesting to note that sprains, strains and dislocation injuries constituted only 6% of admissions for musculoskeletal injuries. Overall, women are 1.5 times more likely to be admitted for fracture than men, mostly from age-related osteoporotic changes. However, in younger age brackets men have a much greater risk of musculoskeletal trauma as a result of transport-, sport- and occupation-related accidents.

Some conditions and medications can increase a person's risk of fracture (see Clinical Box 41.1). Metabolic bone diseases and bone cancer will also increase the risk of fracture (see the chapter 'Bone and joinst disorders').

Fractures may be classified by the mechanism of injury, such as *compression* or *depression*, and also by stability. *Stable fractures* can maintain optimum shape and structure, and may only require splinting and protection for pain relief. *Unstable fractures* will not maintain the correct position without aggressive interventions, such as internal or external fixation (see Figure 41.5).

CLINICAL MANIFESTATIONS

Fractures may cause myriad clinical manifestations, depending on the site of injury, the severity of the trauma and comorbidities. Generally speaking, most people presenting with a fracture will complain of pain, swelling and loss of function. An obvious deformity may be visible either from fracture displacement or significant swelling. Crepitus (a grating sound on movement) may be heard as the ends of bone rub against each other. In the

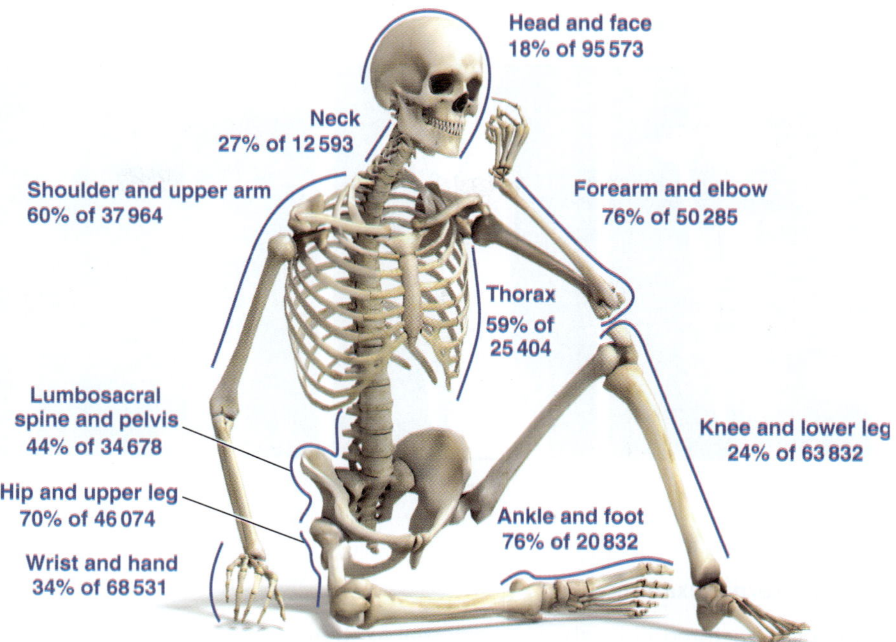

Figure 41.4

Fractures as a percentage of all public hospital admissions for musculoskeletal injuries, per body region in Australia in one year (2020–21)

The percentage is a portion of all admissions for fractures of that particular body part. The whole number is the total number of admissions recorded for musculoskeletal injuries of that body part.

Sources: Developed using data from the Australian Institute of Health and Welfare (2022). Image adapted from © Ralf Juergen Kraft/ Shutterstock.

event of significant blood loss, circulatory shock may manifest (see the chapter 'Vascular disorders and circulatory shock').

CLINICAL DIAGNOSIS AND MANAGEMENT

Diagnosis

Screening for fracture risk prior to a fracture occurring is beneficial but not always achievable. The World Health Organization has developed a tool—the FRAX tool, or fracture risk assessment tool—to predict the 10-year probability of developing a fracture due to low bone mineral density. To calculate the risk of fracture, the tool utilises 12 parameters, including age, sex, the results from dual energy X-ray absorptiometry (DEXA) scans, a history of smoking and selected medication use. This information can be used to determine the need for prophylaxis with calcium supplementation or antiresorptive agents, such as the bisphosphonates (see the chapter 'Bone and joint disorders'). This assessment is especially beneficial in ageing individuals with comorbidities. However, all too often a fracture occurs and the use of a risk assessment tool becomes redundant.

Physical assessment and the collection of a history of the events that contributed to the presentation are important to obtain a clear clinical picture of the potential structural damage and to predict possible adverse events. The most common method for fracture diagnosis is the use of simple medical imaging, such as an X-ray. For more complex injuries or anatomical structures, computed tomography (CT) may be beneficial, as greater detail and a larger array of views are possible.

Management

Management of a fracture will generally include pain relief, and elevation and immobilisation to enable optimum environmental conditions for the bone structure to heal. Specific interventions will vary, depending on the person's clinical presentation, fracture site, mechanism of injury, trauma severity and pre-existing health issues. Promotion of bone healing is the priority.

BONE HEALING

Bone healing processes maintain the continuity of the skeleton once a fracture occurs. Bone healing (or union) remains effective throughout life, but, like other processes, tends to slow with

CLINICAL BOX 41.1

Conditions and medications increasing the risk of fracture

Conditions

- Low bone mineral density due to conditions such as osteoporosis
- Immobility
- Low oestrogen states, such as postmenopause or post-hysterectomy
- Endocrine disorders, such as Cushing's disease
- Congenital disorders, such as hip dysplasia
- Previous fracture

Medications

- Long-term use of corticosteroids
- Proton pump inhibitors
- Antacids
- Some antipsychotic agents (e.g. risperidone and olanzapine)
- Thyroid hormone treatment
- Lithium carbonate (used in the management of mania)
- Methotrexate (an antimetabolite anticancer agent and disease-modifying antirheumatic drug)

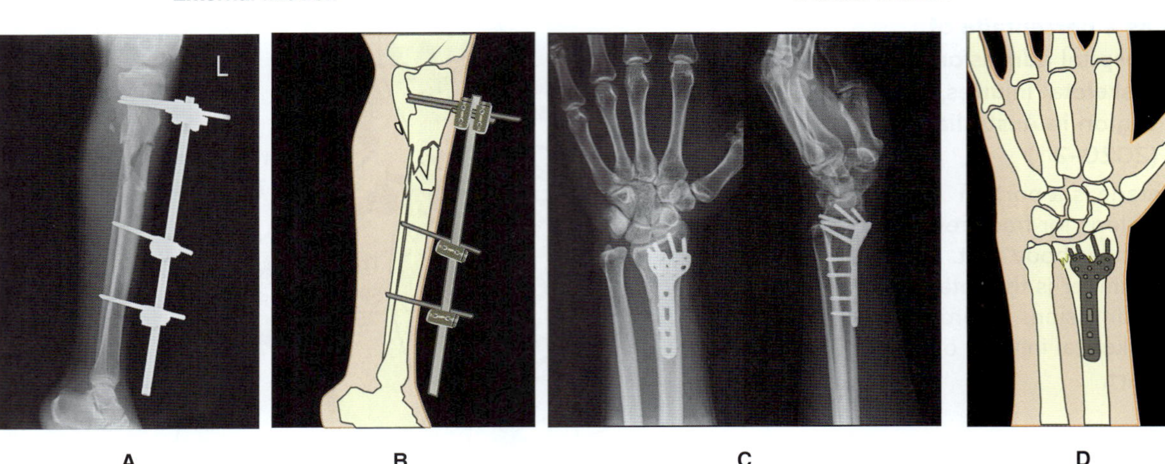

Figure 41.5

External and internal fixation

(A) An X-ray of a fractured tibia, showing external fixation.

(B) An illustration of the fractured tibia, depicting the skin margins to clarify external fixation and anatomical structures (and to demonstrate the fixator configuration).

(C) An X-ray of a fractured radius, showing internal fixation.

(D) An illustration of the fractured radial head, depicting the skin margins to clarify the internal fixation and anatomical structures.

Sources: (A) Jarva Jar/Shutterstock; (B) Sciencopia; (C) MossStudio/Shutterstock; (D) Sciencopia.

advancing age. The healing of a damaged bone occurs in four stages, which are summarised in Table 41.6.

FRACTURE COMPLICATIONS

LEARNING OBJECTIVE 3

Describe the common complications of fracture, including compartment syndrome, delayed union and non-union.

Complications affecting the bone

Various factors may interfere with the speed and degree of bone healing (*union*). **Delayed union** (*a prolonged period of time before bone healing succeeds*) can occur as a result of compromised circulation, infection or immobilisation during bone healing. **Non-union** (*unsuccessful unification of the bone ends*) may develop as a result of tissue loss, compromised circulation, infection, improper splinting and from pathological fractures. **Malunion** (*the misalignment of bone ends*) is most often caused by improper splinting. **Avascular necrosis** is the death of tissue from the loss of blood supply to the area. The areas most at risk of bone loss from avascular necrosis include the head of the femur, the body of the talus (ankle bone) and the scaphoid (a wrist bone). *Osteomyelitis*, an infection of bone, can also occur as a result of fracture (see the chapter 'Bone and join disorders'). The management options for complications to the bone are usually surgical, and often require bone grafts and/or internal fixation.

Complications affecting the limb

Various complications that affect the limb can occur as a result of a fracture. These include compartment syndrome, damage to vascular structures, damage to peripheral nerves or fat embolus syndrome.

Compartment syndrome

Compartment syndrome is a condition occurring as a result of excessive pressure within a muscle compartment. Compartments group muscles are covered by a strong membrane called *fascia*. Normally, the fascia are responsible for maintaining structural shape and keeping the tissues in place; therefore, fascia does not stretch or expand easily.

Aetiology and pathophysiology Inflammation or bleeding into a muscle compartment creates a build-up of pressure within the compartment. Due to the nature of the fascia, the increased pressure is directed inwards, which results in the compression of capillaries, nerves and muscle cells (myocytes). Under these conditions, ischaemia can develop, leading to a reduction in oxygen and nutrients, and a failure to clear toxic waste products, which can damage the cells within the compartment.

Compartment syndrome can develop after a *severe injury*, such as a crush injury, severe haematoma or fracture. *Iatrogenic injury* can be caused when healthcare professionals apply a bandage, splint or cast too tightly; this, too, can ultimately result in compartment syndrome. Less commonly, compartment syndrome can occur in a *chronic form. Exertional (or exercise-induced) compartment syndrome* can occur as a result of

Table 41.6 Stages of bone healing

Stage 1. Haematoma formation

(Immediately after fracture)

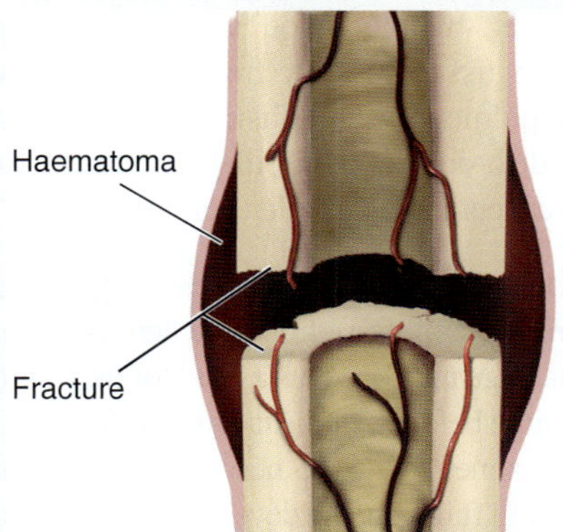

Erythrocytes freely collect in the fractured area as a result of blood vessel rupture from the trauma. Macrophages and neutrophils assist with cleaning the area of debris. Fibroblasts are attracted to assist with rebuilding. Osteoclasts remove necrotic bone.

Dominant cells

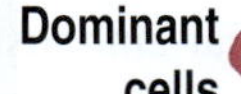

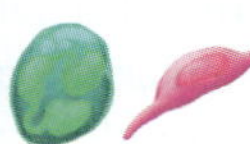
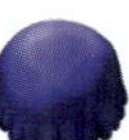

Characteristics

After the initial trauma, blood will collect in the area from lacerated blood vessels, and the osteocytes (bone cells) in the immediate area will die. Within 5 days the large clot—rich with clotting factors, fibrin, fibroblasts, macrophages, monocytes and lymphocytes—will have new blood vessels forming around its periphery and into the fracture site. Osteoblasts (bone-building cells) and osteoclasts (bone-degrading cells) are attracted to the area and begin to proliferate. Within 48 hours the osteoclasts remove the necrotic bone tissue.

Stage 2. Fibrocartilaginous callus formation

(Within 1–2 weeks of fracture)

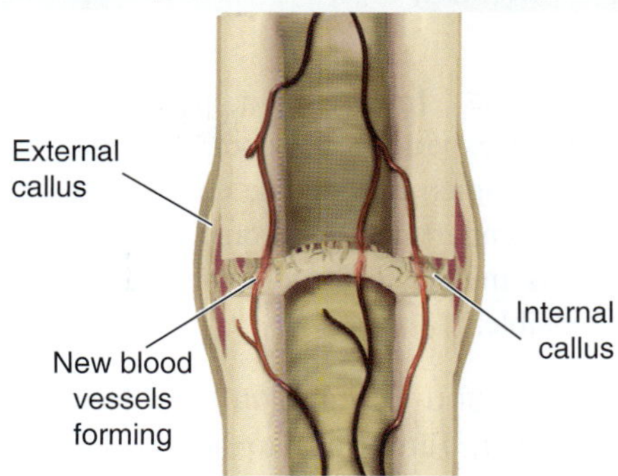

Fibroblasts lay collagen fibres to assist with bridging the ends of the fracture. Chondroblasts lay down cartilage. Some become chondrocytes. Osteoblasts deposit osteoid, the organic bone matrix, that will become bone. The soft callus is comprised of collagen, cartilage and osteoid.

Dominant cells

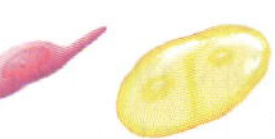
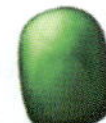

Characteristics

Early granulation tissue is deposited as fibroblasts, and osteoblasts lay collagen fibres, which bridge both sides of the fracture and any bone fragments in the vicinity. Chondroblasts also fabricate patches of cartilage, and osteoblasts then lay an organic bone matrix called osteoid. Within 1 week a soft callus is formed.

Stage 3. Bony callus (ossification)

(Continues for approximately 3 months)

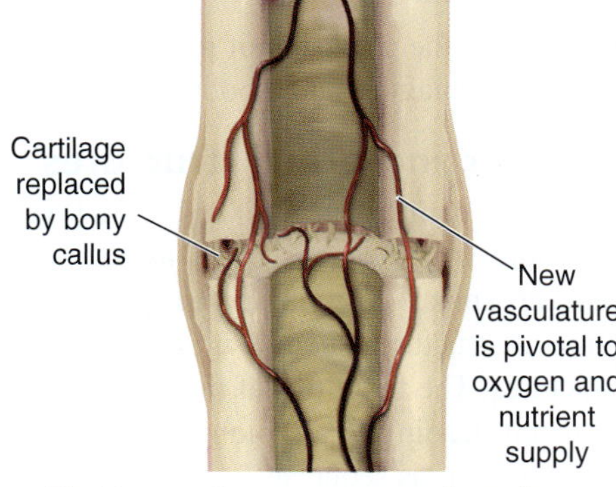

Fibroblasts continue to secrete a matrix of collagen, glycoproteins, and elastic and mesh fibres. Endochondral ossification results in resorption of the cartilaginous callus and replacement with an immature hard callus by osteoblasts.

Dominant cells

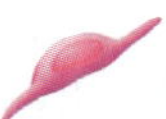
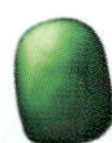

Characteristics

Over the next month the soft callus (osteoid, cartilage and collagen) undergoes mineralisation with calcium and mineral salts. It becomes a hard callus (or 'secondary callus'). This stage continues for approximately 3 months.

Stage 4. Remodelling

(Continues for months to years)

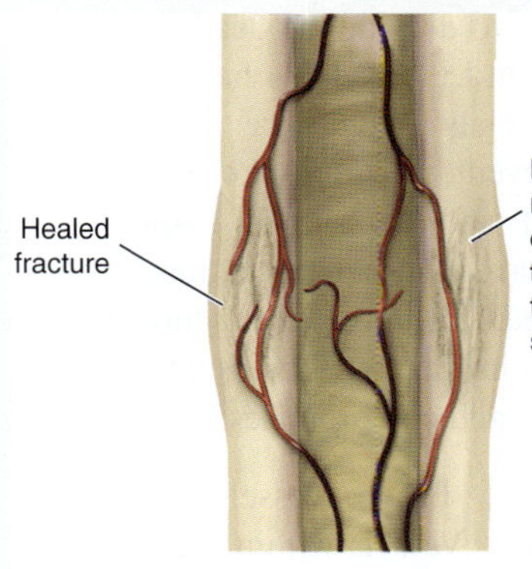

An interplay between the osteoblasts and osteoclasts remodel and reorganise the bone structure for maximal strength. The process is influenced by mechanical stressors stimulating bone formation by osteoblasts and bone resorption by osteoclasts.

Dominant cells

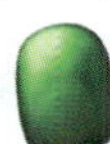
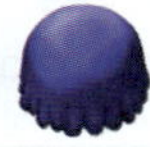

Characteristics

Osteoblasts continue to lay down bone to help strengthen the structure. Osteoclasts begin to remove excess bone and reshape the structure until it resembles its former shape. A new medullary cavity is also shaped by osteoclastic activity. Remodelling may take several years.

Cell key

 RBC
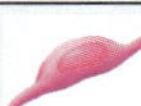 Fibroblast
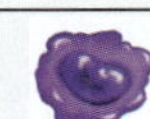 Macrophage
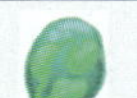 Neutrophil
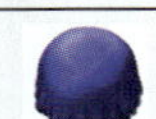 Osteoclast
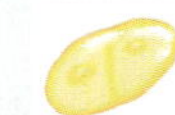 Chondroblast Chondrocyte
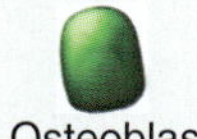 Osteoblast

Source: Illustrations by Averil Bellert © Sciencopia.

excessively increased circulation to a muscle, exceeding the capacity of the fascia to absorb the increased pressure. Exertional compartment syndrome resolves quickly when the activity is ceased.

Clinical manifestations Intense pain, paraesthesia and/or paralysis are commonly experienced in compartment syndrome. Peripherally, the limb digits can become cold and discoloured (cyanosed or white). Compartment syndrome generally develops as a result of serious injury, so evidence of trauma or gross deformity may be visible.

Clinical diagnosis and management Neurovascular observations (see Table 41.3) are critical to the early identification of compartment syndrome. Compartment pressures may be measured, and blood may be drawn to assess other haematological or biochemical parameters. However, in obvious instances treatment should not be delayed, as compartment syndrome can be limb-threatening.

The affected limb should be placed at the level of the heart. Although it would seem that elevation would be appropriate, this will further reduce blood flow and can exacerbate ischaemia. The most important intervention in the management of compartment syndrome is a **fasciotomy** (a cut through the fascia to relieve tension) (see Figure 41.6). Although it is important to quickly correct hypovolaemia (as a result of the trauma), it is critical that a fasciotomy is undertaken urgently. During this surgery, the repair of damaged blood vessels and the stabilisation of fractures can also be achieved. The fasciotomy wound must be left open, as this palliates the compartment pressures. If necrosis develops as a result of the tissue anoxia prior to the fasciotomy, further surgery will be required to debride the dead tissue. The skin cannot be approximated until the oedema has sufficiently reduced; therefore, antimicrobials should be administered prophylactically so as to prevent infection. Postoperatively, the limb should be elevated and appropriate wound care management should be undertaken, as per institutional policy. Analgesia should be provided, and frequent neurovascular observations should continue in case the pressure in other muscle compartments increases and compromises blood flow.

Blood vessel damage Blood vessels are easily damaged as a result of a fracture. Vessels within the bone will certainly be affected, but larger veins and arteries may also be lacerated from bone fragments, compression or the stretching of vessels as a result of the trauma of skeletal deformity. Ischaemia or anoxia in areas serviced by the blood vessels can cause significant problems from tissue loss. A fracture may result in severe blood loss, or pulmonary embolism may occur (see the chapters 'Vascular disorders and circulatory shock' and 'Respiratory infections, cancers and vascular conditions').

Peripheral nerve damage Like blood vessels, peripheral nerves may also be lacerated, compressed or stretched. Neuronal, axonal or myelin sheath damage may occur as a result of the trauma. The severity, location and time before treatment can all influence the result. Possible clinical outcomes related to nerve damage include the restoration of partial or full function, the development of chronic pain, or complete paralysis. Surgical intervention may be needed in an attempt to restore function or control pain.

Fat embolus syndrome When the pelvis or a long bone fractures, there is a risk that fat globules from the bone marrow may inadvertently enter the circulation. Fat embolism syndrome may develop, resulting in serious respiratory compromise, neurological abnormalities and the development of a petechial rash.

Although the pathogenesis is not yet clearly understood, two theories appear to explain the possible process:

1 *mechanical factors* may result in vessel obstruction within a tissue's microcirculation
2 *chemical factors* may damage cells and cause the production of toxic metabolites as a result of the degradation and agglutination of the fat emboli.

Symptom management and the provision of supportive care are the guiding principles of managing fat embolism syndrome.

Complications affecting other structures

Fractures may not only damage nerves and blood vessels, but they can also injure major organs, such as the lungs in rib fractures, brain or spinal cord injury in axial skeleton fractures, or abdominal structures such as urinary or digestive organs in pelvic fractures. The functions of these organs can be compromised as a result, leading to a prolongation of recovery time and, in some cases, serious sequelae.

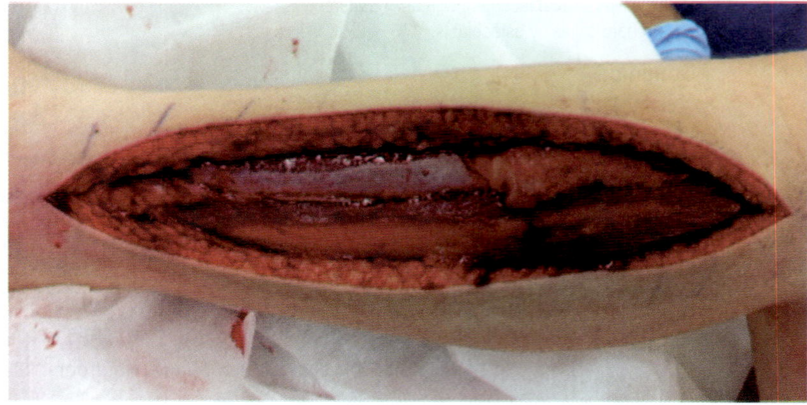

Figure 41.6

Fasciotomy of right lower leg

Medial fasciotomy of the right lower leg for compartment syndrome.

Source: Copyright © 2015 Shane C. O'Neill.

Muscle disorders

LEARNING OBJECTIVE 4

Examine the complexities of disorders resulting in muscle pain such as fibromyalgia and systemic exertion intolerance disease.

FIBROMYALGIA

Fibromyalgia is a somewhat misunderstood condition characterised by *widespread, evolving, episodic muscle pain and tenderness*. Fibromyalgia is not a form of arthritis (joint disease), and does not cause inflammation or damage to joints, muscles or other tissues. Because fibromyalgia can cause chronic pain and fatigue similar to arthritis, some people think of it as a rheumatic condition. The name 'fibromyalgia' is derived from the Latin and Greek root words for 'fibrous tissue' (Latin, *fibro-*), 'muscle' (Greek, *myo-*) and 'pain' (Greek, *algos-*). **Myalgia** is muscle pain and has many causes. Fibromyalgia is a problematic inclusion in this chapter because the aetiology of the condition is unclear. It has not been ascertained that the pathophysiology of fibromyalgia involves damage to the muscular system. Rather, fibromyalgia is a painful condition in which those with it attribute the pain to their muscles.

Aetiology and pathophysiology

Fibromyalgia is really a *syndrome* rather than a disease. The cause of fibromyalgia is unclear. Current research favours the suggestion of *genetic preponderance*; however, genes alone do not appear to cause fibromyalgia. *Catalysts* such as trauma, disease or emotional stressors appear to trigger the development of fibromyalgia in people with the appropriate genetic predisposition. Changes in the central and autonomic nervous, endocrine and immune systems may play a significant role in fibromyalgia. Levels of inhibitory neurotransmitters, such as serotonin and noradrenaline, are decreased, which may contribute to the symptoms of depression and sleep disturbance. Excitatory neurotransmitters, such as glutamate, aspartate and substance P, are increased, which probably contributes to increased pain transmission via primary afferent neurons. When coupled with the autonomic nervous system changes of increased sympathetic tone and decreased parasympathetic tone, and the increase in cytokines from immune system changes, the person will experience pain amplification and central pain sensitisation, resulting in hyperalgesia (see the chapter 'Nociception and pain'). Figure 41.7 explores the probable mechanisms and management principles of fibromyalgia.

Epidemiology

Broad estimates for the prevalence for fibromyalgia range between 2% and 5% of the adult population, with a marked female preponderance. Peak prevalence estimates are considerably higher, particularly among middle-aged women and people with concomitant rheumatological conditions. In 2022, over 15,960 people were admitted for fibromyalgia, with females affected over 11 times more than males. However, admission statistics do not provide a good representation of incidence or prevalence, as the condition can be managed with the assistance of a general practitioner.

Despite lacking an identifiable pathophysiology, fibromyalgia is an important condition because it generates substantial disease and economic burden. In Australia, an estimated 1 million people have fibromyalgia, and it is considered to be almost five times more common than rheumatoid arthritis.

Clinical manifestations

Fibromyalgia is characterised by chronic, widespread pain and **allodynia** (reporting of pain in response to stimuli that would not typically provoke pain; see the chapter 'Nociception and pain'). The International Association for the Study of Pain (IASP) describes pain as '... an unpleasant sensory and emotional experience associated with actual or potential tissue damage, or described in terms of such damage'. This definition of pain is helpful in our consideration of fibromyalgia, because it incorporates both the physical and the psychological experiences of pain, and includes pain perceived in the absence of tissue damage.

Other symptoms, including fatigue, sleep disturbance, joint stiffness, anxiety and depression, and cognition and memory difficulties, complicate the clinical picture of fibromyalgia, and, because not all people experience all symptoms, diagnosis may be difficult and sometimes protracted. Also, because there are no objective, cellular-level tests to confirm fibromyalgia, the diagnosis is contentious.

Clinical diagnosis and management

Diagnosis The diagnosis of fibromyalgia is made taking into account the overall burden of symptoms in people with widespread body pain with no other explanation for the pain. Occasionally, rheumatologists make the diagnosis and rule out other rheumatic diseases, but people with fibromyalgia do not require ongoing specialist rheumatological care.

Laboratory tests and imaging studies may be used to rule out other diseases. In some people fibromyalgia is a diagnosis of exclusion, identified only when other possibilities have been negated. For example, hypothyroidism and polymyalgia rheumatica may mimic fibromyalgia, but blood tests to determine levels of thyroid-stimulating hormone or the erythrocyte sedimentation rate, respectively, can differentiate these conditions from fibromyalgia.

Although tender point examination is widely understood as the key diagnostic feature of fibromyalgia, the examination process is time-consuming, and requires some practitioner training and practice for adequate inter-rater reliability, making it less than ideal as an in-office procedure for general practitioners (i.e. non-rheumatologists and other practitioners not routinely using musculoskeletal examination procedures). Furthermore, some experts argue that reliance on tender points in the diagnostic criteria presents an image of fibromyalgia as a discrete muscle disorder, which under-emphasises other debilitating aspects of the condition (e.g. fatigue, reduced cognitive function, poor memory) and the broad spectrum of variable symptoms, such as paraesthesia and stiffness. Figure 41.8 shows anterior and posterior body maps of the tender points that are assessed in this examination.

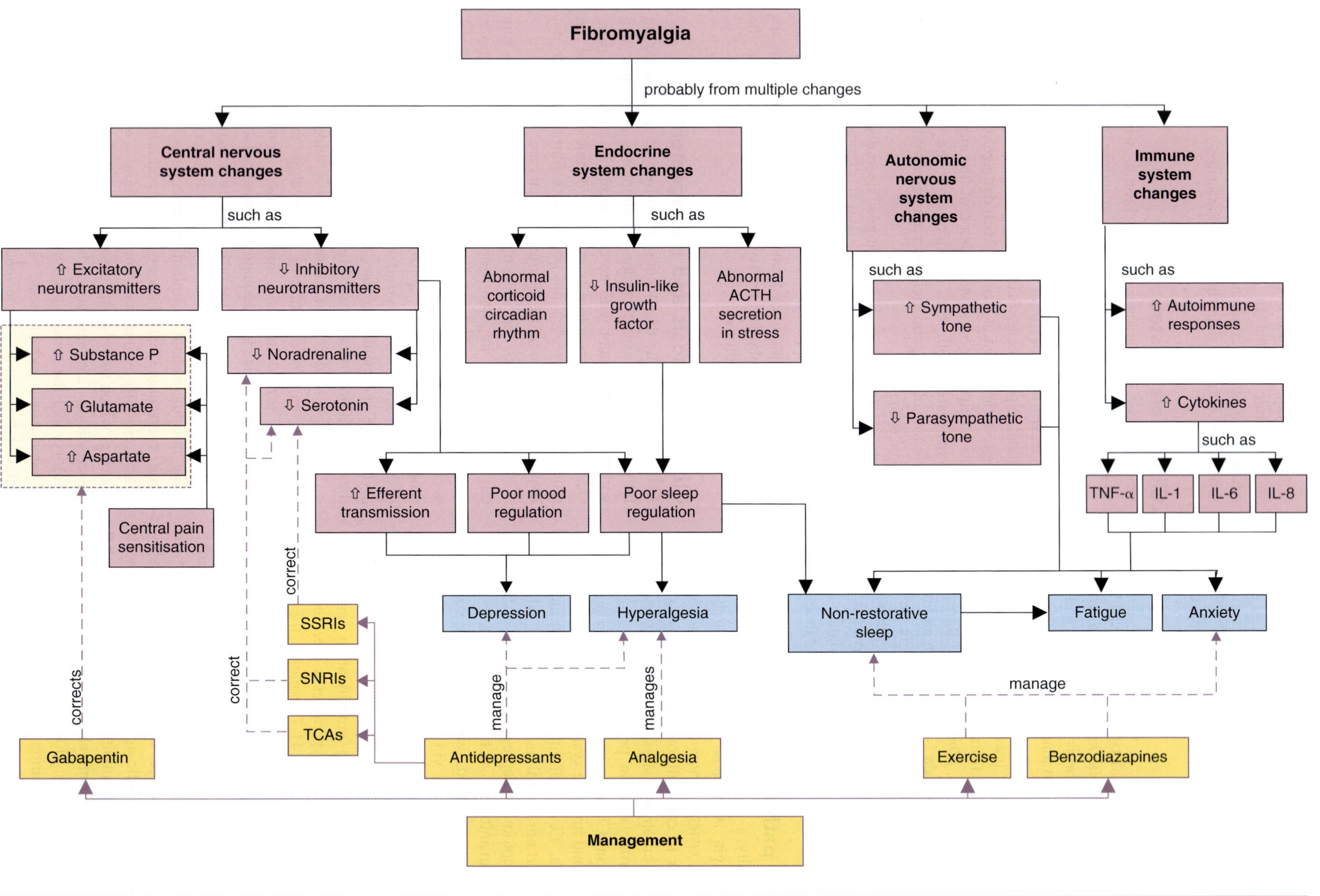

Figure 41.7

Clinical snapshot: Fibromyalgia

↓ = decreased; ↑ = increased; ACTH = adrenocorticotropic hormone; IL = interleukin; SNRIs = selective noradrenaline re-uptake inhibitors; SSRIs = selective serotonin re-uptake inhibitors; TCAs = tricyclic antidepressants; TNF-α = tumour necrosis factor-alpha.

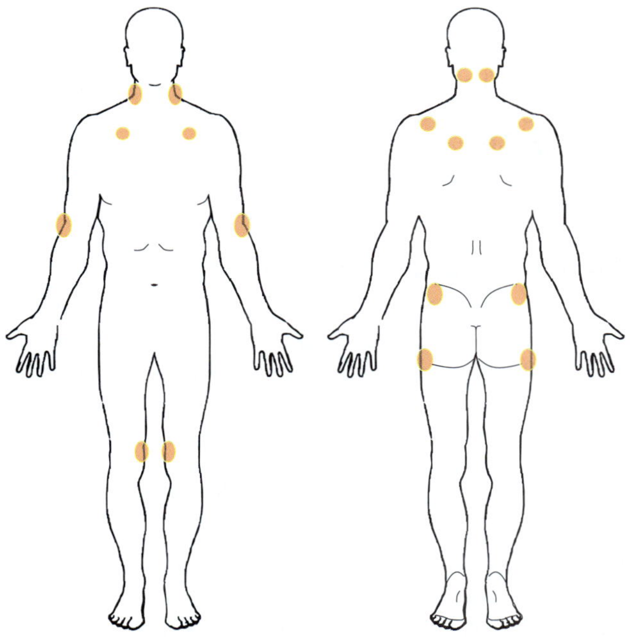

Anterior

Posterior

Figure 41.8

Anterior and posterior body maps of tender point locations in fibromyalgia

In revisions of the diagnostic assessment for fibromyalgia, reliance on tender point examination has been removed. In the revised diagnostic criteria, two symptom-severity scales replace the physical examination of tender points. Pain in all four quadrants of the body for at least three months, and consideration of other multisystem symptoms, are considered diagnostic for fibromyalgia.

Management There is no known cure for fibromyalgia, although the condition may be somewhat self-limiting (point prevalence declines after middle age, suggesting remission in some people). Hence, affected people are guided to expect no cures and to manage fibromyalgia as a chronic condition. Management includes both medication and non-drug treatments to alleviate symptoms.

Three completed Cochrane systematic reviews of treatments for fibromyalgia cover exercise interventions, multidisciplinary rehabilitation and the medication gabapentin for neuropathic pain.

Exercise Although the studies and interventions for fibromyalgia are diverse, the overall conclusions are that supervised aerobic exercise and strength training are beneficial for those with fibromyalgia and improve their physical capacity, but make little difference to tender points or to pain. Therefore, advice suggesting improvements to overall well-being is required, while at the same time ensuring that those affected understand that exact improvements are not the same in everyone and depend partly on the type of exercise undertaken. For people whose primary concerns are pain and tenderness, resistance (strength) training appears to be an important component of an exercise intervention.

It may be difficult for a person with fibromyalgia who is unaccustomed to exercise to determine whether post-exercise tiredness is an aggravation of symptoms or a normal response to exercising, because fatigue is a symptom of fibromyalgia, and tiredness following whole body aerobic exercise is a normal physiological response to having used readily available muscle glycogen stores. Therefore, it may be beneficial for them to consult with clinical exercise healthcare professionals early in their care or for pre-exercise advice, and not only when they are concerned about the adverse effects of exercise.

Multidisciplinary rehabilitation Educational strategies, including behaviour and stress management interventions, combined with physical training, appear to produce some positive effects in the long term, and intuitively appeal to the affected person and practitioners alike.

Medications Several classes of medication are used in the management of fibromyalgia. Currently, antidepressants that alter the reuptake of serotonin and noradrenaline, altering both pain perception and sleep cycles, appear to be effective for many people. Other classes, such as gamma-aminobutyric acid (GABA) analogues, may act by decreasing the release of excitatory and/or pain-generating neurotransmitters and neuropeptides such as glutamate, noradrenaline and substance P.

MYALGIC ENCEPHALOMYELITIS/ CHRONIC FATIGUE SYNDROME (ME/CFS)

Myalgic encephalomyelitis/chronic fatigue syndrome (ME/CFS) (also known as *systemic exertion intolerance disease*) is a long-term disabling and complex condition which has been undergoing many name changes across the past couple of decades. Currently, it is classed under the postviral fatigue syndrome code in the World Health Organization's international ICD-11 classification system. It is characterised by *severe and debilitating fatigue* for a period of at least six months, and is accompanied by *rheumatological, neuropsychological and infection-like symptoms*.

Increasingly, ME/CFS is considered to be a heterogeneous illness involving multiple body systems (neurological, endocrine and immunological) that share similar clinical manifestations. However, the hallmark symptom of this condition is the post-exertional malaise (PEM). ME/CFS can coexist with a number of other illnesses, such as fibromyalgia, irritable bowel syndrome, anxiety disorders and major depression (see the chapter 'Mental health disorders'), multiple chemical sensitivities and temporomandibular joint disorder.

Aetiology and pathophysiology

The aetiology of ME/CFS is complex and multifactorial, with evidence of the involvement of *infectious, immunological and neuropsychological factors*. In terms of genetic factors, ME/CFS may be *familial*, as relatives of people with ME/CFS appear to have higher rates of the condition. Since the COVID-19 pandemic, incidence has increased as many people remain unwell with what appears to be illness similar to ME/CFS.

A comprehensive understanding of the pathophysiology of the condition remains elusive. A number of hypotheses have been tested as to the pathophysiological processes underlying this condition, such as whether ME/CFS is the result of a recognisable infection, an inappropriate immune response that alters central nervous system function, a neuroendocrine disorder, an illness linked to depression, or a psychological response to stimuli in vulnerable people. The evidence pertaining to infectious, immune and neuropsychological parameters is summarised below.

Much effort has been put into the exploration of an immunological basis to ME/CFS. Alterations in immunological parameters have been detected. However, a consistent picture is yet to emerge regarding immune system activation in ME/CFS. A non-specific decrease in lymphocyte proliferation and in natural killer cell cytotoxicity is commonly observed in people with ME/CFS. Increased cytotoxic T cells (Tc cells) bearing specific activation markers have been recorded in people with ME/CFS, as have higher titres of some autoantibodies.

Evidence suggests that certain pathogens such as Epstein–Barr virus, coxsackie B virus, human herpesvirus 6 (HHV-6), and even *Chlamydia pneumoniae* may act as a trigger for ME/CFS, as most people present with elevated titres.

At the level of the central nervous system, changes to neuroendocrine control, sleep maintenance, autonomic nervous system function, motor function, cognition and psychological state have been noted. The activation of the hypothalamic–pituitary–adrenal (HPA) axis is impaired in people with ME/CFS. This suggests an alteration in stress responsiveness. Sleep maintenance is also commonly disrupted, with people with ME/CFS reporting frequent awakenings. It is believed that this disruption may perpetuate the musculoskeletal symptoms in this condition. Disturbances in gait and motor function have also been reported. The normal sympathetic nervous system response to postural changes as measured by tilt-table testing is impaired, leading to hypotension and bradycardia. Alterations in cognitive function are common in people with ME/CFS, manifesting as poor attention, concentration and memory. However, in people with ME/CFS, the changes in biological markers associated with alterations in sleep, the HPA axis and immunity are different from those in people with major depression.

Epidemiology

ME/CFS occurs in both sexes (being marginally more common in women), and is diagnosed in people across the ethnic and socioeconomic spectrum. In Australia within the primary care setting, the prevalence has been estimated at 0.38–0.98%. The typical profile of a person with ME/CFS has been described as an adult between 20 and 50 years of age.

Clinical manifestations

The principal characteristics of ME/CFS include a six-month history of profound fatigue resulting in occupational, personal, educational and social impairment. Other symptoms include post-exertional fatigue unrelieved by rest, an unrefreshing sleep, cognitive impairment, and orthostatic intolerance whereby symptoms are exacerbated by standing. Other manifestations may also occur; however, their nature and presence are more variable in people with ME/CFS. These manifestations include pain and immune system dysfunction, with an increased function of natural killer cells (NK cells) frequently correlating to the severity of illness. Often there may be a concomitant infection and other symptoms associated with immune system activation, such as a sore throat, painful axillary or cervical lymph nodes, and/or a sensitivity to foods or drugs.

Clinical diagnosis and management

Diagnosis Diagnosis is based largely on history and the exclusion of alternative conditions characterised by fatigue and similar clinical manifestations, and the matching of the diagnostic criteria for ME/CFS. A physical examination and laboratory tests may also provide some insight into other possible causes. Conditions that require exclusion are anaemia, thyroid disease, major depression, anxiety states, dementia, connective tissue disease, inflammatory bowel disease, coeliac disease, infection and cancer. Therefore, recommended laboratory tests include a full blood count, erythrocyte sedimentation rate, serum electrolyte, calcium and creatinine levels, liver function tests, thyroid function tests and urinalysis.

Management Once the diagnosis is established, health professionals should develop an individualised plan with the affected person and their family to facilitate rehabilitation—both physical and social—and to promote recovery. The elements of this plan should consist of regular contact with health professionals, education about the condition, access to appropriate services, discouraging excessive rest and social isolation, and evaluating new symptoms and any improvement/deterioration of function.

Inflammatory myopathies

LEARNING OBJECTIVE 5

Explore various inflammatory myopathies, including idiopathic inflammatory myositis and infectious myositis.

Myositis literally means inflammation (*-itis*) of the muscle (*myo-*). Although there are several different types, it is relatively rare. *Idiopathic inflammatory myositis* is the most common group of inflammatory myopathies, and includes *dermatomyositis*, *polymyositis* and *inclusion body myositis*. In Australia, an estimated 3–4 per 100,000 people have inclusion body myositis, and approximately 1–2 per 100,000 people have dermatomyositis or polymyositis. Many other types of myopathies exist, such as *drug-induced myositis*, *infectious myositis* and *myositis ossificans* (where abnormal ossification forms within a muscle). However, this chapter only elaborates on idiopathic inflammatory myositis and infectious myositis.

IDIOPATHIC INFLAMMATORY MYOSITIS

Idiopathic inflammatory myositis is a group of connective tissue disorders that results in *chronic inflammation and muscle weakness in the proximal muscles* (neck, shoulders, hip flexors

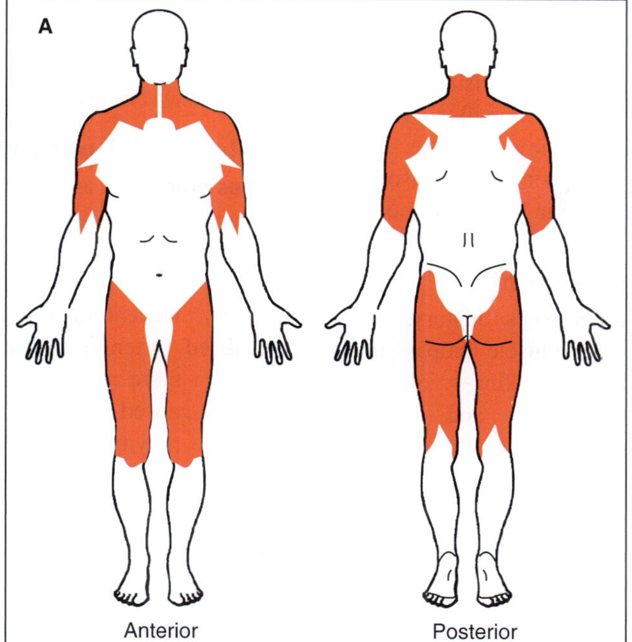

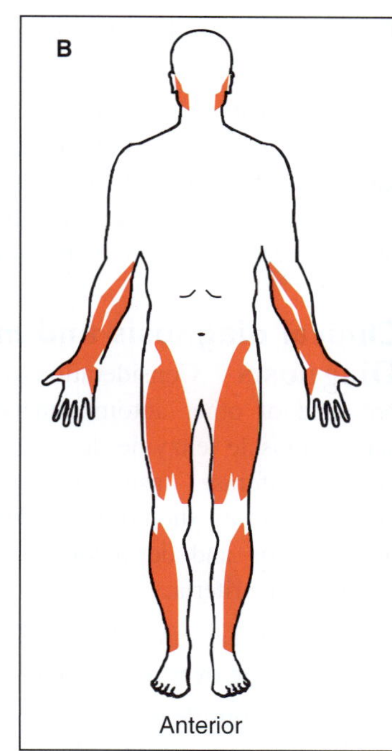

Figure 41.9

The muscles involved in idiopathic inflammatory myositis

(A) Polymyositis and dermatomyositis.
(B) Inclusion body myositis.

and upper legs). The three subclassifications of this systemic connective tissue disorder are polymyositis, dermatomyositis and inclusion body myositis. Figure 41.9 demonstrates the different muscles involved in polymyositis and dermatomyositis compared to inclusion body myositis.

Aetiology and pathophysiology

The term 'idiopathic' suggests that the cause of this disorder is unknown; however, it is thought to be an autoimmune process. Polymyositis and inclusion body myositis result in an *inflammatory response* mediated by Tc cells. The inflammatory process for dermatomyositis appears to be mediated through the complement system, with membrane attack complexes causing vascular destruction and resulting in B cell and dendritic cell infiltration. Chronic inflammation is maintained by a positive feedback loop with the sustained release of inflammatory mediators. Defective energy metabolism systems appear to develop in polymyositis and dermatomyositis, evidence of which is supported by the poor correlation between muscle inflammation and the degree of muscle weakness. This is also supported by the fact that people rarely experience complete recovery of strength with treatment, despite a significant reduction or elimination of inflammatory infiltrates.

Polymyositis

Polymyositis is predominantly seen in females, and commonly diagnosed at about 20 years of age.

Clinical manifestations *Progressive symmetric muscle weakness* develops over weeks to months, and generally affects the large proximal limb muscles and neck extensors. The muscle weakness is often insidious, but can occasionally occur abruptly. People can also complain of myalgia, and the affected muscles are generally tender on palpation. As there is no neural component, sensory and reflex assessments are normal. Polymyositis is also frequently associated with cardiac and interstitial lung disease. Dysphagia and oesophageal dysfunction can be experienced in older people.

Dermatomyositis

Dermatomyositis is seen more commonly in females, with peak prevalence occurring in children at about 7 years of age, and in adults between 30 and 50 years of age.

Clinical manifestations Many of the signs and symptoms of polymyositis occur in dermatomyositis, with the added dimension of cutaneous manifestations. A number of different types of rashes can occur in dermatomyositis; however, these will generally resolve before the onset of muscle weakness:

- *Gottron's papules* is an erythematous, scaly rash over the metacarpophalangeal and interphalangeal joints.
- *Mechanic's hands* is an erythematous, cracking rash on the lateral aspects of the fingernail beds (periungual).
- The *V sign* is an erythematous, macular rash on the anterior neck and chest.
- The *heliotype rash* is a violaceous (violet-coloured) rash over the eyelids. This rash is commonly associated with periorbital oedema.
- *Poikiloderma vasculare atrophicans* is an erythematous rash over the anterior neck, chest, posterior shoulders, back and buttocks.

Inclusion body myositis

Inclusion body myositis is more common in men over 50 years of age. The onset is slow, and the response to therapy tends to be poor.

Clinical manifestations

Inclusion body myositis results in muscle weakness, most often *asymmetrical* in nature. Commonly more distal muscle groups (e.g. wrist and finger flexors, ankle dorsiflexors and knee extensors) are affected early in the clinical course. Jaw muscle weakness and dysphagia are also common. Sensory–neurological assessment is intact, and myalgia is not common.

Clinical diagnosis and management

Diagnosis Consideration of a person's history, the presence of other autoimmune diseases, muscle biopsy and serum muscle enzyme levels (i.e. creatine kinase, alanine aminotransferase, aspartate aminotransferase and lactate dehydrogenase) should be undertaken. The classification of polymyositis and dermatomyositis are commonly used, and include five criteria:

1. Symmetrical muscle weakness in selected locations developing over weeks to months.
2. Positive muscle biopsy:
   dermatomyositis—$CD4^+$ T cells, perivascular infiltration
   polymyositis—$CD8^+$ T cells and B cells
3. Elevation of serum muscle enzyme levels.
4. Electromyographic evidence of changes.
5. For dermatomyositis, the presence of a distinct dermatomyositis-type rash.

In inclusion body myositis, non-necrotic fibres, vacuolated muscle fibres and amyloid deposits are seen on muscle biopsy.

Management Polymyositis and dermatomyositis are both managed with corticosteroids in an attempt to reduce the inflammatory process. Complications associated with chronic corticosteroid use can complicate care and result in issues such as osteoporosis. Myositis can also be associated with cancers, and whether the disease process increases the risk of cancer or whether it can be related to decreased tumour surveillance as a result of immunosuppression, the affected person should be monitored for cancers, including bladder, cervical, ovarian and pancreatic cancer. Non-Hodgkin lymphoma and several respiratory cancers, such as lung and nasopharyngeal cancers, have also been associated with myositis.

Poorer outcomes are associated with later diagnosis and in people with cardiovascular or respiratory illness. Dysphagia complicates recovery as well, and those with cricopharyngeal muscle involvement may develop aspiration pneumonia or other complications associated with dysphagia. Surgical formation of a gastrostomy tube can reduce the risk of pneumonia and improve nutrition.

Unfortunately, inclusion body myositis is incurable, and management is aimed at reducing disease progression. Various immunomodulating agents have been trialled, with varying degrees of failure reported. Although no treatment regimen has been accepted as successful, it is not uncommon for people to receive corticosteroids in an attempt to reduce inflammation and, therefore, disease progression. Participation in exercise programs is also suggested, and may assist with aerobic fitness, but does not appear to improve muscle strength.

INFECTIOUS MYOSITIS

Aetiology and pathophysiology

Infectious myositis is an *infection in the muscle*, which is most often caused by *bacteria*, but can also be caused by *viruses*, *parasites or fungi*. It can result from either haematogenous spread or directly into the muscle in instances of trauma or surgery. Depending on the organism, the infection may be localised (often from bacteria) or it may be widespread, resulting in more multifocal myalgia. Bacterial infections are commonly caused by *Staphylococcus aureus*. However, they can also be polymicrobial. Muscle trauma, bites from insects that become infected, skin infections and the use of illicit drugs by injection increase the risk of infectious myositis, as does being immunocompromised.

Clinical manifestations

The clinical course of **pyomyositis** can be divided into three stages: invasive, suppurative and septicaemic stages. After colonisation, an inflammatory response will occur, and the affected area becomes oedematous and painful. The person may also develop fever and malaise, depending on the severity and the organism causing the infection. This is known as the *invasive stage*. In the *suppurative stage*, an abscess may form and result in the collection of pus, but early on the developing lesion may be confused with muscle strain, haematoma or thrombosis. If the infection becomes systemic, the final stage is *septicaemia*, which can result in septic shock. Infectious myositis caused by a virus or a parasite commonly results in a more diffuse myalgia.

Clinical diagnosis and management

Diagnosis In pyomyositis, the bacterial infection is commonly diagnosed in the suppurative stage, where an abscess can be more readily detected. The large muscle groups of the legs are commonly affected, including the quadriceps and the gluteus group. Aspiration and assessment of the fluid for microscopy, culture and sensitivity may result in identification of the causative bacteria, and the use of ultrasound, computed tomography (CT) or magnetic resonance imaging (MRI) will enable quantification of the size of the abscess. Although pathology results are often of little benefit, leukocytosis is often present, and myositis from parasites will generally result in eosinophilia.

Management Initially, broad-spectrum antimicrobials should be administered. However, as culture and sensitivity information becomes available, more specific, narrow-spectrum antimicrobials should be used. Bacterial myositis can also develop without an abscess. A particularly aggressive and potentially fatal type of infection can be caused by *Streptococcus* spp. Group A streptococcal necrotising myositis is a rapidly developing infection resulting in tissue lysis, bacteraemia and, potentially, multisystem organ failure. Other bacteria can also cause necrosis. 'Gas gangrene' is an infectious myositis caused by *Clostridium* species. It, too, can lead to devastating clinical sequelae. Both of these infections can result in significant tissue loss even with aggressive management. As with most bacterial infections, the administration of antimicrobials is central to their management. Other treatments may include surgical debridement, fasciotomy and, more recently, hyperbaric oxygen therapy.

Viral myositis can be caused by many viruses, but influenza A or B are most commonly involved, although enteroviruses, hepatitis B and C, Epstein–Barr virus and human immunodeficiency virus (HIV) are also associated. Myalgia during a viral infection is relatively common; however, post-influenza myositis causes severe calf pain that may even interfere with ambulation. It is commonly associated with elevations in serum creatine kinase and lactate dehydrogenase. Treatment is most often limited to analgesia, as viral myositis is generally self-limiting. Occasionally, influenza-associated rhabdomyolysis can occur and result in tissue loss, compartment syndrome, renal failure and life-threatening cardiac dysrhythmia. Rhabdomyolysis is associated with damaged skeletal muscle cells releasing myoglobin, electrolytes and other intracellular substances that can enter the circulation and injure vital organs such as the kidneys and heart (for more details, see later in the chapter). Virus-induced rhabdomyolysis is caused by immunological processes initiated by the presence of myotoxic cytokines released as a result of the direct invasion of the virus into the myocyte. Management of virus-induced rhabdomyolysis includes symptom management—such as intravenous fluid support and volume expansion, to correct metabolic anomalies—analgesia and hyperkalaemia management as necessary.

The variety of pathogens that can cause infectious myositis can account for the myriad clinical presentations possible. From localised benign abscess formation through to widespread, generalised problems, such as myalgia, and even to potentially life-threatening consequences such as circulatory shock or rhabdomyolysis, the key to clinical management is related to the causative organism and the presenting and potential signs and symptoms.

Muscular dystrophy

LEARNING OBJECTIVE 6

Discuss the pathophysiology, clinical manifestations and management of muscular dystrophy.

Muscular dystrophy is a group of *inherited muscle disorders* resulting in weakness, loss of function and, ultimately, degeneration of muscles. The weakness is not as a result of central or peripheral nerve involvement, and it is not an inflammatory disorder. Although there are several types of muscular dystrophy, this section focuses only on *Duchenne's muscular dystrophy*. Muscular dystrophy is relatively uncommon in Australia. Of the 3,600 people admitted for myopathies in 2020–21, only 315 people had muscular dystrophy. Muscular Dystrophy Australia estimates approximately 1 baby in 20,000 is born with congenital muscular dystrophy, resulting in a rate of an estimated 0.08% of Australia's population.

AETIOLOGY AND PATHOPHYSIOLOGY

A substance called **dystrophin** is important for cellular stability and is necessary for myocyte integrity. In muscular dystrophy, genetic defects can result in either *a reduction in or an absence of dystrophin*, and intracellular components can leak out of the muscle cells. As necrosis occurs, the tissue is replaced by an infiltrate that may resemble myocyte hypertrophy, but does not result from myocyte growth; rather, it results from a fibrous and fatty substance.

CLINICAL MANIFESTATIONS

Children with Duchenne's muscular dystrophy will have motor difficulties, resulting in a delay in the age at which they first begin to ambulate. Those with muscular dystrophy may, in the early stages, have gait abnormalities, especially a waddling gait with a wide base. As the disease progresses, an increase in the number of falls may be observed. Children will develop difficulty in getting up from a lying or sitting position. Contractures can develop, as can scoliosis. Proximal muscle weakness develops as the disease progresses. The average life expectancy for a person with Duchenne's muscular dystrophy is between 19 and 30 years of age, with death resulting from pulmonary complications or cardiovascular deterioration.

CLINICAL DIAGNOSIS AND MANAGEMENT

Diagnosis

Physical assessment and an evaluation of the personal and family history are important in assessing a child for Duchenne's muscular dystrophy. The Gower's manoeuvre is used to rise from the floor, and is suggestive of proximal muscle weakness. In this manoeuvre, the child must turn prone, place both hands on the floor, walk their legs forward, and then use their hands on top of their thighs to rise from the floor. Blood drawn for biochemical analysis will show an elevated creatine phosphokinase (CPK) level, and these elevations may be high at the beginning of the disease process (as there is more muscle mass). However, as the disease progresses, CPK levels can be significantly reduced as the muscle mass reduces. Genetic investigations using the polymerase chain reaction (PCR) can detect almost all known dystrophin gene deletions.

Management

Currently, there is no cure for Duchenne's muscular dystrophy, and management involves maintenance of muscle function for as long as possible, management of scoliosis with surgery as required, and prevention of cardiovascular and respiratory complications as far as possible. Physiotherapy is pivotal to maintaining muscle strength and function, and to preventing contractures. Ankle–foot orthoses are applied at night to delay contracture formation. Children who lose ambulation early are generally likely to develop respiratory failure more quickly, and ultimately may require mechanical ventilation earlier in their disease process. Nocturnal ventilation by non-invasive methods (such as continuous positive airway pressure [CPAP] or bilevel positive airway pressure [BiPAP]) may be needed to support respiratory function for several years. Prevention of chest infections should be managed with good pulmonary hygiene and regular chest physiotherapy. Influenza vaccination should also be administered annually. Observation for dysphagia is important to prevent the risk of aspiration pneumonia. Enteral feeds through a gastrostomy tube will be required later in the disease, and will also support nutrient needs. If respiratory decline from upper respiratory tract infection occurs, antimicrobials should be commenced as soon as possible.

Although the cause of Duchenne's muscular dystrophy is not inflammatory, some degree of inflammation occurs as a result of muscle destruction. Therefore, corticosteroids are used as the main pharmacological intervention. Unfortunately, drug-associated complications, such as reduced bone mineral density and increased risk of fracture, can develop. Vitamin supplementation and bisphosphonate therapy should be administered to reduce bone loss.

LEARNING OBJECTIVE 7

Explore various muscle conditions, including atrophy, contractures, cramps and delayed-onset muscle soreness.

Muscle atrophy

DISUSE ATROPHY

Aetiology and pathophysiology

Disuse atrophy is a straightforward physiological response to inactivity resulting in the *regression of muscle size and strength*; it is not a pathology per se. *Disuse osteopenia* is similarly regarded. It generally occurs secondary to immobilisation as a result of managing another injury or illness. If muscles or bones are not regularly contracted or loaded, respectively, then these tissues reduce in size and mass. *In muscle*, disuse atrophy occurs as reduction in muscle cross-sectional area. *In bone*, disuse osteopenia presents as reduced bone mineral mass. In both conditions, the underlying architecture of the disused tissue is preserved but the reduced tissue is weakened, and the risk of tissue damage with minor trauma is increased.

Clinical diagnosis and management

Diagnosis Atrophy is expected, and therefore investigation is not necessarily warranted. However, quantification of the extent of disuse atrophy may be ascertained through an examination of the affected limbs with particular attention to size and, if possible, symmetry (when compared to an unaffected limb).

Management Healthcare practitioners do not often see people with uncomplicated disuse atrophy, except when removing casts and splints following the healing of orthopaedic injuries. Management of this condition is through the graduated resumption of activity, taking care not to exceed the load-bearing capacity of the tissues at any stage. More commonly, people come to the attention of healthcare practitioners when disuse atrophy has occurred (perhaps due to a sedentary lifestyle, prolonged rest or bed rest, or the use of a wheelchair), followed by the occurrence of another injury, such as a muscle tear or a tendon rupture under load that would not typically produce that injury. In these cases, management of the traumatic injury is the primary concern, with care, where possible, not to exacerbate the disuse atrophy through the immobilisation of injured limbs.

Because these tissues are alive, and the structural integrity of the tissues persists throughout disuse, these conditions are equally able to be reversed by the resumption of activity. When muscles are used against resistance (strength training), they hypertrophy (increase in cross-sectional area) and become stronger. When bones are placed under weight-bearing load, they increase in cortical density and become stronger.

Unfortunately, the management of disuse atrophy in clinical practice is not quite so simple. Atrophy of both muscle and bone is clinically silent. There is no pain and no perception that tissues are weakening. Age-related decline in muscle and bone strength compounds the tissue loss due to disuse. Moreover, it is a common failing of some people to remember physical triumphs and play down physical declines, leading to a tendency to attempt physical tasks that may exceed their current physical capacities. Injury risk in people with disuse atrophy increases if there is an attempt to restart activity too rapidly.

DENERVATION ATROPHY

Aetiology and pathophysiology

When the nerves supplying skeletal muscle are damaged by disease, trauma, ischaemia, tumours or toxins, muscles innervated by the affected nerve rapidly undergo a significant reduction in muscle mass. The degree of *wasting also depends on the severity of the nerve damage*. If a nerve is only partly injured through compression or partial tear, some function may remain and a diminished stimulus may still get through, resulting in less severe atrophy. In situations such as complete flaccid paralysis from prolonged periods where no neuromuscular stimulation transpires, substantial fibrotic changes to the connective tissue ensheathing the affected muscle (endomysium and perimysium) occur from increased levels of fibronectin, collagen type I and collagen type III.

Many conditions can cause **denervation atrophy**. *Physical trauma* directly to a nerve generally occurs as a result of compression, stretching or severing. This may occur in motor vehicle accidents, falls or sporting injuries. Damage can occur centrally (within the spinal cord) or peripherally (on distal nerves leading to limbs). *Indirect injury* to a nerve from trauma may occur as a result of immense, confined swelling of the tissue that compresses the nerve and results in ischaemia. *Systemic diseases* causing nerve damage include diabetes mellitus, which results in peripheral neuropathy, and renal or hepatic disease, which result in the failure to clear toxic substances from the systemic circulation; these can cause chemical imbalances, resulting in the destruction of nerves. *Tumours, vascular damage, vitamin deficiencies and infections* can all result in nerve damage. Such injury will often result in denervation atrophy.

Clinical manifestations

People will experience loss of muscle mass and report loss of strength or paralysis.

Clinical diagnosis and management

Diagnosis A physical assessment and the collection of a full medical history is a critical place to start. **Electromyography** and nerve conduction velocity studies can be undertaken to determine nerve function. Imaging studies, such as CT or MRI, may indicate the presence of a tumour or a structural anomaly. The presence of systemic disease, such as endocrine, renal or hepatic dysfunction, may be determined by blood analysis.

Management Depending on the cause and potential long-term outcomes, interventions may be attempted. In denervation atrophy, attempting to re-innervate muscle would be the goal. However, often this may not be achievable. In spinal cord injury (see the chapter 'Nerotrauma') or inherited, incurable neuromuscular disease, there is little chance of muscle recovery.

If long-term recovery is possible, the use of a transcutaneous electrical nerve stimulus (TENS) device may be attempted. These appliances are applied to the skin above the target muscle, and deliver electrical stimuli through the skin and into the structures directly beneath the electrode pads. This stimulation can, artificially, sequentially innervate the muscle to cause intermittent contractions and thus prevent permanent atrophy. This type of treatment is called functional electrical stimulation. It will not cure the damaged nerve, but will reduce the atrophy-associated changes in the muscle, in the hope that future treatment modalities can heal nerve tissue; otherwise, after a few years, atrophy-induced muscle changes will render the muscle unsuitable for future advancements.

Muscle contractures

AETIOLOGY AND PATHOPHYSIOLOGY

Contractures involve the *shortening of a muscle–tendon unit or surrounding skin*, reducing the full range of joint movement. Although the mechanism by which they develop is poorly understood, it is known that many conditions can result in contractures. *Trauma or insult to the brain or spinal cord* are common causes. However, *musculoskeletal conditions and burns* can also result in conditions that lead to significantly reduced range of movement in a joint. *Other factors* include incorrect positioning of an immobilised joint, frequent muscle spasm, and absent or inadequate range-of-motion exercises. Contractures have a negative effect on quality of life, causing pain and interfering with activities of daily living. They complicate mobility and positioning, and can result in pressure areas. As children are still undergoing bone growth, sustained pressure from the muscle tone can deform bone and produce abnormal rotation.

Contractures can be neurally- or non-neurally-mediated. *Neurally-mediated contractures* are a result of excessive motor tone, and cause prolonged involuntary reflex muscle contraction. *Non-neurally-mediated contractures* occur as a result of a shortening of skin or connective tissue, such as happens in burns, where, as scar tissue develops, structures underneath the tightening burn scar can inhibit movement and result in muscle-atrophy shortening of associated joint structures, such as tendons and ligaments.

CLINICAL MANIFESTATIONS

The two main signs of contracture are a significant decrease in joint range of motion because of stiff resistance and atrophy of the underlying muscle.

CLINICAL DIAGNOSIS AND MANAGEMENT

Diagnosis

Physical assessment is the cornerstone to the diagnosis of contracture. Assessment of joint range of motion, muscle strength and tone, and peripheral nervous system function should be undertaken.

Management

As with most conditions, prevention is better than cure. It is easier to prevent contracture than it is to manage the care of someone with severe contractures. The use of appropriate positioning, range-of-motion exercises and the application of splinting devices can reduce the risk of contracture development.

Although the interventions for prevention are the same as those for management, more recent research suggests that the current practices involving range-of-motion exercises and stretching are of less benefit than previously considered. A challenge to examine the current management practices is warranted. The complexity and seriousness of contracture development demands research into more effective ways to prevent and manage this problem.

Muscle cramp

AETIOLOGY AND PATHOPHYSIOLOGY

Cramps are *acute, involuntary muscle contractions causing intense myalgia*. They differ from contractures in that they resolve quickly and are generally not associated with significant pathological conditions. Cramps can be divided into skeletal and smooth muscle types.

Most people have experienced *skeletal muscle cramps*, which are commonly associated with *electrolyte imbalance*, such as low sodium, potassium or magnesium levels, *overstretching a muscle* or *muscle fatigue. Reduced peripheral blood flow* resulting from disease processes, such as atherosclerosis, can also result in muscle cramp from reduced nutrient delivery. Although the pathophysiology of skeletal muscle cramps is poorly understood, it is thought that cramps occur as a result of a homeostatic imbalance in the high-energy metabolic pathways.

Smooth muscle cramps can occur in women during menstruation, and can contribute to dysmenorrhoea (see the chapter 'Female reproductive disorders'). It is thought that cramps in a woman's reproductive system during menstruation are a result of *increased levels of pro-inflammatory mediators*, such as prostaglandin, which cause myometrial ischaemia and prolonged uterine contractions.

Smooth muscle cramps also occur in infections of the gastrointestinal system and are sometimes referred to as *spasms. Gastrointestinal and urinary system cramps* are also thought to be caused by the release of inflammatory mediators, which result in the contraction of the muscles of a hollow organ around non-compressible air or fluid, increasing pressures within the lining of the organ, which is then sensed by local baroreceptors and interpreted as pain in the cortex.

CLINICAL MANIFESTATIONS

The location and type of muscle affected (i.e. smooth or skeletal) will influence the type and quality of symptoms experienced; however, one distinctive and common symptom is pain. An example can be seen in gastritis, where cramps from spasmodic contractions of the muscles around the intestines occur from inflammatory mediators released as a result of the presence of a pathogen. Other examples include contractions of the muscles around the gall bladder from infection or blockage, causing the colicky pain renowned in cholecystitis (see the chapter 'Disorders of the liver, the gall bladder and the pancreas'), or dysuria from a urinary tract infection, causing bladder irritation and subsequent detrusor muscle spasm (see the chapter 'Common inflammatory disorders of the kidneys and urinary tract'). Skeletal muscle cramps while exercising can occur in any muscle, but are common in the quadriceps, hamstrings and gastrocnemius muscles. Some people also experience intercostal muscle or abdominal cramps during exercise.

CLINICAL DIAGNOSIS AND MANAGEMENT

Diagnosis

The depth of investigation will depend on the cause of the muscle cramps, and whether they are resulting from smooth muscle or skeletal muscle contraction. A thorough assessment of the conditions surrounding the development of the muscle cramp can be elucidated by the collection of an adequate history. Blood may be drawn for biochemical investigation to determine whether there are any electrolyte imbalances. Other investigations to identify infective processes may also occur, such as an assessment of temperature to determine whether the person is febrile, or the culturing of blood or other appropriate body fluids for the presence of pathogens.

Management

Skeletal muscle cramps can often be prevented by increasing fitness and flexibility in a graded exercise program, including a suitable warm-up and stretching component. It would also be valuable to pay particular attention to the stretching of the specific muscle groups where the person experiences cramping. The management of skeletal muscle cramping during exercise includes stopping the activity that causes the cramps, and if possible applying a gentle stretch to the affected muscle group and holding it until the cramp subsides. If cramp develops after a period of sustained exercise where electrolyte imbalance may be considered a reasonable cause, drinking sports drinks containing electrolyte supplementation may be indicated. Skeletal muscle cramps rarely require further medical assessment or intervention, and subside quickly.

Managing smooth muscle cramps is targeted at the cause. If bacterial infection is identified, the person may require a course of antimicrobials to reduce the cause of the inflammatory response. Smooth muscle cramping associated with menstrual pain can be managed with non-steroidal anti-inflammatory drugs (NSAIDs), which reduce the production of prostaglandin and other pro-inflammatory mediators. This intervention works best if the NSAIDs are taken at early onset of the cramping to reduce the volume of inflammatory substances produced. Further investigation and management may be required if the cause is as a result of serious pathology or is less obvious to the clinician.

Delayed onset muscle soreness (DOMS)

AETIOLOGY AND PATHOPHYSIOLOGY

Delayed onset muscle soreness (DOMS) occurs when people experience *skeletal muscle discomfort following periods of unaccustomed exercise*. There is still debate regarding the mechanism of its development. However, several theories have been posed. Many believe that DOMS is caused by the accumulation of lactic acid in muscles. Empirical evidence does not support this opinion, however. Other theories focus on damage and remodelling as a result of mechanical and biochemical injury. An inflammatory response occurs, and oedema within the muscle tissue may cause pain from pressure and the release of chemical mediators stimulating sensitised pain receptors. C-fibres are distributed throughout a muscle, and action potentials can be elicited by chemical, mechanical and thermal stimuli.

CLINICAL MANIFESTATIONS

Three distinct clinical manifestations occur in DOMS. *Muscle soreness*, *muscle stiffness* and *loss of strength* are the symptoms reported between eight and 48 hours following the activity, and resolve within five to seven days of onset. Muscle strength diminishes during DOMS, and is not proportional to the discomfort experienced. Damage to sarcomeres from mechanical injury and/or fatigue occurs, and is worse in eccentric exercise (exercise that produces the lengthening of a contracted muscle as the external force exceeds the strength of the muscle). Muscle stiffness may occur as a result of altered intracellular calcium homeostasis, owing to either sarcoplasmic reticulum dysfunction or issues with the integrity of the sarcolemma.

CLINICAL DIAGNOSIS AND MANAGEMENT

Diagnosis

A person with DOMS will rarely present to a healthcare practitioner for assessment and management of this condition. However, the collection of a history, including the type, duration and level of intensity of any exercise or manual labour, would be an appropriate approach. There are no diagnostic tests for DOMS.

Management

DOMS is self-limiting, and rarely results in the need for clinical intervention. Research into potential methods to reduce discomfort continues. One of the most effective techniques to reduce DOMS is to lightly exercise the affected muscles. The effects are only temporary, as the soreness returns soon after exercise ceases, yet conditioning of the muscles will occur if the training continues. For élite or professional athletes, some interventions may include the use of compression devices, such as external pneumatic compression equipment, ice-water immersion, massage and the use of pulsed ultrasound to reduce inflammation. Prevention through the use of an appropriately designed, graded exercise program with a focus on repetitive eccentric activity can reduce the effects of unaccustomed exercise.

Rhabdomyolysis

LEARNING OBJECTIVE 8

Identify the causes and management of rhabdomyolysis.

AETIOLOGY AND PATHOPHYSIOLOGY

Rhabdomyolysis is the *destruction of muscle tissue* in response to the *failure of calcium homeostasis inside the myocyte*. When excess extracellular calcium leaks into the myocyte, a cascade begins an abnormal interaction between the actin and myosin, which ultimately destroys the cell. Myocyte destruction results in the release of intracellular contents (including myoglobin, potassium, phosphate, creatine kinase and urate), which may enter systemic circulation. If significant muscle destruction has occurred, a substantial volume of these formerly intracellular agents can cause catastrophic clinical outcomes, including hyperkalaemia, metabolic acidosis and even cardiac arrest. Renal clearance of the free (unbound) myoglobin is overwhelmed and the renal tubules are destroyed, resulting in acute renal failure. Common causes of rhabdomyolysis include crush injury, electrocution, excessive heat stroke, infection and even some medications (e.g. the use of statins and some antipsychotic drugs).

CLINICAL MANIFESTATIONS

Early in the clinical course, there may be little evidence of rhabdomyolysis. The urine may discolour and become more brownish (tea-coloured). Myalgia may be reported, but is not universal; and fever and malaise are common. If the rhabdomyolysis progresses to a more severe occurrence, lower back pain may be reported consistent with renal involvement. Symptoms of decreasing renal function and renal failure may follow, including oliguria or anuria, oedema and electrolyte imbalances. Disseminated intravascular coagulopathy (DIC) can be a complication of rhabdomyolysis, so observations for bleeding or clotting should be undertaken.

CLINICAL DIAGNOSIS AND MANAGEMENT

Diagnosis

Physical assessment and the collection of a thorough history, with a focus on known causes of rhabdomyolysis, are critical. Blood taken for biochemical analysis will demonstrate electrolyte imbalances, including hyperkalaemia, hyperphosphataemia and hypocalcaemia, an increase in creatine kinase, and the renal markers urea and creatinine. As DIC is a possible complication of rhabdomyolysis, a coagulation profile (platelets, prothrombin time, activated partial thromboplastin time) should be collected.

Management

Promoting renal function is critical in the management of rhabdomyolysis. Intravenous hydration with crystalloid fluids to ensure urine output above 200 mL/h may reduce renal damage. The use of diuretics and urinary alkalinisers may also reduce damage to renal tubules. The management of electrolyte imbalance is important. Hyperkalaemia must be controlled through the use of gastrointestinal potassium binders, such as sodium polystyrene sulfonate, insulin–glucose infusion or dialysis as the clinical picture requires. If DIC occurs, management of bleeding should be achieved with fresh frozen plasma, platelets or cryoprecipitate infusions.

INDIGENOUS HEALTH FAST FACTS AND CULTURAL CONSIDERATIONS

FAST FACTS

- *Aboriginal and Torres Strait Islander peoples are more likely to experience facial fractures from assault, whereas the mechanism for non-Indigenous Australians is mostly related to sport or fall.*
- *Aboriginal and Torres Strait Islander men are 1.5 times more likely, and women 1.25 times more likely, than non-Indigenous Australians to experience a hip fracture.*
- *Little information exists regarding myopathy and rhabdomyolysis in Aboriginal and Torres Strait Islander peoples. However, individual case presentations and anecdotal evidence suggest that there is an increased risk of statin-induced myopathy in Indigenous Australians. Further investigation and research are required.*
- *Falls and interpersonal violence were the cause of more facial fractures in Māori and Pacific Islands people than European New Zealanders.*

- *Māori visit a doctor for sprains and strains at similar rates to non-Māori New Zealanders.*
- *Māori and Pacific Islands people are less likely than European New Zealanders to consult a general practitioner for regional pain disorders (including fibromyalgia).*
- *Anecdotal evidence appears to show that muscular dystrophy in Māori and Pacific Islands people is extremely rare, although this has not been confirmed by formal research.*

CULTURAL CONSIDERATIONS

- *Bone health is strongly influenced by diet, and the consumption of a well-balanced diet particularly rich in calcium is most important in the prepubescent years when the child's calcium storage processes are at their peak capacity. Unfortunately, Aboriginal and Torres Strait Islander nutrition is an area of significant disparity, not only in food quality, but also in affordability and availability. Despite many government attempts at program development to address nutritional inequalities, few have succeeded in providing any observable, sustainable or reproducible outcomes to improve nutrition-related health conditions. It is clear that significant, radical and urgent change is needed so the development of culturally competent, sustainable nutrition programs to improve Aboriginal and Torres Strait Islander community nutrition knowledge and access can be found. It appears that these programs would be best derived after significant community consultation, and negotiation with the open-minded, willing purse-string holders of the nation's health dollars. Primary health programs must be at least part of the solution to reduce this significant healthcare gap.*

Sources: Data from Australian Institute of Health and Welfare (2022); Diab et al. (2023); Monk et al. (2022).

CHILDREN AND ADOLESCENTS

- Young children are more prone to fractures than to sprains and strains, because their growth plates are weaker than their ligaments, muscles and tendons.
- Greenstick fractures are common in young children and may take longer to heal, because they occur in the middle of the diaphysis, which heals/grows at a slower rate.
- Injuries to growth plates in prepubescent children may result in limb length discrepancy.
- Duchenne's muscular dystrophy commonly develops in children between 2 and 6 years of age.
- Children rarely report experiences of delayed-onset muscle soreness.
- Until recently, it was thought that children do not develop fibromyalgia. However, now it is thought that between 1% and 7% of children may have a musculoskeletal pain syndrome of some type.

OLDER ADULTS

- Reducing bone mass in ageing results in a significantly increased risk of fracture in the older adult, which is associated with high mortality and morbidity.
- Two-thirds of hospitalisations as a result of falls in people over 65 years of age involve at least one fracture.
- Femur fracture is the most common injury in older adults who fall. It is estimated that 1 in 3 older Australians fall in their home, annually.
- An increased prevalence of fibromyalgia occurs in older adults between 60 and 79 years of age.
- Fibromyalgia symptoms generally increase with age.
- Occulopharyngeal dystrophy is a form of muscular dystrophy, and can affect adults after 40 years of age.
- Treatment of hyperlipidaemia with statins in older adults increases the risk of myopathy, especially if used concomitantly with grapefruit juice, some common cardiovascular medications and macrolide antibiotics.

KEY CLINICAL ISSUES

- Mobility, protection and support are all important roles of the musculoskeletal system. Trauma may interfere with any of these roles.
- Pain, vascular damage and nerve damage may develop as a result of musculoskeletal trauma. Assessments should be sufficiently comprehensive to identify any of these adverse outcomes.
- In cases of fracture, meticulous assessment is required of both the peripheral vasculature (colour, temperature, capillary refill, peripheral pulses and oedema) and neurological systems (sensation, motor function and pain).
- The overall goals of treatment are: anatomical realignment of bone fragments (reduction); immobilisation to maintain realignment; and restoration of normal or near-normal function of the injured part.
- Treatment may include open or closed reduction, traction, casts, external or internal fixation, and analgesia and non-steroidal anti-inflammatory drugs.
- Treatment is directed towards effective pain management, maintenance of nutrition, and prevention of complications associated with the trauma and immobility.
- Trauma to the musculoskeletal system may impair function and contribute to a person's inability to perform activities of daily living (ADLs), such as bathing, dressing and eating, and instrumental activities of daily living (IADLs), such as managing finances, preparing food, managing transportation and housekeeping.
- When dependence occurs, it can result in a loss of self-esteem, the perception of decreased quality of life and depression.
- Health professionals play an important role in public education about the basic principles of safety and accident prevention.
- Health professionals assist people with musculoskeletal trauma and their families to adjust to any restrictions and dependence resulting from their injury.
- Chronic pain conditions cause a physical, emotional and financial burden for those affected. Biopsychosocial assessment is important to ensure that all of the components necessary for management are identified and addressed.
- Disuse atrophy is common in people who are confined to bed or are in immobilising devices. Encouragement to perform appropriate exercises and the provision of analgesia to enable regular completion of the regimen are important in reducing the degree of disuse atrophy.
- Assisting a person with passive or active range-of-motion exercises is one crucial element to reduce contractures. Appropriate positioning when performing pressure area care and the application of splints and orthoses are also important interventions in the prevention of contractures.

CHAPTER REVIEW

- *Musculoskeletal trauma* is an injury to bone, cartilage or soft tissue.
- *Soft tissue injuries* include sprains, strains, dislocations and subluxations. These are usually caused by trauma.
- *Fractures* are described according to type—*open (communication)* or *closed (non-communication)*—in relation to the external environment, and anatomical location. They are classified as *stable* or *unstable*.
- *Clinical manifestations* include immediate localised pain, decreased function and an inability to bear weight or use the affected part. Obvious bone deformity may or may not be present.
- The four stages of fracture healing are: *haematoma formation*; *fibrocartilaginous callus formation*; *ossification*; and *remodelling*.
- *Healing is influenced* by factors such as age, the initial displacement of the fracture, the anatomical location, blood supply to the area, immobilisation, implants, infection and hormones.
- The majority of fractures heal without complications. *Complications* include bone infection, problems with bone union, avascular necrosis, compartment syndrome, venous thrombosis, fat embolism and shock.
- *Fibromyalgia* is a musculoskeletal pain syndrome formerly believed to be more of a psychological issue. Recently, it is clearly becoming known as a physical issue, and further research is now attempting to elucidate the pathophysiology.
- *Management of fibromyalgia* incorporates multiple approaches, including exercise, rehabilitation, and the use of selective serotonin reuptake inhibitors, calcium channel blockers and non-steroidal anti-inflammatory drugs.
- *Myalgic encephalomyelitis/chronic fatigue syndrome (ME/CFS)* is a complex multisystem illness that has an immunological aetiological component.
- There are several different types of myositis, the most common of which are the *idiopathic inflammatory myositis group*. The pathophysiology is unknown with this group of myopathies, and could be due to an autoimmune process, but ultimately results in inflammation and pain in selected muscle groups. Management includes the use of anti-inflammatory agents and other immunomodifying drugs.
- The most common type of muscular dystrophy is *Duchenne's muscular dystrophy*, which mainly affects young boys of 2–6 years of age. This inheritable disorder is untreatable, and causes progressive muscle dysfunction as a result of a reduction in, or absence of, the protein dystrophin, which is required for myocyte stability.
- *Denervation atrophy* is most often chronic, and can only be corrected through re-innervation of the nerve supplying the affected muscles. This is not possible in many types of injuries.
- *Contractures* occur as a result of a shortening of the muscle–tendon unit, which causes significantly reduced range of movement.
- *Cramp* is an intense contraction of a muscle causing significant pain. It generally occurs as a result of transient electrolyte imbalance or inflammatory mediators, depending on whether the cramp is occurring in the smooth or skeletal muscle.
- *Delayed onset muscle soreness (DOMS)* occurs several hours to days after periods of unaccustomed exercise, is benign and will pass without much intervention.
- *Rhabdomyolysis* is a serious, most often acute, destruction of muscle, occurring as a result of the loss of intracellular calcium homeostasis. Rhabdomyolysis can cause substantial adverse clinical outcomes, including renal failure and death.

REVIEW QUESTIONS

1. Differentiate between a strain and a sprain.
2. Mr David Brown has sustained a sprained ankle after he fell awkwardly in a tackle during a football game. It is confirmed that he has only a soft tissue injury. As part of his discharge education he has been told to keep his ankle elevated, reapply the bandage when necessary and apply ice intermittently. He has been given some analgesia and sent home. Explain the mechanism of each of these interventions.
3. Describe the four stages of bone healing.

4 How can neurovascular compromise be assessed? Outline the clinical manifestations of neurovascular compromise.

5 Mr Phillip Grech is a 45-year-old man who fractured his left arm in a motor vehicle accident. An X-ray of the arm reveals a distal fracture extending through the epiphyseal plate. Mr Grech has no previous medical conditions and is otherwise healthy. His fracture requires the insertion of a surgical pin to reattach the distal bone fragment. A cast is applied after surgery. In the early postoperative period, the extremity may swell.
   a Injury to the epiphyseal plate can have extremely serious consequences for prepubescent children. Given that Mr Grech is 45 years of age, what concern will he not have to face?
   b What observations should be undertaken postoperatively?
   c Is Mr Grech at risk of developing compartment syndrome? Explain.
   d What are the manifestations of compartment syndrome?
   e What interventions should be undertaken if it is detected?

6 Describe the following types of fracture:
   a greenstick
   b spiral
   c open
   d comminuted

7 What is the relationship between the signs, symptoms and treatment of fibromyalgia? Outline the clinical manifestations of fibromyalgia, and relate them to either the proposed pathophysiology or the treatment. You may choose to create a diagram to assist you with this task.

8 What is the difference between the three most common forms of idiopathic inflammatory myositis? Create a table with five columns and four rows. In the second, third and fourth columns of the first row, identify one of the three types of idiopathic inflammatory myositis. Label the first column of the subsequent rows, 'Age affected', 'Duration', 'Clinical manifestations' and 'Management'. Complete the table.

9 What is the difference between skeletal muscle and smooth muscle cramp? Design a table that allows you to contrast the clinical manifestations, mechanism and management of cramp.

10 What factors or drugs can cause rhabdomyolysis? Make a list of all the drug groups and factors that increase the risk of someone developing rhabdomyolysis. How can it be detected? How is it managed?

HEALTH PROFESSIONAL CONNECTIONS

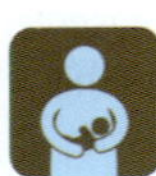

Midwives Although rare, pelvic ring fractures may occur in pregnancy as a result of significant trauma, such as that which may be experienced in a motor vehicle accident. In such situations, if unstable, internal fixation may be required to reduce pain and improve outcomes. Exposure to ionising radiation from X-rays may be required, but, if managed carefully, can be kept to acceptable levels. A history of pelvic fractures may also influence the method of delivery. This decision can be influenced by the injury severity, the degree of deformity and the time since injury. One further issue regarding pelvic injury during pregnancy is the potential of injury to the fetus. Depending on the mechanism of maternal injury, the fetus may also be harmed. In the event of maternal death, the baby is generally lost. Determining factors include the ability of the baby to be delivered within 5 minutes of maternal death, and the neonate's gestational age.

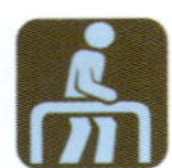

Physiotherapists Physiotherapists are responsible for the rehabilitation and management of soft tissue, dislocation and fracture injuries following initial treatment. Some physiotherapists with advanced training may also cast (or recast) fractures. Physiotherapy may begin during immobilisation, and aims to reduce oedema, improve circulation and maintain muscle function. Physiotherapists also educate people on the use of mobilisation or assistive devices. Physiotherapy after immobilisation aims to regain joint range of motion and muscle strength, and further reduce swelling. The type and severity of injury sustained will dictate the nature, duration and execution of the rehabilitation exercises and the apparatus required. Some techniques may include the use of active or passive exercises, thermotherapy or resistance equipment. Physiotherapists are responsible for assisting with preventing and managing contractures in people with neurological or profound musculoskeletal disability. The education of people, significant others, other healthcare professionals and carers in the protocols and the importance of frequent range-of-motion and stretching exercises will assist to reduce contracture development. Physiotherapists will also work with people in relation to atrophy. It is imperative to understand the cause and potential outcomes of atrophy, as these two factors will significantly influence a management program. In acute disuse injury, an expectation of full recovery is not unreasonable in many situations. However, in severe denervation atrophy, there may be no expectation of even long-term recovery. Management may be directed towards preventing joint deformity, contracture or dislocation. Depending on the presence of other neurological or musculoskeletal injury, long-term goals may focus on attempting to prevent significant atrophy and maintaining the functional structures within the affected muscle groups, in the hope that future research may enable the successful re-innervation of the affected muscles.

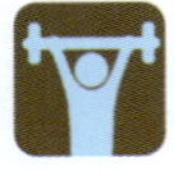

Exercise scientists Exercise is known to increase bone density and reduce fracture risk. However, soft tissue injuries and fractures are not uncommon in many types of sport. While people may be keen to train with injuries, the exercise professional must determine whether doing so is safe. Exercise program modification may be part of the answer. In circumstances of serious injury, medical clearance should be sought before returning to training. Although the absence of all training will result in deconditioning, loss of strength and lost form, returning to training before the injury has fully healed can aggravate the injury and complicate recovery. Other pitfalls include overtraining, resulting in stress fractures, and excessive training in women, leading to loss of excessive body fat, which may result in oestrogen deficiencies, further increasing the risk of stress fractures. Exercise professionals have a duty of care, and considered advice and safe exercise prescription will reduce the risk of injury, soft tissue injury and fracture. Specially designed exercise programs are beneficial for the management of fibromyalgia to reduce pain, increase aerobic capacity, reduce fatigue and depression, and improve sleeping. Various mechanisms contribute to these beneficial effects of exercise in chronic musculoskeletal pain syndromes, including the release of endogenous opioids and the stimulation of cortisol in response to physiological stress, providing some degree of anti-inflammatory effects. Other mechanisms by which exercise is thought to assist in chronic pain disorders are through distraction, as well as the increased endogenous release of tryptophan (the precursor to serotonin). Graded programs must take into account previous levels of fitness, deconditioning, and the degree of fatigue and musculoskeletal stiffness that the person is experiencing. As improvement is realised, it is important to review the program and adjust as necessary.

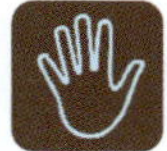

Occupational therapists Occupational therapists will work with people to design and fabricate orthoses to reduce the risk of contractures. Occupational therapists will also assist people to find alternative methods to undertake activities of daily living when their disability complicates self-care. Devices to assist with gripping, lifting or positioning can be provided or invented, depending on the needs of the person.

Nutritionists/Dieticians Nutrition and dietary habits can influence bone mass. The most obvious nutrient is calcium. Inadequate dietary intake of calcium will result in calcium leaching from the bone in order to replenish systemic needs, such as for nerve conduction and blood clotting. Other nutrients important for good bone health include adequate vitamin D to enable calcium absorption from the gastrointestinal tract. Appropriate protein intake is important, but excess protein may increase calcium excretion to manage the increase of sulfate, which is a by-product of protein metabolism. Excess sodium intake increases urinary calcium excretion, so minimal salt should be added to meals. Sufficient sodium intake can occur from the levels already within the diet. Nutrition health professionals need to consider a person's fracture history, and work with other healthcare professionals to ensure that the person's diet will promote bone health. Many diseases of the muscle can result in osteopenia. Ensuring that nutrition and dietary habits promote calcium levels can contribute to reducing the degree of osteopenia experienced. A multidisciplinary team is required to support people with myopathy. Atrophy can cause or be exacerbated by inadequate nutrition. Other nutrients, such as protein, vitamins and minerals, should also be considered when working with someone experiencing muscle pathology.

CASE STUDY

Mr Kim Liu (UR number 727991) is a 28-year-old Korean man who was brought in by paramedics after a motor vehicle accident. He doesn't speak any English. He has suffered an open fracture of the left tibia and fibula. He has left upper quadrant pain, and a seatbelt mark along his left shoulder, neck and chest. Through an interpreter it is determined that he has no known allergies and he has significant pain—9 out of 10—despite intravenous morphine given by the paramedic on site. His observations are as follows:

Temperature	Heart rate	Respiration rate	Blood pressure	SpO_2
37.0°C	100	28	150/86	93% (6 L/min via HM*)

*HM = Hudson mask.

A chest X-ray suggests some stable rib fractures, and leg X-rays reveal crush injuries and comminuted fractures of his left tibia and fibula. An abdominal CT demonstrated a splanchnic haematoma. Mr Liu is going to the operating theatre shortly for an open reduction and internal fixation (ORIF) of his leg fractures, and, depending on his haemodynamic stability, he may also have a laparotomy for the splanchnic haemorrhage. His preoperative pathology results are as follows:

HAEMATOLOGY

Patient location:	Ward 3	**UR:**	527991		
Consultant:	Smith	**NAME:**	Liu		
		Given name:	Kim	**Sex:**	M
		DOB:	23/09/XX	**Age:**	28

Time collected	12:35
Date collected	XX/XX
Year	XXXX
Lab #	3452343

FULL BLOOD COUNT		UNITS	REFERENCE RANGE
Haemoglobin	78	g/L	115–160
White cell count	5.4	$\times 10^9$/L	4.0–11.0
Platelets	190	$\times 10^9$/L	140–400
Haematocrit	0.26		0.33–0.47
Red cell count	3.92	$\times 10^{12}$/L	3.80–5.20
Reticulocyte count	1.8	%	0.2–2.0
MCV	89	fL	80–100
Neutrophils	3.12	$\times 10^9$/L	2.00–8.00
Lymphocytes	3.01	$\times 10^9$/L	1.00–4.00
Monocytes	0.45	$\times 10^9$/L	0.10–1.00
Eosinophils	0.27	$\times 10^9$/L	< 0.60
Basophils	0.11	$\times 10^9$/L	< 0.20
ESR	4	mm/h	< 12
COAGULATION PROFILE			
aPTT	32	secs	24–40
PT	15	secs	11–17
ABG			
pH	7.46		7.35–7.45
$PaCO_2$	32	mmHg	35–45
PaO_2	81	mmHg	> 80
HCO_3^-	23	mmHg	22–26
Oxygen saturations	92	%	> 95

BIOCHEMISTRY

Patient location:	Ward 3	**UR:**	527991		
Consultant:	Smith	**NAME:**	Liu		
		Given name:	Kim	**Sex:**	M
		DOB:	23/09/XX	**Age:**	28

Time collected	12:35
Date collected	XX/XX
Year	XXXX
Lab #	3849721

ELECTROLYTES		UNITS	REFERENCE RANGE
Sodium	139	mmol/L	135–145
Potassium	4.2	mmol/L	3.5–5.2
Chloride	104	mmol/L	95–110
Bicarbonate	24	mmol/L	22–32
Glucose (random)	7.5	mmol/L	3.5–6.9
Iron	16	µmol/L	11–30

CRITICAL THINKING

1. Significant blood loss can occur with fractures. Observe Mr Liu's full blood count, and identify the parameters that would suggest that some blood loss has occurred. What parameters reveal this?
2. Do Mr Liu's observations suggest significant blood loss? Discuss the findings. Consider not only his observations, but also the injury, the sympathetic nervous system responses and the pertinent information gleaned from the full blood count.
3. A coagulation profile was also taken. Is this information valuable? Explain.
4. After surgery, Mr Liu's leg will be bandaged. What observations are required? What complications may occur following a fracture? How can each complication be identified? What interventions should be undertaken in each circumstance? (It may be easier to answer these questions in a table.)
5. Mr Liu may have rib fractures as well. How might this complicate his care? Discuss the effect of rib fractures on ventilation, oxygenation and pain management.

BIBLIOGRAPHY

Antunes, M.D. & Marques, A.P. (2022). The role of physiotherapy in fibromyalgia: current and future perspectives. *Frontiers in Physiology* 13:968292. https://doi.org/10.3389/fphys.2022.968292.

Australian Bureau of Statistics (ABS) (2022). *Causes of death, Australia, 2022.* Canberra: ABS. http://www.abs.gov.au/statistics/health/causes-death.

Australian Institute of Health and Welfare (AIHW) (2020a). *Aboriginal and Torres Strait Islander Health Performance Framework 2020—summary report.* Canberra: Australian Government Department of Health. https://www.indigenoushpf.gov.au/publications/hpf-summary-2020.

Australian Institute of Health and Welfare (AIHW) (2020b). *Australia's children.* Cat. No. CWS 69. Canberra: AIHW. https://www.aihw.gov.au/getmedia/6af928d6-692e-4449-b915-cf2ca946982f/aihw-cws-69-print-report.pdf.aspx?inline=true.

Australian Institute of Health and Welfare (AIHW) (2022a). *Australia's health, 2022: data insights*. Australia's Health series No. 18, Cat. AUS 24. Canberra: AIHW. https://www.aihw.gov.au/reports/australias-health/australias-health-2022-data-insights/about.

Australian Institute of Health and Welfare (AIHW) (2022b). *Principal diagnosis data cubes: separation statistics by principal diagnosis (ICD-10-AM 11th edition), Australia, 2020–21.* Canberra: AIHW. https://www.aihw.gov.au/reports/hospitals/principal-diagnosis-data-cubes/contents/data-cubes.

Australian Institute of Health and Welfare (AIHW) (2023a). *Aboriginal and Torres Strait Islander Health Performance Framework: summary report 2023.* Canberra: AIHW. https://www.indigenoushpf.gov.au/Report-overview/Overview/Summary-Report.

Australian Institute of Health and Welfare (AIHW) (2023b). *Chronic musculoskeletal conditions*. Cat. No. PHE 317.Canberra: AIHW. https://www.aihw.gov.au/reports/chronic-musculoskeletal-conditions/musculoskeletal-conditions/contents/about.

Bauldoff, G., Gubrud-Howe, P.M., Carno, M.-A., Levett-Jones, T., Hales, M., Berry, K., … Stanley, D. (2020). *LeMone and Burke's medical–surgical nursing: critical thinking for person-centred care* (4th [Australian] edn). Sydney: Pearson Australia.

Best, O. & Fredericks, B. (2021). *Yatdjuligin: Aboriginal and Torres Strait Islander nursing and midwifery care* (3rd edn). Port Melbourne, VIC: Cambridge University Press.

Boomershine, C.S. (2021). Fibromyalgia. *Emedicine*. https://emedicine.medscape.com/article/329838-overview.

Bullock, S. & Manias, E. (2022). *Fundamentals of pharmacology* (9th edn). Sydney: Pearson Australia.

Centre for Metabolic Bone Diseases (2023). *FRAX—Fracture Risk Assessment Tool: Oceania.* Sheffield: Centre for Metabolic Bone Diseases, University of Sheffield. https://frax.shef.ac.uk/FRAX/tool.aspx?country=9.

Christidis, R., Lock, M., Walker, T., Egan, M. & Browne, J. (2021). Concerns and priorities of Aboriginal and Torres Strait Islander peoples regarding food and nutrition: a systematic review of qualitative evidence. *International Journal of Equity in Health* 20:220. https://doi.org/10.1186/s12939-021-01551-x.

Diab, J., Flapper, W.J. & Moore, M.H. (2023). Facial fractures in indigenous and non-indigenous populations of South Australia. *Journal of Craniofacial Surgery* 10.1097/SCS.0000000000009195. https://doi.org/10.1097/SCS.0000000000009195.

Dourado, E., Bottazzi, F., Cardelli, C., Conticini, E., Schmidt, J., Cavagna, L. & Barsotti, S. (2023). Idiopathic inflammatory myopathies: one year in review 2022. *Clinical and Experimental Rheumatology* 41(2):199–213. https://doi.org/10.55563/clinexprheumatol/jof6qn.

De Guzman, M.M. (2020). Rhabdomyolysis. *Emedicine*. https://emedicine.medscape.com/article/1007814.

Duan, D., Goemans, N., Takeda, S., Mercuri, E. & Aartsma-Rus, A. (2021). Duchenne muscular dystrophy. *Nature Reviews. Disease Primers* 7(1):13. https://doi.org/10.1038/s41572-021-00248-3.

Galvez-Sánchez, C.M. & Reyes del Paso, G.A. (2020). Diagnostic criteria for fibromyalgia: critical review and future perspectives. *Journal of Clinical Medicine* 9(4):1219. https://doi.org/10.3390/jcm9041219.

Health Quality and Safety Commission | Te Tāhū Hauora (HQSC) (2018). *Falls in people aged 50 and over.* Wellington: HQSCNZ. https://www.hqsc.govt.nz/our-data/atlas-of-healthcare-variation/falls-in-people-aged-50-and-over/.

International Association for the Study of Pain (IASP) (2020). *IASP announces revised definition of pain.* https://www.iasp-pain.org/publications/iasp-news/iasp-announces-revised-definition-of-pain/.

Kedlaya, D. (2022). Postexercise muscle soreness. *Emedicine.* https://emedicine.medscape.com/article/313267-overview.

Leslie, M. & Hudson, S. (2013). *Fibromyalgia: a truly mysterious disease*. Lakeway, TX: National Center of Continuing Education.

Malik, A., Hayat, G., Kalia, J.S. & Guzman, M.A. (2016). Idiopathic inflammatory myopathies: clinical approach and management. *Frontiers in Neurology* 7:64. https://doi.org/10.3389/fneur.2016.00064.

Marieb, E.N. & Hoehn, K. (2019). *Human anatomy and physiology* (11th edn). San Francisco, CA: Pearson Benjamin Cummings.

Monk, J.H.G., Thomson, W.M. & Tong, D.C. (2022). Trends in maxillofacial fractures in Otago-Southland, New Zealand: 2009 to 2020. *New Zealand Medical Journal* 135(1557):76–87.

O'Neill, S.C., Lui, D.F., Murphy, C. & Kiely, P.J. (2015). Lower leg compartment syndrome after appendicectomy. *Case Reports in Orthopedics* 2015:585986. https://doi.org/10.1155/2015/585986.

Orji, N., Campbell, J.A., Wills, K., Hensher, M., Palmer, A.J., Rogerson, M., … de Graaff, B. (2022). Prevalence of myalgic encephalomyelitis/chronic fatigue syndrome (ME/CFS) in Australian primary care patients: only part of the story? *BMC Public Health* 22:1516. https://doi.org/10.1186/s12889-022-13929-9.

Palacios, N., Molsberry, S., Fitzgerald, K.C. & Komaroff, A.L. (2023). Different risk factors distinguish myalgic encephalomyelitis/chronic fatigue syndrome from severe fatigue. *Scientific Reports* 13:2469. https://doi.org/10.1038/s41598-023-29329-x.

Roberts, J.R., Lan, M.L. & Price, M.W. (2020). Chronic fatigue syndrome (myalgic encephalomyelitis) differential diagnoses. *Emedicine*. https://emedicine.medscape.com/article/235980-differential.

Tariq, H., Collins, K., Tait, D., Dunn, J., Altaf, S. & Porter, S. (2022). Factors associated with joint contractures in adults: a systematic review with narrative synthesis. *Disability and Rehabilitation*. https://doi.org/10.1080/09638288.2022.2071480.

Treat-NMD Neuromuscular Network (2023). *New Zealand Neuromuscular Disease Registry (Punaha Io Neurogenetic Research Bank).* https://treat-nmd.org/patient-registry/nmd-registry-new-zealand/.

Vink, M. & Vink-Niese, A. (2023). The draft report by the Institute for Quality and Efficiency in Healthcare does not provide any evidence that graded exercise therapy and cognitive behavioral therapy are safe and effective treatments for myalgic encephalomyelitis/chronic fatigue syndrome. *Diseases* 11(1):11. https://doi.org/10.3390/diseases11010011.

Zengin, A., Shore-Lorenti, C., Sim, M., Maple-Brown, L., Brennan-Olsen, S.L., Lewis, J.R., … Ebeling, P. (2022). Why Aboriginal and Torres Strait Islander Australians fall and fracture: the codesigned Study of Indigenous Muscle and Bone Ageing (SIMBA) protocol. *BMJ Open* 12(4):e056589. https://doi.org/10.1136/bmjopen-2021-056589.

Bone and joint disorders

42

LEARNING OBJECTIVES

After completing this section, you should be able to:

1. Describe the pathophysiological mechanisms, epidemiology, clinical manifestations, diagnosis and management involved in bone and joint developmental disorders.
2. Describe the pathophysiology of arthritic conditions, how they present and how they can be managed.
3. Describe the pathophysiological mechanisms, epidemiology, clinical manifestations, diagnosis and management involved in metabolic bone and joint diseases.
4. Describe the pathophysiological mechanisms, epidemiology, clinical manifestations, diagnosis and management involved in the infective bone disorder osteomyelitis.
5. Describe the pathophysiological mechanisms, epidemiology, clinical manifestations, diagnosis and management involved in osteogenic tumours.

WHAT YOU SHOULD KNOW BEFORE YOU START THIS CHAPTER

Can you describe the principles and major concepts associated with genetic disorders?

Can you describe the process of bone growth and repair?

Can you describe the main stages of inflammation and healing?

Can you differentiate between acute and chronic inflammation?

Can you state the principles associated with infectious disease?

Can you describe the major concepts associated with neoplasia?

Can you identify the normal structure and functions of a joint?

Can you identify and describe the types of joint movements?

Can you describe the major principles and concepts associated with immune disorders?

KEY TERMS

Ankylosing spondylitis
Arthritis
Developmental dysplasia of the hip (DDH)
Disease-modifying antirheumatic drugs (DMARDs)
Ewing's sarcoma
Gout
Kyphosis
Osgood–Schlatter disease (OSD)
Osteoarthritis (OA)
Osteochondroses
Osteomalacia
Osteomyelitis
Osteopenia
Osteoporosis
Osteosarcomas
Paget's disease of the bone
Rheumatoid arthritis
Rickets
Scoliosis
Talipes equinovarus (TEV)
Tophi (tophus)

Introduction

Developmental, metabolic, infectious and neoplastic disorders can affect the musculoskeletal system. As the population ages, musculoskeletal conditions affecting mobility contribute even more to the limitations on independence and to pain and suffering, and further stretch finite healthcare budgets. These disorders can have significant physical, psychosocial and financial ramifications on affected people and their loved ones. Bone and joint developmental disorders, arthritis, metabolic bone diseases, osteomyelitis and bone tumours are discussed in this chapter.

Bone and joint developmental disorders

LEARNING OBJECTIVE 1

Describe the pathophysiological mechanisms, epidemiology, clinical manifestations, diagnosis and management involved in bone and joint developmental disorders.

A number of congenital developmental bone and joint disorders are associated with crippling deformities. In the past, these disorders have stigmatised the children and the families of those affected. Nowadays, with quick identification and early intervention, these conditions can be corrected, but not necessarily cured, greatly improving joint and limb function, and allowing those severely affected children to have more productive lives. In this section, developmental dysplasia of the hip, talipes equinovarus and osteogenesis imperfecta are described.

The other conditions covered in detail in this section, scoliosis and the osteochondroses, may be acquired in childhood (although a congenital form of scoliosis does also exist) and develop due to dysfunction of the immature, growing skeleton.

DEVELOPMENTAL DYSPLASIA OF THE HIP

Aetiology and pathophysiology

Developmental dysplasia of the hip (DDH) is a condition characterised by abnormal growth of the hip joint. The global incidence of the disorder is relatively low, with around 1–20 per 1,000 live births showing the condition. In South Australia the incidence is 7 in 1,000 live births, but in Western Australia it has been reported at 20 per 1,000 births. It is usually identified during the neonatal period, but cases have been diagnosed later in childhood, adolescence and in adulthood. The likelihood of complete correction in older people is reduced, as joint remodelling is more limited. When detected at adolescence and adulthood, the risk of gait disorders, decreased joint strength and the development of degenerative disease is increased.

The aetiology of DDH remains unclear, but a number of genetic and environmental factors are believed to influence the development of the condition (see Table 42.1).

In the past, the condition has been known as *congenital dislocation of the hip*. This terminology has now been discarded, as it is clear that the condition presents with a high degree of variability and progression. The hip joint may be relatively stable, with a mild degree of abnormal femur (ball) and acetabular (socket) development. In this form of dysplasia, the acetabulum usually becomes shallower. The soft tissues of the supporting capsule surrounding the joint may also become lax, contributing to the instability.

In more severe cases, the joint becomes quite unstable, with evidence of potential dislocation, subluxation (partial dislocation) or actual dislocation. The degree of acetabular dysplasia can be significant, causing the femoral head to sit higher up the pelvis. The condition can be *bilateral* or *unilateral*. The latter is more common, and tends to affect the left hip more frequently.

Table 42.1 Genetic and environmental causes of DDH

Cause	Comment
Family history	About one-third of babies with DDH have a blood relative who has had DDH
Female	May be due to the presence of circulating hormone relaxin, inducing lax ligaments
Congenital disorders (e.g. cerebral palsy and myelomeningocele)	Risk of DDH higher in cases where there are nerve or muscle disorders
Oligohydramnios (i.e. reduced intrauterine fluid volume)	Baby in the womb has less space for movement
Breech delivery	Buttock or feet-first presentation results in abnormal mechanical stressors on a newborn's hips
Multiple babies in utero	Decreases intrauterine space
First-time mother	A difficult or prolonged delivery may ensue
Children in cultures that swaddle babies	Forcing an infant's hips to be adducted, leading to a higher rate of hip dysplasia

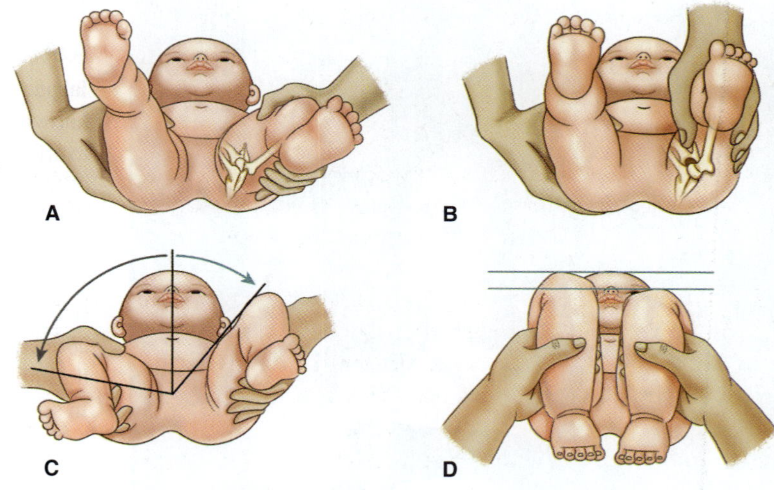

Figure 42.1

Clinical examination for developmental dysplasia of the hip (DDH)

(A) Ortolani's manoeuvre.
(B) Barlow (dislocation) manoeuvre.
(C) Abduction manoeuvre.
(D) Galeazzi manoeuvre.

Source: EJ Roh—Sciencopia.

Clinical manifestations

Common clinical manifestations associated with dislocation of the hip include a turning of the affected leg (or legs) outwards, uneven folds of the skin of the thigh or 'flattened' buttocks, and a widened perineum on the affected side. The affected leg may also appear shorter as the femur sits higher on the pelvis, but this may be hard to see when the condition is bilateral. Limited hip abduction occurs when the hip is fully flexed.

In older children, the child may waddle, walk with a limp or display a toe-walking pattern of ambulation.

Clinical diagnosis and management

Diagnosis The clinical manifestations listed for DDH are not specific for this condition, and may also be associated with a number of other disorders. It is important to take a comprehensive history and perform a thorough clinical examination in order to exclude other conditions.

Two tests are important in the diagnosis of DDH: the Ortolani and Barlow manoeuvres (tests). These tests are used to demonstrate the presence of hip instability. The *Ortolani manoeuvre* is used to relocate the dislocated head of the femur back into the acetabulum. The *Barlow manoeuvre* is used to dislocate the femoral head. Figure 42.1 shows these tests as a part of the clinical examination for DDH. The examination should also be used to reveal evidence of the clinical manifestations, such as limited movement of the hip while fully flexed, apparent shortening of the affected leg, turning of the leg, unevenness of the thigh skin (see Figure 42.2) and flattened buttocks.

Medical imaging can also be used to support a diagnosis of DDH. It can provide a static picture of the structural appearance of the joint, but cannot provide information about joint stability. Ultrasonography is used for the assessment of DDH in infants from birth to around 4 months of age, while X-ray is the usual mode in older babies.

Management Once DDH is diagnosed, prompt intervention tends to produce the best long-term results. Treatment should be directed towards achieving stable reduction of the hip in order to facilitate normal joint development. Splinting the hip in a flexed–abducted position using the Pavlik harness (see Figure 42.3) is regarded as the treatment of choice in babies who are diagnosed early. Surgery is an option for children who are diagnosed after 3 months of age or when the condition remains refractory to splinting.

Once applied, the Pavlik harness remains in place until the hip joint is stable and normally positioned. This is confirmed

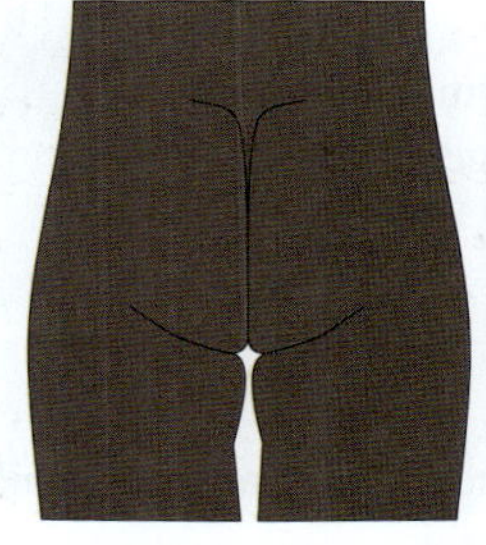

A. Normal symmetry

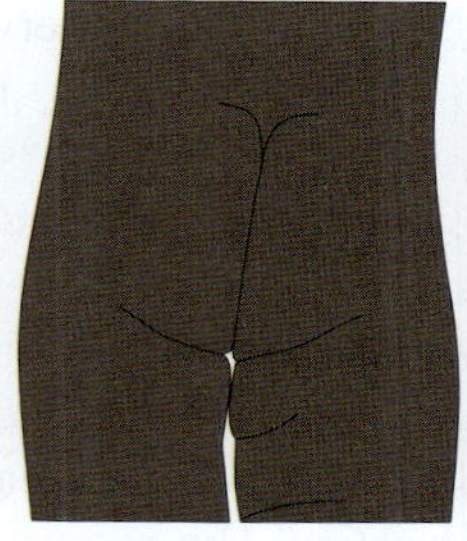

B. Asymmetry of DDH

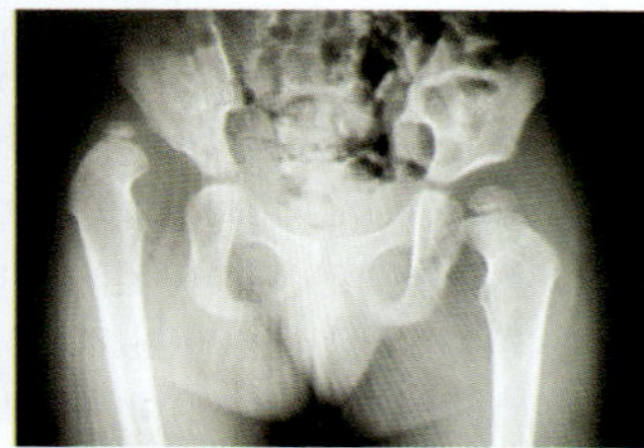

C.

Figure 42.2

Visual asymmetry in DDH

(A) Fat folds in an unaffected child display normal symmetry.
(B) Fat folds in a child with DDH are asymmetrical.
(C) X-ray of a child with hip dysplasia and a dislocated right femur.

Source: (C) Bunsinth-Nan-Pua/Shutterstock.

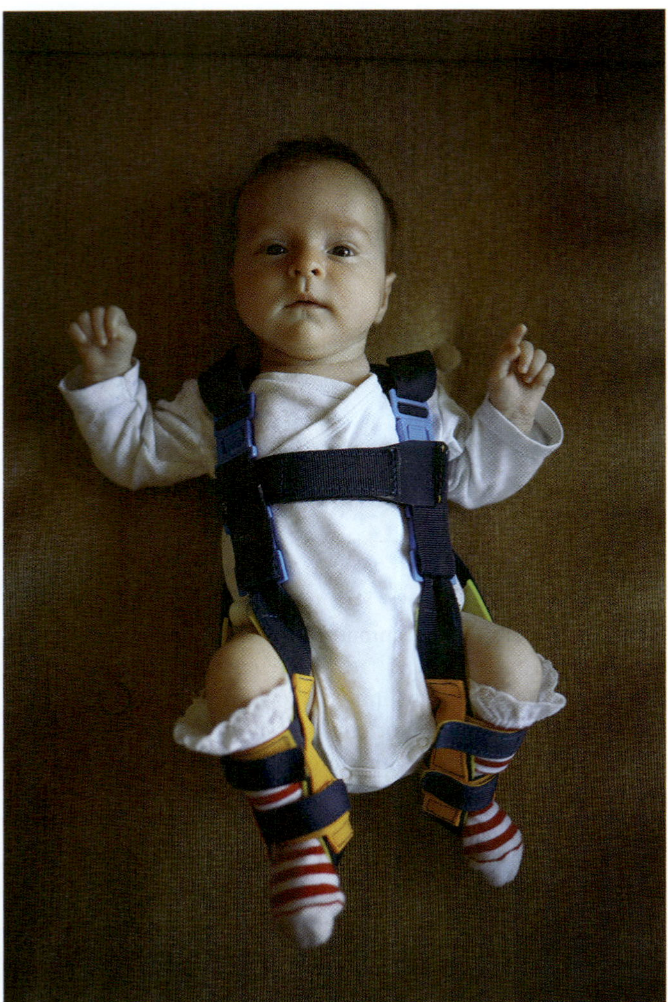

Figure 42.3

The Pavlik harness

The most common treatment for DDH in a child less than 3 months of age is a Pavlik harness. A shirt should be worn under the harness to prevent skin irritation.

Source: Marko Subotin/Shutterstock.

by examination and imaging. The harness can be adjusted as the child grows and the joint stabilises. A complication of this procedure is that pressure on the femoral head can lead to avascular necrosis or temporary palsy of the femoral nerve.

Surgery is directed towards creating a more normal anatomical shape and orientation of the joint. After surgery the child will wear a brace or be placed in a plaster cast for 3–4 months to facilitate reduction.

Conservative treatment may be appropriate in the management of this condition in adolescents and adults. It can include physical therapy, anti-inflammatory drug treatment, activity modification and health education. Hip reconstructive surgery may be required.

TALIPES EQUINOVARUS

Aetiology and pathophysiology

Talipes equinovarus (TEV) is a congenital condition commonly known as *clubfoot*. Its incidence is relatively common, estimated to affect 1–4 live births per 1,000 people. It can occur *unilaterally* or *bilaterally* (see Figure 42.4), although bilateral is more common. Most cases of children born with TEV occur in low- to middle-income countries.

An affected foot is inverted and plantar-flexed at the hindfoot (i.e. turned inwards and downwards at the ankle), while being adducted in the forefoot. Ligaments and muscles associated with the ankle are tight and retracted, and some are severely shortened. In some cases, atrophy and fibrosis of these muscles is observed.

The aetiology of TEV remains unknown; however, a number of factors have been linked to its development. These factors include vascular defects, an aberration in regional growth, early amniocentesis, maternal cigarette smoking, intrauterine enterovirus infection and intrauterine mechanical pressure, as well as neural and/or muscular abnormalities. Genetic factors have also been implicated; first-degree relatives of a child with the idiopathic form of TEV have an increased risk, with monozygotic

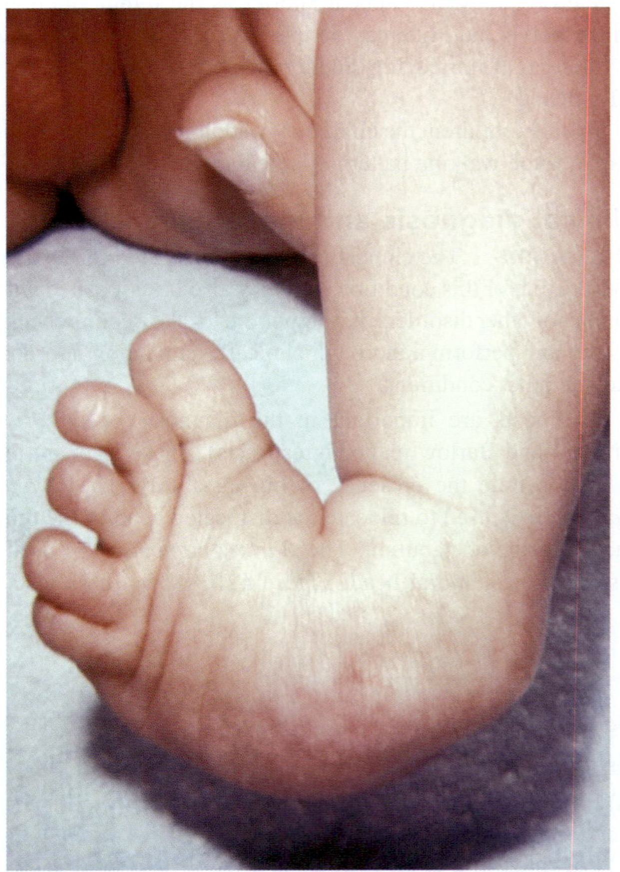

Figure 42.4

Infant with bilateral talipes equinovarus (TEV)

Source: CDC/James W. Hanson, MD, 1973.

twins having an even higher risk. Variations in the genes involved in embryonic muscle structure and function, *HOCA9, TPM1* and *TPM2*, have been identified as risk factors for TEV.

Clinical diagnosis and management

Diagnosis As for DDH, taking a thorough history and an optimal clinical examination are essential in assessing the severity of the deformity and evaluating the progress of the treatment. Classification of the severity of clubfoot is achieved using one of two reliable scored systems: the Pirani score or the Dimeglio score. The *Pirani score* is the simpler test, assessing the degree of foot contracture on the basis of six clinical signs of the condition. The Dimeglio score assesses four parameters according to the degree of stiffness. In both tests, higher scores indicate a more severe condition.

Medical imaging, using sequential fetal ultrasonography, is particularly successful in the antenatal diagnosis of TEV. Ultrasonography and magnetic resonance imaging (MRI) have limited value in the neonatal period, but can be useful in assessing the results of treatment.

Management The aim of treatment is to restore the affected foot to the normal position and prevent recurrence. This can be achieved by surgical or non-surgical (conservative) means. The *surgical approach* involves the release of tight soft tissues in order to produce normal foot positioning.

The two main conservative treatments are the Ponsetti method and the French method. The *Ponsetti method* is considered the gold standard for TEV, and involves the application of serial casts that are in some cases changed weekly. This is followed by the wearing of a brace that holds the foot in an abducted position for a prolonged period. This may be followed by sectioning the Achilles tendon, especially in more severe cases. The *French method* initially involves daily manipulation of the affected foot by a physiotherapist, accompanied by foot immobilisation. After three months, the parents will continue the therapy daily until the child is walking. Correction rates using these non-surgical strategies have been shown to be excellent.

Relapse or recurrence of the deformity can occur following either surgical or non-surgical procedures. Proponents of the Ponsetti method state that relapse is usually associated with parental non-compliance regarding the child wearing the brace. Affected children should be monitored for a period after treatment to assess for relapse. Recurrence after the age of 5 years is rare, and is almost never seen after 7 years of age.

Research indicates that while the use of the Ponseti method leads to some decrease in the range of movement and function at the ankle, the overall functional outcomes were not diminished, and parental satisfaction with treatment was high.

SCOLIOSIS

Aetiology and pathophysiology

Scoliosis is a deformity characterised by *lateral curvature and axial rotation of the spine*. The different forms of scoliosis are known by the terms congenital, neuromuscular and idiopathic. In *congenital scoliosis*, a child is born with the deformity, which is accompanied by defects affecting the heart and kidneys. *Neuromuscular scoliosis* occurs when normal nervous and/or muscle functions are disrupted in diseases such as cerebral palsy or muscular dystrophy, causing alterations in spinal posture.

Idiopathic scoliosis is not associated with other abnormalities. Idiopathic scoliosis consists of subcategories according to the age of onset in the affected child, namely infantile (birth–3 years old), juvenile (4–10 years old) and adolescent (older than 10 years). *Adolescent idiopathic scoliosis (AIS)* is the most common subtype seen in clinical practice in Australia and New Zealand. The aetiology of AIS remains unclear, but it is considered to have a multifactorial basis. Genetic factors have a key role, as there appears to be a familial pattern of inheritance, with a higher risk in families if one member already has the condition.

Epidemiology

AIS has a prevalence rate of 0.47–5.2% in Australia and New Zealand, with girls affected eight to 10 times more than boys, and often more severely. In terms of genetic risk factors, the most likely affected first-degree relative is a maternal female cousin. In New Zealand, a higher incidence of idiopathic scoliosis has been identified in European children than in Pacific Islands children.

Clinical manifestations

The common clinical manifestations of scoliosis are associated with the asymmetrical positioning of the torso caused by the lateral curvature (see Figure 42.5). In severe scoliosis, the curvature can compromise the function of the heart, lungs and gastrointestinal tract. The clinical manifestations of scoliosis include asymmetry of shoulders, scapulae and waist creases, prominence of the thoracic ribs or paravertebral muscles on forward bend, and lateral curvature and vertebral rotation on posteroanterior X-ray. In severe scoliosis, back pain, shortness of breath, anorexia and nausea can develop.

Clinical diagnosis and management

Diagnosis The diagnosis of scoliosis and its cause requires taking a history, performing a clinical examination and considering X-rays of the region. For idiopathic scoliosis, the examination is used to exclude other disorders. The *Adams forward bend test* is a useful assessment tool in the detection of scoliosis. The child is asked to remove their upper garments and bend forwards. A prominence of the ribcage, or large lumbar muscles, on the affected side of the apex will become apparent, suggesting scoliosis. X-ray imaging will confirm the diagnosis. The angle of the curvature, the Cobb angle, is measurable on X-ray and indicates the severity of the condition. Ten degrees or greater is considered scoliosis.

Management The risk of progression of AIS correlates with the severity of the curvature and the child's age at presentation. Affected children about to experience their adolescent growth spurt should be monitored closely, as they are at the most risk of progression. The particular age range of interest is 10–15 years old.

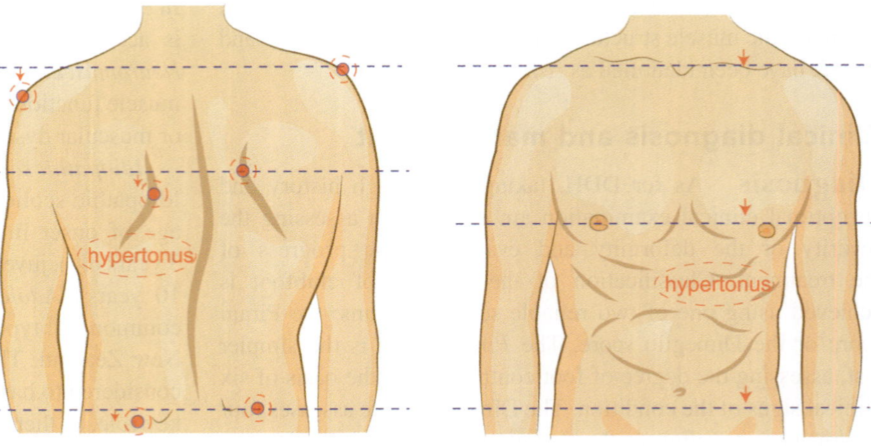

Figure 42.5

Curvature of the spine

(A) Posterior view: Note the disparity in the shoulder, scapula and hip height, and hypertonus around the region of the left latissimus dorsi.
(B) Anterior view: Note the disparity in the clavicle, nipple and hip height, and hypertonus around the upper region of left rectus abdominis.

Source: Artemida-psy/Shutterstock.

The most effective treatments for AIS are the application of a scoliosis brace or surgery. The brace is not curative, but can be used to control and restrict the shape of the curvature. Bracing is often used in cases that are not severe enough to require surgery, or to delay surgery. Surgery is directed towards the internal fixation of the spinal column using rods and hooks to correct the curvature. Spinal fusion of vertebrae may form part of this approach. Figure 42.6 shows a child in a halo brace following surgery. The progress of treatment is monitored using medical imaging.

In terms of prognosis, smaller curvatures are less likely to progress compared to larger ones. Children who present with scoliosis before skeletal maturity are also at greater risk of progression.

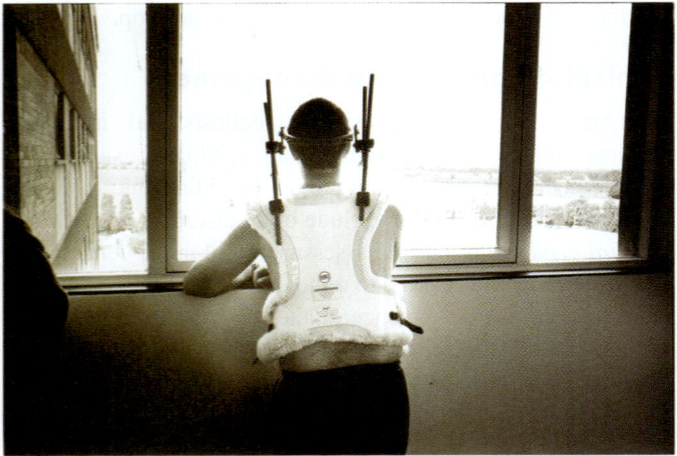

Figure 42.6

Historical image from about 1998 showing a boy wearing a halo brace following three vertebral fractures

Current halo braces differ little from this one of almost three decades ago.

Source: Brian Harris/Independent/Alamy Stock Photo.

OSTEOCHONDROSES

The **osteochondroses** are bone disorders associated with the *immature growing skeleton*. The aetiology of osteochondroses is not well understood, but the onset of these conditions has been linked to injury, mechanical stresses on the epiphyseal growth plate and ossification zones, abnormal skeletal development, vascular interruption to bones, and genetic factors. Common regions of the skeleton affected include the hip, knee, foot, elbow and spine. Osteochrondroses usually resolve once skeletal maturity is reached and the growth plates close.

Osgood–Schlatter disease is the focus of discussion in this section. Legg–Calvé–Perthes disease is another form of osteochondrosis, but is relatively rare.

Osgood–schlatter disease

Aetiology and pathophysiology **Osgood-Schlatter disease (OSD)** is an *inflammatory condition affecting the knee*. In the growing skeleton, the tibial tubercle ossification zone is vulnerable to mechanical stresses. The patellar tendon inserts onto the tibial tubercle. In affected children, the patellar tendon tightens and the tibial tubercle becomes injured; microfractures may also occur. This results in pain, inflammation and swelling of the tubercle.

Epidemiology The incidence rate of OSD in Australia and New Zealand is not readily available. A recent review indicated a prevalence in adolescents between 6.8% and 33%. OSD is usually diagnosed in children between 10 and 14 years of age. More boys than girls are diagnosed with this condition (a case ratio of 14:1), which is thought to be related to differences in the pattern and type of activities between the sexes at this time of life. In 20–30% of cases, the involvement is bilateral. Children who are active and sporty during the adolescent growth spurt appear to be at a greater risk of OSD, as are those who have previously reported a knee injury.

Clinical manifestations The most common clinical manifestation of OSD is anterior knee pain, which is worsened by activities such as jumping, walking up stairs and kneeling. The tubercle may be tender to touch, swollen and quite prominent.

Clinical diagnosis and management

Diagnosis A combination of taking a medical history, a clinical examination and medical imaging is used in the diagnosis of OSD. These diagnostic procedures will assist in ruling out other conditions. X-rays of the knee may show fragmentation of the tibial tubercle and soft tissue swelling.

Management OSD is considered a self-limiting condition that usually resolves as the skeleton matures. Pain associated with the condition responds well to simple analgesic and anti-inflammatory agents, such as paracetamol and the non-steroidal anti-inflammatory drugs (NSAIDs), as well as modification of the child's activity. A physiotherapy program designed to improve the flexibility of the lower limb muscles can also be helpful.

Arthritis

LEARNING OBJECTIVE 2

Describe the pathophysiology of arthritic conditions, how they present and how they can be managed.

Arthritis is a condition generally characterised by *inflammation of the joints*. There are a number of different forms of arthritis, with differing aetiologies and pathogenesis. In this section, we focus on osteoarthritis, rheumatoid arthritis and ankylosing spondylitis. All three forms are *chronic inflammatory diseases* that lead to degeneration of the affected joints and impaired mobility.

OSTEOARTHRITIS

Aetiology and pathophysiology

Osteoarthritis (OA) is a common disorder involving the *degeneration of the synovial joints*. In osteoarthritis, enzymatic degradation of a joint results in loss of cartilage. This occurs mostly in the maximal load-bearing areas. Of the three different types of cartilage—hyaline, elastic and fibrocartilage—*hyaline cartilage* (also known as *articular cartilage*) is most often affected, because it is found in diarthrodial (freely movable) joints. The major components of hyaline cartilage are water, proteoglycans, type II collagen, glycoproteins and minerals. In a joint that is free from disease, the health and structure of the articular cartilage are maintained by a fine balance between pro-inflammatory factors, causing *catabolism* (destruction), and anti-inflammatory factors, causing *anabolism* (synthesis).

In osteoarthritis, a complex interplay of factors, such as genetics, hormones or injury, results in biomechanical stressors that alter this balance, causing an increase in pro-inflammatory factors and a decrease in anti-inflammatory factors.

Matrix metalloproteinases (MMPs) are catabolic enzymes that hydrolyse or destroy the collagen making up the cartilage extracellular matrix. It is thought that pro-inflammatory cytokines—such as interleukins (ILs) (particularly IL-1), tumour necrosis factor-alpha (TNF-α), insulin-like growth factor (IGF) and nuclear factor-κB—induce chondrocytes and synovial cells to synthesise MMPs. Anabolic processes such as chondrocyte proliferation, collagen and proteoglycan synthesis are also inhibited by IL-1 and TNF-α. Therefore, the cartilage is exposed not only to environmental factors that cause its destruction, but also to factors that inhibit its repair. IL-1 and TNF-α also induce *nitric oxide* production, which induces vascular congestion and increased intraosseous pressure, and plays a role in promoting chondrocyte apoptosis. Other inflammatory mediators, such as prostaglandins, continue the joint destruction with flaking and the development of *vertical clefts* (fibrillations) along the cartilage. Excessive articular cartilage degradation ultimately results in denuding of the bone and subchondral bone sclerosis. The subchondral bone plate undergoes change, becoming a dense, hard, ivory-like mass; this process is also known as *eburnation*. In an attempt to overcome cartilage damage in non-pressure areas, cellular proliferation results in bony outgrowths capped with fibrocartilage, known as *osteophytes*. These osteophytes may break off and become loose intra-articular deposits, which are known as *'joint mice'*. Synovial fluid may enter the subchondral bone and form *subchondral cysts* (see Figure 42.7). It is interesting to note that osteophytes can develop early in the disease process; however, subchondral cysts are generally a later sign in severe osteoarthritis.

Changes in osteoblast activity in osteoarthritis under the influence of inflammatory mediators have also been reported, with increased remodelling and reduced mineralisation of the subchondral bone during the early phase of the disease, and increased bone formation and reduced resorption in the later phase.

Although the terms 'primary osteoarthritis' and 'secondary osteoarthritis' have been used historically, this distinction is now less common. When used, the term *secondary osteoarthritis* is often associated with an obvious injury or identifiable contributing condition, and often is associated with osteoarthritis in a younger person, commonly after a knee injury. *Primary osteoarthritis* is considered idiopathic (of unknown cause). Irrespective of whether the osteoarthritis is primary or secondary, the histological effects on the joint are the same (see Figure 42.8).

Epidemiology

Osteoarthritis is the most common form of degenerative joint disease. According to the Australian Institute of Health and Welfare (AIHW), 9.3% of Australians self-reported having osteoarthritis, with approximately 63% of those affected being women. The prevalence is slightly higher in areas of lower socioeconomic status. Thirty-six per cent of people aged over 75 years have osteoarthritis. It is estimated that more than 2.2 million people in Australia have osteoarthritis. In New Zealand, 7.9% of men and 12.7% of women have osteoarthritis. Thirty-six per cent of people aged over 75 years have osteoarthritis. It is estimated that over 400,000 people in New Zealand have osteoarthritis (10.4% of the population).

Some non-modifiable factors that increase the risk of developing osteoarthritis include being of female gender, age and congenital joint anomalies. Modifiable risk factors include obesity, joint injury (e.g. sports injury in young adults), physical inactivity, comorbid conditions and exposure to joint-loading

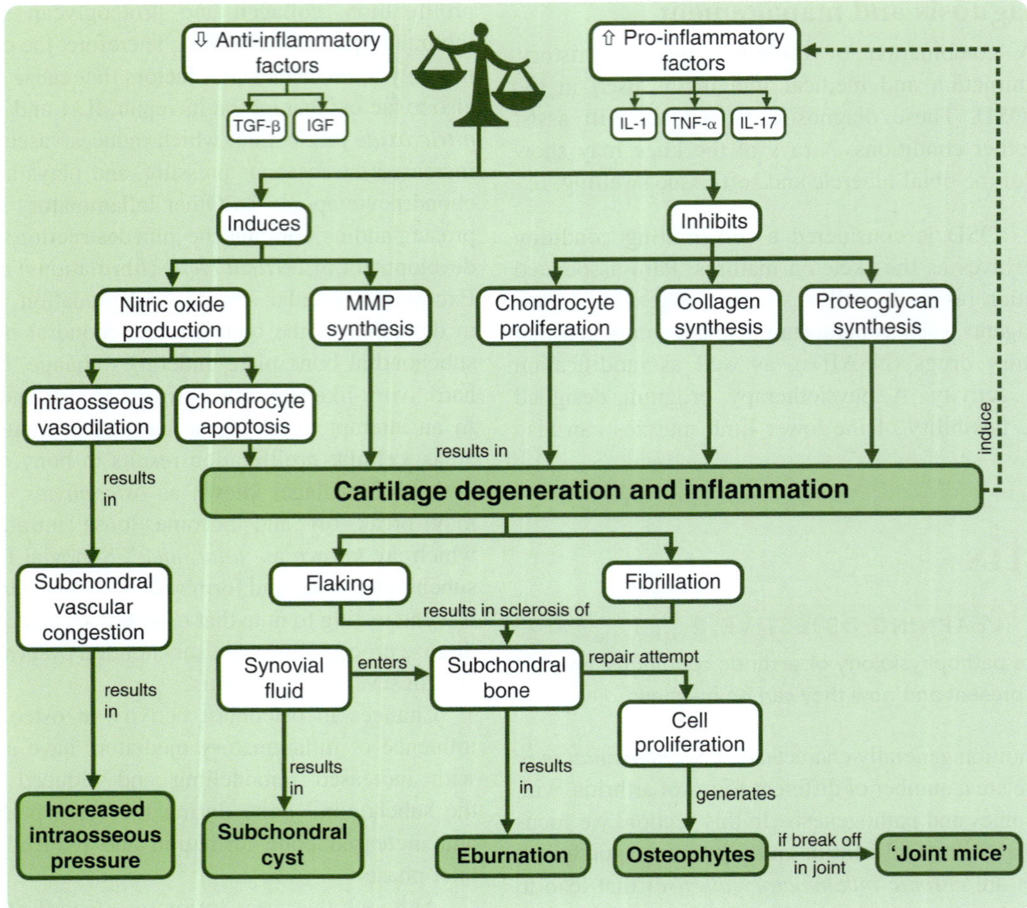

Figure 42.7

Pathophysiology of structural damage to cartilage

↓ = decreased; ↑ = increased; IGF = insulin-like growth factor; IL = interleukin; MMP = matrix metalloproteinase; TGF-β = transforming growth factor-beta; TNF-α = tumour necrosis factor-alpha.

repetitive tasks. Occupations that involve repetitive joint-loading tasks can predispose a person to osteoarthritis.

Clinical manifestations

The most significant clinical manifestations are joint pain and stiffness. Because the onset of osteoarthritis can occur over years, the effect it has on an individual's range of motion and ability to carry out activities of daily living may not be immediately apparent.

Joint pain is often described as a deep ache that becomes worse with overuse. Periods of inactivity can result in joint stiffness, which resolves within 20–30 minutes following activity. The decrease in range of motion can be associated with pain and crepitus. An effusion (collection of fluid) may also occur in the affected joint as a result of synovial fluid accumulation. A difficult cycle of inactivity from pain and altered mobility can cause obesity, which in turn exacerbates osteoarthritis, inducing more pain and altered mobility. Osteoarthritis commonly affects the knees, hips, cervical and lumbar spine, and the hands.

If osteoarthritis affects the hands, Heberden's and Bouchard's nodes may be seen. *Heberden's nodes* are swellings in distal interphalangeal joints (DIPs), whereas *Bouchard's nodes* are swellings in proximal interphalangeal joints (PIPs) (see Figure 42.9B).

Joints may be tender to touch, enlarged and potentially even malaligned. Locking or seizing of a joint during range of motion may be associated with 'joint mice' or fragments of free-floating cartilage. Muscle atrophy may occur as a result of elective disuse because of pain. Figure 42.10 explores the common clinical manifestations and management of osteoarthritis.

Clinical diagnosis and management

Diagnosis The collection of a health history and a physical assessment will provide significant information suggestive of arthritis being involved. The characteristics of the joint pain and stiffness may provide an impression about what type of arthritis is involved. Currently, no blood test exists to assist with diagnosis. An X-ray is an inexpensive, prompt method of determining bony changes within the joint; however, it cannot show cartilage. An assumption about the thickness of the cartilage can be postulated by observing the narrowing of the joint space. Cortical sclerosis will be visible, and the pathology

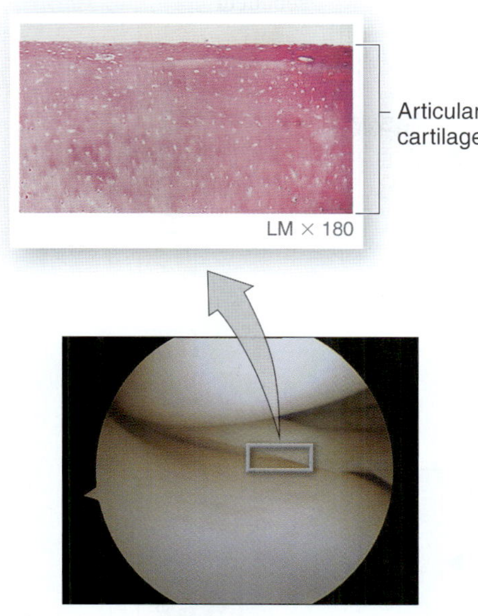

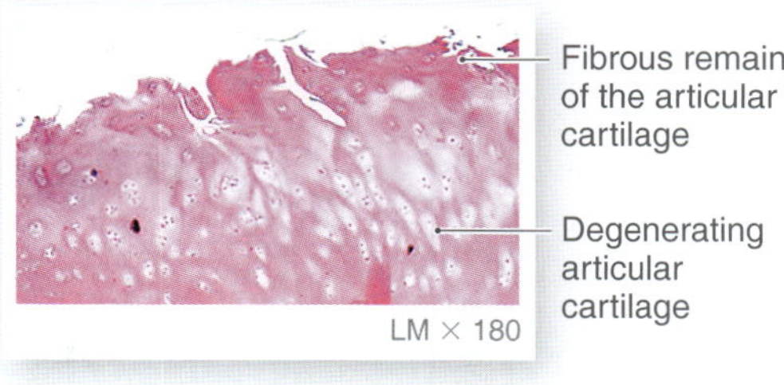

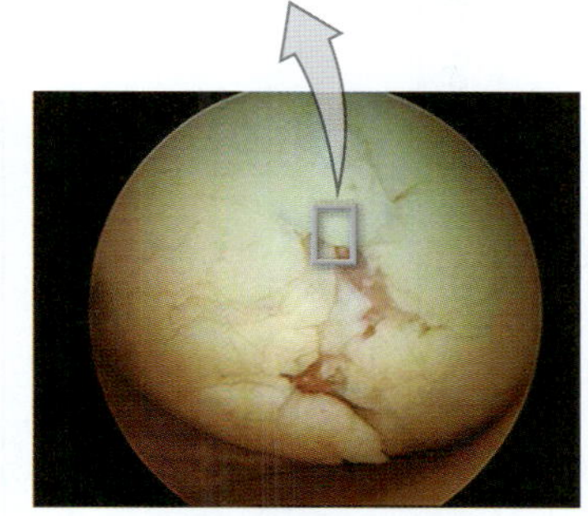

A. Arthroscopic view of normal cartilage

B. Arthroscopic view of damaged cartilage

Figure 42.8

Comparison of a normal and an arthritic joint

(A) Normal joint with smooth articular cartilage.
(B) Joint damaged by osteoarthritis, with articular cartilage flaking, resulting in increased friction and further degradation.

Source: Martini, F.H., Ober, W.C., & Nath, J.L., Visual anatomy and physiology *(1st edn), Box 8.8, p. 274. © 2011. Reprinted by permission of Pearson Education, Inc.*

is generally asymmetric. Osteophytes and subchondral cysts may be visible. The sampling and analysis of the fluid from an effusion may be beneficial to eliminate the presence of septic arthritis or gout. MRI may be beneficial to exclude the presence of osteonecrosis; however, it is expensive and not generally necessary.

Management The primary goals in the management of people with osteoarthritis are the control of pain and the promotion of mobility. Initially, osteoarthritis may be adequately controlled with simple analgesia and over-the-counter non-steroidal anti-inflammatory drugs (NSAIDs). These drugs act to inhibit cyclooxygenase and, hence, reduce the synthesis of

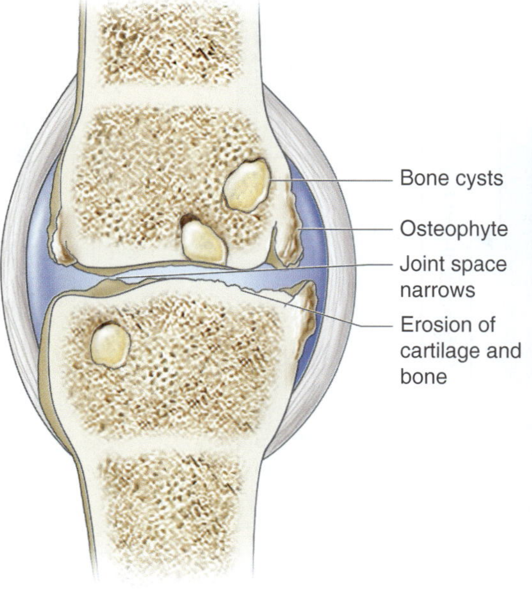

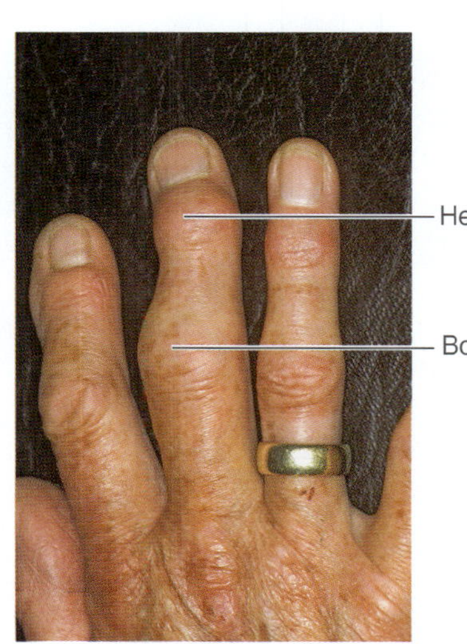

Figure 42.9

Heberden's and Bouchard's nodes

(A) Osteophytes and bone cysts.
(B) Heberden's nodes are nodular masses on the distal interphalangeal joint; Bouchard's nodes are nodular masses on the proximal interphalangeal joint.

Sources: (A) Osborn, K.S., Wraa, C.E. & Watson A. Medical surgical nursing: preparation for practice *(combined volume, 1st edn), Figure 58.1, p. 1834. © 2010. Reprinted by permission of Pearson Education, Inc.; (B) Hercules Robinson/Alamy Stock Photo.*

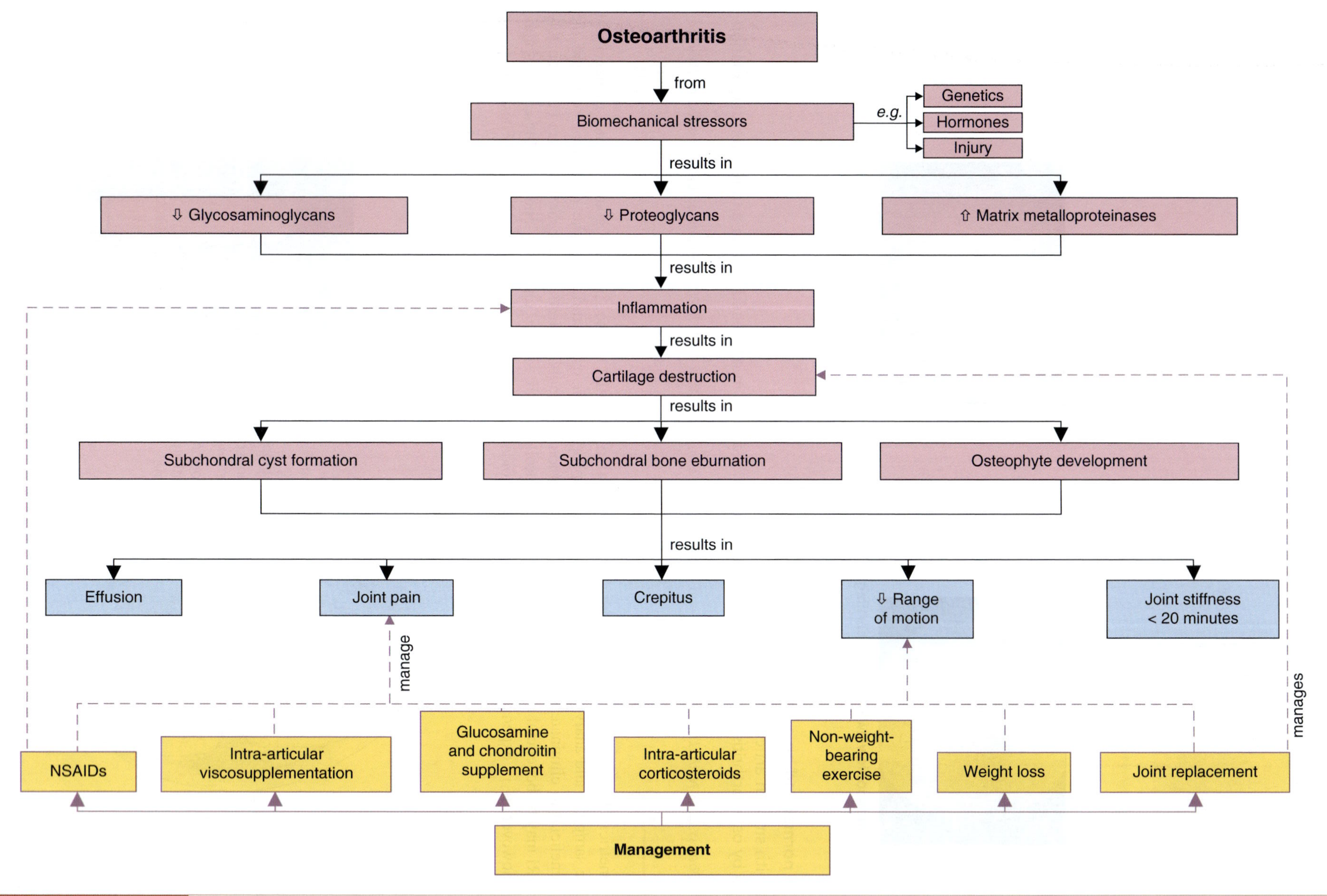

Figure 42.10

Clinical snapshot: Osteoarthritis

↓ = decreased; ↑ = increased; NSAIDS = non-steroidal anti-inflammatory drugs.

prostaglandins. This ultimately reduces pain and inflammation. Topical application of capsaicin, a major component of chilli and a transient receptor potential vanilloid-1 receptor ($TRPV_1$) agonist, may also be effective by interfering with substance-P-mediated pain transmission (see the chapter 'Nociception and pain').

Weight loss and non-weight-bearing exercise will reduce joint strain, improve joint strength and decrease the burden on supporting structures, which can ultimately reduce pain; however, excessive exercise will exacerbate pain and swelling. Research evidence suggests that the regular performance of light exercise, such as Tai Chi, at least twice a week for 60 minutes can significantly reduce pain and improve range of motion.

Some people report improvement with glucosamine and chondroitin supplementation. These products may promote cartilage regeneration; however, the mechanism remains unclear and their true efficacy is still being debated.

The intra-articular injection of corticosteroids or viscosupplementation may be beneficial in the control of pain in some people. Intra-articular corticosteroid administration is known to reduce pain at rest and improve joint range of motion (potentially from the gain in mobility from improved pain management). Local corticosteroid administration has been found to reduce lymphocyte, macrophage and mast cells numbers, thereby diminishing the concentration of pro-inflammatory factors. Intra-articular viscosupplementation is the injection of a glycosaminoglycan such as hyaluronic acid (also known as hyaluronan) into the joint, to augment the diminished synovial fluid volume. As osteoarthritis results in reduced hyaluronic acid within the synovial fluid, the consequent reduction in the viscoelastic properties of the synovial fluid results in increased joint stress. Viscosupplementation has been demonstrated to be effective in reducing pain when the joint is loaded, by increasing the viscoelastic properties of the synovial fluid in the affected joint.

The noradrenaline-serotonin reuptake inhibitor duloxetine has been used in the management of chronic musculoskeletal pain conditions, such as osteoarthritis of the knee. It can be useful as an adjunct to oral NSAID therapy. Serotonin and noradrenaline have a role in the modulation of pain transmission pathways in the brain and spinal cord.

In severe osteoarthritis, the main method of controlling pain and improving function is joint replacement. In Australia and New Zealand, the majority of joint replacement surgeries performed are for osteoarthritis. Arthroplasty (joint replacement) is an elective surgery to remove the diseased joint and replace it with a prosthetic joint that is cemented or screwed into place. Although the viable life expectancy of the prosthesis is only 10 years, the improvement in clinical manifestations can have a significant effect on the individual's quality of life. When a joint replacement wears out, fails or becomes infected, it must be replaced. This revision surgery is more complicated and has a less predictable outcome than the initial surgery.

RHEUMATOID ARTHRITIS

Aetiology and pathophysiology

Rheumatoid arthritis is a chronic inflammatory condition affecting synovial joints. Unlike osteoarthritis, rheumatoid arthritis is an *autoimmune disease* with complex immune system interactions that are still not yet fully understood. This knowledge deficit means that a fully effective, all-encompassing treatment has not yet been developed.

Being an autoimmune disease, rheumatoid arthritis occurs in people with a *defect in the discrimination of self/non-self molecules*. It is thought that the condition also requires a genetic predisposition (a strong association with the human leukocyte antigen [HLA] locus *HLADB1*) and an antigenic stimulus to initiate the chain of immunological events that result in joint destruction and deformity. The disease state develops as a consequence of an interaction between cells within the joint called *fibroblast-like synoviocytes*, the *innate immune system* (macrophages, dendritic cells, neutrophils and mast cells) and the *adaptive immune system* (T and B lymphocytes). Several immune system activities occur, some in parallel and some in sequence, and at this time not all interactions or influences are fully understood. Figure 42.11 summarises the current understanding of the pathophysiology of rheumatoid arthritis. As research into this disease progresses, so will a greater understanding of the pathophysiology.

Following B cell stimulation, autoantibodies such as rheumatoid factor (RF) and anti-citrullinated protein antibody (ACPA) are produced. Some of these become complexed with immunoglobulins such as immunoglobulin G (IgG) or IgM. Autoantibody synthesis stimulates T cell activation, which ultimately results in the synthesis and release of pro-inflammatory cytokines, such as IL-1, IL-6, TNF-α and prostaglandins. Some of these pro-inflammatory cytokines cause macrophages to be attracted into the synovial fluid. This not only causes other white blood cells, such as T cells, mast cells, neutrophils and dendritic cells, to be attracted to the area, but it also promotes angiogenesis. Mast cells and neutrophils ingest the immune complexes and release enzymes that degrade both synovial tissue and articular tissue. The release of receptor activator of nuclear factor κ-B ligand (RANKL), a mediator of osteoclastogenesis (i.e. osteoclast proliferation), along with some other cytokines, results in the increased activity of osteoclasts, causing increased bone destruction, and inhibition of osteoblasts, reducing the volume of bone rebuilding that is occurring. Both of these factors result in bone destruction, atrophy and, ultimately, joint deformity.

Cells within the synovium are called *synoviocytes*. There are two types of synoviocytes: type A are macrophagic cells; type B are fibroblast-like cells that promote synovial hyperplasia and, along with the previously stimulated angiogenesis, form fibrovascular tissue called 'pannus'. Both type A and type B cells induce the synthesis and release of matrix metalloproteinases (MMPs), discussed in the osteoarthritis section above, which cause further cartilage destruction and subsequent inflammation. As the disease progresses, the pannus calcifies and bony alkylosis (i.e. the development of rigidity) occurs, which causes fusion and, ultimately, results in total joint immobility.

As with many autoimmune diseases, pregnancy can influence the disease process. A clear improvement occurs in rheumatoid arthritis during pregnancy. The mechanism underpinning this improvement is unknown; however, theories include an effect

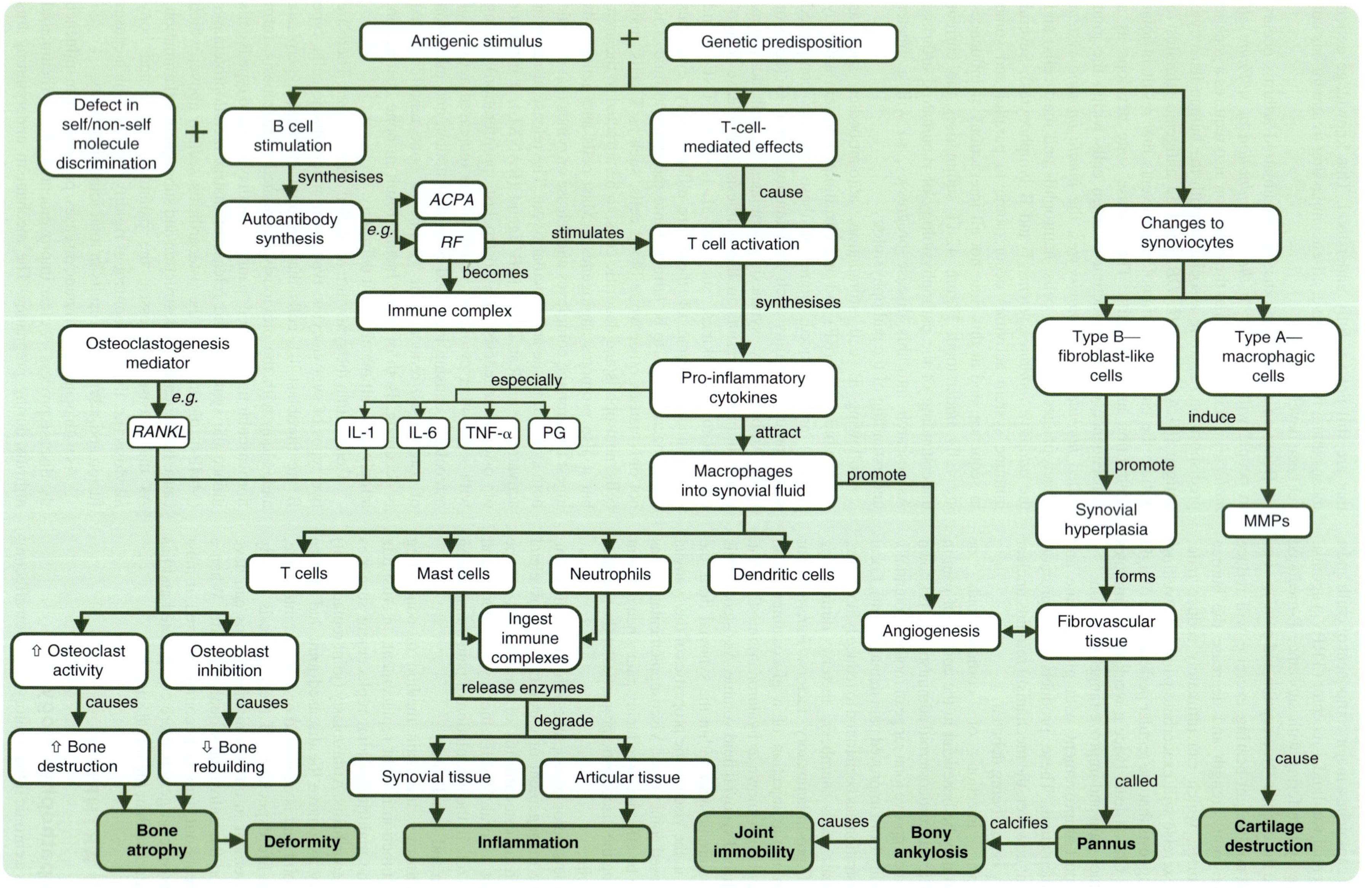

Figure 42.11

Current understanding of the pathophysiology of rheumatoid arthritis

↓ = decreased; ↑ = increased; ACPA = anti-citrullinated protein antibody; IL = interleukin; MMPs = matrix metalloproteinases; PG = prostaglandins; RANKL = receptor activator of nuclear factor κ-B ligand; RF = rheumatoid factor; TNF-α = tumour necrosis factor-alpha.

of the pregnancy hormones on humoral immunity, a pregnancy-induced elevation of anti-inflammatory cytokines and modified neutrophil function. This amelioration is only short-lasting, and postnatal flare-ups are likely. Elevated prolactin levels are pro-inflammatory, and the pregnancy-induced anti-inflammatory cytokines and steroids are lost.

Rheumatoid arthritis can also affect children, and is known as *juvenile idiopathic arthritis* (formerly called *juvenile rheumatoid arthritis*). Juvenile idiopathic arthritis is considered to be more of a group of diseases rather than a single disease. A distinct variation occurs in the presentation of juvenile idiopathic arthritis, which can be limited to fewer than five large joints (*pauciarticular*), more than five joints (*polyarticular*), or significant *systemic* effects, including fever, rash and inflammation of organs such the heart or liver. Fortunately, systemic disease is the least common type of juvenile idiopathic arthritis. Although the mechanism of juvenile idiopathic arthritis is also unknown, it is considered an autoimmune disease, too.

Epidemiology

Rheumatoid arthritis is the second most common form of arthritis. According to the AIHW, 1.9% of Australians (456,000 people) report having rheumatoid arthritis. It is most common in people over 65 years of age. Women are slightly more likely than men to develop rheumatoid arthritis (2.3% of women in the population compared to 1.5% of men). In New Zealand, approximately 100,000 people have rheumatoid arthritis, and women are more likely than men to develop the condition (3.1% women in the population to 2% men).

Some non-modifiable factors that increase the risk of developing rheumatoid arthritis include genetic predisposition, being female and age. Modifiable risk factors include exposure to an infectious agent or some other environmental factor for the antigenic stimulus. Other modifiable factors include cigarette smoking.

Clinical manifestations

The clinical manifestations of rheumatoid arthritis can be divided into those that affect the musculoskeletal system and those that are extra-articular (or systemic) manifestations. Rheumatoid arthritis can affect almost any joint, but it commonly occurs in the hands (see Figure 42.12), feet, ankles, cervical spine, hip, elbow and temporomandibular joints. There is a relatively symmetrical distribution of the affected joints. Figure 42.13 explores the common clinical manifestations and management of rheumatoid arthritis.

Affected joints will commonly be warm and oedematous, with a reduced range of motion. Many with rheumatoid arthritis will complain of discomfort and stiffness that lasts more than an hour after inactivity. As the disease progresses, difficulty in performing activities of daily living and joint deformity develop. Sleep disturbance and fatigue are commonly experienced. Many people also experience depression. Extra-articular manifestations affect the connective tissue and may affect many organ systems (see Figure 42.14).

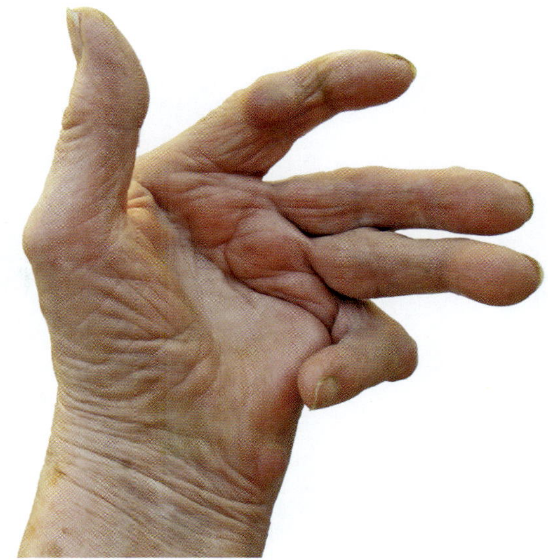

Figure 42.12

A person's hand severely affected by rheumatoid arthritis

Note the swelling and deformity.

Source: peterfactors/Shutterstock.

Clinical diagnosis and management

Diagnosis The Australian Therapeutic Guidelines indicate that a family history of inflammatory arthritis, the presence of joint swelling and pain in five or more joints, symmetrical involvement of the joints involved and/or morning stiffness lasting more than one hour are a strong indication of rheumatoid arthritis. Although there is no definitive test for rheumatoid arthritis, collection of a comprehensive health history and a physical assessment will assist in its accurate diagnosis. Blood tests are performed to exclude other diseases and forms of arthritis, and include a full blood count, which may be useful to detect anaemia or thrombocytosis in the presence of systemic manifestations. The erythrocyte sedimentation rate (ESR) and C-reactive protein (CRP) level, although non-specific, are markers of inflammation. Two antibody tests are also performed: RF and anti-cyclic citrullinated peptide (anti-CCP) antibody levels are measured. Most people with rheumatoid arthritis will have measurable RF antibody levels, and most of these people will also have anti-CCP antibodies; however, even though these are strong indicators of rheumatoid arthritis, along with the history and clinical assessment, they are not diagnostic. An antinuclear antibody (ANA) assay may also be performed, which, along with RF, is a marker of autoantibodies.

X-ray will be necessary to visualise the joint, and demonstrate the degree of disease progression and the presence of subluxation or malalignment. MRI may be done, but is expensive and of limited value other than for cervical spine anomalies. Ultrasound scans are quick, easy and less expensive, and may be of value in distinguishing between Baker's cysts and effusions. Synovial

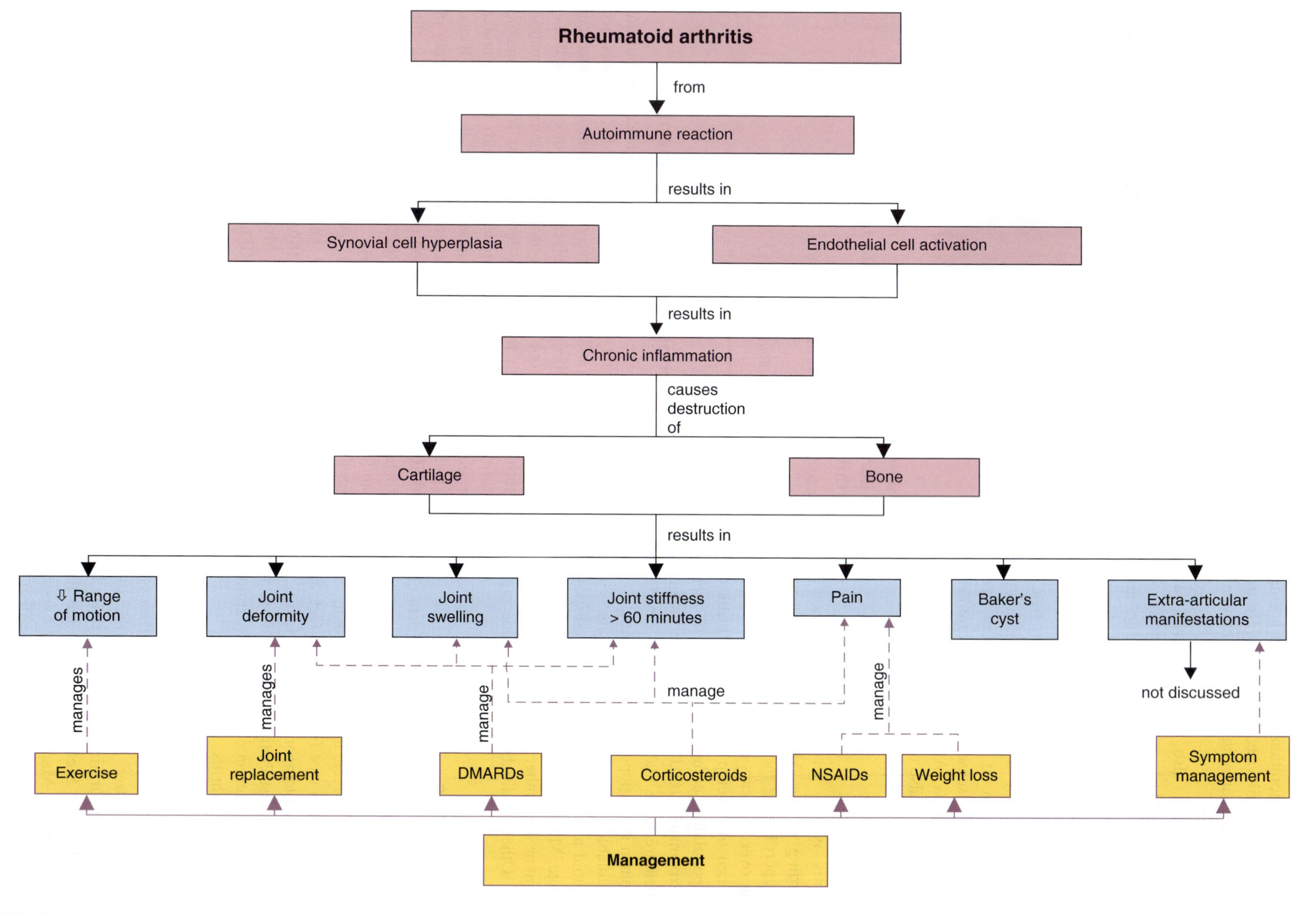

Figure 42.13

Clinical snapshot: Rheumatoid arthritis

↓ = decreased; DMARDs = disease-modifying antirheumatic drugs; NSAIDs = non-steroidal anti-inflammatory drugs.

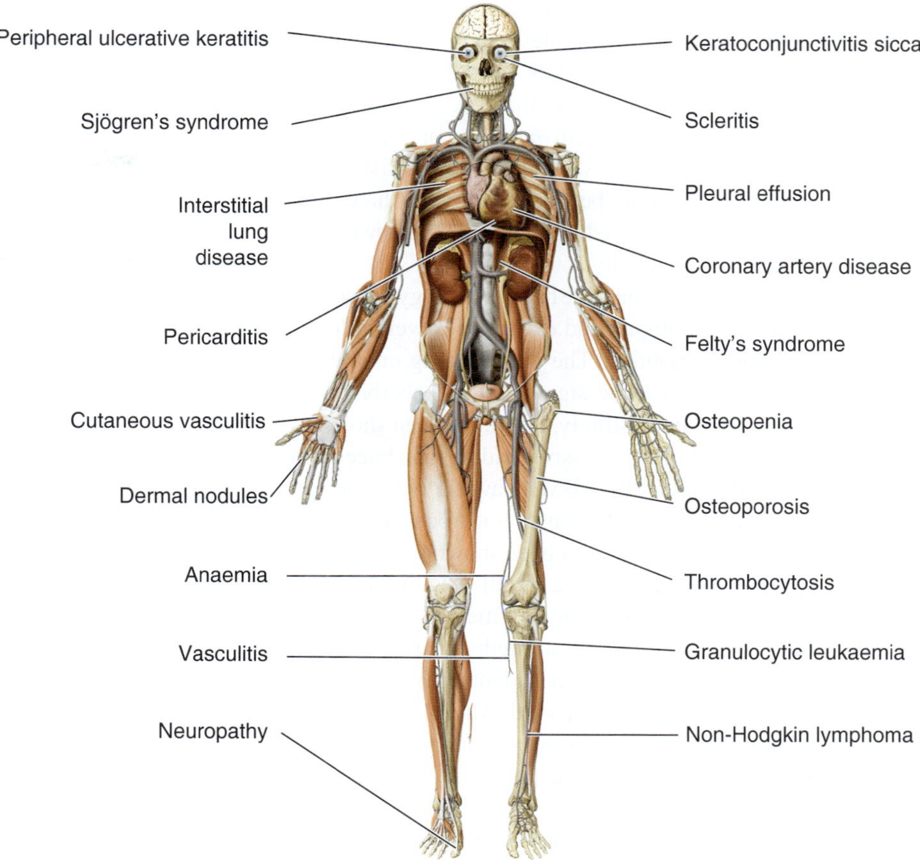

Figure 42.14

Extra-articular (systemic) manifestations of rheumatoid arthritis

Mortality rates in individuals with rheumatoid arthritis are almost three times higher than in healthy individuals, as a direct result of systemic manifestations.

Source: QA International/Universal Images Group North America LLC/Alamy Stock Photo.

fluid analysis may be beneficial to eliminate the presence of infection. Microscopy, culture and sensitivity should be tested. White blood cell counts are generally high, with neutrophils dominating the sample in people with rheumatoid arthritis.

Management Lifestyle management is important in the early stages of rheumatoid arthritis, with the emphasis on exercise, cessation of cigarette smoking and possibly a modification of diet. The latter aspect is controversial, but the most widely supported dietary intervention is the adoption of the 'Mediterranean diet'.

The induction of clinical remission in the form of symptom relief, absence of swollen joints and normalisation of inflammatory markers is a focus of treatment. Early treatment with **disease-modifying antirheumatic drugs (DMARDs)** is very important, and should be initiated by a rheumatologist. Methotrexate or sulphasalazine are two conventional DMARDS commonly used to preserve joint function. Although the mechanism of action of the DMARDs is not well understood, methotrexate is believed to act as a DMARD by increasing the availability of adenosine, thereby interfering with the rapid proliferation of immune system cells involved in the inflammatory response. Sulphasalazine has aspirin-like activity and inhibits prostaglandin synthesis. When DMARDs are used, frequent blood tests (monthly) are required to monitor for signs of toxicity. Generally speaking, DMARDs should not be used in women who are pregnant or who are planning pregnancy within three months.

The use of the *biological DMARDs (bDMARDs)* is indicated when the response to conventional approaches is insufficient. Selected agents can be used as adjunct therapy with methotrexate. Some bDMARDs can block cytokines. Adalimumab, etanercept, certolizumab, golimumab and infliximab inhibit TNF-α. Some agents, such as anakinra, inhibit IL-1, and toclizaumab inhibits IL-6. Other agents are directed at certain cells. Abatacept inhibits a signal that is required for T cell activation, and rituximab inhibits an antigen on B cells. As these drugs target specific mechanisms within the pathogenesis of rheumatoid arthritis, they are more effective than generic anti-inflammatory agents in not only controlling pain but also reducing joint destruction. Currently, only parenteral doses of these agents are available. Given their mechanism of action, these drugs take weeks to months before any obvious benefit is perceived. Education is needed regarding these drugs and, as with any agent, careful observation and monitoring are needed so that any adverse reactions are quickly identified.

During flare-ups, exacerbations, when desiring rapid symptom control or while waiting for the effect of DMARDs to manifest, short-term low-dose corticosteroids may be beneficial. Oral agents may be used, although sometimes severe flare-ups may require intravenous corticosteroid therapy. Intra-articular corticosteroids may be beneficial; however, it is recommended that no more than three injections per year are given to a specific joint.

Residual joint pain during clinical remission can be managed using an NSAID. Risks of gastrointestinal, cardiovascular and renal side-effects from the NSAIDs need to be considered. Gastrointestinal protective agents may be indicated when NSAIDs are used. People with asthma or those taking anticoagulants should not take NSAIDs. Omega-3 fish oils may also be used during this time, but may take up to three months to produce clinical benefits. Fish oils have been shown to have some anti-inflammatory activity.

It is difficult to achieve a balance between energy conservation techniques to manage fatigue, and exercise for weight loss and improvement of joint mobility. The joint loading on knees that occurs in obese people can be significantly exacerbating pain and joint degradation. Interestingly, hips have been shown to be significantly less affected by excessive loading than knees. Those with a healthy body mass index (BMI) have far better outcomes than those with high BMIs. Although functional joint support may be beneficial, splinting has not been shown to be favourable in people with rheumatoid arthritis. Adaptive equipment may be necessary to assist the person with activities of daily living, as joint deformity and loss of muscle strength occur.

Systemic symptoms should be identified and managed as they appear. People at risk of cardiovascular disease may benefit from assessment by a cardiovascular team, as well as from the initiation of prophylactic interventions and lifestyle modifications.

As with osteoarthritis, joint replacement may be necessary. Those with severe deformity may require reconstructive surgery to achieve functional improvement so as to promote independence with activities of daily living. Preparation for surgery should entail weight loss to target bodyweight, ideal nutrition and optimal management of comorbidities.

ANKYLOSING SPONDYLITIS

Aetiology and pathophysiology

In **ankylosing spondylitis**, another form of arthritis, the intra-articular effects are primarily limited to the *vertebral and sacroiliac joints*. Ankylosing means 'rigid' and spondylitis means 'inflammation of the vertebrae'. Ankylosing spondylitis is classified in a larger group of conditions called *spondyloarthropathies*.

Little is known about the cause of ankylosing spondylitis. There does appear to be a genetic predisposition related to the *HLA-B27* gene, as almost 90% of people with the condition have this HLA haplotype. However, more than 100 other conditions also have an association with this gene, and most people with the *HLA-B27* gene haplotype never develop ankylosing spondylitis.

Ankylosing spondylitis is relatively rare, and is two and a half times more common in men than in women. It tends to first manifest in young adults aged 17–35 years.

Current research suggests that three distinct processes caused by various pathways are involved in ankylosing spondylitis (see Figure 42.15). In ankylosing spondylitis, we observe *inflammatory joint erosion* together with *abnormal bony overgrowth*. The *entheses* (the point at which a tendon, ligament or capsule inserts into bone) becomes inflamed due to the action of the pro-inflammatory mediator TNF-α. Joint erosion occurs as a result of products released by osteoclasts, synoviocytes and chondrocytes, which degrade cartilage and bone. Finally, bony growths form that originate from the vertebral enthuses (syndesmophytes). The anomalous bone growth often bridges adjacent vertebrae, fusing the spine and making the affected section immobile.

Clinical manifestations

Initially, dull lower back pain and stiffness are experienced. This may be worse after periods of inactivity, and improve with movement or following a warm shower. Sometimes fever, anorexia and flu-like symptoms may be identified. As the condition becomes chronic, the primary intra-articular effects result in back and neck stiffness. Other musculoskeletal pain may be experienced as a result of changes to posture and gait. Severe ankylosing spondylitis can result in significant spinal fusion that interferes with all facets of activities of daily living.

Ankylosing spondylitis can also be associated with extra-articular conditions, such as iritis or uveitis, and irritable bowel syndromes, such as Crohn's disease or ulcerative colitis. People with iritis (inflammation of the iris, the coloured part of the eye) and uveitis (inflammation of the uvea, the middle layer of the eye) will have a painful, red, watery eye. They may complain of photophobia (light sensitivity) or even blurred vision. Those with irritable bowel syndromes will experience abdominal pain and bloody diarrhoea.

Clinical diagnosis and management

Diagnosis Currently, no definitive diagnostic test exists to confirm ankylosing spondylitis. The collection of a comprehensive health history and a physical examination are important, especially in the context of range-of-motion assessment. An X-ray will generally be taken to observe for structural changes. A full blood count may be performed to exclude comorbidities, and the ESR and/or CRP level may be measured to determine the presence/degree of inflammation. A stool sample may be required to eliminate other enteric diseases or conditions.

Management Ultimately, the goals in management of ankylosing spondylitis are to reduce pain and inflammation, to maintain mobility and to prevent progressive damage. These goals are met through health education to understand the disease and address the psychosocial effects on their lives, an appropriate exercise program, and drug therapy.

The treatment of ankylosing spondylitis is similar to the interventions listed for osteoarthritis and rheumatoid arthritis. Firstly, a combination of simple analgesia, NSAIDs and corticosteroids is recommended. For more severe or unresponsive disease, the bDMARDs (e.g. anti-TNF-α agents) are recommended. The conventional DMARDs have a limited usefulness in ankylosing spondylitis.

Iritis and uveitis must be treated with topical corticosteroid eye drops, and potentially even pupillary-dilating drops. Iritis is a serious complication and can result in loss of sight if not managed quickly. Symptoms of irritable bowel syndrome may be managed with antispasmodic and antidiarrhoeal agents.

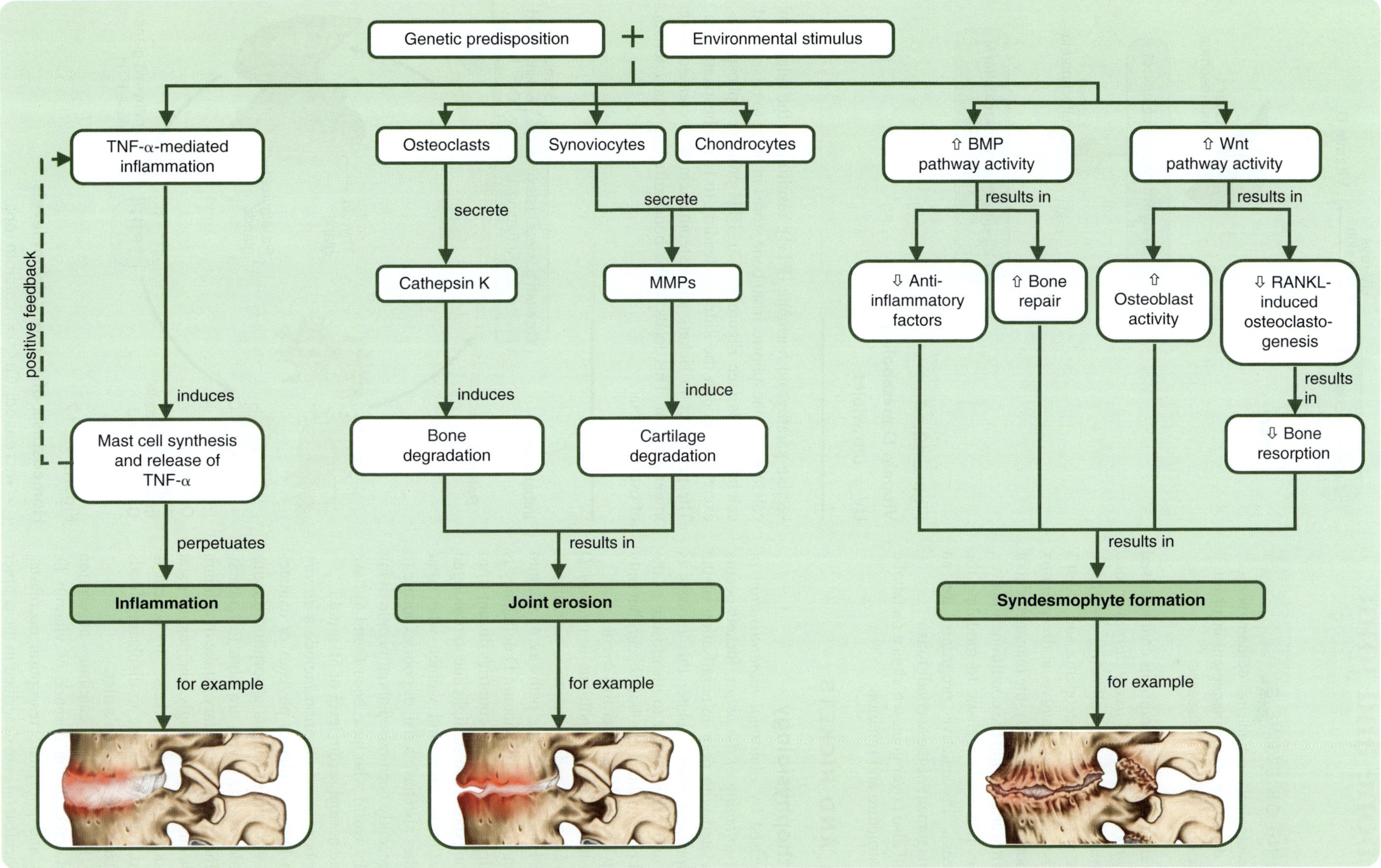

Figure 42.15

Current theories of ankylosing spondylitis pathogenesis

Three distinct processes occur, involving inflammation, joint erosion and syndesmophyte formation.

↓ = decreased; ↑ = increased; BMP = bone morphogenetic protein; MMPs = matrix metalloproteinases; RANKL = receptor activator of nuclear factor κ-B ligand; TNF-α = tumour necrosis factor-alpha; Wnt = molecular name derived from Wingless and Integrase-1.

Source: Vertebral images adapted from stihii/Shutterstock.

Metabolic bone and joint diseases

LEARNING OBJECTIVE 3

Describe the pathophysiological mechanisms, epidemiology, clinical manifestations, diagnosis and management involved in metabolic bone and joint diseases.

Metabolic bone diseases are a family of conditions characterised by *impairment in the process of bone tissue turnover and mineralisation*. The family includes the following disorders: osteomalacia and rickets, osteoporosis, osteopenia and Paget's disease of the bone. The aetiologies involve a diverse mix of environmental and genetic factors. Ideally, the management of these diseases is directed towards curing the condition; however, this may not be possible. It is more realistic to modulate the pathophysiological process. Preventative programs are an important part of the management of these conditions.

In this section, we will also cover gout, which is a metabolic disease that affects joint structure and function.

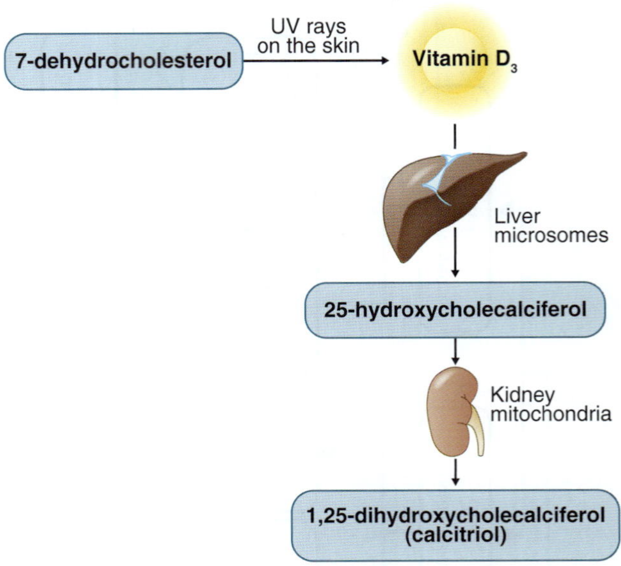

Figure 42.16

Vitamin D metabolism

UV = ultraviolet.

OSTEOMALACIA AND RICKETS

Aetiology and pathophysiology

Osteomalacia is characterised by *abnormal mineralisation of the osseous matrix* and a *softening of the bones*. **Rickets** occurs in children, and is associated with poor mineralisation of the cartilage within the epiphyseal growth plate; this process is known as *endochondral ossification*. Prior to the closure of the growth plate, rickets and osteomalacia can both occur, but only osteomalacia can develop in adulthood after this event.

The most common cause of these conditions is *vitamin D deficiency*. Vitamin D availability and activation is essential in the mineralisation of the bone matrix. The pathway of vitamin D metabolism is shown in Figure 42.16. Vitamin D deficiency is classically associated with people living in countries distant from the equator who have poor exposure to sunlight due to prolonged winters or severe air pollution. Girls and women who wear extensive concealing clothes also have a risk of poor exposure to sunlight. Concerns have recently been raised about people living in the sunniest parts of the world who have been found to have vitamin D levels below the normal serum level of 50 nmol/L.

Other causes of poor bone mineralisation include a *dietary calcium deficiency*. High levels of dietary phylates or oxalates can bind calcium in the gut and impair its absorption. Grains are rich in phylates, while oxalate levels are high in spinach, beans and sweet potato. Increasing the dietary intake of calcium is recommended in such cases. Interestingly, increasing meat intake can reduce the risk of nutritional rickets. The benefit is not yet clearly elucidated, but may be due to displacing foods high in phylates and oxalates in the person's diet.

Activated vitamin D facilitates calcium absorption from the gastrointestinal tract. In the absence of vitamin D, hypocalcaemia develops and phosphate resorption decreases. The effects of severe hypocalcaemia are described in the chapter 'Electrolyte imbalances'. In this state, the parathyroid glands secrete parathyroid hormone (PTH), resulting in the release of calcium and phosphorus from bone stores in order to raise blood calcium levels (see Figure 42.17). PTH promotes phosphorus excretion through the kidneys, leading to hypophosphataemia. The net effect in rickets and osteomalacia is decreased bone mineralisation. This leads to the bone-softening characteristic of osteomalacia.

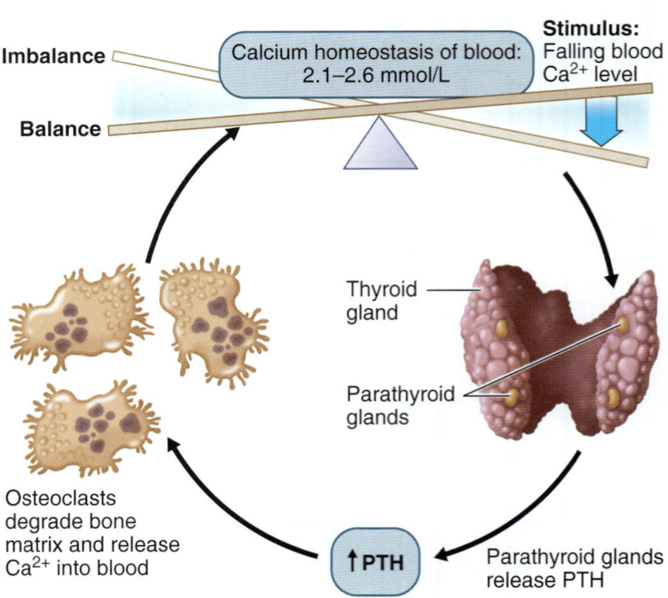

Figure 42.17

Homeostasis of serum calcium levels

↑ = increased; Ca^{2+} = calcium ion; PTH = parathyroid hormone.

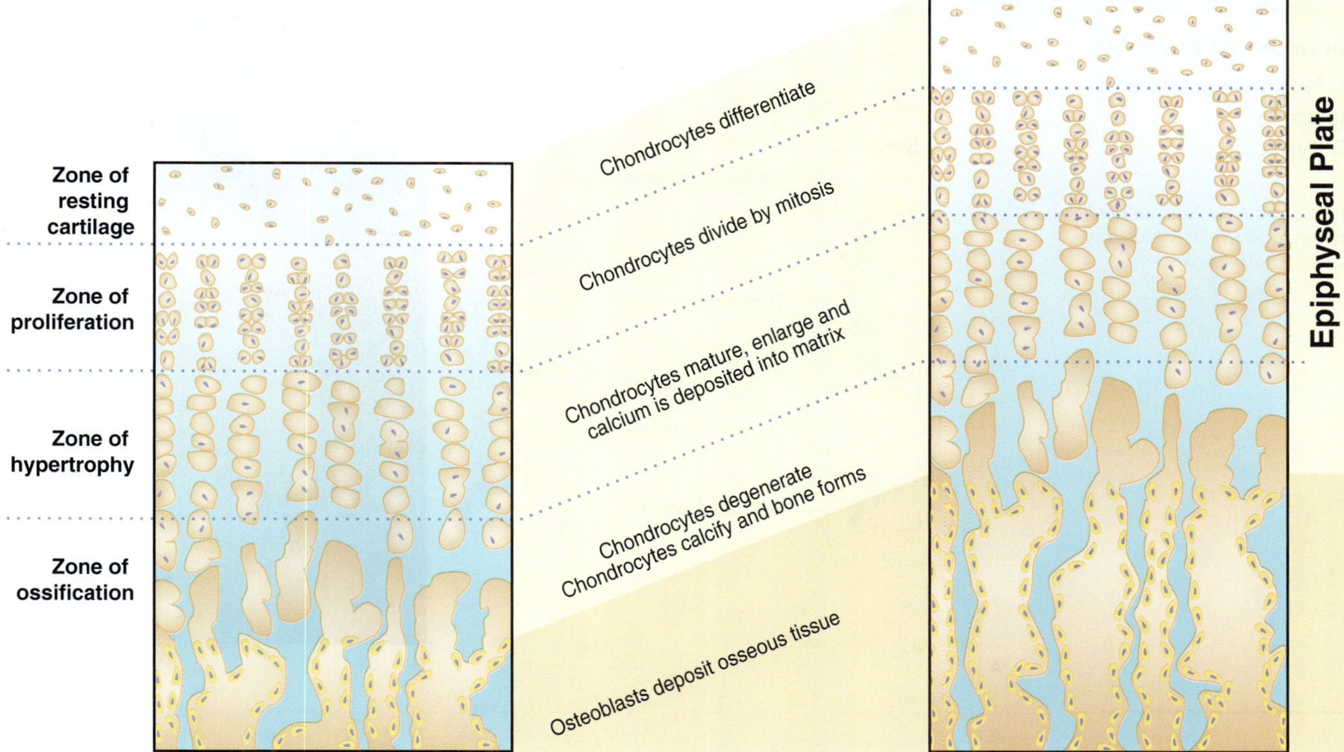

Figure 42.18

Bone development and the four cartilage zones

Normally, the epiphyseal growth plate consists of four distinct cartilaginous zones: the *resting, proliferative, hypertrophic* and *ossification zones* (see Figure 42.18). The cartilage cells of the hypertrophic zone are the focus of ossification. The zone becomes calcified, the cartilage cells undergo apoptosis, the calcified tissue becomes vascularised, and then osteoclasts and osteoblasts migrate into the tissue. In rickets, hypophosphataemia induces a failure in apoptosis of the hypertrophic cartilage cells, leading to an irregular and deformed expansion of the cartilage tissue within the growth plate.

Clinical manifestations

The common clinical manifestations of osteomalacia and rickets are listed in Table 42.2. One manifestation, called *gibbus*

Table 42.2 Clinical manifestations of osteomalacia and rickets

Clinical manifestation	Characteristics
Bone pain	Dull, aching pain, commonly experienced in the ribs, lumbosacral spine, pelvis and legs
Altered mobility and loss of independence	Difficulty rising from a lying position and standing from a sitting position
Muscle weakness	An early sign in severe cases
Pathological fractures	Common in weakened areas; for example, distal radius and proximal femur
Dorsal kyphosis/gibbus deformity	Severe cases
Rickets (children)	Bone growth retardation—decreased longitudinal bone growth, widening of epiphyseal regions
	Joint swelling and pain
	Dental caries and enamel defects
	Delay in developmental milestones
	Gibbus deformity
	Deformity of the lower extremities—bowing of the legs, particularly the tibia

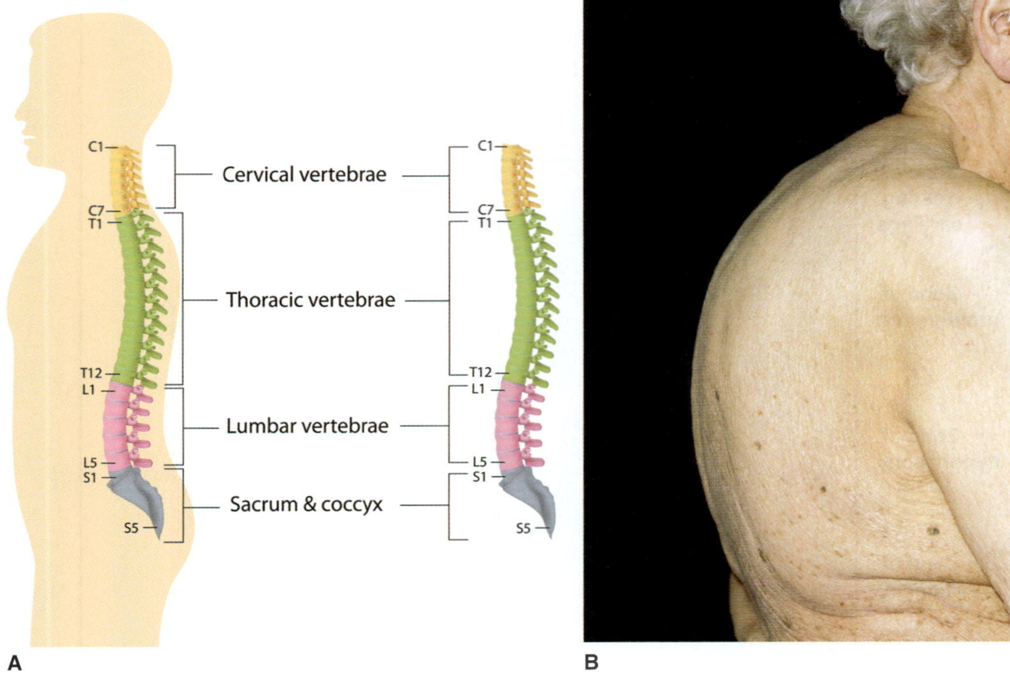

Figure 42.19

Curvature of the spine

(A) Normal curvature of the spine.
(B) Kyphosis.

Sources: (A) Alila Medical Media/ Shutterstock; (B) Dr P. Marazzi/ Science Photo Library.

deformity, is a sharply angled convex deformity of the spine known as **kyphosis** (see Figure 42.19), which involves one or two softened vertebral bodies in the thoracolumbar region. Bowing of the legs of a small child is shown in Figure 42.20.

The systemic signs and symptoms that can develop in children with rickets as a result of the altered availability of calcium and phosphates include convulsions and tetany, hypotonia, constipation, cardiomyopathy and anaemia.

Clinical diagnosis and management

Diagnosis A diagnosis of rickets or osteomalacia can be achieved using clinical examination, laboratory testing and medical imaging. Physical examination is used to assess the clinical manifestations of the condition.

Blood testing of a number of parameters is useful in confirming the diagnosis. The clinical signs of osteomalacia and rickets

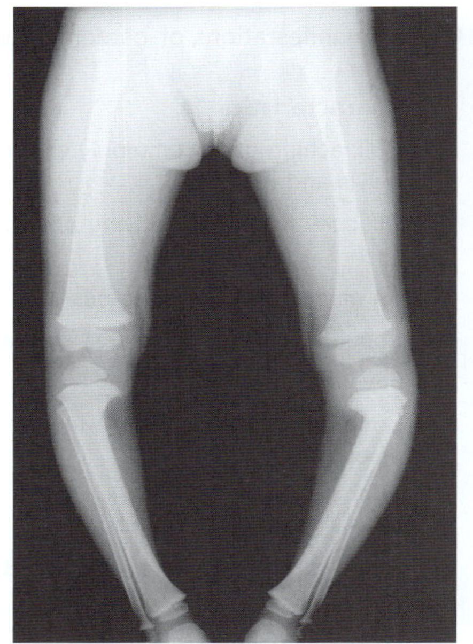

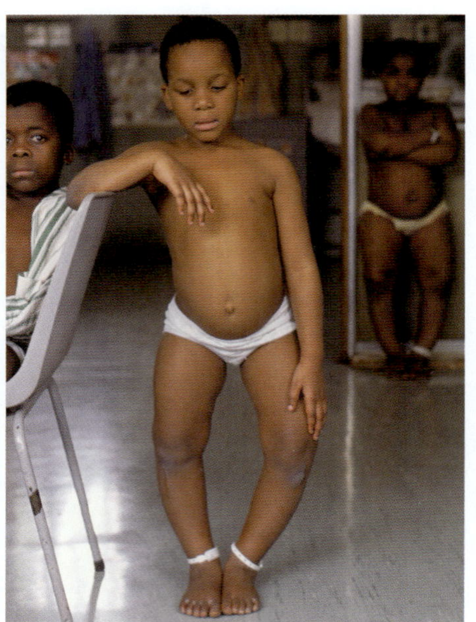

Figure 42.20

The effects of rickets on a small child

(A) X-ray of a child showing some femoral bowing and significant tibial bowing.
(B) Bowed legs in a child affected with rickets.

Sources: (A) Zephyr/Science Photo Library; (B) © Imagestate Media Partners Limited—Impact Photos/Alamy Stock Photo.

are usually observed at activated vitamin D (calcitriol) levels of 25 nmol/L or lower. Serum calcium and phosphate levels are lower than normal, whereas serum PTH levels may be raised. The enzyme alkaline phosphatase is released from overactive osteoblasts into the circulation. Its serum level in these conditions would be expected to be elevated. X-ray imaging may reveal the characteristic linear areas of low density surrounded by sclerosis (*Looser's zones*), osteopenia and coarsened trabecular bone, especially in the femoral neck and shaft. Structural changes may not be obvious on X-ray until well after 30% of bone is lost.

Management Vitamin D supplementation using an inactive form—vitamin D_3—increases body stores of the nutrient and produces relatively rapid alterations in bone structure. Co-therapy with calcium supplements greatly reduces the risk of fractures.

Disease prevention through community education about reasonable exposure to sunlight is vital. In sunny countries like Australia and New Zealand, the balance between appropriate sun protection and exposure to sunlight is important.

OSTEOPOROSIS

Aetiology and pathophysiology

Osteoporosis is characterised by a *significant loss of bone mineral density (BMD)* and a *loss of microstructure*. Bones become brittle and fragile, leading to an increased risk of fractures. Underlying the condition is a change in the *balance between bone formation and resorption*.

This balance is controlled by two populations of bone cells arranged on bone surfaces. *Osteoclasts*, which are derived from bone marrow cells that differentiate along the granulocyte–monocyte pathway, break down bone tissue and facilitate its resorption. *Osteoblasts*, which are specialised fibroblast cells, form new bone. Bone tissue is subject to constant turnover—a process called *bone remodelling*—throughout our lives. Remodelling occurs in response to *environmental influences*, such as mechanical stress or load, as well as the presence of *hormones and other mediators*. Osteoclasts and osteoblasts transform resting bone surfaces into active remodelling sites. These discrete sites throughout the skeleton are known as *bone remodelling units (BMU)*. Osteoclasts in a particular BMU become active, resorbing bone tissue. At the end of this stage, osteoclasts undergo apoptosis. Osteoblasts then migrate to the resorption zones to form a new bone matrix, which becomes mineralised. This cycle of remodelling is represented in Figure 42.21. The rate of turnover is higher in the *trabecular, or cancellous, bone* in the epiphyses of long bones and in the vertebral bodies, than in the *compact bone* found on the metaphyses of long bones.

Osteoclast activity is regulated by a number of chemicals. *Parathyroid hormone, the glucocorticoids and high doses of vitamin D increase activity, while calcitonin, oestrogens and androgens decrease it*. A number of *mediators involved in inflammation* also increase osteoclast activity, including the interleukins and prostaglandins.

Members of the *tissue necrosis factor (TNF) family* and its receptors play a key role in the regulation of osteoclast activation and activity. The key contributors from this family are the

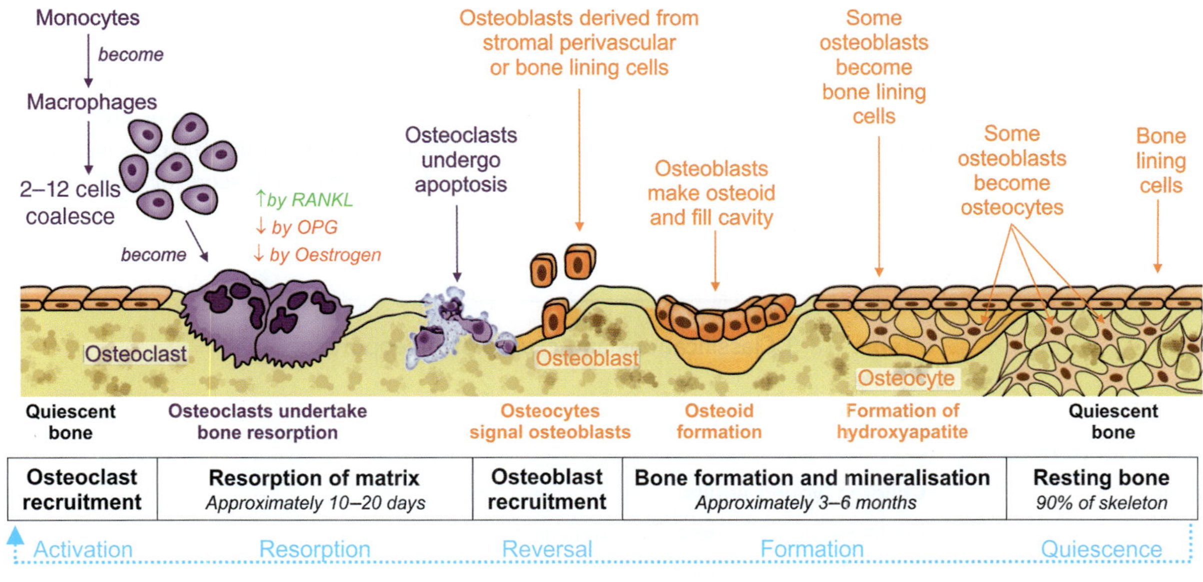

Figure 42.21

Bone turnover cycle

↓ = inhibited; ↑ = stimulated; OPG = osteoprotegerin; RANKL = receptor activator of nuclear factor κ-B ligand.

Source: © Sciencopia.

receptor activator of nuclear factor κ-B ligand (RANKL), the receptor to which this binds, which is called *receptor activator of nuclear factor κ-B (RANK)*, and the endogenous antagonist to RANKL known as *osteoprotegerin (OPG)*. RANK is present on the osteoclast precursor cells. When RANKL interacts with its receptor, osteoclasts proliferate and differentiate, enabling their capacity for bone resorption. OPG is a counter-regulatory substance secreted by osteoblasts that competes with RANKL for binding to RANK, inhibiting osteoclast formation and differentiation. A component of the suppression of oestrogens on osteoclasts is believed to be accounted for by the inhibition of RANKL secretion and promotion of OPG production.

In osteoporosis, the rate of bone resorption dominates its formation due to the relatively greater activation and activity of osteoclasts. This imbalance has been linked to age-related decreases in sex hormones, particularly oestrogens and to a lesser extent androgens, age-related decreases in osteoblasts, and the development of other disease states or the use of drug therapies that induce this condition. These aetiologies give rise to the classification of osteoporosis detailed in Table 42.3. A person with a reduced BMD would be considered to have a pre-osteoporotic condition known as **osteopenia**.

Epidemiology

The most recent data from the Australian Bureau of Statistics (2017–18) estimates 924,000 Australians are living with osteoporosis. In Australia in 2020–21, almost 6,700 people were admitted to public hospitals for osteoporosis-related fractures. Women are predominately affected by this condition, with 29% of women aged 75 years old and over affected, compared to 10% of men. Osteoporosis is more common in the major cities than in rural or regional areas.

In New Zealand, osteoporosis is a major health issue, and its effects on the community are considered to be greater than those of other conditions, such as prostate and breast cancers.

Osteoporosis is considered a preventable condition, and therefore alterations to lifestyle and community education programs, such as falls prevention initiatives, can have a considerable effect on incidence rates. Non-modifiable, modifiable and male-only risk factors for osteoporosis are listed in Table 42.4.

AIHW data also indicate that of all osteoporotic fractures, 32% are to the hip, 13% to the forearm and 13% to the lumbar spine and pelvis. While osteoporosis does not directly cause death, fractures in older adults with osteoporosis have been reported to result in premature death.

Clinical manifestations

A person with osteoporosis is largely asymptomatic, as the pathophysiological process takes place without any overt clinical manifestations. The main manifestation is fractures. These fractures tend to occur under circumstances in which a healthy person of that age would not be expected to experience such an injury. They occur because of the fragile and brittle character of osteoporotic bones. It is common for osteoporotic fractures to occur in the hip, wrist, pelvis, spine and ribs, as these bones have high proportions of cancellous bone, which, as stated earlier, has a relatively higher rate of bone turnover. Multiple asymptomatic vertebral fractures can lead to a change in posture, loss of height and reduced mobility (see Figure 42.22).

Figure 42.23 explores the common clinical manifestations and management of osteoporosis.

Clinical diagnosis and management

Diagnosis Diagnosis for osteoporosis is based on taking a history, a clinical examination and medical imaging in order to establish the differential diagnoses. A history and clinical examination will aid in the assessment of risk factors. In this case, medical imaging is the key confirmatory procedure.

The preferred medical imaging procedure is *dual energy X-ray absorptiometry (DEXA)*. DEXA provides a measurement of BMD. A normal BMD is considered to be no more than 1 standard deviation less than the mean peak bone mass of young, healthy adults. This is represented as a value known as the *T score*; in this case a T score of –1.0 or greater. A diagnosis of osteoporosis is made when the BMD is less than or equal to 2.5 standard deviations: a T score of –2.5 or lower. For a

Table 42.3 Classifications and causes of osteoporosis

Classification	Causes
Primary osteoporosis	
Idiopathic	Children, young adults
Type 1	Postmenopausal—oestrogen deficiency
Type 2	Associated with usual ageing process
Secondary osteoporosis	Results from clinical disorders, hyperthyroidism, hyperparathyroidism, gastrointestinal or renal disorders, and early oophorectomy. Can also occur in association with long-term glucocorticoid use, methotrexate, aluminium-containing antacids, phenytoin or heparin therapy. Other causes are chronic obstructive pulmonary disorder, immobilisation, liver disease, rheumatoid arthritis, sarcoidosis and pregnancy.

Table 42.4 Risk factors for osteoporosis

Non-modifiable risk factors	Modifiable risk factors	Male-only risk factors
Age—increased age brings greater risk	Decrease in bone mineral density	Androgen resistance
Delayed puberty or early menopause	Low bodyweight and low body mass	Androgen deficiency
Absence of oestrogen (menopause)	Sedentary lifestyle or prolonged immobility	Unusually fast decline in testosterone (prostate cancer)
Anorexia causing amenorrhoea	Inability to rise from a chair without using one's arms	Decreased libido and impotence
Small, thin body frame		
Ethnicity—Caucasian and Asian	Diet low in calcium and vitamin D	
Family history of fracture and osteoporosis	Low magnesium levels	
Maternal history of hip fracture	Cigarette smoking	
Malabsorption conditions (coeliac disease, inflammatory bowel disease)	Excessive use of alcohol	
	Excessive sodium intake	
Certain chronic medical conditions (rheumatoid arthritis, chronic renal failure, chronic liver disease)	High caffeine intake*	
	Nulliparity*	
A history of overactive thyroid or parathyroid glands, or treatment with thyroid hormones		
Long-term use of certain medications (corticosteroids and anticonvulsants)		
Fractures after the age of 50 years		
Conditions in which osteomalacia may also be present (osteogenesis imperfecta, Paget's disease of the bone, spinal cord injury)		

**Minor risk factors.*

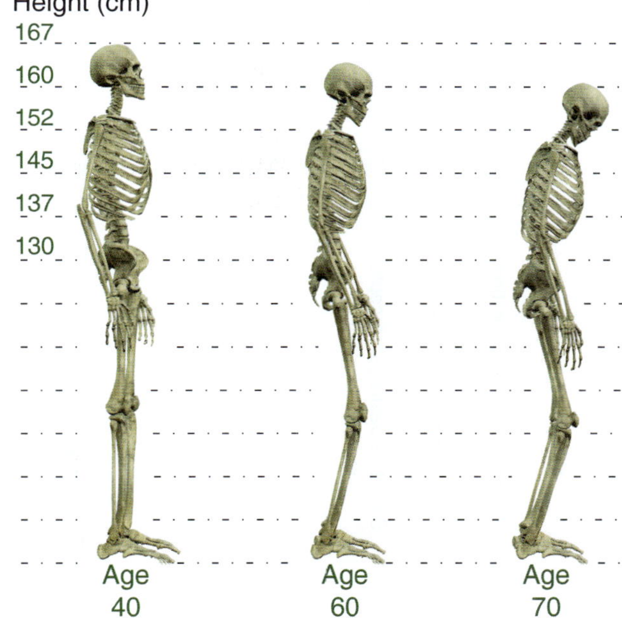

Figure 42.22

Spinal changes associated with osteoporosis

Source: Sciencopia.

measurement between these two scores, the person would be considered to have osteopenia.

Other medical imaging modalities, such as X-ray, computed tomography (CT) scans, MRI and ultrasound, can also be used to assess osteoporosis and osteopenia. An advantage of CT scans is that they can be used to assess BMD in both cancellous and compact bone tissues.

Management The aim of treatment is to reduce the risk of occurrence of osteoporotic fractures. Calcium supplementation is a routine therapy for people at risk of osteoporosis, with vitamin D added where there is evidence of low levels of this nutrient.

The first-line medications in the management of this condition are the antiresorptive agents known as bisphosphonates.

Other medicines used in the management of this condition in postmenopausal women include oestrogens, the selective oestrogen receptor modulator raloxifene, which acts as an oestrogen agonist on bone tissue but as an oestrogen antagonist at its receptors in breast tissue, and the steroid tibolone that has oestrogen-like activity.

The monoclonal antibodies denosumab and romosozumab may also be useful in the management of osteoporosis. Denosumab is directed against RANKL and decreases osteoclast activity. Romosozumab is directed against the protein sclerostin, which inhibits osteoblasts and bone formation. Without the influence of sclerostin, bone formation is enhanced.

Teriparatide is a peptide of the active sequence of parathyroid hormone. When administered intermittently it

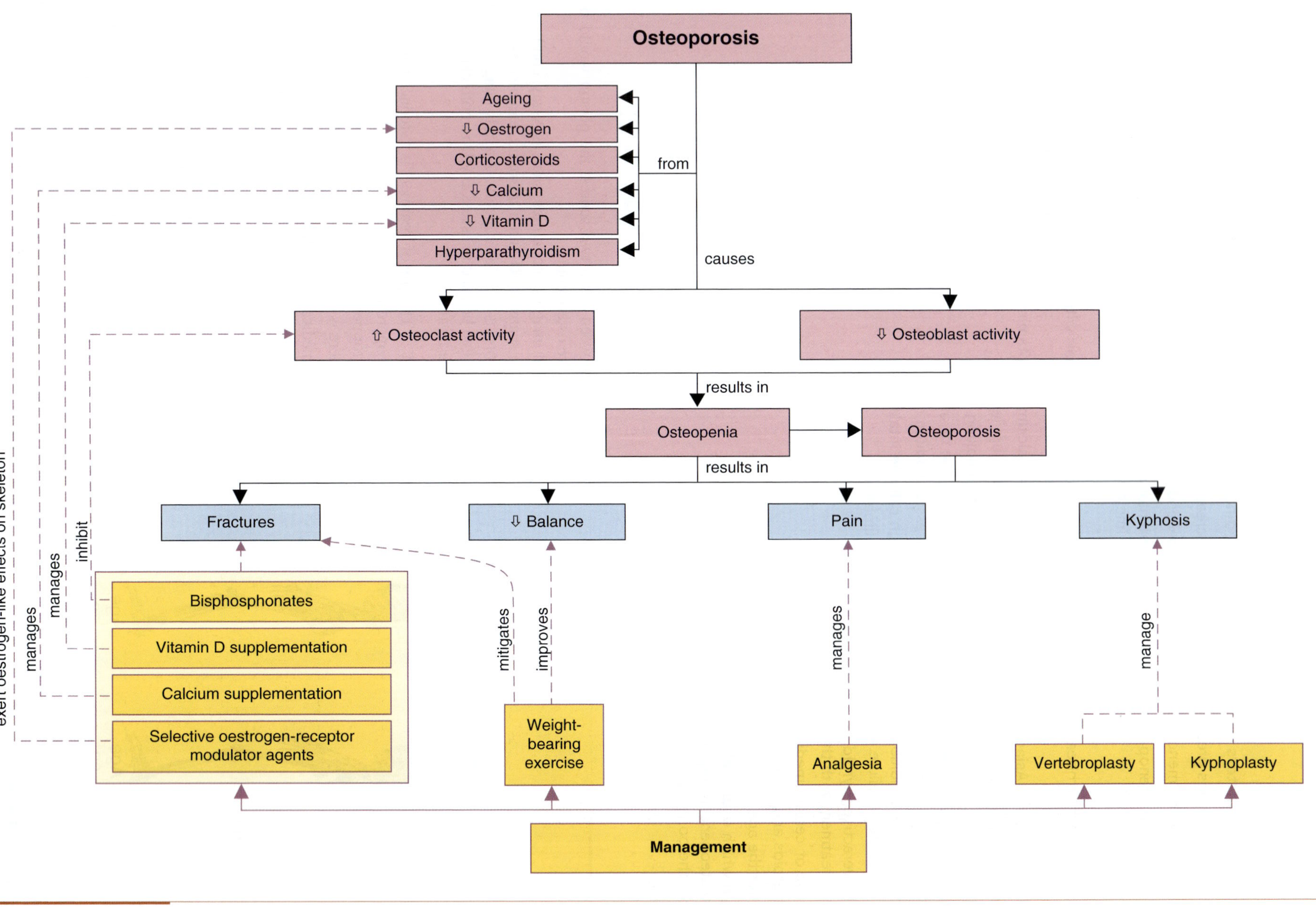

Figure 42.23
Clinical snapshot: Osteoporosis
↓ = decreased; ↑ = increased.

stimulates osteoblasts rather than osteoclasts, thus increasing bone formation.

PAGET'S DISEASE OF THE BONE

Aetiology and pathophysiology

Paget's disease of the bone is characterised by the formation of *disorganised osseous tissue that is weaker than normal*, and therefore more prone to deformity and fracture. It does not affect the whole skeleton, tends to be localised or regional, and may affect only one bone or many.

In this condition, the affected osteoclasts are not only dysfunctional, they are also morphologically abnormal. Cell size and shape is larger than normal, and they possess multiple nuclei. Affected osteoclasts show excessive and accelerated bone resorptive activity (with increased circulating levels of alkaline phosphatase enzyme), but this event is followed by the migration of osteoblasts into the zone and bone formation.

The aetiology of Paget's disease of the bone has been strongly linked to *genetic factors*. The condition develops in family clusters, and within the familial group it displays an autosomal dominant inheritance pattern. However, penetrance is variable. *Environmental factors* are considered to play a role, but their identification remains elusive. An environmental agent that has been implicated in this condition is viral infection, particularly myxoviruses and paramyxoviruses (which includes the measles virus). Other environmental factors that have been suggested include poor dietary calcium intake, mechanical loading of the skeleton and toxin exposure.

Epidemiology

The prevalence of Paget's disease of the bone increases with age, and in Australia has been estimated at 1–2% for people aged over 55 years. In New Zealand, the prevalence rates were comparable, but have declined significantly over the decades. It is rarely seen in people aged younger than 50 years. It is slightly more prevalent in women compared to men (a ratio of 1.6:1). The highest prevalence of the condition in the world is in the northwest of England. Historically Australia and New Zealand, with significant numbers of people with British ancestry, experienced high prevalence rates of this condition.

Clinical manifestations

The common clinical manifestations and their causes are listed in Table 42.5. The common regions of the skeleton affected by Paget's disease of the bone are the pelvis, femur, lumbar region of the spine, skull and tibia.

Clinical diagnosis and management

Diagnosis Diagnosis of this condition comprises a comprehensive history, a clinical examination, medical imaging and laboratory tests. The bone lesions and deformities characteristic of this disorder can be definitively confirmed by X-ray and CT scans. Scintigraphy can be used to assess the extent of skeletal involvement.

Serum levels of the enzyme alkaline phosphatase can be measured to assess the extent of bone turnover. However, the value of this marker is limited when the disorder affects only a few bones of the skeleton.

Management The management of Paget's disease of the bone is similar to that of osteoporosis, with the aim focused on strengthening the bones in order to reduce the risk of fractures. Calcium and vitamin D supplementation is indicated. The use of the bisphosphonate antiresorptive agents is considered the first-line therapy.

Table 42.5 Clinical presentation of Paget's disease of the bone

Symptom	Cause
Bone pain	Joints neighbouring bones with pagetic changes often develop osteoarthritis
Bone deformities	May occur as a result of immature or poorly formed bone
Fractures	Immature or poorly formed bone is unable to withstand the forces that properly developed bone would
Kyphosis, spinal cord compression and paralysis	Pagetic lesions on the spine
Hearing and visual disturbances	Impingement on the cranial nerves
Vertigo	Involvement of the temporal bone can damage cranial nerve VIII
Nerve root compression	Abnormal bone formation can result in nerve root compression
Headache	Pagetic skull bone growth can cause pressure changes within the cranial vault
Hydrocephalus	Pagetic skull bone growth can cause pressure changes within the cranial vault
Dental problems (malocclusion)	Pagetic changes to the mandible or the maxilla can result in loose teeth or jaw deformity

GOUT

Aetiology and pathophysiology

Gout is a relatively common form of arthritis classified as a *crystal-induced arthropathy*. Gout is caused by an *accumulation of uric acid* within the blood, and can occur as a result of its overproduction or underexcretion. Uric acid, an end product of purine metabolism, is formed in the liver and excreted by the kidney. When excessive uric acid remains within the blood, the condition is called *hyperuricaemia*. Retained uric acid can be stored as urate and deposited in soft tissues as crystals. However, a number of people with hyperuricaemia do not go on to develop gout, indicating that *genetic predisposition* plays an important role in the pathogenesis of this condition. This predisposition is most likely linked to purine metabolism.

Purine-rich foods, such as anchovies, liver, mushrooms and legumes, can exacerbate the condition, and are known as *gout flares*. Alcohol ingestion is a major risk factor for gout, and is related to the amount consumed. Interestingly, it is more likely to develop in beer drinkers than in wine or spirits drinkers. Gout often affects men in their fourth or fifth decade of life. People taking diuretics (agents that promote urine output) are at an increased risk of gout because of the chance of dehydration. Some diuretics, such as loop or thiazide diuretics, also promote uric acid retention.

Gouty arthritis occurs when crystals of uric acid are deposited in *synovial joint cavities*. Uric acid crystals can be deposited in the hands, fingers, forearms, knees, elbows or toes. The crystals are phagocytised by macrophages and mast cells that release lytic enzymes and pro-inflammatory mediators. Neutrophils then become activated and acute inflammation ensues. Affected joints become swollen, hot and painful. Pro-inflammatory mediators involved in this reaction include TNF-α, ILs, histamine and prostaglandins.

Clinical manifestations

Gout can cause inflammation and pain in the affected joints (see Figure 42.24). Gouty arthritis of the big toe is a commonly affected joint. Solid lumps of uric acid crystals deposited in tissues are called **tophi**.

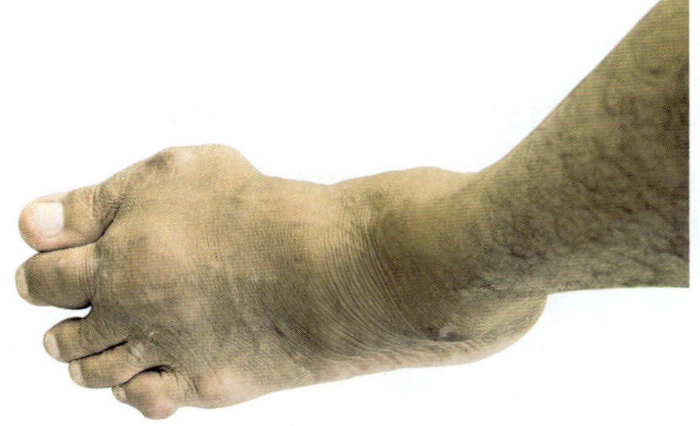

Figure 42.24

Foot with gouty tophi

Source: phokin/Shutterstock.

Clinical diagnosis and management

Diagnosis Collection of a comprehensive health history is important, especially with regards to diet and medications. A full blood count and ESR may be measured to eliminate the presence of other conditions and to assess for systemic inflammation. Serum uric acid levels and renal function tests may also be performed. Concomitant urinary uric acid levels can be measured to determine the volume of uric acid excreted. An X-ray may assist in determining changes to the bone or joint in the affected area, and can demonstrate the findings characteristic of gout, even though these are not diagnostic. Sampling of fluid from the joint (arthrocentesis) may be beneficial to determine the presence of infection, such as septic arthritis.

Management The principles underpinning the management of gout include reducing uric acid stores and the risk of gout flares, and the treatment of acute exacerbations. Education regarding avoidance of purine-rich food is beneficial. Pain from gout flares can generally be managed with simple analgesia and NSAIDs. The anti-inflammatory agent colchicine acts more specifically than the NSAIDs. It is taken up by macrophages and neutrophils, and disables the microtubules that form part of the cell cytoskeleton. The release of lytic enzymes and migration to the site of inflammation can be inhibited.

Assessment of any prescribed medication may be beneficial, to reduce the risk of diuretic-induced gout. Chronic hyperuricaemia can be controlled with agents that lower uric acid, such as probenecid or allopurinol. In those with only one affected joint, the intra-articular administration of corticosteroids may be beneficial; however, it is important to understand that fluid sampled from a joint that has had corticosteroid injections may, microscopically, resemble the crystals seen in gout.

Infective bone disorders

OSTEOMYELITIS

LEARNING OBJECTIVE 4

Describe the pathophysiological mechanisms, epidemiology, clinical manifestations, diagnosis and management involved in the infective bone disorder osteomyelitis.

Aetiology and pathophysiology

Osteomyelitis is an *infection of bone*. Osteomyelitis can be classified as acute or chronic. This classification is based not only on the duration of the infection, but is also linked to the pathological characteristics of the condition (see Figure 42.25). In *acute osteomyelitis*, inflammatory tissue responses are

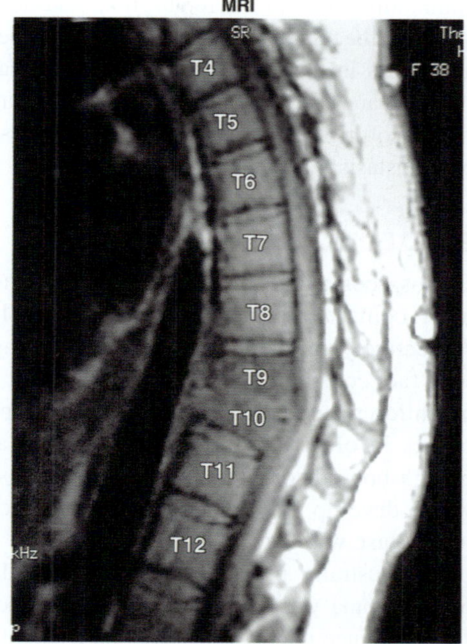

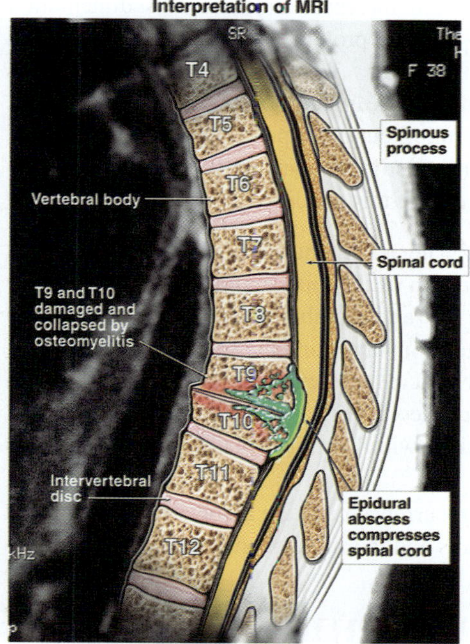

Figure 42.25

Spinal cord compression at T9–10 due to epidural abscess

Source: Nucleus Medical Media Inc/Alamy Stock Photo.

induced by the invading pathogens. In *chronic osteomyelitis*, necrosis is evident.

The most common pathogen in osteomyelitis is *Staphylococcus aureus*. Other microbes can be associated with this type of infection, but it depends on the age of the affected person and how the microbe accessed the bone tissue. In neonates, infection with group B streptococci and *Escherichia coli* is common; in children, the pathogen can be *Streptococcus pyogenes*; and in adults, common pathogens are *Pseudomonas aeruginosa* and other Gram-negative bacteria.

Children, older adults and people who are immunosuppressed are more prone to acute osteomyelitis via blood-borne (*haematogenous*) seeding into long bones. Adults tend to develop chronic osteomyelitis from open or surgical wounds to soft tissue and bone. Osteomyelitis can be a complication of diabetic foot ulcers due to localised tissue ischaemia, and as a result of hip and knee arthroscopy.

Epidemiology

The prevalence of osteomyelitis in wealthy Western countries is estimated at 3–13 in 100,000 people. It is considered one of the more prevalent musculoskeletal infections in children. There has been an increase in incidence of this condition over the decade for both adults and children.

The trends in incidence of acute osteomyelitis by haematogenous spread in Australian and New Zealand children has been previously reported as higher in males than females, and higher in Indigenous children than in those of European backgrounds. (In northern Australia the incidence in 2016 was reported at 82 cases per 100,000 in Indigenous children, compared to 9.2 cases per 100,000 in non-Indigenous children.) There were 9,566 admissions for osteomyelitis in Australian public hospitals in 2021–22.

Risk factors in the development of osteomyelitis are traumatic injury, diabetes mellitus, intravenous drug use and splenectomy.

Clinical manifestations

The common clinical manifestations of acute osteomyelitis include the rapid onset of systemic effects, such as fever, irritability in young children, malaise and fatigue, in addition to localised erythema, swelling, limited movement of the affected joints and bone tenderness.

In chronic osteomyelitis, the clinical manifestations include chronic pain, persistent wound drainage, malaise, chronic fatigue and fever.

Clinical diagnosis and management

Diagnosis A combination of history taking, a clinical examination, imaging, microbial culture and laboratory tests are used in the diagnosis of osteomyelitis. In acute osteomyelitis in children, the rapid onset of the clinical manifestations is important. Blood culture is unreliable.

In chronic osteomyelitis, a good health history can reveal the duration of symptomology. Microbial culture from bone biopsy and histopathological evidence of necrosis assist greatly in diagnosis. An increased erythrocyte sedimentation rate and elevated C-reactive protein level are good markers of inflammation.

Imaging can confirm bone infection in both acute and chronic forms, and assist in ruling out other possible conditions. X-ray, technetium-99m bone scintigraphy and MRI are considered the best modes in diagnosis of this condition.

Management The treatment of osteomyelitis involves the timely administration of the most appropriate antimicrobial agent. The choice of antimicrobial agent depends on the pathogen, or pathogens, involved and the sensitivity test results. Empirical treatment of acute osteomyelitis should be directed to *S. aureus*. In chronic osteomyelitis, surgical removal of necrotic tissue in combination with antimicrobial drug treatment is indicated.

Relatively high recurrence rates are associated with chronic osteomyelitis in adults and in immunocompromised people.

Osteogenic tumours

LEARNING OBJECTIVE 5

Describe the pathophysiological mechanisms, epidemiology, clinical manifestations, diagnosis and management involved in osteogenic tumours.

AETIOLOGY AND PATHOPHYSIOLOGY

Osteogenic tumours are *malignant bone cancers*. They are rare malignancies, but occur most frequently in children and adolescents. This tendency is linked to the adolescent growth spurt, at a time of accelerated bone proliferation. Osteosarcoma and Ewing's sarcoma are the most common osteogenic tumours.

Osteosarcomas can develop in any bone, but most frequently arise in the metaphysis (shaft) of long bones, particularly the distal femur, proximal tibia and proximal humerus. A small percentage of these tumours develop within the axial skeleton, especially the pelvis. The tumours grow in a ball-like mass. As a tumour grows, it presses on the surrounding muscles, forming a pseudocapsular layer. Nodules from the main tumour invade this pseudocapsular layer. The tumour can also irritate the periosteum, which is rich in nerves, and cause pain. Tumour cells will not only invade local surrounding tissues, they can also metastasise to distant body structures. The lungs and other bones are common sites of metastasis. It is rare for osteosarcomas to spread to regional lymph nodes.

Histologically, **Ewing's sarcoma** belongs to a family of neoplasms with small round and blue cells. Non-Hodgkin lymphoma also belongs to this family. The cells are rich in cytoplasmic glycogen, and strongly express a glycoprotein surface antigen called CD99. These features help to differentiate the cells of Ewing's sarcoma from those of other related cancers in this family. Paradoxically, the cells demonstrate low rates of mitosis, despite Ewing's sarcoma being characterised as a very aggressive malignancy. In the majority of cases, Ewing's sarcoma is characterised genetically by a translocation between chromosomes 11 and 22. As in osteosarcoma, the tumour commonly arises in the femur, tibia and humerus. In the axial skeleton, the tumour tends to develop in the pelvis and vertebrae, as well as in the flat bones, such as the scapula, clavicle and ribs. In rare cases, Ewing's sarcoma will arise extraskeletally within soft tissue. The lungs and other bones are common sites of metastasis.

EPIDEMIOLOGY

Osteosarcoma and Ewing's sarcoma are the first and second most common forms of primary solid bone malignancy, respectively, in people under 20 years of age. Osteosarcoma is in fact considered a common malignant cancer (all types) in children and adolescents. A second peak of incidence occurs in older adults over 60 years of age, secondary to benign bone disorders, such as Paget's disease of the bone, which develop into malignancies. Incidence rate is expected to increase with age.

In Australia in 2022 the age-standardised incidence of osteosarcoma was estimated at 8.1 cases per 100,000 people. The incidence rate of osteosarcoma is slightly higher in males (9.2 cases in males, compared to 7.2 cases in females).

CLINICAL MANIFESTATIONS

The clinical manifestations associated with bone neoplasms include dull pain, joint effusion, a decreased range of motion in the affected joint, and hyperpyremia causing the site to be warm, with visible superficial blood vessels.

The common clinical manifestations associated with osteosarcoma include a dull, aching pain, especially at night, which persists for several months before increasing in severity. The sudden severity may be induced by periosteal membrane irritation or, more rarely, because the person has incurred a pathological fracture. Localised clinical manifestations include a decreased range of movement in the affected region, tenderness, swelling or palpable mass, muscle atrophy and limping.

In Ewing's sarcoma, the common signs and symptoms include mild pain that increases in intensity over time as the tumour develops. A palpable mass that is inflamed and tender may be felt. Tumour development in the pelvic or spinal region may lead to neural complications, such as paraesthesias or altered bladder and bowel function.

CLINICAL DIAGNOSIS AND MANAGEMENT

Diagnosis

The assessment of osteosarcoma and Ewing's sarcoma is based on a health history, a clinical examination, radiological investigations, blood tests and histopathological testing.

A combination of radiographic modalities provides valuable information on the development of the tumour. X-rays reveal the pathological changes at the primary bone site, such as bone loss and patchy repair (see Figure 42.26), as well as the presence of nodules in surrounding tissue. MRI and CT scanning can detect the extent of tumour development. Scintigraphic studies can show sites of metastasis.

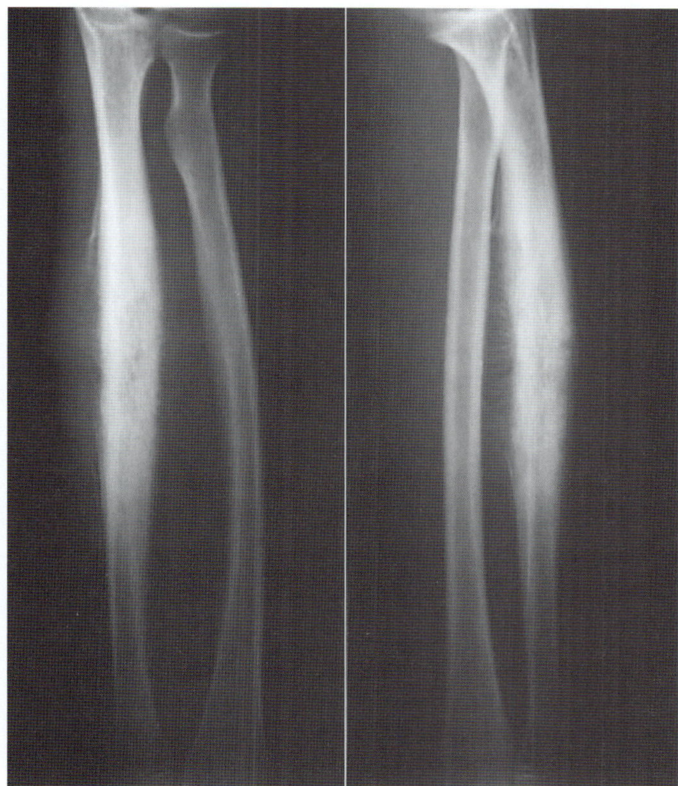

Figure 42.26

X-ray of Ewing's sarcoma of the humerus

This X-ray shows a Ewing's sarcoma in the midshaft of the humerus.

Source: Zephyr/Science Photo Library.

Bone biopsy is the key to confirming the diagnosis, providing information on the grading and staging of the tumour.

A full blood examination may be useful to exclude other disorders. In Ewing's sarcoma, a measurement of the serum lactate dehydrogenase (LDH) level should be obtained as a serum biomarker. Importantly, other conditions can lead to an elevation of LDH, so the result is not specific to Ewing's scarcoma. Serum LDH and alkaline phosphatase (ALP) levels are measured in osteosarcoma. Both may be elevated, but ALP is considered to be more useful in diagnosis, as the levels correlate with the tumour size.

Management

The aim of treatment of these bone malignancies is curative. A combination of chemotherapy, radiotherapy and surgery is used to manage these cancers.

Multiagent chemotherapy has greatly improved the long-term prognosis for people with these conditions. Classic chemotherapeutic agents suitable in the management of osteosarcoma and Ewing's sarcoma may include alkylating agents, cytotoxic antibiotics, plant alkaloids and antimetabolites (see Table 42.6). These drugs induce severe adverse reactions associated with the disruption of cell turnover in normal cell populations, such as nausea and vomiting, alopecia, bone marrow suppression, delayed growth and mouth sores. More targeted drugs such as monoclonal antibodies and protein kinase inhibitors may also be appropriate in therapy.

Surgery may be required in order to remove tumour growths. Tumours in long bones are easier to remove than those associated with the axial skeleton, as it is possible to remove a wider margin around the mass in limbs. Where surgery is less successful or not possible, radiotherapy in combination with chemotherapy is indicated. With the improvements in chemotherapeutic drug treatment, there has been a major shift away from amputating an affected limb to limb 'salvaging' and surgical reconstruction. Better functional and psychosocial outcomes have been shown using this approach.

The prognosis for a person with a bone malignancy is more positive if there is no evidence of metastasis at the time of diagnosis, and where there is less axial skeleton involvement. Relapse of the malignancy often results in a poorer prognosis.

Table 42.6 Mechanisms of action of classic chemotherapeutic agents used to treat malignant bone tumours

Drug grouping	Mechanism of action
Alkylating agents	Form cross-links between DNA bases. The DNA molecule fractures and the cell undergoes apoptosis.
Antimetabolites	Interrupt the synthesis of nucleic acids. Inhibit DNA replication and disrupt the cell cycle.
Plant alkaloids	Disrupt the formation of mitotic spindles, and disrupt mitosis or inhibit topoisomerase involved in DNA repair and replication.
Cytotoxic antibiotics	Generally, this group disrupts protein synthesis and interferes with the cell cycle.

INDIGENOUS HEALTH FAST FACTS AND CULTURAL CONSIDERATIONS

FAST FACTS

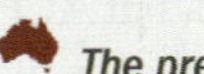

- *The prevalence of rheumatic disease is consistently higher in Indigenous communities, including in Australia and New Zealand.*
- *The prevalence in Australian and Torres Strait Islander peoples was 32%, and 6% in Māori.*
- *Seventeen per cent of Aboriginal and Torres Strait Islander peoples have arthritis, which is slightly more than non-Indigenous Australians (13%).*
- *The prevalence of osteoporosis in Aboriginal and Torres Strait Islander peoples (3.9%) is similar to that of non-Indigenous Australians (3.3%), but is 1.9 times higher in Indigenous males compared to non-Indigenous males.*
- *Māori and Pacific Islands people are less likely than European New Zealanders to experience osteoporosis.*
- *The rate of arthritis in Pacific Islands people is less than half that of European New Zealanders (without age or gender standardisation).*
- *Indigenous Australians have a higher prevalence of gout, at 6.7% in those 20 years and older compared to the crude all-age prevalence at 3.7%.*
- *Indigenous New Zealanders have a higher prevalence of gout compared to non-Indigenous New Zealanders. In 2019, the prevalence of gout was 8.5% in Māori, 14.8% in Pacific Islands people and 4.7% for other New Zealanders.*

CULTURAL CONSIDERATIONS

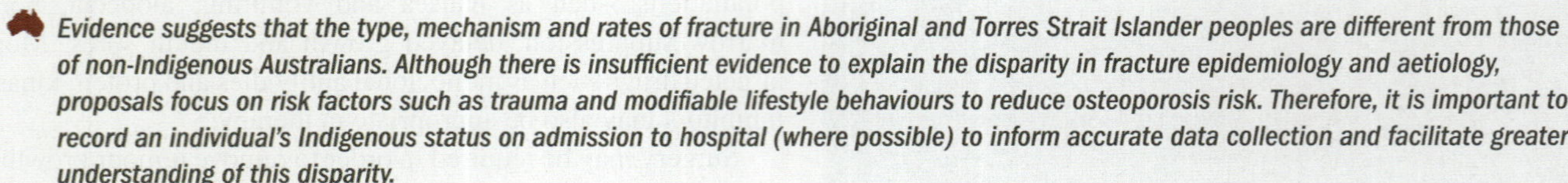

- *Evidence suggests that the type, mechanism and rates of fracture in Aboriginal and Torres Strait Islander peoples are different from those of non-Indigenous Australians. Although there is insufficient evidence to explain the disparity in fracture epidemiology and aetiology, proposals focus on risk factors such as trauma and modifiable lifestyle behaviours to reduce osteoporosis risk. Therefore, it is important to record an individual's Indigenous status on admission to hospital (where possible) to inform accurate data collection and facilitate greater understanding of this disparity.*

Sources: Data from Australian Indigenous HealthInfoNet (2022); Australian Institute of Health and Welfare (2020); Brennan-Olsen et al. (2017); McDougall et al. (2017); Pathmanathan et al. (2021).

CHILDREN AND ADOLESCENTS

- Significant bone growth and turnover occurs during puberty. Sixty per cent of bone mass content is developed during puberty.
- Bone density loss in a pregnant adolescent girl is greater than bone density loss in a pregnant adult woman.
- An increased intake of sweetened beverages in children of 3–7 years of age can potentially reduce bone density through the displacement of milk and calcium intake.
- Children experiencing chronic joint inflammation before the age of 16 years (in one or more joints for a period of six weeks) are considered to have 'juvenile idiopathic arthritis' (also known as 'juvenile arthritis' and formerly known as 'juvenile rheumatoid arthritis').
- Juvenile idiopathic arthritis is most commonly diagnosed in children under 5 years of age. This autoimmune disease is different from rheumatoid arthritis, which is associated with ageing. It is more common in girls than boys.
- Gout is rare in children.

OLDER ADULTS

- Calcium supplementation in older adults can significantly reduce the risk of vertebral fracture.
- Physical exercise is beneficial for older adults, as it not only increases muscle strength and balance, reducing the risk of falls, but it also increases bone density.
- Older adults should have home hazard assessments to reduce the risk of falls. Components of this assessment should include potential trip hazards. However, interventions, such as a reduction in or the elimination of psychotropic agents (where possible), can also reduce the risk of fracture from falls, and should be considered.
- A typical gout flare can present differently in older adults from the way it presents in younger people. Older adults often present with more tophi and with gout of a polyarticular nature.

KEY CLINICAL ISSUES

- Effective care of people with bone disorders includes interventions to maintain the functions of the musculoskeletal system, reducing the risk of injury, fracture and infection, as well as the assessment and monitoring of the individual's body image, and emotional and psychological responses.
- Education for the person and their family is essential to address metabolic bone disorders, lifestyle modifications of risk factors, management and expected outcomes for improving or maintaining bone mineral density.
- Three key essentials to reducing the risk of developing metabolic bone diseases throughout life are appropriate diet, exercise and healthy lifestyle choices.
- Education for people affected by joint disorders is essential in promoting optimum outcomes.
- The mental health of people with joint disorders may also be affected by chronic pain and other physical impairments. Depression is common in those with chronic disease.
- The limitations and restrictions imposed by joint disorders can be detrimental to a person's self-esteem and self-image. Loss of independence can further exacerbate psychological well-being and contribute to stress and depression.
- Promoting mobility and reducing the risk of injury are critical considerations when caring for people with conditions affecting their musculoskeletal system.
- Careful assessment and monitoring of the person's body image and their emotional and psychological responses are also vital aspects of care.

CHAPTER REVIEW

- Developmental dysplasia of the hip, talipes equinovarus, scoliosis and the osteochondroses are *bone and joint developmental disorders* that commonly feature in Australia and New Zealand.
- *Scoliosis* is a deformity characterised by a lateral curvature and axial rotation of the spine. A common form of this condition occurs in adolescents in the absence of other abnormalities, and is called *adolescent idiopathic scoliosis*.
- The *osteochondroses* are a group of disorders that affect the *growing immature skeleton*. Injury, mechanical stresses on the epiphyseal growth plate and ossification zones, abnormal skeletal development, vascular interruption to bones and genetic factors have been linked to their onset. *Osgood–Schlatter disease* affects the knee. Osteochrondroses usually resolve once skeletal maturity is reached and the growth plates close.
- *Arthritis* is *inflammation or degeneration of a joint*, associated with stiffness, oedema and pain. There are dozens of types of arthritis. *Chronic arthritis* includes osteoarthritis, rheumatoid arthritis and gouty arthritis. *Ankylosing spondylitis* is a form of arthritis that damages spinal vertebrae.
- Medication and adjunctive therapies are generally prescribed. Surgical replacement of a damaged joint, most commonly the hip or knee, can be effective when pain and disability are not effectively controlled with non-invasive management.
- *Metabolic bone diseases* affect *bone turnover and mineralisation*. Osteomalacia, rickets, osteoporosis and Paget's disease of the bone are three common metabolic bone disorders in Australia and New Zealand. Fractures are the most common complication of this family of diseases.
- The metabolic bone diseases can result from calcium and phosphate imbalances, vitamin D deficiency, the ageing process, inflammatory mediator action, changes in hormone levels and genetics.
- *Gout* is a *metabolic joint disease characterised by hyperuricaemia and tophi formation in subcutaneous tissues*. The cause of gout is unknown, but a genetic predisposition may be a factor. Excess uric acid in the blood results from either a defect in the metabolism of purines or abnormal retention of uric acid, or both. The onset of an acute episode is generally sudden. The joint is painful, hot, oedematous and red. The joints of the big toe are most commonly affected.
- *Osteomyelitis* may result from a blood-borne pathogen, a contiguous infection or a complication of vascular insufficiency.
- *Bone tumours* can be benign or malignant, primary or metastatic. Bone tumours originate from bone cells, cartilage, fibrous tissue, marrow or vascular tissue.

REVIEW QUESTIONS

1. Sarah Saleh is 14 years old and consumes a diet rich in calcium. However, Sarah rarely receives exposure to sunlight. What condition is she at risk of developing?
2. Briefly outline the differences between benign and malignant tumours.
3. Mr Simon Johnson was admitted for surgical management of chronic osteomyelitis in his right femur.
   a. Outline the methods by which chronic osteomyelitis may develop.
   b. Antimicrobials may not be successful in resolving his osteomyelitis. Why?
   c. What procedure may be undertaken to surgically manage his osteomyelitis?
4. Mrs Sylvia Barton is a frail 76-year-old woman who visits her general practitioner for her annual check-up. Mrs Barton smokes a pack of cigarettes a day, and mainly stays inside. She does no exercise, since she fell last year and fractured her right wrist. Mrs Barton tells you that her mother also had weak bones.
   a. From the history provided, identify the factors that increase Mrs Barton's risk of developing osteoporosis.
   b. A friend wants Mrs Barton to go swimming to help ameliorate her condition. This exercise will be beneficial for her cardiovascular health, but will not greatly assist in reducing the risk of osteoporosis. Why?
   c. What exercises may be more beneficial for Mrs Barton (in relation to osteoporosis risk reduction)? Explain.
5. On examination, it is discovered that Mrs Barton has lost approximately 6 cm in height over the past year.
   a. Explain the mechanism of Mrs Barton's height loss.
   b. What interventions and lifestyle changes would Mrs Barton benefit from to prevent further osteoporosis-related deterioration?
6. Mrs Sonia Green is a 56-year-old primary school teacher. She describes bilateral knee and hand pain that has become worse, is present during rest and is limiting her walking. Mrs Green finds that walking up the two flights of stairs at school increases her pain. Additionally, she finds standing painful. During a physical examination, you note slight ulnar deviation of her fingers and oedema of the

metacarpal, phalangeal and proximal interphalangeal joints. Range of motion is also affected in these joints. Mrs Green has also noticed some instability in her knees. Pathology results demonstrate mild anaemia and a high level of rheumatoid factor. The fluid aspirated from the swelling in her hand was turbid. Knee X-rays demonstrate articular cartilage loss, cystic areas and bony spurs.

a What type of arthritis does Mrs Green have?

b What are the primary objectives in the clinical management of this type of arthritis?

c Identify both pharmacological and non-pharmacological interventions that may assist Mrs Green.

7 Mr David French, aged 56 years, presents to the emergency department with unbearable pain in his right great toe. His toe is red, hot and swollen. Mr French says that this also happened about 18 months ago, although the pain was not as bad then as it is now. He denies any trauma to the extremity, and claims that he wears well-fitting, comfortable shoes. Mr French did mention that he has been drinking a lot of alcohol and attending some lunchtime business meetings in licensed premises this week. Mr French also mentioned that in the past month he commenced taking furosemide.

a Given his clinical presentation and history, what type of arthritis might Mr French be experiencing? Identify all of the factors that contributed to your diagnosis.

b Mr French is to be commenced on medication. What type of medication would be most appropriate for this condition, and how does it work?

c What is the significance of the medication he has commenced taking in the past month?

HEALTH PROFESSIONAL CONNECTIONS

Midwives Midwives are well positioned to assess and determine the presence of congenital bone disorders, such as talipes equinovarus and developmental dysplasia of the hip. A midwife should assess a newborn's hip for hip dysplasia soon after birth, and on follow-up at approximately 1 week old. Other healthcare professionals and child and adolescent healthcare nurses should also periodically check the stability of the child's hip throughout the first year.

Occasionally, midwives will work with pregnant woman who have developed arthritis. Although rheumatoid arthritis symptoms can reduce during pregnancy around the fourth month, they will often flare up within a few months of giving birth. Women with arthritic hips may not be able to deliver vaginally, and a caesarean section may be required. Women with arthritis tend to have an increased risk of miscarriage, premature delivery and neonatal complications. A multidisciplinary team, including a midwife, a rheumatologist and an obstetrician, will be needed to ensure the health of both mother and child.

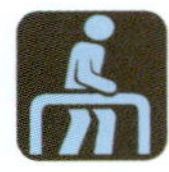

Physiotherapists A physiotherapist will play a large role in rehabilitation, splinting and exercise prescription for most, if not all, bone disorders. Application of Pavlik harnesses, bracing, orthotics and other immobilisation or assistive devices may be required as a component of the management plan. Following the removal of any immobilisation devices, or post-surgery, muscle strengthening and range-of-movement exercises are vital to regain strength and maximal function in the affected body regions. In people with severe scoliosis, compression of the chest cavity can become so serious that tidal volume is significantly reduced. Ventilation can become compromised, and the risk of upper respiratory tract infection increases. Physiotherapists need to assist those with pulmonary hygiene and chest physiotherapy to ensure that lung recruitment is maximal.

Physiotherapists work with people with various types of arthritis. Interventions to assist with maximising function and promoting independent mobility and self-care are a priority. Heat, massage and electrical stimulation are all valuable tools in promoting joint mobility and maximal range of motion. People with arthritis can lose strength from disuse because of pain. Although exercise may initially increase pain, immobilisation will significantly exacerbate pain and loss of function. Therefore, exercise programs to promote functional movement and improve balance, coordination and safety should be developed to assist individual needs.

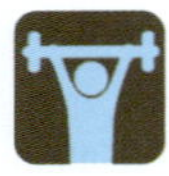

Exercise scientists Weight-bearing exercise aids in stimulating osteoblast activity. Although weight-bearing exercises should be undertaken throughout life, exercise scientists may be responsible for exercise prescription in older populations to reduce the risk of falls and increase bone density. In addition to weight-bearing activity, exercise professionals should also focus on muscle development and balance in order to reduce the risk of fracture.

People with arthritis will benefit from regular, moderate exercise. Exercise professionals working with people who have developed arthritis should initially focus on flexibility and range of motion. As improvement becomes apparent, exercises promoting endurance can be added to the program. It is important to promote activity that the person will enjoy, as this will increase their movement and enhance goal-orientated motivation. Personal choice and disease limitation necessitates the development of individually tailored, realistic programs targeting flexibility, joint range of motion and endurance.

Nutritionists/Dieticians Although a balanced diet made up of appropriate amounts of foods from the five food groups will provide sufficient calcium, people may require further supplementation if they have an absorption issue or a disease process resulting in hypocalcaemia. Foods such as dairy products, including milk, cheese and yoghurt, are a good source of calcium. Other sources include almonds, broccoli and some fortified foods, such as cereal, bread and tofu products. Vitamin D is important, as it is necessary for the absorption of calcium from the gastrointestinal system. Other nutrients that may be required include vitamin K to assist in the use and regulation of calcium, and magnesium, which is an important cofactor for calcitonin and is necessary for the conversion of vitamin D to calcitriol. Sources of vitamin K and magnesium include cauliflower, spinach and Brussels sprouts. Understanding a person's dietary behaviours is imperative in order to determine whether there is an increased risk of bone disorders, such as osteoporosis.

Working with people who have developed gout necessitates focusing on reducing foods that are rich in purine. Although reducing dietary purine will not necessarily cure gout, it can result in reducing the number or severity of flare-ups. Foods high in purine include seafoods such as anchovies, herring and sardines. Some meats are higher in purine, including kidney and liver. Meat extracts can also be purine-rich. Some vegetables, including mushrooms, cauliflower, spinach and asparagus, should be avoided. Finally, gout can also be associated with alcohol intake, and therefore alcohol consumption should be reduced or eliminated from the diet. Although no dietary link can be made with improving arthritis, it is important that those with arthritis are encouraged to keep their weight down to reduce the burden on the lower joints. A well-balanced, healthy diet and moderate exercise will assist with this goal.

CASE STUDY

Mrs Joyce Stevens (UR number 214210) is an 84-year-old woman who is two days postoperative following an elective right hip arthroplasty for rheumatoid arthritis. Mrs Stevens, a widow, is an active member of the community, and performs many hours of volunteer work every week. She still drives, and is responsible for a small area with Meals-on-Wheels. Mrs Stevens also spends three afternoons a week at a local soup kitchen, providing meals for homeless people. On admission, Mrs Stevens reported a two-year history of considerable pain, despite methotrexate, sulphasalazine and diclofenac sodium with misoprostol combination drug. A preoperative X-ray demonstrated medial and superior joint-space narrowing (severe in the right hip), periarticular soft tissue oedema and juxta-articular bony erosions. The surgery was relatively uncomplicated. The prosthesis position is appropriate, although a moderate amount of blood loss occurred postoperatively. Yesterday, she became quite confused (Glasgow coma scale score = 13 [E3, V4, M6]) and today she developed dyspnoea. Her most recent observations are as follows:

Temperature	Heart rate	Respiration rate	Blood pressure	SpO_2
37.5°C	100	30	110/86	93% (RA*)

*RA = room air.

Mrs Stevens is having 1000 mL, q8h intravenous (IV) fluids and IV antimicrobials. As her SpO_2 is decreasing, she has been commenced on oxygen via nasal prongs at 4 L/min. She has been out of bed once since surgery. However, since the confusion has developed she has remained 'rest-in-bed'. Her indwelling catheter remains in situ with a urine output of approximately 45 mL/hour. She is ordered the anticoagulant enoxaparin, and is supposed to be wearing thromboembolic deterrent stockings, but they don't appear to have been reapplied after her postoperative sponge. Mrs Stevens did not have sequential compression devices (SCDs, pronounced 'skuds') applied while she was in bed, as there were no units available. Prior to her deterioration, she was performing q2h incentive spirometry with a Triflow while she was awake. A ventilation/perfusion scan has been booked for Mrs Stevens this afternoon. Her postoperative pathology results are as follows:

HAEMATOLOGY

Patient location:	Ward 3	**UR:**	214210		
Consultant:	Smith	**NAME:**	Stevens		
		Given name:	Joyce	**Sex:**	F
		DOB:	13/08/XX	**Age:**	84

Time collected	07:30
Date collected	XX/XX
Year	XXXX
Lab #	5654654

FULL BLOOD COUNT		UNITS	REFERENCE RANGE
Haemoglobin	87	g/L	115–160
White cell count	5.2	$\times 10^9$/L	4.0–11.0
Platelets	134	$\times 10^9$/L	140–400
Haematocrit	0.29		0.33–0.47
Red cell count	3.70	$\times 10^{12}$/L	3.80–5.20
Reticulocyte count	3.5	%	0.2–2.0
MCV	82	fL	80–100
Neutrophils	3.41	$\times 10^9$/L	2.00–8.00
Lymphocytes	2.54	$\times 10^9$/L	1.00–4.00
Monocytes	0.36	$\times 10^9$/L	0.10–1.00
Eosinophils	0.24	$\times 10^9$/L	< 0.60
Basophils	0.09	$\times 10^9$/L	< 0.20
ESR	14	mm/h	< 12

BIOCHEMISTRY

Patient location:	Ward 3	**UR:**	214210		
Consultant:	Smith	**NAME:**	Stevens		
		Given name:	Joyce	**Sex:**	F
		DOB:	13/08/XX	**Age:**	84

Time collected	07:30
Date collected	XX/XX
Year	XXXX
Lab #	564356345

ELECTROLYTES		UNITS	REFERENCE RANGE
Sodium	146	mmol/L	135–145
Potassium	4.0	mmol/L	3.5–5.2
Chloride	101	mmol/L	95–110
Bicarbonate	23	mmol/L	22–32
Glucose (random)	5.2	mmol/L	3.5–7.7
Iron	7	μmol/L	11–30

CRITICAL THINKING

1. Why does Mrs Stevens require a total hip replacement? What physiological manifestations are apparent to warrant this? Mrs Stevens will require an arthroplasty on the other hip, too. Is it possible to operate on both hips in the same surgery? What would influence this decision?
2. Preoperatively, Mrs Stevens was taking many drugs. What were they? How do they work? Are there any special considerations or precautions needed when taking these medications? Will she need to take these medications following surgery?
3. What do Mrs Stevens's pathology results show? (*Hint:* Look at the red cell count, haemoglobin level and haematocrit.) Is this common following total hip replacement? What can be done to reduce the likelihood of this occurring?
4. Mrs Stevens has deteriorated over the past two days. What may be the cause of this deterioration? Is this a common risk associated with total hip replacements? Explain. What other risks are associated with total hip replacement? How can these be avoided?

BIBLIOGRAPHY

Australian Bureau of Statistics (ABS) (2022). *Health conditions prevalence 2020–21*. Canberra: ABS. https://www.abs.gov.au/statistics/health/health-conditions-and-risks/health-conditions-prevalence/latest-release.

Australian Indigenous Health*Info*Net (2022). *Overview of Aboriginal and Torres Strait Islander health status, 2021*. Perth, WA: Australian Indigenous Health*Info*Net. https://healthinfonet.ecu.edu.au/learn/health-facts/overview-aboriginal-torres-strait-islander-health-status.

Australian Institute of Health and Welfare (AIHW) (2020a). *Arthritis*. Canberra: AIHW. https://www.aihw.gov.au/getmedia/960d8243-95ef-47c1-bc0f-2eecf57ae2e4/Arthritis.pdf.aspx?inline=true.

Australian Institute of Health and Welfare (AIHW) (2020b). *Osteoporosis.* Cat. No. PHE 233. Canberra: AIHW. https://www.aihw.gov.au/getmedia/507c3057-c3cd-4894-83e3-0fb68e357a37/Osteoporosis.pdf.aspx?inline=true#:~:text=Osteoporosis%20is%20a%20condition%20where,to%20be%20classified%20as%20osteoporosis.&text=What%20is%20osteoporosis%3F.

Australian Institute of Health and Welfare (AIHW) (2020c). *Rheumatoid arthritis.* Canberra: AIHW. https://www.aihw.gov.au/getmedia/e9824572-0078-42d5-9669-be2f6efd74cf/Rheumatoid-arthritis.pdf.aspx?inline=true.

Australian Institute of Health and Welfare (AIHW) (2022). *Principal diagnosis data cubes: separation statistics by principal diagnosis (ICD-10-AM 11th edition), Australia, 2020–21.* Canberra: AIWH. https://www.aihw.gov.au/reports/hospitals/principal-diagnosis-data-cubes/contents/data-cubes.

Ball, J.W., Bindler, R.C., Cowen, K.J. & Shaw, M.R. (2017). *Principles of pediatric nursing: caring for children* (7th edn). Upper Saddle River, NJ: Pearson Education, Inc.

Bauldoff, G., Gubrud-Howe, P.M., Carno, M.-A., Levett-Jones, T., Hales, M., Berry, K., … Stanley, D. (2020). *LeMone and Burke's medical–surgical nursing: critical thinking for person-centred care* (4th [Australian] edn). Sydney: Pearson Australia.

Best, O. & Fredericks, B. (2021). *Yatdjuligin: Aboriginal and Torres Strait Islander nursing and midwifery care* (3rd edn). Port Melbourne, VIC: Cambridge University Press.

Brennan-Olsen, S.L., Vogrin, S., Leslie, W.D., Kinsella, R., Toombs, M., Duque, G., … Quirk, S.E. (2017). Fractures in indigenous compared to non-indigenous populations: a systematic review of rates and aetiology. *Bone Reports* 27(6):145–58. https://doi.org/10.1016/j.bonr.2017.04.003.

Britton, C., Brown, S., Ward, L., Rea, S.L., Ratajczak, T. & Walsh, J.P. (2017). The changing presentation of Paget's disease of bone in Australia, a high prevalence region. *Calcified Tissue International* 101(6): 564–69. https://doi.org/10.1007/s00223-017-0312-1.

Bullock, S. & Manias, E. (2022). *Fundamentals of pharmacology* (9th edn). Sydney: Pearson Australia.

Cancer Australia (2023). *Sarcoma*. Sydney: Cancer Australia. https://www.canceraustralia.gov.au/cancer-types/sarcoma/overview.

Corbi, F., Matas, S., Álvarez-Herms, J., Sitko, S., Baiget, E., Reverter-Masia, J. & López-Laval, I. (2022). Osgood–Schlatter disease: appearance, diagnosis and treatment: a narrative review. *Healthcare* 10(6):1011. https://doi.org/10.3390/healthcare10061011.

Davidson, M., London, M. & Ladewig, P. (2020). *Old's maternal-newborn nursing and women's health across the lifespan* (11th edn). Upper Saddle River, NJ: Pearson Education, Inc.

Deloitte Access Economics (2018). *The economic cost of arthritis in New Zealand in 2018.* Wellington: Deloitte Access Economics for Arthritis New Zealand. https://www.arthritis.org.nz/wp-content/uploads/Economic-Cost-of-Arthritis-in-New-Zealand-2018.pdf.

Elam, R.E.W., Jackson, N.N., Machua, W. & Carbone, L.D. (2022). Osteoporosis. *Emedicine.* https://emedicine.medscape.com/article/330598-overview.

Lozada, C.J. & Culpepper Pace, S.S. (2022). Osteoarthritis. *Emedicine.* https://emedicine.medscape.com/article/330487-overview.

Marieb, E.N. & Hoehn, K. (2019). *Human anatomy and physiology* (11th edn). San Francisco, CA: Pearson Benjamin Cummings.

Martini, F.H., Ober, W.C. & Nath, J.L. (2011). *Visual anatomy and physiology* (1st edn). Upper Saddle River, NJ: Pearson Education, Inc.

Marriott, E., Twomey, S., Lee, M. & Williams, N. (2021). Variability in Australian screening guidelines for developmental dysplasia of the hip. *Journal of Paediatrics and Child Health* 57(12):1857–65. https://doi.org/10.1111/jpc.15744.

McDougall, C., Hurd, K. & Barnabe, C. (2017). Systematic review of rheumatic disease epidemiology in the Indigenous populations of Canada, the United States, Australia and New Zealand. *Seminars in Arthritis and Rheumatism* 46(5):275–86. https://doi.org/10.1016/j.semarthrit.2016.10.010.

NCCLEB (2011). *Nursing: a concept-based approach to learning*, Volume 1 (1st edn). Upper Saddle River, NJ: Pearson Education, Inc.

Osborn, K.S., Wraa, C.E. & Watson, A.S. (2010). *Medical–surgical nursing*. Upper Saddle River, NJ: Pearson Education, Inc.

Pathmanathan, K., Robinson, P.C., Hill, C.L. & Keen, H.I. (2021). The prevalence of gout and hyperuricaemia in Australia: an updated systematic review. *Seminars in Arthritis and Rheumatism* 51(1):121–28. https://doi.org/10.1016/j.semarthrit.2020.12.001.

Smith, H.R. & Brown, A. (2020). Rheumatoid arthritis (RA). *Emedicine.* https://emedicine.medscape.com/article/331715-overview.

PART

11

Integumentary system pathophysiology

43 Integumentary system disorders

KEY TERMS

Alopecia
Atopic dermatitis
Bacteraemia
Bullae
Carbuncle
Cellulitis
Contact dermatitis
Depilation
Dermatitis
Dermatophytes
Desquamation
Erythema
Folliculitis
Furuncles
Hyperkeratosis
Incontinence-associated dermatitis
Koilonychia
Leukocytosis
Leukonychia
Leukoplakia
Necrotising fasciitis (NF)
Normal flora
Onychatrophia
Onychauxis
Onychomycosis
Onychorrhexis
Papule
Paronychia
Photoallergic reaction
Photoprotection
Phototoxicity reaction
Psoriasis
Rosacea
Scabies
Sebum
Shingles
Stasis dermatitis
Subungual haematoma
Terminal hair
Urticarial rash
Vasculitis
Vellus hair
Vesicle
Wheal

LEARNING OBJECTIVES

After completing this chapter, you should be able to:

1 Contrast the pathophysiology and management of various types of dermatitis.

2 Identify the various integumentary system changes that occur as a result of psoriasis.

3 Discuss the cutaneous consequences of immune and non-immune-mediated drug eruptions.

4 Examine the pathophysiology and management of various types of bacterial skin infections.

5 Compare and contrast cellulitis and necrotising fasciitis.

6 Describe the consequences of surgical site infections.

7 Discuss other causes of skin disease, including viral and fungal infection.

8 Explain the life cycle of *Sarcoptes scabiei*, and the consequences of a scabies infection.

9 Outline the common pathology of dermal appendages, including hirsutism, alopecia and nail bed conditions.

WHAT YOU SHOULD KNOW BEFORE YOU START THIS CHAPTER

Can you describe the structure and function of the integumentary system?

Can you describe the main stages of inflammation and healing?

Can you outline the principles and major concepts of infectious disease?

Can you describe important principles of infection control?

Can you detail the process of wound healing?

Can you identify the accessory structures of skin?

Introduction

The skin is the largest body organ, and constitutes about 20% of the total weight of the body. Skin and its appendages (e.g. hair, nails and glands) constitute the *integumentary system*. This system is responsible for numerous functions, including temperature and fluid regulation, and vitamin D production, and it plays a significant role in defence against disease, infection or trauma. When skin integrity is compromised, significant negative consequences may occur.

Visible inflammatory conditions commonly manifest as skin lesions. There are numerous types and subtypes of inflammatory conditions affecting the integumentary system. Conditions such as dermatitis, psoriasis and eruptions resulting from drug reactions are common immune reactions. Figure 43.1 explores the common clinical manifestations and management of inflammatory skin conditions. Bites and stings from various insects and other animals can result in painful and significant skin lesions as well; however, these are discussed in the chapter 'Bites and stings'.

Infections of the integumentary system can be caused by numerous pathogens. Skin infections are caused by bacteria, viruses, parasites and fungi. These will be discussed later in the chapter. The complexity of skin infections can be related to many factors, including the number of different organisms involved, the individual's immune function, and the integrity and health of the skin involved. Finally, this chapter also describes the pathology of some dermal appendages, including hirsutism, alopecia and common conditions affecting the nail bed. Other, less common conditions will not be covered in this chapter, and should be researched in dermatology textbooks.

Inflammatory skin conditions

DERMATITIS

LEARNING OBJECTIVE 1

Contrast the pathophysiology and management of various types of dermatitis.

Dermatitis literally means *inflammation of the dermis* (skin) (see Figure 43.2), and can be attributed to many causes. However, the consistent component is an *overreaction of the immune system's non-specific defences*, which results in an excessive inflammatory process. The four common categories of this condition are atopic, contact, stasis and incontinence-associated dermatitis.

Atopic dermatitis

Atopic dermatitis is a chronic condition with intermittent acute episodes or 'flare-ups'. It is characterised by pruritus (itchiness), a history of atopy in personal or family history, eczematous lesions and dry skin. It generally presents in children and, with time, *lichenification* (skin thickening) will occur in affected areas. The condition can resolve after approximately 5 years of age for some of those affected; however, many people can experience a relapse in adolescence or adulthood.

Aetiology and pathophysiology Although not well understood, the two current theories regarding the pathophysiology of atopic dermatitis are an *'inside-out'* progression, where an immune system pathology leads to destruction of the dermal barrier, or an *'outside-in'* progression, where a disruption to the dermal barrier causes an immune system hyperreactivity. More recently, the immune dysfunction has been found to involve an imbalance within the T helper cell (Th cell) subset populations which subsequently result in an increase in interleukins (IL-4, -5 and -13). This increased production results in an increase *immunoglobulin E* (IgE) level by plasma cells. Fortunately, this discovery has enabled the development of monoclonal antibodies as a method of symptom control.

Irrespective of the initial process, there is increased production of both endogenous and exogenous proteases (enzymes that breakdown protein) that results in the further destruction of dermal tissue. Endogenous protease production is increased with the use of cleaning substances that increase skin pH, making it more alkaline, while exogenous proteases can be produced by external agents, such as *Staphylococcus aureus* bacteria or dust mites. Certain individuals have a propensity to develop atopic dermatitis as a result of genetic influences. People with atopic dermatitis tend to have a reduced capacity for protease inhibition. It is also noted that a significant percentage of children who have atopic dermatitis go on to develop other immunoreactive conditions, such as asthma.

Generally speaking, with *IgE sensitisation* and the release of cytokines, interleukins and colony-stimulating factors, the inflammatory mediators cause translocation of fluid, resulting in epidermal fluid loss. The changing dermal environment can become colonised with bacteria and fungi, which is exacerbated by the reduced ability of the keratinocytes to produce antimicrobial peptides. Under certain conditions, colonisation can become infection.

Clinical manifestations Atopic dermatitis commonly occurs first in infancy. The individual can develop pruritic, erythematous and scaly lesions on the cheeks, scalp, peripheries and trunk. If the eruption becomes severe, the affected area may become weepy and crusty. Over time, lichenification can occur, resulting in thickened skin and enhanced markings. An individual with atopic dermatitis may develop a cycle of intermittent acute exacerbations alternating with periods of remission. It is often difficult to identify the precipitating factors that trigger the exacerbations.

Clinical diagnosis and management

Diagnosis There are no beneficial pathology tests to assist with a diagnosis. Visual inspection of the affected area, a history collection and consideration of the individual's age are the key elements to appropriate diagnosis. Mycology or microbiology samples may inform the presence of fungal or bacterial infection. It can be difficult to distinguish atopic dermatitis from several other skin lesions. Consideration of location, history, spread and presentation may assist in this distinction.

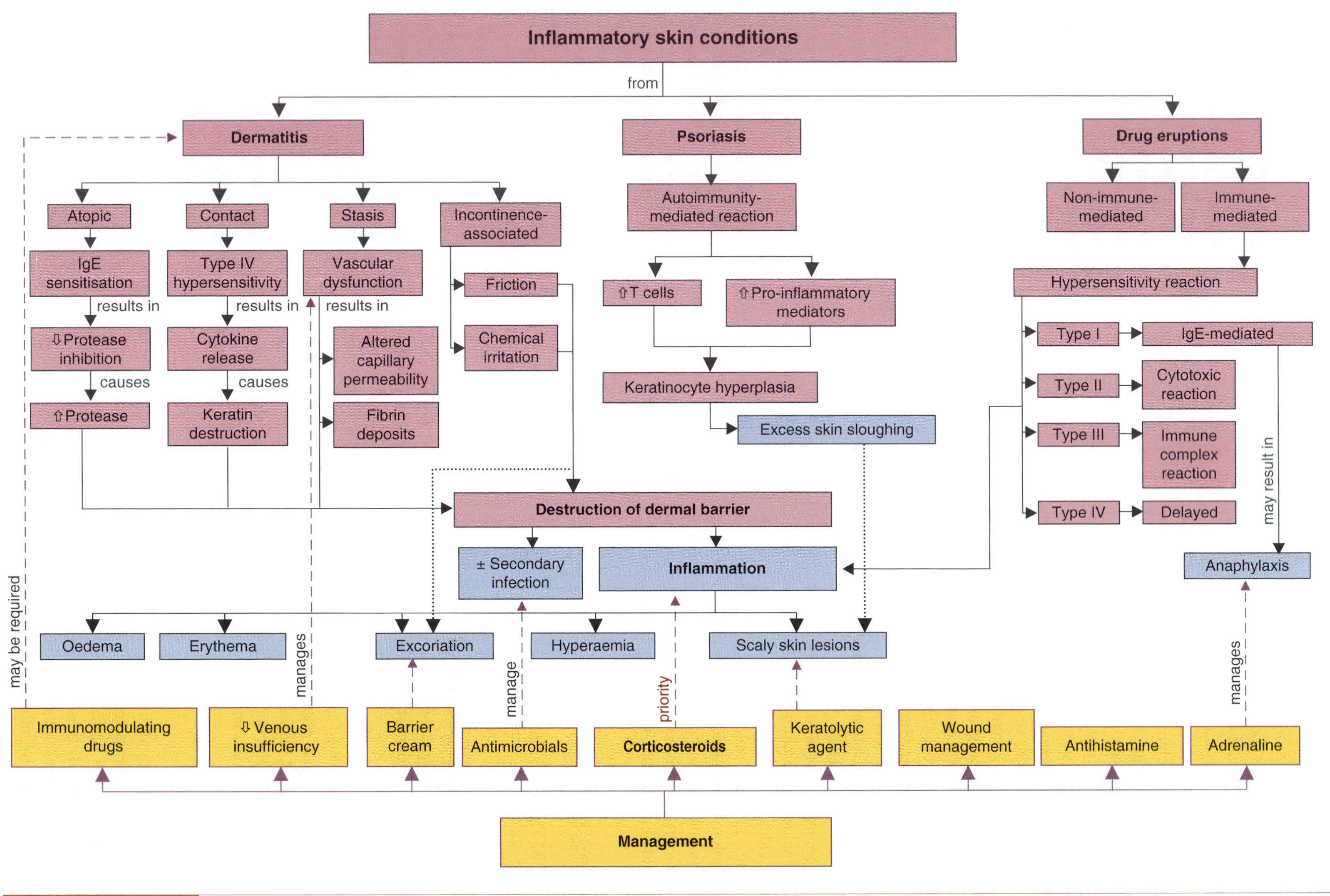

Figure 43.1

Clinical snapshot: Common inflammatory skin conditions

↓ = decreased; ↑ = increased; IgE = immunoglobulin E.

A

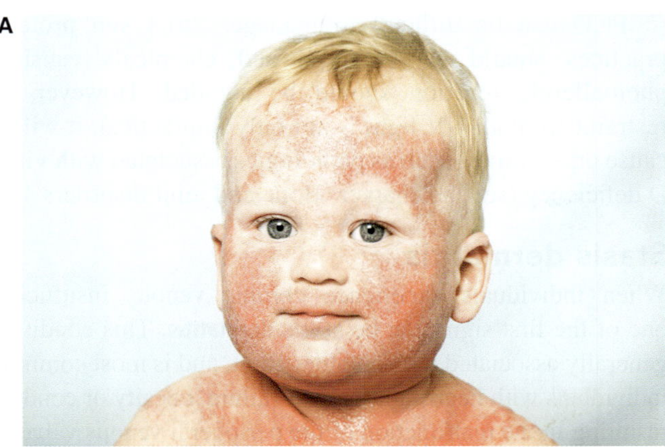

B

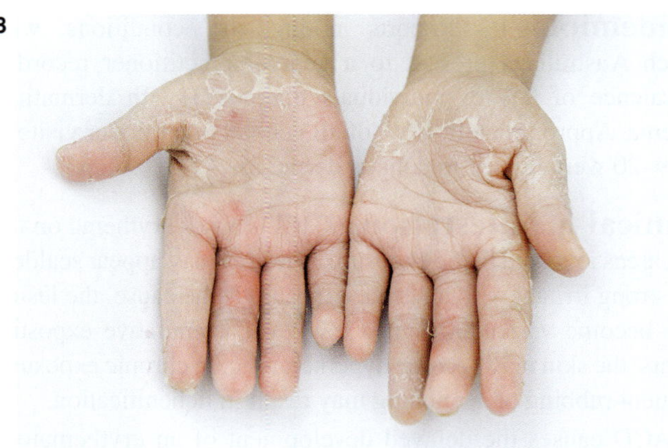

Figure 43.2

Dermatitis

Dermatitis often results in areas of dry, pruritic skin. There may also be areas of erythema. (A) Atopic dermatitis on a baby's face. (B) Contact dermatitis on hands.

Sources: (A) Skylines/Shutterstock; (B) girl-think-position/Shutterstock.

Management Care with hygiene practices is important in the management of this condition, as the compromised dermal layer may become a portal for a more severe progression to systemic infection. pH-Neutral skin preparations should be used, followed by fragrance-free moisturisers. Topical corticosteroid creams are critical in the control of acute flare-ups. Antihistamines can be used to assist an individual in the treatment of pruritus. In the event of a microbial infection, antifungal or antimicrobial agents are necessary.

More recently, systemic immunomodulators, such as monoclonal antibodies (mAbs) have been beneficial in managing symptoms in people with moderate to severe atopic dermatitis (MIMS, 2022). These mAbs block the relevant interleukins from binding to their receptors, decrease signalling, and subsequently result in reduced IgE release. For individuals with severe atopic dermatitis, oral immunosuppressant agents such as ciclosporin, azathioprine or methotrexate can be used; however, these medications come with their own potentially serious side-effects.

Contact dermatitis

Aetiology and pathophysiology

Contact dermatitis can be divided into three subtypes: irritant, allergic and photo contact dermatitis. All three types of contact dermatitis are distinctly different.

Irritant contact dermatitis (ICD) develops in the immediate area after direct contact of the skin with the irritant. No prior sensitisation is necessary. Once the irritant contact occurs, the dermis and epidermis are damaged by denaturing of the keratin and alteration in the structural integrity of the skin, as well as cytokine release. The degree of damage is generally directly proportional to the strength of the irritant, the period of exposure and the location of the contact. The skin irritation can occur either immediately or following a cumulative exposure to the irritant. Cumulative exposure is common with ICD, and is related to frequent hand-washing with low-grade irritants coupled with the friction of the mechanical cleaning. ICD is commonly associated with occupational workplace health and safety claims. Reducing keratinocyte exposure to the irritant can reduce cytokine release and ease the inflammatory response.

Allergic contact dermatitis (ACD) is a type IV delayed (cell-mediated) hypersensitivity reaction (see the chapter 'Immune disorders') that causes cutaneous manifestations. After an initial sensitisation from an allergen, an immune response will begin. This occurs when the *antigen-presenting cells* (e.g. Langerhans cells, dermal dendrocytes and macrophages) attract the antigen and then migrate to the lymph node, where they present it to a Th cell for activation. Memory cells are created, and so are effector T cells. On second exposure, the sensitised T cells release cytokines, resulting in the migration of other leukocytes to the area. In several hours or days an inflammatory process occurs, which results in a delayed reaction.

Photo contact dermatitis (PCD) is less common, and causes a typical dermatitis reaction as a result of combined *exposure to ultraviolet (UV) radiation* and an *interaction with substances* that have been applied to the skin. Chemicals such as sunscreens, fragrances and disinfectants can cause a reaction in some people when activated by the sun (or some other light source). In affected individuals, two reactions are possible. A **phototoxicity reaction** is one in which direct damage occurs, resulting in a lesion similar to sunburn. A **photoallergic reaction** is one in which a cell-mediated response occurs (much like the one described in allergic contact dermatitis—the antigen is the light-activated sensitising agent). This type of reaction causes a typical eczema-type response of **erythema**, lichenification and scaly, pruritic lesions.

Epidemiology Reports noting the conditions with which Australians present to a general practitioner record a prevalence of 7% of individuals diagnosed with dermatitis/eczema. Approximately 1.6% of all general practitioner visits in 2019–20 were related to contact dermatitis.

Clinical manifestations ICD causes erythema on the skin areas involved in the exposure. The area may appear scalded. If a strong irritant with an acute exposure is the cause, the lesion may become vesicular, or if a low-level, cumulative exposure occurs, the skin may become hyperkeratotic. In chronic exposure, frequent rubbing or scratching may result in lichenification.

ACD causes the delayed development of an erythematous area with pruritic **papules** (small, solid, raised skin lesions) and **vesicles** (blister-like skin lesions) generally on the skin areas involved in the exposure. More chronic exposures can result in lichenification, but if the allergen is identified and removed, this is unlikely.

PCD can cause a range of symptoms, but almost always pruritus and erythema in sun-affected areas. Phototoxic reactions cause a burning-type pain. Photoallergic reactions can cause eczematous-type dermatitis and sometimes even hyperpigmentation.

Clinical diagnosis and management

Diagnosis ICD is primarily diagnosed by considering the history and presentation, as well as by undertaking a visual inspection of the affected area. Consultation of the literature for the known irritant is also beneficial (commonly possible, but may not be known). Almost any substance has the capacity to become an irritant given sufficient time and exposure.

ACD is also primarily diagnosed after consideration of the history and presentation, and visual inspection. However, skin patch testing can be beneficial to identify the allergen/s. Skin patch testing involves applying patches with various allergens to the arm or back. After several days, the individual will return to have the patches removed and the results identified. Areas of erythema will demonstrate allergy. This information can then be used to inform the management plan.

PCD can be identified with consideration of the history and presenting signs and symptoms. A skin patch test may be beneficial to eliminate other allergens or isolate the photoallergic chemicals.

Management In an acute exposure resulting in ICD, the immediate treatment is to remove the cause (if known). If the irritant is a solution, it can be managed as a burn (see the chapter 'Skin cancers, burns and scarring'). In the case of more delayed chronic reactions from cumulative exposure, once the irritant is identified and removed, the use of barrier creams and cleaning agents with a pH closer to 5.5 will assist in reducing the inflammation.

ACD is managed through the initial identification of the allergen followed by the application of topical corticosteroid cream. In severe reactions, oral corticosteroids may also be required to control the inflammatory response. Occasionally, individuals experiencing particularly severe episodes of ACD may benefit from immunomodulating drugs.

PCD can be difficult to manage. Strict sun protection practices should be initiated, and chemicals causing a photoallergic reaction should be avoided. However, total restraint from all UV light is not only impractical, it will also cause other issues, such as pathologies associated with vitamin D deficiency (see the chapter 'Bone and joint disorders').

Stasis dermatitis

When individuals experience chronic venous insufficiency, one of the first signs can be **stasis dermatitis**. This condition is generally associated with an older adult, and is most common in individuals with heart failure, liver failure, obesity or conditions resulting in the malfunction of the peripheral venous valves.

Aetiology and pathophysiology As the peripheral venous system becomes dysfunctional, the resulting loss of the valvular function decreases venous return and causes a negative influence on the microcirculation. Alterations in capillary permeability can cause translocation of substances such as fibrinogen into the precapillary tissue. When the fibrinogen converts to fibrin, it can interfere externally with the dermal capillaries and cause hypoxia. As dermal fibrosis occurs and leukocytes become trapped in the tissue, inflammatory mediators and other chemoattractant substances are released, resulting in dermal destruction and subsequent inflammation.

Clinical manifestations Stasis dermatitis can cause a range of symptoms. Generally, the skin becomes oedematous, and the affected area appears a reddish-brown colour from haemosiderin deposits. It is not uncommon for secondary infections to occur. In this situation, the lesion can become pustulous and malodourous. In severe instances, non-infected lesions can weep serosanguinous exudate. The outer area of the lesions may be affected by lichenification. The affected area is generally pruritic. Depending on the severity and degree of hypoxia, local necrosis may occur. Stasis dermatitis can result in skin ulceration when measures to reduce venous insufficiency fail.

Clinical diagnosis and management

Diagnosis No pathology tests definitively identify stasis dermatitis. However, microbiological analysis of the exudate may determine the causative organism from secondary infections. Visual inspection and the collection of a history regarding venous insufficiency or factors resulting in circulatory pathology are important.

Management The primary management principles associated with stasis dermatitis focus on methods to reduce venous insufficiency. These include elevation of the affected limb, compression therapy and wound management. Appropriate and frequent hygiene practices are necessary to prevent infection. If a secondary infection occurs, appropriate antimicrobials should be ordered following microscopy, culture and sensitivity testing. Topical corticosteroid therapy can be used to reduce the inflammatory processes.

Incontinence-associated dermatitis

Incontinence-associated dermatitis has been known by many names, including *nappy rash* and *peri rash*. Skin lesions in the perineal area resulting from urine or faecal incontinence can be excoriated, painful and potentially dangerous. This type of dermatitis is generally associated with the very young or the very old. When associated with aged care, the costs of management can become financially burdensome. However, irrespective of cost, prevention of incontinence-associated dermatitis is important to reduce pain and suffering. The differentiation between dermatitis and skin lesions associated with pressure areas is pivotal in determining the appropriate management of these conditions.

Aetiology and pathophysiology Repeated urine or faecal incontinence results in exposure of the dermal barrier to chemical and physical irritation. An increase in microbial presence also occurs. The chemical irritation is a result of increasing pH from the ammonia. When a person is faecally incontinent, chemical irritation can also be as a result of faecal enzyme activity. Physical irritation can occur as a consequence of the friction of frequent cleaning or the presence of incontinence aids or clothes. These factors initiate the inflammatory process. As inflammation continues, the skin permeability increases and the functional capacity as a barrier is reduced.

Clinical manifestations Early skin changes indicating incontinence-associated dermatitis include erythema and tenderness. As the condition deteriorates, a macerated lesion will develop. The area can become weepy or indurated. If colonisation leads to infection, the area may become pustulous and malodorous.

Clinical diagnosis and management

Diagnosis Apart from sampling exudate for bacterial or fungal infection, no pathology tests confirm the diagnosis of incontinence-associated dermatitis. Visual inspection, a history of incontinence, hygiene practices and the clinical situation will guide the diagnosis of incontinence-associated dermatitis.

Management Prevention is the best management, through the use of topical barrier preparations with antiseptic properties. Obviously, methods to reduce incontinence will be most effective. However, if incontinence-associated dermatitis develops, a regimen of skin cleansing and moisturising is important. Skin preparations with a pH close to that of normal skin are recommended. Moisturising cream is important to reduce erythema and **desquamation** (the shedding of skin epithelium). Newer incontinence aids are being produced from polymer, as research indicates reduced tissue destruction when compared to non-polymer products.

PSORIASIS VULGARIS

LEARNING OBJECTIVE 2

Identify the various integumentary system changes that occur as a result of psoriasis.

Psoriasis (see Figure 43.3) is a *chronic inflammatory skin condition* that occurs as a result of an autoimmune disorder. In approximately 30% of individuals presenting with psoriasis, a positive family history can be identified, which suggests some degree of genetic influence. There are several different types of psoriasis, including plaque, inverse, guttate, erythrodermic and pustular psoriasis. There are also three types of pustular psoriasis.

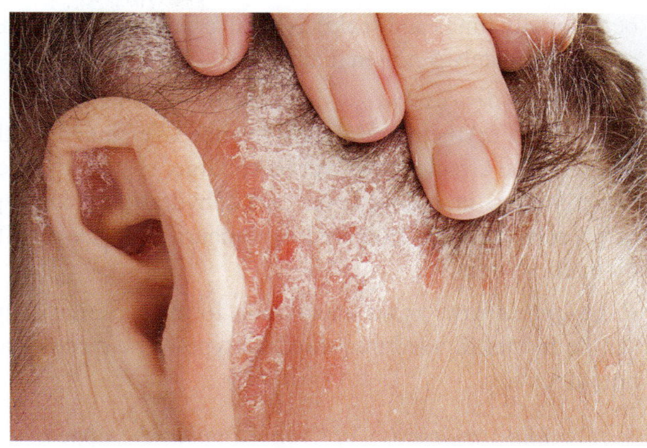

Figure 43.3

Psoriasis

A typical plaque psoriasis of flaking white lesions on an erythematous area in an individual's hairline.

Source: Lipowski Milan/Shutterstock.

Aetiology and pathophysiology

Although not well understood, psoriasis is known to be an *autoimmune disorder* (see the chapter 'Immune disorders'). T cell hyperactivity and increased pro-inflammatory mediators, including tumour necrosis factor-alpha (TNF-α), interferons and interleukins, contribute significantly to the cutaneous manifestations. The affected area experiences a dramatic degree of **hyperkeratosis** (an increase of keratin in the epidermis). Keratinocyte turnover normally occurs at a rate of 22–24 days, but in psoriatic skin, the rate can be as rapid as three to five days. The rapidly produced keratinocytes are immature and poorly formed, retaining their nuclei (parakeratosis). As a consequence, an insufficient amount of lipid is released from these cells so that the corneocytes are less able to adhere to each other and, as a cumulative result, the affected area begins to flake.

Clinical manifestations

The different types of psoriasis have different clinical presentations.

- *Plaque psoriasis* is most common, and results in erythematous areas of flaking skin lesions. The lesions tend to be silvery-white in colour.
- *Inverse psoriasis* (also known as *flexural psoriasis*) appears as smooth erythematous areas under the breast and axilla and in the groin.
- *Guttate psoriasis* can appear soon after an upper respiratory tract infection caused by β-haemolytic *Streptococcus* spp. Guttate psoriasis generally presents on the trunk (and

occasionally limbs and scalp) as small erythematous papules of approximately 5 mm in diameter.

- *Erythrodermic psoriasis* is severe, and appears as widespread erythematous scaly lesions over much of the body. As the affected area can be so large, systemic effects are common, including fever and dehydration. This type of psoriasis may be triggered by sunburn or, occasionally, by medications.
- *Pustular psoriasis* is an uncommon form of psoriasis that can be further divided into three subtypes. The pustules are not infectious.
  - *Pustular psoriasis of von Zumbusch* appears as erythematous and painful lesions over most of the body. Hours after the erythema, vesicular pustulous lesions form. Within one or two days, they dry, peel and then appear smooth. This is followed by further eruptions, coming in waves that may last days to weeks. As the surface area involved in this type of psoriasis is large, it is often associated with systemic symptoms, including fever, dehydration, malaise and tachycardia. This eruption may be triggered by infection, some drugs or pregnancy.
  - *Palmoplantar pustolosis* is another form of pustular psoriasis appearing as erythematous areas underneath pustules on the palms and the soles of the feet. Initially red, the lesions become brown and eventually peel and crust.
  - *Acropustulosis* (also known as *acrodermatitis continua of Hallopeau*) is a rare type of pustular psoriasis appearing on the fingers and toes.

Clinical diagnosis and management

Diagnosis No definitive laboratory investigations are available to assist with the diagnosis of psoriasis. Visual inspection and history analysis are most beneficial. Microbiological analysis for the presence of bacteria or fungus may assist in determining whether infection is a cause or a contributing factor to the lesion.

Management Topical corticosteroid creams assist in reducing the inflammation. Moisturising creams can be beneficial, and are less expensive than corticosteroid creams. Antimicrobial agents and antipruritic preparations (e.g. coal tar) are beneficial. Topical vitamin D analogues are sometimes used with corticosteroids with good effect.

Agents to manage the hyperkeratosis can also be used. Anthralin is a keratolytic agent and is beneficial for reducing scale. Specialised phototherapy treatments of UV light may be available in some institutions, and can occasionally be used at home under strict medical monitoring. The UV light slows the rate of cellular hyperplasia. The risks associated with skin cancer and photodamage are weighed up against the possible benefits of treatment. For some people, with due care, this risk may be warranted.

DRUG ERUPTIONS

LEARNING OBJECTIVE 3

Discuss the cutaneous consequences of immune and non-immune-mediated drug eruptions.

Almost any therapeutic agent can result in cutaneous reactions. Drugs that commonly cause reactions include antimicrobial agents, non-steroidal anti-inflammatory drugs (NSAIDs) and antiseizure agents. Drug eruptions can be divided into two broad categories: *immunologically mediated* and *non-immunologically mediated*. Drug eruptions can be classified by the morphology of the resulting lesions. Some examples are outlined below.

- *Morbilliform rash*—erythematous, macular and papular lesions of approximately 2–10 mm beginning within one or two weeks of commencing the drug. This is the most common cutaneous drug reaction.
- **Urticarial rash**—an intensely pruritic, erythematous rash, with irregularly raised welts (**wheals**). Most lesions subside within 24 hours of ceasing the drug. This is the second most common cutaneous drug reaction.
- *Bullous eruptions*—affected area has vesicles (i.e. is blistered), otherwise known as **bullae**, which may vary in size.
- *Fixed drug eruption*—an erythematous macular skin lesion develops in the same anatomical site on each exposure to the drug. The lesions may progress to bullae on continued exposure. The onset of the rash can occur within hours of administration, and may take a week to subside.
- *Pustular rash*—lesions that are filled with pus, which vary in size and shape.
- *Papulosquamous rash*—eruptions that are erythematous and scaly.
- *Lichenoid rash*—asymmetric lesion with erythematous and generally scaly truncal patches. The oral mucosa can also be affected, causing unilateral lesions of either ulceration or a net-like presentation (reticular).
- *Purpuric rash*—haemorrhages under the skin resulting in bruising/discolouration.
- **Vasculitis**—an erythematous flat rash.

Figure 43.4 shows the terms commonly used to describe skin lesions.

Aetiology and pathophysiology

Using the *Gell–Coombs classification*, immune-mediated drug eruptions can be divided into four types. See the chapter 'Immune disorders' for a detailed discussion on hypersensitivity reactions.

Non-immune-mediated drug eruptions may be classified according to the method by which the reaction occurs. Table 43.1 provides a summary of the pathophysiology and examples of cutaneous manifestations of non-immune-mediated drug eruptions.

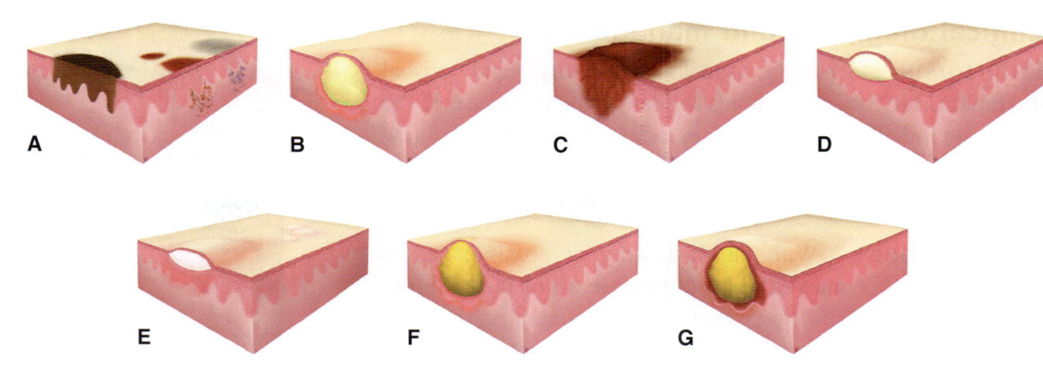

Figure 43.4

Primary skin lesions

(A) Macule.
(B) Papule.
(C) Nodule/tumour.
(D) Vesicle/bulla.
(E) Wheal.
(F) Pustule.
(G) Cyst.

Source: Averil Bellert © Sciencopia

Table 43.1 Non-immune-mediated drug eruptions

Type	Pathophysiology	Examples of cutaneous manifestations
Secondary effects/ adverse reaction	Some drugs may influence the environment, such as destroying normal flora. Some effects cannot be separated from the desired effects of the drug.	Administration of antimicrobials to treat systemic or local infections can cause infections in other areas. Vaginal yeast infections may occur as a result of destruction of normal flora, resulting in loss of control over the fungus that causes candidiasis. Administration of many chemotherapeutic agents can cause alopecia or mucositis.
Accumulation	Prolonged exposure to some drugs can cause skin discolouration.	Prolonged administration of silver nitrate (for epistaxis) can cause argyria (blue discolouration to the nails and skin). Also common with amiodarone (but could be classified as phototoxic, because it is exacerbated by sun exposure).
Overdose	Exaggerated response of the drug as a result of excess (deliberate or accidental).	In the case of an overdose of anticoagulant therapy, petechiae and/or purpura will be seen.
Mast cell mediator release	Some drugs promote a dose-dependent leukotriene and histamine release.	Administration of opioids and non-steroidal anti-inflammatory drugs (NSAIDs) can cause an urticarial rash.
Intolerance	Mechanism unclear, but does not need prior exposure to the drug. Can be exacerbated by pathologies causing an altered metabolism.	Some drugs are not well tolerated and, for certain groups of people or certain classes of drug, intolerance can cause skin eruptions and urticaria.
Jarisch–Herxheimer phenomenon	Release of bacterial endotoxin from antimicrobial-induced microorganism destruction.	Administration of antimicrobials for the treatment of infections (especially from Gram-negative bacteria) can cause macular rash and urticarial eruption as endotoxins are released.
Phototoxic dermatitis	Some drugs, when combined with sun exposure, can cause the production of oxygen free radicals, reactive oxygen species and other inflammatory mediators.	Some photosensitising drugs (including tetracyclines and phenothiazines) can cause erythematous areas with bulla.
Idiosyncratic	Unpredictable and unexplainable.	Any range of cutaneous manifestations possible.

Sources: Data from Blume (2022); Bullock & Manias (2022).

Clinical diagnosis and management

Diagnosis Generally speaking, history and visual inspections are the cornerstones in identifying the cause of the drug eruption. The process may be relatively simple when few drugs are consumed. However, it can become very complex when working with individuals in polypharmacy situations.

Management With the vast array of possible causes and effects, it becomes difficult to explore all of the different management possibilities. Fortunately, general principles apply to most drug eruptions. Primarily, once the offending drug has been identified, administration should be ceased. The resulting cutaneous reactions are commonly treated with corticosteroids to reduce the inflammatory process, and sometimes antihistamines to reduce the pruritus. Avoidance is best if a previous reaction is known. If avoidance is not possible, a desensitisation process may be available, although it is not free from risk. If undertaken, desensitisation must be completed in a controlled environment, with resuscitation and airway management equipment to hand.

ROSACEA

Rosacea is a common chronic, non-infectious skin condition. In Australia, the prevalence is unknown. It is defined by an *erythematous rash persisting on the central portion of the face* for more than three months (see Figure 43.5).

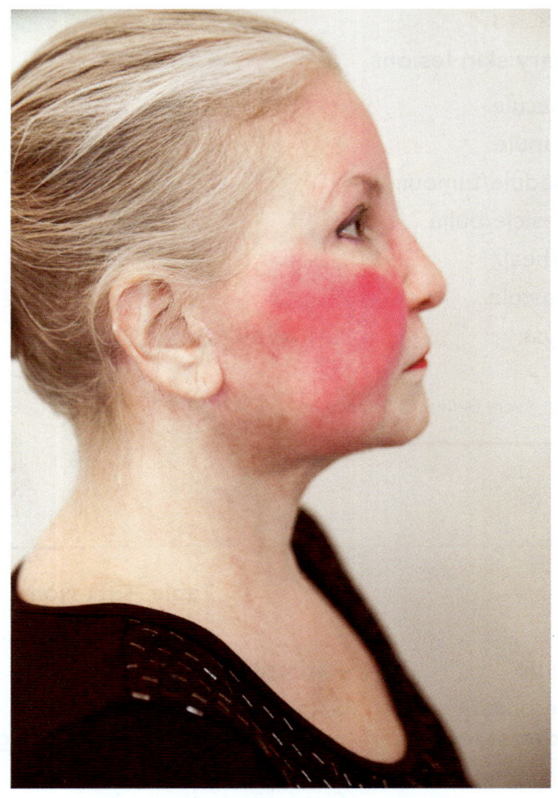

Figure 43.5
Rosacea
An individual with a typical central facial erythematous rash that has lasted more than three months.

Source: Jodi Jacobson/Alamy Stock Photo.

Aetiology and pathophysiology

The pathophysiology of rosacea is unknown; however, there appears to be a strong link to environmental stimuli provoking vascular changes that are probably mediated by the immune system. This is supported by the fact that anti-inflammatory agents can reduce exacerbations. The use of topical antimicrobials may also influence the neutrophil involvement, which is often stimulated by microorganisms common in rosacea. There appears to be a genetic predisposition to rosacea, especially in people with Northern and Eastern European heritage.

Clinical manifestations

Along with the erythema, rosacea may present with areas of telangiectasia (small, dilated blood vessels near the skin surface), and sometimes a papulopustular eruption resembling acne. The erythematous area may also have a painful burning or stinging sensation. The four subtypes of rosacea are outlined below.

1. *Papulopustular rosacea* presents more frequently in women on the central region of the face. The affected area appears erythematous and contains papules with pustules. The lesions are most often follicular in origin, and resemble a sterile cellulitis.
2. *Erythematotelangiectactic rosacea* presents as a burning or stinging central flushing of the face. Visible surface vessels emphasise the erythema. The affected skin may intermittently become scaly as a result of dermatitis. The flushing can be exacerbated by numerous emotional and environmental changes.
3. *Phymatous rosacea* affects the forehead, nose, ears, eyelids and chin, and presents as an erythematous area containing irregular nodules on the surface.
4. *Ocular rosacea* affects tissue in the periorbital area, including the eyelids and conjunctiva. Individuals may complain of dry, inflamed eyes or conjunctivitis several years before the erythematous and telangiectasias changes appear in these areas. This subtype of rosacea may result in vascular inflammation in the sclera, too. Intervention is important in ocular rosacea, as the conjunctival effects may threaten eyesight.

Clinical diagnosis and management

Diagnosis Although history and visual inspection of the affected area will guide diagnosis, a skin biopsy may be performed to exclude systemic lupus erythematosis and sarcoidosis.

Management Identification and elimination (or reduction) of the triggers are a crucial first step in the management of rosacea. **Photoprotection** using hats and sunscreen may reduce exacerbation. Vascular laser therapy is used to reduce visible vessels.

Dermabrasion may be necessary for the nodular lesions.

Skin infections

Infections of the integumentary system can be caused by numerous pathogens. Skin infections are caused by bacteria, viruses, parasites and fungi. The complexity of skin infections can be related to many factors, including the number of different organisms involved, the individual's immune function, and the integrity and health of the skin involved. Figure 43.6 explores the common clinical manifestations and management of skin infections.

BACTERIAL INFECTIONS

LEARNING OBJECTIVE 4

Examine the pathophysiology and management of various types of bacterial skin infections.

A synergistic relationship exists between an individual's skin and mucous membranes, and certain bacteria in specific locations. This non-pathogenic colonisation is called **normal flora**. When different bacteria colonise a region, they may become pathogenic. Also, when normal flora translocate to a region normally considered 'sterile', infection may occur. Figure 43.7 demonstrates the type and location of the most common normal flora.

There are many different types of bacteria, which are most often classified by shape. (See the chapter 'Infectious disease' and Figure 8.2 for an explanation of the different types of bacteria.)

Folliculitis, furuncles and carbuncles

Aetiology and pathophysiology

Folliculitis is *inflammation of the hair shaft*. This inflammation is commonly caused by an infection; however, it can also be caused by chemical irritation or physical injury. Folliculitis is inflammation that remains within the wall of the hair follicle. *Acne* is a form of folliculitis. **Furuncles** are an area of folliculitis involving several follicles, and are generally caused by a staphylococcal infection. Furuncles are often called *boils*. They become red, hot and swollen, and form a pustule. **Carbuncles** are a *collection of furuncles* that extend down to the subcutaneous tissue. They involve many infected hair follicles and form large skin abscesses. They are commonly found on the neck, shoulders, back, hips and thighs. Carbuncles are common in people with diabetes mellitus and those who are immunocompromised. People who live in overcrowded environments, and people with substandard hygiene practices, may be particularly at risk of the development of furuncles or carbuncles. Figure 43.8 shows examples of folliculitis, furuncles and carbuncles.

S. aureus is one of the most common pathogens causing bacterial skin infections. Once a pathogen has colonised the area, it may cause an inflammatory response that results in vasodilation, hyperaemia, chemotaxis, complement activation and pain. Chemotaxis encourages the arrival of neutrophils and macrophages into the skin tissue as they attempt to defend against the offending pathogen. Activation of the complement system results in coating of the pathogen, enhancing phagocytosis. During this time, mast cells within the tissues degranulate and release inflammatory mediators (including histamine), which results in further vasodilation and tissue swelling. Cytokine release from immune cells encourages more inflammatory cells into the affected area of skin, and prostaglandins are released at the site. Prostaglandins irritate the sensory nerve endings in skin tissue, and nociceptive information is transmitted via afferent neurons to the cortex, where it is perceived as pain (see the chapter 'Nociception and pain'). Purulent exudate (pus)—consisting of cellular debris and high levels of protein resulting from the interaction between the neutrophils and the pathogen—accumulates in the affected region.

Clinical manifestations

Folliculitis usually results in an erythematous area, and may demonstrate purulent exudate. Furuncles present as erythematous nodules often contained within a walled cyst. The lesion can contain a large amount of purulent exudate. Consequently, the tissue may erupt and the exudates drain away. Typically, folliculitis and furuncles do not result in systemic inflammatory symptoms. However, carbuncles can cause pyrexia, chills and malaise. Carbuncles will cause a swollen, painful, pustulous and erythematous lesion that may drain from many sites. Not all carbuncles result in systemic symptoms. However, many factors can influence their development, including the level of immunocompromise exhibited by the affected individual, the size of the area involved, and the presence and virulence of multiple pathogens.

Clinical diagnosis and management

Diagnosis Visual inspection will assist in assessing the degree of inflammation and the tissue infection involved. A microbiology sample sent for microscopy, culture and sensitivity (MCS) testing will assist in determining the type of organism and antibiotic sensitivity.

Management Folliculitis is self-limiting, and should be managed with improved hygiene. Depending on the extent and involvement of the furuncles and carbuncles, thorough cleaning and appropriate wound management practices, coupled with a course of antimicrobials, should control the infection.

The appropriate use of antimicrobials, based on the results of the MCS testing, is imperative to ensure optimum efficiency of the treatment, a reduced risk of antimicrobial resistance development and a decreased chance of **bacteraemia** (a bacterial infection within the blood).

Acne vulgaris

Most people have experienced *acne vulgaris*, or simply acne, at some stage of their life, especially during adolescence. After puberty, the degree of acne affecting an individual tends to reduce as they mature into adulthood.

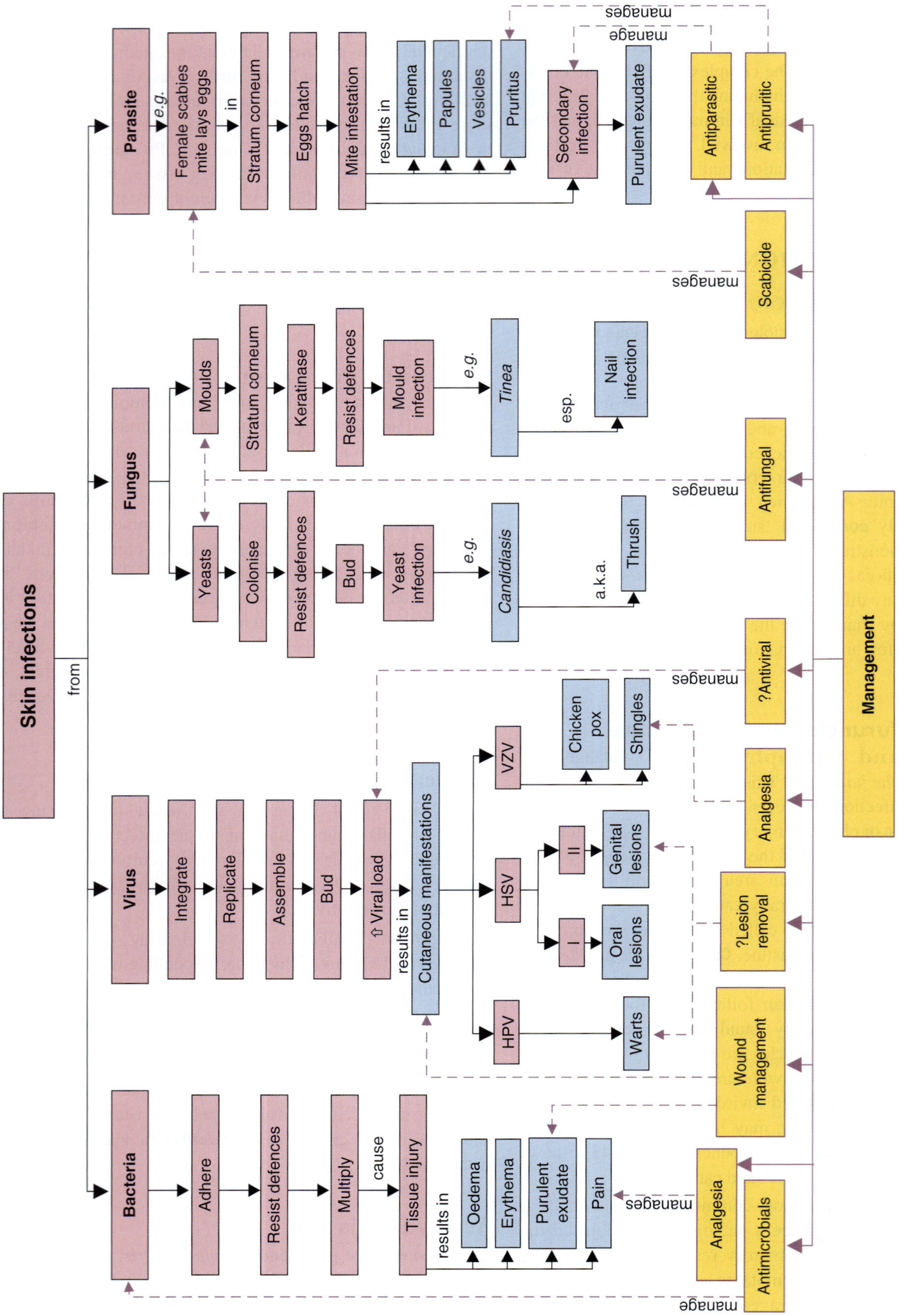

Figure 43.6

Clinical snapshot: Skin infections

↑ = increased; ? = possibly; HPV = human papillomavirus; HSV = herpes simplex virus; VZV = varicella zoster virus.

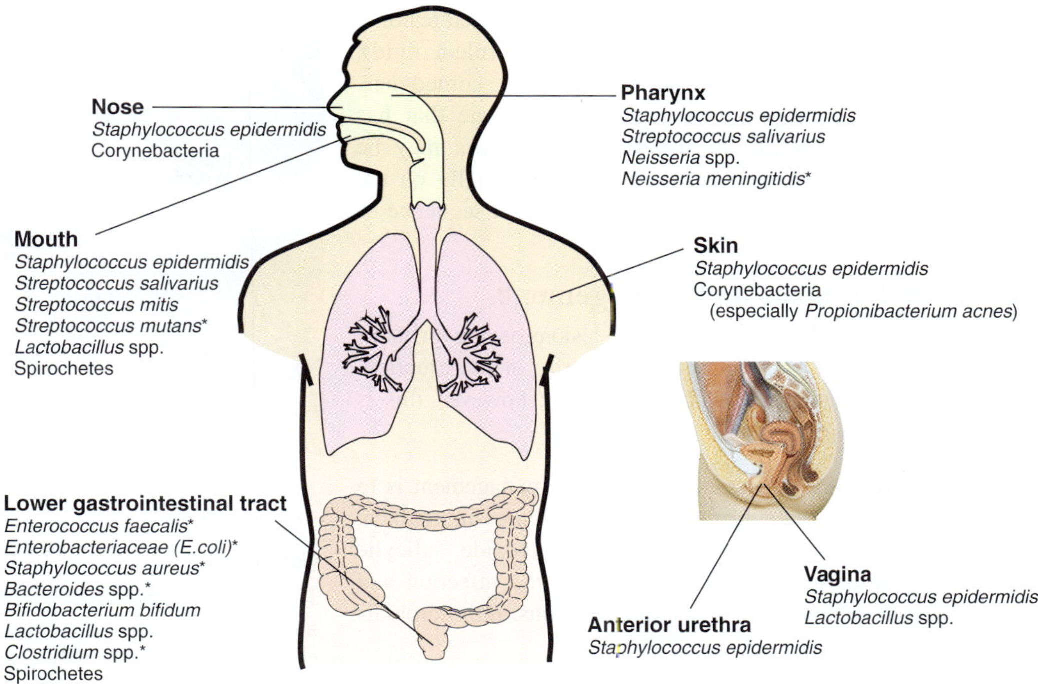

Figure 43.7

Common normal flora: types and location

*Potential pathogen.

Source: Female reproductive system: Sciencopia; tonaquatic19/123RF.

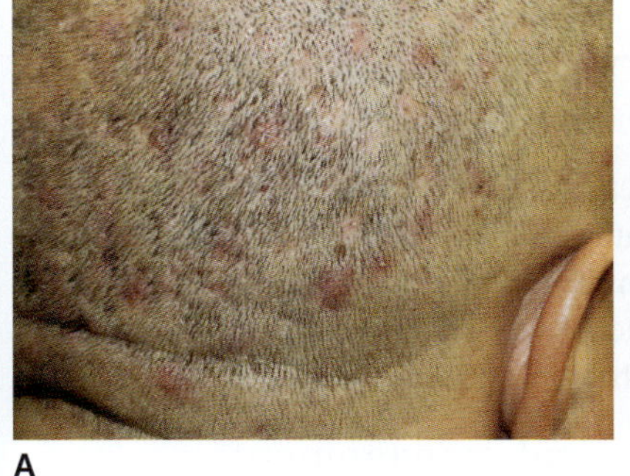
A

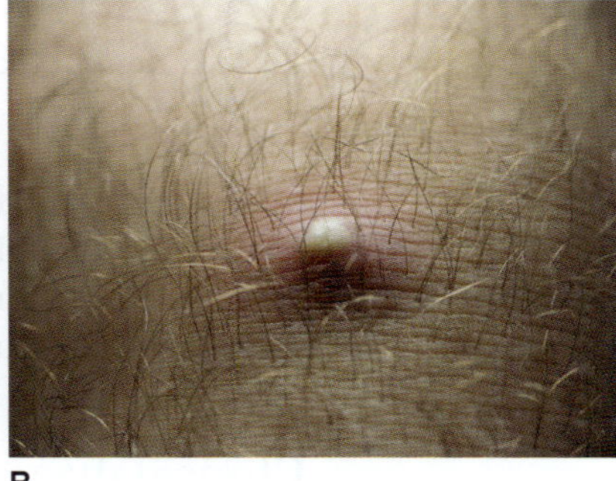
B

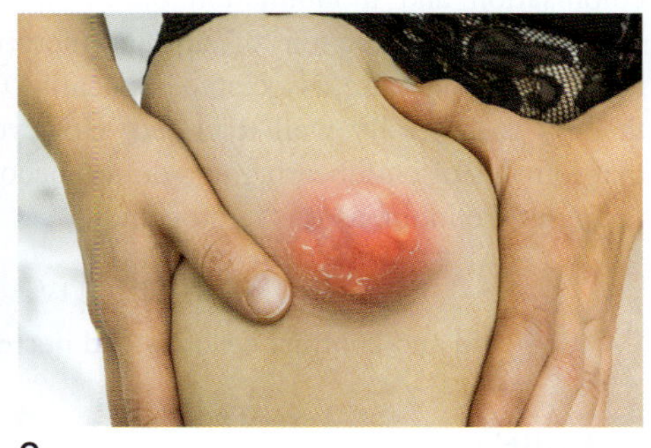
C

Figure 43.8

Three common bacterial skin infections

(A) Folliculitis. (B) Furuncle. (C) Carbuncles.

Sources: (A) Dermatology11/Shutterstock; (B) OMfotovideocontent/Shutterstock; and (C) andriano.cz/Shutterstock.

Aetiology and pathophysiology In acne, the *pilosebaceous unit* (i.e. the follicle and the sebaceous gland) becomes obstructed with **sebum** and desquamated keratinocytes, and mixes with normal flora (commonly *Propionibacterium acnes*). Although there is a migration of normal flora into tissue that is not usually colonised, it is not considered a genuine infection. As a result of the obstruction, there is lysis of sebum into fatty acids, which causes a local inflammatory reaction. Epidermal tissue undergoes hyperproliferation, and hyperkeratosis develops; this contributes to the follicular obstruction. An increase in the volume of sebum produced and the presence of corynebacteria, such as *P. acnes*, further contributes to the development of acne.

Clinical manifestations Acne lesions are called comedones. There are two types of lesions. *Open comedones* are commonly known as *blackheads*, and contain oily debris that is darkened by oxidation. Open comedones have a large follicular orifice. *Closed comedones*, commonly known as *whiteheads*, are small papules with a very small follicular orifice that prevents oxidation; therefore, the material contained within the pilosebaceous unit is white.

Acne may be exacerbated by puberty, trauma, friction, the contraceptive pill or insufficient cleansing after the application of make-up. The lesions can also be classed as inflammatory, non-inflammatory and scars. In the older adult, senile comedones are common in the periorbital region.

Inflammatory lesions have both papules (solid, raised lesions) and pustules (a small, raised collection of purulent fluid), whereas *non-inflammatory lesions* only have comedones. *Scars* are the result of severe or prolonged acne that has left a chronic deformity of the skin. Acne scars may be deep indentations, thickened raised scars (especially on the chest, back and jawline), or appear to be the consequence of 'punching out' skin.

Clinical diagnosis and management

Diagnosis Visual inspection of the lesions is the primary investigative tool. Depending on the severity of the eruption, microbiological samples may be considered; however, this is usually unnecessary.

Management An important part of acne management is to ensure that appropriate hygiene behaviours are undertaken. The use of cleansing agents with benzoyl peroxide, salicylic acid or sulfur may be beneficial to reduce the infection and inflammation. In significant or extreme eruptions, antimicrobials may be useful.

Treatment with a course of retinoids, such as isotretinoin, can be beneficial for individuals experiencing significant effects of acne. Retinoids reduce the amount of sebum, bacterial colonisation and inflammation on the skin. They appear to increase the production of an antimicrobial protein called neutrophil-gelatinase-associated lipocalin (NGAL). Retinoid therapy is generally well tolerated. However, it is imperative that females of childbearing age do not become pregnant while taking isotretinoin, as it is teratogenic.

LEARNING OBJECTIVE 5

Compare and contrast cellulitis and necrotising fasciitis.

Cellulitis

Aetiology and pathophysiology

Cellulitis is an *inflammation of the dermis and subcutaneous tissue* (see Figure 43.9), usually caused by a bacterial infection such as *S. aureus* or *Streptococcus pyogenes*. It usually begins with skin trauma, such as a laceration, a puncture wound or dry, broken skin, which provides pathogens access to the dermis. Ultimately, inflammation occurs as a result of mediator release from the damaged cells. Local cytokine and keratinocyte production contributes to the effect.

People with lymphatic disease, venous insufficiency and obesity are at increased risk of cellulitis. These conditions cause an increased risk of infection as a result of the reduced acid mantle (an acid layer of sebum and sweat that inhibits bacterial and fungal growth).

Epidemiology

In 2020–21, more than 62,000 Australians were admitted to hospital as a result of cellulitis. Eighty-six per cent of these lesions occurred on a limb. However, cellulitis can be more dangerous than the discomfort of symptoms from a skin infection. In 2020, 323 people died as a direct result of cellulitis.

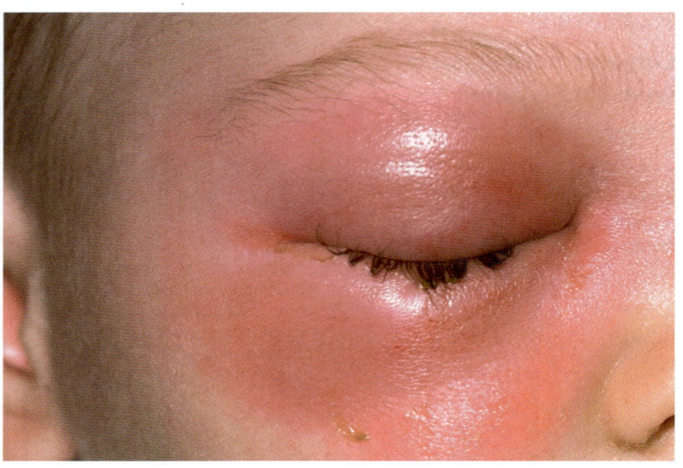

Figure 43.9

Cellulitis

The clinical manifestations of cellulitis are heat over the area, redness, pain and swelling, and occasionally fever, chills and headache. While we often think of cellulitis as typically affecting the legs, it can also occur elsewhere. This is an example of cellulitis in the skin around the eye socket.

Source: Mediscan/Alamy Stock Photo.

Clinical manifestations

The inflamed area becomes erythematous, oedematous and painful. Because of the vasodilation resulting in hyperaemia, the area will be warm to touch. Prostaglandin release will result in pain and, potentially, pyrexia, depending on the concentration of mediator released.

Clinical diagnosis and management

Diagnosis Visual inspection and a consideration of a person's history are critical. Haematology results may demonstrate an increased number of leukocytes. People will have positive blood cultures (bacteraemia) only if the cellulitis was caused via a haematogenous route or the cutaneous infection has also migrated to the circulation. Microscopy culture and sensitivity testing (MCS) may be attempted; however, the lesion usually does not appear pustulous, and bacterial levels in cellulitis can be low, making it difficult to isolate a causative organism.

Management The mainstay of treatment for cellulitis is intravenous antimicrobials and pain management. If MCS testing has elucidated a causative organism, narrow-spectrum antimicrobials can be ordered. However, broad-spectrum antimicrobials may be needed in the early stages. Often, once the inflammation has started to decrease and the infection is controlled, the person can be discharged on oral antimicrobials. Elevation of the affected limb (area) will reduce oedema and, ultimately, pain. Analgesics may also alleviate the discomfort caused by the inflammation. If the cause is determined to be mycological, antifungal preparations are indicated.

Necrotising fasciitis

Necrotising fasciitis (NF) is commonly known by the lay community and media as the *'flesh-eating disease'*. NF can be a very destructive infection, and results in significant tissue loss. The common pathogens associated with necrotising fasciitis are the β-haemolytic bacteria, group A *Streptococcus* (GAS) species. Those most at risk are those with diabetes mellitus and those who are immunocompromised.

Aetiology and pathophysiology Once the causative organism bypasses the integumentary defences, it will spread to the fascia of the subcutaneous tissue. Typical inflammatory responses occur, but the major contributor to the destruction of tissue is related to the *bacterial exotoxins or enterotoxins* produced. As the infection continues, the tissue loss spreads along the fascial planes, with vascular occlusion leading to ischaemia and, ultimately, necrosis.

Clinical manifestations Initially, the lesion may resemble the typical erythema associated with a skin infection. However, the progression generally occurs rapidly, and the tissue may become ulcerated and necrotic within hours. Systemic involvement is typical and presents as pyrexia, tachycardia and hypotension. Septicaemia develops, and an altered level of consciousness may occur. The area can become extremely tender, but as superficial nerves are damaged it can present as less painful than it appears.

Clinical diagnosis and management

Diagnosis Visual inspection of the lesion is important, and quantitative measurements of the involved tissue should be documented. Haematology results may reveal **leukocytosis** (elevated white blood cells). MCS testing of biopsied tissue may be useful in identifying the causative organism and determining the appropriate antimicrobial therapy.

Management As this infection is very aggressive, rapid diagnosis and initiation of treatment is imperative to limit tissue loss. Surgical debridement is critical to control the spread of the pathogen, as well as the destructive enzymes and exotoxins. Unfortunately, amputation may be necessary in order to save life. High mortality rates are associated with increasing tissue destruction. Early surgical intervention can reduce mortality. The administration of intravenous antimicrobials is also imperative to decrease the bacterial load and slow the tissue destruction. Hyperbaric oxygen therapy is also effective, but access is restricted to centres where these facilities are available.

Surgical site infections

LEARNING OBJECTIVE 6

Describe the consequences of surgical site infections.

Nosocomial infections are defined by the *48-hour rule*, whereby only infections that occur 48 hours after admission or within 48 hours of discharge are considered to be hospital-acquired. *Surgical site infections (SSIs)* are those that develop in a surgical wound within 30 days of the operative procedure. They can be classed as *superficial* or *deep*.

> **CLINICAL BOX 43.1**
>
> **Methicillin or multiple resistance?**
>
> Traditionally, the 'M' in MRSA referred to 'methicillin', but more recently the 'M' is considered to mean 'multiple'. This is due to *S. aureus* having developed resistance to more drugs than just methicillin, and because this agent is no longer used in clinical practice.

Aetiology and pathophysiology Currently, the most common organisms causing wound infections in Australia are *S. aureus*, vancomycin-resistant *Enterococcus* (VRE) and several of the extended-spectrum β-lactamase (ESBL)-producing Enterobacteriaceae family.

S. aureus can be either *multi-sensitive (MSSA)* or *multi-resistant (MRSA)* (see Clinical Box 43.1). MRSA is difficult to control, and is generally treated with a drug called vancomycin. However, even this powerful drug is becoming ineffective against the pathogen, as the bacteria are developing a new antibiotic resistance. The strain is called *vancomycin-intermediate S. aureus (VISA)*. This species shows multiple resistance to a range of antibacterial drugs, and has less susceptibility to vancomycin. Although infection rates from VISA in Australia are small at this time, the incidence will increase and, with it, mortality rates will climb.

MRSA can also be classified depending on the source. MRSA strains from people who are not hospitalised are classified as *community-associated (CA-MRSA)*. MRSA that results from healthcare facilities is classified as *hospital-associated (HA-MRSA)*.

Enterococci are normal flora of the gastrointestinal tract and genitalia. *Escherichia coli* is a common species belonging to this group. Enterococci are robust organisms and intrinsically resistant to many antimicrobials. When these organisms translocate to an open wound, they become pathogenic. In Australia, a strain of *Enterococcus* that was not susceptible to the glycopeptide vancomycin was isolated. Since that time, the incidence of vancomycin-resistant *Enterococcus* (also known as *glycopeptide-resistant enterococci [GRE]*) has increased.

An emerging risk is the *ESBL-producing organisms*. This group of bacteria are Gram-negative and produce enzymes that hydrolyse the β-lactam ring in this class of antibiotics. β-Lactam antimicrobials work by inhibiting bacterial cell wall synthesis. They have a β-lactam ring and contain a nucleus in the molecular structure. Penicillins, cephalosporins, monobactams and carbapenems belong to this group of antimicrobials. ESBL-producing organisms include the Enterobacteriaceae family, such as *E. coli* and the *Klebsiella* species.

Irrespective of the mechanism of injury (e.g. surgical site, trauma, ulcer or burn), once the skin integrity is compromised and colonisation occurs, infection can quickly follow. As with all bacterial infections previously discussed, the progression of the inflammatory process and the inter-relationship between the immune system defences and the pathogen will result in purulent exudate and an erythematous, painful wound site. As the wound infection subsides, healing will occur through the three phases of wound healing (see the chapter 'Inflammation and healing').

Epidemiology Almost 79,000 people experienced a hospital-acquired infection in 2020–21. This data accounts for public and private hospital incidence, but not other healthcare facilities such as aged-care or community-care services. Although this number is decreasing as healthcare facilities focus more on prevention, a HAI will invariably complicate a person's recovery, including increases in pain, costs and time to heal.

Clinical manifestations An early sign of wound infection development is an increased amount of pain at the surgical site. Initially, an increase in the volume of serosanguinous fluid may occur; however, this soon develops into purulent exudate. The area will become erythematous and oedematous. The skin can become macerated, and tissue can pull through to suture material or staples, enabling the wound to gape (see Figure 43.10). Depending on the size of the incision, the location and the degree of infection, evisceration may occur. Depending on the bacterial load, the virulence of the pathogen, the degree of immunocompromise and access to the vascular system, the person may develop bacteraemia. Fever, hypotension and tachycardia will result.

Clinical diagnosis and management

Diagnosis MCS testing on sampled exudate or tissue will enable isolation of the causative organisms and selection of the appropriate antimicrobial for optimum effect. With newer but increasingly more common organisms such as *Clostridium difficile*, some laboratories test not for the pathogen but for the toxin produced.

As the tendency to isolate and classify the specific strains increases, DNA sequencing using the polymerase chain reaction continues to grow. This technique is more beneficial for research and epidemiological analysis. These newer techniques can be expensive, and do not necessarily change the clinical management plan. However, identifying new strains can give insight into developing virulence and increasing frequency.

Management Management of wound infections is achieved through MCS testing, followed by administration of the appropriate antimicrobials. Frequent wound redressing to remove the infected wound exudate is also required. However, the most effective management of wound infections is prevention. Prevention processes include a focus on hand hygiene measures and the use of standard precautions. The correct use of personal protective equipment (PPE) and the appropriate removal and disposal of the PPE are paramount to controlling cross-infection.

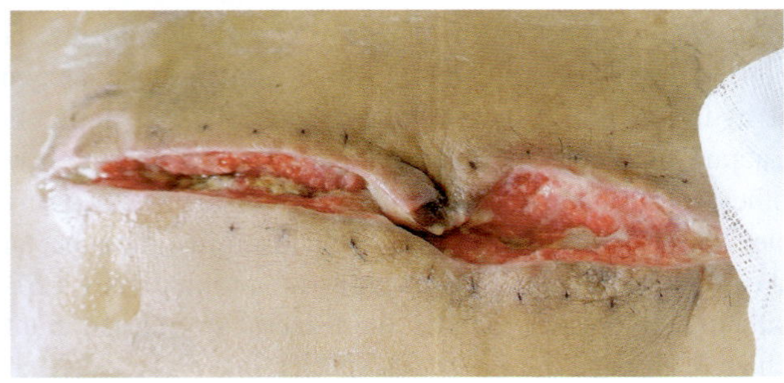

Figure 43.10

Surgical wound infection

Surgical wound dehiscence as a result of wound infection.

Source: Tthawatchai_bandit/Shutterstock.

VIRAL INFECTIONS

LEARNING OBJECTIVE 7

Discuss other causes of skin disease, including viral and fungal infection.

Viruses can cause an array of skin infections and eruptions. Warts, shingles and cold sores are all caused by viruses. These viruses can be very contagious, and, as with many of the infections discussed in this section, direct (or sometimes even indirect) contact with the infected surface or fluid can cause viral transmission.

Human Papillomavirus

Aetiology and pathophysiology

Human papillomavirus (HPV) causes *warts*. There are over 100 strains of HPV, and many different types of warts. Although some HPV strains are associated with cancer, most do not contribute to malignancy development. A few HPV strains are associated with cervical cancer (see the chapter 'Female reproductive disorders').

In 2006, the Australian Government commenced funding for an HPV vaccination program. Children 12–13 years of age are given two injections including a nonavalent vaccine (which protects against nine strains of HPV) at least six months apart. This schedule is considered to be highly effective against the strains that cause the majority of HPV-related cancers and two strains that cause 90% of genital warts (see the chapter 'Female reproductive disorders'). Table 43.2 provides a summary of the types, description and locations of common HPV strains that cause warts.

HPVs are *non-enveloped DNA viruses* (envelopes tend to make it easier for the virus to enter the host cell). Once the virus has made contact with cutaneous or mucosal epithelial cells, it enters the tissue, integrates with it and begins replication. This is followed by reassembly and budding. During this process, it is thought that a protein expressed by the HPV manipulates the control of cell growth, resulting in the deformed lesions, which, depending on the HPV strain, may lead to malignancy.

Clinical manifestations

The morphology of the wart depends on the location and the strain of the virus causing the lesion. Most warts are painless.

Table 43.2 Warts (verruca)

Type	Description	Location	Common HPV strain
Common warts (*Verruca vulgaris*)	Hard Cauliflower-like surface Dome-shaped Skin-coloured Generally localised to one site	Anywhere; commonly: • hands • knees	1, 2, 4, 27, 29
Flat warts (*Verruca plana*)	Flat—slightly raised Reddish-brown or skin-coloured Smooth 2–5 mm in diameter Mostly clustered	Anywhere; commonly • hands • face • lower legs	3, 10, 28, 49
Filiform warts	Long Narrow Skin-coloured Thread-like Individual or clustered Rapid growth	Face; commonly • eyelids • lips • neck	1, 2, 4, 27, 29
Genital warts	Grey/white Large or small Raised or flat Cauliflower-like surface	Penis Vulva Anus	6, 11
Plantar warts	Hard Raised lump With growth may become cauliflower-like May contain black dots	Soles of feet	1, 2
Mosaic warts	Clusters of plantar warts	Hands Soles of feet	1, 2
Periungual	Small Initially smooth, become irregular	In or around toenails and fingernails	1, 2

However, plantar warts may cause discomfort when walking, as the lesion is being forced into the tissue under the foot.

Clinical diagnosis and management

Diagnosis It is unnecessary to obtain histological and serological confirmation of HPV. Visual inspection, and the determination of morphology and location, should sufficiently inform clinical judgment.

Management For non-genital warts, management options range from no treatment through to removal interventions with liquid nitrogen, laser or electrocurettage. The application of topical agents, including salicylic acid or antiviral agents, may be beneficial, depending on the type and location. Injection of chemotherapeutic agents or interferons into the lesion has demonstrated variable results.

Cryosurgery with liquid nitrogen or the use of a carbon dioxide laser is effective, and can be undertaken on pregnant women. Topical therapies containing podophyllin or bichloracetic acid can be effective. A course of interferon injections has also been found to be beneficial. However, destruction of the lesion has been found to be the most effective treatment.

The prevention of genital warts may be achieved through the use of condoms, even if there is no visible lesion. The HPV vaccine, Gardasil, consists of capsid proteins from four strains of the virus. It is recommended for the prevention of cervical cancers. However, once HPV infection occurs, treatment becomes more difficult because of the sensitive area involved.

Human herpesvirus

There are 25 different types of herpesvirus, eight of which cause illness in humans. Table 43.3 presents a summary of the *human herpesvirus (HHV)* types and the conditions associated with infection. The focus of this section is on infection by the herpes simplex virus and the varicella zoster virus.

Herpes simplex virus

Aetiology and pathophysiology *Herpes simplex virus 1 (HSV-1)* causes cold sores. Generally speaking, HSV-1 infections manifest on the mouth, tongue and lips. *Herpes simplex virus 2 (HSV-2)* causes genital herpes. Generally speaking, HSV-2 infections manifest on the penis, the anus and the perineum in men, while in women the infection commonly manifests on the cervix and external genitalia (see the chapters 'Female reproductive disorders' and 'Male reproductive disorders').

The growth cycle of a virus has four stages. In the first instance, the virus will attach to a receptor on the membrane of the cell it invades. On attachment it will then penetrate through fusion or by allowing itself to be engulfed. In the third stage, the virus is transported to the cell's nucleus. The virus directs the nucleus to undertake viral replication, the newly produced parts are assembled, and then the viral copies bud, often taking parts of the cell membrane with them.

With HSV-1, the infection can subside and the virus will travel along the trigeminal ganglia and lie dormant until a stressor causes it to *reactivate*. During latency, there is no evidence of infection. With HSV-2, the infection can become latent by travelling along the lumbosacral ganglia. Stressors causing reactivation can include trauma, stress, immunosuppression or even hormonal fluctuations.

Although, generally speaking, HSV-1 causes perioral infections and HSV-2 causes anogenital infections, there is some crossover, with 10–30% of infections affecting body areas associated with the other strain.

Clinical manifestations HSV-1 will cause painful lesions that cluster around the perioral area (see Figure 43.11A). The vesicular lesions are full of virus and exceedingly contagious. Within a few days, the lesion will dry and form a crust. Inflammation is common, and is associated with erythema and oedema. Viral shedding occurs during active infection, but it can also occur when the individual is asymptomatic.

HSV-2 will cause painful lesions that cluster around the genital area in both males and females (see Figure 43.11B), but can also cause lesions on the buttocks and legs. The affected region will generally be oedematous and erythematous. Other symptoms that may occur with HSV-2 include fever and malaise, and dysuria. Vaginal or penile discharge is also experienced.

Neonates may become infected with facial herpes caused by maternal HSV-2 following a vaginal birth. Intrauterine or perinatal infection is rare; however, the resulting infections can be very serious. Neonatal mortality is significant, so early detection and appropriate management is critical.

HSV can also cause encephalitis. Although HSV-1 encephalitis is more common, HSV-2 encephalitis is also possible. The symptoms can include the obvious neurological manifestations, including headaches and seizures. Early signs may include malaise, nausea and fever.

Clinical diagnosis and management

Diagnosis Although serological assays will determine the specific infection, this may not alter the management plan. Visual inspection and a consideration of the clinical history will be most beneficial.

Management Despite being painful, the lesions that develop are generally self-limiting. Topical or oral antiviral medications are available over the counter. However, these will be most effective if applied before large viral loads have had the opportunity to bud

HSV infections in individuals who are immunocompromised may require more aggressive management, such as admission to hospital, and treatment with antiviral agents, analgesia and intravenous fluids to maintain adequate hydration.

Table 43.3 Summary of human herpesviruses (HHVs) and possible manifestations

HHV type	Virus type	Possible conditions
HHV-1	Herpes simplex virus 1 (HSV-1)	Cold sores, gingivostomatitis, eczema herpeticum, HSV encephalitis
HHV-2	Herpes simplex virus 2 (HSV-2)	Genital lesions, HSV meningitis, HSV proctitis
HHV-3	Varicella zoster virus (VSV)	Chickenpox, shingles
HHV-4	Epstein–Barr virus (EBV)	Infectious mononucleosis, Burkitt's lymphoma
HHV-5	Cytomegalovirus (CMV)	Asymptomatic
HHV-6	Human herpesvirus 6	Asymptomatic, exanthem subitum (roseola infantum), febrile seizures in children, reactivation of HHV-4 or HHV-7
HHV-7	Human herpesvirus 7	Asymptomatic, pityriasis rosea, exanthem subitum (roseola infantum), encephalitis, reactivation of HHV-4, febrile seizures in children
HHV-8	Human herpesvirus 8 (Kaposi's-sarcoma-associated herpesvirus)	Kaposi's sarcoma, primary effusion lymphoma

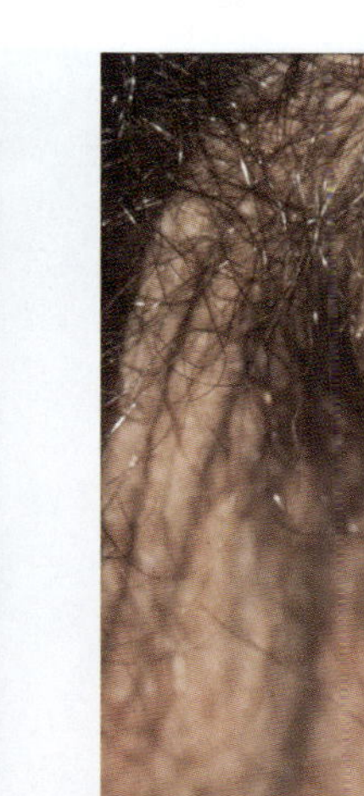

A

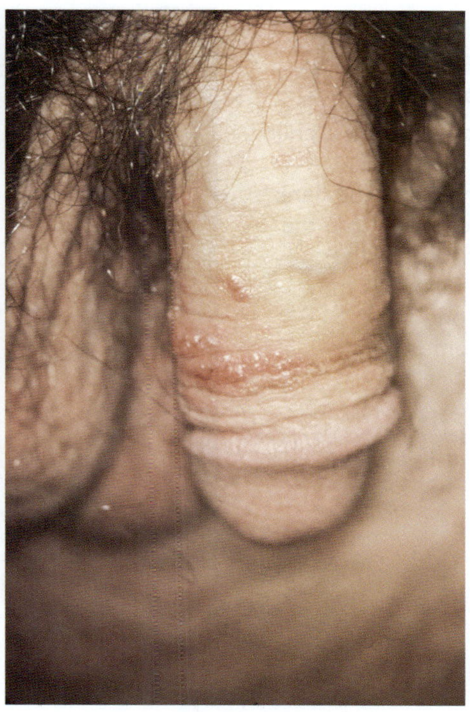

B

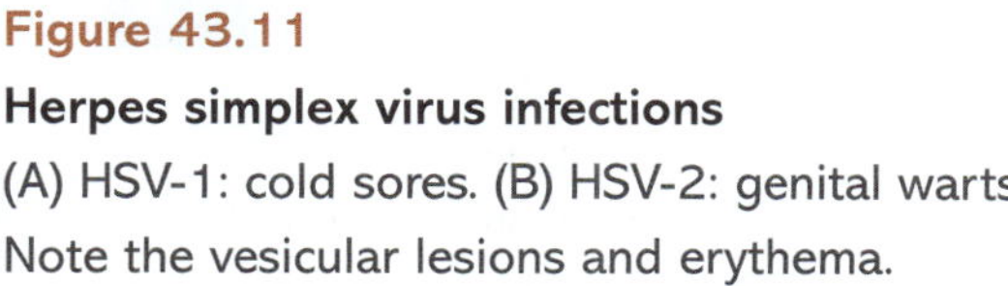

Figure 43.11

Herpes simplex virus infections

(A) HSV-1: cold sores. (B) HSV-2: genital warts. Note the vesicular lesions and erythema.

Sources: (A) Dani Vincek/Shutterstock; (B) CDC/Dr. M.F. Rein.

Varicella zoster virus

Aetiology and pathophysiology

Varicella zoster virus (VZV) is a herpesvirus that causes chickenpox (see Figure 43.12A). Chickenpox is a highly contagious virus that is most common in children (between 5 and 10 years of age). However, adults can still be affected. Transmission of the VZV infection is from *aerosolised viral particles*. VZV incubation time is approximately two weeks. In Australia, VSV is not notifiable in all states and territories. On average, there are approximately 3.3 per 100,000 people admitted per year with VSV to an Australian hospital.

After the primary infection has resolved, individuals can experience a painful, pruritic, vesicular rash that follows the dermatomes (an area of skin supplied by a specific spinal nerve), which can occur many years after the primary infection. Also known as **shingles** (see Figure 43.12B), it is caused by the same virus, and is called *herpes zoster*. The pain associated with this rash is called *post-herpetic neuralgia*, and can be so severe that it requires hospitalisation for significant pain management. Herpes zoster is a *reactivation* of VZV. Herpes zoster can stay latent in the dorsal root ganglia, and when an individual is exposed to a stressor (e.g. trauma, stress, immunosuppression or even hormonal fluctuations) the virus can erupt into a vesicular rash along a dermatome such as the trigeminal nerve and between T3 and L2.

Clinical manifestations

VZV presents as a painful vesicular rash that can start in the truncal area and scalp and move to the peripheries. The individual may experience prodromal symptoms, including malaise, pain and mild fever. Within a period of 8–12 hours, the vesicles will dry and crust. VZV can cause systemic issues, including ophthalmic and neurological complications.

Herpes zoster (shingles) will result in a painful vesicular rash that follows dermatomes. This resulting post-herpetic neuralgia is so painful that it will often require aggressive inpatient management.

Clinical diagnosis and management

Diagnosis Visual inspection and a consideration of relevant history will assist in determining VZV and herpes zoster infections. Swabs sampling the vesicular lesions can be used for nucleic acid detection, and serology can assist with determining the specific infection.

Management Chickenpox (VZV) is most often self-limiting. However, immunocompromised individuals require more supportive interventions. The use of antiviral medications is still debatable, but may be beneficial for some.

Shingles may be treated with antiviral drugs, corticosteroids, or topical and oral analgesics. It is not uncommon for individuals with post-herpetic neuralgia to require tricyclic antidepressants or selective serotonin reuptake inhibitors. Some anticonvulsant medications are also effective against the neuropathic pain associated with this condition (see the chapter 'Nociception and pain'). It is not uncommon for individuals to require opioid therapy in times of extreme pain.

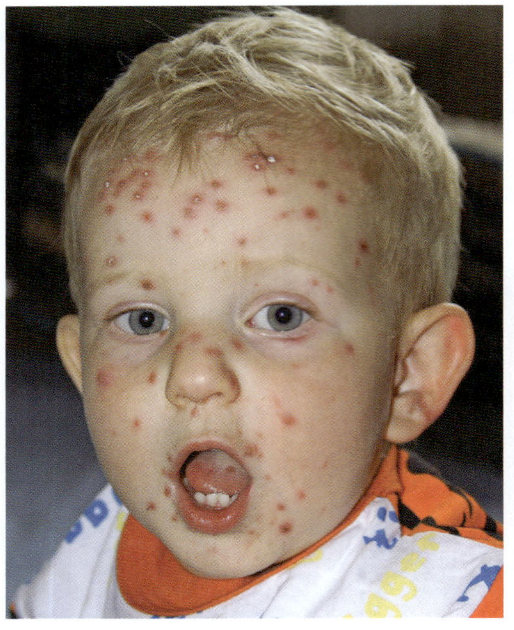

A

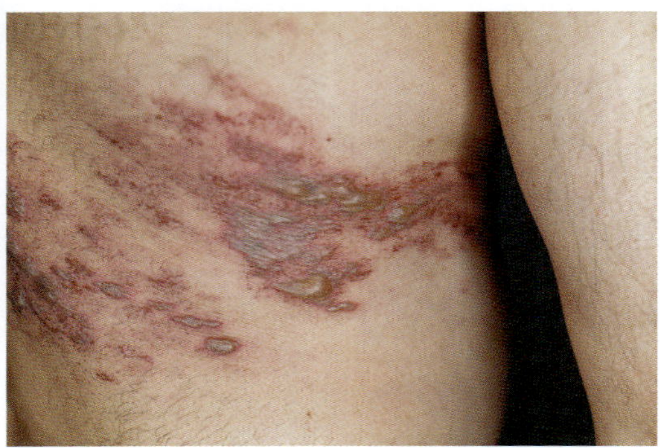

B

Figure 43.12

Varicella zoster virus infection

(A) Chickenpox on a child's face.
(B) Shingles on the flank and abdomen. Note the distinctive path the lesions follow as they track along the dermatomes.

Sources: (A) Complexli/Shutterstock; (B) Felix Fernandez Gonzalez/Getty Images.

FUNGAL INFECTIONS

Fungal growth can cause superficial, cutaneous, subcutaneous or systemic infections; however, this section of the chapter will deal only with superficial and cutaneous infections. Although there are many fungal species, very few are pathogenic to humans. Some fungi are normal flora. *Candida albicans* is a yeast present on the skin, as well as on the mucous membranes of the gastrointestinal and genitourinary tracts of most people. However, it can develop into an opportunistic infection when a person becomes immunocompromised or when a reduction in the other normal flora occurs.

Superficial infections affect the epidermis, hair and nails, while *cutaneous infections* affect the dermis. Cutaneous infections are generally caused by dermatophytes. **Dermatophytes** are the moulds that cause tinea infections. A fungal infection can also be defined as a *mycosis* (pl. mycoses). Figure 43.13 details the common fungal infections.

Yeasts

Aetiology and pathophysiology

Thrush is caused by an overgrowth of yeast (often *C. albicans*). A *Candida* infection can also be called *candidiasis*.

Yeasts are unicellular organisms that reproduce by asexual reproduction (through budding). Although *Candida* generally colonises many mucocutaneous sites in health, environmental changes can result in the organism becoming pathogenic. For infection to occur, several immunological and non-immunological defences must have failed. Defence mechanisms against the fungus include the presence of antimicrobial proteins, keratinocyte-produced cytokines, T cell responses, helper T cell function, environmental pH and the presence of lysozymal enzymes.

Clinical manifestations

Depending on the location, the *Candida* infection can manifest as a macerated, erythematous rash, or a cottage-cheese-like coating or discharge in the focal region. Irrespective of the location, there will generally be pruritus and possibly erythema.

Oral thrush (see Figure 43.14A) presents as a white, cottage-cheese film on the tongue and oral mucosa. If a presentation of white plaques is visible, it is described as *candidal* **leukoplakia** (see Figure 43.14B). If the corners of the mouth crack and become erythematous, it may be called *angular cheilitis* (or *cheilosis*; see Figure 43.15). Vaginal involvement will result in vaginal candidiasis (see Figure 43.16).

Clinical diagnosis and management

Diagnosis A visual assessment and a careful consideration of the history and risk factors are important for diagnosis. Samples from affected sites (skin or nails) can be collected for direct microscopy. Pathology can suggest the presence or absence of systemic infection, and may be beneficial for determining leukocytosis or neutropenia. Blood cultures may be collected to determine systemic infection. Serology can determine the presence of *Candida* antibodies.

Management In people who are immunocompetent, restoration of the normal epithelial barrier (through attention to hygiene behaviours) and treatment with an antifungal agent are important. The formulation used depends on the location: suspensions, suppositories or creams could be used. In those who are immunosuppressed, a prolonged course of treatment may be required. Those with human immunodeficiency virus (HIV) may benefit from antifungal prophylaxis.

Figure 43.13

Common fungal infections

The left side of diagram highlights yeast-like infections, and the right side of diagram highlights conditions caused by dermophytes.

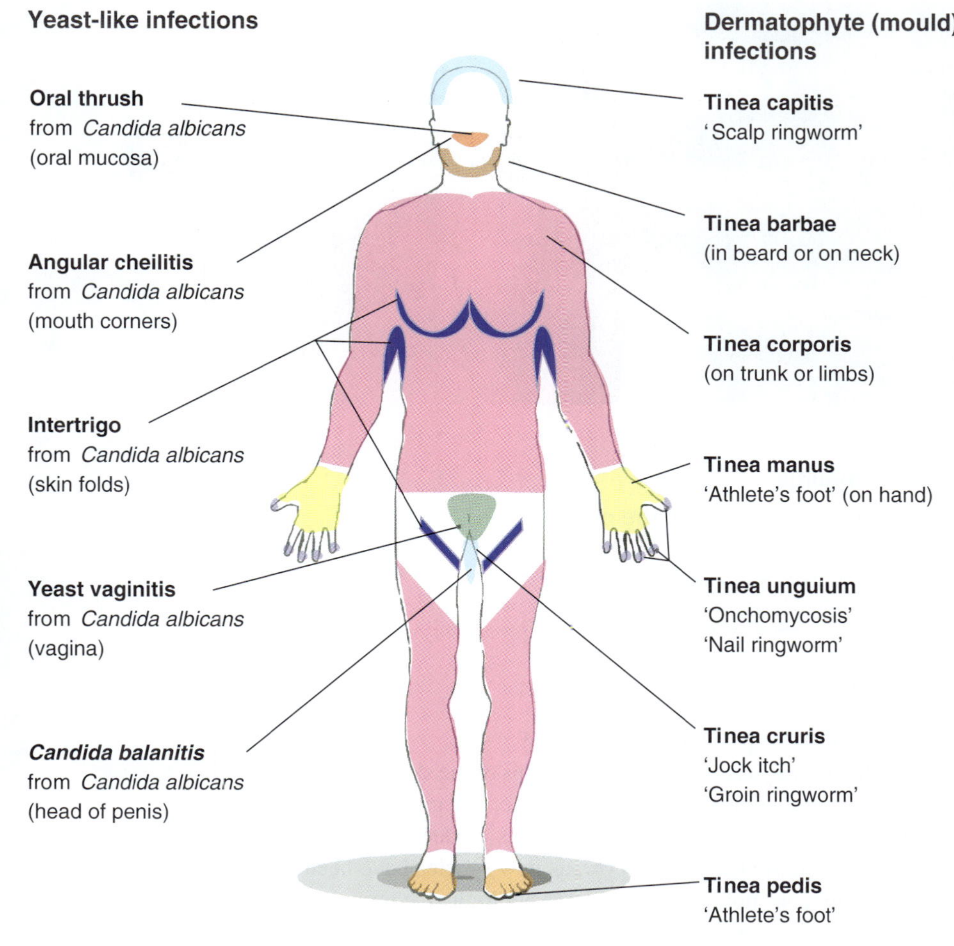

Figure 43.14

Candidiasis

(A) Oral thrush—with white coating on tongue.

(B) Candidal leukoplakia on the tongue.

Sources: (A) Victoria 1/ Shutterstock; (B) Mediscan/ Alamy Stock Photo.

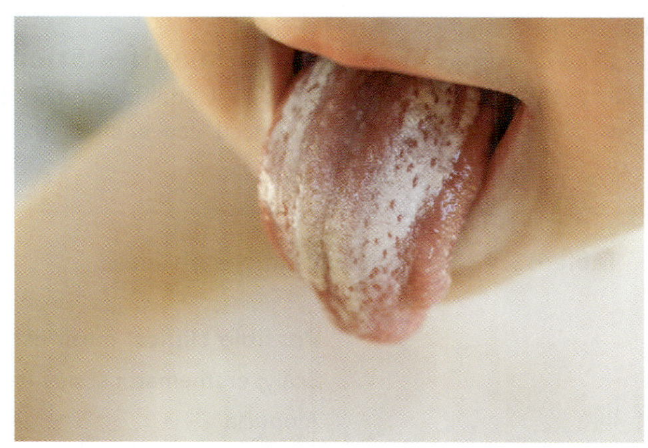

A

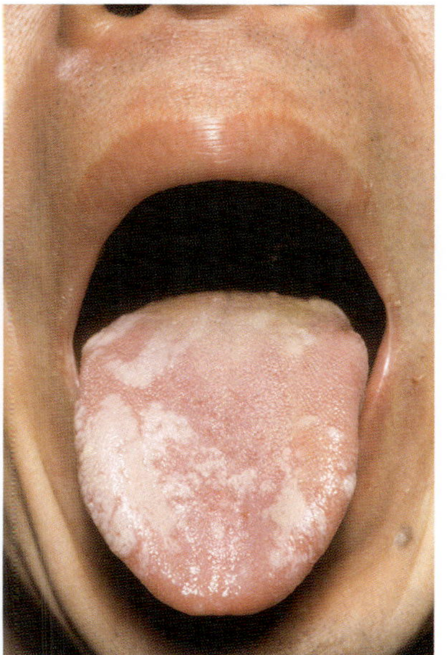

B

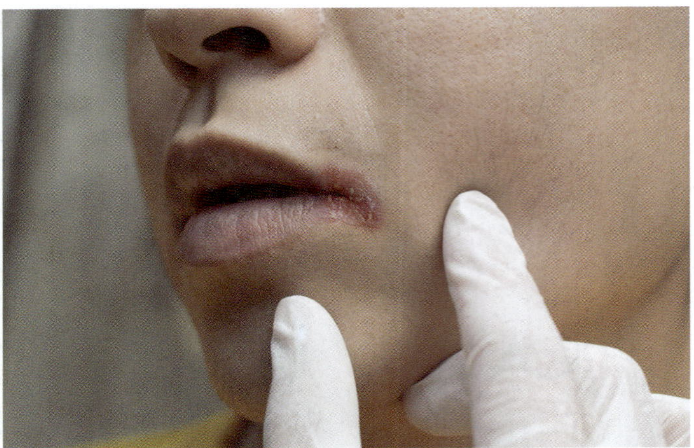

Figure 43.15

Angular cheilitis

Note the cracked edges of the mouth.

Source: Zay Nyi Nyi/Shutterstock.

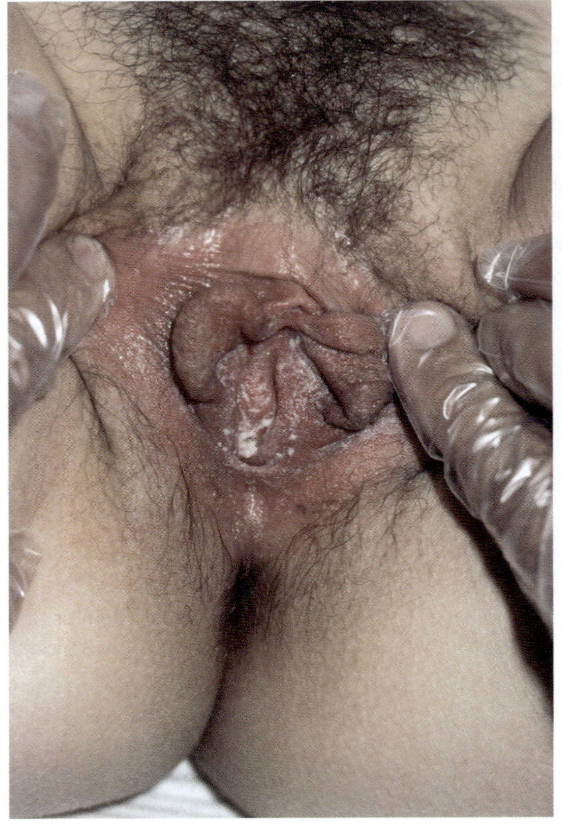

Figure 43.16

Vaginal candidiasis

Note the white cottage-cheese-like discharge between the labia.

Source: Biophoto Associates/Science Source.

Dermatophytes

Aetiology and pathophysiology

Dermatophytes are *fungi* that cause infections of the skin, nails or hair. They require keratin as a nutrient source, and grow on dead skin tissue. There are typically three classes of dermatophytes based on their morphology; however, as new species have been identified, there is now more of a morphological continuum as characteristics overlap. Generally speaking, fungi are eukaryotic, multicellular organisms composed of filaments called *hyphae*. These long, thread-like cells are connected end to end. Dermatophytes reproduce asexually through budding.

The fungus *tinea* causes many infections. Interestingly, the diagnosis name changes depending on the location of the tinea. Tinea is often called *'ringworm'*; however, there is no helminthic (worm) infestation occurring—the dermal manifestations are caused entirely by a fungus.

The fungus responsible for the dermal invasion uses an enzyme called *keratinase* to assist in invading deeper into the stratum corneum skin layer. This proteolytic agent breaks down the dead keratin in the surrounding tissue. The dermatophyte also releases a substance that can inhibit an immune response. Within one to three weeks, the mould will cause a circular lesion. This may cause scaling, shedding or maceration.

Clinical manifestations

Table 43.4 demonstrates the different manifestations experienced, depending on the dermatophyte and the location.

Table 43.4 Clinical manifestations of tinea

Name	Location	Possible clinical manifestations
Tinea barbae	Beard; neck	Scaly; erythematous; pustulous
Tinea capitis	Scalp	Alopecia
Tinea corporis	Trunk (not groin); peripheries	Scaly; pustulous; vesicular; geometric pattern
Tinea cruris	Groin	Erythematous; raised borders
Tinea manum	Palms; between fingers	Scaly; erythematous
Tinea pedis	Feet; between toes	Scaly; macerated; erythematous; pustulous; vesicular
Tinea unguium	Nail	Onycholysis; discoloured; dystrophic

Clinical diagnosis and management

Diagnosis A visual assessment and a careful consideration of history and risk factors are important for diagnosis. Samples from affected sites (e.g. skin, hair or nails) can be collected for direct microscopy.

Management Depending on the location, either topical or oral antimycotic (antifungal) medication is the principal form of management. Discussion of personal hygiene habits is also important. Someone with tinea pedis should be instructed to put socks on before they put their underwear on, so as not to spread the fungal infection via contact between the underwear and the infected foot. For tinea capitis and onychomycosis (an infection of the toenail or fingernail), topical agents are not generally successful.

PARASITIC INFECTIONS

Several parasitic infections cause cutaneous pathology. In Australia, one of the most common infestations is from a mite that burrows into the epidermis. The *Sarcoptes* mite is responsible for causing **scabies**, and is highly contagious.

Scabies (*Sarcoptes scabiei*)

LEARNING OBJECTIVE 8

Explain the life cycle of *Sarcoptes scabiei*, and the consequences of a scabies infection.

Aetiology and pathophysiology

The *Sarcoptes scabiei* mite (see Figure 43.17) is visible to the naked eye. The female mite is approximately 0.4 mm in diameter, and the male is approximately 0.2 mm in diameter. The impregnated female mite burrows approximately 1 mm into the epidermis and lays three to four eggs a day. The male mite will die soon after mating. Each female may lay approximately 80 eggs; however, approximately 90% of all hatched mites die. The life cycle of a scabies mite (about 30 days) is accomplished entirely on the human host (see Figure 43.18). Transmission is from *direct contact* or via *fomites* (an inanimate object capable of transferring infectious organisms), such as bedding or clothes. The risk factors for scabies infections include poor hygiene, overcrowding and malnutrition.

The *S. scabiei* mite uses *protease enzymes* to burrow through the stratum corneum. The developing lesion may be erythematous and hyperkeratotic. Pustules may form as the breach in the integumentary defences results in a *secondary bacterial infection*. The most common pathogens causing the secondary infection are *S. pyogenes* and *S. aureus*. After four to six weeks, a type IV hypersensitivity reaction may occur as a result of exposure to the eggs, their faeces (*scybala*) or the mites themselves. The dermis becomes flooded with lymphocytes and eosinophils. The immune response can result in a *secondary dermatitis*.

Clinical manifestations

Initially, someone with an infestation may be asymptomatic. However, within one to two months the clinical manifestations are visible and the individual becomes contagious. The affected area becomes pruritic and erythematous. The rash may become most irritating at night. The burrows can often be seen, and appear as a thread-like elevation up to 1 cm long. Mites commonly infest the creases of fingers, wrists, elbows and antecubital fossa. The erythematous area contains papules and vesicles.

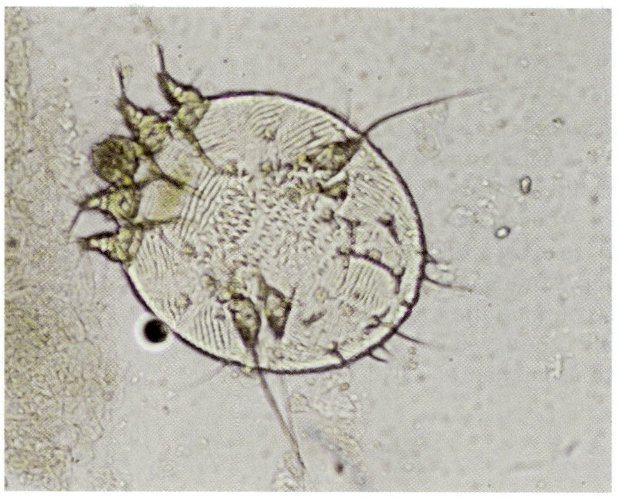

Figure 43.17

Female *Sarcoptes scabiei* mite

Micrograph of approximately 100x magnification.

Source: Toxinmaster/Shutterstock.

Clinical diagnosis and management

Diagnosis Visual inspection may elucidate the thread-like burrows, and skin scrapings of the affected area will be positive for the mite, eggs or scybala. Although there are no definitive laboratory tests, haematology tests may show eosinophilia.

Management Prevention is the best key to scabies control. Promotion of hygiene programs and community scabies education are important. However, in the instance of scabies infection, the rest of the family should also be assessed. Several other people in the family will generally have an infestation as well.

Symptom relief from the pruritus is important for the affected person, who will require the use of an antihistamine. A topical scabicidal agent (permethrin) is necessary to kill the mites. Following a shower, the scabicide cream should be applied from the neck down. The cream should be left on overnight and washed off eight hours later. All clothes and bed linen should be washed in hot, soapy water. They should be dried in the sun or in a hot drier. The treatment should be repeated in seven days for maximum effect.

Dermal appendage disorders

LEARNING OBJECTIVE 9

Outline the common pathology of dermal appendages, including hirsutism, alopecia and nail bed conditions.

HIRSUTISM

Hirsutism is the *excessive growth of hair*. The hair quality tends to be thicker and darker. In women, the characteristic of

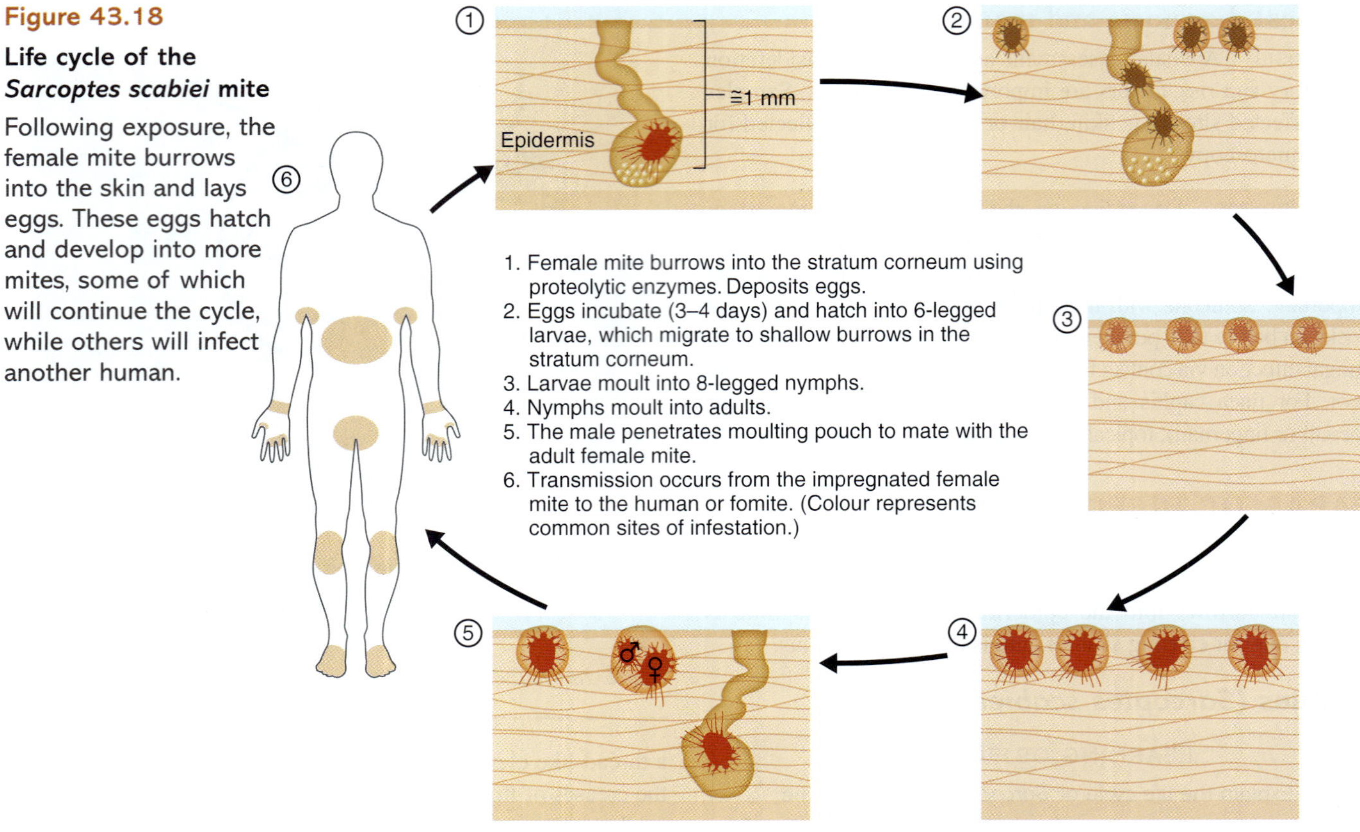

Figure 43.18

Life cycle of the *Sarcoptes scabiei* mite

Following exposure, the female mite burrows into the skin and lays eggs. These eggs hatch and develop into more mites, some of which will continue the cycle, while others will infect another human.

hirsutism is hair development in a male pattern, such as on the face and chest (see Figures 43.19 and 43.20). In men, hirsutism is more difficult to distinguish, but can be proposed for men with overly excessive hair growth. Hirsutism may occur in prepubescent children, and can be a sign of serious endocrine dysfunction.

Aetiology and pathophysiology

The most common cause of hirsutism in women is endocrine dysfunction. *Androgen excess* can be caused by adrenocortical tumours, ovarian disorders or medications. *Androgen-secreting tumours* can produce testosterone and induce virilisation and hirsutism. Androgen excess causes the pilosebaceous units in the axilla, pubic region, sternum and face to convert normal adult vellus hair to thick, darker terminal hair. There is a direct relationship between the circulating androgen level and the degree of hirsutism.

Polycystic ovary syndrome (PCOS) is another cause of androgen excess (see the chapter 'Female reproductive disorders'). The excessive levels of luteinising hormone and insulin caused by PCOS result in an environment that promotes androgen production by the ovaries.

In *congenital adrenal hyperplasia (CAH)* (see the chapter 'Adrenal gland disorders'), an inability to synthesise cortisol and aldosterone leads to excessive androgen production. *Drugs* causing hirsutism include anabolic steroids and high-dose corticosteroids. In some cultures (e.g. Middle Eastern and Mediterranean), excess dark hair is common.

Clinical manifestations

The softer, smaller, lighter **vellus hair** on the chest and face of the individual will change to harder, longer, darker **terminal hair** (see Figure 43.21). The symptoms of common diseases causing hyperandrogenism may be obvious. Some PCOS symptoms include multiple ovarian cysts, infertility, acne, menstrual irregularities or amenorrhoea, insulin resistance and hypertension. CAH symptoms include virilisation and the development of the female external genitalia in male-type pattern.

Clinical diagnosis and management

Diagnosis Visual inspection for terminal hair on the face and chest will confirm the diagnosis. Biochemical investigations to determine the cause of androgen excess are necessary. The measurement of serum testosterone, dehydroepiandrosterone (DHEA), luteinising hormone and follicle-stimulating hormone may confirm an endocrine cause, as may urine cortisol levels. Investigations for PCOS and neoplasms should also be undertaken. A medication history should also be gathered.

Management Management of the underlying cause is important, as hirsutism can be a sign of more serious illness. However, once the cause is established and under control, efforts to manage the aesthetics of the hair growth may be requested. **Depilation** products are available on the market. These products remove hair at the level of the skin. *Epilation* through plucking or waxing removes hair with the root intact and will result in a longer time before the treatment is required again. This method may be more problematic as it may cause skin irritation and

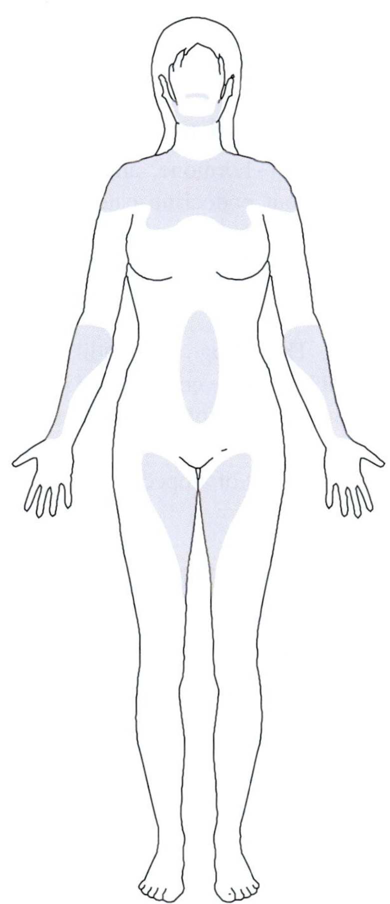

Figure 43.19

Possible sites of excess or unwanted hair in women

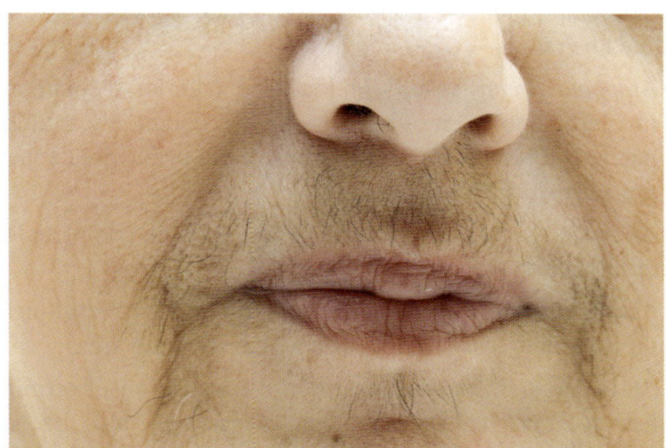

Figure 43.20

Hirsutism in a woman

Source: © Elisa Manzati/Shutterstock.

infection. Permanent removal of hair can also be achieved through laser treatment or electrolysis.

ALOPECIA

Aetiology and pathophysiology

Alopecia means a *loss of hair*. There are several different types of alopecia, and their characteristics are described in the clinical manifestations section below. Normally, there are three phases to a hair growth cycle. *Anagen*, the growth phase, lasts about 1,000 days. In *catagen*, the transition phase, hair growth stops abruptly. Finally, *telogen*, the resting phase, lasts about 100 days, at the end of which time the hair will be shed and replaced with a new hair. In alopecia, anagen can terminate early.

There is limited information regarding the pathophysiology of alopecia. Alopecia can be classified as scarring or non-scarring. *Scarring alopecia* results in damage to the hair follicle. It is thought that an inflammatory process causes follicles to be replaced with scar tissue, resulting in permanent hair loss in the affected area. *Non-scarring alopecia* is temporary hair loss, as the follicle is not damaged. Chemotherapy can cause alopecia, as the agents affect fast-growing cells, such as the hair follicle. This type of hair loss is temporary, although the hair that returns may be a different colour or texture.

Clinical manifestations

Although people shed approximately 50–100 hairs a day, follicular pathology may result in losses of significantly more hairs. The hair loss may be in a common pattern or it may be more random.

The main types of alopecia are alopecia areata, alopecia totalis, alopecia universalis, alopecia androgenetic (both male and female pattern), central centrifugal cicatricial alopecia and

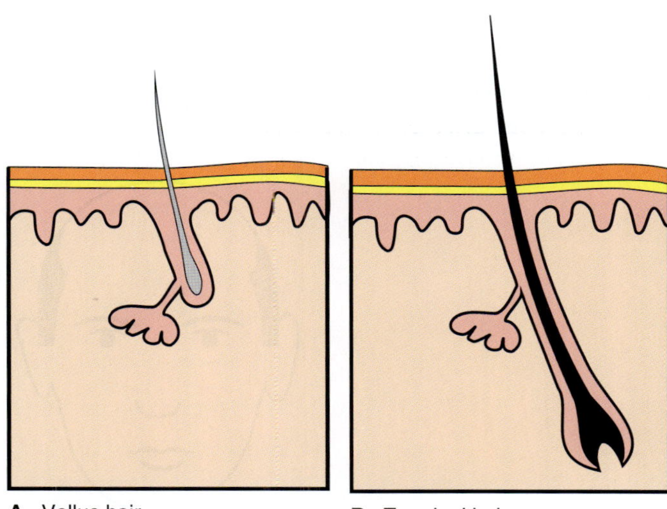

Figure 43.21

Hair types

(A) Vellus hair is softer, smaller and lighter. (B) Terminal hair is harder, longer and darker.

chemotherapy-induced alopecia (see Figure 43.22). These are outlined below.

- *Alopecia areata* results in localised hair loss, commonly involving one patch of hair loss or, less commonly, multiple patches. Individuals with extensive alopecia areata have greater than 50% hair loss.
- *Alopecia totalis* is a rare form resulting in the complete loss of all hair on the scalp.
- *Alopecia universalis* is an even more rare form, resulting in the complete loss of all hair on all hair-bearing areas.
- *Androgenetic alopecia* results in the transition of terminal hair to more vellus scalp hair. Areas may also become completely denuded. The typical female pattern involves loss mostly around the crown. The typical male pattern involves loss mostly on the frontal hairline.
- *Central centrifugal cicatricial alopecia* results in hair loss that spreads from the midline in a symmetric, circular shape outwards. This type of alopecia generally affects African-American women.
- *Chemotherapy-induced alopecia* results in hair loss from alterations to the mitotic and apoptotic processes in the hair follicle. Hair loss is unpredictable and differs depending on many factors, including the agents used and individual variables. Chemotherapy-induced alopecia is temporary, and the hair will return after therapy has finished, although the new hair may be a different colour or texture.

Clinical diagnosis and management

Diagnosis Thyroid hormone and DHEA levels may be beneficial to rule out endocrine causes of alopecia. Poor nutrition may contribute to hair loss, but it is not generally to the extent that can be diagnosed as alopecia. Careful observation for dermatological causes of alopecia is important.

Management The drug minoxidil can be applied topically. It is available over the counter, and is thought to extend the anagen phase and improve follicular perfusion, reducing hair loss. This drug is beneficial for those experiencing hereditary hair loss. For scarring types of alopecia, wigs or hairpieces may be the only option.

DISORDERS OF THE NAIL UNIT

The *nail unit* includes the *nail plate, matrix, cuticle, bed* and *folds*. These components form, support and protect the nail itself. Pathology of the nail unit can result in damaged, abnormal fingernails and toenails. Changes to nails can be as a result of fungal disease, an injury to any portion of the nail unit and some skin conditions. Table 43.5 outlines some common nail disorders.

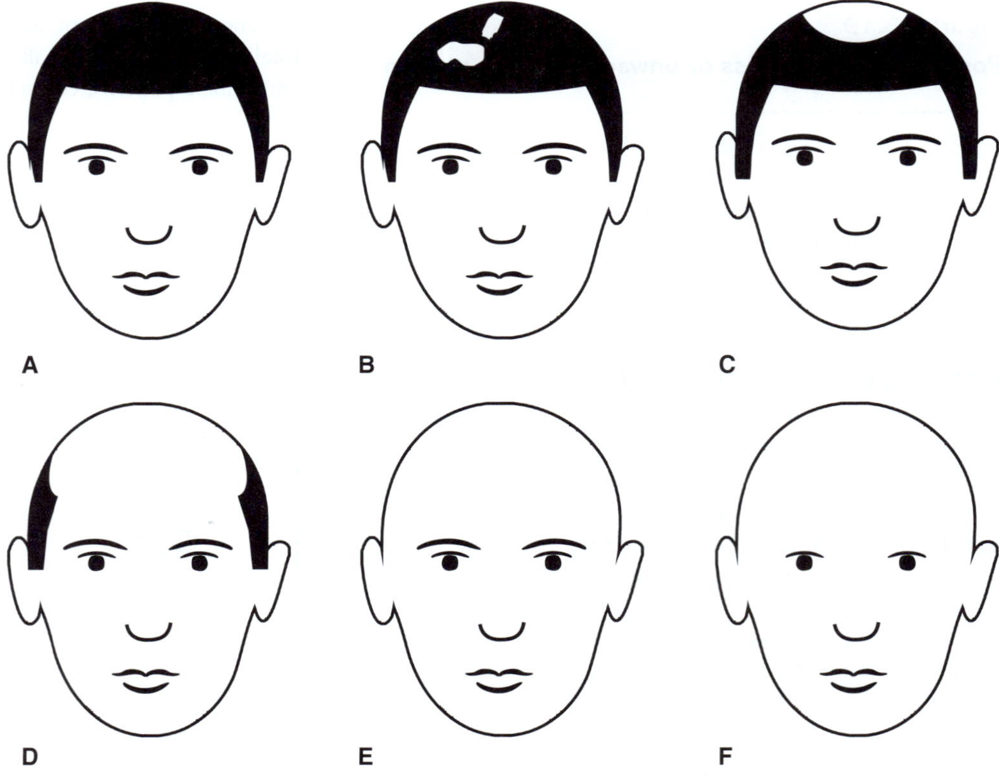

Figure 43.22
Types of alopecia
(A) Normal.
(B) Alopecia areata.
(C) Alopecia androgenetic (female pattern).
(D) Alopecia androgenetic (male pattern).
(E) Alopecia totalis.
(F) Alopecia universalis.

Table 43.5 Common nail disorders

Nail disorder	Pathophysiology	Management
Paronychia 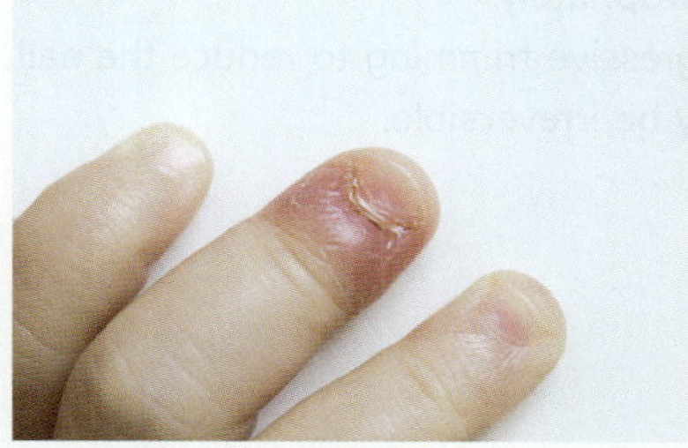	Results from a bacterial or fungal infection in the soft tissue. The pathogen enters the nail crevice (between the nail and the nail fold) and causes an infection around the nail.	Determine the offending pathogen. Oral antimicrobials may be required.
Onychomycosis 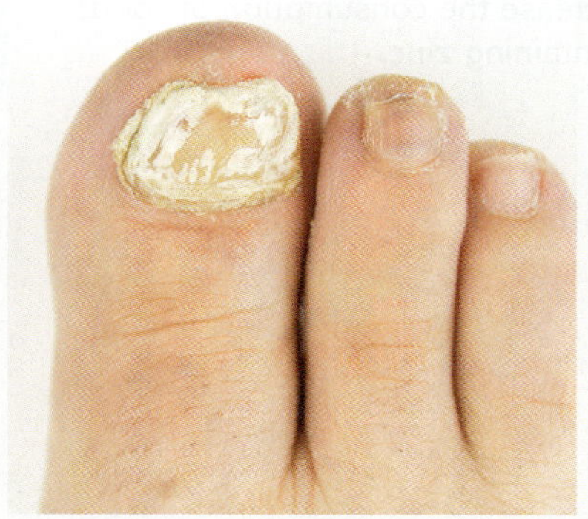	Results from a fungal infection of any component of the nail unit. Also known as *tinea unguium*.	A topical antifungal agent may be used in association with oral antifungal agents. In some cases, nail avulsion may be required.
Onychatrophia 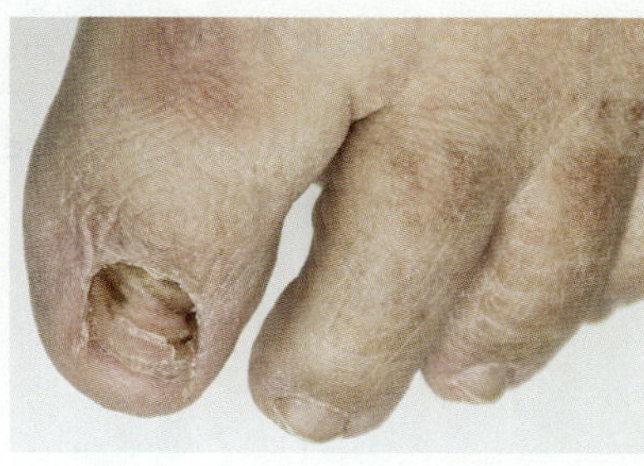	Results from damage to the nail matrix, injury or disease. Results in nail atrophy. The nail may detach.	Investigation for the underlying cause. Management of the underlying cause.
Onychorrhexis 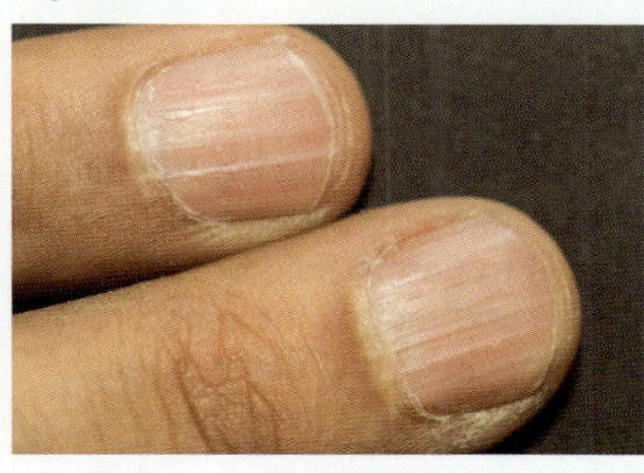	Results from repeated microtrauma of the nail matrix, inflammatory disease or nutritional deficiencies. Results in longitudinal ridging.	Determine the cause and manage appropriately.

Table 43.5 Common nail disorders (*continued*)

Nail disorder	Pathophysiology	Management
Onychauxis 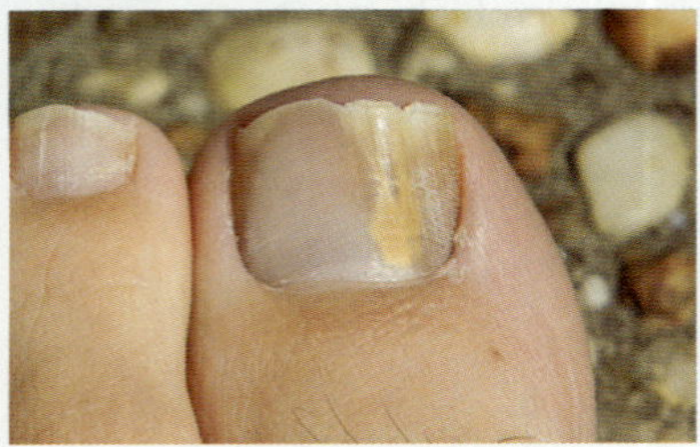	Not well understood, but may result from a chronic inflammatory environment. Results in hypertrophy of the nail.	Determine the cause and manage appropriately. Aggressive trimming to reduce the nail. May be irreversible.
Leukonychia 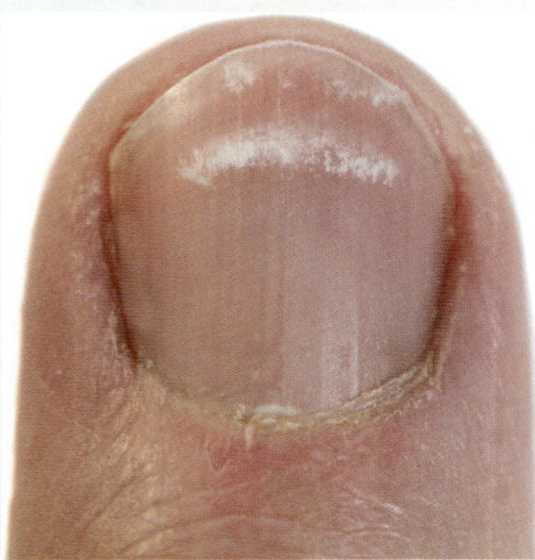	Results from injury to the nail matrix. Causes white marks on nails. Can also be a result of zinc deficiency.	Determine the cause and manage appropriately. Increase the consumption of foods containing zinc.
Koilonychia 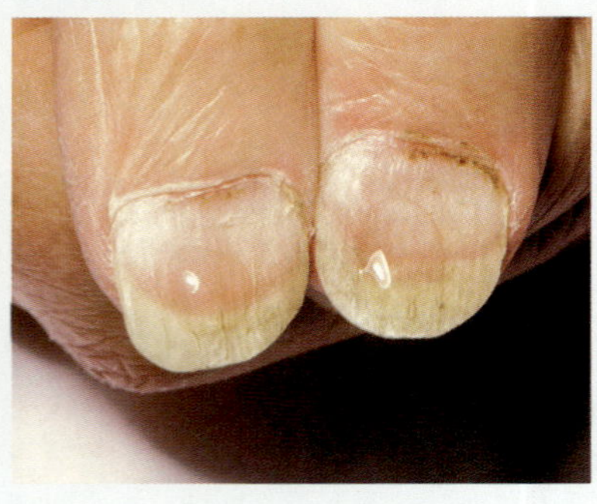	Results from decreased perfusion to the nail unit or any number of systemic diseases (e.g. iron-deficiency anaemia). May also be an inherited disorder. Causes the nail plate to become spoon-like.	Determine the cause and manage appropriately. If due to nutritional deficiency, increase consumption of the deficient nutrient.
Subungual haematoma 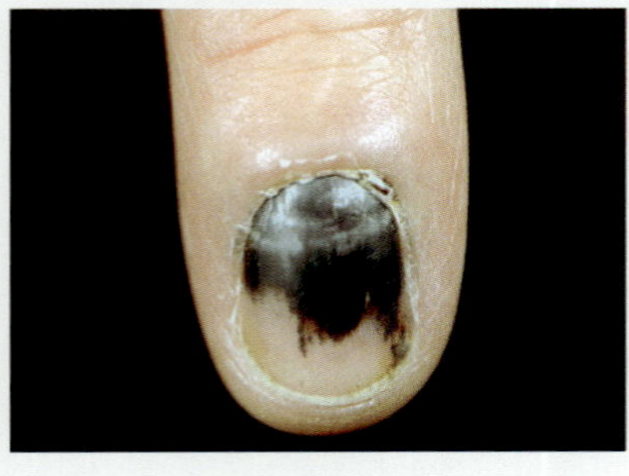	Results from trauma to any component of the nail unit. Is defined as a collection of blood underneath the nail.	If the pressure is producing too much pain, trephining (to make a burr hole in the nail to permit fluid or blood to escape and reduce the pressure under the nail) or nail removal may be required.

Sources: Paronychia—zlikovec/123RF, onychomycosis—Manuel Faba Ortega/123RF; onychatrophia—claudiocaridi/123RF; onychorrhexis—Giuseppe Elio Cammarata/Shutterstock; onychauxis—Youri Appelman/Shutterstock; leukonychia—David Schliepp/Alamy Stock Photo; koilonychia and subungual haematoma—Mediscan/Alamy Stock Photo.

INDIGENOUS HEALTH FAST FACTS AND CULTURAL CONSIDERATIONS

FAST FACTS

- *Aboriginal and Torres Strait Islander peoples experience hospitalisation for cellulitis 1.5 times more than non-Indigenous Australians.*
- *Aboriginal and Torres Strait Islander children are admitted to hospital for management of scabies infestations 15 times more than more than non-Indigenous Australian children.*
- *Scabies can be found in 16–35% of Aboriginal and Torres Strait Islander children living in remote communities.*
- *There is no difference in the rates of dermatitis and eczema between Aboriginal and Torres Strait Islander peoples and non-Indigenous Australians.*
- *Aboriginal and Torres Strait Islander peoples experience psoriasis less frequently than non-Indigenous Australians (0.7:1).*
- *Group A streptococcal infections affect approximately 45% of Aboriginal and Torres Strait Islander children living in remote Australian communities.*
- *Aboriginal and Torres Strait Islander peoples experience infectious and parasitic diseases 3.5 times more than non-Indigenous Australians.*
- *Aboriginal and Torres Strait Islander peoples experience varicella infections resulting in hospitalisation only slightly more than non-Indigenous Australians (1.2:1).*
- *Māori and Pacific Islands children have a higher incidence of severe atopic dermatitis with secondary infection with Staphylococcus aureus than European New Zealand children.*
- *Māori have a higher rates of skin infection than European New Zealanders (1.9:1).*
- *Pacific Islands children have a higher rate of skin infection than European New Zealand children (3.8:1).*
- *Māori women are twice as likely as European New Zealand women to be admitted to hospital with a skin infection.*
- *Pacific Islands people experience hospitalisation for serious skin infections three times more frequently than European New Zealanders.*

CULTURAL CONSIDERATIONS

- *One of the principal reasons for such a significant disparity in the rates for skin infections such as scabies, cellulitis and Group A streptococcal (GAS) infections is overcrowded housing. Eighteen per cent of Aboriginal and Torres Strait Islander peoples live in overcrowded houses, which, although improving, is still too high when compared to non-Indigenous Australians at 5%. It is clear that current programs, mechanisms and levels of government assistance are insufficient, as Aboriginal and Torres Strait Islander peoples are 3.6 times more likely to live in overcrowded houses than non-Indigenous Australians. A greater emphasis is required on community-centred, culturally appropriate, innovative programs to ensure that Indigenous Australians have access to such basic needs as clean, safe accommodation, and this must be a priority for federal, state, territorial and local investment.*

Sources: Data from Australian Indigenous HealthInfoNet (2021); Australian Institute of Health and Welfare (2016a); Cannon & Bowen, (2021); Cure Kids (2021); Davidson et al. (2020); Department of Health (2022); Gramp & Gramp (2021); McCay et al. (2021).

CHILDREN AND ADOLESCENTS

- Atopic dermatitis is uncommon in infants younger than 4 months of age, but commonly arises in children before 2 years of age. It may be at its most severe between 2 and 4 years of age, and usually improves before the teenage years.
- Incontinence-associated dermatitis is common in infants, and was originally known as 'nappy rash'. It can be caused by prolonged exposure to faeces, urine or excessive soap on the clothes. If frequent nappy changes and appropriate perineal hygiene cares are provided and the dermatitis continues, the dermatitis may be an allergic reaction to the nappy or materials, or it may be another skin condition, such as psoriasis, or an infection such as scabies. Further investigation is required in this situation.
- Scabies is highly contagious, and is commonly spread during close physical contact, often in school. Children with active scabies infestation are not permitted to return to school until a weekly treatment with anti-scabies treatment has been performed twice. All members of the household should also be treated.
- Chickenpox is vaccine-preventable, and the Immunise Australia Program provides free vaccinations for children at 18 months of age. Varicella is not part of the New Zealand Ministry of Health National Immunisation Schedule, but can be obtained through general practitioners at a cost.

OLDER ADULTS

- Incontinence-associated dermatitis is common in older adults who have issues with faecal or urinary incontinence. Regular perineal hygiene, the use of barrier creams and regular pressure area care can reduce the incidence of incontinence-associated dermatitis.
- Atopic dermatitis is less common in older adults than it is in children and younger adults, but it is increasing in incidence in developed countries as a result of the ageing population. Senile atopic dermatitis can occur as a result of a recurrence of previous atopic dermatitis, or as a result of continuing atopic dermatitis from adulthood.
- Stasis dermatitis increases with age, and is associated with circulatory issues. Hyperpigmentation, lichenification and oedema are commonly associated with stasis dermatitis, and it is exacerbated by common comorbidities seen in ageing, such as heart failure and peripheral vascular disease. An age-associated decline in cell-mediated immunity may contribute to a significantly higher incidence of shingles in adults older than 50 years of age. A varicella zoster vaccine can be administered to older adults to reduce the incidence of post-herpetic neuralgia.
- The incidence of bacterial skin infections is increased because of age-associated skin senescence and impaired epidermal integrity.
- Administration of antifungal medications to older adults must be undertaken with care because of potential nephrotoxicity and the increased potential for drug–drug interactions from concomitant medication regimens for comorbidities.

KEY CLINICAL ISSUES

- Inflammatory conditions of the skin most often manifest as painful or pruritic rashes. Skin eruptions in skin folds and areas exposed to higher temperatures can be difficult to control. Determination of the cause, thorough cleaning regimens and the application of appropriate agents, such as barrier creams or steroid medications, are pivotal to the management plan.
- It is important to ensure that medicated (e.g. corticosteroid) creams are applied on the appropriate body part. Skin thickness in the areas involved plays an important role in the strength of medication required. Preparations formulated for the face generally have a lower concentration of drug than preparations for the body.
- In relation to contact dermatitis, measures to reduce or eliminate exposure to the irritant are paramount to success in management of the clinical manifestations.
- Incontinence-associated dermatitis can be managed with appropriate and frequent perineal area care. Any individual who is incontinent and unable to communicate should have interventions to prevent this type of dermatitis.
- Psoriasis can be difficult for individuals to cope with, and it can have treatment regimens that are time-consuming, soil clothing and are smelly. Individuals experiencing psoriasis will have a long and difficult clinical course, and need psychosocial support as well as education in order to manage the medication required to manipulate their immune system,
- Allergic reactions to drugs can manifest in the skin. A knowledge of the different types of drug eruptions is important for any healthcare professional responsible for prescribing, providing or administering drugs.
- *Staphylococcus aureus* infections of the skin are common in the community, and also in healthcare institutions. However, bacterial infections developed in hospital have an increased potential to be resistant to more antimicrobials. Healthcare professionals should ensure that they follow infection control procedures to reduce the risk of transmission of infection between individuals.
- An increasing temperature can be a sign of an infection developing. When an individual is febrile, undertake a full assessment, paying particular attention to the potential of skin infections or cellulitis related to wounds, invasive lines or other breaches in integrity. Obtain a sample of any pustulous material for microscopy, culture and sensitivity (MCS) testing before cleaning the purulent site or administering antimicrobials.
- Gram-negative bacteria producing extended-spectrum β-lactamase (ESBL) pose a particularly difficult management challenge, as they can inactivate several types of antimicrobials. MCS testing is important in determining which antimicrobials are effective in the management of this type of infection.
- Care should be taken when reconstituting antimicrobial powders, or administering or discarding antimicrobials, to reduce accidental or frivolous exposure to the environment, in order to reduce the risk of bacteria developing further antimicrobial resistance.
- Antibacterials will have no effect on viruses, but may be administered to control a secondary bacterial infection.
- The post-herpetic neuralgia occurring as a result of shingles can be overwhelming and require significant and varied interventions with analgesic agents and adjuvants.
- The prevention and control of fungal infections can be achieved more readily through the preservation or restoration of a normal epithelial barrier. Frequent assessment and intervention should be undertaken for individuals with continence difficulties.

CHAPTER REVIEW

- *Inflammatory conditions* can cause a wide range of manifestations that develop on the skin.
- An *overactivity of either the innate or the acquired immune system* is responsible for the development of most inflammatory skin conditions.
- There are many types of *dermatitis*. Each type produces different challenges for the individual.
- *Psoriasis* is an autoimmune disorder that results in hyperkeratosis of the affected areas.
- Pharmacological agents can cause inflammatory responses of the skin, which are often called *drug eruptions*.
- *Rosacea* is a common skin condition that results in vascular changes, causing a facial rash.
- *Immunomodifying drugs*, such as corticosteroids, are the mainstay treatment of most cutaneous inflammatory conditions. Often, *antimicrobials* are also required to treat secondary bacterial infections.
- A variety of *pathogens* can cause skin infections.
- *Tissue or exudate samples* may assist the healthcare professional in the selection of appropriate management plans.
- *Bacterial infections* are usually treated with antimicrobials.
- *Viral infections* can result in painful and extensive cutaneous destruction.
- Some viral infections can be present without the person's knowledge, increasing the risk of transmitting the virus through close contact.
- *Fungal infections* are caused by yeasts or moulds.
- *Thrush* is caused by a yeast infection, often resulting in *candidiasis*.
- *Tinea* causes many fungal infections in humans.
- The mite *Sarcoptes scabiei* causes scabies, which is a common skin infection in certain groups of people in Australia.

REVIEW QUESTIONS

1. Define the following terms:
   a. erythema
   b. pruritus
   c. photodamage
   d. vesicle
2. How do the four types of dermatitis differ? Outline their pathophysiology and management.
3. How should the care of someone with incontinence-associated dermatitis be managed?
4. What changes occur to the skin of people with psoriasis?
5. Why are keratolytic agents sometimes used in psoriasis? Outline the mechanism of action of keratolytic agents.
6. How do the pathophysiologies of the four immune-mediated drug eruptions differ from each other?
7. How do the various non-immune-mediated drug eruptions differ from each other?
8. What other conditions need to be ruled out before the diagnosis of rosacea is determined? Why? (*Hint:* What other conditions produce a similar rash?)
9. Compare and contrast the clinical manifestations and management of folliculitis, furuncles and carbuncles.
10. How can normal flora become pathogenic and contribute to a wound infection?
11. What interventions should be undertaken to assist an individual before and after a surgical debridement?
12. Outline the clinical progression of a wound infection from the initial surgical suture line to the infected wound. Identify the pathophysiology, clinical manifestations and management of the wound infection.
13. How does acne develop? Explain the pathophysiology.
14. How can a healthcare professional determine that cellulitis is developing? What interventions should be undertaken to reduce its development?
15. What is surgical debridement? How does it help in the management of necrotising fasciitis? Are there other types of debridement?
16. What two common viruses cause skin infections? What are the infections, and what cutaneous manifestations can occur as result of viral infection?
17. What are the two different types of fungal infection? Explain.
18. Describe the life cycle of the *Sarcoptes scabiei* mite.
19. Identify all of the possible risk factors contributing to a scabies infestation. Explain why each factor increases the risk of scabies infection.
20. What important interventions should be undertaken to manage a scabies outbreak?

HEALTH PROFESSIONAL CONNECTIONS

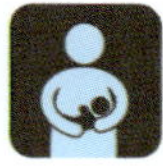

Midwives Incontinence-associated dermatitis (previously known as 'nappy rash') will increase the risk of infection in a newborn. New parents should be taught how to manage the skin of a neonate, including the use of barrier cream, to reduce the risk of dermatitis and secondary skin infection.

Following a caesarean section, vaginal tear or episiotomy, appropriate wound care and adequate hygiene behaviours will reduce the risk of infection. The use of antimicrobials in a breastfeeding woman should be undertaken with care. A number of antimicrobials are safe in the neonate; however, they will sometimes cause diarrhoea or loose stools, as they may influence normal flora levels. A woman with an infection and who is breastfeeding should not receive the antimicrobial chloramphenicol. If no other drug is possible, alternative nutrition options should be undertaken for the baby. Chloramphenicol is known to cause cardiovascular failure, aplastic anaemia, bone marrow suppression and grey baby syndrome in neonates.

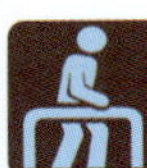

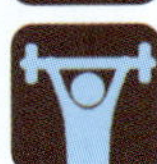

Physiotherapists/Occupational therapists People who require splinting and immobilisation devices are particularly at risk of dermatitis associated with friction and moisture. Splinting devices should be constructed or fitted to reduce the risk of friction. Observations for areas of high pressure should be reviewed, and interventions should be undertaken to modify the splint. Skin integrity should be examined frequently. Depending on the splint construction and design, padding or material should be placed between the splint and the skin to reduce any pressure and moisture that will affect skin integrity.

Exercise scientists Commonly, obese people can develop rashes in their groin or armpits when they begin to exercise. There are many possible causes, including infection from bacteria or fungus. However, the rash may also be caused from excessive friction during the exercise. Individuals should be encouraged to ensure that personal hygiene habits are undertaken. Wearing bike pants underneath sports attire may assist in reducing the friction and moisture within the area. It is important to discuss these concerns and offer potential resolutions so that they may continue their weight loss program. Pain or discomfort related to dermatitis may influence their compliance and commitment to the program.

Nutritionists/Dieticians Malnutrition is a significant variable in the defence against skin infections. Adequate hydration and the consumption of healthy food, including fruit, vegetables, grains, nuts and fish, will assist in promoting skin health and wound healing. Poor nutrition enables skin defences to become less efficient, and secondary skin infections put people at risk for many other conditions.

All allied professionals Conditions resulting in alterations to dermal barriers significantly increase the risk that people will develop a skin infection. Infection control principles and standard precautions should always be practised. The greater the surface area affected, the greater the risk of infection. One of the single most effective ways to reduce the risk of spreading infection is hand-washing. The World Health Organization has developed five moments for hand hygiene. The other serious consideration is preventing equipment from becoming a fomite. Use disposable equipment where possible. If this is not possible, ensure that equipment is cleaned between clients. Small objects such as pens, stethoscopes, neck ties and other personal items are consistently associated with cross-infection. Be mindful of how your actions may affect the morbidity and mortality of those with compromised skin barriers.

CASE STUDY

Mr Allan Barber, a 55-year-old man (UR number 974186), underwent a laparotomy four days ago. He has developed a surgical site infection along his suture line. Mr Barber has type 2 diabetes, for which he takes metformin. His observations were as follows:

Temperature	Heart rate	Respiration rate	Blood pressure	SpO_2
38.3°C	94	24	138/82	98% (2 L/min via NP*)

*NP = nasal prongs.

Mr Barber is receiving intravenous antibiotics q6h. He is ordered paracetamol for when he is febrile, and is to have wound dressings twice a day. Currently, he is having a non-adherent wound dressing with combine applied. He requires a wound review today. The wound has moderate, purulent exudate and 3 cm of cellulitis around the inferior aspect of the laparotomy suture line. The skin is becoming macerated and Steristrips have been used to reduce some of the tension on the suture line. Mr Barber is complaining of pain on the suture site—4/10. He may also have an intra-abdominal abscess. His haematology and microbiology results have returned as follows:

HAEMATOLOGY

Patient location:	Ward 3	**UR:**	974186		
Consultant:	Smith	**NAME:**	Barber		
		Given name:	Allan	**Sex:**	M
		DOB:	12/04/XX	**Age:**	55

Time collected	13:30
Date collected	XX/XX
Year	XXXX
Lab #	3555234

FULL BLOOD COUNT		UNITS	REFERENCE RANGE
Haemoglobin	116	g/L	115–160
White cell count	13.4	$\times 10^9/L$	4.0–11.0
Platelets	160	$\times 10^9/L$	140–400
Haematocrit	0.36		0.33–0.47
Red cell count	3.91	$\times 10^{12}/L$	3.80–5.20
Reticulocyte count	1.3	%	0.2–2.0
MCV	91	fL	80–100
Neutrophils	9.5	$\times 10^9/L$	2.00–8.00
Lymphocytes	2.91	$\times 10^9/L$	1.00–4.00
Monocytes	0.37	$\times 10^9/L$	0.10–1.00
Eosinophils	0.38	$\times 10^9/L$	< 0.60
Basophils	0.09	$\times 10^9/L$	< 0.20
ESR	12	mm/h	< 12

MICROBIOLOGY

Patient location:	Ward 3	**UR:**	974186		
Consultant:	Smith	**NAME:**	Barber		
		Given name:	Allan	**Sex:**	M
		DOB:	12/04/XX	**Age:**	55

Time collected	18:30	**Organisms**	**1.** *E. coli*
Date collected	XX/XX	**Isolated**	**2.** *Staphylococcus aureus*
Year	XXXX		
Lab #	6535345		

Specimen site	Exudate from Laparotomy	**Antimicrobial sensitivities S = Sensitive R = Ressistant**					
Leukocytes	+++	Organism	1	2	Organism	1	2
Erythrocytes	++	Ampicillin		R	Flucloxacillin	R	R
Proteins	trace	Amoxicillin	R	R	Gentamicin	S	S
		Cefotaxime		S	Rifampicin		
		Ceftriaxone	S	S	Sodium fusidate		S
		Cephalothin	S	S	Ticarcillin		R
		Chloramphenicol		R	Timentin		
		Cotrimoxazole	R	R	Trimethoprim	S	R
		Erythromycin		S	Vancomycin	S	S
Gram	**Gram negative**	✔					
stain	**Gram positive**	✔					
	Bacilli	✗					
	Cocci	✔					
	Other	rod					

CRITICAL THINKING

1 Observe the pathology results for Mr Barber. What pathogen/s has/have caused the surgical site infection? What are the characteristics of this/these pathogen/s?

2 At what stage can a surgical site infection be seeded? Explain.

3 Using the history and observations provided, identify and explain all of the data that demonstrate that an infective process has occurred.

4 What risk factors did Mr Barber have that increased the likelihood of a surgical site infection?

5 Explore the microbiology report, with a specific focus on the sensitivity and resistance testing. Which antimicrobials are appropriate for Mr Barber? Why? Which antimicrobials are inappropriate for Mr Barber? Why?

BIBLIOGRAPHY

Auala, T., Zavale, B.G., Mbakwem, A.Ç. & Mocumbi, A.O. (2022). Acute rheumatic fever and rheumatic heart disease: highlighting the role of group a streptococcus in the Global Burden of Cardiovascular Disease. *Pathogens* 11(5):496. https://doi.org/10.3390/pathogens11050496.

Australasian Society of Clinical Immunology and Allergy (ASCIA) (2019). *Atopic dermatitis (eczema)*. Brookvale, NSW: ASCIA. https://www.allergy.org.au/patients/fast-facts/eczema-atopic-dermatitis.

Australian Bureau of Statistics (ABS) (2021). *Causes of death, Australia, 2020.* Canberra: ABS. https://www.abs.gov.au/statistics/health/causes-death/causes-death-australia.

Australian Commission on Safety and Quality in Health Care (ACSQHC) (2021). *AURA 2021: Fourth Australian report on antimicrobial use and resistance in human health.* Sydney, NSW: ACSQHC. https://www.safetyandquality.gov.au/our-work/antimicrobial-resistance/antimicrobial-use-and-resistance-australia-surveillance-system/aura-2021.

Australian Health Ministers' Advisory Council's National and Aboriginal and Torres Strait Islander Health Standing Committee (2016). *Cultural respect framework 2016–2026: for Aboriginal and Torres Strait Islander health—a national approach to building a culturally respectful health system*. Canberra: Australian Government Department of Health. https://nacchocommunique.files.wordpress.com/2016/12/cultural_respect_framework_1december2016_1.pdf.

Australian Indigenous Health*Info*Net (2021). *Overview of Aboriginal and Torres Strait Islander health status, 2020*. Perth, WA: Australian Indigenous Health*Info*Net. https://apo.org.au/sites/default/files/resource-files/2021-03/apo-nid311685.pdf.

Australian Institute of Health and Welfare (AIHW) (2021a). 3.07 Selected potentially preventable hospital admissions. *Aboriginal and Torres Strait Islander Health Performance Framework 2020: online data tables.* Canberra: AIHW. https://www.indigenoushpf.gov.au/measures/3-07-potentially-preventable-hospital-admissions.

Australian Institute of Health and Welfare (AIHW) (2021b). *Aboriginal and Torres Strait Islander Health Performance Framework 2020 summary report*. Cat. No. IHPF 2. Canberra: AIHW. https://www.indigenoushpf.gov.au/publications/hpf-summary-2020.

Australian Institute of Health and Welfare (AIHW) (2022a). Admitted patient care 2020–21. *Table 8.9: Separations (a) with one or more hospital-acquired complications (version 2.0), by complication category, all hospitals, 2020–21.* Canberra: AIHW.

Australian Institute of Health and Welfare (AIHW) (2022b). *Australian Burden of Disease Study: impact and causes of illness and death in Aboriginal and Torres Strait Islander people 2018.* Australian Burden of Disease Study series No. 26. Cat. No. BOD 32. Canberra: AIHW. https://www.aihw.gov.au/getmedia/1656f783-5d69-4c39-8521-9b42a59717d6/aihw-bod-32.pdf.aspx?inline=true.

Australian Institute of Health and Welfare (AIHW) (2022c). *Australia's health, 2022: data insights.* Australia's Health series No. 18. Cat. No. AUS 240. Canberra: AIHW. https://www.aihw.gov.au/getmedia/c91a05ef-307f-4c18-8ed3-dfe33d0c603d/aihw-aus-240.pdf.aspx?inline=true.

Australian Institute of Health and Welfare (AIHW) (2022d). *Principal diagnosis data cubes: separation statistics by principal diagnosis (ICD-10-AM, 11th edition)), Australia, 2020–21.* Canberra: AIHW.

Bauldoff, G., Gubrud-Howe, P.M., Carno, M.-A., Levett-Jones, T., Hales, M., Berry, K., … Stanley, D. (2020). *LeMone and Burke's medical–surgical nursing: critical thinking for person-centred care* (4th [Australian] edn). Sydney: Pearson Australia.

Best, O. & Fredericks, B. (2021). *Yatdjuligin: Aboriginal and Torres Strait Islander nursing and midwifery care* (3rd edn). Port Melbourne, VIC: Cambridge University Press.

Blume, J.E., Ali, L., Ehrlich, M. & Helm, T.N. (2022). Drug eruptions. *Emedicine*. https://emedicine.medscape.com/article/1049474-overview.

Brennan, M., Milne, C., Agrell-Kann, N. & Ekholm, B. (2017). Clinical evaluation of a skin protectant for the management of incontinence-associated dermatitis: an open-label, nonrandomized, prospective study. *Journal of Wound, Ostomy and Continence Nursing* 44(2):172–80. https://pubmed.ncbi.nlm.nih.gov/28267125/.

Bullock, S. & Manias, E. (2022). *Fundamentals of pharmacology* (9th edn). Sydney: Pearson Australia.

Cannon, J.W. & Bowen, A.C. (2021). An update on the burden of group A streptococcal diseases in Australia and vaccine development. *Medical Journal of Australia 215*(1):27–28. https://doi.org/10.5694/mja2.51126.

Cure Kids. (2021). *2021: State of child health in Aotearoa New Zealand*. Auckland: Cure Kids. https://www.curekids.org.nz/downloads/assets/118/1.

Davidson, L., Knight, J. & Bowen, A.C. (2020). Skin infections in Australian Aboriginal children: a narrative review. *Medical Journal of Australia* 212(5):231–37. https://doi.org/10.5694/mja2.50361.

Department of Health (2022). *Communicable Diseases Intelligence 2022. Summary of National Surveillance Data on Vaccine Preventable Diseases in Australia, 2016–2018.* Volume 46. Canberra: Australian Government Department of Health. https://doi.org/10.33321/cdi.2022.46.28.

Flugman, S.L. & Clark, R.A. (2020). Stasis dermatitis. *Emedicine*. https://emedicine.medscape.com/article/1084813-overview.

Gramp, P. & Gramp, D. (2021). Scabies in remote Aboriginal and Torres Strait Islander populations in Australia: a narrative review. *PLoS Neglected Tropical Diseases* 15(9):e0009751. https://doi.org/10.1371/journal.pntd.0009751.

Habashy, J. & Robles, D.T. (2022). Psoriasis. *Emedicine*. https://emedicine.medscape.com/article/1943419-overview.

Helm, T.N. (2022). Allergic contact dermatitis. *Emedicine*. https://emedicine.medscape.com/article/1049216-overview.

Herchline, T.E., Swaminathan, S. & Chandrasekar, P.H. (2022). Cellulitis. *Emedicine*. https://emedicine.medscape.com/article/214222-overview.

Marieb, E.N. & Hoehn, K. (2019). *Human anatomy and physiology* (11th edn). San Francisco, CA: Pearson Benjamin Cummings.

MIMS (2022). *Monthly index of medical specialities*. https://www.mimsonline.com.au/.

National Centre for Immunisation Research and Surveillance (NCIRS) (2022). *Zoster vaccine for Australian adults*. Westmead, NSW: NCIRS. https://www.ncirs.org.au/ncirs-fact-sheets-faqs/zoster-vaccine-australian-adults.

New Zealand Ministry of Health (2014). *Tagata Pasifika in New Zealand*. Wellington: Ministry of Health. https://www.health.govt.nz/our-work/populations/pacific-health/tagata-pasifika-new-zealand.

New Zealand Ministry of Health (2016a). *'Ala Mo'ui progress report: December 2015*. Wellington: Ministry of Health. https://www.health.govt.nz/system/files/documents/publications/ala-moui-progress-report-december-2015-apr16_0.pdf.

New Zealand Ministry of Health (2016b). *Annual update of key results 2015/16: New Zealand health survey.* Wellington: Ministry of Health. https://www.health.govt.nz/publication/annual-update-key-results-2015-16-new-zealand-health-survey.

NPS MedicineWise (2021). *General Practice Insights Report July 2019–June 2020 including analyses related to the impact of COVID-19*. Sydney: NPS MedicineWise. https://www.nps.org.au/assets/NPS/pdf/GPIR-Report-2019-20.pdf.

Rao, J. & Chen, J. (2020). Acne vulgaris. *Emedicine*. https://emedicine.medscape.com/article/1069804-overview.

Royal Australian College of General Practitioners (RACGP) (2021). *General practice: health of the nation 2020*. East Melbourne, Vic: RACGP. https://www.racgp.org.au/getmedia/c2c12dae-21ed-445f-8e50-530305b0520a/Health-of-the-Nation-2020-WEB.pdf.aspx.

Schwartz, R.A. (2022). Dermatologic manifestations of necrotizing fasciitis. *Emedicine*. https://emedicine.medscape.com/article/1054438-overview.

Singhal, H. & Kaur, K. (2023). Wound infection. *Emedicine*. https://emedicine.medscape.com/article/188988-overview.

Stanway, A. & Gomez. J. (2015). *Staphylococcal skin infections*. Retrieved from https://dermnetnz.org/topics/staphylococcal-skin-infection.

Wong, H.K. & Shiver, M. (2020). Urticaria. *Emedicine*. https://emedicine.medscape.com/article/762917-overview.

44 Skin cancers, burns and scarring

KEY TERMS

Avascular
Basal cell carcinomas (BCCs)
Cryotherapy
Curettage
Full-thickness burn
Hypermetabolism
Hypertrophic scar
Keloid scar
Melanin
Melanoma
Partial-thickness burn
Sentinel node
Serosanguineous exudate
Solar keratosis
Squamous cell carcinomas (SCCs)
Superficial burn
Widened scar

LEARNING OBJECTIVES

After completing this chapter, you should be able to:

1 Differentiate between basal cell carcinoma and squamous cell carcinoma.

2 Describe the assessment, identification and management of melanoma lesions.

3 Explain the significance of depth in relation to burn injury.

4 Discuss the various mechanisms of thermal injury.

5 Differentiate between local and systemic responses to burn injury.

6 Discuss the types and pathogenesis of scarring.

WHAT YOU SHOULD KNOW BEFORE YOU START THIS CHAPTER

Can you identify the major structures of the integumentary system and their functions?

Can you describe the main stages of inflammation and healing?

Can you describe the principles and major concepts associated with neoplasia?

Introduction

In this chapter, three important conditions associated with the integumentary system are discussed. Skin cancers, burns and scarring are all conditions that can result in significant disfigurement, and in some cases may even threaten life.

Skin cancers

LEARNING OBJECTIVE 1

Differentiate between basal cell carcinoma and squamous cell carcinoma.

Australia has one of the highest skin cancer rates in the world. Eighty per cent of all newly diagnosed cancers in Australia are skin cancers. Skin cancers are often divided into two types: *non-melanoma skin cancer (NMSC)* and *melanoma*. NMSCs can be further divided into *basal cell carcinoma (BCC)* and *squamous cell carcinoma (SCC)* (see Figure 44.1). Exposure to solar radiation and immunosuppression from drugs or disease increases a person's risk of skin cancer.

BASAL CELL CARCINOMA

Approximately 70% of all NMSCs in Australia are **basal cell carcinomas (BCCs)** (see Figure 44.2A). They are generally slow to grow, and it is unusual for BCCs to metastasise. BCCs mostly form on the head and neck, but may develop on other sites. They are most commonly experienced by older people. It is rare for a child to develop BCC. Basal cells arise from the base of the epidermis and grow upwards and outwards. They may invade the dermis, but are not generally associated with a risk of malignancy.

Determining incidence is difficult as there are no mandatory reporting requirements in Australia. However, previous estimates demonstrate a clear inverse latitude gradient, with Queensland rates averaging 1,355 per 100,000, yet Tasmania and Victoria rates only averaging 482 per 100,00. Unfortunately, the situation is worse when assessed considering lesion incidence, with a rate which is, on average, 11 times higher. This reflects the propensity for those affected to experience numerous BCCs.

Aetiology and pathophysiology

Sun exposure is the major cause of BCCs. Other causes include exposure to arsenic, and certain forms of chemicals and oils used in industry. Host factors which increase the risk of BCCs include light skin (which burns rather than tans), red hair, blue eyes and the increased propensity to freckle easily. It is thought that BCCs arise from *pluripotent stem cells*, and then, because of exposure to some mutagenic factor, the DNA is damaged and cell replication becomes disordered. *Mutations in a gene responsible for cell differentiation* have been identified in almost all types of BCC. One component of this mutation results in the *inability of the cancer cells to shed. Tumour suppressor gene mutations* (e.g. *p53*) are present in approximately 50% of BCC tumours (see the chapter 'Neoplasia' for more details on tumour suppressor genes).

Clinical manifestations

Skin lesions associated with BCCs are generally slow-growing. However, if left untreated, BCCs can become locally destructive and, as these usually form in the head and neck region, result in significant maxillofacial disfigurement. BCCs may take on many forms. The three common growth patterns are superficial, nodular and morphoeic.

- *Superficial* BCCs generally occur on the trunk and limbs. They often present as an erythematous, defined lesion that may be macular or scaly. A pearly type colour may be distributed through the lesion.
- *Nodular* BCCs generally present as a translucent papule or nodule. The lesion may have telangiectasia (i.e. small, dilated vessels close to the skin). As the lesion grows, the borders become rolled. Nodular BCC may ulcerate and bleed and can result in some measure of discomfort.
- *Morphoeic* BCCs generally present as a sclerotic lesion that is pale and scar-like. These lesions may be more aggressive and invade more deeply than other BCCs.

Clinical diagnosis and management

Diagnosis An initial step includes the direct observation of the lesion and comparison to known characteristics. As technology improves, there has been a trend towards artificial intelligence and machine learning to assist dermatologists to increase diagnostic accuracy. Although still in its infancy, some research projects report systems with similar or better accuracy than by dermatologists alone.

The principal method of investigation is biopsy. The variety of presentations that occur with skin lesions make accurate diagnosis difficult, and recent statistics of even experienced dermatologists do not approach 100% accuracy. Therefore, skin biopsies are important to quantify the definitive pathology.

Management Surgical excision of BCCs remains the most appropriate management. Better results are obtained with superficial and nodular types of BCCs, as they are better circumscribed. Unfortunately, morphoeic types result in higher rates of recurrence because the margins are more difficult to define. **Cryotherapy**, **curettage**, diathermy and radiotherapy are less effective than surgical excision.

SQUAMOUS CELL CARCINOMA

Approximately 30% of all NMSCs are **squamous cell carcinomas (SCCs)** (see Figure 44.2B). Many head and neck cancers are SCCs. Although the growth areas differ slightly between men and women, the most common area of SCC development is the face (especially the lips, ears, nose, cheek and eyelids). SCCs are associated with an increased risk of malignancy leading to mortality or significant morbidity (3–7%).

Aetiology and pathophysiology

Sun exposure remains the strongest risk factor in the development of SCCs, as ultraviolet (UV) radiation alters keratinocyte signalling, which induces oxidative stress and subsequently DNA mutation. There appears to be a progression from **solar keratosis** (a thick, warty or callusy skin growth considered a pre-malignant

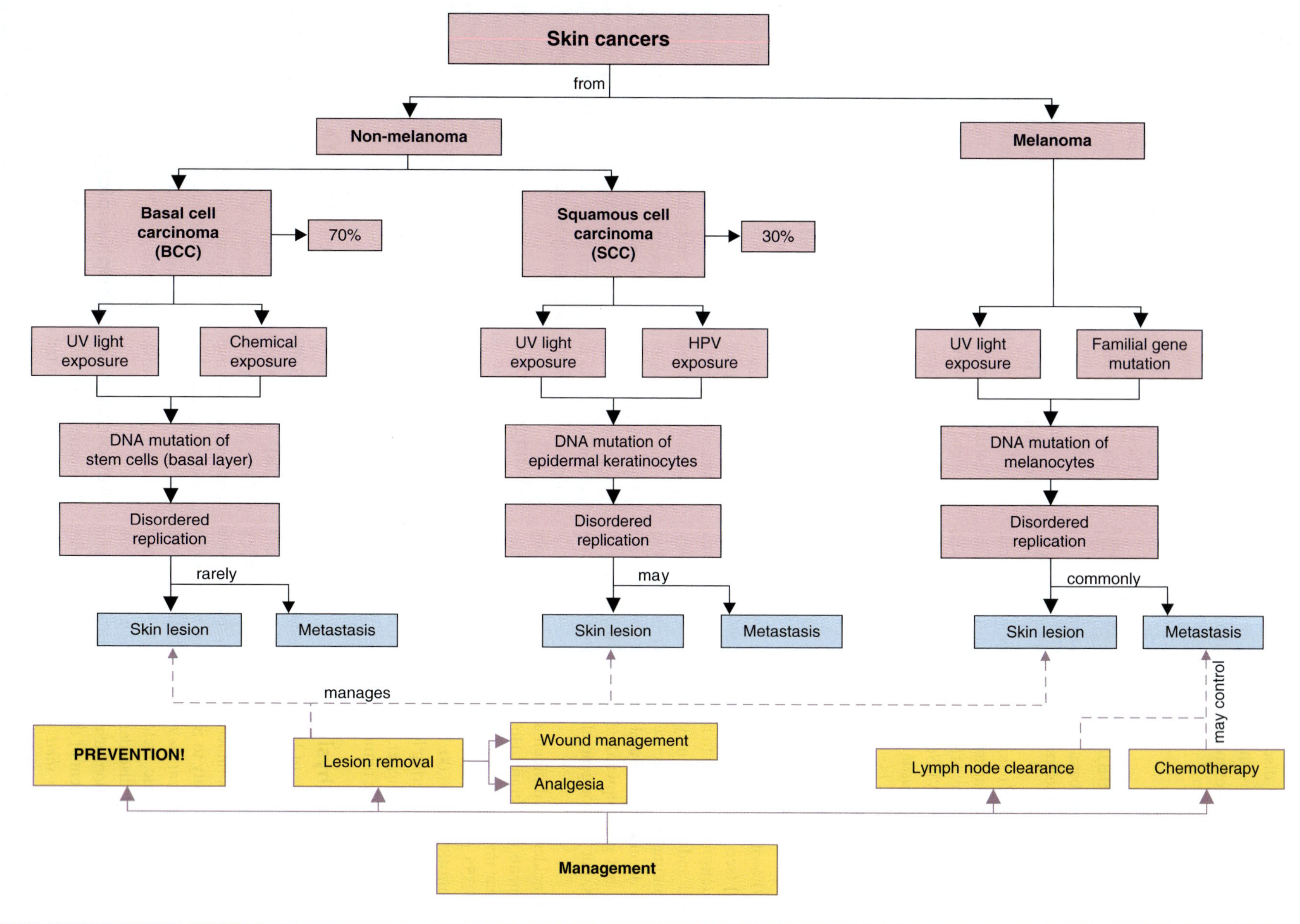

Figure 44.1

Clinical snapshot: Skin cancers

DNA = deoxyribonucleic acid; HPV = human papillomavirus; UV = ultraviolet.

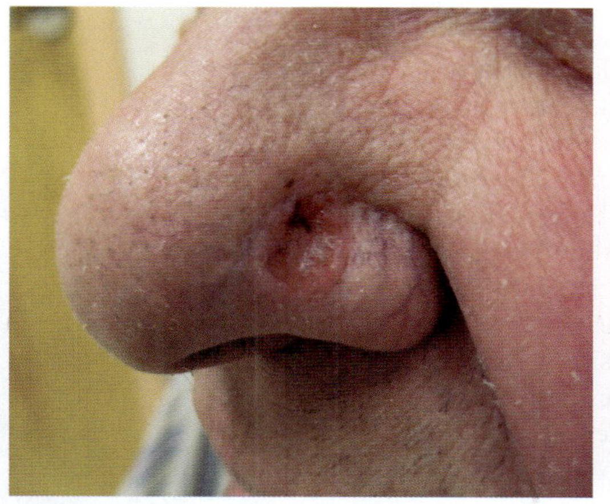
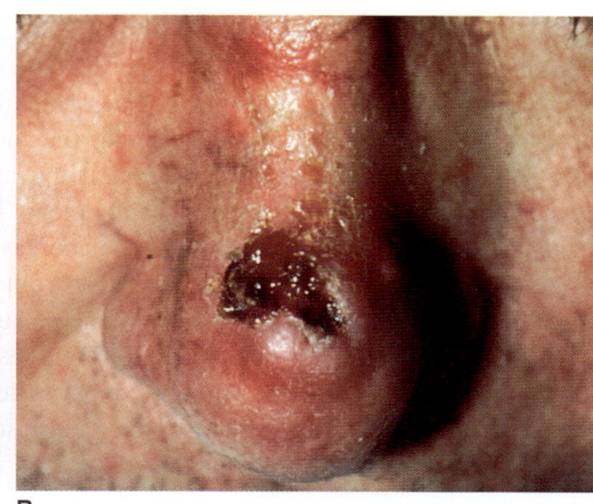

Figure 44.2

Non-melanoma skin cancers

(A) Basal cell carcinoma. (B) Squamous cell carcinoma.

Sources: (A) James Heilman, MD; (B) National Cancer Institute, USA.

neoplasm—also known as actinic keratosis) to SCC. It is important to note that *tumour suppressor gene mutations* (*p53*) are present in almost half of all SCC tumours. Other common gene mutations in SCC involve *NOTCH1* & *NOTCH2* (NOTCH genes are critical in epidermal development and maintenance) and *RAS* mutations (*RAS* genes are critical in control of gene expression impacting directly on cell proliferation, differentiation and survival.

Also, almost one-quarter of all head and neck SCCs have been associated with human papillomavirus (HPV) infection. The mechanism is thought to involve *viral inhibition of DNA repair* and *interference with apoptosis*. Interestingly, HPV-positive SCCs are most often associated with less chance of metastasis and more favourable outcomes than HPV-negative SCCs.

As with BCC, host factors which increase the risk of SCC include light skin, red hair, blue eyes, and the increased propensity to freckle easily. A significant risk factor associated with SCC development is immunosuppression, especially in those taking medications to protect solid organ transplants, those with non-Hodgkin lymphoma (NHL) and those with chronic lymphocytic leukaemia (CML). Furthermore, people with low serum vitamin D levels have a higher risk of developing SCC.

Clinical manifestations

SCC lesions begin as erythematous papules, and many have a degree of hyperkeratosis present. However, a hyperkeratotic lesion is not necessarily an SCC. Over a period of time the lesions may ulcerate, bleed and cause discomfort. As they grow, the lesions may progress to endolymphatic spread. The more nodes involved, the poorer the prognosis. Perineural spread is not common in SCC, and occurs in less than 3% of cases. If haematogenous spread occurs, the prognosis is grim.

Clinical diagnosis and management

Diagnosis Basic skin inspection and dermoscopy (examining the papillary dermis under 10-fold magnification) are the first steps towards diagnosis of skin lesions. Skin biopsies and histopathological examination are important to quantify definitive pathology. However, it can be difficult to distinguish hyperkeratosis from early SCC. Recent statistics of experienced dermatologists do not approach 100% accuracy. Therefore, some new diagnostic modalities are becoming important in the identification of SCCs. High-frequency ultrasonography (HFUS) is a new technology which uses ultrasound to map the vascularity of a skin lesion, and optical coherence tomography (OCT) uses infrared light to produce high-resolution cross-sectional images to locate SCCs. The terminology used in describing lesions consists of *well-differentiated, moderately differentiated* or *poorly differentiated SCCs*.

Management As with BCCs, surgical excision affords a higher rate of success and reduces the risk of recurrence. Depending on the size of the lesion, it may be excised under local anaesthetic at an outpatient's appointment. In the event of a recurrent SCC, the risk of metastasis increases. Radiotherapy may be indicated for recurrent or persistent SCC. Cryotherapy, curettage and diathermy are beneficial for small, well-defined, low-risk lesions. More recently, topical therapies have become available for the non-surgical treatment of superficial lesions such as squamous cells carcinoma in situ (SCC in situ). Application of imiquimod (an immunomodifier which stimulates apoptosis) or fluorouracil (an antimetabolite which inhibits DNA synthesis), can clear the affected area of pre-malignant skin lesions and superficial SCCs. Photodynamic therapy (PDT) with topical pretreatment of 5-aminolevulinic acid or methylaminolevulinate is successfully used in some low-risk in-situ SCCs. The illuminated area undergoes an oxygen-dependent phototoxic reaction, which results in cell death and minimal effects to normal tissue.

MELANOMA

LEARNING OBJECTIVE 2

Describe the assessment, identification and management of melanoma lesions.

According to the Australian Institute of Health and Welfare, approximately 1,300 people died from **melanoma** in 2021. New Zealand mortality statistics are also very high, with over 350 people dying from melanoma a year. As with other skin cancers, the major cause for melanoma is unprotected and prolonged or frequent ultraviolet (UV) radiation exposure. Approximately 80% of all skin cancer deaths are from melanoma, with people over 50 most at risk of diagnosis.

Aetiology and pathophysiology

Melanocytes are epidermal cells that produce melanin. **Melanin** is a protective brown pigment that gives skin its colour and absorbs UV radiation. The less melanin, the more white the skin and the higher the risk of melanoma. It appears that several processes contribute to melanoma development. There is some evidence that approximately 50% of melanomas are *familial*. This may be as a result of gene mutations from several sites, including *tumour suppressor genes* (*p16* and *p53*).

Melanomas have the potential to metastasise to other structures in the region, including lymph nodes, or distant metastases. Common sites of melanoma metastases include the brain, bone, liver and adrenal glands.

Clinical manifestations

As described in Table 44.1, the lesion is most likely to be larger than 6 mm in diameter, with an irregular colour, shape and borders, and may also be bleeding or crusted (see Figure 44.3).

Clinical diagnosis and management

Diagnosis A previous history of significant and severe sun exposure resulting in blisters increases the risk of melanoma development. Collection of a complete history will assist in the diagnosis. Visual inspection of the tumour is undertaken in a structured way using the ABCDE assessment. Extra observations using an EFG assessment can also be undertaken to differentiate from a nodular melanoma (see Table 44.1).

An excisional biopsy is important to reduce the risk of recurrence. Laboratory tests may be beneficial to determine the presence of metastases. Liver function tests may indicate liver involvement. Urea and creatinine levels indicate renal function.

A chest X-ray or computed tomography scan are beneficial in more advanced stages, as the metastases may first be obvious in the lung. Positron emission tomography is beneficial for tracing metastatic disease in soft tissue, the lymph nodes and the liver.

Table 44.1 ABCDE assessment of melanomas

Assessment	Description
Asymmetry	Melanomas often become asymmetrical
Border	The lesion often develops an irregular border
Colour change	The lesions may change colour and be less uniform
Diameter	A lesion larger than 6 mm or one that continues to grow is concerning
Evolving	The surface may change and begin to bleed or it might become raised or crusted
EFG of *nodular melanoma* assessment	
Elevated	May appear newly raised or thickened
Firm	Feels firm (although benign lesions may be firm, too)
Growing	Often grows rapidly over days to weeks

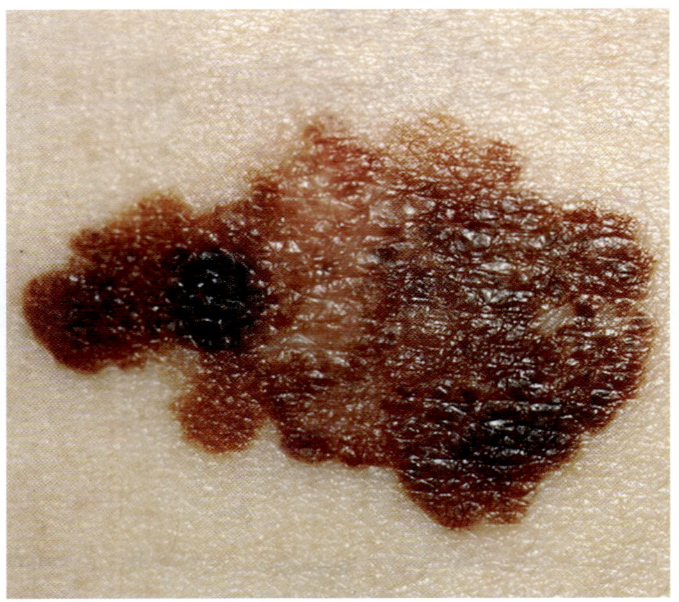

Figure 44.3

Melanoma

Note the lesion's asymmetry, irregular border and variety of colours within the same lesion.

Source: National Cancer Institute, USA.

Management Surgical excision is important, and the removal of large margins should be undertaken. Depending on the staging and progression of the disease, lymph node dissection may also be beneficial. Determination of the **sentinel node** (the node or group of lymph nodes to which the cancer has spread first) is necessary to ensure that regional metastases are not occurring.

Recent management trends have shown that the use of immunomodulators, such as interferon and colony-stimulating factors, may be beneficial. In later stages of disease, chemotherapy may be attempted; however, particular drug combinations have not produced consistent results.

Burns

A burn is an acute *injury to the integumentary system* from *exposure to extreme temperature* (hot or cold), *chemicals, friction, radiation* or *electrical current*. Each year about 6,000 Australians are admitted to hospital for thermal injuries, and approximately 130 of those succumb to their injury. In 2019–20, almost 60% of injuries were caused by contact with heat or hot substances, and 41% from exposure to fire, smoke and flames.

LEARNING OBJECTIVE 3

Explain the significance of depth in relation to burn injury.

Burns can be classified into types by either *cause* or *tissue damage* (see Figure 44.4).

Factors that affect the outcome of a burn include the size of the burn, the age of the person, the location affected and the depth of the burn.

Figure 44.4

Burns classification

(A) A summary of cause and classification related to the tissue damaged.

(B) Classification of burns demonstrating the structures involved. The terminology has been updated: 'first-degree burns' are known as 'superficial burns', 'second-degree burns' are 'partial-thickness burns' and 'third-degree burns' are 'full-thickness burns'.

Source: (B) Nucleus Medical Media Inc/Alamy Stock Photo.

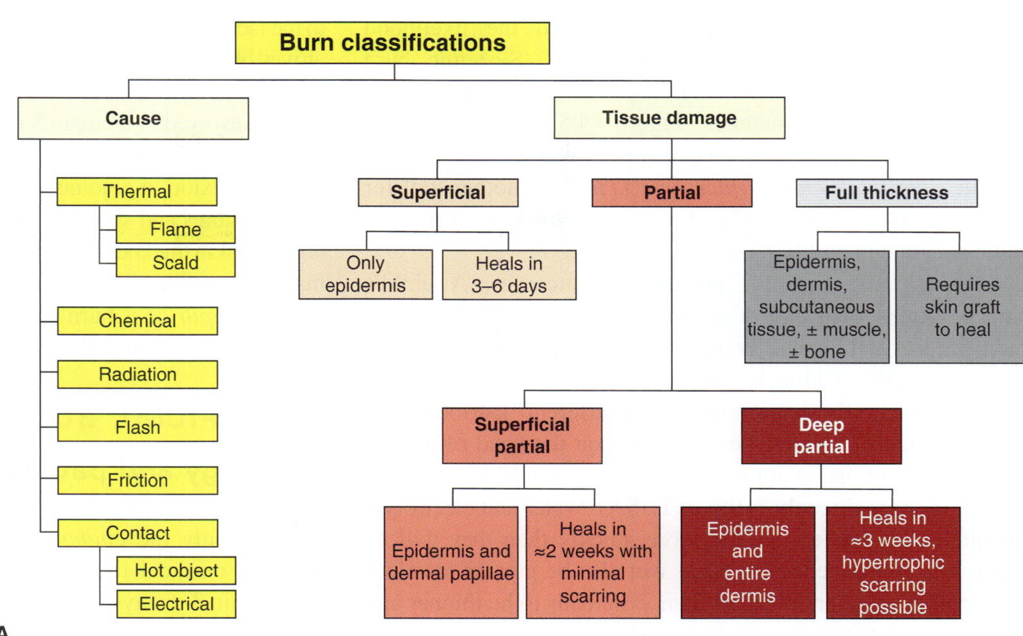

A

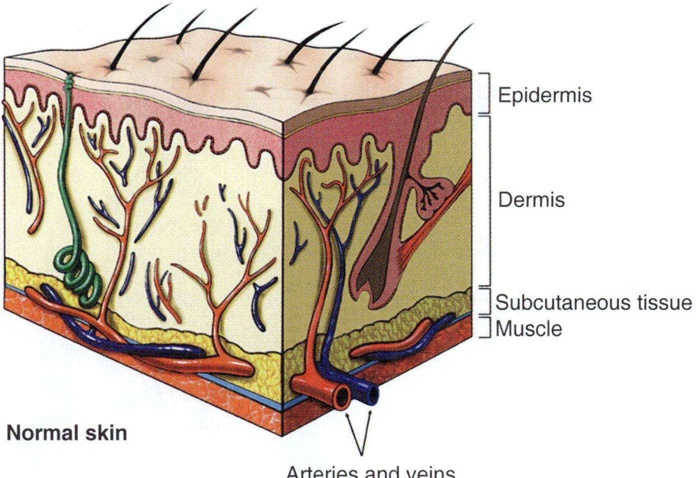

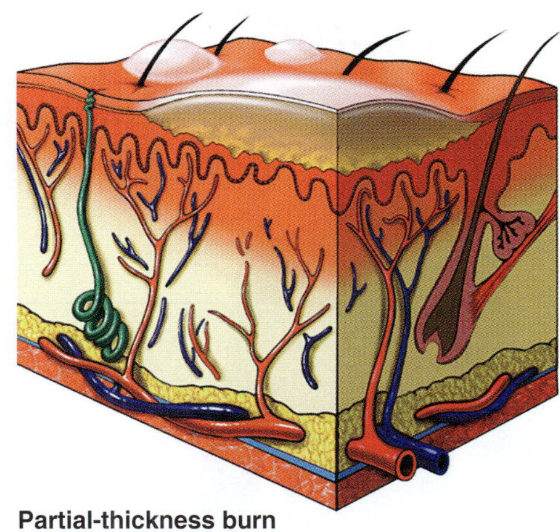

Partial-thickness burn

- Skin blisters
- Involves all of epidermis and some of dermis
- May involve all of dermis

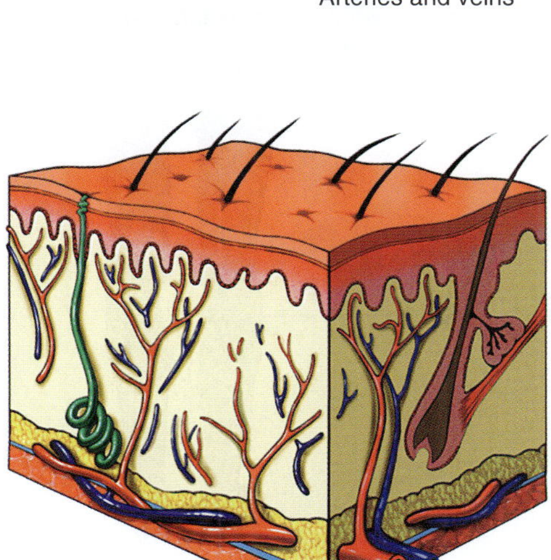

Superficial burn

- Involves top layers of epidermis only

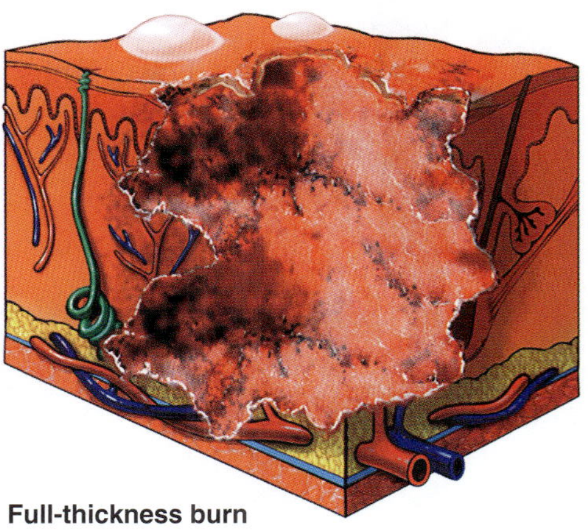

Full-thickness burn

- May extend into deeper tissues

B

An estimate of the *size* of a person's burn is important in determining their clinical management and the likelihood of significant systemic complications (see 'Systemic burn responses', later in this chapter). The size of the burn can be measured by several methods. Figure 44.5 demonstrates the *rule of nines*. The value gained from tallying the percentages is called *the total body surface area (TBSA)*. Another tool for assessing TBSA is the *Lund and Browder chart*. This method is more accurate in children (see Figure 44.6).

Age is another factor influencing outcomes. A child's skin is thinner than that of an adult's, and will burn at lower temperatures and for shorter durations. Scald injuries, especially related to spilt cooking liquids or hot drinks, are common in children. A child's shape results in a different distribution of skin than that of an adult (e.g. the skin on the head of a child under 1 year of age is approximately 19% of TBSA, yet on an adult it is approximately 7–9% of TBSA). Water and electrolyte imbalances will affect a child more quickly than they will an adult. The consequences of burns can also be greater for older people than younger adults, as their skin tends to be thinner and their healing capacity is compromised.

The *location* of a burn also influences the outcome. Burns to the face and neck may result in inflammation that can contribute to airway obstruction. If a burn is circumferential around the chest wall, it may impede chest movement and interfere with oxygenation. If a limb is involved in a circumferential burn, perfusion to that region may be affected and place the extremity at risk. Burns involving areas of flexion (e.g. joints) may develop contractures as the scar tissue matures and shortens. Finally, different body locations have different skin thicknesses and degrees of sensitivity. Some locations may be less affected by temperature or duration than others.

The *depth* of a burn is generally described as *superficial, partial-thickness* or *full-thickness*.

SUPERFICIAL BURNS

Aetiology and pathophysiology

Previously known as a *first-degree burn*, a **superficial burn** involves only the *epidermis* (see Figures 44.4B and 44.7A). There is minimal tissue damage, and the burn will generally heal within 3–6 days without scarring. One of the most common causes of superficial burns is sunburn.

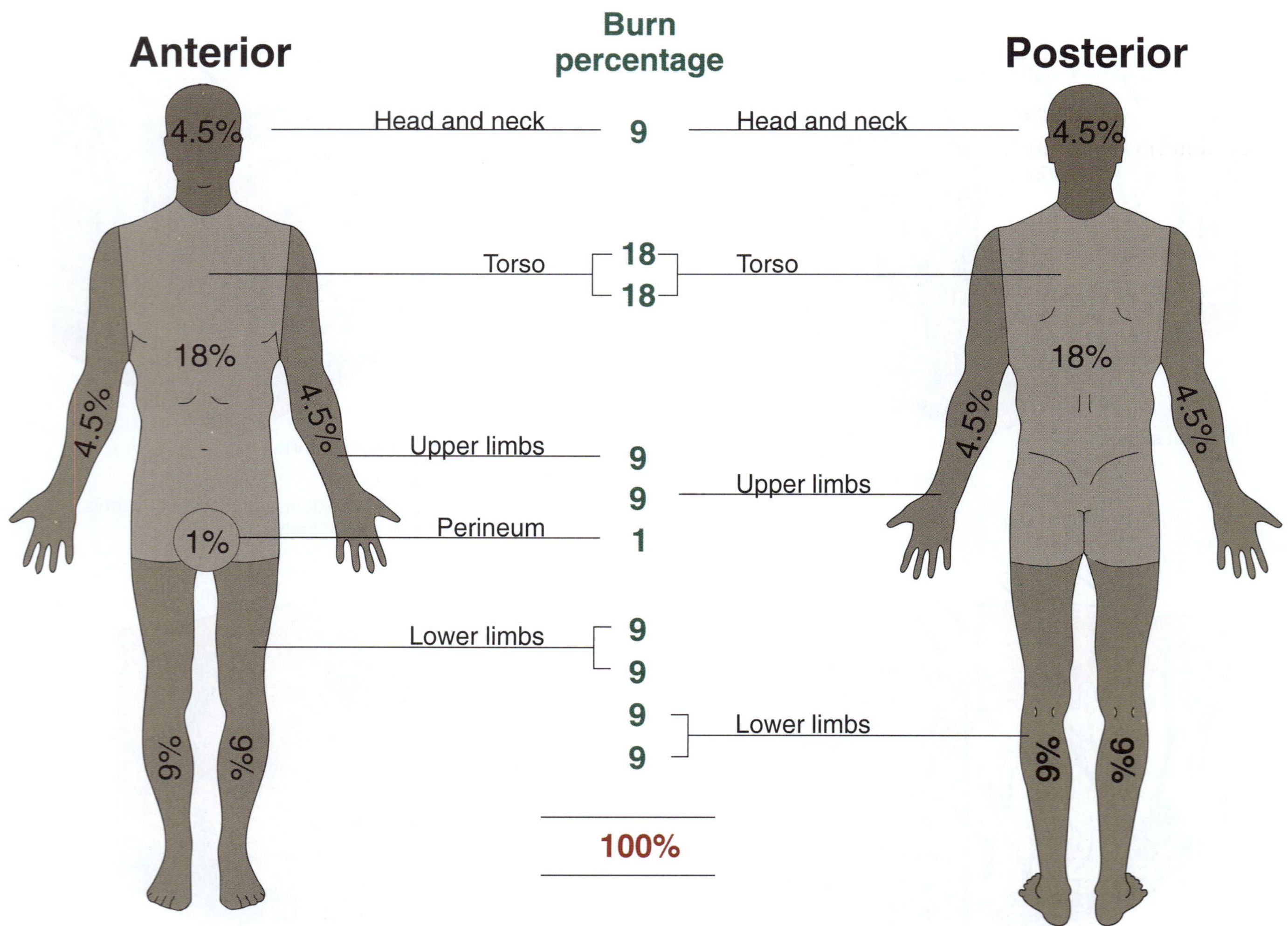

Figure 44.5

Rule of nines chart

Tallying the score representing the area burnt will give an estimation of total body surface area involved.

Area	Age (years)					2nd degree	3rd degree	TBSA% total
	0–1	1–4	5–9	10–15	Adult			
Head	19	17	13	10	7			
Neck	2	2	2	2	2			
Ant. trunk	13	13	13	13	13			
Post. trunk	13	13	13	13	13			
R. buttock	2.5	2.5	2.5	2.5	2.5			
L. buttock	2.5	2.5	2.5	2.5	2.5			
Genitalia	1	1	1	1	1			
R.U. arm	4	4	4	4	4			
L.U. arm	4	4	4	4	4			
R.L. arm	3	3	3	3	3			
L.L. arm	3	3	3	3	3			
R. hand	2.5	2.5	2.5	2.5	2.5			
L. hand	2.5	2.5	2.5	2.5	2.5			
R. thigh	5.5	6.5	8.5	8.5	9.5			
L. thigh	5.5	6.5	8.5	8.5	9.5			
R. leg	5	5	5.5	6	7			
L. leg	5	5	5.5	6	7			
R. foot	3.5	3.5	3.5	3.5	3.5			
L. foot	3.5	3.5	3.5	3.5	3.5			
					Total			

Figure 44.6

Lund and Browder chart

This chart is more accurate than the rule of nines, and is commonly used for assessing burns in children.

ant. = anterior; L. = left; post = posterior; R. = right; R.L. = right lower; R.U. = right upper; TBSA = total body surface area.

A superficial burn does not result in barrier function loss. It is uncommon for a superficial burn to become infected. The damaged cells in the burn area trigger a local inflammatory reaction that is characterised by hyperaemia and oedema.

PARTIAL-THICKNESS BURNS

Aetiology and pathophysiology

Previously known as a *second-degree burn*, a **partial-thickness burn** can be divided into superficial partial-thickness and deep partial-thickness burns. *Superficial partial-thickness burns* involve the *epidermis and some of the dermis* (see Figures 44.4B and 44.7B).

Common causes of this type of burn include contact with hot surfaces, exposure to certain types of dilute chemical agents, or brief exposure to a flame. They may heal without scarring within approximately two weeks of the trauma. *Deep partial-thickness burns* involve *more of the dermis* and may not heal for more than three weeks following the trauma (see Figure 44.7C). They may also result in scarring. Common causes of deep partial-thickness burns include direct contact with flames, intense radiant heat or some chemical agents.

As a superficial partial-thickness burn damages the epidermis and a portion of the dermis, the *superficial vasculature is damaged* and the inflammatory response will result in significant capillary permeability. The *increased capillary permeability* results in a significant amount of **serosanguineous exudate** (a watery, low-protein exudate which is blood-stained). When the extravascular fluid is trapped beneath some skin layers, blisters will form. The pain experienced is generally significant because of the exposure of the nerve endings to air. As not all of the vasculature is damaged, tissue perfusion is not affected and is often hyperaemic because of the local inflammatory mediators released as a direct result of the trauma.

Deep partial-thickness burns involve all of the epidermis and almost all of the dermis. As *more vasculature is damaged, capillary refill is reduced*. Perception to pressure is present, but pain sensation is often less than with superficial partial-thickness burns.

FULL-THICKNESS BURNS

Aetiology and pathophysiology

Formerly known as a *third-degree burn*, a **full-thickness burn** destroys *the dermis and epidermis* (see Figures 44.4B and 44.7D). The burn may also extend down *into subcutaneous tissue, muscle and bone*. This type of burn will not heal without intervention, and will always cause scarring. Common causes of full-thickness burns include direct contact with a flame, chemicals or a high-voltage electric current.

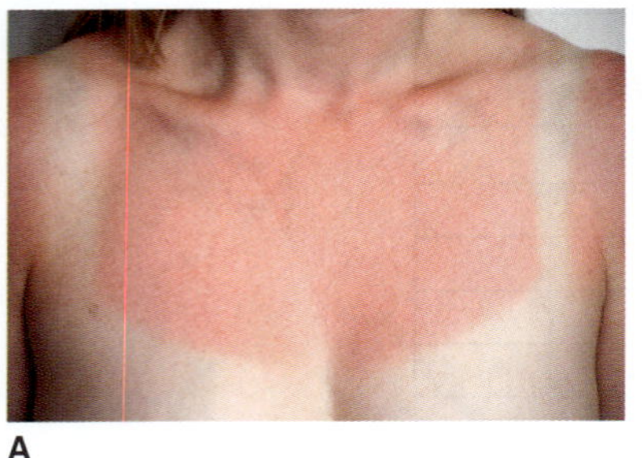
A

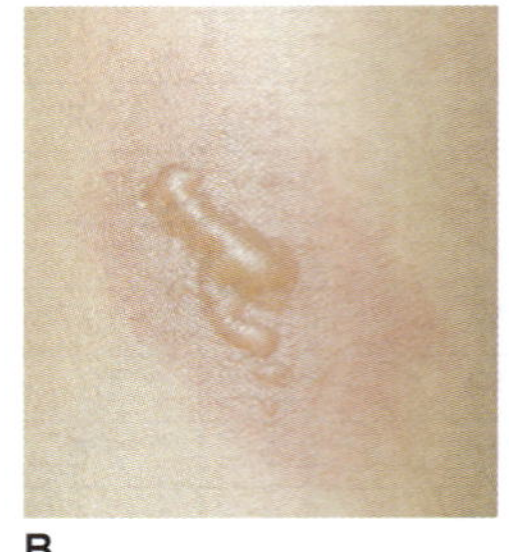
B

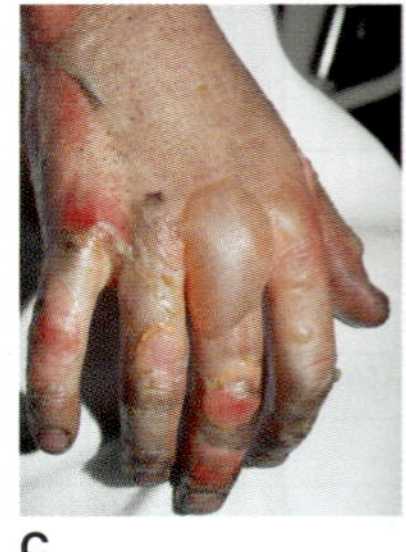
C

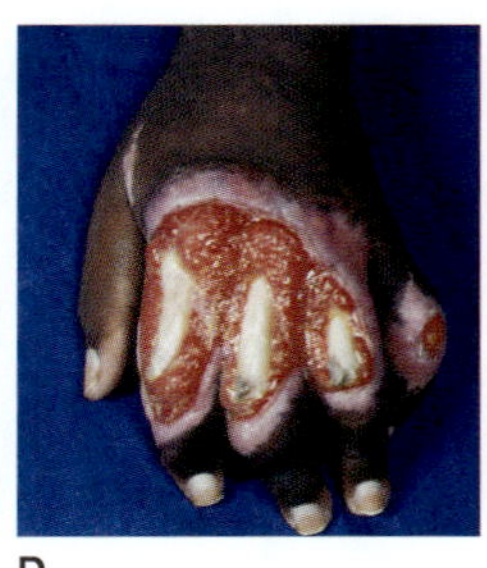
D

Figure 44.7

Types of burns

(A) Superficial burn.
(B) Superficial partial-thickness burn.
(C) Deep partial-thickness burn.
(D) Full-thickness burn.

Sources: (A) DJ40/Shutterstock; (B) Chutchawarn/Shutterstock; (C) James Stevenson/Science Photo Library; (D) Dr M.A. Ansary/Science Photo Library.

As a full-thickness burn destroys the dermis, perfusion to the affected area is lost as the vascular system supplying the area is damaged; as a result, *necrosis* develops. Functions such as *immune defence, temperature regulation and sensation are lost.* Not only is the person at extreme risk of infection, but also fluid balance and temperature regulation are dysfunctional.

The systemic effects of severe burns can be life-threatening. These effects are known to be caused by inflammation, immunosuppression and eschar-derived toxins, and can result in hypothermia, acidosis and coagulopathy. Individually, the effects complicate a person's recovery; however, when combined, these factors contribute to significantly higher mortality rates and are known as the *lethal triad*.

CLINICAL MANIFESTATIONS

The affected area will be erythematous and hyperaemic. The affected tissue will blanch with pressure. Some oedema may be present.

Superficial burns are initially painful and can become pruritic. Sometime later the pain subsides and some of the stratum corneum begins to peel. Superficial burns may involve large areas of skin, and may cause headaches, malaise and chills. Dehydration may contribute to the development of these symptoms.

A superficial partial-thickness burn presents as a moist, erythematous, blistered area. The blisters may form over 24 hours, or they may develop soon after the initial trauma. The burnt person will complain of pain, especially when the burn is exposed to air or changes in temperature. Deep partial-thickness burns may appear pale, erythematous or mottled, and they may be either moist or dry. The deeper the burn, the paler and drier the appearance of the burn.

Burn depth is not the only factor to influence a person's clinical course. As more total body surface area is involved in the burn, clinical manifestations become more complex and dynamic. Thermal injuries exceeding 20% TBSA are accompanied by the severe systemic response.

Observation for, and management of, factors in the lethal triad are clearly critical. The presence of sustained hypothermia ($T^\circ \sim 34.8^\circ C$) increases a person's mortality risk, with time until death occurring more quickly than in those who are normothermic. Burn-induced coagulopathy (BIC) from fibrinolytic dysfunction can manifest as either haemorrhagic or thrombosis. However, within the first 48 hours, a more pro-coagulant potential is generally exhibited, and therefore deep vein thrombosis (DVT) and venous thromboembolism (VTE) are a concern. Conversely, the person with the severe thermal burn may develop disseminated intravascular coagulation (DIC), resulting from platelet and clotting factor depletion. At this time, both bleeding and clotting will complicate the person's recovery, and perioperative blood loss and transfusion requirements significantly increase the risk of poor outcome. Finally, the systemic inflammatory response and excessive volume depletion will result in decreased tissue perfusion. Subsequently, tissue hypoxia ensues and causes metabolic acidosis. If the person develops sepsis, this can exacerbate the acidosis. Therefore, clinicians responsible for caring for people with severe burn injury must consider, observe for, and if possible prevent factors which contribute to acidosis. Coupled with hypothermia and coagulopathy, acidosis will complete the lethal triad and significantly increase mortality risk.

CLINICAL DIAGNOSIS AND MANAGEMENT

Diagnosis

Consideration of the presenting history and a visual inspection of the affected area will assist with diagnosis. An estimate of the size of the burn (TBSA burnt) will contribute to planning its management.

The presence of blisters on sunburn demonstrates a superficial partial-thickness burn instead of merely a superficial burn. A superficial partial-thickness burn will generally blanch with pressure. Assessment of those with darker skin may be difficult. However, evaluation of the presence of eschar (a dry scab or slough), turgor and pain is necessary. Deep partial-thickness burns do not often blanch with pressure. A deeper burn will generally also have more superficial depths of burns on the edges.

The area affected by a full-thickness burn may appear white, yellow, brown or charred. The area is **avascular** and appears waxy. If adipose tissue is involved in a flame burn, the area may appear leathery. Full-thickness burns do not have sensation because the touch and pain receptors have been destroyed. However, areas of lesser burn will generally line the edges of the deep burn, so pain will be experienced. It is important to note, however, that in severe burns the outward appearance of a waxed or charred burn area will most likely disguise the extent of tissue damage beneath it.

Non-cutaneous investigations following burn injury also focus on airway, haematological measures and toxin exposure. Investigations monitoring pulse oximetry and arterial blood gases (for oxygen levels—and other things—see the chapter 'Pulmonary dysfunction'), capnography (for carbon dioxide levels), carboxyhemoglobin levels (carbon monoxide toxicity), and serum lactate (in the context of possible cyanide poisoning—from chemicals released by burning plastic, wools and many other substances).

It should also be noted that conventional coagulation profiles are not reliable in detecting coagulopathy in people with severe thermal injury; therefore, more general tests such as thrombin generation assays (TGAs) provide more detailed information than just a clotting end-point.

Management

The five primary aims in the management of burns are: the management of pain; the protection against infection; the protection against hypothermia; the protection against dehydration; and support of the hypermetabolic state induced by the burn resulting in increased caloric requirements.

Although prevention is best, most healthcare professionals are responsible for caring for people who are already burned.

In a superficial burn, the *four C* approach can guide initial management: **c**ooling, **c**leaning, **c**overing and **c**omfort. An established method of reducing continued tissue damage and minimising the injury zone is to cool the burn under running water (ideally at 15°C for 20 minutes), while cleaning the wound will reduce the risk of infection. Covering the burn will reduce pain and decrease the risk of infection, and comfort can be achieved through analgesia, and splinting if the burn is in the area of a joint. Simple analgesia should be administered for the pain. Fluid replacement should be encouraged, and moisturising cream can be beneficial. If a large surface area is involved in a superficial burn to a child or an older adult, intravenous fluid replacement may be necessary to reduce the effects of dehydration and electrolyte imbalance.

The volume of skin involved in the burn will influence management. People with partial-thickness burns that cover more than 10% of the TBSA should be admitted to a burns unit. Analgesia is critical to the management of partial-thickness burns. For superficial partial-thickness burns, the area should be cleaned and debrided of sloughing epidermis. A silicone dressing with an absorbent dry dressing over the top will reduce pain and assist to reduce exposure to environmental pathogens not already on the affected area. Use of dressings containing silver can reduce bacterial growth, and may be considered. Depending on the location and the size of the burn, skin grafting may be necessary for deep partial-thickness burns. Although deep partial-thickness burns are less painful, areas of lesser burns will be painful. Administration of analgesia should be as frequent as is considered safe and necessary.

In people with full-thickness burns, a long and arduous clinical course with a high risk of complications—such as infection, graft rejection and pain—is often ahead of them.

Pain management from burn injury needs to be aggressive. Despite advances in knowledge, resources and practices, pain control is often suboptimal across the various stages of a person's burn recovery, from dressing changes through to physiotherapy. Depending on the type, location and subsequent interventions required during their recovery, a person may require extremely large doses of opioids and other analgesic agents. Consistent assessment, use of both non-pharmacological and pharmacological approaches, addition of adjuvants and adjustment of dosing regimens are all critical in the management of the person's pain.

Formal fluid resuscitation should occur in those with burns to greater than 15% of their TBSA, to avoid both dehydration and overhydration leading to complications. Large fluid shifts resulting in depletion of intravascular volume occur within the first 24–48 hours in severe burns. Careful fluid resuscitation, accommodating the person's fast-changing clinical requirements, is paramount to avoid complicating recovery with issues associated with over-resuscitation, including multi-organ failure, compartment syndrome and/or respiratory distress.

Chemoprophylaxis to prevent bacterial infection is critical in anyone sustaining more than superficial burn injury. Although there are serious concerns regarding antimicrobial resistance (AMR), many clinicians continue to order prophylactic antimicrobial agents. Currently in Australia, there appears to be continued long-course use of prophylactic antimicrobials, even though the literature remains unconvincing for beneficial clinical outcomes. Therefore, more research in the area would be valuable, enabling expert consensus regarding guidelines for prophylactic antimicrobials use in burns.

As the complexities of burn injury are better understood, it has been discovered that the burn eschar on the surface of those who are severely burned contributes to the severe immunosuppression that they experience. This occurs because the damaged and dying tissue releases molecules known as *damage-associated molecular patterns* (DAMPs), which bind to innate immune system cells and cause a dysregulated inflammatory state. Therefore, 'damage control surgery' is performed not only for debridement to improve wound healing, to release contractures, and decompress compartment syndromes, but also to remove the tissue which is profoundly contributing to the systemic inflammatory response.

Blister management now includes deroofing. Historically, attempts were always made to keep blisters intact. However, best evidence suggests that deroofing improves the ability to assess burn depth, provide pain relief, and remove non-viable tissue. The freely floating or loose epidermis should be trimmed. Deroofing is especially important in the event of opaque blister fluid (suggestive of infection), and any purulent exudate should be swabbed and sent for microscopy, culture and sensitivity (MCS). The wound should then be cleaned and covered.

Recovery time increases with burn depth. Prevention of infection is imperative to reduce the risk of a failed skin graft. Several permanent skin substitute products are available for use, especially in the context of large areas. Synthetic wound dressing products can be used in various circumstances, including reducing wound hydration, the regulation and stimulation of granulation tissue growth, and to reduce the risk of bacterial infection.

- *Silicone gel dressings:* These dressings are generally applied directly to the skin, as they have hydrophobic properties on the wound side which enables atraumatic removal. They are not absorbent, and therefore benefit from the additional placement of an absorbent dressing if a burn is particularly exudative. The silicone is inert and does not react with the tissue, resulting in limited risk of an allergic reaction. They do not have antimicrobial properties.
- *Dressings containing silver ions:* Silver sulfadiazine (SSD) cream was used for many years as an antimicrobial agent for burns; however, newer burns dressings which have elemental silver or a silver-releasing compound impregnated into the dressing are favoured and reduce the need for frequent dressing changes. Some dressings are also made with layers to assist the removal of excess exudate, while others facilitate autolytic debridement of over-granulated areas. The products often need to be moistened either before or once they are applied. Depending on the product, they may require other dressing components for absorbency or adherence.
- *Hydrogels:* Are used in the context of dry or scabbed wounds to moisturise and hydrate. They can often have a cooling effect and provide an atraumatic, non-adhesive quality to wound dressings.

If a full-thickness burn is circumferential around a limb or the torso, the leathery appearance suggests that the skin has lost its capacity to expand. As the burn-induced capillary leak results in progressive oedema (especially after vigorous and appropriate fluid resuscitation), the affected area will direct its compression inwards toward the tissue, effectively causing a compartment-syndrome-like scenario. If the chest is affected by a circumferential burn, the chest wall will become rigid and can impair ventilation, and an escharotomy (an incision through the burnt tissue to relieve the pressure caused by the constrictive, leathery tissue left after full-thickness burns—*eschar*) will be required to enable adequate ventilation. If a limb is affected by circumferential full-thickness burns, the compartment-syndrome-like effects can cause limb-threatening compression, requiring an escharotomy (see Figure 44.8).

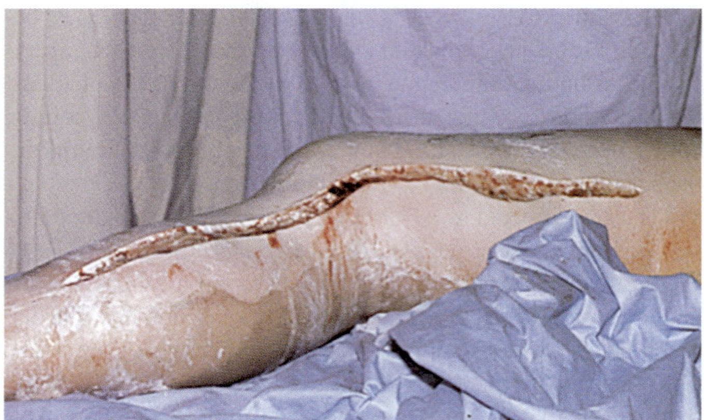

Figure 44.8

Leg escharotomy

Source: Courtesy of William J. Dominic, MD, Leon S. Peters Regional Burn Center, Fresno, California, USA.

BURN MECHANISMS

LEARNING OBJECTIVE 4

Discuss the various mechanisms of thermal injury.

Various mechanisms result in thermal injury, which are commonly divided into temperature, chemical, friction, radiation and electrical causes.

Temperatures exceeding the tolerance of the skin to withstand injury can be caused by scalds or flames. A significant percentage of child and elderly thermal injuries are caused by scalds, whereby a hot liquid (often tap water or oil) contacts the skin. This type of injury mostly involves less than 10% of a person's total body surface area, and often causes superficial wounds (less than one-quarter of these injuries are full-thickness burns). However, 88% of males between 15 and 39 years of age who are hospitalised with burns, have burns caused by highly flammable liquids (such as petrol), with only 22% of these burns sustained while working for an income. In Australia in 2019–20, approximately 20% of hospital admissions for burn injury were caused by fire, yet 74% of deaths resulted from exposure to fire, smoke or flames. This is most likely because more than half of flame burns are associated with inhalational injuries or other accompanying trauma. Interestingly, the national mandated stay-at-home orders resulting from the COVID-19 pandemic had little influence on burn injury statistics during this period.

Chemical injuries can occur from acid or alkali substances coming in contact with the skin, most often as an occupational-related injury. Occasionally, though, these substances are consumed orally (accidentally or on purpose), and subsequent airway and gastrointestinal injuries will ensue (this type of injury will not be discussed here). Alkali burns (e.g. from cement) are often more severe as they can penetrate the skin more easily than acids. Chemical injury first aid management differs from thermal injury, and should include irrigating the area with water for 60 minutes, removing contaminated clothing (if possible), and applying a sterile dressing on the burn. The use of litmus paper may be beneficial to determine if the chemical is acid or alkaline (if unknown), and the use of a neutralising agents, antidotes (eg. calcium gluconate for hydrofluoric acid burns), or chelating agents, such as diphoterine which decontaminates the area of the corrosive or irritant agent, through its absorbent properties. The goal for management of chemical burns is the reduction of tissue inflammation and return of skin to its normal pH (4.7 and 5.5).

Friction injury, although a less frequent mechanism for burns, can nonetheless cause severe injury. These are often caused by treadmills or vacuum cleaners, especially in children. Friction burns from treadmills often cause serious injury, many of which may be as deep as full-thickness burns, and require surgery.

Radiation burns are caused by radio frequency energy or by ionising radiation from sources such as the sun, from iatrogenic causes such as radiation therapy or excessive diagnostic procedures. The term 'radiation burn' is not commonly used by healthcare professionals in radiation therapy, instead often using the term 'radiation dermatitis' or 'radiation-induced skin injury'. Injury may range from relatively superficial cutaneous insult through to severe damage, manifesting in wounds exhibiting erosion, ulceration and/or necrosis.

Electrical injury occurs from either low or high voltage. The electricity is converted to heat and results in a thermal burn. It is important to note that the outward appearance of the cutaneous lesions of this type of injury does not reflect the extent of the trauma to the internal tissues or organs. Depending on the cause, clothes may also catch fire and contribute to further burn injury. Sources of electrical burn may come from power lines, faulty powered devices, or water exposure to powered devices in contact with the affected person, lightning, or electrical weapons such as TASERs. The type of current will influence tissue damage and clinical outcome; for example, *alternating current* (AC) causes more injury than *direct current* (DC). AC current is more common and is used as the power source for building. It causes local muscle contraction and may render the person unable to release the source of the electrical current. DC current is found in lightning and car battery contact, and often throws the person away from the source, which may result in other mechanical injuries. *High-tension* injuries are burns which create two cutaneous injuries—an entry and an exit point (known as contact points), as the current passes through the person. This type of injury will also damage the tissue around the path through which the current has travelled. *Flash* injuries occur from an arc of current from a high-tension voltage source (> 1,000V), where there person can sustain superficial flash burns or thermal injury from clothes catching fire, even though no current actually passes through their body. Each year, approximately 400 people in Australia are injured through exposure to electric current, but this number has been steadily decreasing since 2017. As this type of injury most often occurs in males as a result of occupational accidents, it is likely that the rate reduction may be due to improved education and workplace health and safety regarding electrical risk.

ZONES OF BURN INJURY

LEARNING OBJECTIVE 5

Differentiate between local and systemic responses to burn injury.

Local burn responses

The local response to a burn was first modelled in the 1940s. It describes three burn zones: the zones of hyperaemia, stasis and coagulation. This model still forms the basis of burn pathophysiology today (see Figure 44.9).

- The *zone of hyperaemia* is most distal to the area of maximum damage. In this zone, non-specific inflammatory responses to the trauma of the burn result in vasodilation, hyperaemia and erythema. Recovery of the cells in this area is probable unless further insult, such as secondary infection, occurs.

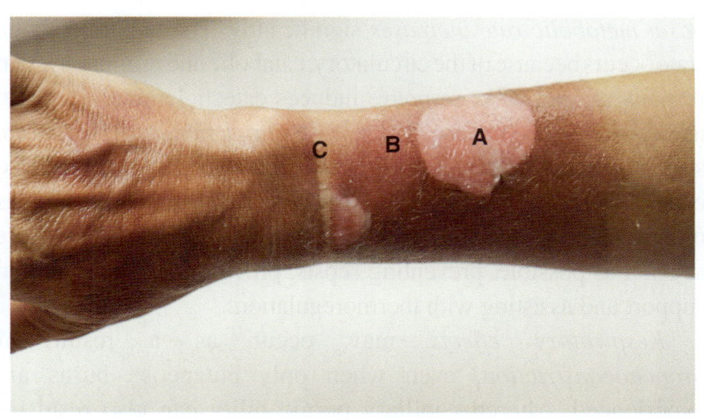

Figure 44.9

The zones of burn injury

(A) The zone of coagulation is extensively damaged, and irreversible tissue loss is expected here (depending on the type of burn).

(B) The zone of stasis is affected by ischaemia, and the injury to cells may progress from chemical mediators. Significant tissue loss is expected here.

(C) The zone of hyperaemia is the least damaged area. Cellular recovery is probable.

Source: Science Photo Library.

- The *zone of stasis* is closer to the area of maximum damage. In this zone, there is decreased perfusion, leading to ischaemia. Injured endothelium causes vasoconstriction, thrombosis and fibrin deposition. Inflammatory mediators are thought to cause progressive injury. Recovery of cells in this area is possible. However, if oedema or prolonged hypoperfusion occurs, this area may still suffer significant tissue loss.
- The *zone of coagulation* is the area of maximum damage. In this zone (depending on the type of burn) there is irreversible tissue loss. The damage is mostly caused by the initial trauma, but may be exacerbated by the coagulation and protein deposition.

Systemic burn responses

Even though a burn may be cutaneous, once the TBSA affected reaches 15%, systemic effects occur. The *systemic vascular effects*, as a result of inflammatory mediators and other cytokines, cause *increased capillary permeability*. The resulting fluid shifts can cause *hypotension*.

Myocardial depressant chemicals and calcium issues can exacerbate the hypotension caused by volume deficit and depress myocardial contraction.

For burns incorporating large surface areas, *fluid and electrolyte issues* are common, as *fluid losses* in the first few hours of the burn can be excessive. These losses can continue for several days post-burn. Adequate fluid and electrolyte replacement are critical to the outcomes of large body surface area burns.

Because of the insult, *metabolic derangement* can occur. The *basal metabolic rate increases* significantly. The hypermetabolic state occurs because of the circulatory, catabolic and immune system responses. The *stress response* induces catecholamine, glucagon and corticosteroid release. The release of *inflammatory mediators*, such as tissue necrosis factor, prostaglandins and leukotrienes, also exaggerates metabolic needs. Important management principles of post-burn **hypermetabolism** include achieving wound closure as soon as possible, preventing sepsis, providing extra nutritional support and assisting with thermoregulation.

Respiratory effects may occur as a result of *bronchoconstriction*, even when only cutaneous burns are experienced. Altered capillary permeability can also result in *respiratory distress syndromes*.

Cell-mediated and humoral pathways of the immune system are challenged, and a generalised *systemic inflammatory response* can occur. The *loss of the integumentary barrier* results in reduced defence against pathogens, and infection can easily occur. Pathogens such as *Staphylococcus aeruginosa* and *Streptococcus pyogenes* are commonly responsible for wound infections.

CLINICAL CONSIDERATIONS RELATED TO THE CAUSE OF BURNS

The burn depth, location and size are important factors associated with clinical outcomes. However, slight variations to presentation, clinical progression and outcome may occur as a direct result of the mechanism by which the burn occurred. Consideration of the cause should always be critical to the clinician. Injury caused by a chemical burn will differ from injuries caused by flame or electrical burns, for example.

Finally, when considering the cause of burns, there may be suspicion of non-accidental injury, especially in burns involving children. In Australia, it is a legal requirement for healthcare providers to report suspected child abuse. Burn injuries that appear to have an obvious pattern (e.g. from cigarettes), burns to the soles of the feet and palms of the hands, or burns to perineal areas should be suspected as potential non-accidental injuries.

Scarring

LEARNING OBJECTIVE 6

Discuss the types and pathogenesis of scarring.

Scarring can be considered as a pathology related to wound healing. Although the process of wound healing is addressed in the chapter 'Inflammation and healing', three common types of scars are addressed here: keloid, hypertrophic and widened scars.

AETIOLOGY AND PATHOPHYSIOLOGY

A keloid scar occurs when the *cellular activity within the wound becomes excessive* and the balance between granulation and apoptosis is lost. Within a year after trauma, the affected tissue develops outside the margins of the original scar. Risk factors for keloid scar formation include being of Aboriginal, Māori, Melanesian or Afro-Caribbean descent, a history of previous keloid formation, prolonged inflammation and healing by second intention. Keloid scars have a thicker epidermal layer than normal scars, and the collagen formation is greater and disorganised.

A **hypertrophic scar** also occurs as a result of *excessive collagen accumulation*. However, the scar growth stays within the confines of the original injury. Unlike keloid formation, skin colour is not a risk factor to hypertrophic scarring.

A **widened scar** occurs as a result of *excess tension on the wound edges* during the wound healing process. The wound may gape, and healing by second intention occurs. Wounds that have experienced an infection are more prone to widened scars.

CLINICAL MANIFESTATIONS

With both keloid and hypertrophic scarring, excess tissue formation along a scar occurs. If the tissue extends beyond the margin of the scar, it is called a keloid scar (see Figure 44.10A); if the tissue remains within the confines of the scar, it is a hypertrophic scar (see Figure 44.10B).

Widened scars present as a scar whose wound edges have not approximated well during healing, and the distance between the wound edges is greater than expected (see Figure 44.10C).

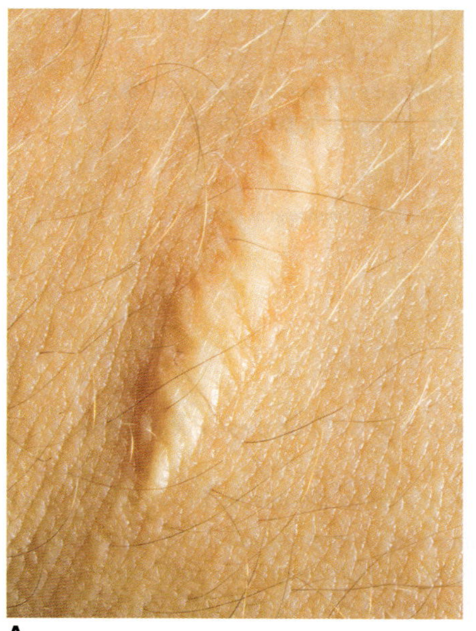
A

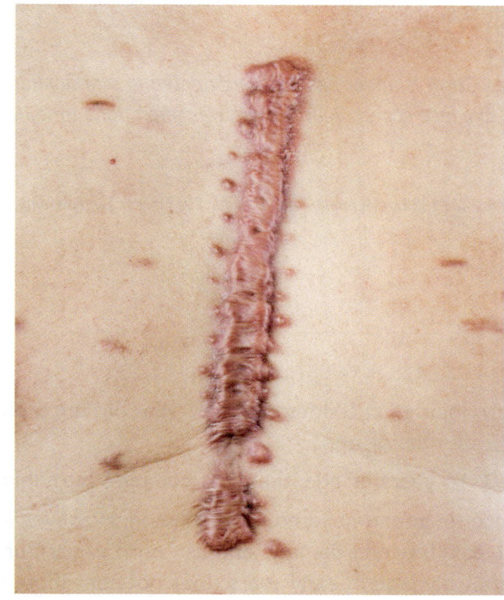
B

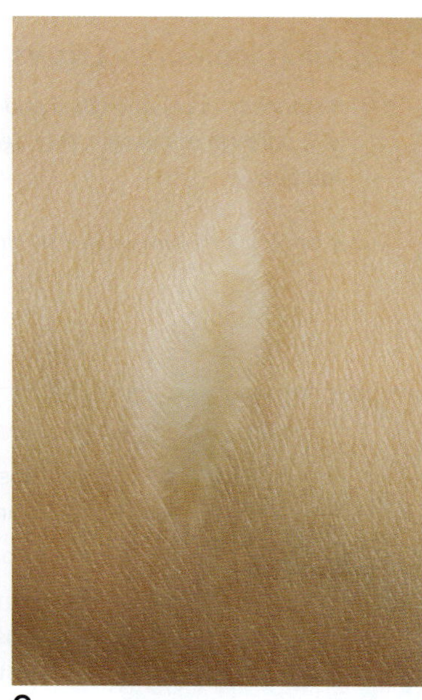
C

Figure 44.10

Types of scars

(A) Keloid scar.
(B) Hypertrophic scar.
(C) Widened scar.

Sources: (A) Fedorov Oleksiy/Shutterstock; (B) supersaiyan3/Shutterstock; (C) Violanda/Shutterstock.

CLINICAL DIAGNOSIS AND MANAGEMENT

Diagnosis

Visual inspection of the wound and a consideration of the history surrounding the initial injury are valuable. Consideration of other risk factors, including race, the mechanism of injury and the person's wound healing history, will also assist in the diagnosis.

Management

Although keloid and hypertrophic scars are self-limiting, those with such scars may request their removal because of issues related to appearance and self-confidence. Some management options include the use of pressure garments, the application of concealing make-up and corticosteroid injections. Excision of keloid scars is not indicated, as the risk of the scar recurring (often larger) is very high.

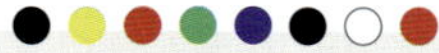

INDIGENOUS HEALTH FAST FACTS AND CULTURAL CONSIDERATIONS

FAST FACTS

- *Aboriginal and Torres Strait Islander Australians are on average 2.9 times more likely than non-Indigenous Australians to be hospitalised for burns and scalds.*
- *Aboriginal and Torres Strait Islander children between 0 and 4 years of age are 3.1 times more likely than non-Indigenous Australian children to be hospitalised for burns and scalds.*
- *Aboriginal and Torres Strait Islander peoples are 3.9 times less likely than non-Indigenous Australians to experience melanoma.*
- *Māori and Pacific Islands people's incidence of melanoma is 4 times lower to that of European New Zealanders. However, early evidence suggests that Māori and Pacific Islands people who do develop melanoma have a higher mortality rate.*
- *Māori children have a higher incidence of burn injury (especially in children under 1 year of age, and 7–13-year-olds) than European New Zealand children.*
- *Pacific Islands children under 4 years of age have a higher incidence of scald injury than European New Zealand children.*

CULTURAL CONSIDERATIONS

Historically, many Aboriginal and Torres Strait Islander peoples participated in scarification (the cutting or chronic rubbing of the skin with abrasive or inflammatory agents to cause scars). Scarification was often done to tell a story of, for example, pain, identity, status or courage.

Sources: Data from Australian Institute of Health and Welfare (2022); Melanoma New Zealand (2017); New Zealand Ministry of Health (2015); Simpson et al. (2017).

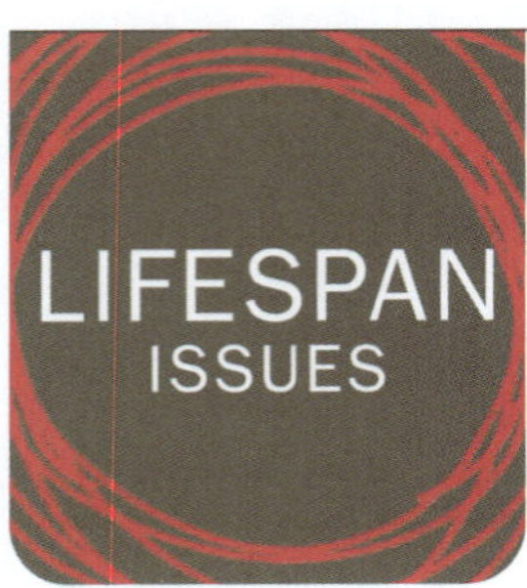

CHILDREN AND ADOLESCENTS

- Most burn injuries in children under 1 year old are scalds, and over 80% of these occur between 7 and 12 months of age.
- In boys 8–14 years of age, the most common burn injury is related to the misuse of petrol.
- Skin cancer in young children is uncommon. However, infants and children have thinner skin that is sensitive to ultraviolet damage and can burn easily. Sun protective behaviours are necessary to ensure that damage in early years does not contribute to melanoma later in life.

OLDER ADULTS

- Scald injuries are common in older adults from 70 years of age, increasing dramatically in adults 85 years and older.
- People who are 75 years or older are five times more likely than a younger person to die from the same burn injury.
- Significant mortality due to squamous cell carcinoma occurs in men around 77 years of age, especially when the site of the primary cancer is on the face, hands, scalp or ears.

KEY CLINICAL ISSUES

- There are three different types of skin cancer. Melanoma is the most lethal and affects younger adults. Squamous cell carcinoma is also dangerous and affects older people. A knowledge of the morphology, incidence and risk factors for each type of skin cancer is important to assist in skin surveillance and referral for further assessment and investigation where necessary.
- Promoting education that encourages children to participate in 'sun smart' behaviours is important to reduce the risk of melanoma and ultraviolet-associated skin cancers in the future.
- Ultraviolet exposure is still necessary to promote vitamin D synthesis. Therefore, protected exposure to the sun in less dangerous times of the day is still important.
- Calculation of the total body surface area burnt is necessary so that fluid resuscitation protocols can be determined.
- Any burns that occur near the face can singe nasal hairs or result in soot on the face, nose or mouth, and so should be considered as airway-threatening injuries. Interventions to obtain an artificial airway and mechanical ventilation should be considered early, to ensure that an airway is secured before oedema complicates this task.
- Burn dressings will differ depending on the mechanism of the burn, the depth and the resulting injury. Generally, covering a burn will reduce the pain and decrease the risk of infection.
- Full-thickness burns will not heal without intervention. This may include surgical debridement and/or skin grafting. New techniques are being developed to increase the amount of skin in a burn-affected area.

CHAPTER REVIEW

- Several types of *skin cancers* occur. Some are *benign* and some are *malignant*.
- Non-malignant skin cancers that are managed quickly can cause few ill effects.
- Non-malignant skin cancers that are not managed well may cause significant damage, resulting in poor aesthetic outcomes.
- *Malignant melanomas* cause approximately 1,300 Australian deaths a year, and over 350 New Zealand deaths a year.
- Melanomas arise from *melanocytes*.
- *Burns* can be caused by many substances and many environments.
- The *depth* of burn will determine the viability of the tissue post-injury. However, the *size and location* of the burn, and the *age* of the person affected, will bear significance on their mortality and morbidity.
- *Scarring* will occur after any cutaneous injury.
- If wound healing is hindered, scarring will occur more readily.

REVIEW QUESTIONS

1 What are the three different types of skin cancers? How can they be distinguished from each other?
2 Can non-malignant skin cancers cause death? Explain.
3 What factors should be assessed in determining whether a skin lesion is a melanoma?
4 What management options are available for the treatment of melanoma?
5 What are the different types of burns? Create a table identifying the different types of burns. Across the top, list the type of burn by burn depth. In the left-hand column, list 'Structures involved', 'Wound appearance', 'Healing and scarring', 'Pain' and 'Notes'. Complete the table.
6 What are the three types of scarring?
7 A person talks to you about the keloid scar that has grown under her chin from a trauma that she sustained when she was a child. She wants to have it removed. What are the options and challenges related to the management of keloid scars?

HEALTH PROFESSIONAL CONNECTIONS

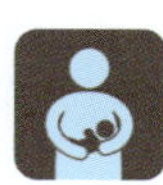

Midwives Scar formation from obstetric or gynaecological procedures can interfere with body image and sexual pleasure, and can complicate future pregnancies. Poorly healing episiotomy scars can cause deformity in the perineal area. Sometimes, scar formation can result in tissue resembling extra labial folds. Episiotomy scars can be painful, interfere with hygiene practices or negatively influence the woman's desire to have intercourse. Topical application of oestrogen, intradermal injection of corticosteroids or surgical interventions may be needed to assist with this issue. Occasionally, uterine scars can rupture or dehisce when a woman has a vaginal birth after a previous birth by caesarean section. This internal rupture increases the risk of maternal and neonatal morbidity and mortality.

Physiotherapists People whose skin integrity has been compromised may develop contractures and an altered range of movement as a result of poor or disorganised wound healing and scar formation. Teamwork should result in a management plan that prevents movement-limiting outcomes. However, if these do occur, interventions to regain range of movement are necessary to reduce morbidity and mortality rates, as well as for functional and aesthetic reasons.

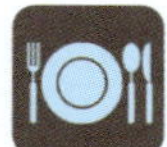

Nutritionists/Dieticians Malnutrition is a significant variable in the defence against skin infections. The hypermetabolic state caused by a burn requires considerable specialised management. People with burns to less than 20% of their body may require high-energy, high-protein diets. Enteral feeds may be required if the person is unable to maintain sufficient nutrient intake. Those with burns to greater than 20% of their total body surface area are unlikely to be able to have their nutrition requirements met orally. The hypermetabolic state induced by a burn injury may last approximately two weeks, and fluctuations are caused by a number of considerations, including the presence of infection. Calorie formulas should be evidenced-based and take the whole clinical situation into account.

CASE STUDY

Mr Craig Peters, who is 45 years of age (UR number 463545), received significant thermal burns from an explosion when he lit a match to see whether there was any petrol in his car's petrol tank. A bystander witnessed the accident and used his coat to extinguish the flames on Mr Peters. Prehospital treatment consisted of oxygen administration, analgesia, initiation of intravenous access and application of water-soaked gauze to the affected sites. The following chart demonstrates the affected areas.

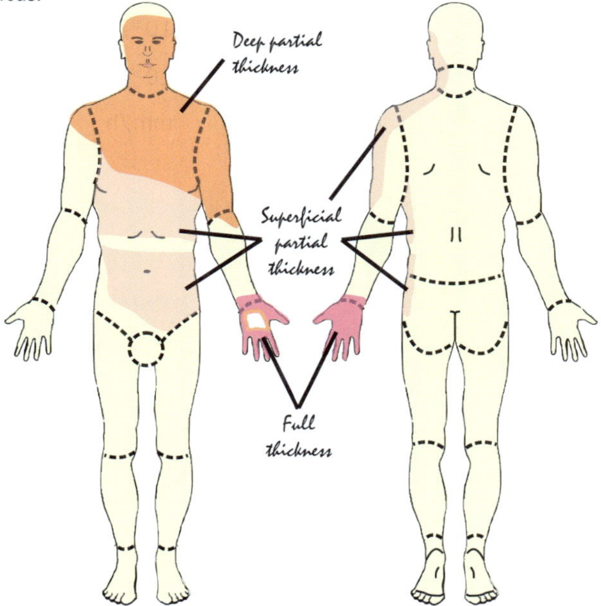

Craig Peters' burn chart

On admission to the emergency department, his observations were as follows:

Temperature	Heart rate	Respiration rate	Blood pressure	SpO_2
36.2°C	108	32	162/84	99% (6 L/min)

As his nasal hairs are singed, it was decided that there was a significant risk of airway involvement, so he was sedated, paralysed and intubated. Blood was also immediately drawn for a full blood count and electrolyte testing. His results are as follows:

HAEMATOLOGY

Patient location:	Burn Unit	**UR:**	463545		
Consultant:	Smith	**NAME:**	Peters		
		Given name:	Craig	**Sex:**	M
		DOB:	04/06/XX	**Age:**	45

Time collected	11:20
Date collected	XX/XX
Year	XXXX
Lab #	5453453

FULL BLOOD COUNT		UNITS	REFERENCE RANGE
Haemoglobin	132	g/L	115–160
White cell count	6.3	$\times 10^9$/L	4.0–11.0
Platelets	320	$\times 10^9$/L	140–400
Haematocrit	0.42		0.33–0.47
Red cell count	3.86	$\times 10^{12}$/L	3.80–5.20
Reticulocyte count	0.9	%	0.2–2.0
MCV	95	fL	80–100
Neutrophils	5.6	$\times 10^9$/L	2.00–8.00
Lymphocytes	3.01	$\times 10^9$/L	1.00–4.00
Monocytes	0.42	$\times 10^9$/L	0.10–1.00
Eosinophils	0.43	$\times 10^9$/L	< 0.60
Basophils	0.11	$\times 10^9$/L	< 0.20
ESR	11	mm/h	< 12

BIOCHEMISTRY

Patient location:	Burn Unit	**UR:**	463545		
Consultant:	Smith	**NAME:**	Peters		
		Given name:	Craig	**Sex:**	M
		DOB:	04/06/XX	**Age:**	45

Time collected	11:20
Date collected	XX/XX
Year	XXXX
Lab #	4534432

ELECTROLYTES		UNITS	REFERENCE RANGE
Sodium	136	mmol/L	135–145
Potassium	3.6	mmol/L	3.5–5.0
Chloride	104	mmol/L	95–110
Bicarbonate	25	mmol/L	22–32
Glucose (random)	6.2	mmol/L	3.5–8.0

CRITICAL THINKING

1 Consult Mr Peters' burn chart and estimate the total body surface area involved in the burn injury. Identify the major risks associated with the severity of his injuries.

2 Describe what is occurring at a cellular level in the three different burn-depth areas. Consider using a table to assist with the explanation. The columns may include headings such as 'Burn type', 'Depth', 'Structures involved' and 'Cellular response'.

3 Note the pathology results. Are any values outside the reference range? Is this expected? Explain.

4 Most of Mr Peters' injuries will not heal without treatment. Identify what interventions will be needed to protect Mr Peters from further adverse outcomes. For each intervention, provide a rationale. Ensure that your answer covers all of the aspects of burn management, including factors such as fluid and electrolyte levels, infection control, analgesia and metabolism.

5 Are there potentially any negative long-term effects of this injury? Explain.

BIBLIOGRAPHY

Australian Health Ministers' Advisory Council's National and Aboriginal and Torres Strait Islander Health Standing Committee (2017). *Cultural respect framework 2016–2026: for Aboriginal and Torres Strait Islander health—a national approach to building a culturally respectful health system*. Canberra: Australian Government Department of Health. https://nacchocommunique.files.wordpress.com/2016/12/cultural_respect_framework_1december2016_1.pdf.

Australian Institute of Health and Welfare (AIHW) (2020). *Aboriginal and Torres Strait Islander health performance framework 2020—summary report*. Cat. No. IHPF 2. Canberra: AIHW. https://www.indigenoushpf.gov.au/publications/hpf-summary-2020.

Australian Institute of Health and Welfare (AIHW) (2021). *Cancer in Australia 2021*. Cancer series No. 133. Cat. No. CAN 144. Canberra: AIHW. https://www.aihw.gov.au/reports/cancer/cancer-in-australia-2021/summary.

Australian Institute of Health and Welfare (AIHW) (2022a). *Australia's health, 2022: data insights*. Australia's health series no. 18. Cat. no. AUS 240. Canberra: AIHW. https://www.aihw.gov.au/reports/australias-health/australias-health-2022-data-insights/about.

Australian Institute of Health and Welfare (AIHW) (2022b). *Injury in Australia: thermal causes.* Canberra: AIHW. https://www.aihw.gov.au/reports/injury/burns-and-other-thermal-causes.

Australian Institute of Health and Welfare (AIHW) (2022c). *Principal diagnosis data cubes: separation statistics by principal diagnosis (ICD-10-AM, 11th edition), Australia, 2020–21.* Canberra: AIHW. https://www.aihw.gov.au/reports/hospitals/principal-diagnosis-data-cubes/contents/data-cubes.

Bader, R.S. (2022). Basal cell carcinoma. *Emedicine*. https://emedicine.medscape.com/article/276624-overview.

Ball, R.L., Keyloun, J.W., Brummel-Ziedins, K., Orfeo, T., Palmieri, T.L., Johnson, L.S., … Shupp, J.W. (2020). Burn-induced coagulopathies: a comprehensive review. *Shock* 54(2):154–67. https://doi.org/10.1097/SHK.0000000000001484.

Baradaran, A., Buchel, E.W. & Vorstenbosch, J. (2021). Thermal burns. *Emedicine*. https://emedicine.medscape.com/article/1278244-overview.

Bauldoff, G., Gubrud-Howe, P.M., Carno, M.-A., Levett-Jones, T., Hales, M., Berry, K., … Stanley, D. (2020). *LeMone and Burke's medical–surgical nursing: critical thinking for person-centred care* (4th [Australian] edn). Sydney: Pearson Australia.

Best, O. & Fredericks, B. (2021). *Yatdjuligin: Aboriginal and Torres Strait Islander nursing and midwifery care* (3rd edn). Port Melbourne, VIC: Cambridge University Press.

Brennan, S., Baird, A.-M., O'Regan, E. & Sheils, O. (2021). The role of human papilloma virus in dictating outcomes in head and neck squamous cell carcinoma. *Frontiers in Molecular Biosciences* 8:677900. https://doi.org/10.3389/fmolb.2021.677900.

Bullock, S. & Manias, E. (2022). *Fundamentals of pharmacology* (9th edn). Sydney: Pearson Australia.

Cancer Council Australia Clinical Guidelines (2021). *Clinical practice guidelines for the diagnosis and management of melanoma.* Sydney: Cancer Council Australia. https://wiki.cancer.org.au/australia/Guidelines:Melanoma.

Chai, H., Chaudhari, N., Kornhaber, R., Cuttle, L., Fear, M., Wood, F. & Martin, L. (2022). Chemical burn to the skin: a systematic review of first aid impacts on clinical outcomes. *Burns* 48(7):1527–43. https://doi.org/10.1016/j.burns.2022.05.006.

Chao, T., Parry, I., Palackic, A., Sen, S., Spratt, H., Mlcak, R.P., … Suman, O.E. (2022). The effects of short bouts of ergometric exercise for severely burned children in intensive care: a randomized controlled trial. *Clinical Rehabilitation* 36(8):1052–61. https://doi.org/10.1177/02692155221095643.

Cushing, T.A. & Wright, R.K. (2020). Electrical injuries in emergency medicine. *Emecidine*. https://emedicine.medscape.com/article/770179-overview.

Das, K., Cockerell, C.J., Patil, A., Pietkiewicz, P., Giulini, M., Grabbe, S. & Goldust, M. (2021). Machine learning and its application in skin cancer. *International Journal of Environmental Research and Public Health* 18(24), 13409. https://doi.org/10.3390/ijerph182413409.

Dreyfuss, I., Kamath, P., Frech, F., Hernandez, L. & Nouri, K. (2022). Squamous cell carcinoma: 2021 updated review of treatment. *Dermatologic Therapy* 35(4):e15308. https://doi.org/10.1111/dth.15308.

Duncanson, M., Oben, G., Adams, J., Richardson, G., Wicken, A. & Pierson, M. (2019). *Health and wellbeing of under-15 year olds in Aotearoa 2018 (National Health and wellbeing of under-15 year olds).* Dunedin: New Zealand Child and Youth Epidemiology Service. http://hdl.handle.net/10523/9641.

Environmental Health Indicators New Zealand (EHINZ) (2021). *Melanoma*. Wellington: EHINZ, Massey University. https://www.ehinz.ac.nz/indicators/uv-exposure/melanoma/.

Gandhi, G., Parashar, A. & Sharma, R.K. (2022). Epidemiology of electrical burns and its impact on quality of life—the developing world scenario. *World Journal of Critical Care Medicine* 11(1):58–69. https://doi.org/10.5492/wjccm.v11.i1.58.

Hedberg, M.L., Berry, C.T., Moshiri, A.S., Xiang, Y., Yeh, C.J., Attilasoy, C., … Seykora, J.T. (2022). Molecular mechanisms of cutaneous squamous cell carcinoma. *International Journal of Molecular Sciences* 23(7):3478. https://doi.org/10.3390/ijms23073478.

Jones, O.T., Matin, R.N., van der Schaar, M., Prathivadi Bhayankaram, K., Ranmuthu, C.K.I., Islam, M.S., … Walter, F.M. (2022). Artificial intelligence and machine learning algorithms for early detection of skin cancer in community and primary care settings: a systematic review. *The Lancet* 4(6), e466–e476. https://doi.org/10.1016/S2589-7500 (22)00023-1.

Long, B., Graybill, J.C. & Rosenberg, H. (2021). Just the facts: evaluation and management of thermal burns. *Canadian Journal of Emergency Medicine* 24):128–30. https://doi.org/10.1007/s43678-021-00222-8.

Lu, P., Holden, D., Padiglione, A. & Cleland, H. (2022). Perioperative antibiotic prophylaxis in Australian burns patients. *Australasian Journal of Plastic Surgery* 5(1):48–55. https://www.researchgate.net/publication/359653585_Perioperative_antibiotic_prophylaxis_in_Australian_burns_patients

Marchalik, R., Rada, E.M., Albino, F.P., Sauerhammer, T.M., Boyajian, M.J., Rogers, G.F. & Oh, A.K. (2018). Upper extremity friction burns in the pediatric patient: a 10-year review. *Plastic and Reconstructive Surgery—Global Open* 6(12):e2048. https://doi.org/10.1097/GOX.0000000000002048.

Marieb, E.N. & Hoehn, K. (2019). *Human anatomy and physiology* (11th edn). San Francisco, CA: Pearson Benjamin Cummings.

Markiewicz-Gospodarek, A., Kozioł, M., Tobiasz, M., Baj, J., Radzikowska-Büchner, E. & Przekora, A. (2022). Burn wound healing: clinical complications, medical care, treatment, and dressing types: the current state of knowledge for clinical practice. *International Journal of Environmental Research and Public Health* 19(3):1338. https://doi.org/10.3390/ijerph19031338.

Menz, B.D., Charani, E., Gordon, D.L., Leather, A.J.M., Moonesinghe, S.R. & Phillips, C.J. (2021). Surgical antibiotic prophylaxis in an era of antibiotic resistance: common resistant bacteria and wider considerations for practice. *Infection and Drug Resistance* 14:5235–52. https://doi.org/10.2147/IDR.S319780.

Najjar, T. (2021). Cutaneous squamous cell carcinoma. *Emedicine*. https://emedicine.medscape.com/article/1965430.

New Zealand Ministry of Health (2021). *New cancer registrations 2019: melanoma—C43 by rate and ethnicity*. Wellington: Ministry of Health. https://www.health.govt.nz/publication/new-cancer-registrations-2019.

Nischwitz, S.P., Luze, H., Popp, D., Winter, R., Draschl, A., Schellnegger, M., … Kamolz, L.-P. (2021). Global burn care and the ideal burn dressing reloaded—a survey of global experts. *Burns* 47(7):1665–74. https://doi.org/10.1016/j.burns.2021.02.008.

Introduction

This chapter focuses on selected bites and stings from various animals. The selection of the spider and snake species discussed is based on the most common bites that cause hospitalisation. Tick bites are also addressed. Wasp and bee stings are discussed, including the reactions experienced after a sting and the appropriate management. Various concepts regarding bites and stings from various marine animals are also examined, including frequency, cause and management, with a particular focus on Irukandji jellyfish.

Although statistics regarding bites and stings are reported by the Australian Institute of Health and Welfare (AIHW), many of those who are bitten or stung manage the injury themselves without ever presenting to a medical facility or healthcare professional for assistance. Therefore, the statistics represented are those of bites and stings that result in hospitalisation.

According to the AIHW, from 2019 to 2020 approximately 25,000 Australians experienced 'contact with living things' (animals, insects and plants) which resulted in injury requiring hospitalisation (more than 50% of these involved dogs). Males received approximately than 57% of the injuries. During 2019–20, 2,465 people were admitted because of toxic effects resulting from bites and stings. Nineteen per cent of these bites were from spiders, with redback spider bites being the most common. Other spiders causing concern include the funnel-web and the white-tailed spiders. Approximately 17% of injuries requiring hospitalisation included envenomation from snakes, such as brown, black and tiger snakes. Wasps and bee stings accounted for more than 26%, and marine animals caused approximately 7% of all hospital presentations. Even though Australia has five of the top 10 most venomous animals in the world and 20 of the 25 most venomous snakes, there are only approximately 20 deaths per year related to envenomation, nationally.

Spider bites

LEARNING OBJECTIVE 1

Discuss the epidemiology related to spider bite hospitalisations in Australia.

Although Australians are more likely to experience a bite from a spider requiring hospitalisation than they are from a snake, statistics from Australian Poisons Information Centres indicate that calls about spider bites are far more frequent than calls about snake bites. While in 45% of spider bites the type of spider remains unidentified, redbacks (see Figure 45.1A) are responsible for 42% of all identified spider bites. The first death from a redback spider bite since 1999 occurred in April 2016, as redback spider bites do not generally result in significant sequelae. It should also be noted that in this incident the cause of death was inconclusive. The white-tailed spider (see Figure 45.1B) is the second most common type of spider bite in Australia (> 7%). Although previously this species was thought to contribute to significant skin ulceration (i.e. necrotising arachnidism), the emerging evidence suggests otherwise. It is highly likely that most, possibly all, of these cases of ulceration attributed to white-tailed spiders were actually from some other cause. Funnel-web spiders (see Figure 45.1C) are responsible for < 4% of bites. This type of spider has generally limited distribution, living mostly around the eastern seaboard. There are over 40 species of funnel-web spider, and potentially all may be dangerous, but only a few species appear likely to bite and significantly envenom humans. Although they have developed a reputation for their deadliness, no deaths have been recorded since 1981 when the **antivenom** became available.

New Zealand has few medically significant venomous spiders. Black widows (Māori: *katipō*—night stinger) and eastern Australian redbacks are the most common species in this country.

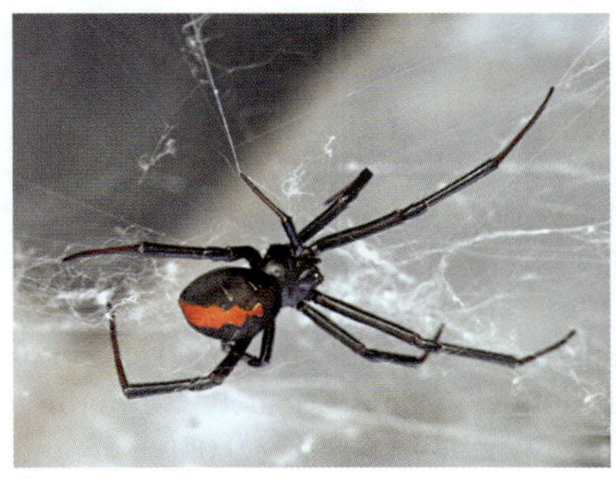
A

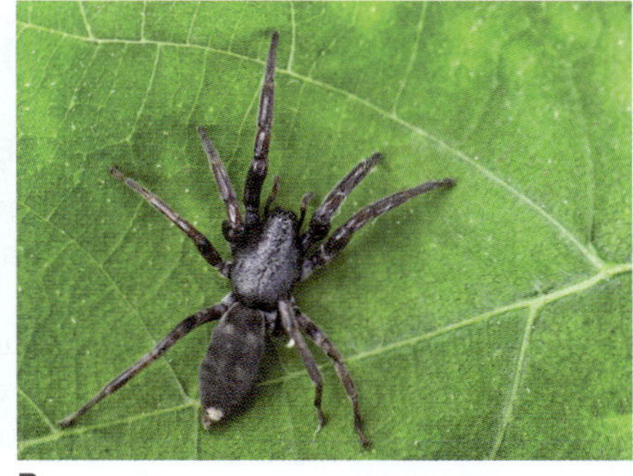
B

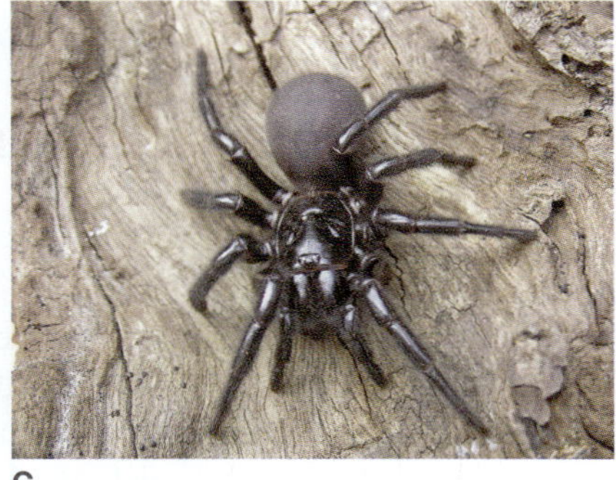
C

Figure 45.1

Spiders whose bites are associated with high rates of hospitalisation

(A) Redback spider. (B) White-tailed spider. (C) Funnel-web spider.

Sources: (A) Peter Waters/Shutterstock; (B) ChameleonsEye/Shutterstock; (C) James van den Broek/Shutterstock.

AETIOLOGY AND PATHOPHYSIOLOGY

LEARNING OBJECTIVE 2

Describe the cutaneous and systemic pathophysiology of common spider envenomations.

Even though redback spider **venom** contains an excitatory **neurotoxin**, and envenoming is common, it is rare for redback spider bites to cause a major clinical threat. Funnel-web spiders have highly toxic venom, and for some species the male spider's venom is significantly more toxic than the female's. The venom contains an excitatory neurotoxin. Fortunately, only a few bites result in **envenomation** (the injection of toxin by the venomous animal into the victim's tissue) and systemic effects. Figure 45.2 explores the clinical manifestations and management of some common spider bites.

CLINICAL MANIFESTATIONS

Redback spider bites begin as a sting and then can progress to severe pain. Bites are commonly associated with a distinctive area of localised sweating, and the skin around the bite may be erythematous or blanched. The pain and sweating may extend over time to involve the whole bitten limb or even the entire body, and there may be associated hypertension. Even if severe, it is unlikely that envenomation will cause death. The bitten person may complain of nausea or malaise, but most instances of redback spider bite do not require hospital admission.

White-tailed spider bites will cause pain and a local inflammatory reaction. Although the venom was once considered to be a necrotising substance, there is strong evidence that it does not damage skin.

Funnel-web spider bites can cause local pain, and often the spider may hang on. However, if systemic envenomation has occurred, a person may develop lip paraesthesia and tongue fasciculation (i.e. twitching) followed by piloerection, diaphoresis, lacrimation and salivation within 10 or more minutes. Tachycardia and hypertension follow quickly. As the systemic effects of a severe envenomation continue, airway obstruction may occur from vomiting, and pulmonary oedema can also develop. Fasciculation and unconsciousness may occur, and ventilatory support is required.

CLINICAL DIAGNOSIS AND MANAGEMENT

Diagnosis

Generally, the diagnosis of spider bites relies on consideration of the history and visual inspection of the affected site. Sometimes, individuals may bring the spider (dead or alive) with them. This may assist in identification, and, as with any other venomous bite/sting, if the suspected offending organism is presented it should be kept for later identification by an expert.

Management

Generally speaking, reassurance and symptom relief is the main management strategy for spider bites. Although only 10–20% of bites result in envenomation, it is important to rule out systemic effects. In cases where the diagnosis is in doubt, observations should be made frequently, and if after about six hours no significant local or systemic effects are detected, the person can be discharged. For known or suspected funnel-web spider bites and mouse spider bites ('big black spider' bites), the affected person should be observed for four hours, and if they have remained asymptomatic throughout they may be safely discharged (as significant envenoming always manifests within the first four hours), but if appropriate first aid has been used (such as application of a pressure bandage and immobilisation of the affected limb), then a longer observation period may be required, to cover a four-hour period from the time of pressure bandage removal. Suspected redback spider bites require observation only if the person is symptomatic, and then for six hours post-bite (longer if they have significant and ongoing symptoms requiring treatment to resolve).

- *Redback* antivenom is available and is the most commonly used antivenom in Australia, with a good safety record. It is used not to save life, but to relieve symptoms resistant to other treatments (analgesia), and for significant or major local, regional or systemic envenoming. Recent reports suggesting that the antivenom may not be effective are inconsistent with decades of experience of treating redback spider bites. Pressure immobilisation is not recommended with a redback spider bite, as it may significantly exacerbate the pain experienced. Ice packs may be beneficial.
- *White-tailed spider* bites rarely require medical attention, but people need reassurance that the common mythology that bites cause skin ulcers is untrue. Occasionally, treatment for a secondary infection may be required. There is no antivenom available for white-tailed spider bites.
- *Funnel-web spider* bites require pressure-immobilisation first aid to retard venom distribution. Basic life support and symptom management is required in severe cases. Generally, only severe envenomations result in systemic effects; however, if not treated, funnel-web spider bites can be fatal. An antivenom exists, and is highly successful and relatively safe.

Snake bites

LEARNING OBJECTIVE 3

Discuss the epidemiology related to snake bite hospitalisations in Australia.

Although there are approximately 5.4 million snakebites worldwide each year resulting in approximately 2.7 million envenomations, Australia experiences only 0.05% of this number. The three most common snake bites in Australia are from the brown snake (genus *Pseudonaja*; multiple species including the dugite and gwardar)—70% of all recorded snake bite deaths in Australia in the past 20 years—the mulga snake/black snake group (genus *Pseudechis*) and the tiger snake group (principally the tiger snake, *Notechis scutatus*, but also related species such as the rough-scaled snake, *Tropidechis carinatus*).

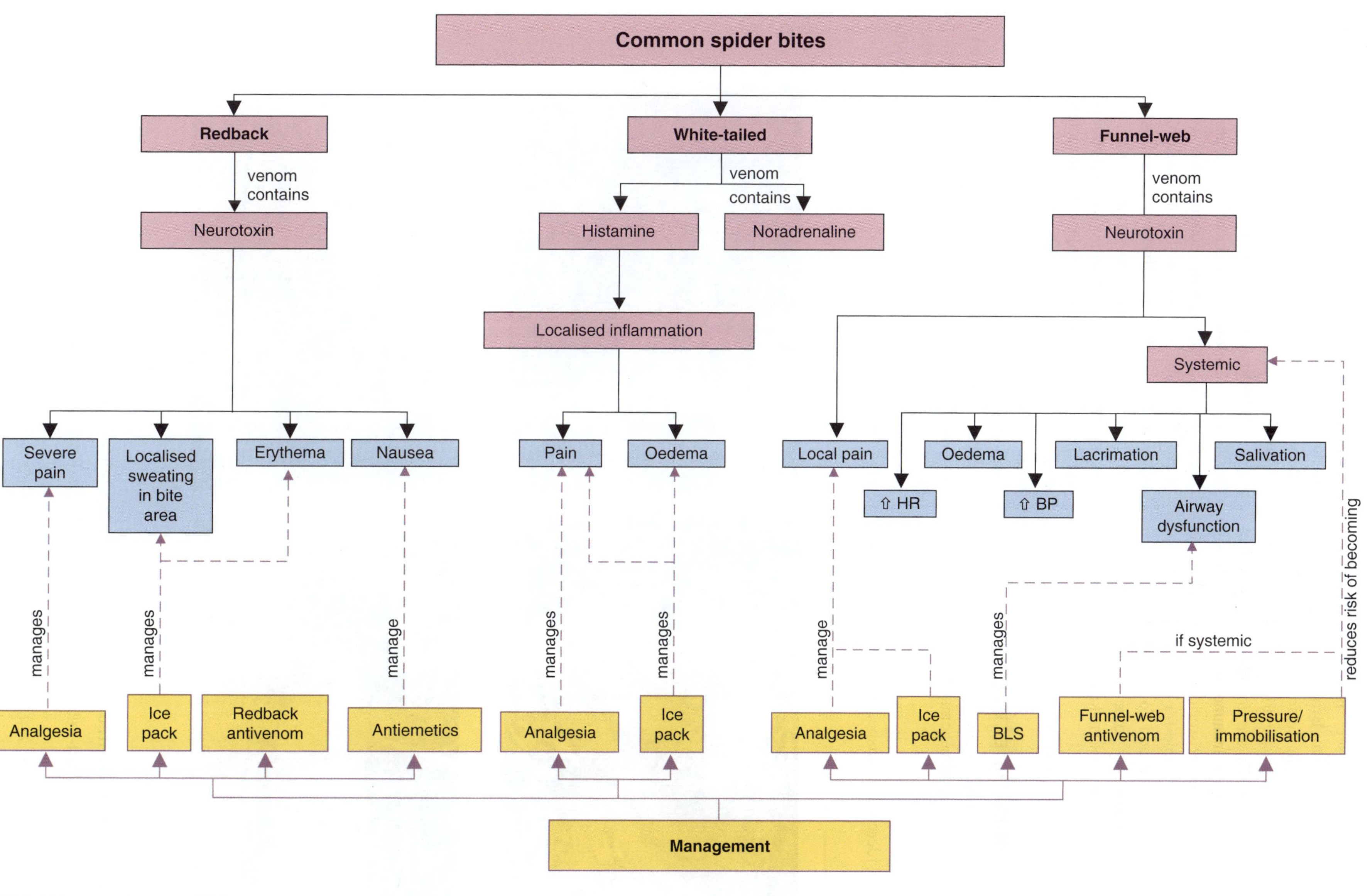

Figure 45.2

Clinical snapshot: Common spider bites

↑ = increased; BLS = basic life support; BP = blood pressure; HR = heart rate.

There are many types of brown snake. Several are endemic to most of Australia. Brown snakes (see Figure 45.3A) are about 1.5 m long, but can grow to over 2 m. Brown snake bites are the leading cause of snake bite death in Australia.

The red-bellied black snake (see Figure 45.3B) and the mulga snake (see Figure 45.3C) are members of the black snake genus and share a common **immunotype** (i.e. have venom that is immunologically similar). Historically, tiger snakes (see Figure 45.3D) have been responsible for many snake bites and fatalities, but changes in habitat and food sources may have reduced numbers significantly in some areas, and they are currently less common as a cause of snake bite.

AETIOLOGY AND PATHOPHYSIOLOGY

LEARNING OBJECTIVE 4

Describe the cutaneous and systemic pathophysiology of common snake envenomations.

Although not all snake bites result in envenomation, all snake bites should be considered as a suspected envenomation until ruled out. Australian snake venoms cause one or more of the following clinical effects in humans, depending on the species: (1) flaccid neurotoxic paralysis caused by pre and post synaptic neurotoxins; (2) systemic myolysis of skeletal muscle caused by myotoxic phospholipases; (3) procoagulant coagulopathy causing defibrination (consumption of the clot-forming protein, fibrinogen), resulting in reduced protection against severe bleeding; (4) anticoagulant coagulopathy causing inhibition of clot formation and potentially increased bleeding; (5) acute kidney injury, usually caused by secondary effects of envenoming, and potentially resulting in severe renal impairment; and (6) a syndrome similar to thrombotic thrombocytopenic purpura and haemolytic uraemic syndrome, characterised by severe thrombocytopenia, intravascular haemolysis, anaemia and renal failure (sometimes called 'MAHA'—*m*icro*a*ngiopathic *h*aemolytic *a*naemia).

The eastern brown snake's venom is considered to be the second most potent in the world, and contains potent procoagulants and neurotoxins. Tiger snake venom is extremely toxic, and contains neurotoxins, myolysins and procoagulants.

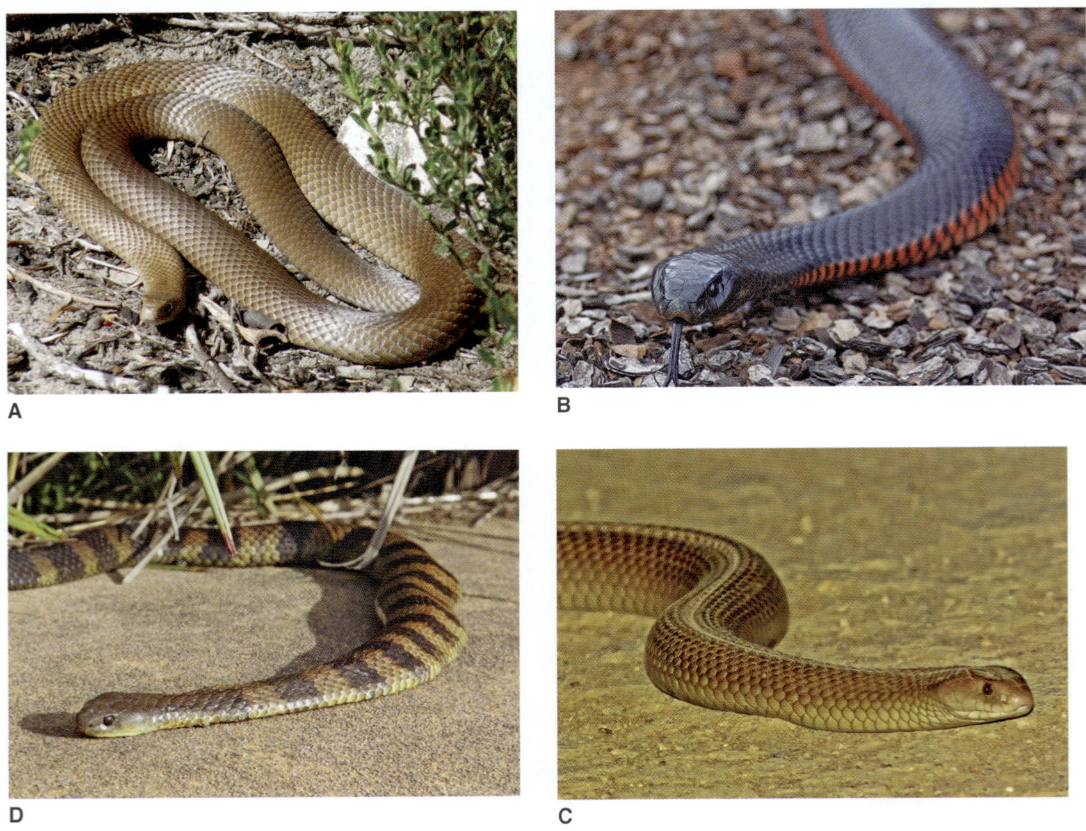

Figure 45.3

Snakes whose bites are associated with high rates of hospitalisation

(A) Eastern brown snake. (B) Red-bellied black snake. (C) Mulga (king brown) snake. (D) Tiger snake.

Sources: (A) © Sylvie Lebchek/Shutterstock; (B) Lakeview Images/Shutterstock; (C) Gypsytwitcher/Shutterstock; (D) dirkr/Shutterstock.

CLINICAL MANIFESTATIONS

LEARNING OBJECTIVE 5

Explain the factors associated with the decision to administer antivenom in snake bite envenomation.

Envenoming by all Australian venomous snakes can cause general non-specific symptoms, including headache, nausea, vomiting, abdominal pain and, less commonly, brief collapse and convulsions. In a small minority of cases the collapse may be cardiac, with dysrhythmias or cardiac arrest, often with a fatal outcome.

Brown snakes have small fangs and limited venom, and initially their bites can often be difficult to detect on the skin. The affected area may not demonstrate erythema, bruising or oedema. The person may complain of non-specific symptoms, such as headache, nausea and abdominal pain, or may be asymptomatic, despite severe defibrination coagulopathy. Defibrination coagulopathy is the classic feature of major envenoming by brown snakes, while paralysis is rare. Urine output should be monitored for signs of kidney damage.

Black snakes (including the mulga snake) can cause significant pain and oedema at the affected bite site, and the area may also be bruised. Local necrosis at the site is rare. They commonly cause non-specific symptoms such as vomiting and abdominal pain. Black snakes occasionally cause significant myolysis and mild anticoagulant coagulopathy, but these features are more common and severe with mulga snake bites.

The tiger snake can cause significant pain, erythema, oedema and bruising at the bite site, and can cause non-specific symptoms such as headache, nausea, abdominal pain, and potentially systemic collapse or seizure. Defibrination coagulopathy, flaccid paralysis and myolysis are all common features of tiger snake envenoming. All may develop within hours unless antivenom is administered, but, as with other snake bites, not every case develops significant envenoming.

CLINICAL DIAGNOSIS AND MANAGEMENT

Diagnosis

Health professionals must take an adequate history in order to assist in determining the likelihood of envenomation and the identification of the type of snake involved. However, in individuals presenting with unconscious collapse, seizures, coagulopathy, myolysis or paralysis, the cause may not necessarily be obvious. Visual inspection is imperative to identify possible bite marks, but if a first aid bandage is in place, do not remove it; just cut a small window over the bite area. Do not wash or clean the bite area, as this interferes with venom detection. If antivenom is required it is preferable to use a 'specific' rather than 'polyvalent' antivenom, but to do this the venom immunotype must be known. This is ascertained by a combination of venom detection (the Commonwealth Serum Laboratories [CSL] Snake Venom Detection Kit [SVDK], see Figure 45.4) and consulting diagnostic algorithms for snakebite (see local policy and procedures). If in any doubt, seek expert advice from a clinical toxinologist (e.g. through CSL, the South Australia Toxinology Service or a Poisons Information Centre).

Management

First aid management for Australian snake bite consists of attempting to reduce the spread of venom. Immobilisation of the limb/affected area is critical. Pressure immobilisation bandages should be applied to reduce venom spread, and medical assistance should be sought immediately. Treatment of envenomation is generally based on clinical circumstances. There is a general approach to managing snake bite, but details of treatment—such as the type and the dose of antivenom

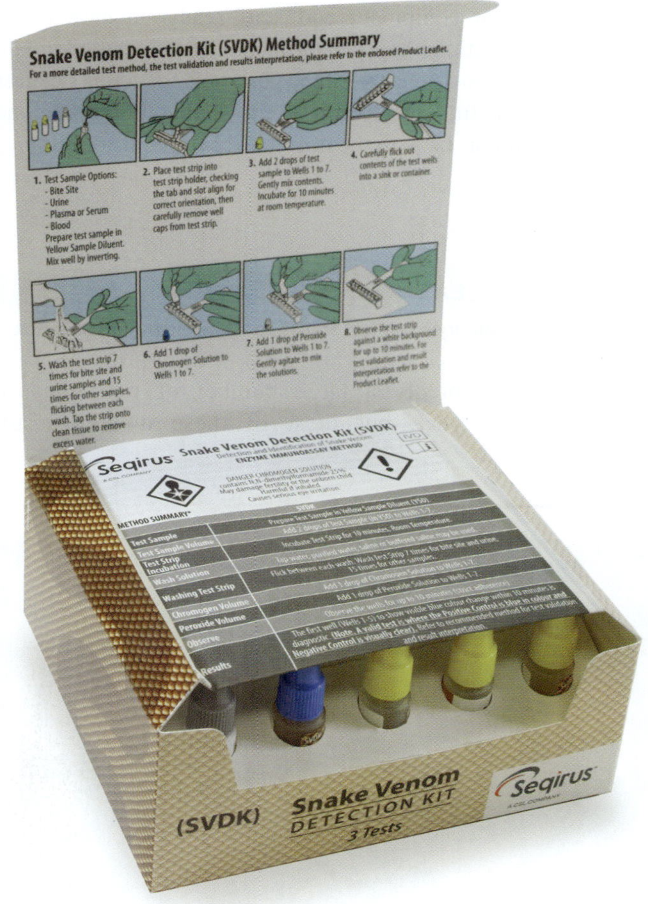

Figure 45.4

Snake Venom Detection Kit (SVDK) test

Source: © Commonwealth Serum Laboratories.

plus ancillary treatments—will vary depending on the type of snake. Snake antivenoms available are brown, black, death adder, Taipan, tiger snake, and a polyvalent snake antivenom (containing antibodies of all five serotypes previously listed) which can be used when symptoms of envenomation are exhibited, but the snake has not be positively identified.

Every suspected snake bite should be managed as a priority; promptly and fully assessed, including appropriate blood tests; and then either treated with antivenom if significantly envenomed, or observed with serial repeat blood tests if apparently non-envenomed. In most areas it is acceptable to discharge someone who has not been envenomed after 12 hours of observation (but do not discharge at night), providing there has been no evidence of envenoming, including repeated blood tests. Those showing evidence of significant envenoming—such as features of one or more of developing paralysis, myolysis, coagulopathy, renal damage or MAHA—will generally require antivenom treatment.

However, while antivenom is potentially life-saving, it does carry some risks and should be used only when indicated, and should not be given to people who have not been envenomed. It should be given only in a hospital setting, with adrenaline and resuscitation equipment and staff ready, in case of an anaphylactic reaction. Any person receiving antivenom should be advised, prior to discharge, of the possibility of **serum sickness** (see the chapter 'Immune disorders'), told what to look for, and instructed to report back to the hospital if symptoms develop.

Tick bites

LEARNING OBJECTIVE 6

Discuss the challenges related to the removal of a paralysis tick.

There are undoubtedly a large number of tick bites in Australia every year, but most of these do not result in hospital attendance. Approximately 170 bites occur each year from the Australian paralysis tick (*Ixodes holocyclus*) (see Figure 45.5), and those bitten do seek medical attention. In a few cases, serious consequences can result from envenomation. Paralysis and, rarely, **anaphylaxis** can develop, and children are at most risk. Tick paralysis has killed more people than funnel-web spider bites. *Zoonotic disease transmission* can also occur; an example of this is Australian tick typhus (spotted fever).

AETIOLOGY AND PATHOPHYSIOLOGY

The saliva of the Australian paralysis tick contains a toxin called *holocyclotoxin*, which interferes with presynaptic transmission in motor neurons. Holocyclotoxin is transferred to a person when the tick feeds on the person's blood, and causes inhibition of acetylcholine release at the neuromuscular junction. This leads to skeletal muscle paralysis. Diaphragmatic paralysis is life-threatening, and should be considered in severe envenomations.

Tick *allergy* is another concern. Allergic reactivity can range from discomfort associated with a local inflammatory response, causing pruritus and erythema (common), to anaphylaxis (rare).

CLINICAL MANIFESTATIONS

Depending on the species of tick, local inflammatory reactions are common and can result in a pruritic, erythematous rash and extensive bruising that lasts for weeks. Secondary skin infections may occur as a result of the break in the integumentary barrier. Localised ulceration can also occur if the mouth part is detached during removal of the tick. However, the greatest concern is an ascending flaccid paralysis (a type of paralysis that begins distally and progresses towards the trunk).

There is no antivenom for tick paralysis, the previous product having been withdrawn from the market, so treatment is

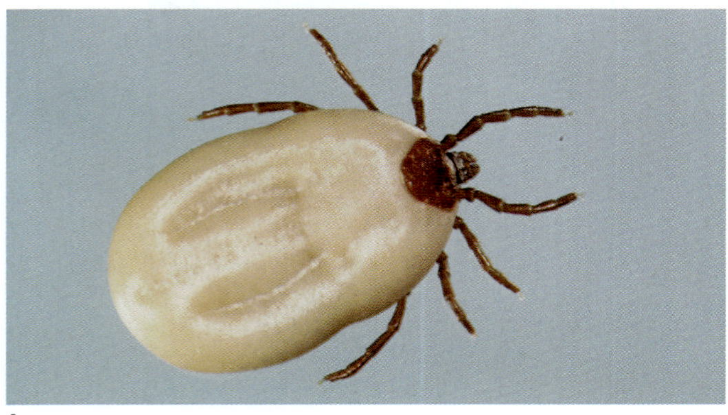

A

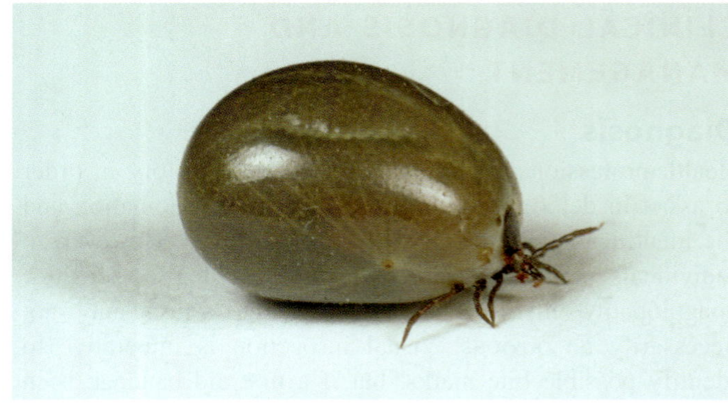

B

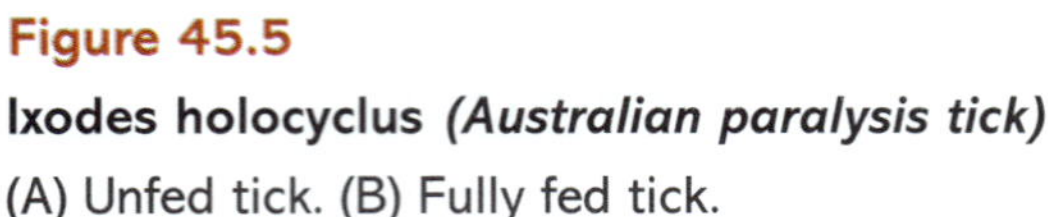

Figure 45.5

Ixodes holocyclus *(Australian paralysis tick)*

(A) Unfed tick. (B) Fully fed tick.

Source: Nigel Cattlin/Alamy Stock Photo.

supportive, including intubation and ventilation if required, and symptomatic. The tick's role as a vector for several bacterial, viral and protozoan diseases can result in Lyme disease and Australian tick typhus (spotted fever). Exacerbation generally occurs when the tick is being removed.

CLINICAL DIAGNOSIS AND MANAGEMENT

Diagnosis

Appropriate consideration of the history and a visual inspection of the affected area are critical. There are no reliable skin tests or laboratory investigations to determine tick allergy.

Management

Prevention of tick exposure is paramount for those who have previously experienced a serious **hypersensitivity reaction** (see the chapter 'Immune disorders'). If a person lives in tick-prone areas, it may also be necessary for them to be issued an adrenaline autoinjector (e.g. EpiPen). When in environments renowned for ticks, measures to reduce tick bite should be instigated. Wearing long-sleeved shirts and trousers, and scanning for ticks is important.

Initial first aid management consists of basic life support and seeking urgent medical assistance. The tick should never be forcefully removed by inexperienced individuals, as this will promote the release of more toxic salivary proteins. Symptomatic treatment and supportive care (intubation and ventilation if there is respiratory paralysis) is the key part of clinical management, plus removal of any embedded ticks. Particularly check the scalp, ears and any areas of skin folds. Ticks should be levered off from around the mouth parts.

Wasp and bee stings

LEARNING OBJECTIVE 7

Compare and contrast the management of a normal reaction and anaphylaxis related to a bee or wasp sting.

Approximately 1,300 stings from wasps and bees requiring hospitalisation occur each year in Australia, and most occur in males. In New Zealand, one person dies every year from wasp or bee stings, and about 2% of the population have a hypersensitivity to bee or wasp venom.

AETIOLOGY AND PATHOPHYSIOLOGY

When a wasp or bee sting penetrates the skin, over *10 different antigens* are injected. Acetylcholine and serotonin are also present in the venom. The *acetylcholine* innervates the dermal nociceptors, causing intense pain, and the *serotonin* causes intense vasospasm. Other substances within the venom cause mast cell degranulation and promote an inflammatory response. The site of the sting becomes erythematous and oedematous, and this may persist for several hours.

Upon sensitisation by past exposure, some individuals may develop an *immunoglobulin-E (IgE)-mediated type I hypersensitivity reaction*, resulting in a dangerous systemic reaction. Urticaria and pruritic wheals may develop. A severe reaction may result in anaphylactic shock.

CLINICAL MANIFESTATIONS

Depending on previous sensitisation, the affected area may develop a painful, erythematous, pruritic wheal (welt) with associated oedema, or the person may develop a hypersensitivity response ranging from mild to anaphylactic. A puncture at the centre of the sting wound may be visible.

With a bee sting, the sting and venom gland usually remain in situ unless scraped off. The sting needs to be scraped away quickly in the opposite direction of its entry, as it can keep delivering venom. Occasionally, a secondary skin infection may occur at the site of the sting.

If an anaphylactic reaction occurs in a previously sensitised person, they may, within minutes, develop hives, angioedema (see Figure 45.6), dyspnoea, nausea and vomiting, and hypotension. This situation is potentially life-threatening.

CLINICAL DIAGNOSIS AND MANAGEMENT

Diagnosis

Attention to the presentation and history should be considered, along with a visual inspection of the affected site. No laboratory test is available to assist in the diagnosis of wasp or bee sting.

Management

The local reaction can be managed with the application of ice to reduce swelling. If the erythema continues for several days or the site becomes pustulous, the sting site may have a secondary

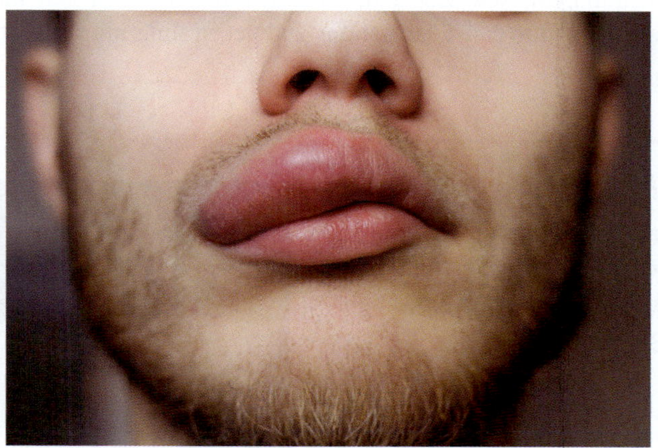

Figure 45.6

Anaphylaxis as a result of a bee sting

Angioedema in a previously sensitised person resulted in an exceedingly swollen lip.

Source: Velimir Zeland/Shutterstock.

bacterial infection and require antimicrobials. Antihistamines may assist with the urticarial reaction.

If anaphylaxis occurs, basic life support principles should be undertaken, followed by advanced cardiac life support. Intramuscularly or intravenously administered adrenaline may be required, depending on the systemic response. Oxygen and ventilator support is important for airway management. The bronchospasm should respond to systemic or nebulised adrenaline or nebulised salbutamol. Intravenous corticosteroids will dampen the immune system reactions.

Marine bites and stings

LEARNING OBJECTIVE 8

Describe the management of the most common marine bites and stings.

According to the AIHW, approximately 393 cases of marine bites and stings result in hospitalisation each year. The most common cause of marine stings is from jellyfish, most commonly the Irukandji jellyfish (*Carukia barnesi*) (see Figure 45.7A). Hence, this is the only marine sting or bite dealt with in this chapter. Other jellyfish are associated with fewer stings requiring hospitalisation. Box jellyfish (see Figure 45.7B) account for less than 3% of stings, while stings from the bluebottle and Pacific man-o-war combined represent less than 2.5% of hospitalised cases. Although these jellyfish are very common on many beaches during summer, they mostly cause only minor cases, and therefore medical intervention is not often sought.

Another marine animal responsible for stings is the stingray. In 2006, Steve Irwin, an Australian environmentalist and television presenter, died within minutes when he was struck by a stingray's barb in the middle of his chest, the barb penetrating his heart. Only three stingray deaths have been recorded in Australia. In New Zealand, stingrays are common and have been known to cause lacerations and penetrating injuries. Most stingray injuries are minor, and trauma from the sting is often more important than venom-induced pain.

AETIOLOGY AND PATHOPHYSIOLOGY

There are approximately 10 species of Irukandji jellyfish, ranging from 1 cm to 10 cm in diameter. They are most commonly found in north Queensland from November to May, but have also been seen in Western Australia. Individuals stung by Irukandji jellyfish can develop Irukandji syndrome. The mechanism of envenomation is not yet clear. However, given the clinical manifestations, it appears that the venom either causes the release of *catecholamines* or contains catecholamines (or catecholamine-like substances), plus **histamine** (and other inflammatory mediators) and possibly *cardiomyotoxins*.

CLINICAL MANIFESTATIONS

About 30 minutes after an Irukandji jellyfish sting, the affected person develops **Irukandji syndrome**. This syndrome includes symptoms such as severe lower back pain, muscle cramps, joint pain, nausea and anxiety, as well as signs such as diaphoresis, vomiting, tachycardia, profound hypertension and oliguria. Cardiac dysfunction and pulmonary oedema may develop.

In many cases, there may be little or no visible evidence of the sting, and the sting site can be small: less than 2 cm in diameter. Cutaneous manifestations of the sting can include an erythematous rash developing papules within five minutes of envenomation. The papules may subside within an hour of the sting, and the erythema may be visible for several days.

CLINICAL DIAGNOSIS AND MANAGEMENT

Diagnosis

The Irukandji jellyfish can be very difficult to see, and occasionally Irukandji syndrome can be misdiagnosed as myocardial infarction, cerebrovascular accident or decompression

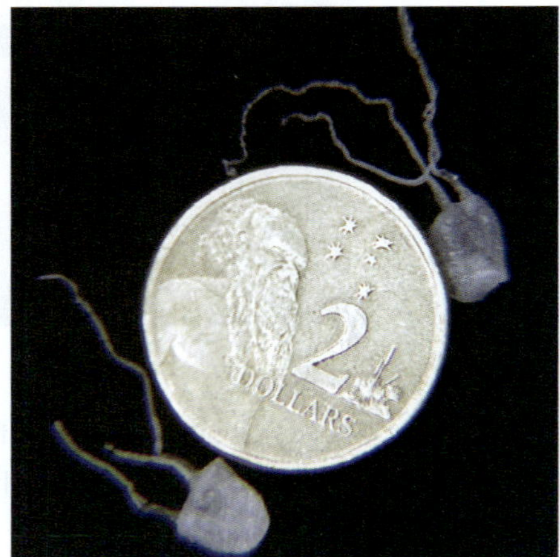

A

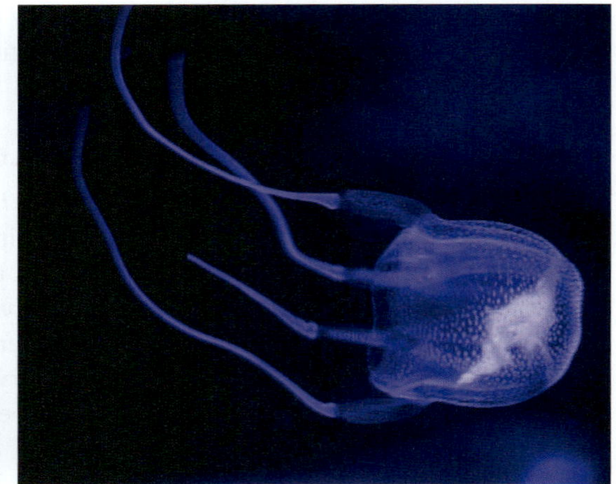

B

Figure 45.7

Jellyfish causing hospitalisation in Australia

(A) Irukandji jellyfish.
(B) Box jellyfish.

Sources: (A) Photographer: Graham Crouch/Newspix; (B) Dewald Kirsten/Shutterstock.

illness. However, the syndrome has two recognised sequelae of pain and catecholamine-like effects. Cardiotoxicity may or may not occur. Consideration of the history, the environment preceding the presentation and the clinical manifestations are the cornerstones of diagnosis of Irukandji syndrome.

Management

The Australian Resuscitation Council recommends that initial first aid should include the application of vinegar to reduce the envenomation, as acetic acid irreversibly inhibits the release of previously undischarged nematocysts (minute stinging capsules that line the tentacles of jellyfish and contain toxin). However, this management is based on limited scientific evidence of efficacy. More recently, attempts to reduce the severe pain through the application of heat have anecdotally provided more success. Research is needed to help with temperature recommendations, and also to confirm the results. Early reports suggest submerging the limb in water at a temperature as hot as the person can tolerate, and refreshing the water as the temperature cools. Early case reports have suggested that there is a significant reduction in pain and scarring following such heat treatment.

Analgesia is essential because of the severe, wave-like pain experienced. The development of profound hypertension may require the administration of antihypertensives in order to prevent a cerebrovascular accident. If pulmonary oedema occurs, airway management and oxygenation may be best achieved with positive pressure ventilation. There is currently no antivenom. The use of IV magnesium sulphate is controversial: some authors/publications suggest that it is effective, whereas emerging evidence suggests that it may offer no benefit. Resolution of this controversy will likely require further clinical trials.

INDIGENOUS HEALTH FAST FACTS AND CULTURAL CONSIDERATIONS

- *Aboriginal and Torres Strait Islander peoples use a variety of flora to relieve pain from bites and stings, such as crushed swamp lily, chewed shoots of grey mangrove (baru-baruga) or warmed bracken leaves.*
- *Māori apply the crushed leaves of the ngaio tree (*Myoporum laetum*) to relieve pain from bites and stings.*

CHILDREN AND ADOLESCENTS

- Children aged 5–14 years experience bites or stings requiring hospitalisation 2.3 times more than children aged 0–4. Boys are bitten or stung almost twice as many times as girls (a statistic that remains throughout all age groups).

OLDER ADULTS

- Older adults require hospitalisation for bites or stings almost as frequently (13 per 100,000) as younger adults (16 per 100,000). Fourteen per cent of people admitted to hospital for bites and stings are 65 years of age or older.

KEY CLINICAL ISSUES

- Most individuals who receive a bite from a spider, bee or wasp never present to an emergency department.
- Depending on the type of spider bite, symptoms may be as simple as mild pain, or as complex and dangerous as sympathetic nervous system reactions requiring intensive intervention. Depending on the envenomation, antivenom may not always be available for a spider bite.
- Globally, not all snake bites have an appropriate antivenom available, but in Australia antivenoms are available to cover all medically important species. The most appropriate management of any type of bite is symptom management; however, for major, potentially lethal envenoming where an antivenom is available (snakebite, funnel-web spider bite, etc.), antivenom therapy is a cornerstone of treatment. Ensure that airway and cardiovascular stability is achieved and sustained before discharge. Discharge education regarding signs and symptoms is also important for the person who has been bitten and for those with whom they are discharged.
- The most common marine bites and stings requiring hospitalisation are from the Irukandji jellyfish. Irukandji syndrome is dangerous and can develop as a result of Irukandji envenomation. Sympathetic nervous system effects are the hallmark of Irukandji jellyfish stings. Severe back pain and cardiovascular symptoms develop. Initial first aid management includes the topical application of vinegar and, later, potentially, intravenous magnesium infusion (although this remains controversial). In the near future, heat may be formally incorporated into management; however, more evidence is required before this technique becomes commonplace.

CHAPTER REVIEW

- *Redback spiders* cause the most spider bites requiring hospitalisation in Australia.
- *Redback spider bites* cause *severe pain* and distinctive *localised hyperhidrosis*.
- *Antivenom* is not available for most types of spiders, but it does exist for the medically important types of spider bites (funnel-web spiders and redback spiders).
- *Pressure immobilisation techniques* should be used for funnel-web spider bites to reduce venom spread, but should not be instituted in redback spider bites, as they may increase the pain by trapping the venom within the local area.
- *Brown snake bites* are the most common snake bite requiring hospitalisation in Australia.
- Not all snake bites result in envenomation.
- Snake venom may contain *neurotoxins, myolysins, anticoagulants* or *procoagulants*.
- *Snake venom detection kits* can be used to determine the immunotype of the snake, ensuring that the correct antivenom is given if available.
- *Tick bites* can cause local inflammatory reactions, pruritus and erythema.
- *Paralysis tick removal* should be performed cautiously.
- *Anaphylaxis* can occur with any bite or sting in a previously sensitised person.
- *Bee stings* must be removed quickly, as the remaining sting and venom gland can continue to deliver toxins.
- In Australia, *jellyfish* are the most common cause of marine stings.

REVIEW QUESTIONS

1. Using appropriate websites and government resources, identify the most current Australian epidemiology relating to common bites and stings for the following:
   a. snake bite
   b. spider bite
   c. marine animal bites and stings
   d. ticks
   e. bees and wasps
2. What types of cutaneous manifestations can occur with spider bites?
3. What types of systemic manifestations can occur with spider bites?
4. How do the management practices for the various common spider bites differ from each other?
5. What factors determine the need for antivenom administration for both snake and spider bites?
6. What is the basic first aid principle related to managing a snake bite?
7. How should paralysis ticks be removed?
8. What interventions should be undertaken when a person presents with a normal reaction to a wasp or bee sting?
9. What immediate and long-term interventions should be undertaken for a person presenting with anaphylaxis related to a bite?
10. How should Irukandji jellyfish stings be managed?

HEALTH PROFESSIONAL CONNECTIONS

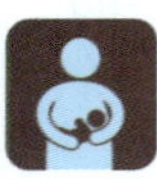

Exercise scientists People are at risk of exposure to bites and stings with boot-camp-style training, beach work and cross-country events. Exercise professionals should be familiar with the first aid management of common bites and stings. First aid equipment should be readily available at all training venues, sporting events and outdoor training sessions.

All allied professionals Bites and stings may still occur in healthcare facilities. It is the responsibility of all healthcare professionals to be mindful of these risks, especially in rural and remote facilities. When visiting people in their own home, the risk of bites and stings increases for the healthcare professional. Ensure that appropriate precautions are taken to protect oneself. Seek assistance where necessary. Report all concerns to supervisors, and follow through to ensure that interventions have occurred to remove the risk before the next visit.

CASE STUDY

Cody Wagner, a 5-year-old boy (UR number 804040), was brought in by his mother with a large localised reaction to a honey bee sting on the ventral side of his right hallux. His mother heard Cody's crying, but did not realise what had happened for several minutes. When she saw Cody's toe, the sting and the venom gland were still in situ. Cody's cries were increasing as time passed. On arrival to the emergency department, Cody was very distressed, holding his foot and crying. His observations were as follows:

Temperature	Heart rate	Respiration rate	Blood pressure	SpO_2
37.2°C	134	38	120/80	97% (RA*)

*RA = room air.

His right hallux was erythematous and oedematous. A small, single skin puncture was visible. An ice pack was applied, but, due to Cody's distress, it was difficult to maintain in place. He was given some oral paracetamol and promethazine elixirs. Over the next 20 minutes Cody became less distressed and went to sleep. He was monitored for a further two hours and discharged into the care of his mother.

CRITICAL THINKING

1 Where is Cody's sting? What is a hallux? Where is the ventral surface?
2 Why did Cody's distress increase for several minutes at the time of the initial injury, even after his mother had come?
3 Analyse Cody's observations. Are they within the reference range for a 5-year-old boy? Explain.
4 Identify all of the interventions undertaken. Explain the rationale for each of the interventions.
5 What discharge teaching does Cody's mother require?
6 Is there a risk that Cody may develop an anaphylactic reaction on the next sting? Explain the mechanism leading to the development of an anaphylactic reaction.

BIBLIOGRAPHY

Arrawarra Sharing Culture Project (2013a). *Fact sheet 14. Useful plants: leaves*. https://www.yumpu.com/s/PxTCdcl3vPjiSmei.

Arrawarra Sharing Culture Project (2013b). *Fact sheet 15. Bush medicine*. https://www.yumpu.com/s/PxTCdcl3vPjiSmei.

Australian Health Ministers' Advisory Council's National and Aboriginal and Torres Strait Islander Health Standing Committee (2017). *Cultural respect framework 2016–2026: for Aboriginal and Torres Strait Islander health—a national approach to building a culturally respectful health system*. Canberra: Australian Government Department of Health. https://nacchocommunique.files.wordpress.com/2016/12/cultural_respect_framework_1december2016_1.pdf.

Australian Institute of Health and Welfare (AIHW) (2021). *Venomous bites and stings 2017–18*. Cat. No. INJCAT 215. Canberra: AIHW. https://www.aihw.gov.au/reports/injury/venomous-bites-and-stings-2017-18/data.

Australian Institute of Health and Welfare (AIHW) (2022a). *Injury in Australia: contact with living things.* Canberra: AIHW. https://www.aihw.gov.au/reports/injcat/213-1/213/contact-with-living-things.

Australian Institute of Health and Welfare (AIHW) (2022b). *Principal diagnosis data cubes: separation statistics by principal diagnosis (ICD-10-AM, 11th edition) Australia, 2020–21.* Canberra: AIHW. https://www.aihw.gov.au/reports/hospitals/principal-diagnosis-data-cubes/contents/data-cubes.

Australian Institute of Health and Welfare (AIHW) & Pointer, S. (2021). *Venomous bites and stings, 2017–18*. Injury Research and Statistics series No. 134. Cat. No. INJCAT 215. Canberra: AIHW. https://www.aihw.gov.au/getmedia/78b416bf-0250-4368-89d6-81e2d9f32528/aihw-injcat-215.pdf.aspx.

Bauldoff, G., Gubrud-Howe, P.M., Carno, M.-A., Levett-Jones, T., Hales, M., Berry, K., ... Stanley, D. (2020). *LeMone and Burke's medical–surgical nursing: critical thinking for person-centred care* (4th [Australian] edn). Sydney: Pearson Australia.

Best, O. & Fredericks, B. (2021). *Yatdjuligin: Aboriginal and Torres Strait Islander nursing and midwifery care* (3rd edn). Port Melbourne, VIC: Cambridge University Press.

Bullock, S. & Manias, E. (2022). *Fundamentals of pharmacology* (9th edn). Sydney: Pearson Australia.

Department of Health (2013). *Arthropod pests of public health significance in Australia*. Canberra: Department of Health. https://www.health.gov.au/sites/default/files/documents/2022/07/enhealth-guidance-arthropod-pests-of-public-health-significance-in-australia.pdf.

Isbister, G.K. (2022). Marine envenomations from corals, sea urchins, fish, or stingrays. *UpToDate*. https://www.uptodate.com/contents/marine-envenomations-from-corals-sea-urchins-fish-or-stingrays.

Leversha, A. & Naylor, D. (2019). *Cellulitis—clinical guidelines*. https://starship.org.nz/guidelines/cellulitis/.

Marieb, E.N. & Hoehn, K. (2019). *Human anatomy and physiology* (11th edn). San Francisco, CA: Pearson Benjamin Cummings.

National Coronial Information System (NCIS) (2020). *NCIS Fact Sheet: animal-related deaths in Australia*. https://www.ncis.org.au/wp-content/uploads/2020/03/NCIS-fact-sheet-Animal-related-deaths.pdf.

Pucca, M.B., Knudsen, C., S. Oliveira, I.S., Rimbault, C., A. Cerni, F.A., Wen, F.H., ... Monteiro, W.M. (2020). Current knowledge on snake dry bites. *Toxins 12*(11):668. https://doi.org/10.3390/toxins12110668.

Rodriguez-Valle, M., McAlister, S., Moolhuijzen, P.M., Booth, M., Agnew, K., Ellenberger, C., ... Tabor, A.E. (2021). Immunomic investigation of holocyclotoxins to produce the first protective anti-venom vaccine against the Australian paralysis tick, *Ixodes holocyclus*. *Frontiers in Immunology* 12:744795. https://doi.org/10.3389/fimmu.2021.744795.

Ryan, R.Y.M., Seymour, J., Loukas, A., Lopez, J.A., Ikonomopoulou, M.P. & Miles, J.J. (2021). Immunological responses to envenomation. *Frontiers in Immunology,* 12:661082. https://doi.org/10.3389/fimmu.2021.661082.

Seqirus (2022). Antivenom range. *Bites and Stings*. https://www.bitesandstings.com.au/sites/default/files/resources/pdf/2020-12/seqirus-antivenom-range-brochure.pdf.

Seymour, J.E. (2017). Are we using the correct first aid for jellyfish? *Medical Journal of Australia* 206(6):249–50. https://www.mja.com.au/journal/2017/206/6/are-we-using-correct-first-aid-jellyfish.

Tibballs, J. (2020). Australian snake antivenom dosing: what is scientific and safe? *Anaesthesia and Intensive Care* 48(2):129–33. https://doi.org/10.1177/0310057X19865268.

White, J. (2022). Snakebites worldwide: management. *UpToDate*. https://www.uptodate.com/contents/snakebites-worldwide-management.

Glossary

Aβ-fibre (A-beta-fibre) Highly sensitive (low-threshold), thickly myelinated, afferent nerve fibres, mechanoreceptors, which are responsible for sensing touch.

Aδ-fibre (A-delta-fibre) A myelinated nerve fibre responsible for transmitting information about sharp pain and temperature from the peripheries to the brain. Considered to be a fast pain transmission.

absence seizure A form of epileptic generalised seizure that causes affected people to lose awareness of their surroundings and display a vacant stare. Also known as 'petit mal'.

acquired brain injury (ABI) An injury to the brain associated with the misuse or abuse of drugs and/or alcohol, or with stroke or tumours.

acquired immune deficiency syndrome (AIDS) The end stages of a disease caused by the human immunodeficiency virus (HIV), which destroys the immune system of infected individuals.

acromegaly A chronic condition caused by a metabolic disorder that results in the gradual elongation of the facial bones. Long bones of the extremities are often affected.

acute coronary syndrome A spectrum of conditions involving myocardial ischaemia, which includes presentations from angina to myocardial infarction with ST segment changes.

acute inflammation A condition involving tissue swelling and oedema that occurs within a short time (second, minutes, hours) of the insult, includes hyperaemia, increased vessel permeability and migration of neutrophils from the capillaries to the interstitial space.

acute kidney injury (AKI) A severe renal impairment that can develop suddenly and rapidly in the course of an acute insult to the kidneys.

acute lymphoblastic leukaemia (ALL) A type of cancer affecting the blood and bone marrow cells that produce lymphocytes. In ALL, an abnormally high production of immature lymphoblasts is produced, crowding the bone marrow.

acute myelogenous leukaemia (AML) The collective name for a group of eight subtypes of blood cell cancer that develop in myeloid cells found in the bone marrow. The myeloid cell line includes erythrocytes, thrombocytes and all leukocytes (except lymphocytes). AML affects very immature cells and develops quickly; therefore, it is classified as acute. (Compare with *chronic myelogenous leukaemia*.)

acute tubular necrosis (ATN) A condition affecting the kidney that results in damage to the renal tubules owing to either hypoxia or toxic substances.

Addison's disease A serious condition caused by the loss of function of the adrenal cortex.

adenoma A benign tumour arising from epithelial tissues in the colon.

adhesions Fibrous bands of scar tissue that connect tissue or organs that are not normally stuck together.

adrenal cortex The outer part of the adrenal gland, it secretes cortisol and androgens.

adrenal insufficiency An inability of the cortex of the adrenal glands (the endocrine gland on top of the kidney) to produce enough cortisol and/or aldosterone to serve the body's needs.

adrenal medulla The inner part of the adrenal gland, it secretes catecholamines such as adrenaline and noradrenaline.

aetiology The study of the cause of a disease.

afterload The resistance that the left ventricle must overcome to eject its contents.

age-related maculopathy The most common cause of loss of vision in older people, it causes a progressive blurring or loss of central vision from damage to the macula.

age-standardised An epidemiological technique adjusting the crude rate of the study population to accommodate for differences in population age structure.

agranulocytosis A significantly decreased number of granulocytes (neutrophils, eosinophils and basophils). Also known as 'neutropenia'.

airway hyperresponsiveness An increased sensitivity of the bronchi and bronchioles to bronchoconstricting stimuli.

aldosterone A mineralocorticoid hormone produced by the adrenal cortex.

allodynia A sensation of pain to a stimulus that would normally be innocuous.

Alma Ata declaration A document signed in 1978 at an international conference on primary healthcare in order to facilitate an acceptable level of health for all by the year 2000.

alopecia Loss of hair to an area of the body as a result of damage to the hair shaft and follicle.

α_1-antitrypsin An antiprotease protein produced by the liver that is responsible for preventing excessive destruction of alveolar cells from neutrophil elastase.

Alzheimer's disease (AD) A progressive and irreversible disease resulting in significant brain damage, causing dementia.

amenorrhoea The absence of a woman's menstrual period.

anaemia An abnormally low level of haemoglobin circulating in the blood. This may be due to a decrease in the production of functional red blood cells, or an increase in the destruction or loss of red blood cells.

analgesic An agent that provides pain relief.

anaphylaxis A potentially life-threatening, multisystem allergic reaction that can occur within 20 minutes of exposure to an allergen. It is classed as a type I hypersensitivity reaction.

anaplastic Pertaining to anaplasia. Anaplasia is the change in a cell to a less differentiated (more primitive) form. Anaplasia occurs in cancer cells, especially in malignancy.

androgens Any hormones of the steroid group responsible for male characteristics.

aneuploidy A variation in the number of chromosomes. There may be fewer (e.g. monosomy: one copy of chromosome 6, as in Turner syndrome) or more chromosomes (e.g. trisomy: three copies of chromosome 21, as in Down syndrome).

aneurysm A dilation in the wall of a blood vessel (generally an artery) from vascular disease, such as atherosclerosis.

angina pectoris A poorly isolated pain in the thorax, most often as a result of myocardial hypoxia.

ankylosing spondylitis A type of arthritis that affects the spine, hip and shoulders, especially the sacroiliac joint. Progression of this disease can lead to the growth of extra bone, which fuses the spine, severely affecting mobility.

anovulation The state where a woman fails to release an egg from her ovaries.

antibiotics See *antimicrobial agents*.

antibodies Immune proteins made by plasma cells, which are derivatives of B lymphocytes, that in binding to antigens induce an immune response. Also known as immunoglobulins. (Compare *antigens*.)

antidiuretic hormone (ADH) A hormone released from the posterior pituitary gland that increases renal tubular reabsorption.

antigens Substances or foreign proteins that cause the production of antibodies by lymphocytes as an immune response to defend the body against the threat. (Compare to *antibodies*.)

antimicrobial drug resistance The ability of a microbe to withstand the effects of antimicrobials, resulting in the proliferation of infectious agents that were once killed by these drugs.

antimicrobial drugs Any agent that can inhibit growth or kill microbes. Common sub-groupings of antimicrobial drugs are antibacterials, antifungals and antivirals. The term 'antimicrobial drug' is sometimes referred to as an 'antibiotic'.

antivenom Agents made from purified antibodies which, when injected, can neutralise toxicity by binding to the circulating venom or venom components.

anuria The inability to produce urine sufficient to remove fluid and wastes from the body. Generally defined as less than 100 mL in 24 hours for an adult, or less than 25 mL in 24 hours for a child. (Compare with *oliguria*.)

anxiety A condition where a person is affected by persistent and excessive apprehension (often with unrealistic concerns) that produces physiological effects, such as a fast heart rate, sweating and/or difficulty breathing.

apnoea A condition resulting in the absence of breathing, which may or may not start again spontaneously.

apoptosis Programmed cell death (cell suicide) that occurs in order for the cell to be replaced by a younger, better functioning cell.

appendicitis An inflammation of the appendix.

arrhythmia See *dysrhythmia*.

arteriovenous (AV) fistula In the context of renal medicine, an AV fistula is a surgical connection of an artery to a vein in order to increase the size of the vein to improve the ease of cannulation access for dialysis.

arteriovenous malformation (AVM) An abnormal connection between arteries and veins in the brain. An AVM is usually congenital.

arthritis A generic term for inflammation of a joint.

arthropods Invertebrate animals with an exoskeleton; includes lice, mites, spiders and insects.

asbestosis An incurable lung condition causing scarring of the lung parenchyma and damage to the pleural membrane as a result of chronic inhalation of asbestos. Symptoms of the condition develop 5–10 years after inhalation.

ascites An abnormal accumulation of serous intraperitoneal fluid.

asthma A chronic, intermittently obstructive lung disease that causes airway hyperresponsiveness, bronchoconstriction and inflammation.

asthma–COPD overlap A term to account for individuals with clinical manifestations of both asthma and chronic obstructive pulmonary disease (COPD).

ataxia A neurological condition resulting in poor coordination and balance.

atelectasis Alveolar collapse resulting in reduced gas exchange.

atherosclerosis A vascular disorder usually associated with ageing, obesity, high cholesterol intake and hypertension. Also known as 'arteriosclerosis'.

athetosis A neurological condition resulting in slow, involuntary movements of the neck, arms, fingers and legs.

atopic dermatitis A condition caused by a hypersensitivity reaction resulting in pruritus and inflammation of the affected skin.

atopy A genetic predisposition to developing an allergic condition, such as food allergy, allergic rhinitis or asthma. Atopy is only a risk factor, and environmental triggers must also be present.

atrial fibrillation A dysrhythmia due to rapid and disorganised electrical activity in the atria.

atrial flutter A type of tachycardia originating in the atria that commonly results in a 'flutter' or 'saw-tooth'-type pattern on an electrocardiograph. The ventricular conduction is typically regular, and is in ratio to the atrial conduction (e.g. 1:2, 1:3 or 1:4). In 'variable' types, the ventricular conduction may not be regular.

atrial septal defect A congenital cardiac anomaly caused by malformation of the atrial septum.

atrial tachycardia (AT) A generic term for rapid dysrhythmias originating from the atria.

atrophy The reduction in the size of a body part (e.g. muscle wasting from disuse, or reduction in the size of an organ from disease).

aura In the context of epilepsy, a sensation that some people may experience warning that a seizure is imminent. An aura may be visual, sensory, psychological or motor.

autoimmune disease A group of more than 80 disorders resulting from an overactive immune system that fails to recognise 'self'. The immune system then attacks and destroys its own tissue.

autonomic dysreflexia A condition occurring in response to a noxious stimulus resulting from an imbalance between the sympathetic and parasympathetic nervous systems in individuals with spinal injury above T6. Autonomic dysreflexia results in profound hypertension and bradycardia, and massive vasodilation and diaphoresis above the spinal injury. Beneath the injury, profound vasoconstriction occurs, as does piloerection and pallor. Autonomic dysreflexia is considered a medical emergency.

autosomal Pertaining to an autosome.

autosomes Any chromosomes that are not sex chromosomes.

avascular The absence of blood vessels in an area.

avascular necrosis Death of bone tissue from the interruption of blood supply to an area of bone.

AVPU scale A rapid neurological assessment technique that is an acronym for Alert, Voice (responds to voice), Pain (responds only to central pain/noxious stimuli), and Unresponsive (is not responsive to pain/noxious stimuli).

avulsion To tear away or tear off a body part. An avulsion fracture is when a ligament or tendon pulls off a piece of bone.

azotaemia The presence of an abnormally high level of nitrogenous substances (i.e. urea and creatinine) in the blood. (Compare with *uraemia*.)

B cells The precursor to plasma cells, which produce antibodies, or memory cells.

bacteraemia When bacteria gain access to the circulatory system.

bacteria Small, prokarytotic, unicellular organisms that can cause infection.

ball-valving Where gas is trapped in alveoli as a result of excess mucus, which has worked its way down to the respiratory airways and acts as a valve that permits air entry on inspiration, but prevents air exiting the alveoli on expiration.

Barrett's oesophagus Barrett's syndrome results in a benign lesion forming on the lining of the lower oesophagus due to chronic irritation of the epithelial tissue from gastric acid reflux.

basal cell carcinoma (BCC) A very common type of non-melanoma skin cancer that develops readily in sun-exposed areas of the body. It develops from basal cells in the skin.

behavioural addiction A disorder similar to substance dependence; however, the repetition is an action rather than the consumption of a substance. This disorder can include any behaviours, such as pathological gambling, kleptomania, compulsive buying, excessive tanning or even sexual addition (to name a few).

benign A generic term referring to the inability of a tumour to metastasise.

benign breast diseases Non-cancerous, painful lumps in breast tissue.

benign prostatic hyperplasia (BPH) A non-cancerous, age-related increase in the size of the prostate gland that may interfere with urinary function.

biliary calculi Stones (choleliths) that form in the gall bladder. (Compare with *cholelithiasis*.)

Biot's breathing A distinctive pattern of breathing generally associated with meningitis or neurological damage, and which is irregular in depth and rate, with periods of apnoea.

bipolar disorder A mental health condition where the person's mood swings between depression and mania.

blood urea nitrogen (BUN) The laboratory measurement of urea levels in the blood.

bradycardia A slow heart rate (less than 60 beats per minute in an adult).

bradykinin An inflammatory mediator that causes vasodilation and increased capillary permeability, and promotes the transmission of pain signals from damaged tissue.

bradypnoea An abnormally slow respiratory rate, generally described as less than 12 breaths per minute in an adult.

brain abscess A serious infection resulting in a localised collection of pus, pathogens (bacteria or fungi), immune cells and other substances within brain tissue.

breast cancer A common neoplasm originating within breast tissue.

bronchiectasis A chronic respiratory condition resulting in permanent changes to the shape and structure of the airways. The bronchi become damaged and widened, an excess of mucus is produced and airway defences are lost.

bronchiolitis Inflammation of the bronchioles.

bronchitis Inflammation of the bronchi.

bruit An abnormal, low-frequency murmur or swishing sound heard when auscultating a vessel.

bullae Raised blisters, each greater than 5 mm, that contain clear fluid (sing. *bulla*).

burden of disease A measure of how life is shortened by illness, injury, disability and premature death in a population.

bursitis Inflammation of a bursa, a fluid-filled sac that cushions a joint.

C-fibre A type of unmyelinated nerve fibre responsible for transmitting information about dull, throbbing pain and temperature from the peripheries to the brain. Considered to be a fast pain transmission.

calcitonin A hormone, produced by the thyroid gland, responsible for the regulation of calcium levels in the blood.

calcium A mineral required for many cellular functions (e.g. neuromuscular functions, coagulation, hormone secretion and impulse transmission).

cancer A generic term describing any condition where abnormal cells divide and invade other tissue unimpeded by normal controls.

carbuncle A skin infection involving many hair follicles, often caused by a staphylococcal bacterial infection.

carcinogen Any substance that has the potential to cause cancer.

carcinogenesis The process of initiating cancer.

cardiomyopathy Any disease or condition affecting cardiac contractility.

carrier In relation to genetics, an individual who has an inherited genetic mutation for a condition or disease but does not express symptoms of that condition. In relation to infectious diseases, a carrier can transmit the infectious agent but does not exhibit symptoms of the disease (e.g. 'Typhoid Mary').

caseous necrosis A condition where dead tissue appears crumbly and cheese-like, commonly seen in tuberculosis lesions.

cataracts An age-related condition resulting in a clouding of the lens in the eye.

cellular immunity Cell-mediated immunity, a type of acquired immunity in which T cells (T lymphocytes) play a dominant role. (Compare with *humoral immunity*.)

cellulitis A bacterial skin infection causing the affected area to become red, hot and painful.

central cord syndrome A condition where the central portion of the spinal cord is affected, causing a disproportionate motor impairment where upper limb function is more affected than lower limb function. This injury is more common in individuals with cervical trauma from a hyperextension injury.

cerebral blood flow (CBF) This refers to the volume of blood supplying brain tissue at any given time. In an average-sized adult, cerebral blood flow is approximately 50 mL/100 g/min (equivalent to approximately 18% of cardiac output).

cerebral infarction Also known as 'stroke'. The death of brain tissue from a lack of blood supply to the area. (Compare with *cerebrovascular accident*.)

cerebral ischaemia Reduced blood flow to an area of the brain, which can be a precursor to a cerebral infarction or may resolve with little to no damage.

cerebral palsy A permanent, non-progressing condition caused by reduced cerebral perfusion occurring in a developing brain, during or around birth.

cerebral perfusion pressure (CPP) A calculated measure of blood flow to the brain. CPP is determined by subtracting intracranial pressure from mean arterial blood pressure.

cerebrovascular accident (CVA) (stroke) The loss of blood supply to an area of brain, which results in tissue death.

cervical cancer Cancer of the cervix, caused by the human papillomavirus (HPV).

chain of transmission Also known as the 'chain of infection', this term refers to a model used to describe all of the steps involved in pathogen spread. Each of the links must be present for an infection to develop.

Cheyne–Stokes breathing A breathing pattern commonly seen in end-of-life care, where the individual alternates between periods of shallow breathing, deep breathing which slows, and apnoea; when breathing starts again, it is fast and shallow.

chlamydia A sexually transmitted infection caused by the bacterium *Chlamydia trachomatis*.

cholangitis Inflammation of the biliary duct system.

cholecystitis Inflammation of the gall bladder.

cholelithiasis The formation of gallstones: cholelithiasis is stones in the gall bladder or bile duct due to pathological formation from cholesterol, calcium salts and bile pigments.

cholesterol A lipid responsible for the absorption and transport of fatty acids. It is the precursor in the synthesis of vitamin D and many hormones, and is an essential component of cell membranes.

chronic fatigue syndrome (CFS) See *myalgic encephalomyelitis/chronic fatigue syndrome (ME/CFS)*.

chronic inflammation A dysfunction of the immune system that develops when an acute inflammatory response does not subside. It results in sustained increased capillary permeability, alterations in blood flow and an accumulation of white blood cells in the affected area.

chronic kidney disease (CKD) The long-term, progressive and permanent damage to the kidneys that can result from renal and systemic disorders.

chronic lymphocytic leukaemia (CLL) A slowly progressing type of leukaemia that affects the B lymphocytes (plasma cells or B cells).

chronic myelogenous leukaemia (CML) A type of blood cell cancer which develops in granulocyte cells found in the bone marrow. Granulocytes are part of the myeloid cell line of white blood cells and include eosinophils and basophils. CML affects partly mature cells, develops gradually (over months to years, and therefore is classified as chronic. (Compare with *acute myelogenous leukaemia*.)

chronic obstructive pulmonary disorders (COPD) A group of lung disorders characterised by difficulty in breathing and obstructed air flow. The two most common conditions associated with COPD are chronic bronchitis and emphysema.

circulatory shock A potentially fatal condition in which a drop in blood pressure is caused by haemorrhage, or the relative loss of circulating blood volume from vasodilation.

cirrhosis A chronic condition resulting in fibrotic tissue and fat infiltration in the liver lobules.

claudication Cramping pain in the lower limbs (often the gastrocnemius) while walking or exercising, due to vascular (ischaemia) or neurogenic (nerve irritation from pressure) causes.

clinical manifestations The signs and symptoms of a condition.

clotting Coagulation of blood.

coagulation Clotting. A blood clot forms as a result of several steps, including platelet aggregation (the clumping of platelets), the laying down of a fibrin network and the presence of calcium.

coagulative necrosis Death of tissue causing fibrous changes to intracellular protein elements, which result in an opaque cellular outline that persists for a prolonged time.

coagulopathy A generic term for any bleeding disorder that results in a person's blood not forming clots appropriately.

coeliac sprue/coeliac disease A chronic condition due to an abnormal immune reaction to the protein gluten. This results in an inflammatory response by the mucosa of the small intestine, leading to nutrient malabsorption. The consumption of a gluten-free diet is the only treatment.

colitis Inflammation of the colon due to infection or an immune system reaction, produces abdominal pain, diarrhoea and bleeding.

colon cancer A condition in which the epithelial cells of the large intestine cease normal cell division and develop cancerous lesions.

colonisation A generic term for the presence and multiplication of a microorganism (generally bacteria) that is not yet causing disease. It is the first stage of infection, when the bacteria have overcome the host's surface defences.

colour blindness Difficulty distinguishing between certain colours as a result of a reduced number or function of the photoreceptor cone cells.

compartment syndrome An increase in pressure within the muscle compartment, owing to swelling or fluid trapped within the fascia.

complement system A system involving a number of specialised proteins that interact to facilitate body defences.

complete lethal gene In the context of genetics, a gene that has mutated such that it results in the death of all individuals carrying the affected gene.

communicable diseases Health conditions caused by microoganisms that can be passed from one human to another.

concentric hypertrophy Growth in width (i.e. as a result of the addition of sarcomeres to a myocyte in parallel). In relation to the heart, this change occurs in response to pressure overload. (Compare with *eccentric hypertrophy*.)

concussion A traumatic brain injury resulting in neurological effects, such as headache, confusion, memory loss or altered level of consciousness.

conduction block Interference of an impulse being transmitted to another area. Most commonly refers to the conduction system of the heart, where a conduction block stops or delays transmission of an impulse.

congenital adrenal hyperplasia (CAH) A genetic endocrine disorder of the adrenal glands causing an excessive production of androgens and an inadequate production of aldosterone and cortisol. This results in abnormal sexual development and sometimes electrolyte disorders.

congenital heart defect A generic term for any structural abnormality of the heart due to inappropriate formation during embryonic or fetal life.

congestive heart failure A condition in which inadequate circulation causes dyspnoea, oedema and fatigue, which ultimately interfere with the ability to cope with the activities of daily living.

congenital malformations A anatomical anomalies that are present at birth, which may be genetic, as a result of exposure to a teratogen (deformity-causing agent) or idiopathic (unknown cause).

congenital or neonatal hypothyroidism A congenital condition resulting from a deficiency of maternal iodine during pregnancy, causing mental retardation, deafness and growth deficiency. Formerly known as 'cretinism'.

conjunctivitis An inflammation of the conjunctiva, commonly caused by infection.

Conn's disease Primary aldosteronism or primary hyperaldosteronism, Conn's disease results in the overproduction of aldosterone, most commonly causing secondary hypertension.

consciousness A state where a person is aware and responds to the environment.

constitutive activity The ability of a receptor to produce a response without ligand binding.

contact dermatitis Inflammation of the skin in response to exposure (touch) to a substance. Contact dermatitis may be caused by either an irritant reaction or an allergic reaction.

contracture An abnormal shortening of a muscle, preventing normal movement.

contrecoup contusions Traumatic brain injuries caused by a blow to the head, which results in damage to the opposite cerebral hemisphere from the effects of transmitted force. (Compare with *coup contusion*.)

conus medullaris A cone-shaped region generally located between thoracic vertebrae 12 and lumbar vertebrae 2 (T12–L2), through which the nerves controlling bladder and bowel function pass. Motor and sensory nerves for the genitals and the lower limbs are also within the region.

coronary artery disease A condition that results in a narrowing of the coronary arteries due to plaques (deposits of cholesterol and fats). This results in angina chest pain caused by a reduced blood supply to the myocardium, and can cause a myocardial infarction. Also known as 'ischaemic heart disease'.

cor pulmonale Right-sided heart failure that occurs as a result of a chronic pulmonary condition.

corpora cavernosa With reference to the penis, the corpora cavernosa is an area of tissue through the length of the penis that fills with blood to facilitate an erection.

corticosteroids A generic term for the steroid hormones, produced by the adrenal cortex.

cortisol A steroid hormone, produced by the adrenal cortex, responsible for significantly reducing inflammation and glucose formation.

coup contusions Traumatic brain injuries at the region of the direct blow to the head. (Compare with *contrecoup contusions*.)

COVID-19 infection A severe acute respiratory disease caused by the SARS CoV-2 virus. The virus can cause systemic illness through direct and indirect injury on other organs such as the brain, heart and liver.

cramps Uncontrollable muscle spasms that may occur in skeletal or smooth muscle.

creatinine A nitrogenous substance formed from the metabolism of creatine. Creatinine is excreted by the kidneys and can be used as a marker of renal function.

Crohn's disease A form of inflammatory bowel disease associated with inflammation of the gastrointestinal tract, often within the small intestine, and which results in pain, diarrhoea and chronic changes to the gastrointestinal tissue.

cryotherapy The use of excessively cold substances or instruments to freeze cells.

cryptorchidism The failure of one (or both) testicles to descend into the scrotum.

curettage A generic term meaning to 'scrape'. Generally used in the context of gynaecological conditions in combination with the word 'dilation' ('dilation and curettage' or 'D&C') to describe the removal of tissue, such as polyps, or an incomplete miscarriage from the uterine wall.

Cushing's disease A condition in which an abnormal increase in the production of adrenocorticotropic hormone, from a tumour in the adrenal cortex or pituitary gland, results in obesity and fatigue.

cyanosis A bluish colouring of the skin that occurs as a result of tissue hypoxia. Can be peripheral (on the fingers and toes) or central (around the mouth and tongue).

cystic fibrosis (CF) A genetic disease caused by faulty chloride transport from defective cell membrane transporters. CF results in abnormally viscous mucus, and causes various significant effects on respiratory, pancreatic and exocrine gland function.

cystitis Inflammation of the urinary bladder.

cystocele A bulging of the bladder into the vagina. Also known as 'anterior vaginal wall prolapse'.

cytokines Substances secreted by immune cells, such as interferons or interleukins, that can alter the activity of other body cells.

debridement The removal of dead or infected tissue to promote wound healing.

deep vein thrombosis (DVT) A blood clot that has formed within a deep vein, often within the legs.

dehydration An imbalance of water intake and output, either from excessive fluid loss or inadequate fluid intake, resulting in an electrolyte imbalance and insufficient fluid volume to support metabolic processes.

delayed after-depolarisations (DADs) Abnormal depolarisations in cardiac myocytes, which interfere with phase 4 of the action potential and can be seen in digoxin toxicity.

delayed onset muscle soreness (DOMS) Pain, discomfort or stiffness in muscles experienced several hours or days after unaccustomed or excessive exercise.

delayed union In the context of bone fracture, the prolonged healing in the ends of a fracture.

deletion In the context of genetics, the loss of some genetic material.

dementia A generic term for the progressive deterioration in an individual's intellectual function, including memory.

denervation atrophy The loss of muscle volume from disuse as a result of an interruption to nerve conduction.

depilation Removal of hair from the surface of the skin.

depression In the context of mental health, depression is the alteration of mood characterised by feelings of sadness and despair, most days, for at least two weeks.

dermatitis A generic term for inflammation of the skin.

dermatophytes Fungi associated with infections of the nails.

descending inhibitory pathway In relation to pain, the nerves in the spinal cord that carry impulses away from the brain and synapse in the dorsal horn, where there is release of endogenous opioids and neurotransmitters. These signals are capable of preventing ascending signals in the spinothalamic tracts, and therefore contribute to the modulation of pain.

desquamation The shedding of superficial epithelium, such as skin or mucosal tissue.

determinants of health Factors such as individual, socioeconomic, sociocultural and environmental conditions that influence the health of a population.

developmental dysplasia of the hip (DDH) Previously known as 'congenital dislocated hip', DDH is either a dislocation or an instability of the hip that can result in hip dysplasia.

diabetes insipidus (DI) A metabolic condition in which a deficiency of antidiuretic hormone results in the excessive loss of fluid; often caused by trauma or a tumour.

diabetes mellitus A heterogenous group of metabolic conditions in which glucose absorption is reduced due to insufficient insulin production or problems with insulin effectiveness, resulting in excessive blood glucose levels. Often referred to by the shortened term 'diabetes'.

diabetic ketoacidosis (DKA) A serious complication of diabetes mellitus resulting in profound hyperglycaemia, dehydration, acidosis and the production of ketones, all of which can contribute to an altered level of consciousness in moderate to severe instances.

diabetic nephropathy A complication of diabetes mellitus. It is a microvascular disease where the glomerular basement membrane of the kidneys become thicker, the glomerulus becomes more permeable to proteins, and glomerulosclerosis (hardening of the glomeruli) eventually develops.

diabetic retinopathy A progressive eye disease that is caused by injury to the retinal blood vessels as a result of hyperglycaemia. The resulting endothelial cell damage causes capillary leak, poor perfusion and angiogenesis of vessels on or out of the surface of the retina.

diarrhoea Excessive and often frequent loss of watery faeces.

diffuse axonal injury (DAI) A traumatic brain injury that results in damage to significant numbers of axons within the brain, causing extensive brain damage and often leaving individuals in persistent vegetative states.

digital clubbing Structural changes to the distal part of fingers (and sometimes toes), resulting in a bulbous and convex shape in the nail bed. It is often associated with chronic pulmonary conditions that result in persistent hypoxia.

diploid A cell with a full set of chromosomes (46). Haploid cells (i.e. gametes) have only half the number of chromosomes (23).

disease-modifying antirheumatic drugs (DMARDs) Drugs that affect the underlying processes that cause inflammation in conditions such as rheumatoid arthritis. DMARDs not only reduce inflammation, they can also slow down joint destruction.

dislocation In the context of the musculoskeletal system, when two bones that normally form a joint are separated by extreme forces placed on the ligaments through some type of traumatic event.

dissecting aneurysm A tear of the inner layer of an arterial wall, resulting in a false pocket. Often associated with the aorta, but can be any artery.

disuse atrophy The loss of muscle volume as a result of inactivity, such as prolonged bed rest.

diverticula Protrusions of part of the intestinal mucosa and submucosa through the muscle layer of the associated intestine, diverticula are common in the sigmoid colon as a result of increased intramural pressure. (See *diverticulitis*.)

diverticulitis Inflammation (or infection) of diverticula.

dominant inheritance In relation to genetics, refers to the trait that will have greater influence in a pair of alleles (e.g. brown eyes are a dominant trait, whereas the other eye colours are recessive traits).

dopamine (DA) A catecholamine that is both a neurotransmitter in the central nervous system and a hormone.

dual diagnosis Used to describe the presence of a mental health issue co-existing in a person with a problematic alcohol, tobacco or other substance use issue.

duodenal ulcers Lesions in the mucous membrane of the duodenum.

duplication In relation to genetics, occurs when an extra, redundant copy of some DNA, an entire gene or a series of genes are accidentally replicated.

dysmenorrhoea Painful menstruation.

dysplasia A generic term for an abnormality in maturation.

dyspnoea Shortness of breath.

dysrhythmias Also known as 'arrhythmias', this is a generic term for an abnormality in the cardiac rhythm.

dystrophin A protein vital for maintaining the structure of skeletal muscle tissue.

dysuria A generic term for difficulty or pain when urinating.

early after-depolarisation (EAD) Abnormal depolarisation in cardiac myocytes that interferes with phase 2 or 3 of the action potential, and which can cause ventricular tachycardia.

eccentric hypertrophy Growth in length (i.e. as a result of the addition of sarcomeres to a myocyte in series). In relation to the heart, this change occurs in response to volume overload. (Compare with *concentric hypertrophy*.)

ectopic hormone secretion A release of hormone from cells or tissues that are not normally responsible for the secretion of that hormone.

ectopic pregnancy A pregnancy occurring outside the uterus, commonly in the fallopian tube, but can occur anywhere in the abdomen.

effusions An abnormal collection of excess fluid, which may develop in any cavity, including in a joint or between the pleura.

electroencephalography (EEG) A measure of brain waves indicating electrical impulses, used in the assessment of the central nervous system for conditions such as epilepsy, sleep disorders and head injury, and in the assessment of brain death.

electrolytes Ions capable of regulating water flow across a cell membrane. Sodium, potassium, magnesium, calcium and chloride ions are important electrolytes in cellular function.

electromyography Measurement of the electrical activity of skeletal muscles.

emphysema A chronic pulmonary condition caused by a loss of elastin and gas trapping, resulting in shortness of breath and hypoxia.

encephalitis Inflammation of the brain commonly associated with infection.

endometriosis A gynaecological condition where uterine tissue is found outside the uterus.

end-stage kidney disease (ESKD) The final stage of chronic renal impairment. Kidney function will not recover.

envenomation The transmission of a poisonous secretion from an animal by a bite or a sting. Usually in reference to a snake, spider or marine animal.

epidemiology The study of the characteristics and distribution patterns of an illness.

epididymitis Inflammation of the epididymis.

epilepsy A neurological condition resulting in an alteration in the person's consciousness, which may be associated with involuntary movement or a seizure.

epileptic focus The region of the cerebral cortex responsible for causing the epileptic event.

epileptogenic Having the capacity to cause an epileptic event.

epispadias In relation to the penis, a congenital malformation that results in the urethra opening on the dorsal surface of the penis.

epithelialisation An early stage of wound healing occurring within the first 24 hours, whereby cells at the base of the wound migrate, proliferate and differentiate to form a temporary protection over the affected area.

erectile dysfunction (ED) Difficulty in sustaining an erection of sufficient quality to satisfy intercourse or sexual activity. Also known as 'impotence'.

erythema A generic term describing an area of red skin caused by dilation of the capillaries. Erythema is a cardinal sign of inflammation, and can be associated with infection.

escape rhythm The rhythm originating from either the atrioventricular node or the His–Purkinje fibres when the normal pacemaker cells higher in the conduction system fail to initiate an impulse.

eukaryotes Organisms containing a clearly defined, membrane-bound nucleus.

eupnoea Normal relaxed breathing.

euvolaemia A state where a person has a normal blood volume.

Ewing's sarcoma A type of malignant bone cancer that develops around puberty.

excitotoxicity A process whereby neurons are overexcited by the neurotransmitter glutamate, causing excess calcium to enter the cells. This enables the activation of enzymes that damage the cell structures, leading to cell death.

extracorporeal shock wave lithotripsy (ESWL) A procedure to disintegrate kidney stones so that they can be passed in the urine. The shock wave is generated outside the body.

extradural haematoma (EDH) A collection of blood between the skull and the dura mater.

extraparenchymal lung disorders Conditions associated with restrictive lung disease that are not caused by lung parenchyma. These conditions include neuromuscular disease affecting the strength of the diaphragm and intercostal muscles, or chest wall deformities such as kyphosis.

exudate The fluid that seeps from a wound.

familial adenomatous polyposis An inherited disorder resulting in the formation of polyps within the large intestine and rectum.

fasciotomy A surgical incision made through the connective tissue that surrounds muscles to relieve high pressures within the compartment.

fat necrosis A type of adipose tissue death where the neutral fats are separated into fatty acids and glycerol, forming a rubbery mass of tissue.

fibrillation An irregular and rapid impulse generation in cardiac fibres, resulting in inadequate contractility and inefficient emptying of the affected chambers. It can occur in the atria (atrial fibrillation) or the ventricles (ventricular fibrillation).

fibroadenoma A type of solid, non-cancerous breast tumour more common in females under 30 years of age.

fibrocystic disease A condition where fluid-filled cystic lumps develop in the ductal tissue of the breast.

fibromyalgia A chronic pain disorder that causes stiffness, myalgia and joint tenderness without detectable inflammation.

fibrosis A generic term for the formation of excess fibrous connective tissue developing in tissue or organs undergoing repair or reactive pathology.

fistula An abnormal communication (connection) between two locations (e.g. internal organs and the skin, hollow organs, or arteries and veins). Most commonly found between the rectum and the urinary tract.

flaccid paralysis A loss of motor control associated with nerve damage causing limp, unresponsive muscles. (Compare with *spastic paralysis*.)

fluid balance The difference between fluid intake and fluid output.

fluid deficit Dehydration; an imbalance in the volume of fluid intake and output, resulting in insufficient fluid volume to support normal function.

fluid excess An imbalance in the volume of fluid intake and output, resulting in too much fluid volume, causing oedema or congestive cardiac failure.

focal cortical dysplasia A common cause of intractable temporal lobe epilepsy, characterised by a GABA-mediated compromise in neuronal inhibition.

focal seizure A form of seizure where the disordered electrical activity of neurons arises in a localised focus within the brain.

folliculitis An inflammation of the hair follicle, commonly associated with infection.

fracture A break in a bone.

fragile chromosomal site An area (locus) of a chromosome associated with breakage or aberration.

full-thickness burn A burn that involves all layers of the skin, and may also include damage to muscle and bone. Previously known as a 'third-degree burn'.

fungi Spore-bearing eukaryotic organisms that can become pathogenic if they bypass normal body defences (sing. fungus).

furuncles Skin infection involving many follicles, commonly caused by staphylococcal bacteria.

gamma-aminobutyric acid (GABA) A chemical messenger substance in the central nervous system which acts as an inhibitory neurotransmitter reducing the excessive firing and excitability of neurons.

gangrene Tissue destruction from hypoxia.

gastric (stomach) ulcers An erosion of the mucosal layer in a localised area of the stomach.

gastroenteritis A generic term for an infection or inflammation of the digestive tract.

gastro-oesophageal reflux disease (GORD) A chronic condition due to an incompetent oesophageal sphincter, which allows in backflow of gastric contents, causing inflammation and mucosal trauma.

general adaptation syndrome A physiological response to physical or emotional stress. The general adaptation syndrome is divided into three stages (alarm, resistance, exhaustion), and defines the body's typical manifestations of continued stress.

generalised seizure A type of seizure whereby both hemispheres of the brain are affected by disordered electrical impulses symmetrically.

genital herpes A sexually transmitted infection caused by the herpes simplex virus (HSV). An infection with HSV-1 generally results in lesions on the mouth and lips, whereas an infection with HSV-2 generally results in lesions on the genitals.

genital warts A sexually transmitted infection caused by the human papillomavirus (HPV).

genotype The genetic make-up of an organism.

giardiasis An intestinal inflammatory condition caused by protozoan infection of *Giardia lamblia*. It is usually due to drinking contaminated water. Giardiasis causes profound fluid loss and electrolyte imbalance from chronic diarrhoea and malabsorption.

gigantism Also known as 'giantism'; an endocrine condition resulting from the excessive secretion of growth hormone from the pituitary gland.

Glasgow coma scale (GCS) A standard measure of neurological function and level of consciousness in which the maximum score is 15 and the minimum score is 3.

glaucoma A condition resulting in irreversible blindness, where the optic nerve is damaged by increased pressures inside the eye and reduced perfusion to the optic nerve.

glomerular filtration rate (GFR) A quantification of the amount of filtrate that the glomeruli can produce in 1 minute. A normal GFR is 100–140 mL/min.

glucocorticoids The steroid hormones produced by the adrenal cortex that influence carbohydrate, protein and fat metabolism. Glucocorticoids also play an important role in reducing inflammation.

gluten A protein found in wheat, rye, barley and oats that causes digestive disorders in people with coeliac disease.

goitre An enlargement of the thyroid gland, manifesting as a prominent swelling in the front of the neck. (Compare with *Graves' disease*.)

gonadocorticoids The steroid hormones secreted by the adrenal cortex that affect sexual organ development (i.e. androgens and oestrogens).

gonorrhoea A sexually transmitted infection that can cause pelvic inflammatory disease in women.

gout A condition caused by the build-up of uric acid crystals, which can be deposited in joints and induce an inflammation.

granulation tissue Collagen-rich, vascular connective tissue forming within a healing wound that replaces the fibrin clot.

granuloma A lesion that forms as a result of chronic inflammation.

Graves' disease A condition in which excessive thyroid hormone is produced. This condition can cause goitre, exophthalmos and tachycardia. (Compare with *goitre*.)

growth hormone (GH) A hormone, secreted by the pituitary gland, that is responsible for linear growth (especially influencing bone growth). GH influences the metabolism of proteins, carbohydrates and lipids.

Guillain–Barré syndrome (GBS) A form of ascending neuromuscular paralysis caused by an immune response that results in the demyelination and inflammation of the peripheral nerves.

haematogenous urinary tract infection An infection in which an infective organism is transported from another site of infection via the bloodstream to infect the kidneys and urinary tract.

haematuria A generic term referring to the presence of blood in the urine.

haemodialysis The artificial filtration of blood using diffusion and ultrafiltration to remove waste products, toxic substances and excess fluid.

haemolysis The destruction of erythrocytes and the subsequent release of haemoglobin; occurs naturally at the end of an erythrocyte's life span (100–120 days).

haemolytic anaemia A condition in which red blood cells are prematurely destroyed.

haemolytic uraemic syndrome A condition in which an infection in the gastrointestinal tract results in the release of substances that destroy the red blood cells. Intravascular thromboemboli are formed in the kidneys, and further platelet aggregation exacerbates the situation.

haemophilia A group of disorders characterised by a deficiency (or absence) of certain clotting factors. All forms of haemophilia are hereditary. The severity of the condition is determined by the extent of the clotting factor deficiency.

haemoptysis Blood-stained sputum.

harm minimisation A framework often used to provide support around issues such as alcohol, tobacco and other drugs. Harm minimisation related to illicit drug use involves reducing supply of, demand for and harm from the drugs.

healing The restoration of lost functional tissue after injury. Tissue repair, where the continuity of a tissue's framework is restored through the formation of scar tissue, is sometimes described as being part of the healing process.

healthcare gap The inadequate provision of health services that permits a disparity in the health measure of a particular cohort within a population.

heart failure A generic term for the inability of the heart to adequately pump fluids through the body to meet its needs.

***Helicobacter pylori* infection** A pathogenic colonisation of the gastric mucosa by the bacterium *H. pylori*, which may lead to the development of gastric ulcers.

helminths Parasitic worms.

hepatic encephalopathy A condition in which toxic nitrogenous substances (including ammonia) enter the systemic circulation, resulting in neurological symptoms ranging from mild, such as forgetfulness and confusion, through to serious, such as seizures, coma and death.

hernia A protrusion of the intestines through the abdominal muscle wall.

heterozygous In the context of genetics, refers to an organism possessing different alleles for a single trait.

high-density lipoprotein (HDL) A class of lipoprotein that transports cholesterol to the liver for excretion or re-utilisation. Also known as 'good cholesterol'.

histamine A chemical mediator that is involved in inflammatory and allergic reactions. The effects induced by this chemical include vasodilation, increased vascular permeability, smooth muscle contraction and prostaglandin synthesis.

Hodgkin lymphoma (HL) A malignant disorder originating in lymphocytes; also known as 'Hodgkin disease'. The distinguishing feature is the Reed–Sternberg cells, which are large, atypically formed macrophages with dysmorphic or multiple nuclei.

homeostasis The maintenance of equilibrium through the continuous adjustment and compensation of physiological processes to deal with constantly changing conditions.

hormone hypersecretion A state of excess hormone levels where the synthesis and release of a hormone from an endocrine gland (or an ectopic source) is increased.

hormone hyposecretion A hormone-deficient state where the synthesis and release of a hormone from an endocrine gland is impaired.

human immunodeficiency virus (HIV) The virus responsible for the acquired immune deficiency syndrome (AIDS). HIV infection has a profound effect on a subgroup of lymphocytes—helper T cells ($CD4^+$ T cells).

human leukocyte antigens (HLA) A group of proteins present on the surface of cells that enable the immune system to distinguish 'self' from 'non-self'.

humoral immunity A type of acquired immunity in which antibodies play a dominant role; also known as 'antibody-mediated immunity'. B cells produce antibodies. (Compare with *cellular immunity*.)

Huntington's disease An autosomal dominant genetic disorder characterised by involuntary writhing movements and progressive dementia.

hydrocele In relation to the testes, a condition characterised by the accumulation of fluid between the layers of the tunica vaginalis covering of the testis.

hydrocephalus A condition characterised by the accumulation of cerebrospinal fluid in the cranium, which can compress the tissue, compromising tissue function and structural integrity.

hydronephrosis Distension of the renal pelvis and calyces due to a urinary tract obstruction that increases renal hydrostatic pressure.

hydrostatic pressure The pressure exerted on the vessel by the volume of blood. (Compare with *osmotic pressure*.)

hyperaemia Excessive blood in an area of the body.

hyperalgesia When an injured part of the body becomes hypersensitive to pain such that minor noxious stimuli induce much greater pain than would be expected.

hypercalcaemia Excessive calcium levels in the blood.

hypercalciuria Too much calcium in the urine.

hypercapnia Elevated levels of carbon dioxide in the blood.

hyperglycaemia Excessive glucose levels in the blood.

hyperinflation An increase in residual lung volume.

hyperkalaemia Excessive potassium levels in the blood.

hyperkeratosis A generic term describing an increase in keratin in the epidermis (stratum corneum).

hypermagnesaemia Excessive magnesium levels in the blood.

hypermetabolism An elevated metabolic rate.

hypernatraemia Excessive sodium levels in the blood.

hyperopia When light entering the eye is focused behind the plane of the retina. Near objects appear out of focus. Also known as 'far-sightedness' or 'long-sightedness'.

hyperoxia A condition in which the oxygen content of the body is elevated above normal.

hyperparathyroidism A condition in which excessive functioning of the parathyroid glands leads to overproduction of parathyroid hormone, resulting in increased extracellular calcium concentrations and hypercalcaemia. Hyperparathyroidism can lead to numerous system clinical manifestations, including fatigue, hypertension, nausea and vomiting, and renal stones.

hyperphosphataemia Excessive phosphate levels in the blood.

hyperplasia An abnormal increase in the number of cells, causing enlargement of the affected organ or tissue.

hyperprolactinaemia Excessive prolactin levels in the blood.

hypersensitivity pneumonitis A condition characterised by a cell-mediated immune reaction directed against the lung parenchyma.

hypersensitivity reaction An inappropriate and disproportionate immune system response to exposure to an antigen. Hypersensitivity reactions are classified by the immune system components mediating the overreaction.

hypertension A chronically elevated blood pressure.

hyperthyroidism A pathologically increased thyroid function, resulting in goitre, exophthalmos and tachycardia. (Compare with *Graves' disease*.)

hypertonic solution A solution containing more dissolved particles relative to cells or the blood.

hypertrophic scar A scar with excessive collagen synthesis, leading to a raised or thickened area contained within the wound margins.

hypertrophy Excessive growth of an organ or tissue as a result of cellular enlargement.

hypocalcaemia Inadequate calcium levels in the blood.

hypocapnia Lower than normal carbon dioxide levels in the blood.

hypoglycaemia Inadequate glucose levels in the blood.

hypokalaemia Inadequate potassium levels in the blood.

hypolactasia Lactose intolerance resulting in an inability to digest milk or milk products.

hypomagnesaemia Inadequate magnesium levels in the blood.

hyponatraemia Where the concentration of sodium within the blood is below normal. This can occur as a result of either insufficient sodium levels or excessive water in the blood.

hypoparathyroidism A condition in which the functioning of the parathyroid glands is abnormally poor, resulting in low calcium and high phosphate levels in the blood. Severe hypoparathyroidism can cause tetany, muscle weakness and neurological issues.

hypophosphataemia Inadequate phosphate levels in the blood.

hypospadias In relation to the penis, a congenital malformation where the urethral opening is on the ventral surface of the penis.

hypothalamus A brain structure that is the major control centre for many critical autonomic nervous system and endocrine functions.

hypothyroidism A pathologically decreased thyroid function, resulting in insufficient production of thyroid hormones; often due to inadequate dietary iodine. (Compare with *Congenital or neonatal hypothyroidism*.)

hypotonic solution A solution containing fewer dissolved particles relative to the cells or the blood.

hypovolaemia Inadequate blood volume. Can be due to dehydration or excessive blood loss.

hypoxaemia Insufficient oxygen in the blood.

hypoxia A state of low oxygen.

idiopathic inflammatory myositis A group of connective tissue disorders characterised by chronic inflammation and muscle weakness in the proximal muscles of the body.

ileus A condition caused by the cessation of peristalsis, resulting in abdominal pain, nausea, vomiting and the absence of passing gas or a stool.

immunity The condition of being resistant to infection by a specific pathogen.

immunodeficiency A condition resulting in an inability of the immune system to resist infection.

immunosuppressants Drugs used to modify (dampen) an immune response. Immunosuppressants are important to prevent organ rejection in transplant surgery.

immunotype Where a substance such as a venom has particular immunological characteristics. Substances with common immunotypes have similar immunological characteristics.

incidence The number of new cases diagnosed within a calendar year.

incontinence-associated dermatitis A painful skin lesion in the perineal region associated with faecal or urine incontinence. Common names for this condition are 'nappy rash' and 'peri-rash'.

infant mortality A measure of the number of children in a population who die before 1 year of age.

infant respiratory distress syndrome (IRDS) An inflammatory interstitial lung disease in premature neonates that develops due to a deficiency in pulmonary surfactant.

infectious disease Any disease caused by a pathogen. Note: not all infectious diseases are communicable (e.g. tetanus).

infectious myositis A localised or widespread muscle infection usually associated with a bacterial cause, commonly *Staphylococcus aureus*.

infertility Defined by the World Health Organization as a couple where the woman is under 34 years of age, who have not conceived after 12 months of unprotected sexual intercourse.

inflammatory bowel disease A collective term for chronic inflammatory conditions thought to be caused by an inappropriate immune response of the intestines to their contents. (See also *ulcerative colitis* and *Crohn's disease*.)

inotropy The process of causing a change in muscular contraction, usually associated with cardiac muscle.

intracranial pressure (ICP) The pressure inside the skull due to the volume of brain tissue, cerebrospinal fluid and blood.

intraocular pressure The pressure within the eyeball due to the volume of aqueous humour.

intravenous pyelogram (IVP) A procedure in which a radio-opaque contrast medium is injected into a blood vessel and X-rays are taken of the pelvic region. The dye concentrates in the renal system and makes the kidneys, ureters and bladder visible on the X-ray.

intussusception A state where the intestines fold in on themselves like a telescope closing. Inside the fold, the intestinal lumen is narrowed and the blood vessels are squeezed.

inverse care law A concept whereby those in the most need of healthcare are the least likely to receive it.

iontopheresis A procedure for the transdermal transport of ions through the skin that is facilitated by an electrical current.

Irukandji syndrome A syndrome of clinical manifestations associated with a sting by the Irukandji jellyfish, including severe lower back pain, muscle cramps, joint pain, nausea and vomiting, anxiety, sweating, tachycardia, hypertension and oliguria.

ischaemia Inadequate blood flow to an organ or tissue.

isotonic solution A solution containing an equivalent number of dissolved particles relative to the cells or the blood.

jaundice A condition in which an individual's skin and sclerae are discoloured yellow.

keloid Pertaining to scarring, it is a raised and fibrous tissue that contains excessive amounts of collagen. A keloid scar enlarges beyond the area of the initial trauma.

keloid scar See *Keloid*.

kernicterus Brain damage caused by an excess of bilirubin as a result of an immature or damaged blood–brain barrier.

kinin–kallikrein system A series of biochemical reactions that leads to the production of kallikrein and the chemical mediators called kinins. The most important kinin is bradykinin, which is involved in inflammation and nociception. Kallikrein is an enzyme that can activate the clotting process.

koilonychia A condition commonly resulting from chronic iron deficiency anaemia, where a finger or tonenail becomes soft, brittle and develops into a spoon-shape as it becomes concave and raised at the edge.

Kussmaul breathing A rapid, deep and often laboured type of breathing; often associated with ketoacidosis.

kyphosis An excessive convex curvature of the thoracic spine.

labyrinthitis An inflammation of the inner ear that affects balance and hearing.

lactase deficiency Lactase deficiency disrupts the conversion of lactose into galactose and glucose. In this state, lactose is fermented in the large bowel, leading to excessive gas within the gut, distending the lumen and stimulating motility. This can result in abdominal discomfort and diarrhoea. The condition is known as 'lactose intolerance'.

lactose intolerance A deficiency in the disaccharidase *lactase (hypolactasia)* results in unmetabolised lactose, which is then fermented by the gut flora, leading to an accumulation of gas in the gut lumen. This can cause abdominal discomfort and increase gut osmotic pressure, leading to diarrhoea.

leukaemia General term for white blood cell cancer.

leukocytosis An increase in white blood cells in the blood, commonly associated with an infection.

leukonychia A condition resulting in a transient white discolouration on the nail plate which may be caused by nutritional deficiency, trauma, infection or systemic disease.

leukopenia An abnormally low number of white blood cells.

leukoplakia White patches on the mucous membranes.

life expectancy A population measure based on the time an average person is anticipated to live.

liquefactive necrosis Cell death associated with a rapid release of lysosomal enzymes and autolysis.

Lou Gehrig's disease A form of motor neurone disease characterised by upper and lower motor neuron degeneration. Also known as 'amyotrophic lateral sclerosis'.

low-density lipoprotein (LDL) A class of lipoprotein that transports cholesterol from the liver to the tissues. Also known as 'bad cholesterol'.

lower respiratory tract infection (LRTI) A respiratory tract infection that develops below the level of the carina caused by viral or bacterial pathogens.

lung cancer A cancer that grows within the tissues of the lower respiratory system.

lymphoma A general term referring to a cancer of the lymphatic tissue.

macrovascular disease Pathology affecting the large blood vessels, ultimately causing complications to the heart (coronary artery disease), limbs (peripheral arterial disease) or brain (stroke).

magnesium The second most abundant cation in intracellular fluid. Magnesium is involved in many processes, including nerve and muscle functioning.

malabsorption An inadequate absorption of nutrients from the gastrointestinal tract.

maldigestion Incomplete digestion.

malformations of cortical development Disorders characterised by abnormalities in the development of the cerebral cortex. Neuronal migration and synaptic connectivity can be greatly disordered, leading to abnormal structure and functioning of the cortex.

malignant A severe condition that tends to become progressively worse. In cancer, a malignant tumour is one that is invasive and tends to spread to distant sites.

malunion The abnormal or incomplete joining of a section of tissue, such as bone or skin, after injury.

mania An affective disorder characterised by increased motor activity, euphoria, racing thoughts, talkativeness, a decreased need for sleep and inflated self-esteem.

mastalgia Pain associated with the breast or mammary glands.

mastitis An inflammation of the mammary glands, usually associated with infection during breastfeeding.

mean arterial pressure (MAP) The average blood pressure for a person during one cardiac cycle. In clinical practice it can be calculated as one-third of the pulse pressure (the difference between the systolic and diastolic pressure readings) plus the diastolic blood pressure reading.

melanin A dark brown pigment produced by melanocytes situated in the epidermis.

melanoma A malignant cancer of skin melanocytes.

meningitis An inflammation of the meninges.

meningocele A herniation of the meninges, where the membranous sac containing cerebrospinal fluid protrudes through the spine.

menorrhagia Excessive bleeding associated with menstruation.

metabolic syndrome A set of risk factors that increase a person's risk of developing diabetes mellitus and cardiovascular disease. Also known as 'syndrome X'.

metaplasia A cellular adaptation where one cell type transforms into another.

metastasis The spread of cancerous cells from a primary tumour to a distant body site via the bloodstream or lymphatic system.

metrorrhagia Abnormal uterine bleeding.

microbes A generic term for organisms that can only be viewed under magnification.

microvascular disease Pathology affecting the small blood vessels, ultimately causing complications to the kidneys (nephropathy), nerves (neuropathy) or eyesight (retinopathy).

microvilli Small projections from a cell's membrane that increase the surface area for absorption or secretion.

mineralocorticoid A steroid hormone secreted by the adrenal cortex that regulates sodium and water balance (e.g. aldosterone).

monosomy A genetic condition where one chromosome has no partner. The diploid number will be one less of a normal set (e.g. 'monosomy 18' means only one chromosome 18 exists in cells, and the 'diploid' number is 45).

mosaic The person's body cells are a mix of different genotypes.

motor neurone disease A degenerative disorder characterised by the deterioration of the motor neurons within the brain and spinal cord, leading to progressive motor weakness and muscle atrophy.

multifactorial inheritance Inheritance where multiple genes, and possibly the environment, interact to determine the particular phenotypical characteristic.

multiple endocrine neoplasia (MEN) A syndrome involving two or more endocrine tumours in one person, which may include the thyroid, parathyroid glands and the pancreas. The inheritance pattern underlying MEN is autosomal dominant.

multiple myeloma A type of malignant cancer originating in plasma cells (B cells) in the bone marrow. These malignant neoplasms typically destroy osseous tissue, causing fractures, bone pain and, subsequently, hypercalcaemia.

multiple sclerosis (MS) A degenerative disorder characterised by the demyelination of central nervous system neurons, leading to multiple white matter plaques within the brain and spinal cord.

muscular dystrophy A genetic condition characterised by a defect in the production of muscle proteins, resulting in progressive muscle weakness and the destruction of muscle tissue.

myalgia Muscle pain.

myalgic encephalomyelitis/chronic fatigue syndrome (ME/CFS) A neurological disorder thought to be caused by many factors, including infection and immunological issues, and which has many manifestations, including overwhelming fatigue, flu-like symptoms that persist for months, and sensitivity to touch, light and sound. Formerly known as *chronic fatigue syndrome* and *systemic exertion intolerance disease*).

mycosis A generic term for a fungal infection.

myelomeningocele A herniation of the meninges and spinal cord tissue, where the membranous sac and nervous tissue protrudes through the spine.

myocardial infarction The death of a region of myocardium resulting from an obstruction in blood flow to the tissue. The condition is commonly known as a heart attack.

myoclonic seizure A seizure characterised by disordered and involuntary twitching and jerking of skeletal muscles.

myopathy A disease affecting muscle tissue.

myopia A visual impairment where an image is focused in front of the retina. This condition is commonly known as 'short-sightedness', where close objects are in focus but distant objects are out of focus.

myositis An inflammation of muscle tissue.

myxoedema A condition caused by reduced thyroid gland function, which results in oedema of the lips and nose, mental deterioration, dry skin and a decreased metabolic rate. This condition is generally associated with low iodine levels in adults. Congenital or neonatal hypothyroidism, formerly known as 'cretinism', is associated with low iodine levels from childhood.

necrosis Unplanned cell death and autolysis associated with injury. Cellular organelles fail, vacuoles appear and the cell membrane pumps seize up, leading to cell rupture.

necrotising fasciitis (NF) A severe and rapidly damaging infection of the soft tissue that results in death of the fascia. The causative organism is normally beta-haemolytic streptococci.

neoplasia The process of new, but abnormal, cellular proliferation. This new growth may be benign or malignant.

neospinothalamic tract An ascending (sensory) spinal tract extending from the spinal cord to the thalamus, and which is important in the transmission of pain, temperature and itching sensations to the brain for processing.

nephritic syndrome A condition resulting in inflammation of the glomerular basement membrane, characterised by hypertension, oliguria, haematuria (blood in the urine), and mild proteinuria (protein in the urine).

nephrolithiasis The formation of a renal calculus (kidney stone).

nephrotic syndrome A condition resulting in damage to the glomerular podocyte, characterised by oedema, hypoalbuminaemia (low blood albumin) and sever proteinuria ((protein in the urine).

nephrotoxicity The state or quality of being damaging to the kidneys.

neural tube defects A condition associated with a disruption of the normal development of the neural tube during the embryonic period.

neuroinflammation An inflammation of nervous tissue.

neuromuscular junction The synapse between the motor neuron and skeletal muscle.

neuropathic pain Pain associated with dysfunction of the nervous system.

neuropathies Dysfunction associated with damage to peripheral, and possibly central, nerves, resulting in pain and/or loss of sensation to the hands or feet.

neurotoxin A substance that damages neurons or nervous tissue.

neutropenia A deficiency of neutrophils within the blood.

nitrite A nitrous acid salt. When measured in urine, an increased nitrite level suggests a urinary tract infection, as bacteria convert urinary nitrates to nitrites.

NO HARM An acronym used to guide the management of soft tissue injury, and which stands for: **NO H**eat, **A**lcohol, **R**unning or **M**assage.

nociception The transmission of sensory information associated with noxious or pain-inducing stimuli.

nociceptive neurons Sensory neurons that transmit pain signals.

non-communicable diseases Health conditions that are not caused by an infectious microoganism and cannot be passed from one human to another.

non-Hodgkin lymphoma (NHL) A malignant tumour involving lymphoid tissue; a diverse group of cancers, including lymphomas, that are not of the Hodgkin type. B and T cell lymphomas account for many of these tumours involving immune system structures.

non-ketotic hyperosmolar coma A coma produced by a high serum osmolarity. The hyperosmolar state leads to polyuria and volume depletion. This condition occurs in people who have diabetes mellitus with some insulin present, so ketosis does not occur.

non-productive pain Pain that does not serve as a warning of injury, where the cause may be difficult to discern.

non-steroidal anti-inflammatory drugs (NSAIDs) A group of drugs that are not steroids, and which cause a reduction in inflammation through reducing prostaglandin formation.

non-union A failure of sections of tissue, such as bone or skin, to heal after injury.

noradrenaline (NA) A chemical messenger substance from the catecholamine family that mediates sympathetic nervous system responses. It can act as a neurotransmitter, mediator or hormone.

normal flora Microorganisms present in or on human bodies that live in a commensal relationship with humans and, under normal conditions, do not cause disease.

nosocomial infection An infection that develops during hospitalisation; also known as 'hospital-acquired infection' (HAI).

obsessive–compulsive disorder (OCD) An anxiety disorder characterised by persistent fearful thoughts and ritualised behaviours.

oedema An excess of interstitial fluid.

oesophagitis Inflammation of the oesophagus.

oliguria The reduced capacity to produce sufficient urine to remove fluid and wastes from the body. Generally defined as urine production of less than 500 mL in 24 hours, or 0.5 mL/kg/hour for children and 30 mL/hour for adults. (Compare with *anuria*.)

oncogene A gene that can potentially induce cancer. The gene controls cell growth and proliferation, but in unusual circumstances may cause normal cells to become malignant.

oncology The biomedical and clinical specialty concerned with an understanding of cancer and its management.

onychatrophia A nail condition resulting in atrophy (wasting) or underdevelopment of the nail as a result of trauma or a number of skin and autoimmune diseases.

onychauxis A nail condition resulting in thicking and often discolouration and deformity. It is commonly associated with ageing.

onychomycosis A fungal infection in a toenail or fingernail.

onychorrhexis A nail condition resulting in thinning, splitting and the development of horizontal or vertical ridges from disordered keratinisation. It is commonly associated with ageing, nutritional deficiencies and hypothyroidism.

opportunistic infection An infection by a normally non-pathogenic organism that has become pathogenic due to an immunosuppressed state in the host.

orchitis An inflammation of a testis or testes. Also known as 'orchiditis'.

orthopnoea Dyspnoea relieved by sitting up or standing erect.

Osgood–Schlatter disease A condition characterised by pain and inflammation of the tibial tubercle in children aged between 10 and 15 years. The patellar tendon tightens and, if this is severe, microfractures of the growth plate at the tibial tubercle may occur.

osmolality The ratio of solutes to fluid.

osmosis The movement of fluid through a semipermeable membrane from a low concentration to a high concentration of solutes.

osmotic pressure The pressure caused by the concentration of a solution to prevent the inward flow of fluid across a semipermeable membrane. (Compare with *hydrostatic pressure*.)

osteoarthritis (OA) A condition characterised by a breakdown of synovial joint cartilage and, in time, the underlying bone.

osteochondroses A group of bone disorders that damage the ossification zones of the immature skeleton of children. The disorders are caused by ischaemia or mechanical stress injury.

osteomalacia A condition associated with abnormal bone mineralisation, resulting in a softening of bones.

osteomyelitis An inflammation of bone tissues, usually associated with an infection.

osteopenia A pre-osteoporotic condition where bone mineralisation density is lower than normal, but not low enough to be regarded as osteoporosis.

osteoporosis A metabolic bone disorder where bone mineralisation density and microstructure are significantly below normal.

osteosarcomas A form of malignant primary bone tumour that tends to occur mostly in children and adolescents.

ovarian cancer A cancer that develops in ovarian tissue.

ovarian cysts Benign tumours that develop as fluid-filled sacs on the surface of the ovary.

oxalate An oxalic acid salt excreted in urine; excessive oxalate may cause kidney stones.

oxidative stress A state where the formation of reactive oxygen species that harm cells exceeds the capacity of the body to inactivate them through the action of antioxidant substances.

oxygen free radicals Highly reactive forms of oxygen that harm cellular structures and body tissues.

Paget's disease of the bone A metabolic bone disorder characterised by the formation of localised or regional disorganised osseous tissue that is weaker than normal and prone to deformity and fracture.

pain The sensation perceived that is triggered by noxious stimuli.

Pain Gate Theory A theory proposed by Melzack and Wall in which sensory information pertaining to touch, pressure and vibration is transmitted along large-diameter myelinated Aβ-afferent fibres, enters the spinal cord and triggers circuits that act to modulate nociceptive inputs from the same body region via peripheral C-fibres, thus suppressing the level of pain felt.

palaeospinothalamic tract A part of the spinothalamic tract associated with the transmission of nociceptive information from the spinal cord to the brain. As well as terminating in the thalamus, this pathway terminates in the midbrain and brainstem, and is involved in the initiation of the emotional, behavioural and visceral components of the pain experience.

pancreatic ductal adenocarcinoma A pancreatic malignant tumour that arises in the epithelium of the pancreatic duct system.

pancreatitis Inflammation of the pancreas.

papule Any small, solid, raised skin lesion of any colour.

paraphimosis Related to the penis, a condition characterised by the foreskin (prepuce) becoming trapped in a retracted position behind the glans penis.

parasites Organisms that take advantage of another without contributing to the host's survival.

parathormone/parathyroid hormone (PTH) Hormone produced by the parathyroid glands, and which is responsible for the regulation of calcium and phosphate.

parathyroid gland Four small glands on the posterior surface of the thyroid gland responsible for the secretion of parathyroid hormone.

parenchyma The functional tissue of an organ, as opposed to supportive or connective tissue.

parenchymal lung disorders A group of restrictive lung disorders that interfere with lung volume and expansion, where the cause is damage to the functional lung tissue itself rather than to other chest structures.

Parkinson's disease A degenerative disorder characterised by rigidity, tremor at rest, postural changes, slowed movements and an absence of spontaneous movement. In this condition, the nigrostriatal pathway within the basal ganglia is damaged.

parkinsonism A group of conditions related to Parkinson's disease that have a similar pathology, but have different aetiologies and clinical presentations.

paronychia An inflammation in a toenail or fingernail often caused by bacterial infection.

partial-thickness burn A type of burn injury where the epidermis and some part of the dermis is damaged.

patent ductus arteriosus A congenital heart defect resulting in a communication between the aorta and the pulmonary artery.

pathogenesis The stages of development of a disorder.

pathogenicity The ability of an organism to become pathogenic (produce disease).

pathophysiology The study of how the functions of cells, tissues and organs are altered in disease or injury.

pelvic inflammatory disease (PID) A condition characterised by an infection of the female reproductive tract that may involve the cervix, uterus, ovaries and fallopian tubes.

penetrance The degree to which the gene/s for a particular characteristic or disorder is/are expressed.

peptic ulcer disease (PUD) An ulcer in the stomach or duodenal mucosa commonly caused by bacteria (*Helicobacter pylori*) or overuse of non-steroidal anti-inflammatory drugs (NSAIDs).

peripheral arterial disease (PAD) See *peripheral vascular disease*.

peripheral vascular disease (PVD) Also known as 'peripheral arterial disease (PAD)', PVD is a condition resulting in peripheral arterial obstruction.

peritoneal dialysis The removal of waste products, toxic substances and excess fluids across the peritoneum (used as a diffusible membrane) by intermittently introducing a solution into the peritoneum and draining it out again.

peritonitis Inflammation of the peritoneum commonly caused by infection.

periventricular heterotopia A condition where neurons do not migrate normally from the grey matter surrounding the ventricles towards the cerebral cortex in early fetal development.

pernicious anaemia Caused by a deficiency of intrinsic factor, which is essential for the absorption of vitamin B_{12}. Vitamin B_{12} (cyanocobalamin) is essential for nuclear maturation and the synthesis of DNA in red blood cells.

phagocytes A generic term for any cell (generally a leukocyte) responsible for engulfing pathogens, waste material and foreign bodies.

phantom limb pain Pain attributed to a missing limb described as shooting, stabbing, pricking, throbbing and/or burning in character.

phenotype The observable characteristics or traits arising out of an interaction between the genotype and the environment.

phimosis In relation to the penis, a condition associated with a non-retractable foreskin.

phlebothrombosis A clot that develops within a vein.

phosphate Phosphoric acid salt; involved in the metabolism, storage and use of energy (in ATP), and the structure of genetic information (in DNA).

photoallergic reaction The delayed cutaneous hypersensitivity reaction to exposure to light (generally sunlight).

photoprotection A management strategy used to reduce an exacerbation of rosacea, a non-infectious skin rash. It involves the wearing of protective clothes, such as hats, or the application of sunscreen.

phototoxicity reaction A reaction associated with the application of a chemical to the skin that reacts with sunlight (or another UV light source) to induce a lesion similar to sunburn; a form of photo contact dermatitis.

pituitary dwarfism Stunted growth as a result of growth hormone deficiency.

pituitary gland An endocrine gland responsible for growth, maturation and metabolism; the hypophysis.

plaque In relation to skin, a scaly patch seen in psoriasis. In relation to vessels, a deposit of fatty material inside the endothelium. In relation to dentistry, a collection of bacteria, food debris and other substances that contribute to the development of gingival disease. In relation to orthopaedics, an area of skeletal muscle attachment to myofilaments. In relation to neurology, a microscopic mass of amyloid and fragmented neural tissue deposited in the cerebrum that contributes to Alzheimer's disease.

pleomorphic A descriptive term used in cancer to indicate the presence of a variety of types of cells in one tumour.

pleura The double-layered membrane on the surface of each lung.

pleurodesis A surgical procedure designed to cause an adhesion of the visceral and parietal layers of the pleural membrane, 'gluing' the pleural cavity in an area of trauma.

pneumoconiosis An occupational lung disorder associated with the inhalation of inorganic dust that causes parenchymal lung disease.

pneumonia An inflammation of lung tissue that impairs gas exchange. It can be caused by an infectious agent or a chemical.

pneumothorax The collapse of a lung, or part of a lung, caused by the accumulation of gas or air in the pleural cavity or in the chest cavity outside the lung.

polycystic kidney diseases Genetic conditions characterised by the formation of multiple kidney cysts that compromise renal function.

polycystic ovary syndrome (PCOS) A condition characterised by irregular or absent ovulation, hyperandrogenaemia and multiple ovarian cysts. The mechanisms involved in its development include insulin resistance and the abnormal functioning of both the hypothalamic-pituitary-gonadal and hypothalamic-pituitary-adrenal axes.

polycythaemias Chronic disease characterised by abnormally high numbers of red blood cells, resulting in hypertension, splenomegaly and hepatomegaly.

polygene traits Genetic characteristics, such as skin colour or height, that are determined by the combination of a number of genes.

polymicrogyria A developmental abnormality that occurs during the formation of the brain that is characterised by an excessive number of small convolutions in the cerebral cortex.

polyploidy A condition characterised by the presence of an additional full set of chromosomes in cells (non-viable in humans).

portal hypertension Excessive blood pressure in the gut and liver vasculature.

post-ictal period A period immediately following a seizure.

post-thrombotic syndrome (PTS) A condition resulting in long-term complications from a venous thromboembolism (clot).

post-traumatic stress disorder (PTSD) An anxiety disorder associated with a traumatic event where the affected person was confronted by death or serious injury.

potassium An electrolyte important for impulse transmission and cell membrane transport.

pre-eclampsia A condition characterised by hypertension and fluid retention in pregnancy.

preload The amount of stretch on heart muscle fibres just prior to contraction. An increase in preload usually results in an increase in volume of blood ejected with each contraction; however, it is influenced by factors such as blood volume, venous return, and the capacity of the ventricles to stretch.

premature ventricular complex An ectopic heart beat originating in the ventricle. Also known as premature ventricular contraction.

presbycusis Age-related hearing loss.

prevalence The total number of cases, both newly diagnosed and existing, of a condition at a particular time.

priapism A condition characterised by prolonged, and sometimes painful, penile erection.

primary brain injury Damage to brain tissues as a direct result of neurotrauma.

productive pain Pain that serves as a warning of tissue injury, which wanes as the injury resolves.

pro-inflammatory chemical mediators Various substances found in the plasma and released from cells in response to immune challenges such as tissue damage. Examples include histamine, serotonin and bradykinin. These substances initiate many of the non-specific immune responses such as vasodilation, increased capillary permeability and chemotaxis.

prokaryotes A generic term for any cellular organisms lacking a distinct nucleus.

prolactin (PRL) A hormone, produced by the pituitary gland, responsible for the stimulation and maintenance of milk secretion.

prolapse A condition where a body structure, such as a vertebral disc or organ, slips out of place from its normal anatomical position.

prostaglandins A paracrine mediator belonging to the family of eicosanoids, 20-carbon fatty acids formed from membrane phospholipids. Prostaglandins have a number of constitutive and inflammatory roles affecting smooth muscle contractility, platelet aggregation, nociception and glomerular filtration, as well as stomach acid and mucus secretion.

prostate cancer A cancer that develops in prostate tissue.

prostatitis An inflammation of the prostate, often associated with urinary tract infections.

protein aggregates The abnormal accumulation of misfolded proteins, or protein fragments, in neurons associated with neurodegenerative disorders such as Parkinson's disease, Alzheimer's disease and Huntington's disease. Protein aggregates associated with these disorders include alpha-synuclein, ubiquitin, beta-amyloid and huntingtin.

proto-oncogene A normal gene which, after mutating, can contribute to cancer development.

protozoa Single-celled eukaryotic organisms that reproduce asexually by cell division.

pruritus Itchiness. A skin irritation resulting in the need to scratch.

psoriasis A chronic autoimmune skin condition characterised by the hyperproliferation of skin cells, leading to areas of erythema and silvery-white scaly patches on the skin.

psychosis A thought disorder characterised by a loss of contact with reality. An affected person shows abnormal behaviour and distorted perception.

pulmonary embolism (PE) An embolism, usually in the form of a clot or foreign matter, arising from the venous circulation, which lodges in and obstructs the pulmonary arterial circulation.

pulmonary hypertension (PH) A condition characterised by increased blood pressure within the pulmonary arteries.

pulmonary oedema The accumulation of fluid within the pulmonary interstitium and alveoli due to an alteration in pulmonary blood pressure or vascular permeability.

pyelonephritis Inflammation of the kidney, generally caused by an infection.

pyomyositis An inflammation of muscle associated with an infection, which is usually caused by bacteria, commonly *Staphylococcus aureus*, and is characterised by abscess formation.

pyuria A generic term for pus in the urine.

Raynaud's syndrome A condition that results in frequent blanching (or cyanosis) of the extremities due to spasm of the digital arteries.

reactive oxygen species (ROS) Free radicals of the oxygen molecule that are highly reactive with cellular structures, such as membranes and DNA, which can lead to gross tissue damage.

recessive inheritance A recessive gene cannot produce the trait it programs for when inherited in combination with a dominant gene. Inheritance of the recessive allele from both parents allows the characteristic to be expressed.

reciprocal translocation A piece of one chromosome changes position with a piece of another chromosome.

rectocele A prolapse of the rectum into the posterior wall of the vagina. The resulting bulge can cause constipation, perineal and vaginal pressure, or even obstruct defecation.

re-entry A mechanism associated with the formation of some cardiac dysrhythmias, in which the electrical signal that excites cardiac muscle cells has the opportunity to excite cells more than once, due to an altered timing of the signal or by it travelling along an alternative pathway through the tissue.

repair A process involved in tissue healing to reduce the size of the damaged area.

respiratory compensation An alteration in respiratory rate in order to shift blood pH towards normal when the cause of the acidosis or alkalosis is metabolic.

respiratory syncytial virus (RSV) A virus considered to be the most common cause of lower respiratory tract infections.

reticular activating system A system formed by a number of brain regions involved in the maintenance of arousal and the waking state, consisting of the brainstem and thalamus, with projections to the hypothalamus.

rhabdomyolysis The destruction of muscle tissue due to a failure of calcium homeostasis.

rheumatic fever A condition characterised by acute inflammation, joint pain, fever and cardiac valve scarring. Rheumatic fever is caused by a previous streptococcal infection.

rheumatic heart disease A condition in which serious and permanent damage has occurred to the heart valve as a result of rheumatic fever.

rheumatoid arthritis A chronic inflammatory autoimmune condition affecting synovial joints.

RICER An acronym, used to guide the management of soft tissue injury, which stands for **R**est, **I**ce, **C**ompress, **E**levate and **R**eferral.

rickets A condition related to osteomalacia. It occurs in children and is associated with poor mineralisation of the cartilage within the epiphyseal growth plate. Associated with a deficiency of vitamin D.

rosacea A common chronic non-infectious skin condition characterised by an erythematous rash on the face and nose.

Rotavirus Any RNA virus from the Reoviridae family. These viruses are known to cause gastroenteritis.

SARS-CoV-2 infection Infection by the virus that causes coronavirus disease-19. This virus is a member of the coronavirus family, and is spread between people mainly through air-borne contact with virus-containing droplets.

scabies A skin infection caused by the *Sarcoptes scabiei* mite.

scar The formation of non-parenchymal tissue that restores the continuity and framework of tissue damaged or destroyed within a wound.

schizophrenia A common form of chronic psychosis where the affected person shows disordered and disorganised thoughts, unusual behaviour, abnormal speech and altered emotions.

scoliosis A deformity characterised by lateral curvature and axial rotation of the spine.

sebum The oily secretion from the sebaceous glands of the skin.

secondary brain injury Brain damage occurring post injury as a result of extracranial causes, such as hypoxia, hypotension or hypoglycaemia, or intracranial causes, such as haemorrhage, swelling or infection.

seizure An episode of inappropriate electrical discharge resulting in disordered brain activity.

self-antigens Cell surface markers that indicate to the immune system that this cell is not to be attacked and destroyed.

senescence The process of ageing. When a cell becomes fully mature and is terminally differentiated.

sentinel node The lymph node to which cancerous cells from a tumour first spread.

sepsis A generic term for the presence of a bacterial infection within the blood.

serosanguineous exudate An accumulation of watery, low-protein fluid in the tissue derived from serum, but which is blood-stained.

serotonin (5-HT) A biogenic amine derived from the amino acid tryptophan that acts as a neurotransmitter, hormone and chemical mediator.

serum sickness A type III hypersensitivity reaction associated with the intravenous administration of antisera from an animal source, which is characterised by the formation of antigen–antibody complexes in the blood that lodge in tissues.

severe acute respiratory syndrome-associated coronavirus 2 (SARS-CoV-2) The virus responsible for the respiratory illness known as COVID-19.

sex chromosomes The one pair of human chromosomes within the set of 23 pairs that determine the sex of the person; X and Y chromosomes.

sex hormones A generic term for the hormones responsible for the development of sex characteristics (e.g. oestrogen, testosterone).

sexually transmitted infections (STIs) These infections are acquired through sexual contact in the form of vaginal, anal or oral sex; also known as 'venereal diseases'.

shingles Shingles occur when the varicella herpes zoster virus that induces chickenpox reactivates after being dormant within the dorsal nerve root ganglia. It erupts as a painful vesicular rash that follows dermatomes.

sickle cell anaemia An incurable type of anaemia in which abnormal haemoglobin produces crescent-shaped red blood cells. The dysmorphic cells are fragile and rupture easily.

sociocultural factors Elements that determine the health and wellness of a person, incorporating aspects such as family, religion, culture, the media or peers.

socioeconomic factors Elements that determine the health and wellness of a person, incorporating aspects such as employment, education or income.

sodium The most common extracellular electrolyte responsible for many important functions, including the maintenance of fluid and electrolyte balance, nerve transmission and muscle contraction.

solar keratosis A thick warty, crusty or callosy skin growth promoted by sun exposure that is considered a pre-malignant neoplasm.

spastic paralysis A loss of motor control associated with central nervous system damage, characterised by involuntary muscle spasms that prevent normal movement. (Compare with *flaccid paralysis*.)

spermatocele An epididymal cyst, which is typically asymptomatic.

spina bifida A condition caused by a failure of the neural tube to close at the caudal end during early embryonic development.

spinal shock The acute transient loss of all reflexive and autonomic function below the level of a spinal cord injury.

spinoreticular tract An ascending tract extending from the spinal cord to the reticular formation associated with the transmission of sensory information, such as pain, promoting arousal and wakefulness.

spinothalamic tract An ascending tract extending from the spinal cord to the thalamus that is associated with the transmission of sensory information, such as pain and temperature. (See also *palaeospinothalamic tract* and *neospinothalamic tract*.)

spirometry The measurement of pulmonary volumes in order to assess lung function and capacity.

sprain A twisting or stretching injury to a ligament.

squamous cell carcinomas (SCCs) A non-melanoma type of skin cancer that occurs as a result of frequent exposure to ultraviolet radiation, such as sunlight.

stasis dermatitis Chronic venous insufficiency leads to the translocation of fibrinogen and the formation of fibrin in the dermal tissue. This causes hypoxia, which leads to dermal tissue destruction and inflammation.

status asthmaticus A medical emergency where an exacerbation of asthma does not respond to therapy.

status epilepticus A medical emergency where an epileptic seizure does not spontaneously resolve or progresses to subsequent seizures without recovery time.

steatorrhoea Excessive fat in the faeces.

strain A stretching or tearing injury to a tendon or muscle.

stress A generic term for a state of extreme pressure causing physical and/or emotional effects.

stressor Something that causes stress.

stroke A cerebrovascular lesion that develops suddenly where a vessel becomes blocked or bleeds and compromises blood supply to an area of the brain.

struvite A mix of magnesium ammonium phosphate crystal with carbonate apatite, found in struvite stones, as a result of urinary tract infections.

subdural haematoma (SDH) The accumulation of blood between the dural and arachnoid meningeal membranes due to an intracranial bleed.

sublethal gene A gene that causes death (before maturity) to less than 50% of the individuals carrying the affected gene. Also known as a sublethal mutation.

subluxation A partial or incomplete displacement of the joint surface.

substance dependence The continued use of a substance despite resulting negative consequences, such as health, financial, relationship or legal problems.

substance P A neuropeptide neurotransmitter and neuromediator associated with nociception and inflammation.

substantia gelatinosa A region of the dorsal horn of the spinal cord involved in the regulation of nociceptive and temperature inputs.

subungual haematoma A nail condition resulting in a collection of blood underneath the nail plate and above the nail matrix, usually resulting from trauma.

superficial burn A skin burn that involves only the epidermis. Previously known as a 'first-degree burn'.

supraventricular tachycardia (SVT) A fast heart rate originating above the ventricles.

surfactant A substance produced by type II alveolar cells that reduces the alveolar surface tension and prevents alveolar collapse.

sympathetic causalgia A condition characterised by a burning pain that is associated with abnormal sympathetic nervous system signalling, due to the sprouting of fibres at the level of dorsal root ganglia or partially denervated skin.

syndrome of inappropriate ADH secretion (SIADH) A condition in which too much antidiuretic hormone (ADH) is released, resulting in excess water retention and hyponatraemia.

syphilis A sexually transmitted infection caused by *Treponema pallidum*.

T cells Specialised lymphocytes produced by the bone marrow and matured in the thymus, which are responsible for cellular-mediated immunity.

tachycardia Fast heart rate (greater than 99 beats per minute in an adult).

tachypnoea A rapid respiration rate.

talipes equinovarus (TEV) A foot deformity characterised by inversion and plantar flexion of the hindfoot; also known as 'clubfoot'.

target tissue responsiveness In an endocrine context, reflects the number and/or sensitivity of the cellular hormone receptors on a tissue.

telomere A region on the ends of each chromosome that prevents the loss of integrity in structure during cell division.

temporal lobe epilepsy Epileptic seizures characterised by involuntary or subconscious behavioural responses.

tendinitis An inflammation of a tendon or tendons, usually associated with injury.

teratoma Tumours arising from precursor cells to the gametes, which, when dissected, may contain hair, teeth, bone, neural tissue or a combination of these.

terminal hair Hair growth characterised by harder, darker, longer hairs.

testicular cancer A cancer that grows in testicular tissues.

tetralogy of Fallot A congenital cardiac condition resulting in four simultaneous malformations: a ventricular septal defect, a misplaced aortic origin, a narrowing of the pulmonary artery and left ventricular enlargement.

thalassaemia A type of anaemia in which haemoglobin synthesis is dysfunctional; it is an autosomal recessive trait.

thromboangiitis obliterans Inflammation and occlusion of the vessels in the legs; also known as Buerger's disease.

thrombocytopenia An abnormally low platelet count.

thrombophlebitis A condition associated with thrombosis formation in response to venous wall inflammation anywhere in the venous circulation.

thyroid gland An endocrine gland located in the anterior neck region, which produces hormones that set the basal metabolic rate and are essential for the normal maturation and maintenance of some body systems, and influence blood calcium ion levels.

thyroid-stimulating hormone (TSH) The hormone produced and released from the pituitary that stimulates the thyroid to release thyroxine and triiodothyronine.

thyrotoxicosis A condition resulting from excessive thyroid hormone production. (See also *Graves' disease*.)

thyroxine (T_4) A prohormone, produced by the thyroid gland, responsible for metabolic homeostasis.

tinnitus A perception of sound with no external stimulus. Persistent tones, clicks, buzzes and ringing noises are sounds commonly experienced.

tonic–clonic seizure Epileptic seizure characterised by three phases: the tonic, clonic and post-ictal phases. Previously known as 'grand mal seizure'.

tonicity A term that reflects the relative osmotic pressure difference in two adjacent compartments.

tophi (sing: tophus) Deposits of uric acid crystals that form lumps in the fingers and toes, hands and knees, forearms and elbows.

transformation In the context of neoplasia, the process of changing normal cells into cancerous cells.

transient ischaemic attack (TIA) A transient form of cerebral ischaemia that produces neurological deficits but resolves completely within 24 hours.

transudate A watery fluid low in protein content that passes through a membrane via filtration pressure without damaging the blood vessel wall.

traumatic brain injury (TBI) A brain injury caused by an external injury to the head. (See also *primary brain injury* and *secondary brain injury*.)

trigeminal neuralgia A condition characterised by episodes of excruciating facial pain.

triglycerides A compound consisting of three fatty acids and a glycerol molecule.

triiodothyronine (T_3) A hormone produced by the thyroid gland responsible for many metabolic process.

triploidy A condition associated with an additional full set of chromosomes, making three sets of 23 chromosomes (not viable in humans).

trisomy A condition characterised by three copies of one particular chromosome.

tropical sprue A condition resulting in malabsorption, which affects people living in tropical and subtropical regions.

true aneurysm A condition in which an artery wall dilates, and which involves all three layers of the artery wall.

tuberculosis A contagious, air-borne, bacterial infection that commonly affects the lungs. *Mycobacterium tuberculosis* is the common agent.

tubulointerstitial nephritis An inflammation of the renal tubules and renal interstitial tissues, due to an immune system cause or toxicity from drugs.

tumorigenesis The process of forming a tumour.

tumour A generic term for any growth, swelling or neoplasm.

tumour markers Substances produced by cancer cells and released into the blood.

tumour suppressor genes Genes that are powerful inhibitors of cell growth. When these genes mutate, cancer may develop.

tumour suppressor proteins Proteins made by tumour suppressor genes that inhibit cell growth.

ulcerative colitis A form of inflammatory bowel disease caused by an abnormal activation of immune processes that leads to inflammation of the epithelium of the large intestine.

upper respiratory tract infection (URTI) An infection of the upper respiratory tract in a region above the level of the carina.

uraemia The presence of too much urea and creatinine in the blood.

urea A nitrogenous end product of protein metabolism that is excreted by the kidneys.

urethritis An inflammation of the urethra, usually associated with an infection.

uric acid A substance resulting from the metabolism of protein. It can be measured in the urine or the blood.

urinary incontinence An involuntary release of urine.

urinary stasis A condition in which urine passage is impaired, resulting in an increased risk of urinary tract infection.

urothelium The transitional epithelium of the renal pelvis, ureters, bladder and urethra.

urticarial rash A red, pruritic skin rash of irregularly raised welts.

uterine (endometrial) cancer A cancer of the endometrial tissues.

uterine fibroids/leiomyomas Benign smooth muscle tumours of the myometrium.

valve regurgitation A condition in which the backflow of blood occurs through an incompetent valve.

valve stenosis A narrowing or constriction of a valve.

varices Distended veins.

varicocele A dilation of the testicular vein.

varicose veins Superficial enlarged and tortuous blood vessels.

vasculitis An inflammation of a blood vessel.

vellus hair Hair growth characterised by softer, smaller and lighter-coloured hair.

venom A toxic substance produced by a poisonous animal that is injected into its prey or attacker.

venous thromboembolism (VTE) A blood clot formed in a vein that breaks away from the vessel wall to travel through the circulation to lodge in smaller blood vessels within the lungs and obstruct blood flow.

ventilation–perfusion (V/Q) mismatch A defect in the matching of the volume of air reaching the alveoli and the volume of blood reaching the vessels supplying the alveoli, expressed as a ratio.

ventilatory failure A condition where both oxygenation and carbon dioxide elimination are compromised; also known as 'type II respiratory failure'.

ventricular fibrillation A severe dysrhythmia that will often result in death due to rapid and irregular impulses occurring in the ventricles. This fibrillation does not permit an appropriate wave-like impulse with a sequential contraction.

ventricular remodelling A change in the size, shape and function of cardiac myocytes as a result of myocardial injury.

ventricular septal defect A condition characterised by a hole in the ventricular septum. A ventricular septal defect is often a congenital cardiac malformation but can have other causes.

ventricular tachycardia (VT) A fast heart rate originating from an ectopic focus in the ventricles.

very-low-density lipoproteins (VLDLs) Large lipoproteins that are a combination of triglycerides, cholesterol and protein. They function to transport lipid from the liver to body cells.

vesicle A generic term for a collection of fluid in a sac-like membrane. In the context of skin, is a fluid-filled lesion (blister-like).

vesicoureteral reflux (VUR) The reflux of urine from the urinary bladder back into the ureters.

Virchow's triad Three factors that are considered to be major contributors to thrombosis development: hypercoagulability, endothelial damage and the character of blood flow.

virulence The ability of a pathogen to cause disease.

viruses Microscopic pathogens, smaller than bacteria, that can only reproduce inside a living host cell.

volvulus The twisting of a loop of intestine through 360 degrees, which occludes its lumen and collapses its blood vessels.

von Willebrand disease An inherited disorder resulting in a deficiency of clotting factor VIII.

vulvar cancer A cancer of the vulva.

vulvovaginitis An inflammation of the vulva and vagina.

wheal A small, swollen skin lesion resulting from an allergic reaction.

wheeze A high-pitched sound, often of a musical quality, caused by a narrowing of the tracheobronchial tree and small airways, most often heard in expiration.

Whipple's disease Intestinal lipodystrophy, it is a rare infectious disease, caused by the Gram-positive bacterium *Tropheryma whipplei*.

widened scar A gaping wound due to excess tension on the wound edges during the healing process. As a result, healing is prolonged.

wind-up In relation to pain perception, as the number of signals through the synapses increases owing to the ongoing inflammatory and neurotransmitter-mediated increase in the sensitivity of the nociceptive neurons, a learning-like process occurs in the dorsal horn. The two cells involved in the synapse change the number and identity of the proteins at the synaptic cleft, increasing the ease with which the signals are transmitted and the strength of those signals at the post-synaptic cell.

wound contraction When the edges of a wound are drawn closer to reduce the area to be repaired.

X-linked A gene carried on an X chromosome.

Zollinger–Ellison syndrome A condition characterised by tumours in the pancreas and/or duodenum, as well as peptic ulcers, due to increased production of gastric acid.

Index

Page numbers in **bold** indicate key terms.

B

E

I